Nadas' Pediatric Cardiology

Nadas' Pediatric Cardiology

Second Edition

Edited by

John F. Keane, M.D.
Professor of Pediatrics, Harvard Medical School
Senior Associate in Cardiology, Department of Cardiology
Children's Hospital Boston
Boston, Massachusetts

James E. Lock, M.D.
Alexander S. Nadas Professor of Pediatrics, Harvard Medical School,
Chairman, Department of Cardiology,
Physician-in-Chief, Children's Hospital Boston,
Boston, Massachusetts

Donald C. Fyler, M.D.
Professor Emeritus of Pediatrics, Harvard Medical School,
Associate Chief of Cardiology Emeritus, Children's Hospital Boston,
Boston, Massachusetts

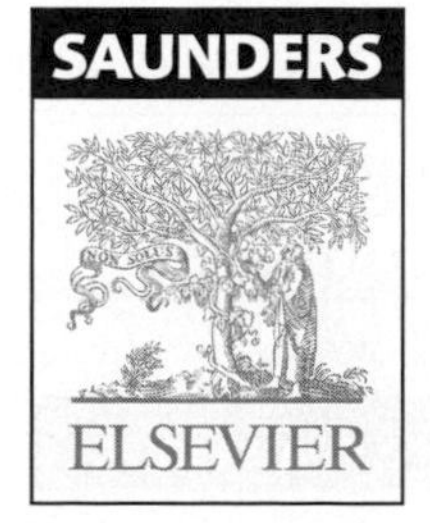

SAUNDERS
ELSEVIER

1600 John F. Kennedy Blvd.
Suite 1800
Philadelphia, Pennsylvania 19103

NADAS' PEDIATRIC CARDIOLOGY
ISBN-13: 978-1-4160-2390-6
ISBN-10: 1-4160-2390-9

Notice

Knowledge and best practice in this field are constantly changing. As new research and experience broaden our knowledge, changes in practice, treatment, and drug therapy may become necessary or appropriate. Readers are advised to check the most current information provided (i) on procedures featured or (ii) by the manufacturer of each product to be administered, to verify the recommended dose or formula, the method and duration of administration, and contraindications. It is the responsibility of the practitioner, relying on his or her own experience and knowledge of the patient, to make diagnoses, to determine dosages and the best treatment for each individual patient, and to take all appropriate safety precautions. To the fullest extent of the law, neither the Publisher nor the Authors assume any liability for any injury and/or damage to persons or property arising out or related to any use of the material contained in this book.

The Publisher

Library of Congress Cataloging-in-Publication Data

Nadas' pediatric cardiology.—2nd ed. / [edited by] John F. Keane
p. ; cm.
Includes bibliographical references and index.
ISBN 1-4160-2390-9
1. Pediatric cardiology. I. Title: Pediatric cardiology. II. Keane, John F., 1934-III. Nadas, Alexander S. (Alexander Sandor), 1913- Pediatric cardiology.
[DNLM: 1. Heart Defects, Congenital. 2. Heart Diseases—Child. 3. Heart Diseases—Infant. WS 290 N1291 2007]
RJ421.N32 2007
617.4′12—dc22

2005057436

Acquisitions Editor: Natasha Andejelkovic
Developmental Editor: Laurie Anello
Project Manager: Mary Stermel
Design Direction: Ellen Zanolle
Marketing Manager: Dana Butler

Printed in (name of country)

Last digit is the print number: 9 8 7 6 5 4 3 2 1

This work is dedicated to

Dr. Nadas' family: his wife, Elizabeth; daughters, Elizabeth Seamans and Trudi Murch; his son, John A. Nadas

The three "Cs": Carol Fyler, Clare Keane, and Carolyn Lock

Contributors

Mark E. Alexander, M.D.
Instructor in Pediatrics, Harvard Medical School; Assistant in Cardiology Department of Cardiology, Children's Hospital Boston, Boston, Massachusetts

Charles I. Berul, M.D.
Associate Professor of Pediatrics, Harvard Medical School; Senior Associate in Cardiology, Department of Cardiology, Children's Hospital Boston, Boston, Massachusetts

Elizabeth D. Blume, M.D.
Assistant Professor of Pediatrics, Harvard Medical School; Associate in Cardiology, Department of Cardiology, Children's Hospital Boston, Boston, Massachusetts

Roger E. Breitbart, M.D.
Assistant Professor of Pediatrics, Harvard Medical School; Associate in Cardiology, Department of Cardiology, Children's Hospital Boston, Boston, Massachusetts

Frank Cecchin, M.D.
Assistant Professor of Pediatrics, Harvard Medical School; Associate in Cardiology, Department of Cardiology, Children's Hospital Boston, Boston, Massachusetts

David E. Clapham, M.D., Ph.D.
Aldo R. Castañeda Professor of Cardiovascular Research and Professor of Neurobiology, Harvard Medical School; Director of Cardiovascular Research, Children's Hospital Boston, Boston, Massachusetts

Steven D. Colan, M.D.
Professor of Pediatrics, Harvard Medical School; Senior Associate in Cardiology, Department of Cardiology and Chief, Non-invasive Laboratories, Children's Hospital Boston, Boston, Massachusetts

Martha A.Q. Curley, RN, Ph.D, FAAN
Director, Cardiovascular and Critical Care Nursing Research, Cardiovascular Program, Children's Hospital Boston, Boston, Massachusetts

Pedro J. del Nido, M.D.
Professor of Surgery, Harvard Medical School; Chairman, Department of Cardiac Surgery, Children's Hospital Boston, Boston, Massachusetts

Michael D. Freed, M.D.
Associate Professor of Pediatrics, Harvard Medical School; Senior Associate in Cardiology, Department of Cardiology and Chief, Inpatient Services, Children's Hospital Boston, Boston, Massachusetts

David R. Fulton, M.D.
Associate Professor of Pediatrics, Harvard Medical School; Senior Associate in Cardiology, Department of Cardiology; Chief, Outpatient Services, Children's Hospital Boston, Boston, Massachusetts

Donald C. Fyler, M.D.
Professor Emeritus of Pediatrics, Harvard Medical School, Associate Chief of Cardiology Emeritus, Children's Hospital Boston, Boston, Massachusetts

Kimberlee Gauvreau, Sc.D.
Assistant Professor of Pediatrics, Harvard Medical School; Assistant Professor of Biostatistics, Harvard School of Public Health; Research Associate in Cardiology Department of Cardiology, Children's Hospital Boston, Boston, Massachusetts

Robert L. Geggel, M.D.
Associate Professor of Pediatrics, Harvard Medical School; Senior Associate in Cardiology, Department of Cardiology, Children's Hospital Boston, Boston, Massachusetts

Tal Geva, M.D.
Associate Professor of Pediatrics, Harvard Medical School; Senior Associate in Cardiology, Department of Cardiology, Children's Hospital Boston, Boston, Massachusetts

Patricia Hickey, M.S., R.N., M.B.A.
Vice President, Cardiovascular/Critical Care Services, Cardiovascular Program Children's Hospital Boston, Boston, Massachusetts

Kathy J. Jenkins, M.D.
Associate Professor of Pediatrics, Harvard Medical School; Senior Associate in Cardiology and Director, Program for Patient Safety and Quality, Department of Cardiology, Children's Hospital Boston, Boston, Massachusetts

John F. Keane, M.D.
Professor of Pediatrics, Harvard Medical School; Senior Associate in Cardiology, Department of Cardiology Children's Hospital Boston, Boston, Massachusetts

Mark T. Keating, M.D.
Professor Department of Pediatrics and Cell Biology, Harvard Medical School; Senior Associate in Cardiology, Department of Cardiology; Investigator, Howard Hughes Medical Institute, Cardiovascular Research, Children's Hospital Boston, Boston, Massachusetts

Ronald V. Lacro, M.D.
Assistant Professor of Pediatrics, Harvard Medical School; Associate in Cardiology, Department of Cardiology, Children's Hospital Boston, Boston, Massachusetts

Michael J. Landzberg, M.D.
Assistant Professor of Medicine, Harvard Medical School; Associate in Cardiology, Department of Cardiology, Children's Hospital Boston; Associate Physician, Cardiovascular Division, Brigham and Women's Hospital, Boston, Massachusetts

Peter Lang, M.D.
Associate Professor of Pediatrics, Harvard Medical School; Senior Associate in Cardiology and Chief, Clinical Training Program, Department of Cardiology, Children's Hospital, Boston, Massachusetts

Peter C. Laussen, M.B.B.S.
D.D. Hansen Professor of Pediatric Anesthesia and Associate Professor of Anesthesia, Harvard Medical School; Senior Associate in Cardiology and Chief, Division Cardiac Intensive Care, Department of Cardiology, Children's Hospital Boston, Boston, Massachusetts

James E. Lock, M.D.
Alexander S. Nadas Professor of Pediatrics, Harvard Medical School, Chairman, Department of Cardiology, Physician-in-chief, Children's Hospital Boston, Boston, Massachusetts

Valerie S. Mandell, M.D.
Radiologist, Walbach 1, Children's Hospital Boston, Boston, Massachusetts

Gerald R. Marx, M.D.
Associate Professor of Pediatrics, Harvard Medical School; Senior Associate in Cardiology and Director of Ultrasound Imaging Research, Department of Cardiology, Children's Hospital Boston, Boston, Massachusetts

John E. Mayer, Jr., M.D.
Professor of Surgery, Harvard Medical School; Senior Associate in Cardiac Surgery, Department of Cardiovascular Surgery, Children's Hospital Boston, Boston, Massachusetts

Mary P. Mullen, M.D.
Instructor in Pediatrics, Harvard Medical School; Assistant in Cardiology, Department of Cardiology, Children's Hospital Boston, Boston, Massachusetts

Jane W. Newburger, M.D., M.P.H.
Professor of Pediatrics, Harvard Medical School; Associate Cardiologist-in-Chief, Department of Cardiology, Children's Hospital Boston, Boston, Massachusetts

Patricia O'Brien, N.P, M.S.N.
Cardiovascular Program, Children's Hospital Boston, Boston, Massachusetts

Frank A. Pigula, M.D.
Assistant Professor of Surgery, Harvard Medical School; Associate in Cardiac Surgery, Department of Cardiovascular Surgery, Children's Hospital Boston, Boston, Massachusetts

Andrew J. Powell, M.D.
Assistant Professor of Pediatrics, Harvard Medical School; Associate in Cardiology, Department of Cardiology, Children's Hospital Boston, Boston, Massachusetts

Jonathan Rhodes, M.D.
Assistant Professor of Pediatrics, Harvard Medical School; Associate in Cardiology, Department of Cardiology, Children's Hospital Boston, Boston, Massachusetts

John K. Triedman, M.D.
Associate Professor of Pediatrics, Harvard Medical School; Senior Associate in Cardiology, Department of Cardiology, Children's Hospital Boston, Boston, Massachusetts

Mary E. van der Velde
Clinical Associate Professor, Pediatrics and Communicable Diseases, Congenital Heart Center, C.S. Mott Hospital, Ann Arbor, Michigan

Richard Van Praagh, M.D.
Professor of Pathology, Emeritus, Harvard Medical School; Research Associate in Cardiology and Cardiac Surgery and Director, Emeritus, Cardiac Registry, Department of Cardiology, Children's Hospital Boston, Boston, Massachusetts

Stella Van Praagh, M.D.
Department of Cardiology, Children's Hospital Boston, Boston, Massachusetts

Edward P. Walsh, M.D.
Associate Professor of Pediatrics, Harvard Medical School; Senior Associate in Cardiology and Chief, Electrophysiology Laboratories, Department of Cardiology, Children's Hospital Boston, Boston, Massachusetts

David L. Wessel, M.D.
Professor of Pediatrics (Anesthesia), Harvard Medical School; Senior Associate in Cardiology, Department of Cardiology; Associate in Cardiovascular Surgery and Anesthesia, Children's Hospital Boston, Boston, Massachusetts

Preface

In 1957, Dr. Nadas first published his text "Pediatric Cardiology." It represented both his experience and opinions in this field, and was intended for "pediatricians, general physicians and medical students." He pointed out it was "not a treatise" on the subject. He felt strongly that since (a) cardiology at Children's Hospital Boston was supported by city, state and federal funds and (b) parents, physicians and local towns depended on the institution for care, it was our obligation to report our experience, including results, regularly. This current edition represents our attempt to continue honoring this obligation, this being the fifth such presentation to date.

The intended audience again includes pediatricians, general physicians and medical students and, in addition, pediatric cardiologists (including those in training), adult cardiologists with an interest in congenital heart disease (who are becoming increasingly necessary as survival continues to improve), interventionalists, and nurses in the field. And, as in the past, it is not a treatise on the subject.

A comparison with the original 1957 version serves to emphasize the enormous strides made, particularly in echocardiography, interventional catheterization, surgery and molecular biology. The number of authors at Children's Hospital has increased from the original "ONE" to 40, rather analogous to the song words "when we started this voyage there was just me and you, but now gathered round us we have our own crew." Some tests and diseases have virtually disappeared, such as phonocardiography and rheumatic fever (in this country), respectively: the decline of the latter in the Boston area was emphasized by the closure of the House of the Good Samaritan some 35 years ago, an institution whose population consisted largely of such patients.

When compared to the most recent edition (1992) a number of new topics have been added, including anesthesia, intensive care, nursing issues, adult congenital heart disease and clinical research, the latter to whet the investigative appetite of the young aspirant in this field. The general template is unchanged in that the table of contents, apart from the above additions, remains the same. We have again used our hierarchical coding system, which despite some limitations, has allowed us to deal with, superficially perhaps, the enormous number (1,375,701) of codes entered from a population that more than doubled over the preceding 14 years. Throughout the clinical chapters we have retained some emphasis on physical diagnosis rather than abandoning this to technology. It has always seemed to us that children (excluding neonates) with noncomplex lesions, unburdened as yet by the acquired diseases of adulthood (including obesity), present us with exquisite physical findings that together with a simple test, such as an electrocardiogram, provide us with enough information to diagnose and quantitate most of these lesions, with later verification (or humiliation) by technological studies. This viewpoint may be expressed another way namely "sticking the neck out is good exercise for the head." As in the last edition, we have included in most of the chapters on specific lesions "Exhibits" which both (a) briefly summarize our own experience from the recent (1988-2002) 14-year period and (b) provide data from the earlier era (1973-1987) for comparison.

Thanks are due to the enormous number of people who have made this book possible, including the physicians and nurses who cared for this patient population. We are also especially grateful to Mairead Sullivan and Joni D'Annolfo (for their humor, patience, and typing skills), Clare Keane (for proofreading par excellence and so much more), Bridget Stewart, Marissa Lory, Gena Coleman; Ellen McCusty and Dr. Kimberlee Gauvreau (for indispensable computer expertise), Alison Clapp (for her literature searches), Bill and Emily Flynn-McIntosh and Emily Harris (for artwork), Bruce Joziatics and Dr. Steven Colan (for echocardiographic pictures and information) and Elsevier for publishing this work. In addition, one of us (JFK) is deeply indebted to Brenda Foster, Drs. John A. Kelly, Arthur M. Levy, and Burton S. Tabakin for help/advice in earlier years without which this endeavor would not have been possible.

John F. Keane M.D.
Donald C. Fyler M.D.
James E. Lock M.D.
Boston, Massachusetts

Contents

Contributors vii

Preface xi

SECTION I

Historical Perspective 1

1A. *The NADAS Years at Children's Hospital* 3
Jane W. Newburger and Donald C. Fyler

1B. *Cardiology at Children's Hospital Boston: Today and into the Future* 7
James E. Lock

SECTION II

Developmental Anatomy 11

2. *Embryology* 13
Richard Van Praagh

3. *Morphologic Anatomy* 27
Richard Van Praagh and Stella Van Praagh

4. *Segmental Approach to Diagnosis* 39
Richard Van Praagh

SECTION III

Dysmorphology 47

5. *Dysmorphology and Genetics* 49
Ronald V. Lacro

SECTION IV

Normal Circulatory Physiology 73

6. *Fetal and Transitional Circulation* 75
Michael D. Freed

SECTION V

Problems Caused by Heart Disease 81

7. *Congestive Heart Failure* 83
Elizabeth D. Blume, Michael D. Freed, and Steven D. Colan

8. *Hypoxemia* 97
Alexander S. Nadas[†] and Donald C. Fyler

9. *Central Nervous System Sequelae of Congenital Heart Disease* 103
Jane W. Newburger

10. *Pulmonary Hypertension* 113
Mary P. Mullen

SECTION VI

Tools of Diagnosis 127

11. *History, Growth, Nutrition, Physical Examination, and Routine Laboratory Tests* 129
Robert L. Geggel and Donald C. Fyler

12. *Electrocardiography and Introduction to Electrophysiologic Techniques* 145
Edward P. Walsh, Mark E. Alexander, and Frank Cecchin

13. *Imaging Techniques: Echocardiography, Magnetic Resonance Imaging, and Computerized Tomography* 183
Tal Geva and Mary E. van der Velde

14. *Cardiac Catheterization* 213
James E. Lock

[†]Deceased

15. *Assessment of Ventricular and Myocardial Performance* 251
Steven D. Colan

16. *Exercise Testing* 275
Jonathan Rhodes

SECTION VII
Allied Disciplines 289

17. *Sedation and Anesthesia in Cardiac Procedures* 291
Peter C. Laussen

18. *Intensive Care Unit* 303
David L. Wessel and Peter C. Laussen

19. *Methodological Issues for Database Development: Trends* 323
John K. Triedman

20. *Methodological Issues in Clinical Research* 337
Kathy J. Jenkins, Kimberlee Gauvreau, and Steven D. Colan

21. *Contemporary Pediatric Cardiovascular Nursing* 347
Patricia O'Brien, Martha A.Q. Curley, and Patricia A. Hickey

SECTION VIII
Acquired Heart Disease 355

22. *Innocent Murmurs, Syncope, and Chest Pain* 357
Jane W. Newburger, Mark E. Alexander, and David R. Fulton

23. *Preventive Heart Disease: Dyslipidemia and Hypertension (Systemic)* 373
Jane W. Newburger

24. *Rheumatic Fever* 387
Donald C. Fyler

25. *Kawasaki Disease* 401
David R. Fulton and Jane W. Newburger

26. *Cardiomyopathies* 415
Steven D. Colan

27. *Pericardial Diseases* 459
Roger E. Breitbart

28. *Infective Endocarditis* 467
Gerald R. Marx

29. *Cardiac Arrhythmias* 477
Edward P. Walsh, Charles I. Berul, and John K. Triedman,

SECTION IX
Congenital Heart Disease 525

30. *Ventricular Septal Defect* 527
John F. Keane and Donald C. Fyler

31. *Pulmonary Stenosis* 549
John F. Keane and Donald C. Fyler

32. *Tetralogy of Fallot* 559
Roger E. Breitbart and Donald C. Fyler

33. *Aortic Outflow Abnormalities* 581
John F. Keane and Donald C. Fyler

34. *Atrial Septal Defect* 603
John F. Keane, Tal Geva, and Donald C. Fyler

35. *Patent Ductus Arteriosus* 617
John F. Keane and Donald C. Fyler

36. *Coarctation of the Aorta* 627
John F. Keane and Donald C. Fyler

37. *D-Transposition of the Great Arteries* 645
David R. Fulton and Donald C. Fyler

38. *Endocardial Cushion Defects* 663
Gerald R. Marx and Donald C. Fyler

39. *Cardiac Malpositions and the Heterotaxy Syndromes* 675
Stella Van Praagh

40. *Mitral Valve and Left Atrial Lesions* 697
Robert L. Geggel and Donald C. Fyler

41. *Hypoplastic Left Heart Syndrome, Mitral Atresia, and Aortic Atresia* 715
Peter Lang and Donald C. Fyler

42. *Pulmonary Atresia with Intact Ventricular Septum* 729
John F. Keane and Donald C. Fyler

43. *Double-Outlet Right Ventricle* 735
John F. Keane and Donald C. Fyler

44. *Single Ventricle* 743
John F. Keane and Donald C. Fyler

45. *Tricuspid Atresia* 753
John F. Keane and Donald C. Fyler

46. *Tricuspid Valve Problems* 761
John F. Keane and Donald C. Fyler

47. *Truncus Arteriosus* 767
John F. Keane and Donald C. Fyler

48. *Total Anomalous Pulmonary Venous Return* 773
John F. Keane and Donald C. Fyler

49. *Aortopulmonary Window* 783
John F. Keane and Donald C. Fyler

50. *Origin of a Pulmonary Artery from the Aorta (Hemitruncus)* 787
John F. Keane and Donald C. Fyler

51. *"Corrected" Transposition of the Great Arteries* 791
John F. Keane and Donald C. Fyler

52. *Vascular Fistulae* 799
John F. Keane and Donald C. Fyler

53. *Coronary Artery Anomalies* 805
John F. Keane and Donald C. Fyler

54. *Vascular Rings and Slings* 811
Andrew J. Powell and Valerie S. Mandell

55. *Cardiac Tumors* 825
Gerald R. Marx and Donald C. Fyler

56. *Adult Congenital Heart Disease* 833
Michael J. Landzberg

SECTION X

Surgical Considerations 843

57. *Neonatal and Infant Cardiac Surgery* 845
Frank A. Pigula and Pedro J. del Nido

58. *Surgical Management of the Patient with the Univentricular Heart* 861
John E. Mayer, Jr.

59. *Minimally Invasive and Robotically Assisted Cardiovascular Surgery, and Extracorporeal Membrane Oxygenation* 869
Pedro J. del Nido

60. *Current and Future Cardiovascular Organ and Tissue Replacement Therapies* 877
John E. Mayer, Jr. and Elizabeth D. Blume

SECTION XI

The Future 889

61. *Cardiac Excitability and Heritable Arrhythmias* 891
David E. Clapham and Mark T. Keating

Appendix

Principal Drugs Used in Pediatric Cardiology 907

Index 911

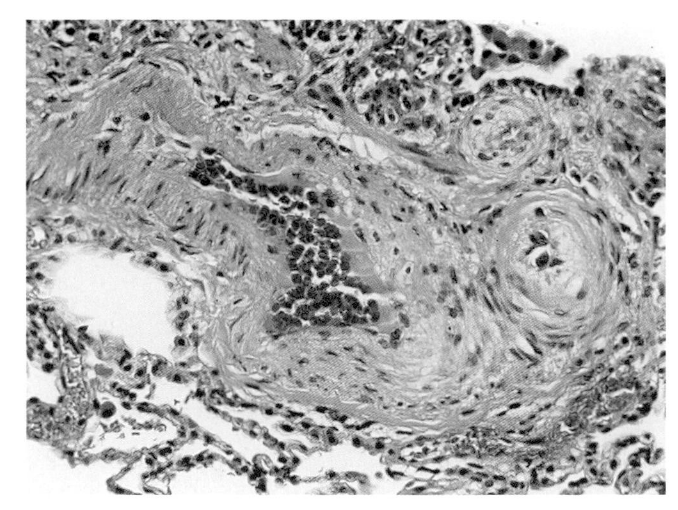

Figure 10-1. Plexiform lesion shows pulmonary artery with medical muscular hypertrophy **(left),** with loss of internal elastic lamina and muscle and replacement by fibrous tissue **(right).** The two small branches **(right)** have fibrous walls and marked intimal thickening. Courtesy of Harry Kozakewich, MD, Children's Hospital Boston.

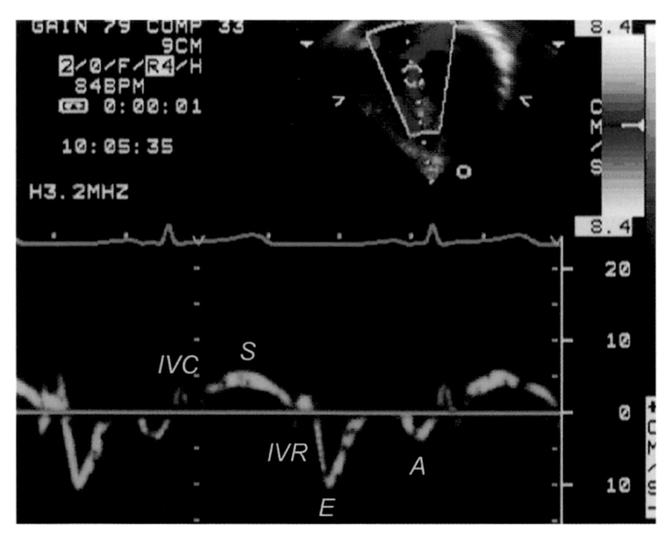

Figure 13-5. Tissue Doppler interrogation of the basal septum from the apical window. A, atrial (late) diastolic phase; E, early diastolic phase; IVC, isovolumic contraction; IVR, isovolumic relaxation.

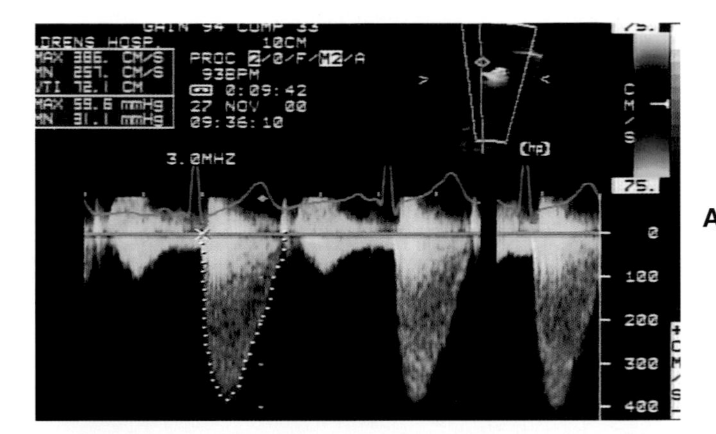

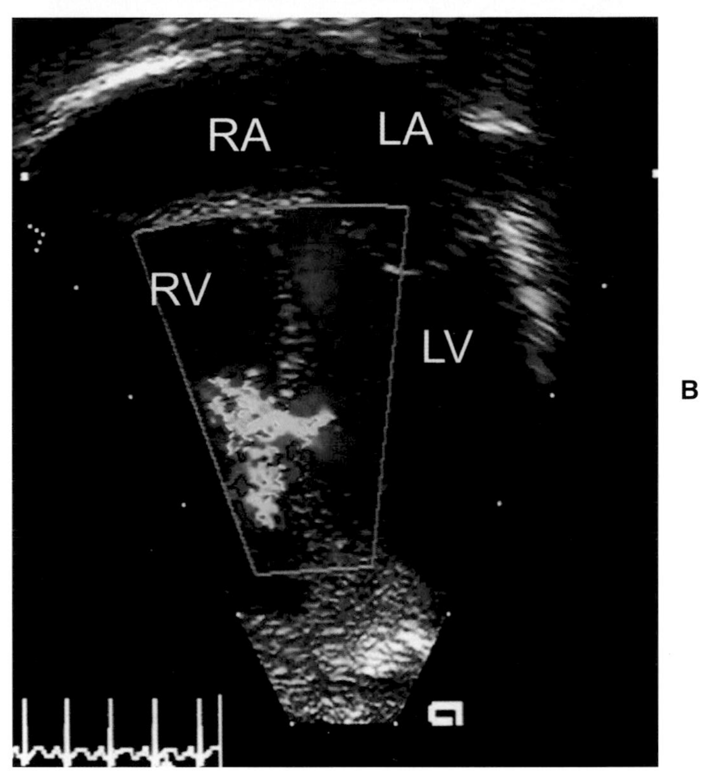

Figure 13-4. Doppler echocardiography. **A,** Interrogation of the left ventricular outflow tract from the apical window with continuous wave Doppler in a patient with subvalvar aortic stenosis. The peak velocity is ~3.9 m/sec and the predicted maximum instantaneous gradient is ~60 mm Hg. Tracing the spectral Doppler signal yields a mean gradient of 31 mm Hg. **B,** Color Doppler flow mapping from the apical window showing a small mid-muscular ventricular septal defect.

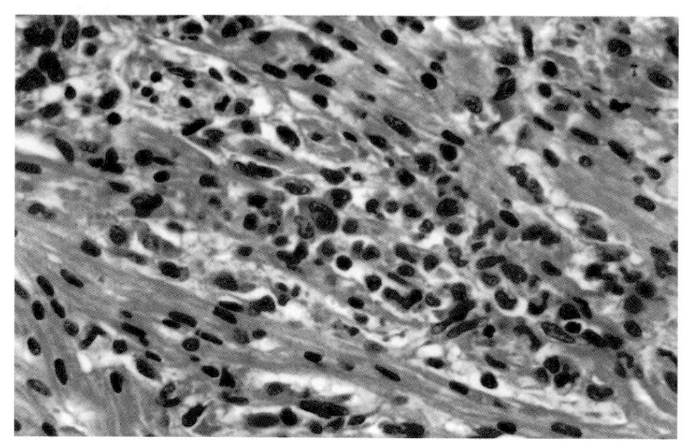

Figure 24-2. Granulomatous stage of an Aschoff nodule showing central necrosis with fibrinoid degeneration and a mixed inflammatory infiltrate of lymphocytes, plasma cells, and large histiocytic cells (Anitschkow cells). Courtesy of Antonio Perez, MD, Children's Hospital Boston.

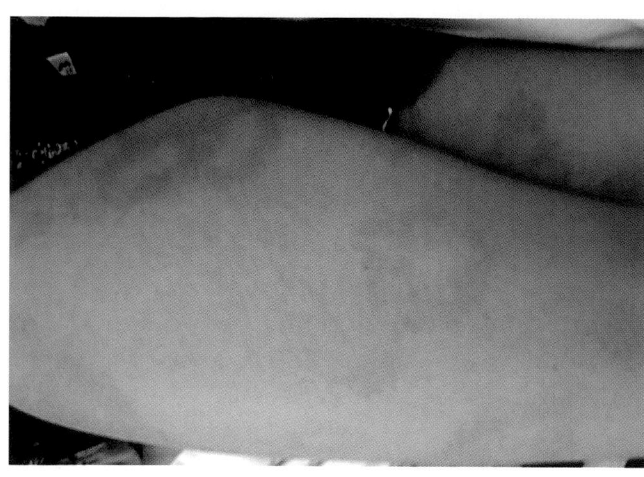

Figure 24-4. Erythema marginatum of the thighs in an 8-year-old boy. Courtesy of John K. Triedman, MD.

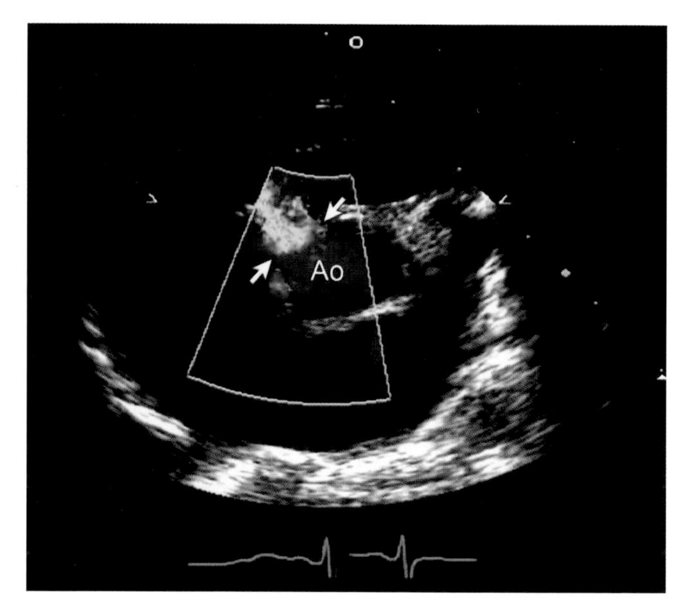

Figure 30-6B. Colorflow Doppler image of a membranous ventricular septal defect (arrows) showing left-to-right flow.

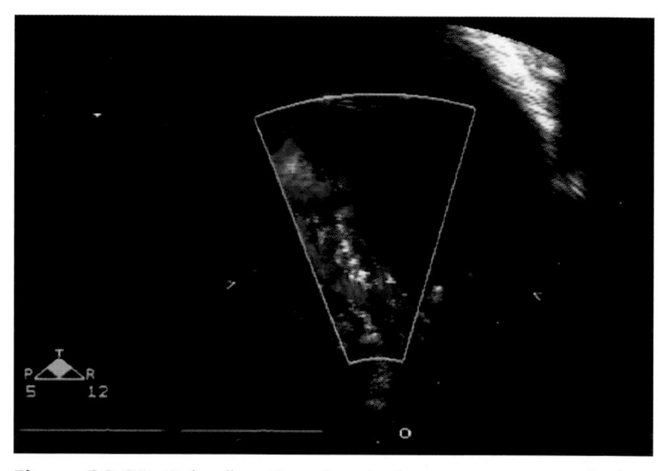

Figure 30-9B. Color-flow Doppler of a large muscular ventricular septal defect clearly shows the two jets (blue) of flow across the interventricular septum.

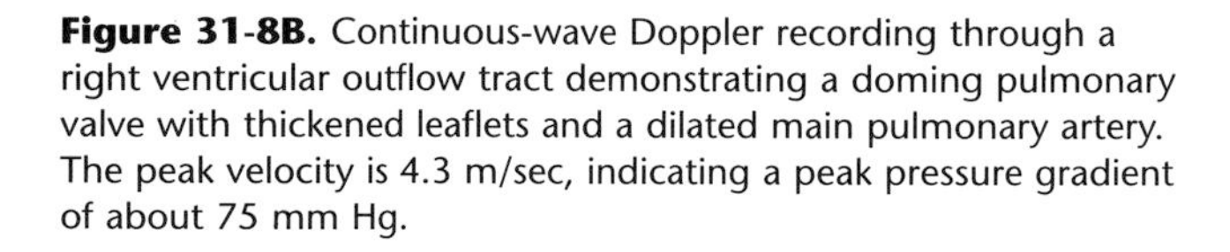

Figure 31-8B. Continuous-wave Doppler recording through a right ventricular outflow tract demonstrating a doming pulmonary valve with thickened leaflets and a dilated main pulmonary artery. The peak velocity is 4.3 m/sec, indicating a peak pressure gradient of about 75 mm Hg.

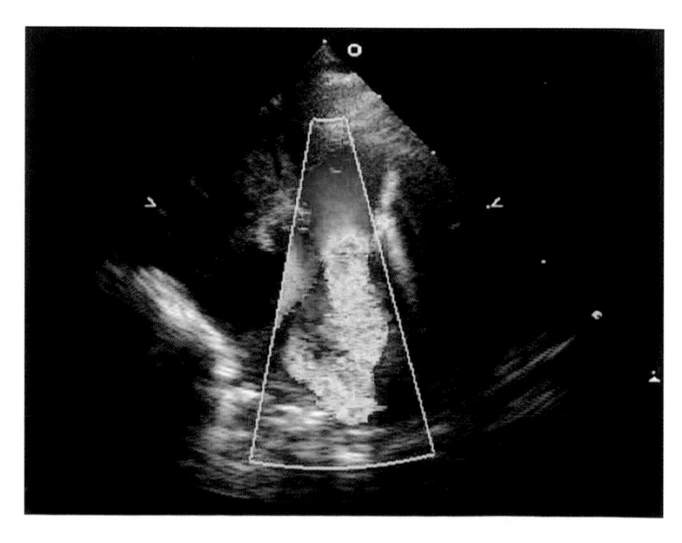

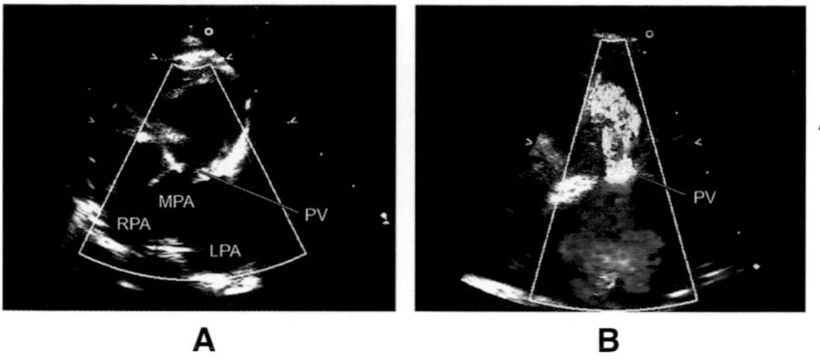

Figure 32-5. Echocardiogram of an infant with tetralogy of Fallot with absent pulmonary valve. **A,** Parasternal short-axis view showing the vestigial pulmonary valve leaflets (PV) and markedly dilated main (MPA), right (RPA), and left (LPA) pulmonary arteries. **B,** Color Doppler mapping corresponding to the image in panel **A,** demonstrating turbulent diastolic flow (multicolor) through the regurgitant pulmonary valve into the right ventricular outflow tract, toward the apex of the scan sector.

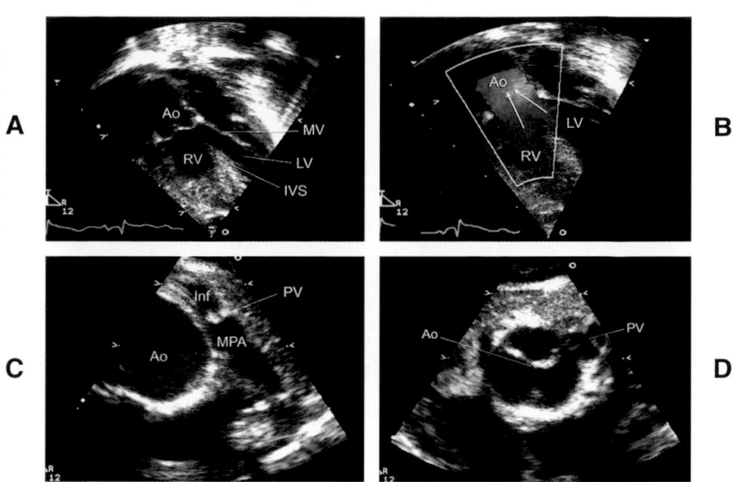

Figure 32-6. Echocardiogram of an infant with tetralogy of Fallot. **A,** Modified apical four-chamber view showing the conoventricular septal defect and dextroposed aorta (Ao) overriding the crest of the muscular interventricular septum (IVS) and related substantially to the right ventricle (RV). Note the absence of subaortic conus, with retained fibrous continuity between the aortic valve and mitral valve (MV), distinguishing tetralogy of Fallot, with preserved left ventricle (LV)-to-aorta continuity, from double-outlet right ventricle. **B,** Color Doppler mapping corresponding to the image in panel **A,** demonstrating systolic flow (blue) from both the left and right ventricles into the aorta (arrows). **C,** Parasternal short-axis view demonstrating the hypoplastic subpulmonary infundibulum (Inf) and small, dysplastic pulmonary valve (PV), small main pulmonary artery (MPA), and large aorta. **D,** Parasternal short axis view demonstrating the hypoplastic pulmonary valve and large aortic valve.

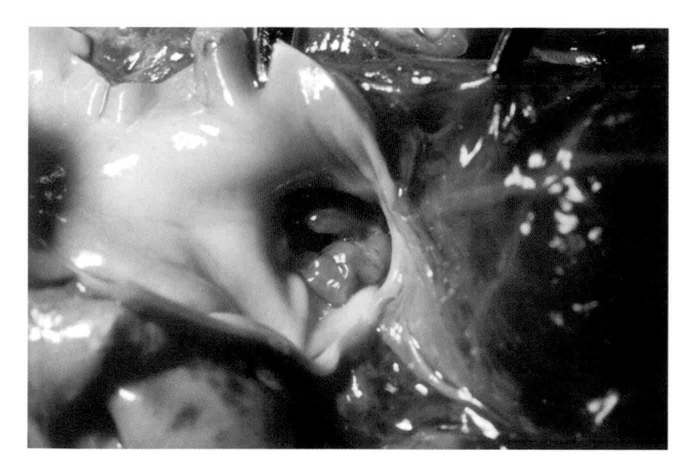

Figure 33-9. Autopsy picture of a nodular primitive-looking critically obstructive valve in a 4-week-old baby who died suddenly at home, undiagnosed. Such valves with survival can mature to become typically bicuspid structures.

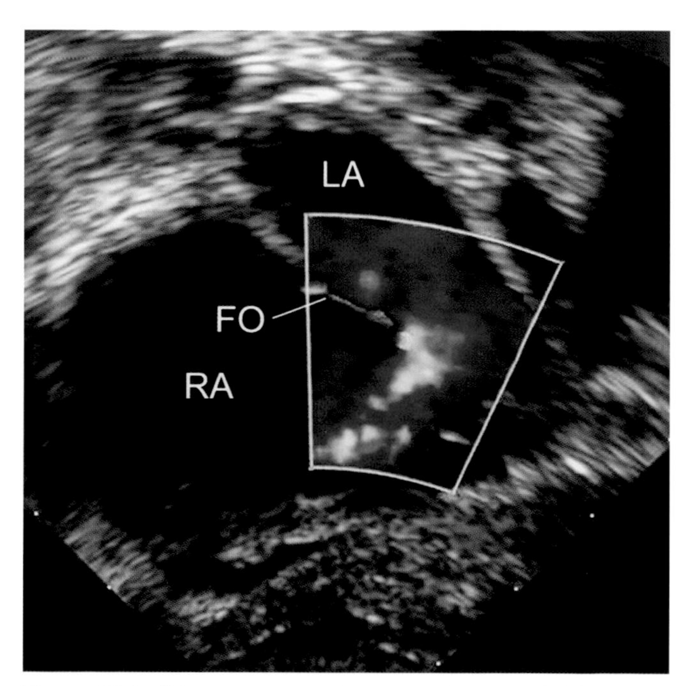

Figure 34-3. Echocardiogram of coronary sinus septal defect outlined by color-flow Doppler. LA, left atrium; FO, foramen ovale; RA, right atrium.

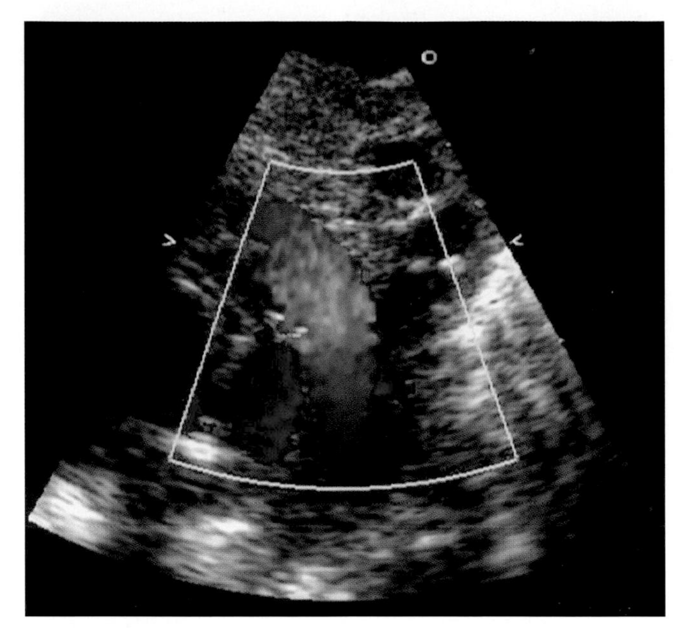

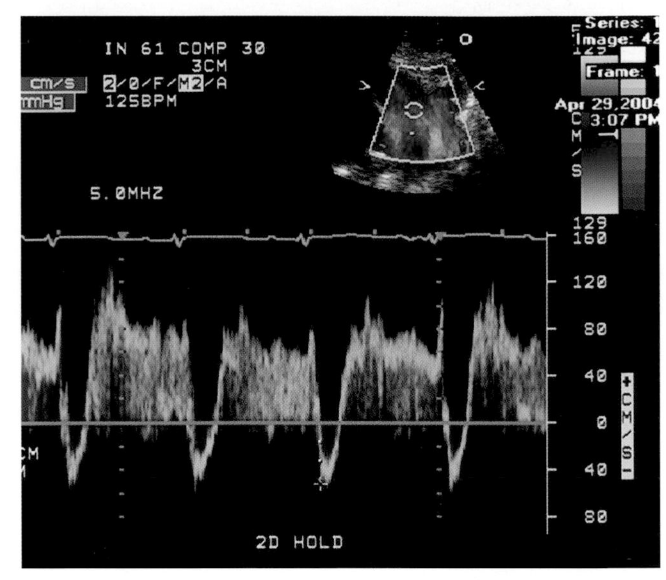

Figure 35-4B. Color-flow Doppler mapping confirms the presence of flow as the red color jet of the PDA flow is seen to enter the MPA. C, Spectral Doppler is used to show the timing and velocity of flow across the PDA. In this case, there is mostly low-velocity left-to-right flow (signal above the baseline indicates a positive Doppler shift reflecting flow toward the transducer) with transient right-to-left flow in early systole (negative Doppler shift).

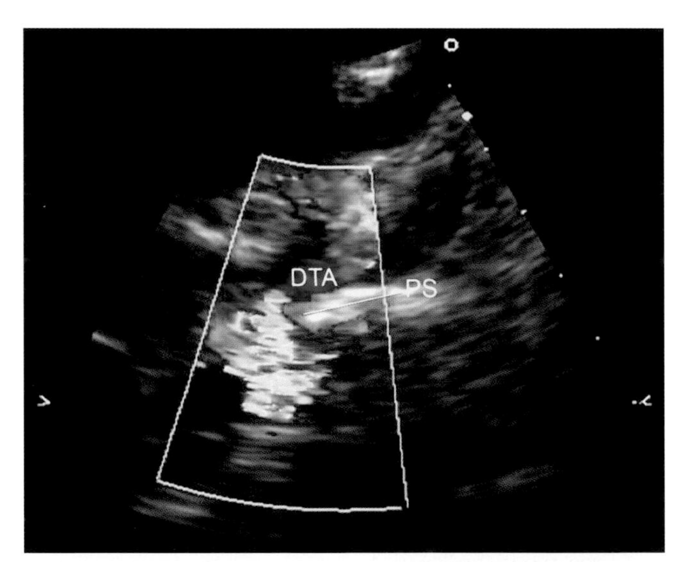

Figure 36-5A. Color Doppler flow mapping of the narrow and tortuous pathway created by the posterior shelf (PS) at the coarctation site between the distal transverse arch (DTA) and the descending aorta. The laminar flow in the transverse arch is indicated by the uniformly blue color Doppler map, whereas turbulent flow begins at the level of the coarctation, as indicated by the mixture of red and blue signals.

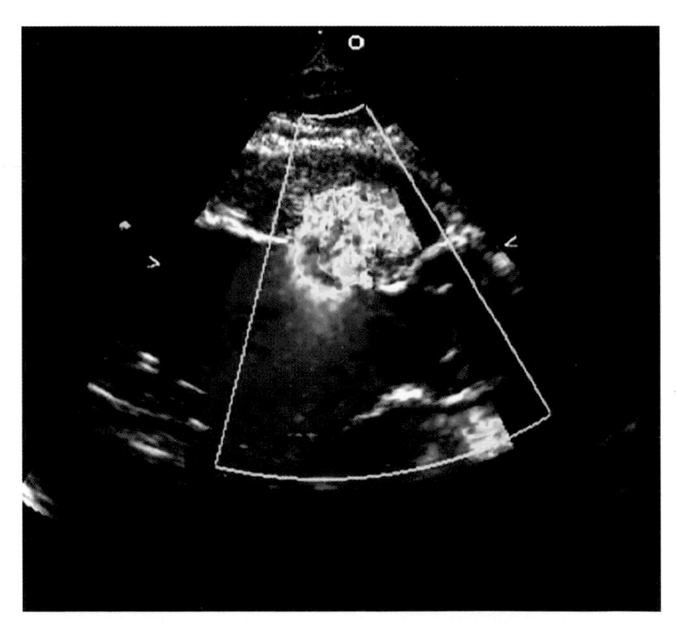

Figure 44-7B. Color Doppler flow mapping with flow acceleration at the level of the inlet to the outflow chamber (so-called bulboventricular foramen) consistent with significant stenosis.

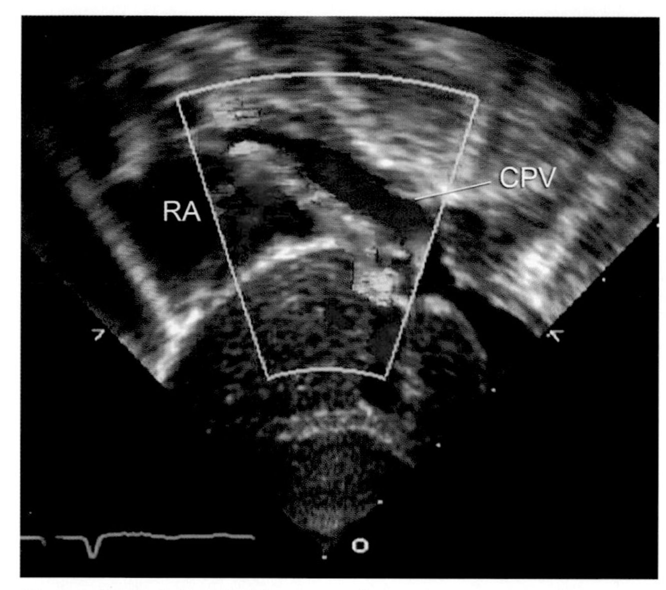

Figure 48-6. Subxyphoid echocardiographic image of obstructed subdiaphragmatic totally anomalous pulmonary venous connection. Color-flow mapping of the CPV shows flow toward the transducer (red) that turns anteriorly and reverses direction (blue) into the RA.

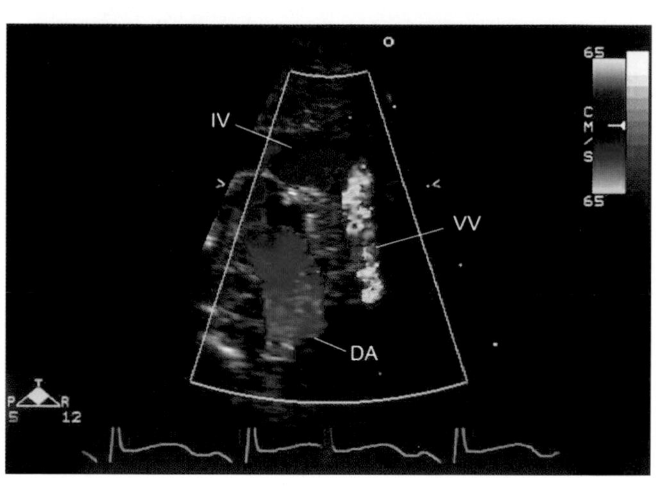

Figure 48-7. Color-flow Doppler image of obstructed supracardiac totally anomalous pulmonary venous drainage. The four pulmonary veins join into a common pulmonary vein that connects to the systemic venous system by means of a vertical vein. The potential for obstruction exists at several levels. In this case, the vertical vein (VV) is the site of obstruction, as reflected by the turbulent flow seen ascending to the left of the descending aorta (DA) and connecting to the innominate vein (IV).

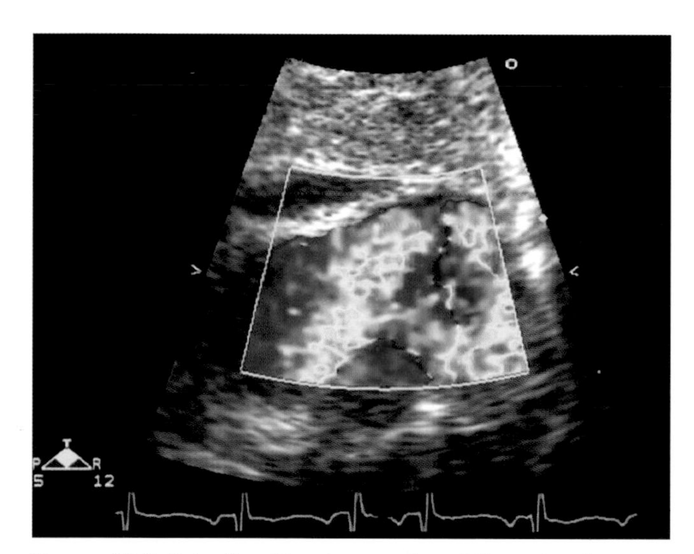

Figure 49-2. Color-flow Doppler mapping of the aortopulmonary window in Fig. 49-1, showing flow toward the transducer (red signal) from the aorta into the pulmonary artery.

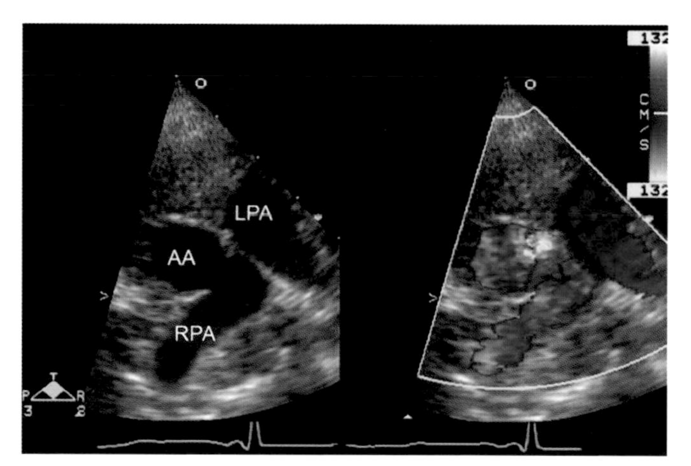

Figure 50-2. Two-dimensional and color-flow Doppler images of origin of the right pulmonary artery (RPA) from the ascending aorta (AA). The left panel shows the anomaly, as well as the left pulmonary artery (LPA) that fails to connect with the RPA. The right panel shows the flow signal connecting the AA to the RPA and the absence of flow between the RPA and LPA. The area of red signal is due to flow acceleration and turbulence at the junction of the AA to the RPA.

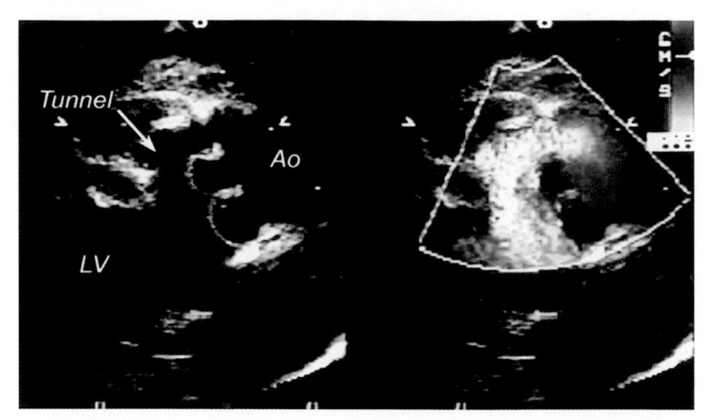

Figure 52-3. Two-dimensional and color-flow Doppler images of a congenital aorta (Ao) to left ventricular (LV) tunnel. The tunnel connects the ascending aorta (above the sinuses of Valsalva) to the LV along the right and anterior aspect of the aorta (left panel). Flow through the tunnel is readily demonstrated by color Doppler (right panel).

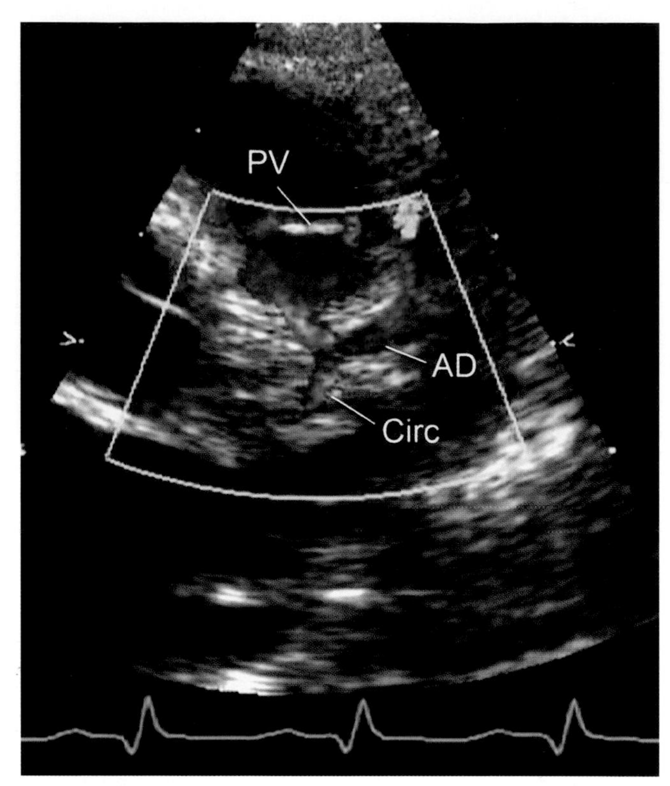

Figure 53-3. Parasternal short-axis color Doppler echocardiogram of anomalous origin of the left coronary artery from the pulmonary artery. Flow in the anterior descending (AD) coronary artery is seen as a blue signal, indicating flow away from the transducer, which in this case is retrograde. Similarly, flow in the circumflex coronary artery (CIRC) is seen as a red signal, consistent with flow toward the transducer, which is also retrograde. The red jet entering the main pulmonary artery just above the level of the pulmonary valve (PV) is the flow signal from the left main coronary artery into the pulmonary root.

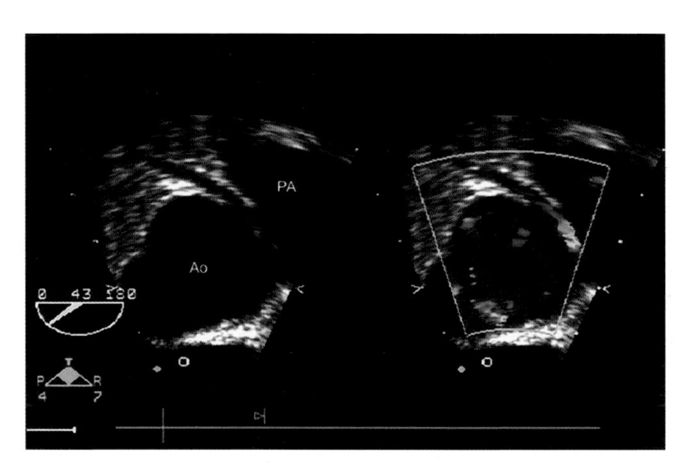

Figure 53-5. Parasternal short-axis view of anomalous origin of the right coronary artery from the left sinus of Valsalva, obtained by transesophageal echocardiography. The right coronary is seen to pass between the aorta (Ao) and pulmonary artery (PA), and flow into the coronary is documented by color-flow mapping.

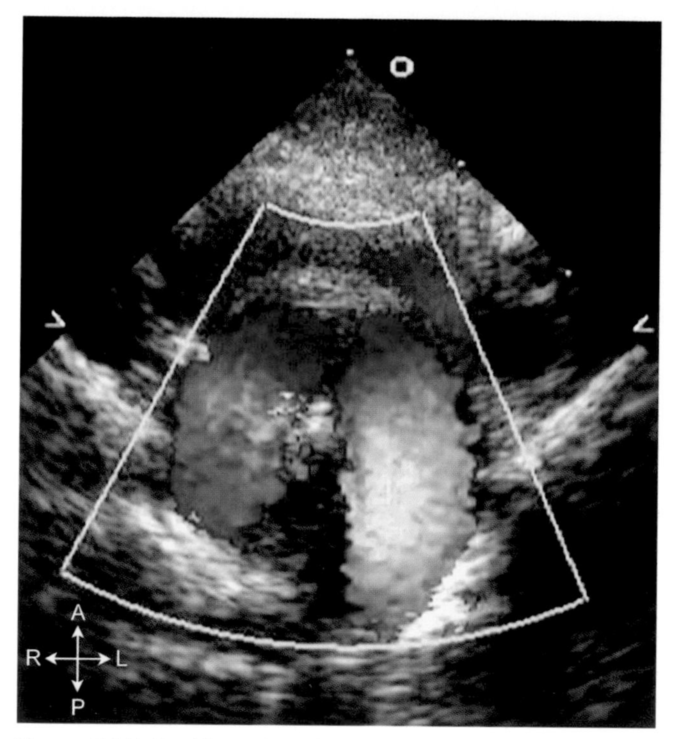

Figure 54-7. Double aortic arch with both arches patent. Echocardiogram from a suprasternal notch view using color Doppler imaging.

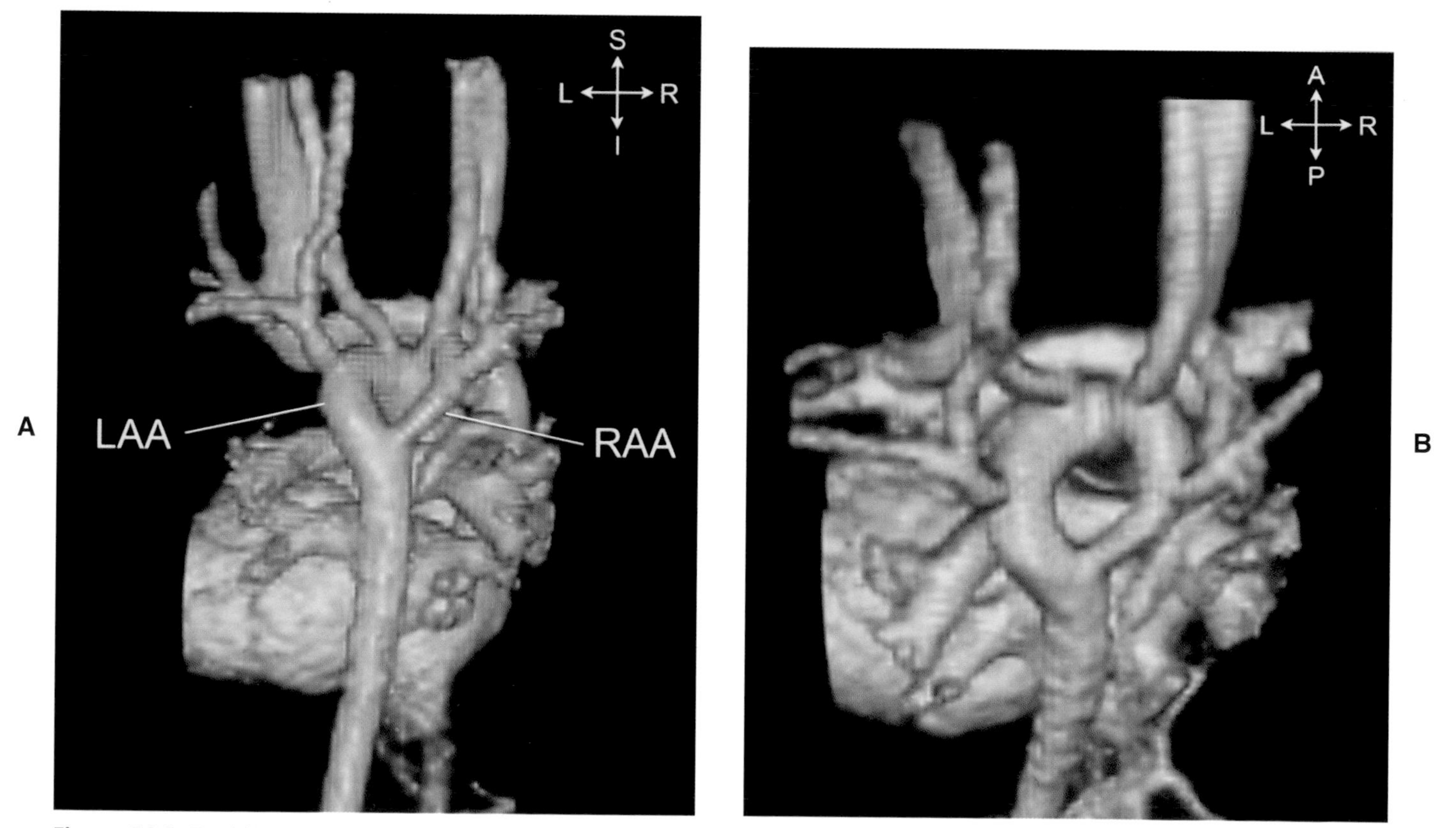

Figure 54-8. Double aortic arch with both arches patent. Volume rendered three-dimensional magnetic resonance angiogram viewed from posterior (A) and superior (B) vantage points. LAA, left aortic arch; RAA right aortic arch.

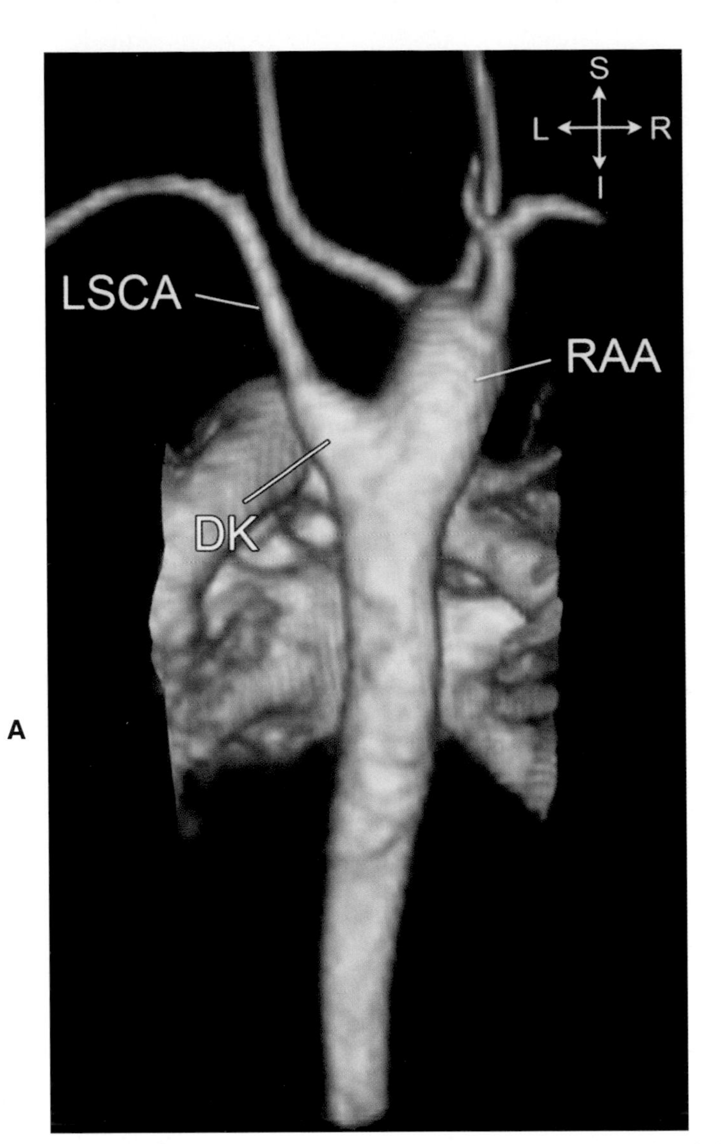

A

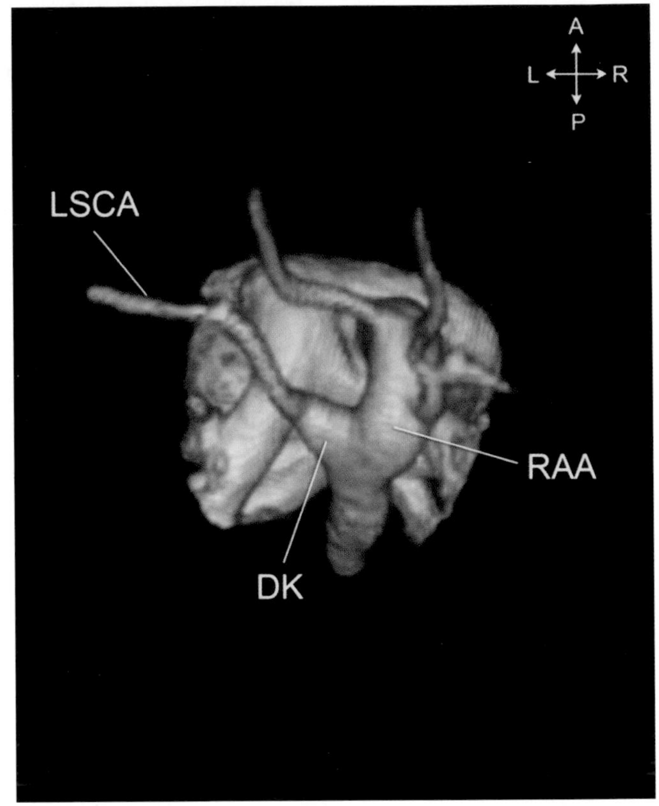

B

Figure 54-9. Right aortic arch with an aberrant origin of the left subclavian artery (LSCA). Volume rendered three dimensional magnetic resonance angiogram viewed from posterior (A) and superior (B) vantage points. DK, diverticulum of Kommerell.

I

Historical Perspective

1A

The NADAS Years at Children's Hospital

JANE W. NEWBURGER, MD, MPH,
AND DONALD C. FYLER, MD

Alexander Sandor Nadas was born in Budapest on November 12, 1913. His mother, Margit, was a prominent milliner in Hungarian society, and his father, Sandor, was a well-known intellectual and writer, who had wanted to be a doctor. In the writing of this textbook, Nadas paid homage to his father by fusing the profession of the writer with that of the physician. Indeed, the small emblem that has appeared at the end of the preface of each edition of this textbook was the trademark of his father's magazine.

Nadas studied medicine at Semmelweis Orvostudomanyi Egyetem in Budapest, from which he graduated in 1937. After 6 months in London studying with Paul Wood, he entered New York City in 1939, as Germany invaded Poland. After passing his entrance certificate for foreign medical graduates, he trained in pediatrics at Children's Hospital in Detroit under the guidance of Dr. Clement Smith, who then chaired its department of pediatrics. He was a resident in pediatrics at the Massachusetts Memorial Hospital in Boston from 1941 through 1942, moving on to become a volunteer pediatric outpatient resident at Children's Hospital Boston, where his outstanding clinical skills were widely noted. When Clem Smith moved to Michigan, he invited Nadas back to become chief resident in pediatrics, a position he held from 1943 to 1945, while also earning another degree as Doctor of Medicine from Wayne State University.

After his stint as chief resident at the Detroit Children's Hospital, Nadas settled down in a private pediatric practice in Greenfield, Massachusetts. In Greenfield, he made news when he was discharged from the staff of a Roman Catholic hospital for his public support of a defeated referendum that would have allowed doctors to give married women contraceptive advice when, in their opinion, pregnancy would have endangered the women's life or health. Even after his return to Boston, Dr. Nadas traveled to Greenfield twice a year to run a pediatric cardiology outreach clinic, always accompanied by one or two cardiology fellows who had the terrifying responsibility of driving his car.

In 1948, after Nadas had been in private practice for about 3 years, Charles A Janeway, then chairman of pediatrics at Children's Hospital Boston, asked him to develop a cardiac service for children comparable to that for adults at the Peter Bent Brigham (now Brigham and Women's) Hospital. Nadas therefore spent 1949 studying adult cardiology at the Brigham, under the tutelage of Samuel A. Levine and Lewis Dexter. By then, Dexter was in the process of developing cardiac catheterization in Boston, while Janet Baldwin, Dickinson Richards, and Andre Cournand were completing the first catheterizations of children in New York.

In 1950, Nadas launched his program in pediatric cardiology at Boston Children's Hospital, with the help of James Dow, a physiologist interested in cardiac catheterization, with whom Nadas had worked at the Brigham. That year, Abraham Rudolph joined the program as its first cardiac fellow, later spending 2 years at Harvard Medical School's physiology department before returning in 1954 to head the cardiac catheterization laboratory. At that time, almost no useful facts were known about cardiac disease in children. Often in the early years, cardiac catheterization in children amounted to accumulation of data on oxygen content and pressure from each heart chamber, these values simply being compared with those reported by Baldwin. A match was considered indicative of a diagnosis—a somewhat tenuous conclusion. Weekly pathology conferences reviewed the anatomic variations of congenital cardiac pathology that had been categorized by Maude Abbott[1] and Helen Taussig.[2]

Nadas made daily auscultatory rounds, assisted by Abe Rudolph, Pat Ongley, and Donald Fyler. He set up a system of dictating detailed bedside observations to the most junior house officer on rounds, these being written on pink slips readily identified in the chart. In the early years, he personally read every electrocardiogram (ECG). After he had obtained a history, detailed auscultation, a 12-lead ECG, and cardiac fluoroscopy, the data were presented, and Nadas then committed himself to a diagnosis and plan of management in public conferences. Over the next day or so, cardiac catheterization would be carried out.

In 1950, 50 children were catheterized, using a fluoroscope located in the Jimmy Fund building. A single blood sample, a pressure recording, and often a spot film were made in each cardiac chamber. Image intensification was not yet available. Exposure to radiation was limited to 10 minutes. Analysis of the blood samples by the Van Slyke technique took hours, great skill, and patience. Delineation of the physiology and anatomy of the various lesions facilitated subsequent operative procedures.

Nadas' detailed notes became the basis for the first edition of this textbook on pediatric cardiology.[3] Whereas the anatomic and fluoroscopic characteristics of congenital cardiac disease had been documented by Helen Taussig,[2] the correlation with auscultatory and ECG characteristics was a major contribution made by Nadas. Books by Ongley on phonocardiography[4] and by Ellison and Restieaux on vectorcardiography[5] documented these efforts.

ACADEMIC PEDIATRIC CARDIOLOGY IN THE NADAS YEARS

Over the ensuing years, the reputation of the units for pediatric cardiology and pediatric cardiac surgery at Boston Children's Hospital grew, and academic pediatric cardiology flourished. Nadas helped devise, and some say dominated, the Natural History Study.[6,7] Findings of the first Natural History Study, in which six centers contributed data from their patients and Harvard School of Public Health served as the data coordinating center, were published as a monograph in 1977.[8] The second Natural History Study followed up these original patients and its findings were published in 1993.[9]

The clinical and academic success of the Nadas enterprise led to recognition by the National Institutes of Health in the form of a large program project grant awarded in 1966. This grant, awarded in competition with programs for adult cardiology, was the first of its size and breadth in pediatric cardiology. The program project included a research unit in which Grier Monroe, Grant LaFarge, and Walter Gamble focused on physiologic questions. Their technique of firing a tiny hollow cylinder, precisely timed by electrocardiography, through the myocardium of rats and into liquid nitrogen for later electron microscopy was ingenious. Gamble used a fiberoptic catheter with a balloon tip filled with saline to visualize the aortic valve in an animal to produce pictures of the valve and was subsequently successfully used to visualize a left ventricle–right atrium (LV-RA) shunt in a teenager. Gamble, a classic inventor with a desk piled high with paper and amazing ideas, was always on hand to solve problems or design new techniques.

LaFarge's special assignment was to help surgeon William Bernhard evaluate the mechanical heart he had implanted in cows. The surreptitious movement of an unconscious cow through the hospital corridors to permit studies in the cardiac catheterization laboratory was a cause for murmuring among the staff, even though these cows were treated with exquisite sterile techniques. The goal was to see how long a cow could be maintained on a mechanical heart so breaks in sterile technique would have been unforgivable. Olli Miettinen, based at the Harvard School of Public Health, provided input on study design, and taught epidemiology and biostatistics to cardiology fellows and faculty. At the New England Primate Center in Southborough, Stephen Vatner studied physiology in intact and unanesthetized animals during normal activities using radiotelemetry.

A cardiac pathology unit was set up and run by Richard and Stella Van Praagh. This unit turned out to be of major value in training pediatric cardiac fellows and surgical residents and, later, invaluable as a basis for the development of cardiac echocardiography and resonance imaging. In the 1950s, Don Fyler was due to go on sabbatical leave from the University of Southern California and when he telephoned Nadas to ask where he thought it would be useful to go, Nadas invited him to come back to Boston and stay. He accepted. Fyler and Gamble set up the first biplane 35-mm General Electric (GE) cineangiographic unit in the country in the sub-basement of Children's Hospital. The hyperbaric chamber was next door, primarily being used by Bill Bernhard for infant cardiac surgery, and occasionally to treat wounded criminals with gas gangrene while the police stood guard. Perhaps because the Nadas' group had grown so large, Janeway declared cardiology to be a hospital department in 1968.

Paul Hugenholtz continued his attempts to measure cardiac output in patients by angiographic techniques, using a digitizing table and a PDP-9 computer. This apparatus, which was used by several groups around the medical school, was the site of storage and management of the data accumulated from the Regional Infant Cardiac Program.[10] Several fellows were sent off to learn new methods, for example Thomas Hougen to work in Thomas Smith's laboratory at the Brigham Cardiology Department, Albert Rocchini to work with Clifford Barger in the Harvard Medical School Department of Physiology, Barry Keane and Edward Walsh to learn electrophysiology at Texas Children's Hospital and the Massachusetts General Hospital, respectively.

By the late 1960s, it was clear that infants with congenital cardiac disease could be accurately diagnosed and, in some cases, helped by surgery. It was also clear, nonetheless, that not all infants with congenital cardiac disease in New England were being recognized and adequately managed. The Regional Infant Cardiac Program was proposed as a way to correct the situation. The Maternal and Child Health Service, along with the National Department of Health, Education and Welfare, agreed and provided funds for an educational program and for the transportation and even hospitalization of patients. All of the hospitals in New England that accepted referred infants with congenital cardiac disease were invited to participate, and all joined. The experiences of this program over nine years have served as a guide for programs of organized care for children with cardiac disease in various parts of the United States of America, and in other countries.[10]

The cardiac surgery section was headed by Robert Gross, who was the first surgeon to successfully ligate a persistently patent arterial duct. Gross's reputation for innovative surgery facilitated development of the Department of Cardiology. With Gross's retirement, Aldo Castaneda was chosen as the next chairman of cardiac surgery, and focused his efforts on reparative heart surgery in young infants. His development of cardiac surgical techniques for infants with cardiac disease succeeded beyond expectations. By the time of Nadas' retirement, three cardiac surgeons were occupied full time.

THE MAN

What permitted Nadas such remarkable success compared to other bright and hard-working physicians? Without doubt, Nadas's greatest advantages came from his spectacular intuition in dealing with and understanding people, his related insight into human behavior and politics, and his gift for language. Together, these gave him an unparalleled ability to "put things in a nutshell." His sharp and sometimes caustic wit diffused many volatile medical discussions and administrative hassles. He never seemed to inhibit verbalizing a thought, which both spiced up medical rounds and caused embarrassment for those fellows who were not in command of the facts. He demanded discipline, hard work, and integrity in those around him. Nadas also took an intense personal interest in the members of his department, regardless of stature, inquiring about their spouses and children, the state of their research, or whatever he thought might be important to them. Little escaped his attention. Above all, Nadas drilled into his trainees the principle that the welfare of the patient was the first priority in all decisions. No compromises were acceptable.

By the time of his retirement in 1982, Nadas had served as Cardiologist-in-Chief at Children's Hospital in Boston for 33 years. In the course of those 33 years, Cardiology had grown to an independent department with over 20 faculty members, three catheterization laboratories, an independent in-patient unit, and a cardiac intensive care unit. His department had become the largest in the world dealing specifically with pediatric cardiology. He was involved in developing subsections of the various national cardiology associations, and was instrumental in developing the pediatric cardiology sub-boards. He had produced over 200 scientific articles; the members of his department added many times more. He had trained over 150 pediatric cardiologists nationally and internationally and had been invited to consult and speak in many countries. Among the numerous honors conferred during his career, he received a Guggenheim fellowship, a Fulbright professorship, the Gifted Teacher Award of the American College of Cardiology, the Edgar Mannheimer Memorial Lecture Award from the European Association for Pediatric Cardiology, and the Paul Dudley White Award of the American Heart Association. Harvard set up the endowed Alexander S. Nadas Chair of Pediatric Cardiology in his honor. He was recognized as a leader not only among pediatricians, but also among adult cardiologists. He had risen from being the "Barefoot Boy from Budapest"—one of his favorite expressions—to being called the "Father of Pediatric Cardiology" by his associates. One evening in his 86th year, after having been honored at the Society for Pediatric Research, he had dinner with old friends at his long-favorite restaurant, the Café Budapest. After an evening of good fellowship, he was escorted home, retired, and died peacefully in his sleep. (Reprinted, in part, with permission from Cardiol Young 14:75, 2004.)

REFERENCES

1. Abbott MES. Atlas of Congenital Cardiac Disease. New York: The American Heart Association, 1936.
2. Taussig HB. Congenital Malformations of the Heart. New York: Commonwealth Fund, 1947.
3. Nadas AS. Pediatric cardiology. Philadelphia: WB Saunders, 1957.
4. Ongley PA. Heart Sounds and Murmurs: A Clinical and Phonocardiographic Study. New York: Grune & Stratton, 1960.
5. Ellison RC, Restieaux NJ. Vectorcardiography in Congenital Heart Disease: A Method for Estimating Severity. Philadelphia: Saunders, 1972.

6. Nadas AS. Report from the Joint Study on the Natural History of Congenital Heart Defects, IV: Clinical course. Introduction. Circulation (Suppl)65:I, 1977.
7. Nadas AS. Report from the Joint Study on the Natural History of Congenital Heart Defects, I: Summary and conclusions. Circulation (Suppl)65:1, 1977.
8. Report from the Joint Study on the Natural History of Congenital Heart Defects. Circulation 65 (Suppl I), 1977.
9. Report from the Second Joint Study on the Natural History of Congenital Heart Defects Eds. Fallon WM, Weidman WH. Circulation 87(Suppl), 1993.
10. Fyler DC. Report of the New England Regional Infant Cardiac Program. Pediatrics 65 (Suppl):375, 1980.

1B

Cardiology at Children's Hospital Boston: Today and Into the Future

JAMES E. LOCK, MD

When Dr. Charles Janeway, physician-in-chief, established the department of cardiology in 1976 under the leadership of Dr. Alexander S. Nadas, the Children's Hospital Boston had articulated three clear-cut missions: To provide truly outstanding clinical care to its patients, to seek to improve the understanding of childhood diseases and develop new cures using research tools and innovative approaches; and to train the future generations of physicians, scientists, and nurses. A description of the current state of the cardiology and its goals and aspirations for the future, can perhaps best be organized around those three missions.

CLINICAL CARE

The goal and expectation of providing unsurpassed clinical care to our patients was the primary mission of this program from its inception, and it remains the core today. An important recent addition to this effort has been the application of rigorous and self-critical methodologies to measure, analyze, and report our results and adverse events, and then to develop tools to improve them as rapidly as possible. The development in the mid 1980s of clinical practice guidelines to assess the postoperative care for children with an increasing number of congenital heart defects has led to reduced hospital stays *and* reduced morbidity.[1,2] The identification and self-critical publication of a series of adverse events ranging from choreoathetosis after surgery,[3] neurologic sequelae of circulatory arrest,[4] vascular trauma in the pulmonary artery bed,[5] myocardial infarctions after repair of pulmonary atresia with intact septum,[6] and others have led directly to improved outcomes. A second revolutionary change in clinical care began two decades ago when the department of cardiology was divided into divisions that permitted highly subspecialized care for the different aspects of patient management. In 1984, 12 cardiologists performed 650 catheterizations per year, but by 1986 only four cardiologists performed nearly 1,000 catheterizations per year. Similarly, all cardiologists took care of their own patients with arrhythmias in 1984, but by 1987 all serious arrhythmias were cared for by three dedicated electrophysiologists. The pediatric cardiac intensive care unit was intermittently staffed by physicians interested in intensive care in 1984; by 1990 the cardiac intensive care unit (CICU), led by David Wessel, was staffed around the clock by physicians specially trained in intensive care. At present, the department of cardiology has six different divisions and three different sections (Table 1). There are seven different faculty cardiologists on call at all times to provide highly specialized cardiac care to a wide range of children and young adults (Boston Adult Congenital Heart Service [BACH]) with cardiovascular diseases.

A third more recent development has allowed us to compare the results of many of our therapeutic surgical and catheter-based procedures to those of other centers around the country. The development of computer tools and algorithms to extract data from many states on the admission of children with cardiac disease has allowed the unbiased assessment of cardiac care across many different centers for the first time.[7] More recently, tools have been developed to adjust for the risk of certain procedures, further improving the assessment of the results of cardiac procedures, especially cardiac surgical procedures.[8, 9] Although these studies may permit brief moments of self-congratulation,

TABLE 1

Division, 2004	Division Chief, 2004	On Call
Invasive Cardiology	J. Lock (Acting)	Yes
Noninvasive Cardiology	S. Colan	Yes
Outpatient Cardiology	D. Fulton	No
Inpatient Cardiology	M. Freed	Yes
Intensive Care	P. Laussen	Yes
Electrophysiology	E. Walsh	Yes
Section	**Section Chief**	
MRI	T. Geva	No
Transplant	E. Blume	Yes
BACH	M. Landzberg	Yes

BACH, Boston Adult Congenital Heart Service; MRI, magnetic resonance imaging.

they also provide clear-cut road maps of ways to improve our own results in certain forms of congenital heart disease. Moving into the next decade, it is increasingly clear that an emphasis on outcomes, patient safety, and adverse event identification and prevention will increasingly dominate the management of the clinical care of all patients, including children with heart disease.

RESEARCH

While descriptive clinical research was always a central part of the department of cardiology during the Nadas era, the basic research remained underdeveloped until the arrival of Bernardo Nadal-Ginard to chair the department in 1983. Although the large and excellent research effort he brought to the institution did not survive his own difficulties of a decade later, the expectation that truly outstanding basic research needed to be a central part of the cardiovascular program did survive. The commitment to an outstanding basic research program is exemplified by the funding in 1996 of the Aldo Castaneda Professorship in Cardiovascular Research. David Clapham is the first incumbent, and Mark Keating, a recent inductee of the National Academy of Science, was recruited several years later. The basic laboratories occupy nearly 15,000 square feet in the Enders Research Building.

The clinical research activities of the department have changed enormously with the development of strong linkages between the department of cardiology and the Harvard School of Public Health led by Jane Newburger, the first director of clinical research. The application of sophisticated clinical research tools and methodology to the field of pediatric cardiology has led to several dozen landmark studies that have markedly improved the evidence that we use to decide how to manage our patients.

Finally, the development of innovative clinical approaches has been perhaps the most characteristic feature of the entire cardiovascular program during the past decade. Many of the surgical-, catheter-, and medical-based therapies, and many of the diagnostic tools that are currently standard throughout our field were developed at the Children's Hospital Boston during the last 25 years. These advances include surgeries for hypoplastic left heart syndrome, primary neonatal arterial switch procedures, fenestrated Fontan procedures, quantitative echocardiography, sophisticated mapping techniques for intracardiac arrhythmias, and a long list of interventional catheter innovations. The commitment to the development of innovative therapies and the active exploration of new approaches remains a central part of the culture of the cardiovascular program at the Children's Hospital Boston, and it will undoubtedly continue into the foreseeable future.

TRAINING

Although medical students, nursing students, interns, and residents all rotate through the cardiovascular program at the Children's Hospital Boston, training is primarily directed at postgraduate training of fellows and senior fellows in advanced clinical and research techniques. The clinical training program, overseen by Peter Lang, currently trains 33 fellows: 19 fellows in their first, second, or third year of clinical cardiology training and 14 fellows in their fourth or fifth year of senior clinical fellowship training in subspecialty areas such as magnetic resonance imaging (MRI), interventional cardiology, or intensive care. Twelve fellows are doing basic research postgraduate work. An innovative program begun nearly 20 years ago is the senior clinical fellowship program: Cardiologists who have graduated from training programs around the world come to Boston for 6 months to a year to study highly specialized aspects of clinical care. Over 100 graduates of the general fellowship program and the senior clinical training program now hold faculty positions in pediatric cardiology around the country, and several dozen lead academic programs around the world.

COLLABORATION

The most important programmatic innovation of the last two decades was the development of the interdisciplinary cardiovascular program for managing children with heart disease. This widely imitated construct brought together leaders from the departments of cardiovascular surgery and cardiology, the division of cardiovascular anesthesia and cardiovascular nursing into an operating committee with rotating leadership. Although the initial functions of this committee were quite limited (assessment of capital budget purchases, development and execution of clinical practice guidelines, maintenance of a unified fundraising activities), the success of this effort has led to an increasing set of responsibilities. Currently, the Cardiovascular Program Operating Committee, chaired by Pedro del Nido, helps oversee a combined research endowment, develops principles for management of patient flow, and helps select the recipient of an annual endowed fellowship. This commitment to a generous spirited collaboration across specialties is an increasingly important requirement for all leaders and members of the cardiovascular program at Children's Hospital Boston.

REFERENCES

1. Laussen P, Roth S. Fast tracking: Efficiently and safely moving patients through the intensive care unit. Prog Pediatr Cardiol 18:149, 2003.
2. Poppleton VK, Moynihan PJ, Hickey PA. Clinical practice guidelines: the Boston experience. Prog Pediatr Cardiol 18:75, 2003.
3. Wong PC, Barlow CF, Hickey PR, et al. Factors associated with choreoathetosis following cardiopulmonary bypass in children with congenital heart disease. Circulation 86:118, 1992
4. Bellinger DC, Wernovsky G, Rappaport LA, et al. Cognitive development of children following early repair of transposition of the great arteries using deep hypothermic circulatory arrest. Pediatrics 87:701, 1991.
5. Baker CM, McGowan FX, Keane JF, et al. Pulmonary artery trauma due to balloon dilation: Recognition, avoidance and management. J Am Coll Cardiol 36:1684–1690, 2000.
6. Giglia TM, Mandell VS, Connor AR, et al. Diagnosis and management of right ventricular dependent coronary circulation in pulmonary atresia with intact ventricular septum. Circulation 86:1516, 1992.
7. Jenkins KJ, Newburger JW, Lock JE, et al. In-hospital mortality for surgical repair of congenital heart defects: preliminary observations of variation by hospital caseload. Pediatrics 95:323, 1995.
8. Jenkins KJ, Gauvreau K, Newburger JW, et al. Consensus-based method for risk adjustment for congenital heart surgery. J Thorac Cardiovasc Surg 123:110, 2002.
9. Jenkins KJ, Gauvreau K. Center-specific differences in mortality: preliminary analysis using the risk adjustment in congenital heart surgery (RACHS-1) method. J Thorac Cardiovasc Surg 124:97, 2002.

II

Developmental Anatomy

2

Embryology[1]

Richard Van Praagh, MD

Embryology is important to pediatric cardiology as a means of understanding. Embryology makes possible the comprehension of complex congenital heart disease, which in turn facilitates its accurate clinical diagnosis. Embryology also helps to clarify both the morphogenesis (pathogenesis) and the etiology (basic causes) of cardiac malformations.

DEFINITION

In man, embryology may be defined as developmental biology from conception to the end of the second month of life (i.e., from conception to the end of the eighth week).

THE FIRST WEEK OF LIFE

The salient events of the first week of life from 0 to 7 days (Fig. 2-1) are (a) ovulation, (b) fertilization, (c) segmentation, (d) blastocyst formation, and (e) the beginning of implantation.

THE SECOND WEEK OF LIFE

The principle developments of the second week of life, from 8 to 14 days (Fig. 2-2), are (a) completion of the implantation, (b) bilaminar disc formation, consisting of ectoderm and endoderm, (c) development of the amniotic cavity, (d) appearance of the yolk sac, and (e) the elaboration of primitive villi of the developing placenta. It is noteworthy that during the first 2 weeks of life, humans have no heart and no vascular system.

THE THIRD WEEK OF LIFE

From the cardiovascular standpoint, the main events of the third week of life, from 15 to 21 days, may be summarized as follows (Figs. 2-3 to 2-5):

1. In humans, the **mesoderm** develops from the ectoderm on the 15th day of life (Fig. 2-3). It is from the mesoderm that the cardiovascular system is formed.
2. The **cardiogenic crescent** of precardiac mesoderm, the immediate precursor of the heart, appears on the 18th day of life (Fig. 2-4A).
3. The **intra-embryonic celom** also develops on the 18th day of life (Fig. 2-5). Cavitation of the mesoderm forms the intra-embryonic celom, from which are derived all of the body cavities—pericardial, pleural, and peritoneal.
4. The **straight heart tube,** or preloop stage, normally develops by 20 days of age (Fig. 2-4B). By analogy with chick embryos, the heartbeat in man probably begins at the straight tube stage, or at the early D-loop or L-loop stage (Fig. 2-4C and 2-4D).
5. **Cardiac loop formation,** normally to the right (D-loop formation) and abnormally to the left (L-loop formation), begins by 21 days of age (Fig. 2-4C and D).

[1]This chapter is based on personal study of embryos from the following sources: the Minot Collection, Harvard Medical School, Boston; the Carnegie Collection, Carnegie Institution, Baltimore; chick embryology, morphologic, and experimental, the Carnegie Institution, Baltimore, and The Children's Hospital, Boston; iv/iv mouse embryology, Dartmouth Medical School, Hanover, New Hampshire; and the literature.

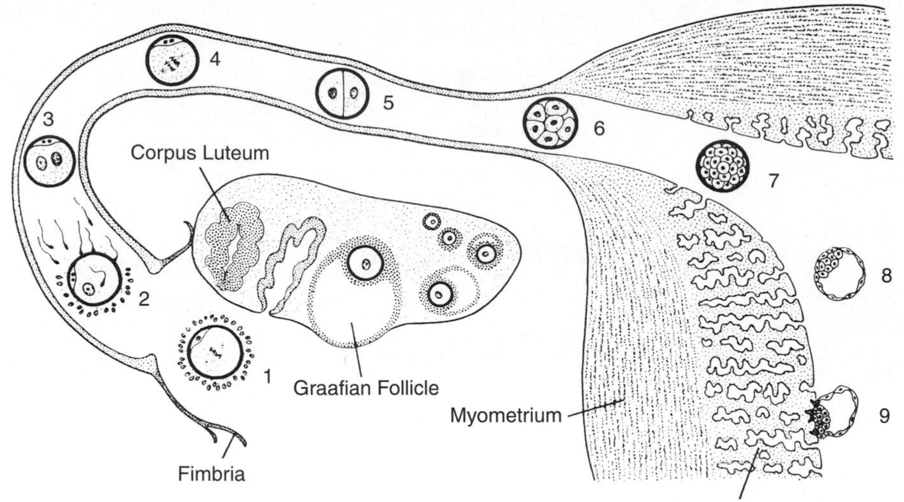

FIGURE 2–1 *Schematic representation of the events taking place during the first week of human development. (1) Occyte immediately after ovulation. (2) Fertilization approximately 12 to 24 hours after ovulation. (3) Stage of the male and female pronuclei. (4) Spindle of the first mitotic division. (5) Two-cell stage (approximately 30 hours of age). (6) Morula containing 12 to16 blastomeres (approximately 3 days of age). (7) Advanced morula stage reaching the uterine lumen (approximately 4 days of age). (8) Early blastocyst stage (approximately 4½ days of age). The zona pellucida has now disappeared. (9) Early phase of implantation (blastocyst approximately 6 days of age).The ovary shows the stages of the transformation between a primary follicle and a graafian follicle as well as a corpus luteum. The uterine endometrium is depicted in the progestational stage.*
From Langman J. Medical Embryology, 2nd ed. Baltimore: Williams & Wilkins, 1969, with permission.

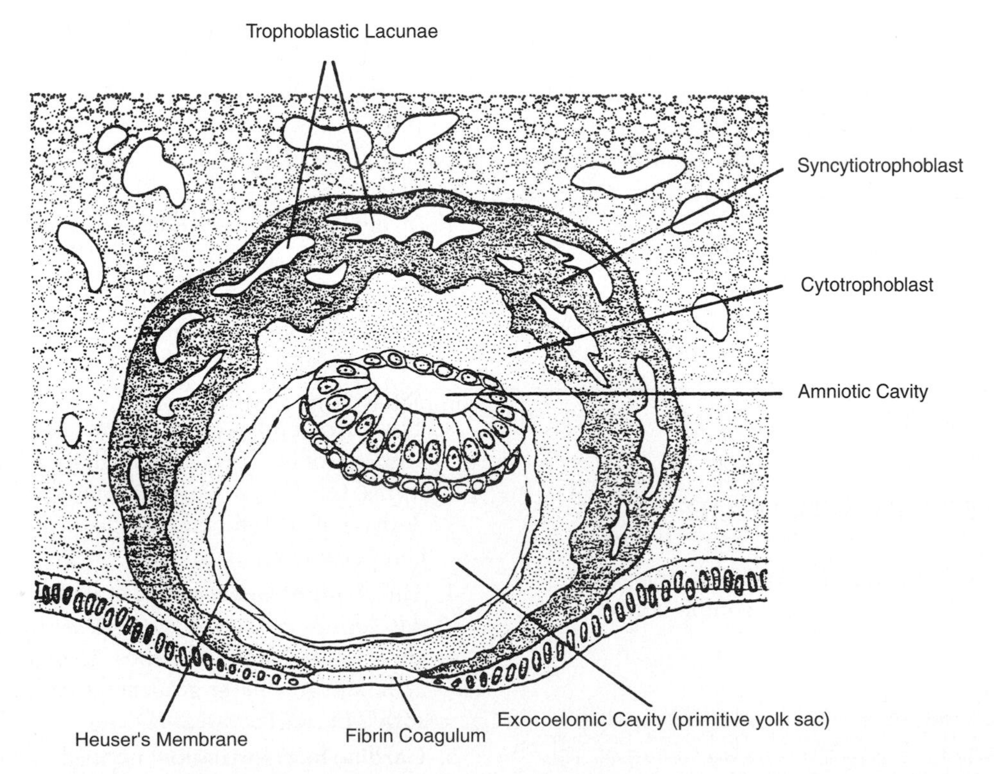

FIGURE 2–2 *The second week of life: the implanted bilaminar disc consisting of the ectoderm and endoderm, before the appearance of the mesoderm.*
From Langman J. Medical Embryology, 2nd ed. Baltimore: Williams & Wilkins, 1969, with permission.

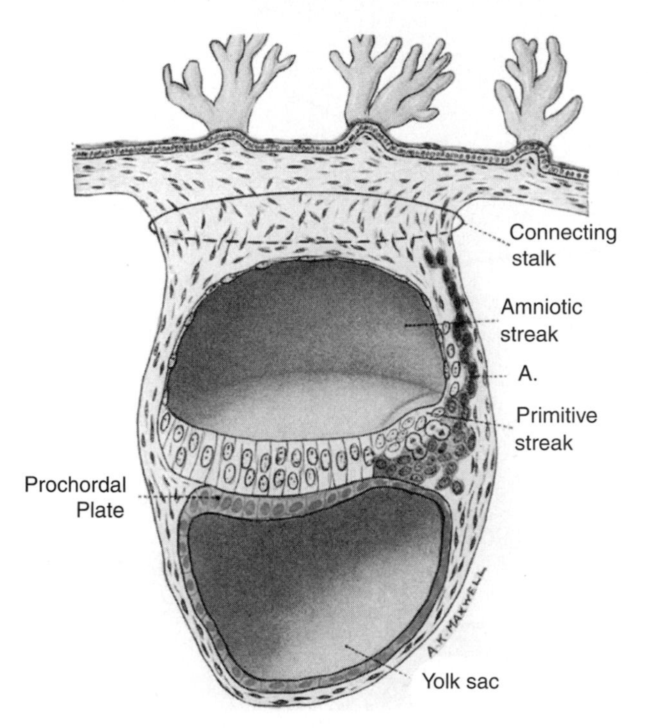

FIGURE 2–3 *The appearance of the mesoderm, from which the cardiovascular system will arise, at 15 days of age. The mesoderm (meaning "middle skin") buds off from the ectoderm.*
From Hamilton WJ, Mossman HW. Human Embryology: Prenatal Development of Form and Function, 4th ed. Baltimore: Williams & Wilkins, 1972, with permission.

THE FOURTH WEEK OF LIFE

The main features of cardiovascular development from 22 to 28 days are the following:

1. Normally, D-loop formation is completed (Fig. 2-6, horizon XI).
2. The development of the morphologically left ventricle and of the morphologically right ventricle begins (Fig. 2-6, horizon XIII).
3. The circulation commences.
4. Cardiovascular septation is initiated.
5. The evolution of the aortic arches begins (Figs. 2-7, 2-8, and 2-9).

Neural crest cells originating from the posterior rhombencephalon (rhombomeres 6–8) begin to migrate into pharyngeal (aortic) arches 3, 4, and 6 (Figs. 2-8 and 2-9) and from there to the heart where they participate in the formulation of conus (including the conal septum), the great arteries (including the aorta, the aortopulmonary septum, the carotids, the subclavians, the ductus arteriosus), and the cardiac ganglia.[1]

Streeter's **horizons,** now often called **stages** (Fig. 2-10), are indicated by Roman numerals in Figure 2-6. Each horizon is a 2-day time interval. To obtain the approximate age of the embryo, double the horizon number. For example, horizon XI indicates a time interval that begins on day 22. Because each horizon is 2 days long, horizon XI extends from days 22 to 24 (Fig. 2-10). Embryonic lengths (in mm) are also given in Figure 2-10, and it is readily possible to convert the length of a normal human embryo into both the developmental stage (horizon) and approximate age.

The left and the right ventricles develop by evagination or outpouching from the primary heart tube, beginning at 22 to 24 days (horizon XI, Fig. 2-6, left side). By 26 to 28 days (horizon XIII, Fig. 2-6, right side), development of the left ventricle is more advanced than that of the right (Fig. 2-6, right side).

True circulation (as opposed to the ebb and flow) is thought to begin in humans at this stage (26–28 days, horizon XIII, Fig. 2-6, right side). This is known as the *in-series circulation* because the blood goes from the morphologically right atrium to the morphologically left atrium, to the left ventricle, to the right ventricle, and the truncus arteriosus (arterial trunk) (Fig. 2-6, right side). The in-series circulation is similar to that which persists in tricuspid atresia.

At the beginning of the fourth week, the first pair of aortic arches has formed (Fig. 2-7). At this stage, the ventricle (future left ventricle) of the D-bulboventricular loop is ventral (anterior) to the proximal bulbus cordis (future right ventricle) (Fig. 2-7, right side). Thus, early in D-loop formation, the left ventricle is anterior to (ventral to) the right ventricle. Hence, among children with congenital heart disease, the anterior ventricle is usually, although not necessarily the right ventricle.

By the 26th day of life, the first pair of aortic arches (earlier mandibular arteries) has involuted completely or nearly completely (Fig. 2-8). The second and third aortic arches have been formed, and the fourth and sixth arches are beginning to form (Fig. 2-8). A large communication between the respiratory and gastrointestinal tracts is present (i.e., a large tracheoesophageal "fistula") is normal at this stage (Fig. 2-8, right side).

By the end of the fourth week (28 days, Fig. 2-9), aortic arches 1 and 2 have involuted. Aortic arches 3 and 4 are present (Fig. 2-9). Aortic arches 5 are incomplete bilaterally. Aortic arches 6 are in the process of forming (complete on the right and incomplete on the left, Fig 2-9). Both pulmonary artery branches are present, as is the common pulmonary vein (Fig. 2-9, left side).

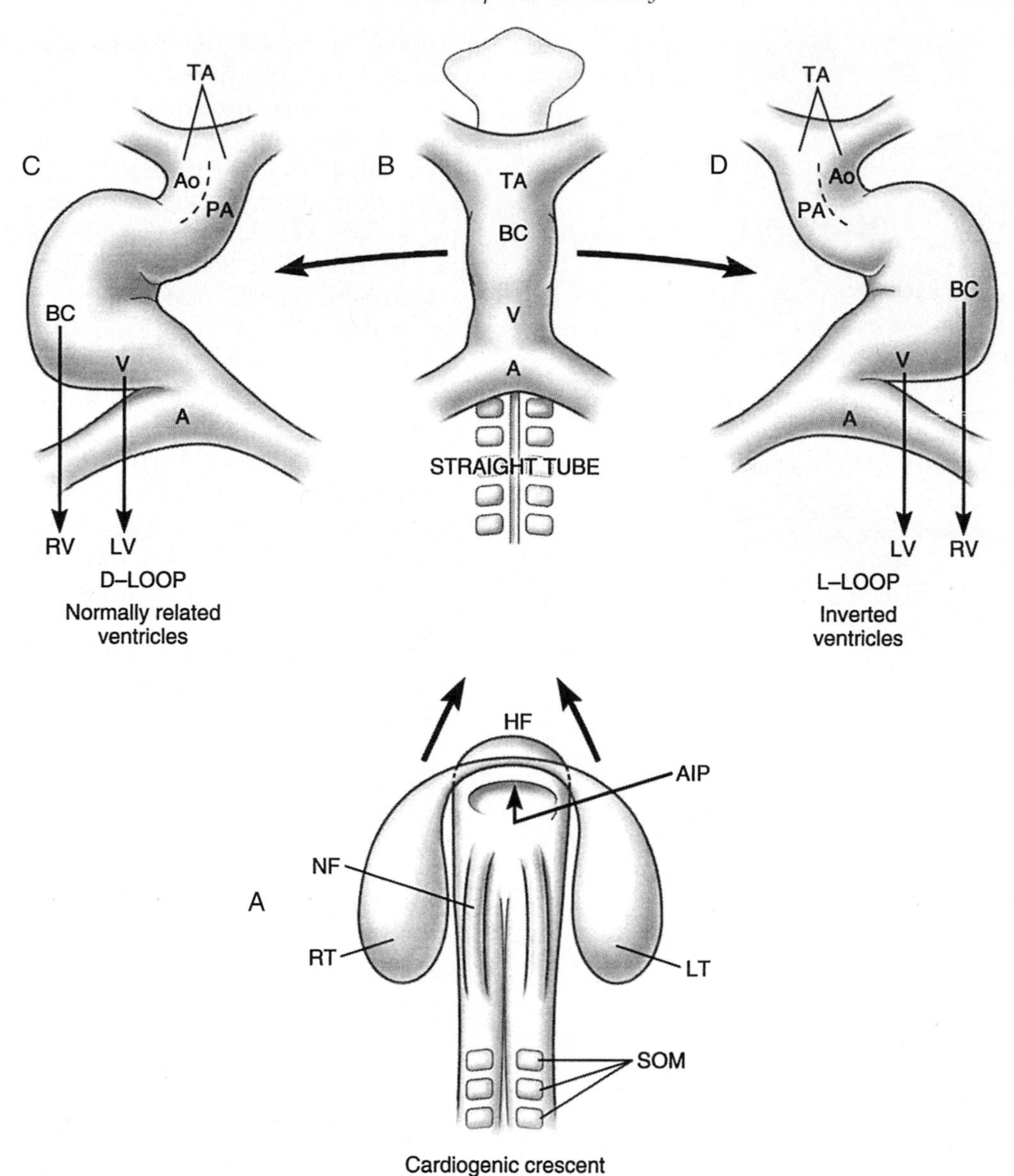

FIGURE 2–4 *Cardiac loop formation.A, Cardiogenic crescent of precardiac mesoderm. B, Straight heart tube or preloop stage. C, D-loop, with solitus (noninverted) ventricles. D, L-loop with inverted (mirror-image) ventricles. A, atrium; AIP, anterior intestinal portal; Ao, aorta; BC, bulbus cordis; HF, head fold; LT, left; LV, morphologically left ventricle; NF, neural fold; PA, (main) pulmonary artery; RT, right; RV, morphologically right ventricle; SOM, somites; TA, truncus arteriosus.*
From Van Praagh R, Weinberg PM, Matsuoka R et al: Malpositions of the heart. In Adams FH, Emmanouilides GC (eds.). Heart Disease in Infants, Children, and Adolescents, 3rd ed. Baltimore: Williams & Wilkins, 1983, with permission.

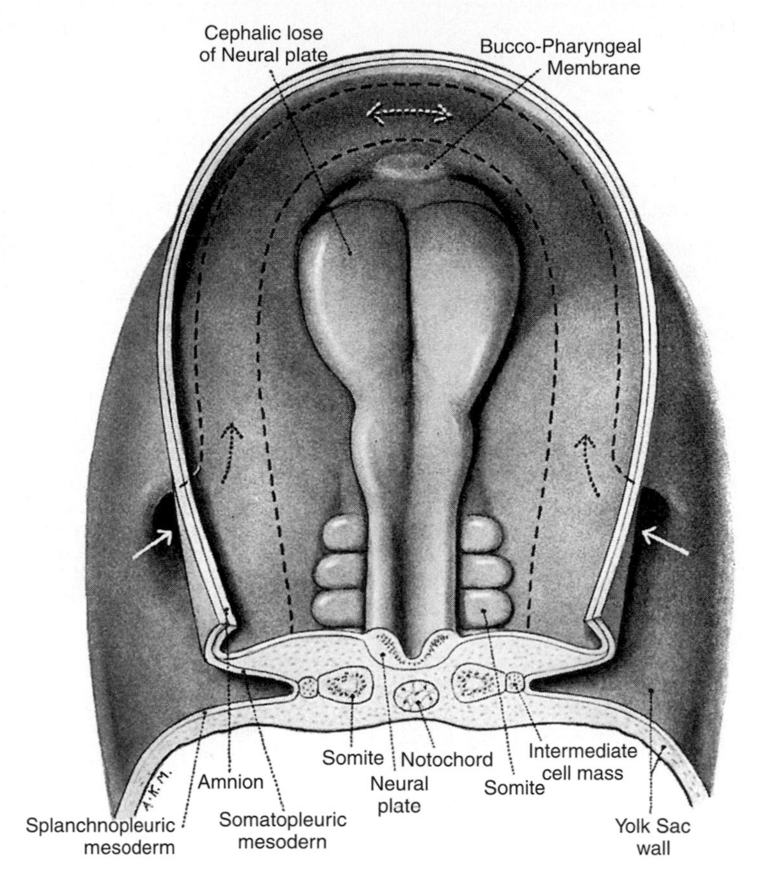

FIGURE 2–5 *Schematic representation of the cranial part of a somite embryo shows the relationships of the intra-embryonic celom, the development of the neural plate, and the continuity between the intrae-mbryonic celom and the extra-embryonic celom. The white arrows indicate the junctions between the two celomata. The dotted arrows are in the intra-embryonic celom.*
From Hamilton WJ, Mossman HW. Human Embryology: Prenatal Development of Form and Function, 4th ed Baltimore: Williams & Wilkins, 1972, with permission.

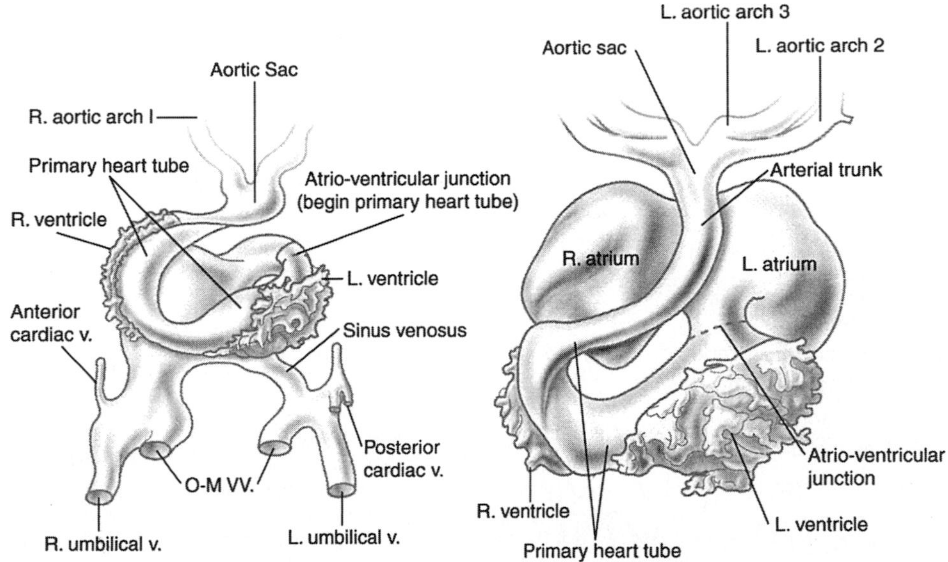

FIGURE 2–6 *Formation of the ventricles. Left, Horizon XI, 22 to 24 days of age. Carnegie embryo No. 2053, original reconstruction of cardiovascular lumen × 60 magnification. Right, Horizon XIII, 26 to 28 days of age, Carnegie embryo No. 836, original reconstruction of cardiovascular luman × 60 magnification. ANT. CARD. V., anterior cardiac vein; ATR.-Ventr. J'CT., atrioventricular junction; L. ATR., morphologically left atrium; LT. Ao. ARCH, left aortic arch; L. UMB. V., left umbilical vein; L. VENTR., morphologically left ventricle; O-M VV., omphalomesentric veins; P. CARD. V., posterior cardiac vein; PRIM., primitive; RT. AO., right aorta; R. ATR., morphologically right atrium; RT. VENTR, morphologically right ventricle; RT. UMBIL. V., right umbilical vein; SIN. VENOSUS, sinus venosus.*
From Streeter GL. Developmental horizons in human embryos, age groups XI to XXIII, vol II. Embryology Reprint. Washington, DC: Carnegie Institution, 1951, with permission.

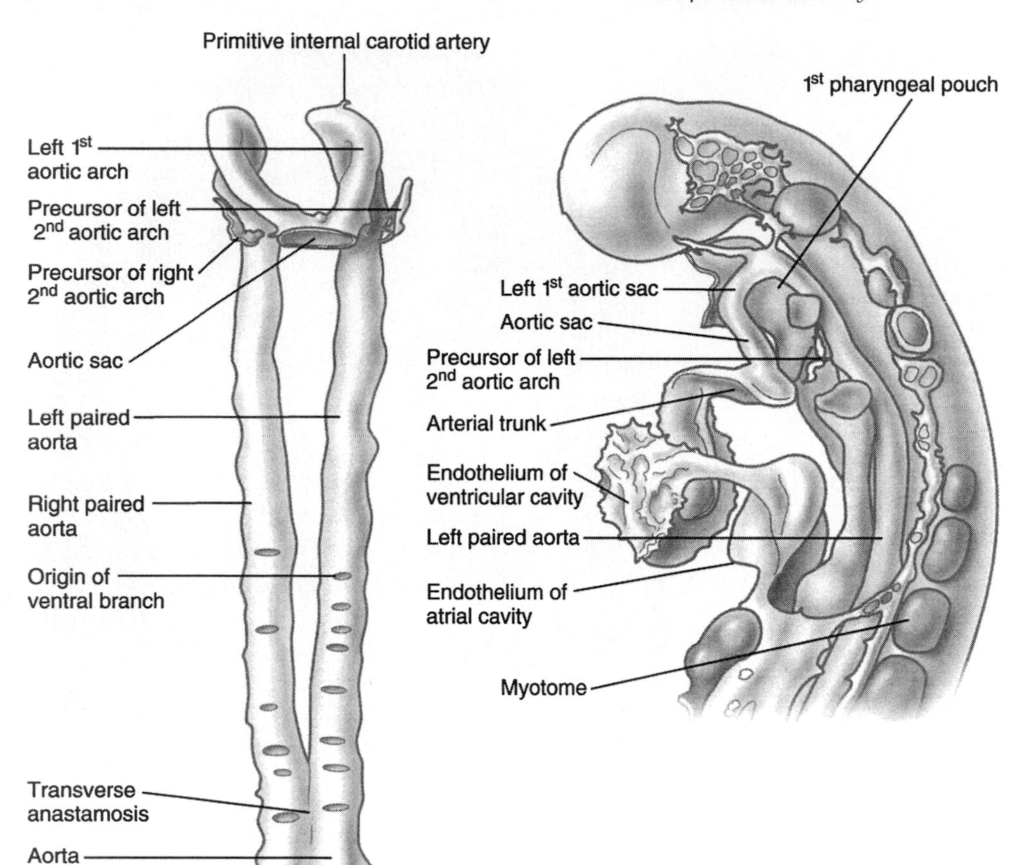

FIGURE 2–7 *First pair of aortic arches arching over (cephalad to) first pair of pharyngeal pouches. Left, ventral view. Right, Left lateral view. Carnegie embryo 2053, horizon XI, 22 to 24 days of age.*
From Congdon ED. Transformation of the aortic-arch system during the development of the human embryo. Contrib Embryol Carnegie Institution 14:47, 1922, with permission.

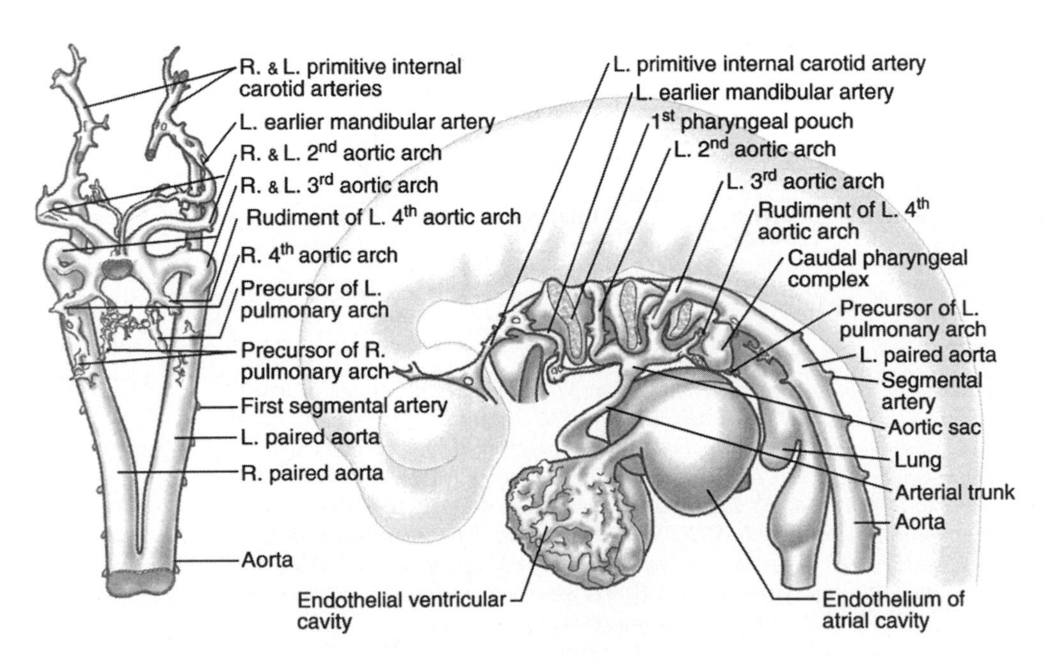

FIGURE 2–8 *Second and third pairs of aortic aches. Left, Ventral view. Right, Left lateral view. Carnegie embryo 836, early horizon XIII, 26 days of age. Each aortic arch passes cephalad to its pharyngeal pouch. Arch 1 is involuting. Arches 4 and 6 are just forming.*
From Congdon ED. Transformation of the aortic-arch system during the development of the human embryo. Contrib Embryol Carnegie Institution 14:47, 1922, with permission.

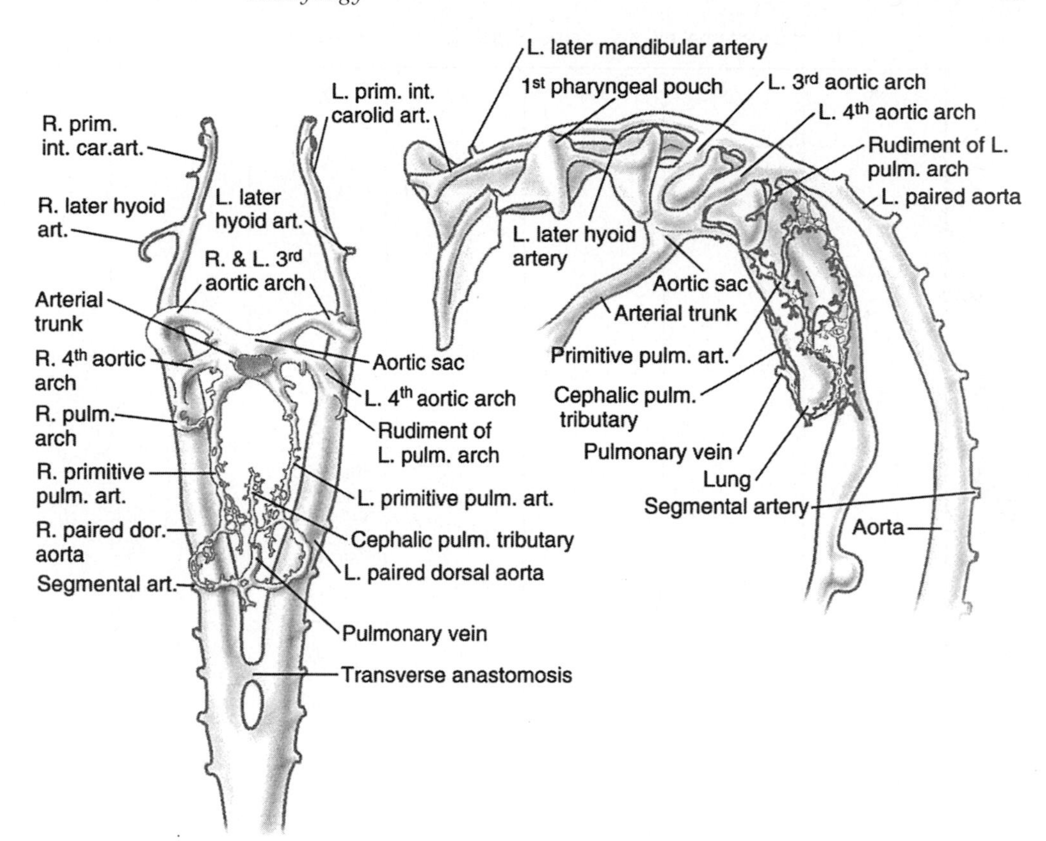

FIGURE 2–9 *Aortic arches 3 and 4. Left, Ventral view. Right, Left lateral view. Carnegie embryo 1380, late horizon XIII, 28 days of age. Aortic arches 1 and 2 have involuted, 2 and 4 are present, 5 is incomplete bilaterally, and 6 is complete on the right but not on the left. Right and left pulmonary artery branches and the common pulmonary vein are present.*
From Congdon ED. Transformation of the aortic-arch system during the development of the human embryo. Contrib Embryol Carnegie Institution 14:47, 1922, with permission.

THE FIFTH WEEK OF LIFE

The major cardiovascular developments between days 29 and 35 may be summarized as follows:

1. The left ventricle, right ventricle, and ventricular septum continue to grow and develop (Fig. 2-11).
2. There is approximation of the aorta to the interventricular foraman, mitral valve, and left ventricle (Figs. 2-11 and 2-12).
3. Separation of the ascending aorta and main pulmonary artery occurs (Fig. 2-12, horizon XVIa, i.e., days 32–33).
4. Separation of the mitral and tricuspid valves is accomplished (Fig. 2-12, horizon XVII, i.e., days 34–36).
5. The right ventricle enlarges (compare Fig. 2-11, left side, with Fig. 2-11, right side).
6. In association with right ventricular enlargement, the muscular ventricular septum moves from right to left beneath the atrioventricular canal (compare Fig. 2-11, left side, with Fig. 2-11, right side).
7. The tricuspid valve now opens into the right ventricle (Fig. 2-11, right, and Fig. 2-12, horizon XVII).
8. The ostium primum is closed by tissue from the endocardial cushions of the atrioventricular canal (Fig. 2-13), thereby separating the atria.
9. The ventricular apex swings horizontally leftward.
10. From days 30 to 36, the pulmonary valve moves from posterior and to the left of the developing aortic valve (30–32 days, horizon XV, Fig. 2-12), to a position beside and to the left of the aortic valve (days 32–33, horizon XVIa, Fig. 2-12), then somewhat anterior and to the left of the aortic valve (days 33–34, horizon XVIb, Fig. 2-12), and finally to its normal anterior position to the left of the aortic valve (days 34–36, horizon XVII, Fig. 2-12).

Hence, the morphogenetic movement of the pulmonary valve is from posterior to anterior, to the left of the aortic valve (Fig. 2-12). The aortic valve moves virtually not at all, except that it keeps on facing the anteriorly moving pulmonary valve (Fig. 2-12). It is thought that the reason for the normal anterior morphogenetic movement of the pulmonary valve is the normal growth and development of the subpulmonary infundibulum, which carries the pulmonary valve superiorly and anteriorly. Conversely, the normal lack of morphogenetic movement of the aortic

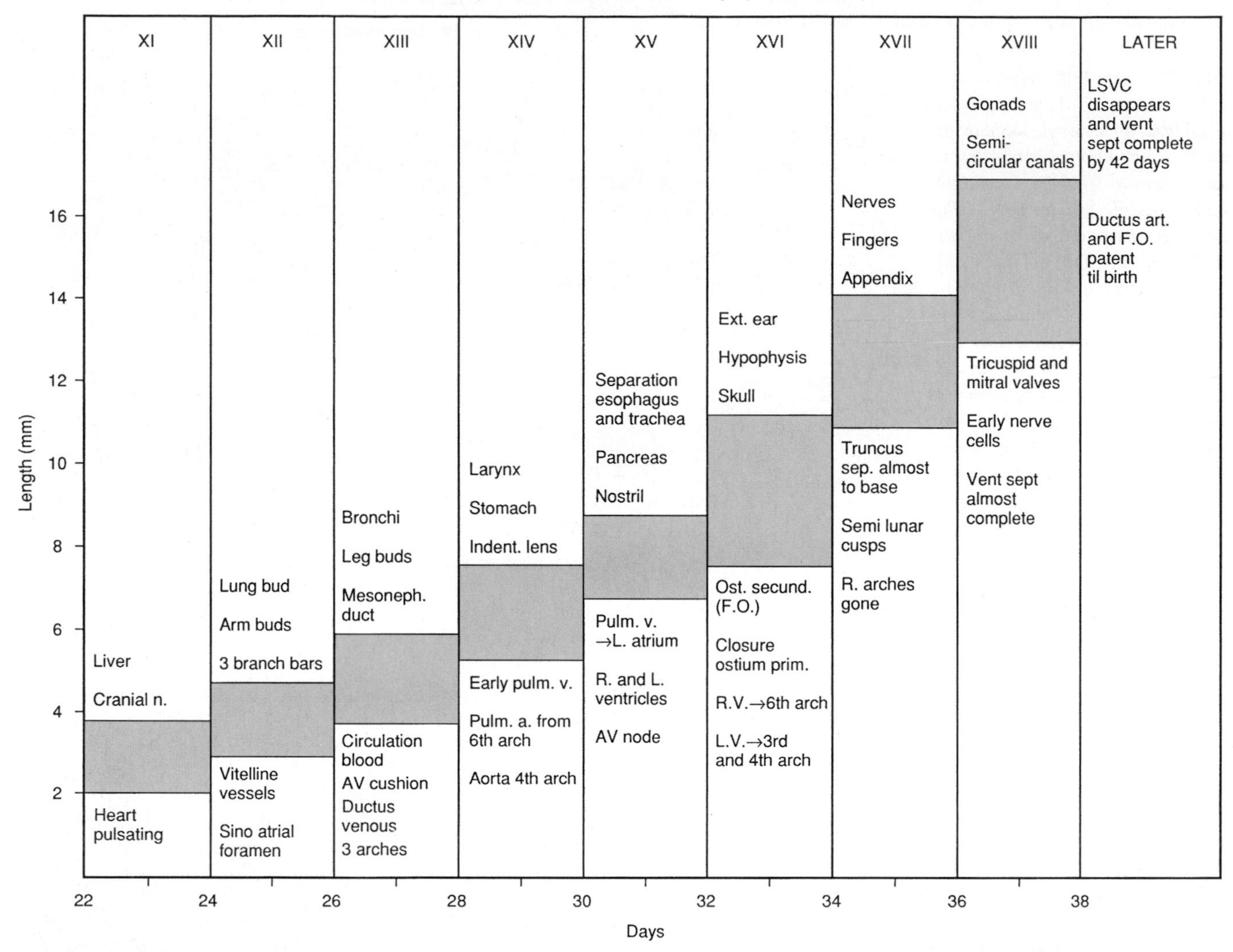

FIGURE 2–10 *Developmental horizons (stages) in the human embryo, modified from Streeter. Horizons are indicated at the top in Roman numerals. Embryonic ages are shown at the bottom in days. Embryonic lengths are given at the left in millimeters (mm). Salient features of each horizon are indicated.*
From Neill CA. Development of the pulmonary veins with reference to the embryology of anomalies of pulmonary venous return. Pediatrics 18:880, 1956, with permission.

valve appears to be due to the normal resorption of the subaortic conal free wall.

The semilunar interrelationship at 30 to 32 days in the human embryo is very similar to that of **D-transposition of the great arteries** (horizon XV, Fig. 2-12). At days 32 to 33, the semilunar interrelationship is side-by-side, similar to that of the **Taussig-Bing malformation** (horizon XVIa, Fig. 2-12). At days 33 to 34, the semilunar interrelationship is similar to that of **tetralogy of Fallot** (horizon XVIb, Fig. 2-12). Because the pulmonary valve has been carried from posterior to anterior on the left-hand side of the ascending aorta, the pulmonary artery must pass in the opposite direction—from anterior to posterior on the left of the ascending aorta—as it passes from the pulmonary valve proximally to the pulmonary bifurcation distally (horizon XVIII, Fig. 2-12). This anterior-to-posterior course of the main pulmonary artery makes it look as though normally related great arteries twist around each other. However, it is thought that the great arteries really are passively **untwisting** about each other as the pulmonary artery passes from the anterior pulmonary valve to the posterior pulmonary bifurcation (horizon XVIII, Fig. 2-12).

Thus, the fifth week is when the primitive, single, in-series circulation, which suffices for water-"breathing" fish, is converted into the definitive, double, in-parallel circulations that characterize air-breathing mammals.

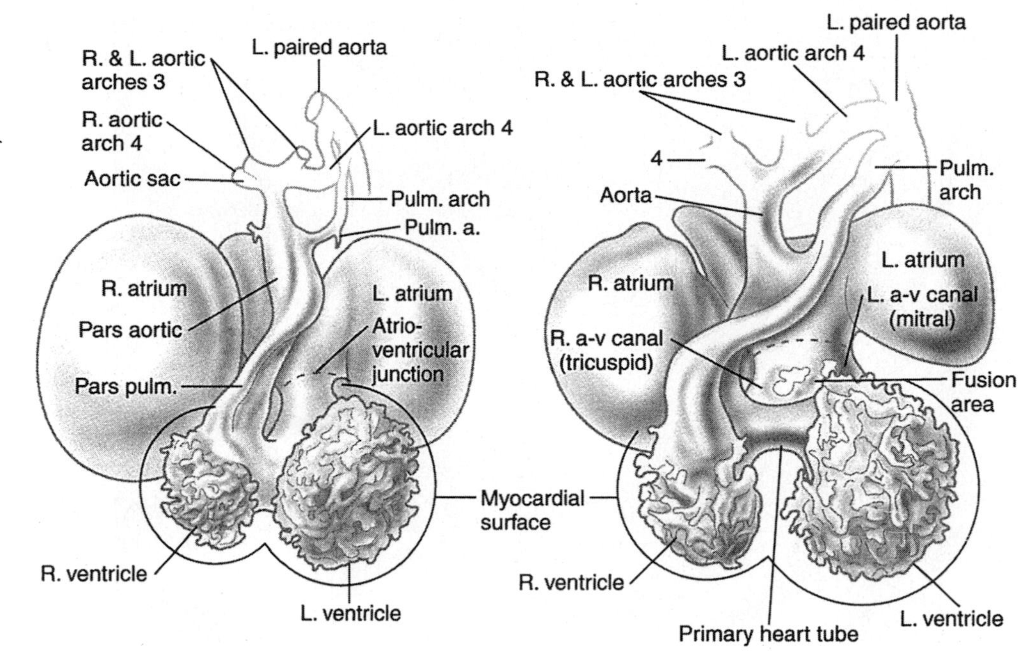

FIGURE 2–11 *Fifth week of life. Left, Horizon XV, 30 to 32 days of age, Carnegie embryo 3385, original reconstruction of cardiovascular lumen × 30. Right, Horizon XVI, Carnegie embryo 6510, original reconstruction of cardiovascular lumen × 30. Abbreviations as in previous figures.*
From Streeter GL. Developmental horizons in human embryos, age groups XI to XXIII, vol II. Embryology Reprint. Washington, DC: Carnegie Institute, 1951, with permission.

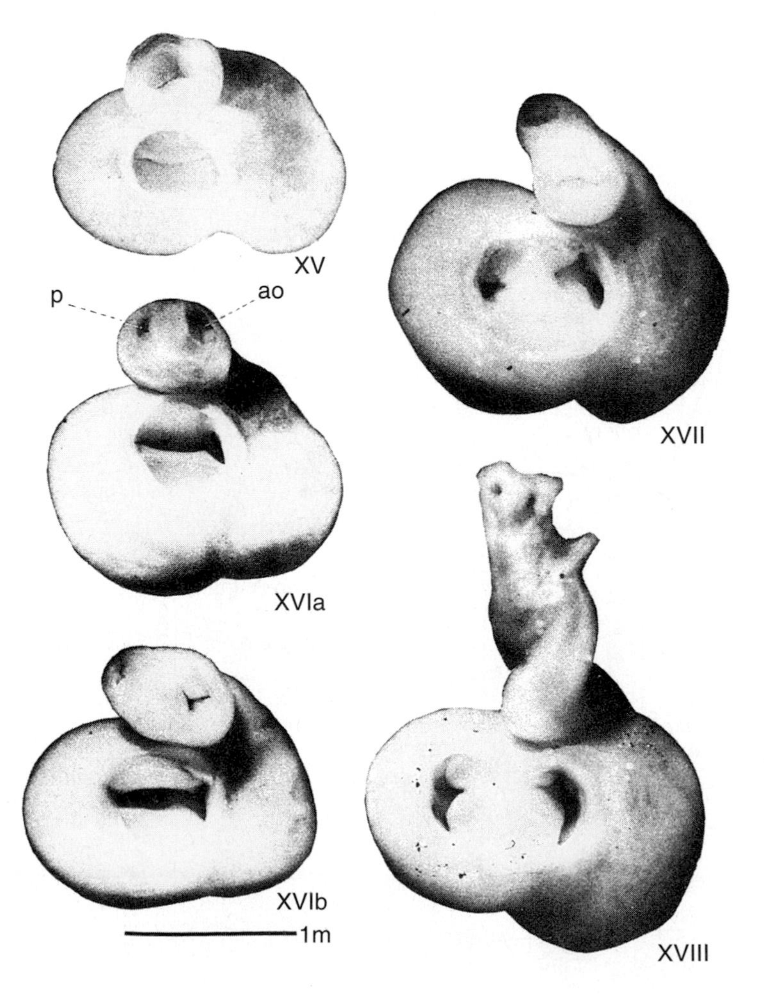

FIGURE 2–12 *Dissections of human embryonic hearts, viewed from above (dorsal aspect), to show positional changes of pulmonary valve (p) relative to aortic valve (ao) from horizons XV to XVIII. Top of figure is ventral (anterior), bottom of figure is dorsal (posterior), the developing pulmonary valve (p) is to the embryo's left, and the developing aortic valve (ao) is to the embryo's right. The atria have been removed to show partitioning of the atrioventricular canal. At the conotruncal junction, the major part of the movement takes place on the pulmonary side of the outlet (p). The aortic valve (ao) keeps on facing the anteriorly migrating pulmonary valve (p), but otherwise the aortic valve moves only slightly.*
From Asami I. Partitioning of the arterial end of the human heart. In Van Praagh R, Takao A (eds): Etiology and Morphogenesis of Congenital Heart Disease. Mount Kisco, NY: Futura Publishing, 1980, p 51, with permission.

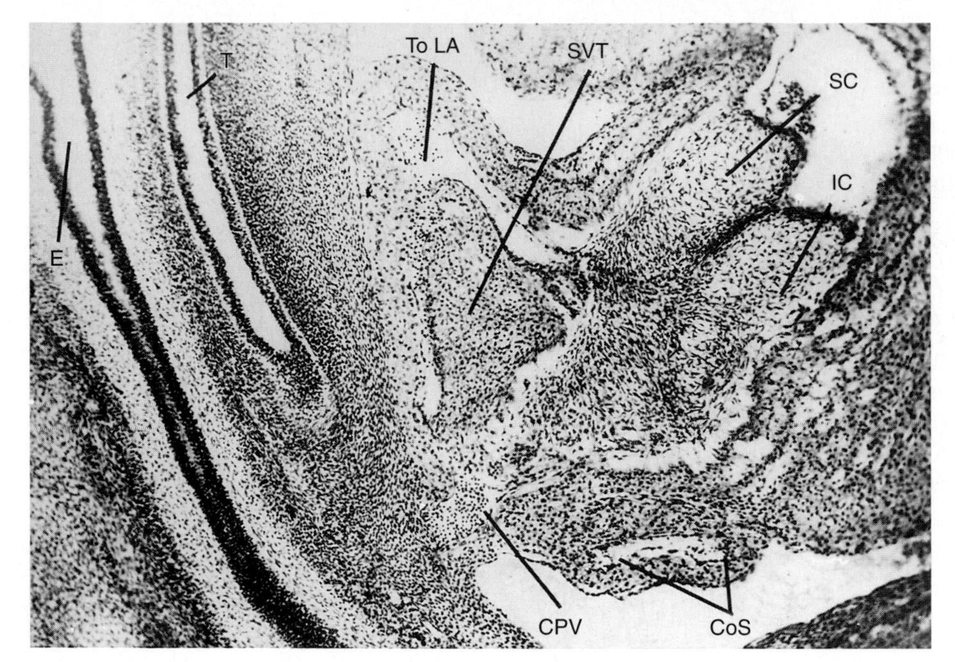

FIGURE 2–13 *Closure of ostium primum by tissue from the endocardial cushions of the atrioventricular (AV) canal, horizon XVI, 33 days of age, Harvard embryo 736, sagittal section number 138, borax carmine and Lyons blue stain, original magnification × 130, right lateral view. Tissue of the superior cushion (SC) and inferior cushion (IC) of the atrioventricular canal has fused with the atrial septum, which is composed of venous or sinus venosus tissue (SVT), this fusion closing the ostium primum. CoS, coronary sinus; CPV, common pulmonary vein; E, esophagus; LA, left atrium; T, trachea.*
From Van Praagh R, Corsini I. Cor triatriatum: pathologic anatomy and consideration of morphogenesis based on 13 postmortem cases and a study of normal development of the pulmonary vein and atrial septum in 83 human embryos. Am Heart J 78: 379–405, 1969, with permission.

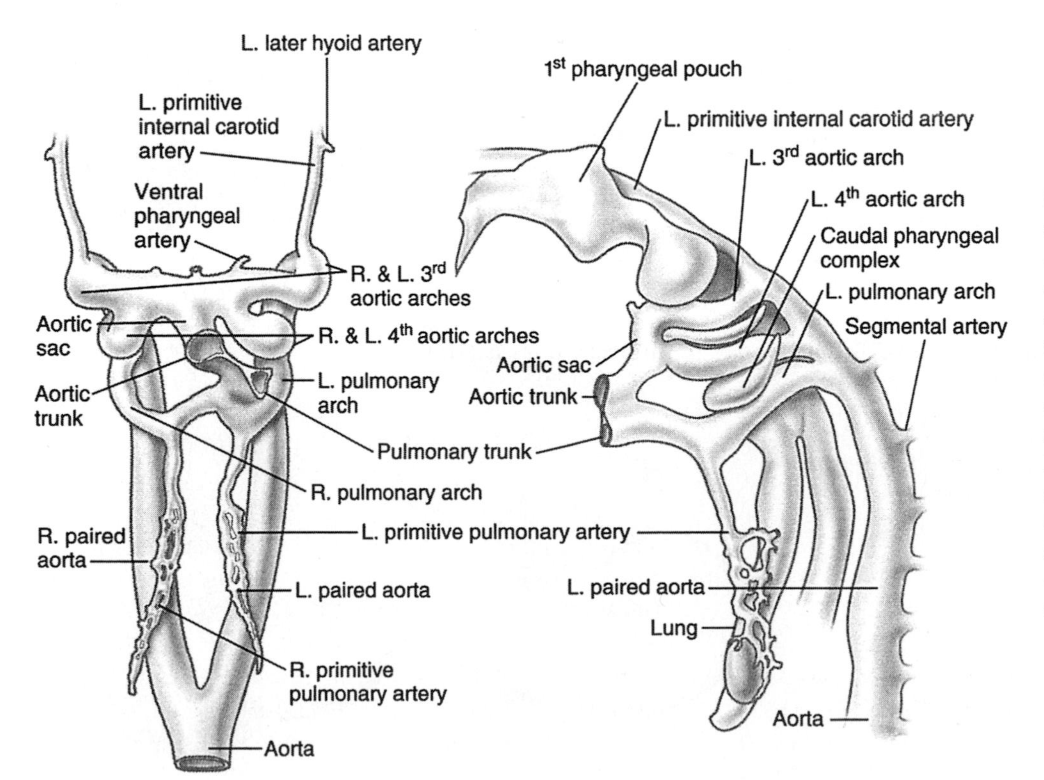

FIGURE 2–14 *Aortic arches 3, 4, and 6. Left, Ventral view. Right, Left lateral view. Carnegie embryo 1121, horizon XVII, 34 to 36 days of age. Distal aortopulmonary separation is well seen (left). Both ductus arteriosi (sixth arches) and both dorsal aortae are still intact.*
From Congdon ED. Transformation of the aortic-arch system during the development of the human embryo. Contrib Embryol Carnegie Institution 14:47, 1922, with permission.

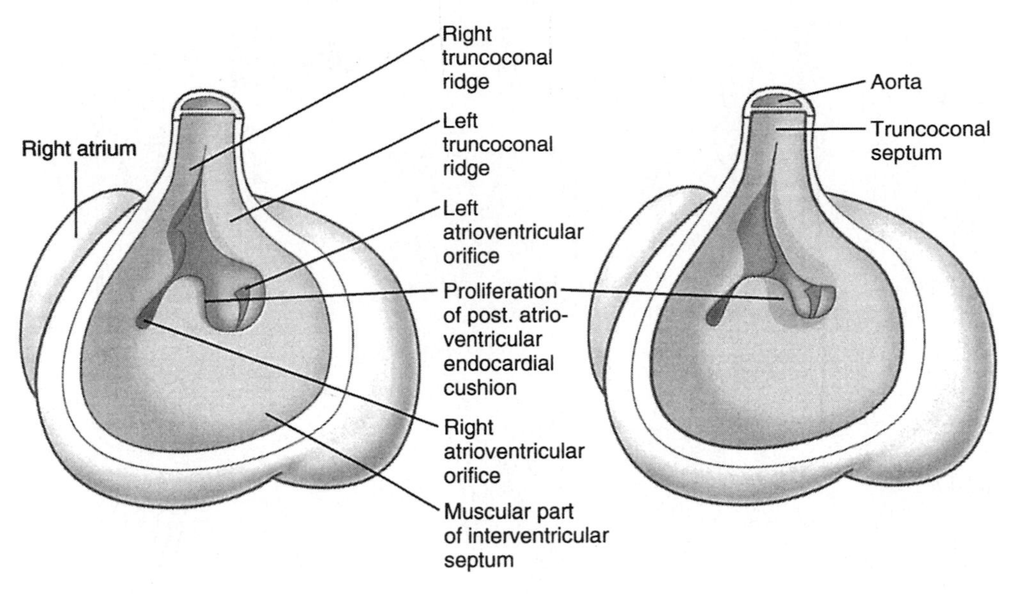

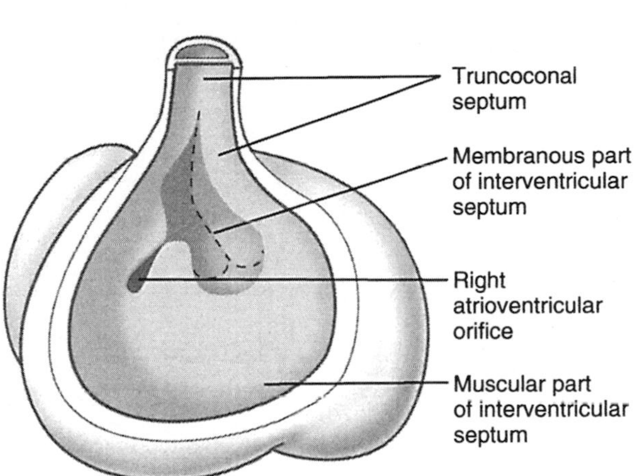

FIGURE 2–15 *Closure of the conal (infundibular) septum and the interventricular foramen. A, 6 weeks. B, Beginning of seventh week. C, End of seventh week.*
From Langman J. Human development-normal and abnormal. In Medical Embryology, 2nd ed. Baltimore: Williams & Wilkins, 1969, with permission.

Cardiovascular separation is nearly completed. However, the interventricular foramen (ventricular septal defect) is still patent.

By the end of the fifth week, aortic arches 3, 4, and 6 are present (Fig. 2-14). Both ductus arteriosi and both dorsal aortae are still intact. During the fifth week, neural crest cells continue to contribute to the development of the infundibulum, the great arteries, and their branches.

THE SIXTH AND SEVENTH WEEKS OF LIFE

The main cardiovascular developments between the 36th and the 49th days of life are (a) closure of the conal (infundibular) septum and (b) closure of the membranous part of the ventricular septum (Fig. 2-15). The ventricular septum usually is closed between 38 and 45 days of age. Closure of the interventricular foramen can be delayed until after birth, when it is known as spontaneous (i.e. surgically unassisted) ventricular septal defect closure.

DEVELOPMENT OF THE AORTIC ARCHES

The evolution of the aortic arches is summarized in Figure 2-16. This diagram is helpful for the understanding of **vascular rings.** In diagram 8 (Fig. 2-16), the asterisks indicate the presence of **fifth arches** bilaterally; these are present in about a third of human embryos at this stage.

There are **four normal interruptions** of the aortic arch system: (a) involution of the right ductus arteriosus or sixth arch (diagram 12, Fig. 2-16); (b) and (c) involution of

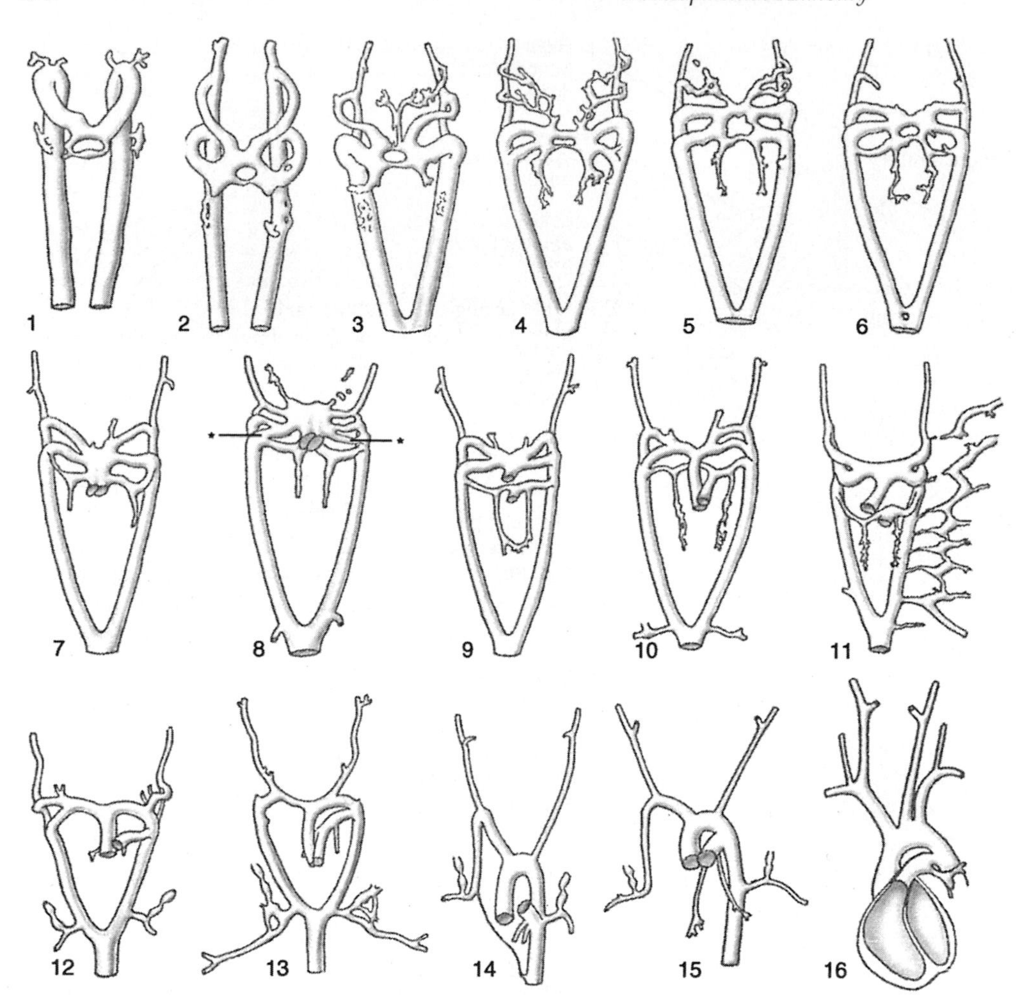

FIGURE 2–16 *Development of the aortic arches. In the earliest stage, only the first arch is present, whereas in the last (full-term fetus), the vessels have acquired nearly their adult form.*
From Congdon ED. Transformation of the aortic-arch system during the development of the human embryo. Contrib Embryol Carnegie Institution 14:47, 1922, with permission.

the ductus caroticus bilaterally (i.e., involution of the dorsal aortae between arches 3 and 4, bilaterally) (diagram 13, Fig. 2-16); and (d) involution of the right dorsal aorta distal to the seventh intersegmental artery (part of the embryonic right subclavian artery), resulting in a left aortic arch (diagram 14, Fig. 2-16).

What determines whether one has a left aortic arch or a right aortic arch? The answer is, whichever **dorsal aorta** persists. If the left dorsal aorta persists, one has a left aortic arch. If the right dorsal aorta persists and the left involutes, one has a right aortic arch. If both dorsal aortae persist, a **double aortic arch** results.

If the right dorsal aorta involutes proximal or cephalad to the seventh intersegmental artery (instead of distal to this artery), the result is an **aberrant right subclavian artery,** which arises as the last brachiocephalic artery from the top of the descending thoracic aorta.

It has often been said (erroneously) that whichever aortic arch is present depends on which fourth aortic arch (left or right) persists. Therefore, it is helpful to know that **both** fourth aortic arches (left and right) normally always persist (Fig. 2-16), regardless of whether a left or a right aortic arch is present. Thus, which aortic arch is present is determined not by the fourth or aortic arches *per se*, but by which dorsal aorta persists and which involutes (diagram 14, Fig. 2-16).

Recently, there has been an explosion of molecular genetics information that is highly relevant to the normal and abnormal development of the human cardiovascular system.[2–4] The interested reader is urged to consult the three textbooks referred to here.[2–4]

SUMMARY

Cardiogenesis begins on the 18th day of life with the formation of the cardiogenic crescent of precardiac mesoderm (Fig. 2-4A) and normally is completed by the 45th day of life with the formation of the membranous part of the ventricular septum (Fig. 2-15). Cardiovascular maturation continues well after birth.

REFERENCES

1. Streeter GL. Developmental horizons in human embryos, age groups XI to XXIII, vol II. Embryology Reprint. Washington, DC: Carnegie Institute, 1951.
2. Clark EB, Nakazawa M, Takao A (eds). Etiology and Morphogenesis of Congenital Heart Disease: Twenty Years of Progress in Genetics and Developmental Biology. Armonk, NY: Futura Publishing, 2000, pp 1–397.
3. de la Cruz MV, Markwald RR (eds). Living Morphogenesis of the Heart. Boston: Birkhäuser, 2000, pp 1–233.
4. Harvey RP, Rosenthal N (eds). Heart Development. San Diego: Academic Press, 1999, pp 1–530.
5. Langman J: Human development-normal and abnormal. In XXX (eds). Medical Embryology, 2nd ed. Baltimore: Williams & Wilkins, 1969.
6. Hamilton WJ, Mossman HW. Human Embryology: Prenatal Development of Form and Function, 4th ed. Baltimore: Williams & Wilkins, 1972.
7. Van Praagh R, Weinberg PM, Matsuoka R, et al. Malpositions of the heart. In Adams FH, Emmanouilides GC (eds): Heart Disease in Infants, Children and Adolescents, 4th ed. Baltimore: Williams & Wilkins, 1983, pp 422–458.
8. Congdon ED. Transformation of the aortic-arch system during the development of the human embryo. Contrib Embryol Carnegie Institution 14:47, 1922.
9. Neill CA. Development of the pulmonary veins with reference to the embryology of anomalies of pulmonary venous return. Pediatrics 18:880, 1956.
10. Asami I. Partitioning of the arterial end of the embryonic heart. In Van Praagh R, Takao A (eds): Etiology and Morphogenesis of Congenital Heart Disease. Mount Kisco, NY: Futura Publishing, 1980, p 51.
11. Van Praagh R, Corsini I. Cor triatriatum: pathologic anatomy and consideration of morphogenesis based on 13 post-mortem cases and a study of normal development of the pulmonary vein and atrial septum in 83 human embryos. Am Heart J 78:379, 1969.

3

Morphologic Anatomy

RICHARD VAN PRAAGH, MD
AND STELLA VAN PRAAGH, MD

An understanding of normal morphologic anatomy is basic to the accurate diagnosis of congenital heart disease. One of the diagnostic problems posed by congenital heart disease is that any cardiac chamber, valve, or vessel can be virtually "anywhere." This means that the diagnostic identification of the cardiac chambers cannot be based on relative position (right-sided or left-sided) or function (venous or arterial, pulmonary or systemic), because position and function are variables in congenital heart disease. A ventricle may be described as left-sided and anterior, but the question then arises, which ventricle is it—the morphologically left or the morphologically right? The diagnostic problem is that a **positionally** left ventricle may be a **morphologically** left ventricle or a **morphologically** right ventricle. Morphologic anatomic identification is the cornerstone of accurate diagnosis.

THE ATRIA

The anatomic features of the morphologically right atrium and the morphologically left atrium are presented in Figures 3-1 to 3-4, and their morphologic anatomic features are summarized in Table 3-1.

The Morphologically Right Atrium

The **external appearance** of the right atrium is highly characteristic (Fig. 3-1). The appendage is broad or triangular. It resembles "Snoopy, looking to his left" (Fig. 3-1). The "bridge of Snoopy's nose" is formed by the tinea sagittalis. Normally, the inferior vena cava and the superior vena cava are also visible externally, returning to the right atrium.

The **internal appearance** of the right atrium is pathognomonic (Fig. 3-2). The **inferior vena cava** connects with the venous (sinus venosus) portion of the right atrium inferiorly, the **superior vena cava** connects with the venous portion superiorly, and the **coronary sinus** opens into the venous portion medially (Fig. 3-2).

The right atrium is that atrium that displays on its septal surface **septum secundum** (Fig. 3-2). The septum secundum is also known as the **limbic ledge,** immediately beneath which a cardiac catheter may be passed into the left atrium, either through a patent foramen ovale or a secundum type of atrial septal defect, or through the septum primum if the fossa ovalis is sealed. Septum secundum's superior limbic band is also called the **crista dividens,** because this is the muscular crest on which the oxygenated blood returning from the placenta up the inferior vena cava in prenatal life divides into two streams, the **via sinistra** flowing into the left heart, and the **via dextra** passing into the right heart. The superior limbic band of the septum secundum is a muscular structure, the **anterior interatrial plica** (fold), which normally lies directly behind the aortic root (Fig. 3-1). It is **medial** to the entry of the superior vena cava (Fig. 3-2).

The **crista terminalis** is a muscular crest that lies **lateral** to the entry of the superior vena cava (Fig. 3-2). The crista terminalis corresponds internally to the **sulcus terminalis** externally, at the sinoatrial junction, where the **sinoatrial node** (the pacemaker of the heart) is located. The crista terminalis marks the termination of the medial sinus venosus or venous part of the right atrium and the beginning of

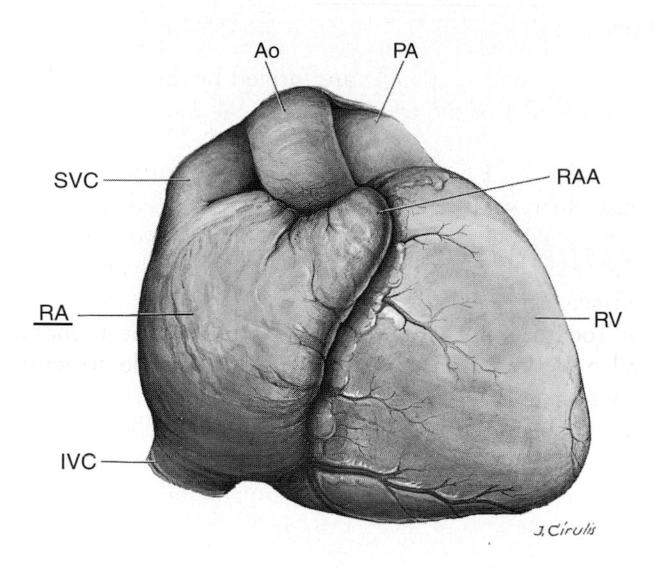

FIGURE 3–1 *Exterior of the morphologically right atrium (RA) (see Table 3-1). RA, right atrium; RAA, right atrial appendage; Ao, aorta; IVC, inferior vena cava; PA, pulmonary artery; RV, morphologically right ventricle; SVC, superior vena cava.*
From Van Praagh R, Vlad P. Dextrocardia, mesocardia, and levocardia. The segmental approach to diagnosis in congenital heart disease. In Keith JD, Rowe RD, Vlad P (eds). Heart Disease in Infancy and Childhood, 3rd ed. New York: Macmillan, 1978, pp 638–695, with permission.

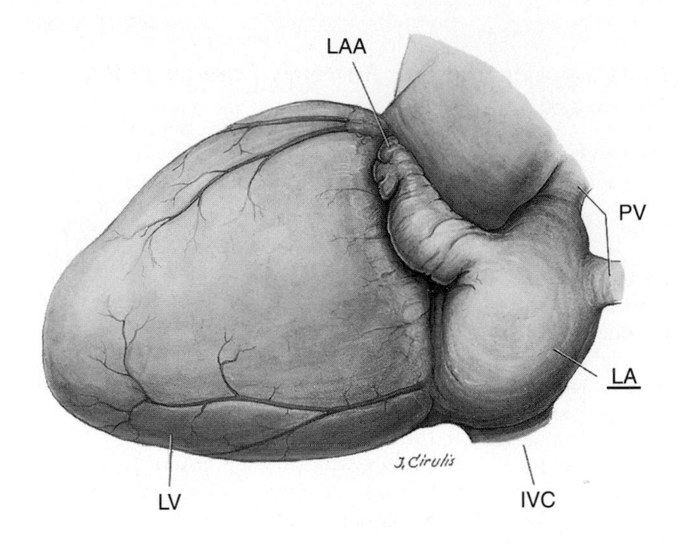

FIGURE 3–3 *Exterior of the morphologically left atrium (LA) (see Table 3-1). IVC, inferior vena cava (connecting with the right atrium); LAA, left atrial appendage; LV, morphologically left ventricle; PV, pulmonary veins.*
From Van Praagh R, Vlad P. Dextrocardia, mesocardia, and levocardia. The segmental approach to diagnosis in congenital heart disease. In Keith JD, Rowe RD, Vlad P (eds). Heart Disease in Infancy and Childhood, 3rd ed. New York: Macmillan, 1978, pp 638–695, with permission.

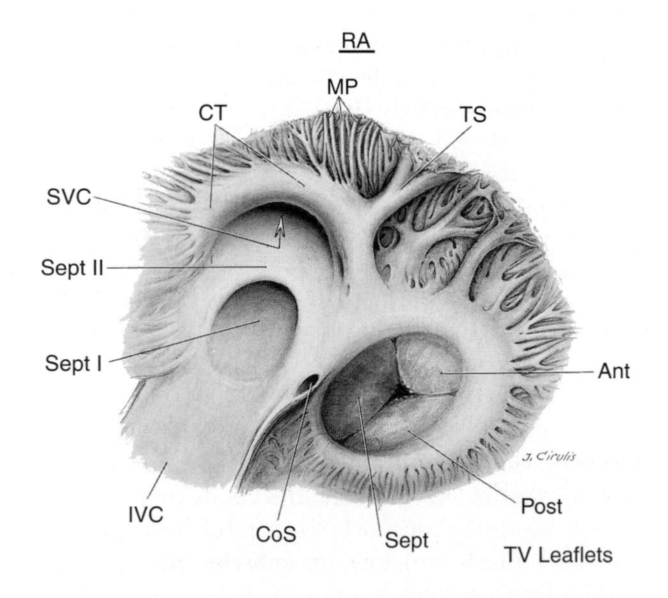

FIGURE 3–2 *Interior of the morphologically right atrium (RA) (see Table 3-1). Ant, anterior; CoS, coronary sinus; CT, crista terminalis; IVC, inferior vena cava; MP, musculi pectinati; Post, posterior; Sept, septal; Sept I, septum primum; Sept II, septum secundum; SVC, superior vena cava; TS, tinea sagittalis; TV, tricuspid valve.*
From Van Praagh R, Vlad P. Dextrocardia, mesocardia, and levocardia. The segmental approach to diagnosis in congenital heart disease. In Keith JD, Rowe RD, Vlad P (eds). Heart Disease in Infancy and Childhood, 3rd ed. New York: Macmillan, 1978, pp 638–695, with permission.

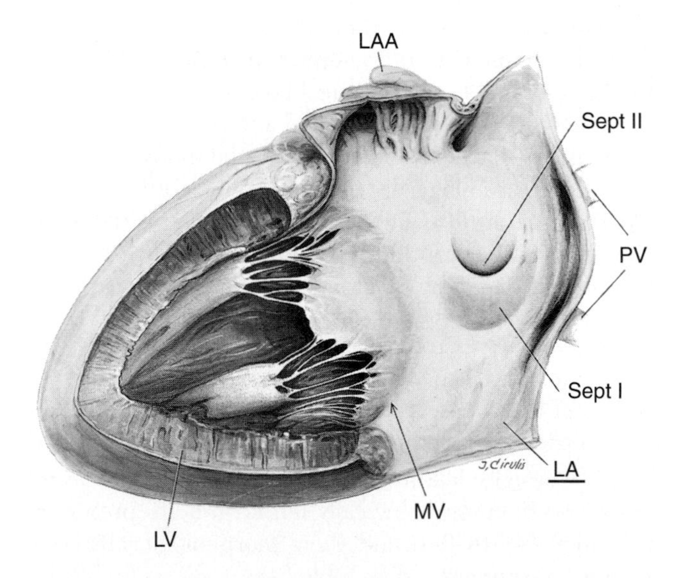

FIGURE 3–4 *Interior of morphologically left atrium (LA) (see Table 3-1). LAA, left atrial appendage; LV, morphologically left ventricle; MV, mitral valve; PV, pulmonary vein; Sept I, septum primum; Sept II, septum secundum.*
From Van Praagh R, Vlad P. Dextrocardia, mesocardia, and levocardia. The segmental approach to diagnosis in congenital heart disease. In Keith JD, Rowe RD, Vlad P (eds). Heart Disease in Infancy and Childhood, 3rd ed. New York: Macmillan, 1978, pp 638–695, with permission.

TABLE 3–1. Morphologic Anatomic Features of Right Atrium and Left Atrium

Anatomic Feature	Right Atrium	Left Atrium
Veins	Inferior vena cava, constant	Pulmonary veins, variable
Superior vena cava, variable		
Coronary sinus, variable		
Appendage	Broad, triangular	Narrow, finger-like
Musculi pectinati	Many	Few
Crista terminalis	Present	Absent
Tinea sagittalis	Present	Absent
Septal surface	Septum secundum	Septum primum
Conduction system	Sinoatrial node	None
Atrioventricular node and bundle		

the more lateral muscular or primitive atrium component of the right atrium. Surgical sutures sunk deeply into the crista terminalis can lead to thrombosis of the artery to the sinoatrial node, resulting in sinoatrial nodal infarction and the sick sinus syndrome. The sinoatrial nodal artery runs through the sinoatrial node like a shish-kabob skewer.

The **musculi pectinati** form approximately parallel ridges that do not crisscross; instead, they are like the bellows of an accordion. The **tinea sagittalis** (Fig. 3-1) intersects the crista terminalis at an approximate right angle (Fig. 3-2). The tip of a cardiac catheter may get lodged behind the tinea sagittalis, leading to perforation of the right atrium.

The **atrioventricular node and bundle** are not grossly visible; hence, it is necessary to know where these structures are to avoid surgically induced or catheter-related heart block. The atrioventricular node is located directly in front of the ostium of the coronary sinus. If one mentally draws a line between the ostium of the coronary sinus and the commissure between the anterior and the septal leaflets of the tricuspid valve (Fig. 3-2), this is where the atrioventricular node and the bundle of His are located. The **pars membranacea septi** (membranous part of the septum) is just medial to the commissure between the anterior and the septal leaflets of the tricuspid valve. The membranous septum has an **atrioventricular portion** between the right atrium and the left ventricle, and an **interventricular portion** between the right and left ventricles. The atrioventricular bundle penetrates just behind the membranous septum to pass from the atrial to the ventricular level, this portion being known as the **penetrating bundle.** The atrioventricular node and bundle consist of specialized muscle (not nerve) tissue. The atrioventricular node and bundle are located within the **triangle of Koch.** The sides of this triangle are formed by the origin of the septal leaflet of the tricuspid valve, the thebesian valve of the coronary sinus, and the tendon of Todaro. The tendon of Todaro is formed by the anterior prolongations of the eustachian valve of the inferior vena cava and the thebesian valve of the coronary sinus, which fuse and run anteriorly as one tendon beneath the right atrial endocardial surface. Thus, although well seen histologically, the tendon of Todaro is not visible grossly. Moreover, the thebesian valve of the coronary sinus is quite a variable structure. Consequently, the most practical way to localize the invisible atrioventricular node and bundle is to draw a line mentally between the ostium of the coronary sinus and the membranous septum at the anteroseptal commissure of the tricuspid valve (Fig. 3-2).

The Morphologically Left Atrium

The **external appearance** of the left atrium is highly characteristic because the left atrial appendage is relatively narrow and long (Fig. 3-3). When straight, the left atrial appendage resembles a pointing finger, or a windsock; when bent or crooked, the appendage resembles a map of Central America. The left atrial appendage remains an appendix to the cavity of the left atrium because the primitive atrial component (the appendage) does not become incorporated into the main cavity of the left atrium (Fig. 3-4), whereas the right atrial appendage does (Figs. 3-1 and 3-2). This is why the shapes of the right and left atrial appendages are so distinctive and so different. The **pulmonary veins** normally connect with the left atrium (Fig. 3-3); however, the pulmonary venous connections are variable, as totally anomalous pulmonary venous connection makes clear.

The **internal appearance** of the left atrium is pathognomonic (Fig. 3-4). The left atrium is the atrium that displays, on its septal surface, the **septum primum** (Fig. 3-4), which is the flap valve of the foramen ovale. In situs solitus of the atria, septum primum lies to the **left** of septum secundum (Fig. 3-5), whereas in visceroatrial situs inversus, septum primum lies to the **right** of septum secundum (Fig. 3-5).

A comparison of the morphologically right and left atria (Figs. 3-1 to 3-4) is summarized in Table 3-1. The right and left atria are a study in contrasts, virtually all details being distinctive and different. This is why, from the diagnostic standpoint, it is readily possible to recognize the morphologically right atrium as opposed to the morphologically left, no matter where either may be located.

Developmentally, each atrium consists of three main components: (a) venous portion, (b) primitive atrium, and (c) atrioventricular canal. The venous component of the morphologically right atrium is the sinus venosus, consisting of the smooth venous component medially formed by the

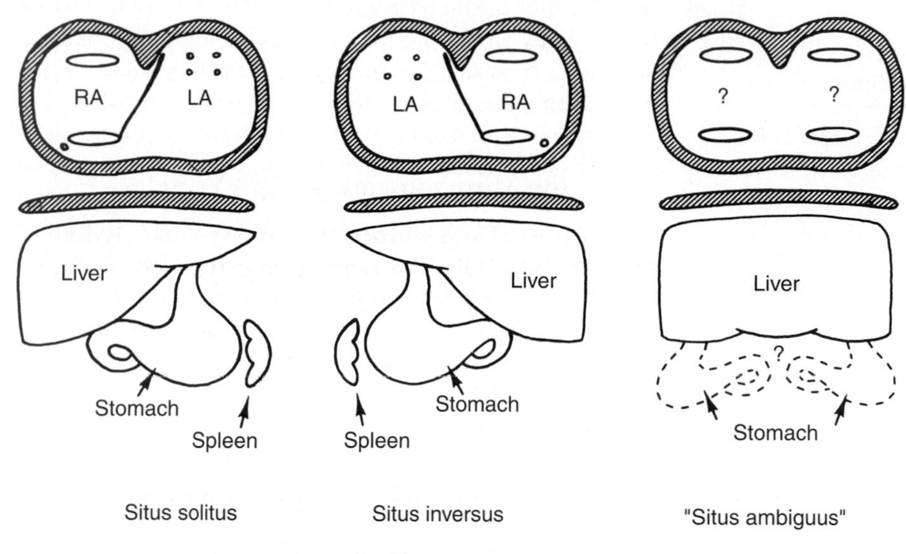

FIGURE 3–5 *The two types of viscero-atrial situs, important diagnostically for atrial localization. In so-called situs ambiguus, the atrial situs is undiagnosed (?). LA, morphologically left atrium; RA, morphologically right atrium. From Van Praagh R. The segmental approach to diagnosis in congenital heart disease. In Bergsma D (ed). Birth Defects: Original Article Series 8:4–23, 1972, with permission.*

entry and confluence of the inferior vena cava, the superior vena cava, and the coronary sinus. The venous component of the morphologically left atrium consists of the common pulmonary vein, which normally is incorporated up to the primary division of each pulmonary venous branch. The primitive atrium component of both atria consists of the appendages, with their characteristic musculi pectinati (pectinate muscles). The atrioventricular canal component of both atria is composed of the atrioventricular valves and the septum of the atrioventricular canal (the atrioventricular septum).

Is it always possible to identify the morphologically right atrium and the morphologically left atrium? Contrary to what has often been said, the authors now believe that the correct answer is "usually yes." The single most highly reliable diagnostic feature of the right atrium[1] is the suprahepatic segment of the inferior vena cava. That atrium with which the inferior vena cava connects almost always is the right atrium (Figs. 3-1 and 3-2), apparent exceptions being very rare. The inferior vena cava rarely can open into an unroofed coronary sinus (i.e., into a coronary sinus with a large coronary sinus septal defect). This creates the impression that the inferior vena cava is connecting with the left atrium. However, the authors believe that, in fact, the inferior vena cava is connecting with the coronary sinus, which normally would drain into the right atrium if the coronary sinus septum were normally formed.[2] Although the inferior vena cava **connects** with the coronary sinus, the inferior vena cava **drains** into the left atrium because of the co-existence of a large coronary sinus septal defect.*

Often in the **polysplenia syndrome,** the renal-to-hepatic segment of the inferior vena cava is absent and there is an enlarged azygos vein that drains normally into the superior vena cava. In such cases with "absence" (i.e., interruption) of the inferior vena cava, the suprahepatic segment of the inferior vena cava serves as an accurate diagnostic marker of the right atrium because the suprahepatic portion of the inferior vena cava is always present.

Even in the so-called **situs ambiguus** of the viscera and atria (Fig. 3-5, right side), which typically is associated with the asplenia and the polysplenia syndromes, recent evidence indicates that the connection of the inferior vena cava identifies the sinus venosus and, hence, the right atrium with accuracy. Typically, the inferior vena cava leads **directly** to the right atrium. Occasionally, the inferior vena cava opens into an "unroofed" coronary sinus, which in turn leads **indirectly** to the right atrium. This means that the inferior vena caval connection usually makes it possible to diagnose the atrial situs in so-called situs ambiguus.[2]

Typically, the appendage of the morphologically right atrium is larger and more anterior than is the appendage of the morphologically left atrium. Thus, both the venous component (the inferior vena cava and the coronary sinus) and the primitive atrial component (the appendage) are

*Whenever the terms right or left are applied to the atria or the ventricles without further qualification, morphologically right and morphologically left is understood.

helpful in the diagnostic localization of the morphologically right atrium.

The concept of **atrial isomerism** is erroneous (i.e., the concept of right atrial isomerism with the asplenia syndrome, and left atrial isomerism with the polysplenia syndrome). Bilateral morphologically right atria and bilateral morphologically left atria have never been documented. For example, a heart with left atrial appendages bilaterally, with a septum primum on both septal surfaces, and with four pulmonary veins bilaterally has never been documented; therefore, to the best of our knowledge, bilateral left atria do not exist. Similarly, a heart with right atrial appendages bilaterally, bilateral inferior and superior venae cavae, coronary sinus entering bilaterally, and having a septum secundum on each septal surface also has never been documented; therefore, bilateral right atria also do not exist. Just as each individual has only one right ventricle and one left ventricle, so too each individual really has only one right atrium and one left atrium. Even though atrial isomerism does not exist, accurately speaking, the appearance suggestive of **isomeric atrial appendages** should certainly make one think of the visceral heterotaxy syndromes: the asplenia syndrome (with right "isomerism" of the atrial appendages), or the polysplenia syndrome (with left "isomerism" of the atrial appendages).

We think that there are really only two types of atrial situs: (a) **situs solitus,** the usual or normal type of atrial arrangement in which the right atrium lies to the right and the left atrium lies to the left; and (b) **situs inversus,** the mirror-image type of atrial arrangement in which the morphologically right atrium is left-sided and the morphologically left atrium is right-sided. We also believe that so-called **situs ambiguus** of the atria indicates those cases in which the atrial situs (solitus or inversus) is undiagnosed. There are really only two types of atrial situs (patterns of anatomic organization), not three (Fig. 3-5).

Is the diagnosis of the atrial situs ambiguus, meaning undiagnosed atrial situs, still necessary? We think that the answer is yes. For example, in visceral heterotaxy with asplenia, a right-sided inferior vena cava (IVC) and a left-sided broad triangular anterior atrial appendage can coexist. In this type of situation, we do not know which datum to "believe"—the right-sided IVC suggesting situs solitus of the atria or the left-sided broad triangular atrial appendage suggesting situs inversus of the atria. When the IVC suggests one type of atrial situs and the appendage morphologies suggest the opposite type of atrial situs, then we invoke the diagnosis of atrial situs ambiguus, meaning that we do not know what the atrial situs is, without stating that atrial (or atrial appendage) isomerism is present, which often is not the case (see Chapter 39).

THE VENTRICLES

The anatomic features of the morphologically right ventricle and the morphologically left ventricle are presented in Figures 3-6 to 3-12 and are summarized in Table 3-2.

The Morphologically Right Ventricle

The **external appearance** of the right ventricle is distinctive (Fig. 3-6). Like the right atrium, the right ventricle also is triangular in shape. The angle between the anterior and diaphragmatic surfaces is typically an acute angle, somewhat less than 90 degrees. Hence, the junction between the anterior and diaphragmatic surfaces of the right ventricle is known as the **acute margin.** The epicardial branches of the **coronary arteries** are highly characteristic, consisting of conal or preventricular branches and the acute marginal branch of the right coronary artery (Fig. 3-6).

The **internal appearance** of the morphologically right ventricle is pathognomonic (Figs. 3-7 to 3-9). The **trabeculae carneae** (muscular trabeculations) are relatively coarse, few, and straight, tending to parallel the right ventricular inflow and the outflow tracts. The **papillary**

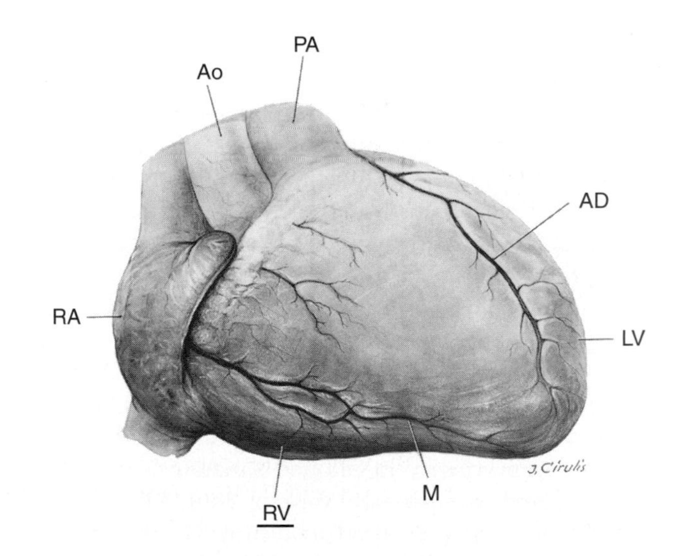

FIGURE 3–6 *Exterior of the morphologically right ventricle (RV). AD, anterior descending coronary artery; Ao, aorta; LV, morphologically left ventricle; M, acute marginal branch of the right coronary artery; PA, main pulmonary artery; RA, morphologically right atrium.*
From Van Praagh R, Vlad P. Dextrocardia, mesocardia, and levocardia. The segmental approach to diagnosis in congenital heart disease. In Keith JD, Rowe RD, Vlad P (eds). Heart Disease in Infancy and Childhood, 3rd ed. New York: Macmillan, 1978, pp 638–695, with permission.

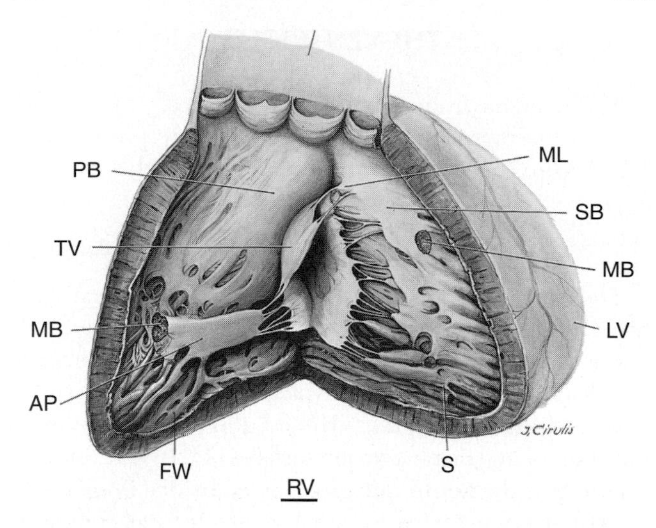

FIGURE 3–7 *Interior of the morphologically right ventricle (RV) (see Table 3-2). AP, anterior papillary muscle; FW, free wall; LV, morphologically left ventricle; MB, moderator band; ML, muscle of Lancisi; PA, main pulmonary artery; PB, parietal band; S, septum; SB, septal band; TV, tricuspid valve.*
From Van Praagh R, Vlad P. Dextrocardia, mesocardia, and levocardia. The segmental approach to diagnosis in congenital heart disease. In Keith JD, Rowe RD, Vlad P (eds). Heart Disease in Infancy and Childhood, 3rd ed. New York: Macmillan, 1978, pp 638–695, with permission.

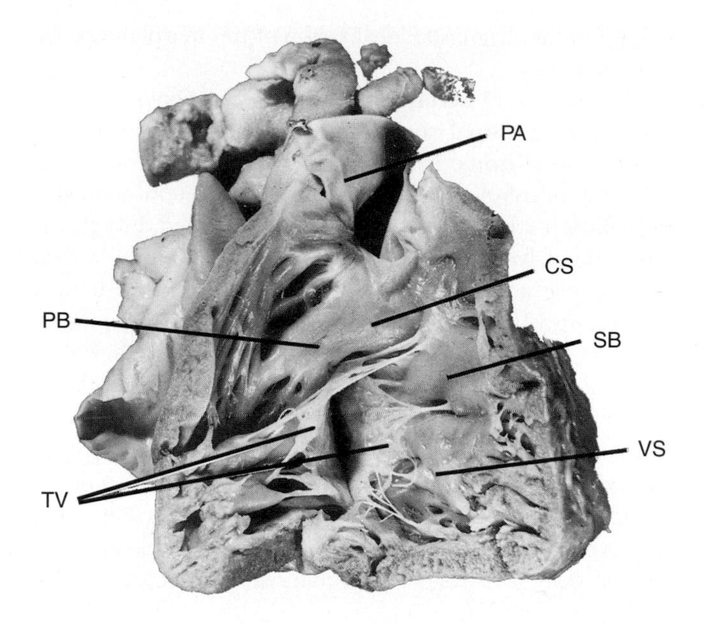

FIGURE 3–8 *Photograph of interior of morphologically right ventricle of young patient (2 months old). Note the "suture" between the crista supraventicularis (CS) of the parietal band (PB) and the septal band (SB). This junction between the parietal band and the septal band, visible in young patients with thin endocardium, is where the parietal band and the septal band dissociate or separate in conotruncal anomalies.*
From Van Praagh R, Van Praagh S, Vlad P, Keith JD. Anatomic types of congenital dextrocardia, diagnostic and embryologic implications. Am J Cardiol 1964;13:510–531, with permission.

muscles of the right ventricle are relatively small (making right ventriculotomy readily possible) and numerous, and they attach both to the septal and to the free wall surfaces. Because of its numerous attachments to the right ventricular septal surface (mostly to the posteroinferior margin of the septal band), the tricuspid valve may be described as "septophilic" (Figs. 3-7 to 3-9).

The number of leaflets of the **tricuspid valve** varies from two in infancy (parietal and septal), to four in old age (anterior, posterior, septal, infundibular). However, throughout most of life, the majority of persons have three leaflets (anterior, posterior, and septal). Nonetheless, in view of the previously mentioned variations, one cannot reliably identify the tricuspid valve by counting its leaflets.

What, then, may be used to distinguish the tricuspid valve from the mitral? The tricuspid leaflets all tend to be approximately the same in depth (Figs. 3-7 to 3-9), although the anterior leaflet often is somewhat deeper than the other two (but without nearly as great a difference in leaflet depth as normally exists in the mitral valve). The tricuspid valve is an inflow valve only, whereas (as will be seen) the mitral valve is both an inflow and an outflow valve (i.e., forming part of both the ventricular inflow and outflow tracts).

The normal definitive right ventricle has a large infundibular or conal component making up its outflow tract (Figs. 3-7 to 3-10). The **infundibulum,** or **conus arteriosus,** is incorporated mainly into the right ventricle, where it forms a conal ring consisting of three components: (a) the **distal conal septum** (Fig. 3-10, component 4), which extends onto the parietal or free wall, forming the **parietal band** (Figs. 3-7 to 3-9); (b) the **septal band,** or **proximal conal septum** (Figs. 3-7 to 3-9, and Fig. 3-10, component 3); and (c) the **moderator band** (Figs. 3-7 to 3-9).

The definitive right ventricle consists of **four anatomic components** (Fig. 3-10): (a) the atrioventricular canal, or junction (Fig. 3-10, component 1); (b) the right ventricular sinus, or body—the pumping portion of the right ventricle (Fig. 3-10, component 2); (c) the septal band, or proximal conus (Fig. 3-10, component 3); and (d) the parietal band, or distal conus (Fig. 3-10, component 4).

The right ventricular inflow tract consists of the atrioventricular canal component and the right ventricular sinus (components 1 and 2, Fig. 3-10). **The right ventricular outflow tract,** or conus, consists of the septal band and the parietal band (components 3 and 4, Fig. 3-10). The apex of the right ventricular sinus lies proximal to the

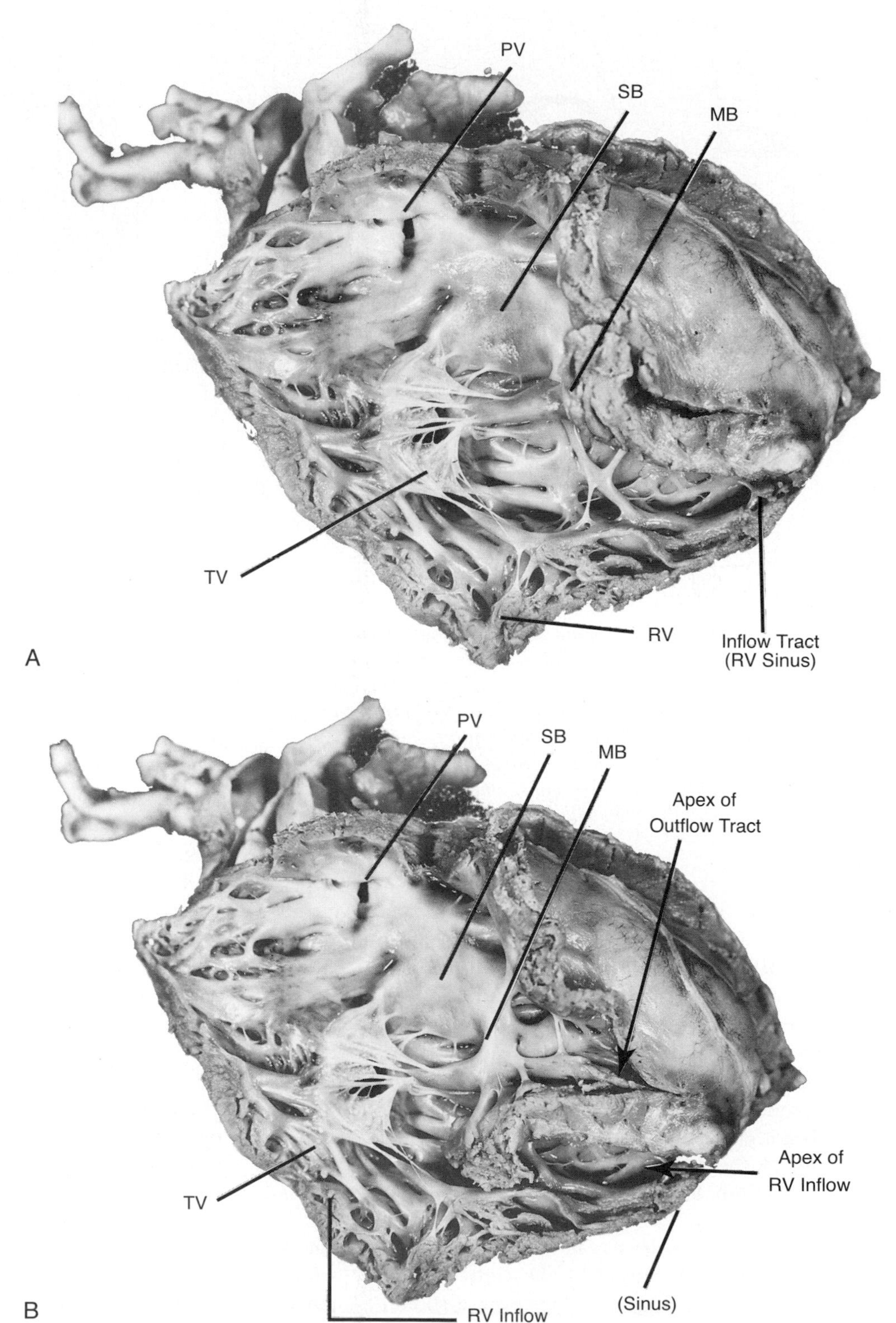

FIGURE 3–9 *Photograph of interior of opened right ventricle and infundibulum. The right ventricular sinus lies inferior and posterior to a ring of infundibular myocardium formed by the parietal band, septal band (SB), and moderator band (MB). The infundibulum (conus) extends from the infundibular ring to the semilunar valve, normally the pulmonary valve (PV). The apex of the right ventricular sinus is proximal to and inferior to the septal band and moderator band (Panel A). The apex of the infundibulum or outflow tract is distal to and superior to the septal and moderator bands (Panel B). The septal band and moderator band belong to the proximal, or apical, or "septal band part" of the infundibulum. The parietal band is part of the distal, or subsemilunar, or "parietal band part" of the infundibulum. Abbreviations are the same as in previous figures.*
From Van Praagh R, Plett JA, Van Praagh S. Single ventricle: pathology, embryology, terminology, and classification. Herz 4:113–150, 1979, with permission.

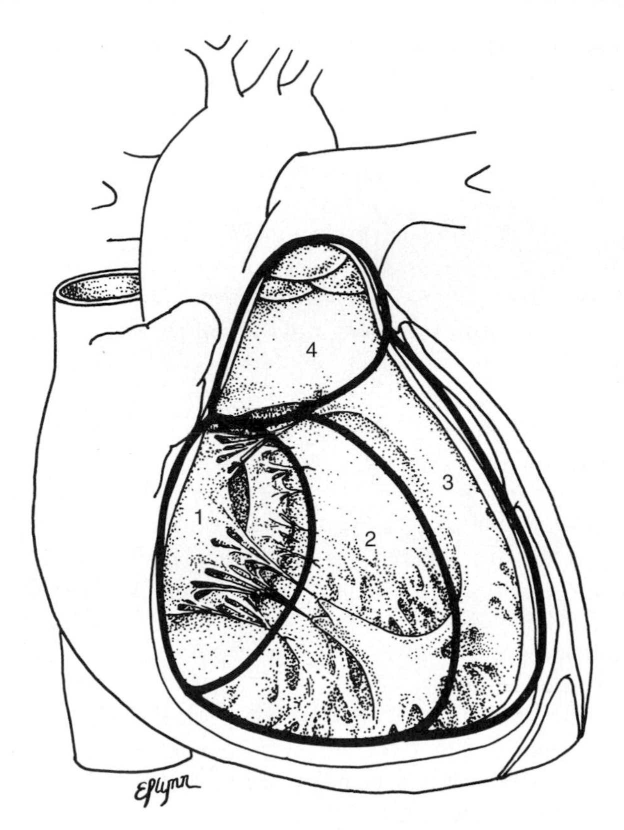

FIGURE 3–10 *The four main anatomic and developmental components of the interventricular septum, right ventricular view; 1, septum of the atrioventricular canal; 2, muscular ventricular septum, or sinus septum; 3, septal band or proximal conal septum; 4, parietal band or distal conal septum.*
From Van Praagh R, Geva T, Kreutzer J. Ventricular septal defects: how shall we describe, name, and classify them? J Am Coll Cardiol 14:1298, 1989, with permission.

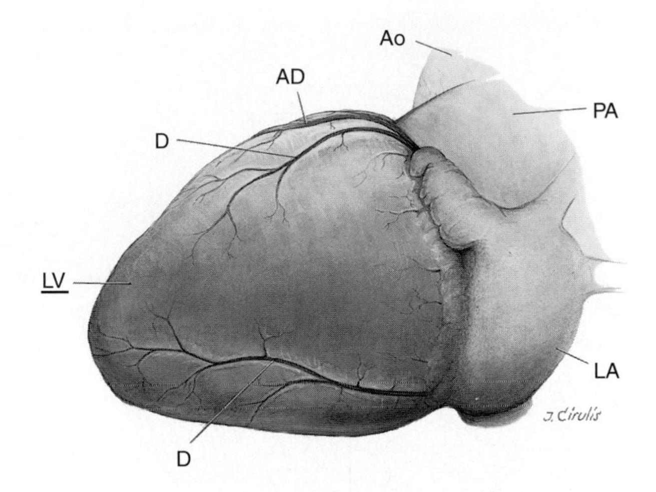

FIGURE 3–11 *Exterior of morphologically left ventricle (LV). AD, anterior descending coronary artery; Ao, aorta; D, diagonal to obtuse marginal coronary artery branches; LA, morphologically left atrium; PA, main pulmonary artery.*
From Van Praagh R, Vlad P. Dextrocardia, mesocardia, and levocardia. The segmental approach to diagnosis in congenital heart disease. In Keith JD, Rowe RD, Vlad P (eds). Heart Disease in Infancy and Childhood, 3rd ed. New York: Macmillan, 1978, pp 638–695, with permission.

moderator band (Fig. 3-9), while the apex of the infundibulum or conus lies distal to the moderator band (Fig. 3-9). Hence, the right ventricle has two apices, proximal and distal to the moderator band.

For the sake of understanding, it is important to appreciate that the **infundibulum (conus)** consists not only of the parietal band (component 4, Fig. 3-10). The septal and moderator bands are also known as the trabecula septomarginalis. An understanding of the four components of the interventricular septum (Fig. 3-10) helps to make the locations of **ventricular septal defects** comprehensible.

The right ventricle may be described as a one-coronary ventricle, being perfused by the **right coronary artery** and its branches (Fig. 3-6). However, it should be understood that the right coronary artery is really the fusion of two arteries: the conus coronary to the conus arteriosus and the right coronary to the right ventricular sinus.

The **conduction system** of the right ventricle (i.e., the right bundle branch) represents the superior radiation. The right bundle emerges just beneath the papillary muscle of the conus (muscle of Lancisi) and runs down the septal band close to its posterior margin and then crosses via the moderator band to the base of the anterior papillary muscle and thence, to the right ventricular free wall (Fig. 3-7). The anterior papillary muscle is the only relatively large papillary muscle in the right ventricle, the others being little more than trabeculae carneae (Fig. 3-7). The conduction system of the right ventricle has no posterior radiation, perhaps because of the absence of a sizable posterior papillary muscle in this ventricle.

The Morphologically Left Ventricle

The **external appearance** of the left ventricle is reminiscent of that of a bullet or a torpedo (Fig. 3-11). Because its external contour is rounded, the left ventricle is said to have an **obtuse margin,** i.e., greater than 90 degrees between the lateral and diaphragmatic surfaces. In addition to the anterior descending branch of the **left coronary artery,** which externally marks the location of the anterior (ventral) portion of the interventricular septum (Figs. 3-6 and 3-11), anterior and posterior obtuse marginal branches of the left coronary artery course across the left ventricular free wall (Fig. 3-11). Also known as

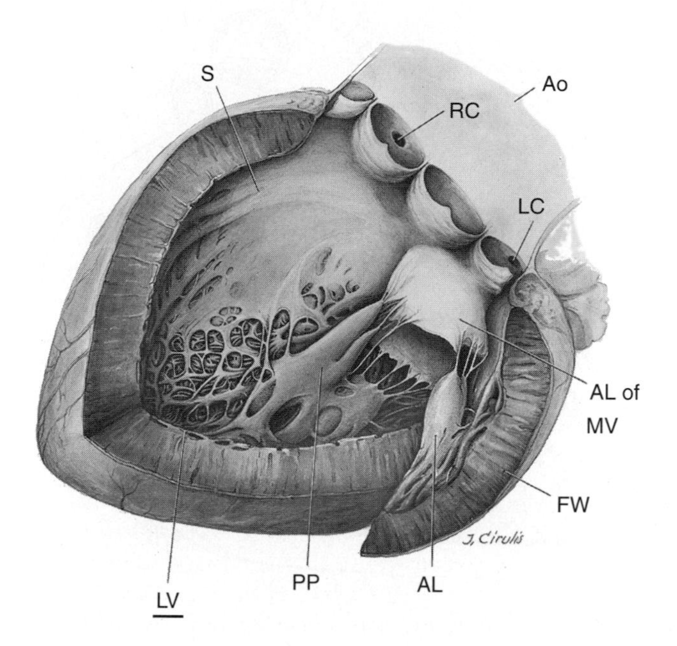

FIGURE 3–12 *Interior of morphologically left ventricle (LV) (see Table 3-2). AL, anterolateral papillary muscle; AL of MV, anterior leaflet of mitral valve; Ao, ascending aorta; FW, free wall; LC, left coronary ostium; PP, posteromedial papillary muscle; RC, right coronary ostium; S, septum.*
From Van Praagh R, Vlad P. Dextrocardia, mesocardia, and levocardia. The segmental approach to diagnosis in congenital heart disease. In Keith JD, Rowe RD, Vlad P (eds). Heart Disease in Infancy and Childhood, 3rd ed. New York: Macmillan, 1978, pp 638–695, with permission.

TABLE 3–2. Morphologic Anatomic Features of the Right Ventricle and Left Ventricle

Anatomic Features	Right Ventricle	Left Ventricle
Trabeculae carneae	Coarse Few Straight	Fine Numerous Oblique
Papillary muscles	Numerous Small Septal and free wall	Two Large Free wall origins only
Atrioventricular valve leaflets	Three Approximately equal depth	Two Very unequal depths
Infundibulum	Well developed	Absent
Semilunar-atrioventricular fibrous continuity	Absent	Present
Coronaries	One (right coronary artery)	Two (left anterior descending and circumflex branch of left coronary)
Conduction system radiations	One	Two

diagonals, these branches supply the large papillary muscles and the adjacent left ventricular free wall.

The interior of the left ventricle is shown in Figures 3-12 to 3-14. The superior portion of the left ventricular septal surface is smooth (nontrabeculated). The inferior portion displays numerous, fine, oblique trabeculae carneae that form a lattice-like mesh. Hence, the **trabeculation** of the left ventricle is fine, very different from the coarse trabeculation of the right ventricle (Figs. 3-7 to 3-9).

There are two **papillary muscles** of the left ventricle: the anterolateral and the posteromedial. The anterolateral is superior and relatively far from the interventricular septum, whereas the posteromedial is inferior and paraseptal. The papillary muscles of the left ventricle are large, arise only from the left ventricular free wall, and cover the interior surface of the free wall to a major degree. Consequently, left ventriculotomy is difficult, except at the left ventricular apex. Because the papillary muscles of the left ventricle do not arise from the left ventricular septal surface, the papillary muscles may be described as "septophobic."

The **mitral valve** has a deep anterior leaflet, and a shallow posterior leaflet—very different from the tricuspid valve. The mitral valve is both an inflow and an outflow valve in the sense that the deep anterior leaflet is an important part of both the inflow and the outflow tracts of the left ventricle.

Normally there is little or no conal musculature beneath the noncoronary and the left coronary leaflets of the aortic valve (Figs. 3-12 and 3-13). This normal absence of conal free-wall musculature permits aortic-mitral fibrous continuity (Figs. 3-12 and 3-13). When the great arteries are normally related, the noncoronary–left coronary commissure of the aortic valve sits directly above the middle of the anterior mitral leaflet (Figs. 3-12 and 3-13). The noncoronary–right coronary commissure sits immediately above the membranous septum, which in turn is located directly above the left bundle branch of the conduction system (Fig. 3-12). The conal septum runs beneath the right coronary leaflet of the aortic valve. The foregoing are highly important landmarks for transaortic therapeutic procedures (balloon dilation or surgery).

The left ventricle may be described as a two-coronary ventricle, supplied by the **anterior descending** and the **circumflex** branches of the left coronary artery.

Typically, the **conduction system** of the left ventricle has two radiations (Fig. 3-12): the superior radiation to the superior (anterolateral) papillary muscle group, and the inferior radiation to the inferior (posteromedial) papillary muscle group.

The left ventricle also consists of **four anatomic components** (Fig. 3-14), which correspond to the four anatomic components that together make up the right ventricle (Fig. 3-10). Ventricular septal defects may

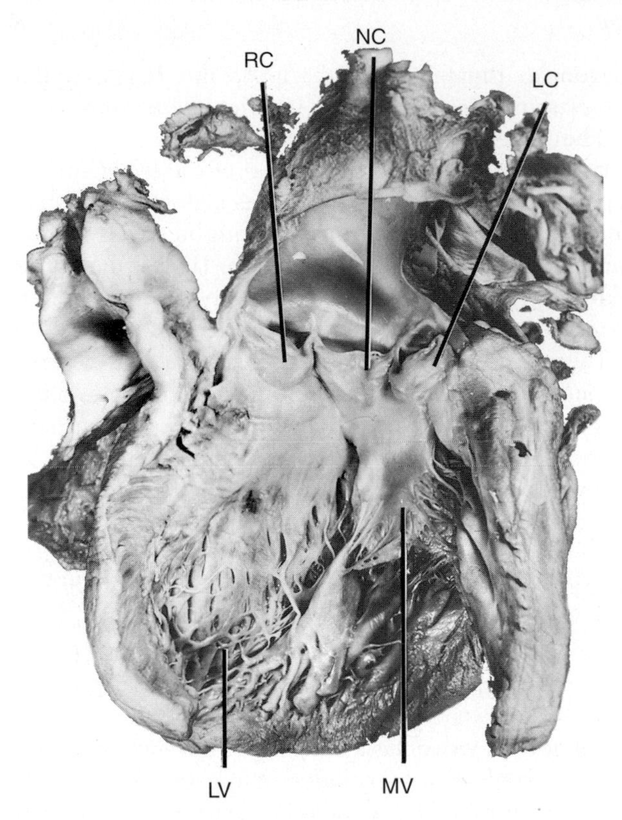

FIGURE 3–13 *Photograph of interior of morphologically left ventricle (LV). LC, left coronary leaflet of aortic valve; MV, anterior leaflet of mitral valve; NC, noncoronary leaflet of aortic valve; RC, right coronary leaflet of aortic valve.*
From Van Praagh R, Van Praagh S, Nebesar RH, et al. Tetralogy of Fallot: underdevelopment of the pulmonary infundibulum and its sequelae. Am J Cardiol 26:25–33, 1970, with permission.

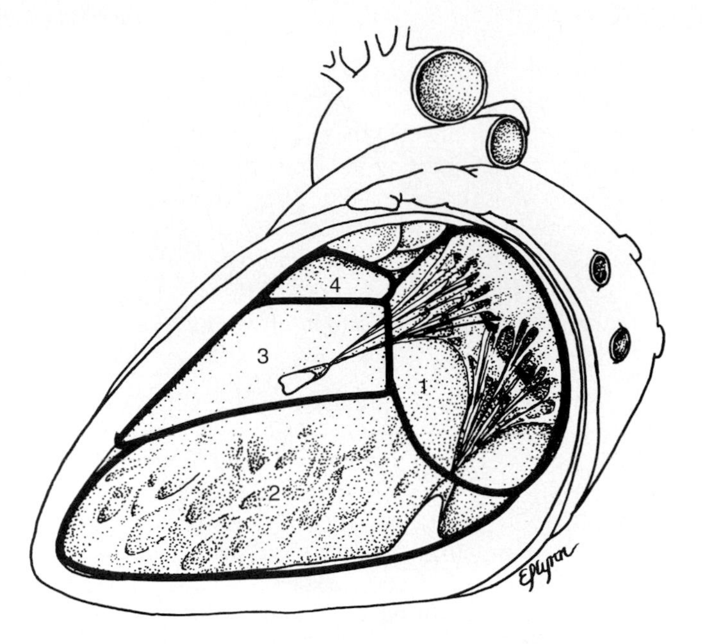

FIGURE 3–14 *The four main anatomic and developmental components of the interventricular septum, left ventricular view. 1, septum of the atrioventricular canal; 2, trabeculated muscular ventricular sinus septum; 3, nontrabeculated muscular septum, corresponding to and continuous with the septal band or proximal conal septum from right ventricular view (Fig. 3-10); 4, parietal band or distal conal septum.*
From Van Praagh R, Geva T, Kreutzer J. Ventricular septal defects: how shall we describe, name, and classify them? J Am Coll Cardiol 14:1298, 1989, with permission.

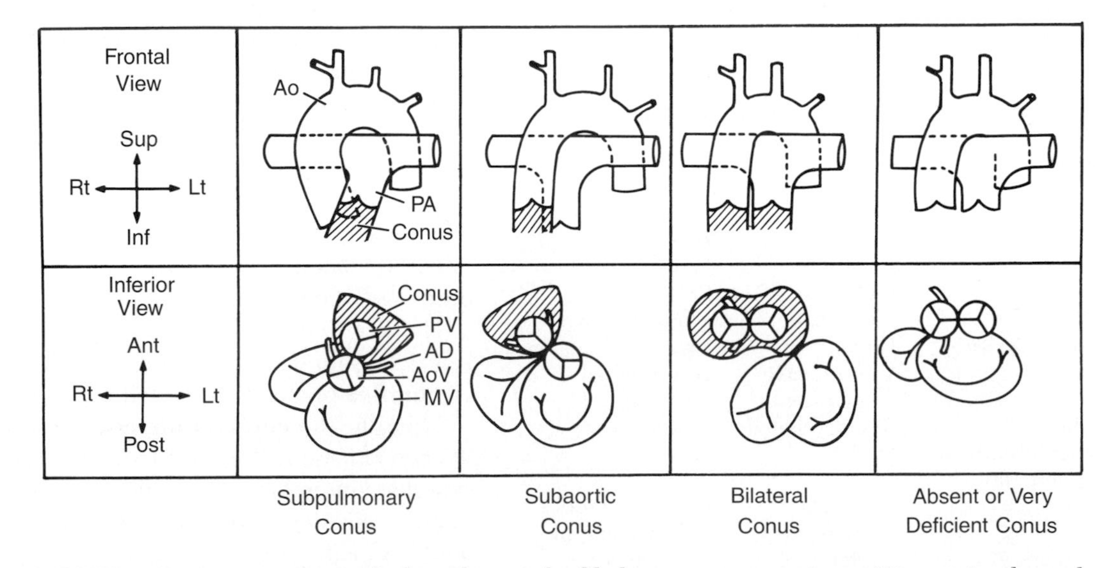

FIGURE 3–15 *Anatomic types of subsemilunar infundibulum or conus arteriosus. AD, anterior descending coronary artery; Ant, anterior; AoV, aortic valve; Inf, inferior; Lt, left; MV, mitral valve; PA, main pulmonary artery; Post, posterior; PV, pulmonary valve; Rt, right; Sup, superior; TV, tricuspid valve.*
Modified from Van Praagh R, Vlad P: Dextrocardia, mesocardia, and levocardia. The segmental approach to diagnosis in congenital heart disease. In Keith JD, Rowe RD, Vlad P (eds): Heart Disease in Infancy and Childhood, 3rd ed. New York: Macmillan, 1978, pp 638–695, with permission.

involve each of these components, and also can occur between them.

Anatomic variations in the conus arteriosus are shown schematically in Figure 3-15. The conus can be: **subpulmonary** with normally related great arteries; **subaortic** with transposition of the great arteries; **bilateral** (subpulmonary and subaortic) typically with double-outlet right ventricle; or **bilaterally absent** (neither subpulmonary nor subaortic) with double-outlet left ventricle.

Comparison and Contrast of the Right and Left Ventricles

The anatomic features of the morphologically right and left ventricles are compared, contrasted, and summarized in Table 3-2. As with the atria (Table 3-1), so too with the ventricles (Table 3-2), virtually all of the anatomic details are distinctive and different. These anatomic features facilitate accurate morphologic diagnosis of the right and left ventricles, regardless of where they are located.

THE IMPORTANCE OF UNDERSTANDING NORMAL MORPHOLOGIC ANATOMY

An understanding of the normal morphologic anatomy of the right and left atria and of the right and left ventricles is not just a baseline or a frame of reference. Instead, an understanding of the morphologic anatomy of the four cardiac chambers is the indispensable key to the diagnosis of much of congenital heart disease: dextrocardia, mesocardia, isolated levocardia, ectopia cordis, superoinferior ventricles, crisscross atrioventricular relations, transposition of the great arteries, double-outlet right ventricle, single ventricle, and so forth. Accurate diagnosis of the aforementioned anomalies—and many more—is based on an understanding of normal morphologic anatomy.

REFERENCES

1. Van Praagh R. The segmental approach to diagnosis in congenital heart disease. In Bergsma D (ed): Birth Defects: Original Article Series 8:4, 1972.
2. Van Praagh S, Kreutzer J, Alday L, et al. Systemic and pulmonary venous connections in visceral heterotaxy, with emphasis on the diagnosis of the atrial situs: a study of 109 postmortem cases. In Clark EB, Takao A (eds): Developmental Cardiology, Morphogensis and Function. Mt. Kisco, NY: Futura, 1990, pp 671–727.
3. Van Praagh R, Vlad P. Dextrocardia, mesocardia, and levocardia. The segmental approach to diagnosis in congenital heart disease. In Keith JD, Rowe RD, Vlad P (eds): Heart Disease in Infancy and Childhood, 3rd ed. New York: Macmillan, 1978, pp 638–695.
4. Van Praagh R, Plett JA, Van Praagh S. Single ventricle: pathology, embryology, terminology, and classification. Herz 4:113, 1979.
5. Van Praagh R, Geva T, Kreutzer J. Ventricular septal defects: how shall we describe, name, and classify them? J Am Coll Cardiol 14:1298, 1989.
6. Van Praagh R, Van Praagh S, Nebesar RA, et al. Tetralogy of Fallot: underdevelopment of the pulmonary infundibulum and its sequelae. Report of a case with cor triatriatum and pulmonary sequestration. Am J Cardiol 26:25, 1970.

4

Segmental Approach to Diagnosis

RICHARD VAN PRAAGH, M.D.

The segmental approach[1–4] (sequential approach,[5,6] systematic approach[7]) to the diagnosis of congenital heart disease[1–15] is based on an understanding of the morphologic and segmental anatomy of the heart. The cardiac segments are the anatomic and embryonic "building blocks" out of which all human hearts—normal and abnormal—are made.

CARDIAC SEGMENTS

The three main cardiac segments are the viscera and atria, the ventricular loop, and the truncus arteriosus. Understanding of the three main cardiac segments is necessary for the diagnostic localization of the atria, the ventricles, and the great arteries (Fig. 4-1).

The two connecting or junctional cardiac segments are the atrioventricular (AV) canal and the infundibulum or conus arteriosus. The atrioventricular canal normally consists of the atrioventricular valves and the atrioventricular septum. The distal or subsemilunar part of the conus arteriosus, or infundibulum, normally consists of a muscular cone or funnel beneath the pulmonary valve, separating the pulmonary valve from both atrioventricular valves (Fig. 4-1, row 1). Normally, there is aortic–mitral fibrous continuity, reflecting the normal absence of subaortic conal free wall myocardium.

Segmental Sets

How many types of human hearts are there? Figure 4-1 provides a partial answer to this question. For each type of heart, the atria, the ventricles, and the great arteries—the three main cardiac segments—may be regarded as the members of a set that are recorded in venoarterial sequence, or blood flow order: {atria, ventricles, great arteries}. Hence, in each segmental set, {1, 2, 3}, the atrial situs is no. 1, the ventricular situs (ventricular loop) is no. 2, and the great arterial situs is no. 3 (Fig. 4-1). Situs denotes the pattern of anatomic organization: solitus (usual or normal) or inversus (a mirror image of solitus).

The types of visceroatrial situs are shown in Figure 4-1: solitus (S), as in {S, -, -}; or inversus (I), as in {I, -, -}; or ambiguus (A), as in {A, -, -} (not shown in Fig. 4-1). In situs ambiguus of the atria, the atrial situs may be indicated by the connections of the suprahepatic segment of the inferior vena cava, the location of the coronary sinus ostium (if present), and the morphology of the atrial appendages. Hence, atrial situs ambiguus, probably basically situs solitus, may be recorded as {A(S), -,-}; and atrial situs ambiguus, probably basically situs inversus, can be denoted as {A(I), -, -}.

The types of ventricular situs are (Fig. 4-1): solitus or D-loop ventricles (D), as in {-, D, -}, the right ventricle being right-handed (Fig. 4-2) and the left ventricle being left-handed;[16,17] or inverted or L-loop (L), as in {-, L, -}, the right ventricle being left-handed (Fig. 4-3) and the left ventricle being right-handed.[16,17]

The types of great arterial situs are (Fig. 4-1): solitus (S), as in solitus normally related great arteries, as in {-, -, S} (row 1, column 1); and inversus (I) as in inverted normally related great arteries, as in {-, -, I} (row 1, column 3).

When the great arteries are abnormally related, the right-sided (dextro, or D) location of the aortic valve relative to the pulmonary valve is symbolized as D, as in {-, -, D}; and the left-sided (levo or L) location of the aortic valve relative to the pulmonary valve is symbolized as L, as in {-, -, L} (Fig. 4-1). D-malpositions of the great arteries are considered to be solitus or noninverted malpositions, the aortic valve normally being right-sided in situs solitus. L-malpositions of

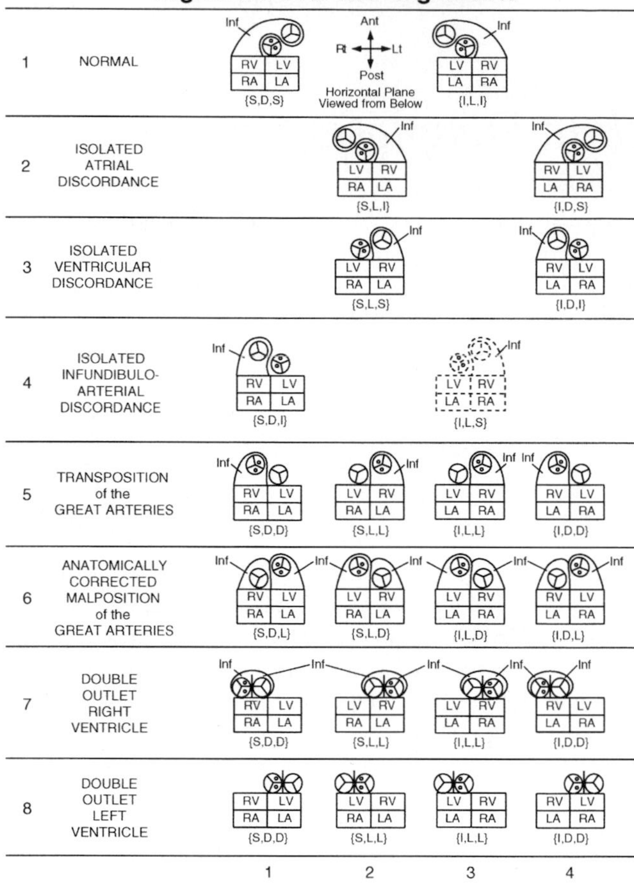

FIGURE 4–1 *Types of human heart: segmental sets and alignments. Heart diagrams are viewed from below, similar to a subxiphoid two-dimensional echocardiogram. Cardiotypes depicted in broken lines had not been documented when this diagram was made. Ant, anterior; Post, posterior; R, right; L, left; RA, morphologically right atrium; LA, morphologically left atrium; RV, morphologically right ventricle; LV, morphologically left ventricle; Inf, infundibulum. The aortic valve is indicated by the coronary ostia; the pulmonary valve is indicated by the absence of the coronary ostia. Braces { } mean "the set of." The segmental sets are explained in the text. Rows 1-4 and 6 have ventriculoarterial (VA) concordance. Row 5, transposition of the great arteries, has VA discordance. Rows 7 and 8 have double-outlet RV and LV, respectively. Columns 1 and 3 have atrioventricular (AV) concordance, {S, D, -} and {I, L, -}, respectively. Columns 2 and 4 have AV discordance, {S, L, -} and {I, D, -}, respectively.*
From Foran RB, Belcourt C, Nanton MA, et al. Isolated infundibuloarterial inversion {S, D, I}: a newly recognized form of congenital heart disease. Am Heart J 116:1337, 1988, with permission.

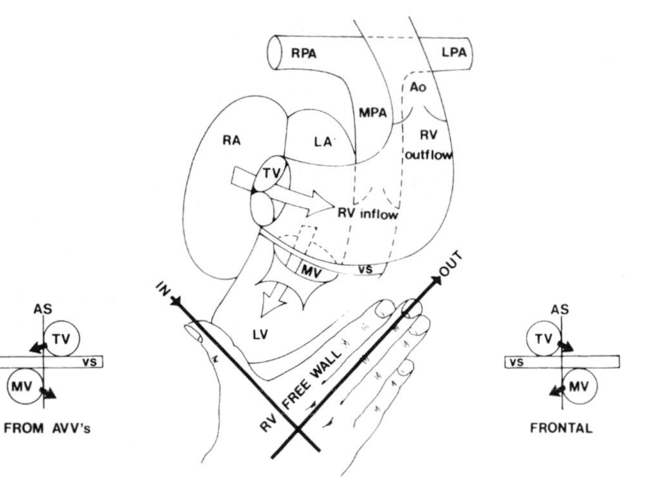

FIGURE 4–2 *The D-loop or solitus right ventricle is right-handed. Figuratively speaking, the thumb of the right hand goes through the tricuspid valve (TV), indicating the RV inflow tract (IN). The fingers go to the right ventricular outflow tract (OUT). The palm of the right hand faces the right ventricular septal surface. The dorsum of the right hand is adjacent to the right ventricular free wall. Abbreviations are as in Figure 1, except: Ao, aorta; AS, atrial septum; AVV's, atrioventricular valves; LPA, left pulmonary artery; MPA, main pulmonary artery; MV, mitral valve; RPA, right pulmonary artery; and VS, ventricular septum. This is a rare case of TGA {S, D, L} with AV concordance and VA discordance, hence physiologically uncorrected (complete) TGA, with crisscross AV relations (arrows), superoinferior ventricles with RV above and LV below and VS approximately horizontal, and with TV superior and to the right relative to the MV which is inferior and to the left. Chirality (handedness) is helpful in diagnosing the type of ventricular loop (D- or L-) when the ventricles are significantly malpositioned in space, as in crisscross AV relations and superoinferior ventricles. Here, the RV is both right-sided and left-sided, and the RV is not to the right of the LV; instead, the RV is above the LV. But note that the TV is to the right of the MV, accurately accurately indicating that D-loop ventricles are present. From Van Praagh S, LaCorte M, Fellows KE, et al. Superioinferior ventricles, anatomic and angiocardiographic finding in 10 postmortem cases. In Van Praagh R, Takao A (eds): Etiology and Morphogenesis of Congenital Heart Disease. Mt. Kisco, NY: Future Publishing, 1980, pp 317–378, with permission.)*

the great arteries are considered to be inverted or mirror-image malpositions because the aortic valve is left-sided relative to the pulmonary valve, as in situs inversus totalis (Fig. 4-1, row 1, column 3). In A-malpositions of the great arteries (not shown in Fig. 4-1), the right–left location of the aortic valve (directly anterior to the pulmonary valve) is equivocal (neither right nor left); hence, A-malpositions may be regarded as of uncertain situs (situs ambiguus of the great arteries).

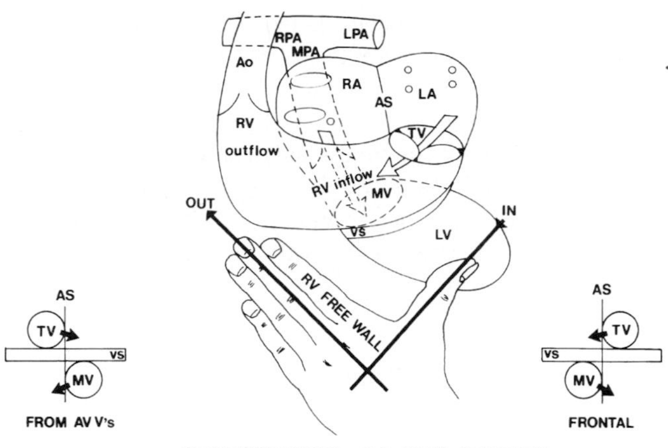

FIGURE 4–3 *The L-loop or inverted right ventricle is left-handed. Figuratively speaking, the thumb of one's left hand goes through the tricuspid valve, indicating the right ventricle inflow tract (IN). The fingers of the left hand go into the right ventricular outflow tract (OUT). The palm of one's left hand faces the right ventricular septal surface and the dorsum of the left hand is adjacent to the right ventricular free wall. Abbreviations are as in previous illustrations. This is a rare case of TGA {S, L, D} with AV discordance and VA discordance, hence physiologically corrected TGA, with crisscross AV relations (arrows), superoinferior ventricles (RV above, LV below), and with TV superior and to the left of the MV (accurately indicating that L-loop ventricles are present). Thus, L-loop ventricles are indicated by AV discordance, left-handed RV (and right-handed LV, not diagrammed), and left-sided TV relative to MV.*
From Van Praagh S, LaCorte M, Fellows KE, et al. Superoinferior ventricles, anatomic and angiocardiographic finding in 10 postmortem cases. In Van Praagh R, Takao A, (eds). Etiology and Morphogenesis of Congenital Heart Disease. Mt. Kisco, NY: Future Publishing, 1980, pp 317–378, with permission.

Consequently, the segmental combinations shown in Figure 4-1 are segmental situs sets. In other words, these segmental combinations (Fig. 4-1) indicate the patterns of anatomic organization (situs) of each of the main cardiac segments {atria, ventricles, great arteries} of any type of congenital heart disease.

Segmental Alignments

Segmental alignments also are shown in Figure 4-1. Atrioventricular alignments are concordant or appropriate when the morphologically right atrium is aligned with, and opens into, the morphologically right ventricle, and the morphologically left atrium is aligned with, and opens into, the morphologically left ventricle. Concordant atrioventricular alignments are shown in vertical columns 1 and 3.

Atrioventricular alignments are discordant or inappropriate when the morphologically right atrium is aligned with, and opens into, the morphologically left ventricle, and the morphologically left atrium is aligned with, and opens into, the morphologically right ventricle. Discordant atrioventricular alignments are shown in vertical columns 2 and 4.

Ventriculoarterial alignments are shown in the horizontal rows (Fig. 4-1). The ventriculoarterial alignments are concordant or appropriate when the morphologically right ventricle is aligned with, and opens into, the pulmonary artery, and when the morphologically left ventricle is aligned with, and opens into, the aorta. Concordant ventriculoarterial alignments are of two types: (1) with normally related great arteries (rows 1 to 4, inclusive); and (2) with abnormally related great arteries (i.e., with anatomically corrected malposition of the great arteries [row 6]).

The ventriculoarterial alignments are abnormal in rows 5 to 8, inclusive. The ventriculoarterial alignments are discordant in transposition of the great arteries (row 5): the morphologically right ventricle is aligned with, and opens into, the aorta, and the morphologically left ventricle is aligned with, and opens into, the pulmonary artery. Other types of abnormal ventriculoarterial alignment include double-outlet right ventricle (row 7) and double-outlet left ventricle (row 8).

Alignments versus Connections

The distinction between segmental alignments and segmental connections should be understood. The atria do not connect directly with the ventricles muscle-to-muscle, except at the atrioventricular bundle of His, because of the interposition of the fibrous atrioventricular canal or junction. Hence, the atria and the ventricle are aligned in various ways (Fig. 4-1), even though they do not connect directly (muscle-to-muscle).

Similarly, the ventricular sinuses (the main pumping portions) do not connect directly with the great arteries, tissue-to-tissue, because of the interposition of the infundibulum or conus arteriosus. Even though the ventricular sinuses do not connect directly with the great arteries, they are aligned in various ways (Fig. 4-1).

The main cardiac segments—the atria, ventricles, and great arteries (Fig. 4-1)—are aligned in various ways, even though they do not connect directly; like "bricks" in a wall, they are connected and separated by the "mortar." The connecting cardiac segments—the atrioventricular junction and infundibulum (conus) —connect the main segments in various ways (Fig. 4-1); the connecting segments are the "mortar." For example, the atria and the ventricles are connected by the fibrous atrioventricular junction; they are also separated, and normally are electrically insulated, from each other by the fibrous atrioventricular junction. If the atria and the ventricles do connect muscle-to-muscle, except at the His bundle, then this is an abnormality of electrophysiologic importance that may result in ventricular pre-excitation, as in the Wolff-Parkinson-White syndrome.

The fact that the atria really do not connect directly with the ventricles also is of great developmental importance. If the right atrium was connected directly with the right ventricle, and if the left atrium was connected directly with the left ventricle, a discordant ventricular L-loop in visceroatrial situs solitus (i.e., {S, L, -}) as in column 2 (Fig. 4-1), probably would be developmentally impossible.

The same principles apply at the ventriculoarterial junction. The facts that the right ventricle (i.e., ventricular sinus) does not connect directly with the pulmonary artery and the left ventricle does not connect directly with the aorta appear to be of great developmental importance. This explains why abnormal ventriculoarterial alignments are developmentally possible (Fig. 4-1)—the ventricles do not connect directly with the great arteries. The development of the conal connector between the ventricular sinuses and the great arteries appears to be of fundamental importance to the type of ventriculoarterial alignment that results (Fig. 4-1).

To summarize, the segmental alignments and connections are distinguished in the interests of anatomic and developmental accuracy. The distinction between alignments and connections is important because they are two different things. Different cardiac segments are involved. Alignments are concerned with the main cardiac segments: atria, ventricles, and great arteries. Connections are concerned with the connecting cardiac segments: the AV canal (junction), and the infundibulum (conus arteriosus). Segmental alignments and connections are both important.

The concepts of concordance and discordance apply well to segmental alignments (Fig. 4-1, columns 1 to 4), but not to connections. The difficulty with connections is that they are Janus-like structures: they "look" proximally and distally at the same time. For example, the right-sided mitral valve in classic physiology corrected transposition of the great arteries; that is transposition of the great arteries {S, L, L} (Fig. 4-1, row 5, column 2), connects the right-sided right atrium with the right-sided left ventricle. This right-sided mitral valve is concordant relative to the right-sided left ventricle, but discordant relative to the right-sided right atrium. The concordant/discordant concept applies unequivocally to alignments because alignments "look" in one direction only—distally (Fig. 4-1).

Associated Malformations

In addition to segmental situs sets and their alignments and connections (Fig. 4-1), associated malformations of the main or connecting cardiac segments are also of great diagnostic importance. Associated malformations are omitted from Figure 4-1 for simplicity. Different segmental sets have distinctive and very different associated malformations: for example, discordant L-loop ventricles have very different associated malformations than do concordant D-loop ventricles.[18] Finally, the functional or physiologic diagnosis is every bit as important as is the aforementioned anatomic diagnosis. How does the segmental set with its alignments and connections (Fig. 4-1), with or without associated malformations, function?

SPECIFIC EXAMPLES

Specific examples of this diagnostic approach, which has been used at Children's Hospital Boston for the past three decades, are summarized as follows (Fig. 4-1).

The Solitus Normal Heart

The solitus normal heart (row 1, column 1) is {S, D, S}, meaning the set of situs solitus of the viscera and atria (S), D-loop or solitus ventricles (D), and solitus normally related great arteries (S). Atrioventricular concordance, ventriculoarterial concordance, and a subpulmonary infundibulum with aortic–mitral direct continuity are present.

In this chapter, whenever the term "concordance" or "discordance" is used without other qualification, it always means **alignment** concordance or discordance, consistent with common usage. Parenthetically, there is another type of concordance or discordance that can be very important, namely **situs** concordance or discordance. One can have {S, D, S} with **straddling tricuspid valve** or **double-inlet left ventricle.** In other words, when the atrioventricular alignments are concordant, as in the normal heart, nothing else need be said diagnostically. If something is not mentioned, one may assume that it is normal, or as expected. However, when the atrioventricular alignments are abnormal, they must be specified, as above. In {S, D, S} with double-inlet left ventricle, there is atrioventricular **situs** concordance (**not** atrioventricular **alignment** concordance): the situs of the atrial segment and of the ventricular segment are both solitus. But the atrioventricular alignments are double-inlet left ventricle.

The Inverted Normal Heart

The inverted normal heart (Fig. 4-1, row 1, column 3) is {I, L, I}—the set or combination of visceroatrial situs inversus (I), L-loop ventricles (L), and inverted normally related great arteries (I). There is a subpulmonary infundibulum with aortic mitral fibrous continuity. Atrioventricular concordance and ventriculoarterial concordance are present.

Ventricular Inversion with Inverted Normally Related Great Arteries in Visceroatrial Situs Solitus

Ventricular inversion with inverted normally related great arteries in visceroatrial situs solitus (Fig. 4-1, row 2, column 2) is {S, L, I}—the set of visceroatrial situs solitus (S), L-loop ventricles (L), and inverted normally related great arteries (I). The infundibulum is subpulmonary. As one would expect from the segmental situs set {S, L, I}, the atrioventricular alignments are discordant and the ventriculoarterial alignments are concordant. Since there is one discordant alignment, the circulations are physiologically uncorrected. In this rare segmental combination, an atrial switch operation (Senning or Mustard) results in an anatomic and a physiologic correction: postoperatively, the left ventricle is the systemic ventricle and the right ventricle is the pulmonary ventricle.

Because the aforementioned name of this anomaly is too long, attempts have been made to shorten it. **Isolated atrial noninversion** has been suggested because only the atria are in situs solitus, the ventricular and great arterial segments both being inverted. The difficulty with "isolated atrial noninversion" is that it is excessively cardiocentric. Although noninversion of the atria may be isolated as far as the heart is concerned, since all of the viscera also are in situs solitus, the atrial noninversion is hardly isolated. However, if understood as a **cardiac** diagnosis, "isolated atrial noninversion" is brief and not inaccurate. The briefest and the clearest diagnosis is, we think, {S, L, I}. This may be spelled out in words if one prefers the longer version.

Isolated Ventricular Inversion

Isolated ventricular inversion is {S, L, S} (Fig. 4-1, row 3, column 2), which means situs solitus of the viscera and atria (S), L-loop ventricles (L), and solitus normally related great arteries (S). As the segmental combination {S, L, S} suggests, there is atrioventricular discordance and ventriculoarterial concordance. Because there is one alignment discordance (i.e., one right–left switching error), the circulations are physiologically uncorrected. This is confirmed by the presence of atrioarterial alignment discordance: the right atrium and the aorta are ipsilateral, both right-sided; and the pulmonary veins and the pulmonary artery are ipsilateral, both left-sided. As in all types of atrioventricular discordance with ventriculoarterial concordance, anatomic repair can be accomplished with an atrial switch procedure.

Isolated Ventricular Noninversion

Isolated ventricular noninversion is {I, D, I} (Fig. 4-1, row 3, column 4)—the set of situs inversus of the viscera and the atria (I), D-loop ventricles (D), and inverted normally related great arteries (I). The infundibulum is subpulmonary, as one would expect with a form of normally related great arteries. As {I, D, I} suggests, there is atrioventricular discordance and ventriculoarterial concordance. Given one discordant alignment, the circulations are physiologically uncorrected. Note the atrioarterial discordance, the right atrium and the aorta being ipsilateral. Again, as in all anatomic types of atrioventricular discordance with ventriculoarterial concordance, an atrial switch procedure results in an anatomic and physiologic correction.

Isolated Infundibuloarterial Inversion

Isolated infundibuloarterial inversion is a newly discovered form of congenital heart disease with the segmental combination of {S, D, I} (Fig. 4-1, row 4, column 1)[19]: situs solitus of the viscera and atria (S), D-loop ventricles (D), and inverted normally related great arteries (I). As {S, D, I} suggests, there is atrioventricular concordance and ventriculoarterial concordance. Consequently, one would expect to have no hemodynamic derangement. Usually, however, the inverted normal type of conotruncus is associated with a **tetralogy of Fallot**–type of malformation. Pulmonary outflow tract obstruction (stenosis or atresia) with a large subaortic ventricular septal defect results in cyanotic congenital heart disease. Also characteristic of tetralogy of Fallot {S, D, I} are dextrocardia, superoinferior ventricles, the appearance of criss-cross atrioventricular relations, small right ventricular sinus (inflow tract), huge ventricular septal defect (confluent ventricular septal defect of atrioventricular canal type with conoventricular ventricular septal defect of the malalignment tetralogy type), and a tendency of the atrioventricular valves to straddle the ventricular septum. The right coronary artery runs across the obstructed pulmonary outflow tract, necessitating the use of an external conduit from the right ventricle to the pulmonary artery, or myocardial resection within the right ventricular outflow tract.[20]

Transposition of the Great Arteries

Transposition of the great arteries (Fig. 4-1, row 5) is a specific type of malposition of the great arteries characterized by ventriculoarterial discordance. Only a few of the segmental combinations that occur with transposition of the great arteries are shown.[18]

Transposition of the Great Arteries {S, D, D}

Transposition of the great arteries {S, D, D} means transposition of the great arteries with the set of visceroatrial situs solitus (S), D-loop ventricles (D), and D-transposition of the great arteries (D). Typically, there is a subaortic infundibulum (conus), with pulmonary-mitral fibrous continuity. There is atrioventricular concordance with ventriculoarterial discordance. There being one segmental alignment discordance, the circulations are physiologically uncorrected: Note the atrioarterial alignment discordance, the right atrium and the aorta being ipsilateral (instead of contralateral as normally). This is the classic form of transposition of the great arteries.

In physiologically uncorrected transposition of the great arteries, the aortic valve can be directly anterior (antero, or A) relative to the pulmonary valve (i.e., transposition of the great arteries {S, D, A} [not shown in Fig. 4-1]). Or the aortic valve can be to the left (levo, or L) relative to the pulmonary valve (i.e., transposition of the great arteries {S, D, L} [Fig. 4-2]). Even though the aortic valve can lie to the left of the pulmonary valve, which may confusingly suggest physiologically corrected transposition of the great arteries, **segmental alignment analysis** clearly indicates that physiologically uncorrected transposition of the great arteries is present: There is only one discordance (right-left switching error) at the ventriculoarterial junction, not two. The vena caval return goes to the aorta (Fig. 4-2).

Transposition of the great arteries {S, D, D} (Fig. 4-1, row 5, column 1) is the classic form of transposition of the great arteries. In 1915, Abbott[21] called this anomaly "**c "complete"** transposition of the great arteries, as opposed to **"partial"** transposition of the great arteries, which is now called **double-outlet right ventricle.** As the term "transposition of the great arteries" is now used, all transpositions (row 5, Fig. 4-1) (physiologically uncorrected and corrected) are complete (as opposed to partial). However, Abbott's usage of complete transposition of the great arteries to mean physiologically uncorrected transposition of the great arteries has stuck. Whenever the term "complete" transposition of the great arteries is used, it means physiologically uncorrected transposition of the great arteries. Transposition of the great arteries {S, D, D} is often simply called **D-transposition of the great arteries,** for convenient brevity. Transposition of the great arteries {S, D, D} is **complete noninverted transposition of the great arteries.** "Complete" means that each artery is placed completely across the ventricular septum, and so arises above the morphologically inappropriate ventricle. "Noninverted" means that the aortic valve is right-sided and the pulmonary valve is left-sided, as is normal in situs solitus: {S, D, S} (row 1, column 1).

Transposition of the great arteries {S, L, L}

Transposition of the great arteries {S, L, L} (Fig. 4-1, row 5, column 2) means transposition of the great arteries with the set of visceroatrial situs solitus (S), L-loop ventricles (L), and L-transposition of the great arteries (L). As {S, L, L} suggests, there is atrioventricular discordance. As transposition of the great arteries indicates, there is ventriculoarterial discordance. This is the classic form of **congenitally physiologically corrected transposition of the great arteries.** The two segmental discordances cancel each other. There is atrioarterial alignment concordance, the left atrium and the aorta being ipsilateral. Transposition of the great arteries {S, L, L} is **complete inverted transposition of the great arteries.** "Complete" means that each great artery is placed completely across the ventricular septum (i.e., that "partial" transposition of the great arteries is not present). "Inverted" means that the semilunar valves are right–left reversed—a mirror image of what is normal in situs solitus (i.e., {S, D, S} [Fig. 4-1, row 1, column 1]). Because transposition of the great arteries {S, L, L} is by far the most common form of L-transposition, this anomaly is often briefly called **L-transposition of the great arteries.** However, {S, L, L} transposition of the great arteries is a little longer and is entirely specific, whereas "L-transposition of the great arteries" does not specify the atrial or the ventricular situs, and consequently is open to misinterpretation.

Transposition of the Great Arteries {I, L, L}

Transposition of the great arteries {I, L, L} (Fig. 4-1, row 5, column 3) denotes transposition of the great arteries with the segmental set of visceroatrial situs inversus (I), L-loop ventricles (L), and L-transposition (L). There is atrioventricular concordance with ventriculoarterial discordance, indicating a physiologically uncorrected circulation (one discordance), the right atrium and the aorta being ipsilateral. Transposition of the great arteries {I, L, L} exemplifies **physiologically uncorrected (complete) transposition of the great arteries in situs inversus.** Transposition of the great arteries {I, L, L} may be viewed as **noninverted transposition of the great arteries for situs inversus,** because the aortic valve usually is left-sided and the pulmonary valve is right-sided in situs inversus totalis (i.e., {I, L, I} [Fig. 4-1, row 1, column 3]). Both in visceroatrial situs solitus and in visceroatrial situs inversus, **physiologically uncorrected transposition** typically is **noninverted transposition of the great arteries** (relative to the semilunar relationship that is usual for the situs, row 1).

Transposition of the Great Arteries {I, D, D}

Transposition of the great arteries {I, D, D} (Fig. 4-1, row 5, column 4) indicates transposition of the great arteries with the segmental combination (set) of visceroatrial situs inversus (I), D-loop ventricles (D), and D-transposition of the great arteries (D). There is atrioventricular discordance, indicating physiologically corrected transposition of the great arteries (two discordances). This is **physiologically corrected transposition of the great arteries in situs inversus.** Transposition of the great arteries {I, D, D} also may be viewed as **inverted transposition of the great arteries for situs inversus:** the semilunar interrelationship is right-left switched compared with the semilunar interrelationship that is usual in situs inversus totalis, i.e., {I, L, I} (row1, column 3). In visceroatrial situs solitus and in visceroatrial situs inversus, **physiologically corrected transposition of the great arteries** typically is **inverted transposition of the great arteries** (relative to the semilunar interrelationship that is usual for the situs, row 1).

Anatomically Corrected Malposition of the Great Arteries

Anatomically corrected malposition of the great arteries (Fig. 4-1, row 6) may be exemplified by the most common form, anatomically corrected malposition of the great arteries {S, D, L} (row 6, column 1), which means anatomically corrected malposition of the great arteries with the segmental set of visceroatrial situs solitus (S), D-loop ventricles (D), and L-malposition of the great arteries (L). As anatomically corrected malposition of the great arteries {S, D, L} suggests, there is atrioventricular concordance and venticuloarterial concordance. A bilateral infundibulum (subaortic and subpulmonary) is more common than is a subaortic infundibulum with pulmonary-mitral fibrous continuity.

Although this form of anatomically corrected malposition of the great arteries has physiologically corrected circulations (the left atrium and aorta are ipsilateral), other forms such as **anatomically corrected malposition of the great arteries {S, L, D}** have physiologically uncorrected circulations, the right atrium and the aorta being ipsilateral (row 6, column 2).

Anatomically corrected malposition of the great arteries also occurs in visceroatrial situs inversus (row 6, columns 3 and 4): **anatomically corrected malposition of the great arteries {I, L, D}** with atrioventricular and venticuloarterial concordance (physiologically corrected); and **anatomically corrected malposition of the great arteries {I, D, L}** with atrioventricular discordance and ventriculoarterial concordance (physiologically uncorrected).

In all forms of anatomically corrected malposition of the great arteries, the ventricles loop in one direction, and the conotruncus twists in the opposite direction (row 6). This may explain why anatomically corrected malposition of the great arteries is so rare. Almost always, the directions of the ventricular looping and infundibuloarterial twisting are the same: both to the right with D-loop ventricles, or both to the left with L-loop ventricles (Fig. 4-1).

The designation **anatomically corrected malposition**[22,23] means that the great arteries are malposed, but despite this fact, the great arteries nonetheless originate above the anatomically correct ventricles: the aorta above the morphologically left ventricle and the pulmonary artery above the morphologically right ventricle. It is in this sense that the malposition of the great arteries is *anatomically* corrected. ACM may or may not be *physiologically* corrected (Fig. 4-1).

Anatomically corrected malposition of the great arteries indicates that the ventriculoarterial concordance and normally related (and normally connected) great arteries are not synonymous. In anatomically corrected malposition of the great arteries, although the ventriculoarterial **alignments** are concordant, the ventriculoarterial **connections** are very abnormal—the conal connector being subaortic and subpulmonary, or subaortic only. In ACM, the great arteries are very abnormally related in space (Fig. 4-1).

Double-Outlet Right Ventricle

Double-outlet right ventricle (Fig. 4-1, row 7) means that both great arteries are entirely or predominantly above the morphologically right ventricle. A few of the segmental sets that occur[24] with double-outlet right ventricle are presented in row 7. For example, double-outlet right ventricle {S, D, D} means double-outlet right ventricle with the set of solitus atria (S), D-loop ventricles (D), and D-malposition of the great arteries (D). Atrioventricular concordance is typical. The ventriculoarterial alignments are, of course, those of double-outlet right ventricle. The segmental anatomy of the other forms of double-outlet right ventricle is self-evident (row 7).

Double-Outlet Left Ventricle

Double-outlet left ventricle (Fig. 4-1, row 8) means that both great arteries are entirely or predominately above the morphologically left ventricle. Some of the segmental combinations that are now known to be associated with double-outlet left ventricle[25] are depicted in row 8 (Fig. 4-1). The most common is double-outlet left ventricle {S, D, D}, which means double-outlet left ventricle with the set of solitus atria (S), D-loop ventricles (D), and D-malposition of the great arteries (D). Typically, the atrioventricular alignments are concordant. By definition, the ventriculoarterial alignments are those of double-outlet left ventricle. Because the segmental anatomy of the other forms depicted should be understood by now, further description will be omitted in the interest of brevity.

SUMMARY

The foregoing is an introduction to the segmental anatomy of congenital heart disease. Diagnosis is based mainly on the following six criteria (Fig. 4-1): segmental situs, alignments, connections, spatial relations, associated malformations, and function.

The segmental approach to the diagnosis of congenital heart disease involves answering the following questions:

1. What type of visceroatrial situs is present?
2. What type of ventricular situs (ventricular loop) is present?
3. What anatomic type of infundibulum and great arteries (conotruncus) does the patient have?
4. What are the atrioventricular alignments?
5. What are the atrioventricular connections?
6. What are the ventriculoarterial alignments?
7. What are the ventriculoarterial connections?
8. Are there any associated malformations?
9. How does the segmental set, with or without associated malformations, function?

The segmental approach to diagnosis is concerned primarily with questions 1 to 8. The **anatomic diagnosis** (questions 1 to 8) is highly relevant to the **physiologic diagnosis** (question 9), and both are important in surgical management.

REFERENCES

1. Calcaterra G, Anderson RH, Lau KC, et al. Dextrocardia-value of segmental analysis in its categorization. Br Heart J 42:497, 1979.
2. Van Praagh R. The segmental approach to diagnosis in congenital heart disease. The Cardiovascular System. Birth Defects: Original Article Series 8:4, 1972.
3. Van Praagh R, Ongley PA, Swan HJC. Anatomic types of single or common ventricle in man. Morphologic and geometric aspects of sixty autopsied cases. Am J Cardiol 13:367, 1964.
4. Van Praagh R, Van Praagh S, Vlad P, et al. Anatomic types of congenital dextrocardia. Diagnostic and embryologic implications. Am J Cardiol 13:510, 1964.
5. Shinebourne EA, Macartney FJ, Anderson RH. Sequential chamber localization: logical approach to diagnosis in congenital heart disease. Br Heart J 38:327, 1976.
6. Tynan MJ, Becker AE, Macartney FJ, et al. Nomenclature and classification of congenital heart disease. Br Heart J 41:544, 1979.
7. Rao PS: Systemic approach to differential diagnosis. Am Heart J 102:389, 1981.
8. Ando M, Satomi G, Takao A. Atresia of tricuspid or mitral orifice: anatomic spectrum and morphogenetic hypothesis. In Van Praagh R, Takao A (eds): Etiology and Morphogenesis of Congenital Heart Disease. Mt. Kisco, NY: Futura Publishing, 1980, pp 421–487.
9. Kirklin JW, Pacifico AD, Bargeron LM, et al. Cardiac repair in anatomically corrected malposition of the great arteries. Circulation 48:153, 1973.
10. Otero Coto E, Quero Jimenez M. Aproximacion segmentaria al diagnostico y clasificacion de las cardiopatias congenitas. Fundamentos y utilidad. Rev Esp Cardiol 30:557, 1977.
11. Stanger P, Rudolph AM, Edwards JE. Cardiac malpositions: An overview based on study of sixty-five necropsy specimens. Circulation 56:159, 1977.
12. Van Praagh R. Terminology of congenital heart disease. Glossary and commentary. Circulation 56:139, 1977.
13. Van Praagh R. Diagnosis of complex congenital heart disease: morphologic anatomic method and terminology. Cardiovasc Intervent Radiol 7:115, 1984.
14. Van Praagh R. The importance of segmental situs in the diagnosis of congenital heart disease. Semin Roentgenol 20:254, 1985.
15. Van Praagh R, Weinberg PM, Foran RB, et al. Malposition of the heart. In Moss AJ, Adams FH, Emmanouilides GC, Riemenschneider TH (eds): Heart Disease in Infants, Children, and Adolescents, 4th ed. Baltimore: Williams & Wilkins, 2001, pp 530–580.
16. Van Praagh R, David I, Gordon D, et al. Ventricular diagnosis and designation. In Godman MJ (ed): Pediatric Cardiology, 1980 World Congress, vol 4. London: Churchill Livingstone, 1981, pp 153–168.
17. Van Praagh S, LaCorte M, Fellows KE, et al. Superioinferior ventricles, anatomic and angiocardiographic finding in 10 postmortem cases. In Van Praagh R, Takao A (eds): Etiology and Morphogenesis of Congenital Heart Disease. Mt. Kisco, NY: Future Publishing, 1980, pp 317–378.
18. Van Praagh R, Weinberg PM, Calder AL, et al. The transposition complexes: how many are there? In Davila JC (ed): Second Henry Ford Hospital International Symposium on Cardiac Surgery. New York: Appleton-Century-Crofts, 1977, pp 207–213.
19. Foran RB, Belcourt C, Nanton MA, et al. Isolated infundibuloarterial inversion {S, D, I}: a newly recognized form of congenital heart disease. Am Heart J 116:1337, 1988.
20. Santini F, Jonas RA, Sanders SP, et al. Tetralogy of Fallot {S, D, I}: successful repair without conduit. Ann Thorac Surg 59:747, 1995.
21. Abbott ME. Congenital cardiac disease. In Osler and McCrae's Modern Medicine, vol 4, 2nd ed. Philadelphia: Lea & Febiger, 1915, p 323.
22. Harris JS, Farber S. Transposition of the great cardiac vessels with special reference to the phylogenetic therapy of Spitzer. Arch Pathol 28:427, 1939.
23. Van Praagh R, Perez-Trevino C, Lopez-Cuellar M, et al. Transposition of the great arteries with posterior aorta, anterior pulmonary artery, subpulmonary conus and fibrous continuity between aortic and atrioventricular valves. Am J Cardiol 28: 621, 1971.
24. Van Praagh S, Davidoff A, Chin A, et al. Double-outlet right ventricle: anatomic types and developmental implications based on a study of 101 autopsied cases. Coeur 13:389, 1982.
25. Van Praagh R, Weinberg PM, Srebro J. Double-outlet left ventricle. In Adams FH, Emmanouilides GC, Riemenschneider TH (eds): Moss' Heart Disease in Infants, Children, and Adolescents, 4th (ed). Baltimore: Williams & Wilkins, 2001, pp 461–485.

III

Dysmorphology

5

Dysmorphology and Genetics

RONALD V. LACRO, MD

In 1966, Smith proposed that the term *dysmorphology* be used to denote the study of abnormalities in morphogenesis, regardless of etiology, timing of origin, or severity.[1] The field has expanded dramatically over the last several decades, as great strides have been made in our understanding of the developmental pathogenesis of many structural defects, including those affecting the cardiovascular system. Congenital anomalies of the cardiovascular system are among the leading causes of morbidity and mortality in infancy and childhood. With an overall incidence between 0.4% and 1% among live-born infants, congenital cardiovascular malformations (CCVMs) or congenital heart defects (CHDs) constitute an etiologically heterogeneous group of birth defects with a variety of known and unknown causes.[2] For most structural cardiovascular malformations, the genetic and biochemical basis for the developmental error is largely unknown. Vigorous research efforts are currently directed at elucidating the genetic, biochemical, and cellular mechanisms involved in normal and abnormal cardiovascular development. An increasing number of specific genes are now implicated in the pathogenesis of congenital cardiovascular malformations in humans and animals. These developments in the dysmorphology and genetics of pediatric heart disease have led to improvements in clinical diagnosis, management, and genetic counseling for individuals and families with congenital heart disease, whether isolated or associated with one or more extracardiac malformations. In this chapter, the etiologic and genetic aspects of congenital cardiovascular malformations will be reviewed, emphasizing those aspects of particular interest to the pediatrician, pediatric cardiologist, and pediatric cardiac surgeon.

APPROACH TO THE CHILD WITH STRUCTURAL DEFECTS

About 4% of all infants have at least one major defect in structural development.[3] A significant proportion of these have congenital cardiovascular malformations, for which the incidence in the general population is between 0.4% and 1%.[2] Furthermore, at least 25% of patients with a congenital heart defect have one or more extracardiac malformations.[4] Cardiologists and cardiac surgeons frequently are involved in the care of patients with multiple malformations involving multiple organ systems. Consultations between the cardiac team and a dysmorphologist or clinical geneticist, play an integral part in the management of affected patients and their families.

A developmental approach to the child with structural defects is depicted in Figure 5-1. The ultimate goal of such an approach is to make a specific diagnosis such that accurate prognosis can be predicted, the recurrence risk can be determined, and an appropriate management plan may be formulated. When evaluating an infant or child with a structural defect, it must first be determined whether the defect has a prenatal or postnatal onset. Usually this distinction can be deduced from a careful history and physical examination. The term **prenatal onset** is used to designate structural abnormalities that are present at birth, whereas **postnatal onset** is used to designate structural abnormalities that are not present at birth, but rather develop postnatally. Some structural defects are categorized as postnatal in onset even though the genetic alteration responsible for them was present prenatally. Once the distinction between prenatal and postnatal onset has been made, a rational

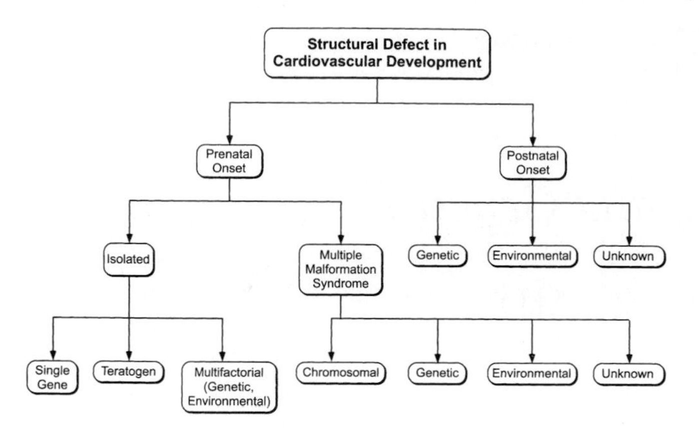

FIGURE 5–1 *A developmental approach to the child with structural defects.*

differential diagnosis can be developed, since this determination narrows the diagnostic possibilities considerably.

The vast majority of structural cardiovascular defects have a prenatal rather than postnatal onset. Congenital heart defects may be the result of *malformation* (abnormal development), *disruption* (interruption of a normal developmental process), or *deformation* (the effects of extrinsic mechanical forces on normal development). Although some isolated defects are caused by single gene mutations (e.g., mutations of the elastin gene, *ELN*, in familial supravalvar aortic stenosis) or known teratogens (e.g., retinoic acid), most currently have no identifiable cause. In the past, most isolated defects were thought to arise from multifactorial influences—a combination of genetic and environmental causes. Recent research efforts have implicated an increasing number of specific genes in the pathogenesis of congenital cardiovascular malformations.

Dysmorphic features and extracardiac malformations are commonly associated with congenital heart defects (25%)[4] and should prompt an evaluation for a possible syndrome. Multiple malformation syndromes arise from chromosomal, genetic, teratogenic (environmental), and unknown causes. For malformation syndromes, the prognosis and recurrence risk for heart disease depend largely on the underlying syndrome diagnosis. In the management of fetuses, infants, children, and adults with congenital cardiovascular malformations, the importance of a genetics evaluation, including consultation with a clinical geneticist and possible cytogenetics evaluation, cannot be overemphasized. When a major cardiovascular malformation is detected prenatally, amniocentesis should be strongly considered, particularly if there is a coexistent extracardiac malformation. In particular, complete atrioventricular canal defects are common in Trisomy 21 syndrome, and conotruncal malformations (truncus arteriosus, tetralogy of Fallot, type B interrupted aortic arch) are common in the chromosome 22 deletion syndrome (velocardiofacial syndrome, DiGeorge sequence), which is associated with genetic abnormalities on the long arm of chromosome 22. In most patients with the chromosome 22 deletion syndrome, a deletion on the long arm of chromosome 22 can be detected by fluorescent in situ hybridization (FISH).

Examples of multiple malformation syndromes of prenatal and postnatal onset are illustrated in Figures 5-2 and 5-3. When structural malformations are present at the time of birth (prenatal onset), the diagnostic possibilities should include chromosomal abnormalities, genetically determined syndromes, and environmental disorders due to prenatal exposure to a teratogen. The child depicted in Figure 5-2 was born to a mother who used the acne medication, *cis*-retinoic acid (Accutane) during her pregnancy.[5]

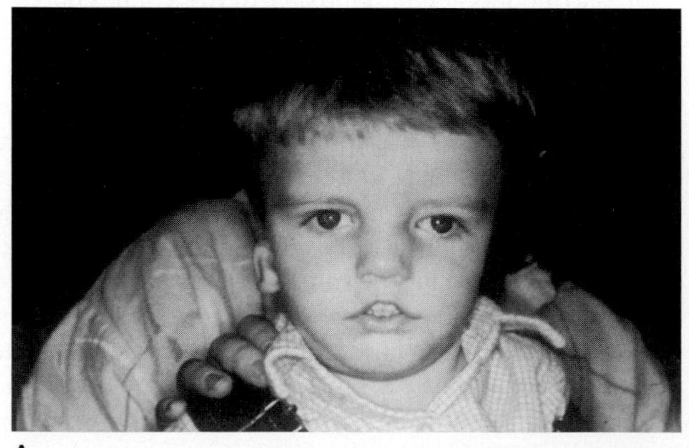

A

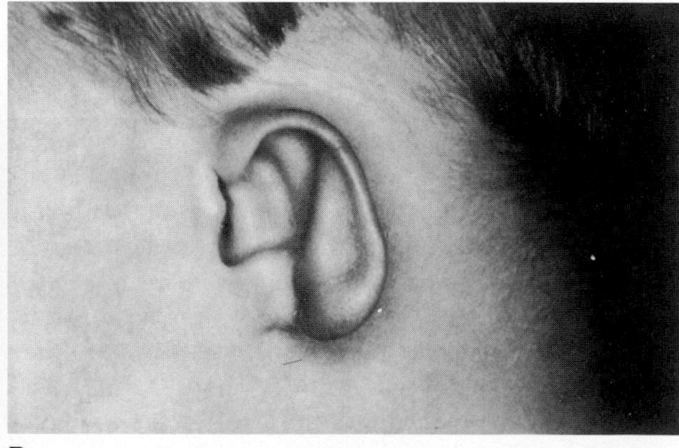

B

Figure 5–2 *Retinoic acid embryopathy in a 2-year-old boy. A, Triangular facies, down-slanting palpebral fissures, and widely spaced eyes. B, Malformed ears. Brain malformations (e.g., hydrocephalus) and conotruncal abnormalities are common. From Fyler DC (ed). Nadas' Pediatric Cardiology. Philadephia: Hanley & Belfus, 1992.*

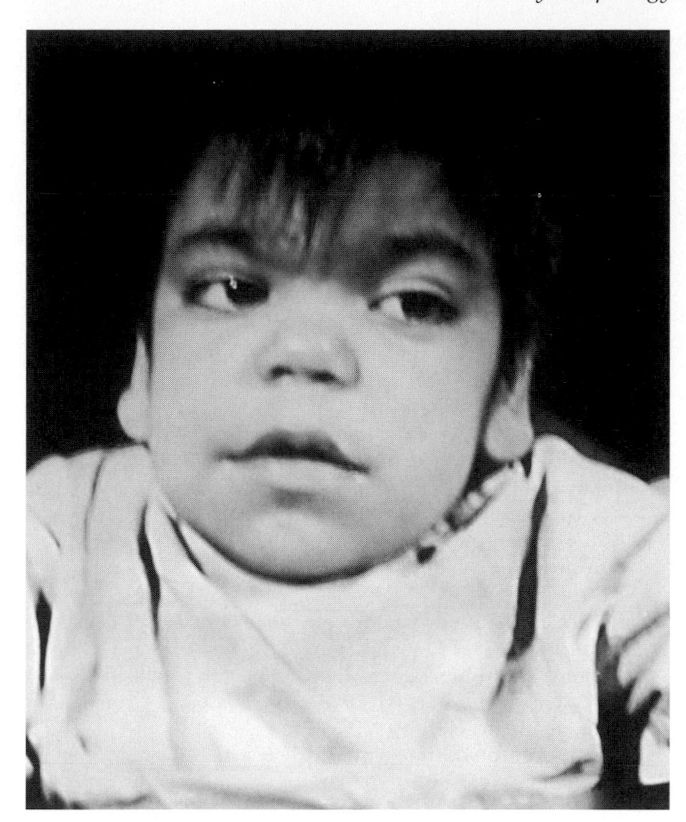

Figure 5–3 *Hurler syndrome (mucopolysaccharidosis I). After birth, the facial features become progressively more coarse. Deposition of mucopolysaccharides leads to cardiac complications including valvar insufficiency, myocardial dysfunction, sudden death from arrhythmia, and diffuse coronary artery disease.*
From Fyler DC (ed). Nadas' Pediatric Cardiology. Philadephia: Hanley & Belfus, 1992.

In these infants, malformations present at birth include craniofacial defects, especially anomalies of the ears and the Robin sequence, defects of the central nervous system including hydrocephalus and microcephaly, thymic abnormalities, and a characteristic spectrum of conotruncal malformations including tetralogy of Fallot, double-outlet right ventricle, supracristal ventricular septal defect, and type B interruption of the aortic arch. The retinoic acid embryopathy is an example of the effect of a teratogen on the developing embryo or fetus. In particular, it demonstrates how a specific teratogen can lead to a characteristic spectrum of cardiac lesions, presumably by acting via a common mechanism interfering with conotruncal development. Disorders caused by environmental agents take on a special significance because prevention prior to conception may be feasible. In general, recognizing that a teratogenic agent was the cause of the structural defect means that the recurrence risk is negligible if the mother avoids the use of that agent during subsequent pregnancies. Other teratogens that are known to cause cardiac malformations in humans include alcohol, anticonvulsants (hydantoins, trimethadione, valproic acid, carbamazepine), lithium, thalidomide, warfarin (Coumadin), the rubella virus, maternal diabetes, and maternal phenylketonuria (see following discussions).

A patient with mucopolysaccharidosis type I (MPS I, Hurler syndrome) is depicted in Figure 5-3. Although the genetic alteration responsible for MPS I syndrome is present prenatally, the structural abnormalities develop postnatally. This child appeared to be normal at birth, having thrived *in utero*. By 18 months of age, coarse facial features, cloudy corneas, poor growth, mental deficiency, and multiple skeletal anomalies became evident. Deposition of mucopolysaccharides in cardiac valve tissue, myocardium, and coronary arteries leads to progressive thickening and stiffening of valve leaflets, valvar insufficiency, myocardial dysfunction, sudden death from arrhythmia, and diffuse coronary artery disease. A small subset of individuals with severe MPS I have an early-onset fatal endocardiofibroelastosis.[6] Postnatal onset of these structural defects should focus the diagnostic evaluation on the etiologic possibilities set forth in Figure 5-1, as they became manifest after birth. They include genetically determined inborn errors of metabolism, degenerative diseases of the central nervous system, and perinatal and postnatal environmental factors such as anoxia, trauma, infection, and drugs.

PATHOGENETIC CLASSIFICATION OF CONGENITAL CARDIOVASCULAR MALFORMATIONS

The traditional nomenclature for classifying structural heart defects is based on presumed embryologic events or on anatomic characteristics and location. Although helpful in naming complex cardiac defects, earlier classification systems may have obscured important pathogenetic relationships. More recently, congenital cardiovascular malformations have been classified by disordered mechanisms (Table 5-1). This newer classification scheme, which is undergoing continuous reassessment and modification, is based on the assumption that there is a limited repertoire of developmental mechanisms and a relatively wide spectrum of phenotypic expression. Clark proposed six major pathogenetic mechanisms that are likely to be involved in the majority of cardiovascular malformations: I, ectomesenchymal tissue migration or neural crest abnormalities (conotruncal and aortic arch anomalies); II, abnormalities of intracardiac blood flow (flow defects); III, cell death abnormalities; IV, extracellular matrix abnormalities (endocardial cushion abnormalities); V, abnormal targeted growth;

TABLE 5–1. Classification of Cardiovascular Malformations by Pathogenetic Mechanisms

Classification
I. Ectomesenchymal tissue migration abnormalities (neural crest defects)
Conotruncal septation defects
Increased mitral–aortic separation (a clinically silent *forme fruste*)
Subarterial or malalignment ventricular septal defect
Double-outlet right ventricle
Tetralogy of Fallot with or without pulmonary atresia
Aorticopulmonary window
Truncus arteriosus communis
Branchial arch defects
Interrupted aortic arch, type B
Double aortic arch
Right aortic arch with mirror image branching
Aberrant subclavian artery
Abnormal conotruncal cushion position
D-transposition of the great arteries
II. Abnormalities of intracardiac blood flow
Left heart defects
Bicuspid aortic valve
Aortic valve stenosis
Coarctation of the aorta
Interrupted aortic arch, type A
Hypoplastic left heart, aortic atresia, and mitral atresia
Right heart defects
Secundum atrial septal defect
Bicuspid pulmonary valve
Pulmonary valve stenosis
Pulmonary valve atresia with intact ventricular septum
Perimembranous ventricular septal defect
III. Cell death abnormalities
Ebstein malformation of the tricuspid valve
Muscular ventricular septal defect
IV. Extracellular matrix abnormalities
Endocardial cushion defects
Ostium primum atrial septal defect
Atrioventricular canal type ventricular septal defect (inflow)
Complete atrioventricular canal defect
Dysplastic pulmonary or aortic valve
V. Abnormal targeted growth
Anomalous pulmonary venous connection
Partially anomalous pulmonary venous connection
Totally anomalous pulmonary venous connection
Cor triatriatum
VI. Abnormal situs and looping
Situs inversus totalis
Isolated
Immotile cilia syndrome, Kartagener syndrome
Heterotaxy
Asplenia syndrome, right isomerism, bilateral rightsidedness
Polysplenia syndrome, left isomerism, bilateral leftsidedness
Looping abnormalities
L-transposition of the great arteries
Ventricular inversion

and VI, abnormal situs and looping (including but not limited to heterotaxy).[7–9]

In the most simple situation (Fig. 5-4), one etiology acts through a single pathogenetic mechanism (A) to produce a single anatomic malformation. However, for many congenital cardiovascular malformations, multiple etiologies may act through a single mechanism (A) to produce a spectrum of anatomic abnormalities.[7] For example, chromosomal deletions involving the long arm of chromosome 22 and prenatal exposure to retinoic acid (multiple etiologies) may act through a single mechanism (disruption of neural crest cell migration) to cause a spectrum of conotruncal malformations, including truncus arteriosus, type B interrupted aortic arch, and tetralogy of Fallot. Although the specific defects within each group are heterogeneous, they share a common disordered mechanism.

Pathogenetic classification is currently being used in some epidemiologic and family studies. Evaluation of cases of congenital heart disease by mechanistic groups can help to clarify relationships among malformations, suggest underlying mechanisms, and elucidate familial patterns and recurrence risks for relatives. Boughman and colleagues[10] found that the risk for congenital heart disease was higher among siblings of individuals with blood flow defects, as compared to other categories of disordered pathogenetic mechanism.

Although Clark's classification system is attractive, some mechanistic groupings have proven more useful than others (e.g., conotruncal malformations, left-sided flow defects, and heterotaxy). Recent studies suggest that the mechanisms and pathways involved in the developmental pathogenesis of cardiovascular malformations are much

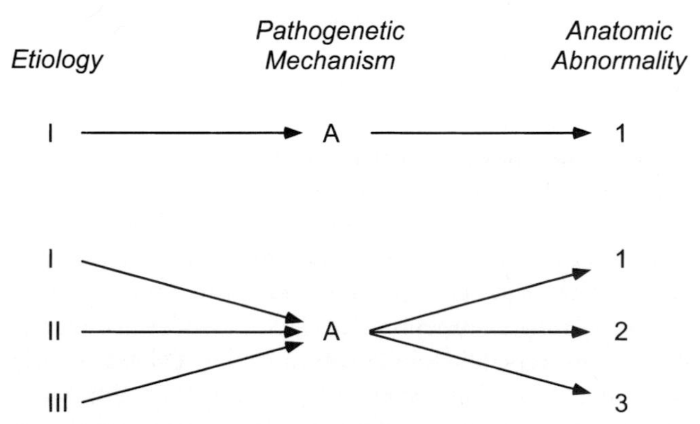

Figure 5–4 *Relationship of etiology, pathogenetic mechanism, and anatomic abnormality (see text).*
From Clark EB. Growth, morphogenesis, and function: the dynamics of cardiovascular development. In Moller JM, Neal WA (eds). Fetal, Neonatal, and Infant Heart Disease. New York: Appleton-Century-Crofts, 1989, pp 1–22, with permission.

more complex than had been predicted by the Clark model. For example, complex interactions between genes and environment and between multiple genes and proteins involved in multiple developmental pathways have been shown to be involved in conotruncal development and the determination of sidedness. Continuing genetic and developmental investigations will lead inevitably to a better understanding of the biologic basis of normal and abnormal morphogenesis. An overview of Clark's classification system is presented here, with the realization that ongoing research will lead to further refinements of the system.

Ectomesenchymal Tissue Migration Abnormalities (Neural Crest Migration Abnormalities/Chromosome 22q11 Deletion Syndrome)

Tissue from the neural crest and branchial arch mesenchyme contributes to the formation and septation of the outflow tract of the heart. Kirby and associates used the quail-chick chimera to show that specific regions of neural crest are major constituents of the conotruncal septation process.[11–13] Ectomesenchymal cells from neural crest are essential for expression of tissue derivatives of each branchial arch and pouch. In addition, neural crest cells course through arches 4, 6, and probably 3 to participate in septation of the conotruncus and aortic sac. Mechanical ablation of small amounts of preotic neural crest produces a spectrum of conotruncal malformations including truncus arteriosus and subarterial ventricular septal defect (Fig. 5-5).[12]

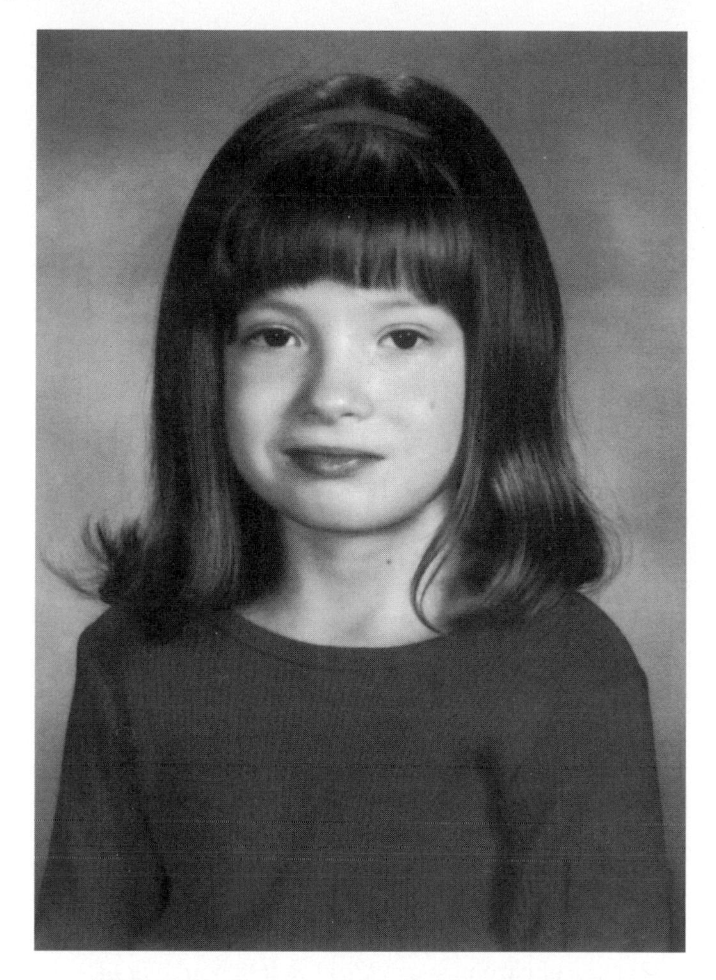

Figure 5–5 *Chromosome 22q11 deletion syndrome.*

Conotruncal malformations, particularly type B interruption of the aortic arch, truncus arteriosus, and tetralogy of Fallot, are overrepresented in patients with DiGeorge sequence, where they are seen in association with hypoplasia or aplasia of the thymus and parathyroid gland, which are derivatives of pharyngeal pouches III and IV. Tetralogy of Fallot is also one of the common cardiac defects in velocardiofacial syndrome, which is characterized by congenital heart defects, palatal abnormalities, learning disability, and a characteristic facies. Previous studies have shown deletions and microdeletions of chromosome 22, within region 22q11, in the majority of patients with DiGeorge sequence and velocardiofacial syndrome, and in some familial cases of congenital heart disease.[14–18] More recently, microdeletions of chromosomal region 22q11 have been identified in patients with nonsyndromic conotruncal cardiac defects[19–20] demonstrating a genetic contribution to the development of some isolated conotruncal malformations and altering our understanding of the risk of heritability of these defects in certain families. DiGeorge sequence, velocardiofacial syndrome, conotruncal anomaly face syndrome, CATCH 22 (an acronym for *c*ardiac defect, *a*bnormal facies, *t*hymic hypoplasia or aplasia and *T*-cell deficiency, *c*left palate, *h*ypoparathyroidism, and *h*ypocalcemia), and some isolated cardiovascular malformations are now included in the chromosome 22 deletion syndrome spectrum.

The first genetic model of the chromosome 22q11 deletion syndrome was a mouse mutant with an engineered deletion of most of the mouse genomic region homologous to the region deleted in human 22q11 deletion patients.[21] These mice, carrying a heterozygous deletion, have aortic arch defects and parathyroid, thymic, and neurobehavioral abnormalities reminiscent of those found in human patients. Additional targeted mutations of the mouse genome allowed investigators to attribute most of these phenotypic findings to haploinsufficiency of a single gene, *Tbx1*.[22–24] Extensive searches for mutations of the *Tbx1* gene in human patients, eventually led to the identification of five patients (three of whom were from the same family) carrying a *Tbx1* gene mutation.[25] Most of these patients had a typical chromosome 22q11 deletion phenotype including heart defects, but did not have learning disabilities. Hence, consistent with mouse genetic results, human *Tbx1* mutation (presumably leading to haploinsufficiency), is sufficient to cause most of the abnormalities observed in the chromosome 22q11 deletion syndrome. A thorough review of the role of *Tbx1* in outflow tract and aortic arch development is beyond the scope of this chapter. Interested readers are referred to a recent review by Baldini.[26]

The chromosome 22q11 deletion syndrome (Fig. 5-5) is common, with an estimated incidence of at least one in 4000.[27] Rarely, an abnormality is detected by standard karyotype. In most cases (approximately 80%), a microdeletion can be demonstrated by FISH.[14–17] In the remainder of cases, there presumably is a mutation or small deletion not detectable with currently available FISH probes. Deletions involving chromosome 10p also have been associated with the chromosome 22 deletion phenotype but are less common.[28] A broad spectrum of clinical manifestations is associated with interstitial chromosome 22q11 deletions, and phenotypic expression is highly variable.[29] Cardiovascular anomalies are present in 75% to 80% of patients with a chromosome 22q11 deletion. When a conotruncal malformation is detected either prenatally or postnatally (tetralogy of Fallot, truncus arteriosus, type B interrupted aortic arch) FISH cytogenetic analysis is recommended to detect a 22q11 deletion.

McElhinney and colleagues[30] have extensively studied the frequency of chromosome 22q11 deletion among patients with various types of cardiovascular defects. They found a chromosome 22q11 deletion in 20 (40%) of 50 patients with truncus arteriosus. Anatomic features that were significantly associated with a deletion included a right aortic arch and/or an abnormal aortic arch branching pattern. There was a trend toward the association of discontinuous pulmonary arteries with a chromosome 22q11 deletion. Interruption of the aortic arch and truncal valve morphology and function did not correlate significantly with the presence of a chromosome 22q11 deletion. In a separate study, they found the chromosome 22q11 deletion in 12 (10%) of 125 patients with conoventricular, posterior malalignment, or conoseptal hypoplasia ventricular septal defect.[31] Anatomic features that were significantly associated with a deletion included abnormal aortic arch sidedness, an abnormal aortic arch branching pattern, a cervical aortic arch, and discontinuous pulmonary arteries. There was no correlation between type of ventral-septal defect (VSD) and chromosome 22q11 deletion. Of 20 patients with an abnormal aortic arch and/or discontinuous pulmonary arteries, 45% had a deletion, compared with only 3% of those with a left aortic arch, normal aortic arch branching, and continuous branch pulmonary arteries. These investigators also found the chromosome 22q11 deletion in 16 (24%) of 66 patients with isolated anomalies of aortic arch laterality and branching, without associated intracardiac defects.[32] These arch anomalies include double aortic arch, right aortic arch with or without aberrant left subclavian artery, and left aortic arch with aberrant right subclavian artery.

While abnormalities of ectomesenchymal migration account for many conotruncal septal defects and branchial arch defects, the pathogenesis of dextro (D)–transposition of the great vessels is thought to involve failure of the conotruncal cushions to spiral.[33] Other human neural crest/branchial arch syndromes which have an overrepresentation of conotruncal malformations and which are associated with abnormalities of branchial arch derivatives include the facio-auriculo-vertebral spectrum (oculo-auriculo-vertebral dysplasia, hemifacial microsomia, Goldenhar syndrome), CHARGE association, thalidomide embryopathy, and retinoic acid embryopathy.

Defects Associated with Abnormalities of Intracardiac Blood Flow

Change in volume distribution of intracardiac blood flow may be a mechanism in the pathogenesis of right and left heart defects. Experimental manipulation of intracardiac blood flow affects cardiac morphogenesis. Reduction in fetal mitral valve inflow produces a spectrum of left ventricular volume ranging from mild left ventricular hypoplasia to hypoplastic left heart syndrome with aortic and mitral atresia.[34] Any event which results in decreased aortic blood flow and increased pulmonary artery and ductal blood flow may lead to one of the defects in the spectrum of left-sided flow defects. For example, in Turner syndrome, where there is deletion of part or all of one of the X chromosome in girls, there is an overrepresentation of left-sided flow defects such as bicommissural aortic valve, coarctation of the aorta, and hypoplastic left heart syndrome,[35] but the link between deletion of the X chromosome and altered blood flow has not been elucidated. The indirect sign of discrepant ventricular size on fetal sonogram (right ventricle larger than left ventricle) can identify fetuses at risk for postnatal development of coarctation of the aorta.[36] It appears likely that blood flow in the developing heart is controlled, at least in part, by genetic factors. During mouse heart development, dHAND and eHAND, which are related basic helix-loop-helix (bHLH) transcription factors, are expressed in a complementary fashion and are restricted to segments of the heart tube fated to form the right and left ventricles, respectively. These factors represent the earliest cardiac chamber-specific transcription factors yet identified.[37]

Extracellular Matrix Abnormalities

The endocardial cushions (atrioventricular and conotruncal) consist primarily of glycosaminoglycans separating the endocardium and the myocardium, and constitute the largest proportion of extracellular matrix in the embryo. Fusion of opposing cushions results in the formation of the tricuspid and mitral orifices at the atrioventricular level, and the pulmonary and aortic orifices in the outflow tract. A thorough discussion of endocardial cushion morphogenesis is beyond the scope of this chapter. A recent excellent review details the advances in the developmental biology of atrioventricular septation and discusses the complex connection between extracellular matrix and growth factor receptor signaling during endocardial cushion morphogenesis[38]:

> *It is becoming clear that converging pathways coordinate early heart valve development and remodeling into functional valve leaflets. The integration of these pathways begins with macro and molecular interactions outside the cell in the extracellular matrix separating the myocardial and endocardial tissue components of the rudimentary heart. Such interactions regulate events at the cell surface through receptors, proteases, and other membrane molecules, which in turn transduce signals into the cell. These signals trigger intracellular cascades that transduce cellular responses through both transcription factor and cofactor activation mediating gene induction or suppression. Chamber septation and valve formation occur from these coordinated molecular events within the endocardial cushions to sustain unidirectional blood flow and embryo viability.*

Clark classified atrioventricular canal defects as defects of extracellular matrix. However, given the complexity of cushion morphogenesis, it can be assumed that defects in many different classes of molecules could contribute to the pathogenesis of atrioventricular canal defects. Our discussion here will be limited to a few genes. The high frequency of atrioventricular canal defects in Down (trisomy 21) syndrome is a clue to the genetic mechanism(s) involved in cushion morphogenesis. Increased adhesion of trisomy 21 cells is the basis of a long-standing model for abnormal atrioventricular canal development. Fetal trisomy 21 fibroblasts explanted from endocardial-cushion-derived structures appear more adhesive *in vitro* than those explanted from normal control fetuses. If the fusion of the atrioventricular cushions is time and location dependent, and the migration of cells in the trisomic embryo is delayed, then there is a greater chance of the process not occurring.[39,40] Type VI collagen may have a role in the pathogenesis of atrioventricular canal defects in trisomy 21 syndrome. The *Col6A1,Col6A2* gene cluster, which encode the alpha-1 and alpha-2 chains for type VI collagen, respectively, fall within the congenital heart defect critical region on chromosome 21. Differences in adhesion to type VI collagen between cultured skin fibroblasts isolated from people with and without trisomy 21 suggest a potential mechanism for developmental defects.[41]

Several families have been reported to have autosomal-dominant atrioventricular canal (AVC) defects with incomplete penetrance,[42] demonstrating that AVC defects can be inherited as a single gene defect. There are two established genetic loci for isolated AVC defects, also known as atrioventricular septal defects (AVSDs), designated AVSD1 and AVSD2, which map to chromosomes 1p31-p21 and 3p25, respectively. The CRELD family consists of two matricellular proteins thought to be involved in cell adhesion processes. Identification and characterization of the *CRELD1* gene on chromosome 3p25 recently led to the establishment of *CRELD1* as the first known genetic risk factor for isolated AVC defects.[43] In a study of 52 people with non–trisomy 21–related AVC defects, approximately 6% of the subjects had missense mutations in the coding region of *CRELD1*.[44] The presence of unaffected family members carrying a *CRELD1* mutation showed that *CRELD1* mutations are neither necessary nor sufficient to cause AVSD, indicating that mutation of *CRELD1* increases susceptibility for AVC defects rather than being a monogenic cause. Characterization of *CRELD1* as a genetic risk factor is consistent with sporadic occurrence of AVC defects in the study population. *CRELD1* has now been assigned to the *AVSD2* locus.

Bone morphogenic protein-4 (Bmp4) is expressed in the endocardial cushions and adjacent tissues of the embryonic mouse heart. Jiao and colleagues[45] developed a transgenic mouse strain using cardiac-specific conditional gene inactivation of a hypomorphic *Bmp4* allele. Deficiency of Bmp4 expression in cardiomyocytes resulted in atrioventricular canal defects, demonstrating that Bmp4 provides a myocardial-derived signal essential for septation. *Bmp4*-deficient mice have a spectrum of atrioventricular canal defects that correlate with the level of *Bmp4* expression. The severity of defect correlated with the level of *Bmp4* expression-the lower the level of Bmp4, the more severe the heart defect.

GATA4 is a transcription factor known to be essential for cardiac development. Garg and colleagues[46] identified mutations in the *GATA4* gene as the monogenic cause of cardiac septal defects in two families with autosomal dominant ostium secundum atrial septal defects. Clinical variability in some affected family members suggests that *GATA4* may be involved in the pathogenesis of other types of congenital heart defects (AVSD, VSD, thickening of the pulmonary valve, or insufficiency of cardiac valves).

CELL DEATH ABNORMALITIES

Controlled cell death is an important molding process in the embryonic heart.[47–48] Ebstein malformation and muscular ventricular septal defect have been postulated to arise from abnormalities in cell death. The tricuspid valve cusps are almost exclusively derived from the interior of the embryonic right ventricular myocardium by a process of undermining of the right ventricular wall.[49] Abnormalities of this process of reabsorption of ventricular myocardium may lead to the Ebstein malformation with displacement of the functional tricuspid valve annulus into the right ventricle. The muscular ventricular septum forms early in development as trabeculations at the apex of the heart coalesce and the margins of the cardiac tube grow toward the endocardial cushions and atrioventricular orifice.[50] Muscular ventricular septal defects may arise from abnormal trabecular organization or secondarily from foci of cellular death that occur during active cardiac remodeling.[7]

Abnormal Targeted Growth

Anomalous pulmonary venous connections are believed to arise from abnormalities in targeted growth. The pulmonary veins form as an outpouching of endothelial-lined mesenchymal tissue from the lung buds, and coalesce into the common pulmonary vein, which bridges across the splanchnic space and fuses with the posterior wall of the primitive left atrium at 5 weeks' gestation.[51] By further remodeling, the common pulmonary vein is gradually absorbed into the posterior wall of the left atrium such that the four pulmonary veins enter the heart individually by eight weeks' gestation. The mechanism is undefined but likely involves an attraction between the pulmonary veins and the left atrium. In the chick embryo, following experimental excision and reimplantation of the lung bud in an inverted orientation, venous connection from lung bud to the left atrium is established in 80% of cases.[52] If connection of the common pulmonary vein to the left atrium does not occur, primitive venous drainage to systemic veins persists (totally anomalous pulmonary venous connection). If absorption of the common pulmonary vein into the left atrium is incomplete, a membrane may persist between the pulmonary veins and the left atrium (cor triatriatum). Bleyl and colleagues[53] have mapped a gene for familial totally anomalous pulmonary venous connection to a locus at chromosome 4q12 in large Utah kindreds, and they have preliminary evidence implicating the gene encoding platelet-derived growth factor receptor alpha (PDGFRA), which is localized in this region.[54]

Situs and Looping Abnormalities

One of the earliest events in cardiac morphogenesis is the formation of the normal d (dextral)-cardiac loop from the previously symmetric, midline cardiac tube. Abnormalities at this stage of cardiac development frequently lead to complex congenital heart disease and associated visceral malformations. In humans, situs abnormalities (heterotaxy syndrome) have been observed in pedigrees consistent with autosomal dominant, autosomal recessive, and X-linked recessive inheritance, suggesting that multiple genes regulate cardiac looping and determine cardiac and visceral situs. Heterotaxy may also be caused by teratogenic exposures, especially maternal diabetes. Isolated congenital heart defects resulting from isomerisms and disturbed looping may be caused by mutations in genes that control early left–right patterning and the earliest steps in cardiogenesis. Belmont and colleagues recently reviewed the complex molecular genetics of heterotaxy syndromes. Genes currently implicated in human heterotaxy include *ZIC3*, *LEFTYA*, *CRYPTIC*, and *ACVR2B*. Roles for *NKX2.5* and *CRELDA* are also suggested by recent case reports.[55]

Genes expressed in dorsal midline cells, specifically notochord cells or adjacent cells induced by the notochord (such as neural tube floorplate), are essential for cardiac left–right development. Several mammalian genes, including transcription factors, dyneins, and cell-cell signaling factors, have been implicated in left–right development either by mutations or by asymmetric expression patterns.[56] Mutations in the gene *ZIC3*, which maps to human chromosome Xq24-27.1, have been identified in humans with X-linked familial situs ambiguous.[57–58] ZIC3 is a member of the ZIC (zinc finger protein of the cerebellum) transcription factor family. In mice and Xenopus, *ZIC3* is expressed in the primitive streak and developing neural tissues, suggesting that it is part of the midline pathway for left–right development. In addition, humans with *ZIC3* mutations have midline defects in addition to cardiac defects.[56–58]

Experiments in the *iv/iv* mouse (*inversus viscerum*) are consistent with a control gene, the presence of which defines the normal relationship of situs solitus. In the absence of the control gene (recessive mutation), there is a random chance of situs inversus or situs solitus.[59] Cardiac abnormalities are found in 40% of developing *iv vivo* and *iv vitro* embryos, and the spectrum of abnormalities is strikingly similar to that seen in humans with heterotaxy syndrome.[60] The IV gene, which has been mapped to the subtelomeric region of mouse chromosome 12, which is syntenic (homologous) with distal human chromosome 14,[61] encodes a novel axonemal dynein, called a left–right dynein, that is expressed in the node and midline. Recent research suggests that dynein, a microtubule-based motor, is involved in the determination of left–right asymmetry and provides insight into the early molecular mechanisms of this process.[62]

Humans with immotile cilia syndrome (Kartagener syndrome, primary ciliary dyskinesia), an autosomal recessive disorder, have ciliary dynein defects and laterality defects, as well as respiratory problems and male infertility.[63] Although situs inversus totalis can be seen in immotile cilia syndrome, situs inversus totalis is generally considered separate from the heterotaxy syndromes. Yet the coexistence of ciliary abnormalities and polysplenia has been reported.[64,65] The precise role of ciliary abnormalities in situs determination in humans has not been fully delineated.

GENETIC COUNSELING FOR CARDIOVASCULAR MALFORMATIONS

When possible, identification of a specific diagnosis or etiology improves accuracy in the prediction of prognosis and the estimation of recurrence risk. The requirements for optimal genetic counseling for cardiovascular malformations include (a) a thorough understanding of the anatomy, management, and outcome of the particular defect, (b) identification of other affected family members and careful pedigree analysis for prediction of familial risks, (c) identification of associated malformations or syndromes, and (d) options for prenatal diagnosis. Ideally, genetic counseling should be provided both by a clinical geneticist or dysmorphologist knowledgeable about cardiac defects and outcome and by a pediatric cardiologist with a keen awareness and interest in genetic issues.[66]

The etiology of congenital heart disease is currently the focus of intense research. Based on the results of this research, our concepts of the causes of congenital heart disease have evolved over the years.[67–69] In the past, genetic counseling for isolated congenital cardiovascular malformations (i.e., without extracardiac malformations or syndromic diagnosis) was transmitted as generalized advice, with the use of an overall recurrence risk for first-degree relatives of 2% to 5%. These malformations were said to be *multifactorial*, which refers to defects caused by the combined effects of one or more alleles at a number of loci interacting with stochastic and/or environmental factors. However, the familial (apparent mendelian or single gene) occurrence of virtually all forms of congenital heart disease has been noted. In the past, the study of familial congenital heart disease in humans has been hindered by a number of factors including reduced penetrance, variable expressivity, genetic heterogeneity, small family size, and decreased survival and reproductive capability especially in those individuals with complex defects. Recent epidemiologic and familial studies suggest that specific *genetic* influences may be more important than previously recognized, and that certain malformations are more likely to have a stronger genetic component.[10,18–20,56–58,66–77]

Clinical and echocardiographic studies of first-degree relatives of patients with complete common atrioventricular canal have detected previously unsuspected congenital heart defects that were clinically less significant than the proband's congenital heart defect but were part of the same mechanistic spectrum (e.g., atrioventricular type of septal defects and left-axis deviation).[78] Brenner and colleagues performed echocardiograms on relatives of 11 infants with HLHS, and observed 5 of 41 first-degree relatives with unrecognized bicommissural aortic valve.[79] In a study designed to define the incidence of cardiac anomalies in first-degree relatives of apparently nonsyndromic children with congenital aortic valve stenosis (AVS), coarctation of the aorta (CoA), and hypoplastic left heart syndrome (HLHS), Lewin and colleagues[80] found bicommissural aortic valve (BAV) in 4.68% of first-degree relatives. Additional relatives had anomalies of the aorta, aortic valve, left ventricle, or mitral valve. Overall, anomalies were found in 20.2% (21 of 104) of mothers, 14.7% (14 of 95) of fathers, 21.6% (8 of 37) of brothers, and 4.8% (2 of 42) of sisters. Echocardiographic anomalies were noted in 10 (35.7%) of 28 AVS families, 22 (42.3%) of 52 CoA families, and 11 (29.1%) of 32 families of HLHS probands, for a total of 33 (29.5%) of 113 families. They concluded that the parents and siblings of affected patients with left-sided obstructive defects should be screened by echocardiography, as the presence of asymptomatic BAV may carry a significant long-term health risk.

The techniques of molecular genetics are becoming increasingly useful for the study of familial congenital heart disease. An increasing number of specific genes are now implicated in the pathogenesis of congenital cardiovascular malformations in humans. These genes are summarized in Table 5-2 and discussed in the following sections. Although the general principles of multifactorial inheritance may still apply in many situations, the recurrence risk may be underestimated in other situations. Therefore, risk projections should be based on the specific congenital heart defect involved as well as the genetic and teratogenic history in an individual family or pregnancy. The recurrence risks for siblings (Table 5-3) and offspring (Table 5-4) are for isolated, nonsyndromic malformations and are based on combined data published during two decades from European and North American populations.[75]

Recent research, accelerated through the Human Genome Project has resulted in the rapid identification of disease genes causing congenital heart defects. Gelb[80] recently reviewed genes relevant for atrial (*GATA4*, *TBX5*,

TABLE 5–2. Known Cardiovascular Gene Defects in Humans

Structural Defects
Thoracic aortic aneurysms and aortic dissection:
11q23.3-q24, 5q13-q14, 3p24.2-p25, genes unknown
Marfan syndrome and related connective tissue disorders:
fibrillin gene mutations, chromosome 15q15.21 (*FBN1*), 5q23-q31 (*FBN2*)
Congenital contractural arachnodactyly, severe form (ventral-septal defect [VSD], atrial-septal defect [ASD], IAA):
Fibrillin 2 gene mutations (*FBN2*), chromosome 5q23-q31
Familial supravalvar aortic stenosis:
elastin gene point mutations (*ELN*), chromosome 7q11.23
Williams syndrome (contiguous gene deletion syndrome):
1- to 2-Mb deletion including elastin (*ELN*) and other genes, chromosome 7q11.23
Alagille syndrome, peripheral pulmonary stenosis, tetralogy of Fallot:
JAG1, Jagged1, a ligand for Notch1 receptor, chromosome 20p12
Rendu-Osler-Weber (hereditary hemorrhagic telangiectasia) syndrome, telangiectasia and pulmonary arteriovenous fistulas:
Endoglin, endothelial cell transforming growth factor-beta binding protein, chromosome 9q33-4
Ehlers-Danlos syndrome, type IV, aortic dilation and aneurysms:
COL3A1 gene, Type III collagen, chromosome 2q31-2
Holt-Oram syndrome/atrial septal defects (heterogeneous):
Chromosome 12q24.1, *TBX5*, a transcription factor
Noonan syndrome (heterogeneous):
Chromosome 12q24.1, *PTPN11*, a tyrosine phosphatase
LEOPARD syndrome (heterogeneous):
Chromosome 12q24.1, *PTPN11*, a tyrosine phosphatase (allelic with Noonan syndrome)
Ellis-van Creveld syndrome:
Chromosome 4p16, *EVC* and *EVC2*
Cornelia de Lange syndrome(heterogeneous):
Chromosome 5p13.1, *NIPBL*, nped-B-like protein
CHARGE syndrome (heterogeneous): chromosome 8q12, *CHD7*
Kabuki syndrome (heterogeneous):
Chromosome 8p22-p23.1 duplication
Familial atrial septal defects (heterogeneous):
CSX gene (*NKX2.5*), transcription factor, chromosome 5q34-35
Chromosome 8p23.1-p22 (*GATA4*), transcription factor
Chromosome 5p, gene unknown
Familial totally anomalous pulmonary venous connection:
Chromosome 4p13-q12, gene unknown, possibly *PDGFRA*
Atrioventricular canal defects:
Chromosome 21q22.2-21q22.3, genes unknown (trisomy 21)
Chromosome 1p31-p21, (*AVSD1*), gene unknown
Chromosome 3p25, (*CRELD1*, *AVSD2*)
Chromosome 8p23.1-p22 (*GATA4*)
Conotruncal defects/CATCH 22 syndrome:
Deletion on chromosome 22q11,*TBX1* and other genes
Deletion on chromosome 10p13, genes unknown
Heterotaxy
ZIC3, transcription factor, chromosome Xq24-27.1
LEFTYA, TGF-beta family of cell-signaling molecules, chromosome 1q42
CRYPTIC, *CFC1*, intercellular signaling molecule, chromosome 2q21.1
ACVR2B, activin A receptor, type IIB, chromosome 3p22
Cardiomyopathies and Arrhythmias
Hypertrophic cardiomyopathy
Cardiac troponin T2, *TNNT2*, on chromosome 1q32
Cardiac troponin T, *TNNI3*, 19q13.4
Beta-myosin heavy chain, *MYH7*, chromosome 14q12
Alpha-tropomyosin, *TPM1*, chromosome 15q22.1
Cardiac myosin binding protein C, *MYBPC3*, chromosome 11p11.2
Essential myosin light chain 3, *MYL3*, chromosome 3p
Regulatory myosin light chain 2, *MYL2*, chromosome 12q23-24.3
Alpha-actin cardiac, *ACTC*, chromosome 15q14
Dilated cardiomyopathy
Dystrophin (XLDC), *DMD*, Xp21; Duchenne and Becker muscular dystrophy and familial X-linked cardiomyopathy
Myotonic dystrophy gene, *DMPK*, a protein kinase, chromosome 19q13.2-13.3
Autosomal dominant gene loci on chromosomes 9q13q22 (*FDC1*), 1q31-q32 (*FDC2*), 10q21-q23 (*FDC3*)
Tafazzin, *TAZ*, Xq28, also neutropenia and short stature
Conduction defects with late development of dilated cardiomyopathy:
Autosomal recessive gene loci on 1q-p1 (*CDDC*) and 3p22-p25 (*CDDC2*)
Isolated dilated cardiomyopathy:
Lamin A/C, *LMNA*, 1q21.1
Myosin binding protein C, Cardiac Type, *MYBPC3*, 11p11.2
Cardiac beta myosin heavy chain, *MYH7*, 14q11
Cardiac troponin T, *TNNI2*, 1q32
Tropomyosin 1, alpha chain, *TPM1*, 15q22.1
Myocardial mitochondrial DNA deletions or mutations
Arrhythmogenic right ventricular dysplasia (ARVD)
Gene loci at chromosomes 14q23-q24, 1q42-q43, 14q12-q22
Long QT syndrome
LQT1, *KCNQ1*, potassium channel gene, chromosome 11p15.5
LQT2, *KCNH2*, potassium channel gene, chromosome 7q35-36
LQT3, *SCN5A*, cardiac sodium channel gene, chromosome 3 p21-24
LQT4, *ANK2*, Ankyrin 2, 4q25-q27
LQT5, *KCNE1*, potassium channel gene, chromosome 21q22.2
LQT6, *KCNE2*, potassium channel gene, chromosome 21q22.1
LQT7, *KCNJ2*, potassium channel gene, chromosome 17q23.1-q24.2
Other conduction defects
Familial heart block, chromosome 19q13.3
Catecholaminergic polymorphic ventricular tachycardia,
AD form: Cardiac ryanodine receptor channel, *RYR2*, 1q42.1-q43
AR form: Calsequestrin, *CASQ2*, 1p13.3-p11
Wolff-Parkinson-White syndrome, linkage of 3 kindreds to 7q3
Mitochondrial cardiomyopathy, associated with skeletal and neuromuscular defects
Missense mutations
Point mutations
Deletion mutations

Table 5–3. Recurrence Risks for Congenital Heart Defects in Siblings

	Percent at Risk	
Defect	One Sibling Affected	Two Siblings Affected
Ventricular septal defect	3	10
Patent ductus arteriosus	3	10
Atrial septal defect	2.5	8
Tetralogy of Fallot	2.5	8
Pulmonary stenosis	2	6
Coarctation of aorta	2	6
Aortic stenosis	2	6
Transposition	1.5	5
Endocardial cushion defects	3	10
Fibroelastosis	4	12
Hypoplastic left heart	2	6
Tricuspid atresia	1	3
Ebstein anomaly	1	3
Truncus arteriosus	1	3
Pulmonary atresia	1	3

From Nora JJ, Nora AH. Update on counseling the family with a first-degree relative with a congenital heart defect. Am J Med Genet 29:137, 1988. Reprinted with permission of John Wiley & Sons, Inc.

NKX2-5) and atrioventricular septal defects (*CRELD1*), patent ductus arteriosus (*TFAP2B*), bicuspid aortic valve and coarctation of the aorta (*KCNJ2*), valvar pulmonary stenosis (*PTPN11*), and branch pulmonary artery stenosis (*JAG1*). These studies provide insights into the molecular genetic causes of congenital heart defects, and suggest that DNA testing may become standard for many forms of congenital heart defects, improving clinicians' ability to anticipate complications for their patients and predict recurrence risk for families of children with congenital heart defects.

Table 5–4. Recurrence Risks for Congenital Heart Defects in Offspring Given One Affected Parent

	Percent at Risk	
Defect	Mother Affected	Father Affected
Aortic stenosis	13–18	3
Atrial septal defect	4–4.5	1.5
Atrioventricular canal	14	1
Coarctation of aorta	4	2
Patent ductus arteriosus	3.5–4	2.5
Pulmonary stenosis	4–6.5	2
Tetralogy of Fallot	2.5	1.5
Ventricular septal defect	6–10	2

From Nora JJ, Nora AH. Update on counseling the family with a first-degree relative with a congenital heart defect. Am J Med Genet 29:137, 1988. Reprinted with permission of John Wiley & Sons, Inc.

Heterozygous mutations in the *NKX2.5* gene, which encodes a DNA transcription factor, were among the first evidence of a genetic cause for congenital heart defects and were initially found in pedigrees with autosomal dominant transmission of cardiac septal defects and atrioventricular conduction abnormalities. *NKX2.5* mutations have subsequently been identified in individuals with ASD, VSD, Ebstein malformation, tetralogy of Fallot, truncus arteriosus, double-outlet right ventricle, L-transposition of the great arteries, interrupted aortic arch, subvalvar aortic stenosis, hypoplastic left heart syndrome, and coarctation of the aorta.[69,70] *NKX2.5* mutations are a rare cause of secundum ASD. Elliot and colleagues[71] found only one *NKX2.5* mutation among 102 individuals with ASD.

GATA4 encodes a transcription factor that was known to play a critical role in cardiogenesis. Garg and colleagues[46] studied a large kindred inheriting a fully penetrant autosomal dominant disorder in which all affected individuals had secundum atrial septal defects. Several also had additional CHDs, including ventricular septal defects, atrioventricular canal defects, and pulmonary valve stenosis. They subsequently identified a second family inheriting secundum atrial septal defects, with a 1–base-pair (bp) deletion in *GATA4*, which results in premature truncation of the protein. These investigators also showed that three genes, *GATA4*, *TBX5*, and *NKX2-5*, which have been associated with secundum atrial septal defects, are now known to produce proteins that form complexes with one another. See further discussion of *CRELD1* under Extracellular Matrix Abnormalities above, and *TBX5*, *PTPN11*, and *JAG1*, in the sections on Holt Oram, Noonan, and Alagille syndromes.

A number of general conclusions can be made based on this exciting research: (a) Whereas in the past it was believed that most cardiovascular malformations were due to multifactorial influences, it is now believed that human congenital heart disease is frequently due to single gene defects and that even sporadic defects may arise from a single gene abnormality; (b) a common genetic defect or pathogenetic mechanism may cause several apparently different forms of congenital cardiovascular malformations. For example, chromosome 22q deletions cause a variety of conotruncal malformations and aortic arch anomalies; (c) the same cardiac malformation can be caused by mutant genes at different loci, indicating that several different, but single, gene defects may cause the same apparent phenotype; (d) the elucidation of the genetic basis of congenital heart disease provides clues to normal cardiovascular developmental biology. As causative or candidate genes are isolated, ablation studies in mice will be essential to define interactions with other genes and to understand the mechanism by which congenital heart disease becomes manifest; (e) interactions of clinical investigators (cardiologists, geneticists, and cardiothoracic surgeons) with basic scientists should allow more rapid progress in defining the genetic basis of congenital cardiovascular malformations. Such research will improve our ability to provide gene-specific treatment for cardiovascular disease with the hope of improved overall prognosis.[67–69]

Known or Presumed Cardiovascular Gene Defects in Humans

The genes implicated in the pathogenesis of cardiovascular malformations *in humans* are summarized in Table 5-2. Such a list is constantly evolving and never complete. Some of the genes listed are relatively well characterized, whereas others have been mapped to a chromosomal location by familial linkage studies but the precise genetic defect remains unknown. Additional studies in animal models, particularly in the mouse, zebrafish, and Xenopus, have added to our understanding of cardiovascular development, but a comprehensive discussion of this research is beyond the scope of this chapter.

Malformation Syndromes Versus Nonsyndromic Defects: A number of the genetic defects listed in Table 5-2 cause malformation syndromes with cardiovascular involvement (e.g., fibrillin mutations cause Marfan syndrome), whereas others cause isolated familial cardiovascular defects (e.g., elastin mutations cause familial supravalvar aortic stenosis). Still others cause malformation syndromes in some individuals and nonsyndromic cardiovascular malformations in other individuals (e.g., chromosome 22q11 deletions).

Familial Cardiomyopathy and Arrhythmias: Genetic mutations in several genes encoding sarcomeric proteins have been associated with hypertrophic cardiomyopathy.[81–83] Mutations in the gene encoding dystrophin not only cause Duchenne and Becker muscular dystrophy, but also cause familial X-linked dilated cardiomyopathy.[84] Other genes for familial cardiomyopathy and familial arrhythmias have been mapped to chromosomal positions but the genes are still unknown.[81–86] Abnormalities in genes encoding cardiac potassium and sodium channels have been linked to long QT syndrome (see Chapter 61).[68,82,86]

Allelic and Nonallelic Heterogeneity: Genetic heterogeneity has been documented or is suspected for a number of conditions. In other words, there can be different causes for the same disease or phenotype. Genetic heterogeneity can be allelic (different mutations at the same gene locus) or nonallelic (mutations at different gene loci causing similar phenotypes), and can explain, at least in part, the variability in clinical phenotype (pattern and severity of expression). For example, many different mutations of the fibrillin gene have been identified in Marfan syndrome and related connective tissue disorders (allelic heterogeneity).[87] In contrast, mutations for several different genes encoding myocardial structural proteins (e.g., β-myosin heavy chain, α-tropomyosin, cardiac troponin T) are associated with hypertrophic cardiomyopathy (nonallelic heterogeneity).[81–83] Similarly, mutations for several different genes encoding cardiac ion channels are associated with long QT syndrome.[82,86] For hypertrophic cardiomyopathy and long QT syndrome, the severity of clinical manifestations and risk for complications such as sudden death depend on the nature of the genetic mutation. Some mutations are associated with mild disease, whereas others are associated with a severe clinical phenotype. Genetic testing is now available for some families with hypertrophic cardiomyopathy and long QT syndrome, and gene-specific therapies are available for some families with long QT syndrome.[81,86]

Mitochondrial Disorders: Cardiomyopathy is a common clinical feature of several well-known mitochondrial syndromes (MELAS [mitochondrial myopathy, encephalopathy, lacticacidosis, stroke] syndrome, MERRF [myoclonic epilepsy and ragged-red fibers] syndrome, NADH-coenzyme Q reductase deficiency, Kearns-Sayre syndrome, MIMyCA [maternally inherited myopathy and cardiomyopathy]). Mitochondrial cardiomyopathy, which is usually accompanied by skeletal and neuromuscular abnormalities, has been attributed to missense mutations, point mutations, and deletion mutations. In addition, isolated dilated cardiomyopathy has been reported associated with myocardial mitochondrial DNA deletions or mutations.[81,84]

MULTIPLE MALFORMATION SYNDROMES WITH CARDIOVASCULAR INVOLVEMENT

Congenital heart defects are common in malformation syndromes. Approximately 70% of spontaneous abortuses and stillborn fetuses with a congenital heart defect and 25% of children with a congenital heart defect have associated extracardiac malformations, often as part of a multiple malformation syndrome. Such syndromes are caused by chromosomal aberrations, teratogens, genetic abnormalities, and unknown causes. For multiple malformation syndromes, the prognosis and recurrence risk for congenital heart disease depend largely on the underlying syndrome. Detection of a congenital heart defect should prompt a search for associated extracardiac malformations and identification of a syndrome. Similarly, individuals with malformation syndromes should be evaluated for the presence of a cardiovascular defect. This discussion will be limited to the more common multiple malformation syndromes and those less common ones in which congenital heart defects are either frequent or distinctive.

Patterns of Syndromic Congenital Cardiovascular Malformations

Since there is a very large number of malformation syndromes with cardiovascular involvement, it is helpful to discuss these syndromes by the patterns of cardiovascular defects associated with them.

Nonspecific Increased Risk: For many malformation syndromes, there is a nonspecific increased risk for congenital cardiovascular malformations (i.e., the overall risk for cardiac defects is higher than the general population risk, but the distribution of types of defects is similar to the general population). In these syndromes, defects that are common are those that are also common in the general population, such as atrial septal defect, ventricular septal defect, and patent ductus arteriosus.

Increased Risk for Specific Defect(s): For some syndromes, there is an increased risk for a specific congenital heart defect. For example, in Noonan syndrome, valvar pulmonary stenosis due to a dysplastic pulmonary valve is common, whereas aortic stenosis is very rare. Hypertrophic cardiomyopathy is seen in approximately 20% to 30% of individuals with Noonan syndrome. In such syndromes, the nature of the cardiovascular malformation can support or contradict the proposed syndrome diagnosis.

Increased Risk for a Specific Family or Spectrum of Defects: For some syndromes, there is an increased risk for a pathogenetic family or spectrum of related defects. For example, in Turner syndrome, the entire spectrum of left heart obstructive/hypoplastic lesions is observed. Although coarctation is most common, the spectrum of defects associated with Turner syndrome ranges from a bicommissural aortic valve without stenosis to hypoplastic left heart syndrome. Similarly, the full spectrum of atrioventricular canal defects is observed in individuals with trisomy 21 syndrome, and conotruncal and aortic arch malformations are overrepresented in the chromosome 22 deletion syndrome.

Defect Pathognomonic for a Specific Syndrome: Occasionally, a specific cardiovascular malformation is virtually pathognomonic for the syndrome. For example, supravalvar aortic stenosis (SVAS) and the associated elastin arteriopathy are relatively uncommon in the general population but are very common in Williams syndrome. When SVAS is diagnosed in a child with dysmorphic features, growth delay, and/or developmental delay, the diagnosis is likely to be Williams syndrome. Fluorescent in situ hybridization (FISH) can differentiate Williams syndrome from familial SVAS (see discussion on Williams syndrome and familial SVAS).

Defect Required for Diagnosis of Syndrome: Finally, in some syndromes, the cardiovascular malformation is required for diagnosis of the syndrome. In other words, the diagnostic criteria for the syndrome include the presence of a cardiovascular abnormality. For example, aortic root dilation or lens dislocation is required to make a diagnosis of Marfan syndrome. Similarly, the diagnosis of Holt-Oram syndrome, an autosomal dominant syndrome of upper limb and cardiac malformations, requires a cardiac defect in at least one member of an affected family.

CHROMOSOMAL SYNDROMES

Given the large number of chromosomal syndromes, this review will be limited to the most common disorders. The incidence of chromosomal abnormalities is about one in 200 at birth and much higher among spontaneous abortions and stillborn fetuses. In a series of spontaneous abortuses and stillborn fetuses with congenital heart defects, a chromosomal abnormality was confirmed in 19% and suspected in up to 36%.[87] Recent studies using high-resolution chromosomal analysis have shown that as many as 13% of all infants with congenital cardiovascular malformations have chromosomal abnormalities.[88] The vast majority of these infants have trisomy 21 syndrome (Down syndrome), which accounts for about 10% of all infants with congenital cardiovascular malformations.

Trisomy 21 Syndrome (Down Syndrome)

Although the classic description of Down syndrome (Fig. 5-6) was published in 1866, the cytogenetic confirmation of its trisomic etiology was not reported until 1959.[89–91] Trisomy 21 syndrome is the most frequent chromosomal aberration affecting live born infants, with an incidence of 1 in 660 live births: 94% are due to nondisjunction, which results in three full copies of chromosome 21 in each cell, 3% are due to parental translocation, and 3% are due to mosaicism.

The phenotype of trisomy 21 syndrome is well recognized. Cardiovascular malformations are found in 40% to 50% of individuals with Down syndrome. There is a distinctive spectrum of cardiac defects with an overrepresentation of endocardial cushion defects (atrioventricular canal defects) compared to the general population. The most common abnormalities (in decreasing order of frequency) include common atrioventricular canal, ventricular septal defect, tetralogy of Fallot, and patent ductus arteriosus. Left-sided obstructive defects such as coarctation and valvar aortic stenosis are rare. Transposition of the great

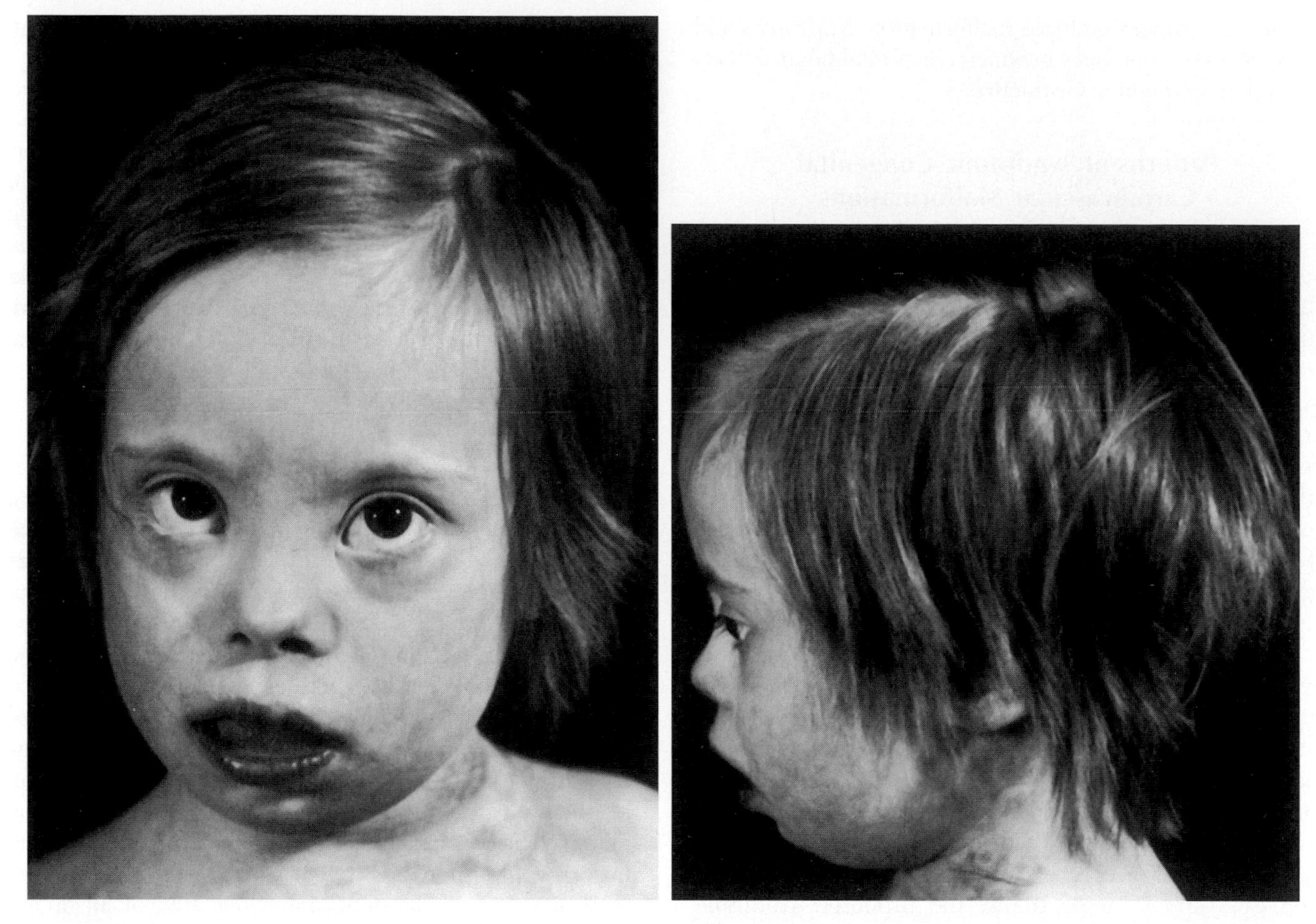

Figure 5–6 *Trisomy 21 (Down) syndrome. Note the flat, expressionless face, small nose, low nasal bridge, bilateral epicanthal folds, and protrusion of the tongue.*
From Fyler DC (ed). Nadas' Pediatric Cardiology. Philadelphia: Hanley & Belfus, 1992.

arteries has not been reported in Down syndrome or any other autosomal trisomy.

Prenatally, trisomy 21 is most often identified when there is advanced maternal age or when maternal serum factors or fetal sonographic findings indicate an increased risk. Prenatal detection of a common atrioventricular canal defect should raise suspicion for Down syndrome, particularly when seen with other sonographic findings suggestive of the syndrome, such as increased nuchal thickness and echogenic foci. Postnatally, the clinical phenotype is so distinctive that cytogenetic analysis is performed primarily to identify cases due to translocation or mosaicism. The risk of recurrence for Down syndrome is 1%, except in rare cases of the translocation carrier parent, when the risk for recurrence will depend on the type of translocation and the sex of the parent that carries it.

Trisomy 18 Syndrome

Trisomy 18 syndrome (Fig. 5-7) is the second most common autosomal chromosomal aberration in humans, with an incidence of one in 3500 newborns.[89–91] The major features found in virtually all affected individuals include intrauterine growth retardation, microcephaly, characteristic craniofacial features (prominent occiput, short palpebral fissures, malformed and low-set ears, small mouth, narrow palate, and micrognathia), clenched hands, a short sternum, a low arch pattern of the dermal ridges on the fingertips, and severe cardiac malformations.

Cardiovascular defects are found in virtually all liveborn infants with trisomy 18 syndrome. Van Praagh et al.[92] reported on the cardiac malformations in 41 karyotyped and autopsied cases of trisomy 18 syndrome. The salient findings included a ventricular septal defect in all cases, polyvalvular disease (malformations of more than one valve) in 93%, a subpulmonary infundibulum in 98%, and a striking absence of transposition of the great arteries and inversion at any level (cardiac or visceral), findings which appear to be characteristic of all autosomal trisomies. The ventricular septal defect was associated with anterosuperior conal septal malalignment in 61% of cases. The malformations of the atrioventricular and semilunar valves were

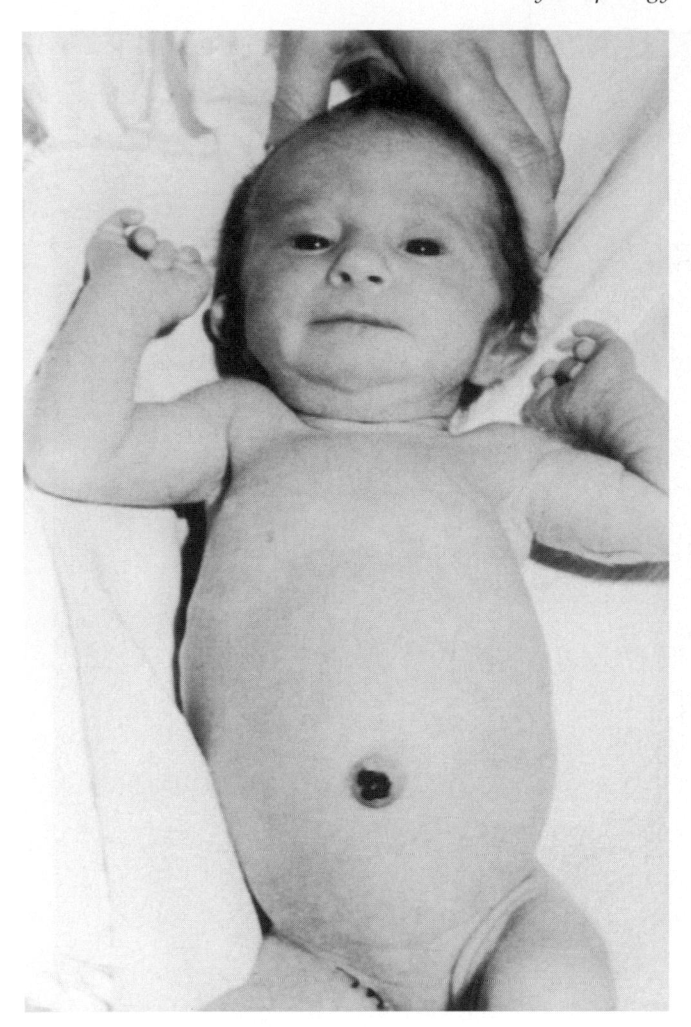

Figure 5–7 *Trisomy 18 syndrome in a newborn infant with complex cardiac defects. Note petite facial features, clenched hands, and short sternum.*
From Fyler DC (ed). Nadas' Pediatric Cardiology. Philadephia: Hanley & Belfus, 1992.

characterized by redundant or thick myxomatous leaflets, long chordae tendineae, and hypoplastic or absent papillary muscles. Other defects included double-outlet right ventricle (10%), all with mitral atresia, and tetralogy of Fallot (15%).

Most infants with trisomy 18 syndrome have severe perinatal difficulties attributable to severe brain dysfunction and severe cardiac defects. Most die within a week of birth, most commonly because of apneic spells. Cardiovascular failure and aspiration pneumonia are common. Survival into the teens and adult age has been reported, but all have been profoundly mentally retarded and completely dependent on care.

Prenatal detection of intrauterine growth retardation, decreased fetal activity, and clenched fists, accompanied by visceral, cardiac, and limb malformation suggests trisomy 18 syndrome. The risk of recurrence for trisomy 18 syndrome is estimated to be less than 1%.

Trisomy 13 Syndrome

Trisomy 13 syndrome has an incidence of about one in 5000 live births.[89–91] The major features include cleft lip and palate; holoprosencephalic defects of the eye, nose, lip, and forebrain; postaxial polydactyly; and localized skin defects of the scalp at the vertex (cutis aplasia congenita). Microphthalmia, colobomata of the iris, and retinal dysplasia are common. Apneic spells, seizures, and severe mental deficiency are hallmarks.

The incidence of cardiovascular malformations is about 80%. The most frequent defects include patent ductus arteriosus (63%), ventricular septal defect (48%), atrial septal defect (40%), abnormal valves (22%), coarctation of the aorta (10%), and dextrocardia (6%). The majority of affected infants (75%) have complex defects.

Infants with trisomy 13 syndrome have a dismally poor prognosis, as in trisomy 18 syndrome. Although long-term survival has been reported occasionally, all survivors are profoundly impaired. Prenatal detection of facial abnormalities, such as holoprosencephaly, cleft lip with or without cleft palate, hand and foot malformations, particularly postaxial polydactyly, and cardiovascular malformations suggests trisomy 13 syndrome. The risk of recurrence is presumed to be less than 1%.

Trisomy or Tetrasomy 22p (Cat-Eye Syndrome)

The small marker chromosome in the cat-eye syndrome is either a tandem duplication of proximal 22q or an isodicentric (22)(pter→q11).[89–91] The classic pattern of malformations includes mild mental deficiency, hypertelorism, down-slanting palpebral fissures, iris coloboma, preauricular pits or tags, and anal and renal malformations, but there is wide variability of phenotypic expression. Cardiovascular malformations have been reported in about 40%, and the occurrence of totally anomalous pulmonary venous connection has been observed in several studies. Additional defects include tetralogy of Fallot, ventricular septal defect, persistent left superior vena cava, interruption of the inferior vena cava, and tricuspid atresia.[98]

Turner Syndrome

The major features of Turner syndrome (Fig. 5-8) include short stature, primary amenorrhea due to ovarian dysgenesis, webbed neck, congenital lymphedema, and cubitus valgus.[89–91] The incidence of Turner syndrome is one in 5000 liveborn female infants. Although common in the first trimester, most 45,X conceptuses are

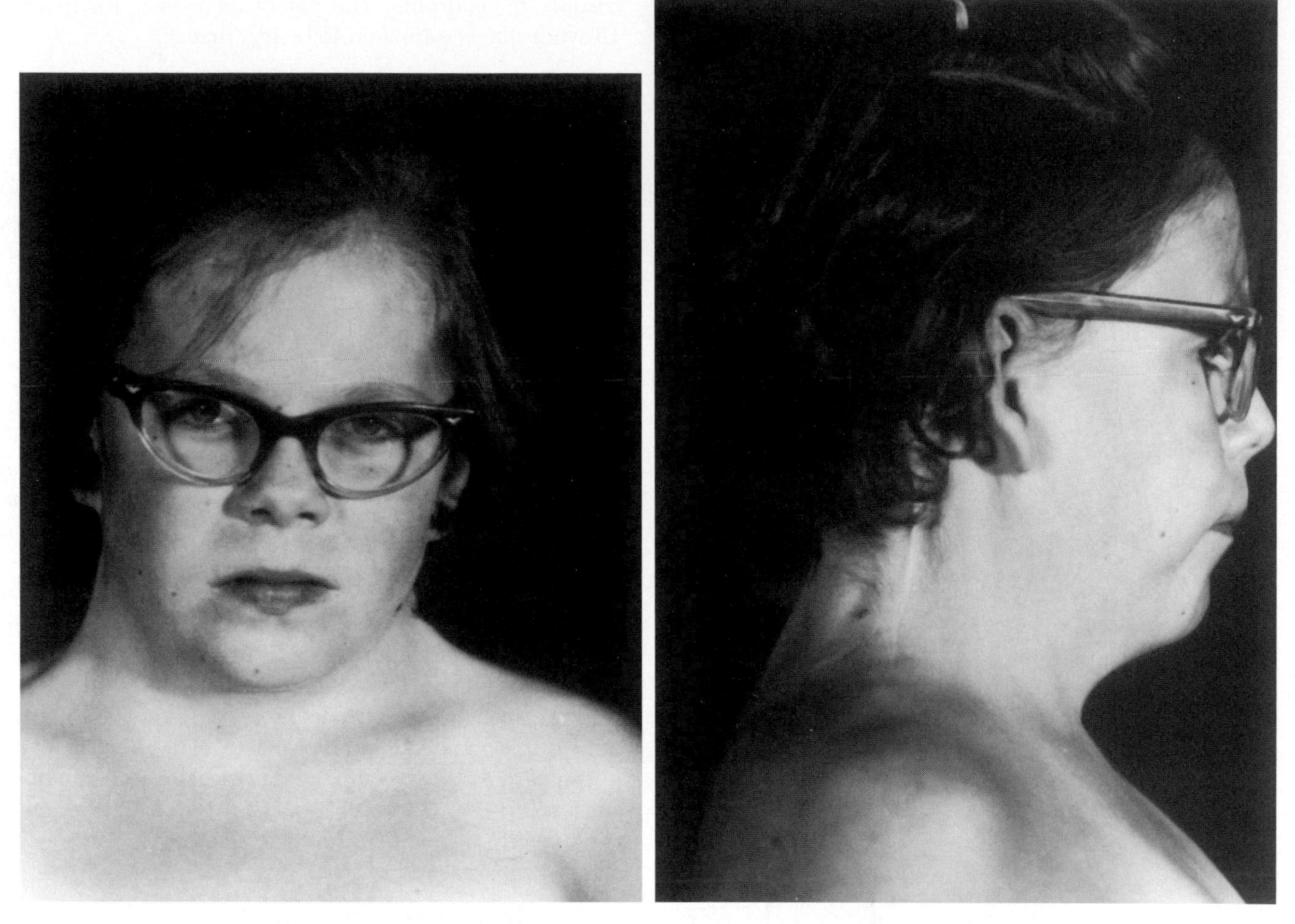

Figure 5–8 *Turner syndrome. Turner syndrome in a young woman with coarctation of the aorta. Note the webbed neck, broad chest, prominent ears, and multiple pigmented nevi.*
From Fyler DC (ed). Nadas' Pediatric Cardiology. Philadelphia: Hanley & Belfus, 1992.

spontaneously aborted. They constitute 25% of spontaneous abortions during the first trimester of pregnancy. More than half of liveborn individuals has a 45,X karyotype without evidence of mosaicism. The remainder show mosaicism and/or more complex rearrangements involving the X chromosome (ring, deletion, isochromosome Xq, isodicentric X, etc.).

Between 20% and 40% of girls with Turner syndrome have significant cardiovascular malformations, most commonly coarctation of the aorta (70%), often bicommissural aortic valve, and aortic stenosis—defects typically not common in girls. In fact, girls with Turner syndrome are prone to a spectrum of left-sided obstructive/hypoplastic defects ranging in severity from asymptomatic bicommissural aortic valve to hypoplastic left heart syndrome. Aortic dilation, dissection, and rupture also have been reported, but the incidence and risk factors for these complications are unclear.[93,94] Systemic hypertension is more common in Turner syndrome than the general population, and should be treated aggressively.

Prenatal recognition of coarctation of the aorta, left-sided hypoplasia, or hypoplastic left heart syndrome in a female infant with hydrops fetalis or cystic hygroma and renal malformation suggests Turner syndrome.

TERATOGENS

Teratogens are chemical, physical, and biologic agents capable of inducing congenital anomalies. Table 5-5 summarizes the known or potential teratogens that involve the cardiovascular system. Some teratogens produce distinct clinical syndromes or recognizable patterns of malformation, the most common of which is the fetal alcohol

Table 5–5. Cardiovascular Abnormalities Caused by Teratogens

Recognizable Phenotypes (Syndromes)	Cardiac Abnormalities
CHEMICAL TERATOGENS	
Fetal alcohol syndrome	Ventricular septal defect, atrial septal defect, tetralogy of Fallot, coarctation of the aorta
Fetal hydantoin syndrome	Ventricular septal defect, tetralogy of Fallot, pulmonary stenosis, patent ductus arteriosus, atrial septal defect, coarctation of the aorta
Fetal trimethadione syndrome	Combined defects
Fetal valproate syndrome	Nonspecific
Fetal carbamazepine syndrome	Ventricular septal defect, tetralogy of Fallot
Retinoic acid embryopathy	Conotruncal malformations
Thalidomide embryopathy	Conotruncal malformations
Fetal warfarin syndrome	Patent ductus arteriosus, peripheral pulmonary stenosis
BIOLOGIC TERATOGENS	
Maternal PKU fetal effects	Tetralogy of Fallot, ventricular septal defect, coarctation of the aorta
Maternal lupus fetal effects	Complete heart block, cardiomyopathy, L-transposition of the great arteries
Fetal rubella syndrome	Patent ductus arteriosus, peripheral pulmonary stenosis, fibromuscular and intimal proliferation of medium and large arteries, ventricular septal defect, atrial septal defect
Nonsyndromic increased risk for malformations	
Lithium	Ebstein anomaly, tricuspid atresia, atrial septal defect
Maternal diabetes	Transposition of the great arteries, ventricular septal defect, coarctation of the aorta, hypertrophic cardiomyopathy

syndrome, whereas other agents cause an increased incidence of single or multiple malformations without a specific syndrome pattern (e.g., maternal ingestion of lithium or maternal diabetes). Biologic teratogens include maternal illnesses (e.g., maternal phenylketonuria or maternal lupus erythematosus) or maternal-fetal infections (e.g., rubella) that can cause birth defects.

Fetal Alcohol Syndrome

One of the most common malformation syndromes, with an estimated frequency greater than one in 1000 live births, the fetal alcohol syndrome (Fig. 5-9) is also one of the most common identifiable causes of mental retardation. The most serious consequence of prenatal alcohol exposure is its effects on brain development and function. About half of all individuals with fetal alcohol syndrome have congenital cardiovascular malformations.[95] By far the most common defect is ventricular septal defect, followed by atrial septal defect and tetralogy of Fallot. Less commonly reported lesions include atrioventricular canal defect, hypoplasia or absence of one pulmonary artery, subaortic stenosis, and complex defects.

SINGLE GENE DISORDERS

Marfan Syndrome

Marfan syndrome is the most common and best characterized of the connective tissue disorders with serious cardiovascular manifestations.[96–98] This condition is an autosomal dominant, multisystem disorder with a wide variability of phenotypic expression involving the skeletal, ocular, cardiovascular, and other systems. Mutations involving the gene, *FBN1*, for the connective tissue protein fibrillin-1, have been documented.[96] Nearly all patients have some cardiovascular involvement, most commonly mitral valve prolapse and aortic root dilation. The risk for aortic regurgitation, dissection, and rupture increases with progressive enlargement of the aortic root. Beta-blockers may retard the rate of dilation of the aortic root and ascending aorta.[97] In adults, replacement of the root and ascending aorta is recommended when the aortic root diameter is greater than 5.5 cm or greater than 5.0 cm if there is a family history of dissection.

Worldwide, surgery for patients with Marfan syndrome is performed by experienced surgeons at a very low risk, with excellent outcomes. Many experienced centers are now

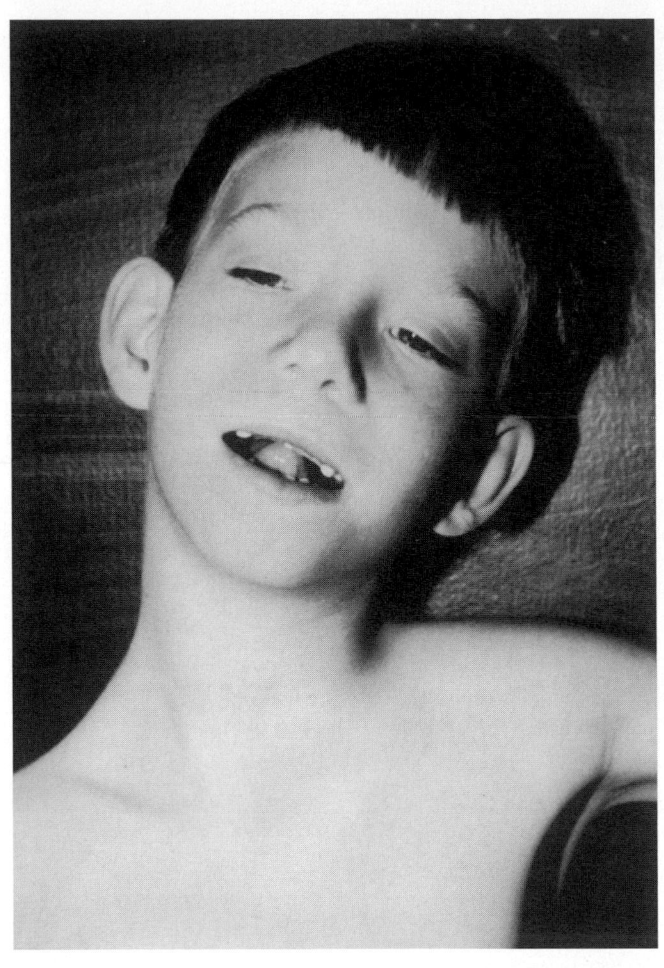

Figure 5–9 *Fetal alcohol syndrome. Typical facies in a child with severe manifestations of prenatal alcohol exposure. Note the short, downslanting palpebral fissures, short upturned nose, long smooth philtrum, and thin upper lip.*
From Fyler DC (ed). Nadas' Pediatric Cardiology. Philadelphia: Hanley & Belfus, 1992.

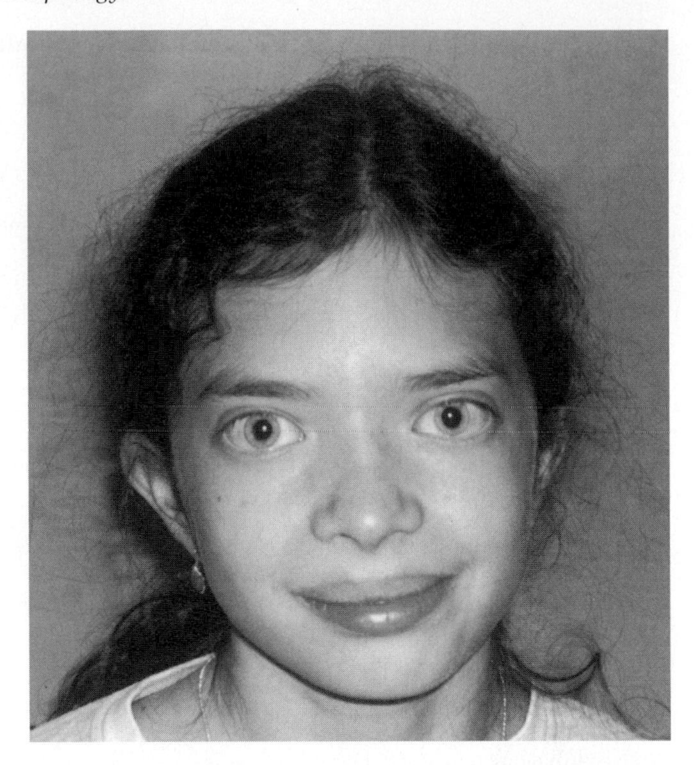

Figure 5–10 *Noonan syndrome.*

routinely offering a valve-sparing aortic root replacement for people with Marfan syndrome, instead of a composite valve graft which involves a prosthetic aortic valve. Because of the low risk of prophylactic aortic root replacement in Marfan syndrome and the devastating effects on short- and long-term survival after dissection, some are now advocating surgery when the aortic root diameter exceeds 45 mm, especially if there is a family history of aortic dissection, when there is a rapid growth of the aorta (i.e., > 5–10 mm/year), or when significant aortic insufficiency is present.[99]

Noonan Syndrome

Noonan syndrome (Fig. 5-10) is a well-known autosomal dominant, multisystem disorder associated with congenital heart defects.[100–102] Based on genetic linkage studies, some families were mapped to chromosome 12q,[103] and in 2001, Tartaglia and colleagues[104,105] reported on their discovery that mutations of the *PTPN11* gene account for about half of the cases with a clinical diagnosis of Noonan syndrome, consistent with genetic heterogeneity. The major features include short stature, seen in about half of affected individuals; mental retardation (usually mild) seen in about 25% of cases; characteristic facial appearance including widely spaced eyes, epicanthal folds, ptosis, and lowset, malformed ears; prominent trapezius muscle with a short webbed neck and low posterior hairline; a shield chest deformity with pectus carinatum superiorly and pectus excavatum inferiorly; cubitus valgus; and cryptorchidism among males. At least 50% of individuals with Noonan syndrome have congenital heart defects. About 75% of those with congenital heart defects have valvar pulmonary stenosis secondary to a dysplastic pulmonary valve with thickened valve leaflets. Particularly unusual is the high incidence of leftward or superior frontal QRS vector, even in the face of severe right ventricular hypertrophy, presumably due to a conduction abnormality. Other defects reported include atrial septal defect (30%, usually associated with pulmonary stenosis), patent ductus arteriosus (10%), and ventricular septal defect (10%). Rare lesions include tetralogy of Fallot, coarctation of the aorta, subaortic stenosis, Ebstein malformation, and complex defects. Hypertrophic cardiomyopathy, which can involve both ventricles, is observed in 10% to 20% of cases.

The *PTPN11* gene encodes SHP-2, a nonmembranous protein tyrosine phosphatase with diverse roles in signal transduction. Particularly relevant to the cardiac involvement in Noonan syndrome, SHP-2 has been shown to act in epidermal growth factor signaling in semilunar valvulogenesis.[69]

Holt-Oram Syndrome

This syndrome of upper limb and cardiovascular malformations (Fig. 5-11) was first described in 1960 by Holt and Oram,[106] who noted the association of radial anomalies with atrial septal defect. It is an autosomal dominant disorder with variable expression, but complete or near-complete penetrance. The gene for Holt-Oram syndrome, mapped to 12q by family linkage studies, encodes a transcription factor, TBX5.[107–109] Other families have not mapped to this locus, consistent with genetic heterogeneity. An affected individual may have isolated upper limb defects, isolated heart defects, or a combination. All gradations of skeletal defects involving the upper limb and shoulder girdle, ranging from mild hypoplasia of the thumb to phocomelia, can occur even within the same family. All patients with involvement of the upper limbs have defects of the thumb. There is no correlation between the severity of the defect of the limb and the cardiac defect.

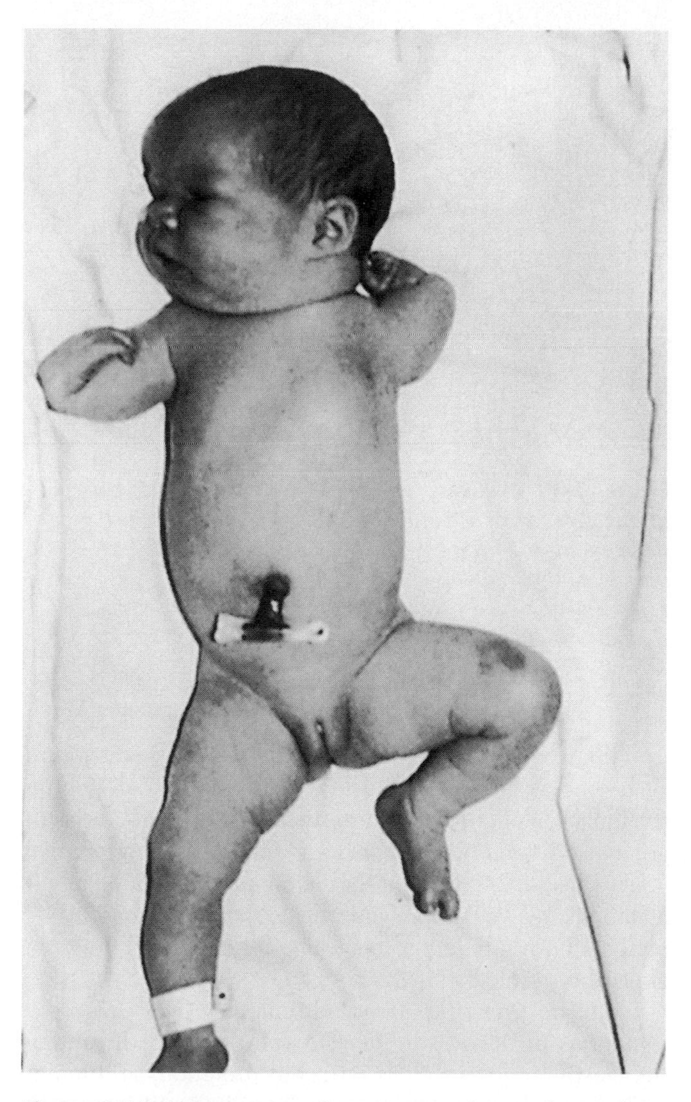

Figure 5–11 *Holt-Oram syndrome in a newborn infant with an atrial septal defect. Note the bilateral deficiency of the upper limbs. From Fyler DC (ed). Nadas' Pediatric Cardiology. Philadephia: Hanley & Belfus, 1992.*

Congenital heart defects are observed in at least half of affected individuals, although there may be an ascertainment bias toward cardiac defects. Atrial septal defect is the most frequent lesion, but a number of cardiac phenotypes have been reported including normal, first-degree atrioventricular block, ostium primum atrial septal defects, isolated ventricular septal defects, and hypoplastic left heart syndrome. Prognosis is dependent on the degree of skeletal deformity and the nature of the cardiac anomaly. Intelligence is normal, and there are no associated visceral malformations.

Alagille Syndrome

The typical manifestations of Alagille syndrome (arteriohepatic dysplasia), an autosomal dominant disorder, include intrahepatic cholestasis due to bile duct paucity, distinctive facies (prominent forehead and chin, deep-set eyes, long nose), anterior chamber abnormalities of the eye, especially posterior embryotoxon, and butterfly hemivertebrae. Peripheral pulmonary artery stenosis is most common, although other defects including tetralogy of Fallot have also been observed.[110] This disorder is caused by mutations or deletions of the *JAG1* gene, which encodes for Jagged 1, a ligand in the Notch intercellular signaling pathway.[69,111–113]

McElhinney and colleagues[114] examined a large cohort of 200 individuals with *JAG1* mutations and/or Alagille syndrome with respect to their cardiac phenotype. They determined that 94% had cardiac involvement. Aside from peripheral pulmonary artery stenosis, which was the most prevalent lesion, other defects included tetralogy of Fallot, pulmonary valve stenosis, atrial septal defect, ventricular septal defect, and assorted other defects at low frequency. A noteworthy finding was that the clinical outcome among those with tetralogy of Fallot was poor, with 43% mortality. Analysis of genotype–phenotype correlation failed to disclose a relationship between the type or location of the *JAG1* mutation and the cardiac phenotype. Overall, this study revealed a relatively high percentage of left-sided defects (11%) and tetralogy of Fallot with apparent excess of those with pulmonary atresia and none with right aortic arch.

Ellis–Van Creveld Syndrome (Chondroectodermal Dysplasia)

Ellis–van Creveld syndrome is an autosomal recessive disorder with the following major features: short stature of prenatal onset (short limbs), ectodermal dysplasia manifested by hypoplastic nails and dental anomalies (neonatal teeth, partial anodontia, small teeth and/or delayed eruption), postaxial polydactyly, narrow thorax, and cardiac defects.[115] About 50% of patients have congenital cardiovascular malformations. Atrial septal defect or common atrium occurs in about half of patients with congenital heart disease. Other less frequent defects include patent ductus arteriosus, persistent left superior vena cava, hypoplastic left heart syndrome, coarctation of the aorta, totally anomalous pulmonary venous connection, and transposition of the great arteries. Most survivors have normal intelligence. Adult stature is in the range of 43 to 60 inches. Dental problems are frequent.

The syndrome has been mapped to chromosome 4p16[116] and mutations of two nonhomologous genes at this locus (*EVC* and *EVC2*) have been identified in affected families.[117,118] For couples with at least one affected child, the recurrence risk is 25% for each subsequent pregnancy.

CONTIGUOUS GENE DELETION SYNDROMES

Williams Syndrome

Williams and colleagues[119,120] described this condition in four unrelated children with mental retardation, an unusual facial appearance, and supravalvar aortic stenosis (Fig. 5-12). Hypocalcemia has been an infrequent finding, particularly beyond the neonatal period. At least half of these individuals have cardiovascular defects. Supravalvar aortic stenosis is the most frequent single defect, but any of the systemic and pulmonary arteries can be affected. Narrowing at the sinotubular ridge can be detected by echocardiography and angiography postnatally, but may be difficult to detect prenatally.

The SVAS complex or elastin arteriopathy can occur as an isolated autosomal dominant disorder (nonsyndromic SVAS) or as part of Williams syndrome.[121] The SVAS complex is a diffuse arteriopathy which can affect all segments of the aorta; any of its branches including the coronary arteries, the brachiocephalic vessels, the mesenteric and the renal arteries, as well as the pulmonary and cerebral arteries. Abnormalities in elastin production are thought to be responsible for the cardiovascular phenotype in both Williams syndrome and nonsyndromic SVAS, so the similarity in vascular abnormalities is predictable. Both conditions link to the elastin gene on chromosome.[7]

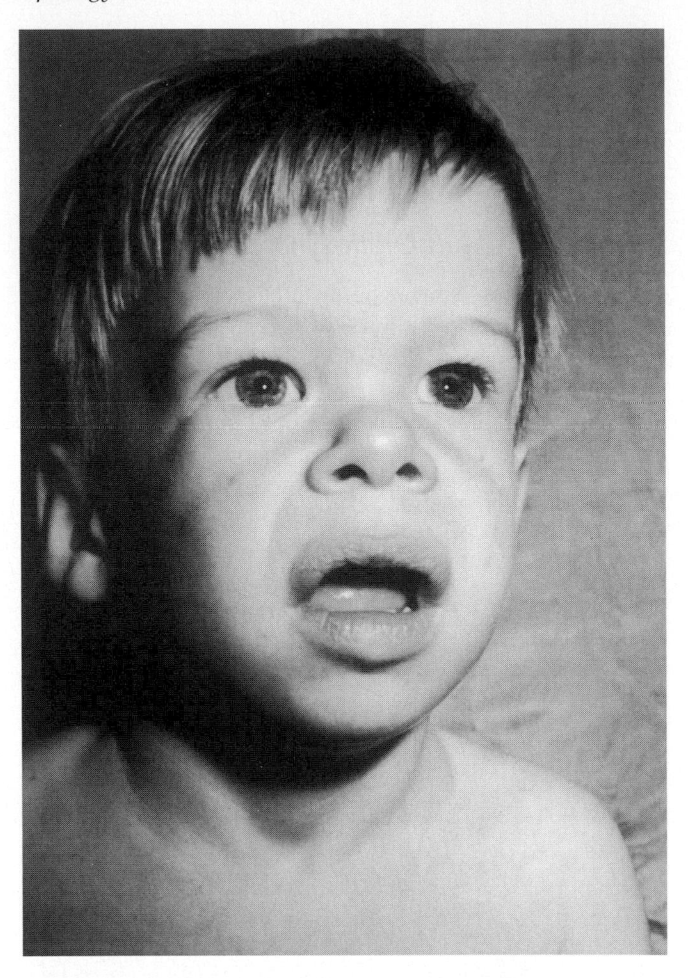

Figure 5–12 *Williams syndrome in a 2-year-old boy with supravalvar aortic stenosis. Note the typical facies including a stellate pattern of the iris, short anteverted nose, long philtrum, prominent lips, and large, open mouth.*
From Fyler DC (ed). Nadas' Pediatric Cardiology. Philadephia: Hanley & Belfus, 1992.

Williams syndrome is a contiguous gene deletion syndrome associated with a 1- to 2-megabase deletion on the long arm of chromosome 7, including the entire elastin gene and 20 additional genes. The loss of these additional genes presumably account for the nonelastin-related manifestations of Williams syndrome. The vast majority of patients have a deletion involving one copy of the elastin gene, detectable by FISH.[121–123]

In contrast, familial (nonsyndromic) SVAS is caused by mutations of the elastin gene. A translocation disrupting the elastin gene as well as intragenic deletions and mutations involving the elastin gene have been identified in nonsyndromic SVAS.[121,124–126] Individuals with familial SVAS typically do not show evidence of a complete deletion of elastin by FISH.

Chromosome 22q Deletions (DiGeorge Sequence, Velocardiofacial Syndrome, CATCH 22)

The DiGeorge sequence, velocardiofacial syndrome, conotruncal face anomaly syndrome, CATCH 22, and some isolated conotruncal malformations are associated with deletions or mutations involving the long arm of chromosome 22 (critical region 22q11.2). The clinical and cardiovascular manifestations are discussed earlier in this chapter under Ectomesenchymal tissue migration abnormalities (neural crest migration abnormalities).

ASSOCIATIONS

An association is a nonrandom occurrence of multiple anomalies not known to be a developmental field defect, sequence, or syndrome. The definition refers solely to statistically (not pathogenetically or causally) related anomalies. A given association, such as the VATER association, can occur in isolation or as part of a broader pattern of malformation, such as in trisomy 18 syndrome or infants born to diabetic mothers.

VATER Association. The VATER association refers to the nonrandom occurrence of defects, including vertebral defects, anal atresia, tracheoesophageal fistula with esophageal atresia, and radial and renal dysplasia. The spectrum has been extended to include cardiac defects, single umbilical artery, and growth deficiency of prenatal onset. Although ventricular septal defects are most common, a wide variety of cardiac lesions has been seen. The etiology of this pattern of malformation is not known. Generally, it has occurred sporadically in an otherwise normal family. Identification of VATER association defects in a particular patient does not, in itself, imply a diagnosis. Rather, the presence of one or more VATER-associated malformations should alert the clinician to the presence of other VATER defects.

CHARGE Association. The CHARGE association is a nonrandom association of congenital anomalies including coloboma, heart disease, atresia choanae, retarded growth and development and/or central nervous system anomalies, genital anomalies and/or hypogonadism, and ear anomalies and/or deafness. Heart defects have been described in 50% to 70% of the patients. Of those with congenital heart disease, 42% had conotruncal anomalies (tetralogy of Fallot, double-outlet right ventricle, truncus arteriosus) and 36% had aortic arch anomalies (vascular ring, aberrant subclavian artery, interrupted aortic arch). Other defects include patent ductus arteriosus, atrioventricular canal, ventricular septal defect, and atrial septal defect. Most patients have some degree of mental deficiency and/or defects of the central nervous system. In some instances, the severity of the malformations has led to death in the perinatal period. Recently Vissers and colleagues[127] detected a microdeletion on chromosome 8q12 in two individuals with CHARGE and mutations in the *CHD7* gene in 10 of 17 individuals with CHARGE.

REFERENCES

1. Smith DW. Dysmorphology (teratology). J Pediatr 69:1150, 1966.
2. Ferencz C, Rubin JD, McCarter RJ, et al. Congenital heart disease prevalence at live birth—the Baltimore-Washington Infant Study. Am J Epidemiol 121:31, 1985.
3. Marden PM, Smith DW, McDonald MJ. Congenital anomalies in the newborn infant including minor variants. J Pediatr 64:357, 1965.
4. Greenwood RD, Rosenthal A, Parisi L, et al. Extracardiac abnormalities in infants with congenital heart disease. Pediatrics 55:485, 1975.
5. Lammer EJ, Chen DT, Hoar RM, et al. Retinoic acid embryopathy. N Engl J Med 313:837, 1985.
6. Clarke LA (Updated 6 August 2004). Mucopolysaccharidosis type I. In GeneReviews at GeneTests: Medical Genetic Information Resource (database online). Seattle: University of Washington, 1997-2005. Available at *http://www.genetests.org*. Accessed 13 March 2005.
7. Clark EB. Growth, morphogenesis, and function: the dynamics of cardiovascular development. In Moller JM, Neal WA (eds.). Fetal, Neonatal, and Infant Heart Disease. New York, Appleton-Century Crofts, 1989, pp 1–22.
8. Rose V, Clark E. Etiology of congenital heart disease. In Freedom RM, Benson LN, Smallhorn JF (eds). Neonatal Heart Disease. London: Springer-Verlag, 1992, pp 3–17.
9. Clark EB. Pathogenetic mechanisms of congenital cardiovascular malformations revisited. Semin Perinatol 20:465, 1996.
10. Boughman JA, Berg KA, Astemborski JA, et al. Familial risks of congenital heart defect assessed in a population-based epidemiologic study. Am J Med Genet 26:839, 1987.
11. Kirby ML, Gale TF, Stewart DE. Neural crest cells contribute to normal aorticopulmonary septation. Science 220:1059, 1983.
12. Kirby ML, Turnage KL, Hays BM. Characterization of conotruncal malformations following ablation of "cardiac" neural crest. Anat Rec 213:87, 1985.
13. Kirby ML, Bockman DR. Neural crest and normal development. A new perspective. Anat Rec 209:1, 1984.
14. Driscoll DA, Budarf ML, Emanuel BS. A genetic etiology for DiGeorge syndrome: consistent deletions and microdeletions of 22q11. Am J Hum Genet 50:924, 1992.
15. Driscoll DA, Spinner NB, Budarf ML, et al. Deletions and microdeletions of 22q11.2 in velo-cardio-facial syndrome. Am J Med Genet 44:261, 1992.
16. Scambler PJ, Carey AH, Wyse RKH, et al. Microdeletions within 22q11 associated with sporadic and familial DiGeorge syndrome. Genomics 10:201, 1991.

17. Scambler PJ, Kelly D, Lindsay E, et al. Velo-cardio-facial syndrome associated with chromosome 22 deletions encompassing the DiGeorge locus. Lancet 339:1138, 1992.
18. Wilson DI, Goodship JA, Burn J, et al. Deletions within chromosome 22q11 in familial congenital heart disease. Lancet 340:573, 1992.
19. Goldmuntz E, Driscoll D, Budarf ML, et al. Microdeletions of chromosomal region 22q11 in patients with congenital conotruncal cardiac defects. J Med Genet 30:807, 1993.
20. Goldmuntz E, Clark BJ, Mitchell LE, et al. Frequency of 22q11 deletions in patients with conotruncal defects. J Am Coll Cardiol 32:499, 1998.
21. Lindsay EA, Botta A, Jurecic V, et al. Congenital heart disease in mice deficient for the DiGeorge syndrome region. Nature 401:379, 1999.
22. Jerome LA, Papaioannou VE. DiGeorge syndrome phenotype in mice mutant for the T-box gene, *Tbx1*. Nat Genet 27:286, 2001.
23. Lindsay EA, Vitelli F, Su H, et al. Tbx1 haploinsufficiency in the DiGeorge syndrome region causes aortic arch defects in mice. Nature 410:97, 2001.
24. Merscher S, Funke B, Epstein JA, et al. TBX1 is responsible for cardiovascular defects in velo-cardio-facial/DiGeorge syndrome. Cell 104:619, 2001.
25. Yagi H, Furutani Y, Hamada H, et al. Role of *TBX1* in human del22q11.2 syndrome. Lancet 362:1366, 2003.
26. Baldini A. DiGeorge syndrome: an update. Curr Opin Cardiol 19:201, 2004.
27. Burn J, Wilson DI, Cross I, et al. The clinical significance of 22q11 deletion. In Clark EB, Markwald RR, Takao A (eds). Developmental Mechanisms of Heart Disease. Armonk, NY: Futura Publishing, 1995, pp 559–567.
28. Daw SCM, Taylor C, Kraman M, et al. A common region of 10p deleted in DiGeorge and velocardiofacial syndromes. Nat Genet 13:458, 1996.
29. Ryan AK, Goodship JA, Wilson DI, et al. Spectrum of clinical features associated with interstitial chromosome 22q11 deletions: a European collaborative study. J Med Genet 34:798, 1997.
30. McElhinney DB, Driscoll DA, Emanuel BS, et al. Chromosome 22q11 deletion in patients with truncus arteriosus. Pediatr Cardiol 24:569, 2003.
31. McElhinney DB, Driscoll DA, Levin ER, et al. Chromosome 22q11 deletion in patients with ventricular septal defect: frequency and associated cardiovascular anomalies. Pediatrics 112:472, 2003.
32. McElhinney DB, Clark BJ, Weinberg PM, et al. Association of chromosome 22q11 deletion with isolated anomalies of aortic arch laterality and branching. J Am Coll Cardiol 37:114, 2001.
33. Van Mierop LHS, Alley RD, Kausel HW, et al. Pathogenesis of transposition complexes, I: embryology of the ventricles and great arteries. Am J Cardiol 12:216, 1963.
34. Harh JY, Paul MH, Gallen WJ, et al. Experimental production of hypoplastic left heart syndrome in the chick embryo. Am J Cardiol 10:127, 1986.
35. Lacro RV, Jones KL, Benirschke K. Pathogenesis of coarctation of the aorta in the Turner syndrome: a pathologic study of fetuses with nuchal cystic hygromas, hydrops fetalis, and female genitalia. Pediatrics 81:445, 1988.
36. Benacerraf BR, Saltzman DH, Sanders SP. Sonographic sign suggesting the prenatal diagnosis of coarctation of the aorta. J Ultrasound Med 8:65, 1989.
37. Thomas T, Yamagishi H, Overbeek PA, et al. The bHLH factors, dHAND and eHAND, specify pulmonary and systemic cardiac ventricles independent of left-right sidedness. Dev Biol 196:228, 1998.
38. Schroeder JA, Jackson LF, Lee DC, et al. Form and function of developing heart valves: coordination by extracellular matrix and growth factor signaling. J Mol Med 81:392, 2003.
39. Kurnit DM, Aldridge JF, Matsuoka R, et al. Increased adhesiveness of trisomy 21 cells and atrioventricular canal malformations in Down syndrome: a stochastic model. Am J Med Genet 20:385, 1985.
40. Kurnit DM, Layton WM, Matthysse S. Genetics, chance, and morphogenesis. Am J Hum Genet 41:979, 1987.
41. Jongewaard IN, Lauer RM, Behrendt DA, et al. Beta 1 integrin activation mediates adhesive differences between trisomy 21 and non-trisomic fibroblasts on type VI collagen. Am J Med Genet 109:298, 2002.
42. Maslen CL. Molecular genetics of atrioventricular septal defects. Curr Opin Cardiol 19:205, 2004.
43. Rupp PA, Fouad GT, Egelston CA, et al. Identification, genomic organization and mRNA expression of *CRELD1*, the founding member of a unique family of matricellular proteins. Gene 293:47, 2002.
44. Robinson SW, Morris CD, Goldmuntz E, et al. Missense mutations in *CRELD1* are associated with cardiac atrioventricular septal defects. Am J Hum Genet 72:1047, 2003.
45. Jiao K, Kulessa H, Tompkins K, et al. An essential role of Bmp4 in the atrioventricular septation of the mouse heart. Genes Dev 15:1, 2003.
46. Garg V, Kathiriya IS, Barnes R, et al. GATA4 mutations cause human congenital heart defects and reveal an interaction with TBX5. Nature 424:443, 2003.
47. Pexieder T. Cell death in the morphogenesis and teratogenesis of the heart. Adv Anat Embryol Cell Biol 51:1, 1975.
48. James TN. Normal and abnormal consequences of apoptosis in the human heart. Annu Rev Physiol 60:309, 1998.
49. Van Mierop LHS, Gessner IH. Pathogenetic mechanisms in congenital cardiovascular malformations. Prog Cardiovasc Dis 15:67, 1972.
50. Ben-Shachar G, Arcilla R, Lucas RV, et al. Ventricular trabeculations in the chick embryo and their contribution to the ventricular and muscular septal development. Circ Res 57:759, 1985.
51. Neill CA. Development of the pulmonary veins with reference to embryology of anomalies of pulmonary venous return. Pediatrics 18:880, 1956.
52. Clark EB, Martini DR, Rosenquist GC. Spectrum of pulmonary venous connections following lung bud inversion in the chick embryo. In Pexieder T (ed). Perspectives in Cardiovascular Research, Mechanisms of Cardiac Morphogenesis and Teratogenesis, Vol 5. New York, Raven Press, 1981, pp 419–430.

53. Bleyl S, Nelson L, Odelberg SJ, et al. A gene for familial total anomalous pulmonary venous return maps to chromosome 4p13-q12. Am J Hum Genet 56:408, 1995.
54. Bleyl SB, Saijoh Y, Klewer SE, et al. Evidence that PDGF signaling is disrupted in human anomalies of the pulmonary veins. (Abstract 1046, presented at American Society for Human Genetics meeting, October 2004, Toronto).
55. Belmont JW, Mohapatra B, Towbin JA, et al. Molecular genetics of heterotaxy syndromes. Curr Opin Cardiol 19:216, 2004.
56. Yost HJ. The genetics of midline and cardiac laterality defects. Curr Opin Cardiol 13:185, 1998.
57. Casey B, Devoto M, Jones KL, et al. Mapping a gene for familial situs abnormalities to human chromosome Xq24-q27.1. Nat Genet 5:403, 1993.
58. Gebbia M, Ferrero GB, Pilia G, et al. X-linked situs abnormalities result from mutations in ZIC3. Nat Genet 17:305, 1997.
59. Brueckner M, McGrath J, D'Eustachio P, et al. Establishment of left-right asymmetry in vertebrates: genetically distinct steps are involved in biological asymmetry and handedness. Ciba Found Symp 162:202, 1991.
60. Icardo JM, de Vega S. Spectrum of heart malformations in mice with situs solitus, situs inversus, and associated visceral heterotaxy. Circulation 84:2547, 1991.
61. Brueckner M, D'Eustachio P, Horwich AL. Linkage mapping of a mouse gene, iv, that controls left-right asymmetry of the heart and viscera. Proc Natl Acad Sci U S A 86:5035, 1989.
62. Supp DM, Witte DP, Potter SS, et al. Mutation of an axonemal dynein affects left-right asymmetry in inversus viscerum mice. Nature 389:963, 1997.
63. Afzelius BA. A human syndrome caused by immotile cilia. Science 193:317, 1976.
64. Teichberg S, Markowitz J, Silverberg M, et al. Abnormal cilia in a child with the polysplenia syndrome and extrahepatic biliary atresia. J Pediatr 100:399, 1982.
65. Schidlow DV, Moriber Katz S, Turtz MG, et al. Polysplenia and Kartagener syndromes in a sibship: association with abnormal respiratory cilia. J Pediatr 100:401, 1982.
66. Lin AE, Garver KL. Genetic counseling for congenital heart defects. J Pediatr 113:1105, 1988.
67. Strauss AW, Johnson MC. The genetic basis of pediatric cardiovascular disease. Semin Perinatol 20:564, 1996.
68. Lewin MB, Glass IA, Power P. Genotype-phenotype correlation in congenital heart disease. Curr Opin Cardiol 19:221, 2004.
69. Gelb BD. Genetic basis of congenital heart disease. Curr Opin Cardiol 19:110, 2004.
70. McElhinney DB, Geiger E, Blinder J, et al. NKX2.5 mutations in patients with congenital heart disease. J Am Coll Cardiol 42:1650, 2003.
71. Elliot DA, Kirk EP, Yeoh T, et al. Cardiac homeobox gene NKX2-5 mutations and congenital heart disease: associations with atrial septal defect and hypoplastic left heart syndrome. J Am Coll Cardiol 41:2072, 2003.
72. Brenner JI, Berg KA, Schneider DS, et al. Cardiac malformations in relatives of infants with hypoplastic left-heart syndrome. Am J Dis Child 143:1492, 1989.
73. Whittemore R, Hobbins JC, Engle MA. Pregnancy and its outcome in women with and without surgical treatment of congenital heart disease. Am J Cardiol 50:641, 1982.
74. Rose V, Gold RJ, Lindsay G, et al. A possible increase in the incidence of congenital heart defects among the offspring of affected parents. J Am Coll Cardiol 6:376, 1985.
75. Nora JJ, Nora AH. Update on counseling the family with a first-degree relative with a congenital heart defect. Am J Med Genet 29:137, 1988.
76. Nora JJ. Causes of congenital heart diseases: old and new modes, mechanisms, and models. Am Heart J 125:1409, 1993.
77. Whittemore R, Wells JA, Castellsague X. A second-generation study of 427 probands with congenital heart defects and their 837 children. J Am Coll Cardiol 23:1459, 1994.
78. Disegni E, Pierpont ME, Bass JL, et al. Two-dimensional echocardiographic identification of endocardial cushion defect in families. Am J Cardiol 55:1649, 1985.
79. Brenner JI, Berg KA, Schneider DS, et al. Cardiac malformations in relatives of infants with hypoplastic left-heart syndrome. Am J Dis Child 140:41, 1986.
80. Lewin MB, McBride KL, Pignatelli R, et al. Echocardiographic evaluation of asymptomatic parental and sibling cardiovascular anomalies associated with congenital left ventricular outflow tract lesions. Pediatrics 114:691, 2004.
81. Malik MSA, Watkins H. The molecular genetics of hypertrophic cardiomyopathy. Curr Opin Cardiol 12:295, 1997.
82. Vincent GM. Role of DNA testing for diagnosis, management, and genetic screening in long QT syndrome, hypertrophic cardiomyopathy, and Marfan syndrome. Heart 86:12, 2002.
83. Seidman JG, Seidman C. The genetic basis for cardiomyopathy. Cell 104:557, 2001.
84. Mestroni L, Giacca M. Molecular genetics of dilated cardiomyopathy. Curr Opin Cardiol 12:303, 1997.
85. Familial Dilated Cardiomyopathy Project Group. Available at *http://www.fdc.to.*
86. Wang Q, Chen Q, Li H, Towbin JA. Molecular genetics of long QT syndrome from genes to patients. Curr Opin Cardiol 12:310, 1997.
87. Lin AE. Congenital heart defects in malformation syndromes. Clin Perinatol 17:641, 1990.
88. Ferencz C, Neill CA, Boughman JA, et al. Congenital cardiovascular malformations associated with chromosome abnormalities: an epidemiologic study. J Pediatr 114:79, 1989.
89. Pierpont MEM, Moller JH (eds). Genetics of Cardiovascular Disease. Boston: Martinus Nijhoff, 1987.
90. Borgaonkar DS. Chromosomal Variation in Man: A Catalog of Chromosomal Variants and Anomalies. New York: Wiley-Liss, 1997.
91. Jones KL. Smith's Recognizable Patterns of Human Malformation. Philadelphia: WB Saunders, 1997.
92. Van Praagh S, Truman T, Firpo A, et al. Cardiac malformations in trisomy 18: a study of 41 postmortem cases. J Am Coll Cardiol 13:1586, 1989.
93. Allen DB, Hendricks SA, Levy JM. Aortic dilation in Turner syndrome. J Pediatr 109:302, 1986.

94. Lin AE, Lippe BM, Geffner ME, et al. Aortic dilation, dissection, and rupture in patients with Turner syndrome. J Pediatr 109:820, 1986.
95. Jones KL, Smith DW, Ulleland CN, et al. Pattern of malformation of offspring of chronic alcoholic mothers. Lancet 1:1267, 1973.
96. Milewicz DM. Molecular genetics of Marfan syndrome and Ehlers-Danlos type IV. Curr Opin Cardiol 13:198, 1998.
97. McKusick VA. The defect in Marfan syndrome. Nature 352:279, 1991.
98. Gray JR, Davies SJ. Marfan syndrome. J Med Genet 33:403, 1996.
99. Braverman AC. Timing of aortic surgery in the Marfan syndrome. Curr Opin Cardiol 19:549, 2004.
100. Mendez HMM, Opitz JM. Noonan syndrome: a review. Am J Med Genet 21:493, 1985.
101. Allanson JE. Noonan syndrome. J Med Genet 24:9, 1987.
102. Allanson JE, Hall JG, Hughes HE, et al. Noonan syndrome: the changing phenotype. Am J Med Genet 21:507, 1985.
103. Jamieson CR, van der Burgt I, Brady AF, et al. Mapping a gene for Noonan syndrome to the long arm of chromosome 12. Nat Genet 8:357, 1994.
104. Tartaglia M, Mehler EL, Goldberg R, et al. Mutations in PTPN11 encoding the protein tyrosine phosphatase SHP-2, cause Noonan syndrome. Nat Genet 29:465, 2001.
105. Tartaglia M, Kalidas K, Shaw A, et al. PTPN11 mutations in Noonan syndrome: molecular spectrum, genotype phenotype correlation, and phenotypic heterogeneity. Am J Hum Genet 70:1555, 2002.
106. Basson CT, Cowley GS, Solomon SD, et al. The clinical and genetic spectrum of the Holt-Oram syndrome (heart-hand syndrome). N Engl J Med 330:885, 1994.
107. Li QY, Newbury-Ecob RA, Terrett JA, et al. Holt-Oram syndrome is caused by mutations in TBX5, a member of the Brachyury (T) gene family. Nat Genet 15:21, 1997.
108. Basson CT, Bachinsky DR, Lin RC, et al. Mutations in human cause limb and cardiac malformation in Holt-Oram syndrome. Nat Genet 15:30, 1997.
109. Mori AD, Bruneau BG. TBX5 mutations and congenital heart disease: Holt-Oram syndrome revealed. Curr Opin Cardiol 19:211, 2004.
110. Krantz ID, Piccoli DA, Spinner NB. Alagille syndrome. J Med Genet 34:152, 1997.
111. Oda T, Elkahloun AG, Pike BL, et al. Mutations in the human Jagged1 gene are responsible for Alagille syndrome. Nat Genet 16:235, 1997.
112. Li L, Krantz ID, Deng Y, et al. Alagille syndrome is caused by mutations in human Jagged1, which encodes a ligand for Notch1. Nat Genet 16:243, 1997.
113. Krantz ID, Colliton RP, Genin A, et al. Spectrum and frequency of jagged1 (JAG1) mutations in Alagille syndrome patients and their families. Am J Hum Genet 62:1361, 1998.
114. McElhinney DB, Krantz ID, Bason L. Analysis of cardiovascular phenotype and genotype-phenotype correlation in individuals with JAG1 mutation and/or Alagille syndrome. Circulation 106:2567, 2002.
115. Ellis RWB, van Creveld S. A syndrome characterized by ectodermal dysplasia, polydactyly, chondro-dysplasia and congenital morbus cordis: report of three cases. Arch Dis Child 15:65, 1940.
116. Polymeropoulos MH, Ide SE, Wright M, et al. The gene for the Ellis-van Creveld syndrome is located on chromosome 4p16. Genomics 35:1, 1996.
117. Ruiz-Perez VL, Ide SE, Strom TM, et al. Mutations in a new gene in Ellis-van Creveld syndrome and Weyers acrodental dysostosis. Nat Genet 24:283, 2000.
118. Ruiz-Perez VL, Tompson SW, Blair HJ, et al. Mutations in two nonhomologous genes in a head-to-head configuration cause Ellis-van Creveld syndrome. Am J Hum Genet 72:728, 2003.
119. Williams JCP, Barratt-Boyes BG, Lowe JB. Supravalvular aortic stenosis. Circulation 24:1311, 1961.
120. Burn J: Williams syndrome. J Med Genet 23:389, 1986.
121. Morris CA: Genetic aspects of supravalvular aortic stenosis. Curr Opin Cardiol 13:214, 1998.
122. Ewart AK, Morris CA, Atkinson D, et al. Hemizygosity at the elastin locus in a developmental disorder, Williams syndrome. Nat Genet 5:11, 1993.
123. Lowery MC, Morris CA, Ewart A, et al. Strong correlation of elastin deletions, detected by FISH, with Williams syndrome: evaluation of 235 patients. Am J Hum Genet 57:49, 1995.
124. Curran ME, Atkinson DL, Ewart AK, et al. The elastin gene is disrupted by a translocation associated with supravalvular aortic stenosis. Cell 73:159, 1993.
125. Ewart AK, Jin W, Atkinson D, et al. Supravalvular aortic stenosis associated with a deletion disrupting the elastin gene. J Clin Invest 93:1071, 1994.
126. Urban Z, Michels VV, Thibodeau SN, et al. Supravalvular aortic stenosis (SVAS): predominance of truncating point mutations within the elastin gene. Am J Hum Genet 63:A390, 1998.
127. Vissers LE, van Ravenswaaij CM, Admiraal R, et al. Mutations in a new member of the chromodomain gene family cause CHARGE syndrome. Nat Genet 36:955, 2004.

IV

Normal Circulatory Physiology

6

Fetal and Transitional Circulation

MICHAEL D. FREED, MD

FETAL CIRCULATION

Most of our modern understanding of the circulation before birth comes from more than 40 years of research on fetal lambs.[1–6]

The fetal circulation is arranged in parallel, rather than in a series, the right ventricle delivering the majority of its output to the placenta for oxygenation, and the left ventricle delivering the majority of its output to the heart, brain, and upper part of the body (Fig. 6-1).[7] However, there is a mixing of the streams at the atrial and great vessel level that diverts blood from the immature lungs to the placenta for oxygen exchange. This parallel circulation permits fetal survival despite a wide variety of complex cardiac lesions.

Normally, blood returning from the placenta via the umbilical venous return splits in the liver; some of it goes into the hepatic veins and the portal system of the liver, whereas the remainder (slightly over half) passes through the ductus venous into the inferior vena cava near its junction with the right atrium. In the right atrium, the blood from the inferior vena cava is divided into two streams by the crista dividens. About 40% of the blood returning from the inferior vena cava (27% of the combined ventricular output) passes across the foramen ovale into the left atrium where it joins with the pulmonary venous return from the lung, passing through the mitral valve into the left ventricle. This blood is then pumped out the ascending aorta where it supplies the coronary, carotid, and subclavian arteries, with approximately a third of this stream (10% of combined ventricular output) passing across the aortic arch into the descending aorta.

Most blood returning from the inferior vena cava joins the superior vena caval drainage and coronary sinus return before passing through the tricuspid valve into the right ventricle and pulmonary artery. Because the fluid-filled lungs and constricted pulmonary arterioles offer a high resistance to flow, most of the blood, almost 90%, passes not to the lungs, but through the open ductus arteriosus into the low-resistance descending aorta and placenta.

The oxygen content of the blood in the fetus is considerably lower than that in the neonate or child, because of the lower efficiency of the placenta compared with the lung as an organ for oxygen exchange (Fig. 6-2). Blood returning from the placenta via the umbilical veins has the highest PO_2 (32–25 mm Hg; oxygen saturation, 70%). The blood that passed into the left ventricle has already mixed with the less saturated vena caval and pulmonary venous return, lowering the PO_2 to 26 to 28 mm Hg (oxygen saturation about 65%) before its distribution to the ascending aorta and upper half of the body.

The umbilical venous return destined for the right ventricle mixes with the superior vena caval return (PO_2 > 12–14 mm Hg; oxygen saturation, 40%), reducing the oxygen content of blood passing into the right ventricle, main pulmonary artery, and descending aorta to about 20 to 22 mm Hg (oxygen saturation, 50%–55%). Thus, blood with the highest oxygen content is diverted to the coronary arteries and brain and that with the lowest oxygen content is diverted to the placenta, increasing the efficiency of oxygen pickup. An additional fetal adaptation to oxygen transport at low oxygen saturations is the presence of high levels of fetal hemoglobin with its high affinity for oxygen and its low p50 (partial pressure of oxygen at the point where 50% of the hemoglobin is oxidized) of approximately 18 or 19 mm Hg. The leftward shift of the oxygen association curve facilitates oxygen uptake at the relatively low PO_2 levels of the placental vasculature.

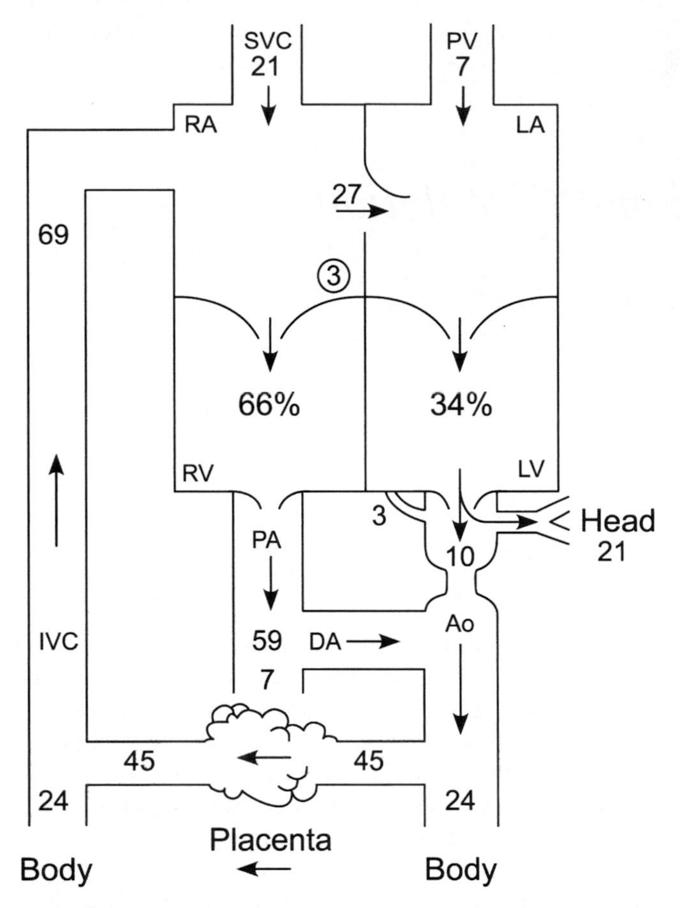

FIGURE 6–1 *The course of the circulation in the late gestation fetal lamb. The numbers represent the percentage of combined ventricular output. Some of the return from the inferior vena cava (IVC) is diverted by the crista dividens in the right atrium (RA) through the foramen ovale into the left atrium (LA), where it meets the pulmonary venous return (PV) and passes into the left ventricle (LV) and is pumped into the ascending aorta. Most of the ascending aortic flow goes to the coronary, subclavian, and carotid arteries, with only 10% of combined ventricular output passing through the aortic arch (indicated by the narrowed point in the aorta) into the descending aorta (AO). The remainder of the inferior vena cava flow mixes with return from the superior vena cava (SVC) and coronary veins (3%) and passes into the right atrium and right ventricle (RV) and is pumped into the pulmonary artery (PA). Because of the high pulmonary resistance, only 7% passes through the lungs (PV), with the rest going into the ductus arteriosus (DA) and then to the descending aorta (AO), to the placenta and lower half of the body.*
Modified from Rudolph AM: Congenital Diseases of the Heart. Armonk, NY: Futura Publishing, 2001, pp 3–44, with permission.

The wide communication between the atria allows for equalization of pressures in the atria (Fig. 6-3); similarly, the patency of the ductus arteriosus results in equalization of pressures in the aorta and pulmonary artery. Because atrial and great vessel pressures are equal, in the absence of pulmonic or aortic stenosis, the ventricular pressures

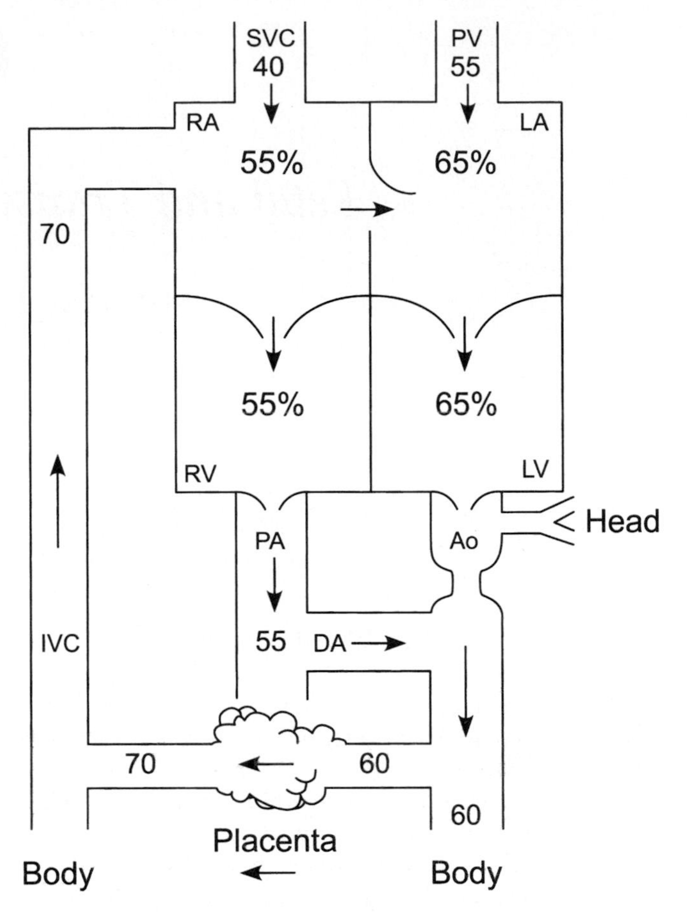

FIGURE 6–2 *The numbers indicate the percent of oxygen saturation in the late gestation lamb. The oxygen saturation is the highest in the inferior vena cava, representing flow that is primarily from the placenta. The saturation of the blood in the heart is slightly higher on the left side than on the right side. The abbreviations in this diagram are the same as in Figure 6-1. Modified from Rudolph AM: Congenital Diseases of the Heart. Armonk, NY: Futura Publishing, 2001, pp 3–44, with permission.*

are equal also, with a systolic pressure of approximately 70 mm Hg, using amniotic pressure as zero.

The fetus has a limited ability to adjust cardiac output. The primary determinants of cardiac output are heart rate, filling pressure (preload), resistance against which the ventricles eject (afterload), and myocardial contractility. Spontaneous changes in heart rate are associated with electrocortical activity as well as with the sleep rate and fetal activity. Using continuous measurements of left and right ventricular output, utilizing electromagnetic flow probes, Rudolph and Heymann[8] have shown that spontaneous increases in heart rate are associated with increasing ventricular output, whereas decreases in heart rate result in a considerable fall of both right and left ventricular output. By electrically pacing the right atrium above the resting level of 160 to 180 beats per minute, the left

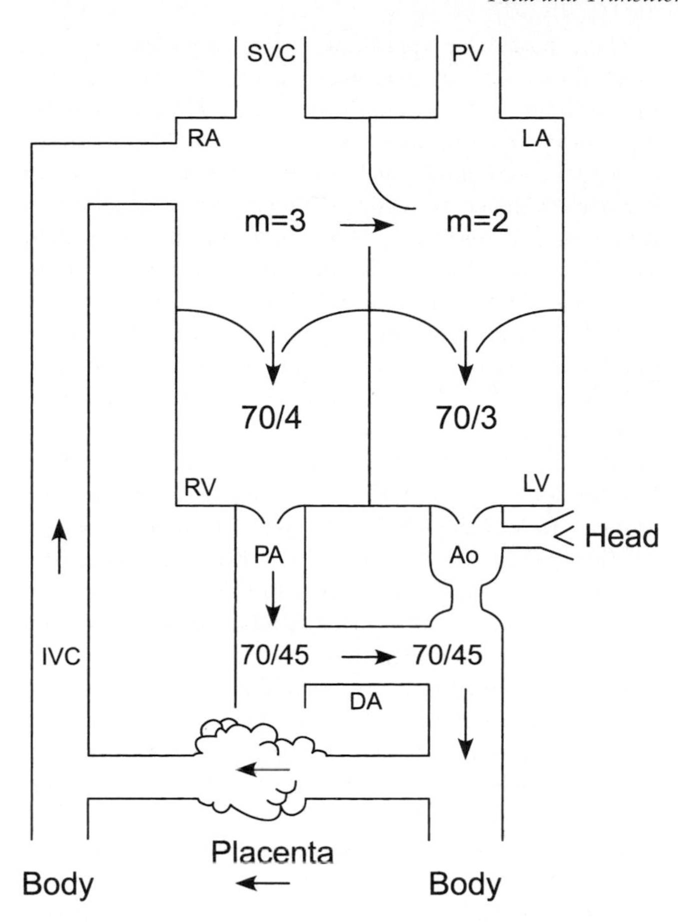

FIGURE 6–3 *The numbers indicate the pressures observed in late gestation lambs. Because large communications between the atrium and great vessels are present, the pressures on both sides of the heart are virtually identical. The abbreviations are the same as in Figure 6-1.*
Modified from Rudolph AM: Congenital Diseases of the Heart. Armonk, NY: Futura Publishing, 2001, pp 3–44, with permission.

ventricular output eventually increases to about 15% above resting levels. Decreasing the heart rate by 50% by vagal stimulation caused a fall in output of approximately 30%.

Contrary to the significant effects of increasing or decreasing heart rate on fetal cardiac output, increasing preload (even to levels as high as a right atrial pressure of 20 mm Hg) produces only very small increases in the ventricular output,[9] suggesting that the fetal ventricle normally functions near the top of its function curve and has little reserve to increase cardiac output. Increasing the work of the heart by increasing afterload (by inflating a balloon in the fetal descending aorta or by methoxamine)[10] produces a dramatic fall in right ventricular output, suggesting that the fetal heart is very sensitive to increases in afterload.

Morphometric studies on the fetal myocardium have demonstrated a significant decrease in myofibrillar content per tissue volume, suggesting that the fetal myocardium has much less contractile tissue than the adult. The active tension produced in excised strips of fetal myocardium was less than that produced by adult myocardium,[11] possibly because of the myofibrillar content, a reduced content of sarcoplasmic reticulum and/or the T-tubule system.[12]

All of the above data suggest that the fetal myocardium is structurally and functionally immature compared with that of the older child or adult. The fetal heart appears to work at the peak of its ventricular function curve, with increases in preload causing little or no change in the cardiac output, and increases in afterload resulting in a marked depression. The limited ability of the fetal heart to respond to stress seems to be mediated primarily through increasing the heart rate.

The structure, hemodynamics, and myocardial function of the fetal circulation have significant consequences in the neonate with congenital heart disease.

1. The parallel circulation, with connections at the atrial and great vessel level, allows a wide variety of cardiac malformations to provide adequate transport of blood to the placenta to pick up oxygen and deliver it to the tissues.
2. The right ventricle performs approximately two thirds of the cardiac work before birth. This is reflected in the size and thickness of the right ventricle before and after birth and may explain why left-sided defects are poorly tolerated after birth, compared with right-sided lesions.
3. Because the normal flow across the aortic isthmus is small (10% of ventricular output), the aortic isthmus is especially vulnerable to small changes in intracardiac flow from various congenital defects. This may account for the relatively high incidence of narrowing (coarctation of the aorta) or atresia (interrupted aortic arch) in this region.
4. Because the pulmonary flow *in utero* is very small compared with that immediately after birth, anomalies preventing normal pulmonary return (total anomalous pulmonary return, mitral stenosis, etc.) may be masked *in utero* when pulmonary venous return is so low anyway.
5. The low levels of circulating oxygen before birth (Po_2, 26–28 mm Hg in the ascending aorta and 20–22 mm Hg in the descending aorta) may account for the relative level of comfort of infants with cyanotic heart disease who may be quite active and comfortable, and may feed well with an arterial Po_2 of 20 to 25 mm Hg, a level that would lead to cerebral and cardiac anoxia, acidosis, and death within a few minutes for the older child or adult.

6. The limited ability of the fetal myocardium to respond to stress makes the hemodynamic consequences of congenital heart disease after birth that much more difficult to tolerate.
7. Birth is a time of stress for the left ventricle. Because of the switch from parallel to serial circulation, there is an increased amount of blood to pump. The ductus arteriosus may, at least briefly, shunt left to right. The work of respiration must be assumed. Of greater importance is the loss of the incubator effect of the uterus; the body metabolism and the circulation must adapt to maintaining body temperature. The possible role of the thyroid in these events has been noted.[13]

TRANSITIONAL CIRCULATION

Within a few moments of birth, profound changes must occur as the newborn rapidly switches from the placenta to the lung as the organ of respiration.[2,14] Failure of any one of a complex series of pulmonary or cardiac events that take place within minutes of birth leads to generalized hypoxemia and brain damage or death.

Soon after the onset of spontaneous respiration, the placenta is removed from the circulation, either by clamping the umbilical cord or, more naturally, by constriction of the umbilical arteries. This suddenly increases the systemic resistance as the lower-resistance placenta is excluded from the circulation. At approximately the same time the onset of spontaneous respiration expands the lungs and brings oxygen to the pulmonary alveoli. Reduction in the pulmonary vascular resistance results from simple physical expansion of the vessels and from the chemo-reflex vasodilation of the pulmonary arteries caused by the high level of oxygen in the alveolar gas.

This sudden increase in systemic vascular resistance and drop in pulmonary vascular resistance causes a reversal of the flow through the ductus arteriosus and an increase in pulmonary flow. Before birth the relative pulmonary and systemic resistances cause 90% of the blood to go through the ductus arteriosus into the descending aorta; by a few minutes after birth 90% goes to the pulmonary arteries, with the pulmonary blood flow increasing from 35 mL/kg/min to 160 to 200 mL/kg/min.

The rapid drop in systemic venous return to the inferior vena cava as the umbilical venous flow is cut off, as well as the increase in pulmonary venous return as the pulmonary blood flow increases, causes the left atrial pressure to rise and the right atrial pressure to fall. When left atrial pressure exceeds right atrial pressure, the flap valve of the foramen ovale closes against the edge of the crista dividens, eliminating left-to-right or right-to-left shunting (Fig. 6-3).

There have been questions in the past regarding how much these marked circulatory changes are influenced by the mechanical changes in the lung parenchyma due to the onset of ventilation, how much by the vasodilatory effects of oxygen, and how much by the increase in systemic vascular resistance, with constriction of the umbilical vessels removing low-resistance placenta from the circulation. Tietel,[15] using monitored fetal sheep near term, found that ventilation alone caused dramatic changes in the central flow patterns, attributable to a large decrease in pulmonary vascular resistance and an associated increase in pulmonary blood flow. Ventilation alone increased the pulmonary venous return from 8% of combined ventricular output to 31%, whereas right ventricular output (which had formerly ejected 90% to the ductus arteriosus) was reduced to less than 50%. Oxygenation further changed the flow patterns so that more than 90% of the flow from the main pulmonary artery went to the lungs rather than through the ductus arteriosus. Umbilical cord occlusion had few additional effects.

Usually, the ductus arteriosus remains patent for several hours or days after birth. Initially, the pulmonary vascular resistance exceeds systemic vascular resistance so that there is a small right-to-left (pulmonary artery-to-aorta) shunt with some systemic desaturation to the lower half of the body. Anything that increases the pulmonary vascular resistance, such as acidosis, hypoxemia, polycythemia, or lung disease, may exacerbate or prolong the normal transient left-to-right shunt. Within a few hours of birth, however, in the normal child, the pulmonary vascular resistance has fallen lower than systemic vascular resistance, resulting in a small "physiologic" left-to-right (aorta-to-pulmonary artery) shunt. Normally, within 10 to 15 hours of birth, the ductus arteriosus has closed, although permanent structural closure may not take place for another 2 to 3 weeks.

The mechanism of closure of the ductus arteriosus is not completely understood. It has been clear for some time that oxygen plays a role.

Coceani and Olley[16] have shown that prostaglandins of the E series are responsible for maintaining patency of the ductus arteriosus during fetal life. It has been possible to keep the ductus open for days, weeks, or months, or even longer in infants with congenital heart disease, by infusion of exogenous prostaglandin E,[17] and it has been possible to close the ductus arteriosus in about 80% of preterm infants weighing less than 1750 g with indomethacin, a nonselective prostaglandin synthetase inhibitor.[18]

Clyman and coworkers[19] observed a decrease in the ability of the ductus arteriosus to dilate and contract within a few hours of postnatal ductal constriction, before the loss of an anatomically patent lumen, in both human newborns and full-term lambs. They postulated that this change reflects early ischemic damage to the inner muscle wall.

Fay and Cooke[20] proposed that irreversibility reflects a mechanical restraint imposed by cellular necrosis, with a loss of intact endothelium leading to constriction from opposing walls until an anatomic lumen is eliminated. The etiology of the necrosis is unknown but it has been postulated that it is caused by interruption of luminal blood flow.

Although some hypoxemia is present soon after birth, because of right-to-left shunting through the ductus arteriosus over the first few hours of life, with continued vasodilation and improved ventilation/perfusion ratios, the normal arterial Po_2 gradually increases from 50 mm Hg at 10 minutes to 62 at 1 hour and 75-83 between 3 hours and 2 days of age. With continued vasodilation the pulmonary pressure gradually falls to about 30 torr within approximately 48 hours. Although further falls in the pulmonary vascular resistance continue for several weeks, the transition to adult circulation is virtually completed within the first few days of life.

REFERENCES

1. Barcroft J. Researches of Pre-natal Life. Springfield, IL: Charles C. Thomas, 1947.
2. Dawes GS. Foetal and Neonatal Physiology: A Comparative Study of the Changes at Birth. Chicago: Year Book Medical Publishers, 1968, pp 90–101, 160–187.
3. Lind J, Wegelius C. Human fetal circulation: changes in the cardiovascular system at birth and disturbances in the post-natal closure of the foramen ovale and ductus arteriosus. Cold Spring Harbor Symposium. Quant Biol 19:109, 1054.
4. Lind J, Stern L, Wegelius C. Human Foetal Neonatal Circulation. Springfield, IL: Charles C Thomas, 1964.
5. Rudolph AM, Heymann MA. The circulation of the fetus in utero. Circ Res 21:163, 1967.
6. Rudolph AM, Heymann MA. Circulatory changes with growth in the fetal lamb. Circ Res 26:289, 1970.
7. Rudolph AM. Congenital Disease of the Heart. Chicago: Year Book Publishers, 1974, pp 1–48.
8. Rudolph AM, Heymann MA. Cardiac output in the fetal lamb: the effects of spontaneous and induced changes of heart rate on right and left ventricular output. J Obstet Gynecol 124:183, 1976.
9. Heymann MA, Rudolph AM. Effects of increasing preload on right ventricular output in fetal lambs in-utero (abstract). Circulation 48(Suppl):37, 1973.
10. Gilbert RD. Effects of afterload and baroreceptors on cardiac function in fetal sheep. J Dev Physiol 4:299, 1982.
11. Friedman WF. The intrinsic properties of the developing heart. In Friedman WF, Lesch M, Sonnenblick EH (eds): Neonatal Heart Disease. New York: Grune and Stratton, 1973, pp 21–49.
12. Hoerter J, Mazet F, Vassort G. Perinatal growth of the rabbit cardiac cell: possible implications for the mechanism of relaxation. J Mol Cell Cardiol 13:725, 1982.
13. Breall JA, Rudolph AM, Heymann MA. Role of thyroid hormone in postnatal circulatory and metabolic adjustments. J Clin Invest 73:1418-1424, 1984.
14. Rudolph AM. Congenital diseases of the heart. Circulation 41: 343 , 1970.
15. Teitel DF, Iwamoto HS, Rudolph AM. Effects of birth related events on central flow patterns. Pediatr Res 22:557, 1987.
16. Coceani F, Olley PM. The response of the ductus arteriosus to prostaglandins. J Physiol Pharmacol 51:220, 1973.
17. Freed MD, Heymann MA, Lewis AB, et al. Prostaglandin E in infants with ductus arteriosus dependent congenital heart disease. Circulation 64:899, 1981.
18. Gersony WM, Peckham GJ, Ellison RC, et al. Effects of indomethacin in premature infants with patent ductus arter-isosus: results of a national collaborative study. J Pediatr 102:895, 1983.
19. Clyman RI, Mauray F, Roman C, et al. Factors determining the loss of ductus arteriosus responsiveness to prostaglandin E. Circulation 68:433, 1984.
20. Fay FS, Cooke PH. Guinea pig ductus arteriosus, II: Irreversible closure after birth. Am J Physiol 222:841, 1972.

V

Problems Caused by Heart Disease

7

Congestive Heart Failure

ELIZABETH D. BLUME, MICHAEL D. FREED,
AND STEVEN D. COLAN

The clinical syndrome of heart failure is the final common pathway of a complex combination of structural, functional, and biologic mechanisms. Compared with adults, children have a markedly different spectrum of etiologies as well as distinct cardiac physiology, clinical presentations, and compensatory mechanisms. The past 35 years have been characterized by a continuous improvement in surgical alternatives and outcomes, and as these patients survive to adulthood, they have created an entire new category of heart disease: the adult with postoperative, otherwise fatal congenital heart disease. This and many other changes in the field of pediatric cardiology limit the availability of disease-specific information concerning the physiology and therapy of congestive heart failure in pediatric congenital and acquired heart disease.

EPIDEMIOLOGY

The incidence of heart failure in children is difficult to estimate. The incidence of the various forms of cardiomyopathy in children has been recently published[1,2] and is presented in Chapter 26, although only a minority of these patients have heart failure. The incidence of heart failure in young children with congenital heart disease has fallen in conjunction with improved surgical options for these patients, including routine neonatal repairs that are undertaken before the onset of symptoms of heart failure. In contrast, the incidence of heart failure in patients who have previously undergone palliative surgery continues to rise as the life expectancy for these children improves. Data concerning the incidence and prevalence of heart failure in children are difficult to compile because the symptom complex is relatively nonspecific and often transient, and patients tend to be categorized according to the underlying disorder rather than the presence or absence of congestive heart failure.

ETIOLOGY

The etiology of heart failure in children is summarized in Tables 7-1 and 7-2. This listing is not comprehensive, but accounts for most cases. In general, the neurohumoral response that eventually results in the variable symptom complex known as *congestive heart failure* is elicited when the hemodynamic demands on the heart exceed the pressure- or flow-generating capacity of the systemic pump due to either inadequate inflow or inadequate outflow. Limited inflow capacity is characteristic of disorders such as pericardial disease, restrictive cardiomyopathy, mitral stenosis, and pulmonary venous obstruction. In contrast to adult populations in whom non–valve-related diastolic heart failure (which has been labeled *heart failure with normal systolic function*) accounts for 40% to 50% of heart failure cases,[3,4] a similar clinical syndrome is virtually unknown in pediatric populations. Limited outflow capacity characterizes disorders such as dilated cardiomyopathy and systemic outflow obstruction. Congestive heart failure in the volume overload lesions (shunts and valvar regurgitation) is typically manifest when a limited diastolic capacity is accompanied by a limited systolic capacity. Congestive heart failure can ensue when normal hemodynamic demands are imposed on myocardium with diminished contractile capacity

TABLE 7–1. Etiology of Heart Failure in the Structurally Normal Heart

Prenatal
Anemia
Arrhythmia
Arteriovenous fistula
Cardiomyopathy
Twin–twin transfusion
Neonates and Infants
Anemia
Arrhythmia
Arteriovenous fistula
Dilated cardiomyopathy
Endocrinopathies
Hypoglycemia
Hypothyroidism
Hypoxic ischemic injury
Hypertension
Infection/sepsis
Kawasaki syndrome
Childhood
Acquired valve disorders
Anemia
Arrhythmia
Dilated cardiomyopathy
Hypertension
Renal failure
Restrictive cardiomyopathy

TABLE 7–2. Etiology of Heart Failure in Patients with Congenital Heart Disease

Prenatal
Atrioventricular valve regurgitation
Mitral stenosis with intact atrial septum
Neonates and Infants
Systemic outflow obstruction
Aortic valve stenosis
Coarctation of the aorta
Subaortic stenosis
Truncal valve stenosis
Systemic inflow obstruction
Cor triatriatum
Mitral stenosis
Pulmonary venous stenosis
Systemic ventricular volume overload
Aortic or mitral regurgitation
Aortopulmonary window
Atrial septal defect
Atrioventricular canal defect
Patent ductus arteriosus
Single ventricle
Totally anomalous pulmonary veins
Truncus arteriosus
Ventricular septal defect
Children
Aortic regurgitation
Mitral regurgitation
Mitral stenosis
Pulmonary vein stenosis

(e.g., cardiomyopathy), when an excess load is imposed on normal myocardium (e.g., arteriovenous fistula), or when a combination of the two occurs. Thus, heart failure may occur with or without *myocardial failure*, a term that specifically refers to contractile dysfunction.

The distinctions as to the presence or absence of congenital heart disease and the presence or absence of myocardial dysfunction are fundamental to the management and prognosis of heart failure in children and young adults. For most forms of congenital heart disease, repair or palliation of the underlying cardiac malformation provides the most salutary effect, whereas alternative methods of managing the symptoms of congestive heart failure are generally less than satisfactory. Similarly, therapy of congestive heart failure that is secondary to nonmyocardial factors such as anemia or renal failure is rarely successful unless the primary cause can be mitigated.

Myocardial dysfunction can be encountered as a consequence of a wide range of disorders that affect the myocardium primarily, such as myocarditis, or as part of a multisystem disorder such as muscular dystrophy. The various forms of cardiomyopathy and the associated disorders are considered in detail in Chapter 26. In addition, a large percentage of children with end-stage heart failure (between 25% and 75%, depending on the age group) have an underlying diagnosis of congenital heart disease.[5] In these patients, even an initially tolerated elevated cardiac workload, if chronically sustained, can lead to cardiac maladaptation and eventual myocardial failure. This situation is by no means unique to pediatrics, having been recognized in patients of all ages with lesions such as chronic severe aortic regurgitation. This chronologic succession of myocardial adaptation followed eventually by myocardial injury and contractile dysfunction has been aptly labeled the *cardiomyopathy of overload*. In contrast to adult patients, in whom ischemic heart disease accounts for two of three cases,[6] children can experience a similar transition without detectable ischemic injury.

The etiology of ventricular dysfunction depends also on the age at presentation. For example, in the newborn period, myocardial dysfunction is rare; however, structural problems that were silent *in utero* secondary to parallel circulations and high pulmonary vascular resistance often present in response to the normal neonatal fall in pulmonary vascular resistance. Similarly, the right ventricle, by way of the ductus arteriosus, can help supply systemic blood flow that would usually derive from the left ventricle. This support mechanism can mask the presence of critical left ventricular outflow obstruction until spontaneous ductal closure, usually during the first week of life. Heart failure from left to right shunts (at the level of the ventricles or the great vessels) typically presents in the third or fourth week. Abnormal heart rate may also lead to congestive heart failure, when the heart rate is either too slow (congenital heart block) or too fast (supraventricular tachycardia). Occasionally, hematologic abnormalities can cause circulatory failure, with severe anemia leading to high output failure and marked polycythemia causing hyperviscosity syndrome. As noted in Table 7-1, other treatable causes of high output failure may be responsible for heart failure in infants with clinical heart failure and preserved or mildly depressed function such as arteriovenous fistulae, hyperthyroidism, and adrenal insufficiency.

By childhood, most congenital lesions have been repaired or palliated. However, congestive heart failure may be seen with chronic valvar regurgitation or progressive ventricular dysfunction. Acquired heart disease, such as myocarditis, endocarditis, idiopathic cardiomyopathy, and complications of other systemic disorders, often first becomes apparent in this age group and is discussed elsewhere in this textbook.

PATHOPHYSIOLOGY

An in-depth review of cardiac pathophysiology is beyond the scope of this text.[7–9] However, because most therapies for congestive heart failure are predicated on interrupting the reflex neurohumoral control mechanisms that account for many of the symptoms of heart failure, it is important to briefly review the physiology of heart failure. As discussed in the foregoing, the unifying feature of the various disparate causes of heart failure is a failure of the heart to keep pace with hemodynamic demands. Although the seminal event is inadequate cardiac output, the cardiovascular system has no flow "sensor" to provide direct feedback to the heart that an increase in flow is required. At the tissue level, flow is controlled by the rate of production and removal of local metabolites. When regional flow is inadequate, the resultant rise in metabolite concentrations stimulates local vasodilation. Flow increases and reduces metabolite concentration, thereby closing the feedback loop. At a system level, the decrease in peripheral resistance causes a fall in blood pressure. Although there are no flow sensors, there are a series of system-level central arterial baroreceptors that respond to the fall in pressure by a series of reflex mechanisms. The sympathetic nervous system (SNS) provides the rapid response reflexes, including adrenergic-mediated tachycardia, stimulation of myocardial contractility, and regional vasoconstriction, in an effort to restore central arterial pressure to normal. The longer-term mechanisms include activation of the renin-angiotensin-aldosterone system (RAAS), which stimulates renal fluid retention to expand vascular volume. The rise in vascular volume improves cardiac filling and restores cardiac output through utilization of preload reserve, again closing the feedback loop. Under normal conditions, these finely tuned control mechanisms maintain pressure, flow, and vascular volume within narrow limits despite significant hemodynamic perturbations. However, when the fall in cardiac output and secondary fall in blood pressure are due to diminished cardiac capacity, utilization of preload reserve may be inadequate to restore cardiac output to normal without an intolerable rise in circulating volume and filling pressure. Under these circumstances, the symptom complex of heart failure, which is primarily a manifestation of systemic and pulmonary venous hypertension, ensues. Ultimately, heart failure is a compromise between the symptoms associated with inadequate cardiac output (euvolemia) and the symptoms associated with venous congestion (hypervolemia).

The SNS and RAAS are critical to sustaining adequate cardiac output, but it has become clear that sustained activation of these systems exacerbates the circulatory disorder. The consequences of chronic volume expansion are well known, with peripheral edema, pulmonary edema, pulmonary hypertension, respiratory insufficiency, and gastrointestinal dysfunction. Less obvious is the potential for these compensatory mechanisms to damage the myocardium directly. For example, aldosterone has been shown to contribute directly to myocyte fibrosis[10] and apoptosis[11] and may thereby contribute to the elevated risk for ventricular arrhythmias and sudden death associated with heart failure. Chronic activation of the SNS is associated with reductions in norepinephrine stores and β-adrenergic receptor density,[12,13] further impairing adrenergically mediated inotropic reserve. The chronic elevation in filling pressure stimulates ventricular remodeling, increasing diastolic capacitance at the expense of elevated systolic wall stress and myocardial oxygen consumption (see Chapter 26). Finally, both the SNS and RAAS stimulate generalized vasoconstriction and redistribution of blood flow, maintaining perfusion of vital organs at the expense of cutaneous, muscular, and renal blood flow.[14,15] Skeletal muscle underperfusion is associated with lactic acidosis secondary to anaerobic metabolism and with symptoms of fatigue and weakness. Diminished renal perfusion causes electrolyte imbalance and nitrogen retention.

The neurohumoral, autocrine, and paracrine alterations associated with heart failure are more pervasive than the foregoing discussion would suggest. In addition to activation of the SNS and RAAS and the counter-regulatory natriuretic peptides, there is augmented release of vasopressin and endothelin, elevated circulating levels of peptide growth factors (e.g., transforming growth factor-α) and inflammatory cytokines (interleukin-1β and tumor necrosis factor-α). These and other local mediators, in conjunction with the autonomic nervous system and circulating hormones, pervasively modulate the function of the cardiovascular system. Additionally, many of these circulating factors impact the growth of cardiovascular tissues and are believed to play an important role in the "remodeling" of myocardium and vasculature.

CLINICAL PRESENTATION

The specific manifestations of heart failure are highly age dependent. Heart failure is fundamentally a constellation of symptoms and physical findings, and although diagnostic testing is crucial for documenting etiology and at times to differentiate heart failure from asthma, pneumonia, or other disorders, such tests do not define the presence or absence of heart failure.

Presentation in Infancy

Feeding difficulties are the most prominent symptoms in infants with heart failure. For the infant, feeding is one of the most physically demanding activities of daily life, and with heart failure, it becomes prolonged, associated with significant tachypnea, tachycardia, and perspiration. The effort of sucking and maintaining a rapid respiratory rate combined with diversion of blood flow to the gut taxes the limited cardiac reserve. Consequently, growth is in many regards the best measure of severity of chronic heart failure in infants. On physical examination, the children are almost invariably tachycardic, with resting heart rates of more than 160 beats/minute in the neonate and more than 120 in the older infant. Tachypnea (a resting respiratory rate greater than 60 breaths/minute in the neonate or greater than 40 in the older infant) is generally noted and is related to increased lung stiffness secondary to increased interstitial fluid from either elevated pulmonary venous pressure (pulmonary edema) or high-flow left-to-right shunts. As heart failure becomes more severe, ventilatory function may become more compromised, and nasal flaring, intercostal retractions, and grunting are seen. Occasionally, examination of the chest shows wheezing that may be confused with bronchiolitis or pneumonia and may be exacerbated by compression of the airways by the distended, hypertensive pulmonary vessels. Rales are rarely audible unless there is coexisting pneumonia, a not infrequent association. The findings at cardiac examination are variable depending on the etiology of the heart failure. Infants with cardiomyopathy usually have a quiet precordium, whereas those with shunt lesions usually have prominent cardiac lifts, and those with obstructive lesions may have a systolic thrill. A mitral regurgitation murmur is common regardless of the underlying disorder. Generally, a third heart sound, even if present, is difficult to appreciate with the rapid heart rates. Distention of the neck veins is rarely noted in neonates but may occasionally be seen in older infants. Hepatomegaly invariably accompanies the elevated systemic venous pressure, but peripheral edema is quite uncommon in infants and is associated with only very severe heart failure. Cool extremities, weakly palpable pulses, and a low arterial blood pressure with narrow pulse pressure may be seen as manifestations of low cardiac output. Mottling of the extremities and slow capillary refill are signs of more severe vascular compromise.

The chest x-ray almost always demonstrates cardiomegaly. Notable exceptions include left atrial obstructive lesions such as cor triatriatum and totally anomalous pulmonary venous connection with obstruction. Excessive pulmonary blood flow is present in those with heart failure secondary to a large left-to-right shunt, and a diffuse haziness secondary to pulmonary venous congestion is found in most of the remainder. Redistribution of pulmonary blood flow to the upper lobes is not diagnostically useful in infants because they spend most of their time supine. Increased lung volumes with hyperexpansion and flattened diaphragms are common, and an enlarged left atrium may cause collapse of the left lower lobe. The electrocardiogram, although almost invariably abnormal, is not useful in assessing heart failure, but it may provide clues to the lesion causing the heart failure. The echocardiogram is the primary diagnostic modality for assessing ventricular function, pericardial effusion, severity of mitral regurgitation, and the presence of associated congenital heart disease.

Presentation in Childhood

The signs and symptoms of congestive heart failure in the older child more closely resemble those in the adult. Breathlessness is a common sign of heart failure in the child. Exertional dyspnea and exaggeration of the usual response of breathlessness on severe exercise are invariably present and correlate in severity with the degree of heart failure. Chronic hacking cough, secondary to congestion of the bronchial mucosa, may also be present in some children. As left atrial pressure increases, the child may develop orthopnea, requiring elevation of the head on several pillows at night. Fatigue and weakness are relatively late manifestations. On physical examination, children with mild or moderate heart failure appear to be in no distress, but those with severe heart failure may be dyspneic at rest. If the onset of heart failure has been relatively abrupt, the child may appear anxious but well nourished; those in whom a more chronic process has occurred usually do not appear anxious but may be malnourished and wasted. Similar to infants, children with more advanced heart failure are usually tachycardic and tachypneic. Low cardiac output may cause peripheral vasoconstriction, resulting in coolness, pallor, and cyanosis of the digits, with poor capillary refill. Increased systemic venous pressure may be detected by distention of the neck veins with venous pulsations visible above the clavicle while the patient is sitting. Hepatomegaly is an early finding, and if the enlargement is relatively acute, there may be flank pain or tenderness owing to stretching of the liver capsule. Although less common than in adults, children may also develop peripheral edema. At first the signs may be subtle, but when there has been a 10% increase in weight, the face, especially the eyelids, begins to appear puffy, and edema develops in dependent parts of the body. Long-standing edema can result in reddening and induration of the skin, usually over the shins and ankles. Exudation of fluid into body cavities may manifest as ascites, pericardial effusion, and, occasionally, hydrothorax. On cardiac examination, there is almost invariably cardiomegaly. The cardiac impulse may be quiet if cardiomyopathy is the cause, but it is usually hyperactive when congestive failure is due to volume overload from a left-to-right shunt or atrioventricular valve regurgitation. A third heart sound occurring in mid-diastole may be a normal finding in children but is more frequently noted in those with heart disease. Pulsus alternans, characterized by a regular rhythm with alternating strong and weak pulsations, can be felt occasionally; however, it is more easily appreciated while measuring blood pressure. Pulsus paradoxus (a fall in blood pressure on inspiration and a rise on expiration), secondary to marked swings in intrapulmonary pressure that affect ventricular filling (as in pericardial tamponade), is seen occasionally in older children.

In children, the chest x-ray almost invariably shows cardiac enlargement. The normal pulmonary arterial flow pattern (i.e., increased flow to the lung bases compared with the apices) is reversed. When the capillary pressures exceed 20 to 25 mm Hg, interstitial pulmonary edema may be seen, causing hazy lung fields, especially in a butterfly pattern around the hila. This may result in Kerley's lines, sharp linear densities in the interlobar septa. In chronic congestive heart failure, proteinuria and high specific gravity of the urine are common findings, and there may be an increase in the blood urea nitrogen and creatinine levels, secondary to reduced renal blood flow. The level of sodium in the urine is usually less than 10 mEq/L. Serum electrolyte values are usually normal before treatment, but hyponatremia, secondary to increased water retention, may be seen in cases of severe, long-standing heart failure. Congestive hepatomegaly and cardiac cirrhosis may lead to abnormalities in liver enzymes or to elevation of bilirubin in rare instances. Although newly discovered congenital heart disease as a cause of congestive heart failure beyond infancy is now rare, the echocardiogram remains the primary diagnostic modality for assessing ventricular function and the contribution of valvar and anatomic abnormalities.

CLASSIFICATION OF SEVERITY OF HEART FAILURE

The New York Heart Association (NYHA) classification is widely used in adult heart failure because of its prognostic value with regard to mortality and symptoms. This scoring system differentiates severity primarily on the basis of activity tolerance and is therefore difficult to apply in young children. Several scoring systems for children have been evaluated. The Ross Classification[16] was developed to score younger children and infants, correlates with plasma norepinephrine levels,[17] has been adopted by the Canadian Cardiovascular Society,[18] and is used in several multicenter pediatric trials. The New York University Pediatric Heart Failure Index is a weighted, linear combination score based on symptoms, signs, and treatment, which appears to correlate with disease in a small group of children compared with normal children.[19] None of these scoring systems have been tested in terms of prognostic capacity for clinical course, response to therapy, or survival. The generalized neuroendocrine activation of heart failure results in measurable elevation of multiple serum markers, and many of these (e.g., norepinephrine, angiotensin, natriuretic peptides type A and B) have been studied to attempt to delineate severity of clinical heart failure.[17,20–23] None has been shown to correlate with survival or need for transplantation in children, however.

DIAGNOSTIC EVALUATION

The diagnostic approach in patients with new-onset heart failure depends in large part on prior probabilities based on the age of the child, presence or absence of congenital heart disease, and coexistent systemic disorders. The most difficult diagnostic dilemmas arise in patients who are free of structural heart disease or other systemic diseases. Electrocardiogram, echocardiogram, and 24-hour Holter monitoring are standard. Most patients undergo evaluation for myocarditis by either endomyocardial biopsy or delayed enhancement cardiac magnetic resonance. In patients with a suspected underlying metabolic disorder or dystrophinopathy, skeletal muscle biopsy is undertaken. Extensive laboratory evaluation to rule out reversible causes of dysfunction are included, such as thyroid function testing, carnitine levels, lactate, and urine organic acids, together with laboratory assessment of severity of heart failure by measurement of natriuretic peptides, serum troponin level, creatinine phosphokinase, and renal and hepatic function tests. As discussed in Chapter 26, the mitochondrial and metabolic disorders represent the most difficult diseases for which to achieve a definitive diagnosis, frequently requiring a time-consuming, stepwise approach.

MANAGEMENT

The successful treatment of congestive heart failure in children is predicated on an understanding of the nature and physiologic consequences of the specific cardiac defect leading to the failure and of the available treatment modalities. For those with structural disease and an associated or aggravating condition that may be the precipitating cause of the heart failure (e.g., fever, dysrhythmias, anemia), prompt recognition and treatment may result in dramatic improvement. If there is a specific anatomic lesion amenable to palliative or corrective surgery, pharmacologic therapy as a bridge to surgical or catheter-based intervention may be warranted. In most other cases of ventricular dysfunction, a variety of general and pharmacologic measures are available to improve the patient's clinical status.

Pharmacologically, the treatment paradigm has been adapted from data acquired in adults with heart failure, based on the documented neurohumoral response and the ability to block this response at several levels. The available pharmacologic agents continue to multiply; thus, any discussion of specific agents becomes rapidly out of date. Furthermore, heart failure is a classic example of the success of polypharmacy, and the relative order of introduction of new medications has evolved and continues to evolve with time.[24] Certain principles, however, are useful in guiding therapy. Afterload reduction is the first line of therapy, escalated to a maximum tolerated dose, with diuretics used primarily to control symptoms of pulmonary insufficiency and peripheral venous congestion. If patients remain symptomatic, digoxin is initiated. An aldosterone-blocking agent is usually added in patients with evidence of dilated cardiomyopathy. If there is severe dysfunction or persistent symptoms, β blockade is added, although the indications for β blockade are evolving rapidly, and it is likely that they will move higher in the list of stepwise therapy.

General Measures

Nutritional intervention is often critical in these patients, who experience an elevated caloric requirement despite a diminished capacity to eat. This includes information from the nutritionist, especially in toddlers who need high-calorie foods. For infants with heart failure, it is crucial to increase the caloric density of the formula or breast milk to aid in growth. Early discussions about gastrostomy tubes are often beneficial. Fluid and dietary salt restriction is generally required in patients with a history of decompensated heart failure. Recommendations as to the level of physical activity are difficult but important. Although there appears to be an increased risk for adverse events associated with intense exercise in patients with moderate to severe ventricular dysfunction, there is nevertheless an overall risk reduction (the so-called paradox of exercise[25]). In general, the benefits of regular exercise participation in terms of survival and improved quality of life outweigh the risks and justify recommending and encouraging exercise for these patients, including organized rehabilitation programs, with certain caveats. Exercise is believed to carry a higher risk in patients with active myocarditis, who are therefore restricted from more than mild levels of exertion during the early phase of the disease.

Angiotensin-Converting Enzyme Inhibitors

As discussed previously, the chronic activation of the SNS and RAAS, although acutely beneficial, contributes to the progression of heart failure over time. The well-documented efficacy of angiotensin-converting enzyme inhibitor (ACEI) therapy in heart failure is related to disruption of the activation of the renin-angiotensin axis and to decreased cardiac adrenergic drive.[26,27] In adults, multiple large clinical trials have shown that therapy with ACEI improves clinical symptoms and survival.[28–31] The SOLVD Treatment Trial[30] showed that enalapril reduced mortality at 2 years by more than 20% in symptomatic patients with low ejection fraction, and the prevention trial showed a decrease of 20% in the composite end point of death and heart failure hospitalizations. Overall, the data in adults indicate that ACEIs improve survival and slow the progression of heart failure, although improvement is often not seen until several weeks after initiation of therapy. These findings have resulted in the recommendation that ACEIs should be used in all patients with heart failure, are intended for long-term use, and should not be stopped unless side effects are intolerable. The experience with ACEIs in children includes several small observational studies[32–36] in infants with heart failure secondary to cardiomyopathy or ventricular volume overload secondary to shunt lesions. Montigny and colleagues[37] found that a single dose of captopril in 12 infants with ventricular septal defects decreased systemic vascular resistance, decreasing the pulmonary-to-systemic flow ratio through an increase in systemic cardiac output, although subsequent studies confirmed this finding only in patients with high systemic vascular resistance at baseline.[38,39]

In the first retrospective data analysis of children with dilated cardiomyopathy treated with ACEIs, Stern and associates[34] showed no change in ejection fraction but a decrease in serum aldosterone. In a larger retrospective analysis of 81 children with dilated cardiomyopathy (mean age 3.6 years), Lewis and coworkers[35] demonstrated increased mortality at 1 year for the patients not taking ACEIs compared with those treated with captopril (30% versus 18%; $P < .05$).

Angiotensin Receptor Blockers

In contrast to the ACEIs, which act by blocking the formation of angiotensin, the angiotensin receptor blockers (ARBs) are competitive antagonists for the angiotensin I (AT_1) receptor. The AT_1 receptors mediate vasoconstriction, aldosterone secretion, sodium resorption, and cell proliferation.[40] The potential advantages to the ARBs include (1) absence of bradykinin breakdown inhibition, which has been implicated in causing the troublesome cough and angioedema that are seen with ACEIs; (2) prevention of "ACE escape"[41–43]; (3) potential for synergism when used in combination with ACEIs; and (4) the theoretical advantage to unopposed AT_2 agonism, which is believed to counter the AT_1 response through vasodilation and antiproliferative effects.[40,44,45] To date, trials in adult patients with heart failure have yielded conflicting results concerning the potential advantage to combination therapy that includes both ARBs and ACEIs.[46–48] ARB therapy appears to represent a reasonable alternative for patients intolerant to ACEIs because rash, chronic cough, and angioedema are not encountered. However, effective doses of ARB represent as much of a risk for hypotension and renal dysfunction as with an ACEI.[49] No safety or efficacy data regarding the use of ARBs in children with heart failure are available. There is very limited reported experience with ARB therapy for pediatric patients.[50] Given the limited pediatric experience, our current practice is to limit the use of these agents to the occasional pediatric patient who is intolerant to ACEIs. In our experience, symptomatic hypotension is rare and can be avoided with careful up-titration of these agents and adjustment of diuretic dosages as necessary on an outpatient basis.

Aldosterone-Blocking Agents

Spironolactone has been in use for many years as a potassium-sparing diuretic, but in 1999, the Randomized Aldactone Evaluation Study (RALES) showed that low-dose spironolactone reduced mortality by 30% in NYHA functional class IV patients. This was not related to the diuretic effect, but rather was specifically due to blockade of aldosterone. This observation is one of many observations over the past 10 years that have implicated aldosterone in a host of adverse biologic effects, including vascular endothelial dysfunction,[51] widespread tissue injury and fibrosis,[52] and myocyte apoptosis.[11] Introduction of ACEIs into standard therapy of heart failure led to reduced use of spironolactone because of the belief that any adverse effects of aldosterone would be prevented by ACEIs and because of concerns that combined use might lead to hyperkalemia. However, although ACEIs induce an acute fall in plasma aldosterone levels, there is a gradual rise in serum concentration that may eventually exceed the pretreatment level, a phenomenon labeled *aldosterone escape*.[53,54] Although confirmation of the survival benefit related to spironolactone therapy in heart failure has not been specifically demonstrated in children, the favorable risk profile justifies its use. The survival benefit of aldosterone blockade in patients with heart failure has also been demonstrated for eplerenone, an aldosterone blocker that does not share spironolactone's affinity for androgen receptors and is therefore not associated with gynecomastia and impotence. There is no reported pediatric experience with eplerenone.

Diuretics

Diuretics are drugs that increase the urinary excretion of salt and water. They act indirectly by increasing renal blood flow or, more commonly, by directly inhibiting solute and water absorption, thereby increasing urine volume. Diuretics may have an effect in the proximal tubule (carbonic anhydrase inhibitors such as acetazolamide), the loop of Henle (furosemide, ethacrynic acid, bumetanide), or the distal convoluted tubule (thiazides, spironolactone). The most commonly used diuretic in pediatrics is furosemide. By blocking the luminal transport in the loop of Henle, reabsorption of sodium and chloride is prevented, and up to 25% of the filtered sodium can be excreted, removing water with it. If given intravenously, the response is usually prompt and impressive when there is an adequate cardiac output. Few data are available concerning the appropriate use of diuretics, but their use is widespread because of the substantial symptomatic relief they provide. Current guidelines in adult patients recommend the use of diuretics in all patients with heart failure and fluid retention in order to achieve a euvolemic state.

Side effects of diuretics therapy must be monitored closely. Hypokalemia can be treated with spironolactone. Hyponatremia should be aggressively treated with restriction of free-water intake because the diuretics are less effective when serum sodium is low. Similarly, metabolic alkalosis secondary to chloride depletion is seen occasionally with the potent loop diuretics and, along with volume contraction, stimulates aldosterone production, which should be avoided. Oral potassium chloride supplements may be effective, but if the alkalosis persists, ammonium chloride may be used for replacement.

Digitalis

The principal myocardial effect of the digitalis glycosides is to increase the force and the velocity of cardiac muscle contraction. This "inotropic" effect is present in cardiac but not skeletal muscle; is dependent on the concentration of a number of ions, including potassium, sodium, calcium, and magnesium; and is entirely independent of the adrenergic system. The inotropic effects result from digitalis binding to, and thereby inhibiting, sodium-potassium (Na-K) adenosine triphosphatase, the enzyme that maintains high intracellular concentrations of sodium in myocardial cells. This poisoning of the sodium pump alters the excitation–contraction coupling, making more calcium available to the contractile elements, increasing the force of contraction.

For children with myocardial failure, this inotropic effect appears to increase cardiac output,[55–57] resulting in a reduction or elimination of symptoms. Low doses of digoxin have been shown to be as effective as higher doses in preventing worsening heart failure in adults,[56] which may reduce the incidence of side effects. Whether it is possible to achieve similar dose reduction in children is unknown, particularly because young patients have long been believed to require and tolerate higher digoxin doses than adults.[58] Despite evidence of symptom relief, several large cohort studies conducted in adults treated for heart failure with digoxin have failed to demonstrate improved survival.[59–62] Virtually no pediatric data are available concerning whether digoxin improves survival in heart failure due to myocardial dysfunction. Digoxin therapy for symptomatic relief of heart failure in infants and children with myocardial dysfunction is generally justified on the basis of controlled trials in adults and limited data in children, along with a strong theoretical base and years of clinical experience.

Despite common usage, the therapeutic utility of digoxin in infants with heart failure due to shunt lesions such as patent ductus arteriosus and ventricular septal defects has a much shakier basis. The symptoms of heart failure in these patients are associated with a diminished forward stroke volume despite normal ventricular function.[63,64] Myocardial contractility appears to be normal in these patients and does not change significantly with digoxin.[65,66] These and other observations have led to considerable skepticism concerning the efficacy of digoxin therapy in these patients.[67–69]

Much of the proven utility of digoxin relates to its electrophysiologic effects, the most important of which is an increase in the effective refractory period of the conduction system, which tends to slow the ventricular response to atrial fibrillation or atrial flutter. In addition, digitalis increases the sensitivity of the arterial baroreceptor reflex, resulting in an increase in vagal and a decrease in sympathetic efferent activity, thereby reducing the resting heart rate.

β Blockade

There is significant clinical and experimental evidence that the stimulation of the sympathetic nervous system contributes to the pathophysiology of chronic heart failure in adults.[21,70,71] The results of multiple clinical trials show a reduction in morbidity and mortality in patients with heart failure treated with β-adrenergic antagonists as adjunctive therapy.[72] Multiple large clinical trials in adults have demonstrated improvements in left ventricular ejection fraction and reductions in rates of hospitalization or listing for transplantation.[73–79] A highly significant 65% reduction in risk for all causes of mortality was noted in a combined analysis of more than 1094 patients enrolled in the U.S. Carvedilol Heart Failure Program.[72,80] Meta-analysis of published, randomized, placebo-controlled trials concluded that β-adrenergic blockade improves ejection fraction and lowers the combined risk for death and hospitalization as a result of heart failure.[81] Studies have also suggested an improvement in functional status, as measured by NYHA classification.[73,74,78,79] Improvements in quality of life or exercise tolerance by treadmill assessment have not been demonstrated.

From a safety standpoint, β-adrenergic antagonists have been used in children for multiple reasons with few side effects. Atenolol has been shown to be safe in healthy children with isolated supraventricular tachycardia in a long-term study,[82] esmolol has been used in postoperative hypertension in children after cardiac surgery,[83] and propranolol has been used safely and effectively in critically ill burn patients.[84] Shaddy and colleagues[85] retrospectively reviewed the effect of metoprolol in four children with dilated cardiomyopathy and found an improvement in ventricular performance and symptoms, with few side effects.

Bruns and associates[86] retrospectively reviewed the use of carvedilol in 46 infants and children with cardiomyopathy (80%) or congenital heart disease (20%) at six centers. All patients were receiving standard treatment with digoxin, diuretics, and ACE inhibitors for at least 3 months before the start of β-blocker therapy. After 3 months of carvedilol, modified NYHA class improved in 67% of patients and worsened in 11%. Side effects, mainly dizziness, hypotension, and headache, occurred in 54% of patients. In a single-center study, Rusconi and coworkers[87] reviewed the results in 24 pediatric patients with dilated cardiomyopathy and showed an improvement in mean left ventricular ejection fraction from 25% to 42% ($P < .001$). The NYHA class improved in 15 patients, 1 patient died, and 3 patients underwent transplantation. In our experience[88] with 20 patients, 12 with dilated cardiomyopathy and 8 with ventricular dysfunction secondary to congenital heart disease at a median age of 8.4 years (range, 7 months to 17 years), median ejection fraction of the treated group improved over the study period (31% to 38%; $P = .08$). In this prospective single-arm study of pediatric patients with dilated cardiomyopathy, the use of adjunct carvedilol improved ejection fraction as compared with untreated controls and trended toward delaying time to transplantation or death. Adverse events included hypoglycemia, bradycardia, and fatigue.

Resynchronization Therapy

Atrioventricular and intraventricular conduction delays adversely affect ventricular function, particularly in patients with dilated cardiomyopathy. Asynchronous contraction impairs systolic function, reduces cardiac output, and elevates end-systolic stress.[89] When contraction is asynchronous, relaxation becomes asynchronous as well, causing both systolic and diastolic dysfunction. Biventricular or left ventricular pacing in patients with heart failure and left bundle branch block lowers ventricular filling pressure,[90] reduces adrenergic activity,[89] and improves systolic function without an increase in myocardial oxygen consumption.[90] A meta-analysis of existing trials, including 809 patients with cardiac resynchronization therapy (CRT) and 825 controls, concluded that CRT results in a 51% reduction in heart failure–associated mortality, although all-cause mortality was not reduced by CRT.[91] Because devices that are capable of both biventricular pacing and defibrillator therapies are now available, it has become common practice to implant these devices,[92] confounding efforts to distinguish which type of intervention is responsible for any survival benefit.

Use of this therapy has primarily relied on the electrocardiographic diagnosis of bundle branch block and QRS prolongation, despite the fact that the relationship between electrical and mechanical dyssynchrony is weak.[93] Direct methods of measuring mechanical noncoherence using Doppler[94] and magnetic resonance imaging[95] methods are being pursued as improved alternatives to patient selection criteria based on electrocardiograms and appear to provide a better predictor of a favorable response to CRT.[96–99]

Application of CRT therapy to children is anecdotal and therefore highly biased toward benefit.[100–106] Many issues remain unresolved in the proper patient selection for this nascent but extremely promising therapy. The risk profile and device longevity are considerably different in pediatric populations compared with adults.[107] Patient selection criteria remain undefined, and many candidate patients have congenital heart disease in conjunction with myocardial failure, increasing the complexity of predicting therapeutic benefit. There appears to be little doubt about the potential for this mode of therapy to become an integral part of the management of children with heart failure, although much work remains to be done to define the disease- and age-specific risk-to-benefit ratios.

Surgery

As discussed earlier, surgical repair of congenital lesions that increase the hemodynamic burden of the patient with heart failure is clearly a priority. However, surgical interventions targeted at improving the function of the failing ventricle have also been explored. In 1997, Batista and associates[108] reported on partial left ventriculectomy as a treatment for patients with end-stage heart failure due to dilated cardiomyopathy. The goal of the surgery is to restore a normal mass-to-volume ratio and wall stress by reducing ventricular volume, and success in this regard has been reported.[109] There also appears to be a salutary effect on ventricular synchrony.[110] This intervention trades an acute reduction in left ventricular capacitance for an acute reduction in systolic wall stress and in this regard is similar to the Myosplint device that is currently undergoing clinical testing.[111] When partial left ventriculectomy is performed in patients with poor ventricular function, there is functional improvement without survival benefit.[112] The primary obstacle to the success of this procedure that has been encountered is a high rate of unmanageable ventricular arrhythmias,[113] severely limiting survival.[114] The experience with this procedure in children is purely anecdotal. Cardiac replacement with heart transplantation has become a standard surgical therapy for end-stage disease and is discussed in detail in Chapter 60.

In summary, treatment of heart failure in infants, children, and young adults is a rapidly evolving field that has completely changed in the past 10 years and promises to continue to do so as our knowledge of pathophysiology and basic science expands. Interventions such as stem cell isolation, modification, and implantation, as well as gene therapy, are already being explored, and their introduction into clinical investigation is on the horizon. Any description of the state of the art in this field is clearly a dated snapshot of the status quo that will be eclipsed as new pharmacologic and surgical therapies continue to evolve.

REFERENCES

1. Lipshultz SE, Sleeper LA, Towbin JA, et al. The incidence of pediatric cardiomyopathy in two regions of the United States. N Engl J Med 348:1647, 2003.
2. Nugent AW, Daubeney PEF, Chondros P, et al. The epidemiology of childhood cardiomyopathy in Australia. N Engl J Med 348:1639, 2003.
3. Gaasch WH, Zile MR. Left ventricular diastolic dysfunction and diastolic heart failure. Annu Rev Med 55:373, 2004.
4. Kessler KM. Is diastolic heart failure synonymous with heart failure with preserved ejection fraction? J Am Coll Cardiol 42:1335, 2003.

5. Boucek MM, Edwards LB, Keck BM, et al. The Registry of the International Society for Heart and Lung Transplantation: Sixth Official Pediatric Report-2003. J Heart Lung Transplant 22:636, 2003.
6. Gheorghiade M, Bonow RO. Chronic heart failure in the United States: A manifestation of coronary artery disease. Circulation 97:282, 1998.
7. Dzau VJ. Autocrine and paracrine mechanisms in the pathophysiology of heart failure. Am J Cardiol 70:4C, 1992.
8. Francis GS, McDonald K, Chu C, et al. Pathophysiologic aspects of end-stage heart failure. Am J Cardiol 75:11A, 1995.
9. Francis GS. Neuroendocrine activity in congestive heart failure. Am J Cardiol 66:33D, 1990.
10. Struthers AD, MacDonald TM. Review of aldosterone- and angiotensin II-induced target organ damage and prevention. Cardiovasc Res 61:663, 2004.
11. Mano A, Tatsumi T, Shiraishi J, et al. Aldosterone directly induces myocyte apoptosis through calcineurin-dependent pathways. Circulation 110:317, 2004.
12. Ungerer M, Böhm M, Elce JS, et al. Altered expression of β-adrenergic receptor kinase and β_1-adrenergic receptors in the failing human heart. Circulation 87:454, 1993.
13. Ungerer M, Hartmann F, Karoglan M, et al. Regional in vivo and in vitro characterization of autonomic innervation in cardiomyopathic human heart. Circulation 97:174, 1998.
14. Leier CV. Regional blood flow in human congestive heart failure. Am Heart J 124:726, 1992.
15. Muller AF, Batin P, Evans S, et al. Regional blood flow in chronic heart failure: The reason for the lack of correlation between patients' exercise tolerance and cardiac output. Br Heart J 67:478, 1992.
16. Ross RD, Bollinger RO, Pinsky WW. Grading the severity of congestive heart failure in infants. Pediatr Cardiol 13:72, 1992.
17. Ross RD, Daniels SR, Schwartz DC, et al. Plasma norepinephrine levels in infants and children with congestive heart failure. Am J Cardiol 59:911, 1987.
18. Johnstone DE, Abdulla A, Arnold JM, et al. Diagnosis and management of heart failure. Canadian Cardiovascular Society. Can J Cardiol 10:613, 1994.
19. Connolly D, Rutkowski M, Auslender M, et al. The New York University Pediatric Heart Failure Index: A new method of quantifying chronic heart failure severity in children. J Pediatr 138:644, 2001.
20. Westerlind A, Wahlander H, Lindstedt G, et al. Clinical signs of heart failure are associated with increased levels of natriuretic peptide types B and A in children with congenital heart defects or cardiomyopathy. Acta Paediatr 93:340, 2004.
21. Buchhorn R, Ross RD, Bartmus D, et al. Activity of the renin-angiotensin-aldosterone and sympathetic nervous system and their relation to hemodynamic and clinical abnormalities in infants with left-to-right shunts. Int J Cardiol 78:225, 2001.
22. Ross RD, Daniels SR, Dolan LM, et al. Determinants of plasma atrial natriuretic factor concentrations in congenital heart disease. Am J Cardiol 62:785, 1988.
23. Ross RD, Daniels SR, Schwartz DC, et al. Return of plasma norepinephrine to normal after resolution of congestive heart failure in congenital heart disease. Am J Cardiol 60: 1411, 1987.
24. Rosenthal D, Chrisant MR, Edens E, et al. International society for heart and lung transplantation: Practice guidelines for management of heart failure in children. J Heart Lung Transplant 23:1313, 2004.
25. Maron BJ. The paradox of exercise. N Engl J Med 343: 1409, 2000.
26. Swedberg K, Eneroth P, Kjekshus J, et al. Hormones regulating cardiovascular function in patients with severe congestive heart failure and their relation to mortality. Circulation 82:1730, 1990.
27. Effects of enalapril on mortality in severe congestive heart failure. Results of the Cooperative North Scandinavian Enalapril Survival Study (CONSENSUS). The CONSENSUS Trial Study Group. N Engl J Med 316:1429, 1987.
28. Cohn JN, Johnson G, Ziesche S, et al. A comparison of enalapril with hydralazine-isosorbide dinitrate in the treatment of chronic congestive heart failure. N Engl J Med 325:303, 1991.
29. The SOLVD Investigators. Effect of enalapril on mortality and the development of heart failure in asymptomatic patients with reduced left ventricular ejection fractions. N Engl J Med 327:685, 1992.
30. Effect of enalapril on survival in patients with reduced left ventricular ejection fractions and congestive heart failure. The SOLVD Investigators. N Engl J Med 325:293, 1991.
31. Packer M. Do angiotensin-converting enzyme inhibitors prolong life in patients with heart failure treated in clinical practice? J Am Coll Cardiol 28:1323, 1996.
32. Leversha AM, Wilson NJ, Clarkson PM, et al. Efficacy and dosage of enalapril in congenital and acquired heart disease. Arch Dis Child 70:35, 1994.
33. Seguchi M, Nakazawa M, Momma K. Effect of enalapril on infants and children with congestive heart failure. Cardiol Young 2:14, 1992.
34. Stern H, Weil J, Genz T, et al. Captopril in children with dilated cardiomyopathy: Acute and long-term effects in a prospective study of hemodynamic and hormonal effects. Pediatr Cardiol 11:22, 1990.
35. Lewis AB, Chabot M. The effect of treatment with angiotensin-converting enzyme inhibitors on survival of pediatric patients with dilated cardiomyopathy. Pediatr Cardiol 14:9, 1993.
36. Mori Y, Nakazawa M, Tomimatsu H, et al. Long-term effect of angiotensin-converting enzyme inhibitor in volume overloaded heart during growth: A controlled pilot study. J Am Coll Cardiol 36:270, 2000.
37. Montigny M, Davignon A, Fouron J-C, et al. Captopril in infants for congestive heart failure secondary to a large ventricular left-to-right shunt. Am J Cardiol 63:631, 1989.
38. Rheuban KS, Carpenter MA, Ayers CA, et al. Acute hemodynamic effects of converting enzyme inhibition in infants with congestive heart failure. J Pediatr 117:668, 1990.
39. Shaddy RE, Teitel DF, Brett C. Short-term hemodynamic effects of captopril in infants with congestive heart failure. Am J Dis Child 142:100, 1988.
40. Unger T. The role of the renin-angiotensin system in the development of cardiovascular disease. Am J Cardiol 89: 3A, 2002.

41. Petrie MC, Padmanabhan N, McDonald JE, et al. Angiotensin converting enzyme (ACE) and non-ACE dependent angiotensin II generation in resistance arteries from patients with heart failure and coronary heart disease. J Am Coll Cardiol 37:1056, 2001.
42. Urata H, Healy B, Stewart RW, et al. Angiotensin II-forming pathways in normal and failing human hearts. Circ Res 66: 883, 1990.
43. Ennezat PV, Berlowitz M, Sonnenblick EH, et al. Therapeutic implications of escape from angiotensin-converting enzyme inhibition in patients with chronic heart failure. Curr Cardiol Rep 2:258, 2000.
44. Gring CN, Francis GS. A hard look at angiotensin receptor blockers in heart failure. J Am Coll Cardiol 44:1841, 2004.
45. McMurray JJ, Pfeffer MA, Swedberg K, et al. Which inhibitor of the renin-angiotensin system should be used in chronic heart failure and acute myocardial infarction? Circulation 110:3281, 2004.
46. Cohn JN, Tognoni G, for the Valsartan Heart Failure Trial Investigators. A randomized trial of the angiotensin-receptor blocker valsartan in chronic heart failure. N Engl J Med 345:1667, 2001.
47. Maggioni AP, Anand I, Gottlieb SO, et al. Effects of valsartan on morbidity and mortality in patients with heart failure not receiving angiotensin-converting enzyme inhibitors. J Am Coll Cardiol 40:1414, 2002.
48. Pfeffer MA, McMurray JJV, Velazquez EJ, et al. Valsartan, captopril, or both in myocardial infarction complicated by heart failure, left ventricular dysfunction, or both. N Engl J Med 349:1893, 2003.
49. Granger CB, McMurray JJ, Yusuf S, et al. Effects of candesartan in patients with chronic heart failure and reduced left-ventricular systolic function intolerant to angiotensin-converting-enzyme inhibitors: The CHARM-Alternative trial. Lancet 362:772, 2003.
50. Tanaka H, Suzuki K, Nakahata T, et al. Combined therapy of enalapril and losartan attenuates histologic progression in immunoglobulin A nephropathy. Pediatr Int 46:576, 2004.
51. Rocha R, Rudolph AE, Frierdich GE, et al. Aldosterone induces a vascular inflammatory phenotype in the rat heart. Am J Physiol Heart Circ Physiol 283:H1802, 2002.
52. Rocha R, Chander PN, Khanna K, et al. Mineralocorticoid blockade reduces vascular injury in stroke-prone hypertensive rats. Hypertension 31:451, 1998.
53. Lee AF, MacFadyen RJ, Struthers AD. Neurohormonal reactivation in heart failure patients on chronic ACE inhibitor therapy: A longitudinal study. Eur J Heart Fail 1:401, 1999.
54. MacFadyen RJ, Lee AFC, Morton JJ, et al. How often are angiotensin II and aldosterone concentrations raised during chronic ACE inhibitor treatment in cardiac failure? Heart 82:57, 1999.
55. Skudicky D, Essop MR, Sareli P. Time-related changes in left ventricular function after double valve replacement for combined aortic and mitral regurgitation in a young rheumatic population: Predictors of postoperative left ventricular performance and role of chordal preservation. Circulation 95:899, 1997.
56. Packer M, Gheorghiade M, Young JB, et al. Withdrawal of digoxin from patients with chronic heart failure treated with angiotensin-converting-enzyme inhibitors. RADIANCE Study. N Engl J Med 329:1, 1993.
57. Adams KF, Jr., Gheorghiade M, Uretsky BF, et al. Clinical benefits of low serum digoxin concentrations in heart failure. J Am Coll Cardiol 39:946, 2002.
58. Kearin M, Kelly JG, O'Malley K. Digoxin "receptors" in neonates: An explanation of less sensitivity to digoxin than in adults. Clin Pharmacol Ther 28:346, 1980.
59. Hood WB Jr., Dans AL, Guyatt GH, et al. Digitalis for treatment of congestive heart failure in patients in sinus rhythm: A systematic review and meta-analysis. J Card Fail 10: 155, 2004.
60. Guyatt GH, Sullivan MJJ, Fallen EL, et al. A controlled trial of digoxin in congestive heart failure. Am J Cardiol 61:371, 1988.
61. Guyatt GH, Devereaux PJ. A review of heart failure treatment. Mt Sinai J Med 71:47, 2004.
62. Jaeschke R, Oxman AD, Guyatt GH. To what extent do congestive heart failure patients in sinus rhythm benefit from digoxin therapy? A systematic overview and meta-analysis. Am J Med 88:279, 1990.
63. Corin WJ, Swindle MM, Spann JF Jr., et al. Mechanism of decreased forward stroke volume in children and swine with ventricular septal defect and failure to thrive. J Clin Invest 82:544, 1988.
64. Gidding SS, Bessel M. Hemodynamic correlates of clinical severity in isolated ventricular septal defect. Pediatr Cardiol 14:135, 1993.
65. Kimball TR, Daniels SR, Meyer RA, et al. Effect of digoxin on contractility and symptoms in infants with a large ventricular septal defect. Am J Cardiol 68:1377, 1991.
66. Kimball TR, Daniels SR, Meyer RA, et al. Relation of symptoms to contractility and defect size in infants with ventricular septal defect. Am J Cardiol 67:1097, 1991.
67. Redington AN, Carvalho JS, Shinebourne EA. Does digoxin have a place in the treatment of the child with congenital heart disease? Cardiovasc Drugs Ther 3:21, 1989.
68. Schmaltz AA. Congestive heart failure in infancy and childhood. Klin Padiatr 211:1, 1999.
69. Hougen TJ. Digitalis use in children: An uncertain future. Prog Pediatr Cardiol 12:37, 2000.
70. Cohn JN. Sympathetic nervous system in heart failure. Circulation 106:2417, 2002.
71. Joseph J, Gilbert EM. The sympathetic nervous system in chronic heart failure. Prog Cardiovasc Dis 41:9, 1998.
72. Packer M, Bristow MR, Cohn JN, et al. The effect of carvedilol on morbidity and mortality in patients with chronic heart failure. US Carvedilol Heart Failure Study Group. N Engl J Med 334:1349, 1996.
73. Waagstein F, Bristow MR, Swedberg K, et al. Beneficial effects of metoprolol in idiopathic dilated cardiomyopathy. Lancet 342:1441, 1993.
74. CIBIS Investigators and Committees. A randomized trial of beta-blockade in heart failure. The Cardiac Insufficiency Bisoprolol Study (CIBIS). Circulation 90:1765, 1994.
75. Australia/New Zealand Heart Failure Research Collaborative Group. Randomised, placebo-controlled trial of carvedilol in

patients with congestive heart failure due to ischaemic heart disease. Lancet 349:375, 1997.
76. Bristow MR, Gilbert EM, Abraham WT, et al. Carvedilol produces dose-related improvements in left ventricular function and survival in subjects with chronic heart failure. Circulation 94:2807, 1996.
77. Packer M, Colucci WS, Sackner-Bernstein JD, et al. Double-blind, placebo-controlled study of the effects of carvedilol in patients with moderate to severe heart failure. The PRECISE Trial. Circulation 94:2793, 1996.
78. Colucci WS, Packer M, Bristow MR, et al. Carvedilol inhibits clinical progression in patients with mild symptoms of heart failure. US Carvedilol Heart Failure Study Group. Circulation 94:2800, 1996.
79. Cohn JN, Fowler MB, Bristow MR, et al. Safety and efficacy of carvedilol in severe heart failure. US Carvedilol Heart Failure Study Group. J Card Fail 3:173, 1997.
80. Fowler MB. Effects of beta blockers on symptoms and functional capacity in heart failure. Am J Cardiol 80:55L, 1997.
81. Lechat P, Packer M, Chalon S, et al. Clinical effects of beta-adrenergic blockade in chronic heart failure: A meta-analysis of double-blind, placebo-controlled, randomized trials. Circulation 98:1184, 1998.
82. Ko JK, Ban JE, Kim YH, et al. Long-term efficacy of atenolol for atrioventricular reciprocating tachycardia in children less than 5 years old. Pediatr Cardiol 25:97, 2004.
83. Wiest DB, Garner SS, Uber WE, et al. Esmolol for the management of pediatric hypertension after cardiac operations. J Thorac Cardiovasc Surg 115:890, 1998.
84. Maykel JA, Pazirandeh S, Bistrian BR. Beta-blockade and severe burns. N Engl J Med 346:707, 2002.
85. Shaddy RE, Olsen SL, Bristow MR, et al. Efficacy and safety of metoprolol in the treatment of doxorubicin-induced cardiomyopathy in pediatric patients. Am Heart J 129:197, 1995.
86. Bruns LA, Chrisant MK, Lamour JM, et al. Carvedilol as therapy in pediatric heart failure: An initial multicenter experience. J Pediatr 138:505, 2001.
87. Rusconi P, Gomez-Marin O, Rossique-Gonzalez M, et al. Carvedilol in children with cardiomyopathy: 3-Year experience at a single institution. J Heart Lung Transplant 23:832, 2004.
88. Blume ED, Canter CE, Spicer RL, et al. Prospective Multi-Center Trial of Adjunct Carvedilol in Pediatric Patients With Moderate Ventricular Dysfunction [abstract]. Circulation 106:II-361, 2004.
89. Leclercq C, Kass DA. Retiming the failing heart: Principles and current clinical status of cardiac resynchronization. J Am Coll Cardiol 39:194, 2002.
90. Nelson GS, Berger RD, Fetics BJ, et al. Left ventricular or biventricular pacing improves cardiac function at diminished energy cost in patients with dilated cardiomyopathy and left bundle-branch block. Circulation 102:3053, 2000.
91. Bradley DJ, Bradley EA, Baughman KL, et al. Cardiac resynchronization and death from progressive heart failure: a meta-analysis of randomized controlled trials. J Am Med Assoc 289:730, 2003.
92. Bradley DJ. Combining resynchronization and defibrillation therapies for heart failure. J Am Med Assoc 289:2719, 2003.
93. Leclercq C, Faris O, Tunin R, et al. Systolic improvement and mechanical resynchronization does not require electrical synchrony in the dilated failing heart with left bundle-branch block. Circulation 106:1760, 2002.
94. Yu CM, Chau E, Sanderson JE, et al. Tissue Doppler echocardiographic evidence of reverse remodeling and improved synchronicity by simultaneously delaying regional contraction after biventricular pacing therapy in heart failure. Circulation 105:438, 2002.
95. Zwanenburg JJM, Götte MJW, Kuijer JPA, et al. Timing of cardiac contraction in humans mapped by high-temporal-resolution MRI tagging: Early onset and late peak of shortening in lateral wall. Am J Physiol Heart Circ Physiol 286: H1872, 2004.
96. Pitzalis MV, Iacoviello M, Romito R, et al. Cardiac resynchronization therapy tailored by echocardiographic evaluation of ventricular asynchrony. J Am Coll Cardiol 40:1615, 2002.
97. Pitzalis MV, Iacoviello M, Romito R, et al. Ventricular asynchrony predicts a better outcome in patients with chronic heart failure receiving cardiac resynchronization therapy. J Am Coll Cardiol 45:65, 2005.
98. Bax JJ, Marwick TH, Molhoek SG, et al. Left ventricular dyssynchrony predicts benefit of cardiac resynchronization therapy in patients with end-stage heart failure before pacemaker implantation. Am J Cardiol 92:1238, 2003.
99. Bax JJ, Bleeker GB, Marwick TH, et al. Left ventricular dyssynchrony predicts response and prognosis after cardiac resynchronization therapy. J Am Coll Cardiol 44:1834, 2004.
100. Bevilacqua LM, Berul CI. Advances in pediatric electrophysiology. Curr Opin Pediatr 16:494, 2004.
101. Blom NA, Bax JJ, Ottenkamp J, et al. Transvenous biventricular pacing in a child after congenital heart surgery as an alternative therapy for congestive heart failure. J Cardiovasc Electrophysiol 14:1110, 2003.
102. Janousek J, Tomek V, Chaloupecky V, et al. Dilated cardiomyopathy associated with dual-chamber pacing in infants: Improvement through either left ventricular cardiac resynchronization or programming the pacemaker off allowing intrinsic normal conduction. J Cardiovasc Electrophysiol 15:470, 2004.
103. Janousek J, Vojtovic P, Hucín B, et al. Resynchronization pacing is a useful adjunct to the management of acute heart failure after surgery for congenital heart defects. Am J Cardiol 88:145, 2001.
104. Nurnberg JH, Butter C, Abdul-Khaliq H, et al. Successful cardiac resynchronization therapy in a 9-year-old boy with dilated cardiomyopathy. Z Kardiol 94:44, 2005.
105. Strieper M, Karpawich P, Frias P, et al. Initial experience with cardiac resynchronization therapy for ventricular dysfunction in young patients with surgically operated congenital heart disease. Am J Cardiol 94:1352, 2004.
106. Zimmerman FJ, Starr JP, Koenig PR, et al. Acute hemodynamic benefit of multisite ventricular pacing after congenital heart surgery. Ann Thorac Surg 75:1775, 2003.
107. Alexander ME, Cecchin F, Walsh EP, et al. Implications of implantable cardioverter defibrillator therapy in congenital heart disease and pediatrics. J Cardiovasc Electrophysiol 15:72, 2004.

108. Batista RJV, Verde J, Nery P, et al. Partial left ventriculectomy to treat end-stage heart disease. Ann Thorac Surg 64:634, 1997.
109. Dickstein ML, Spotnitz HM, Rose EA, et al. Heart reduction surgery: An analysis of the impact on cardiac function. J Thorac Cardiovasc Surg 113:1032, 1997.
110. Schreuder JJ, Steendijk P, Van der Veen FH, et al. Acute and short-term effects of partial left ventriculectomy in dilated cardiomyopathy: Assessment by pressure-volume loops. J Am Coll Cardiol 36:2104, 2000.
111. Guccione JM, Salahieh A, Moonly SM, et al. Myosplint decreases wall stress without depressing function in the failing heart: A finite element model study. Ann Thorac Surg 76:1171, 2003.
112. Kawaguchi AT, Bergsland J, Linde LM. Ventricular volume reduction procedures. J Card Surg 18:S29, 2003.
113. Pastore CA, Arcencio SR, Tobias NM, et al. QT interval dispersion analysis in patients undergoing left partial ventriculectomy (Batista operation). Ann Noninvasive Electrocardiol 9:375, 2004.
114. Bestetti RB. Long-term follow-up of patients undergoing isolated partial left ventriculectomy. Acta Cardiol 59:405, 2004.

8

Hypoxemia

ALEXANDER S. NADAS AND DONALD C. FYLER

Congestive heart failure and hypoxemia are the two principal handicaps that may result from congenital heart disease. Heart failure, as discussed in Chapter 7, is a clinical syndrome (a combination of signs and symptoms) based on certain physiologic phenomena (increased end-diastolic ventricular pressure and inadequate cardiac output to meet the metabolic needs). By contrast, hypoxemia is a biochemical phenomenon (arterial oxygen saturation lower than 90% in room air) that is associated with a number of clinical signs and symptoms. It may be reasonable to state right at the outset that hypoxemia may be due to respiratory causes or to a right-to-left shunt (i.e., the mixture of venous into arterial blood) within or without the heart. The simplest way to differentiate between respiratory and shunt (cardiac) cyanosis is by determining the arterial Po_2 (through an arterial puncture or pulse oximetry) at room air after 100% oxygen has been inhaled for 10 minutes, the "hyperoxia test." The resting, room-air, arterial Po_2 is normally between 90 and 100 mm Hg (+5%). In patients with hypoxemia, arterial Po_2 may vary anywhere from 10 to 80 mm Hg. If the hypoxemia is respiratory in nature, inhalation of 100% oxygen will raise it to between 400 and 500 mm Hg. By contrast, in shunt cyanosis, the Po_2 seldom, if ever, rises above 150 mm Hg in all extremities.

It is a particularly useful test in the newborn nursery, especially when emergency echocardiography service is not available. In this situation, Po_2 transcutaneous values are measured in room air and in oxygen from all extremities. The latter is necessary to take into account arm and leg differences, which may occur depending on the cardiac lesion. For example, in interrupted aortic arch, the right arm values will be normal, whereas those in the lower limbs will be abnormally low because of right to left ductal flow ("differential cyanosis"). In contrast, in the infant with transposition of the great arteries and intact ventricular septum, right arm values are less than those in the lower extremities ("reverse differential cyanosis").

For practical purposes, in the older patient, an oxygen test is not necessary to differentiate between cardiac and respiratory cyanosis. When watching the patient quietly, in the office or at the bedside, the increased respiratory effort of respiratory hypoxemia is usually quite obvious. Plain chest films will also quickly reveal pulmonary pathology and show depressed diaphragms. In rare cases in which the distinction is not clear, the oxygen test is helpful.

CLINICAL CORRELATES OF HYPOXEMIA

Having defined the chemical substrate of hypoxemia and discussed the two principal causes, one should list, briefly, the clinical correlates of hypoxemia. It should be noted that surgical management strategies of the past couple of decades, by emphasizing early repair, have virtually eliminated the incidence of some of these, such as squatting and spells in the young. However, others, such as cyanosis, clubbing, and polycythemia, persist for a variety of reasons.

Cyanosis

Cyanosis is the bluish color of the skin, best noted at the fingernails, toenails, and mucous membranes of the lips and conjunctivae. More than 80 years ago, Lundsgaard and Van Slyke[1] determined that the abnormal color becomes perceptible when 5 g of reduced hemoglobin is present in the capillaries (instead of the normal 2.25 g), corresponding to about 70% saturation with a normal hemoglobin level. The experienced observer can usually detect saturation of

80% to 85%, corresponding, under average circumstances (i.e., hemoglobin, 15 g), to 3 g of reduced hemoglobin.

Cyanosis may be present even if the arterial saturation is normal. This occurs most commonly if the cardiac output is reduced and the arteriovenous difference widens from the usual 40% to as much as 60% or more, giving rise to an increased amount of reduced hemoglobin at the capillary level. The amount of reduced hemoglobin required for this phenomenon is the same as for shunt cyanosis; only the mechanism by which it is created is different. Low-output cyanosis is acrocyanosis: it is most notable (even exclusively so) at the tip of the fingers or the top of the nose, but not so much at the mucous membranes. Patients with acrocyanosis usually have cool extremities and small pulse volume. Clinical conditions resulting in low-output cyanosis include, among others, critical mitral stenosis and pulmonary vascular obstructive disease.

Another instance of visible cyanosis, not associated with arterial unsaturation, is due to polycythemia. In children, this is most common in the newborn period when the hematocrit and hemoglobin are normally very high. The normal arteriovenous difference of about 40% can easily give rise to more than 3 g of reduced hemoglobin in the capillaries of these neonates. All pediatricians, and even obstetricians, are familiar with the plethoric cyanosis of newborns, which sometimes may be hard to differentiate from hypoxemia.

The reciprocal of that phenomenon, the absence of cyanosis in the face of true hypoxemia due to low hematocrit or hemoglobin level, should also be discussed here. For instance, in the case of anemia, with a hemoglobin of 10 g and an average arteriovenous difference of 40%, the amount of reduced hemoglobin in the capillaries may not be more than 2 g; thus, no cyanosis may be detected, although the arterial saturation is 80%.

Therefore, when discussing cyanosis, three factors should be considered: (1) arterial oxygen saturation, (2) oxygen capacity (hemoglobin), and (3) arteriovenous oxygen difference. Cyanosis will be noted if the arterial oxygen saturation is low, if the oxygen capacity is high, or if the arteriovenous difference is increased.

Clubbing

A common and striking concomitant of hypoxemia is clubbing, or hypertrophic osteoarthropathy (see Fig. 11-1 in Chapter 11). In its fully developed form, this consists of widening and thickening of the ends of the fingers and toes accompanied by convex (hourglass-shaped) fingernails. Earlier forms of clubbing consist of shininess and tenseness of the skin over the terminal phalanges, obliterating the wrinkles usually present in this part of the skin. The incipient clubbing is usually accompanied by fiery red finger, a characteristic of early slight arterial unsaturation. Full-blown clubbing in severely cyanotic children may be seen as early as 2 or 3 weeks of age; ordinarily, however, it does not make its appearance until a child is 1 or 2 years old. For some reason, it appears earliest and most pronounced on the thumbs. Physiologic and histologic studies indicate that clubbed fingers have an increased number of capillaries and increased blood flow through a myriad of arteriovenous aneurysms.[2] This is accompanied by an increase in connective tissue in the terminal phalanges.

In children, clubbing almost always indicates congenital heart disease of the cyanotic variety, although occasionally cirrhosis of the liver, infective endocarditis, lung abscess, malabsorption syndromes, or even a familial hereditary condition may be responsible.

Polycythemia

Polycythemia, with increased hemoglobin content, is another consequence of arterial unsaturation. That a low arterial oxygen content acts as a stimulus to bone marrow (through release of erythropoietin from the kidneys) has been amply demonstrated, not only in patients with congenital malformation of the heart but also in people living at high altitudes with low atmospheric tension.[3] The increased oxygen-carrying capacity and oxygen delivery achieved by this means constitute a useful compensatory mechanism until the polycythemia reaches hematocrit levels of 80% or more. At these levels, however, the benefits derived from the increase in available oxygen are probably outweighed by the disadvantages of the high viscosity; actually, capacity increased beyond a "reasonable level" (70% to 75% hematocrit) may result in decreased oxygen delivery. The therapeutic implications of these considerations are discussed later.

Children whose hematocrit level rises during adolescence may become symptomatic. Initially, the symptoms are vague, such as feeling logy, being tired, having a full sensation in the head, and having headaches. Later, the symptoms are no longer vague; the patient simply cannot do what was possible before. Symptoms begin to appear when the hematocrit reaches levels in excess of 70%. Among adults, the hemoglobin manufacturing capacity is quite remarkable, producing amounts to maintain an arterial oximetry value of about 85% at rest. It is important that the hematocrit be measured by the centrifuging technique because the density methods in common use give erroneous readings for these high levels. On examination, murmurs, readily audible before, may no longer be heard, the viscosity having a significant influence on the turbulence required to produce an audible murmur. Symptoms are relieved by reducing the hematocrit. This is best accomplished by a pheresis machine that removes the hemoglobin from the blood and returns the plasma. The hematocrit is continuously monitored and is reduced by 10%; a greater reduction would reduce oxygen-carrying capacity to an uncomfortable degree. The frequency of this procedure at Children's Hospital Boston has decreased significantly from 40 in 1987 to 7 in 2001, reflecting decreasing numbers of both older survivors and earlier diagnosis and surgery. The same result can be attained by removing blood and replacing it with an equal volume of plasma or albumin, as is done occasionally in the cardiac catheterization laboratory. It is important to maintain the blood volume or else the arterial pressure may fall, and in the presence of a ventricular defect, this would result in increased right-to-left shunting and decreased pulmonary blood flow.[4] Phlebotomy, for these reasons, is contraindicated.

The long-term medical problems of hypoxemia, cyanosis, and polycythemia (Fig. 8-1), including renal dysfunction[5,6] and possible implications of elevated natriuretic peptides,[7] are discussed in Chapter 56.

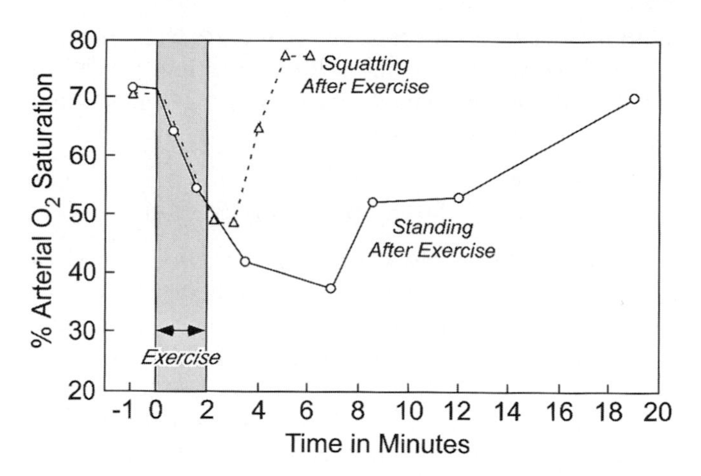

FIGURE 8–2 *Effect of squatting on exercise-induced arterial oxygen unsaturation in a patient with cyanotic heart disease. From Nadas AS, Fyler DC. Pediatric Cardiology. Philadelphia: WB Saunders, 1973.*

Squatting

Squatting is a characteristic posture assumed after exertion by patients with certain types of cyanotic congenital heart disease, specifically tetralogy of Fallot and, less commonly, pulmonary stenosis with an open foramen ovale[8] (Fig. 8-2). It first makes its appearance at 1 or 2 years of age, or when the child starts walking. Usually, although not invariably, social pressure abolishes it at 8 to 10 years of age.

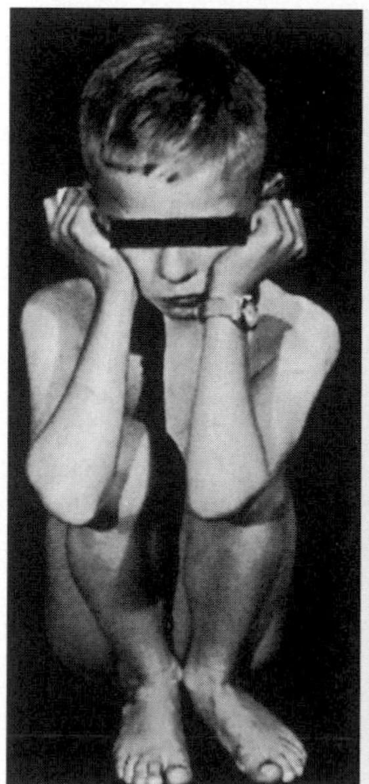
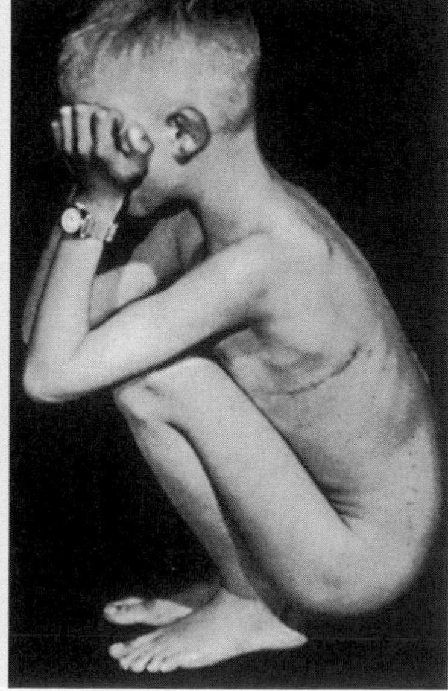

FIGURE 8–1 *Child squatting.*
From Nadas AS, Fyler DC. Pediatric Cardiology. Philadelphia: WB Saunders, 1973.

Detailed studies at Children's Hospital Boston and elsewhere[9] indicate that oxygen saturation, diminished by effort, can be raised to normal more rapidly in a squatting than in a standing position (Fig. 8-3). Probably, this beneficial effect is caused by exclusion of the highly unsaturated lower extremity blood from the circulation, augmenting the peripheral resistance and thus diminishing the degree of right-to-left shunt. That initial increased systemic venous return also occurs in squatting is demonstrated by the fact that immediately after assumption of this characteristic posture, a brief drop in oxygen saturation occurs, corresponding to the "dumping" of highly unsaturated blood from the

Diagnosis

- Tricuspid Atresia
- Transposition of the Great Arteries
- Pulmonary Vascular Obstructive Disease

Age 4 years (1970) - pulmonary artery pressure systemic, deemed inoperable

Age 21 years - HCT 71%; brain abscess - drained surgically

Age 26 years - Gout

Currently age 38 years. Cheerful, marked cyanosis and clubbing, grade 3/6 murmur of pulmonary insufficiency, intermittent episodes of hemoptysis and seizures; Hct 69%, multiple red cell phereses throughout years.

FIGURE 8–3 *Example of problems encountered in a patient with long-standing polycythemia and hypoxia.*

inferior vena cava into the common pool. This, then, is followed by the increase in peripheral saturation due to the shutting out of venous return from the legs and the increase in systemic resistance.

Hypoxic Spells (Cyanotic Spells)

Hypoxic spells are *the* most traumatic consequences of hypoxemia. Ordinarily, they consist of irritability, uncontrollable crying, tachypnea, deepening of cyanosis, disappearance of an ejection murmur, metabolic acidosis, and even loss of consciousness. These spells may affect babies with only mild cyanosis at rest or with no cyanosis at all. They are sudden, episodic phenomena that may occur for no obvious reason, usually early in the morning. Precipitating causes include bowel movements, crying with hunger, or medical interventions (e.g., finger pricks for hemograms or cardiac catheterizations). This experience is frightening, not only for inexperienced parents but also for physicians and nurses.

As a rule, the vicious circle of crying, leading to hypoxemia, leading to more crying, can be interrupted by placing the baby on the shoulder with knees pressed against the abdomen and soothing the infant by quietly patting the back. If the attack is not terminated within minutes, surely within half an hour, morphine should be administered subcutaneously, and oxygen may be administered by face mask to increase the dissolved oxygen in the plasma. Administration of β blockers, presumably to release the infundibular spasm underlying the increase in the right-to-left shunt, may help. If all else fails and the infant is inconsolable, general anesthesia has been administered, and even emergency shunt operations have been performed in years past. Nowadays, the occurrence of a hypoxic spell is an indication for immediate corrective surgery. β Blockers for these episodes are too unreliable and are no longer used.

The spells do not occur in the newborn period; usually, their onset is at 3 to 4 months of age. Careful questioning of new mothers with presumably "pink" infants who have tetralogy of Fallot may elicit a story of morning irritability, attacks of "teething" or momentary "loss of contact." All these symptoms should raise the suspicion for cyanotic spells that might require urgent surgical intervention. These spells may lead to cerebrovascular accidents and even death. Less traumatically, they may lead to decreased intelligence quotients or to more subtle neurologic impairment or learning disability. At Children's Hospital Boston, the present policy is that even one major hypoxic spell is too many and should lead to immediate surgery.

Exercise Intolerance

Exercise intolerance is a less traumatic but equally serious consequence of hypoxemia. The physiologic principle is that the common ejectile chamber, consisting of the right and left ventricles, connected by a large ventricular defect, faces an overriding aorta and an obstructed pulmonary infundibulum in patients with tetralogy of Fallot. Exercise (and this may not be more than sucking a bottle) results in increased demand, which is met by a drop in systemic resistance, and a fixed, and possibly even increased, pulmonary resistance caused by circulating catechols. This results in a decrease in arterial saturation, dyspnea, hyperpnea, and possibly metabolic acidosis. It is interesting to note that older children do not really know how limited their exercise tolerance is because they have never experienced a "normal" exercise tolerance. Occasionally, a high school student or young adult states that his or her exercise tolerance is "normal" when in fact it is severely limited. Not until after successful surgery, curative or palliative, do these patients realize how limited they were. With cardiac surgery early in infancy, these stories of heroism and stoicism are much less common.

Brain Abscess

In a patient with hypoxemia, symptoms of the central nervous system (e.g., headache, focal neurologic signs, convulsions, loss of consciousness) should raise the immediate suspicion of brain abscess because this is the one etiology explaining these symptoms and signs that is clearly treatable (see Fig. 8-1). Vascular lesions of the central nervous system, the alternative possibility, may be manageable but not curable.

Cerebrovascular Accidents

Cerebrovascular accidents not associated with brain abscess and, ranging from transient motor deficit to full-blown hemiplegia, are usually attributable to vascular lesions such as emboli or thrombi or to hypoxic damage occurring as a consequence of hypoxic spells. With current management, the latter have become rarities in this country.

REFERENCES

1. Lundsgaard C, Van Slyke DD. Cyanosis. Medicine 2:1, 1923.
2. Mendlowitz M. Clubbing and hypertrophic osteoarthropathy. Medicine 21:269, 1942.
3. Hurtado A. Aspectos fisiologicos y patologicos de la altura. Lima, Ed. Rimac, 1943.
4. Rosenthal A, Button LN, Nathan DG, et al. Blood volume changes in cyanotic congenital heart disease. Am J Cardiol 27:162, 1971.
5. Flanagan MF, Hourihan M, Keane JF. Incidence of renal dysfunction in adults with cyanotic congenital heart disease. Am J Cardiol 68:403, 1991.

6. Dittrich S, Haas NA, Buhrer C, et al. Renal impairment in patients with longstanding cyanotic congenital heart disease. Acta Paediatr 87(9):949, 1998.
7. Hopkins WE, Chen Z, Fukagawa, et al. Increased atrial and brain natriuretic peptides in adults with cyanotic congenital heart disease: Enhanced understanding of the relationship between hypoxia and natriuretic peptide secretion. Circulation 109:2872, 2004.
8. Lurie PR. Postural effects in tetralogy of Fallot. Am J Med 15:297, 1955.
9. Taussig HB. Congenital Malformations of the Heart, vols. 1 and II. Cambridge, MA: The Commonwealth Fund, Harvard University Press, 1960:1–1019.

9

Central Nervous System Sequelae of Congenital Heart Disease

JANE W. NEWBURGER

Advances in medical, transcatheter, and surgical therapies have reduced mortality rates for virtually all forms of congenital heart disease. Whereas only a few decades ago, 20% of children born with congenital heart disease survived to adulthood, by the 1980s, this figure stood at 85%[1] and has continued to increase. A dramatic increase in the population of school-aged and adult survivors of infant heart surgery has been accompanied by increased recognition of the long-term morbidities associated with congenital heart disease. In particular, it is now recognized that survivors of congenital heart disease frequently suffer adverse neurodevelopmental sequelae, with profound clinical and financial implications.[2]

Adverse neurologic and developmental function among children with congenital heart disease derives from both innate and acquired factors, with cumulative effects. Among innate factors, genetic syndromes (e.g., trisomy 21, 22q11 microdeletion[3–5]) or congenital brain anomalies may contribute to neurodevelopmental impairment. Other neurodevelopmental abnormalities can be acquired through events that accompany heart disease, with or without cardiac surgery. Potential risk factors include severe, chronic hypoxemia or congestive heart failure, episodes of arrhythmia or cardiac arrest, thromboembolic events unrelated to surgery, poor nutritional status, and central nervous system (CNS) infection. Preoperative hemodynamic instability or intraoperative events (discussed later) may cause further CNS damage.[6] In the early postoperative period, cerebral vasoregulatory systems disrupted by hypothermic circulatory arrest and bypass techniques may render the brain to be more vulnerable to hemodynamic fluxes, such as hypotension.[7–9] It is likely that genetic polymorphisms and mutations, preoperative health, operative factors, postoperative events, and sociodemographic variables are each important and interact in their effects on neurodevelopmental outcome.[10]

PATHOLOGY

Neuropathologic and histologic studies of brain of infants and children with congenital heart disease have revealed both focal and diffuse infarction. Focal infarction has been ascribed to thromboembolic events, whereas a diffuse pattern of cerebral injury has been attributed to hypotension and hypoperfusion.[11] More recent neuropathologic autopsy data derived from infants undergoing reparative or palliative cardiac surgery reveal not only that these children are at increased risk for gray matter injury but also that nascent white matter is at risk for injury.[12] In addition to acquired abnormalities, cerebral dysgenesis is reported to occur in 10% to 29% of children with congenital heart disease in autopsy series, with the incidence varying by lesion[13–15]; findings may range from microdysgenesis to gross abnormalities such as agenesis of the corpus callosum, incomplete operculization, and microcephaly.

IMAGING

Despite a compelling body of neuropathologic and neurobehavioral evidence of cognitive and neurologic dysfunction, children with surgically corrected congenital heart disease have been studied comparatively little with magnetic resonance imaging (MRI), especially quantitative

MRI techniques. Most MRI studies have been descriptive in nature and have involved patients with heterogeneous diagnoses. Mahle and colleagues[16] conducted a prospective MRI study of neonates with various types of congenital heart disease before and after surgical correction of their respective lesions. More than 50% of the children in their sample demonstrated evidence of white matter injury after surgery. Strikingly, more than 15% demonstrated evidence of white matter injury and 8% possessed evidence of gray matter injury *before* surgery. Moreover, greater than 50% of the children who received *preoperative* magnetic resonance spectroscopy (MRS) demonstrated elevations of cerebral lactate peaks. McConnell and associates[17] found ventriculomegaly and enlargement of subarachnoid spaces consistent with cerebral atrophy on preoperative MRI in one third of their study sample. MRI performed on patients with congenital heart disease after surgery has revealed findings consistent with both gray matter injury and widely distributed white matter injury.[18] Taken in aggregate, documentation by MRI of brain abnormalities in children with congenital heart disease both before and after corrective surgery is consistent with the hypothesis that the long-term neurodevelopmental outcome of children with congenital heart disease is a product of preoperative condition and perioperative course.

CARDIAC SURGERY

Cardiac surgery may be associated with neurologic complications, including seizures, choreoathetosis,[19] stroke, and hypoxic-ischemic encephalopathy. Prevention of neurologic morbidity has become a major focus of clinical and translational research, with particular attention to methods of vital organ support as detailed later. Recent data at Children's Hospital Boston suggest that acute neurologic morbidity after pediatric open heart surgery occurs in about 2% of patients,[20] compared with an estimated 25% in the past.[21] In calendar year 1998 at our institution, the incidence of clinical seizures in infants undergoing open heart surgery fell to 1%, compared with rates of 9% to 32% in earlier series.[22–24]

Cardiopulmonary Bypass

Prospective studies and clinical trials have particularly focused on adverse neurodevelopmental outcomes caused by perioperative factors, particularly the support techniques used to protect vital organs during cardiac repair.[25] Sources of brain injury from cardiopulmonary bypass itself include microemboli, both particulate and gaseous, macroemboli, and hypoperfusion. In infants and children, the risk for brain injury related to cardiopulmonary bypass may be further influenced by many variables, including duration of total circulation arrest,[26] depth of hypothermia,[27] rate and duration of core cooling,[28] type of pH management chosen during core cooling (alpha stat versus pH stat),[29,30] degree of hemodilution,[31] type of oxygenator (bubble versus membrane), use of arterial filtration, and other aspects of the biochemical milieu.[32,33] Recently, research has focused on the role of genetic polymorphisms mediating the inflammatory response to cardiopulmonary bypass or aspects of cerebral ischemia reperfusion injury during cardiac surgery.[34] In a study of apolipoprotein E alleles, Gaynor and coworkers[35] recently reported that genetic polymorphisms that decrease neuroresiliency and impair neuronal repair after CNS injury are important risk factors for neurodevelopmental dysfunction after infant cardiac surgery. Specifically, Psychomotor Development Index scores were significantly lower among apolipoprotein E ε 2 allele carriers at 1 year of age after infant cardiac surgery.

Deep Hypothermia

Animal experiments and clinical experience have shown apparent safety of hypothermia as low as 15° to 20°C.[36] The protective effect of hypothermia during cerebral ischemia is derived, in part, from a reduction in metabolic activity, reflected in reduced oxygen consumption. Additional mechanisms of hypothermic cerebral protection during ischemia include preservation of intracellular stores of high-energy phosphates and of high intracellular pH, as well as protection against reperfusion injury (including the "no-reflow" phenomenon), calcium influx, and free radical damage.[37]

Total Circulatory Arrest

Since its introduction in the early 1960s, deep hypothermic circulatory arrest (DHCA) has been used widely in open heart surgery for infants.[38,39] A great advantage of this technique is the absence of perfusion cannulas and of blood from the operative field, with reliance on deep hypothermia for protection of the CNS. The use of DHCA for open heart surgery assumes that there is a "safe" duration of total circulatory arrest that is inversely related to body temperature.[36] The organ with the shortest safe circulatory arrest time is the brain. Functional disturbances after circulatory arrest include choreoathetosis[40–45] and transient seizures.[22,41,46] Studies in children who underwent cardiac surgery using DHCA have shown that the likelihood of perioperative seizures and of late neurocognitive deficits are related to duration of DHCA in a nonlinear fashion; circulatory arrest times of less than 30 minutes appear to carry little risk.[26,47]

Acid-Base Management

Arterial carbon dioxide tension (P_{CO_2}) is one of the most important regulatory factors known to affect the level of cerebral blood flow during cardiopulmonary bypass (CPB).[29,48] In the *alpha-stat* strategy, arterial P_{CO_2} is maintained at 40 mm Hg when the sample is measured at 37° C and is not corrected for the patient's temperature. The *pH-stat* strategy adjusts the arterial P_{CO_2} to 40 mm Hg to maintain a pH of 7.40 at the patient's hypothermic temperature. Because brain injury in infants most commonly results from global hypoperfusion during periods of diminished cerebral blood flow or circulatory arrest, *pH stat* is hypothesized to provide better brain protection.[29,30,49]

Hemodilution

Hemodilution during cardiopulmonary bypass is currently almost universal for cardiopulmonary bypass, but the minimum safe hematocrit has been controversial.[50–52] Although hemodilution increases cerebral blood flow,[53] it may limit oxygen delivery by reducing the oxygen carrying capacity of blood, in the setting of the leftward shift of oxyhemoglobin dissociation induced by hypothermia.[50] Infants undergoing reparative open heart surgery using DHCA at lower hematocrit levels (about 20%) have been shown to have worse psychomotor development at age 1 year, compared with children with higher hematocrits. The optimal hematocrit is still being determined in ongoing research studies.

The efficacy of other neuroprotective strategies, such as regional perfusion of the CNS during DHCA, requires evaluation in randomized trials.

POSTOPERATIVE MOVEMENT DISORDERS

Postoperative movement disorders, the most common of which is choreoathetosis, were reported soon after the introduction of deep hypothermic circulatory arrest. The true incidence of these rare disorders is unknown because of underdiagnosis and underreporting. Most often, symptoms of postoperative movement disorders begin 2 to 7 days after surgery, with initial symptoms of confusion, insomnia, and marked irritability, followed by the appearance of abnormal involuntary movement first involving the distal extremities and orofacial muscles and then progressing proximally to involve the girdle muscles and trunk. Severe cases can have violent thrashing.[43] The abnormal movements are most marked when patients are upset and improve during sleep. Symptoms generally worsen over the course of 1 week, stabilize for another 1 or 2 weeks, and then vary in the degree and speed of recovery. The most serious cases have a mortality of about 40%, with survivors showing a high incidence of persistent neurodevelopmental abnormality.[43] Factors hypothesized to be associated with postoperative movement disorders include cyanotic heart disease with systemic to pulmonary collaterals from the head and neck, age at surgery older than 9 months, short cooling durations before onset of deep hypothermic circulatory arrest, deep hypothermia itself, use of alpha-stat strategy of acid base management, and prolonged use of fentanyl and midazolam.[43] Follow-up evaluation of children with postoperative choreoathetosis has been associated with significant deficits in ability (IQ), memory, attention, and language, as well as in motor function, with dyskinesia persisting in about 50%.[19]

POSTOPERATIVE SEIZURES

Seizures after infant heart surgery are presumed to be caused by cerebral hypoxic-ischemic reperfusion injury. Clinically detected seizures are more common in patients with longer durations of total circulatory arrest and occur most frequently in the period between 24 and 48 hours postoperatively.[47] Prospective long-term video electroencephalogram studies have demonstrated that seizures may occur without typical behavioral manifestations; only one in every two or three seizures is apparent clinically,[29,47] related in part to sedative and paralytic agents used in the early postoperative period. The prognosis of seizures in the early postoperative period depends on the underlying etiology. Among patients in whom seizures are related to cerebral dysgenesis or stroke, the risks for chronic epilepsy and significant neurologic and developmental delay are high. In contrast, cryptogenic postoperative seizures generally do not recur after the early postoperative period; hence, infants with postoperative seizures can be discharged without anticonvulsant therapy. However, cryptogenic postoperative seizures are a risk factor for late neurodevelopmental delay.[54]

CARDIAC CATHETERIZATION

The cooperative study on cardiac catheterization monitored complications arising from cardiac catheterization between 1963 and 1965 in 12,367 children and adults.[55] Unfortunately, this study included very small infants, the patients who are most at risk for injury of the CNS. Still, recognized complications of the CNS were reported in about 0.2% of patients. Convulsions, headaches, and impairment of consciousness were reported as late as several hours after catheterization and were usually associated with contrast injection. In 13 patients, focal neurologic injury was presumed to be secondary to embolic events resulting from the use of catheters in the left side of the heart. A more recent review of neurologic complications during catheterization in children reported an incidence of 0.38%, with seizures and stroke being most frequent.[56] Contrast toxicity should be considered in the differential diagnosis of any patient with seizures after cardiac catheterization.[57]

Brain injury from cerebral embolism or hypoxic-ischemic injury can also occur during cardiac catheterization.

CEREBROVASCULAR ACCIDENT (STROKE)

Cerebral infarction may be caused by emboli, thrombosis in situ, or venous thrombosis.[11] Embolic events may occur as a consequence of procedures, such as cardiac surgery, left-sided cardiac catheterization, or catheterization of cyanotic infants. Cerebral emboli can also derive from the heart itself. For example, left-sided prosthetic valves may give rise to emboli. Patients with poor left ventricular function may develop intracardiac thrombus, prompting the need for prophylactic anticoagulation in this setting. Because left atrial thrombus may form during atrial fibrillation, transesophageal echocardiography, anticoagulation, or both are recommended before electrical cardioversion. Infective endocarditis on left-sided structures may lead to septic emboli and cerebral mycotic aneurysms. So-called paradoxical emboli may arise from the systemic veins or right heart structures and travel through an intracardiac communication, such as an atrial septal defect, to the left-sided circulation. Cerebral venous thrombosis may occur in the setting of central venous hypertension, polycythemia, and venous stasis. In addition, it has been proposed that relative anemia is associated with increased blood viscosity and constitutes a risk factor for stroke.[58] An association of cerebrovascular accidents in young children with anemia has also been reported by Molina and colleagues[59] and by Phornphutkul and associates.[60]

NEONATAL INTRACRANIAL HEMORRHAGE

Intraventricular-periventricular hemorrhage occurs with increased frequency in neonates with heart disease who present with acidosis or shock. Because intracranial hemorrhage or hemorrhagic transformation of an ischemic lesion may extend under the conditions of cardiopulmonary bypass, with its use of anticoagulation, increase in fibrinolytic activity, and variation in cerebral perfusion pressure, all neonates with significant preoperative instability should undergo preoperative cranial ultrasound. If intraventricular-periventricular hemorrhage is present, physicians need to balance the risk for continued hemodynamic instability of the infant with that related to worsening hemorrhage on bypass. Surgery involving cardiopulmonary bypass should generally be delayed a minimum of 1 week—and longer for those in whom hemorrhage is intraparenchymal. Subependymal hemorrhage generally should not delay surgery. Elective surgery after intracranial hemorrhage or cerebrovascular accident is generally deferred for 6 weeks.

LATE NEUROLOGIC AND DEVELOPMENTAL OUTCOMES

Cross-sectional and prospective evaluations of children who have undergone repair or palliation of congenital heart defects have identified a number of cognitive, motor, behavioral, and developmental abnormalities.[10,61–69] Whereas test scores of individual patients with congenital heart disease often fall within the normal range, mean performance in the group is lower than that of the general population. Compared with children in the normal population, those who have undergone repair of critical congenital heart disease score lower on tests of IQ, achievement, motor function, speech, language, and behavior, and they often require special services. As children reach school age, they often manifest significant functional limitations in higher-level processing skills, involving attention, executive functions, memory, and visual-spatial skills.[70] One to 3 years after surgery, a test of functional independence revealed that only 21% of congenital heart disease survivors scored within the expected range for age, 40% had difficulty performing activities of daily living, and 53% had socialization difficulties.[67]

In general, children who have undergone repair of simple lesions, such as atrial septal defects, have outcomes similar to those in the normal population,[71,72] whereas those undergoing biventricular repair of more complex lesions, such as D-transposition of the great arteries (D-TGA) or tetralogy of Fallot, have worse developmental outcomes.[69] Children with D-TGA have been studied especially carefully in the Boston Circulatory Arrest Study.[70] At age 8 years, children in whom surgery was performed using longer duration of total circulatory arrest had worse fine and gross motor function, appendicular apraxia, oromotor coordination, and discourse skills. Regardless of the predominant strategy of vital organ support during surgery, D-TGA patients had deficits in motor function (including speech), visual-spatial skills, working memory, hypothesis generation and testing, vigilance and sustained attention, and higher-order language. Although children with D-TGA had normal lower-level skills, such as word reading, they had difficulty with synthesis and integration of information, for example, assembling story elements into a narrative or applying math concepts to solve word problems. At age 8 years, more than one third were receiving remedial services in school. Like other groups of children with congenital heart disease,[73,74] D-TGA patients manifested many of the neurodevelopmental characteristics of "nonverbal learning disabilities."[75]

Children with cyanotic congenital heart disease have lower intelligence quotients and poorer perceptual and gross motor function than children with acyanotic heart disease or well children.[60,76,77] The longer the infant is allowed to remain cyanotic, the greater the potential for measurable deficit at a later age.[60,78–89]

Adverse developmental outcome is most common among those with a single ventricle undergoing the Fontan operation.[61,68] Such patients often have multiple risk factors for neurodevelopmental morbidity, including cyanosis or heart failure, multiple cardiac operations, and use of total circulatory arrest. From among patients with univentricular heart, those with hypoplastic left heart syndrome (HLHS) appear to be at especially high risk.[61,62,90,91] Cerebral dysgenesis is common in this population.[92] In addition, cerebral blood flow is likely to be disturbed *in utero* as the blood of lower-than-usual saturation is supplied to the cerebral circulation through a ductus arteriosus retrograde, often through a hypoplastic aortic arch. Infants in whom HLHS was not diagnosed in the prenatal period may present with shock as the patent ductus arteriosus closes, creating hypoxic-ischemic cerebral injury. Even in stable infants with HLHS awaiting stage I palliation, cerebral oxygen saturation levels assessed by near infrared spectroscopy are lower than in other forms of congenital heart disease.[93] Brain injury can be acquired through intraoperative events, including long duration of deep hypothermic circulatory arrest, or during periods of instability in the postoperative period. Two more operations, a bidirectional Glenn procedure and a Fontan procedure, are then required for complete palliation. With a multitude of risk factors for adverse outcome, a significant fraction of children with HLHS have significantly impaired neurologic and developmental status.[62,91,94,95] Indeed, in a series of school-aged children with HLHS repaired at Children's Hospital of Philadelphia before 1992, Mahle and coworkers[62] reported cerebral palsy in 17%, microcephaly in 13%, IQ scores in the mentally retarded range in 18%, learning disabilities in 14%, and attention deficit hyperactivity disorder in a majority. When HLHS is managed by cardiac transplantation rather than staged palliation, neurodevelopmental outcomes are remarkably similar, with the median full-scale IQ almost 1 standard deviation below average in the normal population.[96]

The emotional adjustment of children facing pediatric heart disease may also present challenges. Among children with D-TGA to whom the Child Health Questionnaire[97] was administered at age 8 years, general physical and psychosocial health status was similar to that of the general population; however, those with lower IQ and academic achievement had worse psychosocial health status.[98] Therefore, it is not surprising that survivors of staged reconstruction for HLHS, a group particularly at risk for neurocognitive morbidity, had diminished overall psychosocial and physical health, with emotional and behavioral difficulties and low self-esteem.[90] Long-term follow-up studies of children with congenital heart disease report elevated rates of psychosocial dysfunction,[99–101] particularly undiagnosed psychiatric illness such as major depressive disorder and panic disorder. Maternal perceptions have been found to be potent predictors of adjustment in school-aged children with pediatric heart disease.[102] In adolescence, many meet some but not all *Diagnostic and Statistical Manual of Mental Disorders* criteria,[103–105] and low self-esteem is common.[106]

INFECTIONS

Neurologic manifestations of *infective endocarditis* include cerebral ischemia or hemorrhage from septic or nonseptic emboli.[107] In addition, mycotic aneurysms of cerebral arteries can occur, presenting catastrophically if they rupture.

Meningitis has been reported to be more common among infants with cyanotic heart disease than among those with acyanotic heart disease or well children.[108,109]

Brain abscess is one of the most serious complications of cyanotic congenital heart disease, with a reported incidence in this population of 2% to 6%; arterial oxygenation is inversely correlated with the incidence, morbidity, and mortality of brain abscess.[110] Indeed, one third to one half of childhood brain abscesses are associated with cyanotic heart disease.[111,112] In patients with cyanotic heart disease, bacteria in venous blood may not pass through the normally effective phagocytic filtering action of the pulmonary capillary bed. In addition, the polycythemia and consequent hyperviscosity associated with chronic hypoxemia reduce capillary blood flow in the brain; microinfarction and reduced tissue oxygenation may then predispose brain tissue to bacterial colonization.[113] Bacterial endocarditis is associated with brain abscess only rarely.[86,114] Brain abscess is exceedingly rare in patients younger than 2 years of age, presumably because they do not yet have periodontal disease.

The classic triad of symptoms of brain abscess (e.g., fever, headaches, and focal neurologic deficit) is present in a minority of patients.[113] Headache is the most common symptom, occurring in about 47% to 82% of patients.[112,115–117] Other common signs and symptoms include fever, seizures, vomiting, stiff neck, and generalized changes in mental status.[112] Symptoms and signs of brain abscess are necessarily dependent on intracranial location. The often subtle symptoms of brain abscess, together with its high morbidity and mortality, mandate a rapid evaluation for this diagnosis in any patient with cyanotic heart disease and possible or definite neurologic findings.

The diagnosis of brain abscess is made using contrast-enhanced computed tomography (CT) or brain MRI.

Examination of peripheral blood is not often helpful; indeed, the white blood cell count is normal in 40% of patients with brain abscess.[86,118,119] Because lumbar puncture in patient with brain abscess may cause clinical deterioration or death,[85,86,120] patients with cyanotic heart disease, fever, and focal neurologic findings should undergo a CT scan or MRI before lumbar puncture is performed.

Brain abscess is treated with antibiotics that have good penetration of the CNS and cover both anaerobic and aerobic bacteria, as well as with image-guided surgical aspiration or surgical excision.[112,121,122] For patients with early cerebritis, therapy with antibiotics alone may be successful. The mortality from brain abscess depends on the location of the lesion, presence of multiple or multiloculated lesions, rupture of the abscess into a ventricle,[123] and the etiologic agent(s), with almost 20% of infections being polymicrobial.[122] The overall mortality of brain abscess in recent series is about 10%,[112,122] but may be lower in the current era.[117] A seizure disorder requiring long-term anticonvulsant medication follows brain abscess in 11% to 35% of cases.[119,122,124]

FUTURE

As survival of children with heart disease has improved, their neurodevelopmental outcomes are of foremost importance in pediatric cardiology today. Children who have undergone reparative or palliative surgery for congenital heart disease should be presumed to be at increased risk, and neurodevelopmental surveillance should be a routine component of their care, so that emerging difficulties can be identified and supportive interventions can be implemented as appropriate. In the future, such outcomes may be improved by advances in technologies (e.g., improved bypass circuits), new drugs and micromolecules guided by pharmacogenomics, and multitiered combination therapies.

REFERENCES

1. British Cardiac Society Working Party. Grown-up congenital heart (GUCH) disease: Current needs and provision of service for adolescents and adults with congenital heart disease in the UK. Heart 88:i1, 2002.
2. Majnemer A, Limperopoulos C. Developmental progress of children with congenital heart defects requiring open heart surgery. Semin Pediatr Neurol 6:12, 1999.
3. Murphy KC. Schizophrenia and velo-cardio-facial syndrome. Lancet 359:426, 2002.
4. Henry JC, van Amelsvoort T, Morris RG, et al. An investigation of the neuropsychological profile in adults with velo-cardio-facial syndrome (VCFS). Neuropsychologia 40:471, 2002.
5. Gerdes M, Solot C, Wang PP, et al. Cognitive and behavior profile of preschool children with chromosome 22q11.2 deletion. Am J Med Genet 85:127, 1999.
6. Cooper MM, Elliott M. Haemodilution. In Jonas RA, Elliott MJ (eds). Cardiopulmonary Bypass in Neonates, Infants, and Young Children. Oxford, UK: Butterworth-Heinemann, 1994:82.
7. Greeley WJ, Ungerleider RM, Smith LR, et al. The effects of deep hypothermic cardiopulmonary bypass and total circulatory arrest on cerebral blood flow in infants and children. J Thorac Cardiovasc Surg 97:737, 1989.
8. Greeley WJ, Kern FH, Ungerleider RM, et al. The effect of hypothermic cardiopulmonary bypass and total circulatory arrest on cerebral metabolism in neonates, infants, and children. J Thorac Cardiovasc Surg 101:783, 1991.
9. Lou H. The "lost autoregulation hypothesis" and brain lesions in the newborn: An update. Brain Dev 10:143, 1988.
10. Limperopoulos C, Majnemer A, Shevell MI, et al. Predictors of developmental disabilities after open heart surgery in young children with congenital heart defects. J Pediatr 141: 51, 2002.
11. Terplan KL. Patterns of brain damage in infants and children with congenital heart disease: Association with catheterization and surgical procedures. Am J Dis Child 125:175, 1973.
12. Kinney HC. Unpublished data.
13. Glauser TA, Rorke LB, Weinberg PM, et al. Acquired neuropathologic lesions associated with the hypoplastic left heart syndrome. Pediatrics 85:991, 1990.
14. Jones M. Anomalies of the brain and congenital heart disease: A study of 52 necropsy cases. Pediatr Pathol 11:721, 1991.
15. Terplan KL. Brain changes in newborns, infants and children with congenital heart disease in association with cardiac surgery. J Neurol 212:225, 1976.
16. Mahle WT, Tavani F, Zimmerman RA, et al. An MRI study of neurological injury before and after congenital heart surgery. Circulation 106:109, 2002.
17. McConnell JR, Fleming WH, Chu WK, et al. Magnetic resonance imaging of the brain in infants and children before and after cardiac surgery: A prospective study. Am J Dis Child 144:374, 1990.
18. Miller G, Mamourian AC, Tesman JR, et al. Long-term MRI changes in brain after pediatric open heart surgery. Child Neuropsychol 9:390, 2001.
19. du Plessis AJ, Bellinger DC, Gauvreau K, et al. Neurologic outcome of choreoathetoid encephalopathy after cardiac surgery. Pediatr Neurol 27:9, 2002.
20. Menache CC, du Plessis AJ, Wessel DL, et al. Current incidence of acute neurologic complications after open-heart operations in children. Ann Thorac Surg 73:1752, 2002.
21. Ferry PC. Neurologic sequelae of open-heart surgery in children. An "irritating question." Am J Dis Child 144:369, 1990.
22. Ehyai A, Fenichel GM, Bender HW. Incidence and prognosis of seizures in infants after cardiac surgery with profound hypothermia and circulatory arrest. JAMA 252:3165, 1984.
23. Miller G, Eggli K, Contant C, et al. Postoperative neurologic complications after open heart surgery on young infants. Arch Pediatr Adolesc Med 149:764, 1995.

24. Castaneda AR, Lamberti J, Sade RM, et al. Open-heart surgery during the first three months of life. J Thorac Cardiovasc Surg 68:719, 1974.
25. Ferry PC. Neurologic sequelae of cardiac surgery in children. Am J Dis Child 141:309, 1987.
26. Wypij D, Newburger JW, Rappaport LA, et al. The effect of duration of deep hypothermic circulatory arrest in infant heart surgery on late neurodevelopment: The Boston Circulatory Arrest Trial. J Thorac Cardiovasc Surg 126:1397, 2003.
27. Schell RM, Stanley T, Croughwell N, et al. Temperature during cardiopulmonary bypass and neuropsychologic outcome. Anesthesiology 77:A119, 1992.
28. Bellinger DC, Wernovsky G, Rappaport LA, et al. Cognitive development of children following early repair of transposition of the great arteries using deep hypothermic circulatory arrest. Pediatrics 87:701, 1991.
29. du Plessis AJ, Jonas RA, Wypij D, et al. Perioperative effects of alpha-stat versus pH-stat strategies for deep hypothermic cardiopulmonary bypass in infants. J Thorac Cardiovasc Surg 114:991, 1997.
30. Bellinger DC, Wypij D, du Plessis AJ, et al. Developmental and neurologic effects of alpha-stat versus pH-stat strategies for deep hypothermic cardiopulmonary bypass in infants [see comments]. [Erratum appears in J Thorac Cardiovasc Surg 2001 May;121(5):893.]. J Thorac Cardiovasc Surg 121: 374, 2001.
31. Jonas RA, Wypij D, Roth SJ, et al. The influence of hemodilution on outcome after hypothermic cardiopulmonary bypass: results of a randomized trial in infants. J Thorac Cardiovasc Surg 126:1765, 2003.
32. Jonas RA. Problems of deep hypothermic circulatory arrest and low-flow perfusion: With particular reference to the paediatric population. In Smith P, Taylor K (eds). Cardiac Surgery and the Brain. London: Edward Arnold, 1993:95–107.
33. Jonas RA. Neurological protection during cardiopulmonary bypass/deep hypothermia. Pediatr Cardiol 19:321, 1998.
34. Tomasdottir H, Hjartarson H, Ricksten A, et al. Tumor necrosis factor gene polymorphism is associated with enhanced systemic inflammatory response and increased cardiopulmonary morbidity after cardiac surgery. Anesth Analg 97:944, 2003.
35. Gaynor JW, Gerdes M, Zackai EH, et al. Apolipoprotein E genotype and neurodevelopmental sequelae of infant cardiac surgery. J Thorac Cardiovasc Surg 126:1736, 2003.
36. Kirklin JW, Barratt-Boyes BG. Cardiac Surgery. New York: John Wiley and Sons, 1986.
37. Hickey PR, Anderson NP. Deep hypothermic circulatory arrest: A review of pathophysiology and clinical experience as a basis for anesthetic management. J Cardiothorac Vasc Anesth 1:137, 1987.
38. Kirklin JW, Dawson B, Devloo RA, et al. Open intracardiac operations: Use of circulatory arrest during hypothermia induced by blood cooling. Ann Surg 154:769, 1961.
39. Weiss M, Piwnica A, Lenfant C, et al. Deep hypothermia with total circulatory arrest. Trans Am Soc Artif Intern Organs 6: 227, 1960.
40. Brunberg JA, Doty DB, Reilly EL. Choreoathetosis in infants following cardiac surgery with deep hypothermic and circulatory arrest. J Pediatr 84:232, 1974.
41. Brunberg JA, Reilly EL, Doty DB. Central nervous system consequences in infants of cardiac surgery using deep hypothermia and circulatory arrest. Circulation 49:62, 1974.
42. Stewart RW, Blackstone EH, Kirklin JW. Neurological dysfunction after cardiac surgery. In Parenzan L, Crupi G, Graham G (eds). Congenital Heart Disease in the First Three Months of Life: Medical and Surgical Aspects. Bologna, Italy: Patron Editore, 1981:431.
43. Wong PC, Barlow CF, Hickey PR, et al. Factors associated with choreoathetosis after cardiopulmonary bypass in children with congenital heart disease. Circulation 85(Suppl 5):II118, 1992.
44. Curless R, Katz D, Perryman R, et al. Choreoathetosis after surgery for congenital heart disease. J Pediatr 124:737, 1994.
45. Wessel DL, du Plessis AJ. Choreoathetosis. In Jonas RA, Newburger JW, Volpe JJ (eds). Brain Injury and Pediatric Cardiac Surgery. Boston: Butterworth-Heinemann, 1996: 353–362.
46. Clarkson PM, MacArthur BA, Barratt-Boyes BG. Developmental progress following cardiac surgery in infants using profound hypothermia and circulatory arrest. Circulation 62:855, 1980.
47. Newburger JW, Jonas RA, Wernovsky G, et al. A comparison of the perioperative neurologic effects of hypothermic circulatory arrest versus low-flow cardiopulmonary bypass in infant heart surgery. N Engl J Med 329:1057, 1993.
48. Burrows F. Con: pH-stat management of blood gases is preferable to alpha-stat in patients undergoing brain cooling for cardiac surgery. J Cardiothorac Vasc Anesth 9:219, 1995.
49. Duebener LF, Hagino I, Sakamoto T, et al. Effects of pH management during deep hypothermic bypass on cerebral microcirculation: Alpha-stat versus pH-stat. Circulation 106:I103, 2002.
50. Cooper MM, Elliott M. Haemodilution. In Jonas RA, Elliott MJ (eds). Cardiopulmonary Bypass in Neonates, Infants, and Young Children. Oxford, UK: Butterworth-Heinemann, 1994:91.
51. Griepp EB, Griepp RB. Cerebral consequences of hypothermic circulatory arrest in adults. J Card Surg 7:134, 1992.
52. Gold JP. Blood conservation for infants and children undergoing surgery for acquired and congenital heart diseases. In Krieger KH, Isom OW (eds). Blood Conservation in Cardiac Surgery. New York: Springer-Verlag, 1998:187–209.
53. Sungurtekin H, Cook DJ, Orszulak TA, et al. Cerebral response to hemodilution during hypothermic cardiopulmonary bypass in adults. Anesth Analg 89:1078, 1999.
54. Bellinger DC, Wypij D, Kuban KCK, et al. Developmental and neurological status of children at 4 years of age after heart surgery with hypothermic circulatory arrest or low-flow cardiopulmonary bypass. Circulation 100:526, 1999.
55. Braunwald E, Gorlin R. Cooperative study on cardiac catheterization: Total population studied, procedures employed, and incidence of complications. Circulation 37: III8, 1968.
56. Liu XY, Wong V, Leung M. Neurologic complications due to catheterization. Pediatr Neurol 24:270, 2001.
57. Torvik A, Walday P. Neurotoxicity of water-soluble contrast media. Acta Radiol Suppl 399:221, 1995.

58. Cottrill CM, Kaplan S. Cerebral vascular accidents in cyanotic congenital heart disease. Am J Dis Child 125:484, 1973.
59. Molina JE, Einzig S, Mastri AR. Brain damage in profound hypothermia: Perfusion versus circulatory arrest. J Thorac Cardiovasc Surg 87:596, 1984.
60. Phornphutkul C, Rosenthal A, Nadas AS, et al. Cerebrovascular accidents in infants and children with cyanotic congenital heart disease. Am J Cardiol 32:329, 1973.
61. Wernovsky G, Stiles KM, Gauvreau K, et al. Cognitive development after the Fontan operation. Circulation 102:883, 2000.
62. Mahle WT, Clancy RR, Moss EM, et al. Neurodevelopmental outcome and lifestyle assessment in school-aged and adolescent children with hypoplastic left heart syndrome. Pediatrics 105:1082, 2000.
63. Mahle WT, Wernovsky G. Long-term developmental outcome of children with complex congenital heart disease [review]. Clin Perinatol 28:235, 2001.
64. Bellinger DC, Jonas RA, Rappaport LA, et al. Developmental and neurologic status of children after heart surgery with hypothermic circulatory arrest or low-flow cardiopulmonary bypass. N Engl J Med 332:549, 1995.
65. Bellinger DC, Rappaport LA, Wypij D, et al. Patterns of developmental dysfunction after surgery during infancy to correct transposition of the great arteries. J Dev Behav Pediatr 18:75, 1997.
66. Bellinger DC, Wypij D, Kuban K, et al. Developmental and neurologic status of children at four years of age after heart surgery with hypothermic circulatory arrest or low-flow cardiopulmonary bypass. Circulation 100:526, 1999.
67. Limperopoulos C, Majnemer A, Shevell MI, et al. Functional limitations in young children with congenital heart defects after cardiac surgery. Pediatrics 108:1325, 2001.
68. Forbess JM, Visconti KJ, Hancock-Friesen C, et al. Neurodevelopmental outcome after congenital heart surgery: Results from an institutional registry. Circulation 106:I95, 2002.
69. Forbess JM, Visconti KJ, Bellinger DC, et al. Neurodevelopmental outcomes after biventricular repair of congenital heart defects. J Thorac Cardiovasc Surg 123: 631, 2002.
70. Bellinger DC, Wypij D, du Plessis AJ, et al. Neurodevelopmental status at eight years in children with dextro-transposition of the great arteries: The Boston Circulatory Arrest Trial. J Thorac Cardiovasc Surg 126:1385, 2003.
71. Visconti KJ, Bichell DP, Jonas RA, et al. Developmental outcome after surgical versus interventional closure of secundum atrial septal defect in children. Circulation 100(Suppl), 1999.
72. Stavinoha PL, Fixler DE, Mahony L. Cardiopulmonary bypass to repair an atrial septal defect does not affect cognitive function in children. Circulation 107:2722, 2003.
73. Tindall S, Rothermel RR, Delamater A, et al. Neuropsychological abilities of children with cardiac disease treated with extracorporeal membrane oxygenation. Dev Neuropsychol 16:101, 1999.
74. Swillen A, Vandeputte L, Cracco J, et al. Neuropsychological, learning and psychosocial profile of primary school aged children with the velo-cardio-facial syndrome (22q11 deletion): Evidence for a nonverbal learning disability? Neuropsychol Dev Cogn Sect C Child Neuropsychol 5:230, 1999.
75. Harnadek MC, Rourke BP. Principal identifying features of the syndrome of nonverbal learning disabilities in children. J Learn Disabil 27:144, 1994.
76. Linde LM, Rasof B, Dunn OJ. Mental development in congenital heart disease. J Pediatr 71:198, 1967.
77. Linde LM, Rasof B, Dunn OJ. Longitudinal studies of intellectual and behavioral development in children with congenital heart disease. Acta Paediatr Scand 59:169, 1970.
78. Newburger JW, Silbert AR, Buckley LP, et al. Cognitive function and duration of hypoxemia in children with transposition of the great arteries. N Engl J Med 310:1495, 1984.
79. Nielsen H, Gyldensted C, Harmsen A. Cerebral abscess: Aetiology and pathogenesis, symptoms, diagnosis and treatment. Acta Neurol Scand 65:609, 1982.
80. O'Dougherty M, Wright FS, Garmezy N. Later competence and adaptation in infants who survive severe heart defects. Child Dev 54:1129, 1983.
81. Rahn H, Reeves RB, Howell BJ. Hydrogen ion regulation, temperature and evolution. Am Rev Respir Dis 112:165, 1975.
82. Rebeyka IM, Coles JG, Wilson GJ. The effect of low-flow cardiopulmonary bypass on cerebral function: An experimental and clinical study. Ann Thorac Surg 43:391, 1987.
83. Richter JA. Profound hypothermia and circulatory arrest: Studies on intraoperative metabolic changes and late postoperative development after correction of congenital heart disease. In deLange S, Hennis PJ, Kettler D, et al (eds). Cardiac Anesthesia: Problems, Innovations. New York: Nijhoff, 1986:121–142.
84. Rossi R, Ekroth R, Lincoln C. Detection of cerebral injury after total circulatory arrest and profound hypothermia by estimation of specific creatinine kinase isoenzyme levels using monoclonal antibody techniques. Am J Cardiol 58: 1236, 1986.
85. Samson DS, Clark K. A current review of brain abscess. Am J Med 54:201, 1973.
86. Scheld MW, Winn RH. Brain abscess. In Mandell GL, Douglas RG, Bennett JE (eds). Principles and Practice of Infectious Diseases. New York: John Wiley and Sons, 1985: 585–591.
87. Settergren G, Ohqvist Gun Lundberg S. Cerebral blood flow and cerebral metabolism in children following cardiac surgery with deep hypothermia and circulatory arrest. Clinical course and follow-up of psychomotor development. Scand J Thor Cardiovasc Surg 16:209, 1982.
88. Shaw PJ, Bates D, Cartlidge NEF. Neurologic and neuropsychological morbidity following major heart surgery: Comparison of coronary artery bypass and peripheral vascular surgery. Stroke 18:700, 1987.
89. Silbert A, Wolff PH, Mayer B, et al. Cyanotic heart disease and psychological development. Pediatrics 43:192, 1969.
90. Williams DL, Gelijns AC, Moskowitz AJ, et al. Hypoplastic left heart syndrome: Valuing the survival. J Thorac Cardiovasc Surg 119:720, 2000.

91. Goldberg CS, Schwartz EM, Brunberg JA, et al. Neurodevelopmental outcome of patients after the Fontan operation: A comparison between children with hypoplastic left heart syndrome and other functional single ventricle lesions. J Pediatr 137:646, 2000.
92. Glauser TA, Rorke LB, Weinberg PM, et al. Congenital brain anomalies associated with the hypoplastic left heart syndrome. Pediatrics 85:984, 1990.
93. Kurth CD, Steven JL, Montenegro LM, et al. Cerebral oxygen saturation before congenital heart surgery. Ann Thorac Surg 72:187, 2001.
94. Rogers BT, Msall ME, Buck GM, et al. Neurodevelopmental outcome of infants with hypoplastic left heart syndrome. J Pediatr 126:496, 1995.
95. Kern JH, Hinton VJ, Nereo NE, et al. Early developmental outcome after the Norwood procedure for Hypoplastic Left Heart Syndrome. Pediatrics 102:1148, 1998.
96. Ikle L, Hale K, Fashaw L, et al. Developmental outcome of patients with hypoplastic left heart syndrome treated with heart transplantation. J Pediatr 142:20, 2003.
97. Landgraf JM, Abetz L, Ware JE Jr. Child Health Questionnaire (CHQ). Boston: The Health Institute, New England Medical Center, 1996.
98. Dunbar-Masterson C, Wypij D, Bellinger DC, et al. General health status of children with D-transposition of the great arteries after the arterial switch operation. Circulation 104:I138, 2001.
99. Bjornstad PG, Spurkland I, Linberg, HL. The impact of severe congenital heart disease on physical and psychosocial functioning in adolescents. Cardiol Young 5:56, 2002.
100. Spurkland I, Bjornstad PG, Lindberg H, et al. Mental health and psychosocial functioning in adolescents with congenital heart disease: A comparison between adolescents born with severe heart defect and atrial septal defect. Acta Paediatr 82:71, 1993.
101. Utens EM, Verhulst FC, Meijboom FJ, et al. Behavioural and emotional problems in children and adolescents with congenital heart disease. Psychol Med 23:415, 1993.
102. DeMaso DR, Campis LK, Wypij D, et al. The impact of maternal perceptions and medical severity on the adjustment of children with congenital heart disease. J Pediatr Psychol 16:137, 1991.
103. Brandhagen DJ, Feldt RH, Williams DE. Long-term psychologic implications of congenital heart disease: A 25-year follow-up [see comments]. Mayo Clin Proc 66:474, 1991.
104. Bromberg JI, Beasley PJ, D'Angelo EJ, et al. Depression and anxiety in adults with congenital heart disease: A pilot study. Manuscript submitted for publication, 2002.
105. Horner T, Liberthson R, Jellinek MS. Psychosocial profile of adults with complex congenital heart disease. Mayo Clin Proc 75:31, 2000.
106. Salzer-Muhar U, Herle M, Floquet P, et al. Self-concept in male and female adolescents with congenital heart disease. Clin Pediatr 41:17, 2002.
107. Ferrieri P, Gewitz MH, Gerber MA, et al. Unique features of infective endocarditis in childhood. Circulation 105: 2115, 2002.
108. Sotaniemi KA. Cerebral outcome after extracorporeal circulation: Comparison between prospective and retrospective evaluations. Arch Neurol 40:75, 1983.
109. Stevenson J, Stone E, Dillard D, et al. Intellectual development of children subjected to prolonged circulatory arrest during hypothermic open heart surgery in infancy. Circulation 49:54, 1974.
110. Shu-yuan Y. Brain abscess associated with congenital heart disease. Surg Neurol 31:129, 1989.
111. Aebi C, Kaufmann F, Schaad U. Brain abscess in childhood: Long-term experiences. Eur J Pediatr 150:282, 1991.
112. Ciurea AV, Stoica F, Vasilescu G, et al. Neurosurgical management of brain abscesses in children. Childs Nerv Syst 15:309, 1999.
113. Fischer EG, McLennan JE, Suzuki Y. Cerebral abscess in children. Am J Dis Child 135:746, 1981.
114. Morgan H, Wood M, Murphey F. Experience with 88 consecutive cases of brain abscess. J Neurosurg 38:698, 1973.
115. Jadavji T, Humphreys RP, Prober CG. Brain abscesses in infants and children. Pediatr Infect Dis 4:394, 1985.
116. Wong TT, Lee LS, Wang HS, et al. Brain abscesses in children: A cooperative study of 83 cases. Childs Nerv Syst 5:19, 1989.
117. Tekkok IH, Erbengi A. Management of brain abscess in children: Review of 130 cases over a period of 21 years. Childs Nerv Syst 8:411, 1992.
118. Carey ME. Brain abscesses. Contemp Neurosurg 3:1, 1982.
119. Fischbein CA, Rosenthal A, Fisher EG, et al. Risk factors in brain abscess in patients with congenital heart disease. Am J Cardiol 34:97, 1974.
120. Heinneman HS, Braude AI. Anaerobic infection of the brain: Observations on eighteen consecutive cases of brain abscess. Am J Med 35:682, 1963.
121. Saez-Llorens X. Brain abscess in children. Semin Pediatr Infect Dis 14:108, 2003.
122. Roche M, Humphreys H, Smyth E, et al. A twelve-year review of central nervous system bacterial abscesses: Presentation and aetiology. Clin Microbiol Infect 9:803, 2003.
123. Takeshita M, Kagawa M, Yato S, et al. Current treatment of brain abscess in patients with congenital cyanotic heart disease. Neurosurgery 41:1270, 1997.
124. Garvey G. Current concepts of bacterial infections of the central nervous system: Bacterial meningitis and bacterial brain abscess. J Neurosurg 59:735, 1983.

10

Pulmonary Hypertension

Mary P. Mullen

The pulmonary circulation, normally a site of low resistance to blood flow, is subject to physiologic changes as well as a variety of disease processes influencing pulmonary arterial pressures. Without therapy, sustained elevation in pulmonary vascular resistance may result in progressive right ventricular dysfunction and death. Recent advances in the understanding of molecular genetics, cell biology, pathophysiology and treatment strategies have revolutionized the care of children with pulmonary vascular disease, resulting in improved survival and increased quality of life.[1–6] The pediatric cardiologist plays a critical role in the diagnosis and management of the child with pulmonary hypertension. This chapter deals with a general approach to pulmonary hypertension and excludes specific management of lesions secondary to structural cardiac defects.

PULMONARY VASCULAR DEVELOPMENT

The mechanisms involved in pulmonary vascular formation during lung development are complex and remain incompletely understood. It is known that vessel formation begins at the earliest stages of lung development and involves cell–extracellular matrix and cell–cell interactions.[7,8] Various growth factors have been implicated in the vascular development of the pulmonary circulation, including members of the vascular endothelial growth factor, angiopoietin, and ephrin families.

The pulmonary circulation undergoes important physiologic and anatomic changes in the first hours, weeks, and months of life. *In utero*, the pulmonary arteries are relatively thick walled, and pulmonary vascular resistance is very high, limiting pulmonary blood flow to less than 10% of combined right and left ventricular output.[9] At birth, the combined effects of mechanical expansion of the lung, increased oxygen tension, and shear stress lead to an increase in prostacyclin[10] and nitric oxide (NO) synthesis[11] and to the release of humoral substances such as bradykinin and adenosine, resulting in an acute decrease in pulmonary vascular resistance and allowing pulmonary blood flow to accommodate 100% of cardiac output.[9]

PATHOPHYSIOLOGY OF PULMONARY HYPERTENSION

Elevated pulmonary arterial pressure arises from three well-characterized vascular changes: vasoconstriction, thrombus formation, or proliferation of smooth muscle or endothelial cells in the pulmonary vessels.[12] Thus, pulmonary hypertension is associated with conditions causing chronic vasoconstriction, thrombosis, or abnormalities of vessel function.

Recent advances in molecular biology have allowed for the identification of several key mediators of vascular function in the pulmonary vasculature.[12] Arachidonic acid metabolites such as prostacyclin and thromboxane A_2 are active in the pulmonary vessels, associated with vasodilation and vasoconstriction, respectively. In addition, prostacyclin is a platelet inhibitor and is capable of inhibiting endothelial cell proliferation, whereas thromboxane A_2 is a platelet activator. Endothelin-1 is a vasoconstrictor that causes smooth muscle proliferation in pulmonary vessels.[13] Vasodilation is induced by NO, which is produced by endothelial cells, through a cyclic guanosine monophosphate

TABLE 10–1. Factors Involved in Mediating Pulmonary Hypertension

Factor	Pulmonary Vascular Tone Effects	Hemostatic Effects	Cellular Effects	Clinical Observations
Prostacyclin (arachidonic acid metabolite)	Vasodilator	Inhibits platelet function	Inhibits proliferation of smooth muscle/endothelial cells	Decreased production in PH patients
Thromboxane A_2 (arachidonic acid metabolite)	Vasoconstrictor	Activates platelet function		Increased levels in PH patients
Endothelin-1 (21 amino-acid peptide)	Vasoconstrictor		Smooth muscle mitogen	Increased levels in PH patients; levels inversely correlate with cardiac output
Nitric oxide	Vasodilator	Inhibits platelet function	Inhibits proliferation of smooth muscle/endothelial cells	Decreased levels of NO synthase in pulmonary vessels of patients with PH

(cGMP)-dependent pathway,[14] and which additionally inhibits platelet function and smooth vessel proliferation.

Clinical studies suggest imbalances in these potent vasoactive factors, as well as in other vasoactive compounds, such as vascular endothelial cell growth factor, adrenomedullin, serotonin, and vasoactive peptides, in patients with pulmonary hypertension. These findings are summarized in Table 10-1. With great consistency, patients with pulmonary hypertension have been found to have altered homeostatic balances of these factors, tending toward prothrombotic, vasoconstrictive physiology. These clinical findings suggest that acquired alterations in normal vascular physiology contribute to the onset of pulmonary hypertension.

Other conditions that contribute to chronic changes in the pulmonary vasculature include hypoxemia and small vessel thrombosis. Chronic hypoxemia contributes to pulmonary vasoconstriction. Thrombotic events in the microvasculature contribute to hypoxia and also release acute mediators that contribute to vasoconstriction.

The pathologic vascular changes associated with pulmonary hypertension were described by Heath and Edwards[15] in patients with pulmonary hypertension secondary to congenital septal defects. Classic initial changes (Heath and Edwards grades 1 and 2) include medial hypertrophy, smooth muscle extension into nonmuscular arteries, and intimal cell proliferation from smooth muscle thickening. Progressive changes include intimal fibrosis and eventual thinning of the media with dilation of the vessels (grades 3 and 4). Eventually, medial fibrosis and necrotizing arteritis changes (grades 5 and 6) arise in the pulmonary vessels (Fig. 10-1).

These observations suggest that the pathophysiology of pulmonary hypertension is governed by alterations in the normal function of vascular tone, hemostatic activity, and vascular cell biology. Imbalances between vasodilators and vasoconstrictors, platelet activation and inhibition, and endothelial and smooth muscle cell proliferation and inhibition conspire to cause chronic pathologic changes in pulmonary vessels and worsening clinical symptoms (Fig. 10-2). Importantly, these contributing factors to the pathophysiology of pulmonary hypertension also serve as emerging targets for treatment. Strategies that reverse these underlying contributors to pulmonary hypertension appear able to improve clinical function in patients.

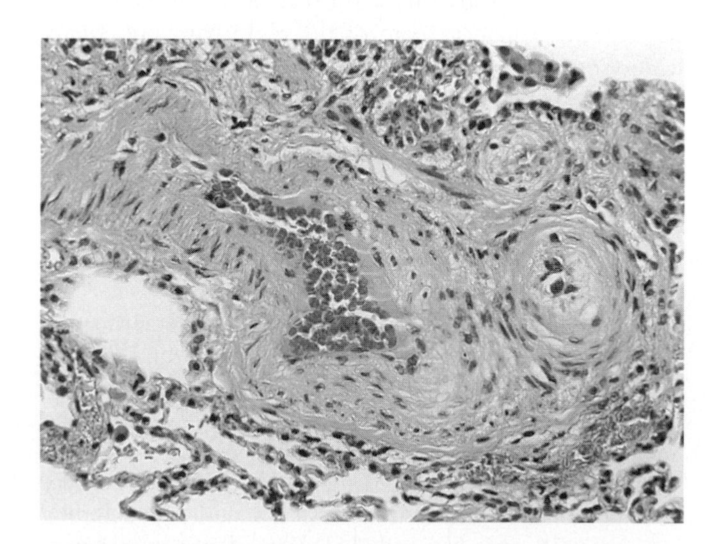

FIGURE 10–1 *Plexiform lesion shows pulmonary artery with medical muscular hypertrophy* ***(left)****, with loss of internal elastic lamina and muscle and replacement by fibrous tissue* ***(right)****. The two small branches* ***(right)*** *have fibrous walls and marked intimal thickening.*
Courtesy of Harry Kozakewich, MD, Children's Hospital Boston.

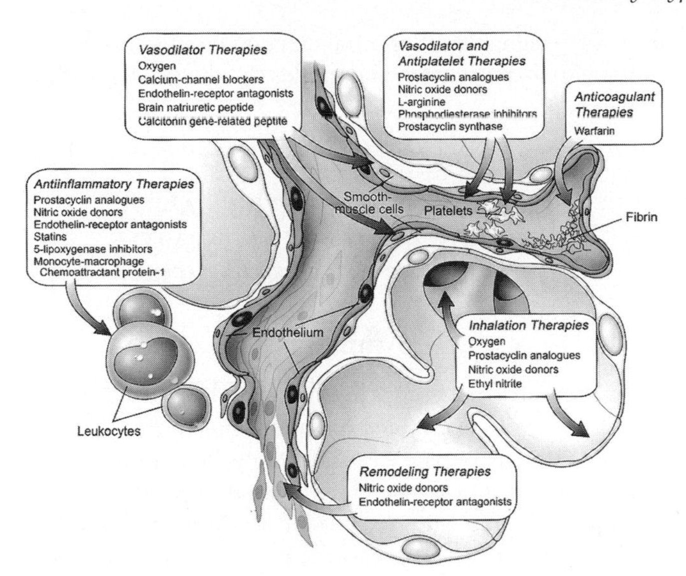

FIGURE 10–2 *Pathophysiologic factors and therapeutic targets in pulmonary hypertension.*
Adapted from Farber HW, Loscalzo J. Pulmonary arterial hypertension. N Engl J Med 351:1655, 2004, copyright © 2004, Massachusetts Medical Society. All rights reserved.

GENETIC CAUSES OF PULMONARY HYPERTENSION

Clinical descriptions of familial cases of pulmonary hypertension date back to the 1950s. However, recent genetic studies have allowed characterization of specific, inherited mutations that predispose patients to pulmonary hypertension. Family registry data and DNA linkage analyses have led to the identification of two specific genes—bone morphogenetic protein receptor type 2 (*BMPR2*) and activin-like kinase type 1 (*ALK1*)—that are associated with pulmonary hypertension.[16–19] These defects are autosomal dominant, although there is incomplete penetrance, meaning that the development of symptoms in affected individuals is highly variable. *BMPR2* and *ALK1* are both members of the transforming growth factor-β (TGF-β) receptor family. *BMPR2* was linked to pulmonary hypertension through familial studies and classic genetic linkage analyses. The gene is located on chromosome 2q33. A variety of mutations in the receptor, including mutations in the extracellular, transmembrane, and intracellular kinase domains, have been characterized, all of which are associated with pulmonary hypertension, although different families possess unique mutations. Most mutations give rise to frameshift or nonsense mutations that truncate the protein.

Clinical studies of families with hereditary hemorrhagic telangiectasia (HHT) led to identification of another gene, *ALK1*, associated with both HHT and familial pulmonary hypertension. HHT families with missense and nonsense mutations in *ALK1* had cases of pulmonary hypertension identical in clinical and pathologic appearance to those seen among patients with *BMPR2* mutations.

To date, it seems that about 10% of idiopathic cases of pulmonary hypertension arise from mutations in *BMPR2*, which accounts for roughly half of all cases of familial pulmonary hypertension.[20] Among *BMPR2* mutation carriers, the lifetime risk for pulmonary hypertension is estimated to be between 15% and 20%. The prevalence and penetrance for *ALK1* mutations in pulmonary hypertension are not well established.

Patients diagnosed with pulmonary hypertension merit a thorough family history to explore whether hereditary factors may contribute to their risk for disease. At present, genetic testing for these specific mutations remains an investigational tool available only through research laboratories.

One important outcome of these genetic findings has been the implication of the TGF-β signaling pathway in the pathogenesis of pulmonary hypertension. It is believed that changes in TGF-β receptor signaling contribute to endothelial and smooth muscle cell proliferation in the pulmonary vasculature[21] (Fig. 10-3). The low incidence of pulmonary hypertension in individuals with known mutations in *BMPR2* and *ALK1* supports the concept that in addition to hereditary predisposition, additional triggers such as acquired events or environmental exposures are needed to give rise to the clinical syndrome of pulmonary hypertension. It seems likely that the known genetic

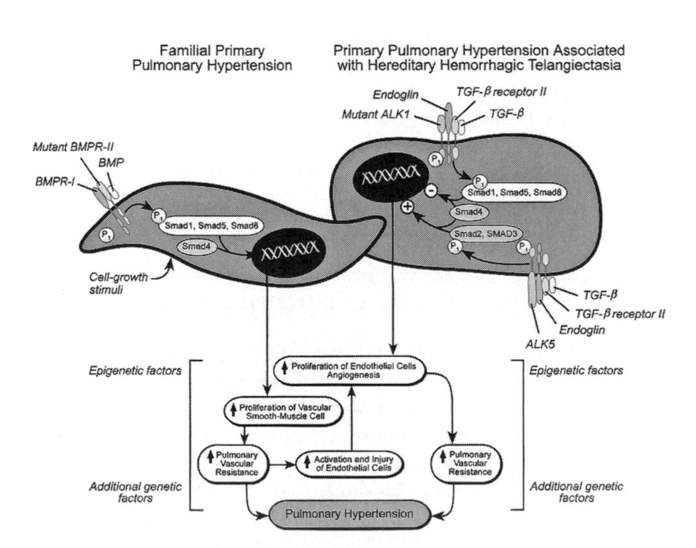

FIGURE 10–3 *Pathophysiology of genetic predisposition to pulmonary hypertension.*
Adapted from Loscalzo J. Genetic clues to the cause of primary pulmonary hypertension. N Engl J Med 345:367, 2001. copyright © 2001, Massachusetts Medical Society. All rights reserved.

contributions alter one aspect of the triad of endothelial cell biology, vasoconstriction, and thrombosis by predisposing to cellular proliferation in the pulmonary arteries. Additional injury in the other domains is necessary for pulmonary hypertension to develop.

CLINICAL CLASSIFICATION OF PULMONARY HYPERTENSION

All pulmonary hypertension is classified according to World Health Organization revised criteria (2003), which reflect the underlying etiology believed to be the primary contributor to disease[22] (Table 10-2). Major causes in this classification are (1) primary pulmonary arterial changes from idiopathic or familial causes, or acquired from a variety of other medical conditions, toxic exposures, or congenital systemic-to-pulmonary vascular shunts; (2) pulmonary hypertension with major venous or capillary involvement; (3) persistent pulmonary hypertension of the newborn; (4) pulmonary venous hypertension arising from left-sided heart disease; (5) pulmonary hypertension arising from chronic lung diseases associated with hypoxia; (6) pulmonary hypertension in association with chronic thrombotic-embolic disease; and (7) pulmonary hypertension arising in the setting of miscellaneous disorders that are associated with extrinsic compression of the vasculature. This classification provides a valuable differential diagnosis to the problem of pulmonary hypertension and guides the diagnostic workup of patients.

CLINICAL PRESENTATION AND EVALUATION OF PATIENTS WITH PULMONARY HYPERTENSION

Symptoms

The pediatric patient with pulmonary hypertension may be referred with symptoms including shortness of breath, exercise intolerance, and easy fatigability. Patients may experience chest pain, chronic cough, vomiting, and recurrent syncope. Children with right-to-left shunting in the setting of elevated right-sided pressures may have been noted to be intermittently cyanotic. Infants may be irritable, exhibit poor feeding, or display tachypnea. These findings are all nonspecific and require thoughtful evaluation before a diagnosis of pulmonary hypertension can be established. Based on the clinical history, the patient is assigned to a functional class (I to IV) according to World Health Organization Guidelines, which are a modification of the New York Heart Association heart failure classification[23] (Table 10-3). This classification scale allows prognosis of long-term outcomes and provides treatment recommendations.

TABLE 10–2. Diagnostic Classification of Pulmonary Hypertension

I. Pulmonary arterial hypertension
- Idiopathic
- Familial
- Associated with
  - Collagen vascular disease
  - Congenital ventricular to pulmonary shunts
    - Atrial and ventricular septal defect
    - Patent ductus arteriosus, Atrioventricular septal defects
    - Aortopulmonary window, Truncus arteriosus
    - Single ventricle with unobstructed pulmonary blood flow
  - Portal Hypertension, HIV infection, Pertussis
  - Drugs and toxins (cocaine, methamphetamine, tryptophan, rapeseed oil, anoregixens such as aminorex fumarate, fenfluramine, dexfenfluramine)
  - Other (thyroid disorders, glycogen storage disease, Gaucher disease, hereditary hemorrhagic telangiectasia, hemoglobinopathies such as sickle cell anemia and β-thalassemia, myeloproliferative disorders, splenectomy)

II. Associated with significant venous or capillary involvement
- Pulmonary veno-occlusive disease
- Pulmonary capillary hemangiomatosis

III. Persistent pulmonary hypertension of the newborn

IV. Pulmonary hypertension with left heart disease
- Left-sided atrial or ventricular heart disease
  - Pulmonary vein stenosis, Cor-triatriatum

V. Pulmonary hypertension associated with lung diseases and/or hypoxemia
- Chronic obstructive pulmonary disease, Interstitial lung disease
- Bronchopulmonary, Alveolar capillary dysplasia
  - Congenital diaphragmatic hernia
  - Obstructive sleep apnea
  - Chronic tonsillar hypertrophy, Craniofacial disorders
  - Alveolar hypoventilation disorders, Residence at high altitude
- Developmental abnormalities

VI. Pulmonary hypertension due to chronic thrombotic and/or embolic disease

VII. Miscellaneous
- Sarcoidosis, histocytosis X, lymphangiomatosis, compression of pulmonary vessels

(Modified from Simonneau et al: Clinic classification of pulmonary hypertension. J Am Coll Cardiol 43:55, 2004.)

TABLE 10–3. Functional Classification of Pulmonary Hypertension

A. Class I—Patients with pulmonary hypertension but without resulting limitation of physical activity. Ordinary physical activity dose not cause undue dyspnoea or fatigue, chest pain or near syncope
B. Class II—Patients with pulmonary hypertension resulting in slight limitation of physical activity. They are comfortable at rest. Ordinary physical activity causes undue dyspnoea or fatigue, chest pain or near syncope
C. Class III—Patients with pulmonary hypertension resulting in pronounced limitation of physical activity. They are comfortable at rest. Less than ordinary activity causes undue dyspnoea or fatigue, chest pain or near syncope
D. Class IV—Patients with pulmonary hypertension with inability to carry out any physical activity without symptoms. These patients manifest signs of right heart failure. Dyspnoea and/or fatigue may even be present at rest. Discomfort is increased by any physical activity

Functional classification of pulmonary hypertension modified after the New York Heart Association functional classification according to the World Health Organization, 1998. From British Cardiac Society Guidelines and Medical Practice Committee. Recommendations on the management of pulmonary hypertension in clinical practice. Heart 86 (Suppl 1):11, 2001.

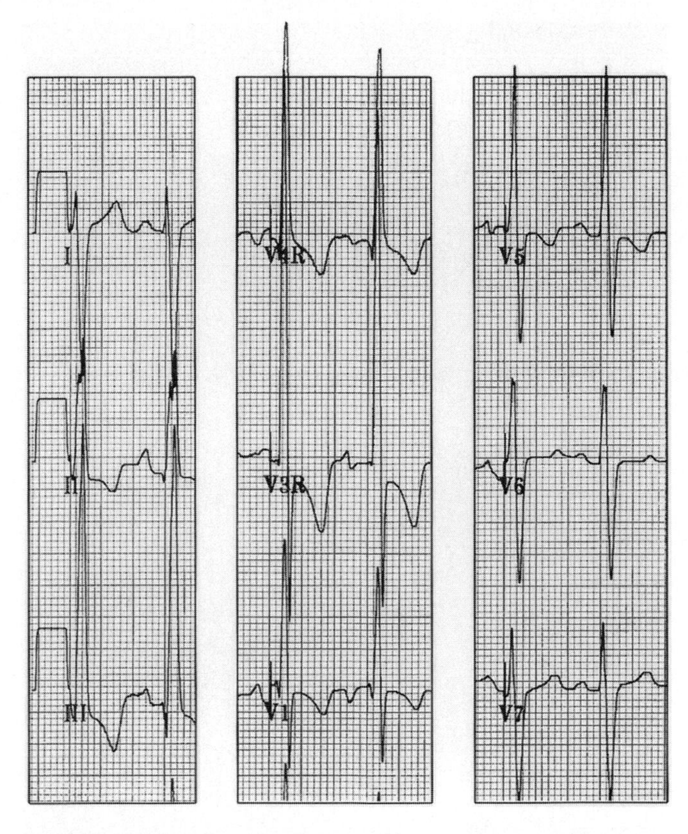

FIGURE 10–4 *Electrocardiogram from a 10-year-old patient with severe idiopathic pulmonary hypertension and systemic-level pulmonary resistance unresponsive to vasodilators, showing marked right ventricular hypertrophy.*

Physical Examination

Initial examination of patients with pulmonary hypertension may reveal tachypnea and cyanosis. Cardiac exam may reveal a right ventricular heave and palpable second heart sound. Auscultation may disclose that the latter is single or narrowly split with an accentuated pulmonary component, reflecting elevated pulmonary artery pressure. There may be a soft blowing systolic murmur of tricuspid regurgitation along the left sternal border, and there may be an early high-frequency diastolic murmur of pulmonary regurgitation, both due to the elevated right-sided pressures. The child with right heart failure may have increased jugular venous pressure, hepatomegaly, ascites, or pedal edema.

Electrocardiogram

The electrocardiogram typically displays right axis deviation and right ventricular hypertrophy. There may be depressed S-T segments and inverted T waves in the anterior and lateral chest leads consistent with increased right ventricular strain[24] (Fig. 10-4).

Chest Radiograph

The chest radiograph may show cardiac enlargement with a prominent main pulmonary artery segment. There may be decreased vasculature in the peripheral lung fields due to paucity of pulmonary blood flow (Fig. 10-5). Computed tomography is important in every patient with pulmonary hypertension to exclude primary lung disease.

Cardiac Evaluation

When the diagnosis of pulmonary hypertension is suspected, a thorough initial cardiovascular evaluation is warranted to establish the diagnosis and to exclude structural cardiac lesions, as well as to characterize the patient's hemodynamics and potential response to drug therapy.

Echocardiography

The echocardiographic evaluation is essential to evaluate cardiac anatomy, rule out contributing causes such as left-sided structural heart disease, pulmonary vein stenosis, and shunt lesions. Patients with pulmonary hypertension can have right ventricular systolic pressure estimated through use of Doppler echocardiography if some tricuspid regurgitation is present. Other imaging findings include right atrial and ventricular enlargement as well as pulmonary artery dilation and regurgitation.

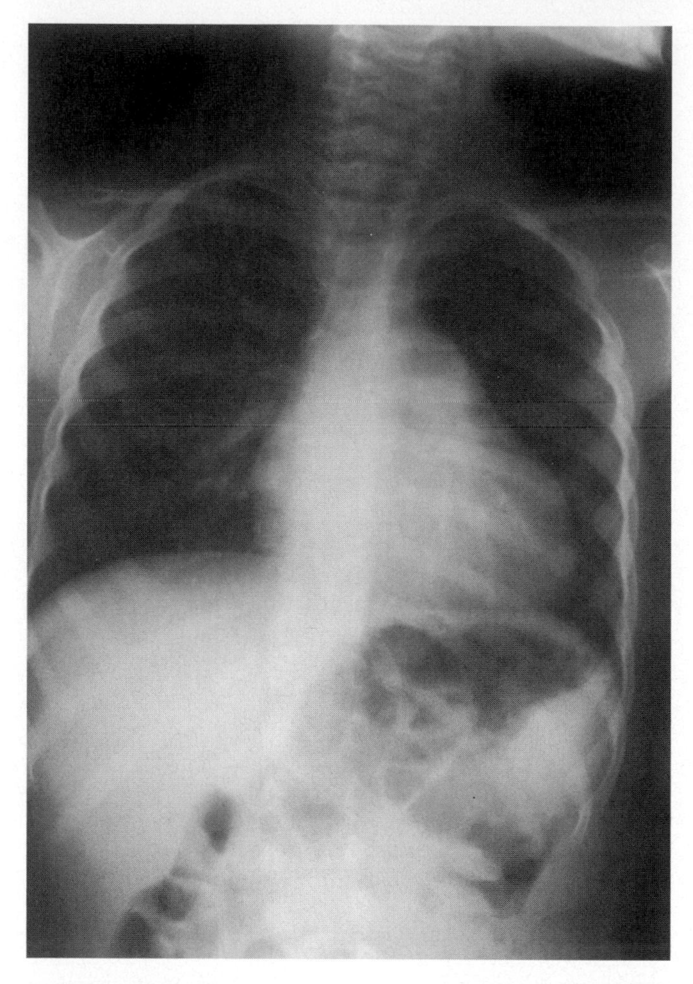

FIGURE 10–5 *Chest x-ray in a 3-year-old with idiopathic pulmonary hypertension. Note the prominent main pulmonary artery segment.*
From Fyler DC [ed]. Nadas' Pediatric Cardiology. Philadelphia: Hanley and Belfus, 1992.

Cardiac Catheterization

Catheterization of the child with pulmonary artery hypertension is essential for diagnosis and evaluation of therapeutic options and must be carefully planned with coordinated care both before and after the procedure by catheterization and anesthesia staff. Patients must be adequately sedated without incurring hypoventilation to avoid respiratory acidosis. Scrupulous attention should be paid to the patient's hydration status before catheterization. Hemodynamic measurements at the time of catheterization establish the diagnosis of pulmonary hypertension, defined as a mean pulmonary artery pressure (mPAP) greater than 25 mm Hg at rest or greater than 30 mm Hg with exercise, with a pulmonary capillary wedge pressure or left ventricular end diastolic pressure of 15 mm Hg or less and pulmonary vascular resistance greater than 3 units.[25] Cardiac output measurements are determined by thermodilution in patients without shunting or by the Fick method with measured oxygen consumption in those with a patent foramen ovale and minor shunting in either direction.

Pulmonary vasodilator testing at the time of catheterization with a short-acting pulmonary vasodilator is critical to deciding on therapeutic options for the child with pulmonary hypertension. Patients can be challenged with inhalation of 100% oxygen or use of short-acting agents such as inhaled NO, or by intravenous adenosine or prostacyclin to determine whether the vasculature is responsive to vasodilator therapy. Response is defined as reduction in mPAP of at least 10 mm Hg to achieve mPAP of 40 mm Hg or less while maintaining normal or high cardiac output. This subset of patients may benefit from long-term calcium channel blocker therapy.[26] The rate of response to acute vasodilator therapy ranges from 40% to 60% in children (Fig. 10-6; Exhibit 10-1), with younger patients being more likely to have a better response.[27]

Angiography is performed after hemodynamic assessment, with great care being taken to avoid precipitating a pulmonary hypertensive crisis. Selective, preferably distal, pulmonary artery contrast injections are used to visualize the pulmonary vasculature. Distal stenotic lesions, whether congenital or acquired owing to recanalization of thrombotic lesions, are carefully balloon-dilated. In addition, an aortogram is included to exclude aortopulmonary connections. After cardiac catheterization, patients are observed carefully for hypoventilation after sedation, which may contribute to acidosis and precipitate a pulmonary hypertensive crisis.

DIAGNOSTIC EVALUATION OF PATIENTS WITH PULMONARY HYPERTENSION

When a diagnosis of pulmonary hypertension has been made, a thorough diagnostic investigation is mandatory, this to include all possible underlying, and in some instances, reversible causes. Our own detailed diagnostic algorithm employed at Children's Hospital Boston is shown in Table 10-4. Based on clinical history, family history, and presenting symptoms, tests including ventilation-perfusion scans or high-resolution computed tomography to rule out chronic thromboembolic disease, pulmonary function testing, exercise testing, sleep study, liver function tests and liver ultrasound, thyroid function tests, evaluation for collagen vascular disease, human immunodeficiency virus testing, hypercoagulability workup, and genetic and metabolic screening are undertaken. Given the increased morbidity and mortality risks associated with lung biopsy, this procedure

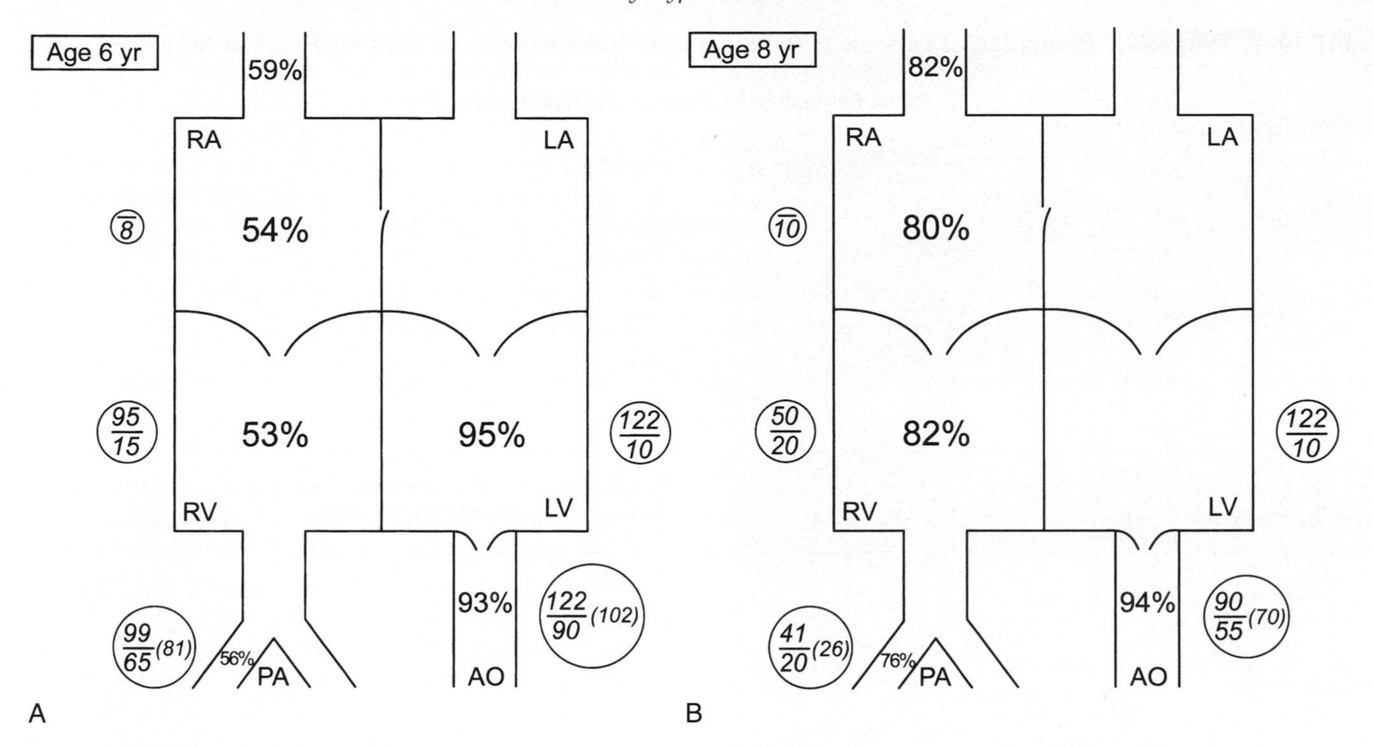

FIGURE 10–6 *Catheterization data in a patient with idiopathic pulmonary hypertension.* ***A,*** *At age 6 years, before treatment, showing severe pulmonary hypertension with resistance (29 Wood units), low cardiac output (2.5 L/min/m^2), responding to 100% O_2 and nitric oxide.* ***B,*** *At age 8 years, after 2 years of intravenous prostacyclin, showing significant reduction of pulmonary artery pressure and resistance (3.4 Wood units) and improved cardiac output (4.7 L/min/m^2); right ventricular hypertrophy had also significantly decreased on electrocardiogram. AO, aorta, LA, left atrium; LV, left ventricle; PA, pulmonary artery; RA, right atrium; RV, right ventricle.*

Exhibit 10-1
Children's Hospital Boston Experience
1988-2002

Pulmonary Hypertension with Dermal Heart

Over 14 years, 55 patients (71% female) with pulmonary artery hypertension and a structurally normal heart were seen. Of these, a thrombotic etiology was considered the underlying cause in 28 and idiopathic in the other 27 patients. There were no instances of pulmonary veno-occlusive disease or vasculitis encountered in this search.

Groups	*N*	*%F*	*Cath Age*	*Rp*	*Median Follow-up*
Thrombotic	28	64	28-79 yr (median, 48)	4-35 (median, 13)	2 yr
Idiopathic	27	78	2 mo-39 yr (median, 14)	8-60 (median, 30)	2 yr

In the idiopathic group, some reduction in pulmonary resistance (Rp) with vasodilators occurred in 47% (dramatic in 15%; see Fig. 10-6), one had alveolar dysplasia on a lung biopsy, and another underwent bilateral lung transplantation at age 4 yr and repeated at age 8 yr. There were 6 known deaths in the idiopathic group at ages 2-35 yr (median, 30 yr and Rp 32 Wood units), unresponsive to vasodilators.

N, Patient number; F, Female.

TABLE 10–4. Diagnostic Evaluation of Patients with Pulmonary Hypertension at Childrens Hospital Boston

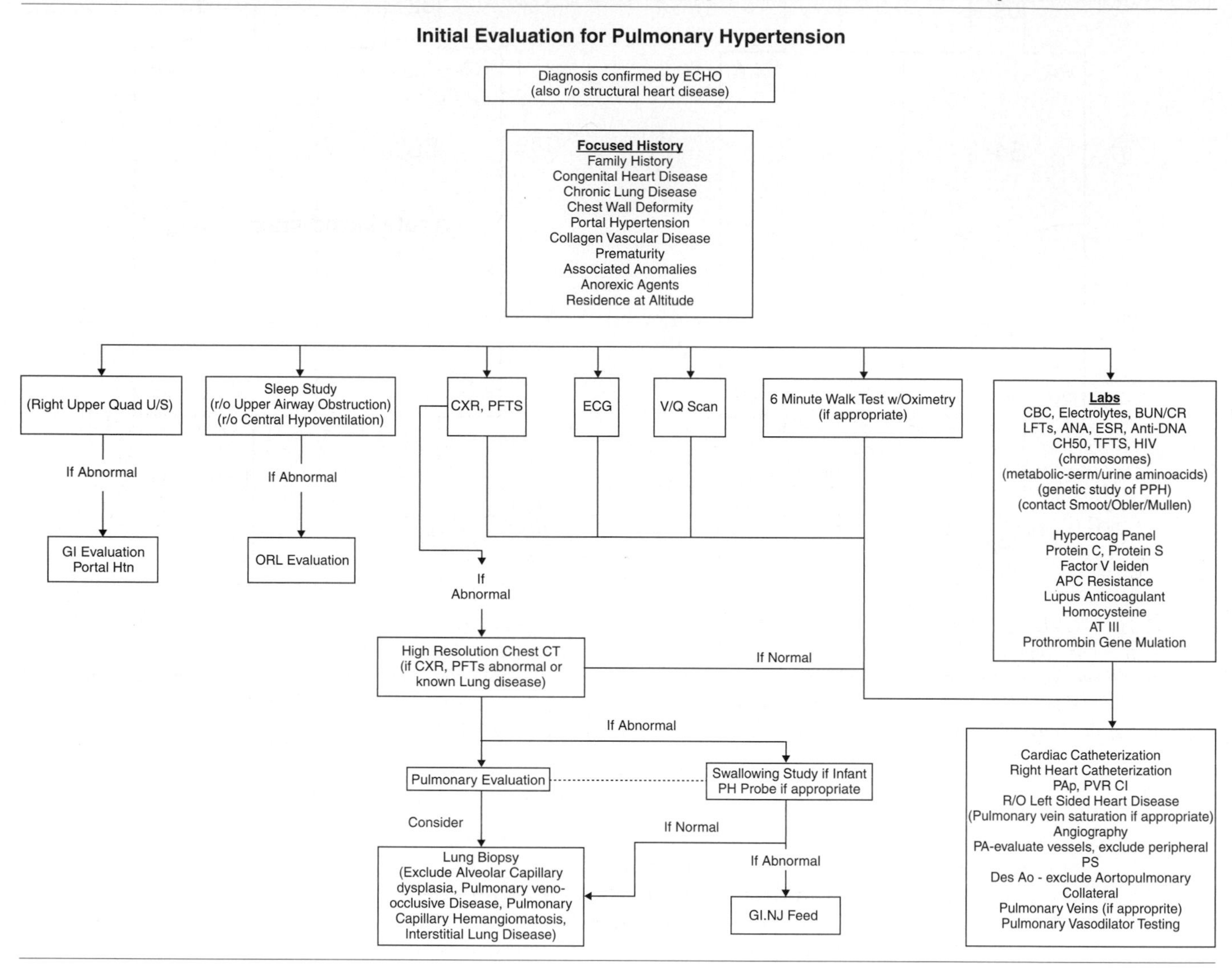

is reserved for the diagnosis of diseases that may change therapy, including vasculitis, granulomatous lung disease, pulmonary veno-occlusive disease, pulmonary capillary hemangiomatosis, alveolar capillary dysplasia, and various interstitial lung diseases.[28–30]

NATURAL HISTORY AND THERAPY FOR PULMONARY HYPERTENSION

The true incidence of pulmonary hypertension is not known. Estimates suggest 1 to 2 cases per 1 million people in the population. There is a predominance of cases in girls and women, with a female-to-male ratio of 1.7 or 1.8 to 1.[31] As recently as the 1980s, pulmonary hypertension carried a grave prognosis in children, with a median life expectancy of less than 1 year.[32] Recent advances in diagnosis and treatment have improved the natural history of pulmonary hypertension in children, which in the past was dismal. Indeed, recent data suggest a median survival well in excess of 5 years in patients with access to vasodilator therapy such as prostacyclin and calcium channel blocker treatment[33] (Fig 10-7). Prolonged survival is particularly observed among those who respond favorably to vasodilator treatment. This finding places a premium on the correct classification of patients as responders or nonresponders to acute vasodilator testing.

There are several unique challenges when interpreting the treatment literature for pulmonary hypertension.

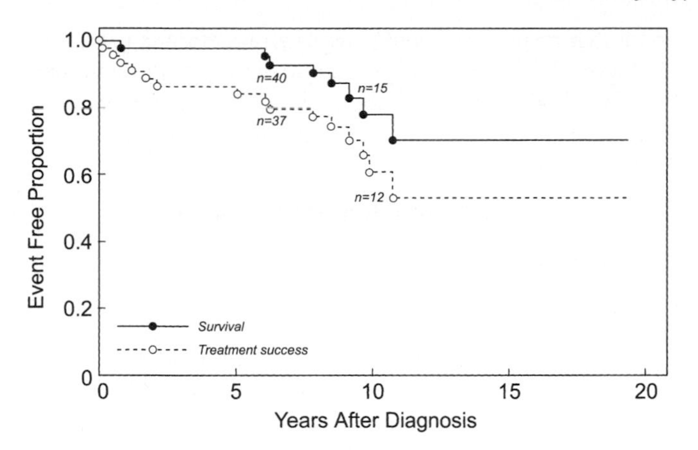

FIGURE 10–7 *Survival of pediatric patients with pulmonary hypertension in the modern treatment era. Data show Kaplan-Meier analyses for treatment success and transplant-free overall survival for pediatric patients with pulmonary hypertension treated with prostacyclin and/or calcium blocker therapy.*
From Young D, Widlitz AC, Rosenzweig EB, et al. Outcomes in children with idiopathic pulmonary arterial hypertension. Circulation 110(6):660, 2004.

First, pulmonary hypertension is a heterogeneous disorder, arising from many different etiologic factors, not all of which are known. This diversity complicates the understanding of the treatment and expected outcomes for patients. Second, pulmonary hypertension, particularly in the pediatric population, is a relatively rare disorder. Thus, treatment principles for children are often derived from observations in adults, without large clinical experiences in younger people to confirm independently the same observations. There are reasons that data from adults may not be easily extrapolated to children, including the different natural life expectancy, different etiologies for pulmonary hypertension, different intrinsic pulmonary vascular reactivity, and historically worse natural history of the disease in children. Third, the critical end points for clinical trials are widely debated. Many trials have reported on mean changes in 6-minute walking distance[34] or changes in hemodynamic parameters. Both of these may be challenging in younger children. Beyond these technical challenges, there are relatively few studies that have reported on long-term clinical outcomes such as survival, or on quality of life or functional status, which may be crucial measures for children and their families. For all these reasons, treatment of children with pulmonary hypertension remains individualized. Although many algorithms have been promulgated to guide treatment choices, the exact sequence, duration, combination, and timing of treatments have not been characterized.[22,35,36]

The therapeutic approach to the child with pulmonary hypertension begins with a thorough identification of underlying causes and with first treatments directed at these factors.[37] These may include such measures as supplemental oxygen for patients with parenchymal lung disease, anti-inflammatory therapies for patients with collagen vascular disease, continuous positive airway pressure therapy and tonsillectomy for patients with obstructive sleep apnea,[38,39] and anticoagulation and potential thromboendarterectomy for chronic thromboembolic disease.

Acute Vasodilator Testing

As noted earlier, the initial evaluation for treatment of pulmonary hypertension is assessment of response to acute vasodilator therapy with inhaled NO, intravenous prostacyclin, or other short-acting vasodilator. Patients with a significant hemodynamic response to acute vasodilator testing during cardiac catheterization (a decrease of at least 20% in mPAP to 40 mm Hg or less, with no change or an increase in cardiac output) are defined as "responders." They are likely to respond to calcium channel blockade and other vasodilator therapies, whereas in contrast, nonresponders are unlikely to respond to calcium channel blocker therapy, and indeed their use in such patients is dangerous[40] (Fig. 10-8). An overview of treatment for pulmonary hypertension based

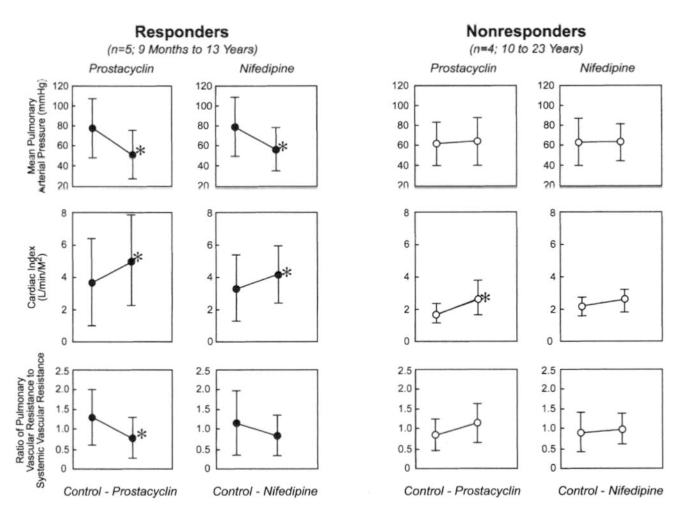

FIGURE 10–8 *Acute vasodilator testing: sensitivity of responders and nonresponders to calcium channel blocker therapy. Nine patients with primary pulmonary hypertension underwent acute testing with prostacyclin (9–38 ng/kg/min) and nifedipine (0.5–2.0 mg/kg). Those who responded to prostacyclin had a 20% or greater decrease in mean pulmonary arterial pressure, a rise in cardiac index, and no change or a decrease in the pulmonary-to-systemic vascular resistance ratio. Patients who responded to a prostacyclin also showed similar hemodynamic improvement with nifedipine. Those who responded (mean age, 5 years) were considerably younger than those who did not (mean age, 17.3 years).*
From Barst RJ. Pharmacologically induced pulmonary vasodilation in children and young adults with primary pulmonary hypertension. Chest 89:497, 1986.

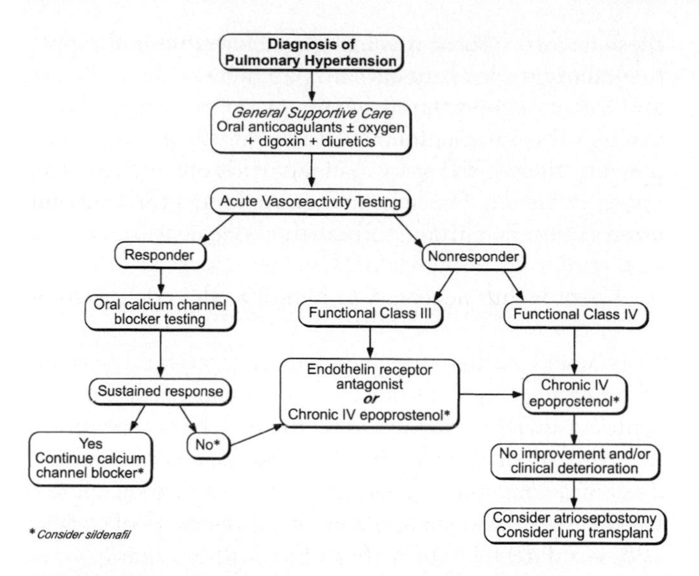

FIGURE 10–9 *Algorithm for treatment of pulmonary hypertension. (Adapted from the World Symposium on Pulmonary Arterial Hypertension, 2003.)*
From Badesch DB, Abman SH, Ahearn GS, et al. Medical therapy for pulmonary arterial hypertension: ACCP evidence-based clinical practice guidelines. Chest 126(1 Suppl):355, 2004.

on initial response to acute vasodilator testing is presented in Figure 10-9. Table 10-5 lists some of the agents commonly used in children with pulmonary hypertension and includes dosage data, mechanisms of action, and side effects.

Calcium Channel Blockers

Historical experience with use of calcium channel blockers as vasodilator therapy suggested that these drugs can prolong survival in patients who respond.[1] To date, there are no randomized clinical trials involving calcium channel blockers for pulmonary hypertension. Because of the potential for severe hemodynamic collapse during initial challenge with calcium channel blockers, these drugs are not appropriate as first-line treatment during diagnostic challenge. Instead, acute vasodilator testing is done with oxygen, NO, or prostacyclin.[41] Patients who respond to such therapies are candidates for initiation of calcium channel blocker treatment, performed with close hemodynamic monitoring. Patients who tolerate initiation of calcium channel blockers and who have sustained hemodynamic benefit are continued on oral therapy. Patients without sustained benefit during initiation of therapy should have treatment with calcium channel blockers discontinued. Fewer than 20% of adults have a favorable clinical response to such therapy, compared with nearly 40% of children.[27,42] Dosage is cautiously titrated to optimize cardiac output and minimize pulmonary hypertension.

TABLE 10–5. Common Therapeutic Agents for Pediatric Patients with Pulmonary Hypertension

Agent	Mechanism of Action	Dose/Therapeutic Range	Side Effects
Oxygen	Vasodilator	Titrate to provide symptom relief, reduce hypoxemia or standard nocturnal dose	
Warfarin	Anticoagulant	Standard prophylaxis: INR 1.5 to 2. Patients prone to trauma, such as toddlers: INR < 1.5; Patients with known hypercoaguable state: INR 2.5 to 3.5	Bleeding
Digoxin	Positive inotrope; anti-arrhythmic	8 to 10 mcg/kg QD or BID depending on age for management of right heart failure	Dysrhythmia
Diuretics		Titrate to manage volume in patients with right heart failure	Hypotension; electrolyte disturbance
Nifedipine	Calcium channel blocker vasodilator	Titrated dose based on decrease in pulmonary pressures with maintenance of cardiac output and pulmonary wedge pressure	Hypotension, hemodynamic compromise
Inhaled Nitric oxide	Vasodilator	Titrated to effect	Rebound hypertension with cessation of therapy; methemoglobinemia
Sildenafil	Phosphodiesterase inhibitor	Investigational, off-label use IV/PO	Headache; flushing; nasal congestion
Bosentan	Endothelin receptor antagonist	Titrated BID oral dose	Transaminase elevations/hepatic toxicity; flushing; syncope; teratogen; anemia
Prostacyclin	Vasodilator and inhibitor of platelet aggregration	IV: epoprostenol SQ: treprostinil PO: beraprost Inhaled: iloprost } titrate to effect	Headache, diarrhea, jaw pain, leg pain, rash, nausea, flushing, syncope, catheter complications (IV)

Prostacyclin

Prostacyclin therapy has been widely studied in the treatment of pulmonary hypertension. Because of its potent vasodilatory activity in the pulmonary vasculature, it is a useful drug for such patients, although the precise mechanism of action is not known. It has been shown to improve hemodynamic function, exercise tolerance, quality of life, and survival for patients with primary pulmonary hypertension.[6,43] Prostacyclin (epoprostenol) is most commonly administered as a continuous intravenous infusion through a central venous catheter. The initial dose is 0.5 to 1 ng/kg, which is carefully titrated over time based on patient tolerability and response. It can be effective regardless of clinical response to acute pulmonary vasodilator testing. Because it requires continuous intravenous access, patients are subject to a variety of complications, including catheter sepsis and, if treatment is interrupted inadvertently, significant hemodynamic changes. Children can thrive on this drug over long periods of time. Resistance or tolerance to prostacyclin therapy can occur, the mechanisms of which are unknown. A variety of prostacyclin formulations have been developed such that oral (beraprost), inhaled (iloprost), and subcutaneous (treprostinil) routes of administration are now available.

Endothelin Receptor Antagonists

Endothelin-1, a potent vasoconstrictor, mediates its activity through two types of endothelin receptors, ET_A and ET_B. Newer treatments for pulmonary hypertension include the dual-receptor antagonist Bosentan and the ET_A selective receptor antagonist, sitaxsentan.[44] Bosentan has been shown in randomized clinical trials to improve functional capacity and hemodynamics in adults with pulmonary hypertension,[45,46] and similar results have been identified in children.[47] This drug has induced elevation of liver function tests and anemia, both of which are reversible. Thus, careful monitoring of transaminases and hemoglobin levels is necessary during treatment. In addition, Bosentan is a potential teratogen. Young patients need to be counseled as to these effects and use effective forms of contraception.

Inhaled Nitric Oxide

This is a selective pulmonary vasodilator with a brief half-life and rapid inactivation by hemoglobin.[48,49] Additional beneficial effects include improvement of oxygenation in the setting of ventilation-perfusion mismatch, inhibition of platelet aggregation, decreased proliferation of vascular smooth muscle, and promotion of vascular remodeling.[50,51] Treatment studies have demonstrated that NO is effective in acute vasodilator testing in the catheterization laboratory, in treating persistent pulmonary hypertension of the newborn,[52–54] and in managing postoperative pulmonary hypertension after repair of congenital heart disease[55] and after lung and heart transplantation.[50,56] Several reports have also described the beneficial effects of chronic administration of inhaled NO in ambulatory patients.[57,58] Patients treated with NO should be monitored for methemoglobin levels. They are at risk for rebound pulmonary hypertension with abrupt discontinuation of therapy. Careful weaning of treatment is thus necessary to minimize this complication.

Type 5 Phosphodiesterase Inhibitors

Sildenafil is a selective inhibitor of type 5 phosphodiesterase, which breaks down cGMP and limits cGMP-mediated NO vasodilation. Elevated amounts of type 5 phosphodiesterase are found in the pulmonary vasculature. Because sildenafil can prolong the activity of NO, it has been used to prevent the rebound hypertension that can be observed with discontinuation of NO therapy.[59] It has also been shown to decrease hypoxic pulmonary vasoconstriction in adults.[60] A number of small studies to date suggest encouraging results with improvement in hemodynamic and functional parameters. In addition, administration in combination with prostacyclins is being evaluated.

General Supportive Care

Anticoagulation

Warfarin therapy in adults with primary pulmonary hypertension is associated with improved survival.[1,61] It is known to be beneficial in those with chronic thromboembolism[62]; therefore, it is thought that because microvessel thrombosis may contribute to the ongoing pathogenesis of pulmonary hypertension, anticoagulation may help minimize damage to the vasculature even in the absence of overt hypercoagulable states or proven thromboembolism. The optimal dose of warfarin in children is uncertain, but currently a target international normalized ratio (INR) of 1.5 to 2.0 is sought. For toddlers or patients at risk for bleeding, lower INR levels of less than 1.5 are used. In those with documented thromboembolism, hypercoagulable states such as positive cardiolipin or lupus anticoagulant tests, or known inherited thrombotic disorders, higher INR levels are used.

Oxygen

Supplemental oxygen therapy can be valuable in certain patients with pulmonary hypertension to alleviate chronic hypoxemia or to minimize nocturnal desaturation. Such patients include those with sleep apnea or other hypoventilation syndromes, patients with intrinsic lung disease or acute respiratory infection, and patients with exercise-induced hypoxia. Patients with advanced right heart failure and resting oxygen desaturation may also benefit from oxygen therapy.[63]

Management of Right Heart Failure

Patients with pulmonary hypertension and right heart failure may benefit from cardiac glycosides such as digoxin and from diuretic therapy. Because these patients are vulnerable to reductions in cardiac preload, the initiation of diuretic therapy needs to be done cautiously to avoid excessive volume depletion and hypotension.

Prophylaxis Measures

Because patients with pulmonary hypertension are vulnerable to the effects of respiratory inflammation, they should be vaccinated against influenza and pneumococcal pneumonia, and respiratory infections should be managed aggressively.

Refractory Pulmonary Hypertension

Despite advances in medical management of pulmonary hypertension, patients may be either nonresponsive to such therapies or develop treatment-refractory disease. These patients, who often have marked symptoms of right heart failure or the particularly ominous recurrent syncope, have limited treatment options. By facilitating right-to-left shunting, atrial septostomy can improve cardiac output and may contribute to improved survival for patients with refractory pulmonary hypertension.[64,65] This procedure may also serve as a bridging technique to transplantation. Single and bilateral lung transplantation, as well as heart-lung transplantation, have been performed in patients with refractory pulmonary hypertension. Results to date are highly variable, and neither the optimal transplantation procedure nor patient selection criteria are established.[66,67] In practice, patients with medically refractory pulmonary hypertension should be referred for evaluation at a lung transplantation center.

SUMMARY

The causes of pulmonary hypertension in children, often referred to in the past as *primary* or *idiopathic*, have been identified in increasing numbers in recent years. Recent advances have illuminated the pathophysiology of this disorder and enabled the development of more effective treatment options. As a consequence, children have experienced remarkable progress in both function and life expectancy. Because of the rarity of pulmonary hypertension, complex physiology, and limited available treatment facilities, these patients merit evaluation and treatment at comprehensive medical centers with experience in the medical, interventional, and surgical management of pulmonary hypertension. Treatment recommendations are guided by the symptom profile of the patient, by identification of any etiologic factors, and by the response to various therapeutic options. With judicious management, patients can expect considerable improvement in their functional status. Ongoing clinical trials and new agents promise better therapeutic options in the years ahead.

REFERENCES

1. Rich S, Kaufmann E, Levy PS. The effect of high doses of calcium-channel blockers on survival in primary pulmonary hypertension. N Engl J Med 327:76, 1992.
2. Higenbottam T, Wheeldon D, Wells F, et al. Long-term treatment of primary pulmonary hypertension with continuous intravenous epoprostenol (prostacyclin). Lancet 1(8385): 1046, 1984.
3. Barst RJ, Rubin LJ, McGoon MD, et al. Survival in primary pulmonary hypertension with long-term continuous intravenous prostacyclin. Ann Intern Med 121:409, 1994.
4. Adatia I. Recent advances in pulmonary vascular disease. Curr Opin Pediatr 14:292, 2002.
5. Wessel D. Current and future strategies in the treatment of childhood pulmonary hypertension. In Barst R (ed). Progress in Pediatric Cardiology. Shannon, Ireland: Elsevier Science Ireland Ltd., 2001:289.
6. Rosenzweig EB, Kerstein D, Barst RJ. Long-term prostacyclin for pulmonary hypertension with associated congenital heart defects. Circulation 99(14):1858, 1999.
7. Stenmark KR, Gebb SA. Lung vascular development: Breathing new life into an old problem. Am J Respir Cell Mol Biol 28:133, 2003.
8. Copland I, Post M. Lung development and fetal lung growth. Paediatr Respir Rev 5:S259, 2004.
9. Ghanayem NS, Gordon JB. Modulation of pulmonary vasomotor tone in the fetus and neonate. Respir Res 2:139, 2001.
10. Leffler CW, Hessler JR, Green RS. The onset of breathing at birth stimulates pulmonary vascular prostacyclin synthesis. Pediatr Res 18:938, 1984.
11. Shaul PW, Farrar MA, Magness RR. Pulmonary endothelial nitric oxide production is developmentally regulated in the fetus and newborn. Am J Physiol 265(4 Pt 2):H1056, 1993.
12. Farber HW, Loscalzo J. Pulmonary arterial hypertension. N Engl J Med 351:1655, 2004.
13. Hassoun PM, Thappa V, Landman MJ, et al. Endothelin 1: Mitogenic activity on pulmonary artery smooth muscle cells and release from hypoxic endothelial cells. Proc Soc Exper Biol Med 165, 1992.
14. Palmer RMJ, Ashton DS, Moncada S. Vascular endothelial cells synthesize nitric oxide from L-arginine. Nature 333:664, 1988.
15. Heath D, Edwards JE. The pathology of hypertensive pulmonary vascular disease: A description of six grades of structural changes in the pulmonary arteries with special

attention to congenital cardiac septal defects. Circulation 18: 533, 1958.
16. Lane KB, Machado RD, Pauciulo MW, et al. Heterozygous germline mutations in BMPR2, encoding a TGF-beta receptor, cause familial primary pulmonary hypertension. The International PPH Consortium. Nat Genet 26:81, 2000.
17. Thomson JR, Machado RD, Pauciulo MW, et al. Sporadic primary pulmonary hypertension is associated with germline mutations of the gene encoding BMPR-II, a receptor member of the TGF-beta family. J Med Genet 37(10):741, 2000.
18. Trembath RC, Thomson JR, Machado RD, et al. Clinical and molecular genetic features of pulmonary hypertension in patients with hereditary hemorrhagic telangiectasia. N Engl J Med 345:325, 2001.
19. Deng Z, Morse JH, Slager SL, et al. Familial primary pulmonary hypertension (gene PPH1) is caused by mutations in the bone morphogenetic protein receptor-II gene. Am J Hum Genet 67(3):737, 2000.
20. Newman JH, Trembath RC, Morse JA, et al. Genetic basis of pulmonary arterial hypertension: Current understanding and future directions. J Am Coll Cardiol 43:33S, 2004.
21. Loscalzo J. Genetic clues to the cause of primary pulmonary hypertension. N Engl J Med 345:367, 2001.
22. Simonneau G, Galie N, Rubin LJ, et al. Clinical classification of pulmonary hypertension. J Am Coll Cardiol 43:5S, 2004.
23. British Cardiac Society Guidelines and Medical Practice Committee. Recommendations on the management of pulmonary hypertension in clinical practice. Heart (British Cardiac Society) 86(Suppl 1):I1, 2001.
24. Bossone E, Paciocco G, Iarussi D, et al. The prognostic role of the ECG in primary pulmonary hypertension. Chest 121(2):513, 2002.
25. Barst RJ, McGoon M, Torbicki A, et al. Diagnosis and differential assessment of pulmonary arterial hypertension. J Am Coll Cardiol 43:S40, 2004.
26. Sitbon O, Humbert M, Ioos V, et al. Who benefits from long-term calcium-channel blocker therapy in primary pulmonary hypertension? Am J Respir Crit Care Med 167: A440, 2003.
27. Barst RJ, Maislin G, Fishman AP. Vasodilator therapy for primary pulmonary hypertension in children. Circulation 99:1197, 1999.
28. McGoon M, Gutterman D, Steen V, et al. Screening, early detection, and diagnosis of pulmonary arterial hypertension: ACCP evidence-based clinical practice guidelines. Chest 126(1 Suppl):14S–34S, 2004.
29. Nicod P, Moser KM. Primary pulmonary hypertension. The risk and benefit of lung biopsy [see comment]. Circulation 80(5):1486, 1989.
30. Jaklitsch MT, Linden BC, Braunlin EA, et al. Open-lung biopsy guides therapy in children. Ann Thorac Surg 71:1779, 2001.
31. Loyd JE, Butler MG, Foroud TM, et al. Genetic anticipation and abnormal gender ratio at birth in familial primary pulmonary hypertension. Am J Respir Crit Care Med 152(1):93, 1995.
32. D'Alonzo GE, Barst RJ, Ayres SM, et al. Survival in patients with primary pulmonary hypertension: Results from a national prospective registry. Ann Intern Med 115(5):343, 1991.
33. Young D, Widlitz AC, Rosenzweig EB, et al. Outcomes in children with idiopathic pulmonary arterial hypertension. Circulation 110(6):660, 2004.
34. Guyatt GH, Sullivan MJ, Thompson PJ, et al. The 6-minute walk: A new measure of exercise capacity in patients with chronic heart failure. Can Med Assoc J 132(8):919, 1985.
35. Galie N, Seeger W, Naeije R, et al. Comparative analysis of clinical trials and evidence-based treatment algorithm in pulmonary arterial hypertension. J Am Coll Cardiol 43:81S, 2004.
36. Humbert M, Sitbon O, Simonneau G. Treatment of pulmonary arterial hypertension. N Engl J Med 351:1425, 2004.
37. Badesch DB, Abman SH, Ahearn GS, et al. Medical therapy for pulmonary arterial hypertension: ACCP evidence-based clinical practice guidelines. Chest 126(1 Suppl):35S, 2004.
38. Gozal D, O'Brien LM. Snoring and obstructive sleep apnea in children: Why should we treat? Paediatr Resp Rev 5:S371, 2004.
39. Blum RH, McGowan FX Jr. Chronic upper airway obstruction and cardiac dysfunction: Anatomy, pathophysiology and anesthetic implications. Paediatr Anaesth 14:75, 2004.
40. Barst RJ. Pharmacologically induced pulmonary vasodilatation in children and young adults with primary pulmonary hypertension. Chest 89(4):497, 1986.
41. Sitbon O, Brenot F, Denjean A, et al. Inhaled nitric oxide as a screening vasodilator agent in primary pulmonary hypertension: A dose-response study and comparison with prostacyclin. Am J Respir Crit Care Med 151(2 Pt 1):384, 1995.
42. Sandoval J, Bauerle O, Gomez A, et al. Primary pulmonary hypertension in children: Clinical characterization and survival. J Am Coll Cardiol 25(2):466–474, 1995.
43. Barst RJ, Rubin LJ, Long WA, et al. A comparison of continuous intravenous epoprostenol (prostacyclin) with conventional therapy for primary pulmonary hypertension. The Primary Pulmonary Hypertension Study Group. N Engl J Med 334: 296, 1996.
44. Rich S, McLaughlin VV. Endothelin receptor blockers in cardiovascular disease. Circulation 108:2184, 2003.
45. Channick RN, Simonneau G, Sitbon O, et al. Effects of the dual endothelin-receptor antagonist bosentan in patients with pulmonary hypertension: A randomised placebo-controlled study. Lancet 358:1119, 2001.
46. Rubin LJ, Badesch DB, Barst RJ, et al. Bosentan therapy for pulmonary arterial hypertension. N Engl J Med 346: 896, 2002.
47. Barst RJ, Ivy D, Dingemanse J, et al. Pharmacokinetics, safety, and efficacy of bosentan in pediatric patients with pulmonary arterial hypertension. Clin Pharmacol Ther 73(4):372, 2003.
48. Rimar S, Gillis CN. Selective pulmonary vasodilation by inhaled nitric oxide is due to hemoglobin inactivation. Circulation 88:2884, 1993.
49. Adatia I, Perry S, Landzberg M, et al. Inhaled nitric oxide and hemodynamic evaluation of patients with pulmonary hypertension before transplantation. J Am Coll Cardiol 25:1656, 1995.
50. Adatia I, Lillehei C, Arnold JH, et al. Inhaled nitric oxide in the treatment of postoperative graft dysfunction after lung transplantation. Ann Thorac Surg 57(5):1311, 1994.

51. Roberts JD, Polaner DM, Lang P, et al. Inhaled nitric oxide in persistent pulmonary hypertension of the newborn. Lancet 340:818, 1992.
52. The Neonatal Inhaled Nitric Oxide Study Group. Inhaled nitric oxide in full-term and nearly full-term infants with hypoxic respiratory failure. N Eng J Med 336:597, 1997.
53. Wessel DL, Adatia I, Van Marter LJ, et al. Improved oxygenation in a randomized trial of inhaled nitric oxide for persistent pulmonary hypertension of the newborn. Pediatrics 100(5):E7, 1997.
54. Kinsella JP, Neish SR, Shaffer E, et al. Low-dose inhalational nitric oxide in persistent pulmonary hypertension of the newborn. Lancet 340:819, 1992.
55. Wessel DL, Adatia I, Giglia TM, et al. Use of inhaled nitric oxide and acetylcholine in the evaluation of pulmonary hypertension and endothelial function after cardiopulmonary bypass. Circulation 88:2128, 1993.
56. Girard C, Durand PG, Vedrinne C. Inhaled nitric oxide for right ventricular failure after heart transplantation. J Cardiothorac Vasc Anesth 7:481, 1993.
57. Ivy DD, Griebel JL, Kinsella JP, et al. Acute hemodynamic effects of pulsed delivery of low flow nasal nitric oxide in children with pulmonary hypertension. J Pediatr 133:453, 1998.
58. Mullen MP, Thomas K, Almodovar MC. Ambulatory inhaled nitric oxide for pediatric patients with pulmonary hypertension provides sustained reduction in pulmonary artery pressures. Circulation 104(11), 679. 2001.
59. Atz AM, Wessel DL. Sildenafil ameliorates effects of inhaled nitric oxide withdrawal. Anesthesiology 91:307, 1999.
60. Zhao L, Mason NA, Morrell NW, et al. Sildenafil inhibits hypoxia-induced pulmonary hypertension. Circulation 104(4): 424, 2001.
61. Fuster V, Steele PM, Edwards WD, et al. Primary pulmonary hypertension: Natural history and the importance of thrombosis. Circulation 70(4):580, 1984.
62. Fedullo PF, Auger WR, Kerr KM, et al. Chronic thromboembolic pulmonary hypertension. N Engl J Med 345: 1465, 2001.
63. Ngai P, Basner R, Yoney A, et al. Nocturnal oxygen desaturation predicts poorer pulmonary hemodynamics in children with primary pulmonary hypertension. Am J Respir Crit Care Med 165:A99, 2002.
64. Kerstein D, Levy PS, Hsu DT, et al. Blade balloon atrial septostomy in patients with severe primary pulmonary hypertension. Circulation 91(7):2028, 1995.
65. Klepetko W, Mayer E, Sandoval J, et al. Interventional and surgical modalities of treatment for pulmonary arterial hypertension. J Am Coll Cardiol 43:73S, 2004.
66. Doyle RL, McCrory D, Channick RN, et al. Surgical treatments/interventions for pulmonary arterial hypertension: ACCP evidence-based clinical practice guidelines. Chest 126(1 Suppl):63S–71S, 2004.
67. Mendeloff EN, Meyers BF, Sundt TM, et al. Lung transplantation for pulmonary vascular disease. Ann Thorac Surg 73(1):209; discussion, 217, 2002.

VI

Tools of Diagnosis

11

History, Growth, Nutrition, Physical Examination, and Routine Laboratory Tests

ROBERT L. GEGGEL AND DONALD C. FYLER

The quality of patient care depends on a thorough bedside assessment of the patient's status. A complete history and physical examination enables the physician to compile an appropriate differential diagnosis, order tests in a suitable manner, and efficiently care for the patient. The physician must remember that all tests, even those viewed as noninvasive, such as echocardiography and chest radiography, are a concern to parents and patients. The ability to manage patients without overtesting is one of the features of the excellent clinician.

HISTORY

The pediatric history requires obtaining information from the care providers and, after infancy and early childhood, also from the patient. Parents who bring their children to a pediatric cardiologist even for evaluation of an innocent murmur are typically anxious[1]; therefore, it is important to establish a trusting and empathetic relationship with the family. As outlined in a previous edition of this book,[2] it is helpful to conduct the interview in a relaxed manner so that information can be recalled and shared with the physician.

Pertinent issues to be addressed in the history depend on the age of the patient and the clinical concern. The following topics need to be considered.

1. **Prenatal testing:** The results of any fetal ultrasounds performed during pregnancy can identify structural disease before birth. In a 12-month review of the in-patient cardiology consult service at Children's Hospital Boston (July 2001 to June 2002), 85% of infants with cyanosis caused by structural heart disease were identified before birth.[3]

2. **Pregnancy history:** Maternal use of medication can influence the likelihood of congenital heart disease developing in the fetus (see Chapter 5). Maternal diabetes mellitus is associated with an increased incidence of transposition of the great arteries, hypertrophic cardiomyopathy, coarctation, and ventricular septal defect. Maternal systemic lupus erythematosus is associated with fetal complete atrioventricular block.[4] Maternal exposure to infectious agents can contribute to cardiac defects in the neonate: rubella with peripheral pulmonary stenosis, patent ductus arteriosus, or ventricular septal defect; and Coxsackie virus with myocarditis (see Chapter 5).

3. **Perinatal history:** Maternal history of premature rupture of membranes, fever, or use of sedatives or anesthetics raises concern about sepsis and decreased respiratory effort. For infants with cyanosis, gestational age, Apgar scores, and history of meconium aspiration are useful to determine the likelihood of hyaline membrane disease, perinatal asphyxia, persistent hypertension of the newborn, or pneumonia. The response to oxygen helps to distinguish a cardiac from pulmonary basis for cyanosis.[5]

4. **Other birth defects:** A variety of syndromes are associated with congenital heart disease[6] (see Chapter 5). Commonly encountered syndromes and the frequency and most common type of congenital heart disease include trisomy 21 (45%; atrioventricular canal defect, ventricular septal defect, tetralogy of Fallot); VACTERL syndrome (*v*ertebral defects, *a*nal atresia, *c*ardiac defect, *t*racheo-esophageal fistula, *r*enal anomaly, *l*imb anomaly) (50%; ventricular septal defect, tetralogy of Fallot), trisomy 13 or 18 (more than 80%; ventricular septal defect), Noonan's syndrome (50%; pulmonary stenosis, hypertrophic cardiomyopathy),

Turner's syndrome (35%; aortic stenosis, cardiomyopathy, coarctation), Williams syndrome (50%; supravalvar aortic stenosis, coarctation, peripheral pulmonary stenosis), and Marfan syndrome (nearly all patients; aortic dilation, mitral valve prolapse, mitral regurgitation, aortic regurgitation).

5. **Family history:** Congenital heart disease affecting a previous child or a parent increases the risk for structural heart disease in the infant.[7] Early myocardial infarction in first-degree relatives (younger than 50 years for men, younger than 60 years for women) merits screening for hyperlipidemia (see Chapter 22). Sudden death is associated with various genetic diseases, including cardiomyopathy, prolonged QT interval, Brugada syndrome, Marfan syndrome, or arrhythmogenic right ventricular dysplasia.[8] Hypertension in the extended family should lead to close monitoring of this variable, especially in adolescence when essential hypertension may initially develop.

6. **Initial detection of murmur:** Knowledge of the time a murmur was initially detected leads a clinician to consider different categories of cardiac disease. For neonates, murmurs detected in the first 6 hours of life typically involve valve regurgitation (tricuspid valve from perinatal stress, mitral valve from cardiac dysfunction) or valve stenosis, whereas murmurs detected after 6 hours of age can also represent shunt lesions that present as pulmonary vascular resistance falls (e.g., atrial or ventricular septal defect, patent ductus arteriosus, peripheral pulmonary stenosis). It is important to note that some neonates may only be examined by a physician after 6 hours of age, and others may have both valve stenosis and septal defects (e.g., tetralogy of Fallot). Systolic murmurs detected initially at 2 to 4 years of age frequently are innocent but can represent structural heart disease if the patient was frequently uncooperative for earlier examinations, had progression in the severity of the lesion, or developed an acquired condition. During childhood, a new murmur of mitral or aortic regurgitation raises the possibility of rheumatic heart disease so that inquiry should be made about a history of streptococcal pharyngitis, unexplained fever, arthritis, chorea, and rashes.

7. **Growth and development:** The normal infant gradually eats a larger volume of food at increasing intervals. This pattern is not observed in infants with lesions associated with poor cardiac function, pulmonary edema, or significant left-to-right shunting (ratio of pulmonary to systemic flow greater than 2:1). Lesions associated with large shunts gradually become symptomatic as pulmonary vascular resistance decreases over the first 2 to 8 weeks of life. Infants with lesions associated with shunting at the ventricular or great vessel level are generally more symptomatic than those with only atrial-level shunting. Symptoms consist of tachypnea, diaphoresis, and feeding difficulties of early fatigue and decreased oral intake. Such infants can have failure to thrive and delays in developmental milestones.

8. **Cyanosis:** Cyanosis can have a cardiac, pulmonary, central nervous system, or hematologic basis. A full discussion can be found in Chapter 8. Cyanosis is often initially detected by experienced nurses in the newborn unit. The characteristics of fetal hemoglobin and the presence of darker skin pigmentation make the detection of mild cyanosis more difficult.

Infants with tetralogy of Fallot can have cyanotic spells (see Chapter 32). A single well-documented episode is an indication to proceed with surgical repair or palliation. In regions of the world where screening or infant surgery is not available, older children without prior intervention can have squatting episodes to relieve these cyanotic spells.

A common occurrence, especially in fair-skinned infants, is the transient development of peripheral cyanosis involving the distal extremities and perioral region. This appearance often occurs with cold exposure, such as after a bath, and represents vasomotor instability, a normal finding in infancy.

9. **Common issues evaluated in childhood and adolescence:** Although a variety of symptoms lead to cardiac consultation, several issues are frequently encountered.

a. *Endurance:* Parents, other adults such as teachers or coaches, or the patient may note decreased exercise tolerance compared with peers. Activity limitations may have a cardiac basis or be caused by poor general conditioning, obesity, exercise-induced reactive airway disease, other pulmonary disease, or neuromuscular disease. Determining the severity, duration, and progression of limitations and the associated symptoms helps to distinguish among these possibilities. The occurrence of limitations associated with obstructive lesions such as aortic stenosis or pulmonary stenosis is an indication for intervention.

b. *Chest pain:* Chest pain is a frequent symptom in children and has a cardiac basis in only 1% to 6% of patients.[9] Heart conditions include structural heart disease, such as left ventricular outflow obstruction, aortic dissection, ruptured sinus of Valsalva aneurysm, or coronary anomalies; acquired heart diseases, include pericarditis, myocarditis, Kawasaki disease, or arrhythmias, most commonly supraventricular tachycardia.

In children, chest pain typically has a musculoskeletal or idiopathic basis and is self-resolving. Musculoskeletal issues include costochondritis, myodynia, rib fracture, or slipping rib syndrome. Slipping rib syndrome involves the 8th, 9th, and 10th ribs, whose costal cartilages do not attach to the sternum; these ribs are attached to each other by fibrous tissue that is susceptible to trauma.[10] If these fibrous connections are weakened, the ribs can rub together, irritating the intercostal nerve and producing pain. Patients can describe "something slipping or giving away," "a popping sensation," or "hearing a clicking sound." Musculoskeletal pain typically is sharp in quality, is located at the costochondral junction or insertion site of the pectoralis major muscle group, and frequently increases during inspiration. There often is a history of activity that can lead to muscle injury, such as sports, weight lifting, use of a knapsack to carry heavy school books, or direct trauma.

Other causes of chest pain include hyperventilation; psychiatric disorders; breast disease; respiratory disease, including pneumonia, pneumothorax, pneumomediastinum, or reactive airway disease; pulmonary hypertension; pulmonary embolism; gastrointestinal disorders; and exposure to toxins (cocaine, cannabis, cigarettes). A full discussion can be found in Chapter 22. In the absence of associated symptoms of illness, positive physical examination findings related to the cardiac or respiratory systems, or symptoms during exertion, a serious organic cause is unlikely.[9]

c. *Syncope:* Syncope is more common during adolescence than in childhood and frequently has a vasovagal or orthostatic basis. These episodes are often preceded by symptoms of diaphoresis, nausea, or development of tunnel vision. Consciousness is usually regained quickly upon becoming supine. There often is a history of dehydration, exposure to a warm environment (crowded auditorium, hot summer day, warm shower), or standing for prolonged periods of time. Syncope can be precipitated by hair combing, cough, painful stimulation, fear, hyperventilation, micturition, or defecation. Orthostatic changes in blood pressure can be exacerbated by a variety of medications, including diuretics or vasoactive agents.

Syncope can also be caused by neurologic disorders, including seizures, breath-holding spells, or migraine headaches. Seizures can be associated with tonic-clonic movements and postepisode fatigue. Breath-holding spells often occur with sudden fright, pain, or frustration in children between 18 months and 5 years of age. Cardiac causes include right or left obstructive heart disease, pulmonary hypertension, and arrhythmia, including prolonged QT syndrome and bradyarrhythmia or tachyarrhythmia. The occurrence of symptoms during or shortly after exercise can be associated with a vasovagal mechanism but increases the risk for an underlying cardiac basis.[11,12] A review of syncope can be found in Chapter 22.

d. *Palpitations:* Awareness of palpitations may represent an abnormality in rate or rhythm. Sinus tachycardia associated with anxiety or activity usually has a gradual onset and resolution. Supraventricular tachycardia typically has a sudden onset and end as the circuit responsible for supporting the arrhythmia opens and closes. Other tachyarrhythmias (atrial flutter, atrial fibrillation, ventricular tachycardia) can have a similar pattern. Prolonged episodes of these arrhythmias can be associated with dizziness or syncope. Tachyarrhythmia occurring with exercise may represent catecholamine-sensitive ventricular tachycardia. Irregular rhythms can represent atrial, junctional, or ventricular premature beats. Some patients with rare premature beats note every single one, whereas others with thousands of daily premature beats report no symptoms and come to medical attention when an irregular rhythm is noted on physical examination.

PHYSICAL EXAMINATION

The physical examination needs to be complete because heart disease can affect multiple organ systems. The order of the examination will vary depending on the age of the patient. For infants and toddlers, it is often best to perform auscultation first when the patient is more likely to be quiet. Many portions of the physical examination can be performed with the infant or toddler in the parent's lap, which can aid in the level of patient cooperation. Infants can be fed or given a pacifier to achieve a quiet state.

General Examination

General inspection of the child will give clues to the state of health, cyanosis, or anemia. Height and weight measurements are important; plotting these values on growth curves aids in determining the presence of failure to thrive. Heart disease associated with large left-to-right shunts, pulmonary edema, or ventricular dysfunction can impair growth. In such patients, weight typically is affected before height. Infants should gain about 20 g/day; weight gain less than this amount caused by heart disease is an indication for adjustment in medication (diuretics, digoxin, correction of anemia if present) and use of caloric-supplemented food. If these methods are insufficient, surgical intervention is necessary. A normal infant can grow while receiving 100 calories/kg/day; infants whose growth is impaired by heart disease typically require 130 to 140 calories/kg/day. Expressed breast milk or formula contains 20 calories/ounce; each can be supplemented in stages with carbohydrate or fat to provide 30 calories/ounce so that caloric needs are fulfilled even if the infant has reduced volume of intake. For the mother interested in maintaining breast-feeding and depending on the degree of failure-to-thrive, some feedings can occur at the breast, whereas others can consist of supplemented expressed breast milk. An approach to caloric supplementation is outlined in Table 11-1.

General inspection also gives clues to the presence of syndromes that frequently are associated with specific heart disease. Extracardiac anomalies occur in about 20% of patients with congenital heart disease.[13] Multiple syndromes have characteristic facies (see Chapter 5). A webbed neck and short stature are seen in Turner's syndrome. Arachnodactyly, pectus deformity, scoliosis, and arm span exceeding height are features of Marfan syndrome. Radial dysplasia is a component of Holt-Oram syndrome.

TABLE 11–1. Caloric Supplementation for Infant with Failure to Thrive

	Formula	Breast Milk
Caloric concentration	13 ounces concentrated formula* 8 ounces water	3 ounces breast milk
24 cal/ounce	No additives	1 tsp infant formula powder†
26 cal/ounce	1½ tbsp Polycose powder	1½ tsp infant formula powder†
28 cal/ounce	3 tbsp Polycose powder	1½ tsp infant formula powder† 1 tsp Polycose powder
30 cal/ounce	3 tbsp Polycose powder 1 tsp corn oil	1½ tsp infant formula powder† 1½ tsp Polycose powder
Days 1–3: 24 cal/ounce formula or breast milk		
Days 4–6: 26 cal/ounce formula or breast milk		
Days 7–9: 28 cal/ounce formula or breast milk		
Days 10–12: 30 cal/ounce formula or breast milk		

*Need to emphasize concentrated rather than ready-mixed formula.
†Any commercially available formula powder (e.g., Enfamil, Prosobee, Nutramigen, Pregestimil)
cal, calorie; tbsp, tablespoon; tsp teaspoon.

A large-for-gestational-age neonate suggests maternal diabetes mellitus.

Vital Signs

Review of the vital signs enables the clinician to form a general appraisal of the patient and consider certain diagnostic possibilities.

Pulse

The pulse is examined with respect to rate, rhythm, prominence, and variation.[14]

Rate. Sinus tachycardia occurs in a variety of conditions, including anxiety, fever, pain, anemia, large left-to-right shunts, decreased cardiac contractility, cardiac tamponade, sepsis, pulmonary disease, or hyperthyroidism. Supraventricular tachycardia in infants or children typically occurs at a rate that is too rapid to count by an observer (more than 220 beats/minute). Bradycardia occurs in high-level athletes and in children with eating disorders (anorexia nervosa, bulimia), hypothyroidism, or heart block. The average resting heart rate in the first week of life is 125 beats/minute, at 1 year is 120 beats/minute, at 5 to 8 years is 100 beats/minute, and at 12 to 16 years is 85 beats/minute.[15]

Rhythm. A phasic variation related to the respiratory cycle (faster during inspiration) is characteristic of sinus arrhythmia. This pattern is more common in young children than in adults and is a normal variant. The variation in heart rate occasionally can be profound, but review of an electrocardiogram leads to the diagnosis. Occasional premature beats can represent atrial, ventricular, or junctional premature beats. Nonconducted atrial premature beats are the most common cause of a "pause" in the well-newborn nursery[16] and typically resolve during the first month of life. Isolated ventricular premature beats are common in adolescence; resolution with exercise performed in the examination room (jumping jacks) suggests a benign etiology.

Prominence. Bounding pulses are present in febrile states, hyperthyroidism, exercise, anxiety, severe anemia, or complete heart block and with aortic runoff lesions that produce increased pulse pressure (aortic regurgitation, patent ductus arteriosus, arteriovenous malformations, aortopulmonary window, truncus arteriosus). The prominent pulse classically associated with aortic regurgitation has been termed *Corrigan's pulse* or *water hammer pulse*. Such prominent pulses also produce visible ebbing and flowing of the capillary pulse that can be observed by partially compressing the nail bed, a phenomenon termed *Quincke's pulse*.[14]

Generalized decreased pulses are associated with low cardiac output. This can be caused by acquired heart disease such as myocarditis, with congenital heart disease such as obstructive lesions or cardiomyopathy, and with pericardial tamponade or constrictive pericarditis. A rare form of vasculitis affecting the large arteries, Takayasu's arteritis, can be associated with decreased pulses and is termed *pulseless disease*.

Differential prominence of pulses is present in several conditions. The most common is coarctation of the aorta, which usually is associated with easily palpable upper extremity pulses (if left ventricular function is normal) and reduced or absent femoral pulses. If there is a large coexisting patent ductus arteriosus and right-to-left ductal shunting, the lower extremity pulses may be normal, although in such circumstances, there may be differential oxygen saturation levels between the upper and lower body. In infants with large thighs, the femoral pulse occasionally can be difficult to locate. The leg should be abducted; the femoral artery is located in the groin region along the line that joins the knee with the umbilicus. Coarctation usually occurs in the aortic isthmus just distal to the origin of the left subclavian artery. In some infants, the origin of the left subclavian artery can be involved, so that the pulse in the left arm is weaker than the pulse in the right arm. In rare cases, there can be anomalous origin of the right subclavian artery from the descending aorta in an infant with coarctation, so that the pulses in all four extremities are reduced; in such patients, the carotid pulse will be more prominent. A second condition associated with differential pulses is supravalvar aortic stenosis, a lesion often present in patients with Williams syndrome. In these patients, the pulse in the right arm can be more prominent than the pulse in the left arm; this discrepancy is produced by the Coanda effect, which increases flow to the innominate artery. Finally, Takayasu's aortitis can preferentially affect the individual brachiocephalic arteries or portions of the aorta with resultant differences in extremity pulses.[17]

Variation. Variable pulse impulse in the same location occurs in several conditions. Pulsus paradoxus involves an exaggerated decrease in inspiratory systolic pressure of more than 10 mm Hg and is associated with pericardial tamponade or severe respiratory distress (see discussion of blood pressure below). Pulsus alternans consists of a decrease in systolic pressure on alternate beats and indicates severe left ventricular dysfunction. This variation is more easily appreciated when observing intravascular blood pressure recordings than by palpating the pulse.[2] Pulsus bisferiens consists of a pulse with two peaks separated by a plateau and can occur in patients with either obstructive left ventricular cardiomyopathy or large left ventricular stroke volumes.[14]

Blood Pressure

While four extremity blood pressures are often obtained, with the rare exceptions of aortitis or aberrant origin of the subclavian artery in a patient with coarctation, obtaining the blood pressure in the right arm and one leg provides sufficient screening. The right arm is preferred because the origin of the left subclavian artery can be stenosed in some patients with coarctation. Unless a femoral artery was injured in a previous catheterization, the pressure should be similar in each leg.

Accuracy of blood pressure measurement depends on selection of a properly sized cuff, in infants and toddlers on a quiet and cooperative state, and in older children and adolescents on assessment of the presence of anxiety (white-coat hypertension). The inflatable bladder should have a length sufficient to fully encircle the circumference of the extremity and a width to cover about 75% of the distance between the joints on either end of the portion of the extremity around which the cuff is placed.[18] If the cuff is too small, artificially high values are obtained. The cuff needs to be applied snugly around the extremity because a loose-fitting cuff needs higher pressure to occlude the artery.[14] Agitation leads to elevation in blood pressure. A coarctation can be missed if the infant is quiet while the arm pressure is obtained and crying during measurement of the leg pressure. In many clinics, the blood pressure is measured by assistants, and note is not made of patient behavior. If the femoral pulses are diminished and the blood pressure values demonstrate no arm–leg discrepancy, the physician should repeat the measurements when the infant is observed to be cooperative to confirm the values. If hypertension is noted in children or adolescents who are anxious, it is helpful to repeat the measurements at the end of the examination when the patient may be more relaxed.

There are several techniques available to measure blood pressure, including palpation and the Doppler method, each of which estimates systolic pressure; auscultation, which is technically difficult in an infant or toddler; and the oscillometric method, which is the most commonly used technique in clinics and medical wards. Another method, the flush technique, is rarely used and yields values closer to the mean pressure. The techniques are reviewed in Chapter 23. The lower extremity systolic pressure can be 5 to 10 mm Hg greater than the upper extremity value because of the standing wave effect, with successive heart beats adding to the pressure downstream. Systolic pressure in the upper extremity that is more than 10 mm Hg higher than that in the lower extremity is a sign of coarctation of the aorta.

The pulse pressure is the difference between systolic and diastolic values. The pulse pressure is increased in conditions associated with bounding pulses and decreased in states associated with diminished pulses (see pulse description given earlier).

When checking for pulsus paradoxus, the auscultation method must be used. Finding a manometric blood pressure cuff occasionally is difficult on wards accustomed to the use of oscillometric equipment. Initially, the systolic pressure is estimated by quickly deflating the inflated cuff. The cuff is then reinflated about 20 mm Hg above this value and slowly deflated (1 to 2 mm Hg per beat). The systolic pressures at which the Korotkoff sound is initially auscultated intermittently and then consistently are noted; the difference in these values is the pulsus paradoxus. A pulsus paradoxus of more than 10 mm Hg is abnormal and is a feature of pericardial tamponade or severe respiratory disease.

Respirations

Tachypnea is present with pulmonary parenchymal disease, pulmonary edema, large left-to-right shunts that elevate pulmonary venous pressure, and conditions causing metabolic acidosis. In infants at rest, persistent respiratory rates of more than 60 breaths/minute are abnormal; transient increases can occur after eating or agitation.[14] Quiet tachypnea is often present in left-to-right shunt lesions, whereas labored tachypnea is observed in patients with pulmonary disease.[2] Both can be accompanied by intercostal or subcostal retractions, flaring of the alae nasi, or audible wheezing. Orthopnea is a sign of left ventricular dysfunction or severe elevation in pulmonary venous pressure.

Venous Pressure

In the cooperative child or adolescent, venous pressure can be estimated by examination of the jugular vein. When the patient is sitting or reclining at a 45-degree angle, the jugular vein should not be visible above the level of the clavicle. Measuring the difference in the height of the jugular vein with a parallel line drawn through the level of the manubrium yields central venous pressure (Fig. 11-1).

The venous pulsation is undulating and nonpalpable, decreases with inspiration, and changes in height with patient position. Distinguishing the various components (a, c, and v waves; x and y descents) is difficult in children, both because of neck size and the presence of tachycardia. Prominent jugular venous waves are present in a variety of conditions, including atrial contraction into a stiff right ventricle or against a closed tricuspid valve (tricuspid atresia; complete heart block, in which case prominent pulsation is intermittent), tricuspid regurgitation, pericardial disease (pericardial tamponade, constrictive pericarditis), vein of Galen malformation, or superior vena cava obstruction.[14]

Cardiac Examination

The cardiac examination includes inspection, palpation, and auscultation. The classic description by Osler also included percussion of the cardiac border, which is currently rarely done and is not as reliable in detecting cardiomegaly as the readily available imaging techniques of radiography or echocardiography.

Inspection

A visible apical impulse can be seen in left ventricular volume overload lesions, including significant mitral or aortic regurgitation, or lesions associated with large left-to-right shunts. A visible parasternal impulse is associated with right ventricular volume overload lesions, including tetralogy of Fallot, absent pulmonary valve associated with severe pulmonary regurgitation or severe tricuspid regurgitation

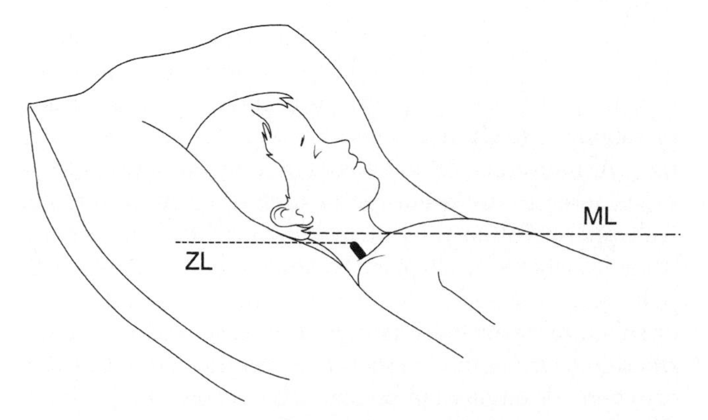

FIGURE 11–1 *Clinical estimation of venous pressure. With the patient lying at approximately 45 degrees, the pressure (ZL) in the right atrium does not rise above the manubrium (ML).*
From Lewis T. Diseases of the Heart Described for Practitioners and Students, 2nd ed. New York: Macmillan, 1937.

associated with Ebstein's anomaly, and large arteriovenous malformations.

Palpation

Palpation involves evaluation of ventricular impulses, thrills, and heart sounds. The apical impulse is best appreciated using the tips of the index and middle fingers and is normally located in the left midclavicular line in the fourth or fifth intercostal space. The apical impulse is displaced laterally and is more prominent in left ventricular overload lesions such as severe aortic or mitral regurgitation or lesions associated with large left-to-right shunts at the ventricular or great vessel level. The apical impulse is right-sided in dextrocardia or displaced in a rightward direction in dextroposition in conditions including left-sided congenital diaphragmatic hernia, left lobar emphysema, or scimitar syndrome. The right ventricular impulse is best detected by placing the hand on the chest with the heads of the metacarpals along the left costochondral junctions. A prominent lift indicates right ventricular hypertension or right ventricular volume overload. The right ventricular impulse can also be assessed in the epigastric area. The palm of the right hand is placed on the abdomen so that the index and middle fingers can slide under the xiphoid process; the tips of the fingers can palpate the right ventricular impulse.

Precordial thrills indicate the presence of a murmur of at least grade 4. The timing and location of thrills should be noted. Systolic thrills at the left lower sternal border usually are caused by ventricular septal defects that may be small and associated with a high interventricular pressure gradient or large and associated with a large left-to-right shunt. Occasionally, a thrill in this region is caused by tricuspid regurgitation if there is right ventricular hypertension. Mitral, aortic, and pulmonary thrills are located at the apex, right upper sternal border, and left upper sternal border, respectively. Aortic valve thrills can sometimes also be detected over the carotid artery or in the suprasternal notch. A suprasternal notch thrill is rarely associated with pulmonary stenosis and helps to distinguish aortic stenosis from pulmonary stenosis. Thrills associated with aortic or pulmonary stenosis indicate significant degrees of obstruction. Although most thrills occur in systole, diastolic thrills can occur at the apex with mitral stenosis, or along the left sternal border with aortic or pulmonary regurgitation.

A palpable second heart sound usually indicates severe pulmonary hypertension but can also be present in conditions in which the aorta has an anterior location, such as transposition of the great arteries. A palpable first heart sound can be present in hyperdynamic states.[14]

Auscultation

Thorough auscultation requires the examiner to follow a simple rule: listen to one sound at a time. Components to be evaluated or assessed to be present include S_1, S_2, S_3, S_4, ejection click, opening snap, pericardial rub, and murmurs (systolic, diastolic, continuous). Some congenital cardiac lesions can produce multiple abnormal sounds and murmurs, and a system of auscultation is required so that all available data are collected and a reliable diagnosis is made. For example, a soft systolic murmur at the left upper sternal border may represent an innocent flow murmur. If there is also a widely fixed split S_2, the murmur may represent an atrial septal defect, or if there is a variable systolic ejection click in the same region, the murmur may represent valvar pulmonary stenosis.

For auscultation to be completed, the proper environment and tools must be used. The examination room should be quiet without extraneous noises from the patient, relatives, or heating or air-conditioning system. The stethoscope should have a bell to detect low-frequency sounds and a diaphragm for high-frequency sounds. In infants, an adult-sized diaphragm covers most of the precordium so that a pediatric-sized version aids in localizing sounds. The tubing should be no longer than 16 to 18 inches with a bore of 1/8 inch. There should be no leak from the chest piece to ear piece so that sound transmission is optimized.[19] The patient should be evaluated in more than one position, including supine, sitting, and standing, depending on the diagnosis, because some heart sounds change or are more easily appreciated with different patient posture.

First Heart Sound (S_1). S_1 is produced by mitral and tricuspid valve closure and is coincident with the QRS complex on the electrocardiogram (Fig 11-2). S_1 is usually perceived as a single sound because the mitral and tricuspid valve components are nearly simultaneous.[20] In the pediatric age range, however, some patients can have a perceptibly split S_1 that typically is most easily detected over the tricuspid area at the left lower sternal border. If the split is detected at the apex, consideration must be given to an early systolic ejection click associated with a bicuspid aortic valve, and echocardiography may be needed for differentiation. S_1 also can be split in right bundle branch block owing to delay in tricuspid valve closure.[21]

The intensity of S_1 is increased in high cardiac output states because of greater velocity of leaflet closure and in conditions associated with greater mitral valve excursion during closure, including short PR interval and mild mitral stenosis (because the elevated left atrial pressure maintains the valve in a more open position). The intensity of S_1 is decreased in conditions associated with low cardiac output, elevated ventricular end-diastolic pressure, mitral regurgitation due to failure of valve coaptation, or decreased valve excursion present in patients with prolonged PR interval or severe mitral stenosis.[20] Patients with complete heart block have variable intensity of S_1.[2]

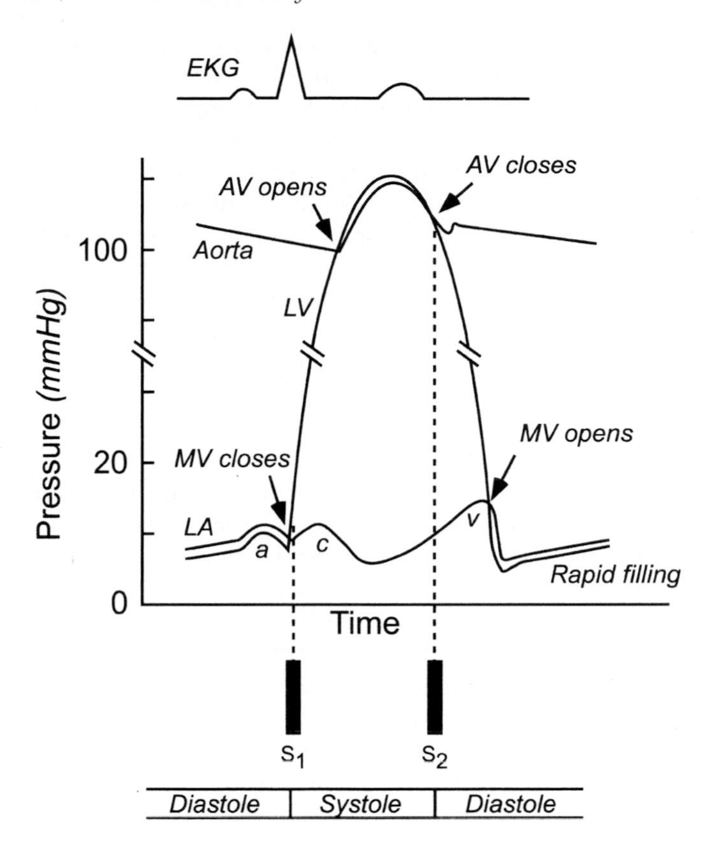

FIGURE 11–2 *The normal cardiac cycle depicted for left-sided chambers. Similar relationships exist for the right-sided chambers. Substitute right atrium for left atrium (LA), right ventricle for left ventricle (LV), and pulmonary artery for aorta. The a wave of the atrial pulse coincides with the P wave on the electrocardiogram (ECG). The mitral valve (MV) closes as left ventricle pressure exceeds atrial pressure and produces the first heart sound (S1). This coincides with the QRS complex on the ECG. Mitral valve closure increases atrial pressure and produces the c wave on the atrial pressure curve. The aortic valve (AV) subsequently opens as ventricular pressure exceeds aortic pressure. The aortic valve closes during ventricular relaxation and produces the second heart sound (S_2). This roughly coincides with the end of the T wave on the ECG. Atrial pressure rises (v wave) owing to filling of the atria while the mitral valve is closed. The mitral valve opens as left ventricular pressure falls below left atrial pressure.*
From Marino BS, Goldblatt A. Heart sounds and murmurs. In Lilly LS [ed]. Pathophysiology of heart disease. Philadelphia: Lea & Febiger, 1992:18.

Second Heart Sound (S_2). S_2 is produced by closure of the semilunar valves and is typically best appreciated at the left upper sternal border. The quality of S_2 yields important information on cardiac physiology and provides a framework for the remainder of the auscultatory examination. The pulmonary valve normally closes after the aortic valve because of relative delayed electrical activation of the right ventricle and lower pulmonary impedance.

The respiratory cycle has different effects on the pulmonary and systemic circulations. Inspiration increases venous return to the right heart and lowers pulmonary impedance, which prolongs right ventricular systole, and reduces pulmonary venous return to the left heart, which shortens left ventricular systole. During inspiration, the aortic and pulmonary valve components of S_2 split by about 0.05 seconds. These effects are reversed in expiration, so that S_2 typically becomes single. Detecting splitting of S_2 is always challenging. If the split is easily detected, the split is often wide. In infants with tachycardia and tachypnea, correlating S_2 with the respiratory cycle is impossible. The best the examiner can do is to detect variability with a split present in some beats and not in others.

A widely fixed split S_2 occurs with right ventricular volume overload lesions, the most common of which is atrial septal defect. The less common conditions of total or partial anomalous pulmonary venous connection or large arteriovenous malformation can produce a similar feature. In these conditions, the persistent right ventricular volume overload delays pulmonary valve closure so that the split is greater than 0.05 seconds, often as long as 0.10 seconds. Wide inspiratory splitting with respiratory variation occurs with right bundle branch block, pulmonary stenosis, or idiopathic dilation of the main pulmonary artery due to delayed activation or prolonged contraction of the right ventricle.[14] As pulmonary stenosis progresses, splitting becomes difficult to detect owing to a softer pulmonary closure sound and prolongation of the murmur beyond the aortic component. Wide splitting can also occur with significant mitral regurgitation due to shortened left ventricular ejection time and earlier closure of the aortic valve.[21] Paradoxical splitting is uncommon in children and involves detecting two components to S_2 in expiration and a single sound in inspiration; this can occur with delayed or prolonged left ventricular contraction in patients with left bundle branch block, aortic stenosis, or some forms of Wolff-Parkinson-White syndrome.[14]

The intensity of S_2 depends on the pressure closing the semilunar valves and the anterior-posterior position of the great arteries. The most common cause of a loud S_2 is pulmonary hypertension, which can arise from a variety of causes.[22] Pulmonary hypertension can be caused by increased pulmonary flow or elevated pulmonary vascular resistance; evaluation of murmurs often helps to distinguish between these two mechanisms, with the former being associated with diastolic rumbles across the atrioventricular valve that receives increased flow. Increased intensity of S_2 is also present in patients with transposition of the great arteries because of the anterior location of the aorta, and often in tetralogy of Fallot.

S_2 is single in patients with severe pulmonary hypertension because the elevated diastolic pressure in the pulmonary circulation closes the pulmonary valve sooner. Mild or moderate pulmonary hypertension is associated with a narrowly split S_2. S_2 is also single when there is atresia of one the semilunar valves.

Third Heart Sound (S_3). The third heart sound is produced during the rapid filling phase of the ventricle in early diastole and is best heard with the bell of the stethoscope. This sound produces a gallop rhythm that has the cadence of the syllables of "Ken-tuc-ky." The last component of this sequence represents the third heart sound.[20] This sound can be detected in some normal children, although this is not very common. Cardiac diseases associated with a third heart sound include myocardial dysfunction or volume overload conditions, especially those created by large left-to-right shunts. In the latter, the sound is followed by a diastolic murmur created by increased flow across the affected atrioventricular valve. A third heart sound produced by the left ventricle is detected in the apical region, whereas that from the right ventricle is noted at the left lower sternal border. Right ventricular sounds often increase during inspiration because of increased flow.[21]

Fourth Heart Sound (S_4). The fourth heart sound is produced by atrial contraction in late diastole and is also best heard with the bell of the stethoscope. This sound produces a gallop rhythm that has the cadence of the syllables of "Ten-nes-see." The first component of this sequence represents the S_4.[20] This sound is abnormal and is seen in conditions associated with decreased ventricular compliance so that increased atrial contractile force is required to fill the ventricle. These conditions include those produced by myocardial ischemia or ventricular hypertrophy such as hypertrophic cardiomyopathy, systemic hypertension, and valvar aortic or pulmonary stenosis. An S_4 is not produced if there is coexisting atrial fibrillation or junctional tachycardia because of absent atrial contraction.[2,21]

When both an S_3 and S_4 are present, there is a quadruple rhythm. In such a situation, if there is tachycardia and resulting shortening of diastole, the two extra sounds may become superimposed and create a summation gallop.[20,23,24]

Opening Snap. An opening snap is a high-frequency sound associated with mitral stenosis. As the degree of mitral stenosis progresses, the opening snap occurs earlier in diastole because of elevated atrial pressures and becomes softer because of decreased leaflet mobility.

Clicks. Ejection clicks are brief, high-frequency, sharp sounds that have a quality distinct from S_1 and S_2. They usually are associated with abnormal valve structure. Evaluation of location, timing (early versus mid-systolic), and nature (constant versus variable) enables the examiner to determine the affected valve (Table 11-2). In patients with mitral valve prolapse, the click may be associated with a murmur of mitral regurgitation that is only present or louder

TABLE 11–2. Qualities of Clicks Associated with Valve Disorders

Valve	Location	Timing in Systole	Nature
Mitral	Apex	Mid to late	Constant
Aortic	Apex	Early	Constant
Pulmonary	LUSB	Early	Variable
Tricuspid	LLSB	Mid to late	Constant

LLSB, left lower sternal border; LUSB, left upper sternal border.

in the standing than supine position because of reduced left ventricular volume that produces a greater degree of prolapse. An analogy is observing the mainsail on a sailboat. When fully hoisted, the sail "prolapses" through the plane of the boom and mast. If one climbed the mast and cut off the top 15 feet (correlating with the reduced left ventricular volume in the standing than supine position) and hoisted the sail again, it would "prolapse" to a greater degree.

The click associated with aortic stenosis or bicuspid aortic valve is best detected at the apex rather than the aortic valve region at the right upper sternal border. At times, it is difficult to distinguish a split S_1 (normal variant) from an aortic valve ejection click, and echocardiography is needed for differentiation. The click associated with pulmonary stenosis is located at the left upper sternal border and is variable and louder in expiration because of greater systolic valve excursion in this phase of the respiratory cycle.[21] Clicks associated with semilunar valve stenosis become softer as the degree of obstruction progresses because of reduced valve mobility. Ebstein's anomaly of the tricuspid valve can be associated with a systolic click at the left lower sternal border.

Clicks occasionally occur in conditions associated with dilation of the aorta or pulmonary artery. The latter can occur with pulmonary hypertension, patent ductus arteriosus, or idiopathic dilation of the main pulmonary artery. In neonates with left-to-right shunting across a patent ductus arteriosus, there may be multiple systolic clicks at the left upper sternal border that sound like rolling a pair of dice in one's hand. This sound may be produced by wavelike expansion of the pulmonary artery. Clicks can also be produced by membranous ventricular septal defects associated with aneurysm of the ventricular septum and are located at the left lower sternal border.

Pericardial Friction Rub. A pericardial friction rub is created when inflamed visceral and parietal pericardial surfaces contact each other. The sound is similar to rubbing two pieces of sandpaper together and has a grating quality. The rub may be auscultated in systole, diastole, or continuously and is best heard with the diaphragm. The rub is typically loudest along the left sternal border with the patient sitting and leaning forward and often has inspiratory accentuation. It commonly is present after surgery involving entry into the pericardial space and in pericarditis. The sound is not present if there is a moderate to large pericardial effusion because the two surfaces of the pericardium cannot rub together.

Murmurs. Various features of a murmur need to be evaluated to fully assess this finding.[14,21]

Intensity. The intensity of a murmur is graded on a scale of 1 through 6[25] (Table 11-3). Murmurs grade 4 or greater are associated with a palpable thrill. The loudness depends on both the pressure gradient and the volume of blood flowing across the site creating the murmur. For example, the murmur associated with moderate neonatal pulmonary stenosis or large ventricular septal defect increases in the first few weeks of life as pulmonary vascular resistance decreases, producing a larger pressure gradient in the former and an increased left-to-right shunt in the latter.

Timing. Systolic murmurs are created by flow through stenotic semilunar valves or regurgitant atrioventricular valves, other stenotic regions (coarctation, double chamber right ventricle, subvalvar or supravalvar semilunar valve obstruction, peripheral pulmonary stenosis), or increased cardiac output across normal semilunar valves associated with tachycardia or anemia. The innocent Still's murmur is discussed separately in Chapter 22.

Diastolic murmurs are caused by regurgitant flow across semilunar valves or turbulent flow across atrioventricular valves. The latter can represent true stenosis, as in mitral stenosis, or relative stenosis that is seen in patients with large left-to-right shunt lesions or significant atrioventricular valve regurgitation. The normal atrioventricular valve can accommodate twice the normal stroke volume nonturbulently.

TABLE 11–3. Grading of Intensity of Heart Murmurs

Grade 1: faintest sound that can be detected; often detected by cardiologists but not by general physicians
Grade 2: soft murmur that is readily detectable
Grade 3: louder than grade 2 but not associated with a palpable thrill
Grade 4: easily detected murmur associated with a palpable thrill
Grade 5: very loud murmur audible with the stethoscope placed lightly on the chest
Grade 6: extremely loud murmur audible with the stethoscope off the chest

From Marino BS, Goldblatt A. Heart sounds and murmurs. In Lilly LS (ed): Pathophysiology of Heart Disease. Philadelphia: Lea & Febiger, 1992: 18–29; and Freeman AR, Levine SA. The clinical significance of the systolic murmur: A study of 1,000 consecutive "non-cardiac" cases. Ann Intern Med 6:1371, 1933.

Larger blood flows create a murmur. Left-to-right shunt lesions associated with pulmonary-to-systemic flow ratio (Qp/Qs) greater than 2:1 in patients with an atrial septal defect will produce a diastolic murmur across the tricuspid valve at the left lower sternal border and in patients with a ventricular septal defect will create a diastolic murmur across the mitral valve at the apex; similar murmurs are present with moderate to severe tricuspid and mitral regurgitation, respectively. Such murmurs are low velocity, best heard with the bell of the stethoscope, and usually of low intensity (grade 1 or 2).

Continuous murmurs begin in systole and persist through S_2 into early, mid, or all of diastole. Such murmurs often are audible throughout the cardiac cycle but can have phasic variation in intensity depending on the pressure gradient in systole and diastole. They are produced when there are connections between the following:

1. Systemic and pulmonary arterial circulations: surgically created Blalock-Taussig, Waterston, Potts, or central shunts, patent ductus arteriosus, aortopulmonary collateral artery, aortopulmonary window, anomalous left coronary artery arising from the main pulmonary artery
2. Systemic arteries and veins: arteriovenous malformation
3. Systemic arteries and cardiac chambers: coronary arteriovenous fistula, ruptured sinus of Valsalva aneurysm
4. Disturbed flow in arteries: collateral circulation associated with severe coarctation
5. Disturbed flow in veins: venous hum

A continuous murmur is distinguished from a to-and-fro murmur, which consists of two murmurs, one that occurs in systole and the other that occurs in diastole. A to-and-fro murmur does not continue through S_2 but instead has peak intensity earlier in systole. Examples include patients with combined aortic stenosis and aortic regurgitation (as can occur after balloon dilation of a stenotic bicuspid valve), combined pulmonary stenosis and pulmonary regurgitation (as can occur after repair of tetralogy of Fallot), or ventricular septal defect, prolapsed aortic cusp, and aortic regurgitation.

Timing also includes whether the murmur occurs in early, mid, or late systole or diastole. An early systolic murmur at the left lower sternal border is characteristic of a small muscular ventricular septal defect; in this condition, as the ventricle contracts, the septal defect closes so that the murmur is not holosystolic. A mid to late systolic murmur at the apex is characteristic of mild mitral regurgitation associated with mitral valve prolapse; as the ventricle decreases in size during systole, a mitral valve with either redundant valve tissue or lengthened chordae tendineae can become incompetent.

Location and Radiation. The region where a murmur is loudest and direction of radiation provide additional clues to the diagnosis. Aortic valve stenosis has maximal intensity at the right upper sternal border and may radiate to the suprasternal notch and carotid arteries. Aortic valve regurgitation is most easily detected at the left upper sternal border with the patient sitting, leaning forward, in expiration. Pulmonary stenosis and regurgitation are maximal at the left upper sternal border. The severity of aortic or pulmonary regurgitation correlates with the amount of radiation: mild limited to the left upper sternal border, moderate being audible also at the left midsternal border, and severe radiating to the left lower sternal border. The systolic murmur of peripheral pulmonary stenosis common in infancy is maximal at the left upper sternal border and radiates to the infraclavicular and axillary regions and to the back. Systolic murmurs at the left lower sternal border usually represent a ventricular septal defect but can be associated with tricuspid regurgitation. The murmur of tricuspid regurgitation usually increases during inspiration. Mitral valve disease is best heard at the apex with the patient in the lateral decubitus position. Mitral regurgitation typically radiates to the axilla.

Sites other than the precordium need to be auscultated as well. Coarctation is best heard in the intrascapular region on the back. Long-standing severe coarctation can produce collateral circulation audible as continuous murmur over the ribs where the intercostals arteries course. Arteriovenous malformations may be audible over the affected body region, for example, the cranium for vein of Galen malformations or right upper quadrant for hepatic source.

Shape. Diamond-shaped murmurs occur with ventricular obstructive lesions (semilunar valvar, subvalvar, or supravalvar stenosis, coarctation) or hyperdynamic states (anemia, hyperthyroidism, fever). These murmurs begin after S_1 and end before the component of S_2 (aortic or pulmonary) associated with the side of the heart from which the murmur originates.[21] Holosystolic murmurs have a plateau shape and are characteristic of ventricular septal defects other than small muscular defects or with atrioventricular valve regurgitation. These murmurs begin with S_1 and end with the aortic or pulmonary component of S_2, depending on whether they are left- or right-sided in origin. Decrescendo murmurs decrease in intensity during the cardiac cycle and include the diastolic murmurs of aortic regurgitation and pulmonary regurgitation.

Quality. Harsh murmurs are characteristic of murmurs caused by ventricular outflow tract obstruction or hyperdynamic states. Blowing murmurs are typical of valve regurgitation. A rumbling quality is a feature of diastolic turbulence across atrioventricular valves. A vibratory, musical, or humming property is associated with the innocent Still's murmur.

Chest Examination

Chest Deformity

Congenital heart disease associated with cardiomegaly can produce prominence of the left chest due to the effects of cardiac contraction against an elastic rib cage.[2] Pectus carinatum is a feature of Marfan syndrome. Pectus excavatum is associated with mitral valve prolapse; the mitral valve prolapse often improves after surgical correction of the chest wall deformity.[26] An asymmetric precordial bulge can also be seen in pulmonary conditions, including atelectasis, pneumothorax, emphysema, and diaphragmatic hernia.[27]

Chest Wall Examination

Chest pain in children frequently has a musculoskeletal basis, including costochondritis, slipping rib syndrome, or myodynia. The diagnosis of musculoskeletal pain can be confirmed by an ability to reproduce a similar quality of discomfort by palpation of the chest. The examination should include palpation of the costochondral junctions, the insertion site of the pectoralis major muscle group by grasping the head of the muscle between the examiner's fingers and thumb, the inframammary area, and other regions of the chest where pain is reported. Although one would expect the right and left costochondral junctions to be equally affected, the left-sided junctions are more typically involved.[28] In patients with slipping rib syndrome, the examiner can perform the "hooking" maneuver by placing fingers around the lower costal margin and lifting anteriorly to elicit a click and reproduce pain.[10] The demonstration of pain reproduction and an explanation of the anatomic basis are reassuring to the family and patient and help allay concerns about the heart.

Pulmonary Auscultation

Lesions associated with excessive pulmonary flow or left-sided dysfunction or obstruction can be associated with inspiratory rales or expiratory wheezing. These features are also present in patients with reactive airway disease or pneumonia.

Abdomen Examination

Palpation of the liver yields information about visceral situs and central venous pressure. A right-sided liver indicates normal situs of the abdominal viscera, a left-sided liver indicates situs inversus, and a midline liver indicates the presence of situs ambiguous and heterotaxy. Hepatomegaly is present in conditions associated with elevated central venous pressure. Percussion of the liver size helps to distinguish patients with "false" hepatomegaly caused by inferior displacement by a flattened diaphragm caused by hyperinflation. Palpation of the liver is easier when the abdomen is soft. Flexing the knees can relax the abdominal musculature. In infants, the liver can normally be palpated about 2 cm below the costal margin in the mid-clavicular line. In children, the liver can be palpated 1 cm below the right costal margin. An engorged liver is usually tender to palpation. A pulsatile liver is palpated in patients with elevated right atrial pressure, most commonly associated with significant tricuspid regurgitation.

In infants, a spleen tip can normally be palpated under the costal margin. Location of the spleen also aids in determination of visceral situs. Elevated central venous pressure usually does not produce splenomegaly. An enlarged spleen is a feature of bacterial endocarditis, and in a known cardiac patient with fever or new regurgitant murmur, this physical finding should prompt thorough evaluation of that complication.

Ascites is an uncommon feature of congenital heart disease. Placing one hand in each flank and detecting a fluid wave with one hand created by pressure applied by the other can determine its presence.

Extremities Examination

Edema

Pitting edema in infants generally has a renal rather than cardiac basis. In children and adolescents, edema can be caused by cardiac dysfunction, and in patients with a modified Fontan procedure, it can be caused by protein-losing enteropathy, a complication that occurs with high venous pressure. Swelling of the face, neck, and arms can occur with superior vena cava obstruction that occasionally is seen after Senning or Mustard repair for transposition of the great arteries, bidirectional Glenn shunt for palliation of functional single ventricle, intravascular thrombosis associated with an indwelling central venous catheter, or obstructing mediastinal mass. Obstruction of the inferior vena cava or iliac or femoral veins occasionally occurs secondary to *in utero* thrombosis or as a complication of catheterization and can produce edema of the abdomen and lower extremities. Doughy, nonpitting swelling of the hands and feet represents lymphedema that is seen in some infants with Turner's syndrome.

Clubbing

Clubbing is a feature of chronic cyanosis and is uncommon in early infancy. The change in appearance of the distal portion of the digit consists of rounding or convexity of the nail bed and thickening and shining of the skin at the base of the nail (Fig. 11-3). With marked clubbing, the terminal phalange becomes bulbous. Mild cases can be detected by dividing the diameter of the finger at the base of the nail bed by the diameter at the distal interphalangeal joint; clubbing is present when the value is greater than 1.[14,29]

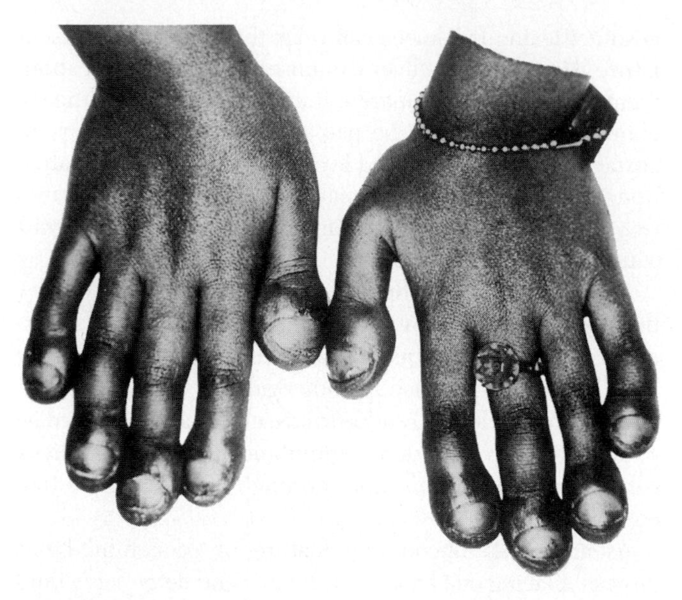

FIGURE 11–3 *Clubbed fingers.*
From Fyler DC (ed). Nadas' Pediatric Cardiology. Philadelphia: Harley & Belfus, 1992.

Differential Cyanosis

Certain congenital heart defects create an effect of differential cyanosis in which the upper half of the body is pink and the lower half blue, or vice versa. Systemic-level pulmonary vascular resistance and a patent ductus arteriosus need to be present for this phenomenon to occur. The oxygen saturation can be higher in the upper extremity in patients with normally related great arteries if there is right-to-left shunting at the level of the ductus arteriosus. This can occur in infants with either persistent pulmonary hypertension of the newborn, severe coarctation of the aorta, or interrupted aortic arch. The differential effect is reduced if there is also right-to-left shunting at the level of the foramen ovale, or if there is left-to-right shunting across a coexisting ventricular septal defect.[30] The lower portion of the body can be more cyanotic than the upper segment in older patients with Eisenmenger syndrome caused by a persistent large patent ductus arteriosus. In patients with transposition of the great arteries associated with either coarctation or pulmonary hypertension, differential cyanosis can be reversed with lower levels of oxygen saturation in the upper extremity.

ROUTINE LABORATORY TESTS

A variety of laboratory tests may be required for appropriate management of children with congenital heart disease. Selective aspects of these tests are mentioned below.

Hematology Tests

Leukocytosis

The white blood cell count may be elevated in infectious diseases (acute rheumatic fever, bacterial endocarditis, pericarditis), airway disease associated with excessive pulmonary flow or pulmonary venous congestion, or inflammatory conditions (aortitis, collagen vascular disease). Leukocytosis can also occur in patients with urinary tract infections, common in those with renal anomalies, or in patients with sinusitis, which can be a complication of chronic use of a nasogastric tube for nutritional support.

Hematocrit

The hematocrit is elevated in patients with cyanotic heart disease. In such patients, it is important to also check the mean corpuscular volume (MCV) to rule out relative anemia. Patients with microcytic anemia (MCV less than 80) are at increased risk for thrombotic complications, including cerebrovascular accidents.[31] The normal red blood cell has a biconcave surface membrane structure; the microcytic red blood cell has a less redundant membrane and is more likely to lodge in rather than pass through the capillary bed. In such patients, low-dose iron therapy should be instituted and the hematocrit response carefully monitored to avoid excessive polycythemia. Hematocrit levels greater than 70% are associated with exponential increases in blood viscosity and decreased cardiac output that can produce symptoms of decreased exercise tolerance, headache, cerebrovascular accident, and chest pain.[32] If such symptoms are present in patients with this degree of polycythemia, partial erythropheresis should be performed. The amount of whole blood to remove can be calculated from the following formula:

$$\text{Blood volume to remove (mL)} = \text{Estimated blood volume (mL)} \times (\text{Hct}_i - \text{Hct}_d)/\text{Hct}_i,$$

where Hct_i is the initial central venous hematocrit and Hct_d is the desired central venous hematocrit.

The blood volume in a neonate is 85 mL/kg, in a child is 70 mL/kg, and in an adult is 65 mL/kg. The hematocrit should not be reduced by more than 10% because such patients require increased oxygen carrying capacity for adequate oxygen delivery to the tissues. It is safest to do an isovolumetric exchange, replacing blood withdrawn with an equal volume of normal saline, fresh frozen plasma, or 5% salt-poor albumin.

Platelets

Polycythemia is frequently associated with thrombocytopenia (platelet levels, 50,000 to 80,000/mm^3) because megakaryocytes are "crowded out" by red blood cell precursors in the bone marrow. Thrombocytosis is a feature of Kawasaki disease, with platelet counts occasionally exceeding 1 million/mm.[3]

Howell-Jolly Bodies

Patients with heterotaxy syndrome can have asplenia. Microscopic evaluation of the peripheral blood smear will demonstrate Howell-Jolly bodies. Howell-Jolly bodies can normally be present in the first few weeks of life. A liver-spleen scan with technetium-99m or abdominal ultrasound can confirm the absence of a spleen.

The erythrocyte sedimentation rate (ESR) is elevated in inflammatory conditions and in bacterial endocarditis. The ESR correlates with the severity of congestive heart failure and is lower in patients with lower cardiac output or elevated right atrial pressure.[33]

Urinalysis

Hematuria can be a feature of bacterial endocarditis. The specific gravity yields information on fluid status. Pyuria can be associated with urinary tract infections or inflammatory conditions such as Kawasaki disease.

Blood Chemistries

Serum levels of sodium, potassium, chloride, calcium, magnesium, and phosphorous are monitored for patients receiving diuretics or those presenting with arrhythmias, especially if ventricular in origin. Serum levels of various antiarrhythmic or antiseizure medication can be determined. Digoxin levels should be drawn 8 to 12 hours after an oral dose to determine peak serum levels. Anticoagulation can be monitored by determining plasma heparin levels if this medication is used. The normal value is 0.3 to 0.5 U/mL. The infusion rate is adjusted to achieve this level. For those receiving warfarin sodium (Coumadin), the international normalized ratio (INR) is monitored. The goal for the INR value for patients with a prosthetic mechanical valve is 2.5 to 3.5, and for cerebrovascular accident prophylaxis for those with atrial fibrillation, cardiomyopathy, or right-to-left atrial level shunting, 2.0 to 2.5. Special precautions are required for obtaining an INR in patients with polycythemia and hematocrit greater than 55% to 60%. The typical tubes used for the assay contain a set amount of diluent that assumes a normal plasma volume. Patients with significant polycythemia need some of the diluent removed or else an artificially elevated INR value will be obtained. The laboratory should be contacted to determine the amount of diluent to remove for a given hematocrit level.

Blood Cultures

Blood cultures for bacterial and fungal pathogens are required for the evaluation of endocarditis. Ideally, a minimum of three cultures from separate venipunctures are obtained on the first day to definitively evaluate this condition; if there is no growth by the second day, an additional two cultures may be obtained[34] (see Chapter 28).

Level of Oxygenation

Transcutaneous oxygen saturation from preductal and postductal sites identifies patients with cyanosis, including those with differential cyanosis as described in an earlier section. Transcutaneous oxygen saturation is also useful in establishing the response to prostaglandin E_1 infusion. The oxygen dissociation curve is steep for values less than 70 mm Hg; thus, for lower levels, small decreases in oxygen tension are associated with large decreases in oxygen saturation.[35]

Additional information is obtained from arterial blood gas measurement. An elevated arterial P_{CO_2} value indicates the presence of pulmonary disease. A reduced pH level raises concern about poor cardiac output. The combination of severe hypoxemia, metabolic acidosis, and marked hypercarbia can also occur in patients with D-transposition of the great arteries when there is inadequate mixing at the atrial, ventricular, and great vessel level. A combination of low oxygen saturation and normal oxygen tension is present in methemoglobinemia. In this uncommon condition, blood has a chocolate-brown color and does not become red when exposed to air.[36]

The hyperoxia test is useful in distinguishing cardiac from pulmonary causes of cyanosis. In cyanotic heart disease associated with intracardiac right-to-left shunting, blood in the pulmonary veins is fully saturated with oxygen in ambient air. Administering higher concentrations of inspired oxygen increases the amount of dissolved oxygen but has minimal effect on systemic oxygen saturation or oxygen tension levels. Conversely, patients with pulmonary disease have pulmonary venous desaturation. Administering supplemental oxygen typically increases pulmonary venous oxygen levels and improves systemic oxygenation. The hyperoxia test is performed by placing the patient in 100% oxygen for 10 minutes either using an Oxyhood or endotracheal tube if already intubated. An arterial blood gas should be obtained from a preductal source (right arm); alternatively, transcutaneous P_{O_2} monitors can be used. Patients with cyanotic heart disease rarely have the preductal oxygen tension exceed 150 mm Hg, whereas patients with pulmonary disease usually exceed this value.[37] The level of arterial P_{O_2} in 100% oxygen helps to distinguish the various types of cyanotic heart disease (Table 11-4).

The interpretation of the hyperoxia test requires determination of both the arterial P_{O_2} and oxygen saturation. Because of the characteristics of the oxygen dissociation curve, a patient receiving a fractional inspired oxygen concentration of 1.0 could have 100% oxygen saturation

TABLE 11–4. Typical Results of Hyperoxia Test

	FiO_2 = 0.21		FiO_2 = 1
	PaO_2	PaO_2	$PaCO_2$
Normal	>70 (>95)	>300 (100)	35
Pulmonary disease	50 (85)	>150 (100)	50
Neurologic disease	50 (85)	>150 (100)	50
Methemoglobinemia	>70 (<85)	>200 (<85)	35
Cardiac disease			
Parallel circulation*	<40 (<75)	<50 (<85)	35
Mixing with reduced PBF†	<40 (<75)	<50 (<85)	35
Mixing without restricted PBF‡	40-60 (75-93)	<150 (<100)	35
Preductal Postductal			
Differential cyanosis§	70 (95)	<40 (<75)	variable, 35–50
Reverse differential cyanosis¶	<40 (<75)	>50 (>90)	variable, 35–50

*Transposition of the great arteries with or without ventricular septal defect.
†Tricuspid atresia with pulmonary stenosis, pulmonary atresia, critical pulmonary stenosis with intact ventricular septum, or tetralogy of Fallot.
‡Truncus arteriosus, total anomalous pulmonary venous connection without obstruction, hypoplastic left heart syndrome, single ventricle without pulmonary stenosis of pulmonary atresia.
§Persistent pulmonary hypertension of the newborn, interrupted aortic arch, severe coarctation.
¶Transposition of the great arteries associated with either coarctation or suprasystemic pulmonary vascular resistance.
Adapted from Marino BS, Bird GL, Wernovsky G. Diagnosis and management of the newborn with suspected congenital heart disease. Clin Perinatol 28:91, 2001.

associated with an arterial Po_2 of 75, a value that is abnormal. It is important to note that systemic oxygen tension can increase in some patients with cyanotic heart disease if there is coexisting airway disease (e.g., pulmonary edema or pneumonia) or mixing lesions involving both right-to-left and left-to-right shunting. In the latter situation (e.g., truncus arteriosus or single ventricle with patent ductus arteriosus), supplemental oxygen may decrease pulmonary vascular resistance, thereby increasing pulmonary flow, which when mixing with a fixed amount of systemic venous return, produces a higher level of aortic oxygenation. For such patients, the chest radiograph typically demonstrates cardiomegaly and prominent pulmonary vascularity. Nevertheless, even though the preductal oxygen tension may increase over ambient air levels in these conditions, the value rarely exceeds 150 mm Hg.[37] Also, some patients with severe lung disease may have minimal improvement with supplemental oxygen. In these patients, however, the chest radiograph and arterial Pco_2 level aid in establishing the underlying disorder.

Chest Radiograph

The chest radiograph provides information on heart size, pulmonary blood flow, situs of the aortic arch, and pulmonary disease (pulmonary hypoplasia, pneumonia, emphysema, atelectasis, pneumothorax or pneumomediastinum, and pleural effusion). The normal heart size is less than 50% of the cardiothoracic diameter. In infants, a large overlying anterior thymus can give the impression of cardiomegaly. The thymus has a nonsmooth, frequently undulating border that distinguishes it from a cardiac chamber.

Left-to-right shunt lesions have increased pulmonary arterial markings, whereas cyanotic lesions associated with obstructive right-sided lesions typically have dark, underperfused lung fields. Some patients with D-transposition of the great arteries can have asymmetric blood flow with more prominent markings in the right lung because the long axis of the left ventricle is more in line with the right than left pulmonary artery. Because of the relationship of the bronchi with the pulmonary arteries and left atrium, the left main, left upper, and right middle bronchi are more susceptible to compression by enlarged vessels or chambers (Fig. 11-4). Depending on the degree of obstruction, emphysema or atelectasis is produced.[38]

The tracheal air shadow has an indentation on the side of the aortic arch (Fig. 11-5). A right aortic arch is present in about 25% of patients with tetralogy of Fallot and in 30% of patients with truncus arteriosus.

Radioisotope Scans

Nuclear perfusion scans are helpful in determining the percentage of perfusion to the right and left lungs and aid in determining the effect of intervention

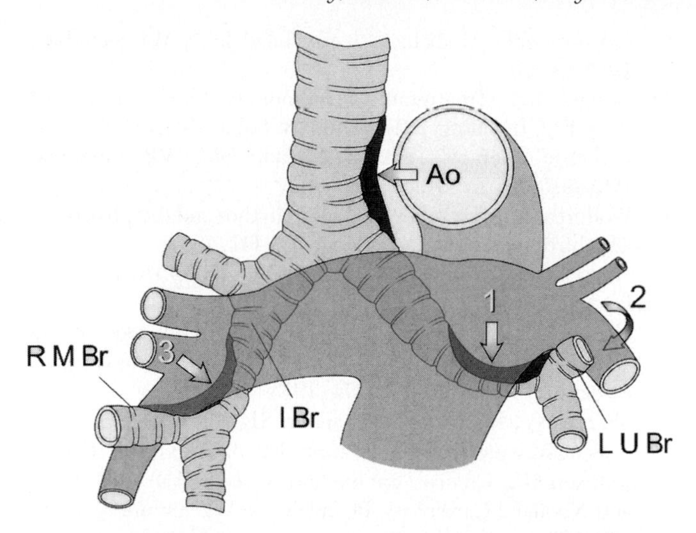

FIGURE 11–4 *Portions of the tracheobronchial tree at increased risk for compression from enlarged pulmonary arteries or left atrium. The left pulmonary artery courses superior to the left main bronchus (L. Br.)[1] and hooks around the left upper bronchus (L.U. Br.).[2] The distended left pulmonary artery pushes the aorta (Ao) medially and accentuates the indentation of the trachea made by a left aortic arch. The left recurrent laryngeal nerve lies in this area and can be compressed. The branch of the right pulmonary artery that supplies the right lower lobe crosses the junction of the intermediate bronchus (I. Br.) and right middle bronchus (R.M. Br.). The left atrium lies below the tracheal bifurcation. Enlargement of the left atrium increases the angle of the tracheal bifurcation mainly by upward deflection of the left main bronchus.*
From Stranger P, Lucas RV Jr, Edward JE. Anatomic factors causing respiratory distress in acyanotic congenital heart disease. Pediatrics, 43:760, 1969.

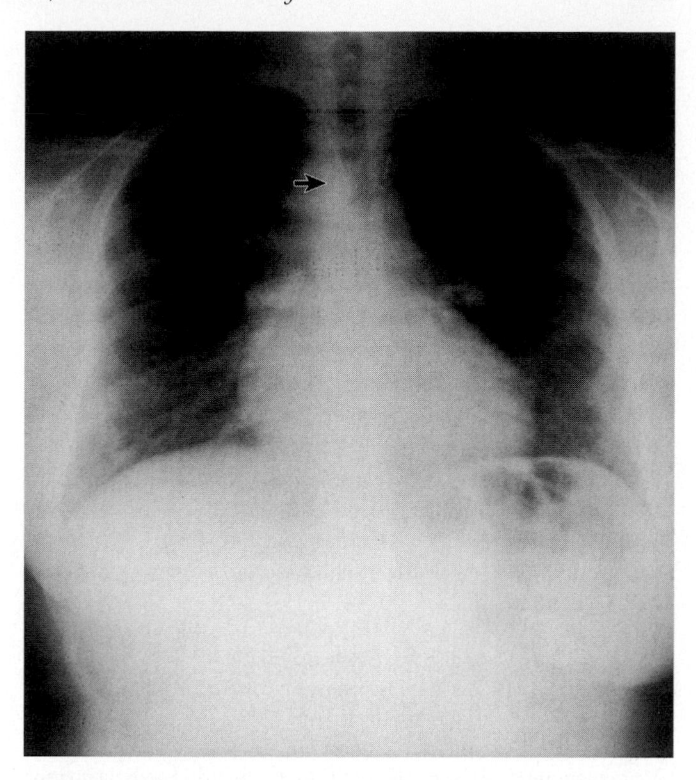

FIGURE 11–5 *Right aortic arch in a patient with tetralogy of Fallot. Note the indentation on the right side of the trachea made by the aortic arch (black arrow).*
From Fyler DC (ed). Nadas' Pediatric Cardiology. Philadelphia: Harley & Belfus, 1992.

(surgical or catheterization) for peripheral pulmonary stenosis. Quantitative nuclear angiography can also estimate the degree of left-to-right shunting; this noninvasive measurement assists the clinician in determining whether a significant sized shunt is present.[39] Myocardial perfusion scans evaluate ventricular function and are discussed in Chapter 15.

Arrhythmia Evaluation

Various recording devices are available to record the heart rhythm on an outpatient basis. A 24-hour Holter monitor is able to record every beat but is somewhat cumbersome to wear. This test is helpful to quantitate the amount and degree of ventricular ectopy or extent of bradycardia; intermittent symptoms frequently do not occur on the day this type of monitor is used. Intermittent symptoms can be recorded with the use of an event monitor or loop recorder. The former consists of a small unit about twice the size of a typical pager unit; at the time of symptoms, the unit is placed directly on the left precordium, and the rhythm is recorded. The latter consists of a small unit with wire attachments to three chest electrodes. The heart rhythm is recorded for several minutes, and then a new interval is recorded over the former tracing; at the time of symptoms, the unit is activated to save the current tracing. Both the event and loop monitor tracings can be sent over the telephone and permit correlation of symptoms with cardiac rhythm. These units are helpful in the diagnosis of intermittent tachyarrhythmias, the former for episodes that last for more than 1 minute and the latter for shorter episodes. In patients with recurrent syncope, palpitations, or dizziness for whom an arrhythmia cannot be ruled out by these devices, an insertable loop recorder can be used. This device is inserted under local anesthesia in the upper chest and can continuously record the heart rate and rhythm for up to 14 months.[40]

REFERENCES

1. Geggel RL, Horowitz LM, Brown EA, et al. Parental anxiety associated with referral of a child to a pediatric cardiologist for evaluation of a Still's murmur. J Pediatr 140:747, 2002.

2. Fyler DC, Nadas AS. History, physical examination, and laboratory test. In Fyler DC (ed). Nadas' Pediatric Cardiology. Philadelphia, Hanley & Belfus, 1992:101–116.
3. Geggel RL. Conditions leading to pediatric cardiology consultation in a tertiary academic hospital. Pediatrics 2004 (in press).
4. Frohn-Mulder IM, Meilof JF, Szatmari A, et al. Clinical significance of maternal anti-RO/SS-A antibodies in children with isolated heart block. J Am Coll Cardiol 23:1677, 1994.
5. Geggel RL, Armsby LB. Evaluation and initial management of cyanotic heart disease in the newborn. Retrieved from UpToDate at http://www.uptodate.
6. Marino BS, Bird GL, Wernovsky G. Diagnosis and management of the newborn with suspected congenital heart disease. Clin Perinatol 28:91, 2001.
7. Whittemore R, Wells JA, Castellsague X. A second-generation study of 427 probands with congenital heart defects and their 837 children. J Am Coll Cardiol 23:1459, 1994.
8. Wren C. Sudden death in children and adolescents. Heart 88:426, 2002.
9. Geggel RL. Evaluation of pediatric chest pain. Retrieved from UpToDate at http://www.uptodate.
10. Heinz, GJ III, Zavala, DC. Slipping rib syndrome: Diagnosis using the hooking maneuver. JAMA 237:794, 1977.
11. Wolff GS, Young ML, Tamer DF. Syncope: Diagnosis and management. In Deal B, Wolff G, Gelband H (eds). Current concepts in diagnosis and management of arrhythmias in infants and children. Armonk, NY: Futura, 1998:223–239.
12. Johnsrude CL. Current approach to pediatric syncope. Pediatr Cardiol 21:522, 2000.
13. Greenwood RD, Rosenthal A, Parisi L, et al. Extracardiac anomalies in children with congenital heart disease. Pediatrics 55:485, 1975.
14. Duff DF, McNamara DG. History and physical examination of the cardiovascular system. In Garson A Jr, Bricker TM, Fisher DJ, Neish SR (eds). The Science and Practice of Pediatric Cardiology. Baltimore: Williams & Wilkins, 1998: 693–713.
15. Davignon A. Percentile charts: ECG standards for children. Pediatr Cardiol 1:133, 1980.
16. Marriott HJL. Atrial arrhythmias. In Marriott HJL (ed). Practical Electrocardiography, 5th ed. Baltimore: Williams & Wilkins, 1975:128–152.
17. Subramanyan R, Joy J, Balakrishnan KG. Natural history of aortoarteritis (Takayasu's disease). Circulation 80:429, 1989.
18. Report of the Second Task Force on Blood Pressure Control in Children—1987. Pediatrics 79:1–25, 1987.
19. Rappaport MB, Sprague HB. Physiologic and physical laws that govern auscultation, and their clinical application. Am Heart J 21:257, 1941.
20. Marino BS, Goldblatt A. Heart sounds and murmurs. In Lilly LS (ed). Pathophysiology of Heart Disease. Philadelphia, Lea & Febiger, 1992:18–29.
21. Perloff JK. Heart sounds and murmurs: physiologic mechanisms. In Braunwald E (ed). Heart Disease: A Textbook of Cardiovascular Medicine, 4th ed. Philadelphia: WB Saunders, 1992:43–63.
22. Geggel RL. Treatment of pulmonary hypertension. In Burg FD, Ingelfinger JR, Wald ER, Polin RA (eds). Current Pediatric Therapy, 16th ed. Philadelphia: WB Saunders, 1999:597–601.
23. Wolferth CC, Margolies A. Gallop rhythm and the physiological third heart sound. Am Heart J 8:441, 1933.
24. Warren JV, Leonard JJ, Weissler AM. Gallop rhythm. Ann Intern Med 48:580, 1958.
25. Freeman AR, Levine SA. The clinical significance of the systolic murmur: A study of 1,000 consecutive "non-cardiac" cases. Ann Intern Med 6:1371, 1933.
26. Shamberger RC, Welch KJ, Sanders SP. Mitral valve prolapse associated with pectus excavatum. J Pediatr 111:404, 1987.
27. Johnson GL. Clinical examination. In Long WA (ed): Fetal and Neonatal Cardiology. Philadelphia: WB Saunders, 1990: 223–235.
28. Brown RT. Costochondritis in adolescents. J Adolesc Health Care 1:198, 1981.
29. Sly R. Objective assessment of digital clubbing in Caucasian, Negro, and Oriental subjects. Chest 64:687, 1973.
30. Lees MH. Cyanosis of the newborn infant. J Pediatr 77:484, 1970.
31. Phornphutkul C, Rosenthal A, Nadas AS, et al. Cerebrovascular accidents in infants and children with cyanotic congenital heart disease. Am J Cardiol 32:329, 1973.
32. Ammash N, Warnes CA. Cerebrovascular events in adult patients with cyanotic congenital heart disease. J Am Coll Cardiol 28:768, 1996.
33. Haber HL, Leavy JA, Kessler PD, et al. The erythrocyte sedimentation rate in congestive heart failure. N Engl J Med 324:353, 1991.
34. Ferrieri P, Gewitz MH, Gerber MA, et al. Unique features of infective endocarditis in childhood. Circulation 105:2115, 2002.
35. Rudolph AM. Oxygen uptake and delivery. In Rudolph AM (ed). Congenital Diseases of the Heart. Armonk, NY: Futura, 2001:85–119.
36. Jaffe ER. Methemoglobinemia in the differential diagnosis of cyanosis. Hosp Pract 20:92, 1985.
37. Jones RWA, Baumer JH, Joseph MC, et al. Arterial oxygen tension and response to oxygen breathing in differential diagnosis of congenital heart disease in infancy. Arch Dis Child 51:667, 1976.
38. Stanger P, Lucas RV Jr, Edwards JE. Anatomic factors causing respiratory distress in acyanotic congenital cardiac disease. Pediatrics 43:760, 1969.
39. Maltz DL, Treves S. Quantitative radionuclide angiocardiography: Determination of Qp:Qs in children. Circulation 47: 1049, 1973.
40. Krahn A., Klein G, Yee R., et al. Final results from a pilot study with an implantable loop recorder to determine the etiology of syncope in patients with negative non-invasive and invasive testing. Am J Cardiol 82:117, 1998.

12

Electrocardiography and Introduction to Electrophysiologic Techniques

EDWARD P. WALSH, MARK E. ALEXANDER, AND FRANK CECCHIN

Of the benefits which graphic methods have conferred upon practical medicine, it is my desire to speak but briefly. These records have placed the entire question of irregular or disordered mechanism of the human heart upon a rational basis..., they have influenced prognosis..., they have potentially abolished the promiscuous administration of certain cardiac poisons, and have clearly shown the line which therapy should follow.[1]

Thomas Lewis, 1924

Electrocardiography, accurate physical examination, and radiology form the tripod on which rests the clinical diagnosis in pediatric cardiology. Omission of, unfamiliarity with, or misinterpretation of any of these three tools spells disaster.[2]

Alexander S. Nadas, 1957

The optimism of Sir Thomas Lewis and the cautions of Dr. Nadas regarding the electrocardiogram (ECG) remain valid even in this day of sophisticated echocardiography, Doppler flow analysis, and magnetic resonance imaging. Although it must be admitted that fine details of cardiac anatomy are now best evaluated with these modern techniques, the ECG is not (and never will be) obsolete. It is still the quickest, safest, and least expensive diagnostic tool in cardiology and is unparalleled in its ability to register arrhythmias and conduction defects. With proper interpretation, the ECG also offers a useful reflection of cardiac position, chamber enlargement, myocardial damage, and certain metabolic disorders. It has clearly proven its worth after more than a century of continuous clinical use.

This chapter is intended as a review of electrocardiography as it applies to the pediatric patient. Rather than simply catalogue a litany of rules for ECG interpretation, we have expanded the discussion here to encompass the basic cellular events underlying cardiac electrical activity, along with a survey of invasive and noninvasive techniques used for in-depth analysis of cardiac rhythm and conduction patterns. This information is intended not only to clarify the origin of ECG signals recorded from the body surface but also to serve as an introduction to the broader topic of cardiac arrhythmias that will be addressed further in Chapter 29 of this text.

BASIC ELECTROPHYSIOLOGY

Cellular Action Potential

The ECG is several steps removed from electrical activity at the cellular level, but the two are intimately related. Cellular events can be recorded directly using microelectrodes equipped with tips that are small enough to pierce individual cell membranes. When a microelectrode invades a normal cardiac cell, it encounters a field of net negative charge relative to the outside environment. This is the *diastolic resting potential* of the cell, which is maintained by the selective permeability of membrane channels to certain ions, as well as the operation of membrane ion pumps. If the cell interior becomes slightly depolarized (i.e., less negatively charged), it may reach a critical value referred to as the *threshold potential.* At this point, an abrupt change in membrane channel properties allows a sudden flood of positive ions to enter the cell, and an *action potential* develops.

Two general types of cardiac action potentials can be observed. The most common, known as the *fast response* or *sodium channel* type, normally occurs in cells of atrial muscle, ventricular muscle, His-Purkinje cells, and probably accessory atrioventricular (AV) conduction tissue (e.g., Wolff-Parkinson-White syndrome). These cells generally register a resting potential at about −90 mV and depend on sodium ions as the positive charge carrier for their initial rapid phase 0 depolarization (Fig. 12-1). Immediately after phase 0, there is a complex sequence of activation and deactivation for the various ion channels involved with potassium, sodium, chloride, and calcium flux. This proceeds in an orderly pattern that initially maintains the net intracellular charge in balance with the outside environment for a period known as the phase 2 *plateau*, but eventually progresses to phase 3 *repolarization* to restore the cell back to its phase 4 resting state.

A second variety of action potential, referred to as the *slow response* or *calcium channel* type, occurs predominantly in cells of the sinoatrial (SA) node and the AV node. It is distinguished by a resting potential of about −60 mV and has a less acute upstroke for the initial phase 0 depolarization. These cells utilize calcium along with some sodium to provide the inward ionic current for depolarization (Fig. 12-2). An important feature of slow response cells is the property of *automaticity*. Spontaneous upward drift of the diastolic potential during phase 4 enables the cell to reach threshold of its own accord and thereby act as a natural pacemaker for the heart (Fig. 12-3). Some fast response cells are also capable of spontaneous automaticity, but at much slower rates.

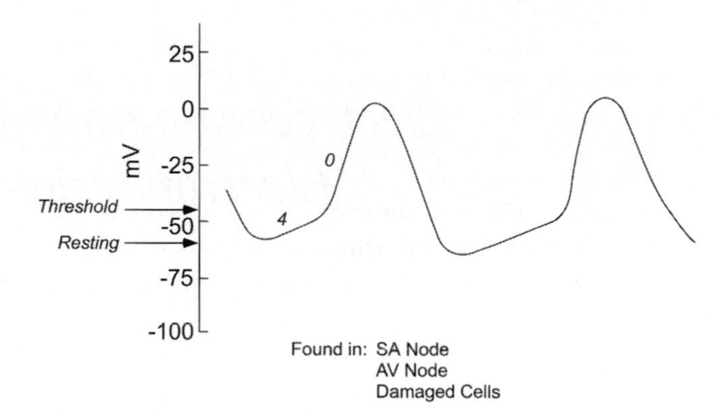

FIGURE 12–2 *Diagrammatic action potential of a slow response cardiac cell. The depolarization during phase 0 is due predominantly to calcium influx. Note gradual spontaneous depolarization during phase 4 which imparts the property of automaticity to such cells.*
From Fyler DC. Nadas' Pediatric Cardiology. Philadelphia: Hanley & Belfus, 1992.

Cell-to-Cell Conduction

When a cardiac cell depolarizes, it usually stimulates neighboring tissue in such a fashion that the activation sequence is transmitted from cell to cell throughout the heart.

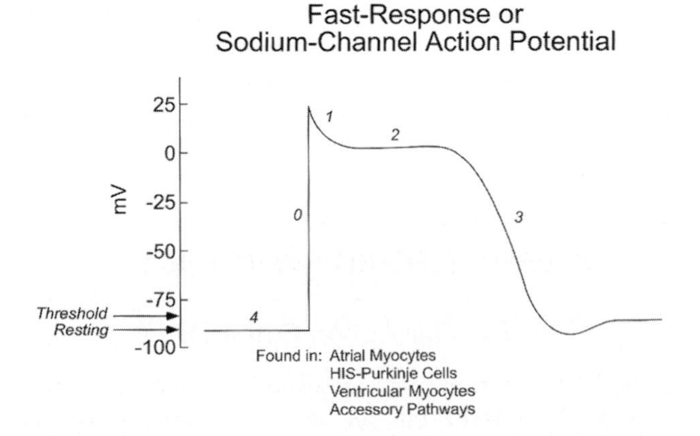

FIGURE 12–1 *Diagrammatic action potential of a fast response cardiac cell. The rapid depolarization during phase 0 is caused by sodium influx.*
From Fyler DC. Nadas' Pediatric Cardiology. Philadelphia: Hanley & Belfus, 1992.

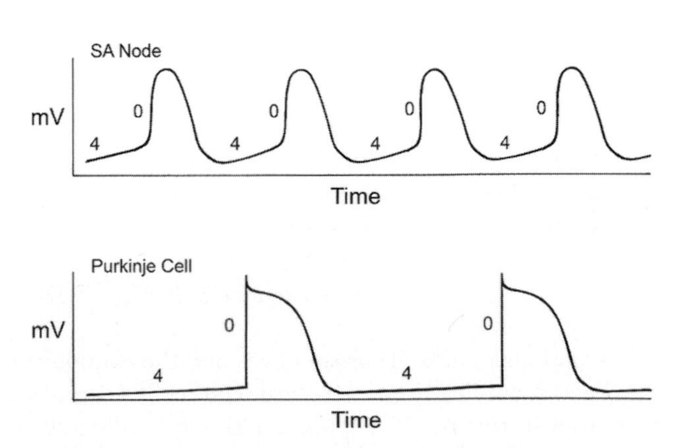

FIGURE 12–3 *Comparison of the rate for spontaneous automaticity of a slow response cell (e.g., sinus node) with that of a fast response cell (e.g., Purkinje cell); differences are due to the slope of phase 4 depolarization.*
From Fyler DC. Nadas' Pediatric Cardiology. Philadelphia: Hanley & Belfus, 1992.

For this process to repeat smoothly, cells must have sufficient time to repolarize and recover between stimuli. If the initiating impulse is premature, the cells may not be prepared, or may be only partially prepared, for reactivation. The time needed to recover from a prior stimulus is known as the *refractory period*, which usually lasts until cells have nearly completed their repolarization process (late phase 3 or early phase 4). During the *absolute* refractory period, a cell does not respond in any way to a new impulse, regardless of the stimulus strength. During the *relative* refractory period, a cell may respond occasionally, but only if the premature stimulus is sufficiently strong. During the early phase of the relative refractory period, a cell sometimes responds to a premature stimulus with an incomplete and low-amplitude action potential that is too weak to propagate any further to cells downstream. This is designated as the *effective* refractory period (ERP). The distinction between absolute and effective refractoriness is subtle but important because the ERP may be measured in the intact heart with clinical electrophysiologic techniques. For practical clinical purposes, the effective and absolute refractory periods can be considered similar (Fig. 12-4).

Conduction through the Intact Heart

A normal heartbeat begins with the spontaneous depolarization of a cell in the SA node, located at the junction of the superior vena cava and right atrium in the area of the sulcus terminalis. This event then activates adjacent atrial muscle cells so that a wave of depolarization spreads out from high in the right atrium like ripples in a pond. The wavefront reaches the lower parts of the right atrium after about 30 msec and finishes at the lateral part of the left atrium after about 80 msec. The electrical activity from SA node depolarization is too small to be recorded from the body surface, but atrial muscle cell depolarization is clearly registered as the P wave on the ECG. The P wave corresponds to phase 0 of the action potentials from individual atrial myocytes and reflects the leading edge of the depolarization wavefront as it travels from cell to cell. Once all atrial cells have undergone their initial rapid depolarization and entered the phase 2 plateau, the P wave is complete. Phase 3 repolarization of atrial cells causes a very small deflection on the surface ECG, referred to as the T_A wave. This wave is rarely seen because it is usually obscured by the QRS complex, but under special conditions such as heart block, the atrial repolarization wave may be appreciated (Fig. 12-5).

As the atrial activation wavefront passes through the lower right atrium, depolarization of the AV node is initiated. This node is a complex interface consisting predominantly of slow response cells located in an anatomic region referred to as the *triangle of Koch* (Fig. 12-6). Conduction velocity within the AV node is relatively slow, and it varies according to the timing of atrial impulses. Premature beats or accelerated atrial rhythm exaggerate AV nodal delay in a gradual and progressive manner described as *decremental conduction*, which can ultimately produce the stereotypic sequence of conduction block that is easily recognized as *Wenckebach* periodicity (Fig. 12-7). This pattern is rather specific to slow response cells. Conduction through fast response cells, by contrast, tends to be all or none, with a fairly fixed conduction velocity.

Electrical activity within the AV node is not directly registered on the surface ECG. One must rely on upstream events (P wave) and downstream events (QRS complex) as indirect measures of the process. On the surface ECG, the

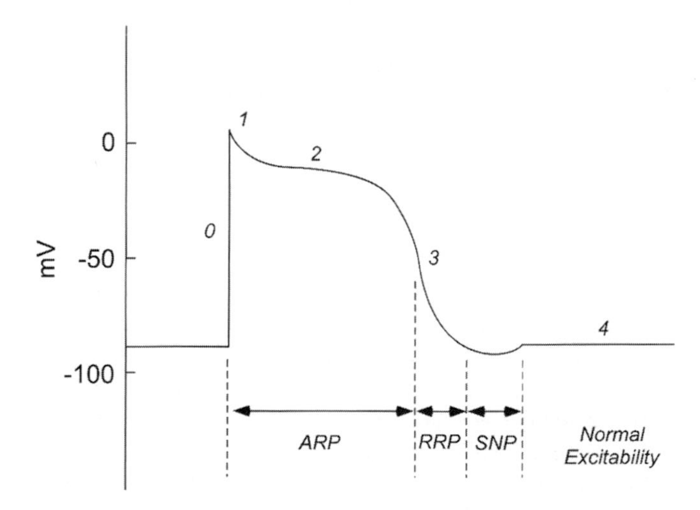

FIGURE 12–4 *Diagrammatic fast response action potential showing the time course of refractoriness and excitability. During the absolute refractory period (ARP), the cell cannot be re-excited regardless of stimulus strength. During the relative refractory period (RRP), only large-amplitude stimuli can re-excite the cell. Some cells may display a supernormal period (SNP) at the end of phase 3, which permits excitability with low-amplitude stimuli. From Fyler DC. Nadas' Pediatric Cardiology. Philadelphia: Hanley & Belfus, 1992.*

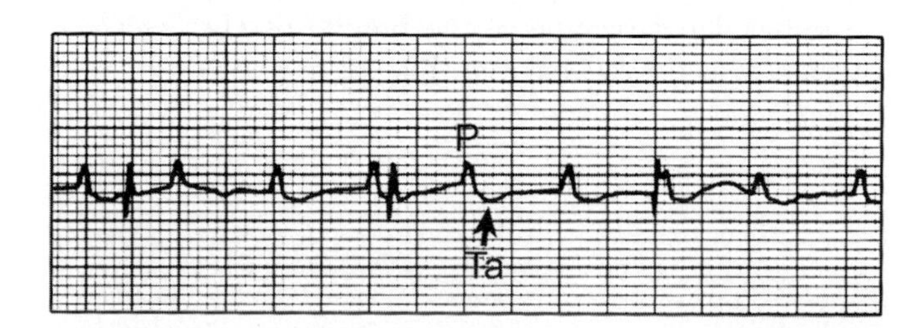

FIGURE 12–5 *The T_A wave of atrial repolarization clearly seen in a patient with complete heart block and atrial enlargement. From Fyler DC. Nadas' Pediatric Cardiology. Philadelphia: Hanley & Belfus, 1992.*

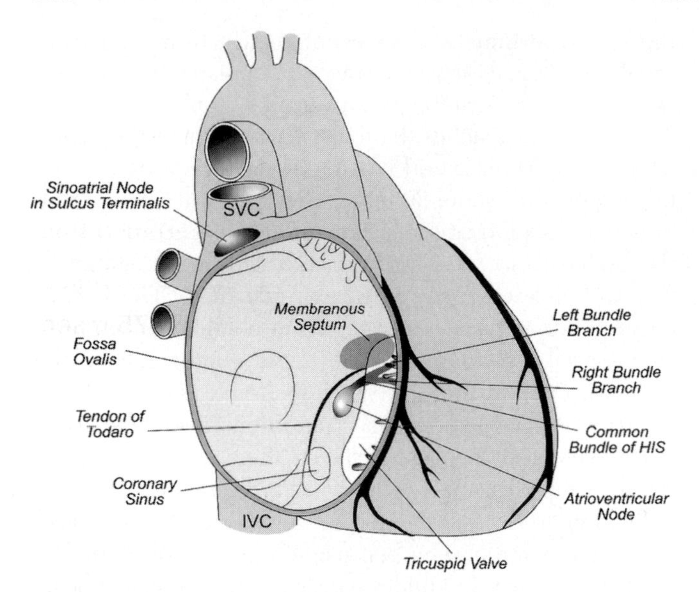

FIGURE 12–6 *Schematic view of the interior of the right atrium emphasizing the landmarks of the normal conduction system. The AV node lies within the triangle of Koch. The apex of this triangle lies at the membranous septum, with its long sides marked by the tendon of Todaro and the rim of the tricuspid valve; its base is at the coronary sinus.*
From Fyler DC. Nadas' Pediatric Cardiology. Philadelphia: Hanley & Belfus, 1992.

PR interval provides a rough estimation of AV node conduction, but there is actually much more to this interval than AV node activity alone. To be precise, the PR interval includes conduction times: (1) from high to low in the right atrium, (2) in the AV node proper, and (3) in the His-Purkinje system. To dissect the PR interval into these individual components, an intracardiac electrode catheter can be positioned across the medial aspect of the tricuspid valve as part of an electrophysiologic study to straddle an area near the bundle of His. This specialized recording reveals localized low right atrial activation, followed by a small deflection from the common bundle of His, and finally the local right ventricular activation. An index of true AV node conduction time can be obtained by measuring the interval between low right atrial depolarization and the initial depolarization of the bundle of His, which is referred to as the *AH interval* (Fig. 12-8).

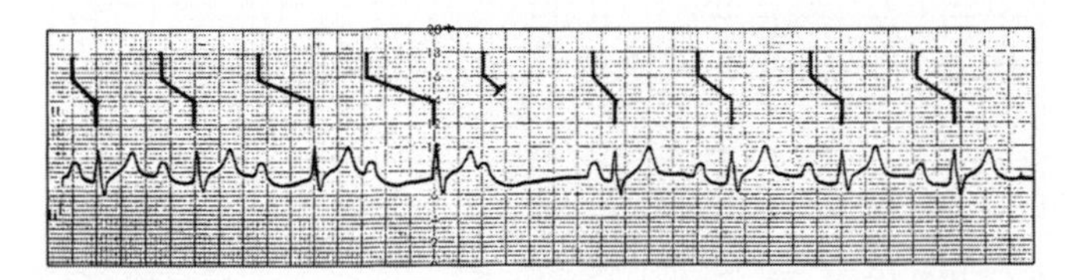

FIGURE 12–7 *Lead II rhythm strip and laddergram demonstrating AV nodal Wenckebach phenomenon.*
From Fyler DC. Nadas' Pediatric Cardiology. Philadelphia: Hanley & Belfus, 1992.

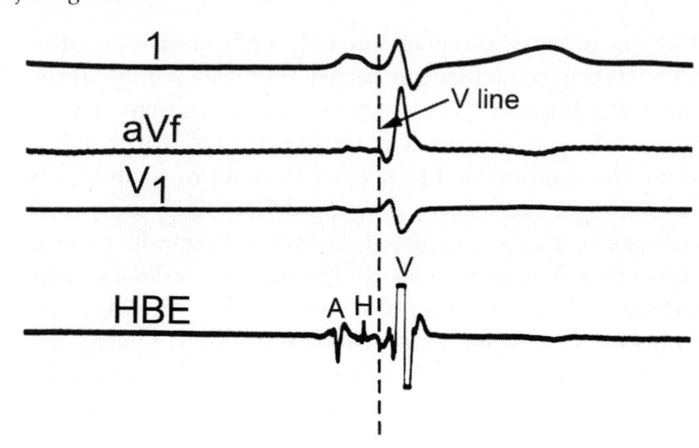

FIGURE 12–8 *Simultaneous surface ECG leads and the His bundle electrogram (HBE). The A-H interval is measured from the beginning of the A deflection to the beginning of the H deflection. The H-V interval is measured from the beginning of the H deflection to the V line, which marks the earliest ventricular activation in any lead.*
From Fyler DC. Nadas' Pediatric Cardiology. Philadelphia: Hanley & Belfus, 1992.

Beyond the AV node, the excitation process enters the common bundle of His. This bundle crosses the AV junction on the right ventricular side, just beneath the membranous septum (see Fig. 12-6). Cells of the His-Purkinje system have fast response action potentials, and generally rapid conduction velocity. The propagated impulse traverses the common bundle of His, splits into right and left bundle branches, and quickly exits from the terminal Purkinje fibers to begin activation of ventricular myocytes, all in about 40 msec. On the intracardiac His recording, the time from the initial His deflection to the beginning of ventricular activation (*HV interval*) is an accurate measure of His-Purkinje conduction time (see Fig. 12-8).

Conduction along the His-Purkinje network occurs as the cells are depolarizing (i.e., during phase 0). Their repolarization begins long after the excitation wavefront has passed on to ventricular muscle. Indeed, final repolarization of His-Purkinje cells tends to be one of the last electrical events during a cardiac cycle and probably contributes to some portion of the small terminal U wave seen occasionally on the normal ECG.

As the excitation wavefront leaves the His-Purkinje system, phase 0 of ventricular myocyte depolarization begins. The His-Purkinje system is highly arborized in its terminal portion, and these multiple exit sites promote depolarization of several different ventricular regions at one time, a process that is further complicated by the heart's three-dimensional geometry. To better visualize ventricular activation, it is useful to divide events into small time segments and examine the order of regional depolarization. A simplification of the sequence is shown in Figure 12-9, beginning with left-to-right septal activation, followed by

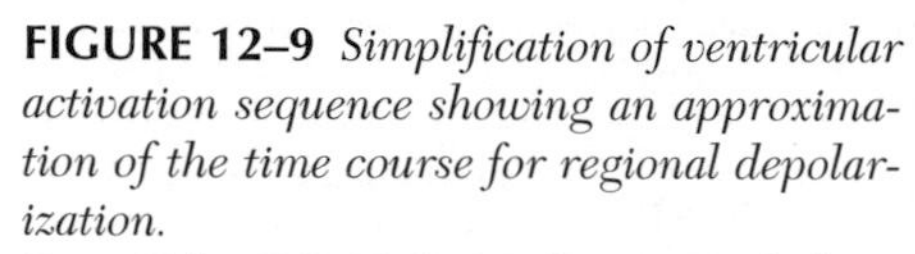

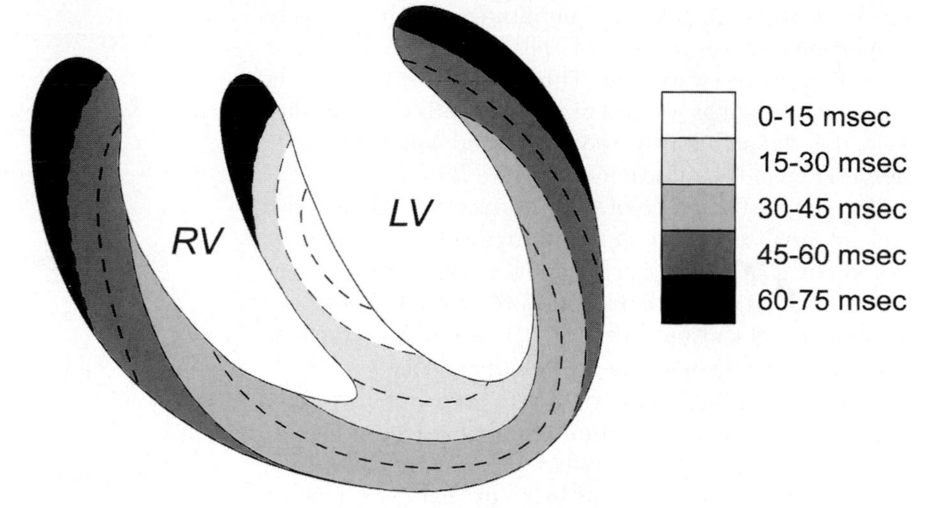

FIGURE 12–9 *Simplification of ventricular activation sequence showing an approximation of the time course for regional depolarization.*
From Fyler DC. Nadas' Pediatric Cardiology. Philadelphia: Hanley & Belfus, 1992.

activation of the left and right apex, the endocardium of the right and left ventricular free walls, the free wall epicardium, the base of the left ventricle, and finally, the right ventricular outflow tract. The advancing wavefront in each region generates a signal that can be recorded from the body surfaces as the QRS complex.

The QRS is complete once all ventricular cells have depolarized (usually within 90 msec). The ST segment is registered while the cells remain at the phase 2 plateau. At the onset of phase 3 repolarization, inscription of the T wave begins. Repolarization is less homogeneous than depolarization; hence, there is a relatively protracted duration for the T wave compared with the QRS. Additionally, the repolarization sequence is just the opposite of depolarization and appears to follow the reverse direction of epicardium toward endocardium. When all ventricular myocytes are back to phase 4, the T wave is complete.

Graphic Recording of Cardiac Electrical Activity

It should be apparent from the preceding discussion that the signal registered on the surface ECG occurs during abrupt changes in cellular conditions, with the P wave and QRS complex marking the acute phase 0 transition from resting potential to the fully depolarized state, and the T_A, T, and U waves marking phase 3 repolarization back to the diastolic resting potential. In fact, when all cells in a given cardiac chamber are either fully depolarized (phases 1 and 2) or fully repolarized (phase 4), the signal recorded from the body surface has the same isoelectric appearance even though intracellular conditions differ dramatically. Thus, what is measured with an ECG is not cellular voltage, but rather the current that arises at the boundary between depolarized and repolarized cells as activation and deactivation wavefronts move through a cardiac chamber. This boundary acts as a dipole, which generates current because of the presence of opposing charges in front and behind. Movement of this dipole relative to an ECG electrode produces the electrocardiographic signal (Fig. 12-10). During depolarization, the leading edge of the activation wavefront is charged positive, and the trailing edge negative. Movement toward a recording electrode results in an upward deflection on the ECG, and movement away results in a downward deflection. Repolarization wavefronts have a negative leading edge and generate signals with just the opposite deflections. In addition to direction, electrocardiographic signals

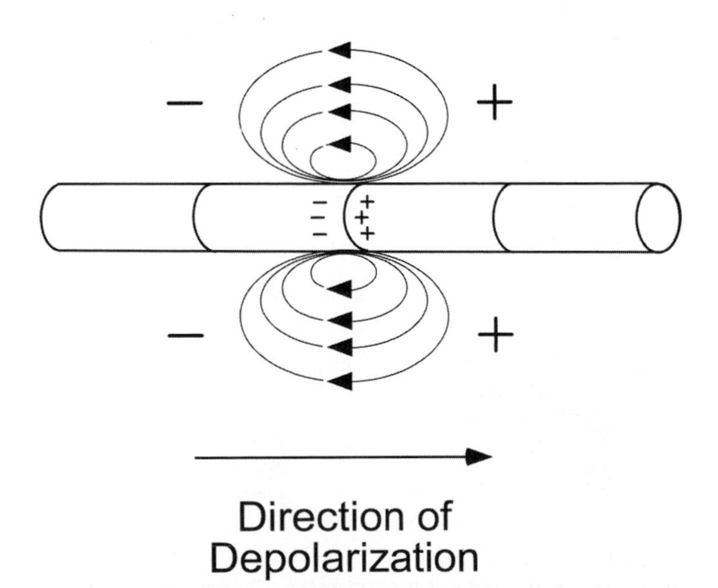

FIGURE 12–10 *The dipole created by advancing depolarization along a series of cardiac cells generates fields of extracellular current. From Fyler DC. Nadas' Pediatric Cardiology. Philadelphia: Hanley & Belfus,1992.*

can be further qualified by amplitude, which is largely proportional to the number of cells being stimulated at a given time by the wavefront. Thus, these electrical events can be described as a series of vectors, with directionality reflecting the path for the wavefront, and amplitude (voltage) reflecting the muscle mass involved.

The simplest example of body surface recording is the cycle of atrial activation, shown in Figure 12-11 with three hypothetical ECG leads on the left arm, right arm, and leg. The normal atrial depolarization wavefront advances from the upper right atrium, resulting in a mean vector that inscribes positive P waves in the left arm and leg leads, with a negative deflection in the right arm lead. Repolarization follows in the same path after a short isoelectric period, generating a T_A of opposite polarity.

The ventricular cycle results in a more complex series of vectors (Fig. 12-12). The process begins with septal activation, which generates a small negative deflection (Q wave) in the left arm lead and a small positive deflection in the leg lead. The right arm, being nearly at right angles to this vector, records little activity at this point. With left apex depolarization, the vector abruptly shifts leftward and inferior, beginning the inscription of an R wave in the left arm, further increasing the positive amplitude of the leg recording, with a negative deflection now appearing in the right arm lead. As events proceed to the ventricular free walls, there is competition between the simultaneous vectors of left- and right-sided depolarization. In a normal heart, the left ventricle wins out by virtue of its larger muscle mass, and the resultant net vector continues leftward. Final depolarization of the left base and right outflow tract generates superior and rightward vectors, causing inscription of a negative S wave in the left arm and leg leads, with a positive deflection in the right arm lead.

The repolarization process of the ventricle is even more involved. Unlike the atrium, the vectors of repolarization do not exactly retrace the same steps as depolarization because ventricular myocytes generally repolarize in an

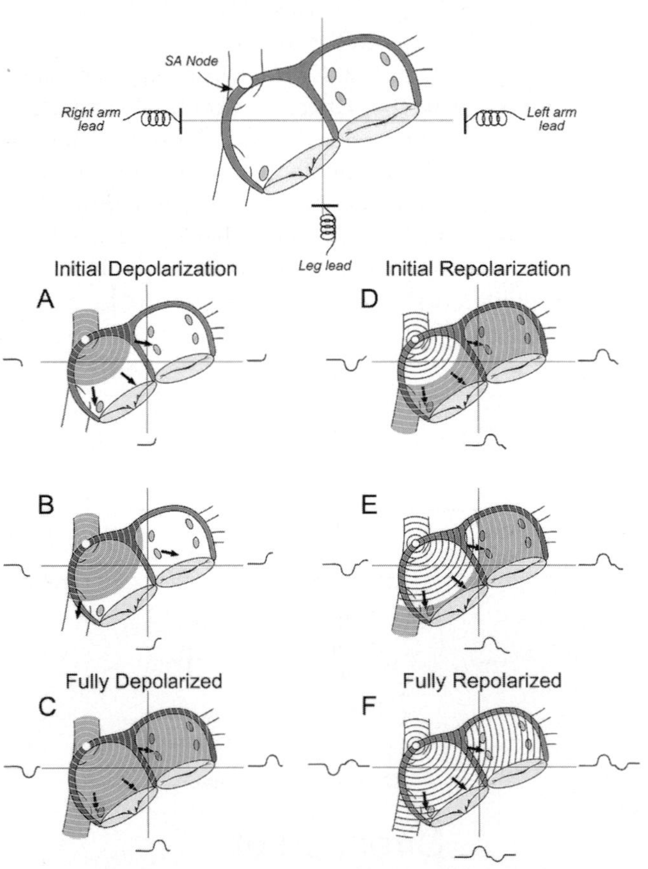

FIGURE 12–11 *Genesis of the P wave and Ta wave:* ***A****, Onset of the P wave.* ***C****, Completed P wave.* ***D****, Onset of Ta.* ***F****, Completion of P-Ta.*
From Fyler DC. Nadas' Pediatric Cardiology. Philadelphia: Hanley & Belfus, 1992.

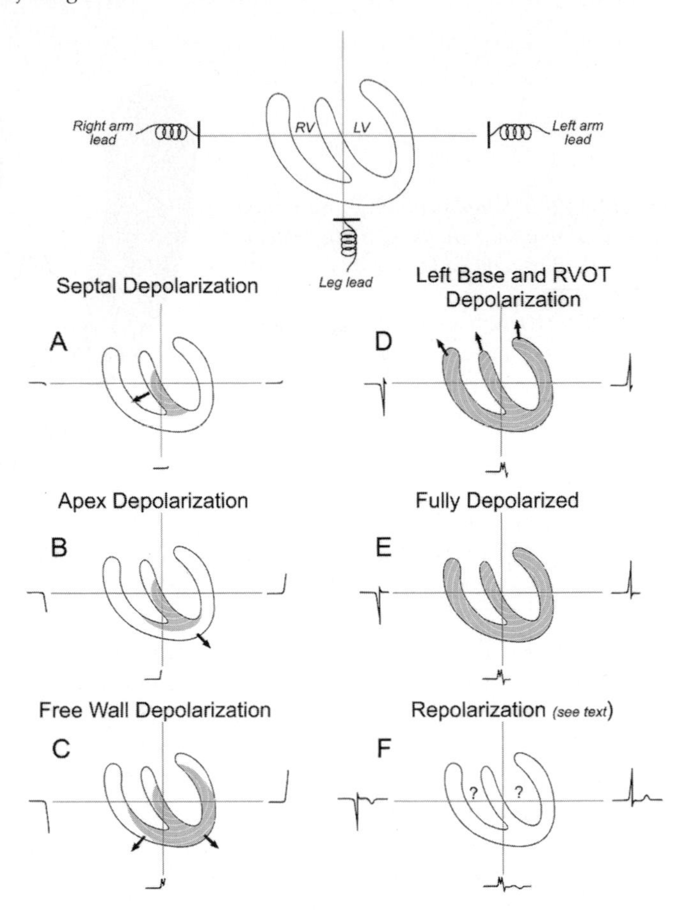

FIGURE 12–12 *Genesis of the QRS. Ventricular repolarization is a more complex process than atrial repolarization (see text).* ***A–E****, Segmental spread of ventricular depolarization generating the QRS.* ***F****, Repolarization (T wave).*
From Fyler DC. Nadas' Pediatric Cardiology. Philadelphia: Hanley & Belfus, 1992.

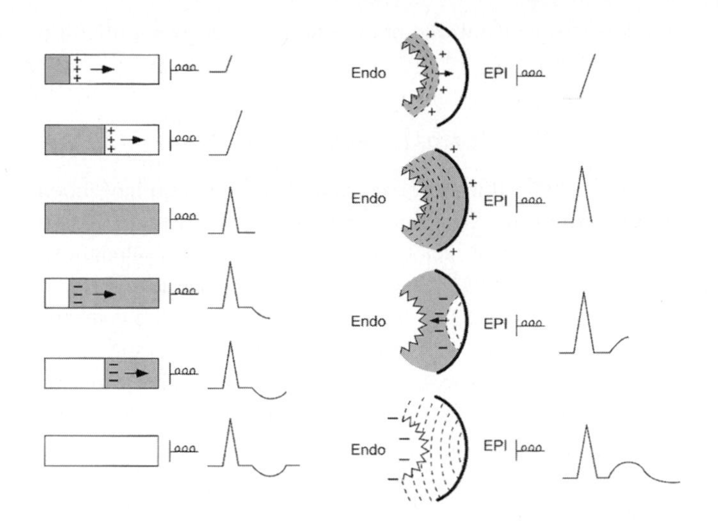

FIGURE 12–13 *Comparison of depolarization and repolarization along a hypothetical strip of ventricular muscle (where the T wave is inverted) and the proposed sequence of repolarization for the intact heart (which generates a T wave with the same polarity as the QRS). ENDO, endocardium; EPI, epicardium.*
From Fyler DC. Nadas' Pediatric Cardiology. Philadelphia: Hanley & Belfus, 1992.

epicardial to endocardial direction. For this reason, the direction of the T wave is similar to that of the QRS, and not reversed as in the case of atrial tissue or simple experimented models of isolated cardiac muscle fibers (Fig. 12-13).

The basic principles of cardiac excitation and recording are summarized in Figure 12-14. The interested reader is referred to several comprehensive reviews[3–8] for further details of these topics.

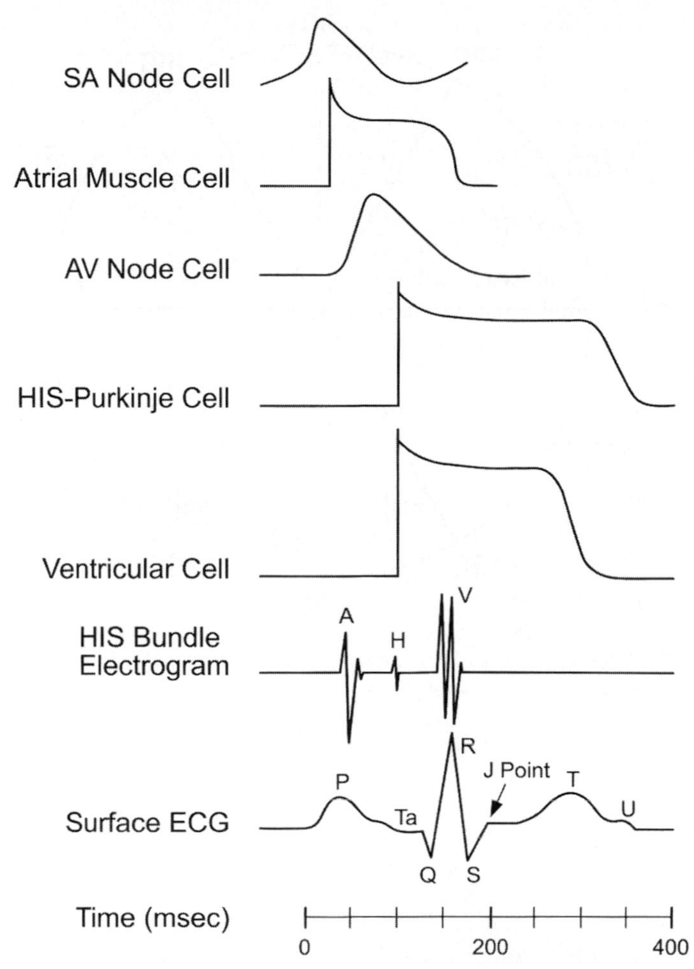

FIGURE 12–14 *Comparative time course of cellular action potentials, intracardiac electrograms from the bundle of His, and the surface ECG.*
From Fyler DC. Nadas' Pediatric Cardiology. Philadelphia: Hanley & Belfus, 1992.

THE ELECTROCARDIOGRAM

Lead Systems and Technique

The standard ECG evolved from a three-lead system introduced by Einthoven to a 15-lead tracing in current use for pediatric recording. The two major lead groupings include the limb leads and the precordial leads. The limb leads can be further divided into Einthoven's standard bipolar system (I, II, and III), and an "augmented" variation of Wilson's unipolar lead system (aV_R, aV_L, and aV_F). Einthoven's leads record potentials between electrode pairs: left arm (positive) to right arm (negative) = lead I; left leg (positive) to right arm (negative) = lead II; and left leg (positive) to left arm (negative) = lead III. Wilson's leads record from a single limb in reference to a zero potential central terminal: right arm (positive) = aV_R; left arm (positive) = aV_L; and left leg (positive) = aV_F. A wavefront moving toward the positive terminal of one of these leads registers a positive deflection on the ECG. These leads form a compass around the frontal plane, which is divided into 360 degrees, with lead positions and degree coordinates as shown in Figure 12-15.

The precordial leads (V_{4R} through V_7) view the electrical activity in the horizontal plane. They are all unipolar (positive) and are referenced to a zero potential central terminal, but without augmentation. Electrode placement is slightly modified in pediatric studies to obtain lead positions far out on the right side of the chest and laterally on the left side of the chest (Fig. 12-16).

Routine recordings are made with a chart paper speed of 25 mm/sec and are usually standardized with an amplitude response of 1 mV/10 mm. If a patient's ventricular voltages are exceptionally large, the amplitude response should be reduced to 1 mV/5 mm or even 1 mV/2.5 mm to avoid QRS overshoot and superimposed signals. However, whenever nonstandard amplification is used for ECG display, the

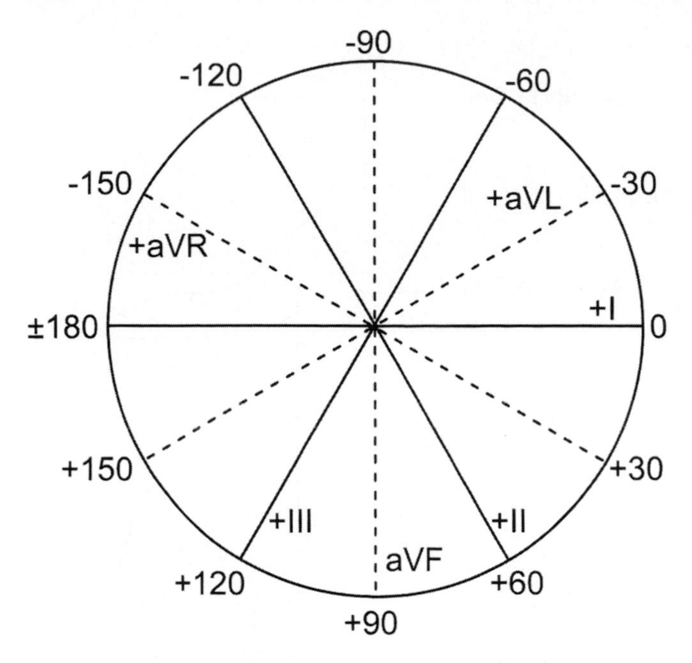

FIGURE 12–15 *Degree coordinates and positive pole of the limb ECG leads in the frontal plane.*
From Fyler DC. Nadas' Pediatric Cardiology. Philadelphia: Hanley & Belfus, 1992.

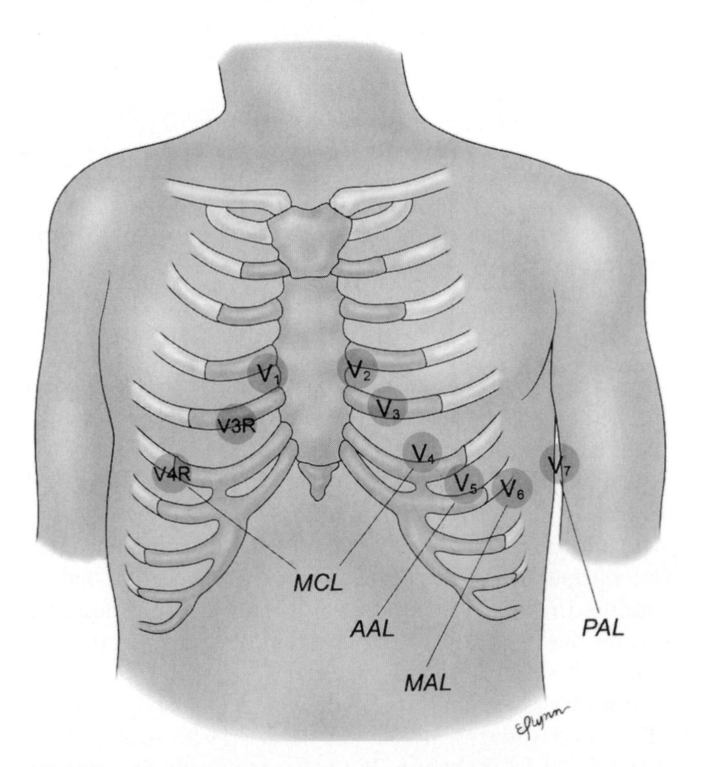

FIGURE 12–16 *Location of the precordial leads for pediatric ECG recording. MCL, midclavicular line; AAL, anterior axillary line; MAL, midaxillary line; PAL, posterior axillary line.*
From Fyler DC. Nadas' Pediatric Cardiology. Philadelphia: Hanley & Belfus, 1992.

appropriate calibration mark must be clearly highlighted on the recording.

The Normal Electrocardiogram

The normal values referred to in this discussion have been drawn from our experience at Children's Hospital Boston and the classic publications of Davignon and colleagues,[8] Garson,[9] and Fisch.[10] Data are abstracted for quick reference in Table 12-1. The ECG should be read in a systemic fashion, beginning with measurements of axes and intervals, followed by waveform analysis, all of which must be synthesized into a final impression based on history and physical examination.

Axis

The electrical axis refers to the predominant direction (or mean vector) of a waveform in the frontal plane. By identifying the limb lead with the largest positive deflection for the waveform in question, and remembering the coordinates for this lead on the frontal compass face, one can assign a value in degrees for the mean axis. The easiest example involves the P wave. Because normal atrial activation begins at the SA node and spreads through the atrium high-to-low and right-to-left, the wavefront of depolarization flows toward the southeast quadrant of the frontal plane. Lead II (+60 degrees) best records this area and usually registers the largest positive P wave. A lead from the northwest quadrant (aV_R) simultaneously registers a deep negative P wave. Leads that record at nearly right angles to the P-wave vector (aV_L and III) are equiphasic or isoelectric, with relatively low amplitude. The P-wave axis for a normal heart in sinus rhythm should be between 0 and +90 degrees regardless of the patient's age. An abnormal axis can be seen in ectopic atrial rhythms or atrial malpositions.

The mean QRS axis is calculated in a similar fashion by identifying the limb lead with the largest positive R wave and assigning the corresponding degree value. In contrast to the P-wave axis, the normal QRS axis has wide age-dependent variation. In the case of newborns, for whom the right ventricle is relatively hypertrophied by virtue of its intrauterine workload, the axis is directed rightward, usually about 120 degrees. As the left ventricle becomes relatively more dominant during the first 6 months of life, the axis gradually shifts toward +60 degrees and should remain between about 0 and +90 degrees thereafter. An abnormal QRS axis can be seen with ventricular hypertrophy, malpositions, intraventricular conduction disturbances, and infarction.

The T-wave axis is usually concordant with the QRS in the frontal plane. There may be some discrepancy in the early months of life, but by the time the child is 6 months old, the QRS and T axes should not differ by more than 60 degrees. An abnormal T-wave axis can be seen in marked

TABLE 12–1. Normal Range and Mean Value for Selected Electrocardiogram Measurements in Children*

AGE	0-7 days	1 wk–1 mo	1 mo-6 mo	6 mo-1 yr	1 yr-5 yr	5-10 yr	10-15 yr	>15 yr
Rate (beats/min)	90-160 (125)	100-175 (140)	110-180 (145)	100-180 (130)	70-160 (110)	65-140 (100)	60-130 (90)	60-100 (80)
QRS axis (degrees)	70-180 (120)	45-160 (100)	10-120 (80)	5-110 (60)	5-110 (60)	5-110 (60)	5-110 (60)	5-110 (60)
PR lead II (msec)	80-150 (100)	80-150 (100)	80-150 (100)	80-150 (100)	80-150 (120)	80-150 (120)	90-180 (140)	100-200 (160)
QRS duration (msec)	40-70 (50)	40-70 (50)	40-70 (50)	40-70 (50)	45-80 (65)	45-80 (65)	50-90 (70)	60-90 (80)
Maximum QTc† (msec)	450 max	450 max	450 max	450 max	440 max	440 max	440 max	430 max
QRS V_1 Q (mm)	0	0	0	0	0	0	0	0
R (mm)	5-25 (15)	3-22 (10)	3-20 (10)	2-20 (9)	2-18 (8)	1-15 (5)	1-12 (5)	1-6 (2)
S (mm)	0-22 (7)	0-16 (5)	0-15 (5)	1-20 (6)	1-20 (10)	3-21 (12)	3-22 (11)	3-13 (8)
QRS V_5 Q (mm)	0-1 (0.5)	0-3 (0.5)	0-3 (0.5)	0-3 (0.5)	0-5 (1)	0-5 (1)	0-3 (0.5)	0-2 (0.5)
R (mm)	2-20 (10)	3-25 (12)	5-30 (17)	10-30 (20)	10-35 (23)	13-38 (25)	10-35 (20)	7-21 (13)
S (mm)	2-19 (10)	2-16 (8)	1-16 (8)	1-14 (6)	1-13 (5)	1-11 (4)	1-10 (3)	0-5 (2)
QRS V_6 Q (mm)	0-2 (0.5)	0-2 (0.5)	0-2 (0.5)	0-3 (0.5)	0-4 (1)	0-4 (1)	0-3 (1)	0-2 (0.5)
R (mm)	1-12 (5)	1-17 (7)	3-20 (10)	5-22 (12)	6-22 (14)	8-25 (16)	8-24 (15)	5-18 (10)
S (mm)	0-9 (3)	0-9 (3)	0-9 (3)	0-7 (3)	0-6 (2)	0-4 (2)	0-4 (1)	0-2 (1)
T-wave V_1 (mm)	*0-4 days* = −3 to +4 (0) *4-7 days* = −4 to +2 (−1)	−6 to −1 (−3)	−6 to −1 (−3)	−6 to −1 (−3)	−6 to −1 (−3)	−6 to +2 (−2)	−4 to +3 (−1)	−2 to +2 (+1)

Adapted from references 8-10.

*Values reported as 2nd-98th percentile (mean), except for QTC (maximum value only) and >15 yr data, which report ± 1 SD.

†QTc as corrected by Bazett's formula (QTc = QT ÷ square root RR).

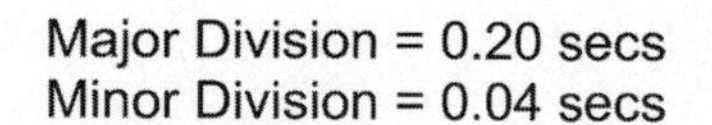

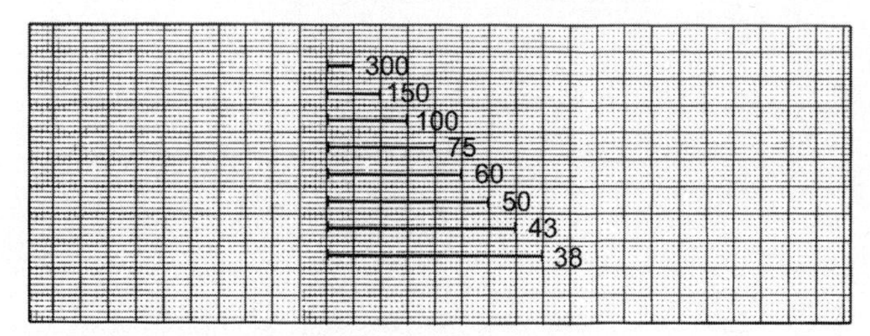

FIGURE 12–17 *At chart paper speed of 25 mm/sec, each major division = 0.20 sec, and each minor division = 0.04 sec. Heart rate in beats per minute can be determined from the number of large divisions between the QRS complexes.*
From Fyler DC. Nadas' Pediatric Cardiology. Philadelphia: Hanley & Belfus, 1992.

hypertrophy with ventricular strain, ischemia, myopathy, and some intraventricular conduction disturbances.

Rhythm and Rate

Cardiac excitation arising from the SA node generates a P wave with a normal axis at a rate within the limits for age (see Table 12-1). Rate determination is usually a straightforward exercise (Fig. 12-17). *Respirophasic sinus arrhythmia* is a normal finding in healthy children, as is the observation of a *shifting atrial pacemaker*, where a subsidiary P wave with a different axis than sinus rhythm takes over during episodic slowing of the SA node.

P Wave

The contour and amplitude of the P wave are an indirect measure of atrial size. The normal P wave should have a smooth dome shape in lead II and should never be taller than 0.3 mV or wider than 0.12 second in duration. Occasionally, there may be a small notch in the P wave of lead II, but this is acceptable if amplitude and duration fall within the normal range.

T_A Wave

The shallow wave of atrial repolarization is rarely seen on the normal ECG because of its low amplitude and superimposition of the QRS complex. It may be seen occasionally in patients with heart block when the QRS is delayed or dissociated. The normal T_A wave is directed opposite from the P wave and is usually less than 0.1 mV in depth. Atrial enlargement or inflammation distorts the T_A wave.

PR Interval

The PR interval is measured from the beginning of the P wave to the initial deflection of ventricular activation (it is more precisely a PQ interval). As noted earlier, the PR includes several electrical events, with AV node conduction accounting for the major portion. The normal PR interval is less than 0.16 second in young children or 0.18 second in adolescents and adults. A prolonged PR interval can be due to enhanced vagal tone, cardiac medications (digoxin and antiarrhythmic agents), or disease involving either the AV node or the His-Purkinje system. A short PR interval (less than 0.08 second) may be observed in Wolff-Parkinson-White syndrome.

QRS Complex

Registration of the QRS begins when cardiac excitation leaves the His-Purkinje system and the ventricular myocytes begin to depolarize. The QRS complex is evaluated for its morphology, amplitude, and duration.

QRS morphology is dictated by the sequence of regional ventricular activation, and the balance (right versus left) of ventricular muscle mass, as previously discussed. The normal heart leaves a characteristic QRS shape in each lead of the ECG, which may change because of distorted activation sequence or hypertrophy. Beyond infancy, the normal pattern is one of a small Q wave, followed by a large R and a small S wave in left-sided leads (I, II, or aV_L, V_3–V_6), whereas right-sided leads (aV_R, III, V_{4R}–V_2) typically register a small R followed by a deep S wave.

QRS amplitude is a more quantitative measure of ventricular mass and compliments QRS morphology when evaluating a trace for hypertrophy. Normal values are established for R-wave amplitude, as well as for Q- and S-wave amplitudes, in each individual lead. Measurements in the precordial leads are particularly sensitive indicators of an abnormality. Normal amplitude values vary widely with patient age, and tables of normal data should be on hand during review of all pediatric ECGs.

The duration of the QRS complex is related to the speed of conduction within the His-Purkinje system, as well as from myocyte to myocyte within the ventricles. Duration increases slightly with age. In normal infants, the QRS width should be less than 0.08 second, and in those older than 6 months, less than 0.10 second. Prolongation of the QRS may be seen with block of His-Purkinje conduction (bundle branch block), slow myocyte conduction (due to muscle injury, drugs, or electrolyte disturbances), severe ventricular hypertrophy, and some cases of preexcitation.

ST Segment

Ventricular muscle cells are in the plateau phase of their action potential (phase 2) during the ST segment. Because no electrical wavefronts are advancing or retreating through the heart, the body surface recording is normally isoelectric. The *J point* at the termination of the S wave marks the beginning of the ST segment and should not deviate more than about 1 mm from the baseline.

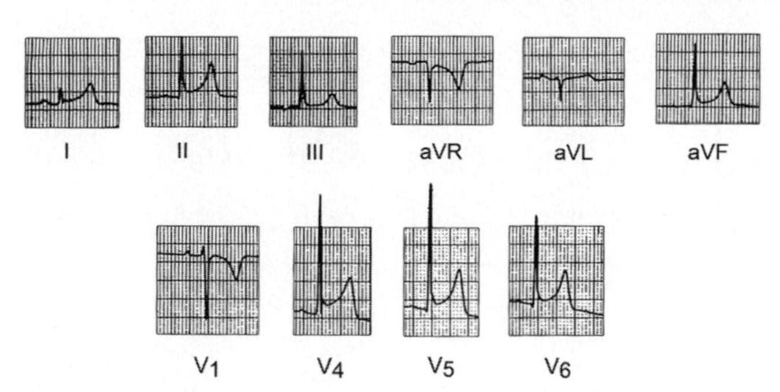

FIGURE 12–18 *A dramatic example of early repolarization in a healthy athletic 15-year-old boy.*
From Fyler DC. Nadas' Pediatric Cardiology. Philadelphia: Hanley & Belfus, 1992.

Deviations in ST level may be caused by ischemia, inflammation, severe hypertrophy, and some medications. One normal variant is the *early repolarization* pattern, seen occasionally in healthy adolescent patients, where the J point can be elevated 2 to 4 mm. Usually, this elevation is observed in the lateral (V_4–V_6) and inferior (II, III, aV_F) leads and is accompanied by strikingly tall T waves in the same leads (Fig. 12-18). The diagnosis of benign early repolarization should not be made if the elevation is more than 4 mm or the T wave is of low amplitude.

T Wave

The T wave corresponds to phase 3 repolarization of ventricular myocytes. The normal T-wave amplitude is variable and is not routinely quantitated. On the other hand, the direction of the T wave deserves careful attention. As mentioned, the T-wave axis should follow the same net direction as the QRS in the frontal plane within about 60 degrees, and discordance of the axis in the limb leads may suggest pathology. The precordial leads follow somewhat different rules for T-wave direction. Over the left chest, the T wave is still normally concordant with the QRS, but there are important age-dependent variations in the rightward leads. From birth to 4 to 7 days of age, the T wave is upright in all precordial leads. After this, the T wave becomes negative over the right chest (V_{4R}–V_1), while remaining positive in the left chest leads. This pattern persists until adolescence, when the T waves tend to resume an upright direction in all chest leads. This sequence is critical to remember during analysis of ECGs in children because an upright T wave in the right precordial leads between the age of 7 days and early adolescence is a potential indicator of right ventricular hypertrophy.

QT Interval

The QT interval is a reflection of the total action potential duration for ventricular myocytes. It is measured from the onset of the QRS to the point of T-wave termination. Because the normal QT interval varies with heart rate (longer at slow rates, shorter at fast rates), the measurement is adjusted with the formula: QT (seconds)/square root R-R (seconds). This rate-corrected interval (QT_c) should be less than 0.45 second in infants, 0.44 second in children, and 0.43 second in adults. A prolonged QT_c interval can be of dramatic clinical significance. The hereditary *long QT syndromes* are potentially fatal disorders, and early detection on an ECG is imperative. The QT_c is also prolonged by many antiarrhythmic drugs and by some electrolyte imbalances.

U Wave

The U wave is thought to reflect the relatively late repolarization process of His-Purkinje cells and certain left ventricular myocytes. It is not always seen on the ECG of normal patients. When present, a normal U wave is of low amplitude (less than one fourth the height of the T wave) and has the same polarity as its T wave. When the U wave is abnormally prominent (more than half the height of the T wave), it should be included in the measurement of the QT interval. Occasionally, the amplitude of the U wave may become accentuated secondary to hypokalemia, antiarrhythmic drugs, and some forms of long QT syndrome.

The Abnormal Electrocardiogram

The ECG should never be interpreted in isolation, and there should always be specific questions to answer when the test is ordered regarding rhythm, hypertrophy, myocardial injury, and so forth. Additionally, one should constantly bear in mind that a child can have serious heart disease with a normal-appearing ECG, particularly in the first few days of life.

Rate and Rhythm

Cardiac rhythm should be the first item scrutinized on the ECG tracing. If the rhythm is abnormal, many of the assumptions regarding hypertrophy, malpositions, ischemia, and so forth will become invalid. To evaluate these issues accurately, the ECG needs to be repeated after sinus rhythm is restored. A detailed discussion of cardiac arrhythmias is presented in Chapter 29.

Cardiac Malpositions

Chamber orientation is reflected on the ECG by the axis and the morphology of the P wave and the QRS complex. Atrial situs is determined with considerable accuracy by deciding which side of the atrium contains the SA node. In situs solitus, the SA node activates high in the right atrium, and the resultant atrial depolarization wavefront generates a P-wave axis of about +60 degrees, whereas in situs inversus, the activation emanates from high in the left-sided atrium,

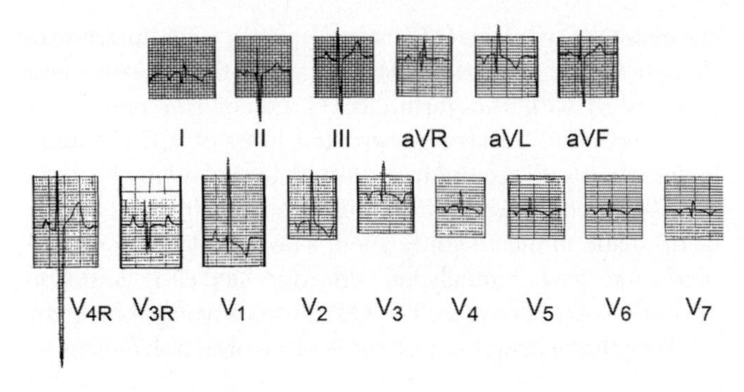

FIGURE 12–19 *ECG from a 6-year-old patient with documented situs inversus and a P-wave axis of +150 degrees. Dextrocardia is also present.*
From Fyler DC. Nadas' Pediatric Cardiology. Philadelphia: Hanley & Belfus, 1992

so that the P axis is about +120 degrees (Fig. 12-19). Variable patterns may be seen in the heterotaxy syndromes. For example, patients with asplenia may have bilateral SA nodes, and the P-wave axis may alternate or fuse between +60 and +120 degrees. In polysplenia, there may not be a true SA node, and such patients usually rely on a subsidiary atrial pacemaker focus that can have a variable location.

Gross ventricular orientation is best estimated from the precordial leads. Normal levocardia has a characteristic pattern of relatively low (or predominately negative) voltage in the right chest leads (V_{4R}–V_2) with positive forces of higher amplitude in the mid and left chest leads. In *dextrocardia* (Figs. 12-19 and 12-20), the pattern is classically reversed. Further insight into ventricular anatomy may be gained by determining the embryologic ventricular looping. The normal *D-loop* orientation has an anatomic right ventricle and tricuspid valve located on the right side of the heart. In an *L-loop* anomaly, the ventricular relationship is inverted; hence, the septal activation wavefront must travel right-to-left. This changes the QRS morphology to one of initial Q waves in right-sided limb or precordial leads, with small initial R waves on the left side (see Fig. 12-20).

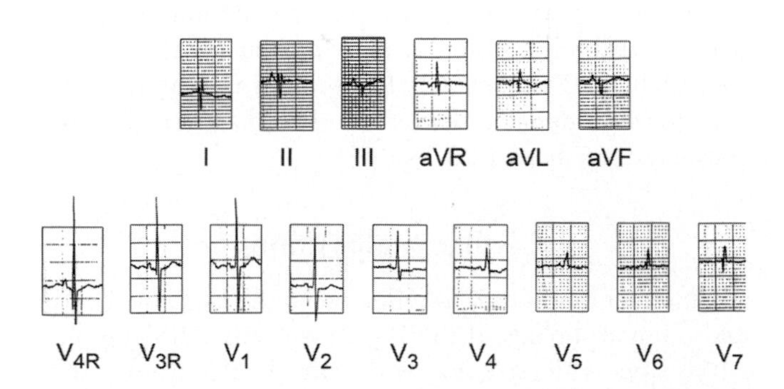

FIGURE 12–20 *ECG from a patient with L-looped ventricles (note the RSR pattern in V_4–V_7 and the QRS pattern in V_{4R} and V_{3R}) and dextrocardia (note prominent voltage in the right chest leads).*
From Fyler DC. Nadas' Pediatric Cardiology. Philadelphia: Hanley & Belfus, 1992.

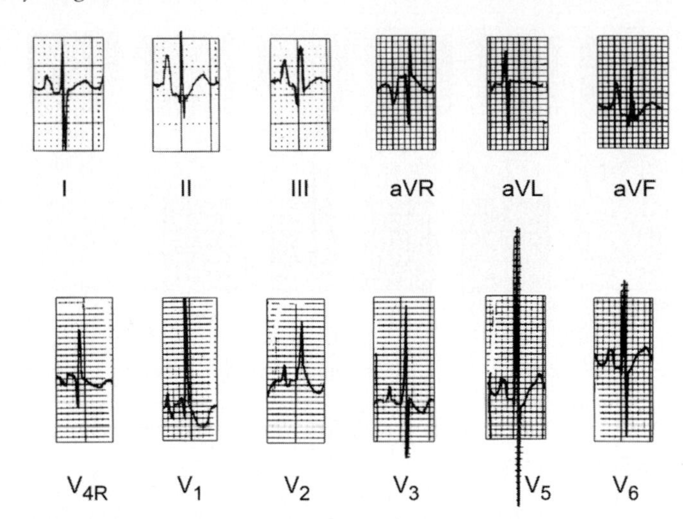

FIGURE 12–21 *ECG showing right atrial enlargement.*
From Fyler DC. Nadas' Pediatric Cardiology. Philadelphia: Hanley & Belfus, 1992.

Atrial Enlargement

The surface ECG is a fair indicator of atrial enlargement. Because the right atrium is the first to depolarize, indicators of right-sided enlargement are found in the early portions of the P wave. The diagnostic criterion for isolated *right atrial enlargement* is the presence in lead II of a peaked narrow P wave greater than 0.30 mV in amplitude, accompanied by either a tall P wave or a biphasic P wave with an early deep negative deflection in lead V_1 (Fig. 12-21). *Left atrial enlargement* is reflected in the terminal portion of the P wave. The classic findings include a broad, notched P wave in lead II (duration greater than 0.10 to 0.12 second) or a deep slurred terminal portion of a biphasic P wave in V_1 (Fig. 12-22). A combination of the above amplitude and duration criteria is indicative of *biatrial enlargement* (Fig. 12-23).

Ventricular Hypertrophy

Identification of ventricular hypertrophy from the surface ECG is far from a perfect science. Although criteria are generally accurate for right ventricular hypertrophy (RVH), the diagnosis of left ventricular hypertrophy (LVH) is sometimes difficult until the process is far advanced.

Right Ventricular Hypertrophy

Screening for RVH is particularly important in children because the more common congenital defects impose an

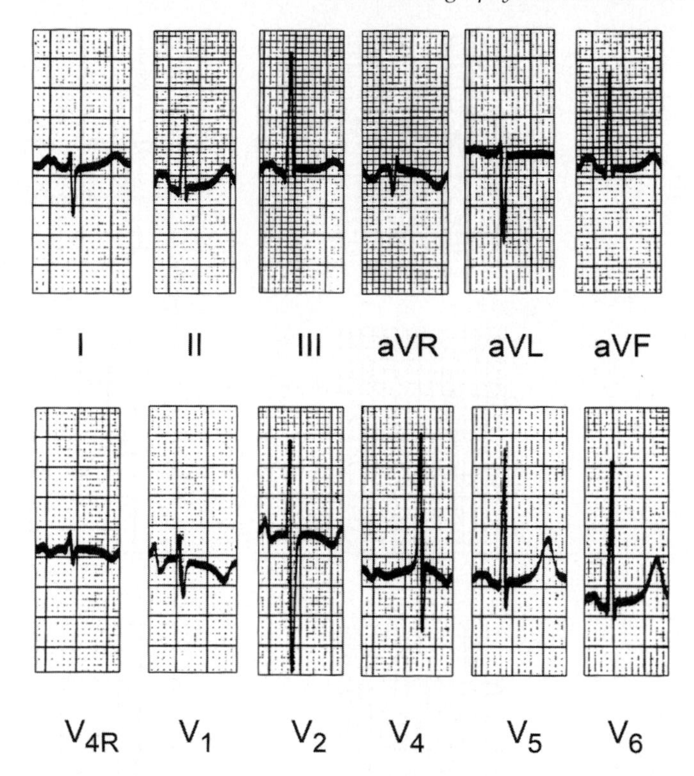

FIGURE 12–22 *ECG showing left atrial enlargement.*
From Fyler DC. Nadas' Pediatric Cardiology. Philadelphia: Hanley & Belfus, 1992.

increased work load on this chamber. Fortunately, the criteria that have evolved are fairly sensitive.

R-Wave Amplitude in V_1 Higher than the 98th Percentile for Age. This finding is very specific outside the newborn period. The height of the R wave in this lead correlates well with right ventricular systolic pressure and is sufficiently quantitative to allow prediction of right ventricular pressure for isolated pulmonary valve stenosis using the formula: R-wave height (in millimeters) × 5 = peak systolic pressure (mm Hg).

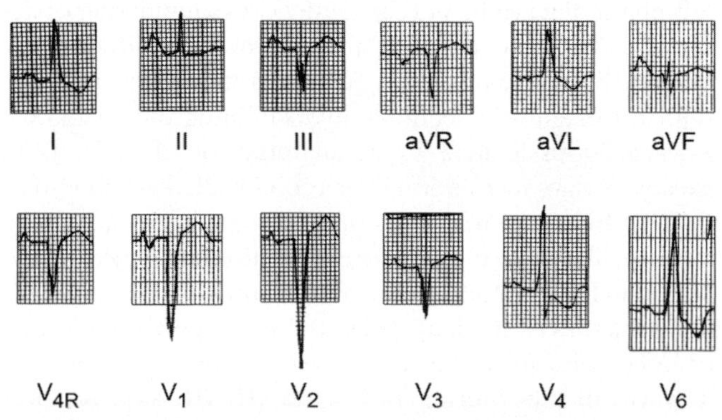

FIGURE 12–23 *ECG showing biatrial enlargement.*
From Fyler DC. Nadas' Pediatric Cardiology. Philadelphia: Hanley & Belfus, 1992.

Abnormal T-Wave Direction in V1. As previously mentioned, the T-wave direction in lead V_1 changes with time: it is upright in newborns, negative beyond the age of 7 days, and positive again in adolescents and adults. A persistently upright T wave after the seventh day of life is a sensitive indicator of elevated right ventricular pressure, and when combined with R-wave amplitude, even greater precision is possible. Mild degrees of RVH may show a normal R-wave amplitude but an upright T wave in V_1. Moderate RVH is characterized by abnormal height of the R wave in conjunction with the upright T wave. In marked RVH, the R wave remains excessive, but the T wave may now be deeply inverted in what is referred to as a *strain* pattern (Fig. 12-24).

S-Wave Depth in V_6 Lower than the 98(th) Percentile for Age. This measurement is useful in patients with increased right ventricular pressure secondary to chronic lung disease. Respiratory disorders such as cystic fibrosis can lower the voltage pattern recorded from the right chest because of heart rotation and hyperexpansion of the lungs. Despite low anterior forces, RVH can still be diagnosed when the lateral S wave is deep. This pattern of RVH, when associated with right atrial enlargement in a

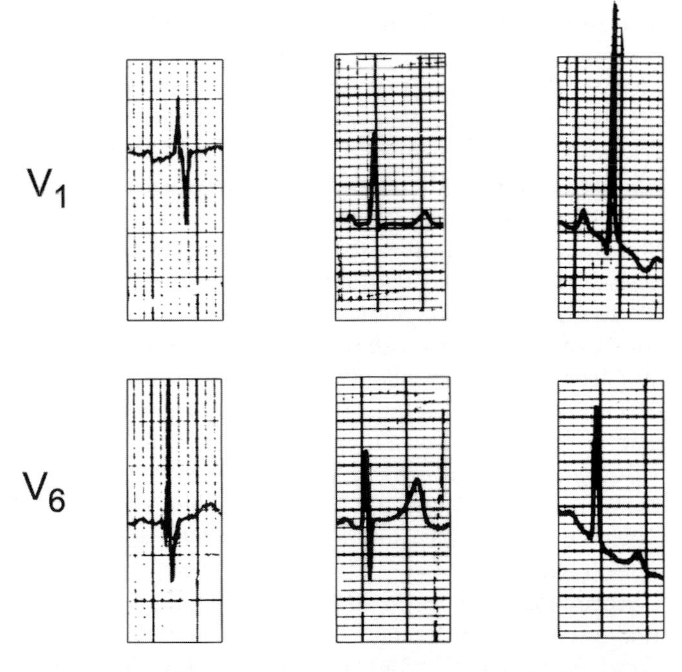

FIGURE 12–24 *ECG patterns with varying degrees of right ventricular pressure load hypertrophy.* ***A****, Mild RVH in a 9-month-old suggested by an upright T wave in V_1, but without excess R-wave voltage.* ***B****, Moderate RVH in a 4-year-old with an upright T wave and excess R-wave voltage in V_1.* ***C****, Marked RVH in a 7-year-old showing a very tall R wave with an inverted T wave ("strain" pattern) in V_1.*
From Fyler DC. Nadas' Pediatric Cardiology. Philadelphia: Hanley & Belfus, 1992.

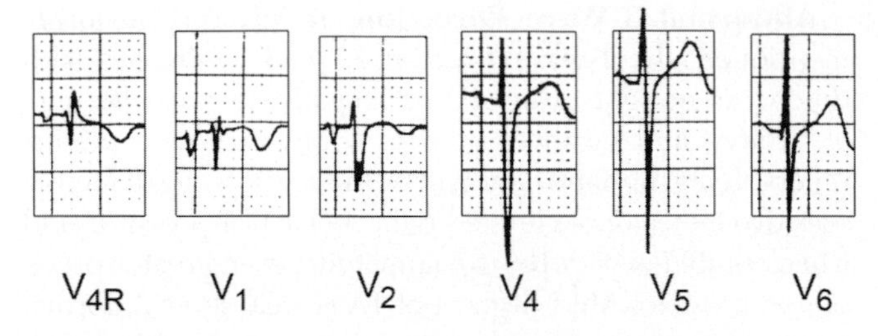

FIGURE 12–25 *The pattern of RVH seen in chronic lung disease (cystic fibrosis in this case), characterized by deep, lateral S waves and by normal voltages in the right chest.*
From Fyler DC. Nadas' Pediatric Cardiology. Philadelphia: Hanley & Belfus, 1992.

patient with severe pulmonary disease, is characteristic of *cor pulmonale* (Fig. 12-25).

Right Axis Deviation. Isolated right axis deviation is not specific for RVH and may be observed in conduction disturbances such as left posterior hemiblock. When present in conjunction with other RVH criteria, it lends additional support for the diagnosis.

QR Pattern in V_1. This criterion is likewise not absolute for RVH but is supportive evidence when associated with a tall R wave in the right chest leads. A QR pattern may also be seen with L-loop ventricles and anterior infarction.

RSR′ Pattern in V_1. It is important to understand the significance and limitations of this finding in children. Increased right ventricular volume loads imposed by common lesions such as an atrial septal defect may create a pattern of V_1 of a small initial R wave, followed by an S wave, terminating with a tall R′ wave (Fig. 12-26). A diagnosis of RVH should be made only when the secondary R′ wave is large in amplitude. Some normal children may have a similar pattern with a lower-amplitude R′ wave. It is also useful to examine the distribution of the RSR′ pattern in multiple precordial leads because large right ventricular volume loads may cause the RSR′ pattern to extend from V_{4R} all the way across V_3 or V_4, whereas the pattern does not usually extend beyond V_1 in normal children. An RSR′ pattern may also be caused by incomplete right bundle branch block.

Abnormal R/S Ratio in V_1 or V_6. Normal values for R/S ratios are well established, and these data can be drawn on when the decision regarding RVH is questionable. However, it is rare to see abnormal ratios as an isolated finding, and one should hesitate to make a firm diagnosis of RVH on the basis of this criterion alone.

Left Ventricular Hypertrophy

It is difficult to predict LVH with certainty from the ECG. The diagnosis is best entertained when multiple criteria are fulfilled.

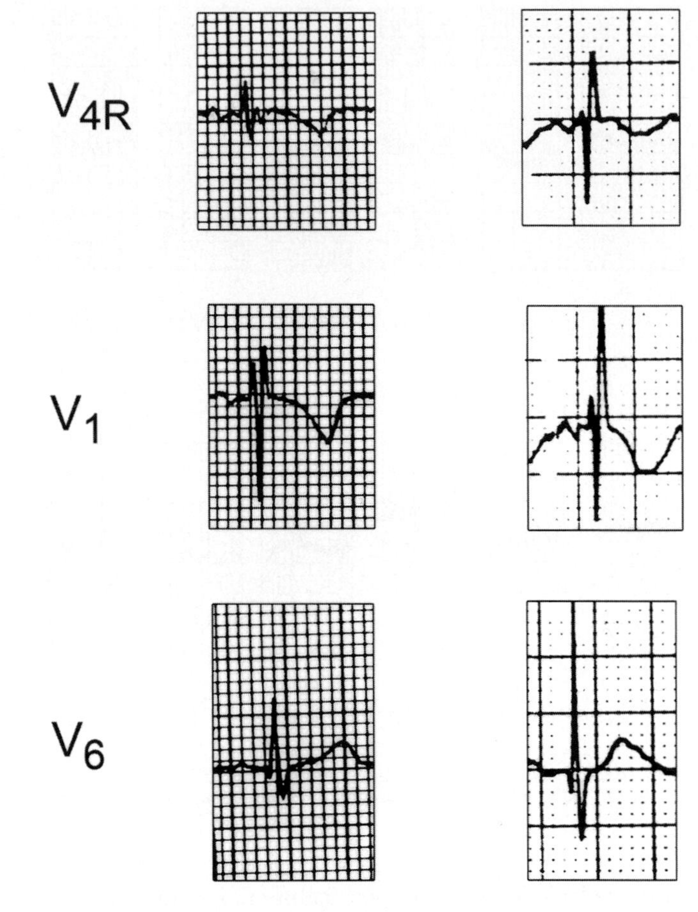

FIGURE 12–26 *The RSR′ pattern in lead V_1:* ***A****, Normal patient without heart disease.* ***B****, Patient with increased RV volume load due to large atrial septal defect. Note the taller R′ wave in the abnormal trace.*
From Fyler DC. Nadas' Pediatric Cardiology. Philadelphia: Hanley & Belfus, 1992.

R-Wave Amplitude in V_5–V_6 Greater than the 98th Percentile for Age. The voltage criteria for LVH are not very exact. Hypertrophy may be present with normal left precordial forces, and in some normal children (particularly athletic teenagers), the R-wave amplitude may exceed the 98th percentile. Attempts have been made to improve diagnostic accuracy by examining the reciprocal S-wave depth in lead V_1 as an indicator of LVH using isolated S-wave measurement or a combination of S in V_1 plus R in V_6, but there remain limitations to voltage data alone.

Lateral T-Wave Inversion (Strain Pattern). In the Natural History Study of congenital aortic stenosis, T-wave abnormalities were identified as the most specific indicators of LVH. Left ventricular strain presents a pattern of inverted T waves in the inferior limb leads (II, III, aV_F) and left precordial leads (V_5 and V_6), sometimes associated with depression of the ST segment. There may or may not be voltage indications of LVH (Fig. 12-27). Although the

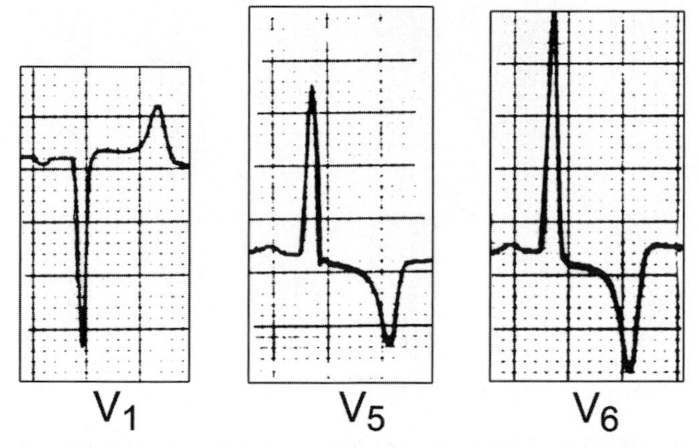

FIGURE 12–27 *LVH with "strain" pattern in a patient with aortic stenosis. The T-wave inversion is dramatic even though the R-wave voltage does not exceed normal limits.*
From Fyler DC. Nadas' Pediatric Cardiology. Philadelphia: Hanley & Belfus, 1992.

presence of these T-wave changes usually suggests advanced degrees of hypertrophy, the presence of ischemia or myocardial inflammation must bc cxcluded before this criterion can be applied with certainty.

Left Avis Deviation. An abnormal leftward axis is supportive evidence for LVH. The utility of this criterion is best appreciated in the neonate, in whom the QRS axis is normally directed rightward. The presence of a *mature* axis in the 0 to +90 degree range or a *superior* axis in the 0 to –90 degree range in early infancy suggests a definite cardiac abnormality. Left axis deviation may also be due to conduction disturbances such as left anterior hemiblock.

Abnormal Lateral Q Wave. The Q wave in leads V_5 and V_6 (septal depolarization) may be distorted if the left ventricle is very dilated or markedly thick. There can be deviation and rotation of septal position, and increased competition from vectors of left apex and left free-wall depolarization. As a broad generalization, a dilated volume-loaded left ventricle tends to have an abnormally deep Q wave in the leftward leads in lesions such as aortic regurgitation, patent ductus, or ventricular septal defect (Fig. 12-28). Concentric hypertrophy from a pressure load such as aortic stenosis is more likely to be associated with a small or absent Q wave (Fig. 12-29).

Single Ventricle Hypertrophy

There are no firm criteria to apply for hypertrophy of a single ventricle in complex congenital anomalies. What is

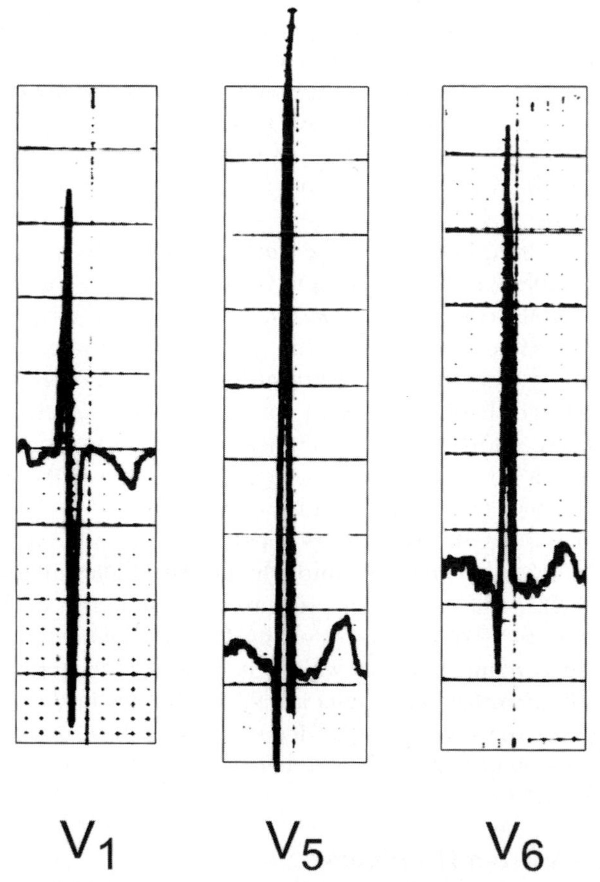

FIGURE 12–28 *The typical ECG pattern for LVH due to a large volume load, with deep Q waves in V_5 and V_6 in an infant with a large ventricular septal defect.*
From Fyler DC. Nadas' Pediatric Cardiology. Philadelphia: Hanley & Belfus, 1992.

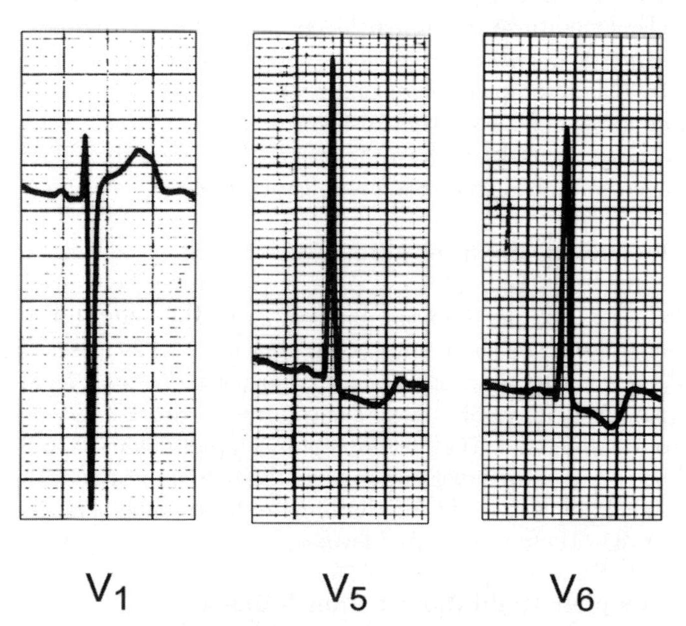

FIGURE 12–29 *The typical ECG pattern for LVH due to increased pressure load in a patient with aortic stenosis, showing minimal Q waves in V_5 and V_6.*
From Fyler DC. Nadas' Pediatric Cardiology. Philadelphia: Hanley & Belfus, 1992.

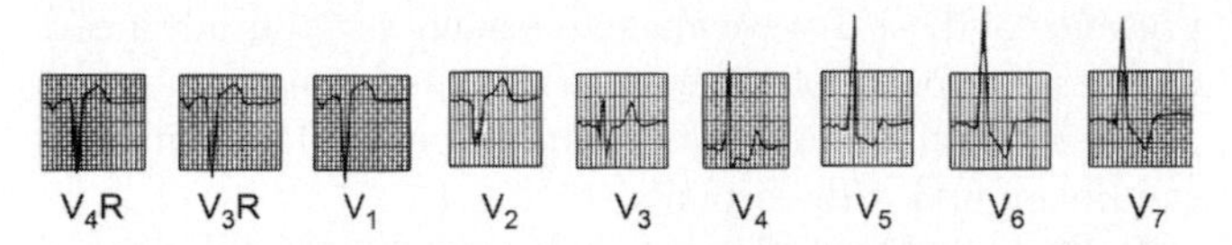

FIGURE 12–30 *Absent RV forces (no R wave in right precordial leads) in a patient with tricuspid atresia.*
From Fyler DC. Nadas' Pediatric Cardiology. Philadelphia: Hanley & Belfus, 1992.

most surprising is that an ECG in such conditions can look deceptively normal at times, at least for the newborn. However, voltage criteria for single ventricles generally exceed those for either RVH or LVH in some precordial lead as the children age. The exact QRS morphology is variable, depending on the presence and location of the ventricular septum, which anatomic ventricle is indeed present, and the rotation of the abnormal heart in the thorax. One may be able to predict which ventricle is absent by noting which side of the precordium has deficient positive voltage (Fig. 12-30). Absent ventricle (or hypoplastic ventricle) may also be suspected if a septal Q wave is not seen in any precordial lead.

Intraventricular Conduction Abnormalities

From the common bundle of His, intraventricular conduction fibers divide into the right and left bundle branches. The left bundle actually fans out along the entire left ventricular septal surface, but may be considered to split into two major divisions: the left anterior and left posterior fascicles. Partial or complete block at any one of these sites creates delay in regional ventricular activation and a characteristic change in QRS pattern. Likewise, the presence of an accessory conduction pathway distorts regional activation.

Incomplete Right Bundle Branch Block

An RSR′ pattern in the right precordial leads with normal QRS duration may indicate an incomplete conduction disturbance in the right ventricle. However, an identical pattern may be seen in healthy normal individuals or in patients with right ventricular volume overload, as previously discussed. The diagnosis of incomplete block should be reserved for situations in which RSR′ is associated with a slightly prolonged QRS duration in the absence of a left-to-right shunt at the atrial level.

Complete Right Bundle Branch Block

When transmission is interrupted along the right bundle branch, the septum and left ventricle can activate normally, but the right ventricle must depend on slower cell-to-cell activation spreading left to right. The resultant QRS complex has prolonged duration (greater than 0.10 second for infants, greater than 0.12 second for older patients) and

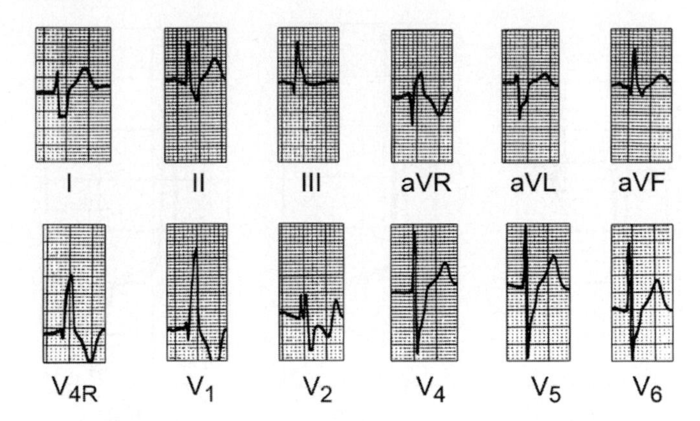

FIGURE 12–31 *ECG pattern of complete right bundle branch block.*
From Fyler DC. Nadas' Pediatric Cardiology. Philadelphia: Hanley & Belfus, 1992.

a characteristic morphology that reflects the late, slow activation wavefront spreading toward the right heart. The initial portion of the QRS is generated by the usual septal and initial left ventricular depolarization and thus is quite similar to normal (small R wave in V_1, QR in V_6). The subsequent slow wavefront traveling toward the right heart inscribes a tall slurred R′ wave in V_1 and an equally sluggish S wave in V_6 (Fig. 12-31). A pattern of complete right bundle branch block is a frequent observation after surgical repair of ventricular septal defects and tetralogy of Fallot. Of interest, the classic electrocardiographic picture of complete right bundle branch block can be seen with interruption of either the *peripheral* portions of the right His-Purkinje network or central right bundle branch itself. Although the surface electrocardiographic patterns are indistinguishable, by using an intracardiac electrode catheter, normal conduction times to the right ventricular apex can be measured in the former condition, whereas apex activation is delayed with a central injury.

The ability to diagnose ventricular hypertrophy on the ECG is lost in complete bundle branch block. Attempts to correlate right ventricular pressure with the height of the R′ wave in V_1, or with the extent of RSR′ distribution across the precordium, have met with limited success. Additionally, bundle branch block results in diffuse changes in the S-T segment, the T wave, and QT interval, so that the usual electrocardiographic markers of ischemia, strain, and prolonged QTc are lost.

Left Anterior Hemiblock

Conduction block in the left anterior fascicle produces a shift in QRS axis to the range of −60 degrees, without prolongation of QRS duration. Whereas the anterior-superior and posterior-inferior portions of the normal left ventricle are usually depolarized simultaneously by their respective fascicles, block in the anterior limb changes the sequence.

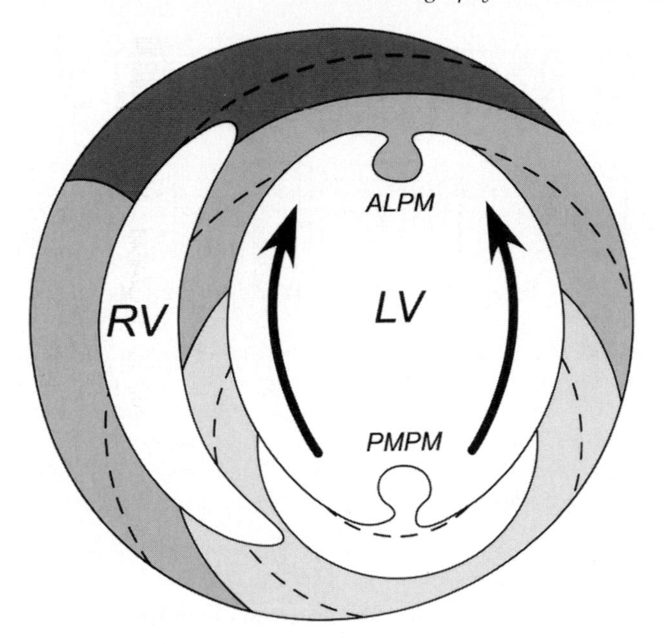

FIGURE 12–32 *Axis shift in left anterior hemiblock. Depolarization of the LV spreads from inferior to superior, generating a superior axis. ALPM, anterolateral papillary muscle; PMPM, posteromedial papillary muscle.*
From Fyler DC. Nadas' Pediatric Cardiology. Philadelphia: Hanley & Belfus, 1992.

The inferior regions activate normally, but the depolarization wavefront must then spread upward, producing a superiorly directed vector in the frontal plane (Fig. 12-32). Isolated block in the anterior fascicle is rare in children but may occur with myocardial inflammation, ischemia, and surgical or catheter trauma.

Certain congenital cardiac anomalies, notably endocardial cushion defects and tricuspid atresia, have electrocardiographic patterns with a leftward *superior QRS axis* that mimic left anterior hemiblock. The abnormal axis is not due to true conduction defects in these cases, but instead results from the abnormal anatomic location of the conduction fibers in cushion defects (Fig. 12-33) or the unusual left ventricular shape and orientation in tricuspid atresia (Fig. 12-34).

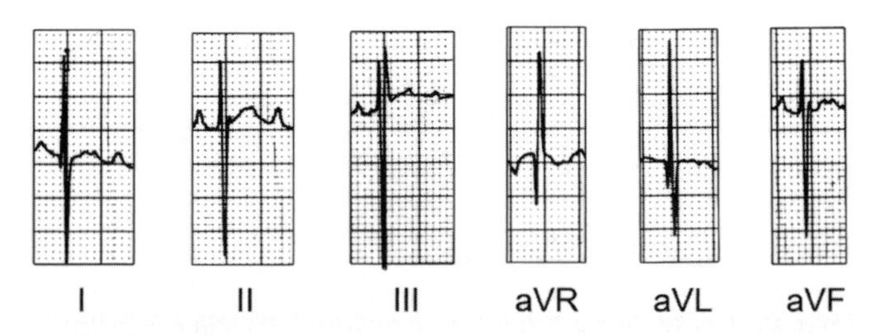

FIGURE 12–33 *Superior QRS axis (−90 degrees) in a patient with AV canal defect.*
From Fyler DC. Nadas' Pediatric Cardiology. Philadelphia: Hanley & Belfus, 1992.

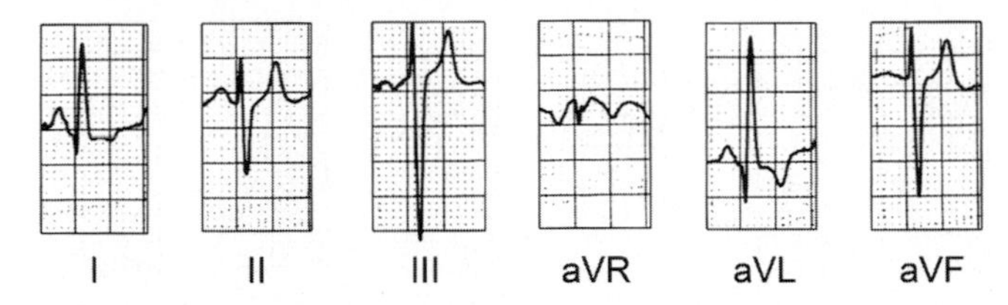

FIGURE 12–34 *Superior axis (−60 degrees) in a patient with tricuspid atresia.*
From Fyler DC. Nadas' Pediatric Cardiology. Philadelphia: Hanley & Belfus, 1992.

Left Posterior Hemiblock

The QRS duration remains normal, but the axis is shifted right and inferior to about +120 degrees when the posterior fascicle is interrupted. The activation pattern in the left ventricle is just the reverse of anterior hemiblock (Fig. 12-35). Because right axis deviation is seen commonly in infants and children with right ventricular hypertrophy, the label of posterior hemiblock should be reserved for instances when an abrupt and dramatic axis shift has occurred between serial ECGs.

Complete Left Bundle Branch Block

When the main left bundle branch is interrupted, ventricular activation begins solely through the right bundle. The septum must now depolarize right to left, and the left ventricle must rely on late transmission of the activation wavefront, which is directed leftward and posterior.

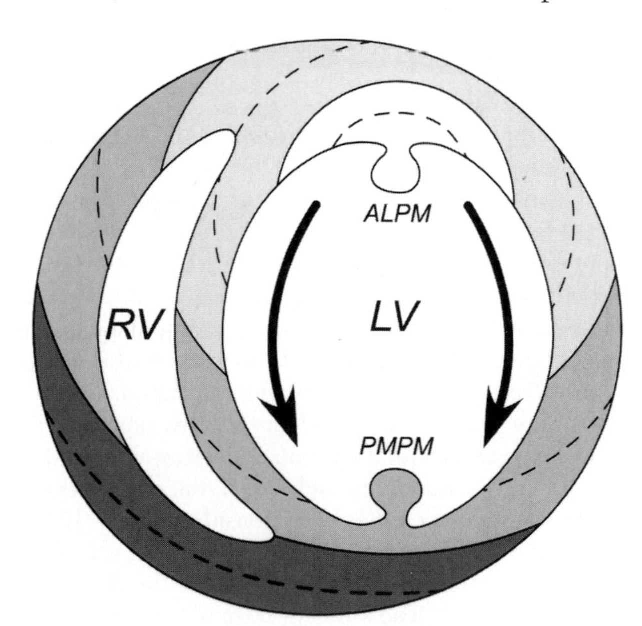

FIGURE 12–35 *Axis shift in left posterior hemiblock. Depolarization of the LV spreads from superior to inferior. ALPM, anterolateral papillary muscle; PMPM, posteromedial papillary muscle.*
From Fyler DC. Nadas' Pediatric Cardiology. Philadelphia: Hanley & Belfus, 1992.

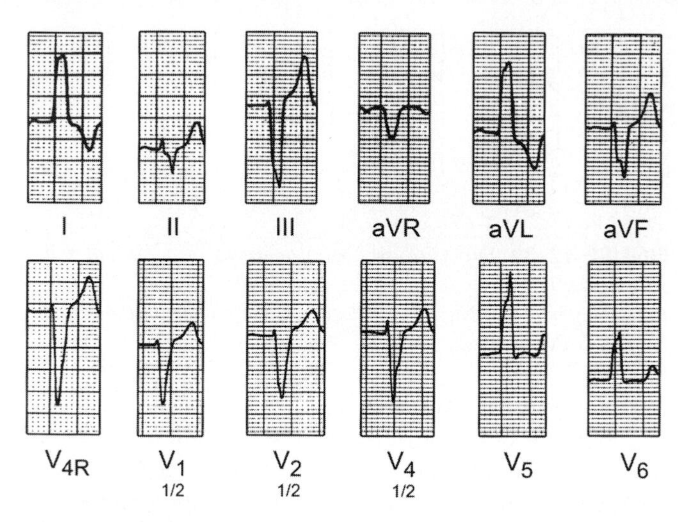

FIGURE 12–36 *ECG pattern of complete left bundle branch block. From Fyler DC. Nadas' Pediatric Cardiology. Philadelphia: Hanley & Belfus, 1992.*

The QRS is prolonged, slurred, and directed away from the right chest leads (mostly negative in V_1) and toward the lateral precordial leads (positive in V_5–V_7) (Fig. 12-36). As with complete right bundle branch block, ventricular hypertrophy, ischemic changes, and QT prolongation cannot be interpreted easily from ECGs. Very advanced degrees of concentric left ventricular hypertrophy can produce an electrocardiographic pattern identical to that of complete left bundle branch block, and the two conditions may be impossible to distinguish by ECG recordings.

Bifascicular Block

The combination of complete right bundle branch block and left anterior hemiblock may occur after surgical correction of congenital heart defects. For example, following repair of tetralogy of Fallot, bifascicular block of this type is present in 10% of patients. The electrocardiographic pattern is essentially a combination of the findings for the two individual conduction defects. Recall that in right bundle branch block, the initial portion of the QRS reflects the normal pattern of septal and left ventricular activation. If a new shift to a superior axis is detected for this early portion of the QRS in conjunction with the terminal slurring characteristic of complete right bundle branch block, the coexistence of left anterior hemiblock should be considered (Fig. 12-37).

Combined right bundle and left posterior fascicular block is less common in children and is difficult to diagnose from the ECG. The initial portion of the QRS, representing septal and left ventricular activation, is shifted rightward in this case. Because children undergoing cardiac surgery often have preexistent right axis deviation from right ventricular hypertrophy, it may be impossible to appreciate this particular conduction change in the postoperative period.

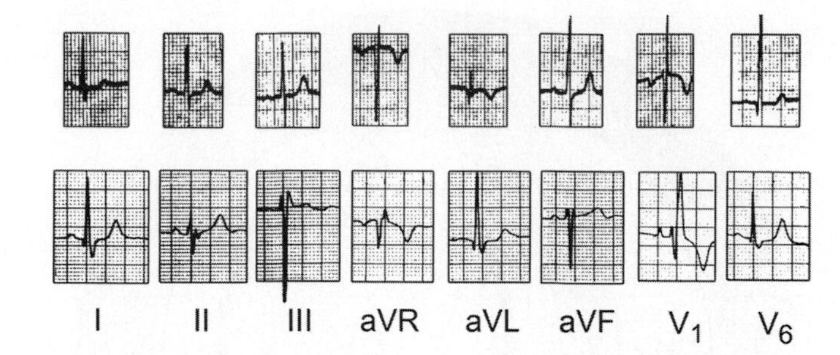

FIGURE 12–37 *Preoperative (**A**) and postoperative (**B**) ECG recordings from a patient with tetralogy of Fallot, showing postoperative right bundle branch block and a superior shift in the axis for initial LV depolarization consistent with left anterior hemiblock. From Fyler DC. Nadas' Pediatric Cardiology. Philadelphia: Hanley & Belfus, 1992.*

Preexcitation

Preexcitation implies that a portion of ventricular tissue is being activated ahead of schedule relative to normal His-Purkinje conduction. In *Wolff-Parkinson-White (WPW) syndrome,* this early activation occurs over an accessory connection between atrial and ventricular muscle located anywhere along the right or left AV grooves. As an atrial depolarization wavefront approaches the ventricles, it may advance over the accessory pathway, the normal AV node, or both. Normal AV nodal conduction is relatively slow, but the accessory pathway transmits rapid activation to a focal ventricular segment. The region of early activation generates a *delta wave* on the ECG (Fig. 12-38) with a short PR (actually a P-delta) interval. Because some portion of ventricular activation still occurs over the normal His pathway, there is fusion between preexcitation and the normal depolarization sequence.

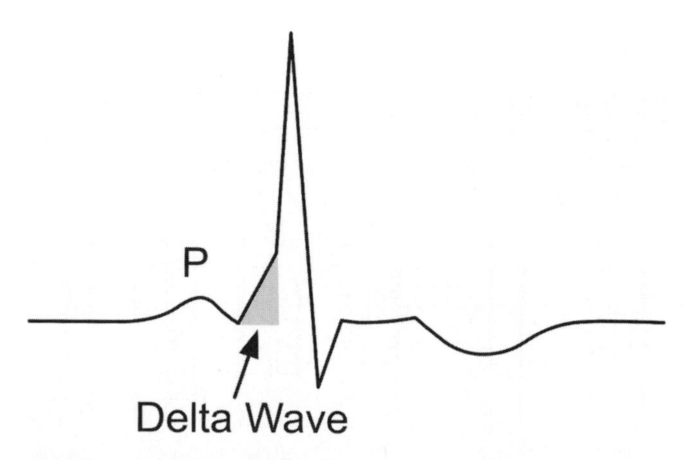

FIGURE 12–38 *Short P-R interval and the delta wave of ventricular preexcitation.*
From Fyler DC. Nadas' Pediatric Cardiology. Philadelphia: Hanley & Belfus, 1992.

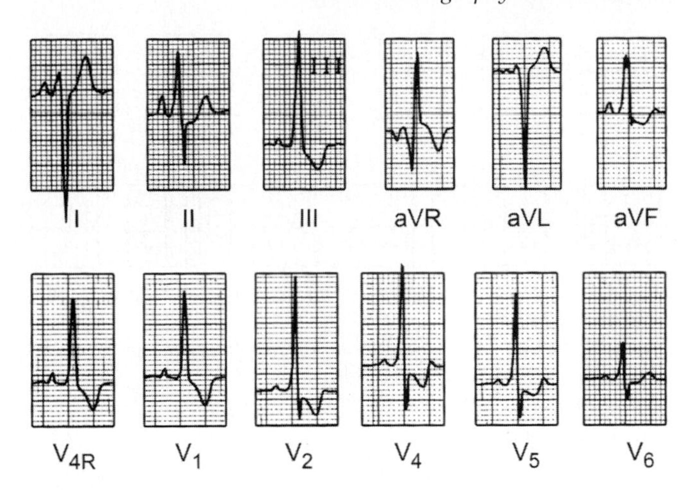

FIGURE 12–39 *ECG showing Wolff-Parkinson-White syndrome in a patient with a left posterolateral accessory pathway. The precordial pattern is akin to right bundle branch block.*
From Fyler DC. Nadas' Pediatric Cardiology. Philadelphia: Hanley & Belfus, 1992.

The electrocardiographic patterns in the WPW syndrome are variable, depending on the location of the accessory pathway and its conduction characteristics. At the most simplistic level, left-sided accessory pathways can be expected to produce negative delta waves in the left-sided ECG leads (I, aV_L, V_5, V_6) and positive delta waves in the right-sided leads (aV_R, V_{4R}–V_1) because the early activation vector is traveling left to right. For the most part, the right ventricle is activated by the normal AV node, but only after the usual nodal time delay, thus generating a gross QRS morphology reminiscent of right bundle branch block (Fig. 12-39). Right-sided accessory pathways, by comparison, are usually associated with positive delta waves in the left-sided leads (Fig. 12-40) and a QRS pattern more closely resembling left bundle branch block. Electrophysiologists who deal with WPW syndrome on a regular basis have developed several ECG algorithms[11,12] that provide far more exacting estimates of accessory pathway location based on fine details of delta wave polarity and QRS shape (see Chapter 29).

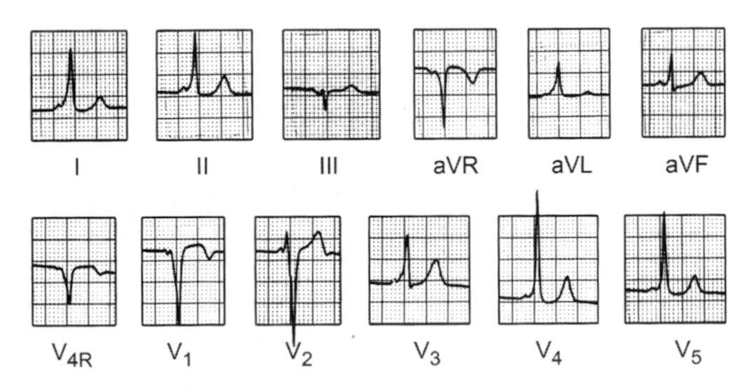

FIGURE 12–40 *ECG showing Wolff-Parkinson-White syndrome in a patient with a right lateral accessory pathway. The precordial pattern is akin to left bundle branch block.*
From Fyler DC. Nadas' Pediatric Cardiology. Philadelphia: Hanley & Belfus, 1992.

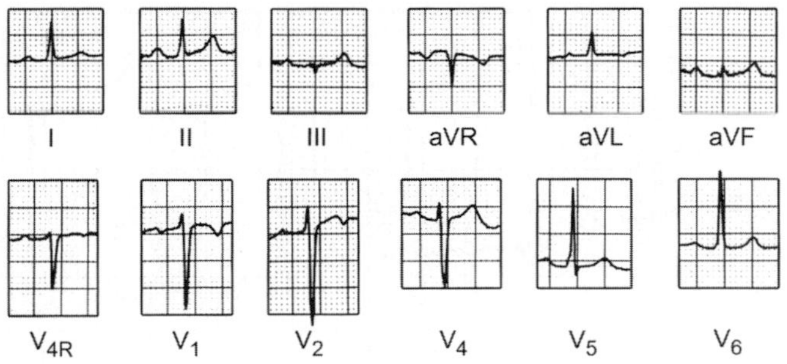

FIGURE 12–41 *Delta waves (best seen in leads II, V_5) with a normal P-R interval in a patient with a Mahaim fiber proven at electrophysiologic study.*
From Fyler DC. Nadas' Pediatric Cardiology. Philadelphia: Hanley & Belfus, 1992.

A less common form of preexcitation is associated with the presence of a *Mahaim fiber.* Until fairly recently, these fibers were thought to represent accessory connections running from the AV node into right ventricular muscle, but they are now better understood as long and slowly conducting accessory pathways running from the anterolateral tricuspid ring to the anterior surface of the right ventricle where they may join the terminal portions of the right bundle branch.[13] Because conduction through the Mahaim fiber is rather slow, the PR interval remains fairly normal on the ECG. However, activation through the Mahaim pathway can still preexcite a small portion of the right ventricle to generate a delta wave (Fig. 12-41). Mahaim fibers are rare and may require intracardiac electrophysiologic study to confirm their presence or distinguish them from the WPW syndrome.

In both WPW and Mahaim preexcitation, the ability to use the ECG for evaluation of hypertrophy, changes in the ST segment and T wave, and QT measurement is lost (similar to bundle branch block).

Changes in the ST Segment and T Wave

No other aspect of ECG interpretation is as dependent on good clinical history as the evaluation of abnormalities of the ST segment and T wave. Unfortunately, pathologic changes are often nonspecific. Elevation or depression of the J point and changes in the T wave can be seen in almost any condition involving myocyte injury, pericardial inflammation, abnormal ion channel function, or certain electrolyte disturbances.

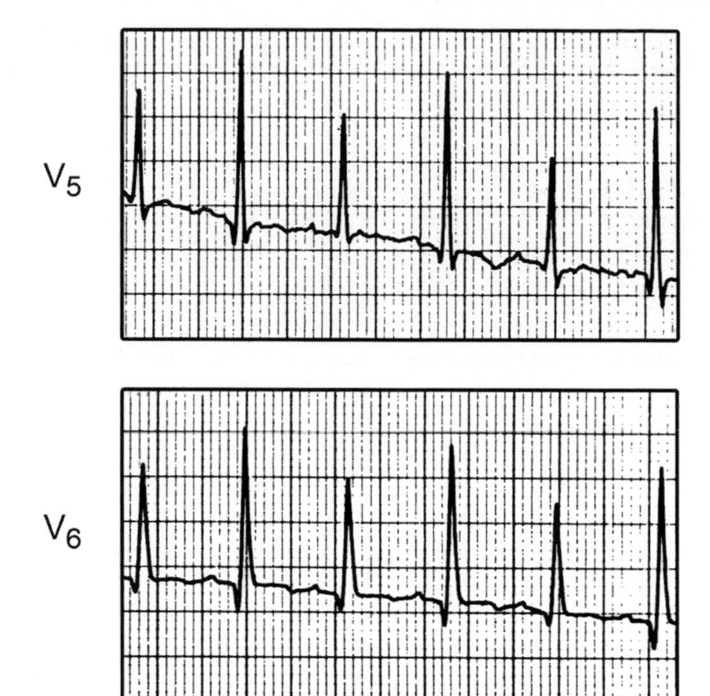

FIGURE 12–42 *Electrical alternans in a teenage boy with large pericardial effusion. Note also the nonspecific flattening of the T wave in V_5 and V_6.*
From Fyler DC. Nadas' Pediatric Cardiology. Philadelphia: Hanley & Belfus, 1992.

Pericarditis and Pericardial Effusion

Pericardial inflammation produces a sequence of changes in the ST segment and T wave that evolve as the disorder progresses. The earliest finding is elevation of the ST segment with preservation of normal T-wave amplitude and direction. Later, the ST segment returns to the baseline, but the T wave becomes flattened and, ultimately, inverted. As opposed to the focal changes in the ST segment and T wave that are seen in ischemic syndromes, the electrocardiographic findings in pericarditis are diffuse and usually involve all leads, except perhaps aV_R and the right precordium. Additionally, pericarditis influences both atrial and ventricular surfaces, such that noticeable depression of the T_A wave may sometimes be observed. Occasionally, the presence of a large effusion in the pericardial space results in diminished ventricular voltages and a pattern of QRS amplitude variation known as *QRS alternans* (Fig. 12-42).

Myocarditis

The electrocardiographic findings in myocarditis are variable but usually involved diminished ventricular voltages and T-wave inversion during the acute illness. Atrioventricular and intraventricular conduction disturbances, along with ventricular arrhythmias, are common (Fig. 12-43).

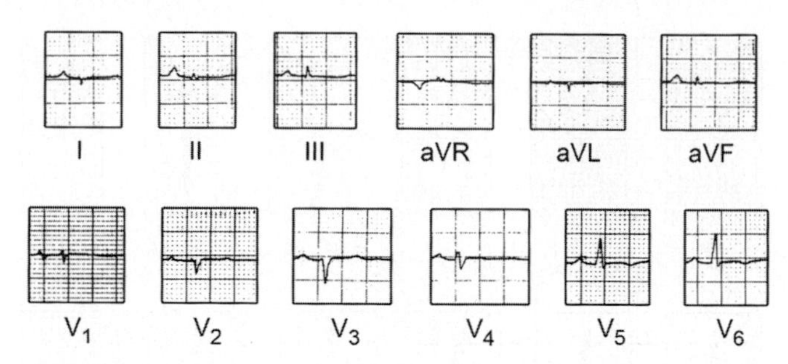

FIGURE 12–43 *Dramatically low QRS voltage in a patient with dilated myopathy from myocarditis.*
From Fyler DC. Nadas' Pediatric Cardiology. Philadelphia: Hanley & Belfus, 1992.

Hypertrophic Cardiomyopathy

The changes in the ST segment and T wave seen in hypertrophic cardiomyopathy are similar to the left ventricular strain pattern that occurs with advanced hypertrophy from any cause. The lateral T waves are inverted, and the J point may be depressed. Voltage criteria for LVH are usually present (Fig. 12-44). About 30% of patients also have prominent Q waves in the lateral and inferior leads and may display left axis deviation. A somewhat high percentage of patients with hypertrophic myopathy have also been found to have preexcitation from accessory AV pathways (WPW syndrome). The PR interval may appear short in some cases of hypertrophic myopathy even when such pathways are absent; hence, a formal electrophysiology study may sometimes be needed to distinguish pseudopreexcitation from true WPW.

Dilated Cardiomyopathy

There are no specific electrocardiographic findings to aid in the diagnosis of the dilated myopathy, although the ECG is rarely normal in such cases. Because the etiology

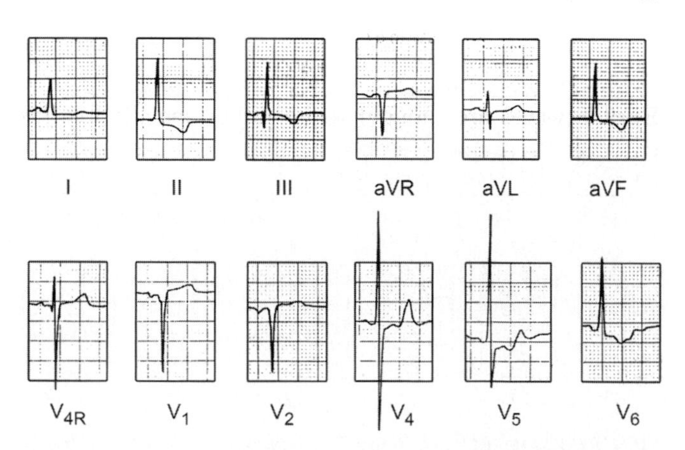

FIGURE 12–44 *ECG from a patient with hypertrophic obstructive cardiomyopathy showing LVH and "strain."*
From Fyler DC. Nadas' Pediatric Cardiology. Philadelphia: Hanley & Belfus, 1992.

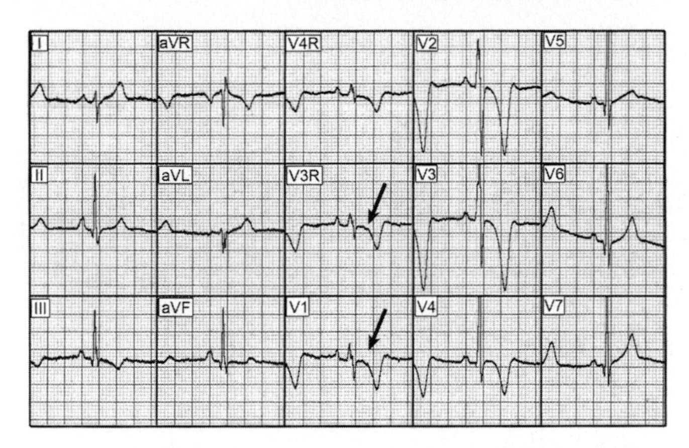

FIGURE 12–45 *ECG from a teenage patient with familial arrhythmogenic RV dysplasia who had documented ventricular tachycardia as well as a dilated RV on echocardiogram. Note the deeply negative precordial T waves and the subtle epsilon wave in the right chest leads (**arrows**).*

is so variable, the ECG can include almost any of the patterns seen with inflammatory disease or hypertrophy, although ST depression (rather than elevation) is most common.

Arrhythmogenic Right Ventricular Dysplasia

This familial disease involving right ventricular myopathy and recurrent ventricular tachycardia can be extremely difficult to diagnose by any testing modality. The ECG actually seems to be one of the most reliable tools for establishing its presence. The classic findings[14] include variable degrees of right ventricular conduction delay, a pattern of inverted precordial T waves extending from V_{4R} all the way out beyond V_2, and ventricular ectopy. Most importantly, a so-called epsilon wave (Fig. 12-45) can sometimes be detected in the right precordial leads as a small high-frequency spike during the early portion of ST segment. Epsilon waves are thought to be rather specific for this disease.

Long QT Syndrome

As mentioned, a QTc that exceeds normal limits may indicate a membrane channelopathy associated with one of the heredity long QT syndromes. Because of the serious prognosis attached to this disorder, it is imperative that the QT interval be scrutinized carefully on all ECG recordings, particularly in leads II, V_5, and V_6 where prolongation seems to be most dramatic.[15] In addition to prolonged duration, long QT syndrome can also produce abnormal contours for repolarization signals, such as *notched T waves* and gross alterations in T-wave direction known as *T-wave alternans* (Fig. 12-46).

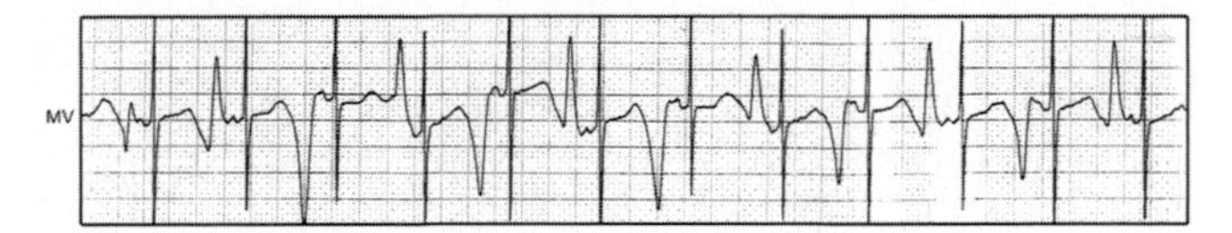

FIGURE 12–46 *Dramatic T-wave alternans in a patient with a severe form of long QT syndrome.*

Brugada Syndrome

Brugada syndrome is a more recently recognized hereditary channelopathy causing ventricular tachycardia,[16] which is usually associated with right bundle branch block and dramatic ST elevation in leads V_1 through V_3 (Fig. 12-47). The QTc tends to be normal. These findings can wax and wane in a given patient to the point that the ECG appears rather normal at times. Provocative challenges with certain antiarrhythmic drugs may be needed to uncover the abnormalities.

Short QT Syndrome

A new familial condition known as short QT syndrome has now been described.[17] This rare disorder is associated with ventricular arrhythmias similar to long QT syndrome, but the patients demonstrate strikingly short QTc values of less than 0.30 second, along with very tall peaked T waves.

Ischemia

Myocardial ischemia is a rare problem in pediatric practice, but it may occur with certain congenital anomalies or inflammation of the coronary arterial vasculature. Hypoxic insults result in an evolution of electrocardiographic findings, which tend to parallel cellular events. During the initial *ischemic phase,* the most dramatic changes occur in the T wave, which becomes tall and peaked in those leads that record near the affected myocardial segment. These changes are usually accompanied by some deviation of the

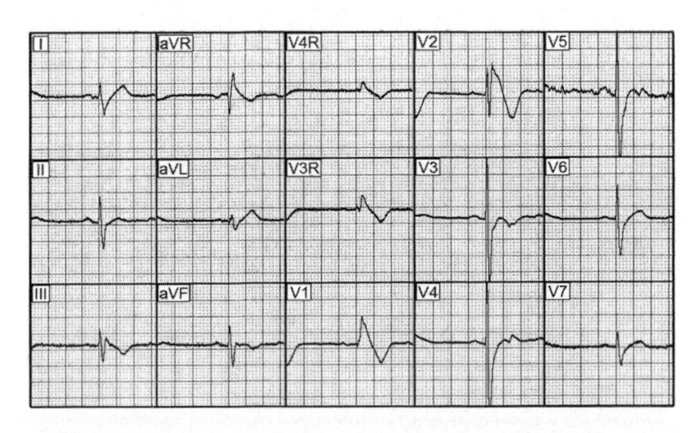

FIGURE 12–47 *ECG from a young boy with recurrent VT due to Brugada syndrome. Note unusual appearance of the ST segment and T waves in the right precordium.*

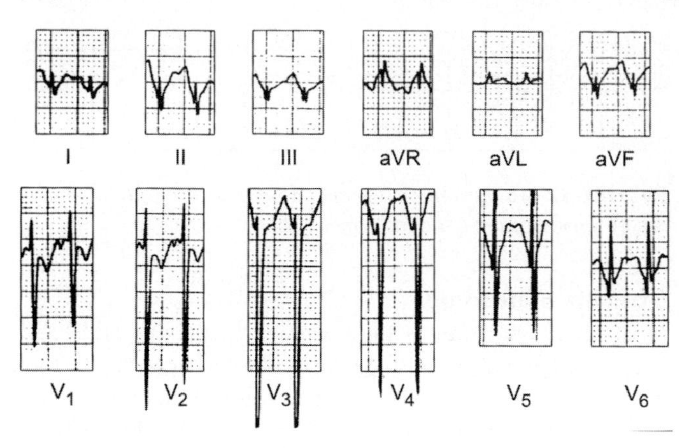

FIGURE 12–48 *ECG showing acute ischemia with lateral (V_4–V_6) and inferior (aV_F) elevation of the S-T segment.*
From Fyler DC. Nadas' Pediatric Cardiology. Philadelphia: Hanley & Belfus, 1992.

ST segment (Fig. 12-48). If the pathologic process is promptly reversed, these changes can resolve. However, if the insult persists, the *injury phase* commences and may be seen on the ECG as a more dramatic shift in the ST segment. The ST deviation may be upward or downward, depending on whether the injured cells are epicardial or endocardial (Fig. 12-49). During the injury phase, correction of the underlying cause may still result in reversion to a normal ECG. When the injury persists, cell death *(infarction phase)* follows, reflected on the ECG as a diminution of R-wave voltage and the appearance of Q waves in those leads facing the infarcted segment (Fig. 12-50).

The most common cause of myocardial ischemia in pediatric practice involves anomalous origin of the left coronary from the pulmonary artery. At initial presentation, variable degrees of injury or infarction are apparent, typically involving ventricular muscle in the distribution of

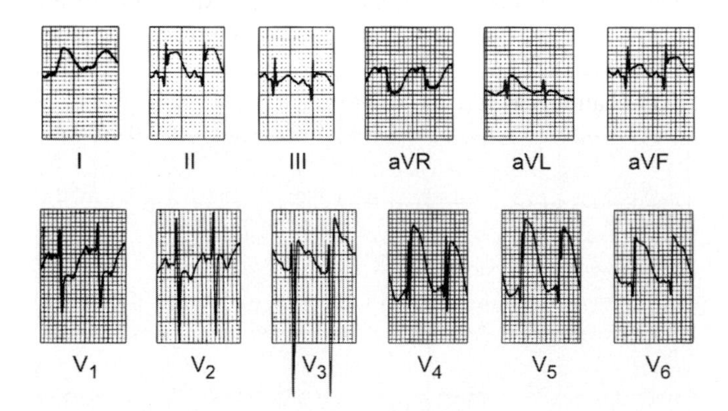

FIGURE 12–49 *Follow-up ECG from the same patient as in (Figure 12-48) several hours later, now showing marked changes in the S-T segment caused by myocardial injury.*
From Fyler DC. Nadas' Pediatric Cardiology. Philadelphia: Hanley & Belfus, 1992.

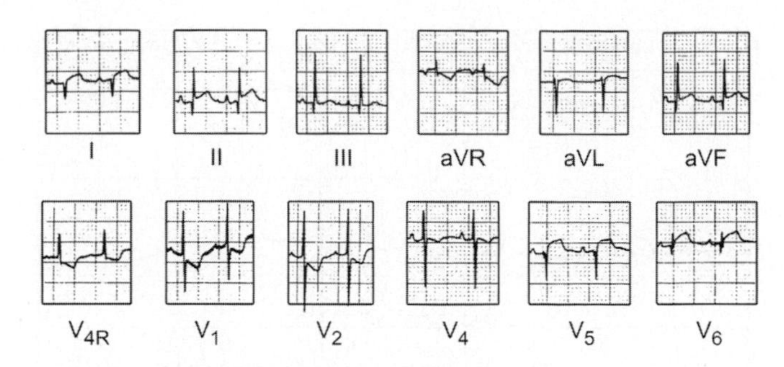

FIGURE 12–50 *ECG showing lateral myocardial infarction with a deep Q wave and loss of the R wave in lead V_5.*
From Fyler DC. Nadas' Pediatric Cardiology. Philadelphia: Hanley & Belfus, 1992.

the left anterior descending artery (i.e., anterior and septal areas). The electrocardiographic findings in severely afflicted infants include deep Q waves in leftward and lateral leads (I, aV_L, V_3–V_6) and loss of the mid-precordial R wave (V_3–V_5), with a normal QRS axis (Fig. 12-51). Children who present beyond infancy are more likely to have left axis deviation, smaller Q waves in the leftward and lateral leads, and increased voltages suggestive of LVH (Fig. 12-52).

Electrolyte Abnormalities

Significant changes may occur on the surface ECG with certain electrolyte disturbances, most notably potassium, calcium, and magnesium imbalance. With *hyperkalemia,* the electrocardiographic findings are quite specific for anything more than mild abnormalities. Moderate elevation of serum potassium concentration (greater than 6.0 mEq/L) causes tall, peaked T waves, along with some widening of the QRS complex (Fig. 12-53). Marked elevation (more than 8.0 mEq/L) causes profound widening of the P wave and QRS complex, resulting in a pattern for sinus rhythm

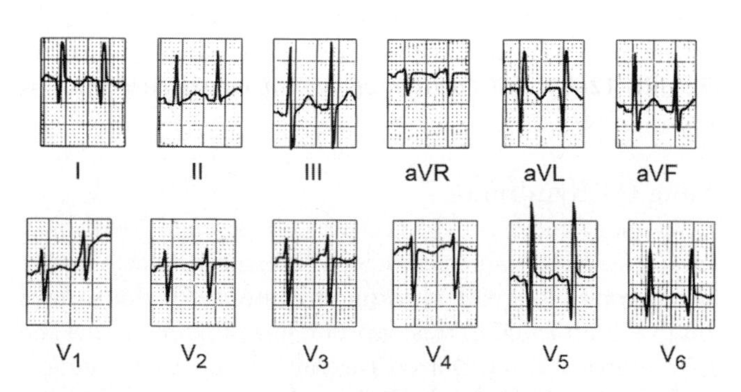

FIGURE 12–51 *ECG from infant with origin of the left coronary artery from the pulmonary artery who arrived at the hospital in shock. Note the deep, wide Q waves in V_5 and V_6, and the small R wave in V_4.*
From Fyler DC. Nadas' Pediatric Cardiology. Philadelphia: Hanley & Belfus, 1992.

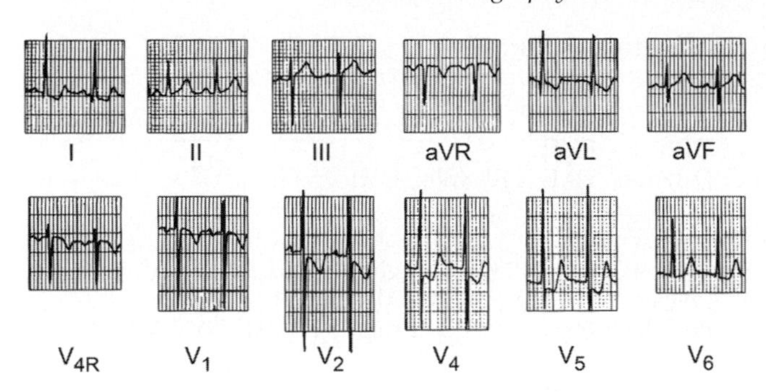

FIGURE 12–52 *ECG from an asymptomatic 12-year-old with the origin of the left coronary artery from the pulmonary artery. Except for mild left axis deviation, borderline LVH, and nonspecific changes in the S-T segment, the trace is deceptively unimpressive.*
From Fyler DC. Nadas' Pediatric Cardiology. Philadelphia: Hanley & Belfus, 1992.

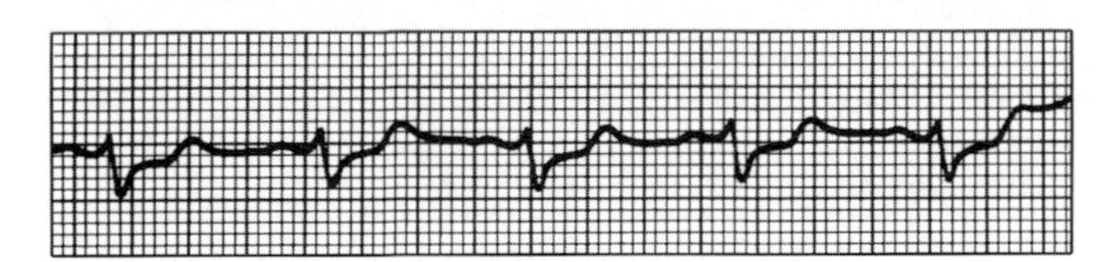

FIGURE 12–53 *ECG pattern of moderate hyperkalemia (K+ = 7.0). Note the widening of the QRS.*
From Fyler DC. Nadas' Pediatric Cardiology. Philadelphia: Hanley & Belfus, 1992.

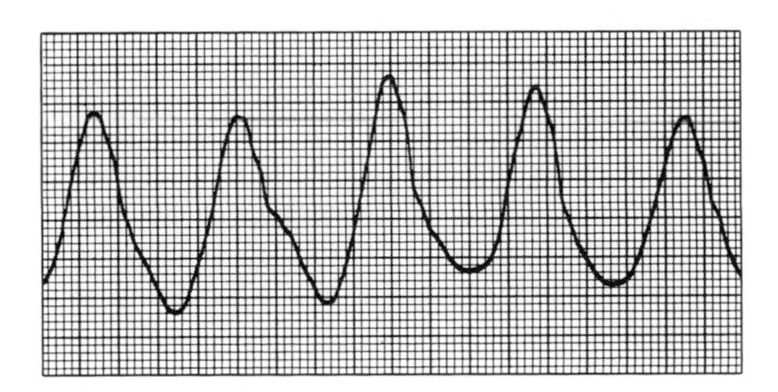

FIGURE 12–54 *ECG pattern of marked hyperkalemia (K+ = 8.9) showing a "sine wave" pattern.*
From Fyler DC. Nadas' Pediatric Cardiology. Philadelphia: Hanley & Belfus, 1992.

that resembles a sine wave or mimics wide ventricular tachycardia (Fig. 12-54). Fibrillation and asystole can result from acute severe elevations of serum potassium. *Hypokalemia* (less than 3.0 mEq/L) results in a low-amplitude, flattened T wave, with the appearance of prominent U waves.

Calcium and *magnesium* predominantly influence speed of cellular repolarization. Low levels of either ion prolong the QT interval, whereas high serum levels may shorten the QT slightly.

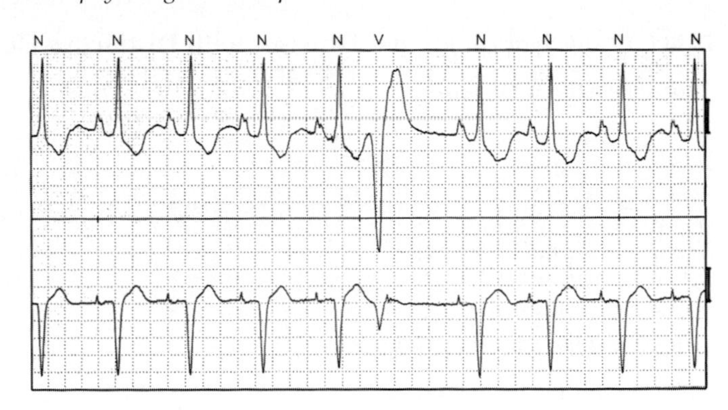

FIGURE 12–55 *Example of printout from a Holter scanning device showing a ventricular premature beat. N, normal complex; V, ventricular premature beat.*
From Fyler DC. Nadas' Pediatric Cardiology. Philadelphia: Hanley & Belfus, 1992.

Pathognomonic Electrocardiographic Patterns

Table 12-2 lists some cardiac conditions and syndromes in which the ECG findings are sufficiently specific to allow rapid diagnosis. These disorders are discussed individually elsewhere in this text but are abstracted here for quick reference.

HOLTER MONITORING AND EVENT RECORDING

Unless one is fortunate enough to have an ECG hooked up during a clinical arrhythmia episode, alternate techniques for long-term rhythm recording must be employed. The most familiar tool for this purpose is the *Holter monitor,* which provides 24-hour continuous rhythm recording from adhesive electrodes on the chest. Modern Holter equipment involves a lightweight battery-powered device that stores data to a digital file. Two or three simultaneous ECG channels are usually recorded and synchronized to a 24-hour clock. The patient and family maintain a written diary to correlate activity or symptoms with rhythm status. The recording is later played back on a high-speed analysis system by a technician using computerized arrhythmia detection templates. Paper copies of interesting events can then be printed for physician review (Fig. 12-55). Most analysis systems also provide data on heart rate trends (minimum, maximum, mean, and degree of variability) along with quantitation of supraventricular and ventricular ectopy.

The Holter monitor is suitable only if an arrhythmia occurs at a frequency greater than once in 24 hours. For patients who go many days or weeks between events, a long-term *event recorder*, which the patient keeps for a period of 30 to 60 days, is a far more appropriate tool.[18]

TABLE 12–2. Syndromes and Diseases with Distinctive Electrocardiogram Features

Anatomic Heart Disease	
AV canal defect	Superior QRS axis, RVH
Tricuspid atresia	Superior QRS axis, BAE, ↓RV volts, LVH
Situs inversus	P axis +120°
Dextrocardia	↑RV volts, ↓↓LV volts
L-loop ("inverted") ventricles	RSR on left (I, aV_L, V_5, V_6), QR on right (aV_R, V_1), AVB
Origin LCA from PA	Deep Q wave and ↓ volts V_3- V_5, ± LAD, ± LVH
Hypertrophic myopathy	LVH "strain," deep Q wave V_3–V_6, ± short PR, LAE, SVT, VT
Congenital Conduction Disorders	
Wolff-Parkinson-White syndrome	Short PR, delta wave, SVT
Mahaim fiber	Normal PR, delta wave, SVT
Maternal lupus (fetal exposure)	AVB
Familial Arrhythmia Disorders	
Long QT (Romano-Ward)	↑QTc, notched T wave, VT, (normal hearing)
Long QT (Jervell & Lange-Nielsen)	↑↑QTc, notched T wave, T-wave alternans, VT, (deafness)
Short QT	↓↓QTc (< 0.30), VT
Brugada syndrome	RVCD, dramatic ST elevation V_1 – V_3, VT
Arrhythmogenic RV dysplasia	Epsilon wave, T wave inversion V_1-V_3, RVCD, VT
Catecholaminergic VT	VT with exercise
Anderson's syndrome	VT, periodic paralysis
Systemic Disorders	
Pompe's disease	Short PR, ↑↑ ventricular volts, ± deep Q waves
Friedreich's ataxia	Sinus tachy, LVH, SVT, VT
Becker's muscular dystrophy	IVCD, AVB, SVT
Duchenne's muscular dystrophy	RVH, deep Q (I & aV_L), SVT, VT
Myotonic dystrophy	Sinus brady, IVCD, AVB, SVT
Kearns-Sayre syndrome	IVCD, AVB
Lyme disease	AVB
Chagas' disease	AVB
Hypothyroidism	Sinus brady, AVB
Hyperthyroidism	Sinus tachy, SVT
Hypokalemia	Low-amplitude T wave, prominent U wave, ± long QTc
Hyperkalemia	Peaked T wave, IVCD, "sine wave" pattern, VT
Hypothermia (severe)	Osborn or "J" wave, sinus brady, AVB, IVCD, ↑QTc, VT

AVB, atrioventricular block; AV, atrioventricular; BAE, biatrial enlargement; IVCD, intraventricular conduction disturbance; LAE, left atrial enlargement; LCA, left coronary artery; LVH, left ventricular hypertrophy; PA, pulmonary artery; RV, right ventricle; RVCD, right ventricular conduction disturbance; RVH, right ventricular hypertrophy; SVT, supraventricular tachycardia; VT, ventricular tachycardia.

Some event recording devices are intended to be worn on an episodic basis, whereas others are designed to be worn continuously to capture fleeting arrhythmic events (Fig. 12-56). When either device is activated, a rhythm strip is recorded for 1 minute or so and stored in memory. The recording is later played back as an oscillating audio signal that is easily decoded back into an electrocardiographic waveform with appropriate equipment. One major advantage of this technology is that the audio signals can be sent long distance over a standard telephone to a central decoding station, thus saving the patient travel time while also hastening detection of potentially serious rhythm disorders. Event recorders are useful for the diagnosis of episodic palpitations of undetermined etiology, or for evaluation of vague symptoms (e.g., dizziness or chest pain) when an arrhythmia is part of the differential diagnosis. Implantable event recorders that are inserted subcutaneously in the pectoral area have also been developed in recent years and may be indicated in select cases.

EXERCISE TESTING FOR RHYTHM EVALUATION

Manipulation of autonomic tone can provide information regarding rhythm status that is not always available on a resting ECG. Enhancement of sympathetic drive during dynamic exercise permits analysis of sinus node function, intracardiac conduction, and certain tachyarrhythmias. The two primary exercise techniques used in pediatrics are

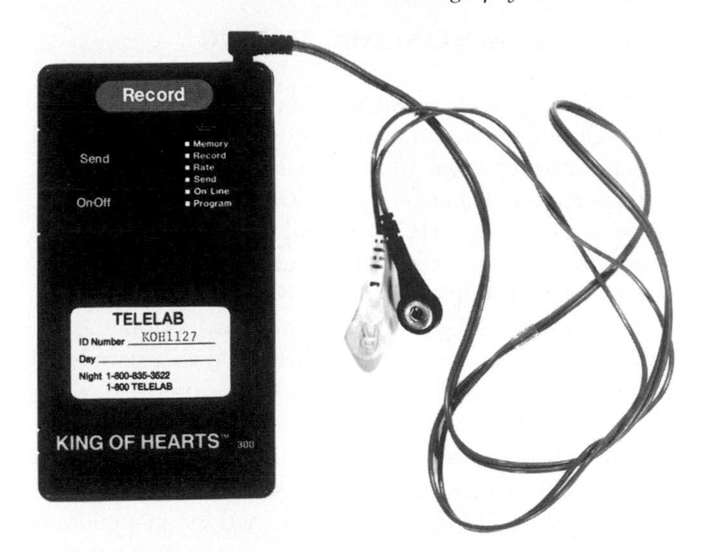

FIGURE 12–56 *An event recorder with a memory loop that records the preceding 30 sec of rhythm and a subsequent 30 sec when the device is activated.*
From Fyler DC. Nadas' Pediatric Cardiology. Philadelphia: Hanley & Belfus, 1992.

the Bruce protocol on a treadmill, and the stationary bicycle protocol (see Chapter 16). The treadmill has an increased static component to its workload and generally produces higher peak heart rates, although bicycle exercise can provide higher fidelity electrocardiographic tracings because there is less body motion to generate baseline artifact. Both techniques are relatively straightforward to use for rhythm evaluation in patients as young as 6 years old. Although exercise testing in children is safe, the personnel need to be prepared for arrhythmias and other unexpected indications for test termination. Of 3120 consecutive studies analyzed from our center, 5% (n = 156) were terminated prematurely for findings other than fatigue, including worrisome ventricular arrhythmias (n = 59), syncope or marked presyncope (n = 44), supraventricular tachycardia (SVT; n = 27), or exercise heart rate approaching detection rates for an automatic implantable defibrillator shock (n = 15).

Chronotropic incompetence from sinus node dysfunction can be assessed reasonably well with exercise testing by comparing the maximum achieved heart rate with norms for age. For patients with various degrees of AV block, exercise may be used to assess changes in conduction pattern, evaluate escape rates, or look for the development of ventricular ectopy at peak exercise.[19] Such data may assist in determining timing for permanent pacemaker insertion. For patients with a pacemaker already in place, exercise studies can be used to adjust the degree of rate responsiveness and evaluate upper rate limit settings of the device.

Ventricular arrhythmias are a fairly common indication for exercise testing. It is generally believed that suppression of ventricular ectopy at peak exercise portends a benign prognosis, although there are certainly exceptions to this rule. More to the point, ventricular ectopy that either fails to extinguish at elevated heart rates or is exacerbated with exercise[20,21] suggests clinically important disease (Fig. 12-57). Exercise testing may also be used to provide a spectrum of QT intervals for review at varied heart rates[22] or to detect exercise-induced arrhythmias in suspected cases of long QT syndrome.

Supraventricular arrhythmias do not generally lend themselves to evaluation by exercise testing, with the notable exception of WPW syndrome, in which the anterograde conduction characteristics of the accessory pathway can be assessed. When patients with clear delta waves and

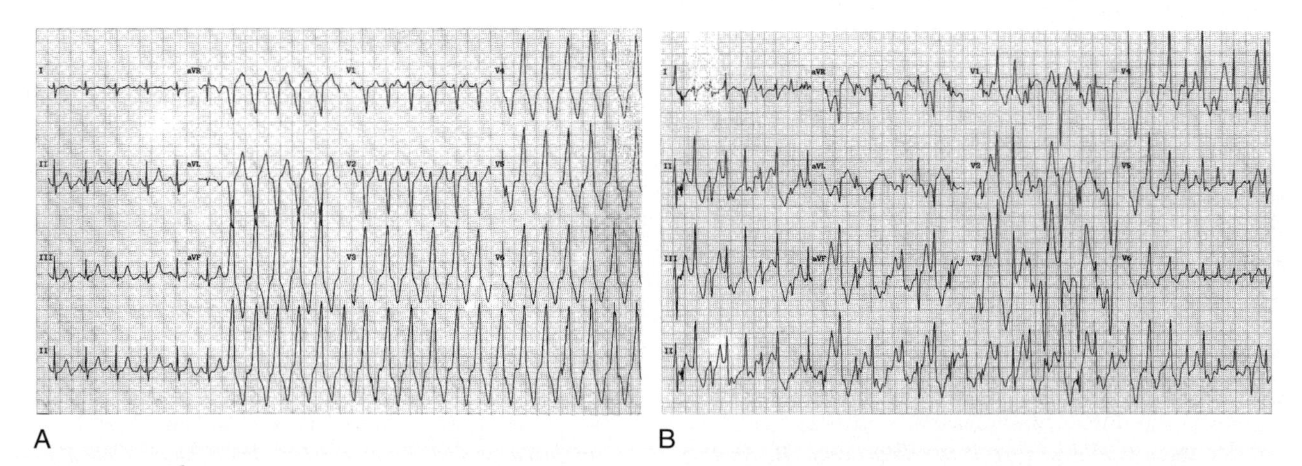

FIGURE 12–57 ***A**, Abrupt onset of sustained monomorphic ventricular tachycardia with treadmill exercise in a 15-year-old with palpitations. **B**, Nearly sustained, somewhat polymorphic, ventricular tachycardia at peak exercise in an adolescent female with recurrent syncope.*

short PR intervals develop sinus tachycardia in response to exercise, an atrial rate may be reached whereby the capacity of the accessory pathway to conduct anterograde is exceeded, so that all ventricular activation occurs over the AV node. At this point, the QRS complex and the PR interval normalize (Fig. 12-58). The sinus rate at which anterograde preexcitation is blocked correlates fairly well with conduction measurements for the accessory pathway obtained at electrophysiologic study and may help predict the potential risk for rapid anterograde conduction should the patient ever develop atrial fibrillation. The unequivocal loss of preexcitation in response to sinus tachycardia can usually be interpreted to indicate a patient is at relatively low risk for rapid preexcited atrial fibrillation.[23]

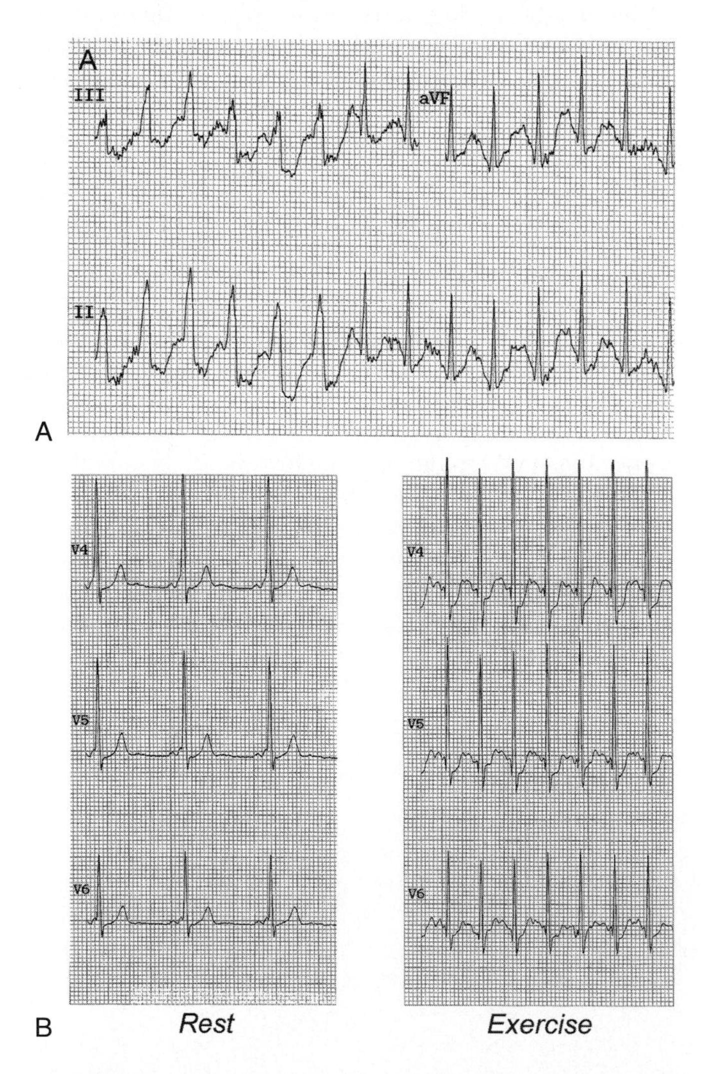

FIGURE 12–58 *A, Treadmill exercise testing on a 16-year-old with palpitations and Wolf-Parkinson-White syndrome. At a heart rate of 189, there is abrupt loss of the delta wave.* ***B****, Another patient with Wolf-Parkinson-White syndrome who has progressive QRS fusion but maintains a subtle delta wave up to maximum sinus rates of 189.*

AUTONOMIC TESTING

Dynamic exercise testing permits observation of rhythm status during enhanced sympathetic state, but controlled manipulation of vagal tone is more difficult to achieve. Perhaps the best technique currently available for this purpose is the *head-up tilt* (HUT) procedure, during which the complex orthostatic reflexes involved with vasomotor regulation and heart rate control can be assessed.[24–26]

The basic technique for HUT involves positioning the patient supine on a motorized tilt table with a peripheral intravenous line in place, and monitoring the ECG along with noninvasive arterial blood pressure. After a 15 minute period of baseline observation in the supine position, the patient is tilted to a nearly upright posture (60 to 70 degrees), and the patient's physiology is reassessed for an additional 15 minutes. If no symptoms or arrhythmias occur, the patient is returned to the supine position, and the entire sequence is repeated during an isoproterenol infusion (Fig. 12-59).

A positive HUT test may suggest a benign, neurally mediated mechanism as the etiology for recurrent syncope, or for episodic arrhythmias such as sinus bradycardia,

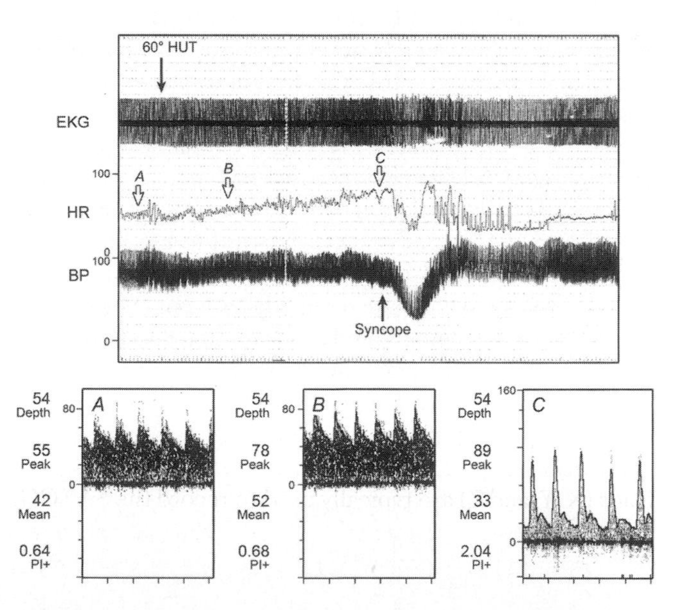

FIGURE 12–59 *Composite data from a head-up tilt test in a patient with intermittent syncope. Condition (****A****) is supine baseline before tilt. With initial head-up tilt (****B****), there is a minor increase in heart rate and narrowing of pulse pressure.* ***The bottom panel*** *shows preserved cerebral blood flow velocity. With longer-duration 60-degree tilt, there are increasing, cyclic swings in heart rate and blood pressure, eventually associated (****C****) with presyncopal symptoms, decreased cerebral blood flow velocity, and then a marked decrease in both heart rate and blood pressure associated with syncope. In recovery, the heart rate remains relatively slow for several minutes before abruptly returning to a more normal pattern.*

transient AV block, or exaggerated orthostatic sinus tachycardia. However, because of the relatively high incidence (up to 40%) of false-positive responses to HUT testing in asymptomatic children,[27,28] the results need to be interpreted with caution. Inducing vasovagal syncope or a reflex bradycardia simply cannot be viewed as excluding other disease. Studies are only useful if the physiologic data correlate cleanly with symptoms, and the possibility of more serious cardiac disorders has been dismissed by other techniques.

SIGNAL AVERAGING

Signal averaging produces a high-resolution, high-amplitude electrical recording from the body surface that allows one to view subtle electrical events that are too small to be seen on a traditional ECG. This is accomplished by recording a hundred or more consecutive waveforms that are superimposed in the computer memory of the recording device, producing a composite or average signal from the multiple beats. Random electrical noise that is not part of the composite waveform is easily subtracted, and the resultant signal is amplified to permit a glimpse at low-voltage events that usually go undetected on the routine ECG.

Signal-averaging technology is used primarily as a risk-assessment tool for ventricular arrhythmias. The standard *signal-averaged electrocardiogram (SAECG)* involves a highly amplified QRS complex focused on the depolarization process.[29,30] During normal ventricular depolarization, healthy myocytes activate quickly and inscribe the sharp QRS complex, but areas of diseased myocardium may have sluggish cell-to-cell conduction that continues to generate small-amplitude signals lasting beyond the normal QRS duration. The amplitude of these *late potentials* is typically too small to be appreciated through ambient electrical noise, but they can be uncovered by the SAECG during the terminal portion of the QRS (Fig. 12-60). Three orthogonal leads (X, Y, and Z) are typically used to record the SAECG, which are then summed and a vector magnitude obtained that transforms all net ventricular voltages into positive values. Commercial systems usually allow these data to be obtained in about 5 to 10 minutes. The transformed signal is then analyzed for three principle variables; total QRS duration, the root mean squared amplitude of the terminal 40 msec of the signal (RMS40), and the duration of high-frequency signals with low amplitude (HFLA). Longer-filtered QRS durations, the presence of low-amplitude signals in the terminal portion of the QRS, and longer duration of those low-amplitude signals each represents characteristics of late potentials.

A second signal-averaging test focuses on the repolarization process by searching for alterations in T-wave amplitude between successive heartbeats, known as *T-wave alternans* (TWA). Although some patients with severe forms of long QT syndrome may occasionally demonstrate gross T-wave alternans on a conventional ECG recording, far more subtle T-wave alterations can occur in other forms of heart disease.[31] These small changes involve measurements in the range of microvolts, which would be far beneath the usual millivolt resolution available on the standard ECG. Microvolt TWA is detected by using specialized skin electrodes, collecting 128 consecutive beats that are averaged to allow spectral analysis of oscillations in T-wave amplitude. The patient's heart rate is also raised with exercise, atrial pacing, or medication, and the measurements are repeated. Results are considered abnormal in the presence of TWA greater than 1.9 μV at rest, or the appearance of specific amplitude alternans at heart rates between 100 and 130 beats/minute (Fig. 12-61).

Pediatric data remain limited regarding the significance of late potentials or microvolt T-wave alternans. Furthermore, both tests may have reduced value in the presence of bundle branch block. At present, these tests are used primarily as confirmatory or supportive data for young patients with a normal QRS duration who already have other concrete risk factors for ventricular arrhythmias.

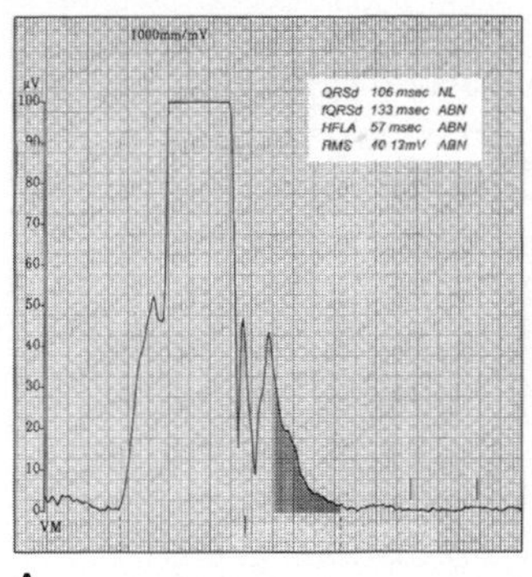

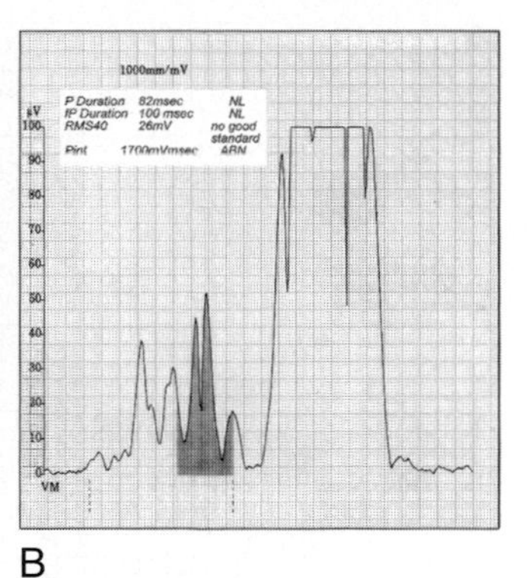

FIGURE 12–60 **A**, *Signal-averaged QRS in a 15-year-old with ventricular fibrillation triggered during an argument with his brother. The filtered QRS duration is prolonged at 133 msec with late potentials consisting of both prolonged high-frequency/low-amplitude (HFLA) signals less than 40 μV and abnormally low, root mean square and mean voltages in the terminal 40 msec.* ***B***, *Signal-averaged P wave in an adolescent with mitral stenosis and atrial fibrillation. While the filtered and unfiltered P wave durations are normal, the integral of the P wave (Pint) is markedly prolonged (upper limits of normal, 800 μV/msec). There are not good standards for the RMS voltage of the terminal 40 msec. fQRSd: filtered QRS duration; HFLA: duration of high frequency, low-amplitude signals in the terminal 40 msec of the filtered QRS; Pint: time-voltage integral of the P-wave amplitude/duration; RMS40: root mean square amplitude of late potentials within the terminal 40 msec*

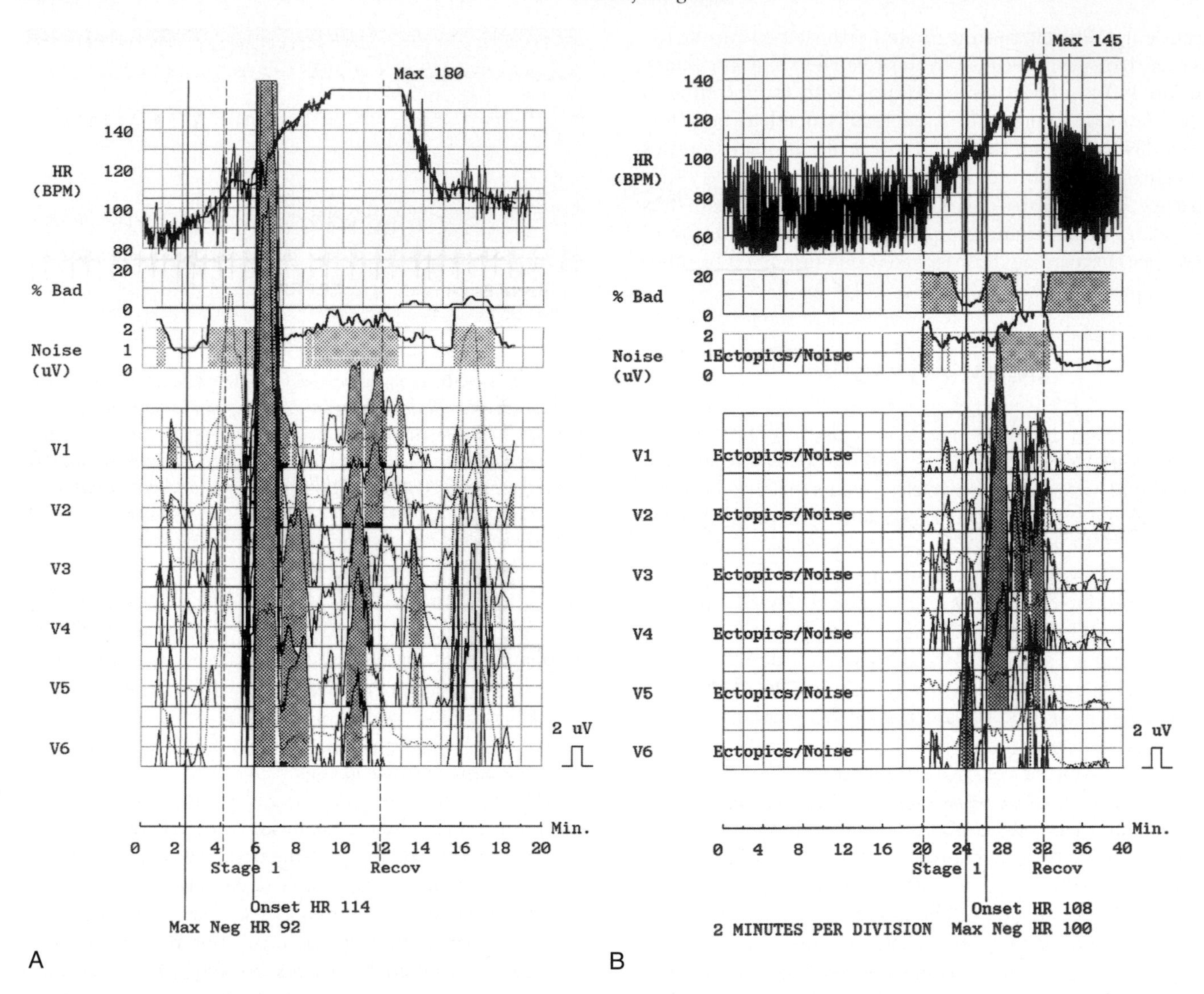

FIGURE 12–61 *Treadmill exercise development of microvolt t-wave alternans.* ***A****, A 13-year-old with hypertrophic cardiomyopathy and cardiac arrest who develops high-amplitude TWA (lead X; Valt, 9.52; ratio, 34.93) in multiple leads with an onset heart rate of 114.* ***B****, Treadmill development of t-wave alternans in an asymptomatic 11-year-old with nonsustained ventricular tachycardia and a large, isolated, left ventricular fibroma. The frequent single premature ventricular beats and sinus arrhythmia at rest preclude analysis until resolution at a heart rate of 108, when there is high-amplitude sustained microvolt t-wave alternans.*

TRANSESOPHAGEAL RECORDING AND PACING

The proximity of the esophagus to the left atrium allows a recording and pacing electrode to be placed immediately adjacent to atrial muscle without requiring vascular entry. A properly positioned esophageal lead will record a sharp, high-amplitude atrial electrogram that is far superior to a surface ECG signal for identifying atrial timing during complex arrhythmias. Flexible bipolar pacing wires specifically designed for esophageal use are easily inserted with the same technique used for nasogastric tube placement. Proper lead positioning is important to obtain a high-quality electrogram and achieve an acceptable threshold for pacing. The position may be checked by moving the lead up and down the middle portion of the esophagus and looking for the site that records the largest atrial electrogram (Fig. 12-62), or by consulting published charts that correlate ideal insertion depth with body size.[32] Any device capable of registering electrophysiologic signals can be used to display the electrogram from an esophageal lead (Fig. 12-63), including conventional ECG equipment. An esophageal electrogram is exceedingly helpful for recording atrial activity during arrhythmias when the mechanism is

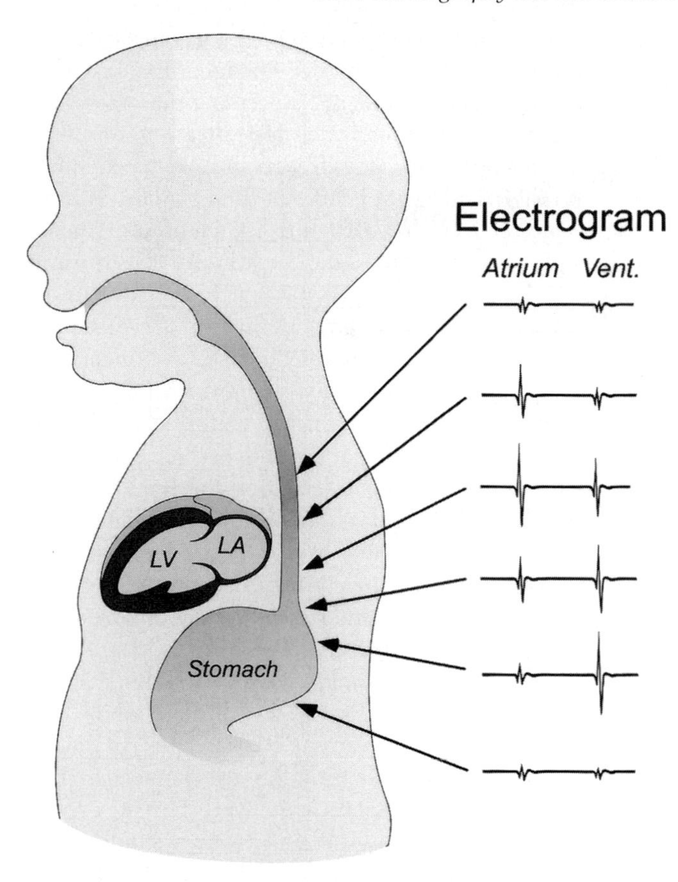

FIGURE 12–62 *The anatomic relationship of the infant esophagus to atrial muscle. The ideal electrogram at mid-esophagus has an atrial spike that is equal to, or larger than, the ventricular signal. LV, ventricle; LA, left atrium.*
From Fyler DC. Nadas' Pediatric Cardiology. Philadelphia: Hanley & Belfus, 1992.

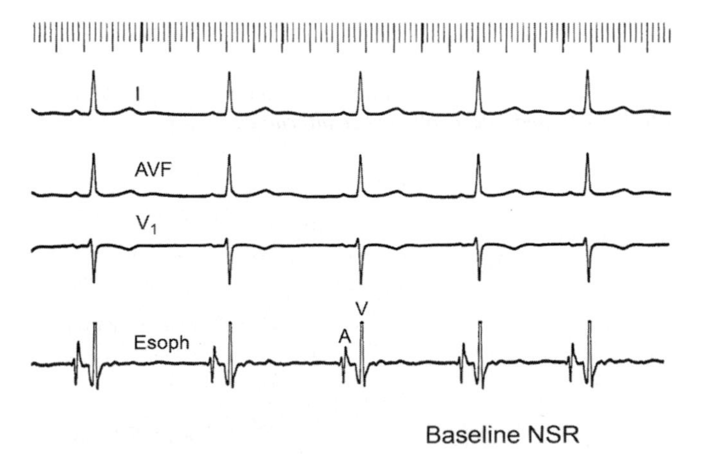

FIGURE 12–63 *Esophageal electrogram and three simultaneous ECG recordings during normal sinus rhythm.*
From Fyler DC. Nadas' Pediatric Cardiology. Philadelphia: Hanley & Belfus, 1992.

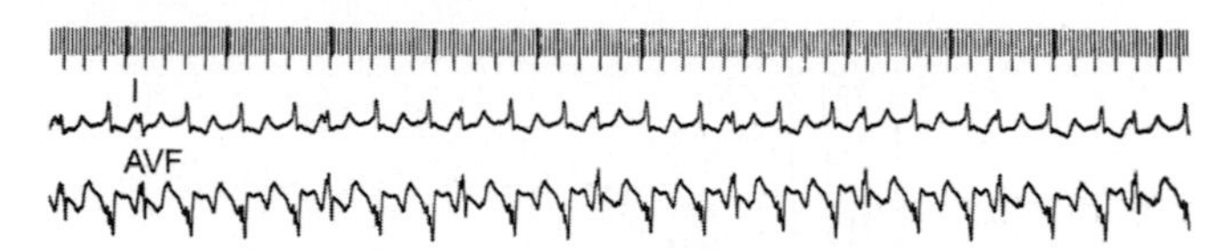

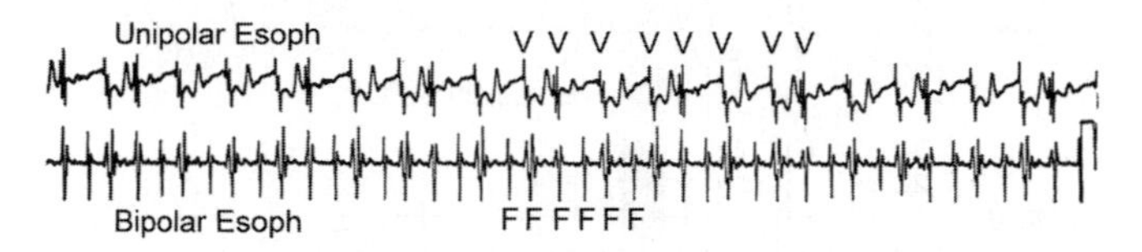

FIGURE 12–64 *Two surface ECG leads (I and aV_F) recorded simultaneously with esophageal electrograms in a patient with atrial flutter and alternating 2:1 and 3:2 conduction. Note how the bipolar esophageal signal clarifies atrial activity. A unipolar esophageal recording will highlight only ventricular activity.*
From Fyler DC. Nadas' Pediatric Cardiology. Philadelphia: Hanley & Belfus, 1992.

unclear on a surface ECG. A classic example is atrial flutter with 2:1 conduction to the ventricles, in which the esophageal electrogram can uncover a hidden flutter wave (Fig. 12-64) that might otherwise have been obscured by the QRS on a standard ECG.

Transesophageal pacing requires a higher pacemaker output than is used for an electrode in direct contact with atrial tissue. Whereas intracardiac pacing is routinely done at a pulse width of about 2.0 msec, the capacity for wider pulses of up to 10.0 msec is needed for transesophageal pacing. The expanded pulse width permits atrial capture at amplitude settings of about 10 to 15 mA. Except for very rare instances, ventricular pacing is not possible with an esophageal electrode. Atrial pacing through the esophageal lead can be used for temporary correction of sinus bradycardia, but it is more frequently employed for short bursts of rapid overdrive pacing of the atrium to interrupt reentry SVT. The overdrive technique is extremely successful in converting reentry circuits within the AV node or those involving an accessory pathway (Fig. 12-65), and it may be successful in as many as 80% of cases involving atrial flutter.

INTRACARDIAC ELECTROPHYSIOLOGIC STUDIES

Intracardiac electrical recording has evolved rapidly during the past 35 years from simple analysis of His bundle signals[33] to complex three-dimensional maps of endocardial propagation.[34] The systematic use of these intracardiac recordings, coupled with programmed stimulation to induce arrhythmias under controlled conditions, has expanded our understanding of the mechanism and risk for just about

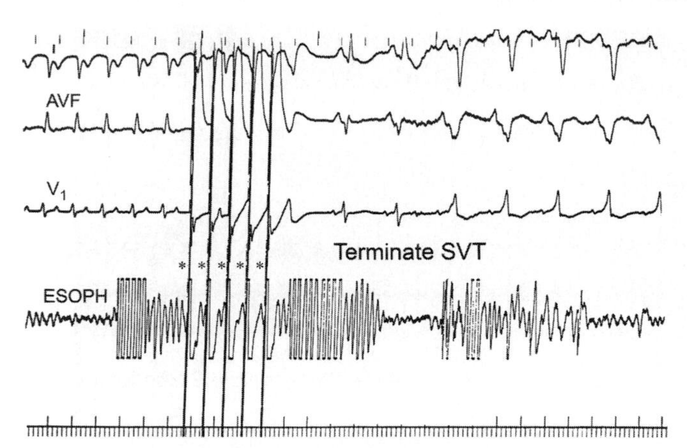

FIGURE 12–65 *Termination of supraventricular tachycardia with 5 beats of esophageal burst pacing in a patient with the Wolff-Parkinson-White syndrome. Note that full preexcitation returns after the second sinus beat.*
From Fyler DC. Nadas' Pediatric Cardiology. Philadelphia: Hanley & Belfus, 1992.

every type of arrhythmia in man. Electrophysiologic study (EPS) has also laid the groundwork for the use of transcatheter ablative techniques that have revolutionized tachycardia management in patients of all ages. Although diagnostic EPS and catheter ablation are usually combined in a single procedure in the current era (Fig. 12-66), this section focuses exclusively on diagnostic techniques, with discussion of ablation reserved for Chapter 29.

Equipment

The basic equipment needed to perform EPS includes an imaging system for catheter localization, an electrophysiologic recording system, and a stimulator for cardiac pacing.[35] Intracardiac electrograms are filtered and displayed on a multichannel recorder along with simultaneous surface ECG leads (most often I, aV_F, V_1, and V_6). The recording system is usually computerized with digital processing that allows for real-time analysis at various sweep speeds (anywhere from 25 to 400 mm/sec), along with freeze and playback, annotation, and digital storage of the recorded signals. Studies are performed in a cardiac catheterization laboratory using fluoroscopic imaging to guide catheter navigation. Nonfluoroscopic catheter navigation techniques are now being introduced to many laboratories that can decrease radiation exposure and create virtual electrical activation maps of the heart. The other essential requirements for EPS are standard resuscitation equipment, reliable defibrillation equipment, and most importantly, an experienced staff. The type of sedation utilized for EPS is based on the type of study, patient's age, and arrhythmia mechanism. General anesthesia is frequently used for children who are undergoing EPS combined with ablation, but conscious sedation is usually sufficient for purely diagnostic procedures in children.

Studies are performed with catheters ranging in size from 2 to 9 French. These are equipped with variable arrays of electrodes at the distal tip (Fig. 12-67) through which one can pace and record from various cardiac sites. Standard percutaneous techniques are used for vascular access. The number and types of catheters employed depend on the specific goals of the study, ranging from a single atrial catheter to induce supraventricular arrhythmias, to four or five catheters for a complete electrophysiologic survey of the heart. The standard pacing and recording sites are shown in Figure 12-68 and include the high right atrium, the bundle of His, the coronary sinus (CS), and the right ventricular apex.

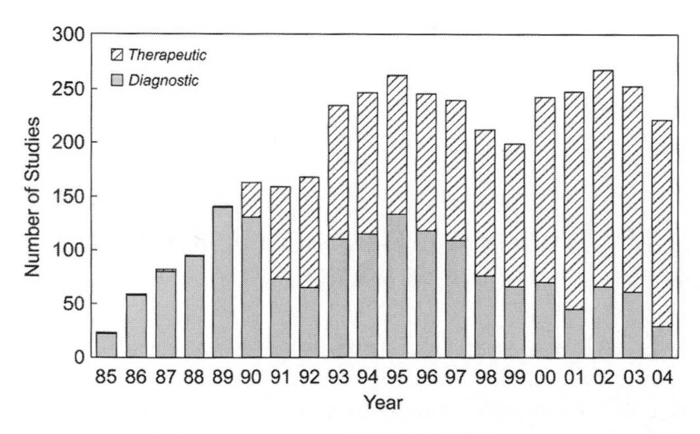

FIGURE 12–66 *The yearly numbers of invasive diagnostic and therapeutic intracardiac electrophysiology studies done at Children's Hospital Boston from 1985 to 2004. The percentage of purely diagnostic studies dropped from nearly 100% in the late 1980s to only 12% in 2004.*

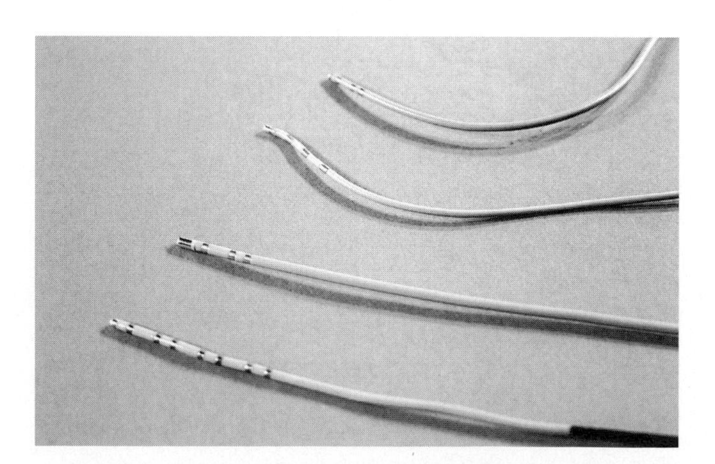

FIGURE 12–67 *Example of electrode catheters for intracardiac electrophysiologic study. Shown here (from top to bottom) are a 4 Fr quadripolar catheter, 5 Fr HBE catheter, 7 Fr deflectable quadripolar catheter with a 4-mm tip (used for ablation), and a 7 Fr deflectable octapolar catheter (used for coronary sinus recording).*

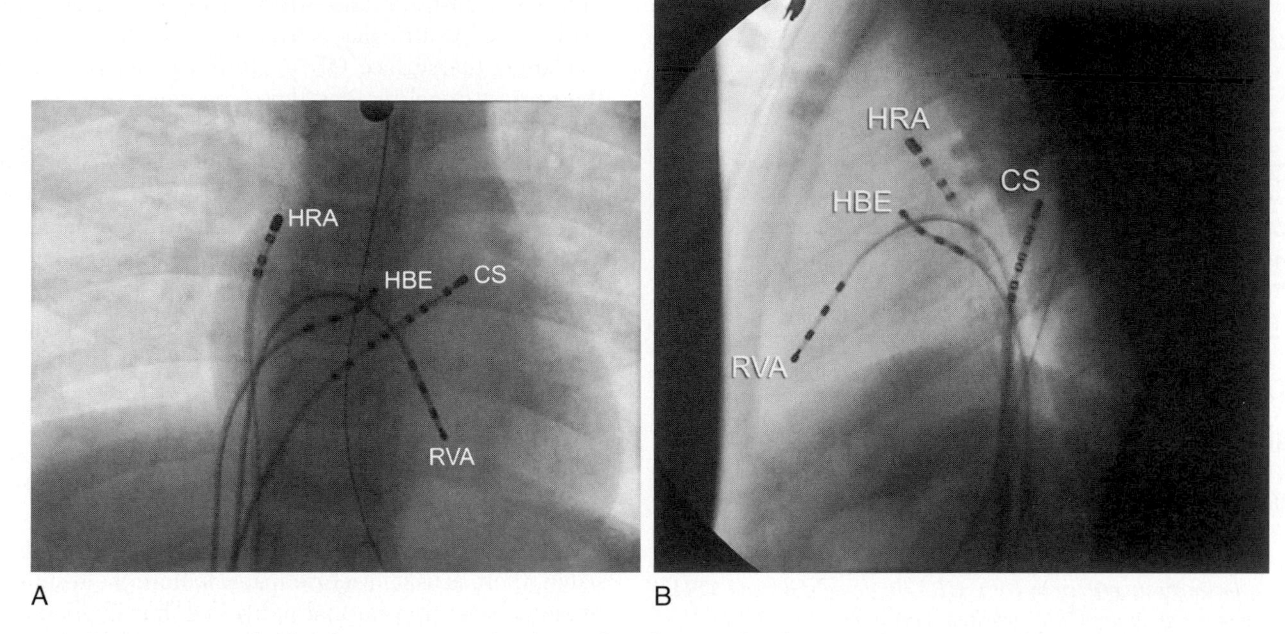

FIGURE 12–68 *Standard catheter positions for electrophysiologic study, shown in the AP (**A**) and lateral (**B**) fluoroscopic projections. HRA, high right atrium; HBE, His bundle electrogram; CS, coronary sinus; RVA, right ventricular apex.*

High Right Atrium

The high right atrium (HRA) site is located at the superior vena cava–right atrial junction, in close proximity to the SA node. Sometimes this catheter is placed in the right atrial appendage instead, to improve stability during long procedures and ablations. Right atrial pacing is used for assessing SA and AV node function, inducing supraventricular arrhythmias, and on rare occasions, inducing idiopathic ventricular tachycardias.

His Bundle Electrogram

The His bundle electrogram (HBE) is obtained by positioning the catheter just across the tricuspid valve at its medial and superior rim, near the area of the common bundle of His. Because the catheter straddles the valve ring, it records local right atrial depolarization and local right ventricular depolarization, along with a distinct His deflection. The HBE dissects AV conduction into AV node and His-Purkinje components. It is a crucial recording site for analysis of AV conduction disturbances and for determining the supraventricular origin of an arrhythmia.

Coronary Sinus

A catheter in the CS records both atrial and ventricular signals from the left heart. This electrode is usually positioned from a femoral vein approach using a tip-deflecting mechanism built into the catheter shaft. If CS entry proves difficult, a CS angiogram may be performed to guide electrophysiologic catheter placement. Occasionally, a large Eustachian ridge guards the CS ostium, and a superior approach is needed. This can be accomplished through the right internal jugular vein, subclavian vein, or brachial vein. The CS catheter is mandatory for evaluation of SVT, particularly if an accessory pathway is suspected.

Right Ventricular Apex

The right ventricular apex (RVA) provides a stable site for ventricular pacing and recording. It is used during evaluation of SVT to examine retrograde conduction, as well as for the study of ventricular arrhythmias. An additional ventricular pacing site in the right ventricular outflow tract (RVOT) may be included in some cases.

DIAGNOSTIC MANEUVERS

Diagnostic EPS involves three general categories of data: (1) baseline rhythm, (2) pacing maneuvers to evaluate functional characteristics, and (3) programmed stimulation with a series of premature beats to initiate tachycardias. A comprehensive EPS will involve systematic collection of all these items, as outlined below.

Baseline Recording

Resting rhythm is examined to determine conduction times and activation sequence throughout the heart (Fig. 12-69). In normal sinus rhythm, the HRA catheter is

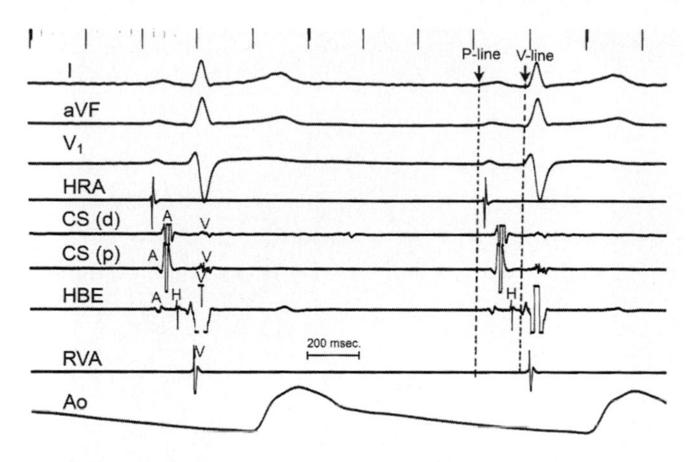

FIGURE 12–69 *Baseline signals during sinus rhythm, including three surface ECG leads, along with multiple intracardiac recordings. Atrial activation is indexed against a P line and shows earliest intracardiac activation in HRA near the sinus node. Ventricular activation is indexed against the V line, and normally shows the earliest activity in RVA. HRA, high right atrium; CSd, distal coronary sinus; CSp, proximal coronary sinus; HBE, His bundle electrogram; RVA, right ventricular apex; Ao, arterial blood pressure.*
From Fyler DC. Nadas' Pediatric Cardiology. Philadelphia: Hanley & Belfus, 1992.

the first to register electrical activity by virtue of its close proximity to the SA node, followed by the low right atrium (first signal on HBE catheter) 20 to 25 msec later, and finally the lateral left atrium (first signal on distal CS catheter) after about 60 msec. Ectopic foci or other supraventricular arrhythmias will shift the atrial activation sequence in favor of the site of origin of the abnormal rhythm.

Conduction time within the AV node may be determined by measuring the AH interval of the HBE recording. The normal AH interval varies between 40 and 100 msec in children. A prolonged AH interval can be observed in patients taking certain antiarrhythmic drugs, those with high vagal tone, and those with disease of the AV node. It is shortened under conditions of high circulating catecholamines.

The HV interval, representing conduction time in the His-Purkinje system, is also recorded by the HBE catheter and should be between 35 and 55 msec in normal children. Prolonged resting HV intervals usually suggest His-Purkinje pathology. A short HV may be observed in the preexcitation syndromes, including WPW syndrome and Mahaim fibers.

The final baseline measurements come from regional ventricular activation times. The standard catheter positions provide ventricular activation from three locations, including the apex of the right ventricle (RVA catheter), right ventricular inflow (last signal on HBE catheter), and left ventricular base (last signal on CS catheter). Measurements are indexed against a V line, which is marked at the earliest evidence of ventricular activation in any recording lead (including the surface QRS). Normally, the RVA displays the earliest signals among these recording sites, about 10 to 35 msec after onset of the QRS. Block in the central right bundle branch can cause delayed RVA activation (more than 50 msec). In WPW syndrome, preexcitation through a right-sided accessory pathway may promote early activation of the right ventricular inflow area, or conversely, a left-sided pathway may cause the left ventricular base along the CS to activate ahead of schedule.

Functional Characteristics of the SA Node

The principal maneuver used to evaluate SA node status during EPS is the *sinus node recovery time* (SNRT). This involves pacing the HRA for 30 to 60 seconds at rates above resting rhythm. When pacing is abruptly terminated, there is usually a brief pause before the resumption of sinus beats in a normal individual, but if the pause is protracted, SA node dysfunction is suggested. The recovery time is usually "corrected" by subtracting the resting cycle length (i.e., the time between two normal sinus beats) from the recovery cycle length (i.e., the time from the last paced beat to the first spontaneous sinus beat) to yield a corrected sinus node recovery time (CSNRT). Normal values for CSNRT should be less than about 275 msec for children.[36] When there is advanced disease of the SA node, the abnormal SNRT is usually quite blatant (Fig. 12-70).

Functional Characteristics of the AV Node

The most straightforward technique for evaluation of AV conduction involves short bursts of pacing in the HRA

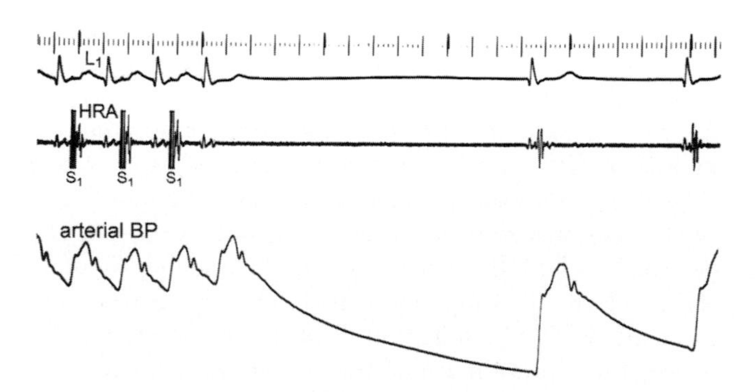

FIGURE 12–70 *An example of prolonged sinus node recovery. After 60 sec of pacing (S_1) in HRA at a rate of 150 beats/min (cycle length, 150 msec), pacing abruptly terminated. There is a pause of nearly 3.0 sec before a junctional escape beat restores the rhythm. HRA, high right atrium.*
From Fyler DC. Nadas' Pediatric Cardiology. Philadelphia: Hanley & Belfus, 1992.

while observing the ventricular response. The pacing cycle length is decreased in 10-msec steps until a rate is encountered at which the Wenckebach phenomenon occurs. For normal children, Wenckebach is not usually observed until the pacing cycle length has been decreased to less than about 350 msec (i.e., rate faster than 171 beats/min).

More precise evaluation of the AV node is performed with the introduction of single premature beats at the HRA, delivered at an interval that is progressively shortened in 10-msec steps (Fig. 12-71). As the stimulus is moved earlier, a gradual and progressive increase in the A-H interval is seen related to the normal decremental properties of the slow response cells in the AV node. Eventually, a stimulus can be delivered early enough to block at the AV node. This registers on the HBE electrogram as an atrial signal without a His or ventricular deflection. The premature interval at which this conduction fails to occur is defined as the ERP for the AV node and normally ranges from 240 to 320 msec in children. As the stimulus timing is adjusted to a shorter coupling interval, a point will eventually be reached at which the atrial tissue no longer depolarizes. This is designated the atrial muscle ERP and is encountered between 170 and 240 msec in normal children.

Functional Characteristics of His-Purkinje Conduction

Function of the His-Purkinje system may likewise be evaluated with the single extrastimulus technique. Normally, the HV interval tends to remain constant, and the QRS complex tends to remain narrow during premature atrial stimulation. Some patients may develop QRS aberration due to rate-related bundle branch block in response to early beats, but this is usually a benign finding. More significant is the observation of block in the bundle of His in response to an early stimulus, which registers on the HBE as an atrial signal followed by a His deflection, but without conduction to the ventricles. When the ERP of the common bundle of His is encountered ahead of the AV node ERP in a young patient, His-Purkinje disease may be suggested.

Functional Characteristics of Ventricular Tissue

The ERP can also be measured for ventricular muscle, using the single extrastimulus technique. This information is most useful during the study of ventricular arrhythmias, when one might wish to compare baseline conditions to the alteration in ERP related to antiarrhythmic drugs. The longest premature interval at which a stimulus fails to capture the ventricular arrhythmia is defined as the ventricular muscle ERP, and normally occurs at 180 to 260 msec. Ventricular stimulation is also used to evaluate the pattern of retrograde conduction to the atrium.

Evaluation of Supraventricular Tachycardia

Many patients with SVT can be managed without a formal EPS. However, if the arrhythmia has been refractory to first-line management or is associated with serious

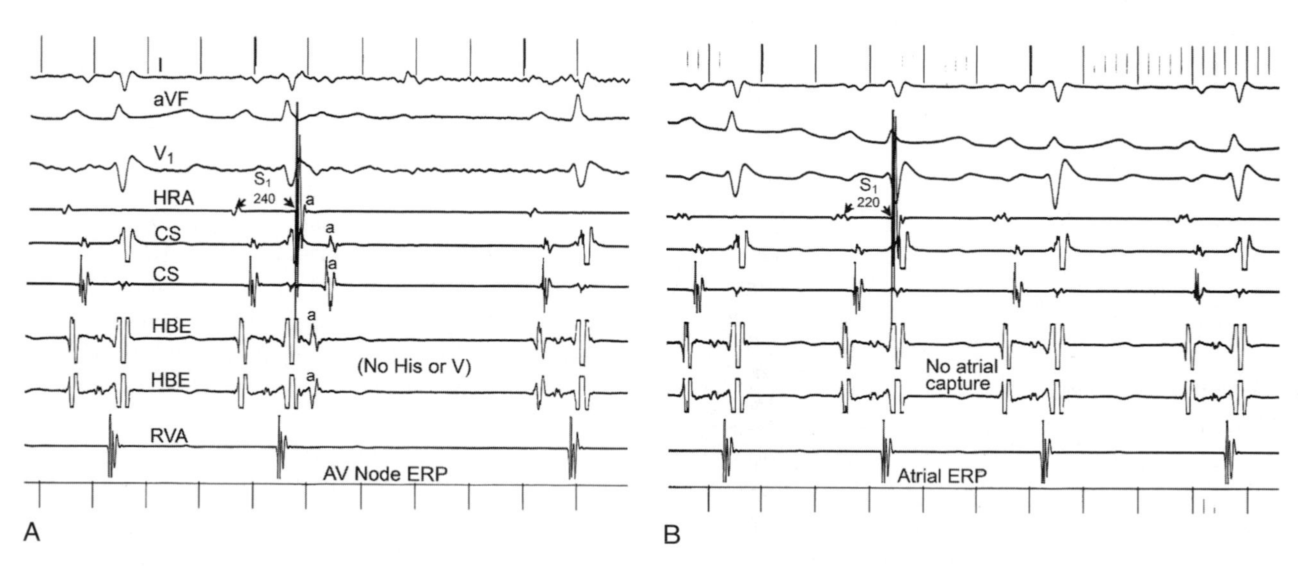

FIGURE 12–71 *The effective refractory periods of the AV node (**A**) and atrial muscle (**B**). In panel **A**, the premature beat captures the atrium but blocks at the AV node such that no His bundle signal is seen. In **B**, a slightly earlier beat fails to capture the atrium entirely. HRA, high right atrium; CS, coronary sinus; HBE, His bundle electrogram; RVA, right ventricular apex. From Fyler DC. Nadas' Pediatric Cardiology. Philadelphia: Hanley & Belfus, 1992.*

symptoms, an intracardiac EPS is usually indicated to determine the mechanism and to map the substrate with a view toward catheter ablation.

Studies for SVT require catheters at the four standard recording sites. Resting rhythm is first examined for the atrial activation pattern and any evidence of preexcitation. A routine evaluation of the functional status of the entire conducting system is then performed as described previously. During these maneuvers, or with more aggressive stimulation, SVT may be induced.

There is a long list of mechanisms for pediatric SVT (see Chapter 29), but as a starting point, one may divide them into the broad categories of *automatic foci* or *reentry* circuits. The automatic variety tend to occur spontaneously or in response to increased catecholamine levels but generally are not induced or terminated with pacing techniques. Reentry, by far the more common mechanism in children, is easily induced by carefully timed premature beats during EPS and can usually be interrupted by overdrive pacing.

Mapping of SVT begins by determining whether the AV node and ventricle are critical components of the disorder. Those forms of SVT that arise from within atrial muscle *(primary atrial SVT)* usually display intermittent block at the AV node that does not modify the atrial rate. By comparison, tachycardias with a fixed 1:1 AV relationship *(AV reciprocating SVT)* terminate promptly whenever this ratio is disturbed. The latter is typical behavior for SVT owing to accessory pathways, as well as for most cases of AV node reentry.

Precision mapping of an arrhythmia location is possible with attention to the atrial activation sequence during SVT. Localization of both automatic foci (Fig. 12-72) and accessory pathways (Fig. 12-73) is accomplished by carefully noting the site of the earliest atrial signal.

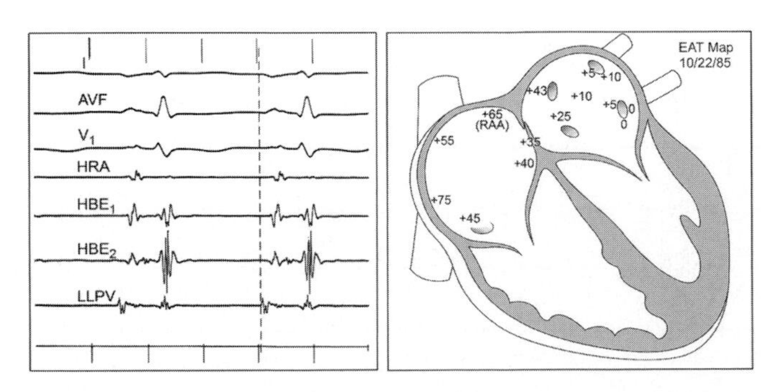

FIGURE 12–72 *An example of atrial activation sequence mapping in a patient with ectopic atrial tachycardia. The earliest atrial activity was found mapping near the left lower pulmonary vein (LLPV). HBE, His bundle electrogram; HRA, high right atrium.* *From Fyler DC. Nadas' Pediatric Cardiology. Philadelphia: Hanley & Belfus, 1992.*

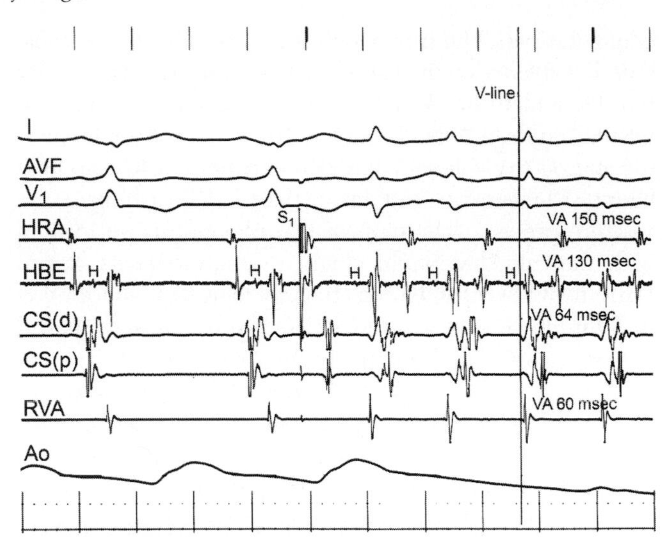

FIGURE 12–73 *Mapping during orthodromic reentrant tachycardia in Wolff-Parkinson-White syndrome. Tachycardia is induced with a single premature beat (S_1) that conducts to the ventricle over the AV node and returns to the atrium through the accessory pathway. The shortest VA time (i.e., the earliest retrograde signal) is seen in the proximal coronary sinus, corresponding to a left-sided accessory pathway. HRA, high right atrium; CSd, distal coronary sinus; CSp, proximal coronary sinus; HBE, His bundle electrogram; RVA, right ventricular apex; Ao, arterial blood pressure.* *From Fyler DC. Nadas' Pediatric Cardiology. Philadelphia: Hanley & Belfus, 1992.*

Evaluation of Ventricular Arrhythmias

Ventricular stimulation studies are performed with three major goals in mind. First, some tachyarrhythmias that appear to be ventricular tachycardia (VT) because of a wide QRS on surface ECG are actually SVT with aberration or preexcitation. Because the prognosis and treatment differ so drastically for SVT and VT, EPS is usually indicated to establish the exact mechanism whenever uncertainty exists. Second, EPS can be used to help elucidate the mechanism and location of a patient's VT, which can assist the clinician in choosing among drug therapy, ablation, or an implantable defibrillator for long-term management. Finally, programmed stimulation can sometimes be used as a tool for stratifying a patient's risk for spontaneous VT by observing the patient's response to a standard ventricular pacing protocol.[37]

A complete VT study begins with baseline recording from at least three sites, including the HRA, HBE, and RVA. Atrial stimulation is then performed to evaluate functional characteristics of the conducting system and to rule out atypical SVT as the cause of the clinical arrhythmia. A ventricular stimulation protocol is then carried out in an attempt to induce VT. Protocols for ventricular stimulation vary, and it must be remembered that a point can be reached at which the stimulation becomes so provocative that an induced arrhythmia is nonspecific and bears little resemblance to the clinical tachycardia. Additionally, some forms of VT may involve a mechanism other than classic reentry, and normal stimulation techniques may be unsuccessful in reproducing the disorder. At most centers, ventricular stimulation studies usually involve the following protocol:

1. Stimulation at the RVA with an 8-beat drive train ($S_1 \times 8$) followed by one or more extrastimuli (S_n) delivered at progressively premature intervals (shortened in 10-msec decrements) until local ventricular muscle is refractory
   a. Single premature beats following 8 beats of ventricular pacing ($S_1 \times 8$, S_2) using at least two different cycle lengths for S_1 (usually 600, 500, or 400 msec)
   b. Double premature beats following 8 beats of pacing ($S_1 \times 8$, S_2, S_3) using at least two different cycle lengths for S_1
   c. Triple premature beats following 8 beats of ventricular pacing ($S_1 \times 8$, S_2, S_3, S_4) using at least two different cycle lengths for S_1
2. Stimulation at a second site, usually the RVOT, with an identical sequence
3. Repetition of RVA and RVOT stimulation during isoproterenol infusion
4. Optional additions to the protocol:
   a. The standard sequence at a third site such as the left ventricular apex
   b. Stimulation with four premature beats ($S_1 \times 8$, S_2, S_3, S_4, S_5)
   c. Burst ventricular pacing at progressively rapid rates

The possible responses to ventricular stimulation are shown in Figure 12-74. Whenever sustained arrhythmias are induced and result in hemodynamic compromise, the team must react quickly to terminate the condition. For monomorphic VT, this can often be accomplished with a short burst of overdrive pacing in the ventricle (Fig. 12-75), but rapid polymorphic VT or ventricular fibrillation needs to be terminated promptly with a DC shock.

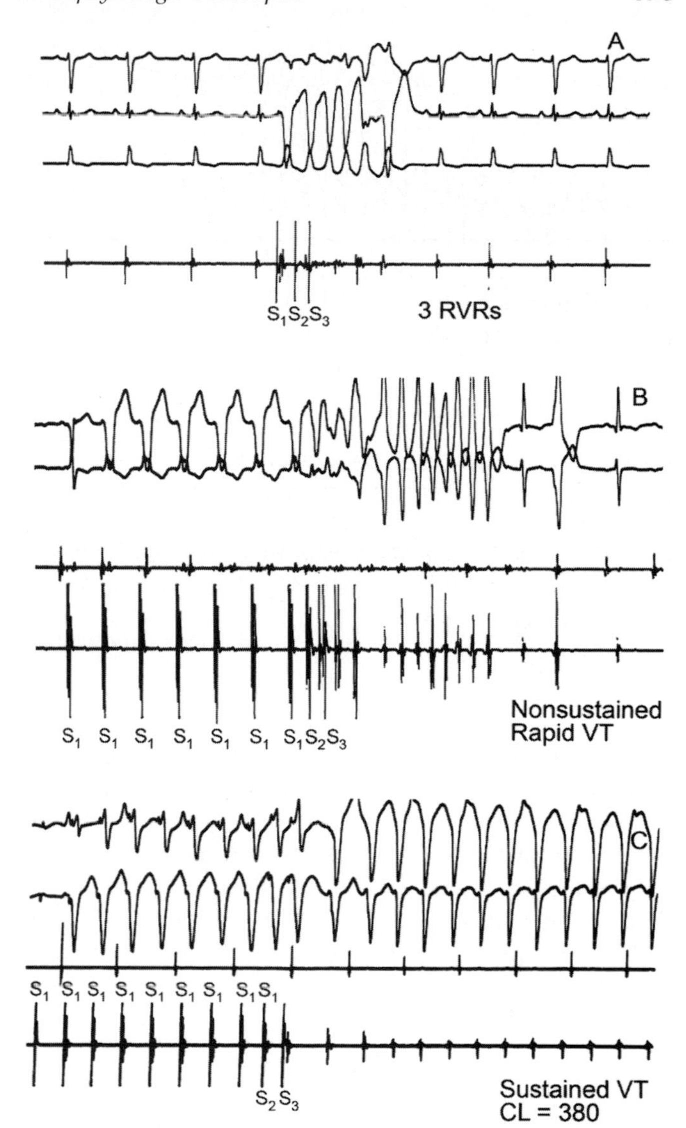

FIGURE 12–74 *Examples of possible responses to ventricular programmed stimulation.* ***A****, Repetitive ventricular responses (RVRs).* ***B****, Nonsustained ventricular tachycardia.* ***C****, Sustained ventricular tachycardia.*
From Fyler DC. Nadas' Pediatric Cardiology. Philadelphia: Hanley & Belfus, 1992.

Ancillary Tests

During investigation of select ventricular arrhythmias, the EPS procedure may be coupled with hemodynamic assessment, angiography, endomyocardial biopsy, voltage mapping, and drug challenges. Hemodynamic data may reveal abnormalities not apparent on echocardiography, such as pulmonary hypertension or restrictive cardiomyopathy. Angiography may be indicated to delineate coronary anomalies, ventricular morphologic changes, and chamber aneurysms. When new-onset cardiomyopathy or myocarditis is suspected, an endomyocardial biopsy is useful to confirm the diagnosis. Voltage mapping is a relatively new procedure during which automated measurements of local electrogram voltage from one or both ventricular chambers is displayed on a virtual three-dimensional cardiac chamber map. Areas of very low voltage may correspond to scar or diseased myocardium. This technique may help in the diagnosis of certain cardiomyopathies, including arrhythmogenic right ventricular dysplasia. Finally, provocative drug challenges with adenosine, catecholamines,

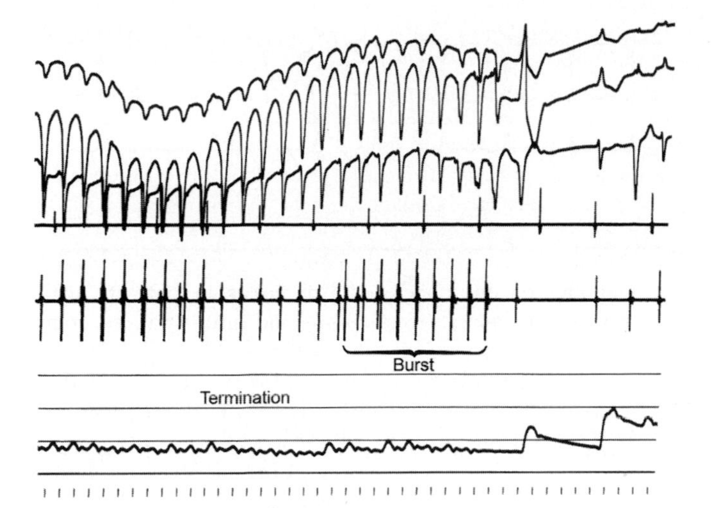

FIGURE 12–75 *Termination of an induced episode of sustained monomorphic ventricular tachycardia with burst pacing during electrophysiologic testing.*
From Fyler DC. Nadas' Pediatric Cardiology. Philadelphia: Hanley & Belfus, 1992.

or procainamide can uncover certain underlying electrical abnormalities. Adenosine is useful to expose cryptic preexcitation during sinus rhythm or to reveal the presence of a unidirectional retrograde accessory pathway during ventricular pacing. An isoproterenol infusion is frequently used to induce various types of catecholamine-sensitive VT. Procainamide infusion can be used to uncover evidence of certain membrane channelopathies, such as Brugada syndrome.

REFERENCES

1. Lewis T. The Mechanisms and Graphic Registration of the Heart Beat [preface]. London: Shaw and Sons, 1925:vi.
2. Nadas AS. Electrocardiography. In Pediatric Cardiology. Philadelphia: WB Saunders, 1957:42.
3. Garson A. Recording the sequence of cardiac activity. In The Electrocardiogram in Infants and Children. Philadelphia: Lea & Febiger, 1983:19–48.
4. Gilmore RF, Zipes DP. Cellular basis for cardiac arrhythmias. Cardiol Clin 1:3, 1983.
5. Plonsey R. The biophysical basis for electrocardiography. In Liebman J, Plonsey R, Gillette RC (eds). Pediatric Electrocardiography. Baltimore: Williams & Wilkins, 1982:1–14.
6. Zipes DP. Genesis of cardiac arrhythmias: Electrophysiological considerations. In Braunwald E (ed). Heart Disease. Philadelphia: WB Saunders, 1984:605–620.
7. Mullen MP, VanPraagh R, Walsh EP. Development and anatomy of the cardiac conduction system. In Walsh EP, Saul JP, Triedman JK (eds). Cardiac Arrhythmias in Children and Young Adults with Congenital Heart Disease. Philadelphia: Lippincott Williams & Wilkins, 2001:93–111.
8. Davignon A, Rautaharju PM, Boisselle E, et al. Normal ECG standards for infants and children. Pediatr Cardiol 1:123, 1979.
9. Garson A. Chamber enlargement and hypertrophy. In The Electrocardiogram in Infants and Children. Philadelphia: Lea & Febiger, 1983:99–118.
10. Fisch C. Electrocardiography and vectocardiography. In Braunwald E (ed). Heart Disease. Philadelphia: WB Saunders, 1984:200–222.
11. Arruda MS, McClelland JH, Wang X, et al. Development and validation of an ECG algorithm for identifying accessory pathway ablation site in Wolff-Parkinson-White syndrome. J Cardiovasc Electrophysiol 9:2, 1998.
12. Fitzpatrick AP, Gonzales RP, Lesh MD, et al. New algorithm for the localization of accessory atrioventricular connections using a baseline electrocardiogram. J Am Coll Cardiol 23:107, 1994.
13. Klein LS, Hackett FK, Zipes DP, et al. Radiofrequency catheter ablation of Mahaim fibers at the tricuspid annulus. Circulation 87:738, 1993.
14. Nasir K, Bomma C, Tandri H, et al. Electrocardiographic features of arrhythmogenic right ventricular dysplasia/cardiomyopathy according to disease severity: a need to broaden diagnostic criteria. Circulation 110:1527, 2004.
15. Schwartz PJ, Priori SG, Spazzolini C, et al. Genotype-phenotype correlation in the long-QT syndrome: Gene-specific triggers for life-threatening arrhythmias. Circulation 103:89, 2001.
16. Brugada J, Brugada P. Further characterization of the syndrome of right bundle branch block, ST segment elevation, and sudden cardiac death. J Cardiovasc Electrophysiol 8:325, 1997.
17. Gaita F, Giustetto C, Bianchi F, et al. Short QT syndrome: Pharmacological treatment. J Am Coll Cardiol 43:1494, 2004.
18. Saarel EV, Stefanelli CB, Fischbach PS, et al. Transtelephonic electrocardiographic monitors for evaluation of children and adolescents with suspected arrhythmias. Pediatrics 113:248, 2004.
19. Karpawich PP, Gillette PC, Garson A Jr, et al. Congenital complete atrioventricular block: Clinical and electrophysiologic predictors of need for pacemaker insertion. Am J Cardiol 48:1098, 1981.
20. Weigel TJ, Porter CJ, Mottram CD, et al. Detecting arrhythmia by exercise electrocardiography in pediatric patients: Assessment of sensitivity and influence on clinical management. Mayo Clin Proc 66:379, 1991.
21. Leenhardt A, Lucet V, Denjoy I, et al. Catecholaminergic polymorphic ventricular tachycardia in children: A 7-year follow-up of 21 patients. Circulation 91:1512, 1995.
22. Takenaka K, Ai T, Shimizu W, et al. Exercise stress test amplifies genotype-phenotype correlation in the LQT1 and LQT2 forms of the long-QT syndrome. Circulation 107:838, 2003.
23. Gaita F, Giustetto C, Riccardi R, et al. Stress test and pharmacologic tests as methods to identify patients with Wolff-Parkinson-White syndrome at risk of sudden death. Am J Cardiol 64:487, 1989.
24. Salim MA, Ware LE, Barnard M, et al. Syncope recurrence in children: Relation to tilt-test results. Pediatrics 102:924, 1998.

25. Stewart JM, Gewitz MH, Weldon A, et al. Patterns of orthostatic intolerance: The orthostatic tachycardia syndrome and adolescent chronic fatigue. J Pediatr 135:218, 1999.
26. Ross BA, Hughes S, Anderson E, et al. Abnormal responses to orthostatic testing in children and adolescents with recurrent unexplained syncope. Am Heart J 122:748, 1991.
27. de jong-de Vos van Steenwijk CC, Wieling W, Johannes JM, et al. Incidence and hemodynamic characteristics of near-fainting in healthy 6- to 16- year old subjects. J Am Coll Cardiol 25:1615, 1995.
28. Lewis DA, Zlotocha J, Henke L, et al. Specificity of head-up tilt testing in adolescents: Effect of various degrees of tilt challenge in normal control subjects. J Am Coll Cardiol 30:1057, 1997.
29. Davis AM, McCrindle BW, Hamilton RM, et al. Normal values for the childhood signal-averaged ECG. Pacing Clin Electrophysiol 19:793, 1996.
30. Breirhardt G, Borggrefe M. Recent advances in the identification of patients at risk of ventricular tachyarrhythmias: role of ventricular late potentials. Circulation 75:1091,1987.
31. Bloomfield DM, Steinman RC, Namerow PB, et al. Microvolt T-wave alternans distinguishes between patients likely and patients not likely to benefit from implanted cardiac defibrillator therapy: A solution to the Multicenter Automatic Defibrillator Implantation Trial (MADIT) II conundrum. Circulation 110:1885, 2004.
32. Benson DW, Dunnigan A, Benditt DG, et al. Transesophageal cardiac pacing: History, application, technique. Clin Prog Pacing Electrophysiol 2:360, 1984.
33. Scherlag BJ, Lau SH, Helfant RA, et al. Catheter technique for recording His bundle activity in man. Circulation 39:13, 1969.
34. Triedman JK, Alexander ME, Berul CI, et al. Electroanatomic mapping of entrained and exit zones in patients with repaired congenital heart disease and intra-atrial reentrant tachycardia. Circulation 103:2060, 2001.
35. Pass RH, Walsh EP. Intracardiac electrophysiologic testing in pediatric patients. In Walsh EP, Saul JP, Triedman JK (eds). Cardiac Arrhythmias in Children and Young Adults with Congenital Heart Disease. Philadelphia: Lippincott Williams & Wilkins, 2001:57–94.
36. Yabek SM, Jarmakani JM, Roberts NK. Sinus node function in children: Factors influencing its evaluation. Circulation 53:28, 1976.
37. Alexander ME, Walsh EP, Saul JP, et al. Value of programmed ventricular stimulation in patients with congenital heart disease. J Cardiovasc Electrophysiol. 10:1033, 1999.

13

Imaging Techniques: Echocardiography, Magnetic Resonance Imaging, and Computerized Tomography

TAL GEVA, MD AND MARY E. VAN DER VELDE

Diagnostic imaging of the cardiovascular system has evolved dramatically over the past several decades. Until the advent of cardiac ultrasound in the 1970s, cardiac catheterization and angiography were the principle methods used to image the heart and great vessels. During the second half of the 1970s, M-mode echocardiography—the first generation of cardiac ultrasound—provided limited anatomic information insufficient to replace angiography in most patients with congenital heart disease (CHD). During the 1980s, however, the rapid evolution of two-dimensional (2D) echocardiography transformed the field. Advances in transducer design, image processing and display, and development of novel imaging planes allowed accurate and complete diagnosis of complex congenital defects with increasingly high-quality images.[1–4] The introduction of Doppler ultrasound to investigate blood flow added the ability to perform comprehensive hemodynamic assessment. By the mid to late 1980s, much of the necessary anatomic and hemodynamic information required for patient management could be obtained noninvasively, eliminating the need for diagnostic catheterization in many patients. In the 1990s, further advances in the field of pediatric cardiac imaging included three-dimensional (3D) echocardiography and the application of magnetic resonance imaging (MRI) to CHD. By the end of the 1990s, cardiac catheterization assumed an increasingly therapeutic (as opposed to diagnostic) role in pediatric patients. More recently, the advent of multidetector computed tomography has further expanded the arsenal of noninvasive imaging tools. This chapter reviews the principles and clinical application of the major noninvasive diagnostic imaging modalities used to evaluate congenital and acquired heart disease in pediatric patients: echocardiography, cardiovascular magnetic resonance imaging (CMR), and cardiovascular computed tomography (CCT).

ECHOCARDIOGRAPHY AND DOPPLER ULTRASOUND

Echocardiographic examination provides extensive anatomic and hemodynamic information noninvasively, in real time, and at relatively low cost. Current imaging systems can easily be relocated to the intensive care unit, operating room, or catheterization laboratory as needed; newer handheld systems provide easy portability and reasonably good image quality. Table 13-1 summarizes some of the common indications for echocardiography.

Technical Background

The imaging surface of an ultrasound transducer is comprised of multiple electronic elements containing piezoelectric crystals. When excited by an electrical impulse sent from a pulse generator, the molecules within the crystal vibrate, producing an ultrasound wave that travels through soft tissue at approximately 1540 m/second. When the ultrasound wave encounters an interface between tissues with different acoustic properties (e.g, blood and myocardium), a portion of the ultrasound energy is reflected back to the

TABLE 13–1. Common Indications for Echocardiography in Pediatric Patients

Congenital heart disease (known or suspected)
Kawasaki disease
Rheumatic heart disease
Primary or secondary cardiomyopathy
Cardiotoxic medications (such as anthracycline chemotherapy)
Pericardial disease or effusion
Suspected endocarditis
Persistent pulmonary hypertension of the newborn
Primary pulmonary hypertension
Cerebrovascular infarct (embolic)
Chest pain
Syncope
Rhythm and conduction abnormalities
Genetic syndromes and multiple congenital anomalies
Cardiac and paracardiac tumors
Arteriovenous malformations (high-output state)

transducer and the remainder continues forward until it encounters the next tissue interface. Returning ultrasound energy absorbed by the piezoelectric crystals is converted into electrical energy, which then goes through a series of electronic processes, including amplification, filtering, post-processing, and display. The distance of a reflecting surface from the transducer is calculated on the basis of the time it takes the energy to reach the structure and return to the transducer. This information then determines the location of dots representing that structure on a display screen. This process is repeated approximately 1000 times per second (1000 Hz) to create an image.

When directed at a highly reflective tissue such as air-filled lung, bone, or scar tissue, most or all of the ultrasound energy is reflected back and structures beyond the reflective interface cannot be imaged. Images are obtained via various acoustic *windows*, which provide relatively unimpeded access to the heart and vessels. Standard echocardiographic windows and views are described in a subsequent section.

The diagnostic quality of echocardiographic images depends on multiple factors, many of which can be adjusted by the operator, including spatial (axial and lateral), temporal, and contrast resolution.[4] Axial resolution distinguishes as separate two adjacent points along the axis of the ultrasound beam, and lateral resolution distinguishes between two adjacent points on a line perpendicular to the beam. Temporal resolution distinguishes sequential events from each other (for assessment of moving targets), and contrast resolution distinguishes differences in tissue density. The degree of resolution is determined by, among other factors, the frequency of the ultrasound wave, its width, transducer size and shape, focus, transmit and receive gains, and the depth of the image. Modern ultrasound transducers provide a wide range of frequencies that can be adjusted to optimize image quality in patients with widely differing body sizes and acoustic windows.

M-Mode Echocardiography

M-mode echocardiography provides an *ice pick* view of the heart in real time, demonstrating tissue interfaces at varying distances along a single narrow line or beam on the *y*-axis, and time on the *x*-axis (Fig. 13-1). This spatially one-dimensional image of the heart is characterized by excellent temporal and axial resolutions but provides limited anatomic information. Having been replaced by 2D echo imaging, M-mode is no longer practical for anatomic imaging of the heart, but is used primarily for evaluation of left ventricular dimensions and function. When superior temporal resolution is required, 2D-directed M-mode may be useful for assessing motion of certain structures such as native and prosthetic valve leaflets.

Two-Dimensional Echocardiography

In current clinical practice, 2D echocardiography is the primary tool for anatomic imaging. The ultrasound beam is swept rapidly in an arc, creating multiple linear M-mode images, which are then aligned sequentially to create a cross-sectional image of the heart (Fig. 13-2). Mechanical transducers rotate or rock the ultrasound crystal, while phased array transducers electronically sweep the beam through multiple piezoelectric crystals. Individual lines within the 2D image are constructed at a rate termed the "pulse repetition frequency" (PRF).[5] The speed of ultrasound in tissue and the depth of the image, in turn, govern the pulse repetition rate. Compared with adults, the shorter

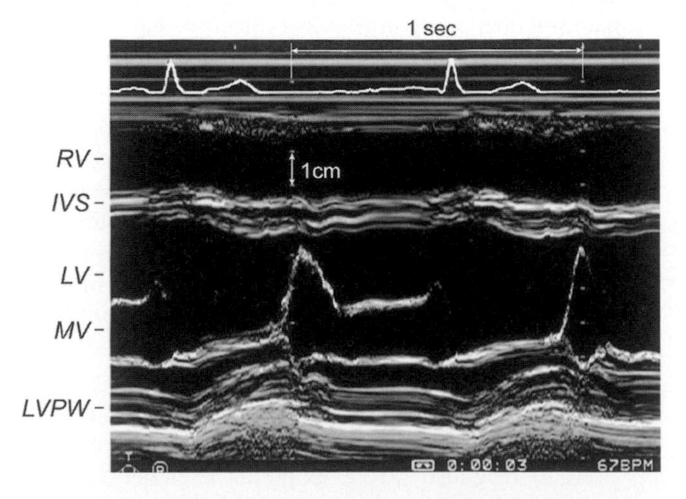

FIGURE 13–1 *M-mode tracing of the ventricles. IVS, interventricular septum; LV, left ventricle; LVPW, left ventricular posterior wall; MV, mitral valve; RV, right ventricle.*

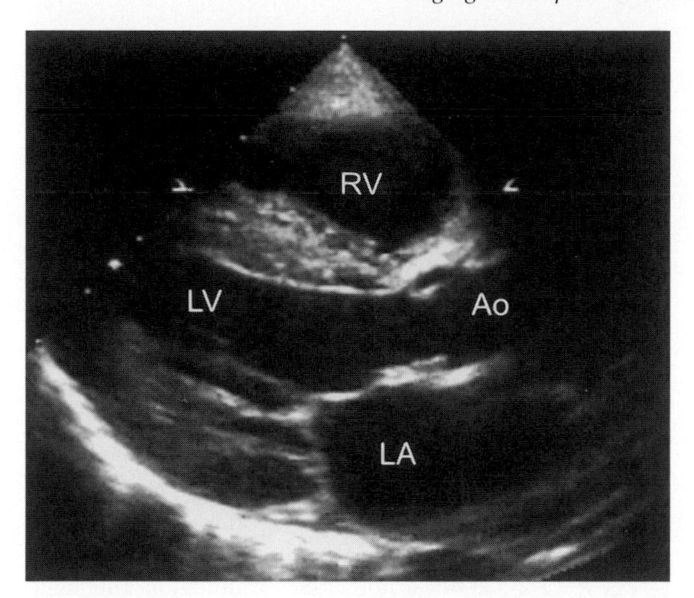

FIGURE 13–2 *Two-dimensional echocardiogram in the parasternal long-axis view. Ao, aorta; LA, left atrium; LV, left ventricle; RV, right ventricle.*

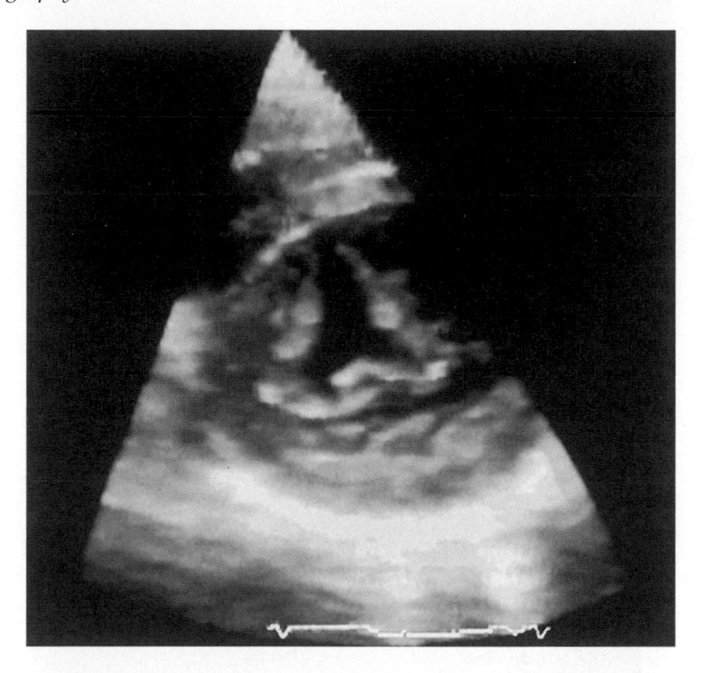

FIGURE 13–3 *Three-dimensional echocardiogram. Diastolic frame showing a cleft anterior mitral leaflet in a patient with primum atrial septal defect.*

distance between the transducer and the heart in infants and children allows higher pulse repetition frequency and results in better image quality. PRF influences frame rate, which is an important determinant of temporal resolution and is a vital contributor to good image quality in pediatric patients with their relatively rapid heart rates. Recent advances such as parallel processing allow very high frame rates (>200 Hz), greatly enhancing temporal resolution.[6]

Three-Dimensional Echocardiography

An experienced examiner or observer can mentally construct a 3D image of the heart from serial 2D tomographic echocardiographic images obtained by sweeping the transducer across the chest. Three-dimensional echocardiography provides an alternative means of displaying echocardiographically obtained information about cardiovascular structures and their interrelations, and may give a clearer picture of the anatomy for those less familiar with 2D imaging. Early 3D echo imaging was based on computer reconstruction of contiguous 2D cross-sectional images, and was hampered by difficulties in accurately registering the ultrasound image data in time and space and by long image processing time. Development of gating techniques, improved computer technology and software, and refinement of the user interface have resulted in shorter acquisition and reconstruction times and improved image quality.[7] The introduction of real-time 3D echocardiography (RT-3DE) allows the technology to complement, and enhances its potential to eventually replace 2D echocardiography, in clinical practice. RT-3DE sends and receives a pyramidal set of ultrasound energy data from several thousand piezoelectric transducer elements, producing a 3D image using parallel image processing techniques (Fig. 13-3).[7,8] Although spatial and temporal resolution of current RT-3DE technology are still somewhat limited, given the rapid evolution of the technology, image quality is certain to approach that of 2D echo in the near future.

Doppler Echocardiography

Doppler ultrasound assessment of normal and abnormal hemodynamics is a fundamental part of the echocardiographic examination.[2–4] Two-dimensional–guided Doppler interrogation has greatly enhanced the clinical utility of this technology, allowing evaluation of flow characteristics virtually anywhere within the heart and great vessels. Spectral and color-coded Doppler flow mapping are routinely used to measure velocity and direction of blood flow in healthy and diseased hearts (Fig. 13-4). Doppler-derived calculations provide quantitative estimation of flow (such as stroke volume and cardiac output), pressure gradients, cross-sectional flow area, and prediction of intracardiac pressures. Doppler technology also allows qualitative and semiquantitative assessment of valve regurgitation, intra- and extracardiac shunts, and myocardial motion (tissue Doppler imaging).

Doppler technology is based on the knowledge that when a propagated sound wave encounters a moving target,

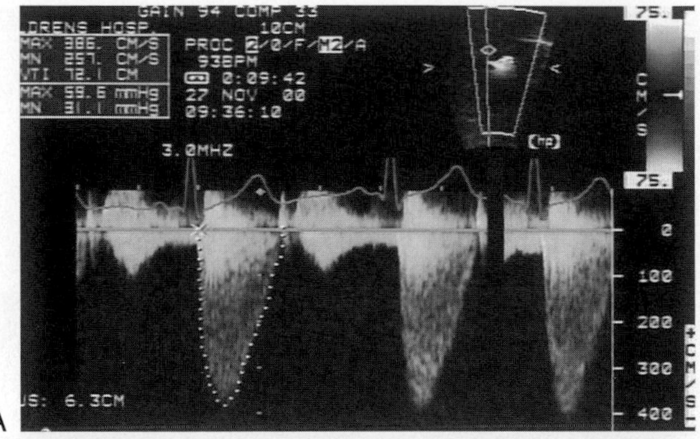

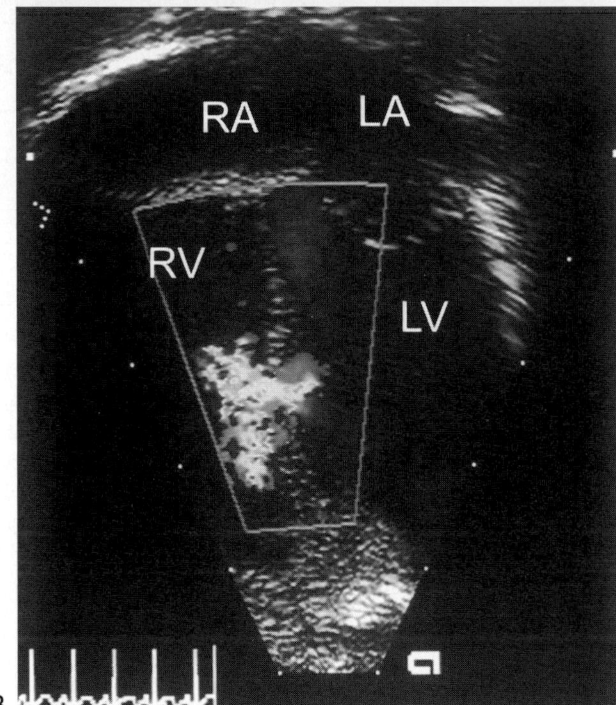

FIGURE 13–4 *Doppler echocardiography. A, Interrogation of the left ventricular outflow tract from the apical window with continuous wave Doppler in a patient with subvalvar aortic stenosis. The peak velocity is ~3.9 m/sec and the predicted maximum instantaneous gradient is ~60 mm Hg. Tracing the spectral Doppler signal yields a mean gradient of 31 mm Hg. B, Color Doppler flow mapping from the apical window showing a small mid-muscular ventricular septal defect.*

the frequency of the reflected sound wave changes in a predictable fashion, shifting in proportion to the velocity of the target relative to the transducer. The frequency shift, known as Doppler shift (Δf), is related to the transmitted frequency (Fo), the average velocity of sound (C) in tissue at 37 degrees centigrade (1540 m/sec), the velocity (V) and the direction of the target relative to the ultrasound beam (ϕ), according to the formula

$$\Delta f = \frac{2Fo \cdot V \cdot \cos\phi}{C}$$

This equation can be rearranged to solve for the velocity of the moving target: $V = \frac{C \cdot \Delta f}{2Fo \cdot \cos\phi}$. The cosine function in the Doppler equation predicts that when the ultrasound beam is parallel to the direction of the moving target (angle of incidence = zero), the Doppler frequency shift is maximal (cosine 0 degrees = 1), whereas when the target is moving perpendicular to the ultrasound beam (cosine 90 degrees = 0), no frequency shift will be detected regardless of the target's true velocity. It is important to recognize that the angle of incidence has three dimensions, whereas image display is 2D and the third dimension is not assessed. In 2D echocardiographic examination, the angle of incidence can be estimated but not confirmed, and the direction of flow may be unpredictable, particularly in high-velocity lesions such as aortic stenosis. As long as the angle of incidence relative to the actual direction of flow does not exceed 20 degrees, the true velocity will be underestimated by 6% or less (cosine 20 degrees = 0.94). When the angle of incidence exceeds 20 degrees, the degree of underestimation of flow velocity rapidly increases. Therefore, when performing a Doppler examination every effort is made to align the ultrasound beam with the target flow jet so that the highest available spectral signals and corresponding velocities are recorded and the accompanying audio signals reach the highest pitch. Color Doppler flow mapping allows imaging of the target jet and helps minimize the angle of incidence.

Continuous-Wave Doppler: This method uses two separate transducer elements, allowing continuous, simultaneous transmission and detection of the Doppler signal. As a result, all reflectors along the path of the ultrasound beam contribute to the recorded signal, and it is impossible to discern the location of the highest flow velocity, a phenomenon termed "range ambiguity." The advantage of this method is that virtually any peak velocity within the physiologic range can be recorded unambiguously. Continuous wave Doppler is most useful in assessing high velocity flow jets and gradients at easily identifiable locations, as in semilunar valve stenosis and restrictive ventricular septal defects (Fig. 13-4A).

Pulsed Doppler: In this method, a brief burst of ultrasound energy is emitted by the transducer, which then *listens* for the returning waves for a predetermined period of time. By superimposing the range-gated Doppler beam on the 2D image, the operator can choose the region to be interrogated, limiting the timing and duration of reception to allow only the returning signals from a discrete, specific location to be processed. According to the sampling theorem, the maximum measurable frequency shift in one direction is half the sampling rate (or pulse repetition rate). In other words, the maximum velocity or Doppler shift that can be unambiguously recorded is limited by a finite sampling rate, and decreases with increasing distance from the transducer. The further the interrogated region is from the transducer, the longer it takes for the ultrasound wave to reach it and return. To avoid range ambiguity, the transducer must wait for the returning signal before emitting a new one. When the sampling rate is less than twice the frequency shift, *aliasing* results. The highest frequency shift (i.e, velocity) that can be unambiguously displayed is termed the "Nyquist limit." The lower the transducer frequency, the higher the Nyquist limit.

High-Pulse Repetition Frequency (HPRF) Doppler: This method is intermediate between continuous and pulsed wave Doppler. Instead of waiting for the returning pulse before emitting the next one, the system sends a subsequent pulse during the "listening period" for the original one. By doing so, pulse repetition frequency is increased and the Nyquist limit is extended. The price is paid in range ambiguity; the examiner cannot be certain at which of several locations along the beam path the maximal recorded velocity was actually detected.

Color-Coded Doppler Flow Mapping: In color Doppler, the returning ultrasound signals from multiple locations along the scan line are assessed for frequency shift. For each gate assessed, the frequency shifts are averaged, and the mean velocity and direction of flow are color-coded and assigned to pixels within the display (Fig. 13-4*B*). By convention, flow toward the transducer is coded red and flow away from the transducer is coded blue. The intensity of the color display is proportional to the averaged frequency shift and flow velocity. A second color, typically green or yellow, is assigned to pixels depending on the statistical variance of the frequency shifts within each gate. A color-coded Doppler flow image is constructed by combining adjacent lines of processed Doppler information, and superimposed on the gray-scale 2D image. Color Doppler flow mapping is particularly useful in pediatric echocardiography because it greatly enhances the ability to identify and investigate sources of abnormal flow such as septal defects, stenotic and regurgitant valves, coronary artery fistulae, patent ductus arteriosus, and so forth.

Tissue Doppler: Tissue Doppler imaging is a relatively new technique for assessing myocardial velocity, strain, and function.[9] The technique is based on the differences in velocity and amplitude between flowing blood and the myocardium. Whereas the velocity of moving blood is relatively high and the amplitude of the Doppler signal is low, the velocity of the contracting and relaxing myocardium is low and the amplitude of the Doppler signal is high. By filtering out the higher velocity, low-amplitude signals from the blood, myocardial velocities are readily measured. Tissue Doppler imaging is used to assess longitudinal (base-to-apex) and radial (short-axis) myocardial velocities as well as time intervals such as isovolumic contraction and relaxation times, ejection time, and others (Fig. 13-5).

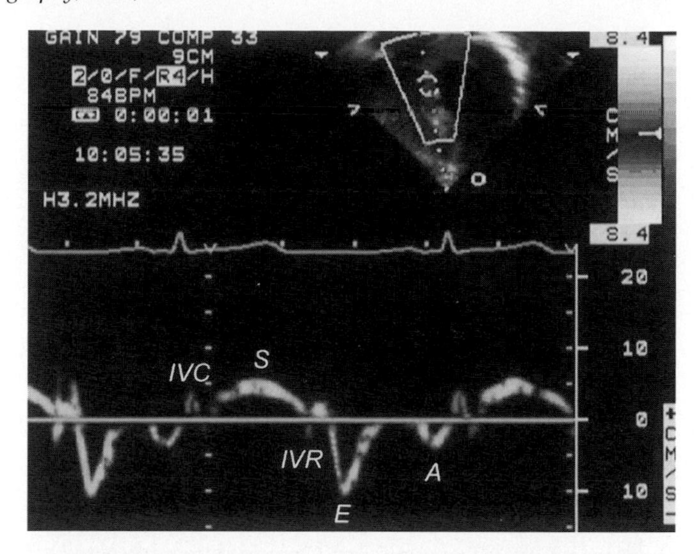

FIGURE 13–5 *Tissue Doppler interrogation of the basal septum from the apical window. A, atrial (late) diastolic phase; E, early diastolic phase; IVC, isovolumic contraction; IVR, isovolumic relaxation.*

Contrast Echocardiography

As early as the late 1960s, Gramiak et al.[10] noted that intravascular injections of solution resulted in a contrast effect detectable by ultrasound. Initially, this technique was used to identify structures on M-mode images. Contrast echocardiography has been used to detect systemic[11] and pulmonary venous anomalies[12] and to detect intracardiac and great artery level shunts.[2,13] A bolus of agitated saline injected in a peripheral vein creates contrast that opacifies the right heart, but essentially completely dissipates in a single pass through the capillaries of the pulmonary vascular bed. Appearance of contrast in the left heart indicates a probable intracardiac or intrapulmonary right-to-left shunt. In pediatric echocardiography, contrast studies are primarily used to investigate suspected intracardiac shunts not detectable by color Doppler or in patients with limited echocardiographic windows, baffle leaks after cardiac surgery, and pulmonary arteriovenous malformations. Newer ultrasound contrast agents cross the pulmonary capillaries and opacify the left heart chambers. These agents are used to improve visualization of the left ventricular cavity in patients with poor acoustic windows and are being investigated as a tool for assessment of myocardial perfusion.[14]

Objectives of the Echocardiographic Examination

The echocardiographic examination is tailored to the individual patient on the basis of physical examination and history, results of previous testing, clinical status, and expected level of cooperation. The first echocardiogram should ideally include a comprehensive survey of all components of the central cardiovascular system. Subsequent examinations may be targeted to answer specific clinical questions. It is often prudent, however, to perform a relatively complete study at follow-up, even in patients with previous comprehensive echocardiograms, because of the dynamic nature of congenital and acquired heart disease.[15–19]

Examination Technique

A comprehensive anatomic examination includes determination of visceral situs, cardiac position, atrial situs, systemic and pulmonary venous connections, ventricular situs, atrioventricular and ventriculoarterial alignments and connections, great arterial anatomy, and proximal coronary artery pattern. Color and spectral Doppler examination of the valves, great vessels, and atrial and ventricular septae is an important component of the basic examination, as is at least a qualitative assessment of ventricular function. The examiner should proceed through the study in an orderly fashion, preferably obtaining views in a predetermined, customary sequence to ensure local standardization of studies and facilitate subsequent review. It is helpful to go through a mental checklist of anatomic and functional information needed, both during and at the end of the exam, to ensure that a complete study has been obtained. In patients who are sedated and may awaken before the study is completed, and in those who are critically ill or unstable, it is often advisable to prioritize the elements of the study and obtain the most important information first.

Mental 3D reconstruction of cardiac anatomy is facilitated by recordings of complete sweeps through the heart and vessels, from one side or end of the heart to the other, from each view. This method also increases the likelihood that subtle findings overlooked during image acquisition will be detected on subsequent review of the images.

After each imaging sweep is completed and recorded, focused color and spectral Doppler interrogation of the atrial and ventricular septa, valves, and vessels should be performed. To maximize color Doppler quality and frame rate, rather than trying to examine all structures in the field of view simultaneously, each relevant structure should be examined individually using as narrow a region of interest as possible. Color Doppler should be used to align the pulsed or continuous wave Doppler beam with the flow jet being examined. Images of important findings, and color and spectral Doppler of normal and abnormal flow jets, should be recorded so that an interpreting physician who did not perform the examination nonetheless has enough information to confidently report the findings.

Sedation

To perform a complete echocardiographic examination in infants and uncooperative children, sedation is often necessary. The sedative should be chosen based on the time needed to obtain all of the necessary information. Adequate sedation for a complete echocardiographic examination can be accomplished with one of several medications. Oral chloral hydrate (50–80 mg/kg up to a maximum dose of 1000 mg) provides deep sedation usually lasting 60 to 120 minutes, which should be adequate for a complete study in a child with complex congenital heart disease.[20–22] Intranasal midazolam provides lighter, conscious sedation, rendering the patient cooperative for a shorter period of time.[22–24] Intravenous midazolam or narcotics may be preferable in some situations, particularly in the intensive care unit. Institutional guidelines for conscious and deep sedation, including nothing by mouth (NPO) restrictions and availability of resuscitation equipment, should be adhered to, and qualified medical personnel not involved in performing the echo should be responsible for monitoring the patient's cardiorespiratory status. The American Academy of Pediatrics has published guidelines for monitoring and management of pediatric patients during and after sedation for diagnostic and therapeutic procedures.[25]

Equipment

A variety of commercially available echocardiographic systems are suitable for examination of pediatric patients. For the degree of image resolution necessary for diagnosis of congenital anomalies, it is important that high-frequency transducers be available. For 2D imaging, one should use the highest frequency transducer capable of obtaining good images of the structures being examined; a lower frequency may be needed for color and spectral Doppler examination of the same structures. Multifrequency transducers expedite the acquisition of information.

Echocardiographic Views

Standard Imaging Planes and Image Display: Standard echocardiographic imaging planes include *long axis* planes paralleling the major (long) axis of the left ventricle (LV), and *short axis* planes perpendicular to the major axis of the LV. These views are obtained from subxiphoid (subcostal) and parasternal windows; a *four-chamber* view is obtained over the cardiac apex. Additional standard imaging planes include that paralleling the long axis of the aortic arch, and coronal views from the suprasternal notch. In addition, specialized views to optimally display the atrial septum, branch pulmonary arteries, ductus arteriosus, and coronary arteries are components of a complete anatomic survey.

Unconventional imaging planes and windows are often necessary to obtain complete anatomic information, especially in the setting of complex congenital defects and distorted intrathoracic anatomy (as in diaphragmatic hernia, for example). The examiner must be flexible, improvising as needed to obtain the necessary information.

The transducer is oriented so that images are displayed in an *anatomically correct* orientation, as if the patient were facing the viewer; right-sided structures are displayed on the left side of the screen and visa versa. To prevent confusion during interpretation and review, it is critical to follow this rule, whatever the position of the cardiac apex (levo- or dextrocardia). The exception to this is the parasternal long axis view, which, by convention, is displayed so that cranial structures are on the right side of the image and the cardiac apex is on the left side of the image, regardless of the position of the heart.

Subxiphoid (Subcostal) View (Fig. 13-6*A*): Sweeps from the subxiphoid window provide a wide-angle view of the entire heart and great vessels. This view is particularly useful in infants and small children, because of the proximity of the transducer to the heart and lack of intervening bone or lung tissue. Beginning with subcostal sweeps is the most efficient way to assess cardiac position, visceral and atrial situs, obtain an overview of the intracardiac and great vessel anatomy, and determine the relationships between structures. Once the basic anatomy is determined, systematic investigation of details of anatomy and valve function can be performed using other views.

Imaging from the subxiphoid window is performed with the patient lying flat on his or her back. Bending the knees helps relax the abdominal muscles. Beginning with a cross-sectional view of the abdomen from just below and often slightly lateral to the xiphoid process, a cross-section of the abdominal aorta and inferior vena cava (IVC), and their relationship to each other and the spine, is displayed. The position of the stomach is usually evident due to highly reflective air within it. Angling slightly superiorly demonstrates the hemidiaphragms and their motion with respiration. The transducer plane is swept superiorly through the diaphragm, from the posterior inferior surface to the anterior surface of the heart, ending with a coronal slice through the right ventricular outflow tract (Fig. 13-6*A*). Turning the transducer 90 degrees clockwise provides a subxiphoid short-axis view (Fig. 13-6*B*). Beginning with a plane demonstrating the superior and inferior vena cavae, the transducer plane is swept through the heart from one side to the other, ending at the cardiac apex. In patients with a good subxiphoid window, these two sweeps demonstrate the systemic and pulmonary venous connections, atrial septum, atrioventricular (AV) valve morphology, ventricular septum, both outflow tracts, proximal great arteries, and descending aorta. In patients with poor or inaccessible apical and parasternal windows, a nearly complete examination (with the exception of optimal images of the aortic arch and coronary artery origins) can be performed from the subxiphoid window.

If images are good from this view, the atrial and ventricular septa, pulmonary veins, and outflow tracts should be examined with color Doppler. This window also provides a good angle for spectral Doppler interrogation of the outflow tracts, superior and inferior vena cavae, and abdominal aorta.

Apical View (Fig. 13-6*C*): Apical imaging is usually best with the patient lying approximately 45 degrees up on the left side (for levocardia), bringing the apex closer to the chest wall and displacing the lung. Positioning the transducer over the cardiac apex, one obtains a four-chamber view of the heart, displaying both atria, both AV valves at their maximum lateral dimensions, and both ventricles in long axis. Sweeping posteriorly, the coronary sinus and posterior ventricular septum are imaged. Sweeping anteriorly, the left and right ventricular outflow tracts are imaged. The pulmonary veins are visible but individual veins are usually better evaluated on other views. Rotating the transducer clockwise approximately 90 degrees displays a *two-chamber* view of the left ventricular inflow and outflow tracts.

Color Doppler interrogation of the AV valves, muscular ventricular septum, and left ventricular outflow tract (LVOT) should be performed from the apical view, which also provides good angles for spectral Doppler interrogation of AV valves, LVOT, aortic valve, and the right upper pulmonary vein. Moving the transducer slightly medially toward the left lower sternal border often allows imaging and Doppler evaluation of the right ventricular outflow tract and pulmonary valve.

Parasternal Views (Fig. 13-6*D,E*): Parasternal views are obtained just lateral to the sternum, usually in the third or fourth left intercostal space. It is helpful to have the patient rolled up on his or her left side. The initial long axis image is obtained with the transducer plane oriented from the patient's right shoulder to the left hip. With proper orientation, the left atrium, mitral valve, left ventricle, posterior LV free wall and septum, LV outflow tract, aortic valve, and ascending aorta are displayed (Fig. 13-6*D*). Sweeping inferiorly and rightward toward the right hip images the right atrium, tricuspid valve, and right ventricular (RV) inflow, and sweeping superiorly and leftward displays the RV outflow tract, pulmonary valve, and main pulmonary artery. This view provides another opportunity for color Doppler interrogation of the AV valves, ventricular septum, outflow tracts, and semilunar valves.

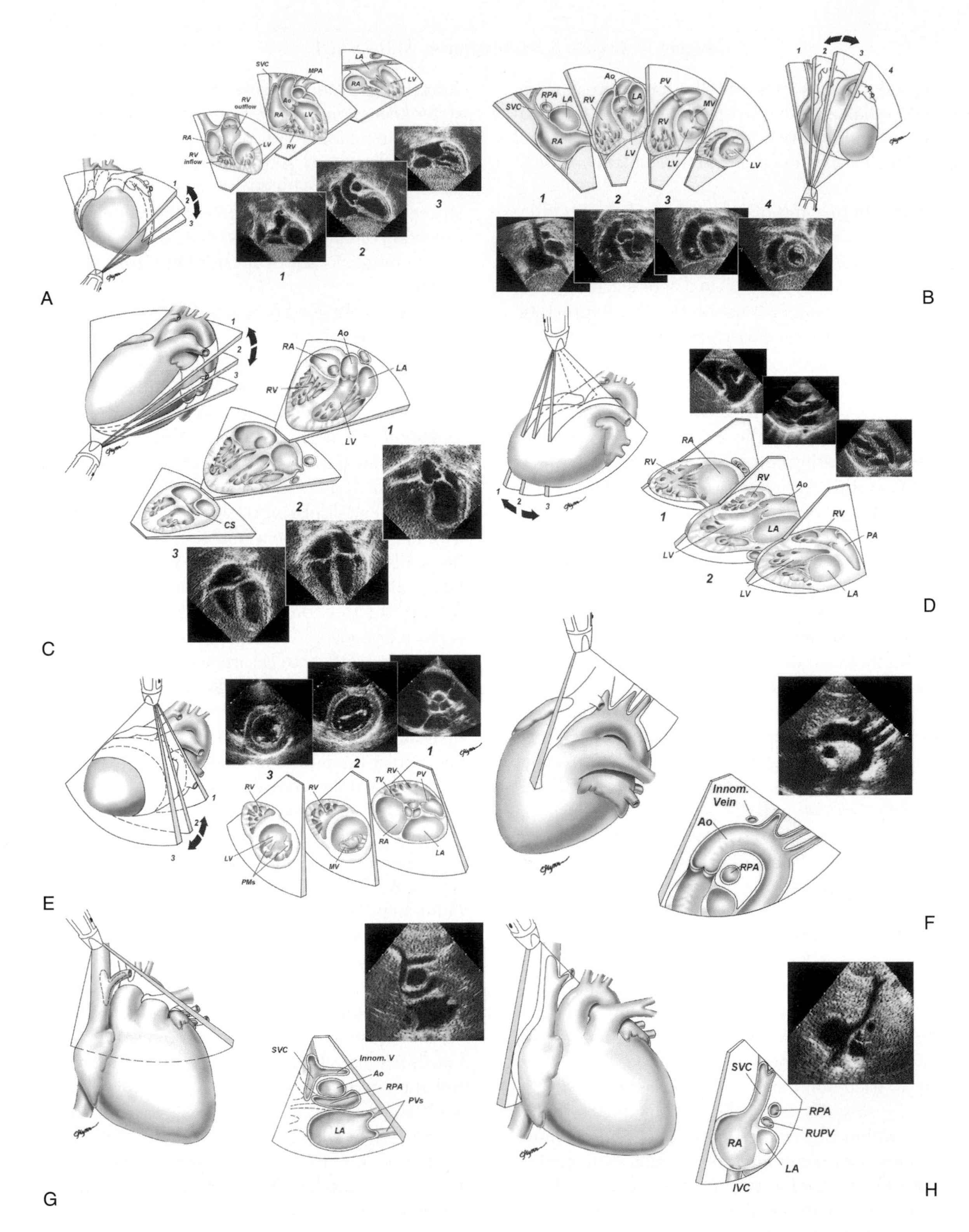

FIGURE 13–6 *Two-dimensional echocardiographic imaging planes (see text for details). A, Subxiphoid long-axis. B, Subxiphoid short axis. C, Apical four-chamber. D, Parasternal long axis. E, Parasternal short-axis view. F, Suprasternal notch view: long axis of aorta. G, Suprasternal notch view: transverse view. H, Right parasternal view. Ao, aorta; Innom, innominate; IVC, inferior vena cava; LA, left atrium; LV, left ventricle; MPA, main pulmonary artery; MV, mitral valve; PMs, papillary muscles; PV, pulmonary valve; PVs, pulmonary veins; RA, right atrium; RV, right ventricle; RPA, right pulmonary artery; RUPV, right upper pulmonary vein; SVC, superior vena cava; TV, tricuspid valve. From Geva T. Echocardiography and Doppler ultrasound. In Garson, A, Bricker, JT, Fisher, DJ, Neish SR (eds). The Science and Practice of Pediatric Cardiology. Baltimore: Williams & Wilkins, 1997, pp 789, with permission.*

The parasternal short-axis view is obtained from the same window, with the transducer rotated 90 degrees clockwise (Fig. 13-6*E*). Beginning with a cross section of the LV at the level of the mitral valve, RV inflow and outflow tracts, sweeping apically scans the LV chamber and the muscular ventricular septum. Sweeping up toward the base of the heart, the aortic valve is imaged in cross section, along with the coronary origins, the atrioventricular canal, membranous and conoventricular septa, pulmonary valve and main pulmonary artery. Color Doppler and, if indicated, spectral Doppler interrogation of the ventricular septum and pulmonary veins is typically performed from this view, as is Doppler examination of the pulmonary valve.

The pulmonary artery bifurcation is usually best seen from one or two interspaces higher, with slightly more clockwise rotation. Rotating counterclockwise approximately 90 degrees allows imaging of a ductus arteriosus in long axis. A right parasternal view is often helpful for imaging the atrial septum and superior vena cava (SVC), and provides a good angle for Doppler examination of the aortic valve and ascending aorta (Fig. 13-6*H*).

Suprasternal Notch View (Fig. 13-6*F*,*G*): For suprasternal notch imaging, it is usually helpful to have the patient lie flat on his or her back with a roll under the shoulders, hyperextending the neck and turning the head to the side to provide better exposure. This position may make younger children apprehensive, and repositioning sleeping infants and children may awaken them. It is sometimes possible to obtain satisfactory suprasternal notch views, or similar images from the top of the sternum or the right or left infraclavicular space, without repositioning the patient.

Beginning with the transducer plane oriented from left to right and aimed inferiorly in a coronal plane, one sees a cross-section of the ascending aorta, the long axis of the right pulmonary artery, and a cross-section of the SVC (Fig. 13-6*G*). In infants and many children, most or all of the pulmonary veins can also be imaged from this view. Sweeping cranially through the ascending aorta and SVC, one obtains a long axis of the left innominate vein and transverse aortic arch, and further cranial angulation demonstrates the brachiocephalic arteries. Color Doppler interrogation of the innominate vein (to assess for a persistent left SVC) and pulmonary veins is typically performed from this view.

Counterclockwise rotation of the transducer images the entire aortic arch in long axis (Fig. 13-6*F*), allowing color and spectral Doppler examination of the ascending and descending aorta. To demonstrate a right aortic arch, some echocardiographers rotate the transducer clockwise to display the descending aorta on the left side of the screen.

Interpretation and Reporting

Interpretation of pediatric echocardiographic examinations requires thorough knowledge of normal cardiac morphology and the myriad of potential congenital and acquired anomalies. While reviewing the images, the interpreter builds a mental 3D image of the anatomy and systematically runs down a checklist to ensure that cardiac relationships and structures are clearly delineated, and any potential anomalies are either clearly demonstrated or excluded. The reader is referred to the earlier sections on morphologic anatomy (see Chapter 3) and segmental approach to diagnosis (see Chapter 4), and subsequent chapters on acquired and congenital anomalies, for detailed descriptions.

Reports should be unambiguous in the description of the segmental anatomy and atrioventricular and ventriculoarterial relationships so that the reader has no doubt as to the sidedness of structures and looping. It is preferable to refer to the ventricles by their morphology rather than the side of the body on which they are located; to eliminate ambiguity, in a patient with L-looped ventricles (ventricular inversion) for example, one might describe the "right-sided morphologic left ventricle."

QUANTITATIVE ANALYSIS

Cardiovascular structures can be measured on still-frame 2D echocardiographic images with reasonable accuracy. Measurements of individual structures can be compared to published normal values to determine whether they fall within the expected range for the patient's somatic size, and if not, the extent of deviation from normal.

Description of Technique

Measurement of linear dimension (such as vessel or valve annulus diameter), cross-sectional area (such as valve area) or 3D volume (ventricular volume or mass) helps to determine the severity of disease and predict natural history and prognosis. Unlike in adult cardiology, because of the wide variation in size of pediatric patients and the considerable growth of cardiovascular structures between birth and adulthood, it is critical that measurements be adjusted to body size to allow meaningful comparison between patients.

The growth of cardiac structures may not have a linear relationship to body surface area, height, weight, or age. In fact, most linear dimensions (such as valve and vessel diameters) are best indexed to the square root of body surface area.[26,27] This is expected since the heart and great vessels grow much more rapidly during the first 2 to 4 years of life compared with later childhood and adolescence. For example, when the aortic valve annulus diameter is indexed to the square root of the body surface area, the mean annulus diameter in the normal population is 1.51 $cm/m^{0.5}$ in all children, from newborn to adult size. It follows that cross-sectional measurements are best indexed to body surface area.[27] Colan et al. suggest that left ventricular volume should be indexed to the body surface area raised to the 1.28 power, and left ventricular mass should be indexed to the body surface area raised to the 1.23 power (unpublished data).

Comparison of measurements between individuals is simplified by the use of Z values. The Z value indicates the deviation of a measurement relative to the regression line of a normal data set, and is expressed as the number of standard deviations from the expected mean. It is calculated as:

$$\text{Z value} = \frac{\text{Measured value} - \text{Mean value of normal population}}{\text{Standard deviation of healthy population}}$$

Expression of measurements as Z values allows comparison between patients and the normal population, regardless of body size.

Assessment of the volume of the left ventricular chamber is an integral component of the echocardiographic evaluation of patients with suspected LV hypoplasia and those with lesions causing LV volume overload. Algorithms for calculating LV volume based on various geometric models have been developed and are reviewed in more detail elsewhere.[2–4] The biplane Simpson's rule is among the most reliable of these methods. The left ventricle is imaged in two orthogonal views, which share a common long axis: for example, the apical four- and two-chamber views (Fig. 13-7A). Left ventricular volume is calculated using the formula:

$$V = \frac{\pi}{4} \times \sum_{i=1}^{N} ai \times bi \times \frac{L}{N}$$

where a_i = slice radius in the apical two-chamber view, b_i = slice radius in the apical four-chamber view, L = left ventricular length, N = number of slices and V = volume. The biplane area–length method uses the formula $V = 5/6 \times$ cross-sectional area of the LV in short axis × LV length in long axis (Fig. 13-7*B*). Measurement of left and right ventricular volumes using 3D reconstruction indicates that it is more accurate than 2D echocardiographic techniques.[28,29]

Left ventricular myocardial volume (and therefore mass) can be measured using 2D or 3D echocardiography by calculating the total volume of the left ventricle including the myocardium, and subtracting the chamber volume. Left ventricular mass is calculated by multiplying the myocardial volume by the density of muscle (1.055 g/mL).

Since it is not influenced by acoustic windows and does not require prediction of chamber geometry, MRI is an excellent alternative to echocardiography for measuring volume and mass and is considered the reference standard to which other techniques are compared.[28,30] This is discussed further in a subsequent section.

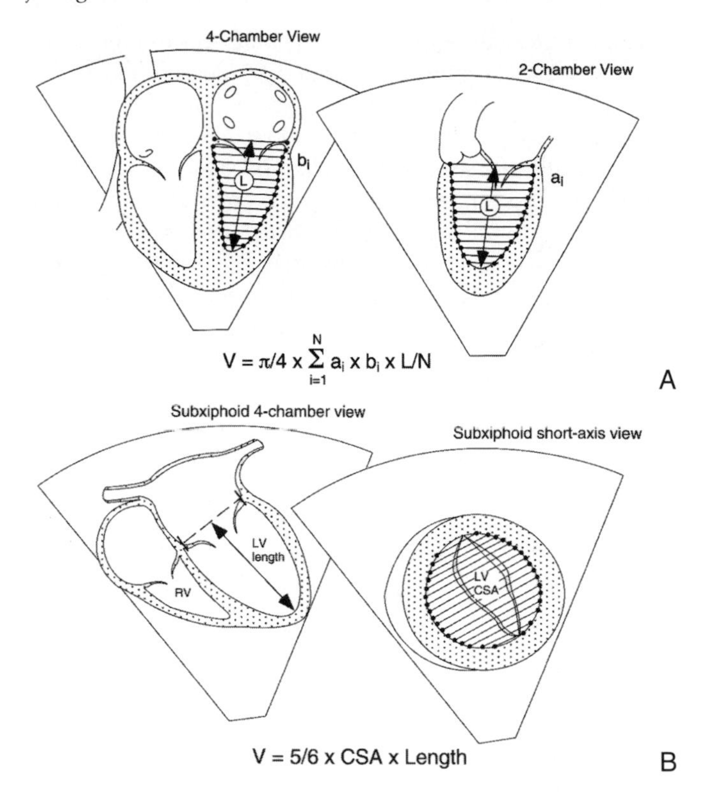

FIGURE 13–7 *Left ventricle volume calculation. A, Simpson rule. B, Area–length method.*
From Geva T. Echocardiography and Doppler ultrasound. In Garson, A, Bricker, JT, Fisher, DJ, Neish SR (eds). The Science and Practice of Pediatric Cardiology. Baltimore: Williams & Wilkins, 1997, pp 789, with permission.

Ventricular Function

Commonly used indices of ventricular function, including shortening fraction, fractional area change, ejection fraction, velocity of circumferential fiber (VCF) shortening, peak dp/dt, and systolic time intervals, measure global pump function. These indices are, however, unable to distinguish between the effects of altered loading conditions and intrinsic abnormalities in myocardial contractility. Acutely decreasing preload or increasing afterload will depress the shortening and ejection fractions, which may be incorrectly interpreted as being due to an intrinsic abnormality of myocardial contractility. Conversely, normal shortening or ejection fractions may be measured even in the setting of abnormal myocardial contractility, given the right loading conditions. The advantage of most of these indices is their relative simplicity and ease of acquisition. Load-independent assessment of left ventricular systolic function requires a more sophisticated analysis. The interested reader is referred to the subsequent chapter on Assessment of Ventricular and Myocardial Performance (see Chapter 15).

Doppler Evaluation of Pressure Gradients

Because congenital heart defects frequently result in elevated pressure in one or more cardiac chambers or vessels, it is valuable to have a noninvasive means of estimating pressure. Doppler technology allows estimation of pressure across valves and between chambers, in many cases eliminating the need for hemodynamic cardiac catheterization and helping to determine the timing of surgical or catheter intervention. The most common uses of Doppler pressure gradient estimation in pediatric cardiology include assessment of right ventricular and pulmonary artery pressures in the setting of a ventricular septal defect, and evaluation of outflow tract obstruction. Determination of the systolic pressure gradient between the right ventricle and right atrium can be estimated by Doppler interrogation of a tricuspid regurgitation jet; using an assumed right atrial pressure, right ventricular and pulmonary artery systolic pressures can be predicted. This is useful not only in numerous forms of congenital cardiac disease both before and after repair, but also in noncardiac disease such as primary pulmonary hypertension and cor pulmonale.

Calculation of Pressure Gradients

In the 1700s, Daniel Bernoulli investigated the forces present in moving fluid. His principle, which was originally derived by considering the conservation of mechanical energy within the fluid, states that as the speed of moving fluid increases, the pressure within the fluid decreases. The Bernoulli equation allows prediction of the pressure difference (ΔP) between two points separated by a distance (s) using the velocity at the two points (V_1 and V_2), the fluid density (for blood, ρ = 1060 kg/m^3), and the velocity-dependent viscous friction according to:

$$\Delta P = \underbrace{\frac{1}{2}\rho(V_2^2 - V_1^2)}_{\text{convective acceleration}} + \underbrace{\rho\int_1^2 \frac{d\vec{V}}{dt}d\vec{s}}_{\text{flow acceleration}} + \underbrace{R(\vec{V})}_{\text{viscous friction}}$$

For most clinical applications of the Bernoulli equation, the convective acceleration component of the formula is considered the most significant. The combination of values for blood density and conversion of pressure units into millimeters of mercury (mm Hg) and velocity units into meters per second (m/seconds), yields a coefficient value of 3.98, which for all physiologically relevant clinical situations can be rounded to 4. The second term of the equation, representing the pressure drop generated by flow acceleration during the brief lag between the onset of the velocity and pressure curves is clinically unimportant and is dropped. The third term describes the force necessary to overcome viscous friction, which, for pressure drops across a discrete orifice, is negligible. For most clinical applications, a simplified formula is used based on the following assumptions: (a) The velocity proximal to the obstruction (V_1) is negligible compared with the velocity just distal to the obstruction (V_2); (b) peak flow acceleration occurs in early systole when the pressure gradient is irrelevant and can be ignored; (c) viscous friction is trivial; and (d) the flow is laminar. The Bernoulli equation can therefore be simplified to the following:

$$\Delta P = 4(V_2)^2$$

This simplified formula has been proven valid in *in vitro* flow models[31] and in a variety of clinical settings.[32] However, the assumptions allowing simplification of the Bernoulli equation may not always be correct. For example, in long-segment narrowing such as a Blalock-Taussig shunt, ignoring the viscous friction term of the Bernoulli equation may result in significant underestimation of the pressure drop. The limitations leading to errors in estimation of pressure gradient are reviewed in more detail elsewhere.[2–5,33]

SPECIAL ECHOCARDIOGRAPHIC PROCEDURES

Transesophageal Echocardiography

Echocardiographic imaging from the esophagus provides high-quality images of intracardiac structures in almost every patient, because of the absence of intervening structures, like lung and bone, which interfere with the transmission of acoustic energy. Transesophageal echocardiography (TEE) is particularly useful in patients in whom transthoracic acoustic windows are poor or inaccessible. Technological advances since the introduction of TEE, such as multiplane imaging capability and miniaturization of probes for pediatric patients, have greatly expanded its role in pediatric cardiology.

Indications: Preoperative TEE can elucidate anatomic details that may have been incompletely evaluated on preoperative transthoracic studies and may alter the surgical plan.[34,35] The most important role of TEE in hospital-based pediatric cardiovascular programs, however, is likely to be the postoperative evaluation of cardiac surgical results in the operating room. Although TEE can be performed while the patient is still on cardiopulmonary bypass, low flow limits the ability to assess hemodynamics. Once bypass flow is reduced or stopped, hemodynamics approach those expected after separation from bypass, and surgical results can be assessed with more accuracy and confidence.

TEE is particularly helpful for assessing the efficacy of septal defect repair, patent ductus arteriosus closure, relief of outflow tract obstruction, valvuloplasty for regurgitation, and intracardiac baffles and can identify residual lesions not otherwise suspected.[35–37] If unsatisfactory results or significant residual lesions are identified by TEE, bypass can be resumed, and the repair can be revised and then reassessed. TEE also provides a real-time assessment of myocardial function during the rapidly changing hemodynamic state immediately after discontinuing bypass.

TEE offers high-quality imaging of patients who otherwise pose a challenge to the echocardiographer, particularly larger patients and those with inaccessible acoustic windows (e.g, patients with open chest after surgery, undergoing interventional cardiac catheterization, or with bandages covering the chest wall). Structures that are particularly well suited to TEE examination are those located closest to the esophagus, including the atrial septum, pulmonary veins, superior vena cava, AV valves, left ventricular outflow tract, aortic valve, coronary artery origins, and surgically created atrial baffles. TEE evaluation of prosthetic AV valve function, regurgitation, and perivalvar leaks is usually far superior to that obtained by transthoracic imaging. More anterior structures, such as the right ventricular outflow tract, pulmonary valve, and anterior muscular septum, and those obscured by adjacent airways (such as the left pulmonary artery) can be more difficult to evaluate. TEE is superior to transthoracic imaging for ruling out intracardiac thrombus and vegetation, particularly in larger patients and those with suboptimal surface windows.

TEE has proven invaluable in guiding interventional catheterization procedures such as device closure of atrial and ventricular septal defects, especially when the defect is large or the intracardiac anatomy or cardiac position is atypical. TEE is also useful during less commonly performed interventions, such as balloon dilation and stenting of a venous baffle or complex outflow tract obstruction.[38]

Equipment and Technique: A variety of TEE probes are commercially available for most echocardiographic imaging systems, including probes small enough for patients weighing as little as 2 kg, and multiplane probes capable of 180-degree rotation of the imaging plane. TEE is performed using local anesthesia, conscious sedation, or general anesthesia, depending on the patient's ability to cooperate, clinical status, and concomitant procedures. Experienced medical personnel should insert the probe to avoid injury to the patient's teeth, posterior pharynx, airway, or esophagus. Use of bite guards and probe sleeves minimizes damage to the probe and prevents transmission of infection. If sedation is used, dedicated medical personnel should be responsible for monitoring the patient's cardiorespiratory status during the exam.

Although the questions to be answered by TEE may be limited, once these have been addressed a comprehensive examination of intracardiac structures and great vessels for additional unsuspected findings is advisable, assuming patient status is not prohibitive. In particular, the study should include careful examination of structures that are often difficult to assess transthoracically, specifically the atrial septum, pulmonary veins, and coronary artery origins.

Figure 13-8 shows representative TEE views. A comprehensive TEE examination often begins with the probe tip in the stomach, where anteflexion provides views of the left and right ventricles for assessment of myocardial function, AV valve morphology, and the muscular ventricular septum. The best angles for Doppler interrogation of right and left ventricular outflow tract gradients are usually obtained from the stomach. This view, however, cannot usually be obtained in patients whose heart is not on the same side as the stomach. Withdrawal of the probe into the lower and mid-esophagus provides excellent images of the atrial septum, pulmonary veins, atrial appendages, AV valves, LV outflow tract, aortic and pulmonary valves, and coronary arteries. Straightening or retroflexion of the probe results in a four-chamber view, and anteflexion images the ventricles and aortic valve in cross-section. A higher esophageal view allows examination of the main and branch pulmonary arteries, ductus arteriosus, transverse aortic arch, and superior vena cava. Rotating the probe's imaging face posteriorly demonstrates the descending aorta. Examination of the heart from the stomach and multiple levels in the esophagus with a multiplane imaging probe provides nearly as many imaging planes as a transthoracic echocardiographic examination, without interference from lung and bony tissues. Standards for image display vary among institutions; displaying the TEE images with the same orientation as corresponding transthoracic images in the same plane, however, helps orient viewers more familiar with transthoracic images. The interested reader is referred to guidelines for transesophageal echocardiography in children published by the American Society of Echocardiography in 1992.[39]

Patient Selection and Safety: Although in experienced hands TEE is very safe, complications such as oropharyngeal and esophageal injury and compression of airways and vascular structures can occur.[40–43] Contraindications to TEE include unrepaired tracheoesophageal fistula, significant esophageal stricture, active upper gastrointestinal bleeding, and an uncontrolled airway in a patient with significant respiratory or cardiac compromise. Relative contraindications might include previous esophageal surgery, esophageal varices or diverticulum, cervical spine instability, immobility, or deformity, and severe coagulopathy.[2,39]

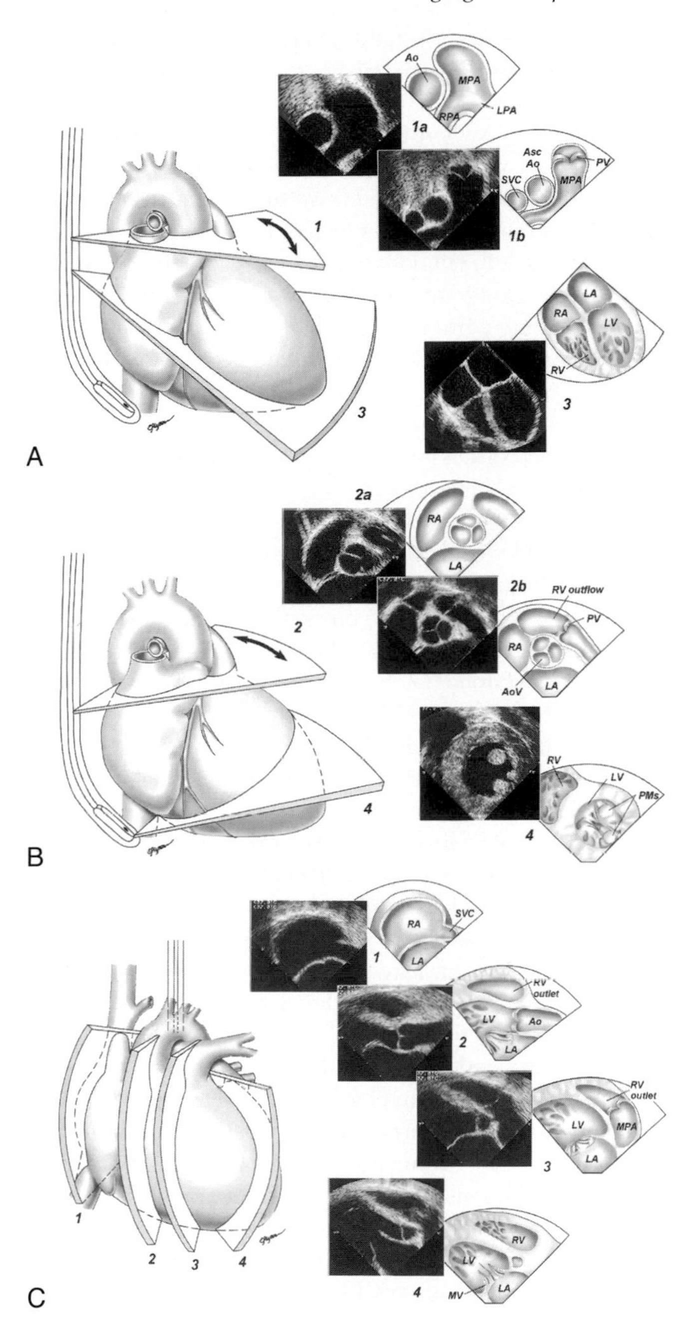

FIGURE 13–8 *Transesophageal imaging. A, Transverse plane: cross-sectional view at level 1a depicts the proximal ascending aorta (Ao), main pulmonary artery (MPA), and left and right pulmonary arteries (LPA and RPA, respectively). A rightward tilt of the transducer shows the RPA as it passes behind the superior vena cava (SVC) and ascending aorta (Asc Ao). To obtain a four-chamber view (level 3), the transducer is advanced in the esophagus with slight retroflexion of the scope. B, Level 2 is parallel to the transthoracic parasternal short-axis view. In level 2a, the atrial septum is imaged by a slight rightward tilt of the transducer. In level 2B, the aortic valve (AoV) is seen in cross-section in the center of the image, the left atrium (LA), right atrium (RA), tricuspid valve, right ventricular outflow (RV outflow), pulmonary valve (PV), and the proximal main pulmonary artery are seen. By advancing the transducer into the lower esophagus and anteflexing the scope, a cross sectional view of the left ventricle (LV), mitral valve, and papillary muscles is obtained (level 4). Note that image orientation is the same as in transthoracic echocardiography. C, Vertical (longitudinal) plane: The sweep begins at a plane that crosses the SVC, LA, RA, and atrial septum (level 1). Next, a leftward tilt of the transducer shows an image parallel to the transthoracic parasternal long-axis view of the LA, mitral valve, LV, left ventricular outflow tract and proximal aorta (Ao) (level 2). Further leftward tilt of the transducer (level 3) shows the right ventricular outflow tract (RV outlet), pulmonary valve, and main pulmonary artery (MPA). The sweep continues leftward to show the leftward aspects of the left atrium, mitral valve, and left ventricle (level 4). Further leftward tilt depicts the left atrial appendage and the left pulmonary veins (not shown). Note that image orientation is the same as in transthoracic echocardiography.*
From Geva T. Echocardiography and Doppler ultrasound. In Garson, A, Bricker, JT, Fisher, DJ, Neish SR (eds). The Science and Practice of Pediatric Cardiology. Baltimore: Williams & Wilkins, 1997, pp 789, with permission.

FETAL ECHOCARDIOGRAPHY

History: Early attempts to use M-mode echocardiography to diagnose abnormalities of fetal cardiac structure and rhythm were met with limited success.[44] With the advent of high-resolution 2D imaging in the 1980s, detailed examination of fetal cardiac anatomy and accurate diagnosis of even very complex congenital heart defects became possible (Fig. 13-9).[45,46] Today, fetal echocardiography performed via the maternal abdomen can reliably diagnose congenital heart defects as early as 14 weeks of gestation. Transvaginal ultrasound can provide reasonable images of the fetal heart as early as 10 weeks of gestation.[47,48]

Detection of Congenital Heart Disease on Routine Ultrasound: The detection rate of congenital heart disease on routine screening obstetrical ultrasound is highly variable and operator-dependent. Documentation of a four-chamber view alone has proven inadequate to rule out most fetal heart disease.[49,50] When accompanied by a view of the great arteries, the detection rate increases significantly.[51–53] However, the defects most likely to be detected on routine ultrasound screening are those in which there is a significantly hypoplastic ventricle or great artery, large ventricular septal defect, obvious abnormality of the AV valves (absent or common AV valve), significant cardiomegaly, or nonimmune hydrops. Particularly in fetuses thought to be at low risk for congenital heart disease, defects such as isolated semilunar valve stenosis, hypoplastic aortic arch with coarctation, transposition of the great arteries, and anomalies of the pulmonary and systemic veins are less likely to be detected except by well-trained, meticulous, and motivated

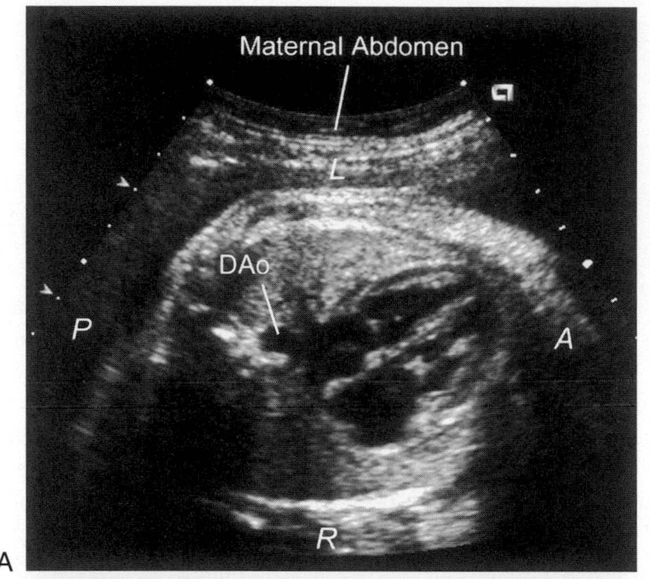

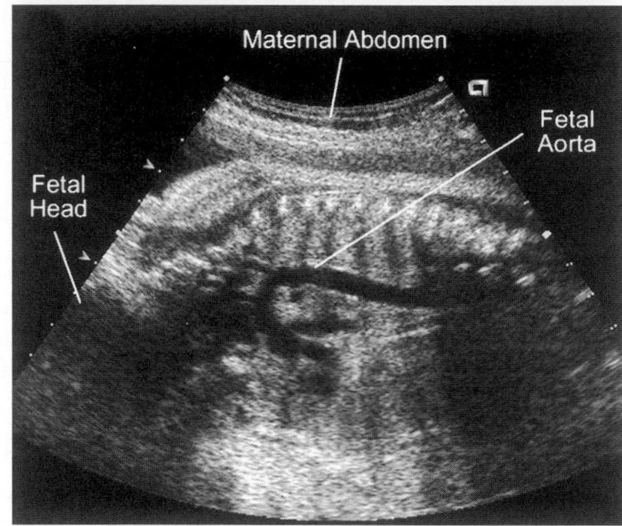

FIGURE 13–9 *Fetal echocardiogram. A, Four-chamber view. B, Oblique sagittal view of the thoracic and abdominal aorta. A, anterior; Dao, descending aorta; L, left; LA, left atrium; P, posterior; R, right; RA, right atrium; RV, right ventricle.*

obstetrical sonographers.[53] Indications for fetal echocardiography are summarized in Table 13-2. The initial scan in fetuses at risk for congenital heart defects should be performed at 14 to 18 weeks of gestation. Although image resolution is better later in gestation in most instances, later detection of major heart disease reduces options for termination, while increasing the maternal morbidity associated with that procedure.

Fetal Circulation and Natural History of Congenital Heart Disease: Accurate diagnosis of fetal congenital heart defects requires knowledge of the wide variety of possible lesions and their echocardiographic appearance as well as familiarity with the fetal circulation and the effects of structural and functional heart disease on this unique system.

In fetal life, oxygen is provided by the mother via the placenta and umbilical vein; much of this relatively well-oxygenated blood is shunted from the right atrium into the left heart across the foramen ovale. Because the fetal lungs are not expanded, pulmonary vascular resistance is high and most of the right ventricular output bypasses the lungs to the descending aorta through the ductus arteriosus. Right and left ventricular, aortic, and pulmonary artery pressures are equal in the healthy fetal circulation, and the right and left sides of the heart operate in parallel rather than in series. More detailed discussion of the fetal circulation is provided in Chapter 6.

Evidence suggests that decreased flow through heart chambers and vessels slows and even arrests their growth. For example, in the setting of severe aortic or pulmonary valve stenosis with an intact ventricular septum, the ventricle on the affected side of the heart has diminished diastolic filling and poor systolic function; growth of this ventricle slows or stops, which may render the ventricle severely hypoplastic by the third trimester.[54–56] Flow is redirected at the atrial level to the nonaffected side of the heart, increasing the volume load and causing it to dilate.

In the setting of severe aortic or pulmonary valve stenosis or atresia with a significant ventricular septal defect, however, the ventricles will maintain equal, normal pressures and in the absence of AV valve abnormalities, both will continue to grow normally. The great artery of the affected valve will usually be hypoplastic, again presumably due to decreased antegrade flow.

The volume and direction of flow at the foramen ovale and ductus arteriosus can change in the setting of structural and hemodynamic abnormalities. With significant reduction of antegrade flow through the right heart and pulmonary valve (as in pulmonary atresia), the direction of flow at the ductus arteriosus will reverse toward the pulmonary artery. In critical aortic stenosis or aortic atresia, flow in the aortic arch and ascending aorta will be mostly or entirely retrograde from the ductus arteriosus. In mitral atresia, flow across the atrial septum reverses, shunting from left atrium to right atrium. If the foramen ovale is small or absent when septum primum is pushed toward the right, left atrial and pulmonary venous hypertension will ensue, which may have deleterious effects on development of the pulmonary vascular bed.[57,58]

Technique: Fetal echocardiography should be performed by sonographers or physicians who are experienced in echocardiographic examination of congenital heart defects and understand how these individual defects alter the circulation differently in the fetus than in a newborn. Basic familiarity with the examination of fetal structures outside the

TABLE 13–2. Indications for Fetal Echocardiography

Fetal risk factors
- Suspected cardiac anomaly on level I scan
- Abnormal visceral situs
- Abnormal cardiac position or axis
- Extracardiac structural anomalies associated with CHD, including:
  - Two-vessel cord
  - Nuchal thickening/lucency
  - Diaphragmatic hernia
  - Duodenal atresia
  - Tracheoesophageal fistula
  - Cystic hygroma
- Chromosomal abnormalities including:
  - Trisomy 21
  - Chromosome 22q11 microdeletion (velocardiofacial syndrome, VCFS)
  - Turner syndrome
  - Fetal dysrhythmias
  - Irregular rhythm
  - Tachyarrhythmia
  - Bradyarrhythmia
  - Intrauterine growth retardation
  - Nonimmune hydrops fetalis
- Structural anomaly affecting cardiovascular physiology, including:
  - Sacrococcygeal teratoma
  - Twin–twin transfusion
  - Acardiac twin
  - Vein of Galen aneurysm
  - Congenital cystic adenomatous malformation of the lung

Maternal risk factors
- Congenital heart disease
- Exposure to teratogen (sample list only)
- Lithium carbonate
- Alcohol
- Phenytoin
- Other anticonvulsants
- Trimethadione
- Isoretinoin
- Thalidomide
- Amphetamines (?)
- Diabetes
- Phenylketonuria
- Maternal infection
- Parvovirus
- Toxoplasmosis
- Coxsackie virus
- Cytomegalovirus
- Mumps virus
- Maternal autoantibodies

Familial risk factors
- Congenital heart disease
- Syndromes
- Trisomy 21 (Down)
- Marfan
- Noonan
- Tuberous sclerosis
- Velocardiofacial/DiGeorge

heart, including the ability to recognize significant lung hypoplasia, thoracic masses, and the signs of hydrops fetalis and fetal distress are useful.

The mother should lie in a comfortable position on the examining table, with her head elevated at a height that is comfortable for her. She may be more comfortable lying slightly on her left side, which is also beneficial for the fetus, particularly later in gestation; compression of the maternal inferior vena cava by the uterus decreases venous return to her heart, which may cause hypotension and decreased placental perfusion. It is not necessary for the mother's bladder to be full and, for comfort, she should be encouraged to empty her bladder before the examination.

The fetal echocardiographer has little control over fetal position, which may change frequently during the examination; one learns to reorient as the position of the fetus changes, using fetal cardiac landmarks. After first assessing the position of the fetus in the uterus, one can identify the fetal right and left sides. The position of the fetal cardiac apex and stomach are determined, and these can then be used as side locators as the fetus changes position. Adverse fetal position may be altered by having the mother turn on her side or take a walk or by stimulating the fetus to move by gently shaking the mother's abdomen.

Although a segmental approach to diagnosis is important, it is often difficult to obtain images of fetal cardiac structures in a predetermined sequence; it is more time-efficient to image structures as they present themselves, eventually evaluating the entire heart. It is helpful to maintain a mental checklist of all of the components of a complete study, ensuring that all items are addressed before completing the examination. In addition to assessment of cardiac morphology, spectral and color Doppler assessment of valve function, measurement of cardiac structures, assessment of heart rate and rhythm, and qualitative assessment of ventricular function are all part of a comprehensive fetal echocardiographic examination. Normal dimensions of fetal cardiac structures with respect to gestational age have been published.[59–62] An assessment of fetal size, using measurements of the head, femur, and abdomen, is useful for interpreting cardiac measurements, particularly if the fetus is large or small for gestational age.

Fetal Arrhythmia: Evaluation of fetal arrhythmias begins with an assessment of rate and regularity, followed by determination of the potential mechanism of arrhythmia. Simultaneous M-mode interrogation of contraction of the atrial wall (preferably the atrial appendage) and a ventricular wall or the aortic valve can demonstrate timing of contraction of the atria and ventricles and their relationship to each other, but can be technically difficult to obtain. Simultaneous Doppler interrogation of the LV inflow and outflow can provide similar information and is usually easier to obtain. Another technique that allows evaluation of fetal cardiac rhythm is color-coded tissue Doppler.[63] Finally, careful 2D imaging of the contraction of the appendages and ventricles can give clues as to the nature of the arrhythmia, distinguishing complete AV block from sinus bradycardia, for example. Determination of cardiac anatomy and ventricular and valve function, as well as an assessment for signs of hydrops (pleural and pericardial effusion, ascites, skin thickening) are part of a comprehensive evaluation of any fetal arrhythmia.

Limitations of Fetal Echocardiography: Despite high-quality images of the fetal heart, there are some cardiac abnormalities that cannot be excluded in fetal life. These include small ventral septal defects, mild valve abnormalities, coronary artery anomalies, some atrial septal defects, and persistent patency of the ductus arteriosus. Although reasonably accurate predictors of postnatal coarctation of the aorta have been described,[64–66] potential coarctation cannot be ruled out with certainty in any fetus. There are some situations in which a complete examination cannot be performed, usually due to maternal body habitus or persistently suboptimal fetal position.

Counseling: Physicians or medical professionals who counsel parents about the results of fetal echocardiography must be knowledgeable about the defect in question, including *in utero* and postnatal natural history, expected postnatal course, anticipated surgical or catheter interventions and their success rates, and expected quality of life, as well as the range of possible outcomes from best to worst case scenario. In addition, because many congenital heart defects are associated with syndromes or chromosomal anomalies, the counselor must have a basic knowledge of these associations to provide the parents with a comprehensive picture of the disease and its implications for the child's life. The limitations of the echocardiogram and of fetal echocardiography in general should be explained.

A team approach is useful in preparing parents and families for perinatal and postnatal events. Early involvement of pediatric cardiologists, obstetricians, neonatologists, social workers, cardiothoracic surgeons, genetic counselors, and cardiac nurses may be beneficial in helping families to obtain the information and resources they need. Meeting with various members of the medical team who will be caring for the infant after birth, and a tour of the nursery or intensive care unit where the infant will be taken, helps parents cope with the diagnosis of heart disease in their child and mentally prepares them for postnatal events, thereby reducing anxiety.[67]

Clinical Implications: Prenatal diagnosis allows planning of delivery in a tertiary care center where pediatric cardiologists, intensivists, cardiac surgeons, neonatologists, and other specialists are available to care for the infant. Postnatal management strategies can be planned and discussed with the parents in advance. Prostaglandin E_2 can be instituted for ductus-dependent lesions, preventing harmful levels of hypoxia and acidosis in most instances.

In addition, if urgent postnatal catheter or surgical therapy is anticipated, delivery can be coordinated to ensure that the necessary personnel are present. In rare instances there may be a role for an *EXIT to ECMO* (extracorporeal membrane oxygenation) strategy, in which the newborn is placed on an extracorporeal membrane oxygenator in the delivery room before separation from the placenta.

Although reports conflict as to whether prenatal diagnosis of congenital heart disease lowers mortality, evidence shows that morbidity is reduced.[68–71] Increased and earlier prenatal detection of the most severe types of congenital heart disease may result in decreased prevalence of these diseases in newborn populations in some countries, due to elective terminations.[72,73]

Prenatal diagnosis can affect management during pregnancy. Fetal tachyarrhythmias may be treated by administration of medication to the mother;[74–76] this in turn may prevent development of hydrops fetalis and the need for early delivery. Autoimmune congenital heart block may be prevented or diminished by maternal administration of steroids,[77] again reducing the risk of hydrops and early delivery. Hydrops caused by structural or functional cardiac abnormalities may also prompt early delivery, if the fetus is deemed more likely to survive *ex utero*. Finally, there may be an increasing role for prenatal catheter and surgical interventions.

Early attempts at transcatheter balloon dilation of the aortic valve in fetuses with critical aortic stenosis were largely unsuccessful.[78] More recently, investigators at Children's Hospital in Boston have had high rates of technical success for prenatal interventional procedures in critical aortic stenosis, critical pulmonary stenosis, premature closure of the foramen ovale, and hypoplastic left heart syndrome with intact or nearly intact atrial septum.[79,80] The effect of transcatheter interventions on *in utero* natural history and short and long-term outcome awaits further study.

SAFETY AND COMPLICATIONS

To date, no pre- or postnatal adverse effects resulting from diagnostic ultrasound have been reported. Medical personnel using this technology must however be cognizant that ultrasound is a form of mechanical energy which under certain conditions can cause damage to exposed tissue. This injury can result from conversion of mechanical energy to heat or from creation of gaseous microcavitations.

Thus far, biologic damage has been observed only in nonclinical laboratory conditions. The American Institute of Ultrasound in Medicine has stated that

> *No confirmed biologic effects on patients or instrument operator caused by exposure at intensities typical of present diagnostic ultrasound instruments have ever been reported. Although the possibility that such biologic effects may be identified in the future, current data indicate that the benefits to patients of the prudent use of diagnostic ultrasound outweigh the risks, if any, that may be present.*[81]

MAGNETIC RESONANCE IMAGING

Although MRI has been used for evaluation of the cardiovascular system since the early 1980s, its clinical implementation has been initially slow due to long scan time and limited diagnostic information, which was predominantly confined to morphology. Rapid developments in hardware design, computer sciences, and imaging sequences during the 1990s led to a dramatic expansion of the clinical utility of cardiovascular magnetic resonance (CMR) in patients with congenital and acquired heart disease.[82–84] CMR complements echocardiography, provides a noninvasive alternative to x-ray angiography, and avoids many of the limitations of these modalities. For example, in contrast to echocardiography, acoustic windows and body size do not limit CMR, and, unlike cardiac catheterization, CMR does not use ionizing radiation. In today's clinical practice, CMR is increasingly used in concert with other imaging modalities (most commonly echocardiography) for assessment of cardiac anatomy and function,[85] measurements of blood flow,[86] tissue characterization,[87,88] and, more recently, for evaluation of myocardial perfusion and viability.[89] The following section reviews basic CMR techniques, indications and contraindications to CMR, and special considerations in patients with congenital heart disease.

CMR Imaging Techniques and Their Clinical Applications

Background: The primary source of signal used to construct MR images is derived from hydrogen protons (^{1}H). In MRI, the ^{1}H protons are often referred to as *spins* because their angular momentum results in a precession (spinning) around the axis of the primary magnetic field. The highest concentrations of ^{1}H protons are in water and fat. Through the use of a strong static magnetic field, much weaker but rapidly varying magnetic field gradients, and short pulses of radiofrequency (RF) energy, the ^{1}H protons (spins) in selected regions of the body are stimulated to emit RF waves. These RF waves are then used to construct MR images. The strength of the static magnetic field in most clinical scanners used for CMR is 1.5 Tesla (T) (1 Tesla = 10,000 gauss [G]; the strength of earth's magnetic field at its surface is approximately 0.5G). More recently, MRI scanners with static field strength of 3T have become available.

As with any other diagnostic modality, an in-depth knowledge of the underlying MRI physics is essential for maximizing its utility and understanding its pitfalls and limitations. This, in turn, enhances the quality of the interpretation of the imaging data. A detailed discussion of MRI physics is beyond the scope of this chapter and can be found in other sources.[90,91]

Cardiac and Respiratory Gating: Because most CMR techniques acquire data over multiple heartbeats, cardiac and respiratory motions during image acquisition result in image blurring. Several techniques have been developed to overcome this problem. The most common approach to compensate for cardiac motion is to synchronize image acquisition with the cardiac cycle, either by electrocardiographic (ECG) gating or with a pulse oximetry trace (called *peripheral gating*). Electrocardiographic gating can be accomplished with a high-quality standard ECG trace or with a vectorcardiogram (VCG) signal.[92] Recently, a new technique called *self-gating*, which relies on cardiac motion and avoids the use of ECG triggering altogether has been described.[93] Blurring due to respiratory motion can be avoided either by having the patient hold his or her breath for periods of 5 to 10 seconds during data acquisition or by synchronizing image data acquisition to the respiratory and cardiac cycles. Another approach that reduces blurring from respiratory motion is to repeat the image acquisition several times and average the data. Respiratory motion can be tracked by either a bellows device placed around the abdomen or by MR navigator pulse that concurrently tracks the position of the diaphragm or cardiac border.[94]

A fundamentally different approach to avoid motion-induced image blurring is to acquire the MR data fast enough so that cardiac and respiratory motions are *frozen* in time. Recent advances in gradient coil performance, parallel acquisition techniques, and image display methods have allowed real-time CMR at 20 to 30 frames per second, albeit at the expense of spatial resolution.[95–98] This technology, which is now commercially available on some clinical scanners, may obviate the need for ECG and respiratory triggering.

CMR Examination Techniques: The building blocks of any MRI examination are called *pulse sequences*. An MRI pulse sequence describes the way the magnetic field gradients and RF pulses are applied to produce images with particular characteristics. Some of the pulse sequences used in clinical CMR practice are described in the following paragraphs. During the course of a CMR examination, the examiner selects the pulse sequences and prescribes imaging locations and planes to acquire the image data in order to address specific clinical questions.

Spin Echo: The MR signal is produced by applying a brief RF pulse that tips the spins 90 degrees relative to the axis of the main magnetic field, followed by a 180-degree refocusing RF pulse. Because of the relatively long time interval between spin excitation and data sampling, flowing blood will leave the image plane by the time the signal is sampled. The result is an image in which flowing blood appears black whereas more stationary tissues produce MR signals displayed in varying shades of gray or white (*black blood* imaging) (Fig. 13-10A). Other features of spin echo (SE) pulse sequences include a single image per cardiac cycle (static imaging), high tissue contrast, and, compared with gradient echo pulse sequences, relative insensitivity to inhomogeneities in the magnetic field. In clinical practice, such inhomogeneities are mostly due to ferromagnetic implants such as sternal wires, prosthetic heart valves, stents, coils, and so forth. SE sequences can also be modified to alter tissue contrast and characterize abnormal structures (e.g, T1- and T2-weighting) (Fig. 13-10*B*). Standard SE requires several minutes (usually 2–4 minutes depending on heart rate and imaging parameters) to acquire an image data set. Fast spin echo (FSE) (also called *turbo*) requires a much shorter image acquisition time because instead of acquiring a single phase encoding line for each 90-degree RF pulse, multiple phase encoding lines are acquired in rapid succession (called *echo train*). As a result, image acquisition can be completed during 10 to 15 seconds of breath holding. In FSE sequence, the blood signal is *nulled* by an inversion pulse (called *double inversion recovery*) rather than relying on blood flow alone.

Standard SE used to be the *work horse* of CMR during the 1980s. In today's clinical practice, standard SE has been largely replaced by FSE with double inversion recovery.[90] Examples of clinical applications include assessment of tissue characteristics (e.g, cardiac tumors, arrhythmogenic right ventricular dysplasia, myocardial noncompaction, and ventricular aneurysm), vessel wall imaging (e.g, aortic dissection), evaluation of the pericardium, and anatomic imaging in patients with metallic implants.

Gradient Echo: Gradient echo MR is a class of pulse sequences that produce bright blood images. The fundamental difference between SE and gradient echo sequences is that in the latter the initial RF pulse tips the spins at an angle (called *flip angle*) smaller than 90 degrees. Gradient echo sequences are generally faster than SE sequences because the time between spin excitation and signal detection (called *echo time* or TE) is much shorter. The signal from stationary or relatively slow-moving tissues (such as the myocardium) is gray because the spins within the selected slice are partially saturated by the rapid repetition of the

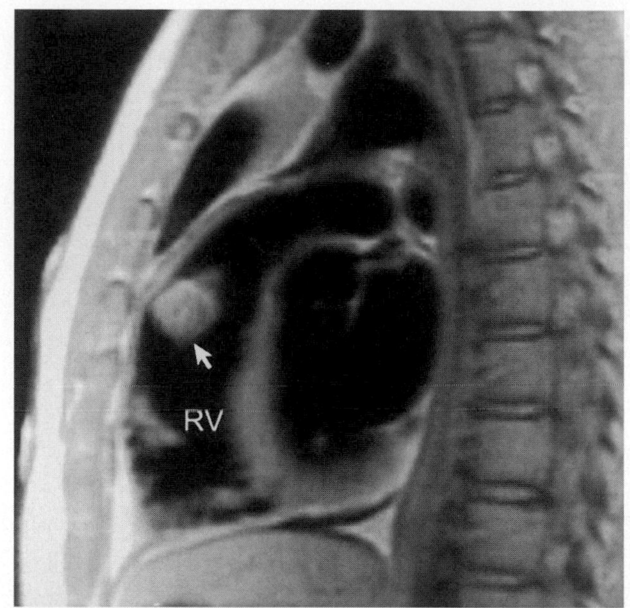

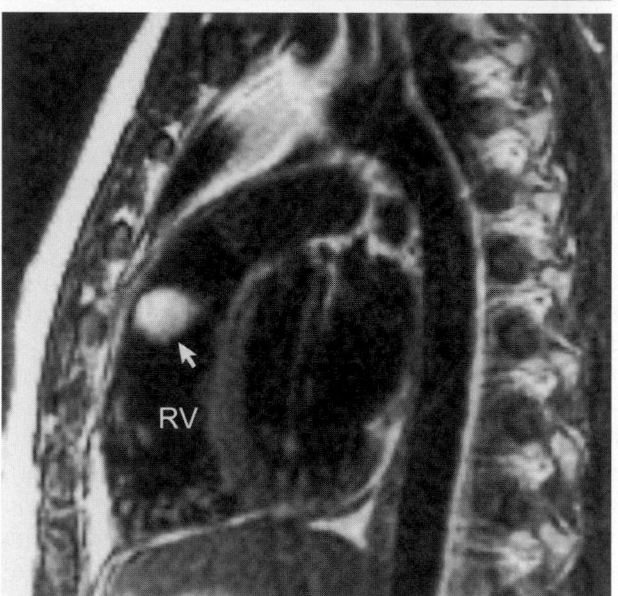

FIGURE 13–10 *Black blood imaging of a cardiac tumor (arrow) in the right ventricular outflow tract (RV) using fast spin echo with double inversion recovery pulse sequence. A, T1-weighted image; B, T2-weighted image showing increased signal intensity of the tumor, consistent with hemangioma (confirmed by histology).*

RF pulse. In other words, the spins do not have sufficient time to return to their original unexcited state during the short interval between RF pulses, which result in a relatively weak signal. On the other hand, blood that flows into the slice contains unsaturated spins that produce relatively strong signals, hence the term *bright blood* imaging (Fig. 13-11). An important feature of gradient echo sequences is high imaging speed, which allows reconstruction of multiple images during the cardiac cycle that can be displayed in

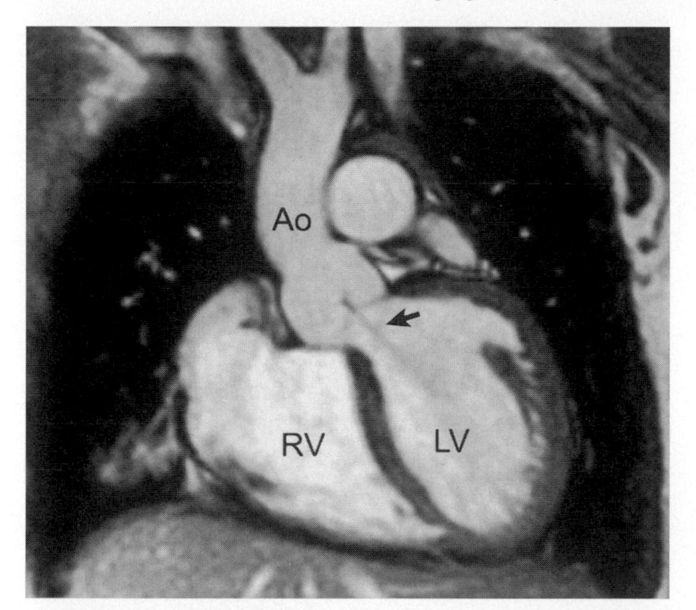

FIGURE 13–11 *Diastolic frame of electrocardiogram-triggered gradient echo (steady-state free precession) cine magnetic resonance imaging in the coronal plane. Note the small jet of aortic regurgitation (arrow).*

cine loop format. Compared with SE techniques, gradient echo sequences have a relatively low tissue contrast and are more susceptible to inhomogeneities in the magnetic field. Examples of some common clinical applications include assessment of cardiovascular anatomy, ventricular dimensions and function, valve regurgitation, and myocardial perfusion and viability.

Assessment of Ventricular Function: Ventricular dimensions and function are assessed by obtaining a series of contiguous images across the ventricles. The principle CMR sequence used for quantitative evaluation of ventricular function is gradient echo cine MRI. The most common imaging sequence used today is cardiac-triggered steady-state free precession.[99,100] This sequence is known by several proprietary names, including true fast imaging with steady precession (trueFISP), balanced fast field echo (bFFE), and fast imaging employing steady state acquisition (FIESTA). It requires a short acquisition time (typically 4–10 seconds for each location, depending on heart rate and imaging parameters), provides a sharp contrast between the blood pool and the myocardium, and has minimal motion-induced blurring during systole. Its main disadvantage is its sensitivity to inhomogeneities in the magnetic field, mostly from implanted metallic devices.

The technique used for evaluation of ventricular dimensions and function is shown in Fig. 13-12.[101–103] By tracing the blood–endocardium boundary, the volume of the slice is calculated as the product of its cross-sectional area and thickness, assuming an equal slice area throughout its thickness.

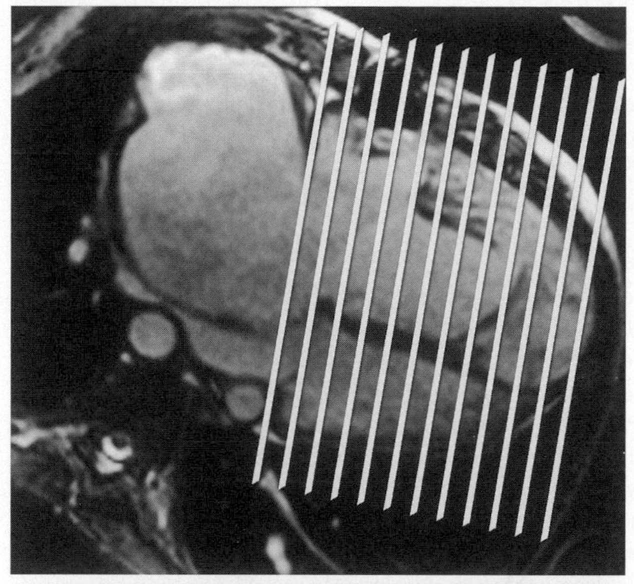

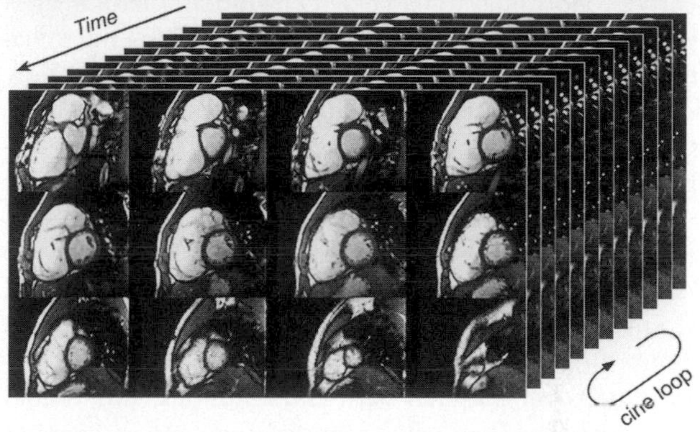

FIGURE 13–12 *Magnetic resonance imaging assessment of ventricular function in a patient with repaired tetralogy of Fallot and right ventricular dilatation. A, A diastolic frame of an electrocardiogram-triggered steady state free precession cine magnetic resonance imaging in the four-chamber plane is used to prescribe multiple contiguous slices perpendicular to the long-axis from the base through the apex. B, Multiple (usually 12) short-axis slices displayed in cine loop format.*

Ventricular volume is then determined by summation of the volumes of all slices. The process can be repeated for each frame in the cardiac cycle to obtain a continuous time-volume loop or may be performed only on a diastolic and a systolic frame to calculate diastolic and systolic volumes. From this data one can calculate left and right ventricular ejection fractions and stroke volumes. Since the patient's heart rate at the time of image acquisition is known, one can calculate left and right ventricular output. Ventricular mass is calculated by tracing the epicardial borders, subtracting the endocardial volumes, and multiplying the resultant muscle volume by the specific gravity of the myocardium (1.05 g/mm^3).

Multiple studies have demonstrated that measurements of ventricular dimensions and function by CMR are highly accurate and reproducible.[104–108] Advantages of this technique include a 3D data set, clear distinction between the blood pool and the myocardium, high spatial and temporal resolutions, and no reliance on a geometric model.

Several CMR techniques can be used for assessment of regional wall motion and myocardial mechanics. The most common method is myocardial tagging in which dark stripes are placed across the image at the onset of the R wave of the ECG. As the myocardium moves during the cardiac cycle, the tags follow it and their rotation, translation, and deformation can be tracked allowing for calculation of myocardial strain and strain rate.[109–112]

Velocity Encoded Cine MRI: This gradient echo sequence is based on the principle that the signal from spins flowing through specially designed magnetic field gradients accumulates a predictable phase shift that is linearly proportional to its velocity. Multiple phase images are constructed during the cardiac cycle in which the signal amplitude of each voxel is proportion to the mean flow velocity within that voxel. Blood flow is measured by defining a region of interest around a vessel, integrating the velocities of the enclosed voxels, and multiplying the product by the vessel's cross-sectional area (Fig. 13-13). *In vivo* and *in vitro* studies show that measurements of blood flow by velocity encoded cine MRI (VEC MRI) are accurate and reproducible.[86,113–116] Examples of clinical applications include measurements of pulmonary-to-systemic flow ratio (Qp/Qs) in patients with shunt lesions, differential pulmonary blood flow, valve regurgitation, and assessment of flow patterns in patients with Fontan palliation.

Contrast-Enhanced 3-Dimensional MR Angiography: This is a gradient echo technique in which the administration of a T1-shortening contrast agent, typically a gadolinium (Gd) chelate such as Gd-DTPA, markedly increases the contrast between vascular and nonvascular structures (Fig. 13-14*A*).[117–119] This method of angiography is less prone to flow-related artifacts than other MR techniques and has a short acquisition time. Contrast-enhanced 3D magnetic resonance angiography (CE 3D MRA) is usually performed without cardiac gating using a 3D fast gradient echo acquisition lasting 10 to 25 seconds. Patients hold their breath during image acquisition to minimize respiratory motion artifacts. Two or more image data sets are usually acquired and the entire procedure takes only a few minutes to perform. Recently developed parallel processing techniques and improved sequence design allow shortening the acquisition time to 3 to 5 seconds, thus opening the door to time-resolved 3D MRA.[120] The 3D data set can be navigated on a computer workstation using a variety of image display techniques, including rapid construction of intuitive 3D models (Fig. 13-14*B*).[121]

Myocardial Perfusion and Viability: CMR can assess myocardial perfusion by detecting the transit and distribution of a contrast agent through the heart. Using ultrafast multislice imaging with an echo-planar gradient echo pulse sequence, the first pass of a bolus of gadolinium-based MR contrast agent (usually Gd-DTPA) is observed. Myocardial regions with decreased perfusion exhibit delayed or lack of signal enhancement.[122,123] Stress perfusion imaging, which has improved sensitivity and specificity for detection of coronary artery stenosis over rest perfusion alone, can be achieved by administering a coronary vasodilator (e.g, adenosine or dipyridamole) or by dobutamine or other vasoactive drugs.[124,125] The principle advantages of CMR perfusion over nuclear techniques include superior spatial resolution and lack of ionizing radiation.[126] An alternative method for detection of myocardial ischemia is to induce regional wall motion abnormalities with dobutamine stress (with or without atropine). Comparison between first-pass myocardial perfusion and dobutamine stress MRI with regard to the ability of these techniques to detect coronary artery stenosis in adults is the subject of ongoing investigations.[127–129]

Myocardial viability can be assessed by CMR using a modified gradient echo technique 10 to 20 minutes after administration of Gd-DTPA. Using an inversion pulse, the signal from viable myocardium is suppressed whereas nonviable myocardium exhibits high signal intensity (hyperenhancement) due to retention of the contrast agent (Fig. 13-15). Studies of myocardial infarction in animal models as well as a growing number of human clinical studies have demonstrated that this technique (called *myocardial delayed enhancement*) is both sensitive and specific for detection of irreversible myocardial injury.[130–133] Other studies have shown that this method allows detection of inflammation (myocarditis and pericarditis[134,135]) and myocardial fibrosis (e.g, in hypertrophic cardiomyopathy[136]).

Approach to Magnetic Resonance Imaging Evaluation of Congenital Heart Disease

Detailed pre-examination planning is crucial given the wide array of imaging sequences available and the often complex nature of the clinical, anatomic, and functional issues in patients with CHD. The importance of a careful review of the patient's medical history, including details of all cardiovascular surgical procedures, interventional catheterizations, findings of previous diagnostic tests and current clinical status, cannot be overemphasized. As is the case with echocardiography and cardiac catheterization, CMR is an interactive diagnostic procedure that requires online review and interpretation of the data by the supervising physician. The unpredictable nature of the anatomy and hemodynamics often require adjustment of the examination protocol, modification of imaging planes, adding, deleting,

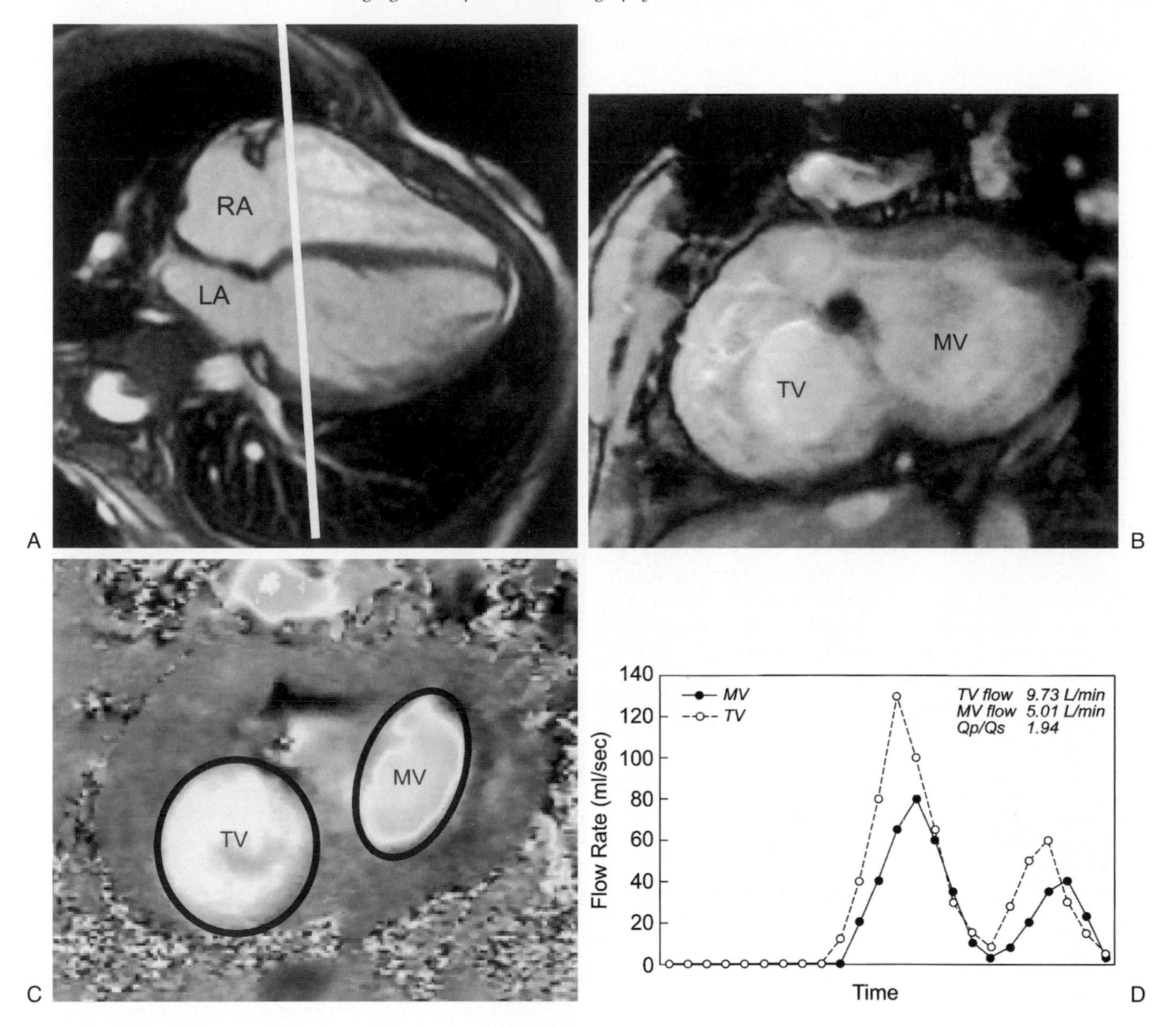

FIGURE 13–13 *Magnetic resonance imaging measurements of blood flow through the atrioventricular valves in a patient with left-to-right shunt from a secundum atrial septal defect. A, An image in the four-chamber plane is used for placement of the electrocardiogram-triggered phase contrast cine magnetic resonance imaging sequence perpendicular to plane of the atrioventricular valves. B, Magnitude image reconstructed from the amplitude of the magnetic resonance radiofrequency signal provides anatomic depiction. C, Phase image reconstructed from the phase difference of the magnetic resonance radiofrequency signal provides information on flow velocity and direction. A region of interest is drawn around the flow signals in the atrioventricular valves. D, Instantaneous flow rates (mL/sec) are calculated by integration of the velocities across the regions of interest. The areas under the flow curves represent stroke volumes.*

or changing sequences, and adjustment of imaging parameters. Reliance on standardized protocols and post-hoc reading alone in these patients might result in incomplete or even erroneous interpretation.

Indications: CMR is now used to obtain diagnostic information in a wide range of congenital and acquired pediatric heart disease. It is usually performed in concert with other tests, including echocardiography, cardiac catheterization, computed tomography, and nuclear scintigraphy. The most common clinical scenarios in which CMR is requested involve one or more of the following: (a) when the existing diagnostic information is incomplete

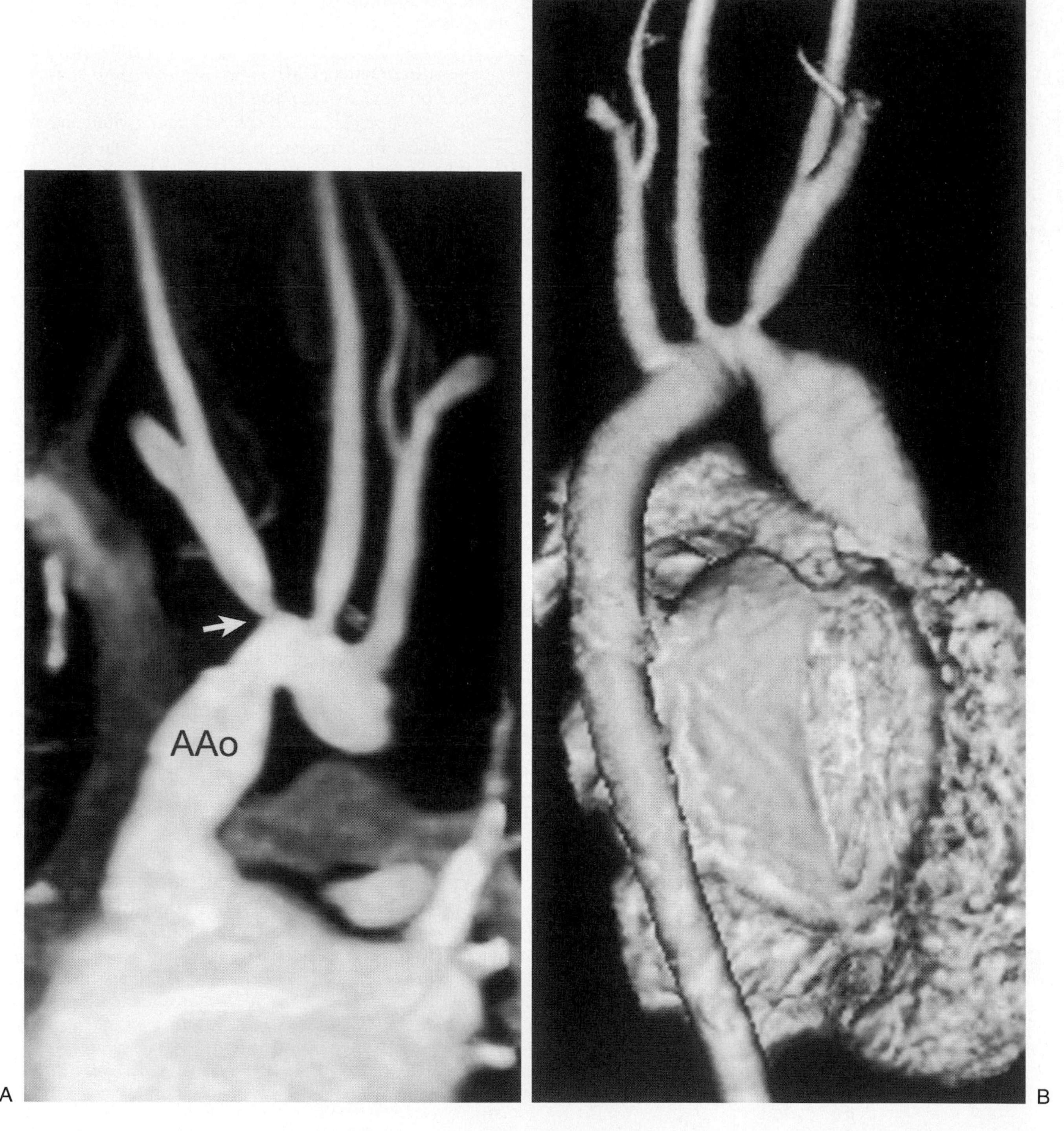

FIGURE 13–14 *Gadolinium-enhanced three-dimensional magnetic resonance angiogram in a patient with Williams syndrome who underwent patch repair of supravalvar aortic stenosis. A, Maximum intensity projection image showing stenosis of the origin of the right innominate artery (arrow) as well as mild narrowing and an acute angle between the ascending aorta and transverse arch. B, Three-dimensional volume rendering.*

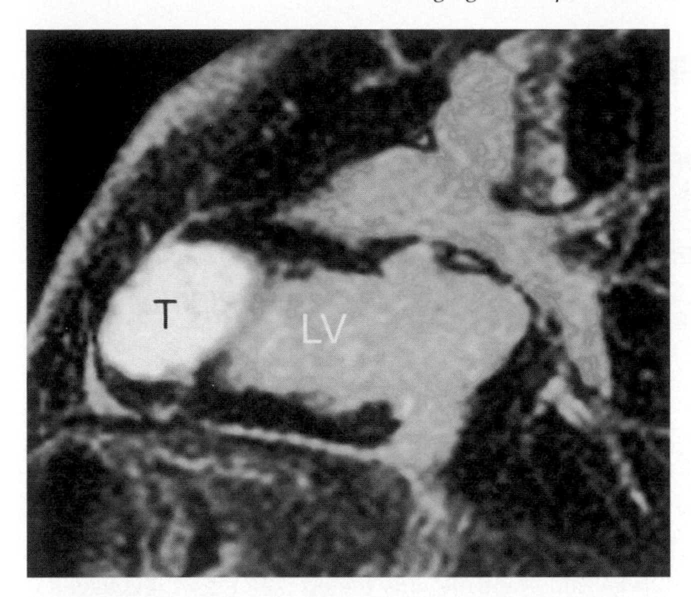

FIGURE 13–15 *Delayed myocardial enhancement sequence approximately 12 minutes after administration of gadolinium DTPA (0.2 mmol/kg) in a patient with cardiac tumor. The signal in the tumor (T) is bright indicating retention of the contrast agent within the tumor, consistent with fibrosis (typical for cardiac fibroma). Note that the signal of the remainder of the left ventricular myocardium is dark since the contrast has cleared from the viable myocardium.*

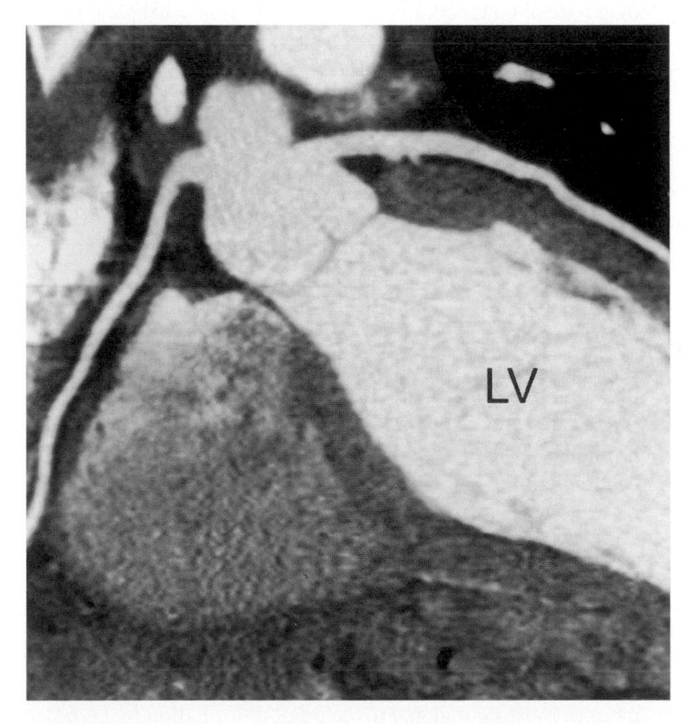

FIGURE 13–16 *Contrast-enhanced electrocardiogram-triggered 16-row detector computed tomography angiogram (CTA) of the coronary arteries showing origin of the right coronary artery just above the right aortic sinotubular junction.*

or inconsistent; (b) to avoid diagnostic catheterization with its associated risks; and (c) for the unique capabilities of CMR (e.g, site-specific flow measurements, tissue characteristics). In practice, CMR is increasingly used in patients with suboptimal echocardiographic windows, a relatively common problem in adolescents and adults with congenital heart disease, for assessment of ventricular dimensions and function, and for quantification of valve regurgitation. The most common referral diagnoses for CMR at Children's Hospital Boston in 2002 and 2003 were postoperative tetralogy of Fallot (23% of studies), followed by anomalies of the aorta (16%), complex two-ventricle (e.g, postoperative transposition of the great arteries) (13%), single ventricle (10%), and quantitative evaluation of ventricular dimensions and function as the primary reason for referral (7%).

Contraindications and Safety: There are no known deleterious biologic effects caused by the static magnetic fields used in 1.5T clinical MRI scanners.[137] Standards developed by the Food and Drug Administration (FDA) set strict limits on the energy deposited by the various imaging sequences. Nevertheless, safety rules must be strictly observed in the MRI suite to prevent injury. Patients and any accompanying individuals should be carefully screened for metallic objects or medical devices before entering the MRI suite.[138] Monitoring equipment, oxygen tanks, intravenous poles, and any other medical or transport devices must be MRI compatible. Loops of ECG or any other monitoring cables can cause skin burns and must be avoided. Earplugs or other protective devices should be used to prevent acoustic damage.

Implanted medical devices can cause hazards in the MRI environment. Devices can potentially undergo undesirable torquing movements if the magnetic field is sufficiently strong and if they contained sufficient ferromagnetic material. Another potential hazard is heating of devices due to energy deposited by the rapidly switched magnetic field gradients and RF pulses. Electronic devices such as pacemakers and implanted defibrillators can malfunction in the MRI environment. Fortunately, most implants used in patients with heart disease (e.g, sternal wires, heart valves, stents, and occluding devices and coils) are not considered a contraindication to MRI.[139,140] Several devices are considered either a relative or an absolute contraindication to MRI. Most centers deem the presence of a cardiac pacemaker to be an absolute contraindication to MRI. This assertion, however, has recently been challenged.[141] Information regarding the safety of individual devices can be determined either by consulting a published source on MRI safety or by contacting the manufacturer.

Sedation and Anesthesia

Acquisition of diagnostic-quality CMR images requires the patient to lie still in the scanner for up to 1 hour.

In general, we have found that patients younger than 7 years cannot usually cooperate with a typical CMR examination and require sedation or anesthesia. Some patients between 7 and 10 years old are capable of cooperation, whereas most children older than 10 years can undergo a CMR study without sedation provided their mental development is age-appropriate and they are not claustrophobic. Sedation administered via oral, rectal, or intravenous routes can be safe and effective in preventing patient movement and is a reasonable choice for CMR.[142] However, it carries the risk of an unprotected airway, particularly in an infant with significant cardiac disease and little hemodynamic reserve and does not address the issue of respiratory motion. General anesthesia is safe when performed by experienced practitioners and has the added benefit of the ability to suspend respiration during image acquisition. For these reasons, our center has opted to use general anesthesia, performed by anesthesiologists specializing in pediatric cardiac patients, in almost all cases requiring sedation.[143]

The potential need for sedation or anesthesia should be assessed well in advance of the procedure. The patient's developmental age and maturity are the primary consideration in the decision, but other factors, such as the length of the anticipated examination and prior experience with procedures should be considered.

COMPUTED TOMOGRAPHY

Computed tomography uses rapidly rotating x-ray beams and detectors to create an image. The radiation that is not absorbed by the tissue passes into multiple detectors in the scanner's gantry and is converted into digital signals, which are then combined by a computer program to form a cross-sectional image. Images are acquired in the axial (transverse) plane and can be viewed on a computer workstation using several techniques. CT technology has witnessed a remarkably rapid evolution in recent years, which has led to improved spatial and temporal resolutions and shorter scan times. For example, the spatial resolution of a 16-detector row CT is up to $0.5 \times 0.5 \times 0.6$ mm and the temporal resolution is 105 to 210 milliseconds.[144] At present, the temporal resolution of CT lags behind that of MRI but as 32- and 64-row detector CT scans are becoming commercially available and the technology continues to improve, higher temporal resolution is expected.

CT angiography (CTA) of the cardiovascular system is performed during injection of nonionic iodinated contrast agent. Breath-holding during image acquisition is important to eliminate blurring due to respiratory motion.[145] The use of ECG triggering reduces image blurring due to cardiac motion but results in an increased radiation dose. In general, ECG triggering is required for coronary imaging, and for high-quality cine imaging of intracardiac anatomy (Fig. 13-16). CTA of the aorta, pulmonary arteries, and venous structures generally does not require ECG triggering.

CTA is capable of providing excellent quality static anatomic imaging of cardiovascular structures and is an excellent noninvasive alternative to cardiac catheterization. Its advantages include high spatial resolution, good contrast between vascular and nonvascular structures, short imaging time, reduced need for sedation (as compared with MRI), and additional diagnostic information regarding parenchymal lung disease.[84] Disadvantages of CT include exposure to a significant dose of ionizing radiation,[146] little or no functional information, relatively low soft-tissue contrast (as compared with MRI), and risks associated with the use of iodinated contrast agents (e.g, nephrotoxicity, allergic reaction). In clinical practice, CTA has an important role in selected patients with congenital heart disease who have contraindications to MRI (e.g, pacemaker, implantable defibrillator) or in others who would have limited evaluation by MR due to artifacts from metallic objects such as stainless steel coils.

REFERENCES

1. Sanders S. Echocardiography and related techniques in the diagnosis of congenital heart disease, I: Veins, atria and interatrial septum. Echocardiography 1:185, 1984.
2. Snider AR, Serwer GA, Ritter SB. Echocardiography in Pediatric Heart Disease. St. Louis: Mosby, 1997.
3. Silverman NH. Pediatric Echocardiography. Baltimore: Williams & Wilkins, 1993.
4. Geva T. Echocardiography and Doppler ultrasound. In Garson A, Bricker, JT, Fisher, DJ, Neish SR (eds). The Science and Practice of Pediatric Cardiology. Baltimore: Williams & Wilkins, 1997, p 789.
5. Feigenbaum H. Echocardiography. Philadelphia: Lea & Febiger, 1994.
6. Rein AJ, Nadjari M, Bromiker R, et al. Detection of an obstructive membrane in the ductus arteriosus of a fetus using high frame rate echocardiography. Fetal Diagn Ther 13:250, 1998.
7. Espinola-Zavaleta N, Munoz-Castellanos L, Attie F, et al. Anatomic three-dimensional echocardiographic correlation of bicuspid aortic valve. J Am Soc Echocardiogr 16:46, 2003.
8. Sitges M, Jones M, Shiota T, et al. Real-time three-dimensional color doppler evaluation of the flow convergence zone for quantification of mitral regurgitation: Validation experimental animal study and initial clinical experience. J Am Soc Echocardiogr 16:38, 2003.
9. Edvardsen T, Gerber BL, Garot J, et al. Quantitative assessment of intrinsic regional myocardial deformation by Doppler strain rate echocardiography in humans: validation against three-dimensional tagged magnetic resonance imaging. Circulation 106:50, 2002.

10. Gramiak R, Shah PM, Kramer DH. Ultrasound cardiography: contrast studies in anatomy and function. Radiology 92:939, 1969.
11. Cohen BE, Winer HE, Kronzon I. Echocardiographic findings in patients with left superior vena cava and dilated coronary sinus. Am J Cardiol 44:158, 1979.
12. Snider AR, Silverman NH, Turley K, et al. Evaluation of infradiaphragmatic total anomalous pulmonary venous connection with two-dimensional echocardiography. Circulation 66:1129, 1982.
13. Allen HD, Sahn DJ, Goldberg SJ. New serial contrast technique for assessment of left to right shunting patent ductus arteriosus in the neonate. Am J Cardiol 41:288, 1978.
14. Jeetley P, Swinburn J, Hickman M, et al. Myocardial contrast echocardiography predicts left ventricular remodelling after acute myocardial infarction. J Am Soc Echocardiogr 17:1030, 2004.
15. Kleinert S, Geva T. Echocardiographic morphometry and geometry of the left ventricular outflow tract in fixed subaortic stenosis. J Am Coll Cardiol 22:1501, 1993.
16. Wong PC, Sanders SP, Jonas RA, et al. Pulmonary valve-moderator band distance and association with development of double-chambered right ventricle. Am J Cardiol 68:1681, 1991.
17. Manganas C, Iliopoulos J, Chard RB, et al. Reoperation and coarctation of the aorta: the need for lifelong surveillance. Ann Thorac Surg 72:1222, 2001.
18. Matitiau A, Geva T, Colan SD, et al. Bulboventricular foramen size in infants with double-inlet left ventricle or tricuspid atresia with transposed great arteries: influence on initial palliative operation and rate of growth. J Am Coll Cardiol 19:142, 1992.
19. McMahon CJ, Gauvreau K, Edwards JC, et al. Risk factors for aortic valve dysfunction in children with discrete subvalvar aortic stenosis. Am J Cardiol 94:459, 2004.
20. Lipshitz M, Marino BL, Sanders SP. Chloral hydrate side effects in young children: causes and management. Heart Lung 22:408, 1993.
21. Napoli KL, Ingall CG, Martin GR. Safety and efficacy of chloral hydrate sedation in children undergoing echocardiography. J Pediatr 129:287, 1996.
22. Krauss B, Green SM. Sedation and analgesia for procedures in children. N Engl J Med 342:938, 2000.
23. Latson LA, Cheatham JP, Gumbiner CH, et al. Midazolam nose drops for outpatient echocardiography sedation in infants. Am Heart J 121:209, 1991.
24. Davis PJ, Tome JA, McGowan FX Jr, et al. Preanesthetic medication with intranasal midazolam for brief pediatric surgical procedures: effect on recovery and hospital discharge times. Anesthesiology 82:2, 1995.
25. American Academy of Pediatrics Committee on Drugs: Guidelines for monitoring and management of pediatric patients during and after sedation for diagnostic and therapeutic procedures. Pediatrics 89:1110, 1992.
26. Tanner J. Fallacy of per-weight and per-surface area standards, and their relation to spurious correlation. J App Physiol 2:1, 1949.
27. Gutgesell HP, Rembold CM. Growth of the human heart relative to body surface area. Am J Cardiol 65:662, 1990.
28. Jenkins C, Bricknell K, Hanekom L, et al. Reproducibility and accuracy of echocardiographic measurements of left ventricular parameters using real-time three-dimensional echocardiography. J Am Coll Cardiol 44:878, 2004.
29. Arai K, Hozumi T, Matsumura Y, et al. Accuracy of measurement of left ventricular volume and ejection fraction by new real-time three-dimensional echocardiography in patients with wall motion abnormalities secondary to myocardial infarction. Am J Cardiol 94:552, 2004.
30. Altmann K, Shen Z, Boxt LM, et al. Comparison of three-dimensional echocardiographic assessment of volume, mass, and function in children with functionally single left ventricles with two-dimensional echocardiography and magnetic resonance imaging. Am J Cardiol 80:1060, 1997.
31. Valdes-Cruz LM, Yoganathan AP, Tamura T, et al. Studies in vitro of the relationship between ultrasound and laser Doppler velocimetry and applicability to the simplified Bernoulli relationship. Circulation 73:300, 1986.
32. Yoganathan AP, Valdes-Cruz LM, Schmidt-Dohna J, et al. Continuous-wave Doppler velocities and gradients across fixed tunnel obstructions: studies in vitro and in vivo. Circulation 76:657, 1987.
33. Smith MD, Dawson PL, Elion JL, et al. Correlation of continuous wave Doppler velocities with cardiac catheterization gradients: an experimental model of aortic stenosis. J Am Coll Cardiol 6:1306, 1985.
34. Gentles TL, Rosenfeld HM, Sanders SP, et al. Pediatric biplane transesophageal echocardiography: preliminary experience. Am Heart J 128:1225, 1994.
35. Randolph GR, Hagler DJ, Connolly HM, et al. Intraoperative transesophageal echocardiography during surgery for congenital heart defects. J Thorac Cardiovasc Surg 124:1176, 2002.
36. Rosenfeld HM, Gentles TL, Wernovsky G, et al. Utility of intraoperative transesophageal echocardiography in the assessment of residual cardiac defects. Pediatr Cardiol 19:346, 1998.
37. Muhiudeen Russell IA, Miller-Hance WC, Silverman NH. Intraoperative transesophageal echocardiography for pediatric patients with congenital heart disease. Anesth Analg 87:1058, 1998.
38. van der Velde EA. Echocardiography in the catheterization laboratory. In Lock JE, Keane JF, Perry SB (eds). Diagnostic and Interventional Catheterization in Congenital Heart Disease. Norwell, MA: Kluwer Academic Publishers, 2000, pp 355.
39. Fyfe DA, Ritter SB, Snider AR, et al. Guidelines for transesophageal echocardiography in children. J Am Soc Echocardiogr 5:640, 1992.
40. Greene MA, Alexander JA, Knauf DG, et al. Endoscopic evaluation of the esophagus in infants and children immediately following intraoperative use of transesophageal echocardiography. Chest 116:1247, 1999.
41. Stevenson JG. Incidence of complications in pediatric transesophageal echocardiography: experience in 1650 cases. J Am Soc Echocardiogr 12:527, 1999.
42. Savino JS, Hanson CW 3rd, Bigelow DC, et al. Oropharyngeal injury after transesophageal echocardiography. J Cardiothorac Vasc Anesth 8:76, 1994.

43. Frommelt PC, Stuth EA. Transesophageal echocardiographic in total anomalous pulmonary venous drainage: hypotension caused by compression of the pulmonary venous confluence during probe passage. J Am Soc Echocardiogr 7:652, 1994.
44. Kleinman CS, Hobbins JC, Jaffe CC, et al. Echocardiographic studies of the human fetus: prenatal diagnosis of congenital heart disease and cardiac dysrhythmias. Pediatrics 65:1059, 1980.
45. Kleinman C. Fetal echocardiography: diagnosing congenital heart disease in the human fetus. In ACC Educational Highlights, Bethesda, MD, 1996.
46. Allan LD, Crawford DC, Anderson RH, et al. Echocardiographic and anatomical correlations in fetal congenital heart disease. Br Heart J 52:542, 1984.
47. Achiron R, Rotstein Z, Lipitz S, et al. First-trimester diagnosis of fetal congenital heart disease by transvaginal ultrasonography. Obstet Gynecol 84:69, 1994.
48. Budorick NE, Millman SL. New modalities for imaging the fetal heart. Semin Perinatol 24:352, 2000.
49. Buskens E, Grobbee DE, Frohn-Mulder IM, et al. Efficacy of routine fetal ultrasound screening for congenital heart disease in normal pregnancy. Circulation 94:67, 1996.
50. Montana E, Khoury MJ, Cragan JD, et al. Trends and outcomes after prenatal diagnosis of congenital cardiac malformations by fetal echocardiography in a well defined birth population, Atlanta, Georgia, 1990-1994. J Am Coll Cardiol 28:1805, 1996.
51. Achiron R, Glaser J, Gelernter I, et al. Extended fetal echocardiographic examination for detecting cardiac malformations in low risk pregnancies. BMJ 304:671, 1992.
52. Kirk JS, Riggs TW, Comstock CH, et al. Prenatal screening for cardiac anomalies: the value of routine addition of the aortic root to the four-chamber view. Obstet Gynecol 84:427, 1994.
53. Bromley B, Estroff JA, Sanders SP, et al. Fetal echocardiography: accuracy and limitations in a population at high and low risk for heart defects. Am J Obstet Gynecol 166:1473, 1992.
54. Simpson JM, Sharland GK. Natural history and outcome of aortic stenosis diagnosed prenatally. Heart 77:205, 1997.
55. Hornberger LK, Sanders SP, Sahn DJ, et al. In utero pulmonary artery and aortic growth and potential for progression of pulmonary outflow tract obstruction in tetralogy of Fallot. J Am Coll Cardiol 25:739, 1995.
56. Hornberger LK, Sanders SP, Rein AJ, et al. Left heart obstructive lesions and left ventricular growth in the midtrimester fetus: a longitudinal study. Circulation 92:1531, 1995.
57. Vlahos AP, Lock JE, McElhinney DB, et al. Hypoplastic left heart syndrome with intact or highly restrictive atrial septum: outcome after neonatal transcatheter atrial septostomy. Circulation 109:2326, 2004.
58. Rychik J, Rome JJ, Collins MH, et al. The hypoplastic left heart syndrome with intact atrial septum: atrial morphology, pulmonary vascular histopathology and outcome. J Am Coll Cardiol 34:554, 1999.
59. Sharland GK, Allan LD. Normal fetal cardiac measurements derived by cross-sectional echocardiography. Ultrasound Obstet Gynecol 2:175, 1992.
60. Gembruch U, Shi C, Smrcek JM. Biometry of the fetal heart between 10 and 17 weeks of gestation. Fetal Diagn Ther 15:20, 2000.
61. Shapiro I, Degani S, Leibovitz Z, et al. Fetal cardiac measurements derived by transvaginal and transabdominal cross-sectional echocardiography from 14 weeks of gestation to term. Ultrasound Obstet Gynecol 12:404, 1998.
62. Achiron R, Zimand S, Hegesh J, et al. Fetal aortic arch measurements between 14 and 38 weeks' gestation: in-utero ultrasonographic study. Ultrasound Obstet Gynecol 15:226, 2000.
63. Rein AJ, O'Donnell C, Geva T, et al. Use of tissue velocity imaging in the diagnosis of fetal cardiac arrhythmias. Circulation 106:1827, 2002.
64. Hornberger LK, Sahn DJ, Kleinman CS, et al. Antenatal diagnosis of coarctation of the aorta: a multicenter experience. J Am Coll Cardiol 23:417, 1994.
65. Hornberger LK, Weintraub RG, Pesonen E, et al. Echocardiographic study of the morphology and growth of the aortic arch in the human fetus. Observations related to the prenatal diagnosis of coarctation. Circulation 86:741, 1992.
66. Benacerraf BR, Saltzman DH, Sanders SP. Sonographic sign suggesting the prenatal diagnosis of coarctation of the aorta. J Ultrasound Med 8:65, 1989.
67. Sklansky M, Tang A, Levy D, et al. Maternal psychological impact of fetal echocardiography. J Am Soc Echocardiogr 15:159, 2002.
68. Copel JA, Tan AS, Kleinman CS. Does a prenatal diagnosis of congenital heart disease alter short-term outcome? Ultrasound Obstet Gynecol 10:237, 1997.
69. Tworetzky W, McElhinney DB, Reddy VM, et al. Improved surgical outcome after fetal diagnosis of hypoplastic left heart syndrome. Circulation 103:1269, 2001.
70. Kumar RK, Newburger JW, Gauvreau K, et al. Comparison of outcome when hypoplastic left heart syndrome and transposition of the great arteries are diagnosed prenatally versus when diagnosis of these two conditions is made only postnatally. Am J Cardiol 83:1649, 1999.
71. Bonnet D, Coltri A, Butera G, et al. Detection of transposition of the great arteries in fetuses reduces neonatal morbidity and mortality. Circulation 99:916, 1999.
72. Allan LD, Cook A, Sullivan I, et al. Hypoplastic left heart syndrome: effects of fetal echocardiography on birth prevalence. Lancet 337:959, 1991.
73. Daubeney PE, Sharland GK, Cook AC, et al. Pulmonary atresia with intact ventricular septum: impact of fetal echocardiography on incidence at birth and postnatal outcome. UK and Eire Collaborative Study of Pulmonary Atresia with Intact Ventricular Septum. Circulation 98:562, 1998.
74. Copel JA, Friedman AH, Kleinman CS. Management of fetal cardiac arrhythmias. Obstet Gynecol Clin North Am 24:201, 1997.
75. Copel JA, Liang RI, Demasio K, et al. The clinical significance of the irregular fetal heart rhythm. Am J Obstet Gynecol 182:813, 2000.
76. Oudijk MA, Ruskamp JM, Ververs FF, et al. Treatment of fetal tachycardia with sotalol: transplacental pharmacokinetics and pharmacodynamics. J Am Coll Cardiol 42:765, 2003.

77. Brackley KJ, Ismail KM, Wright JG, et al. The resolution of fetal hydrops using combined maternal digoxin and dexamethasone therapy in a case of isolated complete heart block at 30 weeks gestation. Fetal Diagn Ther 15:355, 2000.
78. Kohl T, Sharland G, Allan LD, et al. World experience of percutaneous ultrasound-guided balloon valvuloplasty in human fetuses with severe aortic valve obstruction. Am J Cardiol 85:1230, 2000.
79. Tworetzky W, Wilkins-Haug L, Jennings RW, et al. Balloon dilation of severe aortic stenosis in the fetus: potential for prevention of hypoplastic left heart syndrome: candidate selection, technique, and results of successful intervention. Circulation 110:2125, 2004.
80. Marshall AC, van der Velde ME, Tworetzky W, et al. Creation of an atrial septal defect in utero for fetuses with hypoplastic left heart syndrome and intact or highly restrictive atrial septum. Circulation 110:253, 2004.
81. Bioeffects considerations for the safety of diagnostic ultrasound. American Institute of Ultrasound in Medicine. Bioeffects Committee. J Ultrasound Med 7:S1, 1988.
82. Geva T. Introduction: magnetic resonance imaging. Pediatr Cardiol 21:3, 2000.
83. Geva T, Sahn, DJ, Powell AJ. Magnetic resonance imaging of congenital heart disease in adults. Progress in Pediatric Cardiology 17:21, 2003.
84. Boxt LM. Magnetic resonance and computed tomographic evaluation of congenital heart disease. J Magn Reson Imaging 19:827, 2004.
85. Sahn DJ, Vick GW 3rd. Review of new techniques in echocardiography and magnetic resonance imaging as applied to patients with congenital heart disease. Heart 86(Suppl 2):II41, 2001.
86. Powell AJ, Geva T. Blood flow measurement by magnetic resonance imaging in congenital heart disease. Pediatr Cardiol 21:47, 2000.
87. Kiaffas MG, Powell AJ, Geva T. Magnetic resonance imaging evaluation of cardiac tumor characteristics in infants and children. Am J Cardiol 89:1229, 2002.
88. Anderson LJ, Holden S, Davis B, et al. Cardiovascular T2-star (T2*) magnetic resonance for the early diagnosis of myocardial iron overload. Eur Heart J 22:2171, 2001.
89. Prakash A, Powell AJ, Krishnamurthy R, et al. Magnetic resonance imaging evaluation of myocardial perfusion and viability in congenital and acquired pediatric heart disease. Am J Cardiol 93:657, 2004.
90. Mulkern RV, Chung T. From signal to image: magnetic resonance imaging physics for cardiac magnetic resonance. Pediatr Cardiol 21:5, 2000.
91. Axel L. Physics and technology of cardiovascular MR imaging. Cardiol Clin 16:125, 1998.
92. Chia JM, Fischer SE, Wickline SA, et al. Performance of QRS detection for cardiac magnetic resonance imaging with a novel vectorcardiographic triggering method. J Magn Reson Imaging 12:678, 2000.
93. Larson AC, White RD, Laub G, et al. Self-gated cardiac cine MRI. Magn Reson Med 51:93, 2004.
94. Spuentrup E, Buecker A, Stuber M, et al. Navigator-gated coronary magnetic resonance angiography using steady-state-free-precession: comparison to standard T2-prepared gradient-echo and spiral imaging. Invest Radiol 38:263, 2003.
95. Wetzel SG, Lee VS, Tan AG, et al. Real-time interactive duplex MR measurements: application in neurovascular imaging. AJR Am J Roentgenol 177:703, 2001.
96. Buecker A, Adam GB, Neuerburg JM, et al. Simultaneous real-time visualization of the catheter tip and vascular anatomy for MR-guided PTA of iliac arteries in an animal model. J Magn Reson Imaging 16:201, 2002.
97. Plein S, Smith WH, Ridgway JP, et al. Measurements of left ventricular dimensions using real-time acquisition in cardiac magnetic resonance imaging: comparison with conventional gradient echo imaging. Magma 13:101, 2001.
98. Sampath S, Derbyshire JA, Atalar E, et al. Real-time imaging of two-dimensional cardiac strain using a harmonic phase magnetic resonance imaging (HARP-MRI) pulse sequence. Magn Reson Med 50:154, 2003.
99. Carr JC, Simonetti O, Bundy J, et al. Cine MR angiography of the heart with segmented true fast imaging with steady-state precession. Radiology 219:828, 2001.
100. Plein S, Bloomer TN, Ridgway JP, et al. Steady-state free precession magnetic resonance imaging of the heart: comparison with segmented k-space gradient-echo imaging. J Magn Reson Imaging 14:230, 2001.
101. Lorenz CH, Walker ES, Morgan VL, et al. Normal human right and left ventricular mass, systolic function, and gender differences by cine magnetic resonance imaging. J Cardiovasc Magn Reson 1:7, 1999.
102. Lorenz CH. The range of normal values of cardiovascular structures in infants, children, and adolescents measured by magnetic resonance imaging. Pediatr Cardiol 21:37, 2000.
103. Alfakih K, Plein S, Thiele H, et al. Normal human left and right ventricular dimensions for MRI as assessed by turbo gradient echo and steady-state free precession imaging sequences. J Magn Reson Imaging 17:323, 2003.
104. Bellenger NG, Davies LC, Francis JM, et al. Reduction in sample size for studies of remodeling in heart failure by the use of cardiovascular magnetic resonance. J Cardiovasc Magn Reson 2:271, 2000.
105. Bellenger NG, Marcus NJ, Davies C, et al. Left ventricular function and mass after orthotopic heart transplantation: a comparison of cardiovascular magnetic resonance with echocardiography. J Heart Lung Transplant 19:444, 2000.
106. Pattynama PM, Lamb HJ, van der Velde EA, et al. Reproducibility of MRI-derived measurements of right ventricular volumes and myocardial mass. Magn Reson Imaging 13:53, 1995.
107. Natale L, Meduri A, Caltavuturo C, et al. MRI assessment of ventricular function. Rays 26:35, 2001
108. van der Geest RJ, Buller VG, Jansen E, et al. Comparison between manual and semiautomated analysis of left ventricular volume parameters from short-axis MR images. J Comput Assist Tomogr 21:756, 1997.
109. Power TP, Kramer CM, Shaffer AL, et al. Breath-hold dobutamine magnetic resonance myocardial tagging: normal left ventricular response. Am J Cardiol 80:1203, 1997.

110. Ungacta FF, Davila-Roman VG, Moulton MJ, et al. MRI-radiofrequency tissue tagging in patients with aortic insufficiency before and after operation. Ann Thorac Surg 65:943, 1998.
111. Reichek N. MRI myocardial tagging. J Magn Reson Imaging 10:609, 1999.
112. Fogel MA, Gupta KB, Weinberg PM, et al. Regional wall motion and strain analysis across stages of Fontan reconstruction by magnetic resonance tagging. Am J Physiol 269:H1132, 1995.
113. Mohiaddin RH, Gatehouse PD, Henien M, et al. Cine MR Fourier velocimetry of blood flow through cardiac valves: comparison with Doppler echocardiography. J Magn Reson Imaging 7:657, 1997.
114. Niezen RA, Doornbos J, van der Wall EE, et al. Measurement of aortic and pulmonary flow with MRI at rest and during physical exercise. J Comput Assist Tomogr 22:194, 1998.
115. Oyre S, Ringgaard S, Kozerke S, et al. Accurate noninvasive quantitation of blood flow, cross-sectional lumen vessel area and wall shear stress by three-dimensional paraboloid modeling of magnetic resonance imaging velocity data. J Am Coll Cardiol 32:128, 1998.
116. Powell AJ, Maier SE, Chung T, et al. Phase-velocity cine magnetic resonance imaging measurement of pulsatile blood flow in children and young adults: in vitro and in vivo validation. Pediatr Cardiol 21:104, 2000.
117. Carr DH. Paramagnetic contrast media for magnetic resonance imaging of the mediastinum and lungs. J Thorac Imaging 1:74, 1985.
118. Rajagopalan S, Prince M. Magnetic resonance angiographic techniques for the diagnosis of arterial disease. Cardiol Clin 20:501, 2002.
119. Prince MR. Contrast-enhanced MR angiography: theory and optimization. Magn Reson Imaging Clin N Am 6:257, 1998.
120. Du J, Carroll TJ, Wagner HJ, et al. Time-resolved, undersampled projection reconstruction imaging for high-resolution CE-MRA of the distal runoff vessels. Magn Reson Med 48:516, 2002.
121. Greil GF, Powell AJ, Gildein HP, et al. Gadolinium-enhanced three-dimensional magnetic resonance angiography of pulmonary and systemic venous anomalies. J Am Coll Cardiol 39:335, 2002.
122. Schwitter J, Nanz D, Kneifel S, et al. Assessment of myocardial perfusion in coronary artery disease by magnetic resonance: a comparison with positron emission tomography and coronary angiography. Circulation 103:2230, 2001.
123. Nagel E, al-Saadi N, Fleck E. Cardiovascular magnetic resonance: myocardial perfusion. Herz 25:409, 2000.
124. Nagel E, Klein C, Paetsch I, et al. Magnetic resonance perfusion measurements for the noninvasive detection of coronary artery disease. Circulation 108:432, 2003.
125. Zenovich A, Muehling OM, Panse PM, et al. Magnetic resonance first-pass perfusion imaging: overview and perspectives. Rays 26:53, 2001.
126. Wagner A, Mahrholdt H, Holly TA, et al. Contrast-enhanced MRI and routine single photon emission computed tomography (SPECT) perfusion imaging for detection of subendocardial myocardial infarcts: an imaging study. Lancet 361:374, 2003.
127. Nagel E, Lehmkuhl HB, Bocksch W, et al. Noninvasive diagnosis of ischemia-induced wall motion abnormalities with the use of high-dose dobutamine stress MRI: comparison with dobutamine stress echocardiography. Circulation 99:763, 1999.
128. Baer FM, Crnac J, Schmidt M, et al. Magnetic resonance pharmacological stress for detecting coronary disease. Comparison with echocardiography. Herz 25:400, 2000.
129. Trent RJ, Waiter GD, Hillis GS, et al. Dobutamine magnetic resonance imaging as a predictor of myocardial functional recovery after revascularisation. Heart 83:40, 2000.
130. Klein C, Nekolla SG, Bengel FM, et al. Assessment of myocardial viability with contrast-enhanced magnetic resonance imaging: comparison with positron emission tomography. Circulation 105:162, 2002.
131. Kuhl HP, Beek AM, van der Weerdt AP, et al. Myocardial viability in chronic ischemic heart disease: comparison of contrast-enhanced magnetic resonance imaging with (18)F-fluorodeoxyglucose positron emission tomography. J Am Coll Cardiol 41:1341, 2003.
132. Kim RJ, Fieno DS, Parrish TB, et al. Relationship of MRI delayed contrast enhancement to irreversible injury, infarct age, and contractile function. Circulation 100:1992, 1999.
133. Kim RJ, Hillenbrand HB, Judd RM. Evaluation of myocardial viability by MRI. Herz 25:417, 2000.
134. Laissy JP, Messin B, Varenne O, et al. MRI of acute myocarditis: a comprehensive approach based on various imaging sequences. Chest 122:1638, 2002.
135. Mahrholdt H, Goedecke C, Wagner A, et al. Cardiovascular magnetic resonance assessment of human myocarditis: a comparison to histology and molecular pathology. Circulation 109:1250, 2004.
136. Kim RJ, Judd RM. Gadolinium-enhanced magnetic resonance imaging in hypertrophic cardiomyopathy: in vivo imaging of the pathologic substrate for premature cardiac death? J Am Coll Cardiol 41:1568, 2003.
137. Wolff S, James TL, Young GB, et al. Magnetic resonance imaging: absence of in vitro cytogenetic damage. Radiology 155:163, 1985.
138. Sawyer-Glover AM, Shellock FG. Pre-MRI procedure screening: recommendations and safety considerations for biomedical implants and devices. J Magn Reson Imaging 12:92, 2000.
139. Shellock FG, Crues JV 3rd. MR Safety and the American College of Radiology White Paper. AJR Am J Roentgenol 178:1349, 2002.
140. Ahmed S, Shellock FG. Magnetic resonance imaging safety: implications for cardiovascular patients. J Cardiovasc Magn Reson 3:171, 2001.
141. Martin ET, Coman JA, Shellock FG, et al. Magnetic resonance imaging and cardiac pacemaker safety at 1.5-Tesla. J Am Coll Cardiol 43:1315, 2004.
142. Didier D, Ratib O, Beghetti M, et al. Morphologic and functional evaluation of congenital heart disease by

magnetic resonance imaging. J Magn Reson Imaging 10:639, 1999.

143. Odegard KC, DiNardo JA, Tsai-Goodman B, et al. Anaesthesia considerations for cardiac MRI in infants and small children. Paediatr Anaesth 14:471, 2004.
144. Pannu HK, Flohr TG, Corl FM, et al. Current concepts in multi-detector row CT evaluation of the coronary arteries: principles, techniques, and anatomy. Radiographics 23 Spec No:S111, 2003.
145. Lee EY, Siegel MJ, Hildebolt CF, et al. MDCT evaluation of thoracic aortic anomalies in pediatric patients and young adults: comparison of axial, multiplanar, and 3D images. AJR Am J Roentgenol 182:777, 2004.
146. Frush DP. Review of radiation issues for computed tomography. Semin Ultrasound CT MR 25:17, 2004.

14

Cardiac Catheterization

JAMES E. LOCK, MD

Stephen Hales' measurement of equine arterial pressure,[1] Werner Forssman's celebrated auto-cannulation,[2] and Andre Cournand's assessment of pulmonary arterial pressures in human disease[3] mark the known beginnings of cardiac catheterization. The first cardiac catheterization in a case of congenital heart disease was reported in 1946.[4] Until that time, the notion that an atrial septal defect resulted in a left-to-right shunt was surmised from the anatomic findings of a large right heart. This hypothesis was supported by the case of a 32-year-old woman with an atrial septal defect who had superior vena caval oxygen content of 10.4 mL per 100 mL, an inferior vena caval content of 9.5 mL per 100 mL, and a right atrial oxygen content of 12.1 mL per 100 mL.

The first therapeutic cardiac catheterization procedures in congenital heart disease were described in the remarkable reports from the Institute for Cardiology from Mexico City where Rubio-Alvarez and his colleagues used their own blade-equipped catheter (Fig. 14-1).[5,6] Using this device in a 32-year-old woman, they reduced the systolic pulmonary valve gradient from 90 to 30 mm Hg. Despite such successes, transcatheter therapy remained dormant until the lifesaving balloon septostomy technique for transposition of the great arteries by Rashkind and Miller.[7]

Since these pioneering studies, the capabilities of cardiac catheterization in children have increased enormously. All parts of the normal and abnormal circulation are routinely cannulated. Many forms of heart disease that previously required operative management are now corrected with transcatheter techniques (some on an outpatient basis) and some diseases that previously were inoperable can be effectively managed at cardiac catheterization.[8]

INDICATIONS FOR CARDIAC CATHETERIZATION

Because of their capability for showing excellent anatomic detail and the possibility for repeated examinations, echocardiography and magnetic resonance imaging have largely supplanted angiography as the prime source for examining cardiac anatomy. Angiography is still needed when there are poor echocardiographic windows, when there is intervening bone or air-filled lung (e.g., scoliosis or abnormalities of the peripheral pulmonary arteries), or when fine vascular detail is required. The physiologic estimates based on indirect echocardiographic observations are statistically valid but less precise than those obtained at cardiac catheterization. Nonetheless, the easy ability to repeat observations makes the echocardiogram the prime tool in following physiologic abnormalities (e.g., pressure gradients or myocardial function).

Catheterization continues to become safer and more precise. New, smaller catheters, more flexible shafts, flow-directed balloons, less toxic contrast agents, improved anatomic understanding provided by precatheterization evaluation, and imaging systems that offer superior resolution with less radiation have all contributed to this improved safety.

In general, cardiac catheterization is used (a) when precise physiologic measurements are needed (e.g., in documenting the severity of aortic or mitral stenosis or studying the feasibility of a Fontan procedure); (b) when the anatomic features are poorly visualized by echocardiography (e.g., peripheral pulmonary arterial or venous structures);

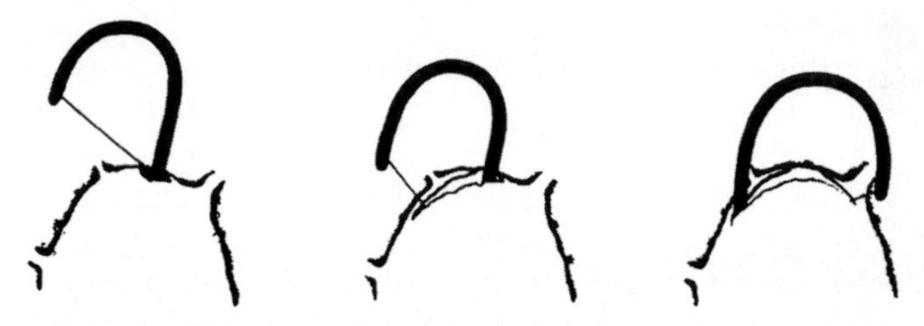

FIGURE 14–1 *Diagram of the first interventional catheter used by Rubio-Alvarez in 1953 to successfully open a stenotic pulmonary valve.*
Reprinted from Arch Institut Cardiol, Mexico 23:183, 1953.

(c) when electrophysiologic studies are needed; or (d) when therapeutic catheterization is planned.

Given the enormous variabilities in congenital heart disease, skill at echocardiographic diagnosis, surgical approaches, and experience at interventional techniques, a listing of the indications for cardiac catheterization that would apply to each cardiac institution simply is not possible. Table 14-1 summarizes the indications used at Children's Hospital Boston in 2005 on a lesion-by-lesion basis. Further discussion of indications will be presented in the chapters on individual lesions.

RISKS OF CATHETERIZATION

Although the frequency of complications from catheterization has decreased, they still occur, particularly in sick infants and patients undergoing certain high-risk interventions. Published major complications were noted in about 30% of infants classified as high risk, 14% in the medium-risk group and 4% of those in the low-risk category when reviewed 20 years ago.[9] In addition, the incidence of complications requiring treatment was 12% in infants younger than 4 months old, compared with 1.5% in the older infants. Careful prospective studies of adverse events in the intervention era are still pending, although we are now analyzing preliminary data.

TABLE 14–1. Indications for Cardiac Catheterization - 2005

Diagnosis	Catheterization Usually Indicated?	Potential or Real Indication for Catheterization
Atrial Septal Defect Secundum	Yes	Transcatheter closure of moderate and large central defects
Patent Ductus Arteriosus	Yes	Transcatheter closure of most defects
Coarctation in Infancy	No	Dilation for palliation of complex disease
Coarctation, Older Children and Young Adults	Yes	Balloon angioplasty and/or stent implantation
Transposition of the Great Arteries in Infancy	Yes	Balloon septostomy, coronary anatomy and relief of pulmonary artery obstruction post-operatively
Ventricular Septal Defect	No	Transcatheter closure of residual or muscular defects
Pulmonary Stenosis	Yes	Balloon valvotomy
Tetralogy of Fallot, pre-op	No	Rule out collaterals, muscular VSD's and/or distal PA anatomy
Tetralogy of Fallot Pulmonary Atresia	Yes	Pulmonary artery anatomy, possible intervention to coil collaterals or enlarge pulmonary arteries
Complete AV Canal	No	Cath rarely indicated
Aortic Stenosis	Yes	Balloon valvotomy
Hypoplastic Left Ventricle, pre-op	No	Dilation or stenting of restricted atrial septum
Hypoplastic Left Ventricle, post-op	Yes	Arch obstruction, collateral vessels, pulmonary artery obstruction
Single Ventricle, pre-op	No	Central pulmonary artery and arch anatomy, rule out collateral
Single Ventricle Prior to Glenn	Yes/No	Resistances, pulmonary artery anatomy, collaterals
Single Ventricle Fenestrated Fontan	Yes	Fenestration closure, collateral closure, pulmonary artery anatomy, optimization of anatomy
Truncus Arteriosus	No	Truncal valve anatomy, pulmonary artery anatomy, hemodynamics of truncal stenosis or regurgitation
Pulmonary Atresia Intact Septum	Yes	Pulmonary artery anatomy, coronary artery anatomy, possible valve perforation
Total Anomalous Pulmonary Venous Connection - Pre-operatively	No	Assess anatomy of mixed venous drainage
Cardiac Transplantation	Yes	Cardiac biopsies, coronary artery anatomy, hemodynamics
Coronary Arteriovenous Fistula	Yes	Transcatheter closure
Primary Pulmonary Hypertension	Yes	Drug testing, possible creation of atrial septal defect

Deaths

When deaths occurring within 24 hours of cardiac catheterization, including those after cardiac surgery, were analyzed 21 years ago, mortality was higher in neonates than in older children.[10] The average rate was reported at 16.0% in the first week of life, 9.7% in neonates younger than 1 month and 4.5% in those younger than 1 year, the overall mortality for all ages being 2.0%. In another study mortality was 3.8% within 24 hours and 8.3% within 48 hours of cardiac catheterization in the first year of life.[9] When lesions, such as hypoplastic left heart, and surgical deaths were excluded, no deaths directly attributable to catheterization occurred during the first 24 hours, and the mortality within 48 hours was 0.3%. Of note, these studies included only diagnostic catheterizations.

The 1980 to 1988 overall mortality rate within 48 hours of catheterization in 6101 studies at the Boston Children's Hospital was 1.7%, ranging from 10.2% in the first week of life to 0.5% in patients older than 1 year. Rarely, death has been reported in patients with primary pulmonary hypertension.[11] More recently, we have developed a risk-adjusted measure of catheterization laboratory deaths and adverse events. In that preliminary study, the risk of death attributable to catheterization was 0.3%.

Risks from Diagnostic Catheterization

Arterial and Venous Complications

Most catheterizations at the Children's Hospital Boston are carried out percutaneously via the femoral vessels. With this approach, arterial occlusion is rare beyond infancy, although subclinical iliac obstruction may be underdiagnosed. In the first 6 months of life, using a 4-French (4F) pigtail catheter for retrograde arterial catheterizations, temporary or permanent pulse loss occurred in 10% of the babies. Pulse loss occurred less frequently if a smaller (3F) pigtail catheter was used.[12] The use of heparin,[13] and, more recently, streptokinase[14] has been effective in achieving recovery of pulses in most of these infants.

Thrombosis of the inferior vena cava or iliac vein in the first 6 months of life is a recognized problem of uncertain magnitude. In early years, vena caval occlusion was identified in 16% of babies following a percutaneous study, compared with 1.2% using the cut-down approach.[15] No definite risk factors other than the technique used were identified, although other investigators have implicated the use of balloon septostomy catheters.[15,16] In the 1980s, the incidence of vena caval occlusion after percutaneous studies in infants decreased to 7%. At subsequent catheterization, the iliac vein has been patent in 59% and occluded in 15%, whereas patency of the iliac vein was uncertain in the other 26%.[17]

Arrhythmias

Catheter-related atrial or ventricular premature beats are frequent and usually insignificant. Sustained atrial tachycardias are generally easily terminated by catheter-induced atrial or ventricular extrasystoles, by overdrive atrial pacing, or by electrical cardioversion if necessary. Ventricular tachycardia or fibrillation is rare, usually occurs in critically ill infants and responds to countershock and appropriate medical management. Atrioventricular conduction disturbances occur but are almost invariably transient in nature.

Myocardial Stain and/or Perforation

Since the advent of pigtail and balloon catheters, these complications of angiography are now rarely seen. Most stains now occur when side-hole catheters are forced against a vessel wall by a stiff intraluminal guide wire during injections.

Apnea and Airway Obstruction

Apnea is a known and troublesome side effect of the use of prostaglandin palliation, and may occur during catheterization. Airway obstruction may result from sedation and somnolence, and produces characteristically wide respiratory swings in atrial tracings.

Air Emboli

Air emboli are associated with angiography or interventional procedures. Usually, the bubbles are small and can be prevented by inserting a transparent section of tubing between the catheter and the injector. At the Children's Hospital Boston there have been three instances of large air emboli associated with an open sheath in the right atrium, without permanent sequelae. This problem can be prevented by using sheaths with diaphragms.

Other Complications

Transient neurological deficits are rare and are presumably embolic in origin, although contrast induced seizures or adverse drugs events may occur. **Transient fevers** are not uncommon during the first few hours following catheterization and are generally of uncertain etiology. **Endocarditis** is extremely rare: In recent years we have seen two cases after prolonged interventional procedures via umbilical vessels in newborns who were not on antibiotic therapy.

Complications of Interventional Catheterizations

Complications are more common during interventional catheterizations, and include balloon or device damage to vessels, valves, and other cardiac structures, cardiac perforation or even rupture; damage to remote structures because of embolizations or thrombus, and other adverse events.

Although not all events are preventable or possibly preventable, many are avoidable, and a compulsive prospective study of catheter-based adverse events in the current era is overdue. At Children's Hospital Boston during the year 2004, 3.3% of procedures were complicated by serious or somewhat serious adverse events that were judged to be avoidable or possibly avoidable by our own faculty. A careful review of these data will undoubtedly improve patient care.

HEMODYNAMIC EVALUATION

A complete description of the methods used to evaluate physiologic variables in congenital heart disease is beyond the scope of this book and has been discussed elsewhere.[8,18] What follows is an overview designed to help the reader to gain understanding of the techniques being used.

Pressure Measurements

Recording systems consist of a fluid-filled catheter, a pressure transducer, an amplifier and a computer. The fluid-filled catheter transmits the pressure wave from the heart to a transducer, which converts the energy of pressure to an electrical impulse through mechanical displacement of a movable diaphragm. This electrical impulse is proportional to the displacement of the diaphragm and, therefore, to the pressure. The electrical signal generated is small and must be amplified and then converted to an analog of the pressure wave in the computer. Each component from the catheter to the recorder can contribute to error in measurement.

The demands on a recording system vary with heart rate. At a heart rate of 60 beats per minute (bpm), a system capable of recording 10 Hz (cycles per second) is adequate, but at a heart rate of 180 bpm, a rate not unknown in infants, a system capable of recording 30 Hz is required.

The response of the system depends, in part, on damping (i.e., anything that dissipates energy and changes the amplitude of oscillations in the diaphragm). Underdamping (which causes an artificial increase in pressure fluctuation) can occur when the catheter tip or shaft is moved during recording. Overdamping (artificial reduction in pressure fluctuation) is more common. Overdamping increases as the catheter diameter decreases and its length and compliance increase. Overdamping due to small catheter diameter is especially relevant when catheterizing infants. Damping is also increased by the presence of air, blood, and clots in the system or loose connections (e.g., between the catheter and transducer).

There are other sources of error. By convention, the pressure at the level of the heart is set at 0 mm Hg by opening the transducer to air at the level of the heart and adjusting the recorder to read zero. It is assumed that the heart is at mid chest for this setting. Using a manometer, the transducer is then calibrated over a range of pressures appropriate for the procedure, usually 0 to 200 mm Hg. Failure to adjust the height of the transducer and calibrate the equipment properly leads to inaccurate pressure recordings. The stability or drift of a system is defined by its tendency, once calibrated, to change over time. Although the drift of most systems should be minimal, it is prudent to check the calibration during a catheterization, usually by switching transducers when recording nearly equal pressures (e.g., left ventricle and femoral artery).

Pressure recorders allow pressures to be displayed or recorded at different attenuations; that is, the scale of the pressure tracing can be changed. Pressures are also displayed or recorded as phasic or mean pressures. A phasic recording shows the instantaneous fluctuations in a pressure and is important for determining systolic and diastolic pressures and the presence of normal and abnormal waves. Modern pressure recorders automatically determine and display the mean pressure using electronic damping. The mean pressures of atria and arteries are routinely recorded and used, for example, to calculate vascular resistance.

The ideal catheter for recording pressures is stiff, large and short. Catheter selection is also determined by the size of the patient and the vessel to be entered. The number and position of holes are also important. Endhole catheters are required to record pulmonary capillary or venous wedge pressures and are optimal for localizing gradients. Occlusion of the end hole by the wall of the heart is not uncommon but easily recognized. Also, endhole catheters, especially balloon-tipped catheters, can become entrapped (for example, in the atrial appendage, ventricular apex, or trabeculae), leading to falsely elevated pressure. Because such tracings often have a normal contour, entrapment can be difficult to recognize. The use of catheters with multiple side holes reduces the problem of entrapment. However, they cannot be used for wedge pressures and are not optimal for localizing gradients. Double-lumen catheters, with a single end hole and a second single side hole, can be useful for recording gradients.

Right Atrial Pressure

The normal right atrial pressure consists of the a, c, and v waves and x and y descents (Figs. 14-2 and 14-3). The a wave is associated with atrial contraction at the end of diastole. It is usually the dominant wave in the right atrium. The c wave, a small notch on the descending side of the a wave, is clinically unimportant, and is associated with displacement of the tricuspid valve toward the right atrium in early systole. The v wave peaks during late systole and is related to continued atrial filling against the closed tricuspid valve. The x descent is the fall in pressure following the a and c waves due to a decrease in pericardial pressure and movement of

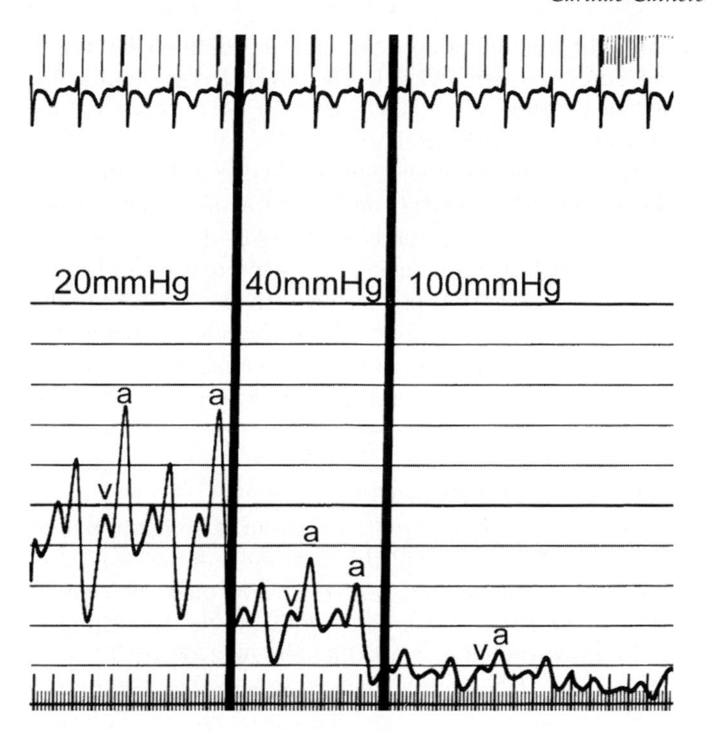

FIGURE 14–2 *Right atrial tracing at three different attenuations. In addition to phasic intracardiac changes, the pressure falls during inspiration.*
From Fyler DC (ed). Nadas' Pediatric Cardiology, Philadelphia: Hanley & Belfus, 1992.

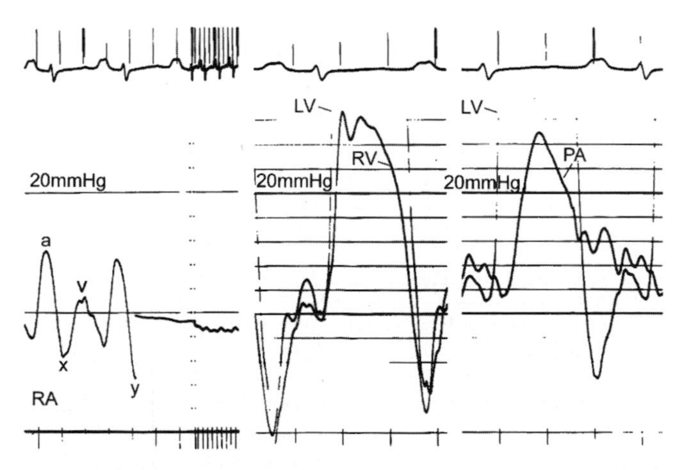

FIGURE 14–3 *Normal pressure tracings. RA, right atrial pressure tracing; RV, right ventricular pressure tracing; PA, pulmonary artery tracing; LV, left ventricular tracing, which is only partially seen. Note the similarity of the right ventricular and pulmonary artery systolic trace and the similarity of the right and left ventricular diastolic pressure tracings.*
From Fyler DC (ed). Nadas' Pediatric Cardiology, Philadelphia: Hanley & Belfus, 1992.

the tricuspid valve away from the right atrium during ventricular ejection. They descent is the decrease in pressure following the v wave and is due to opening of the tricuspid valve at the beginning of diastole.

Flow in the venae cavae is greatest during the x and y descents and ventricular filling is greatest during early diastole, with only about 30% of filling associated with atrial contraction. Pressure and flow also vary with respiration. Right atrial pressure is highest at the end of expiration and drops during inspiration, because of variation in intrathoracic pressure. This normal variation becomes exaggerated during periods of airway obstruction. Because of the low pressure, right atrial and ventricular filling are increased during inspiration. By convention, right atrial pressure is measured at the end of expiration.

Normally, the mean right atrial pressure is 3 + 2 mm Hg. The a wave is the dominant wave, commonly 2 to 3 mm Hg higher than the v wave. Abnormalities of right atrial pressure include changes in mean pressure and changes in the normal pattern and relationships among the waves and troughs. Increases in right atrial mean pressure are associated with right ventricular dysfunction (decreased compliance) and outflow obstruction (tricuspid stenosis or atresia associated with a restrictive interatrial communication). In tricuspid regurgitation, the v wave may be dominant.

Superior and Inferior Vena Caval Pressure

Pressures in the superior and inferior venae cavae have contours similar to the right atrial pressure, and are not recorded routinely, except in any patient suspected of having caval obstruction.

Left Atrial Pressure

The a, c, and v waves and x and y descents are also seen in the left atrial pressure tracing. In contrast to right atrial pressure, the v wave is dominant in the normal left atrium. The mean left atrial pressure is normally 8 mm Hg. Elevations in left atrial pressure occur in patients with left ventricular dysfunction and in those with outflow obstruction (mitral stenosis or atresia with a restrictive interatrial communication). The v wave is increased in mitral regurgitation and decreased in total anomalous pulmonary venous return.

Pulmonary Artery "Wedge" Pressure

The pulmonary artery wedge pressure is measured by advancing an endhole catheter, with or without a balloon, into a branch of the pulmonary artery until the vessel is occluded by the catheter or, more commonly, by inflating the balloon. The pressure recorded through the end hole reflects distal pressure, that is, the left atrial pressure. The wedge pressure is routinely recorded simultaneously with the left ventricular end diastolic pressure; normally there is no gradient. Differences in pressure suggest disease, improperly calibrated transducers, or a defective wedge pressure. The latter occurs when the catheter is *overwedged* or only *partially wedged*. The wedge pressure should look like a left atrial tracing, demonstrate respiratory variation, and be lower than the pulmonary artery pressure. The *wedge* position of the catheter can be confirmed by checking that the blood is fully saturated, or by injecting a small amount of contrast, which will not wash out if the catheter is properly wedged. Because of the intervening capillaries and pulmonary veins, the wedge pressure is delayed and damped, compared with direct measurement of the left atrial pressure. When important left atrial gradients are suspected, they should be measured directly.

Pulmonary Vein Pressure

Normal pressure tracings of pulmonary veins are similar to left atrial tracings. Abnormal elevation of pulmonary vein pressure in the presence of a normal left atrial valve suggests stenosis of the pulmonary veins. However, if only one or two of the veins are stenotic, flow within the lungs is redistributed and a minimal gradient may be measured across the stenotic veins.

Pulmonary Vein "Wedge" Pressure

If a catheter is wedged in a pulmonary vein, with or without a balloon, the pressure measured may reflect pulmonary artery pressure. This technique is conceptually similar to that used to measure pulmonary arterial wedge pressure. Achieving proper wedge position involves similar attention to detail. Although not employed routinely, obtaining pulmonary vein wedge pressure is the only way to estimate pulmonary artery pressure when the pulmonary arteries cannot be measured directly (e.g., patients with pulmonary atresia without shunts or with shunts that cannot be crossed). Although the wedge pressure estimate tends to be lower than actual pulmonary artery pressure, it is relatively accurate in patients with low or normal pulmonary artery pressure.

Right Ventricular Pressure

Normal ventricular pressures are easily distinguishable from atrial and arterial pressures. The right ventricular pressure wave consists of a rapid upstroke during isovolumic contraction, a systolic plateau, and a fall to near zero during isovolumic relaxation. There is, then, a gradual increase in pressure during diastole with a late diastolic increase associated with the a wave of atrial contraction (Fig. 14-3). The peak systolic and end-diastolic pressures, which vary with respiration, are measured routinely. *End-diastole* is identified as the point where the right atrial and ventricular tracings cross at the end of diastole or at the junction of the a wave and the rapid upstroke in the ventricular tracing. The former is the most accurate, but because simultaneous right atrial and right ventricular pressures are not routinely recorded, the latter is often utilized. The normal right ventricular systolic pressure is less than 30 mm Hg and the end-diastolic pressure is about 5 mm Hg.

Abnormal elevation of right ventricular systolic pressure occurs in outflow obstruction (e.g., pulmonary valve stenosis, pulmonary artery bands, or stenosis of the pulmonary artery branches), pulmonary artery hypertension, or lesions such as ventricular septal defects. In double-chambered right ventricle, anomalous muscle bundles obstruct the outflow portion of the right ventricle and create a proximal high-pressure chamber and a distal low-pressure chamber (Fig. 14-4).

Left Ventricular Pressure

The left ventricular pressure contour is similar to that of the right ventricle except the upstroke is more rapid, the systolic plateau flatter, and the a wave more prominent (Fig. 14-5). End-diastolic pressure varies with respiration and is measured as described for the right ventricle.

Normally, left ventricular systolic pressure equals the aortic systolic pressure; both increase with age. The end-diastolic pressure is normally less than 12 mm Hg and is slightly higher than the left atrial mean pressure.

Pulmonary Artery Pressure

The normal systolic pressure in the pulmonary artery equals the right ventricle, but the diastolic pressure is

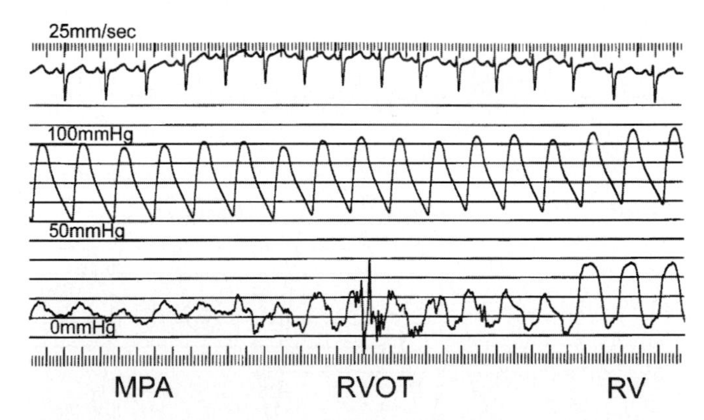

FIGURE 14–4 *Pressure pullback in a patient with double-chambered right ventricle. Upper tracing, Electrocardiogram. Middle tracing, Arterial pressure. Lower tracing, Obtained from the catheter as it was withdrawn from the pulmonary artery to the right ventricle. Note that the pressure gradient occurs within the ventricle. MPA, main pulmonary artery; RV, right ventricle. Stenosis below the pulmonary valve will produce a characteristic pressure tracing in the right ventricular outflow tract (RVOT), with a further gradient into the body of the right ventricle.*
From Fyler DC (ed). Nadas' Pediatric Cardiology, Philadelphia: Hanley & Belfus, 1992.

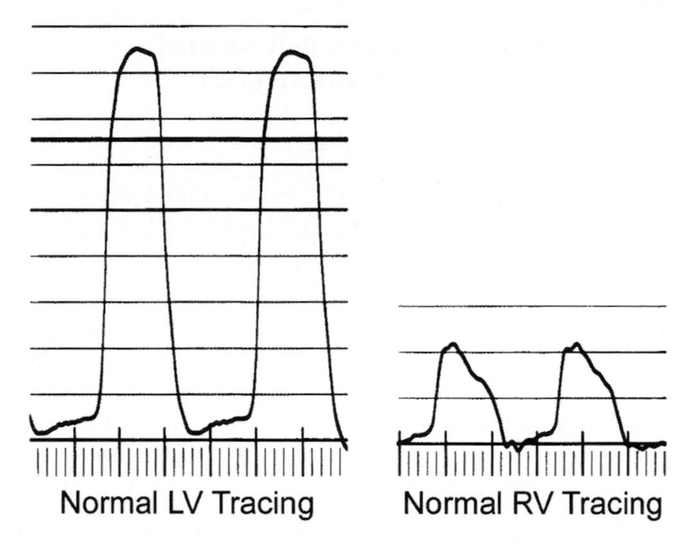

FIGURE 14–5 *Normal right and left ventricular pressure tracing. A normal left ventricular pressure tracing has a flattened systolic pressure phase and very rapid upslopes and downslopes. From Fyler DC (ed). Nadas' Pediatric Cardiology, Philadelphia: Hanley & Belfus, 1992.*

higher because of closure of the pulmonary valve. Respiratory variation is common and, by convention, pressures are measured at the end of expiration. Normal mean pulmonary artery pressure is less than 20 mm Hg.

Aortic Pressure

The normal central aortic pressure wave consists of a systolic rise and a plateau, with a dicrotic notch on the downstroke. Closure of the aortic valve causes the diastolic pressure to remain well above the ventricular diastolic pressure. The aortic pressure and contours of the tracing vary, depending on where the pressure is measured. As the catheter is moved more peripherally (e.g., in the brachial or iliac arteries), the systolic pressure increases and the diastolic pressure decreases owing to "standing wave" amplification of the pulse. Thus, for example, when measuring gradients across the aortic valve, it is improper to compare left ventricular systolic pressure directly with femoral artery systolic pressure.

Aside from systemic hypertension or hypotension, abnormalities in aortic pressure usually are related to the presence of gradients (e.g., supravalvar aortic stenosis or coarctation of the aorta) or a wide pulse pressure (e.g., aortic regurgitation, shunts such as a patent ductus arteriosus, systemic arteriovenous malformations and decreased systemic resistance), or a narrow pulse pressure due to low output.

Gradients

A pressure gradient is the difference in pressure between two sites in the cardiovascular system and can be measured as a **mean gradient,** a **peak gradient** or an **instantaneous gradient.** The severity of stenotic lesions commonly is described in terms of pressure gradients, although, in fact, the gradient depends on both the cross-sectional area of the obstruction and the flow across it. Thus, a severe narrowing may be associated with only a minimal gradient if the flow across the lesion is low.

Most commonly, a catheter is withdrawn across the obstruction while the pressure is being continuously recorded. Although this provides nearly simultaneous pressure recordings and allows easy measurement of peak and mean gradients, determination of instantaneous gradients requires that the two tracings be superimposed.

When assessing gradients, it is vital to assess flow across the lesion. In aortic or mitral valve stenosis, one should always estimate cardiac output. However, some lesions are so complex that accurate assessment of severity, using gradients and flows, becomes nearly impossible. For example, in stenosis of multiple branches of the pulmonary artery, it is not possible to measure flow across each lesion. In such situations, assessment of obstruction must rely on imaging techniques, lung scan data, or both.

OXYGEN CONTENT AND SATURATION

The oxygen content, or the saturation of the blood from the various chambers of the heart and great vessels, detects and quantifies shunts and, when combined with oxygen consumption, determines cardiac output. **Oxygen saturation** is the percent of hemoglobin that is present as oxyhemoglobin and it can be measured using reflectance oximetry. **Oxygen content** is defined as the total amount of oxygen present in the blood, both as oxyhemoglobin and that dissolved in the plasma. Formerly, it was measured directly, using the method of Van Slyke, but now oxygen sensing cells are used. Oxygen content per liter of blood may be calculated from oxygen saturation:

$$O_2 \text{ content} = (O_2 \text{ Sat} \times 1.36 \times 10 \times \text{Hgb concentration})$$

The O_2 Sat is the percent of oxygenated hemoglobin. The value of 1.36 is the amount of O_2 a gram of hemoglobin will carry when fully saturated. The 10 is used to convert 100 mL to liters. The contribution of dissolved O_2 is small and commonly ignored except when the pO_2 is very high, such as when 100% oxygen is being administered.

Oxygen contents (O_2 con) and oxygen consumption (VO_2) are used to calculate blood flow using the equations:

$$\text{Pulmonary blood flow} = \frac{VO_2 \text{ (mL/min)}}{\text{PV } O_2 \text{ con} - \text{PA } O_2 \text{ con}}$$

$$\text{Systemic blood flow} = \frac{VO_2\ (\text{mL/min})}{\text{SA } O_2 \text{ con} - \text{MV } O_2 \text{ con}}$$

where PV is pulmonary vein, PA is pulmonary artery, SA is systemic artery, and MV is mixed (systemic) venous.

If complete mixing of inferior vena caval, superior vena caval, and coronary sinus blood occurred, the right atrial, right ventricular, and pulmonary arterial oxygen saturations would equal the mixed venous content. In fact, studies have shown that variability in oxygen content is greatest in the right atrium[19] and least in the pulmonary artery, owing to incomplete mixing in the right atrium. Thus, in the absence of shunts, the pulmonary arterial saturation is used as the mixed venous oxygen saturation. In the presence of left-to-right shunts (see below), mixed venous oxygen contents must be obtained proximal to the site of the shunt.

In the absence of right-to-left shunts, mixing in the left side of the heart is insignificant because there is little variation in the oxygen content in the various pulmonary veins. In the presence of right-to-left shunts, the oxygen content must be measured proximal to the site of the shunt to calculate pulmonary blood flow.

Shunts

Both extracardiac and intracardiac defects allow shunting of blood between the pulmonary (right-sided) and systemic (left-sided) circulations. Shunts may be left-to-right, right-to-left, or bidirectional. Shunts can be localized using angiography, Doppler echocardiography, or a variety of indicators, including oxygen saturation, radionucleotides, and indocyanine green dye. This section will focus on detection and quantification of shunts using oxygen content or saturations.

Left-to-Right Shunts

In a left-to-right shunt, the flow of blood from the left side of the heart to the right leads to an increase in oxygen saturation in the right side of the heart. To detect this increase, samples are drawn from each right heart chamber. Significant increases in saturation between chambers must exceed the normal variation for that chamber.[19] Thus, the saturation in the right atrium varies 5% even without a shunt; a rise would be diagnostic only if the right atrial saturation exceeded superior vena caval saturation by at least 6%.

Right-to-Left Shunt

With a right-to-left shunt, oxygen saturation decreases in the left heart. Unlike evidence for a left-to-right shunt, virtually any consistent decrease in oxygen saturation is diagnostic. For practical purposes, any decrease from normal arterial saturation (i.e., 95%) is considered as evidence of a right-to-left shunt in a child with heart disease until proven otherwise.

CALCULATIONS IN CARDIAC CATHETERIZATION

Shunts

A left-to-right shunt ($Q_{L\text{-}R}$) increases pulmonary blood flow (Q_p) compared with systemic blood flow (Q_s), and the shunt can be quantified by the equation:

$$Q_{L\text{-}R} = Q_p - Q_s$$

Usually, in children, the superior vena caval (SVC) oxygen content is taken as the mixed venous oxygen content. In discussing shunts it is common to refer to the pulmonary-to-systemic flow ratio (Q_p/Q_s).

$$\frac{\dfrac{\text{Oxygen Consumption}}{\text{PV } O_2\% - \text{PA } O_2\%}}{\dfrac{\text{Oxygen Consumption}}{\text{SA } O_2\% - \text{MV } O_2\%}} = \frac{Q_p}{Q_s} = \frac{\text{SA } O_2 - \text{MV } O_2}{\text{PV } O_2 - \text{PA } O_2}$$

Thus, the Q_p/Q_s can be determined without measuring or assuming an oxygen consumption, using only oxygen saturations.

In addition to pulmonary and systemic flows, the concept of effective flow (Q_{EFF}) is useful in calculating shunts. The effective pulmonary blood flow is the volume of unoxygenated blood flowing to the lungs (i.e., the amount of blood that picks up oxygen on passing through the lungs). For example, with a pure left-to-right shunt, effective pulmonary blood flow (Q_{EFF}) would equal the total pulmonary blood flow (Q_p) minus the shunt flow ($Q_{L\text{-}R}$) which equals systemic blood flow (Q_s). In bidirectional shunts, the left-to-right shunt is calculated as $Q_p - Q_{EFF}$, and the right-to-left shunt is calculated as $Q_s - Q_{EFF}$.

When quantifying shunts, saturations should be obtained as nearly simultaneously as possible to reduce hemodynamic variation. If the values of two series are different or if they suggest a shunt of borderline significance, more series are performed or another indicator is used. In general, shunt size measurements are estimates. To suppose that one can distinguish Q_p/Q_s ratios of 2 versus 2.2 or 1.8 is to ignore the variations inherent in the measurements. Thus, if the superior vena cava saturation is 80, the pulmonary artery saturation 95, and the systemic artery saturation 100, the Q_p/Q_s is (100 – 80)/(100 – 95) or 4. If the oximetry run is repeated and the superior vena cava saturation is 78, the pulmonary artery saturation 96, and systemic artery saturation 99, the Q_p/Q_s ratio is (99 – 78)/(99 – 96) or 7.

In certain lesions it may be impossible to obtain adequately mixed samples to calculate shunt size. With a patent ductus arteriosus, the left pulmonary artery saturation is commonly higher than the right, and it is not possible to obtain truly mixed pulmonary arterial saturations. Averaging the values assumes that flow to both lungs is equal. With total anomalous pulmonary venous connections it may be impossible to obtain mixed venous saturations.

Finally, some patients have more than one defect associated with left-to-right shunts. Thus, a patient may have an atrial septal defect, a ventricular septal defect, and a patent ductus arteriosus. Analyzing saturations from oximetry runs in a stepwise fashion, one might attempt to calculate the magnitude of the left-to-right shunt associated with each lesion. This assumes, incorrectly, complete mixing at each level. It also assumes that the increase at each level is due to only the lesion at that level. This may not be the case if, for example, the ventricular septal defect is associated with a left ventricular-right atrial shunt or there is tricuspid regurgitation.

Calculations for right-to-left shunts are fundamentally similar to calculations for left-to-right shunts. A right-to-left shunt ($Q_{R\text{-}L}$) leads to a decrease in left-sided saturations at or distal to the site of the shunt, and systemic blood flow (Q_s) is higher than pulmonary blood flow. It can be calculated as:

$$Q_{R-L} = Q_p - Q_s$$

$$Q_P/Q_S = \frac{SA\ O_2 - MV\ O_2}{PV\ O_2 - PA\ O_2}$$

In addition to right-to-left shunts, left-sided desaturation can be caused by pulmonary venous hypoxemia in a patient with lung disease. If the left atrium and pulmonary veins can be entered, the pulmonary venous saturation should be measured in as many pulmonary veins as possible. If the measurements are low, lung disease is suggested and 100% oxygen administered to the patient will significantly increase the pulmonary venous saturation. If the intrapulmonary shunt is due to a pulmonary arteriovenous malformation, the low saturation will increase modestly. Alternatively, if there is an atrial septal defect, an attempt should be made to occlude the defect with a balloon and measure the left atrial or systemic arterial saturation, which will normalize if the desaturation is due to a right-to-left shunt through the defect.

Cardiac Output

Cardiac output is the volume of blood pumped into the systemic circulation by the heart, expressed as liters per minute. When corrected for body surface area (liters/minute, m^2), cardiac output is referred to as the *cardiac index*. In patients with no shunts, pulmonary, systemic, and effective blood flows are equal (ignoring the minimal contribution of the bronchial circulation), and under stable conditions the term *cardiac output* can be used without confusion. However, in the presence of shunts, pulmonary, systemic, and effective blood flows may be unequal. In these patients, the more specific terms *pulmonary, systemic*, and *effective* blood flows are used.

Measurements or estimates of cardiac output, resistances, and valve areas are a routine part of most cardiac catheterizations. Indicator-dilution measurements are most commonly used to measure cardiac output. In general, if one knows the amount of indicator (I) added to (or subtracted from) a flowing fluid and the concentration of the indicator before (upstream) (C_b) and after (downstream) (C_a) its addition, one can calculate the volume of fluid (V) from the equation.

$$V = \frac{I}{C_a - C_b}$$

Assuming constant flow during the period of measurement, flow (Q) can be calculated by the introduction of a time term (t) into the equation:

$$Q = \frac{I}{(C_a - C_b)t}$$

Numerous indicators have been used to measure cardiac output. The most common methods currently used are thermodilution (the indicator is cold saline) and the Fick method, when the indicator is oxygen. The use of indocyanine green dye has been replaced by thermodilution.

Thermodilution Cardiac Output

The cardiac output is calculated as:

$$CO = \frac{V \times D_i \times S_i \times (T_b - T_i)}{dT \times t \times D_b \times S_b \times 1000/60}$$

where CO = cardiac output, V = volume injected minus dead space, D_i = density of injectate, S_i = specific heat of injectate, T_b = temperature of blood, T_i = temperature of injectate, dT = average temperature change, t = duration of temperature change (sec), D_b = density of blood, S_b = specific heat of blood, and 1000/60 = 1000 mL per 50 seconds.

The indicator is cold saline, commonly injected in the right atrium, and a thermistor in the pulmonary artery measures blood temperature. The measured flow is equal to pulmonary blood flow and, in the absence of shunts, to the systemic blood flow. Thermodilution catheters have two lumens with a thermistor at the distal end. Various sizes are available so that when the thermistor is in the pulmonary artery, the proximal port, which is in the right atrium, can be used for injection. A curve shows the change in temperature with time at the thermistor, and calculations of output are made by dedicated computers.

The term $dT \times t$ in the denominator is the area under the curve, and cardiac output is inversely proportional to this area. The temperature at the thermistor is determined by the temperature of the blood, the temperature of the injectate, and the flow. The higher the flow, the more the injectate will be warmed, reducing the cold signal. However, the injectate is also warmed by contact with the catheter and the vessel walls. If the thermistor is in direct contact with a vessel wall, warming is increased, and cardiac output will be overestimated. Thermodilution techniques have been used to measure flows in specific vessels or organs by positioning the thermistor and injection port at appropriate sites. For example, blood flow to the right lung in a patient with a Glenn anastomosis can be measured by injecting the superior vena cava with the thermistor in the right pulmonary artery. This technique, which assumes complete mixing of the thermal bolus, has been supplanted by newer MRI techniques (see Chapter 13).

Fick Method

Using the Fick method, the indicator is oxygen and cardiac output or flow (Q) is calculated from oxygen consumption/minute (VO_2) divided by the difference in oxygen content between arterial (C_a) and venous (C_v) blood.

$$Q = \frac{VO_2 \text{ (L/min)}}{(C_a - C_v)}$$

As above, in the absence of shunts, pulmonary blood flow equals systemic blood flow. That is, the amounts of blood pumped by the right and left ventricles are equal. Pulmonary blood flow (Q_p) is:

$$Q_p \text{ (L/min)} = \frac{VO_2 \text{ (L/min)}}{PV\,O_2 \text{ con} - PA\,O_2 \text{ con}}$$

where PV O_2 con and PA O_2 con are the pulmonary venous and the pulmonary arterial oxygen contents. Similarly the systemic blood flow (Q_s) is:

$$Q_s \text{ (L/min)} = \frac{VO_2 \text{ (L/min)}}{SA\,O_2 \text{ con} - MV\,O_2 \text{ con}}$$

where SA O_2 con and MV O_2 con are the systemic arterial and mixed venous oxygen contents.

Several devices are available for measuring oxygen consumption. Often, the entire volume of air expired gas is determined, as well as the relative volumes of oxygen, nitrogen, and/or carbon dioxide. Comparing the concentrations of gases in inspired (room air) and expired air allow calculation of the oxygen consumption.

The second method does not involve collecting all the expired air, but uses a hood and a pump to withdraw air from the hood to an oxygen sensing device. If air is withdrawn from the hood at a rate (V_m) so that the fractional content of O_2 at the oxygen sensor remains constant at 0.122, O_2 consumption can be estimated.

Vascular Resistance

Calculations of vascular resistance (R) are made by relating the mean pressure change (delta P) across a circuit to the flow (Q) across the circuit, using the equation:

$$R = \frac{\text{delta P}}{Q}$$

Thus, systemic vascular (SVR) and pulmonary vascular (PVR) resistances are calculated:

$$SVR = \frac{Ao - RA}{Q_s} \qquad PVR = \frac{PA - LA}{Q_p}$$

where Ao is the mean aortic pressure, RA is the mean right atrial pressure, PA is the mean pulmonary artery pressure, and LA (or pulmonary capillary wedge) is the mean left atrial pressure. The pressures are in mm Hg and the flows in liters/minute and, thus, resistance is expressed as mm Hg/l/min (or Wood units). Resistance is commonly normalized for body surface area (BSA) by multiplying the calculated resistance by the BSA.

Valve Areas

The most commonly used formulas for calculating valve areas are based on the work of Gorlin and Gorlin[20] in 1951. The first is $A = V/VC_c$, where A is the valve area, F is the flow rate, V is the velocity of flow, and C_c is the coefficient of orifice contraction. The second, which relates velocity to pressure gradient, is $V = C_v$ 2gh, where C_v is the coefficient of velocity, g is acceleration due to gravity (980 cm/sec/sec), and h is the pressure gradient. Combining these equations yields:

$$\text{Valve area} = \frac{F}{(C)\,(44.3)\,h}$$

where C is a constant. Flow across a valve occurs during diastole at the mitral and tricuspid valves, and during systole at the aortic and pulmonary valves. The final formula takes this into account by including the diastolic filling period (DFP, seconds per beat) or the systolic ejection period (SEP, seconds per beat) and the heart rate (HR beats sec).

$$A = \frac{CO/(DFP \text{ or } SEP)\ HR}{44.3\ (C)}$$

where A is the area in cm^3, CO is the cardiac output in cm^3/min, and delta is the mean pressure gradient. The beginning and end of the diastolic filling period are the points where the atrial and ventricular pressure tracings intersect; the intersections of ventricular and arterial tracings at the beginning and end of systole define the systolic ejection period. When determined in this way, the constant, C, is 0.85 for the mitral valve and 1 for the aortic, pulmonary, and tricuspid valves.

The equations predict that, for any given valve area, decreasing the flow across the valve decreases the gradient and increasing the flow increases the gradient. Therefore, it is logical to classify severity of valvar stenoses in terms of valve area. Because most children with stenosis of pulmonary or aortic valves have normal cardiac outputs, the flow term in the equation tends to be a constant and severity varies directly with the gradient.

ANGIOGRAPHIC EVALUATION

Image Production

Basic equipment for image production includes the generator, the x-ray tube, and image chain mounted opposite each other on a fixed stand or C-arm. The image chain consists of an image intensifier and a high-quality television camera on traditional equipment or a flat plane detector on newer technology (Fig. 14-6). Cine cameras have been replaced by digital recording and processing systems. For pediatric studies, simultaneous biplane cineangiography is often necessary to provide sufficient anatomic information with minimal contrast material.

The x-ray generator supplies and controls three variables: kilovoltage (kv) (which determines the energy spectrum of the x-rays), milliAmperes (mA, the tube current that determines the number of x-ray photons produced), and milliseconds (msec, the length of exposure or pulse width in cineangiography). Inside the x-ray tube a thin tungsten filament, the cathode, boils off electrons at a rate controlled by the current applied. When a high-voltage current is applied, electrons accelerate across the tube and strike the rotating anode, causing x-ray photons to be emitted.

During standard fluoroscopy and cineangiography, x-rays are delivered in short pulses instead of continuously. Radiation is delivered at a much higher level during angiography. The length of each pulse, or *pulse width*, determines the exposure for each individual frame. Pulse widths should be kept short to prevent blurring, but need to be long

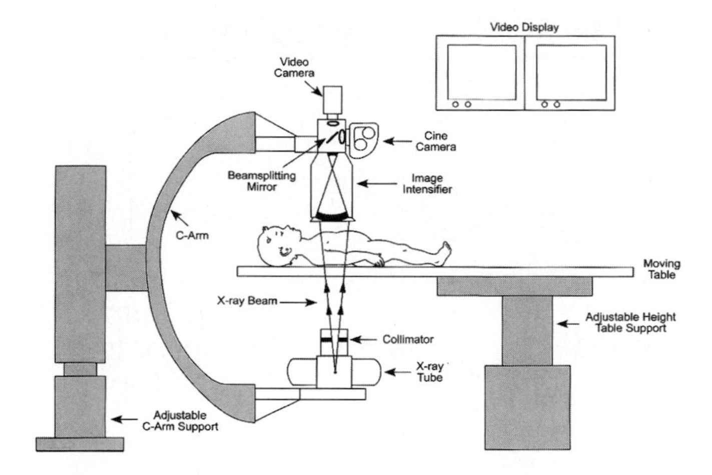

FIGURE 14–6 *Schematic representation of a single C-arm with x-ray tube, image intensifier, and cine camera over moving table top. From Fyler DC (ed). Nadas' Pediatric Cardiology, Philadelphia: Hanley & Belfus, 1992.*

enough to provide a sufficient number of photons so that the image will not be too grainy. The pulse width in cineangiography should not exceed 5 msec in pediatrics and 10 msec in adults.[22]

The image intensifier in the traditional image chain is the large canister mounted above or to the side of the patient. Its broad circular face, closest to the patient's body, contains the *input phosphor*, a screen of cesium iodide crystals that produces visible light when struck by x-ray photons. The distribution of light produced by the phosphor corresponds to the spatial information formed by the attenuation of the x-rays by the patient's heart or by contrast agents used in angiocardiography. Light produced by the phosphor is detected by an immediately adjacent photocathode that generates low-energy electrons; these electrons are accelerated, and then focused by electronic lenses to produce a bright but modified image on the output phosphor at the other end of the image intensifier (Fig. 14-7). The intensification of the image is produced by minification (that is, by concentrating the light into a smaller, brighter area) and by electronic gain, thereby using the lowest possible x-ray dose. The total gain in brightness achieved by modern image intensifiers is 2000- to 6000-fold.[21]

The effective input phosphor varies from 4 to 14 inches. Because the output phosphor is the same size regardless of the input phosphor, the image obtained at the face of a 6-inch input field will be magnified more than the image obtained at the face of a 9-inch input field size. Thus, a 9-inch image intensifier may be electronically switched to input the image from a 6-inch field and the image will be magnified. A small input phosphor field size is important for infant cardiography to provide adequate magnification and spatial resolution, whereas a large input phosphor is vital to image adults with congenital heart disease.

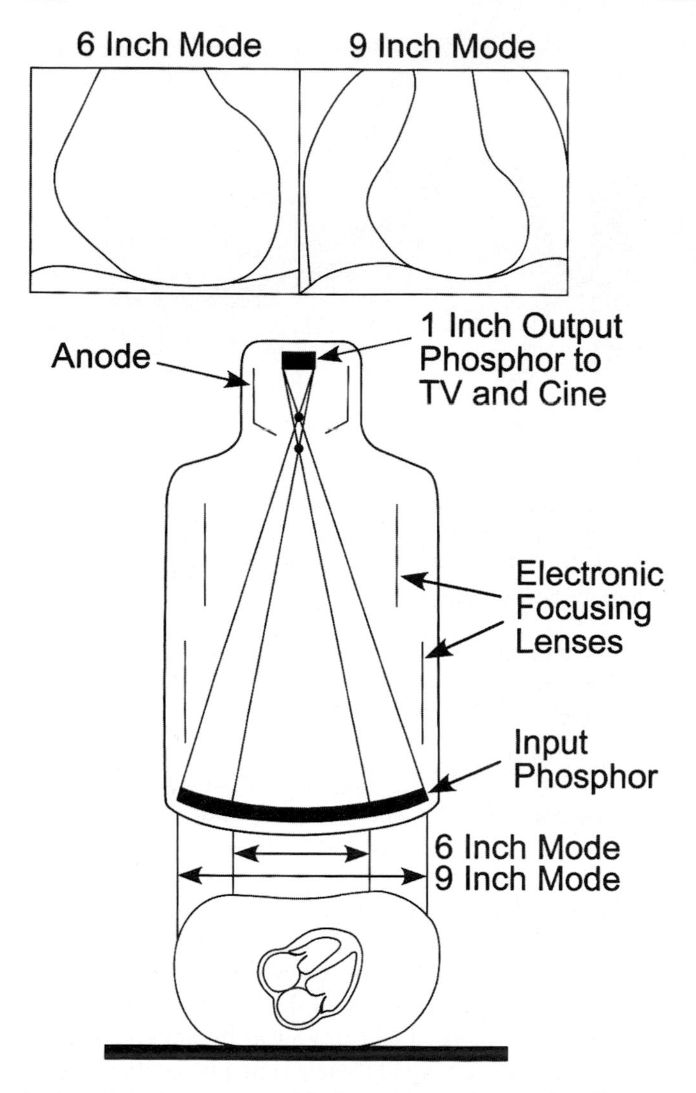

FIGURE 14–7 *Drawing of dual-mode image intensifier illustrating the principles involved in magnification modes.*
From Fyler DC (ed). Nadas' Pediatric Cardiology, Philadelphia: Hanley & Belfus, 1992.

Image Recording and Processing

The light from the image produced by the output phosphor is split during angiography: Some goes to the monitor and some goes to the recorded image. Pulsed fluoroscopy is performed at tube currents of 5 to 100 mA; when the cine pedal is depressed, the current is boosted about 10-fold. The TV camera allows the operator to monitor the actual injection and simultaneously record the injection on a high quality video disc. An additional television monitor for each plane can provide a freeze-frame image of the injection. Although film-based angiography can provide magnificent images with a resolution up to four line pairs per mm, the improvements in computer enhancement of digital images and the ease of handling such images has made film-based angiography virtually obsolete.

Modern images of all types, including those obtained at cardiac angiography, are viewed and processed digitally. The analog image is converted to digital information (pixels) that can be mathematically manipulated. Contrast enhancement, edge enhancement or smoothing, digital subtraction, and computed tomography provide advantages in selected situations. As network systems and storage systems for digital information improve and increase, major changes in handling of cardiovascular images continue to occur. Recently, flat-panel detectors that serve the same purpose as the image intensifier and television camera have been introduced. These devices are more compact and directly convert the x-ray pattern in space exiting the patient into digital format.

Radiation Exposure and Protection

Conventional radiation units include the roentgen (R), a unit of radiation exposure; the rad, a unit of absorbed dose; and the rem, a unit of dose equivalent (rads multiplied by a quality factor to measure biologic effect). The last two units have recently been replaced by grays and sieverts respectively.

Fluoroscopic patient exposure to the skin is usually about 0.5 to 1.0 R/mA per minute of conventional fluoroscopic time. For cineangiography of an adult, the skin dose is about 20–30 mR per frame.[23] Thus, the total dose to the patient, and the total scatter dose to personnel is determined by the length of fluoroscopic time (usually recorded in minutes), by the length of angiographic time, the angiographic frame rate, and the patient girth. Of course, total exposure is doubled for biplane usage. By comparison, 1 second of cineangiography at 30 frames per second is equivalent to 10 seconds of fluoroscopy.[24] Usually, in a routine diagnostic study, the major exposure to both patient and operator occurs during angiography rather than fluoroscopy. In interventional cases, lengthy fluoroscopic times can result in total fluoroscopic exposures to the patient and personnel in excess of the angiography exposures.

Cooperative studies have reported patient exposure for a complete adult cardiac catheterization of 20 to 47 R.[25–28] To put this dose range into perspective, it can be compared with doses for other x-ray studies on adults: chest x-ray, 0.03 to 0.04 R; intravenous pyelogram, 2 to 3 R; barium enema, 2 to 4 R. Naturally occurring background radiation is about 0.3 R per year.[29,30]

Personnel exposure is largely due to scattered x-ray photons, the x-ray dose being inversely related to the square of the distance from the source of the scatter: The point on the patient irradiated by primary x-rays. Wraparound lead aprons are necessary; thyroid shields are recommended.[28,31]

In a review of radiation exposures from different laboratories, Reuter reported the dosage to the operator from a single catheterization procedure to be in the following range[28]: 4.6 to 154 mR to the hand of the angiographer, 3.5 to 33 mR to the thyroid, and 6.4 to 30 mR to the eye. The National Council on Radiation Protection and Measurement (NCRP) and the International Commission on Radiological Protection have set up guidelines for permissible yearly exposure. NCRP recommends a limit of radiation per year of 5 rem to the whole body, 75 rem to the hands, and 15 rem to the thyroid.[32]

Good habits for fluoroscopy should be taught and practiced consistently. The image receptor should be as close as possible to the patient's chest; fluoroscopic time should be reserved for catheter manipulations and test injections, and biplane fluoroscopy should be used only when necessary. All operators of fluoroscopic equipment in the catheterization laboratory should receive specific training and demonstrate competency in sound radiation protection principles.

Contrast Agents

Contrast agents used in cardiac angiography are water-soluble, complex organic compounds, sharing in common the basic building block of three iodine atoms bound to a benzene ring. Modern contrast agents can be either high-osmolality or low-osmolality agents. Both types of contrast, using an equivalent concentration of iodine, produce angiographic images which are of equal radiographic contrast. Low-osmolality agents cause less patient discomfort, may be safer, and are now routinely used.

Chemistry. High-osmolality ionic agents are salts of tri-iodinated benzene derivatives of diatrozoic or iothalamic acid (the anions), which are bound to sodium or methylglucamine (the cations; Fig. 14-8). When in solution, the number of particles is immediately doubled; this results in a solution that is extremely hypertonic, with osmolality six to seven times that of blood. The hypertonicity of these agents not only causes the pain and warmth that the patient feels, but is responsible in part for a number of other adverse physiologic responses.

Nonionic contrast is formulated by replacing the carboxyl group of the benzene ring with a nonionizing side chain, so that the compound does not dissociate in solution; thus, its osmolality is half as great as an ionic compound (Fig. 14-8). Nonionic agents include iohexol and iopamidol.[33]

Osmolality may also be reduced by linking two tri-iodinated benzoic acids together to form a dimer (Fig. 14-8). This is prepared as a salt of sodium or meglumine, which then dissociates in solution into two particles as conventional ionic agents do. Because each anionic particle contains six rather than three iodine atoms (as in conventional contrast), fewer particles are needed for a given iodine concentration, and the osmolality is reduced by half.[34,35]

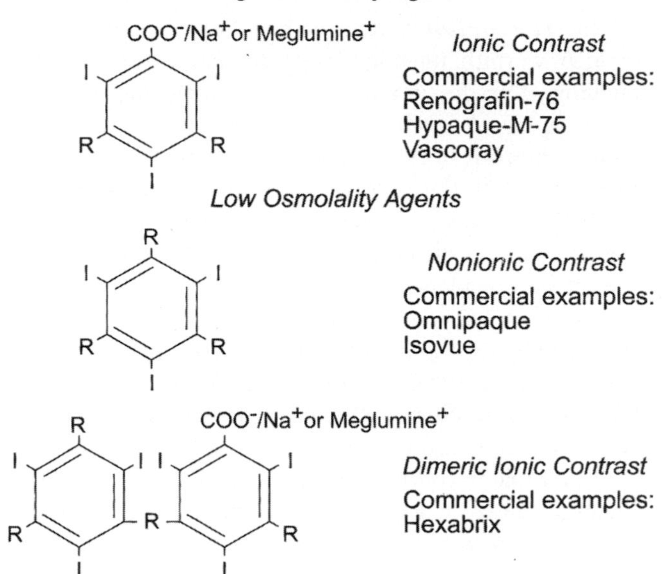

FIGURE 14–8 *Chemical composition of various contrast agents. From Fyler DC (ed). Nadas' Pediatric Cardiology, Philadelphia: Hanley & Belfus, 1992.*

Physiology. When contrast agents are injected, there is a shift of fluid from interstitial and intracellular spaces into the intravascular space, causing volume expansion, a slight drop in hematocrit, and a change in electrolyte concentration.[36–38] Thus, important pressure and flow measurements should always be made prior to contrast injections. With normal renal excretion, values can be expected to return to baseline within a few minutes, but newborns, fragile infants, and any patient with severely compromised cardiac function will be adversely affected.[39,40]

Injection of contrast into the pulmonary vascular bed causes a rise in pulmonary artery pressure owing to a combination of vasospasm[33,40] and elevation of left atrial pressure.[36] The release of histamine from mast cells and basophils, platelet dysfunction, and sludging of distorted red cells may play a role also.

Reflex tachycardia occurs in response to contrast-induced hypotension, and with increased intravascular volume, there is transient increase in cardiac output, along with a rise in ventricular diastolic pressure.[41] In the already compromised patient, this depressant effect, combined with volume expansion secondary to injection of the contrast, may precipitate pulmonary edema. Low-osmolality agents may produce less systemic hypotension, less tachycardia, and less ventricular dysfunction.[43,44] Finally, high-osmolality contrast decreases the threshold for ventricular fibrillation.[45]

Other toxic effects of high-osmolar contrast agents include decreased red cell pliability and increased viscosity, osmotic diuresis, proteinuria, hematuria, and, occasionally, renal failure.

Adverse reactions. Arterial injection of contrast agent produces warmth; injection into pulmonary vessels produce coughing. Life-threatening reactions, including bronchospasm, laryngeal edema, and vascular collapse, have been reported in from 1/3000 to 1/14,000 patients; most patients are resuscitated, the reported mortality being 1/10,000 to 1/40,000.[46,47] These reactions probably have some allergic basis, as patients with any history of allergy have a two to three times greater incidence of reaction than does the nonallergic population.[46,48] However, one reaction does not foretell a second, with or without pretreatment, although from 15% to 60% of patients with a previous history of a severe contrast reaction have another severe reaction when catheterization is repeated. Increased production of bradykinin may play a significant role in contrast reaction in patients with a history of allergy. Severe reactions may be less frequent with low-osmolality contrast.

Contrast toxicity. Advanced catheter management of certain defects (e.g., multiple severe peripheral pulmonary artery stenoses, *Swiss cheese* ventricular septal defects, brachiocephalic arteriopathy) may require, for optimum patient management, contrast dosages that were unheard of a decade ago. While newer contrast agents have superior safety profiles, the risks of contrast toxicity in these long, complicated procedures remain unclear. A recent study at our hospital of very-high-contrast dosing suggests that, although these procedures are more dangerous, the enhanced risk is primarily due to unfavorable anatomy (Table 14-2).

TABLE 14–2. Relation Between Contrast Dose and Adverse Events at Pediatric Cardiac Catheterization July 2002 - July 2003

	Cases with Adverse Events		
Contrast Dose	**# of Cases**	**# of AE's**	**AE/Procedure**
< 4 cc/kg	736	95	13%
4-8 cc/kg	324	94	29%
> 8 cc/kg	87	33*	38%

*Eight of these 33 AE's (adverse events) were moderately serious or serious. 5 of these 8 were due to vessel trauma, 2 due to embolization, and the other possibly attributable to contrast (seizures post cath of unclear etiology).

Angiocardiography

The first step in any selective angiography is vascular access to the necessary chamber with an appropriate catheter. Usually, femoral vessels are used for percutaneous vascular access in nearly all forms of congenital heart disease, with the umbilical, subclavian, jugular, and upper limb vessels available for special circumstances. In general, angiograms are performed with sidehole catheters adequate to deliver a large volume of contrast rapidly (e.g., up to 1.5 mL/kg in a second or less); the volume and speed are determined by multiple factors, including chamber size and flow. A more complete discussion of angiographic techniques in general, and special procedures such as balloon occlusion angiography, wedge angiography, and coronary angiography in children, is available elsewhere.[8]

Modern biplane C-arm equipment has facilitated the acquisition of the axial views, introduced in the late 1970s, which accurately delineate various parts of the cardiac anatomy.[49–52] Because in most cases today the basic diagnosis has been established by echocardiography before arrival in the catheterization laboratory, each angiographic view can be chosen to answer a specific anatomic question.

Axial angiography was developed to profile specific parts of the heart along the x-ray beam. For example, the ventricular septum runs neither in the sagittal nor the coronal plane, but obliquely such that a left anterior oblique view shows the midportion of the curved ventricular septum better than a simple lateral view does. Thus, the long axis of the heart is between horizontal and vertical, the bifurcation of the pulmonary artery is horizontal and the aortic arch runs obliquely from front to back. Axial views were developed to take these anatomic facts into account and provide specific information about each chamber or vessel. However, simple frontal and lateral views are still useful, or even preferred, for demonstration of certain anatomic areas or when the abnormalities are so deranged that a preliminary view is desired.

The most common and useful views are (a) posterior-anterior, (b) lateral, (c) long axial oblique, and (d) hepatoclavicular. A long axial oblique view is obtained by placing the intensifier at 70-degree left anterior oblique with a 20-degree cranial angulation. Usually this is combined with the orthogonal right anterior oblique view (Fig. 14-9*A*). In left ventriculography, the long axial oblique projection provides good visualization of the mid and apical muscular septum, the membranous septum, and the subaortic area (Fig. 14-9*B*). This enables the viewer to see the motion of the anterior leaflet of the mitral valve, and the ventricular wall motion in the septal, apical, and posterior aspects, as well as mitral regurgitation and left ventricular-right atrial shunts. The aortic valve, the coronary arteries, and the arch and great vessels are well displayed. The right anterior oblique, orthogonal view provides information about anterior muscular septal and subpulmonary defects (Fig. 14-9*C*), both of which are difficult to pinpoint on other views. In tetralogy of Fallot, the infundibulum,

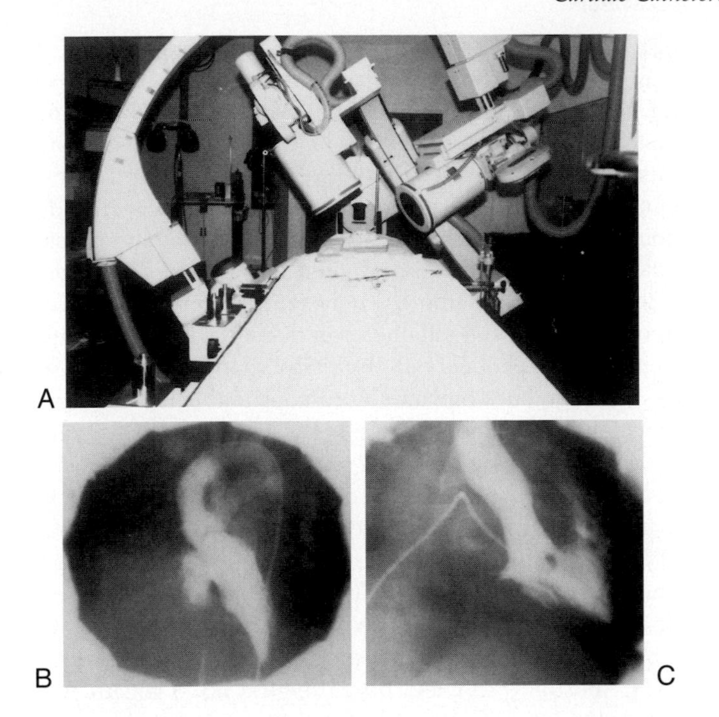

FIGURE 14–9 *A, View of biplane equipment positioned for long axial oblique and right anterior oblique views. B, Left ventriculogram taken in the long axial oblique view illustrating a perimembranous ventricular septal defect. C, Left ventriculogram taken in the right anterior oblique view illustrating an anterior muscular ventricular septal defect.*
From Fyler DC (ed). Nadas' Pediatric Cardiology, Philadelphia: Hanley & Belfus, 1992.

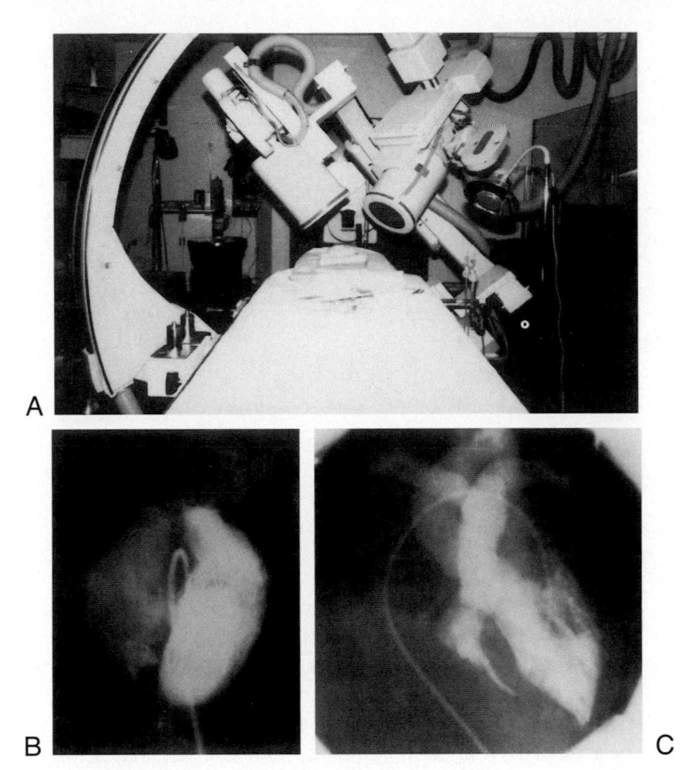

FIGURE 14–10 *A, View of biplane equipment positioned for hepatoclavicular and right anterior oblique views. Note that the obliquity is less steep and has more cranial angulation than that used in Figure 14-9 for the long axial oblique view. B, Left ventriculogram taken in the hepatoclavicular view illustrating a common atrioventricular canal defect. C, Left ventriculogram taken in the hepatoclavicular view illustrating anatomy in a patient with tricuspid atresia.*
From Fyler DC (ed). Nadas' Pediatric Cardiology, Philadelphia: Hanley & Belfus, 1992.

pulmonary valve, and right pulmonary artery are nicely demonstrated.

The hepatoclavicular view was so named to describe the direction of the x-ray beam from the liver below to the left clavicle above. Technically, it is a shallower (40 degree) long axial oblique view with steeper (40 degree) cranial angulation compared with the long axial oblique (Fig. 14-10*A*). This view focuses on the posterior aspect of the ventricular septum, in the region of the atrioventricular canal. In this projection, one can actually visualize a common atrioventricular valve, rather than infer its presence by an angiographic sign such as the *gooseneck* (Fig. 14-10*B*). This view is also called the four-chambered view because both atria and both ventricles can be seen in each of four quadrants of the image, so that valvular regurgitation, defects from the left ventricle to the right atrium and left or right overriding or atresia of the atrioventricular valves can be recognized (Fig. 14-10*C*).

The frontal view with 40-degree cranial angulation (Fig. 14-11*A,B*) is particularly useful for displaying the pulmonary artery bifurcation. The complementary orthogonal lateral view of the right ventricle (Fig. 14-11*C*) displays the pulmonary infundibulum and valve as well as the main and left pulmonary artery in profile. In tetralogy, septal alignment is particularly well illustrated, as the conal septum is profiled in its excessively anterior position (Fig. 14-11*C*).

The most common angiographic views and the diagnoses and injected chambers in which they are most helpful are displayed in Table 14-3.

INTERVENTIONAL CATHETERIZATION

In recent years the introduction of interventional techniques in the management of patients with congenital heart disease has revolutionized pediatric cardiac care (Exhibit 14-1). Many techniques have become accepted

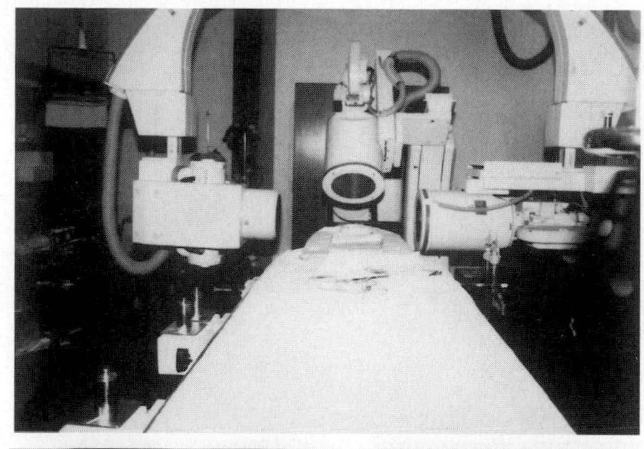

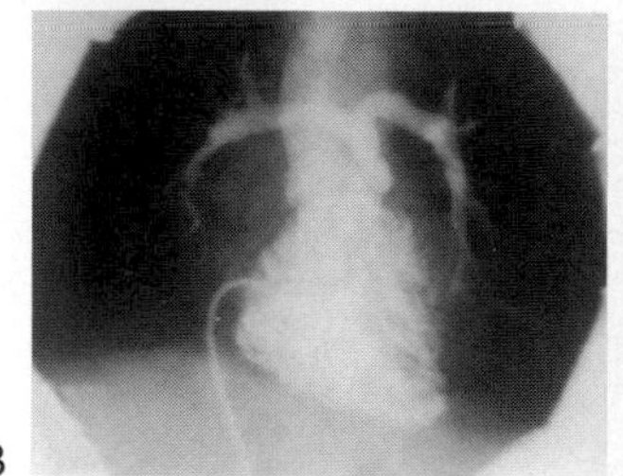

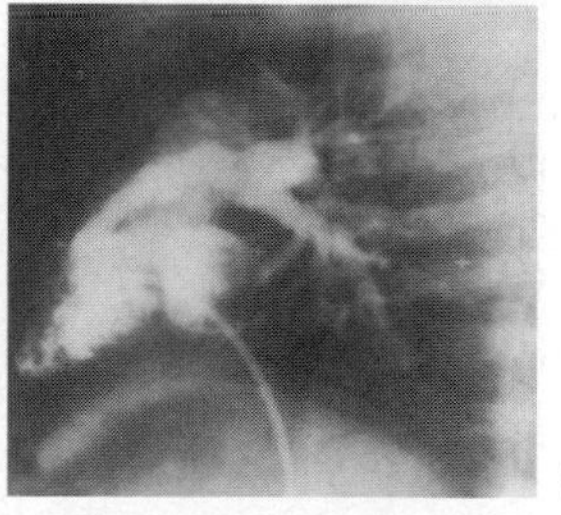

FIGURE 14–11 *A, View of biplane equipment positioned for a frontal view with cranial angulation and a lateral view. B, Right ventriculogram in a frontal projection with cranial angulation demonstrating the pulmonary artery bifurcation in a patient with tetralogy of Fallot. C, Right ventriculogram in the lateral projection demonstrating anterior malalignment of the conal septum with resulting infundibular narrowing and a ventricular septal defect in a patient with tetralogy of Fallot.*
From Fyler DC (ed). Nadas' Pediatric Cardiology, Philadelphia: Hanley & Belfus, 1992.

as standard therapy; others are under development. This chapter will emphasize the more common and clinically useful interventional procedures with a brief outline of fetal interventions at the conclusion.

Myocardial Biopsy

Despite years of improved noninvasive diagnosis for the management of congenital and acquired heart disease, endocardial biopsy[53] in children remains the mainstay in the diagnostic management of post–heart transplantation cellular rejection. The biopsy is carried out before or after transplantation as part of a defined diagnostic process. Before transplantation, diagnostic studies in addition to biopsies may include the administration of nitric oxide (70–80 ppm) to test reactivity of the pulmonary vascular bed. Extensive blood work often accompanies the pretransplantation evaluation. Following transplantation, a careful review of the clinical history will outline the presence of vascular anomalies that may persist following transplantation. Our current protocol for posttransplantation surveillance biopsy is weekly for the first 4 weeks, every other weeks for the next 3 months, monthly for the next 2 months, every 3 months for the next 6 months, and every 6 months after that indefinitely. In addition, we perform selective coronary angiography 1 year following transplantation, and annually thereafter. We obtain at least five biopsies from the right ventricular septum, equal to or greater than a millimeter in diameter, in all patients. In infants and patients with decreased ventricular wall thickness, we use both biplane fluoroscopy and echocardiography to guide our biopsies. Using these techniques we have had five cases of myocardial perforation in 4000 biopsies performed at our institution, all prior to transplantation in patients with thin-walled dilated cardiomyopathies, and four of five patients were younger than 1 year. Although bioptomes vary from 3F to 7F, we used 5F bioptomes in all procedures to obtain adequate size sample. The Sparrowhawk bioptome has been used for most of our biopsies recently (ATC, Boston, MA), and fits through a no. 5 sheath. We access the femoral or subclavian vein in patients less than 15 kg, and in older patients we use the right internal jugular vein, allowing the patient to ambulate immediately after the procedure. After obtaining vascular access, the long sheath and bioptome are both preformed such that the sheath and bioptome are directed toward the right ventricular septum. Biplane fluoroscopy and, when necessary, angiography demonstrates the right ventricular anatomy. Following completion of the biopsies, we heparinize the patient and advance a wedge catheter into the heart to record baseline hemodynamics. When necessary, further studies are performed. Myocardial perforation remains the most common complication, while arrhythmias, heart block, tricuspid valve damage, air and clot emboli, and puncture of and entry into other vascular chambers may occur but have been extremely rare in our experience.[54]

BALLOON VALVOTOMY

Valvar Pulmonary Stenosis

Following the initial report of Kan and associates in 1982,[55] using a noncompliant balloon to treat valvar pulmonary stenosis, this therapy quickly became widespread. It is effective and safe, providing excellent relief of obstruction in children[56,57] and in neonates.[58] Valvar pulmonary stenosis is well tolerated for some years, and because large catheters are often needed for effective relief, elective procedures are done at 3 to 9 months of age, except for neonates with critical obstruction.

TABLE 14–3. Views Used to Demonstrate the Anatomy of Congenital Heart Lesions

Long Axial Oblique 70° LAO, 20° Cranial	Hepatoclavicular Four-Chamber View 40° LAO, 40° Cranial	Rao or Orthogonal View to Long Axial Oblique or Hepatoclavicular	Frontal and Lateral
Left Ventriculogram	*Left Ventriculogram*	*Left Ventriculogram*	*Pulmonary Arteriogram*
VSD - midmuscular apical membranous	VSD - post muscular common AV canal type	VSD - subpulmonary anterior muscular	TAPVR - venous regurn Distal branch PA anatomy
Tetralogy - malalignment VSD multiple VSD's	Tricuspid Atresia - size of VSD size of *RV* outflow	Tetralogy - pulmonary infundibulum	*Innominate Vein* Persistent LSVC
D-TGA - subpulmonary area and VSD	Straddling Tricuspid Valve	Mitral valve - mitral insufficiency mitral prolapse	
DORV - VSD location and size	Single Ventricle	LV function - anterior wall motion apical wall motion inferior wall motion	*Right Ventriculogram*
Sub AS - LV outflow and mitral valve	*Right Ventricutogram*	*Aortogram*	Pulmonary stenosis
LV function - septal wall posterior wall	Tetralogy - PA bifurcation proximal LPA	Coronary arteries	Pulmonary atresia - intact septum
Aortogram	*Pulmonary Arteriogram*	*Pulmonary Arteriogram*	DORV
PDA	Tetralogy - PA bifurcation (postop.) proximal LPA	Right pulmonary artery	*Inferior Vena Cava or Superior Vena Cava*
Tetralogy - coronary arteries	*Aortogram*	Frontal view with cranial angulation	Complex ventricular anatomy
AS - aortic valve morphology aortic insufficiency	Similar to long axial oblique	*Right Ventriculogram*	Heterotaxy syndromes
Arch abnormalities - hypoplasia coarctation	Frontal view with caudal angulation 30°-40° caudal	Tetralogy - PA bifurcation	*Pulmonary Vein Injection*
	Aortogram (balloon occlusion)	*Pulmonary Arteriogram*	Pulmonary atresia - to find true PA (wedge injection)
	Coronary Arteries in Transposition	Tetralogy - postop. bifurcation	Anomalous venous drainage

AS = aortic stenosis
DORV = double outlet right ventricle
D-TGA = D-transposition of the great arteries
LAO = Long axial oblique
LPA = Left pulmonary artery
LSVC = left superior vena cava
LV = left ventricle
PA = pulmonary artery
PDA = patent ductus arteriosus
RAO = right axial oblique
RV = right ventricle
TAPVR = total anomalous pulmonary venous return
TGA= Transposition of the great arteries
VSD = Ventricular septal defect
(From Nadas' Pediatric Cardiology, (ed) Fyler DC, Hanley & Belfus, Philadelphia, 1992).

Older Patients

Technique

Following routine catheterization of the right heart, the pulmonary valve annulus is measured from a lateral right ventriculogram. A balloon diameter 120% + 10% of the size of the annulus is chosen and positioned over a guide wire (preferably advanced to the left lower lobe) across the stenotic valve. It is inflated with dilute contrast until the waist is abolished (Fig. 14-12), and then rapidly deflated. Occasionally, among older patients, two balloons are used,[63] both of which may be introduced via the same femoral vein. The hemodynamic parameters are then reassessed; care is taken to measure any residual gradients at valvar as well as infundibular levels, after which a right ventricular cineangiogram is made.

Results

Balloon valvuloplasty for pulmonary stenosis is becoming an increasingly smaller part of the interventional catheter volume at Children's Hospital Boston for several reasons: Results are excellent in virtually all centers and

Exhibit 14-1
Children's Hospital Boston Experience Interventional Cardiac Catheterization Procedures and Numbers/Yr. (N/Yr.)

Procedure	Years	
	1984-1987 N/Yr.	1988-2002 N/Yr.
Myocardial Biopsy	22	119
Peripheral Pulmonary Stenosis	26	107
Coil Vessel Occlusion	22	64
Stent Placement	0	59
Atrial Septal Defect Closure	2	42
Pulmonary Valve Plasty	29	33
Rashkind Procedure	22	28
Patent Ductus Closure	10	28
Aortic Valve Plasty	26	25
Coarctation of Aorta Dilation	20	24
Ventricular Septal Defect Closure	1	17
Mitral Valve Dilation	1	5

While the total number of yearly catheterizations has increased (from 950 in 1987 to 1375 in 2001), the interventional proportion increase has been particularly dramatic (from 33% in 1987 to 76% in 2001) with purely diagnostic studies decreasing from 67% to 24% in these same years.

long-distance referrals are quite uncommon, restenosis is quite rare outside of the newborn period and thus a single valvotomy is likely to last decades, if not a lifetime, and patients with moderate stenosis (e.g., gradients between 30 and 45 mm Hg) who had formerly been followed medically have all by now had successful balloon valvotomies. The safety of the procedure, including the absence of mortality and the rarity of hemodynamic instability and cardiac trauma remain unchanged, as does the average gradient reduction of about 65%, leaving a mean final gradient across the valve itself of 12 to 13 mm Hg. We have, somewhat arbitrarily, slightly reduced the size of the balloon to annulus ratio in the last decade from 130% to 140% of annulus size[57] to 120% of annulus size, based on the unproven notion that gradient relief will be almost the same but pulmonary regurgitation would be less.

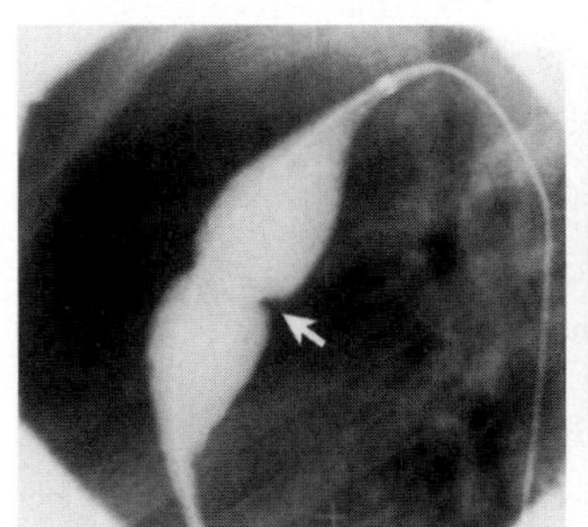

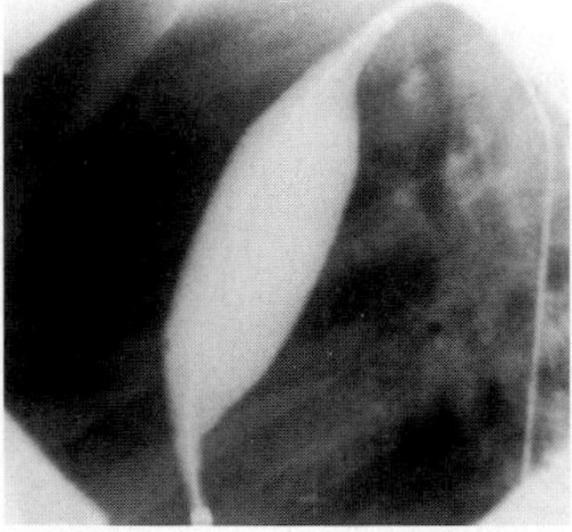

FIGURE 14–12 *Pulmonary valve dilation using the static balloon technique of Dr. Jean Kan. A waist (arrow) appears in the 18-mm balloon at 2 atm and disappears at 4 atm.*
From Fyler DC (ed). Nadas' Pediatric Cardiology, Philadelphia: Hanley & Belfus, 1992.

Finally, there is a subset of patients who have partially dysplastic valves with a smaller than normal annulus, and thicker than normal valves. The response of balloon angioplasty to these patients is less satisfactory than that seen in typical valvar pulmonary stenosis. However, the use of very high pressure balloons (16–20 atm) will cause enlargement of both the annulus and the valvar orifice, thereby reducing or eliminating the need for surgery, with right ventricular outflow patch reconstruction.

Neonates with Critical Obstruction

Technique

Virtually all of these babies are cyanotic because of right to left atrial shunting and many are intubated and receiving prostaglandin E.[58] Following right heart catheterization, the size of the annulus is measured from a right lateral ventricular cineangiogram. The valve can be crossed with difficulty using a 5F balloon endhole catheter. The easiest technique is to advance a 3F or 4F Judkins right coronary catheter into the body of the right ventricle over the bent end of a stiff guide wire and then turn the catheter clockwise into the right ventricular infundibulum. A small (0.014 inch) guide wire is then passed via a patent ductus arteriosus to the descending aorta or to a lower lobe pulmonary artery. A low profile 2- to 4-mm balloon is used first to dilate the valve (Fig. 14-13), followed by a larger balloon (120% the annulus size). Hemodynamic parameters are remeasured after which a right ventricular cineangiogram is made.

Results

This procedure has become technically simpler and safer with advancements in catheter and wire production. Most neonates with critical pulmonary stenosis have relatively soft valves that are easy to split, and thus the use of larger, stiffer high pressure balloons is rarely necessary. Coronary balloons up to 4 to 5 mm are ideal for obtaining the initial dilation and stabilizing the patients, and a low-profile (3F) balloon such as the Tyshak Mini in sizes up to 8 mm is often completely satisfactory for producing excellent gradient relief. Restenosis of these valves is quite common, does not seem to be related to the technique used, and should be expected in 25% to 50% of cases in the first year of life. Late gradients are similar to those obtained in older patients. A small but not trivial percentage of

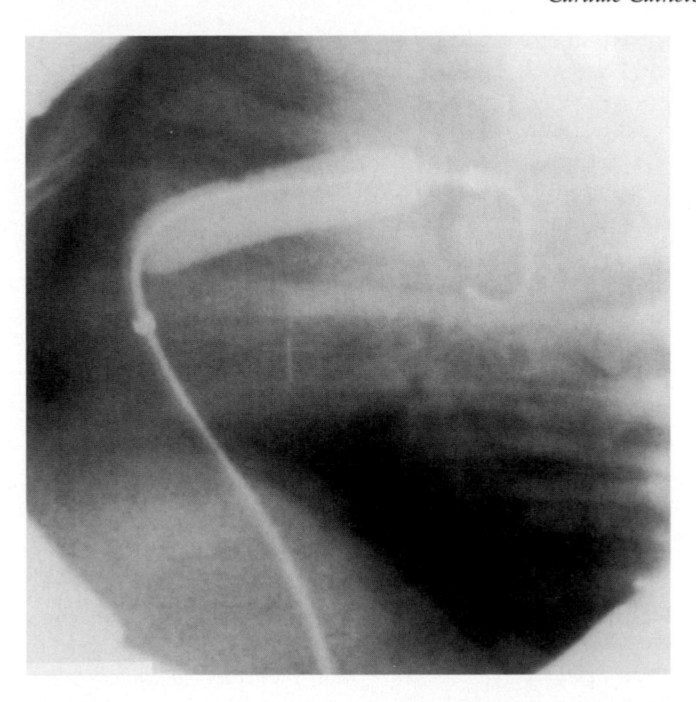

FIGURE 14–13 *The first balloon being inflated in neonate with a critically stenotic pulmonary valve. The right ventricular outflow is shorter, more curved, and there is less room for an inflated balloon. From Fyler DC (ed). Nadas' Pediatric Cardiology, Philadelphia: Hanley & Belfus, 1992.*

neonates with critical pulmonary stenosis will have associated tricuspid stenosis. This diagnosis may be very difficult to make in the neonatal period due to poor right ventricular compliance, and decreased flow across the tricuspid valve, lower-than-systemic right ventricular pressures, persistent cyanosis, or symptoms persisting more than 2 weeks following the procedure should prompt the suspicion of associated tricuspid valvar stenosis.

Complications

Complications among the first 33 patients included a late death from sepsis, two successfully managed right ventricular perforations, and injury to the iliac vein.[58] This procedure has become safer in the past two decades (Table 14-4) with a single death associated with the procedure in the last 77 patients. In general, the consistent, safe, and effective dilation of critical pulmonary stenosis in the neonate is one hallmark of a high-quality pediatric interventional catheterization laboratory.

Pulmonary Atresia with Intact Septum

Although many neonates with this condition have right ventricular–dependent coronary circulation and are directed down the Fontan pathway,[60] and some have a small annulus that needs surgical management, some infants with PA/IVS are good candidates for transcatheter valve perforation and subsequent valve dilation.[61]

TABLE 14–4. Balloon Dilation For Isolated Valvar PS Children's Hospital Boston

	Age	Number	Early Deaths	Mortality
1/85 - 11/04	< 1 month	135	7	5.2%
	1-12 months	120	0	0.0%
	1-10 years	191	0	0.0%
	10 years +	70	0	0.0%
	Total	516	7	1.4%
1/85 - 12/94	< 1 month	58	6	10.3%
1/95 - 11/04	< 1 month	77	1	1.3%

Mortality (30 day) for dilation of critical neonatal valvar pulmonary stenosis (PS) has decreased over past 2 decades (10.3% to 1.3%).

The decision of when to perforate an atretic pulmonary valve in the catheterization laboratory (as opposed to recommending surgical enlargement) depends on the size of the annulus, and whether or not valve perforation alone will result in subsequent adequate gradient relief. Excellent relief of obstruction seems to be required for long-term growth of the right ventricle, and if the annulus is small, balloon dilation alone is unlikely to result in adequate gradient relief.

For those patients with adequately sized right ventricles, and an annulus at least 3 to 4 mm in diameter, perforation is an excellent alternative to surgery. The technique is very similar to that described for pulmonary valve dilation, with three important exceptions. First, the outflow tract and main pulmonary artery tend to be more horizontal on a lateral fluoroscopy than in standard pulmonary stenosis. Thus, the catheter angle frequently needs to point straight backward in order to effectively enter the valve orifice. A 4F Judkins left catheter that has been cut off to a total angle of 120 degrees is often preferable to a Judkins right. Second, during the radiofrequency perforation of the valve, it is imperative to have a catheter in the aorta and main pulmonary artery through the ductus in order to perform angiograms, which are essential to ensure that you are approaching the pulmonary artery in both planes with the catheter and wire tip in order to avoid perforation. Finally, the valve is frequently best perforated with a radiofrequency wire. This wire may or may not be adequate to allow a balloon catheter to pass over it once it enters the pulmonary artery, and since the tip is relatively stiff, it can produce vascular damage if it is not inserted in the right place. Often, it is easier to perforate the valve, get a catheter to follow that wire, and then switch to an 0.14 exchange wire to allow subsequent dilations to occur easily.

The results of this procedure are less satisfactory than that for critical pulmonary stenosis. Complication rates are higher: One patient in our series developed a perforation of the right ventricular outflow tract which required active resuscitation and urgent surgical management for a satisfactory outcome. Cyanosis frequently persists for days or longer, necessitating prolonged management on the intensive care unit with prostaglandins. Although the results of this procedure are not demonstrably better than surgical management, there is a theoretical advantage in that gradient relief may be adequate without the need for a transannular patch and subsequent substantial pulmonary regurgitation. The actual benefits of this procedure over surgical management remain, for the moment, uncertain.

Valvar Aortic Stenosis

Soon after the report of balloon valvotomy for congenital pulmonary stenosis, use of this technique in the management of aortic stenosis was described.[62] It is clear that, in comparison with pulmonary stenosis, dilating the aortic valve is more difficult and dangerous, particularly in adults and infants, and gradient reduction is less effective.[63–68] From experimental data in lambs[64] it is evident that balloon sizes 20% larger than the valve annulus result in significant valvar and perivalvar damage.

At the present time, balloon valvotomy is undertaken in children and adolescents with peak systolic ejection gradients greater than 45 to 50 mm Hg without severe aortic regurgitation[68] and is undertaken in infants with critical obstruction regardless of the gradient value.[69]

Older Patients

Technique

Following routine right and left heart catheterization, including aortography, a pigtail catheter is often placed in the contralateral femoral artery for subsequent pressure measurement and angiography. The valve annulus is measured from a left ventricular angiogram taken in the long axial oblique view (Fig. 14-14). A balloon, preferably 3 to 4 cm long and with a diameter less than 90% of the annulus, is advanced over an exchange wire, the distal end of the wire having been looped in the ventricle. The balloon is positioned across the valve and inflated to abolish the (hopefully) subtle waist, and deflated immediately. We generally dilate aortic valves two to five times, progressively increasing both the inflation pressure and the size of the balloon to increase the effective dilation diameter by 1-mm increments or less, until the residual gradient has been reduced by 50% or more or aortic regurgitation has increased modestly. In some older patients it may be necessary to use two balloons and extra-stiff wires.

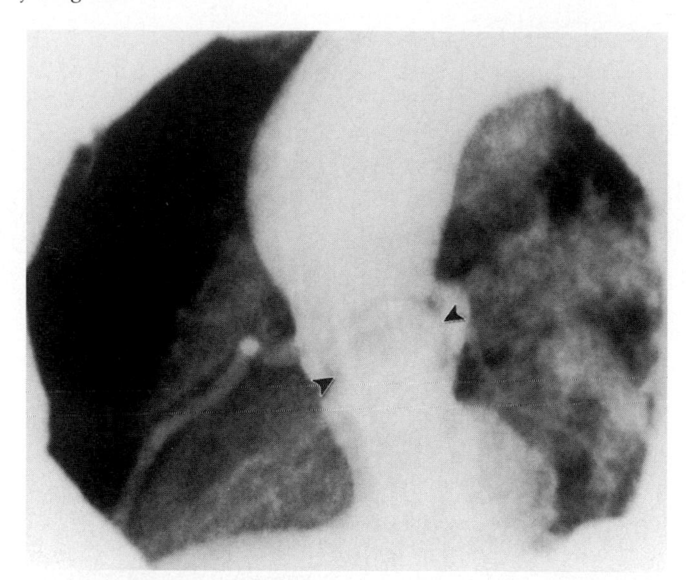

FIGURE 14–14 *Measurement of an annulus size is taken from the valve hinge points (arrows).*
From Fyler DC (ed). Nadas' Pediatric Cardiology, Philadelphia: Hanley & Belfus, 1992.

Neonates with Critical Obstruction

Technique

These babies are particularly fragile, are prone to ventricular fibrillation, and often have low gradients across the valve because of diminished cardiac output. The size of the left ventricular cavity is less than normal in some. The usually patent foramen ovale allows constant monitoring of the left ventricular pressure. While the initial hemodynamic and angiographic evaluation may be carried out quickly in many via the umbilical vessels, prolonged use of the umbilical artery for the dilating procedure can be hazardous. Thus, if the initial approach through the umbilical artery is not easy, a femoral artery is used. A 3F pigtail is passed via a 3F sheath to the left ventricle using a .0014-inch wire. The valve is dilated with a Tyshak miniballoon 1 cm long, with the first dilation at 80% to 85%. Serial gradually increasing balloon sizes are even more important in these patients. Hemodynamic measurements are carried out as for older patients.

Results

A total of 544 patients have undergone aortic valve dilation at the Children's Hospital Boston in the last 20 years, with the numbers being approximately equally distributed throughout that period. On average, gradient reduction has been 55%, and some degree of increase in aortic regurgitation has occurred in 60% to 80% of the patients. The overall mortality rate for the entire series has been 3.7%.

There are, however, two striking changes that have occurred during the past 20 years. The first is a substantial reduction in mortality: the mortality rate from 1985 to 1994[70] approached 7%. Most of the mortality occurred in neonates with an occasional death outside of the neonatal period. The increased mortality in neonates is not surprising: the patients are sicker, the procedure is more technically difficult, and neonates frequently have associated serious heart disease such as coarctation, mitral stenosis or ventricular defects which add to the hemodynamic burden of the aortic stenosis. In the last decade, the mortality rate has fallen to 0.7%, with 2 deaths in 60 neonates, and no mortality after 30 days of age (Table 14-5). These improved results reflect improved catheter technology, meticulous attention to detail, and undoubtedly an adoption of the strategy of multiple serial dilations with small changes in balloon diameter to reduce the risk of severe aortic regurgitation. Thus, dilation of aortic stenosis in children has clearly become the initial procedure of choice in managing this patient population.

Other Complications

Mitral regurgitation was evident at the conclusion of the procedure in two children, both very early in our experience, both of whom required surgical plication of tears in the anterior mitral leaflet. At the time of both surgeries it was noted that the aortic valves had been adequately and appropriately opened by the balloon valvotomy. This should be a preventable complication. Ventricular fibrillation can occur but responds to cardioversion, and transient left bundle branch block is common. Arterial pulse loss immediately following the procedure occurred in 15% to 25% in our earlier series of patients, nearly all infants. In one infant who weighed 4 kg, the external iliac artery was ruptured during attempts to introduce a 7F sheath, mandating uneventful surgical repair. Following the administration of heparin, with or without streptokinase therapy, pulses return in two-thirds of the patients. However, the incidence of subclinical arterial obstruction is uncertain.

Subaortic Stenosis

To date, our limited experience with attempts to dilate discrete or diffuse varieties of this lesion has not resulted in lasting relief of the gradient, although early success in some discrete forms has been reported.[71]

Mitral Valvar Stenosis

Balloon valvotomy for rheumatic mitral stenosis was first reported in children in 1985[72] and 1986.[73] Extensive worldwide experience has established this procedure as the initial treatment of choice for rheumatic mitral valve stenosis under most circumstances. The incidence of rheumatic mitral stenosis in the United States in children continues to decline despite occasional recent outbursts of rheumatic fever. This indication for mitral valvotomy in childhood has become exceedingly rare.

In contrast, the use of balloon angioplasty to dilate congenital mitral stenosis has emerged as a very successful palliation for this otherwise serious disease.[74,75] Since 1986, more than 100 children have undergone catheter management of congenital mitral stenosis at our institution.

Technique

In general, our indications for intervention in patients with severe congenital mitral stenosis include (a) systemic or higher pulmonary artery pressures, (b) failure to thrive or frequent respiratory infections requiring intensive medical management, or (c) mean mitral gradients greater than 15 mm Hg. Noninvasive assessment of transmitral valve gradients in patients with congenital mitral stenosis is less reliable than that for aortic or pulmonary stenosis, perhaps in part due to the fact that the cause of the obstruction is usually complex in these patients.

Following standard right and left catheterization, the left atrial pressure is measured directly with a Brockenbrough needle, and a 7F balloon-tipped catheter is advanced from the left atrium to the left ventricle. Care is taken to be sure

TABLE 14–5. Mortality (30 Day) After Valvuloplasty for Aortic Stenosis

Children's Hospital Boston							
1984-1994				1995-2004			
Age	#Pts	Deaths	Mortality Rate	Age	#Pts	Deaths	Mortality Rate
< 1 mo	55	15	29.1%	< 1 mo	57	2	3.5%
1-12 mo	74	1	1.4%	1-12 mo	68	0	0%
1-10 yrs	80	1	1.3%	1-10 yrs	69	0	0%
10-30 yrs	86	1	6.4%	10-30 yrs	60	0	0%
Total	295	19	6.4%		274	2	0.7%

Mortality (30 day) for dilation of valvar aortic stenosis has decreased, particularly in neonates, in the past 2 decades.

that the balloon is at least partially inflated when it crosses the left ventricular inflow in order to avoid passing through a very small intratrabecular space. Left ventriculography prior to crossing the valve in an RAO view demonstrates the plane of the mitral valve and establishes the degree of pre-existing mitral regurgitation. An 0.18 to 0.35 guide wire is advanced into the apex of the left ventricle, using preformed curves to ensure a stable position, and a balloon is inflated across the mitral leaflet tips (Fig. 14-15). As is the case with aortic stenosis, we use multiple inflations using smaller balloon sizes to begin with, and differing inflation pressures to modulate balloon diameter, allow reasonable gradient reduction without producing severe mitral regurgitation. Since the anatomic substrate of obstruction is unpredictable, we start with balloons that are related to BSA rather than annulus size: 8 mm for BSA 0.4 to 0.8 m^2, 10 for BSA 0.8 to 1.2 m^2, and 12 mm for BSA > 1.2 m^2. Gradients are measured before and after every dilation, hoping to reduce the gradient by at least 50%, although reducing the mean gradient by 25% to 30% is frequently clinically significant. Angiography will often demonstrate mitral regurgitation when a wire is across the valve, but once the wire is removed the mitral regurgitation is reduced. Thus, these patients undergo an average of almost 4 different dilations in order to obtain an adequate clinical result.

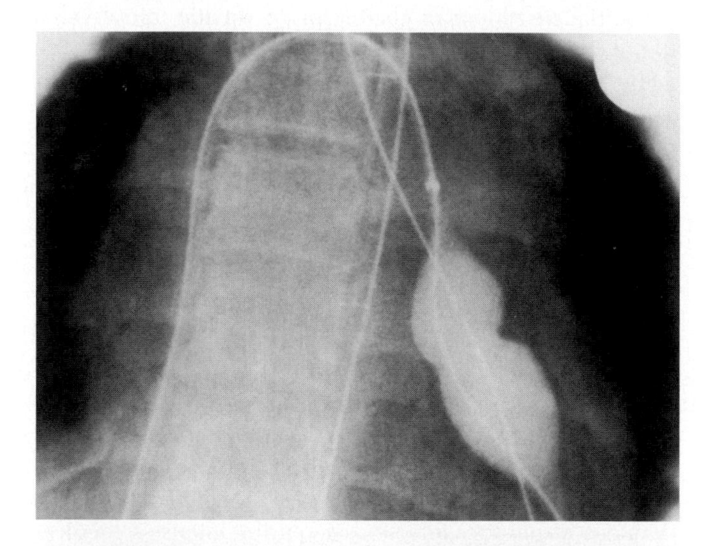

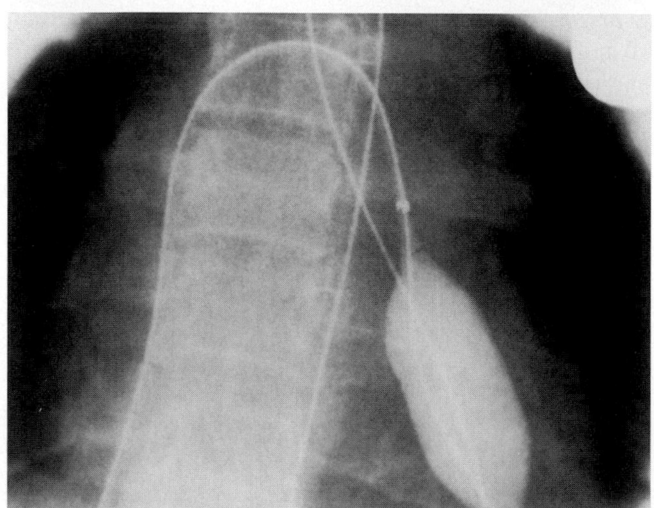

FIGURE 14–15 *From the first successful transseptal dilatation of a mitral valve in a child. The initial balloons were short (3 cm) to avoid damage to the atrial septum and left ventricular apex, a precaution that proved unnecessary. Top, The waist. Bottom, The waist has disappeared.*
From Fyler DC (ed). Nadas' Pediatric Cardiology, Philadelphia: Hanley & Belfus, 1992.

Results

Early in our experience, we demonstrated that patients with supravalvar mitral stenosis had a higher degree of mitral regurgitation than other forms of congenital mitral stenosis.[74] Those patients are now referred directly to surgery. If a patient with typical congenital mitral stenosis undergoes surgical management as the primary strategy, the reported early mortality rate can be high, whereas balloon dilation in our center is associated with an early procedural mortality less than 2%, and defers the need for surgical management of the valve by an average of more than 4 years. In the most recent decade, 5-year survival using balloon dilation as the initial strategy for patients with severe congenital mitral stenosis is greater than 90%, indicating a substantial improvement in the management of these patients (Fig. 14-16).

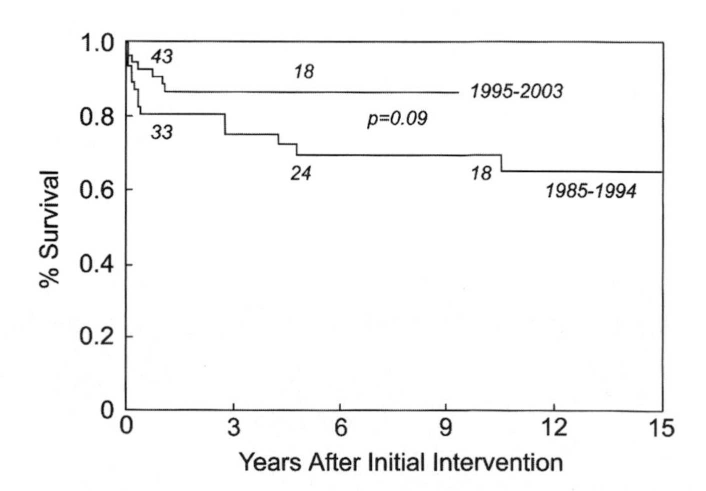

FIGURE 14–16 *Survival of infants with severe congenital mitral stenosis after intervention (balloon dilation, surgery) although showing improvement in 1995–2003 (58 infants) compared with 1985–1994 group (52 infants) mortality remains significant. Courtesy of Dr. McElhinney.*

Prosthetic Valve Stenosis

Attempts to dilate stenotic bioprosthetic valves within right heart conduits have not been very successful.[76] We have taken this approach in fewer than 25 patients ranging in age from 3 to 22 years, 9 of whom had porcine valves in conduits, and the rest had homografts. The gradient was reduced by more than 20 mm Hg in fewer than half the patients. While unsuccessful in most patients, this procedure will allow postponement of conduit or valve replacement in some patients for 6 to 18 months.

BALLOON ANGIOPLASTY

Pulmonary Arteries

Surgical enlargement of narrowed central pulmonary arteries is essential to the management of many patients with tetralogy of Fallot and similar lesions; usually this procedure is successful, restenosis is uncommon, and patch enlargement may extend into the pulmonary artery branches for a short distance with success. However, more distal obstructions and long-segment stenosis (so-called *hypoplastic pulmonary arteries*) are refractory to standard operative management. Balloon angioplasty is now the procedure of choice for these patients and is a very common interventional procedure at our institution. Stenosis of pulmonary artery branches is the most common abnormality found at catheterization after repair of tetralogy of Fallot (Fig. 14-17), and many patients with other arteriopathies have severely obstructed pulmonary arteries.

Initial animal studies indicated that dilation of narrowed pulmonary artery branches was feasible and produced long-lasting success.[77] Preliminary and recent clinical studies[78–80] have demonstrated that most forms of pulmonary arterial narrowings can be dilated. The procedure is not without risk; hemodynamic instability and vascular rupture have resulted in significant morbidity and occasional mortality.[81]

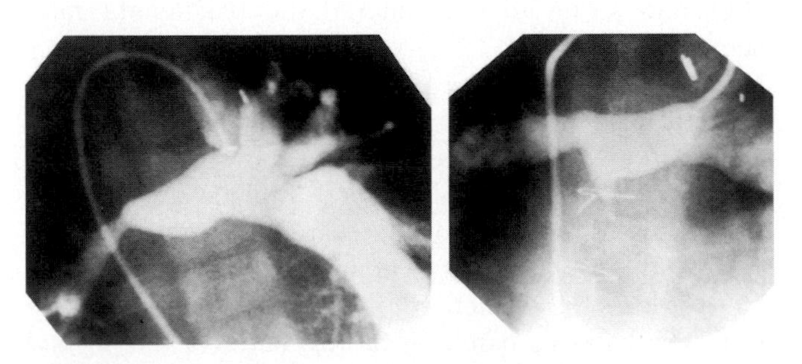

FIGURE 14–17 *Successful dilatation of a right pulmonary artery via a left Blalock-Taussig shunt.*
From Fyler DC (ed). Nadas' Pediatric Cardiology, Philadelphia: Hanley & Belfus, 1992.

Technique

Precatheterization evaluation of these patients includes estimates of the severity of right ventricular outflow obstruction (murmur intensity, right ventricular hypertrophy on the electrocardiogram, septal position, and regurgitant jets by echocardiography), and an estimate of the flow distribution to the two lungs. In any child with bilateral disease, the lung with the least flow has the greatest degree of obstruction, and should be dilated first.

The need for pulmonary arterial dilation is assessed by routine right and left heart catheterization. Candidates should have one or more of the following abnormalities attributable, at least in part, to the arterial narrowings: (a) cyanosis, (b) signs or symptoms of right heart failure, (c) more than half systemic right ventricular pressures, (d) less than 20% to 25% of the cardiac output directed to one lung, (e) pulmonary hypertension in unobstructed lobes, or (f) moderate distal obstruction in the setting of severe pulmonary regurgitation. Pulmonary arterial anatomy is determined from selective biplane right and left pulmonary arteriograms; care is taken to outline distal as well as proximal arterial anatomy. The worst, most distal lesion is dilated first; distal lesions are the most difficult to reach but can be occluded without major hemodynamic instability. An appropriate catheter is advanced into the largest vessel distal to the obstruction (usually the lower lobe artery), taking care to avoid small branches. The guiding wire should be as stiff and as large as possible, and needs to be shaped to allow balloon catheters to track successfully.

After wire positioning, an initial balloon about 3.0 to 3.5 times the size of the narrowed vessel is selected if a small patient is being dilated or about 2.5 to 3 times for an adolescent or adult. If a modest (about 75% to 90% of the balloon diameter) waist is seen, the balloon is inflated to 8 to 10 atm until the waist disappears. If a tighter waist is seen, the balloon is removed, and a smaller one inserted. If no waist is seen, larger balloons or better balloon positions are needed. Care is taken when crossing a recently dilated arterial site; angiograms and pressure measurements may be repeated without losing distal wire position if Y-adaptors are used. Generally, multiple narrowings along the same artery are dilated at one sitting (in the so-called *hypoplastic* artery). We routinely dilate both right and left pulmonary arteries in the same catheterization. In severe forms of diffuse arteriopathy, many (eight or more) vessels must be dilated at the same procedure to avoid deleterious abnormalities of flow distribution.[84] Postdilation angiograms delineate success or failure, identify postdilatation tears and aneurysms, and outline any residual lesions (Figs. 14-18 and 14-19).

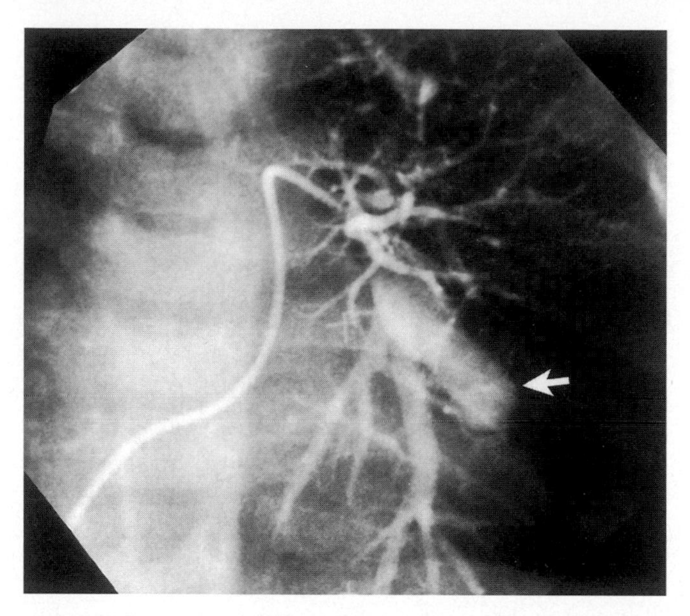

FIGURE 14–18 *Postdilation aneurysm in a left pulmonary artery (arrow). Increased experience and improved technique have made this an avoidable complication.*
From Fyler DC (ed). Nadas' Pediatric Cardiology, Philadelphia: Hanley & Belfus, 1992.

Finally, the recent extension of cutting balloon technology to the obstructed pulmonary artery has produced very encouraging preliminary results.[82,83] The size of the required balloon is small (no more than 0.5–1.0 mm larger than the persistent waist at 8 atm),[83] and in a prospective randomized trial just being completed, cutting balloon angioplasty produces better anatomic improvement than high-pressure (> 15 atm) dilation.

Pulmonary arterial angioplasty has proven to be essential as part of the rehabilitation of diminutive pulmonary arteries.[84] After establishment of right ventricular-pulmonary arterial continuity with small (8–10 mm) homografts during infancy, balloon dilatation is used to relieve the distal stenoses that invariably remain. Transcatheter closure of remaining collaterals and surgical relief of remaining obstructions, along with closure of any ventricular septal defect, complete the process and permit successful repair of these patients (Fig. 14-20).[85]

Results

Given that it is difficult, if not impossible, to measure flow in small branch pulmonary arteries, we have mostly defined successful balloon angioplasty in branch pulmonary arteries as a 50% or larger increase in the diameter of the vessel. Using this criterion, the frequency of successful balloon angioplasty, initially 60%, has increased with the advent of high pressure angioplasty and improved catheter and wire techniques, to about 75%.[79] Since each obstructed vessel contributes a relatively small proportion of the hemodynamic load to a patient with multiple branch pulmonary artery obstructions, it is often difficult to assess the short term clinical results of dilation angioplasty of these vessels. Nonetheless, using lung scans, dilations invariably demonstrate increased flow to lung segments perfused by successfully dilated vessels.

Complications

Mortality for this procedure has fallen steadily since it was introduced more than two decades ago. Four of the first 200 children died due to the procedure, but only 1 of the last 400, for a mortality approaching 0.2%.[81] Morbidity includes hemoptysis due to vessel trauma, unilateral pulmonary edema, and aneurysms. Aneurysms in the pulmonary artery tree following angioplasty have been generally benign so long as the perfusion pressure is low. The patient with pulmonary artery obstructions in the early postoperative period has vessels that are particularly fragile, and in such patients, the use of small-diameter stents have largely replaced standard balloon angioplasty.

Unrepaired Coarctation of the Aorta

Dilation of unrepaired aortic coarctation produces less than complete initial gradient relief, with frequent restenosis in infants.[86] Successful procedures succeed by tearing the vascular intima and part or all of the media and may result in aneurysms both in experimental animals and in children.[87,88] Thus, the role of balloon dilation in the management of the infant or child with an uncomplicated, unrepaired aortic coarctation remains unclear, despite more than 20 years of experience. There is no doubt, however, that balloon dilation can be a useful procedure in the infant or child who may be at high risk for standard surgical management. Stent technology has renewed interest in transcatheter therapy for coarctation in the older child, and seems to have altered the risk/benefit ratio (see below).

Technique

With few exceptions, vascular access is obtained percutaneously via the femoral arteries. Biplane angiography outlines the dimensions of the coarctation and the aorta above and below the obstruction. Initially, balloons about 2.5 to 3 times the diameter of the narrowing are used. We never use balloons based on the diameter of the *normal* aorta, because of cases we have reviewed from other institutions when such a practice can result, when a tight waist is seen, in catastrophic aortic damage. Frequently, larger balloons are required when no improvement is seen on the initial postdilation angiogram. To avoid injuring normal

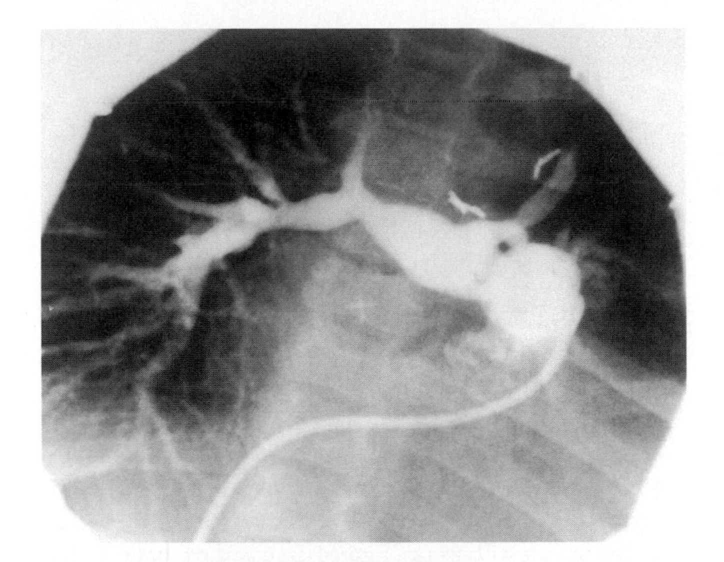

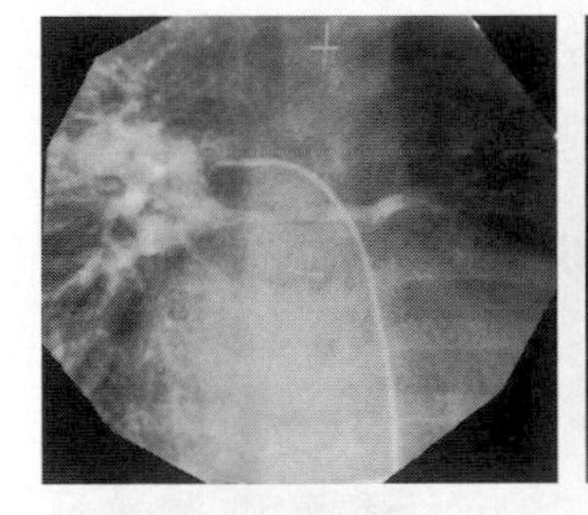

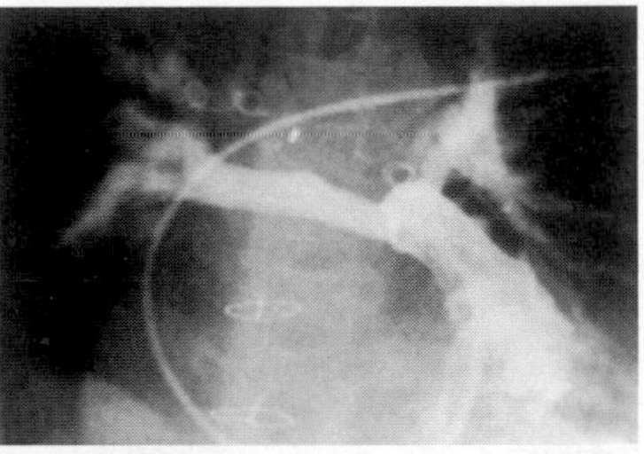

FIGURE 14–20 *A, Patient with tetralogy of Fallot with pulmonary atresia and excess collaterals. Note the tiny right and left pulmonary arteries which were opacified by injection into a right collateral vessel. B, Same patient after coil occlusion of collaterals, surgical opening of the outflow tract, and balloon dilatation of the pulmonary arteries.*
From Fyler DC (ed). Nadas' Pediatric Cardiology, Philadelphia: Hanley & Belfus, 1992.

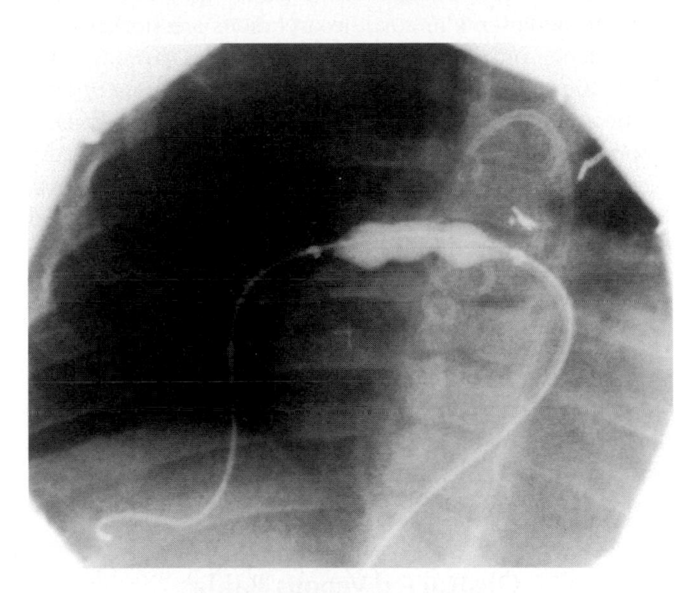

aorta, long balloons (more than 3 cm) and balloons more than 50% larger than the unaffected aorta are avoided. As with pulmonary arteries, if a tight waist is seen in the balloon at low (1–2 atm) pressure, the balloon must be removed without proceeding to full inflation to avoid major vessel damage.

Results

Initial results in dilating unrepaired neonatal coarctations demonstrated a recurrence rate approaching 100% in the first 6 months after dilation.[86] More recent reports have noted long-lasting gradient relief in children, with lower morbidity than seen after surgery.[89,90] but residual gradients remain a significant problem.

In general, catheter management is more successful if there is a thin curtain of endothelial thickening in the coarctation where the aortic diameter itself is relatively normal. Under such circumstances, balloon angioplasty alone can provide quite acceptable gradient relief with a modest risk to the patient. Patients in whom the coarctation is somewhat more diffuse and associated with a reduced aortic outer diameter are much less likely to get a good result from balloon angioplasty alone. At this time, our most common indication for coarctation angioplasty alone is in children or adults with very severe coarctations in whom balloon angioplasty by itself can produce a moderate degree of gradient relief. When the vessel heals, over the course of 3 to

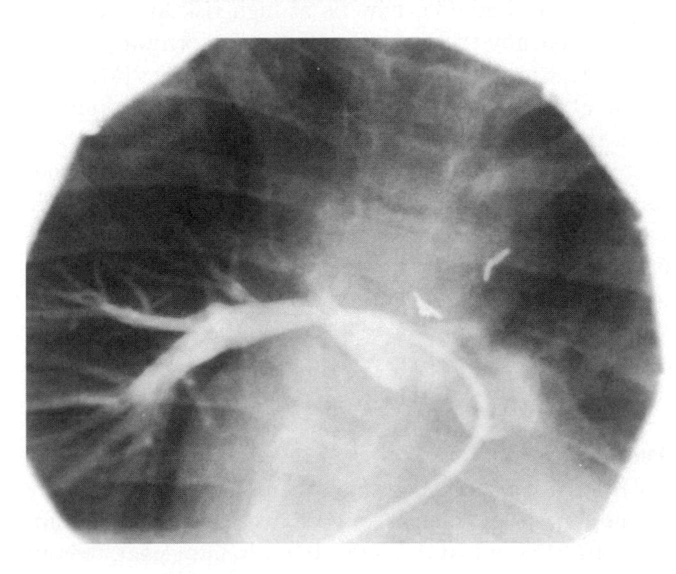

FIGURE 14–19 *Dilation of two obstructions in the right pulmonary artery. The distal right lower lobe is enlarged, but the proximal, shunt-related lesion is unchanged.*
From Fyler DC (ed). Nadas' Pediatric Cardiology, Philadelphia: Hanley & Belfus, 1992.

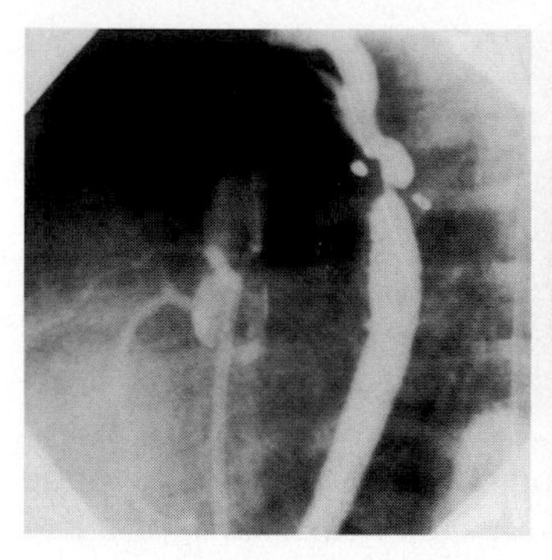
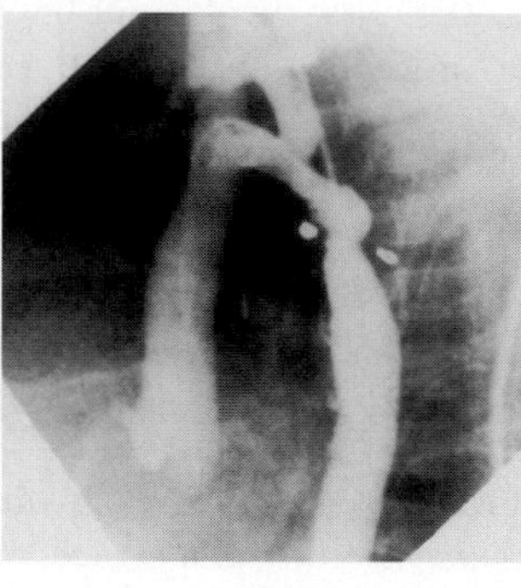

FIGURE 14–21 *Successful dilatation of a recurrent coarctation following subclavian flap repair.*
From Fyler DC (ed). Nadas' Pediatric Cardiology, Philadelphia: Hanley & Belfus, 1992.

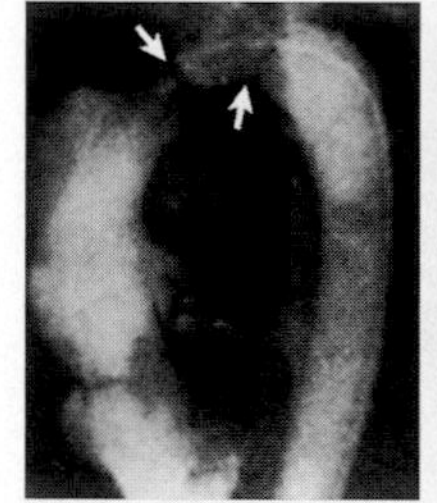
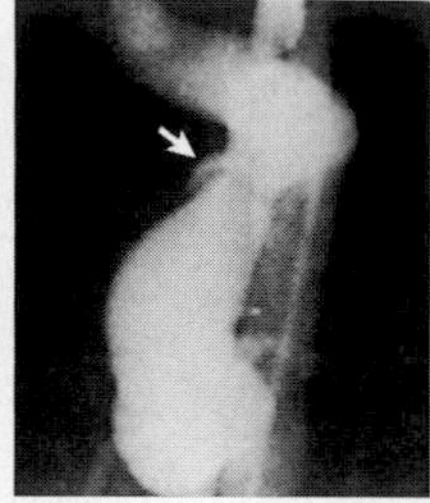
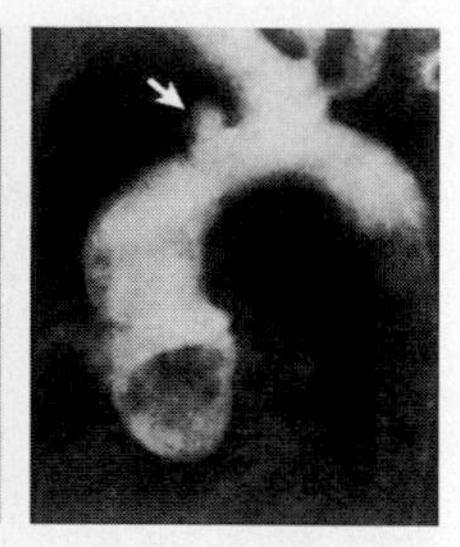

FIGURE 14–22 *Balloon dilatation of arch obstruction which persisted after repair of interrupted aortic arch. Late aneurysm (arrows) seen 1 year later.*
From Fyler DC (ed). Nadas' Pediatric Cardiology, Philadelphia: Hanley & Belfus, 1992.

12 months, it can then be safely stented to a much larger diameter without producing serious vascular injury.

Postoperative Coarctation of the Aorta

Unlike unrepaired aortic coarctation, postoperative aortic obstruction can be a formidable surgical challenge: Mortality rates are higher, morbidity can be considerable, and gradient relief frequently is incomplete. Balloon angioplasty has been a very useful tool in the management of arch obstructions that remain after repair of aortic coarctations (Fig. 14-21), interrupted aortic arches, and the hypoplastic left heart syndrome.[91]

Technique

The procedure is quite similar to that outlined for unrepaired aortic coarctation. Initially, balloon size is chosen to be 2.5 to 3 times the size of the obstruction, but the final balloon size frequently is larger. The use of a long sheath (to allow frequent measurement of gradients and angiographic diameters) is helpful in deciding when a large enough balloon has been used.

Results

The results of balloon angioplasty of postoperative aortic coarctation are very similar to that of native aortic coarctations. In general, gradients fall substantially, with an average gradient reduction above 50%. With the advent of stents for coarctation, we only dilate postoperative lesions primarily as noted above when the obstruction is extremely tight as part of a staged procedure.

Complications

As with pulmonary artery angioplasty, the risks from dilation of native or recurrent coarctations at our hospital have fallen with experience. Despite these reduced risks, aneurysms can still occur (Fig. 14-22), and we believe that dilations and stents in aortic coarctations are perhaps the most dangerous interventional procedure in congenital heart disease. There are more than a dozen cases of fatal or near fatal aortic trauma surrounding these cases. Although very few, if any, cases have been reported in the medical literature, the trauma appears secondary to areas within the coarctation complex that are noncompliant and thin-walled. This rare (1%–2%) kind of coarctation may rupture when an otherwise *appropriate*-sized balloon is used for dilation or stenting, especially if the balloon is chosen based on the diameter of the *normal* aorta. Test dilation of the area that produces a tighter than expected waist in the balloon should prompt immediate balloon deflation, and redilation with a smaller balloon. Using these precautions, we have had no catastrophic aortic ruptures or deaths in over 200 procedures.

Obstructed Venous Baffles

Until recently the mainstay of surgery for transposition of the great arteries, the atrial inversion operations (Mustard, Senning) can be complicated by obstructions in the limbs of the systemic or pulmonary venous baffle. Generally, these obstructions are at the level of the old atrial septum, a structure that can be dilated successfully.[92] Balloon angioplasty has become an attractive alternative to surgical revision of the baffle. As transvenous pacing and AICD leads are increasingly used in survivors of Mustard or Senning surgery, the frequency of superior vena caval baffle obstruction also seems to increase, perhaps due to increased recognition in otherwise mildly symptomatic patients.

Technique

These lesions are extremely compliant and generally require very large balloons, or even two balloons. Successful dilations occur when the obstruction is at, or near, the old

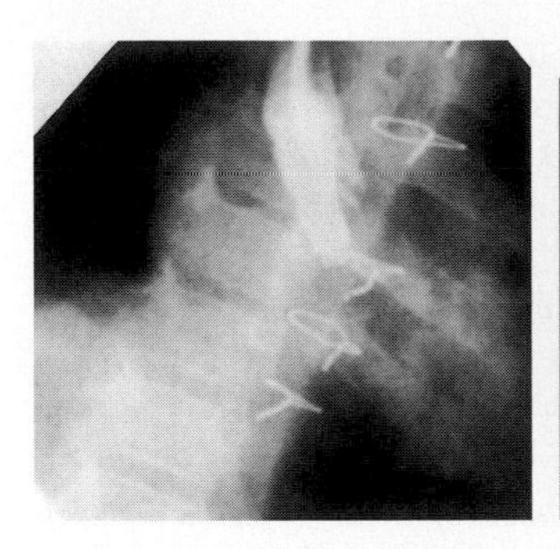
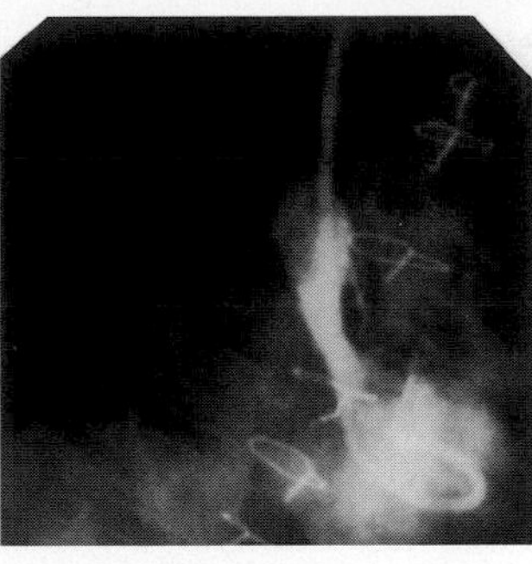

FIGURE 14–23 *Successful dilatation of an obstructed venous baffle following the atrial inversion procedure.*
From Fyler DC (ed). Nadas' Pediatric Cardiology, Philadelphia: Hanley & Belfus, 1992.

atrial septum; thus, predilation definition of the anatomy is important. Initially, balloons about five times the diameter of the narrowing are inflated to low pressures (1–2 atm). Larger and larger balloons are used until a waist is seen at low pressures and disappears at high pressures. Balloons as much as 10 times larger than the narrowed segment may be needed. Indeed, the need for such large balloons in this lesion resulted in the early use of the double-balloon technique in children. After successful dilatation, pressure measurements and angiography are repeated (Fig. 14-23). In general these procedures remain helpful, especially when a functioning pacemaker wire crosses the area of narrowing, making stent implantation impractical. Gradients are generally reduced by 50%. Although we have had no significant morbidity in patients with simple obstructions, patients with total occlusions can develop nonfatal aneurysms after recanalization and simple dilation.

PULMONARY VENOUS OBSTRUCTIONS

Unlike older patients with obstructed pulmonary venous baffles, most infants and children who have obstructions of pulmonary veins appear to have a different disease. It is either a primary pulmonary venous obstruction, or obstruction that follows shortly after surgery for total anomalous pulmonary venous connection, or partial anomalous pulmonary venous connection associated with heterotaxy syndrome. These patients appear to have diffuse disease in their small, medium and large pulmonary veins that has recently been attributed to myofibroblasts rather than simple scar tissue or endothelial thickening. The veins respond acutely to a dilation, but invariably restenose in several hours, days or weeks following the procedure.[97] Thus, the use of interventional cardiology has not, to our knowledge, been life-saving in these infants.

Recently, an attempt has been made at our institution to treat these patients with antineoplastic agents, pursuing the hypothesis that this disease is a diffuse tumor rather than straightforward congenital heart disease. While most patients treated in this fashion have died within 1 or 2 years of diagnosis, there are now four long-term (> 2 years) survivors. In those patients, the use of simple pulmonary vein angioplasty, cutting balloon angioplasty, atherectomy catheters, or stents coated with antiproliferative agents may help the patient to survive long enough for a chemotherapeutic approach to succeed. A more complete analysis of this approach is pending. Nonetheless, it is our belief that, in the absence of systemic therapy, interventional catheter techniques have never been successful in producing prolonged survival in infants with obstructed pulmonary veins.

Neonatal Balloon Atrial Septostomy

Balloon atrial septostomy, introduced by Rashkind and Miller in 1966, remains the standard method of creating an atrial septal defect in the newborn.[7] Although intracardiac complications occurred during the early years, these complications have virtually disappeared, although limitations became evident: the duration of septal patency was temporary in many infants, and septostomy was usually ineffective in infants older than 1 month. Nonetheless, balloon septostomy remains the procedure of choice in the newborn with transposition of the great arteries, being particularly useful in the baby with d-transposition in whom an arterial switch procedure can be carried out within days of birth.

Technique

In recent years, we have used the Miller septostomy catheter (American Edwards Laboratories), introduced through a 7F sheath with a diaphragm. Entry, preferably through an umbilical venous site, allows the balloon to be inflated with 2.5 to 3.5 mL of dilute contrast in the left atrium, provided that the cavity is large enough to accept this inflated size (smaller amounts are necessary in premature or low birth weight infants). The balloon is then rapidly jerked two to three times across the septum, and the defect is then assessed echocardiographically. We formerly used the Park blade in older infants with reasonable results and acceptable morbidity.[96] However, 4- to 8-mm premounted stents that will fit through 4F or 5F sheaths has simplified creation of durable atrial defects in older patients, and have replaced the Park blade.

STENTS

The development of stent technology in the last decade, driven primarily by the accelerated use of stents in coronary artery disease in adults, was also applied to iliac artery and bile duct obstructions. Stents developed for these indications have become increasingly applicable to children with congenital heart disease, and stent implantation is a rapidly growing management of congenital heart disease at cardiac catheterization.

The most commonly used locations for stents in congenital heart disease are branch pulmonary arteries, conduits after surgery for tetralogy of Fallot, and aortic coarctations. Less common, but highly useful, indications for stents include management of tunnel subaortic stenosis, maintenance of atrial septal patency in patients with single ventricle physiology, palliation of certain patients with hypoplastic left heart syndrome, and management of systemic venous and pulmonary venous baffle obstructions.

Stents in Pulmonary Arteries

The first use of stents in congenital heart disease occurred in pulmonary arteries,[94] and it remains perhaps the most common indication for this device in pediatrics.[95–97] Stents are well suited to managing central pulmonary artery obstructions, since angioplasty works by stretching the vessel to its maximum diameter, and then inducing a partial tear, allowing the vessel to heal in an open position. The initial stretch, which frequently doubles the diameter of the vessel, recoils and is lost following angioplasty alone. Thus, stent implantation can provide a much larger diameter increase than angioplasty alone. In addition, vessels that are kinked rather than anatomically obstructed can only be successfully managed at catheterization with a stent.

Three disadvantages to implanting stents continue to limit their use. If an arterial side branch of an artery is *jailed* by the stent, especially a relatively soft side branch, that branch can become compressed and obstructed, and may be very difficult to reopen. We are fanatical in our efforts to avoid *jailing* side branches in pulmonary arteries, especially in patients with a limited vascular bed. Stents can only be implanted once, and can rarely if ever be repositioned or removed once implanted, except with surgery. Thus, a stent in a growing child will not grow as the child grows. While late redilation can frequently increase the diameter of stents as long as 5 to 10 years after the initial implantation, anatomy and stent characteristics may limit the ultimate size that a stent can reach. Thus, implanting stents in growing children must take into consideration the impact of growth. Finally, stents are very difficult to remove if positioned incorrectly, unlike other cardiac implants: misplaced stents frequently wind up occupying more or less benign positions in the vena cava or descending aorta.

Technique

Precise angiography demonstrates not only the diameter in both planes of the area to be stented, but also the presence or absence of side branches. It is always safest to *test dilate* an area that needs to be stented to (a) assess the compliance of the lesion (if the lesion is highly compliant, the first stent one may put in will actually be too small to stay stable and embolize inadvertently), (b) to assess balloon migration during inflation, and (c) understand the way the geometry changes with balloon inflation, which may well alter the angle at which one deposits the stent. Not all lesions require test predilation: When multiple interventions are required, the patient is hemodynamically unstable, or catheter access is very difficult, clinical judgment may well decide against pre-dilation. In general, the stent length should be somewhat smaller than the length of the balloon, and it should be crimped onto the balloon securely. We tend to mount stents onto catheters inside of sheaths outside the body, and then advance the entire sheath and stent-balloon combination to the lesion in order to avoid migration of the stent during passage through the sheath. The use of a long sheath is particularly helpful to allow frequent test injections during stent implantation to ensure precise location. Once the stent is fully expanded, the ideal angiographic appearance is a subtle hour-glass shape to the stent, indicating that it is centered on an obstruction (Fig. 14-24), and thus is very unlikely to migrate.

Results and Complications

In an attempt to get an updated understanding of transcatheter therapy for branch pulmonary artery stenosis, we recently reviewed more than 100 angioplasties and stent implantations at our institution. These results demonstrate that stents are mostly utilized in compliant main, left or right pulmonary arteries, and in those locations produce a near doubling of the size of the branch pulmonary arteries. Jailing of side branch pulmonary arteries was uncommon. Stents that were implanted in more distal pulmonary artery locations were more frequently used to *salvage* obstructive intimal flaps or aneurysms that were associated with reduced flow. No mortality was associated with stent implantation in pulmonary arteries since the inception of

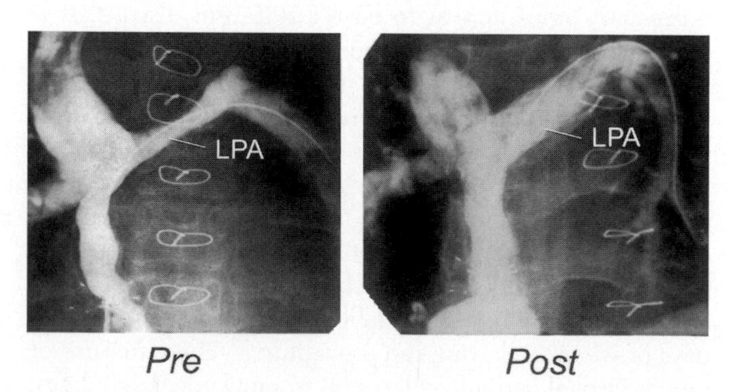

FIGURE 14–24 *Left pulmonary artery (LPA) hypoplasia PRE, with enlargement POST stent placement.*

this procedure. Morbidity was primarily related to the adverse events already described for angioplasty alone. Stent-specific morbidity was due to stent migration or jailing of side branches. Although the former was almost always managed by repositioning the stent in a *benign* location, jailing of side branches by pulmonary artery stents, while often benign, can be a very devastating complication in children with limited vascular beds.

Stents in Aortic Coarctation

The techniques for stents in aortic coarctations are similar to those for pulmonary arteries, except that test dilation is more necessary in this lesion. As noted previously, coarctations can have a highly variable compliance, and one needs to inspect the shape and tightness of a waist in order to be sure that full inflation of the balloon does not produce catastrophic vascular trauma, especially in postoperative or calcified lesions. If the very first inflation of a balloon in a coarcted aorta is during primary stenting, one cannot assess the presence of a tight coarctation waist, and full expansion may produce vascular rupture.

Stents are ideally suited to manage mild coarctations in older children (Fig. 14-25). Coarctations in older patients are frequently associated with surprisingly high left atrial and left ventricular end diastolic pressures, indicating left ventricular diastolic dysfunction, even with relatively mild disease.[98] For that reason, we have increasingly used stents to palliate patients with coarctations and gradients as low as 10 to 20 mm Hg, provided that the anatomy is suitable (i.e., distal to the brachiocephalic vessels), and that a stent large enough to expand to at least 20 mm can be deployed.

Results and Complications

In our first 33 patients, stenting of aortic coarctations produced an 80% reduction in gradient from 25 to 5 mm Hg, with a minimal lumen diameter increase from 8 to 13 mm.

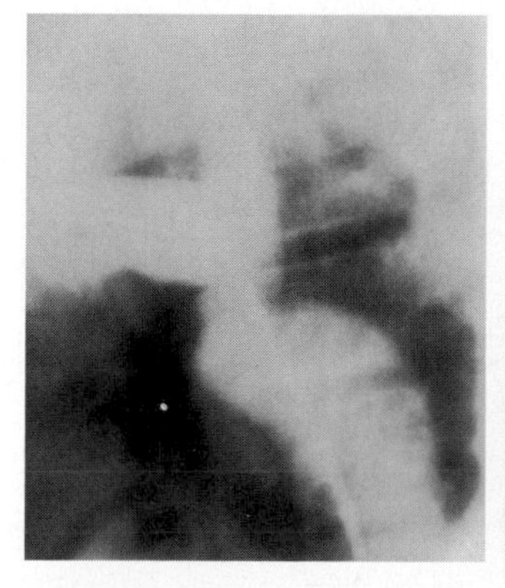
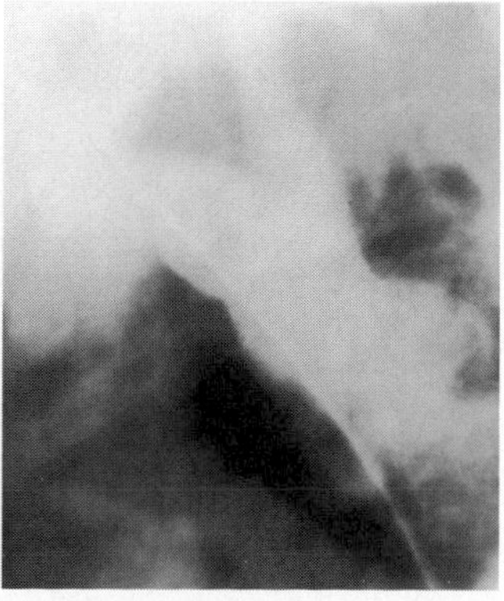

FIGURE 14–25 *Showing mild residual postoperative coarctation, lateral view, in a 14-year-old relieved by stent placement with abolition of 20 mm Hg peak systolic gradient.*

There were no aneurysms determined angiographically in this group of patients. Subsequent to that, over 140 patients have been admitted for stent implantation in coarctations at Children's Hospital Boston, with similar gradient results. Although small areas of aortic irregularity have been seen, there has been no mortality, and no patients have developed aneurysms requiring medical or surgical management. There was a small increase in gradient at follow up, although a second catheterization and dilation returned the average gradient to baseline levels or lower in all patients. One patient, the third in our series, had a myocardial infarction due to a wire that was inadvertently left in a distal left anterior descending branch during extensive catheter, balloon and stent manipulations. A second patient developed transient bundle branch block, and a third patient developed transient neurologic events associated with a relatively long procedure. There was no mortality in the series, and no patient required surgical or medical management of significant aneurysms. Several patients did have stent malposition, with subsequent re-expansion in the thoracic aorta without subsequent sequelae. One such stent fractured late, but remained in situ and produced no sequelae. Based on this favorable risk-benefit ratio, stents remain our procedure of choice for managing older patients with coarctations and recurrent coarctations, although considerable care must be taken to avoid serious aortic injury.

Stents in Right Ventricular Conduits

Nearly all children who receive bioprosthetic conduits to palliate tetralogy of Fallot or truncus arteriosus develop obstruction of those bioprostheses. Sometimes due to physical shrinkage of the conduit, and sometimes due to compression or kinking, early restenosis may force a child to undergo three, four, or five conduit change operations in childhood, presumably increasing the risk of cumulative myocardial or neurologic damage. Stents have been shown to delay the need for conduit change in our initial series by an average of 44 months,[99] and improvements in technology have improved this result in our more recent experience. The technique is similar to that employed in branch pulmonary arteries, with two exceptions. First, one needs to try to avoid trapping the pulmonary valve leaflets in the conduit, especially if there is residual functioning of those leaflets. We assess pulmonary regurgitation with MRI and by measuring diastolic pressure in the main pulmonary artery and the right ventricle simultaneously. If those pressures are identical, we assume the patient has free pulmonary regurgitation; if the pressures are separated, we assume some residual valve function. Second, the anatomy and location of coronary arteries must be clearly established before implanting stents into conduits. A stent can be expanded and compress a coronary artery, producing acute myocardial ischemia. Indeed, test dilation in the conduit using a balloon filled with very dilute contrast material and simultaneous injection in a coronary artery demonstrated serious coronary obstruction in three patients. All three were referred to surgery.

Other Uses of Stents

Finally, stents have been used successfully to manage obstructions of the atrial septum, especially in infants with hypoplastic left heart syndrome,[100] obstructions to brachiocephalic vessels in diffuse arteriopathies,[101] and tunnel subaortic stenosis. In all of these cases, the results of the procedure appear quite promising, although the numbers are small and statistical inferences are not available. We have little direct experience with stents in a ductus arteriosus because of our institutional bias to pursue early reparative or palliative operations, but the results reported from other centers are encouraging.

CLOSURE TECHNIQUES

Coil Embolization of Aortopulmonary Vessels

Aortopulmonary collateral vessels are encountered frequently in tetralogy of Fallot and other forms of congenital heart disease. Their anatomy is highly variable; they may arise from head and neck vessels, the abdominal aorta, or coronary arteries, as well as from the descending thoracic aorta. Their courses within the thorax are unpredictable, and intraoperative recognition may be difficult. Patients with single ventricles and long-standing cyanosis may develop enlarged *normal* intercostal vessels that provide competitive, inefficient pulmonary blood flow after a Fontan. Coil embolization at catheterization is the treatment of choice for both lesions.[102,103]

Technique

Precise angiographic definition is mandatory to identify the optimum coil size and location. Because the course of the vessel is often tortuous, multiple views and selective injections are needed. We avoid closing collaterals where no second source of blood to the affected lung is evident, to avoid losing pulmonary vascular bed. However, even when a collateral is the only source, closure is well tolerated. Coils are chosen to be 10% to 30% larger than the diameter of the vessel to be closed; smaller coils are nonocclusive and larger coils may extrude back into the aorta (Fig. 14-26). Frequently, multiple coils are needed to close high-flow lesions; larger coils are used as a framework and smaller coils subsequently, to retard flow. The vessels are usually closed using a retrograde percutaneous technique with

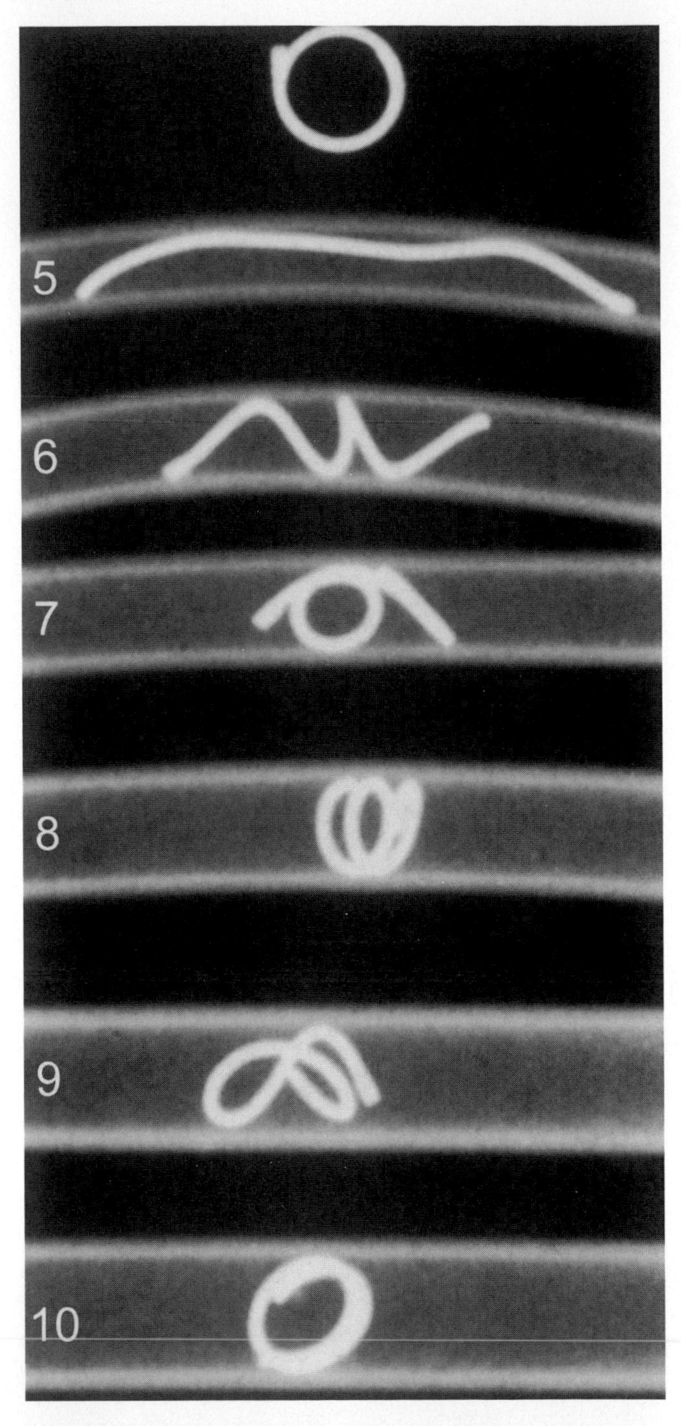

FIGURE 14–26 *Coils placed in tubes of varying size. Oversized coils (top) will be nonocclusive; undersized coils (bottom) will encircle in mid-channel and allow flow on either side.*
From Fyler DC (ed). Nadas' Pediatric Cardiology, Philadelphia: Hanley & Belfus, 1992.

catheters that provide a straight course to the vessel and allow careful control of the tip during coil placement.

Results and Complications

Although initially designed primarily for use in patients with tetralogy of Fallot, coil embolization of aortopulmonary collaterals is now used primarily in children prior to or following a Fontan operation who have enlarged chest wall collaterals that compete with venous blood in its passage through the lungs as part of our institutional approach to maximize Fontan circulations on an elective basis. Closure rates exceed 95%. There has been no mortality associated with the procedure, and significant morbidity is rare. Inadvertent coil embolization to the lung is rare, and most often the coil can and should be retrieved. Even without retrieval, the incorrectly positioned coil does not cause symptoms.

Coil Embolization of Other Vessels

In addition to their use in aortopulmonary vessels, coils have been useful for closing Blalock-Taussig shunts, systemic arteriovenous (AV) fistulae, pulmonary arteriovenous fistulae producing cyanosis, and venous malformations producing right-to-left shunts. An important special circumstance is the closure of coronary AV fistulae (Fig. 14-27). Although each use, by itself, is not common, in aggregate they demonstrate the versatility of coils to achieve vessel closure.

The use of coils to close these various lesions is similar to that described for aortopulmonary vessels. As above, coils need to be 10% to 30% larger than arterial-stretched diameters; the vessel will not stretch if it is a modified synthetic Blalock shunt but a systemic vein may stretch by 50% or more.

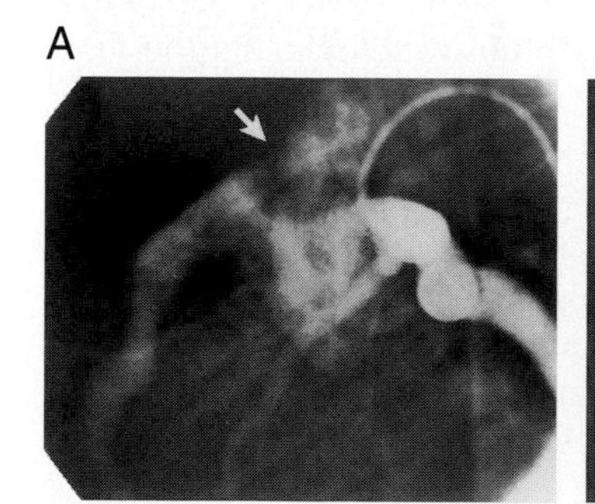

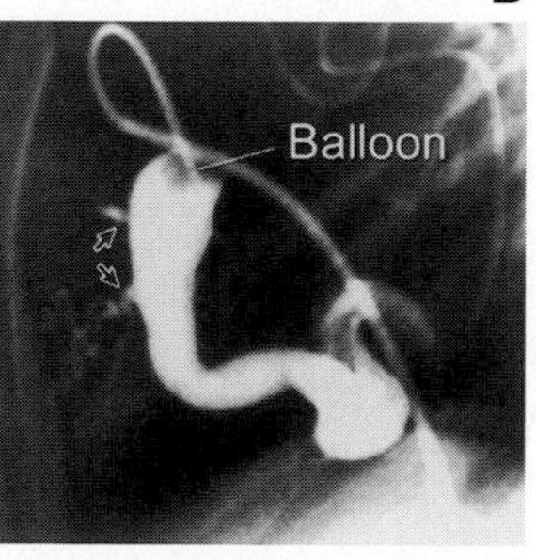

FIGURE 14–27 *Frames from cineangiogram, lateral view in 12-year-old patient with coronary artery fistula. A, There is a single left coronary artery selectively injected via a retrograde catheter from the aorta showing the orifice of the fistula opening into the right ventricular outflow tract (arrow): (B) when the fistula is occluded by a transvenous balloon catheter contrast injected into the distal fistula identifies important right ventricular free wall branches not seen on (A): (open arrows): this fistula was closed in the region of the balloon with coils, leaving these branches open.*

Results and Complications

In general, the results and complications of coil occlusion of these vessels are similar to those encountered in aortopulmonary collaterals. In addition, we have reported a total of 33 coronary arteriovenous fistulae undergoing closure since 1988.[104] Most of those closures used coils, and most of those coils were advanced retrograde from the femoral artery to the very distal end of the fistula. The results of this procedure have been excellent, with 85% of the fistulae successfully closed, and no deaths, documented early myocardial infarctions, or evidence of other significant morbidity.

Catheter Closure of Patent Ductus Arteriosus

Although use of the Portsmann plug[105] and the original Rashkind device[106] to close patent ducts were never approved by the Food and Drug Administration, and therefore never made it to routine clinical use, the successful experience with those techniques prompted the development of both coils[107] and, more recently, dedicated ductal closure plugs.[108] At the present time, the large majority of patent ductus arteriosi in children and adults can be closed at cardiac catheterization without the need for surgical management, the current exceptions being those in premature infants and large window-like ducts in younger patients. The technique for closure depends on whether one uses coils or Amplatzer plugs. Coils are generally delivered retrograde from the femoral artery, with two thirds of the first coil loop delivered in the pulmonary artery, and the other 2.5 to 3.5 loops of coil delivered in the aortic ductal ampulla. Larger ducts may require two coils, or the use of a snare or bioptome to hold the first coil in place while a second coil is delivered. The multiple coil technique has become less necessary with the development of Amplatzer PDA plugs. When using an Amplatzer PDA plug, the ductus is crossed from the pulmonary artery side, the distal end of the catheter is positioned in the descending aorta, and the Amplatzer plug, with its larger aortic cap, is deployed in the aorta, pulled back against the aortic ampulla, and the rest of the body of the plug is deployed within the ductus so that a small part of the plug extrudes toward the pulmonary end of the ductus (Fig. 14-28). Both the lateral tension of the nitinol mesh and aortic pressure keeps the Amplatzer plug in place, and the same thing is true for coils.

Results

The results of PDA closure with coils remain excellent, although we have had two coils embolize to the pulmonary

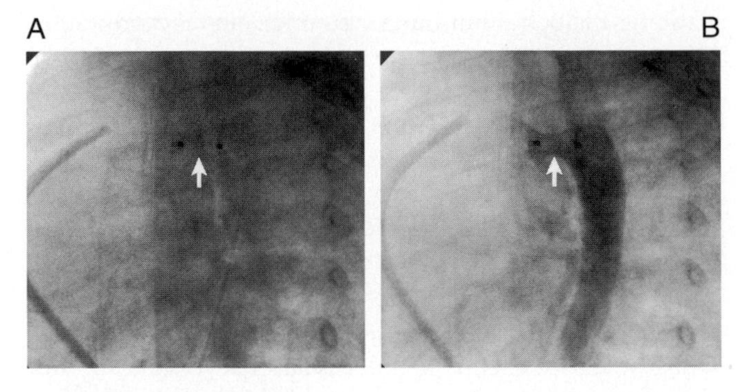

FIGURE 14–28 *Amplatzer, size 8/6 mm (arrows), in patent ductus arteriosus in 1-year-old, lateral view, without (A) and with contrast injection (B) in thoracic aorta.*

artery in the last 100 patients that could not be retrieved and were left in situ. In both cases, there were no clinical sequelae. To date, our own experience with the Amplatzer plug has been limited to several dozen cases, although the results seem to be quite good. In the manuscript published by Bilkis et al.,[108] more than 200 patients were reported with a 98% complete closure rate at 6 months, with morbidity including embolizations and mild aortic narrowing in fewer than 4% of cases.

Transcatheter Closure of Atrial Septal Defects

As with patent ductus arteriosus, an atrial septal defect was first closed using ingenious transcatheter techniques 30 years ago by King and Mills.[109] Although the first four cases were successfully performed, the size of the sheath (23F) and a significant incidence of residual leaks prevented this technique from being adopting for widespread use. Since then, a large number of devices have been developed to close atrial septal defects, including the hooked device of Rashkind, the original Clamshell device, the Angelwings device, the Asdos device, the Helix device, and others. At present, only two devices are approved in this country for closure of atrial defects: the Amplatzer device, which is approved for certain patent foramina ovalia and atrial septal defects; and the CardioSEAL device, which is approved for some types of patent foramina ovalia. Although work continues on the design and application of atrial septal defect closure devices, most of the data that are available come from those two devices.

The Amplatzer device uses a novel technique of stenting open the atrial septal defect itself to reduce the instability of the device, and fills the hole with a combination of nitinol mesh and fibers which promote clotting and subsequent closure.[110,111] Because the device relies on stretching the defect as part of the closure technique, it is larger than other devices for any given hole size, and has been more commonly associated with early and late atrial arrhythmias,[112] or distortion of cardiac structures. Despite these complications, which are generally not life threatening, the Amplatzer device has achieved widespread use because of its ease of implantation and relatively high closure rates.[113] The technique is similar to that which was developed for earlier devices: we estimate the size of the atrial septal defect by balloon sizing: the balloon is minimally inflated so as to avoid disrupting the atrial septum, and once the balloon is found to occlude the defect either echocardiographically or angiocardiographically, the internal diameter of the Amplatzer device is chosen to be the same as, or 1 mm larger or smaller, than the diameter of the defect itself. We do not oversize Amplatzer devices in order to reduce the risk of both late atrial arrhythmias and interference with other cardiac structures. Once the device size is chosen, a 9F to 12F sheath is advanced through the atrial defect, the distal dome of the Amplatzer device as well as the central portion are exposed in the left atrium, snugged into the atrial defect with a fair amount of backward traction, and then the proximal disc is exposed. In this device, the most common source of misplacement is to have the inferior segment of the right atrial disc partially on the left atrial side. Unless a serious error has been made in estimating atrial septal defect size, displacement of part of the left atrial disc through the defect and into the right atrium is quite uncommon. Once both discs have been opened, the device is still attached to the delivery guide wire and can be jiggled back and forth to ensure a level of stability. The attachment technique of the Amplatzer device is a threaded coaxial screw mechanism into the device which does not allow the device to rotate on the tip of the catheter, and thus the device will distort the atrial septum before release. Once the device is released, it lines up against the atrial septum well, although the discs can frequently protrude for millimeters or more into either the left or right atrial cavity (Fig. 14-29). This protrusion tends to diminish with time, as the discs of the device enlarge and flatten over the course of weeks and months. Different authors have used fluoroscopy alone, transesophageal echo or intracardiac echo to aid in placement of the devices, and each of these imaging techniques has its own advantages and disadvantages.

The results of Amplatzer implantation into atrial defects are generally quite good. In the largest series published that was used to support approval of the device,[110] the frequency of a successful procedure (a combination of almost complete or complete closure and the absence of major complications) was 95%, which compared favorably to surgery. Although surgical closure rates are higher than the closure rates for any of the transcatheter device techniques, the incidence of significant complications has been somewhat higher with surgery, most especially pericardial effusions and

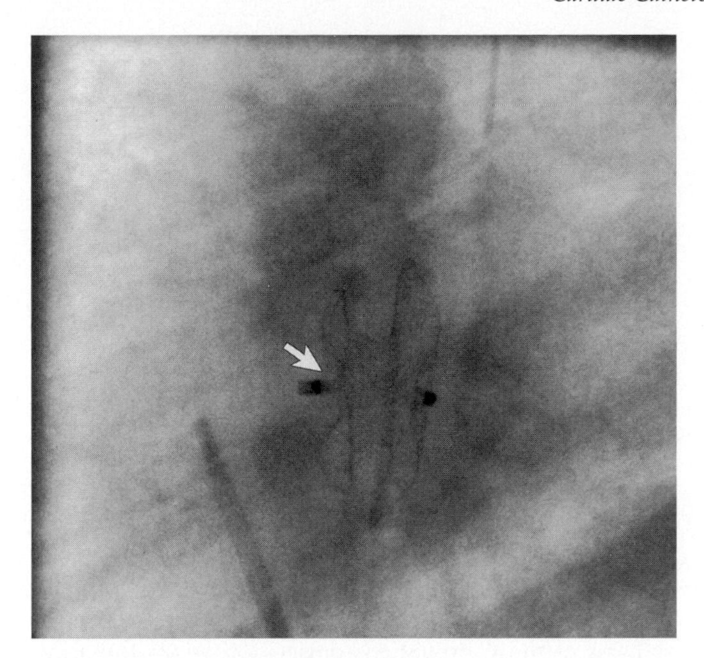

FIGURE 14–29 *Amplatzer, size 14 mm (arrow) in atrial septal defect in 5-year-old, lateral view.*

atrial arrhythmias. Thus, catheter closure of atrial septal defects is an attractive alternative to surgery and, in many centers including ours, it has become the procedure of choice for patients with moderate or large sized, centrally located atrial defects.

Complications

As noted above, the major complications from the Amplatzer device have been atrial arrhythmias and interference with other cardiac structures. More recently, however, a series of nearly 3 dozen cases of late erosion of Amplatzer atrial devices producing serious or catastrophic events have occurred during postmarket evaluation of the device.[113,114] These late erosions (as late as 3 years after implantation) are much more common than encountered with other devices, although they are still rare and probably occur in fewer than 5 of 1000 cases. Nonetheless, they remain a source of concern and help stimulate efforts to improve this device and others.

The other widely used atrial device is the CardioSEAL, and its more recent modification, the STARFlex device. For atrial septal defects, the CardioSEAL device is much less widely used than the Amplatzer device because of the ease of implantation of the Amplatzer device, and the retrievability of the Amplatzer device if the device is misplaced prior to release. The technique for implanting the CardioSEAL and STARFlex device is similar to that for the Amplatzer device except that the left and right atrial discs are smaller, spring-loaded arms with attached Dacron. Thus, the CardioSEAL device has a much lower profile inside the

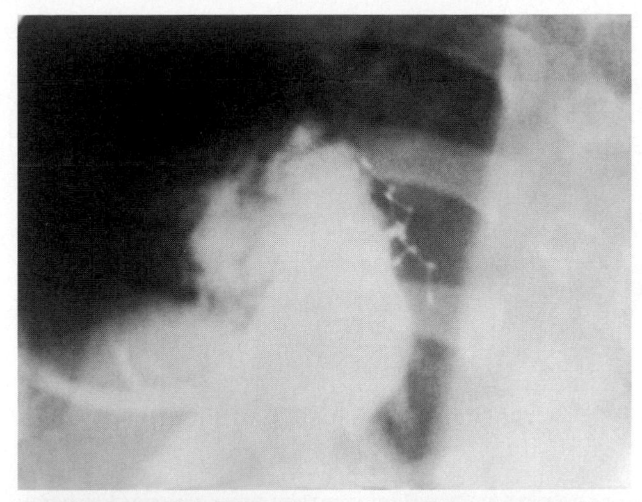

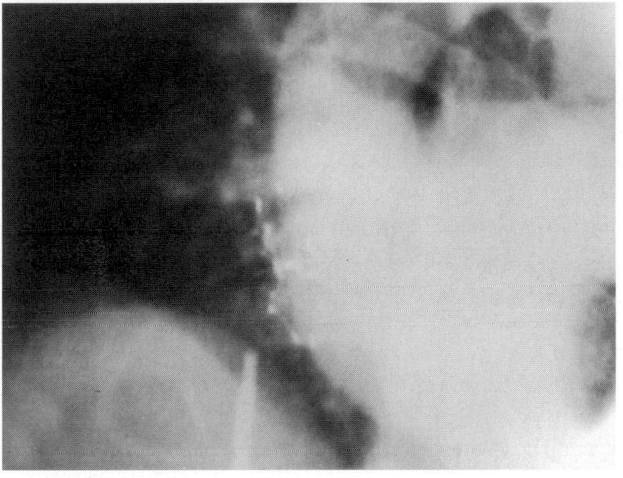

FIGURE 14–30 *Umbrella closure of an atrial septal defect. A, Right atrial angiogram shows no right-to-left shunt. B, Levophase shows no left-to-right shunt.*
From Fyler DC (ed). Nadas' Pediatric Cardiology, Philadelphia: Hanley & Belfus, 1992.

heart (Fig. 14-30), and has been associated with fewer late arrhythmias or interference with other cardiac structures. Since the CardioSEAL and STARFlex devices do not fill the atrial defect with material, the closure rate has been lower in some studies than that of the Amplatzer device, although a recent study from our hospital indicates that, in our experience, the closure rate from STARFlex for moderate sized (< 18 mm) defects is at least as good as the Amplatzer, with lower complications (Table 14-6). For these reasons, given the absence of late erosions and arrhythmias with the CardioSEAL and STARFlex, we have tended to use that device for small to moderate atrial defects, or multiply fenestrated defects, and have used the Amplatzer device for larger atrial defects, especially in older patients and adults.

TABLE 14–6. Rates of Closure and Severe Complications in Simple Atrial Septal Defects Comparing STARFlex and Amplatzer Devices and Surgery. (Courtesy of Dr. Alan Nugent)

	Closure Rate	Residual Shunt	Severe Complications
STARFlex™	98%	2%	0%
Amplatzer Septal Occluder (ref. 111)	99%	1%	1%
Surgery (ref. 111)	100%	0%	5%

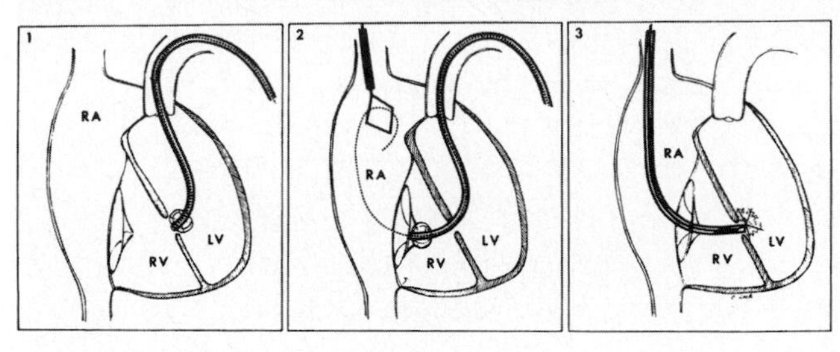

FIGURE 14–31 *Original technique for transcatheter closure of ventricular septal defects.*
From Fyler DC (ed). Nadas' Pediatric Cardiology, Philadelphia: Hanley & Belfus, 1992.

Transcatheter Closure of Patent Foramen Ovale

For the most part, patent foramen ovale closure has been used to prevent strokes in adult patients who are at risk for multiple neurologic events, or who have had more than one neurologic event associated with a patent foramen ovale.[115] The CardioSEAL was the first device approved for closure of patent foramen ovale and is the most widely used device in this country for this indication.[116] The technique is similar to that for closure of atrial septal defects, although, in general, foramen catheter closure is much more straightforward and easier than closure of atrial septal defects. Although a recent report[117] has suggested an increased incidence of clot formation in patients who have received CardioSEAL devices for closure of a patent foramen ovale, the authors in that study used an unusual technique of reversing heparinization at the end of the catheterization with Protamine, a technique which should probably be avoided whenever intracardiac devices are implanted. We have rarely (< 0.5%) encountered significant clots on CardioSEAL devices after foramen closure.

Transcatheter Closure of Ventricular Septal Defects

Catheter closure of muscular, post-operative, or fenestrated defects is now an accepted and standard practice at our institution,[118] with more than 200 defects having been successfully closed.[119] The technique is much more complicated than that for closure of atrial septal defects, and requires careful attention to vascular access, catheter course, and associated intracardiac structures. In general, the technique has become more standardized with time, and catheter approaches depend on the location of the defect. We try to cross ventricular septal defects from the left side of the heart to the right side using balloon tipped catheters and flow to go through the largest channel of the defect whenever possible, and then snare a guide wire in the right atrium or a pulmonary artery, producing a through-and-through vascular loop (Fig. 14-31) as described in the initial manuscript.[120] A 10F sheath is then advanced over the guide wire, presteamed if necessary to avoid kinking, to cross the ventricular septal defect. In general, it is safer to open the right ventricular arms first, and the left ventricular arms of the CardioSEAL device second. If the arms that are opened first are ensnared in myocardium near the defect, this is less important on the right side of the heart, whereas if the proximal arms are opened and become ensnared in myocardial tissue they can be stretched open while holding the device prior to release, by readvancing the sheath, and splaying the arms open on the left side of the septum. Once the device is in excellent location, it can be released. If more defects are present, two, three or four of them can be closed at the same catheterization, or one can oversize the device and *blanket* the left side of the septum.

Results

Although this is one of the more difficult and complex of the interventional catheter procedures, we successfully implanted 168 of 170 devices, with a significant decrease in flow in more than 90% of patients and, more importantly, improved clinical status in a similar percentage. Thus catheter closure of post-operative or muscular VSDs is now an approved procedure and, in most patients, is the procedure of choice at our hospital. We also use this technique to close fenestrated ventricular defect patches in patients with tetralogy of Fallot and restrictive pulmonary beds.[85] Recently, a muscular Amplatzer ventricular septal defect device has been used to close defects with the same principle as the Amplatzer atrial defect device.[120] We have no experience with this device. While the reported experience regarding closure status has been good, the clinical improvement associated with device implantation remains unreported.[121]

Catheter closure of perimembranous ventricular defects has recently been approached using a novel Amplatzer device which has an asymmetric disc on the left and right ventricular side, permitting the device to be positioned closer to the aortic and tricuspid valve than would be the case for any other ventricular defect closure devices.[122] Although the preliminary results have indicated that the incidence of complete heart block is higher than that for surgical procedures, the success rate has generally been good.

Transcatheter Closure of Miscellaneous Defects

Closure devices have now been used to close a variety of clinically significant vascular communications including coronary arteriovenous fistulae, paravalvar leaks, abnormal venous channels, pulmonary and systemic arteriovenous malformations, and other lesions. A complete description of each of these closure techniques is beyond the scope of this chapter, and is available elsewhere.[8] In general, each of these has proven to be clinically quite useful, with a favorable risk-benefit ratio for most patients at our institution. We are especially interested in catheter closure of paravalvar leaks,[123] with an encouraging experience in over 40 cases.

Transcatheter Implantation of Pulmonary Valves

Experimental work began more than a decade ago on using stent mounted valves to correct regurgitant lesions, especially in the pulmonary vascular bed, in children with congenital heart disease. The animal work has been done by Bonhoeffer and colleagues.[124] Although the preliminary work used extremely large catheter shafts, continuous refinement in tools and techniques has made this a much more feasible procedure in the last few years, with the first patient series being reported in 2002.[125] It is likely that a clinical trial of this device will begin in 2005. Although the indications for such a technique, and the late results remain unclear, a considerable amount of effort is likely to be spent in the next decade to make transcatheter pulmonary valve replacement a common procedure in the management of tetralogy of Fallot.

FETAL INTERVENTION

Serial fetal echocardiographic studies during pregnancy have documented progression of severe pulmonary and aortic valvar obstruction to atresia accompanied by growth failure of associated ventricular structures. In earlier years, results of attempts to dilate these in a small number during pregnancy have been somewhat disappointing.[126–129] In a revisit of this complex procedure, requiring simultaneous participation of multiple specialists, 20 fetuses with severe aortic obstruction underwent dilation at our institution.[130] It was noted that left heart structures grew following dilation and a third of the babies delivered alive have been two ventricle survivors.

REFERENCES

1. Hales S. Statical Essays Containing Haemastaticks West End of St. Paul's. London: W. Innys and R. Manby, 1733.
2. Forssman W. Die Sondierung des rechten Herzens. Klin Wschr 8:2085, 1929.
3. Cournand AF, Ranges HS. Catheterization of the right auricle in man. Proc Soc Ex Biol Med 46:42, 1941.
4. Brannon ES, Weens HS, Warren JV. Atrial septal defect: study of hemodynamics by the technique of right heart catheterization. Am J Med Sci 210;480, 1946.
5. Rubio-Alvarez V, Limon RL. Comisurotomia tricuspidea por medio e un cateter modificado. Arch Inst Cardiol Mexico 25:57, 1953.
6. Rubio-Alvarez V, Limon RL, Soni J. Valvulotomias intracardias pormedico de un cateter. Arch Inst Cardiol Mexico 23:183, 1953.
7. Rashkind WJ, Miller WW. Creation of an atrial septal defect without thoracotomy: A palliative approach to complete transposition of the great vessels. J Am Med Assoc 1996:991, 1966.
8. Lock JE, Keane JF, Perry SB (eds). Diagnostic and Interventional Catheterization in Congenital Heart Disease. Norwell, MA: Kluwer Academic Publishers, 2000.
9. Cohn HE, Freed MD, Hellenbrand WF, et al. Complications and mortality associated with cardiac catheterization in infants under one year: a prospective study. Pediatr Cardiol 6:123, 1985.
10. Stoermer J, Hentrich F, Galal D, et al. Risks der Herzkatheterisierung und angiokardiographic in sauglings und kindersalter. Klin Padiatr 196:191, 1984.
11. Keane JF, Fyler DC, Nadas AS. Hazards of cardiac catheterization in children with primary pulmonary vascular obstruction. Am Heart J 96:556, 1978.
12. Keane JF, Fellows KE, Lang P, et al. Pediatric arterial catheterization using a 3.2 French catheter. Cathet Cardiovasc Diagn 8:201, 1982.
13. Freed MD, Keane JF, Rosenthal A. The effect of heparinization to prevent arterial thrombosis after percutaneous cardiac catheterization in children. Circulation 50:565, 1974.
14. Wessel DL, Keane JF, Fellows KE, et al. Fibrinolytic therapy for femoral arterial thrombosis following cardiac catheterization in infants and children. Am J Cardiol 58:347, 1986.
15. Keane JF, Lang P, Newburger JW, et al. Iliac vein inferior caval thrombosis after cardiac catheterization in infancy. Pediatr Cardiol 1:257, 1980.
16. Beitzke A, Suppan C, Justich E. Complications in 1000 cardiac catheter examinations in childhood. Rontgenblatter 35:430, 1982.
17. Matthews RA, Park SC, Neches WH, et al. Iliac venous thrombosis in infants and children after cardiac catheterization. Cathet Cardiovasc Diagn 5:67, 1979.
18. Rudolph AM. Congenital Diseases of the Heart. Chicago: Year Book Medical Publishers, 1974, pp 49–167.

19. Freed MD, Miettinen OS, Nadas AS. Oxymetric detection of intracardiac left-to-right shunts. Br Heart J 42:690, 1979.
20. Gorlin R, Gorlin G. Hydraulic formula for calculation of stenotic mitral valves, and central circulatory shunts. Am Heart J 41:1, 1951.
21. Curry TS, Dowdy JE, Murry RC. Christensen's Introduction to the Physics of Diagnostic Radiology, 3rd ed. Philadelphia: Lea & Feigner, 1984.
22. Friesinger G, Adams DF, Bourassa MG, et al. Report of the Inter-society Commission for Heart Disease Resources. Optimal resources for examination of the heart and lungs: cardiac catheterization and radiographic facilities. Circulation 68:893a, 1983.
23. Levin D, Dunham L. Angiography: principles underlying proper utilization of radiologic and cineangiographic equipment. In Grossman W (ed). Cardiac Catheterization and Angiography, 2nd ed. Philadelphia: Lea & Febiger, 1980.
24. Moore RE. The Physics of Cardiac Angiography. Riverside, CA: Myrle, 1985.
25. Balter S, Sones FM, Brancato R. Radiation exposure to the operator performing cardiac angiography with U-arm systems. Circulation 58:925, 1978.
26. Leibovic SJ, Fellows KE. Patient radiation exposure during pediatric cardiac catheterization. Cardiovasc Intervent Radiol 6:150, 1983.
27. Miller SW, Castronove FP. Radiation exposure and protection in cardiac catheterization laboratories. Am J Cardiol 55:177, 1985.
28. Reuter FG. Physician and patient exposure during cardiac catheterization. Circulation 58:134, 1978.
29. Freeman LM, Blaufox MD (eds). Physicians' Desk Reference for Radiology and Nuclear Medicine 1979/1980. Oradell, NJ: Medical Economics, 1979.
30. Hall EJ. Radiation and Life, 2nd ed. New York: Pergamon Press, 1987.
31. Richman AH,Chen B, Katz M. Effectiveness of lead lenses in reducing radiation exposure. Radiology 121:357, 1976.
32. Shapiro J. Radiation Protection: A Guide for Scientists and Physicians. Cambridge, MA: Harvard University Press, 1972.
33. Almen T. Development of nonionic contrast media. Invest Radiol 20(suppl):2, 1985.
34. Swanson DP, Thrall JH, Shetty PC. Evaluation of intravascular low-osmolality contrast agents. Clin Pharm 5:877, 1986.
35. Dawson P. New contrast agents: chemistry and pharmacology. Invest Radiol 19(Suppl):293, 1985.
36. Fischer HW. Hemodynamic reactions to angiographic media; a survey and commentary. Radiology 91:66, 1968.
37. Friesinger G, Schaffer J, Cooley JM, et al. Hemodynamic consequences of the injection of radiopaque material. Circulation 31:730, 1965.
38. Iseri L, Kaplan A, Evans MJ, et al. Effect of concentrated contrast media during angiography on plasma volume and plasma osmolality. Am Heart J 69:154, 1965.
39. Sagy M, Aladjem M, Shem-Tov A, et al. The renal effect of radiocontrast administration during cardioangiography in two different groups with congenital heart disease. Eur J Pediatr 141:2336, 1984.
40. Dawson P. Chemotoxicity of contrast media and clinical adverse effects: a review. Invest Radiol 20(Suppl):84, 1985.
41. Hayward R, Dawson P. Contrast agents in angiocardiography. Br Heart J 52:361, 1984.
42. Anthony CL, Tonkin ILD, Marin-Garcia J, et al. A double-blind randomized clinical study of the safety, tolerability and efficacy of Hexabrix in pediatric angiocardiography. Invest Radiol 19 (Suppl):335, 1985.
43. McClennan BL. Low osmolality contrast media: premises and promises. Radiology 162:1, 1987.
44. Reagan K, Bettman MA, Finkelstein J, et al. Double-blind study of a new nonionic contrast agent for cardiac angiography. Radiology 167:409, 1988.
45. Wolf CL, Draft L, Kilzer K. Contrast agents lower ventricular fibrillation threshold. Radiology 129:215, 1978.
46. Shehadi WH. Adverse reactions to intravascularly administered contrast media: a comprehensive study based on a prospective survey. AJR 124:145, 1975.
47. Shehadi WH. Contrast media adverse reactions. Occurrence, recurrence and distribution patterns. Radiology 43:11, 1982.
48. Lasser EC. A coherent biochemical basis for increased reactivity to contrast material in allergic patients: a novel concept. AJR 149:1281, 1987.
49. Bargeron LM, Elliot LP, Soto B, et al. Axial cineangiography in congenital heart disease, I: Concept, technical and anatomic considerations. Circulation 56:1075, 1977.
50. Elliot LP, Bargeron LM, Bream PR, et al. Axial cineangiography in congenital heart disease, II: Specific lesions. Circulation 56:1084, 1977.
51. Fellows KE, Keane JF, Freed MD. Angled views in cineangiography of congenital heart disease. Circulation 56:484, 1977.
52. Soto B, Coghlan CH, Bargeron LM. Present status of axially angled angiocardiography. Cardiovasc Intervent Radiol 7: 154, 1984.
53. Lurie PR, Fujita M, Neustein HB. Transvascular endomyocardial biopsy in infants and children: description of a new technique. Am J Cardiol 42:453, 1978.
54. Pophal SG, Sigfusson G, Booth KL, et al. Complications of endomyocardial biopsy in children. J Am Coll Cardiol 34 (7):2105, 1999
55. Kan JS, White RI, Mitchell SE, et al. Percutaneous balloon valvuloplasty: a new method for treating congenital pulmonary valve stenosis. N Engl J Med 307:540, 1982.
56. Lababidi ZA, Wu JR. Percutaneous pulmonary valvuloplasty. Am J Cardiol 52:560, 1983.
57. Radtke W, Keane JF, Fellows KE, et al. Percutaneous balloon valvotomy of congenital pulmonary stenosis using oversized balloons. J Am Coll Cardiol 8:909, 1986.
58. Colli AM, Perry SB, Lock, JE, et al. Balloon dilation of critical valvar pulmonary stenosis in the first month of life. Cath Cardiovasc Diag 34:23, 1995.
59. Yeager SB. Balloon selection for double balloon valvotomy. J Am Coll Cardiol 9:467, 1987.
60. Giglia TM, Mandell VS, Connor AR, et al. Diagnosis and management of right ventricular dependent coronary circulation in pulmonary atresia with intact ventricular septum. Circulation 86 (5):1516, 1992.

61. Agnoletti G, Piechaud JF, Bonhoeffer P, et al. Perforation of the atretic pulmonary valve. Long term follow up. J Am Coll Cardiol 41:1339, 2003
62. Lababidi Z, Wu J, Wallis JT. Percutaneous balloon aortic valvuloplasty: results in 23 patients. Am J Cardiol 53:194, 1984.
63. Cribier A, Savin T, Berland J, et al. Percutaneous transluminal balloon valvuloplasty of adult aortic stenosis: report of 92 cases. J Am Coll Cardiol 9:381, 1987.
64. Helgason H, Keane JF, Fellows KE, et al. Balloon dilation of the aortic valve: studies in normal lambs and in children with aortic stenosis. J Am Coll Cardiol 9:816, 1987.
65. McKay RG, Safian RD, Lock JE, et al. Balloon dilation of calcific aortic stenosis in elderly patients: postmortem, intraoperative and percutaneous valvuloplasty studies. Circulation 74:119, 1986.
66. Rupprath G, Neuhaus KL. Percutaneous balloon aortic valvuloplasty in infancy and childhood. Am J Cardiol 55:1855, 1985.
67. Waller BF, Girod DA, Dillon JC. Transverse aortic wall tears in infants after balloon angioplasty for aortic valve stenosis. J Am Coll Cardiol 4:1235, 1984.
68. Sholler GF, Keane, JF, Perry SB, et al. Balloon dilation of congenital aortic stenosis: results and influence of technical and morphologic features on outcome. Circulation 78:351, 1988.
69. Egito E, Moore P, O'Sullivan J, et al. Transvascular balloon dilation for neonatal critical aortic stenosis: Early and late results. J Am Coll Cardiol 29 (2):442, 1997.
70. Moore P, Egito E, Mowrey H, et al. Mid term results of balloon dilation of congenital aortic stenosis: Predictors of success. J Am Coll Cardiol 27 (5):1257, 1996.
71. DeLezo JS, Pan M, Sancho M, et al. Percutaneous transluminal balloon dilation for discrete subaortic stenosis. Am J Cardiol 58:619, 1986.
72. Lock JE, Khalilullah M, Shrivastava S, et al. Percutaneous catheter commissurotomy in rheumatic mitral stenosis. N Eng J Med 313:1519, 1985.
73. Kveselis DA, Rocchini AP, Beekman R, et al. Balloon angioplasty for congenital mitral stenosis. J Am Coll Cardiol 57:348, 1986.
74. Spevak PJ, Bass JL, Ben-Shachar G, et al. Balloon angioplasty for non-rheumatic mitral stenosis in children. Am J Cardiol 66:472, 1990.
75. Moore P, Adatia I, Spevak PJ, et al. Severe congenital mitral stenosis in infants. Circulation 89:2099, 1994.
76. Lloyd TR, Marvin WJ Jr, Mahoney LT, et al. Balloon dilation valvuloplasty of bioprosthetic valves in extracardiac conduits. Am Heart J 114:268, 1987.
77. Lock JE, Niemi T, Einzig S, et al. Transvenous angioplasty of experimental branch pulmonary artery stenosis in newborn lambs. Circulation 64:886, 1981.
78. Lock JE, Castaneda-Zuniga WR, Fuhrman BP, et al. Balloon dilation angioplasty of hypoplastic and stenotic pulmonary arteries. Circulation 67:962, 1983.
79. Gentles T, Lock JE, Perry S. High pressure balloon angioplasty for branch pulmonary artery stenosis: Early experience. J Am Coll Cardiol 22:867, 1993.
80. Geggel RL, Gauvreau K, Lock JE. Balloon dilation angioplasty of peripheral pulmonary stenosis associated with Williams syndrome. Circulation 103:2165, 2001.
81. Baker CM, McGowan FX, Keane JF, et al. Pulmonary artery truma due to balloon dilation: Recognition, avoidance and management. J Am Coll Cardiol 36:1684, 2000.
82. Rhodes J, Lane G, Mesia F, et al. Cutting balloon angioplasty for children with small vessel pulmonary artery stenoses. Cath Cardiovasc Diag 55:73, 2002.
83. Bergersen LJ, Perry SB, Lock JE. Effect of cutting balloon angioplasty on resistant pulmonary artery stenois. Am J Cardiol 91:185, 2003.
84. Rome JJ, Mayer JE, Castaneda AR, et al. Tetralogy of Fallot with pulmonary atresia: Rehabilitation of diminutive pulmonary arteries. Circulation 88(4):1691, 1993.
85. Marshall AC, Love BA, Lang P, et al. Staged repair of tetralogy of Fallot and diminutive pulmonary arteries using a fenestrated ventricular septal defect patch. J Thorac Cardiovasc Surg 126:1427, 2003.
86. Lock JE, Bass JL, Amplatz K, et al. Balloon dilation angioplasty of coarctations in infants and children. Circulation 68:109, 1983.
87. Lock JE, Niemi T, Burke BA, et al. Transcatheter angioplasty of experimental aortic coarctation. Circulation 66:1280, 1982.
88. Marvin WJ, Mahoney LT, Rose EF. Pathologic sequelae of balloon dilatation angioplasty for unoperated coarctation of the aorta in children (abstract). J Am Coll Cardiol 7:117A, 1986.
89. Ovaert C, McCrindle BW, Nykanen, D, et al. Balloon angioplasty of native coarctation: Clinical outcomes and predictors of success. J Am Coll Cardiol 35:988, 2000.
90. Shaddy RE, Boucek MM, Sturtevant JE, et al. Comparison of angioplasty and surgery for unoperated coarctation of the aorta. Circulation 87 (3):793, 1993
91. Saul JP, Keane JF, Fellows KE, et al. Balloon dilation angioplasty of postoperative aortic obstructions. Am J Cardiol 59:943, 1987.
92. Lock JE, Bass JL, Castaneda-Zuniga W, et al. Dilation angioplasty of congenital or operative narrowings of venous channels. Circulation 70:457, 1984.
93. Mendelsohn MD, Bove EL, Lupinetti FM, et al. Intraoperative and percutaneous stenting of congenital pulmonary artery and vein stenosis. Circulation 88:210, 1993.
94. O'Laughlin MP, Perry SB, Lock JE, et al. Use of endovascular stents in congenital heart disease. Circulation 83:1923, 1991.
95. O'Laughlin MP, Slack MC, Grifka, RG, et al. Implantation and intermediate-term follow-up of stents in congenital heart disease. Circulation 88:605, 1993.
96. Fogelman R, Nykanen D, Smallhorn JF, et al. Endovascular stents in the pulmonary circulation. Clinical impact on management and medium term follow-up. Circulation 92:881, 1995.
97. Rothman A, Perry SB, Keane JF, et al. Early results and follow-up of balloon angioplasty for branch pulmonary artery stents. J Am Coll Cardiol 15:1109, 1990.

98. Marshall AC, Perry SB, Keane JF, et al. Early results and medium term follow up of stent implantation for mild residual or recurrent aortic coarctation. Am Heart J 139:1054, 2000.
99. Powell AJ, Lock JE, Keane JF, et al. Prolongation of RV-PA conduit life span by percutaneous stent implantation: Intermediate term results. Circulation 92 (11):3282, 1995.
100. Vlahos AP, Lock JE, McElhinney DB, et al. Hypoplastic left heart syndrome with intact or highly restrictive atrial septum. Circulation 109:2326, 2004.
101. Siwik ES, Perry SB, Lock JE. Endovascular stent implantation in patients with stenotic aorto-arteropathies: Early and medium term results. Cath Cardiovasc Intervent 59:380, 2003.
102. Fuhrman BP, Bass JL, Castaneda-Zuniga W, et al. Coil embolization of congenital thoracic vascular anomalies in infants and children. Circulation 70:285, 1984.
103. Perry SB, Radtke W, Fellows KE, et al. Coil embolization to occlude aortopulmonary collaterals and shunts in patients with congenital heart disease. J Am Coll Cardiol 13:100, 1989.
104. Armsby LR, Keane JF, Sherwood MC, et al. Management of coronary artery fistulae: Patient selection and results of transcatheter closure. J Am Coll Cardiol 39:1026, 2002.
105. Portsmann W, Wierny L, Warnke H, et al. Catheter closure of patent ductus arteriosus: 62 cases treated without thoracotomy. Radiol Clin North Am 9:203, 1971.
106. Rashkind WJ, Mullins CE, Hellenbrand WE, et al. Nonsurgical closure of patent ductus arteriosus: clinical application of the Rashkind PDA occluder system. Circulation 75:583, 1987.
107. Moore JW, GeorgeI, Kirkpatrick SE, et al. Percutaneous closure of the small patent ductus arteriosus using occluding spring coils. J Am Coll Cardiol 23:759, 1994.
108. Bilkis AA, Alwi M, Hasri S, et al. The Amplatzer duct occluder: Experience in 209 patients. J Am Coll Cardiol 37:258, 2001.
109. King TD, Mills NL. Secundum atrial septal defect: nonoperative closure during cardiac catheterization. JAMA 235:2506, 1976.
110. Masura J, Gavora P, Formanek A, et al. Transcatheter closure of secundum atrial septal defects usign the new self-centering Amplatzer septal occluder: Initial human experience. Cath & Cardiovasc Diag 42:388, 1997
111. Zhong-Dong D, Hijazi ZM, Kleinman CS, et al. Comparison between transcatheter and surgical closure of secundum atrial septal defect in children and adults. J Am Coll Cardiol 39:1836, 2002.
112. Hill SL, Berul CI, Patel HT, et al. Early ECG abnormalities associated with transcatheter closure of atrial septal defects using the Amplatzer septal occluder. J Inervent Cardiac Electrophysiology. 4:469, 2000.
113. Amin Z, Hijazi ZM, Bass JL, et al. Erosion of Amplatzer septal occluder after closure of secundum atrial septal defects. Review of registry of complications and recommendations to minimize future risk. Cath & Cardiovasc Intervent. 63(4): 496, 2004.
114. Divekar A, Gaamargwe T, Shaihk N, et al. Cardiac perforation after device closure of atrial septal defects with the Amplatzer septal occluder. J Am Coll Cardiol 45:1213, 2005.
115. Bridges ND, Hellenbrand W, Latson L, et al. Transcatheter closure of patent foramen ovale after presumed paradoxical embolism. Circulation 86:1902, 1992.
116. Hung J, Landzberg MJ, Jenkins KJ, et al. Closure of patent foramen ovale for paradoxical emboli: Intermediate-term risk of recurrent neurological events following transcatheter device placement. J Am Coll Cardiol 35(5):1311, 2000.
117. Krumsdorf U, Ostermayer S, Billinger K, et al. Incidence and clinical course of thrombus formation on atrial defect and patent foramen ovale clousre devices in 1,000 consecutive patients. J Am Coll Cardiol Jan 21;43(2):302, 2004.
118. Lock JE, Block PC, McKay RG, et al. Transcatheter closure of ventricular septal defects. Circulation 78:361, 1988.
119. Knauth AL, Lock JE, Perry SB, et al. Transcatheter device closure of congenital and post-operative residual ventricular septal defects. Circuation 110:501, 2004.
120. Amin Z, Gu X, Berry JM, et al. New device for closure of muscular ventricular septal defects in canine model. Circulation 100:320, 1999.
121. Holzer R, Balzer D, Cao QL, et al. Device closure of ventricular septal defects using the Amplatzer muscular ventricular septal defect occluder: immediate and mid-term results of a U.S. registry. J Am Coll Cardiol 43: 2004.
122. Hijazi ZM, Hakim F, Haweleh AA, et al. Catheter closure of perimembranous ventricular septal defects using the new Amplatzer membranous VSD occluder: initial clinical experience. Catheter Cardiovasc Interv 56:508, 2002.
123. Hourihan MB, Perry SB, Mandell VS, et al. Transcatheter umbrella closure of valvular and paravalvular leaks. J Am Coll Cardiol 20:1371, 1992.
124. Bonhoeffer P, Boudjemline Y, Saliba Z, et al. Transcatheter implantation of a bovine valve in pulmonary position: a lamb study. Circulation 102:813, 2000.
125. Bonhoeffer P, Boudjemline Y, Qureshi SA, et al. Percutaneous insertion of the pulmonary valve. J Am Coll Cardiol 39:1664, 2002.
126. Tulzer G, Arzt W, Franklin CG, et al. Fetal pulmonary valvuloplasty for critical pulmonary stenosis or atresia with intact septum. Lancet 360:1567, 2002.
127. Maxwell D, Allan L, Tynan MJ: Balloon dilatation of the aortic valve in the fetus: a report of two cases. Br Heart J 65:236, 1991.
128. Lopes LM, Cha SC, Kajita LJ, et al. Balloon dilatation of the aortic valve in the fetus: a case report. Fetal Diagn Ther 11:296, 1996.
129. Kohl T, Sharland G, Allan LD, et al. World experience of percutaneous ultrasound-guided valvuloplasty in human fetuses with severe aortic valve obstruction. Am J Cardiol 85:1230, 2000.
130. Tworetzky W, Wilkins-Haug L, Jennings RW, et al. Balloon dilation of severe aortic stenosis in the fetus. Circulation 110:2125, 2004.

15

Assessment of Ventricular and Myocardial Performance

STEVEN D. COLAN

The field of pediatric cardiology has undergone a fundamental transition over the past 25 years wherein myocardial function has moved from a secondary to a primary issue for most forms of heart disease diagnosed during childhood. This transformation, which is attributable to the dramatically improved outlook for these diseases, has been engendered by improvements in diagnostics, interventional catheterization, surgery, anesthesia, and postoperative care. This success has resulted is a sharp increase in survival and therefore in the prevalence of postoperative childhood heart disease. An unanticipated consequence has been the creation of a cohort for whom the health of myocardium has now become the principle determinant of their long-term clinical management, quality of life, and survival. Despite the importance of this aspect of cardiovascular care and the large number of diagnostic modalities that are available to evaluate ventricular function, the available tools remain suboptimal. Congenital heart disease remains one of the most challenging areas for the evaluation of ventricular performance because of complicating factors such as (a) age- and size-related changes in myocardial and vascular performance, (b) the nearly universal presence of abnormal volume and/or pressure loads in structural heart disease, (c) high prevalence of ventricular morphologies that do not lend themselves to standard geometric models, and (d) technical issues related to the increased risk and difficulty in obtaining invasive data from these patients, the need for sedation in small children, and the limited ability of infants and children to cooperate. The intent of this discussion is to review the general issues related to the assessment of myocardial contractility and loading conditions and to focus attention on those aspects of particular importance to the field of congenital heart disease. The data that are used to evaluate ventricular and myocardial function include measurements of pressure, flow, volume, and fiber shortening, each of which can be obtained using an ever-expanding and improving battery of techniques that includes catheterization, echocardiography, magnetic resonance, radionuclide imaging, positron emission tomography, and computed tomography. The technical aspects of data acquisition and methods of measurement for the various techniques are discussed in detail elsewhere and will not be repeated here. Rather, the physiologic basis for the analysis and interpretation of the data will be emphasized, independent of the particular method by which elemental data are acquired.

CARDIAC VERSUS MYOCARDIAL FUNCTION

The heart may be viewed as a pump designed to move blood from a low-pressure venous reservoir to the high-pressure arterial tree. From this perspective, cardiac function can be considered normal as long as adequate flow rates at acceptable venous and arterial pressures are maintained. This can be likened to a *black box* approach, wherein the external performance of a pump is examined with no attention to the internal workings of the machine. This is the approach taken by the dependent organ systems, which exert control over the cardiovascular system through autonomic and hormonal systems that respond to changes in pressure and flow, but have no *sensor* that directly reflects the state of the myocardium. The success of this approach is attested to by the common practice of monitoring arterial and venous pressures and cardiac output in the postoperative intensive care unit. Unfortunately, the view of the heart as a pump provides very limited information about the status of the myocardium. For example, it is commonly observed that relatively severe myocardial dysfunction may coexist with normal arterial and venous pressures and normal cardiac output. Evaluation of the health of the myocardium requires of myocardial function rather than cardiac function, an approach that has been described as viewing the heart as a muscle. From this point of view, the function of the myocardium is to variably lengthen and shorten against a load. This can be effectively divided into diastole, during which the muscle must attain a certain length by the application of a physiologically tolerable force, and systole, during which an adequate magnitude of shortening and force generation is required. The assessment of these two phases of the cardiac cycle will be considered individually, although the intimate relationship between systolic and diastolic performance makes their separate consideration somewhat artificial.

ASSESSMENT OF SYSTOLIC PERFORMANCE

Despite advances in the understanding of myocardial mechanics and the recognized limitations of the technique, ejection fraction and shortening fraction remain the most common clinical methods of assessing systolic function. Both are calculated in a similar fashion. Ejection fraction represents the fraction of blood expelled with each beat, and is calculated from end-diastolic volume (EDV) and end-systolic volume (ESV) as (EDV – ESV)/EDV. Shortening fraction is similarly calculated from end-diastolic dimension (EDD) and end-systolic dimension (ESD) as (EDD – ESD)/EDD. Although used less commonly, it is also possible to calculate the fractional area change from end-diastolic cross-sectional area (EDA) and end-systolic cross-sectional area (ESA) as (EDA – ESA)/EDA. At the myocardial level, systolic function is represented by the magnitude of systolic shortening of the individual myofibers, and each of these indices provides an estimate of the percent of systolic fiber shortening (the absolute amount of systolic fiber shortening normalized for the end-diastolic fiber length). Percent of shortening is a global descriptor of pump performance that incorporates arterioventricular and venoventricular interactions as well as the inotropic state and, as such, has become firmly entrenched as a clinically useful tool. Although it has long been understood that the magnitude of shortening is the final product of a complex interplay of factors, which include vascular and hormonal influences, cardiac hypertrophy and geometry, and myocardial function,[1–4] it is common clinical practice to equate the percent of shortening with myocardial contractility. Among the factors that account for this simplification is the clinical observation that depressed contractility is a common cause of reduced fiber shortening. However, reduced fiber shortening sufficiently severe to cause congestive heart failure may be present despite normal contractility[5] and, conversely, normal fiber shortening may be present despite abnormal contractility, although these situations are less common. Hence, for most patients, use of more complex methods of evaluating ventricular performance that have the capacity to quantify contractility may appear to be unnecessary. Unfortunately, it is clear that assessment of shortening alone fails to accurately reflect the contractile state of the myocardium in all subjects because of the additional effects of preload and afterload on the process of fiber shortening and these limitations can only be detected through the use of load-independent techniques.

Endocardial, Mid-Wall, and Global Fiber Shortening. Ejection fraction, fractional area change, and shortening fraction are calculated as the fractional change in chamber volume, endocardial area, and endocardial diameter, respectively. Each provides an estimate of endocardial fiber shortening, that is, the shortening of myofibers lying on the endocardial surface. The clinical practice of relying on endocardial indices is based on a number of factors. The endocardium demarcates ventricular volume, and therefore stroke volume and cardiac output, which are indices of considerable importance for evaluating pump function. Endocardial indices can be calculated from contrast and radionuclide angiography, but epicardial borders cannot. Although endocardial indices are appropriate for evaluation of pump function, they do not adequately measure global fiber shortening. Geometrically, the circumferentially oriented myofibers closer to the endocardial surface shorten the furthest, with progressively lower magnitude shortening through the wall to the level of the epicardium. Endocardial indices would provide a reasonable surrogate for global fiber shortening if there was a constant relationship between the two, but the magnitude of misrepresentation varies as a function of the thickness-to-dimension ratio and the absolute endocardial shortening fraction.[6]

Global average fiber shortening can be estimated by several methods. Mid-wall fiber shortening can be calculated directly based on geometric considerations. The position of a myofiber positioned halfway between the endocardium and the epicardium is tracked to its position at end-systole as it moves closer to the epicardium over the course of systole, and from these calculated mid-wall diameters, the mid-wall circumferential fiber shortening is calculated.[7–9] Because of the nonlinear fall in fiber shortening across the ventricular wall, this method underestimates average circumferential transmural fiber shortening by 1% to 5% and fails to account for longitudinal fiber shortening.

Endocardial and epicardial surface rendering from three-dimensional echocardiographic or magnetic resonance imaging data can be used to geometrically estimate global average fiber shortening, although this method is not commercially available. Magnetic resonance–based myocardial tissue tagging techniques provide data concerning regional and global myofiber shortening,[10,11] but these techniques are not widely available.

Reliance on endocardial indices of fiber shortening has been found to result in clinically important overestimation of fiber shortening in patients with left ventricular hypertrophy.[6,12] This has resulted in underdiagnosis of myocardial dysfunction in patients with left ventricular hypertrophy[8,13] and misrepresentation of cardiac mechanics in patients with congenital aortic stenosis and postoperative coarctation of the aorta. Because the magnitude of misrepresentation relates directly to the thickness-to-dimension ratio, this issue is less important in conditions characterized by relatively thin-walled ventricles, such as dilated cardiomyopathy.

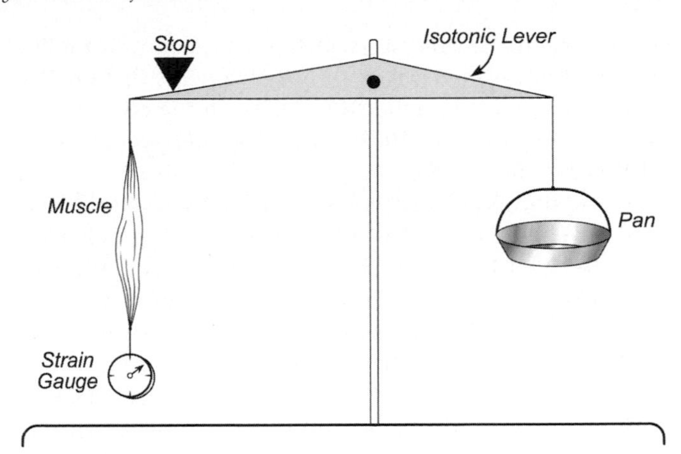

FIGURE 15–1 *Illustration of an isolated cardiac muscle apparatus. The strip of muscle is attached at one end to a movable lever and is fixed at the other end to a force transducer that records the strength and speed of contraction. The movable lever monitors muscle length and transmits force due to weights added to a pan on the opposite end of the lever. Weight is added to the pan to stretch the muscle to the desired end-diastolic length, following which a stop is placed to prevent further lengthening. Because the muscle is exposed to this weight prior to contraction, it is known as "preload." Further weight can then be added to the pan but because of the mechanical stop mechanism, the muscle is not exposed to this force until contraction ensues, and this is therefore known as "afterload." The total weight in the pan represents the force resisting shortening.*
From Fyler DC [ed.]. Nadas' Pediatric Cardiology. Philadelphia: Hanley & Belfus, 1992.

Factors Influencing Fiber Shortening

Frequently, the terms *afterload, preload*, and *contractility* are used in a conceptual rather than specific meaning. These terms were introduced on the basis of studies of isolated cardiac muscle and their meaning to the physiology of the intact heart can only be understood in this frame of reference. Much of our understanding of cardiac muscle physiology derives from studies performed using isolated strips of cardiac muscle in a setup similar to that illustrated in Figure 15-1, and this body of work has been reviewed in detail by Braunwald and Ross.[4] The isolated muscle preparation has generated a wealth of information. Reproducible relationships between the speed, strength, and degree of shortening and the loading conditions (afterload and preload) can be obtained using this system. The responses to changes in afterload and/or preload are considered to represent external factors, whereas effects not ascribable to altered load are assumed to reflect intrinsic properties of the muscle, which are subsumed under the label *contractility*. This very useful working definition must be modified to accommodate experimental observations which indicate that loading status and contractility are not entirely independent factors, as is discussed subsequently.

Preload

In the isolated muscle, preload refers to the force needed to attain the desired precontraction length. Increasing this length while other conditions (afterload and contractility) are held constant results in increased total shortening, increased peak generated force, and higher peak velocity of shortening, properties known as the Frank-Starling relationship due to the seminal work on this phenomenon performed by Otto Frank and E. H. Starling. At the molecular level, the sliding-filament model of contraction predicts the preload effect on the basis of a length-dependent variation in the number of interacting cross bridges between contractile proteins.[14] Accordingly, an increase in end-diastolic fiber length (EDFL) alters the degree of myofilament overlap and proportionally increases the extent of shortening. Although, due to its origins, the concept of a force is intrinsic to the word preload, at the fiber level, preload is best represented by EDFL. Although the normally compliant muscle has a predictable force-length relationship, many pathologic processes disrupt this relationship, and therefore EDFL is the only reliable index of preload.

Length-Dependent Activation. It should be noted that experiments in isolated hearts have shown that changes in sarcomere length cannot fully account for the preload effect.[15] If the preload effect was entirely related to the mechanical consequence of an increase in fiber length, the change in shortening should be precisely proportional to the increase in end-diastolic fiber length. In fact, the increase in shortening is in excess of what is anticipated, a phenomenon ("length-dependent activation") that appears secondary to enhanced excitation-contraction coupling at longer muscle lengths.[16,17] Thus, it appears that preload modulates the contractile state, although the contribution is small compared with the contractility-independent effects of a change in EDFL.

At the fiber level, preload is best represented by EDFL, but extrapolation to the intact ventricle is problematic because EDFL cannot be directly measured. Although preload in the intact ventricle is often estimated by parameters such as end-diastolic pressure, volume, or wall stress, each of these fails as a true representation of fiber length under certain conditions. Under normal circumstances, a rise in end-diastolic pressure results in greater EDFL. If there are external constraints (e.g., pericardial effusion or constriction or restrictive cardiomyopathy), this pressure–length relationship will be disturbed. Perhaps more problematic is the variability of pressure-volume relationships (that is, chamber compliance), making pressure an unreliable parameter for comparing preload among patients. Although atrial filling pressures are usually monitored in the postoperative period, in part as a measure of preload status, it is particularly under these circumstances that pressure may not accurately reflect EDFL because of (a) altered myocardial compliance after cardiopulmonary bypass, (b) abnormal external constraint (mechanical ventilation, mediastinal edema, pericardial effusion), or (c) increased ventricular interaction due to elevation in right ventricular pressure (reactive pulmonary hypertension).

End-diastolic volume more directly reflects EDFL over the short term, but the ability of the ventricle to remodel and add fibers in series prevents this from being a useful index for comparisons between patients or for longitudinal assessment over more than a few days. End-diastolic stress provides a measure of the force distending the ventricle, but provides an accurate estimate of EDFL only when myocardial compliance is normal. Numerous conditions are known to invalidate this assumption (ischemia, fibrosis, drug therapy, effects of cardiopulmonary bypass). Thus, each of these indices fails as an adequate measure of preload. Because EDFL cannot be directly measured *in vivo*, some alternative approach must be taken. An approach based on analysis of the stress-shortening and stress-velocity relationships, which will be presented in more detail subsequently, relies on measuring the functional consequences of the existing preload conditions. In brief, because the magnitude of shortening depends on afterload, preload, and contractility, if afterload, contractility, and shortening can be directly measured, then preload can be calculated. Stated more intuitively, if the degree of shortening can be adjusted for the other factors that influence the contraction process, then the adjusted shortening will directly represent the EDFL, or preload.

Afterload

In the isolated muscle preparation, afterload refers to the weight or load that is faced by the contracting muscle, that is, the force resisting shortening. Clinically, arterial pressure, resistance, and impedance are often used as measures of afterload, but these parameters fail to account for the geometric relationship between sarcomere shortening and force generation.[18] In the isolated muscle preparation, force is exerted in a linear fashion. However, the muscle fiber embedded in the ventricular wall shortens tangentially and generates a force directed toward the cavity, creating significant complexity in the estimation of the forces in the wall and at the fiber level. Based on the Laplace relationship, it is possible to calculate the relationship between wall tension (T), pressure (P), and the radius of curvature (R) for thin-walled circular chambers where $T = P \times R$ (Fig. 15-2). Because there are multiple fibers across the ventricular wall and the force on each fiber is of interest, the force must be adjusted for wall thickness (h) by calculating wall stress (force per unit area) as stress = $T/h = (P \times R)/h$. This, of course, is a mathematic simplification, because the radius of curvature of the inner wall in a thick-walled vessel is different from that of the outer wall. Therefore, it is customary to use midwall radius and to calculate the stress as a mean transmural value.

The heart is also nonspherical, so the radius of curvature is not uniform and, in fact, is different in the short-axis (circumferential) and long-axis (meridional) directions even in the normal heart. It is not believed to be possible to directly measure ventricular wall stress,[19] although interesting

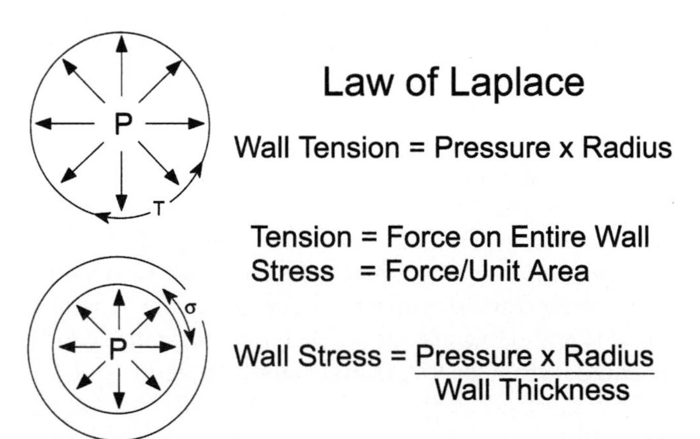

FIGURE 15–2 *The Laplace relationship describes the relationship between the radius of curvature, transmural pressure, and wall tension. Division of tension by wall thickness provides a measure of the force per unit of cross sectional area.*
From Fyler DC [ed.]. Nadas' Pediatric Cardiology. Philadelphia: Hanley & Belfus, 1992.

possible methods have been reported.[20] As a consequence, the correct method of calculating wall stress remains controversial. Certain geometric assumptions are necessary before a representative value for meridional and circumferential stress can be estimated, and several formulas have been proposed. Although quantitatively dissimilar, yielding different absolute values for wall stress, the relative values obtained with these methods are comparable.[21] Thus, it appears to be of greater importance to consider the assumptions made in the derivation rather than the exact formula that is used. In each instance, the primary data from which these calculations are performed are the transmural pressure, the radius of curvature of the wall, and wall thickness. The radius and thickness data can be obtained from any of several modalities, including cineangiographic or radionuclide ventriculograms, echocardiograms, or magnetic resonance imaging. Similarly, pressure data can be obtained from invasive or noninvasive means. Noninvasive aortic pressure can be obtained by recording indirect carotid (or axillary in young children) pulse waveforms calibrated with peripheral blood pressure.[22–24] If arterial pressure is not representative of left ventricular pressure because of aortic stenosis, end-systolic pressures in the aorta and left ventricle are still equal and, therefore, end-systolic stress can still be calculated.[25] In addition, Doppler measurement in the ascending aorta can be used to calculate the instantaneous transvalvar pressure gradient, which, when added to aortic pressure, equals left ventricular pressure.[26] Thus, even in the presence of aortic stenosis it is possible to calculate wall stress throughout systole.

Of course, there are alternative approaches to assessing afterload. In particular, if one is interested in characterizing the pump performance of the heart, the arterial impedance (that is, the force resisting ejection) provides more meaningful information.[27] However, recognizing that it may seem rather counterintuitive to characterize afterload in terms of measurements performed on the ventricle itself, it is worthwhile emphasizing that the intent is to quantify the factors that control myocardial performance, and hence we are interested in determining the afterload faced by the myofibrils rather than the ventricle as a whole. For the myocardium, it is the force opposing shortening within the wall which is the most direct measure of afterload. Although factors external to the heart (vascular resistance, capacitance, compliance, etc.) affect ventricular performance secondarily, but the means by which they affect myocardial performance is through their influence on wall stress.[18]

The transition from afterload as a constant weight in the isolated muscle preparation to afterload as wall stress in the intact ventricle introduces another level of complexity to the analysis, because wall stress is not constant during the course of the cardiac cycle. As shown in Figure 15-3, with the rise and fall of ventricular pressure, the decrease in ventricular dimension, and the increase in wall thickness during the contraction phase, wall stress rises rapidly to a peak value in early ejection, falls in a near-linear fashion to the end of ejection, and then drops more rapidly to diastolic levels. The cyclic variation in wall stress raises the issue as to which phase of the process of stress development and decay is the most important determinant of fiber shortening. Various investigators have used peak, mean, total systolic (stress-time integral) and end-systolic stress as indices of afterload. Each of these components has a different physiologic significance, and the appropriate index of afterload depends on the question that is to be addressed. That is, because myocardial oxygen consumption correlates more closely with total stress (stress-time integral) than with other stress indices,[28,29] this is the appropriate index when using wall stress to predict myocardial substrate utilization. Similarly, peak wall stress correlates most closely with the magnitude of hypertrophy[25,30–33] and, thus, is the appropriate stress index when assessing a stimulus to hypertrophy or the adequacy of hypertrophy. However, the measure of afterload that relates most closely to systolic performance is the stress at end-systole. That is, end-systolic stress is the force that determines the extent of systolic shortening and is the index of afterload that is most relevant to the assessment of ventricular function. Because this is by no means intuitively obvious, and because alternative measures of afterload are frequently used in assessing ventricular performance, it is worthwhile to review the evidence that this is

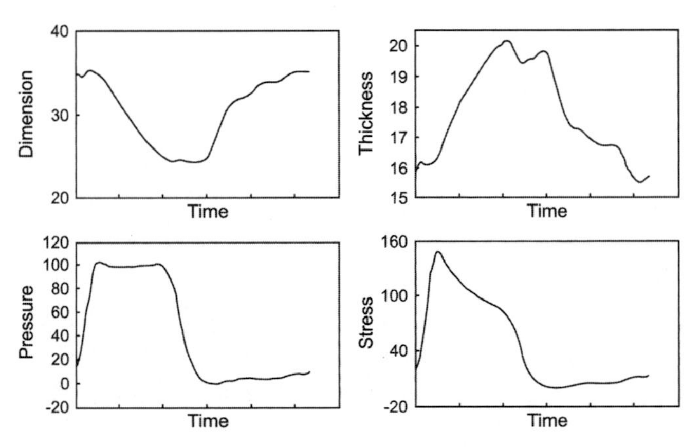

FIGURE 15–3 *With the rise and fall of ventricular pressure, the fall in ventricular dimension, and the rise in wall thickness during the contraction phase, wall stress rises rapidly to a peak value in early ejection, falls in a near-linear fashion to end-ejection, and then drops more rapidly to diastolic levels.*
From Fyler DC [ed.]. Nadas' Pediatric Cardiology. Philadelphia: Hanley & Belfus, 1992.

in fact the case. A series of observations in isolated muscle preparations and whole ventricles have revealed several fundamental properties of cardiac muscle that are relevant to this discussion.

Based on work in isolated cardiac muscle preparations and isolated hearts, the fundamental observation is that end-systolic stress determines end-systolic length at a constant contractile state. When the isolated cardiac muscle is allowed to shorten isotonically (Fig. 15-4) or shortens against a variable load from a fixed end-diastolic length (Fig. 15-5), a linear end-systolic force-length relation is observed regardless of the end-diastolic length.[34,35] Equivalent relationships are present in the intact ventricle, where a linear end-systolic stress-volume or pressure-volume relation is found in both isovolumic and ejecting ventricles.[36] Conceptually, the myocardium continues to contract until the critical force-length relation is encountered, at which time relaxation ensues. The force–length relation is relatively independent of the events earlier in the cardiac cycle (the ejection force–length trajectory), or, in other words, it is relatively history independent.[37] The limitations on this history-independence will be discussed later, but within the confines of these limits, end-systolic force is the determinant of end-systolic length for any constant contractile state.

Wall stress at all phases of systole except end-systole can be altered without associated change in net myocardial shortening. When isolated heart preparations are held at a fixed end-systolic and end-diastolic volume (therefore, by necessity, end-systolic and end-diastolic wall thicknesses are constant also), the ejection conditions can be varied widely and the same end-systolic pressure will be attained (Fig. 15-6).[37] Thus, a constant magnitude of fiber shortening is observed as long as end-systolic wall stress is constant, even though peak and mean ejection pressure and peak, mean, and total wall stress are variable.

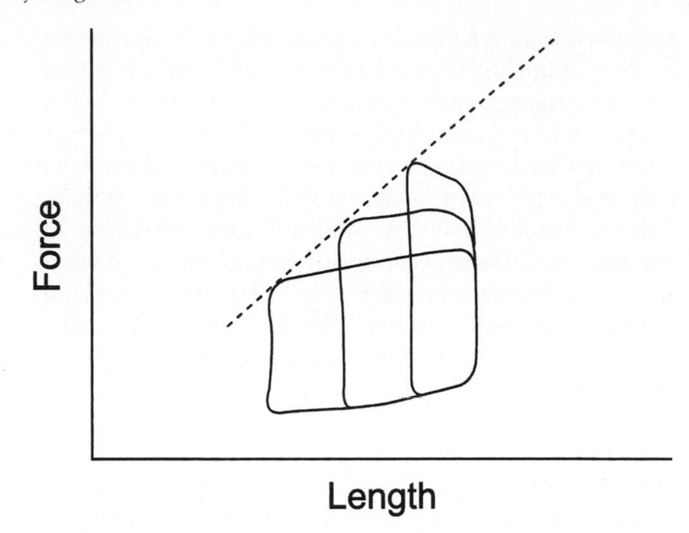

FIGURE 15–5 *When isolated cardiac muscle shortens against a variable load from a fixed end-diastolic length, the end-systolic force-length relationship is linear and is the same as that observed with isotonic contractions.*

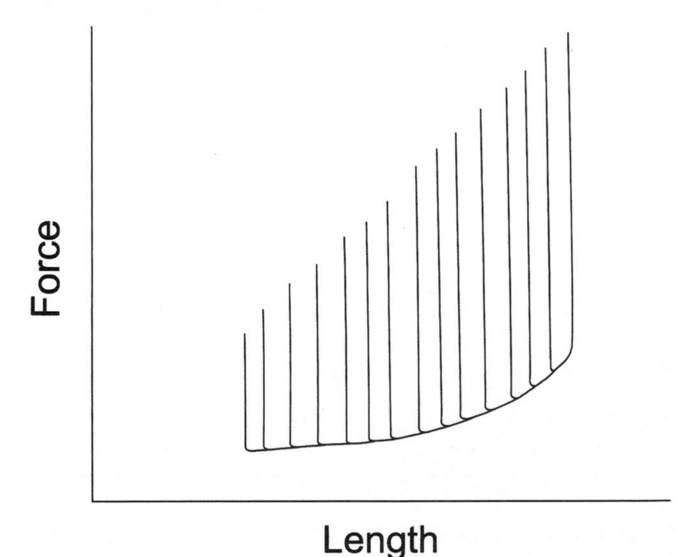

FIGURE 15–4 *When isolated cardiac muscle is allowed to shorten isotonically, the determinant of the rise in force is seen to be the end-systolic length, because a linear end-systolic force-length relation is maintained independent of the end-diastolic length.*

From Fyler DC [ed.]. Nadas' Pediatric Cardiology. Philadelphia: Hanley & Belfus, 1992.

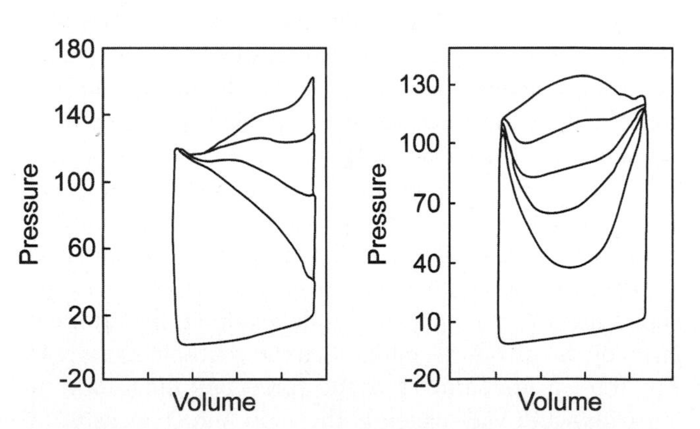

FIGURE 15–6 *When isolated heart preparations are held at a fixed end-systolic and end-diastolic volume (and therefore by necessity end-systolic and end-diastolic wall thicknesses are also invariant), the ejection conditions can be varied widely and the same end-systolic pressure is attained. Thus, wall stress varies substantially at all points in the cardiac cycle without affecting end-systolic volume and ejected volume, providing end-systolic pressure is constant.*

Modified from Suga H, Kitabatake A, Sagawa K. End-systolic pressure determines stroke volume from fixed end-diastolic volume in the isolated canine left ventricle under a constant contractile state. Circ Res 44:238, 1979, with permission.

Shortening Deactivation. As would be expected, there are limits to the degree to which end-systolic force determines end-systolic fiber length. In particular, if the isometric end-systolic length–tension relationship is compared with the end-systolic length–tension relationship found when shortening is permitted, the end-systolic length is longer in the latter situation.[38,39] In essence, the length attained when the muscle shortens is less than would be predicted based on the isometric relation. This phenomenon has been labeled "shortening deactivation" and represents an actual loss of the maximum force-generating capacity (contractility) of the muscle caused by the process of shortening.[40] Because this fall in contractility is proportional to the overall magnitude of shortening, and because shortening is dependent on end-systolic stress, this represents at least a potential means by which changes in afterload may alter contractility. Of course, this disturbs the conceptual framework of afterload, preload, and contractility as independent determinants of ventricular function. Similarly, the preload-related phenomenon of "length-dependent activation" is representative of a process by which loading conditions may modulate contractile state. Although the magnitude of these effects is not clear, in the intact heart length-dependent activation and shortening deactivation appear to counterbalance each other to a large extent.[15,41–43]

Wall Stress versus Fiberstress. Wall stress is the force within the myocardium, and is intrinsically directional. During diastole, this force is exerted on all of the elements within the wall. During systole, the myofiber is the active, energy-consuming element that produces the shortening force, and the force within the myofibers is known as *fiberstress*. The fiberstress is not equivalent to wall stress.[44] The hydrostatic forces within the myocardium are not taken into consideration by wall stress formulas, and therefore wall stress underestimates fiberstress.[45] Fiberstress can be calculated as a global parameter, dependent solely on ventricular mass, volume, and transmural pressure.[46] Although in many circumstances the quantitative differences between wall stress and fiberstress do not introduce significant artifact to the understanding of myocardial mechanics, fiberstress is the more important determinant of systolic function and the differences are of particular importance in the presence of significant hypertrophy.[47]

Contractility

As previously defined, contractility refers to the intrinsic properties of cardiac muscle, that is, those contractile characteristics that are not secondary to afterload or preload. Although this distinction is somewhat artificial inasmuch as preload and afterload may, in fact, influence contractility under certain circumstances, the concept is very useful in the understanding of cardiovascular physiology, providing the limits are understood. Various indices have been reported to provide relatively load-independent measures of contractility, each of which has advantages and limitations. Rather than a comprehensive review, only those methods that have a significant body of confirmatory research will be discussed here.

End-Systolic Pressure-Volume Relationship. Much of our current understanding of the physiology of myocardial contractility is based on examination of myocardial force–length relationships and their equivalent in the intact heart and in the ventricular pressure-volume and stress–volume curves. As detailed in the discussion of afterload, for any given contractile state, there is a unique end-systolic force–length (or pressure-volume) relationship that is linear, at least within the physiologic range of ventricular volumes. The end-systolic pressure-volume relationship (ESPVR) shown in Figures 15-7 and 15-8 illustrates this point. Elastance is the ratio of pressure to volume, and this ratio achieves a maximum value at end-systole. The slope of the line connecting the end-systolic elastance at various levels of afterload (the ESPVR) was named "maximum elastance" (E_{max}) by Suga in his seminal work in this area.[48] When the contractile state is augmented (for example, during catecholamine infusion), the degree of shortening is increased for any end-systolic pressure, and the attained end-systolic pressure is higher for any end-systolic volume.[49] In effect, the ESPVR has a steeper slope and is shifted to the left (Fig. 15-7). The opposite effect is seen with a fall in contractility, which results in a rightward shift and a shallower slope

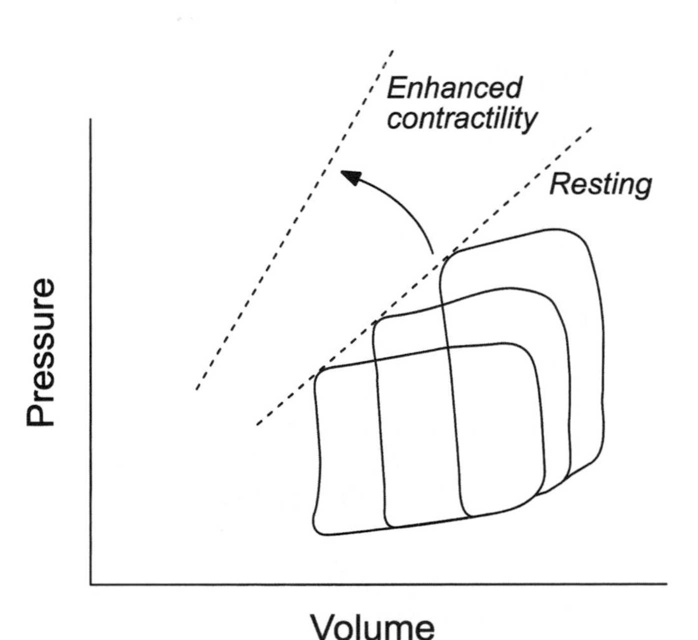

FIGURE 15–7 *Augmentation of myocardial contractility (for example, during catecholamine infusion) results in a shift of the end-systolic pressure-volume relation to the left with a higher slope.*
From Fyler DC [ed.]. Nadas' Pediatric Cardiology. Philadelphia: Hanley & Belfus, 1992.

to the ESPVR. Because the ESPVR is independent of preload (within limits to be discussed) and because afterload is directly incorporated, the ESPVR provides a relatively load-independent measure of the contractile state.[36,50,51]

Calculation of the ESPVR involves the collection of pressure-volume or pressure–dimension data over a range of end-systolic pressures at a constant contractile state (Fig. 15-8). Alteration of end-systolic pressure can be performed by several methods, including transient occlusion of the inferior vena cava, pharmacologic manipulation of load with vasoconstrictors or vasodilators, or partial aortic occlusion. Although several invasive and noninvasive methods for clinical assessment of the ESPVR have been reported, several problems with this analysis have not been fully overcome. The ESPVR, although linear and load-independent in the isolated dog heart model,[48,49,52] has been shown to be nonlinear under other conditions, both from a theoretical approach[53] and from experimental observations,[42,54–56] and it is not entirely load-independent[43,57–60] Because the degree of nonlinearity is variable, data must be gathered over a wide range of pressure values for any meaningful curve-fitting calculations. Although the position and steepness of the relation can be used to detect changes in contractile state in the same subject, the slope of the ESPVR is dependent on absolute ventricular size[61,62] making comparison of subjects with differences in ventricular size uncertain. Because data must be obtained over a range of end-systolic pressures, there is considerable opportunity for reflex alteration in autonomic tone in response to the elevation or reduction of blood pressure, thereby potentially altering the inotropic state during data collection, which would invalidate the data analysis. The need for pressure manipulation prevents frequent repetition of the test, precludes reassessment over short intervals, and renders the test, at best, cumbersome and, at worst, unusable for routine clinical use.

Several indices, theoretically based on the end-systolic pressure-volume relationship but obtainable without the need for afterload manipulation, have been reported. If the assumption is made that the line of the end-systolic pressure-volume relationship passes through the origin (Fig. 15-9), then any single end-systolic pressure-volume ratio can be used as an index of contractility. Although this type of single-point analysis has been used by many

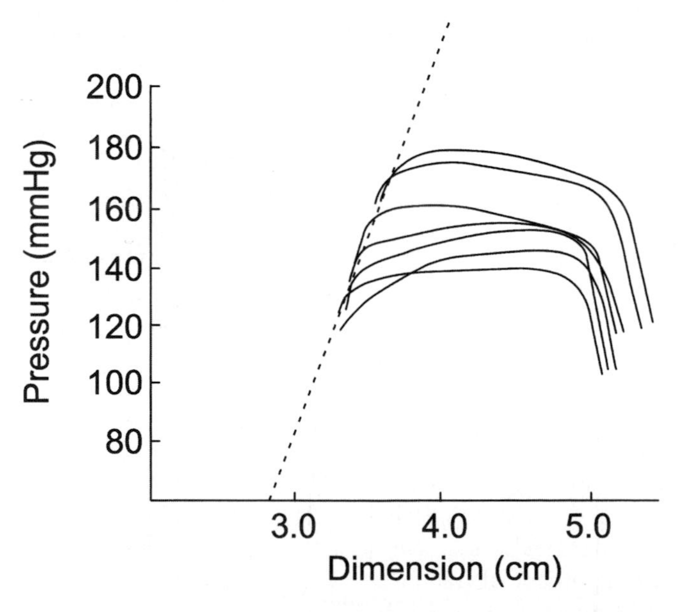

FIGURE 15–8 *The end-systolic pressure-volume relation can be obtained clinically, either invasively or noninvasively, by collecting pressure-volume or pressure-dimension data over a range of end-systolic pressures at a constant contractile state.*
From Colan SD, Sanders SP, Ingelfinger JR, Harmon W. Left ventricular mechanics and contractile state in children and young adults with end-stage renal disease: effect of dialysis and renal transplantation. J Am Coll Cardiol 10:1085–1094, 1987, with permission.

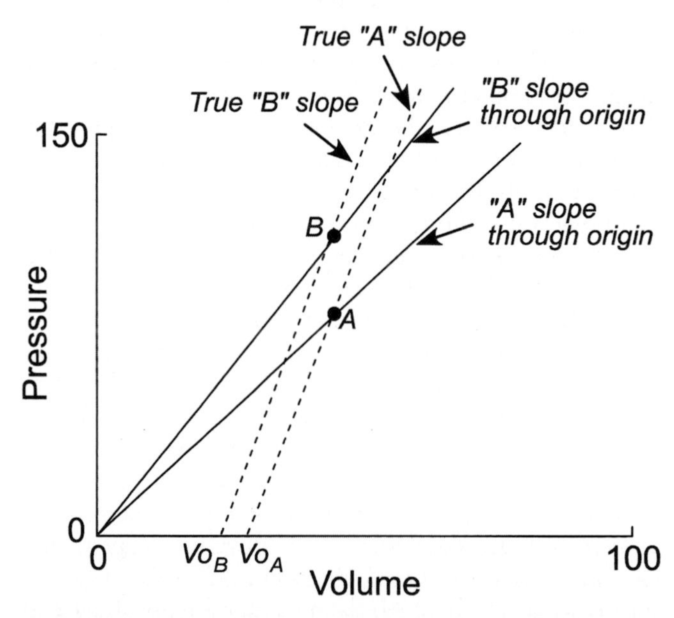

FIGURE 15–9 *Significant potential error is incurred by the use of the end-systolic pressure-volume ratio as an index of contractility. Use of this index assumes that the end-systolic pressure-volume relationship passes through the origin. When the single end-systolic pressure-volume value is used to estimate E_{max}, the conclusion is reached that the contractile state for point B is better than for point A, because the slope through the origin is steeper (solid lines). However, the possibility also exists that these represent ventricles with different zero-pressure volumes, but equal contractility because the true E_{max} values (dotted lines) are equal.*
From Fyler DC [ed.]. Nadas' Pediatric Cardiology. Philadelphia: Hanley & Belfus, 1992.

investigators, the limitations should be recognized. Essentially, this type of comparison forces the end-systolic pressure-volume relation through zero. The error incurred is the greatest in large ventricles, where a steep ESPVR with a large volume intercept will be misrepresented as a shallow ESPVR (Fig. 15-9), leading to the misdiagnosis of reduced contractility.

Preload-Adjusted dP/dt. The maximum rate of rise in ventricular pressure (dP/dt_{max}) is a sensitive index of contractility, the utility of which is limited by preload dependence. A number of methods of adjusting dP/dt_{max} for preload effects have been explored, including division by pressure at the time of dP/dt_{max} or some fixed point earlier in isovolumic systole[63] and adjustment for end-diastolic volume.[64] As predicted based on the E_{max} relationship, dP/dt_{max} has a linear relationship to left ventricular end-diastolic volume, and the slope of this relationship (Fig. 15-10) is a load independent index of contractility.[64] The primary limitations to this index are not dissimilar to the limitations inherent in the measurement of both dP/dt and the ESPVR. Data must be acquired invasively using a high-fidelity catheter over a broad range of end-diastolic volumes to provide a valid estimate of the slope value. There is significant potential for autonomically mediated changes in contractility during the manipulation of end-diastolic volume, such as occlusion of the inferior vena cava. Perhaps most important, adjustment of dP/dt_{max} for end-diastolic volume is intrinsically dependent on absolute volume, invalidating comparisons between individuals with different heart size. The limitations of EDV as an index of preload (see discussion of preload earlier in this chapter) are primarily responsible for the limitations to the use of EDV as a means of adjusting for preload.

Preload-Recruitable Stroke Work. Ventricular stroke work (SW) can be calculated as the integral of the pressure–volume loop. Although SW is highly preload-dependent, it demonstrates a linear relationship to end-diastolic volume (EDV), the slope of which is sensitive to contractility and relatively independent of loading conditions (Fig. 15-10). Similar to preloaded-adjusted dP/dt, manipulation of end-diastolic volume permits generation of data over multiple cardiac cycles from which the slope of this linear relation can be calculated.[65] Several authors have taken advantage of the fact that pressure-volume data obtained over a range of variably preloaded beats obtained in conscious animals can be used to calculate the ESPVR, preload-adjusted dP/dt_{max}, and preload-recruitable SW and have compared these indices in left and right ventricles.[65–68] These studies have not uniformly demonstrated a significant advantage to one or the other of these indices, although preload-recruitable SW appears to manifest a more linear relationship over the rather large range of EDV achieved under these experimental conditions (usually a 100% increase from minimum EDV). Most of the objections concerning the limitations of E_{max} and preload-adjusted dP/dt_{max} are also applicable to preload-recruitable SW, including the range of EDV that must be evaluated, the extent of preload-independence,[69] and whether the preload-recruitable SW is dependent on absolute EDV.

Preload-Adjusted Maximal Ventricular Power. Ventricular power is the rate of change of energy transfer (work), and instantaneous power can be calculated as the product of instantaneous pressure and flow. Flow can be obtained as the rate of change in volume (dV/dt), permitting derivation of power from pressure-volume loops. However, flow can also be derived from Doppler, potentially providing a noninvasive index of global ventricular contractility that has no reliance on ventricular geometry. Although several indices of contractility based on power have been reported, maximal ventricular power (PWR_{max}) has received the most attention. PWR_{max} is an early systolic event that is largely independent of afterload but is highly dependent on preload.[70] Therefore, a number of investigators have evaluated methods to adjust PWR_{max} for preload, primarily examining methods of adjustment of PWR_{max} for EDV. Studies by Schenk et al.[71] have indicated that, similar to preload-adjusted dP/dt_{max} and preload-recruitable SW, the relationship between PWR_{max} and EDV is linear with a slope value that is sensitive to contractility. Thus, the approach to preload adjustment for each of these indices includes the need to define the volume intercept of the regression, a requirement that results in a dependence of the normalized index on absolute ventricular size. In addition, if preload-adjusted PWR_{max} requires measurement of ventricular volume, the index cannot be obtained from pressure and flow measurements alone, diminishing its appeal.

Stress-Shortening and Stress-Velocity Analysis. Preload-adjusted dP/dt, preload-recruitable stroke work, and preload-adjusted maximal ventricular power are each methods of estimating load-independent contractility by evaluating a preload-dependent index of contractility and adjusting for the effect of preload. In addition to the limitations due to use of end-diastolic volume as an index of preload, derivation of each of these indices requires load manipulation. As an alternative, the possibility of fully accounting for the influence of loading conditions on standard indices of ejection performance has been explored. Both percent of fractional shortening (FS) and the mean velocity of shortening (VCF) are indices of contractility known to be dependent on loading status. When end-systolic stress is used to assess afterload, FS and VCF are found to fall in an inversely linear fashion during afterload augmentation (Fig. 15-11).[72] Of particular interest, the slopes of the stress-velocity and stress-shortening relations are the same in different individuals (Fig. 15-12), and the slope in any individual parallels the mean population regression (Fig. 15-13). The stress-shortening and stress-velocity

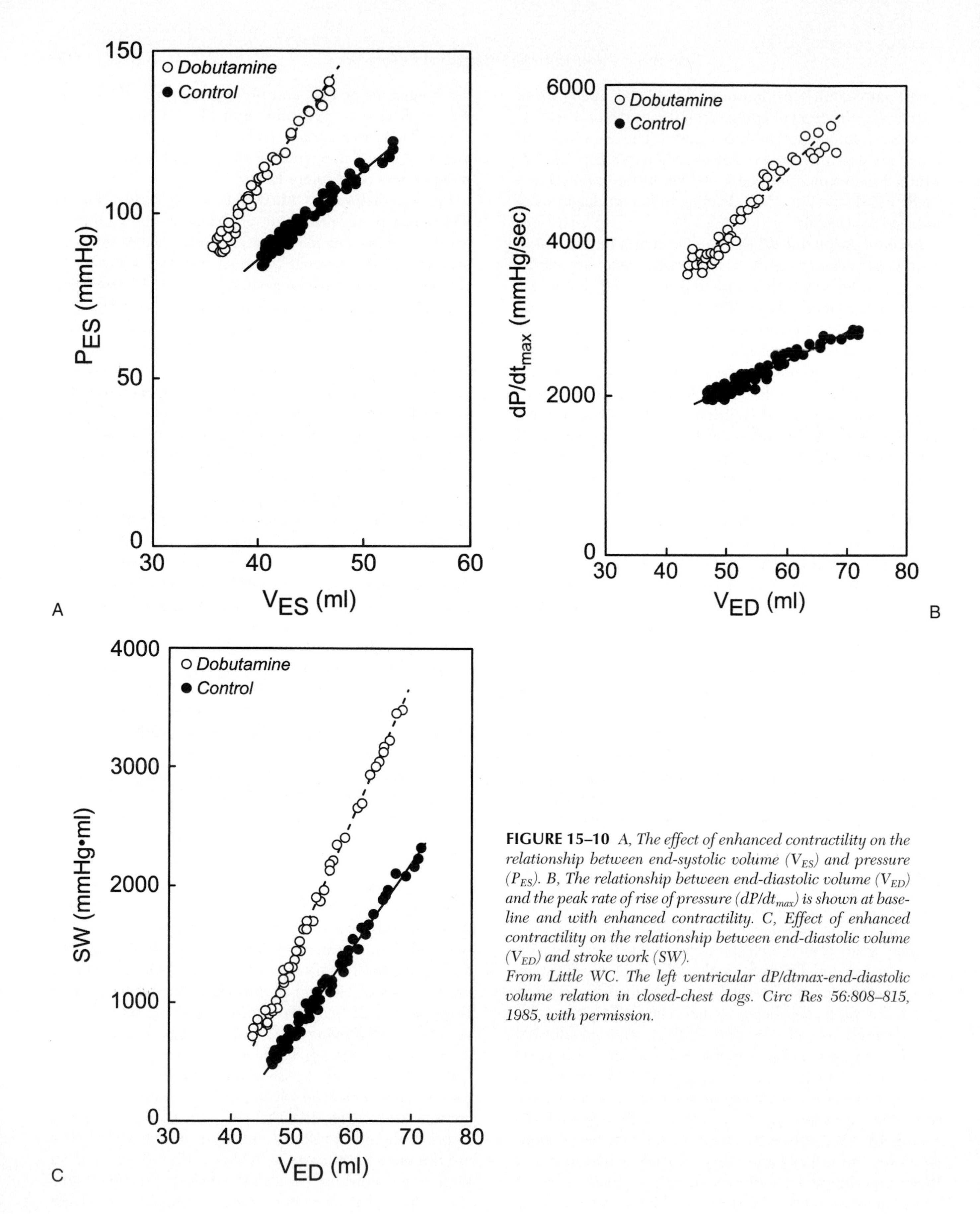

FIGURE 15–10 *A, The effect of enhanced contractility on the relationship between end-systolic volume (V_{ES}) and pressure (P_{ES}). B, The relationship between end-diastolic volume (V_{ED}) and the peak rate of rise of pressure (dP/dt_{max}) is shown at baseline and with enhanced contractility. C, Effect of enhanced contractility on the relationship between end-diastolic volume (V_{ED}) and stroke work (SW).*

From Little WC. The left ventricular dP/dtmax-end-diastolic volume relation in closed-chest dogs. Circ Res 56:808–815, 1985, with permission.

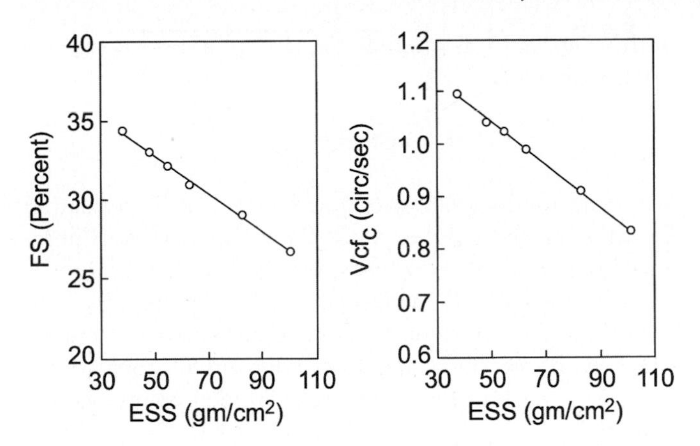

FIGURE 15–11 *Data obtained in a single individual during infusion of the alpha-adrenergic agent, methoxamine. End-systolic stress and ventricular performance, assessed by either fractional shortening or the velocity of shortening, are closely related in an inversely linear fashion.*
From Fyler DC [ed.]. Nadas' Pediatric Cardiology. Philadelphia: Hanley & Belfus, 1992.

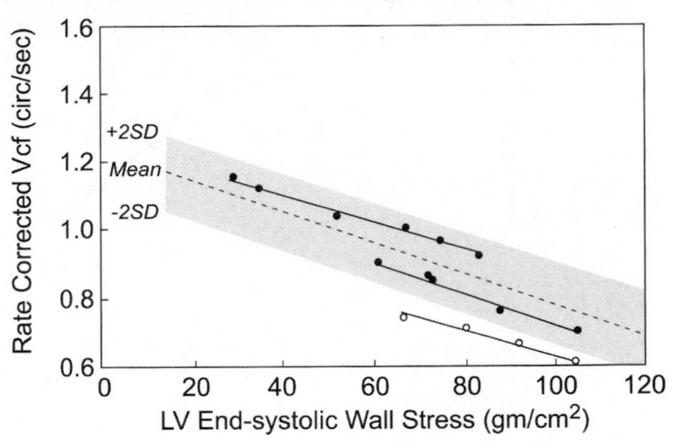

FIGURE 15–13 *The slope of the stress-velocity relationship in any individual (solid lines) runs parallel to the slope of other individuals and to the slope of the population regression.*
From Fyler, DC [ed.]. Nadas' Pediatric Cardiology. Philadelphia: Hanley & Belfus, 1992.

relationships are sensitive to contractility (Fig. 15-14) and, thus, represent afterload-adjusted indices of contractility. Numerous examples of the clinical application of these indices have been reported.[5,25,30,73–95]

Although either of these indices permits assessment of contractility independent of afterload effects, it is through the combination of the two that a complete description of the factors influencing cardiac performance can be obtained because of the differential effects of preload on VCF and FS. Increased preload is known to augment fiber shortening and therefore FS. The effect of changes in preload on the stress-shortening relation is predictable (Fig. 15-15) and mimics the effect of changes in contractility. Thus, the stress-shortening relation fails to distinguish the effects of altered preload from altered contractility. In contrast, VCF is not dependent on preload.[72,96–99] Although there are almost certainly limits to the extent of this preload-independence, variations in preload within the physiologic range do not significantly alter VCF. The lack of effect of EDFL on both end-systolic stress and VCF accounts for the preload-independence of the stress-velocity relation (Fig. 15-15).[72] Thus, the stress-velocity relation represents

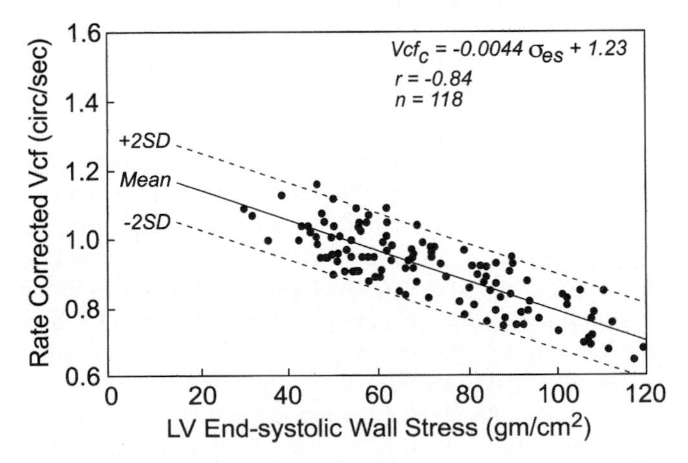

FIGURE 15–12 *A similar inversely linear relationship between end-systolic stress and velocity of shortening is also noted when the results from a large number of individuals are combined.*
From Fyler DC [ed.]. Nadas' Pediatric Cardiology. Philadelphia: Hanley & Belfus, 1992.

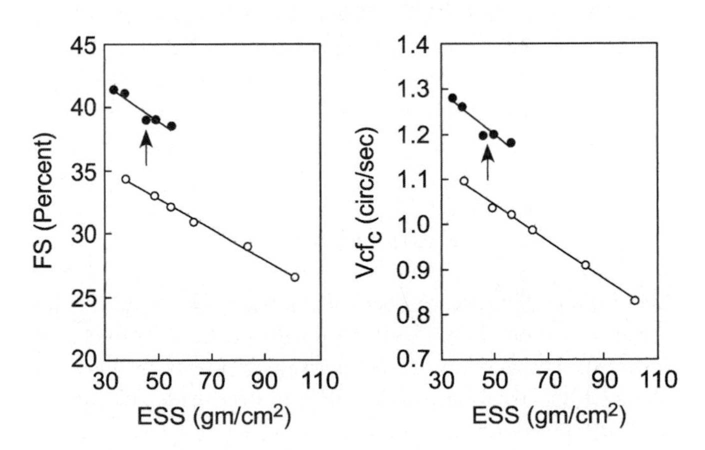

FIGURE 15–14 *Infusion of dobutamine results in an upward shift of the stress-shortening and stress-velocity relationships. Thus, for any level of afterload, enhanced contractility results in higher magnitude and velocity of shortening.*
From Fyler, DC [ed.]. Nadas' Pediatric Cardiology. Philadelphia: Hanley & Belfus, 1992.

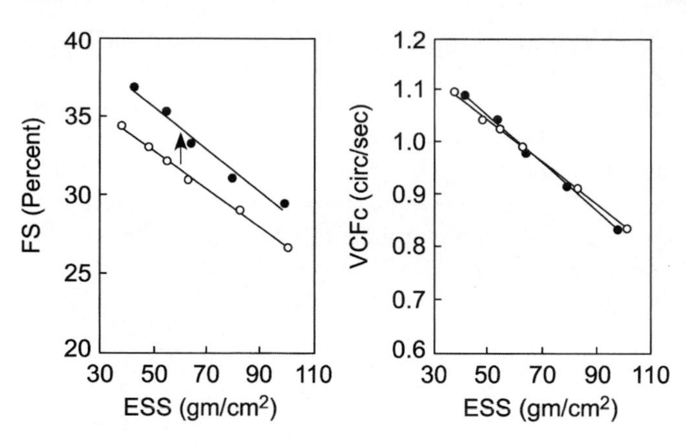

FIGURE 15–15 *The effect of preload augmentation on the stress-shortening and stress-velocity relationships in one subject is shown. The effect of changes in preload on the stress-shortening relation is predictable and mimics the effect of changes in contractility. The lack of effect of end-diastolic fiber length on both end-systolic stress and mean velocity of shortening accounts for the preload independence of the stress-velocity relation. From Fyler, DC [ed.]. Nadas' Pediatric Cardiology, Philadelphia: Hanley & Belfus, 1992.*

a preload-independent index of contractility that incorporates afterload. When stress-velocity analysis is combined with stress-shortening analysis, abnormalities in fiber shortening not related to afterload or contractility (as assessed by the stress-velocity relation) can be recognized as being secondary to preload effects.

It is also possible to address these calculations in a more analytic fashion. Because percent of fiber shortening depends on the EDFL (preload), the force resisting shortening (afterload), the frequency of contraction (heart rate), and contractility, it is possible to express quantitatively the percent of fiber shortening (ΔL) as a function (F) of preload (λ), afterload (σ), heart rate (ν), and contractility (c) as follows:

$$(1)\ \Delta L = F(\lambda, \sigma, \nu, c)$$

The effect of the frequency of contraction on shortening appears to be mediated primarily through effects on contractility, whereby it is possible to express observed contractility (c′) as a function (F″) of heart rate (ν) and the rate-independent contractile state (c):

$$(2)\ c' = F'(\nu, c)$$

Then, formula (1) can be rewritten as:

$$(3)\ \Delta L = F(\lambda, \sigma, c')$$

Furthermore, VCF is a function (F″) of afterload (σ) and contractility (c):

$$(4)\ VCF = F''(\sigma, c)$$

Afterload (end-systolic stress) and VCF can be measured directly; and F″ can be solved for c. The observed heart rate (ν) and calculated contractility (c) can then be substituted in formula (2) to calculate c′. Finally, the observed values for fiber shortening (ΔL) and end-systolic stress (σ) along with the calculated rate-independent contractility (c′) can be substituted in equation (3) to yield preload (λ) directly.

The stress-shortening relation has been used as an index of contractility by a number of authors[100–102] without adjustment for preload effects. This simplification can be justified when preload effects are unlikely to be significant. Under normal circumstances, the left ventricle operates near the peak of the Frank-Starling mechanism, particularly when measurements are performed with the patient in the supine position.[103] This accounts for the absence of preload augmentation during supine exercise, in contrast to the utilization of preload reserve that accompanies upright exercise.[104] Thus, the assumption has been made that preload effects are negligible under usual physiologic circumstances in humans.[103,105] Certainly, there are circumstances under which this assumption is invalid. For example, during hemodialysis there is a striking reduction in preload manifested as a disproportionate fall in shortening compared with changes in the velocity of shortening (Fig. 15-16).[5] Similarly, long-distance runners manifest a reduction in the stress-adjusted shortening fraction secondary to reduced preload when assessed at rest.[30] This finding can be understood as a ventricle adapted to a large volume load that is assessed when the volume load is not present, that is, in the preload-reduced state. Postoperative patients in whom fluid administration is restricted who are also undergoing treatment with diuretics manifest reduced preload.[80] Preload-related changes in myocardial shortening have been shown to have a significant impact on the assessment of ventricular performance in the presence of aortic or mitral regurgitation.[53,106] Although it may be possible to define those physiologic states in which preload effects can safely be ignored, it is almost certainly preferable to measure them directly through the use of combined stress-shortening and stress-velocity analysis.

There are a number of limitations to these indices. The calculations for wall stress and the indices of ventricular function (FS and VCF) assume a symmetric ventricular configuration and pattern of contraction. In the normally shaped ventricle, the radius of curvature of the posterior wall along both the major and minor axes can be measured directly from long- and short-axis imaging data. If there are

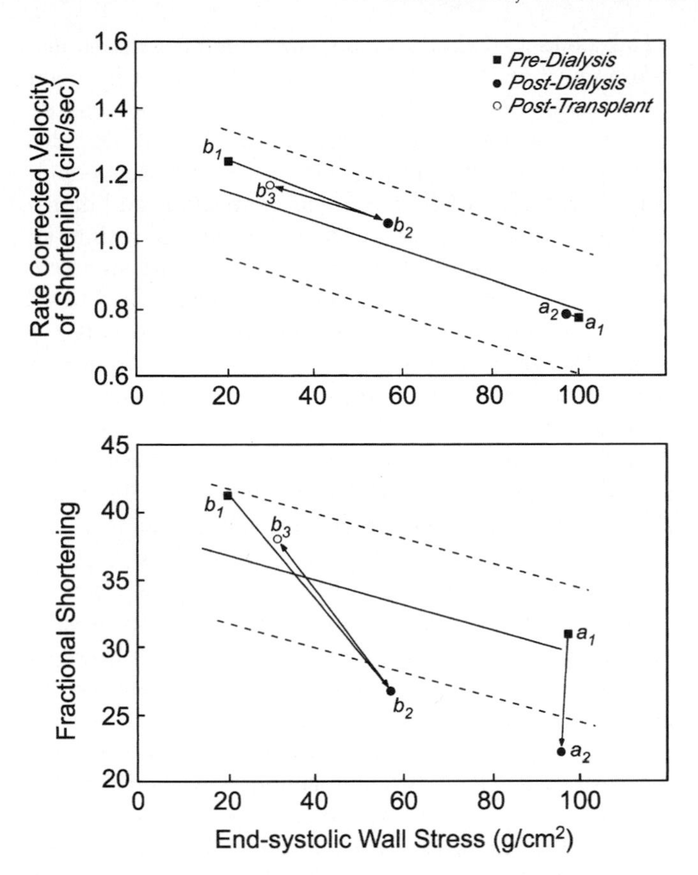

FIGURE 15–16 *Two subjects evaluated before and after dialysis and/or transplantation. Subject "a" experienced a marked reduction in fractional shortening in spite of little change in afterload (end-systolic stress is unchanged) and no change in contractility (the stress-velocity relation is unchanged). These findings are consistent with preload effects alone. Subject "b" experienced a rise in afterload (higher end-systolic stress) after dialysis with secondary and proportional reduction in the velocity of shortening, indicating no change in contractility. The disproportionate fall in fractional shortening is indicative of reduced preload. From Fyler, DC [ed.]. Nadas' Pediatric Cardiology, Philadelphia: Hanley & Belfus, 1992.*

regional abnormalities in shape or if the ventricle is distorted because of septal displacement (right ventricular pressure or volume overload) the major and minor axes will not accurately reflect the radius of curvature of the posterior wall and the standard formulas for calculation of wall stress cannot be used.

The assumptions concerning ventricular geometry which underlie the stress calculations are equally applicable to the indices of ventricular performance. Both FS and VCF are reliable indices of global fiber shortening only in ventricles with a symmetric pattern of contraction and a circular cross-sectional configuration. That is, because these calculations use changes in dimension to estimate alteration in fiber length, there must be a constant and known geometric relation between circumference and dimension. Although these indices have been calculated in subjects in whom the left ventricular configuration and change in systolic shape during contraction are clearly abnormal,[107] because there is no reliable relation to myofiber shortening or contractility in this situation these indices are not valid under such circumstances.

ASSESSMENT OF DIASTOLIC PERFORMANCE

Abnormalities of ventricular filling, although less commonly recognized than systolic dysfunction, constitute an active area of basic and clinical investigation. It has become apparent in recent years that the failure to recognize diastolic dysfunction is more frequently due to inadequate means of detection and quantification than to the rarity of the disorder. Although the available methods for assessing diastolic function are expanding, clinical assessment of diastole still has not attained the level of ease, accuracy, and routine associated with evaluation of systolic function.

Typically, diastole is taken to encompass that period from cessation of ejection to the time of mitral valve closure at the onset of the rapid rise in pressure during contraction. Hemodynamically, this period encompasses isovolumic relaxation, rapid filling, diastasis, and atrial contraction. From the aspect of myocardial mechanics, the primary event is muscle lengthening in response to a combination of effects that inhibit or promote lengthening. It is customary to divide discussions about diastole into an early, active phase of relaxation, when changes in force and length are primarily the result of changes within the myocardium, and a later, passive phase, during which changes in force and length are primarily the result of external forces. Therefore, abnormalities of diastolic performance are generally related to the corresponding processes of active relaxation and passive myocardial compliance. These represent distinct properties of the myocardium which may vary independently from each other.[108] However, because the process of relaxation is not completed until after the onset of filling, these events overlap in time to a variable degree. Although it is instructive to discuss relaxation and compliance as separate phenomena, it must be recognized also that this period of overlap is of considerable importance when clinical indices of diastolic performance are considered.

Ventricular Relaxation

Abnormal relaxation has been identified in association with a number of cardiac disorders. In particular, ischemia has been noted to result in profound alteration in the rate at which pressure falls during isovolumic relaxation.[109–111] In the presence of ischemia, abnormalities of relaxation are detectable before any changes in systolic performance, a finding that is not unexpected when the energetics of contraction and relaxation are considered.[112] The mechanisms involved in relaxation of cardiac muscle are believed to relate to both activation-controlled and load-controlled force decay mechanisms. The activation-controlled loss of force within the ventricular wall, which occurs early in diastole, is an active, energy-consuming process, accounting for as much as 15% of the total energy utilized by the beating heart.[113,114] Adenosine triphosphate–dependent calcium sequestration by the sarcoplasmic reticulum results in actin-myosin dissociation caused by reduction of the Ca^{++} concentration in the region of the myofilament below the level needed for myofibrillar adenosine triphosphatase activation.

Indices of Relaxation

Generally, the measurement of relaxation in the intact ventricle is based on indices calculated from ventricular pressure–time relations during isovolumic relaxation. During this period of the cardiac cycle, ventricular volume is constant, and therefore, it may be assumed that dimension and wall thickness are also constant. If these assumptions are valid, decreases in wall tension, wall stress, and pressure are parallel processes and changes in pressure accurately reflect changes in force. In fact, because of alteration of ventricular conformation during isovolumic relaxation, changes in pressure and stress are not strictly equivalent. That is, as discussed earlier, wall stress relates to the local radius of curvature. During systole, the ventricle shortens proportionally more in the short than in the long axis, assuming a more elliptical shape. Diastolic lengthening is temporally and spatially nonuniform,[115,116] resulting in some change in shape even during isovolumic diastole. However, because the change in shape is small compared with the change in pressure, it is generally neglected. The pressure-based indices that have been used are based on the observation that during isovolumic relaxation pressure falls in an exponential fashion. Because the peak rate of pressure decrease [$(dP/dt)_{min}$] nearly always occurs after completion of ejection, the pressure trace from $(dP/dt)_{min}$ to the time of mitral valve opening (pressure crossover point for left atrial and left ventricular pressure) can be fit to a curve of the form $P_t = P_0 e^{-t/t} + P_b$, where P_t = pressure as a function of time, P_0 = pressure at the time of $(dP/dt)_{min}$, t = time, t = time constant of relaxation, and P_b = asymptotic pressure. Mathematically, the time constant t represents the time required for the pressure at $(dP/dt)_{min}$ to be reduced by 1/e.

Calculation of the time constant of relaxation requires use of a high-fidelity catheter positioned in the left ventricle. This limits the use of this technology, particularly in children. Alternative indices of relaxation include those based on analysis of the early diastolic filling phase, which are discussed in subsequent sections of this chapter, and the isovolumic relaxation time (IRT). IRT is the length of time between aortic valve closure and mitral valve opening, and can be noninvasively measured through m-mode and Doppler techniques.[117] The length of this time period depends in part on the rate of fall of ventricular pressure, and therefore IRT correlates with the time constant of relaxation. However, the IRT also depends on arterial pressure, as a determinant of the pressure at which the aortic valve closes, and left atrial pressure, as a determinant of the pressure at which the mitral valve opens. Reduced arterial pressure in conjunction with elevated left atrial pressure can easily counterbalance the impact of a slowed rate of fall of pressure during isovolumic relaxation, resulting in a normal IRT despite impaired relaxation. Thus, although readily available, IRT is at best a weak index of relaxation.

Factors Affecting Relaxation

Differentiation of intrinsic myocardial relaxation abnormalities from those secondary to external influences requires a consideration of the factors that are known to influence this process. Most prominent among these are load-dependent mechanisms of relaxation, which have been extensively described in isolated muscle preparations. Although the presence of load-controlled decay mechanisms in cardiac muscle has been widely documented, the physiologic importance of these mechanisms for the intact ventricle remains controversial. In principle, the effects of load-dependent control of relaxation could be mediated by hemodynamic loading during late ejection, during isovolumic relaxation, and during the period of rapid filling. There has been substantial disagreement concerning the effect of altered load on ventricular relaxation in animal studies,[118] with relatively few studies available in humans. However, in a study by Starling and associates,[118] moderate alterations in load were not found to affect the process of isovolumic relaxation in humans.

Because ventricular relaxation indices rely on the global parameter of chamber pressure rather than on events at the sarcomere level, nonuniform contraction and relaxation causes prolongation of t and altered early filling patterns in animals[119] and humans.[120,121] This mechanism contributes importantly to the impaired relaxation indices observed in association with ventricular paced rhythms and bundle branch block. Under these circumstances, ventricular relaxation may be impaired even though myocardial relaxation is normal.

Usually, changes in contractility and systolic shortening are associated with significant changes in relaxation and appear to act through similar mechanisms. Because the inactivation mechanism is distinct from the activation mechanism involved in contraction, changes in relaxation do not always parallel changes in contractility. Thus, isoproterenol increases contractility and the rate of relaxation, but an increase in calcium concentration impairs relaxation while augmenting contractility. The number of cross bridges and the duration of their cycles can be altered by various mechanisms, which, in turn, play a major role in determining the decline in force during relaxation. These mechanisms act either by *sensitizing the contractile protein*, resulting in a slower and later decline in force, or by *desensitization of the contractile protein*, resulting in an earlier and faster decline in force.[122] In addition to pharmacologic agents, some mechanical control mechanisms, such as the magnitude of shortening, may also act in this fashion. In isolated muscle preparations, the affinity of troponin-C for calcium appears to relate inversely to the magnitude of shortening.[123–125] The reduction in bound calcium that results from the process of shortening enhances the rate of relaxation and the load-induced rapid lengthening. Thus, the rate of relaxation is dependent on the total magnitude of shortening, whether altered by preload, afterload, or contractility. The physiologic significance of shortening enhancement of relaxation, independent of changes in contractility, is uncertain.

In addition to sarcomeric deactivation, elastic recoil plays an important role in force decay during the isovolumic relaxation period. Elastic recoil is secondary to release of elastic forces stored during systole that manifest as restoring forces early in diastole.[126] This phenomenon can result in ventricular pressure falling below atmospheric pressure during early diastole, thereby facilitating filling through a process of diastolic suction.[76,126–129] The degree of negativity attained is inversely proportional to the end-systolic volume.[76] The importance of restoring forces varies with respect to the hemodynamic and the myocardial status.[76,130] Under normal conditions, elastic recoil appears to be a major determinant of the peak rate of fiber relengthening.[129] In the presence of myocardial dysfunction with an elevated end-systolic volume, the stored forces are relatively less and recoil plays a reduced role in ventricular filling. Elastic recoil is one of the forces that acts during the period of isovolumic relaxation. Therefore, the process of relaxation as quantified by t includes the effects of both inactivation and restoring forces. An important implication of diastolic suction is the intrinsic linkage between systolic and diastolic function. Diminished force of contraction results in a reduced rate of relaxation, regardless of whether intrinsic diastolic myocardial properties are abnormal or not.

VENTRICULAR AND MYOCARDIAL COMPLIANCE

In contrast to the active process of inactivation in the early part of diastole, the pressure-volume relation of the ventricle later in diastole is predominantly determined by the passive elastic properties of the myocardium. However, many nonmyocardial factors contribute, and the distinction between chamber and myocardial properties is challenging. Chamber stiffness (change in pressure/change in volume = dP/dV) and compliance (change in volume/change in pressure = dV/dP) refer to analysis of the pressure–volume relation of the ventricle and, as such, encompass a variety of factors including myocardial properties, ventricular geometry, pericardial restraint, coronary filling, incomplete relaxation, and interventricular interaction.[131] The magnitude of the influence of each of these features under various hemodynamic circumstances has been the subject of considerable interest.[131] Although chamber stiffness and compliance are measures of the ability of the ventricle to distend under pressure, myocardial stiffness refers to the ability of the muscle to stretch when exposed to a lengthening force. The force can be quantified as wall stress (s). Strain (e) is defined as the change in length with respect to a reference length, ideally with the reference being the resting length, that is, length at a stress of zero. Thus, chamber properties are represented by the pressure–volume relation and myocardial properties are represented by the stress-strain relation, defined as myocardial stiffness (ds/de) and myocardial compliance (de/ds). If the myocardium were a purely elastic material, the change in length would depend only on the elongating force. However, the force required to induce rapid changes in length exceeds that required for more gradual stretching. Thus, myocardial stress is a function of both strain and strain rate (rate of change in length) and the myocardium is, therefore, a viscoelastic material. The viscous properties are most evident during periods of rapid lengthening, such as the rapid filling phase and atrial systole. Although the magnitude of the viscous effects is controversial, most investigators have incorporated viscous effects in their mathematic models or limited the analysis to periods in diastole when viscous effects are expected to be minimal (at the middle and end of diastole). Myocardial compliance contributes to ventricular compliance, but is only one of many contributing factors, and is often a minor determinant. Therefore, abnormal ventricular compliance, similar to abnormal ventricular relaxation, cannot be assumed to reflect abnormal diastolic myocardial properties.

Indices of Myocardial Compliance

Many approaches to quantitative analysis of myocardial compliance have been described. In general, a mathematic model developed from predicted material properties and geometric considerations is used to calculate the best-fit equation for the pressure-volume or stress-strain data in mid and late diastole. For example, if an exponential stress–strain relationship is assumed, the equation for a purely elastic material is $\sigma = \alpha(e^{\beta\varepsilon} - 1)$, where σ = stress, ε = strain, and α and β are the descriptive parameters that describe the exponential stress-strain properties of the myocardium.

If a viscoelastic model is used, it becomes necessary to incorporate the velocity of change in fiber length (strain rate = $d\varepsilon/dt$) and a parameter that represents the magnitude of the viscoelastic properties (η) into the equation, as $\sigma = \alpha(e^{\beta\varepsilon} - 1) + \eta(d\varepsilon/dt)$.

Although this approach has been used by a number of authors,[132] there is substantial controversy as to the correct method for the calculation of stress and the stress-strain relationship.[53,106,133] These controversies relate to the correct equation used to describe the material properties of the myocardium and the correct method for normalizing forces and dimensions to account for differences in geometry. Regardless of which equations are used, several methodologic problems are common to the stress-strain calculations:

1. The reference length for strain calculations is best taken at zero stress, that is, at a transmural pressure of zero. Because this is difficult to obtain as a static measurement (to eliminate viscous effects) in clinical situations, it is generally estimated by extrapolation of the observed stress-strain relationship or else another reference point is selected.
2. Adjustment for the nonzero external constraining forces from the pericardium and thorax is necessary to obtain myocardial compliance, necessitating either direct or indirect measurement of transmural pressure. In animals[134] and humans,[135] right atrial pressure has been found to provide a good estimate of pericardial pressure. Studies of this sort have not been performed in patients with congenital heart disease, in whom the right ventricular transmural filling pressure would be expected to be nonzero because of the frequent finding of right ventricular hypertrophy.
3. The available methods for determining ventricular volume yield relatively few data points per beat, with sampling every 25 to 35 msec. The number of data points available for the curve fit is small, particularly at high heart rates. Few data points result in large variance and broad confidence intervals for the derived indices, particularly when nonlinear curve fits are used. In infants and young children, diastolic periods of 60 to 80 msec may be encountered (Fig. 15-17), precluding any meaningful mathematic analysis of pressure-volume data.
4. One must either include viscous effects in the model or exclude periods of rapid filling from the analysis. The latter approach further limits the number of data points per beat available for the curve fit, augmenting the problem referred to above.
5. The full range of physiologic stress-strain relations should be included for the most meaningful analysis, because extrapolation beyond the observed data range introduces large errors. To obtain the full physiologic range for end-diastolic pressure, interventions that raise and lower left ventricular filling pressure must be performed.

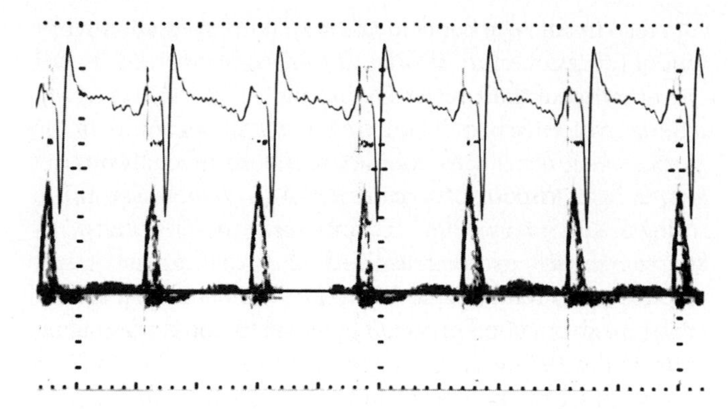

FIGURE 15–17 *Mitral valve Doppler tracing in an infant with critical aortic stenosis, illustrating the very short diastolic filling periods (50–60 msec) that may be encountered in this age group and the absence of separate early and atrial flow waves. From Fyler, DC [ed.]. Nadas' Pediatric Cardiology, Philadelphia: Hanley & Belfus, 1992.*

These technical obstacles have seriously impeded efforts to define normal and abnormal passive myocardial properties. Few data exist in children and certainly there are no methods that have made it into clinical use. The indices of relaxation that are commonly used are typically noninvasive indices that rely on analysis of filling behavior to infer passive ventricular properties and thereby secondarily infer passive myocardial behavior. The filling indices are discussed below.

Overlap of Active and Passive Periods of Diastole

The amount of fiber lengthening that occurs during isovolumic relaxation is minimal, allowing the passive myocardial properties to be neglected during this portion of diastole. By mid-diastole, relaxation is generally complete and only passive myocardial properties are influential. Although normally complete shortly after mitral valve opening, in some pathologic conditions relaxation may not be completed until later in diastole. Even in the normal heart, pressure continues to decline during early rapid filling in spite of increasing dimension, indicating that both active and passive processes are influential during this time. Pasipoularides and coworkers[136] postulated that measured left ventricular pressure represents the summation of components due to relaxation and passive filling. Potentially, an analytic approach of this sort could account for the observed pressure-volume or stress-strain relation throughout diastole. A meaningful model for the period of diastole during which active and passive myocardial properties interact is clearly desirable because it coincides with rapid filling, during which most of the filling occurs. In addition to potential confounding effects from viscous properties of the myocardium, there may be some influence of lengthening on relaxation. In isolated muscle, a load applied after relaxation ensues results in augmentation of relaxation.[137] In contrast, canine ventricles were found to have slower relaxation during filling compared with nonfilling beats.[128] A model that can account for the observed pressure-volume relationship throughout diastole remains elusive.

Diastolic Filling

The major physiologic consequences of abnormal relaxation and/or compliance are mediated through altered or impaired filling. At the whole organ level, filling is the primary event during diastole, and diastolic dysfunction is primarily of importance when disordered filling is the result. Most of the available methods for noninvasive assessment of diastolic function are based on assessment of the pattern of diastolic filling. Although normal or abnormal patterns of filling are relatively easy to document using these methods, it must be understood that because of the interaction of relaxation and compliance and the influence of external factors, abnormal filling may occur in spite of normal relaxation and compliance, and normal filling may occur in spite of abnormal myocardial diastolic properties. This section will focus on diastolic filling dynamics and their relation to myocardial properties and external factors.

Diastolic Filling Indices

The timing of diastolic filling events has been studied by a number of authors.[138–140] The onset of filling begins with unloading of the mitral valve during isovolumic relaxation. At moderate heart rates, this process is readily visible on two-dimensional echocardiography, where the frame preceding mitral valve opening shows some apical movement of the anterior mitral leaflet without separation of the valve leaflets. When ventricular pressure falls below left atrial pressure (first atrioventricular pressure crossover), rapid filling ensues. Ventricular pressure continues to decline during early rapid filling as the relaxation rate continues to exceed the filling force. After minimum pressure is attained, the effect of filling exceeds that of relaxation and ventricular pressure begins to rise. At or near the time of the peak rate of mitral inflow, ventricular pressure exceeds atrial pressure (second atrioventricular pressure crossover), and deceleration of the early filling wave begins. The entire deceleration phase occurs against an adverse pressure gradient, which provides the decelerating force. At lower heart rates, atrial filling from venous flow leads to a rise in atrial pressure until mid-diastolic atrial and ventricular pressure are essentially equal, and transmitral flow nearly ceases (diastasis). The late filling wave is due to atrial systole, which at higher heart rates merges with the early filling wave. At normal atrioventricular conduction intervals, the atrial filling wave continues beyond the QRS complex until the onset of ventricular contraction leads to ventricular pressure in excess of atrial pressure, subsequent valve closure, and cessation of flow.

The pattern of diastolic filling can be quantitatively assessed by numerous invasive and noninvasive means, including angiography, computed tomography, radionuclide scintigraphy, echocardiography (m-mode, two-dimensional, and three-dimensional), and Doppler ultrasonography. With the exception of Doppler, each of these methods provides a measure of the relation of left ventricular volume or dimension to time, from which the rate of change of volume or dimension can be obtained as a measure of flow rate. These volumetric methods all rely on some means of identification of ventricular borders in a user-interactive fashion. For these modalities, flow is derived as the first derivative of the time–volume curve, a calculation that introduces substantial and unpredictable amplification of any error in measurement. Doppler ultrasonography measures left ventricular filling velocity directly, eliminating the problems involved in the calculation of the time derivative.

The peak rate of flow, the time to peak flow, and some ratio of early and late filling are indices derived from all of these techniques. In addition, a number of variables derived from the Doppler time-velocity curve have been examined, including the ratio of the peak early versus the peak late velocity, the ratio of early versus late flow, the rate at which peak early flow is attained (acceleration time) and the rate of deceleration. It should be noted that although indices based on the ratio of early diastolic–to–late diastolic events have received a great deal of attention, at the higher heart rates that are normal in infants and children these events may merge (Fig. 15-17), precluding these calculations.

Relation of Diastolic Filling to Myocardial Properties

Diastolic filling generally proceeds in two phases, with an early diastolic filling wave (E wave) and a late diastolic filling wave following atrial contraction (A wave) usually separated by a period of minimal flow. The E wave occurs during the period of overlap between ventricular relaxation and early filling and is therefore determined by relaxation and compliance.[141] The A wave is a late diastolic phenomenon and is determined by numerous factors, including ventricular compliance. The most common interpretation is that the peak E velocity is determined primarily by ventricular relaxation and the peak A velocity is determined by ventricular compliance. Elevated E/A is generally taken to imply abnormal compliance, reduced E/A is interpreted as abnormal relaxation, and normal E/A interpreted as either normal or as secondary to abnormalities in both relaxation and compliance ("pseudo-normalization"). Incorporation of additional measurements enables the phenomenon of pseudo-normalization to be partially overcome. The deceleration phase of the E wave generally takes place after completion of relaxation and is therefore primarily determined by ventricular compliance. Similarly, duration of the A wave and the duration of flow reversal in the pulmonary veins depend on ventricular compliance. A scoring system based on the combination of these indices has been proposed as a means of using diastolic filling dynamics to detect and grade diastolic ventricular properties.[141] Many authors have reviewed the limitations to these indices.[142,143]

The ***rate of ventricular flow propagation*** (V_P) is an alternative index of early diastolic function.[144] The rate at which the early diastolic bolus of flow propagates toward the ventricular apex has a significant negative correlation with the time constant of relaxation (t), indicating that a short value of t promotes more rapid flow toward the ventricular apex.[145] Although several methods can be used to measure flow propagation, m-mode color Doppler appears to be the most practical.[142] Flow propagation velocity can exceed peak early-inflow velocity, reflecting the effect of elastic recoil in the creation of intraventricular pressure gradients[142] and documenting the important contribution of elastic recoil to the process of ventricular relaxation. In contrast to pulsed Doppler indices of relaxation, V_P appears to be insensitive to atrial filling pressure. Because of the sensitivity of relaxation to heart rate, afterload, contractility, and disordered conduction, V_P is anticipated to be influenced by these factors although this issue has not been adequately explored.

Tissue-Doppler Diastolic Indices. Doppler samples obtained directly from myocardium can be used to assess the instantaneous velocity of tissue motion relative to the ultrasound transducer. These indices do not directly assess inflow, elastic recoil, relaxation, or compliance, but rather represent the directional tissue velocity resulting from the complex interplay of these factors. The diastolic tissue Doppler pattern parallels the mitral inflow pattern with an early diastolic phase (E_M) and a late diastolic wave (A_M) corresponding to the atrial filling wave (Fig. 15-18). However, the determinants of tissue motion are somewhat different from the determinants of flow. Long-axis tissue motion as measured from an apically positioned transducer position manifests an early diastolic tissue Doppler wave during the acceleration phase of the early inflow wave, and a late diastolic tissue Doppler wave during the acceleration phase of the late inflow wave (Fig. 15-18). Although late diastolic tissue motion is passive, and therefore relates closely to filling in response to atrial contraction, E_M reportedly correlates with the time constant of relaxation and is relatively independent of left atrial pressure.[146,147] For this reason, E_M has been considered a surrogate index for t,[148] whereas the ratio of the peak early transmitral flow velocity (E) to the peak early myocardial tissue velocity (E/E_M) predicts filling pressure.[149]

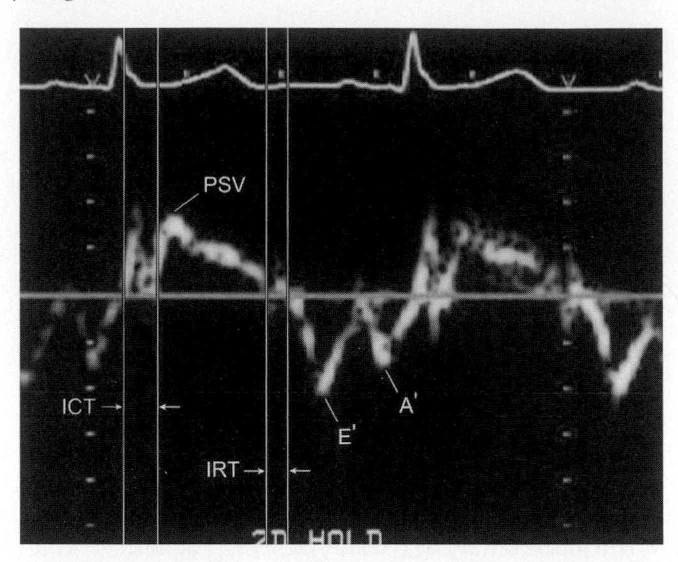

FIGURE 15–18 *Example of tissue Doppler from the lateral mitral valve annulus sampled from an apical window. Isovolumic contraction time (ICT) is characterized by biphasic motion, first toward the apex and then away. Motion during systole is exclusively directed toward the apex, usually with peak velocity (PSV) early in systole. During isovolumic relaxation time (IRT), the ICT motion is reversed, with motion initially away from the apex followed by motion toward the apex. There are usually two distinct apically directed peaks during diastole, one early in diastole (E′) and one following atrial contraction (A′).*

Clinical Interpretation of Noninvasive Diastolic Indices. Despite intense investigation, the debate as to the meaning of Doppler-based diastolic indices persists.[150] This dilemma is in part a consequence of a limited ability to discern myocardial from ventricular diastolic properties. Additionally, verification of the physiologic significance of the Doppler indices has been in large measure based on correlation analysis, which demonstrates association but not causation. The primary limitation of correlation analysis is the potential failure to recognize the primary role played by covariants. As recently reviewed by Maurer et al.,[143] the filling abnormalities demonstrated by Doppler echocardiography are primarily a manifestation of elevated left atrial pressure and do not directly reflect intrinsic myocardial abnormalities. The predictive capacity of the Doppler indices for the diagnosis of impaired ventricular compliance is determined by the degree to which the elevation in filling pressure is secondary to abnormalities in ventricular compliance.

Regardless of whether a causal relation exists, impaired compliance is commonly accompanied by elevated filling pressure because there is colinearity between filling pressure, ventricular compliance, and filling dynamics. However, abnormal filling pressure, although an important contributor to clinical status, is an extremely unreliable index of intrinsic myocardial properties because of its dependence on a myriad of confounding factors and the ease with which it is modified by therapeutic interventions. Thus, the validity of these indices in the assessment of myocardial diastolic properties is questionable.

One of the important areas of clinical application of the Doppler-derived indices of diastolic function has been in the adult population with diastolic heart failure, so called *heart failure with a normal ejection fraction*.[150,151] This clinical syndrome of congestive heart failure with preserved systolic function accounts for a significant percentage of heart failure in older adults, but is very uncommon in children and young adults. Causes include left ventricular diastolic dysfunction; valvular heart diseases such as mitral stenosis; pericardial diseases such as tamponade; and volume overload situations such as severe anemia. It is desirable to detect abnormalities of diastolic dysfunction secondary to cardiomyopathy (hypertrophic, restrictive, and infiltrative disorders); for purposes of disease diagnosis and for treatment optimization. The sensitivity and specificity of the noninvasive indices of diastolic function have not been critically evaluated in this population, particularly in the pediatric population, significantly limiting the confidence with which they can be used.

REFERENCES

1. Ross Jr. J. Afterload mismatch and preload reserve: A conceptual framework for the analysis of ventricular function. Prog Cardiovasc Dis 18:255, 1976.
2. Weber KT, Janicki JS, Hunter WC, et al. The contractile behavior of the heart and its functional coupling to the circulation. Prog Cardiovasc Dis 24:375, 1982.
3. Elzinga G, Westerhof N. How to quantify pump function of the heart. The value of variables derived from measurements on isolated muscle. Circ Res 44:303, 1979.
4. Braunwald E, Ross Jr. J. Control of cardiac performance. In Berne RM, Sperclakis N, Geiger SR, (eds). Handbook of Physiology, 2: The Cardiovascular System, vol. 1. Baltimore: Williams & Wilkins, 1979, pp 533–580.
5. Colan SD, Sanders SP, Ingelfinger JR, et al. Left ventricular mechanics and contractile state in children and young adults with end-stage renal disease: effect of dialysis and renal transplantation. J Am Coll Cardiol 10:1085, 1987.
6. Gentles TL, Sanders SP, Colan SD. Misrepresentation of left ventricular contractile function by endocardial indexes: clinical implications after coarctation repair. Am Heart J 140: 585, 2000.
7. Wachtell K, Papademetriou V, Smith G, et al. Relation of impaired left ventricular filling to systolic midwall mechanics in hypertensive patients with normal left ventricular systolic chamber function: The Losartan Intervention for Endpoint Reduction in Hypertension (LIFE) study. Am Heart J 148: 538, 2004.
8. Dong SJ. Midwall fractional shortening in physiologic and pathologic left ventricular hypertrophy. Am J Hypertens 16:792, 2003.
9. Moran AM, Friehs I, Takeuchi K, et al. Noninvasive serial evaluation of myocardial mechanics in pressure overload hypertrophy of rabbit myocardium. Herz 28:52, 2003.
10. Van der Toorn A, Barenbrug P, Snoep G, et al. Transmural gradients of cardiac myofiber shortening in aortic valve stenosis patients using MRI tagging. Am J Physiol Heart Circ Physiol 283:H1609, 2002.
11. Moulton MJ, Creswell LL, Downing SW, et al. Spline surface interpolation for calculating 3-D ventricular strains from MRI tissue tagging. Am J Physiol Heart Circ Physiol 270:H281, 1996.
12. Walker RE, Moran AM, Gauvreau K, et al. Evidence of adverse ventricular interdependence in patients with atrial septal defects. Am J Cardiol 93:1374, 2004.
13. Verdecchia P, Schillaci G, Reboldi G, et al. Prognostic value at midwall shortening fraction and its relation with left ventricular mass in systemic hypertension. Am J Cardiol 87:479, 2001.
14. Appleton CP, Hatle LK, Popp RL. Demonstration of restrictive ventricular physiology by Doppler echocardiography. J Am Coll Cardiol 11:757, 1988.
15. Hunter WC. End-systolic pressure as a balance between opposing effects of ejection. Circ Res 64:265, 1989.
16. Konhilas JP, Irving TC, De Tombe PP. Frank-Starling law of the heart and the cellular mechanisms of length-dependent activation. Pflugers Arch Eur J Physiol 445:305, 2002.
17. Reyes M, Freeman GL, Escobedo D, et al. Enhancement of contractility with sustained afterload in the intact murine heart: blunting of length-dependent activation. Circulation 107:2962, 2003.
18. Lang RM, Borow KM, Neumann A, et al. Systemic vascular resistance: an unreliable index of left ventricular afterload. Circulation 74:1114, 1986.
19. Huisman RM, Elzinga G, Westerhof N, et al. Measurement of left ventricular wall stress. Cardiovasc Res 14:142, 1980.
20. Lunkenheimer PP, Redmann K, Florek J, et al. The forces generated within the musculature of the left ventricular wall. Heart 90:200, 2004.
21. Huisman RM, Sipkema P, Westerhof N, et al. Comparison of models used to calculate left ventricular wall force. Med Biol Eng Comput 18:133, 1980.
22. Colan SD, Borow KM, Neumann A. Use of the calibrated carotid pulse tracing for calculation of left ventricular pressure and wall stress throughout ejection. Am Heart J 109:1306, 1985.
23. Colan SD, Borow KM, MacPherson D, et al. Use of the indirect axillary pulse tracing for noninvasive determination of ejection time, upstroke time, and left ventricular wall stress throughout ejection in infants and young children. Am J Cardiol 53:1154, 1984.

24. Colan SD, Fujii A, Borow KM, et al. Noninvasive determination of systolic, diastolic and end-systolic blood pressure in neonates, infants and young children: comparison with central aortic pressure measurements. Am J Cardiol 52:867, 1983.
25. Borow KM, Colan SD, Neumann A. Altered left ventricular mechanics in patients with valvular aortic stenosis and coarctation of the aorta: effects on systolic performance and late outcome. Circulation 72:515, 1985.
26. Sholler GF, Colan SD, Sanders SP, et al. Noninvasive estimation of the left ventricular pressure waveform throughout ejection in young patients with aortic stenosis. J Am Coll Cardiol 12:492, 1988.
27. Latham RD, Rubal BJ, Sipkema P, et al. Ventricular/vascular coupling and regional arterial dynamics in the chronically hypertensive baboon: Correlation with cardiovascular structural adaptation. Circ Res 63:798, 1988.
28. Suga H, Goto Y, Nozawa T, et al. Force-time integral decreases with ejection despite constant oxygen consumption and pressure-volume area in dog left ventricle. Circ Res 60: 797, 1987.
29. Laskey WK, Reichek N, St John Sutton M, et al. Matching of myocardial oxygen consumption to mechanical load in human left ventricular hypertrophy and dysfunction. J Am Coll Cardiol 3:291, 1984.
30. Colan SD, Sanders SP, Borow KM. Physiologic hypertrophy: effects on left ventricular systolic mechanics in athletes. J Am Coll Cardiol 9:776, 1987.
31. Aoyagi T, Fujii AM, Flanagan MF, et al. Transition from compensated hypertrophy to intrinsic myocardial dysfunction during development of left ventricular pressure-overload hypertrophy in conscious sheep. Systolic dysfunction precedes diastolic dysfunction. Circulation 88:2415, 1993.
32. Boutin C, Jonas RA, Sanders SP, et al. Rapid two-stage arterial switch operation: Acquisition of left ventricular mass after pulmonary artery banding in infants with transposition of the great arteries. Circulation 90:1304, 1994.
33. Van Empel VPM, De Windt LJ. Myocyte hypertrophy and apoptosis: a balancing act. Cardiovasc Res 63:487, 2004.
34. Sonnenblick EH. Instantaneous force-velocity-length determinant in contraction of heart muscle. Circ Res 16:441, 1965.
35. Huntsman LL, Rondinone JF, Martyn DA. Force-length relations in cardiac muscle segments. Am J Physiol 244: H701, 1983.
36. Suga H. Cardiac energetics: from E(max) to pressure-volume area. Clin Exp Pharmacol Physiol 30:580, 2003.
37. Suga H, Kitabatake A, Sagawa K. End-systolic pressure determines stroke volume from fixed end-diastolic volume in the isolated canine left ventricle under a constant contractile state. Circ Res 44:238, 1979.
38. Landesberg A. End-systolic pressure-volume relationship and intracellular control of contraction. Am J Physiol Heart Circ Physiol 270:H338, 1996.
39. Van der Velde ET, Burkhoff D, Steendijk P, et al. Nonlinearity and load sensitivity of end-systolic pressure-volume relation of canine left ventricle in vivo. Circulation 83:315, 1991.
40. Lakatta EG. Starling law of the heart is explained by an intimate interaction of muscle length and myofilament calcium activation. J Am Coll Cardiol 10:1157, 1987.
41. Sugiura S, Hunter WC, Sagawa K. Long-term versus intrabeat history of ejection as determinants of canine ventricular end-systolic pressure. Circ Res 64:255, 1989.
42. Kass DA, Beyar R, Lankford E, et al. Influence of contractile state on curvilinearity of in situ end-systolic pressure-volume relations. Circulation 79:167, 1989.
43. Baan J, Van der Velde ET. Sensitivity of left ventricular end-systolic pressure-volume relation to type of loading intervention in dogs. Circ Res 62:1247, 1988.
44. Regen DM. Myocardial stress equations: fiberstresses of the prolate spheroid. J Theor Biol 109:191, 1984.
45. Regen DM. Calculation of left ventricular wall stress. Circ Res 67:245, 1990.
46. Arts T, Bovendeerd PHM, Prinzen FW, et al. Relation between left ventricular cavity pressure and volume and systolic fiber stress and strain in the wall. Biophys J 59:93, 1991.
47. Gentles TL, Colan SD. Wall stress misrepresents afterload in children and young adults with abnormal left ventricular geometry. J Appl Physiol 92:1053, 2002.
48. Suga H, Sagawa K. Instantaneous pressure-volume relationships and their ratio in the excised, supported canine left ventricle. Circ Res 35:117, 1974.
49. Suga H, Sagawa K, Shoukas AA. Load independence of the instantaneous pressure-volume ratio of the canine left ventricle and effects of epinephrine and heart rate on the ratio. Circ Res 32:314, 1973.
50. Takaoka H, Suga H, Goto Y, et al. Cardiodynamic conditions for the linearity of preload recruitable stroke work. Heart Vessels 10:57, 1995.
51. Tanaka N, Nozawa T, Yasumura Y, et al. Oxygen consumption for constant work is minimal at lowest working contractility in normal dog hearts. Jpn J Physiol 43:627, 1993.
52. Taylor RR, Covell JW, Ross JJr. Volume-tension diagrams of ejecting and isovolumic contractions in left ventricle. Am J Physiol 216:1097, 1969.
53. Mirsky I, Tajimi T, Peterson KL. The development of the entire end-systolic pressure-volume and ejection fraction-afterload relations: a new concept of systolic myocardial stiffness. Circulation 76:343, 1987.
54. Su JB, Crozatier B. Preload-induced curvilinearity of left ventricular end-systolic pressure-volume relations: Effects on derived indexes in closed-chest dogs. Circulation 79:431, 1989.
55. Little WC, Cheng C-P, Peterson T, et al. Response of the left ventricular end-systolic pressure-volume relation in conscious dogs to a wide range of contractile states. Circulation 78: 736, 1988.
56. Burkhoff D, Sugiura S, Yue DT, et al. Contractility-dependent curvilinearity of end-systolic pressure-volume relations. Am J Physiol 252:H1218, 1987.
57. Spratt JA, Tyson GS, Glower DD, et al. The end-systolic pressure-volume relationship in conscious dogs. Circulation 75:1295, 1987.
58. Maughan WL, Sunagawa K, Sagawa K. Effects of arterial input impedance on mean ventricular pressure-flow relation. Am J Physiol 247:H978, 1984.
59. Freeman GL, Little WC, O'Rourke RA. The effect of vasoactive agents on the left ventricular end-systolic pressure-volume relation in closed-chest dogs. Circulation 74:1107, 1986.

60. Crottogini AJ, Willshaw P, Barra JG, et al. Inconsistency of the slope and the volume intercept of the end-systolic pressure-volume relationship as individual indexes of inotropic state in conscious dogs: presentation of an index combining both variables. Circulation 76:1115, 1987.
61. Suga H, Hisano R, Goto Y, et al. Normalization of end-systolic pressure-volume relation and Emax of different sized hearts. Jpn Circ J 48:136, 1984.
62. Belcher P, Boerboom LE, Olinger GN. Standardization of end-systolic pressure-volume relation in the dog. Am J Physiol 249:H547, 1985.
63. Davidson DM, Covell JW, Malloch CI, et al. Factors influencing indices of left ventricle contractility in the conscious dog. Cardiovasc Res 8:299, 1974.
64. Little WC. The left ventricular dP/dtmax-end diastolic volume relation in closed-chest dogs. Circ Res 56:808, 1985.
65. Feneley MP, Skelton TN, Kisslo KB, et al. Comparison of preload recruitable stroke work, end-systolic pressure-volume and dP/dt_{max}-end-diastolic volume relations as indexes of left ventricular contractile performance in patients undergoing routine cardiac catheterization. J Am Coll Cardiol 19:1522, 1992.
66. Rahko PS. Comparative efficacy of three indexes of left ventricular performance derived from pressure-volume loops in heart failure induced by tachypacing. J Am Coll Cardiol 23:209, 1994.
67. Karunanithi MK, Michniewicz J, Copeland SE, et al. Right ventricular preload recruitable stroke work, end-systolic pressure-volume, and dP/dt_{max}-end-diastolic volume relations compared as indexes of right ventricular contractile performance in conscious dogs. Circ Res 70:1169, 1992.
68. Little WC, Cheng C-P, Mumma M, et al. Comparison of measures of left ventricular contractile performance derived from pressure-volume loops in conscious dogs. Circulation 80:1378, 1989.
69. Lester SJ, Shin H, Lambert AS, et al. Is PA-PWRmax truly a preload-independent index of myocardial contractility in anesthetized humans? Cardiology 102:77, 2004.
70. Kass DA, Beyar R. Evaluation of contractile state by maximal ventricular power divided by the square of end-diastolic volume. Circulation 84:1698, 1991.
71. Schenk S, Popovic ZB, Ochiai Y, et al. Preload-adjusted right ventricular maximal power: concept and validation. Am J Physiol Heart Circ Physiol 287:H1632, 2004.
72. Colan SD, Borow KM, Neumann A. Left ventricular end-systolic wall stress-velocity of fiber shortening relation: a load-independent index of myocardial contractility. J Am Coll Cardiol 4:715, 1984.
73. Lang RM, Fellner SK, Neumann A, et al. Left ventricular contractility varies directly with the blood ionized calcium. Ann Intern Med 108:524, 1988.
74. Lang RM, Borow KM, Neumann A, et al. Role of the $beta_2$ adrenoceptor in mediating positive inotropic activity in the failing heart and its relation to the hemodynamic actions of dopexamine hydrochloride. Am J Cardiol 62(Suppl 5):46C, 1988.
75. Lang RM, Borow KM, Neumann A, et al. Adverse cardiac effects of acute alcohol ingestion in young adults. Ann Intern Med 102:742, 1985.
76. Hori M, Yellin EL, Sonnenblick EH. Left ventricular diastolic suction as a mechanism of ventricular filling. Jpn Circ J 46: 124, 1982.
77. Graham TP, Franklin RC, Wyse RK, et al. Left ventricular wall stress and contractile function in transposition of the great arteries after the Rastelli operation. J Thorac Cardiovasc Surg 93:775, 1987.
78. Graham TP, Jr., Franklin RCG, Wyse RKH, et al. Left ventricular wall stress and contractile function in childhood: normal values and comparison of Fontan repair versus palliation only in patients with tricuspid atresia. Circulation 74:I-61, 1986.
79. Feldman T, Borow KM, Sarne DH, et al. Myocardial mechanics in hyperthyroidism: importance of left ventricular loading conditions, heart rate and contractile state. J Am Coll Cardiol 7:967, 1986.
80. Colan SD, Trowitzsch E, Wernovsky G, et al. Myocardial performance after arterial switch operation for transposition of the great arteries with intact ventricular septum. Circulation 78:132, 1988.
81. Colan SD. Noninvasive assessment of myocardial mechanics: a review of analysis of stress-shortening and stress-velocity. Cardiol Young 2:1, 1992.
82. Holzman RS, Van der Velde ME, Kaus SJ, et al. Sevoflurane depresses myocardial contractility less than halothane during induction of anesthesia in children. Anesthesiology 85:1260, 1996.
83. Williams RV, Lorenz JN, Witt SA, et al. End-systolic stress-velocity and pressure-dimension relationships by transthoracic echocardiography in mice. Am J Physiol Heart Circ Physiol 274:H1828, 1998.
84. Boutin C, Wernovsky G, Sanders SP, et al. Rapid two-stage arterial switch operation: evaluation of left ventricular systolic mechanics after an acute pressure overload stimulus in infancy. Circulation 90:1294, 1994.
85. Colan SD, Parness IA, Spevak PJ, et al. Developmental modulation of myocardial mechanics: age- and growth-related alterations in afterload and contractility. J Am Coll Cardiol 19:619, 1992.
86. Colan SD. Mechanics of left ventricular systolic and diastolic function in physiologic hypertrophy of the athlete heart. Cardiol Clin 10:227, 1992.
87. Fishberger SB, Colan SD, Saul JP, et al. Myocardial mechanics before and after ablation of chronic tachycardia. Pacing Clin Electrophysiol 19:42, 1996.
88. Gentles TL, Colan SD, Wilson NJ, et al. Left ventricular mechanics during and after acute rheumatic fever: Contractile dysfunction is closely related to valve regurgitation. J Am Coll Cardiol 37:201, 2001.
89. Lipshultz SE, Easley KA, Orav EJ, et al. Cardiac dysfunction and mortality in HIV-infected children: the prospective P^2C^2HIV multicenter study. Circulation 102:1542, 2000.
90. Lipshultz SE, Colan SD, Gelber RD, et al. Late cardiac effects of Doxorubicin therapy for acute lymphoblastic leukemia in childhood. N Engl J Med 324:808, 1991.
91. Lipshultz SE, Easley KA, Orav EJ, et al. Left ventricular structure and function in children infected with human immunodeficiency virus - The prospective P^2C^2 HIV multicenter study. Circulation 97:1246, 1998.

92. Moran AM, Newburger JW, Sanders SP, et al. Abnormal myocardial mechanics in Kawasaki disease: Rapid response to gamma-globulin. Am Heart J 139:217, 2000.
93. Moran AM, Lipshultz SE, Rifai N, et al. Non-invasive assessment of rejection in pediatric transplant patients: serologic and echocardiographic prediction of biopsy-proven myocardial rejection. J Heart Lung Transplant 19:756, 2000.
94. Schwartz ML, Jonas RA, Colan SD. Anomalous origin of left coronary artery from pulmonary artery: Recovery of left ventricular function after dual coronary repair. J Am Coll Cardiol 30:547, 1997.
95. Sluysmans T, Sanders SP, van der Velde M, et al. Natural history and patterns of recovery of contractile function in single left ventricle after Fontan operation. Circulation 86: 1753, 1992.
96. Rumberger JA, Weiss RM, Feiring AJ, et al. Patterns of regional diastolic function in the normal human left ventricle: An ultrafast computed tomographic study. J Am Coll Cardiol 14:119, 1989.
97. Quinones MA, Gaasch WH, Alexander JK. Influence of acute changes in preload, afterload, contractile state and heart rate on ejection and isovolumic indices of myocardial contractility in man. Circulation 53:293, 1976.
98. Nixon JV, Murray RG, Leonard PD, et al. Effect of large variations in preload on left ventricular performance characteristics in normal subjects. Circulation 65:698, 1982.
99. Mahler F, Ross J, O'Rourke RA, et al. Effects of changes in preload, afterload, and inotropic state on ejection and isovolumic phase measures of contractility in the conscious dog. Am J Cardiol 35:626, 1975.
100. Gunther S, Grossman W. Determinants of ventricular function in pressure-overload hypertrophy in man. Circulation 59:679, 1979.
101. Schulman DS, Remetz MS, Elefteriades J, et al. Mild mitral insufficiency is a marker of impaired left ventricular performance in aortic stenosis. J Am Coll Cardiol 13:796, 1989.
102. Carabello BA, Green LH, Grossman W, et al. Hemodynamic determinants of prognosis of aortic valve replacement in critical aortic stenosis and advanced congestive heart failure. Circulation 62:42, 1980.
103. Parker JO, Case RB. Normal left ventricular function. Circulation 60:4, 1979.
104. Poliner LR, Dehmer GJ, Lewis SE, et al. Left ventricular performance in normal subjects: a comparison of the responses to exercise in the upright and supine positions. Circulation 62:528, 1980.
105. Ross JJr. Mechanism of cardiac contraction. What roles for preload, afterload, and inotropic state in heart failure. Eur Heart J 4(Supp A):19, 1983.
106. Mirsky I, Corin WJ, Murakami T, et al. Correction for preload in assessment of myocardial contractility in aortic and mitral valve disease: Application of the concept of systolic myocardial stiffness. Circulation 78:68, 1988.
107. Maroto E, Fouron JC, Douste-Blazy MY, et al. Influence of age on wall thickness, cavity dimensions, and myocardial contractility of the left ventricle in simple transposition of the great arteries. Circulation 67:1311, 1983.
108. Hoit BD, Lew WYW, LeWinter M. Regional variation in pericardial contact pressure in the canine ventricle. Am J Physiol 255:H1370, 1988.
109. Ross J, Jr. Is there a true increase in myocardial stiffness with acute ischemia. Am J Cardiol 63:87E, 1989.
110. Nakamura Y, Sasayama S, Nonogi H, et al. Alterations in left ventricular relaxation, early diastolic filling and passive viscoelastic properties during postpacing ischemia. Am J Cardiol 63:72E, 1989.
111. Greenberg MA, Menegus MA. Ischemia-induced diastolic dysfunction: New observations, new questions. J Am Coll Cardiol 13:1071, 1989.
112. Katz AM. Sarcoplasmic reticular control of cardiac contraction and relaxation. In Grossman W, Lorell BH, (eds). Diastolic Relaxation of the Heart. Boston: Martinus Nijhoff, 1988, pp 11–16.
113. Nayler WG, Williams AJ. Relaxation in the mammalian heart muscle: some ultrastructural and biochemical considerations. Fourth Workshop on Contractile Behavior of the Heart, Utrecht, The Netherlands, 4–6 Sept. Eur J Cardiol 7(Suppl):35, 1978.
114. Langer GA. Ion fluxes in cardiac excitation and contraction and their relation to myocardial contractility. Physiol Rev 48:708, 1968.
115. Shapiro B, Marier DL, St. John Sutton MG, et al. Regional non-uniformity of wall dynamics in normal left ventricle. Br Heart J 45:264, 1981.
116. Lew WYW, LeWinter MM. Regional circumferential lengthening patterns in canine left ventricle. Am J Physiol 245:H741, 1983.
117. Tham EB, Silverman NH. Measurement of the Tei index: a comparison of M-mode and pulse Doppler methods. J Am Soc Echocardiogr 17:1259, 2004.
118. Starling MR, Montgomery DG, Mancini J, et al. Load independence of the rate of isovolumic relaxation in man. Circulation 76:1274, 1987.
119. Lew WYW, Rasmussen CM. Influence of nonuniformity on rate of left ventricular pressure fall in the dog. Am J Physiol 256:H222, 1989.
120. Kumada T, Katayama K, Matsuzaki M, et al. Usefulness of negative dP/dt upstroke pattern for assessment of left ventricular relaxation in coronary artery disease. Am J Cardiol 63: 60E, 1989.
121. Bonow RO, Vitale DF, Bacharach SL, et al. Effects of aging on asynchronous left ventricular regional function and global ventricular filling in normal human subjects. J Am Coll Cardiol 11:50, 1988.
122. Winegrad S. Regulation of cardiac contractile proteins: correlation between physiology and biochemistry. Circ Res 55:565, 1984.
123. Pan BS, Howe ER, Solaro J. Calcium binding to troponin-C in loaded and unloaded myofilaments of chemically skinned heart muscle preparations. Fed Proc 42:574, 1983.
124. Housemans PR, Lee NKM, Blinks JR. Active shortening retards the decline of the intracellular calcium transient in mammalian heart muscle. Science 221:159, 1983.
125. Balfour IC, Covitz W, Arensman FW, et al. Left ventricular filling in sickle cell anemia. Am J Cardiol 61:395, 1988.

126. Yellin EL, Hori M, Yoran C, et al. Left ventricular relaxation in the filling and nonfilling intact canine heart. Am J Physiol 250:H620, 1986.
127. Suga H, Goto Y, Igarashi Y, et al. Ventricular suction under zero source pressure for filling. Am J Physiol 251:H47, 1986.
128. Nikolic S, Yellin EL, Tamura K, et al. Passive properties of canine left ventricle: Diastolic stiffness and restoring forces. Circ Res 62:1210, 1988.
129. Caillet D, Crozatier B. Role of myocardial restoring forces in the determination of early diastolic peak velocity of fibre lengthening in the concious dog. Cardiovasc Res 16:107, 1982.
130. Suga H, Sagawa K, Kostiuk DP. Controls of ventricular contractility assessed by pressure-volume ratio, Emax. Cardiovasc Res 10:582, 1976.
131. Gilbert JC, Glantz SA. Determinants of left ventricular filling and of the diastolic pressure-volume relation. Circ Res 64: 827, 1989.
132. Nakamura T, Abe H, Arai S, et al. The stress-strain relationship of the diastolic cardiac muscle and left ventricular compliance in the pressure-overload canine heart. Jpn Circ J 46: 76, 1982.
133. Mirsky I. Assessment of diastolic function: suggested methods and future considerations. Circulation 69:836, 1984.
134. Smiseth OA, Frais MA, Kingma I, et al. Assessment of pericardial constraint: the relation between right ventricular filling pressure and pericardial pressure measured after pericardiocentesis. J Am Coll Cardiol 7:307, 1986.
135. Tyberg JV, Taichman GC, Smith ER, et al. The relationship between pericardial pressure and right atrial pressure: an intraoperative study. Circulation 73:428, 1986.
136. Pasipoularides A, Mirsky I, Hess OM, et al. Myocardial relaxation and passive diastolic properties in man. Circulation 74:991, 1986.
137. Brutsaert DL, Rademakers FE, Sys SU. Triple control of relaxation: implications in cardiac disease. Circulation 69: 190, 1984.
138. Stoddard MF, Pearson AC, Kern MJ, et al. Left ventricular diastolic function: Comparison of pulsed Doppler echocardiographic and hemodynamic indexes in subjects with and without coronary artery disease. J Am Coll Cardiol 13:327, 1989.
139. Norman A, Thomas N, Coakley J, et al. Distinction of Becker from limb-girdle muscular dystrophy by means of dystrophin cDNA probes. Lancet 1:466, 1989.
140. Courtois M, Kovács SJ, Jr., Ludbrook PA. Transmitral pressure-flow velocity relation: Importance of regional pressure gradients in the left ventricle during diastole. Circulation 78:661, 1988.
141. Nishimura RA, Tajik AJ. Evaluation of diastolic filling of left ventricle in health and disease: Doppler echocardiography is the clinician's rosetta stone. J Am Coll Cardiol 30:8, 1997.
142. Garcia MJ, Thomas JD, Klein AL. New Doppler echocardiographic applications for the study of diastolic function. J Am Coll Cardiol 32:865, 1998.
143. Maurer MS, Spevack D, Burkhoff D, et al. Diastolic dysfunction: can it be diagnosed by Doppler echocardiography? J Am Coll Cardiol 44:1543, 2004.
144. Garcia MJ, Smedira NG, Greenberg NL, et al. Color M-mode Doppler flow propagation velocity is a preload insensitive index of left ventricular relaxation: animal and human validation. J Am Coll Cardiol 35:201, 2000.
145. Brun P, Tribouilloy C, Duval A-M, et al. Left ventricular flow propagation during early filling is related to wall relaxation: A color M-mode Doppler analysis. J Am Coll Cardiol 20:420, 1992.
146. Oki T, Tabata T, Yamada H, et al. Clinical application of pulsed Doppler tissue imaging for assessing abnormal left ventricular relaxation. Am J Cardiol 79:921, 1997.
147. Hung KC, Huang HL, Chu CM, et al. Evaluating preload dependence of a novel Doppler application in assessment of left ventricular diastolic function during hemodialysis. Am J Kidney Dis 43:1040, 2004.
148. Kato T, Noda A, Izawa H, et al. Myocardial velocity gradient as a noninvasively determined index of left ventricular diastolic dysfunction in patients with hypertrophic cardiomyopathy. J Am Coll Cardiol 42:278, 2003.
149. Nagueh SF, Middleton KJ, Kopelen HA, et al. Doppler tissue imaging: A noninvasive technique for evaluation of left ventricular relaxation and estimation of filling pressures. J Am Coll Cardiol 30:1527, 1997.
150. Burkhoff D, Maurer MS, Packer M. Heart failure with a normal ejection fraction - Is it really a disorder of diastolic function? Circulation 107:656, 2003.
151. Gaasch WH, Zile MR. Left ventricular diastolic dysfunction and diastolic heart failure. Ann Rev Med 55:373, 2004.

16

Exercise Testing

JONATHAN RHODES, MD

The primary task of the cardiopulmonary system is to provide blood flow (and oxygen) in quantities sufficient to support the metabolic needs of the body. This system is maximally stressed when the body's metabolic rate is increased, a condition that occurs most commonly during physical activity or exercise. Most of the clinical tests used by the pediatric cardiologist assess the cardiopulmonary system when the patient is at rest, lying on a table. Although valuable, these tests do not necessarily predict the manner in which the cardiopulmonary system will respond to the demands of exercise, nor do they reliably inform the clinician regarding a patient's true capacity to perform physical activities.[1] Conclusions based on a patient's (or a patient's family's) subjective account of his or her exercise function are also unreliable, as these reports can often be distorted and misleading.[2] Formal exercise testing, however, provides physicians with an opportunity to gain valuable, objective insights into these and other clinically important aspects of a patient's cardiopulmonary function.

PHYSIOLOGY OF EXERCISE

Interpretation of exercise data, and an appreciation of the capabilities of this technology, requires an understanding of the physiology of exercise and the mechanisms by which the cardiovascular system normally meets the metabolic demands of exercise. This chapter will therefore begin with a review of some basic exercise physiology.

The energy required to perform the mechanical work of exercise is derived from the hydrolysis of adenosine triphosphate (ATP). At rest, skeletal muscle possesses only limited quantities of ATP and other high-energy phosphate molecules. If exercise is to be continued for more than a brief period of time, ATP must be continually replenished through the metabolism of fuels (e.g., fats and carbohydrates). The aerobic metabolism of fuels produces large quantities of ATP per molecule of substrate, but requires an adequate supply of oxygen. This oxygen must be delivered to the exercising skeletal muscle by the cardiovascular system. The mechanisms by which the cardiovascular system delivers oxygen to the skeletal muscles are best understood from consideration of the Fick equation:

$$\begin{aligned} \acute{\upsilon}_{O2} &= [\text{C.O.}] \times [\text{oxygen extraction}] \\ &= [\text{HR} \times \text{SV}] \times [C_aO_2 - C_vO_2] \\ &= [\text{HR} \times \text{SV}] \times [1.36(\text{Hgb})(S_aO_2 - S_vO_2)] \end{aligned}$$

($\acute{\upsilon}_{O2}$: oxygen consumption; C.O.: cardiac output; HR: heart rate; SV: stroke volume; C_aO_2: arterial oxygen content; C_vO_2: venous oxygen content; Hgb: hemoglobin concentration; S_aO_2: arterial oxygen saturation; S_vO_2: venous oxygen saturation)

Normally, during exercise, each of these variables is altered so as to maximize oxygen delivery.

Heart Rate

During exercise, heart rate rises up to threefold from resting values of 60 to 80 bpm to ~200 bpm at peak exercise.[3,4] This rise is mediated primarily by the autonomic nervous system via an increase in sympathetic activity and a reduction in parasympathetic activity.[5]

Stroke Volume

During a progressive upright exercise test, stroke volume rises rapidly during the early phases of exercise and, at a relatively early point in the study, plateaus at a level one-and-a-half to two times greater than baseline.[6] (Thereafter, increases in cardiac output are due primarily to increases in heart rate.) The increase in stroke volume is mediated by (a) increased cardiac contractility secondary to increased adrenergic stimulation; (b) decreased afterload secondary to a dramatic decline in systemic and pulmonary vascular resistance during exercise; (c) enhanced ventricular filling secondary to the pumping action of the skeletal muscles;[7] and (d) improved lusitropic function.[8] Hence, peak exercise is typically associated with a five fold increase in cardiac output (HR × SV).

Oxygen Extraction

Normally, at rest, arterial oxygen saturation approaches 100% and mixed venous oxygen saturation is approximately 70%. Hence, the body extracts only 30% of the oxygen delivered to it. At peak exercise, however, the exercising muscles extract a much greater percentage of the oxygen delivered to them. Mixed venous oxygen saturation typically falls to less than 30% and total body oxygen extraction more than doubles at peak exercise.[9]

Hence from consideration of the Fick equation, it can be seen that the cardiovascular adaptations to exercise permit the oxygen consumption at peak exercise to increase more than 10-fold over resting values.

In addition to consuming oxygen, the aerobic metabolism of fuels produces carbon dioxide. For each carbon atom of glucose that is metabolized, one molecule of oxygen is consumed and one molecule of carbon dioxide is produced:

$$\text{H-C-OH} + O_2 \rightarrow H_2O + CO_2$$

(6 ATP generated/carbon atom)

The respiratory quotient (i.e., the stoichiometrically determined ratio of the number of moles of carbon dioxide produced in this chemical reaction divided by the number of moles of oxygen consumed by this reaction) is 1.0.

The aerobic metabolism of each carbon atom from the hydrocarbon chain of a free fatty acid consumes 1½ molecules of oxygen and produces one molecule of carbon dioxide:

$$\text{H-C-H} + 1\tfrac{1}{2}\,O_2 \rightarrow H_2O + CO_2$$

(8 ATP generated/carbon atom)

The respiratory quotient for this chemical reaction is 0.67.

Consequently, during aerobic metabolism, when a mixture of fats and carbohydrates are consumed, the respiratory exchange ratio (RER; the ratio of the *measured* carbon dioxide production divided by the *measured* oxygen consumption) is typically approximately 0.80 (i.e., between 0.67 and 1.0).

Although the aerobic metabolism of fuels produces large quantities of ATP, the amount of ATP that a muscle cell may derive from aerobic metabolism is limited by the amount of oxygen that is delivered to the cell. As the intensity of exercise increases, the energy requirements of the muscle cell rise and may, if oxygen delivery is limited, ultimately exceed that which can be produced by aerobic metabolism. Under these circumstances, the muscle cell may begin to rely on anaerobic metabolism of glucose to provide a portion of its energy needs:

$$\underset{\text{glucose}}{C_6H_{12}O_6} \rightarrow \underset{\text{lactic acid}}{2(CH_3CHOHCOOH)}$$

(0.3 ATP generated/carbon atom)

Anaerobic metabolism does not produce as much ATP as aerobic metabolism, but it does not require oxygen. Anaerobic metabolism also produces lactic acid, which reacts with bicarbonate to produce carbon dioxide:

$$\underset{\text{lactic acid}}{CH_3CHOHCOOH} + \underset{\text{bicarbonate}}{HCO_3^-} \rightarrow \underset{\text{lactate}}{CH_3CHOHCOO^-} + H_2O + \underset{\text{carbon dioxide}}{CO_2}$$

Hence, when the muscles begin to rely on anaerobic metabolism to generate some of the ATP required to perform the mechanical work of exercise, serum lactate levels abruptly rise and an increase in carbon dioxide production, out of proportion to the concomitant increase in $\acute{\upsilon}_{O2}$, is observed. During a progressive exercise test, the point at which these phenomena are detected is called the lactate threshold or anaerobic threshold or, perhaps most appropriately when only expiratory gases are measured, the ventilatory anaerobic threshold. Although some controversy exists concerning the mechanisms and physiology that underlie it,[10,11] most exercise physiologists agree that the anaerobic threshold is a clinically useful and valid concept that informs our understanding of many of the phenomena encountered in the exercise physiology laboratory.[12–14]

The elimination of carbon dioxide is another important function of the cardiopulmonary system that may be maximally stressed during exercise. The mechanisms used by the lungs to excrete the large quantities of carbon dioxide produced during exercise are best understood from the alveolar ventilation equation:

$$\acute{\upsilon}_{CO2} = \acute{\upsilon}_A \times P_ACO_2/P_B$$

This equation states that the amount of carbon dioxide eliminated by the lungs ($\acute{\upsilon}_{CO2}$) is equal to the alveolar ventilation ($\acute{\upsilon}_A$, L/minute) times the partial pressure of carbon dioxide in the alveolar gas (P_ACO_2) divided by the barometric pressure (P_B). The alveolar ventilation is equal to the alveolar volume (V_A, the volume of air participating in gas exchange with each breath; l/breath) times the respiratory rate (RR; breaths per minute). Hence

$$\acute{\upsilon}_{CO2} = \acute{\upsilon}RR \times V_A \times P_ACO_2/P_B$$

However, V_A is equal to the tidal volume minus the volume of the physiologic dead space ($V_T - V_D$). Substituting this term for V_A yields:

$$\begin{aligned}\acute{\upsilon}_{CO2} &= RR \times (V_T - V_D) \times P_ACO_2/P_B \\ &= RR \times V_T\,(1 - V_D/V_T) \times P_ACO_2/P_B\end{aligned}$$

Under idealized conditions, the alveolar pCO_2 equals the arterial pCO_2 ($P_ACO_2 = PaCO_2$) and the equation may be rewritten:

$$\acute{\upsilon}_{CO2} = RR \times V_T(1 - V_D/V_T) \times PaCO_2/P_B$$

In a manner analogous to that encountered with regard to the delivery of oxygen, the physiologic variables of this equation are altered so as to optimize carbon dioxide elimination during exercise.

Respiratory Rate

During a progressive exercise test, a normal subject's respiratory rate rises slowly initially. During later, more intense stages of exercise, however, the respiratory rate rises more rapidly and, at peak exercise, may increase to more than three times resting values.[15]

Tidal Volume

During a progressive exercise test, tidal volume rises rapidly at first and, at a relatively early stage of exercise, tends to plateau at a level approximately three times greater than resting values.[15]

Dead Space/Tidal Volume Ratio

Anatomic dead space (i.e., the volume of air in the trachea, bronchi and other airways that does not participate in gas exchange) does not change appreciably during exercise. Physiologic dead space may actually decline secondary to improved matching of ventilation and perfusion. Hence, during exercise the dead space/tidal volume ratio falls rapidly (as tidal volume rises and dead space remains unchanged or declines slightly) and then levels off at a level one third to one half of the resting value.[15–17]

CENTRAL HEMODYNAMICS

It is instructive to consider the changes in central hemodynamics that occur during exercise, and the hemodynamic burdens that these changes impose upon the right and left ventricles. Invasive data concerning exercise-related changes in central hemodynamics are not available from children. However, data are available from normal young adult subjects. In these individuals systemic arterial pressure rises steeply as the intensity of exercise is increased. At peak exercise, systolic blood pressure typically exceeds resting values by 50% to 75%. In contrast, diastolic pressure changes little during exercise. Consequently, mean arterial pressure increases modestly, rising only 25% to 30% above resting values. The relatively modest rise in mean arterial pressure, despite the four- to fivefold increase in cardiac output that accompanies strenuous exercise, indicates that systemic vascular resistance falls dramatically during exercise, typically falling to levels 30% to 40% of resting values. Most of the fall in systemic vascular resistance is due to dilation of blood vessels in the exercising muscles and the cutaneous vascular beds.[18]

Left ventricular filling pressures also rise during exercise. At peak exercise, they may exceed resting values by 5 to 10 mm Hg, an increase of approximately 100%.[18]

In young adults, pulmonary artery systolic pressure rises progressively as the intensity of exercise is increased. Near peak exercise, pulmonary artery systolic pressures are typically 100% greater than resting values. Pulmonary artery diastolic pressures change little during exercise. Mean pulmonary artery pressures rise to levels approximately 10 mm Hg (~70%) above resting values. Almost all of the increase in mean pulmonary artery pressure is due to the rise in left-sided filling pressure. The transpulmonary gradient changes little during exercise, indicating that the four to fivefold increase in pulmonary blood flow during exercise is accompanied by an almost reciprocal fall in pulmonary vascular resistance.[18] This fall is mediated by dilation of pulmonary resistance vessels and by recruitment of pulmonary vascular beds that are normally closed or only partially perfused at rest.[19]

It can be seen from this analysis that the hemodynamic work performed by the left ventricle at peak exercise (pressure × flow) is more than six times greater than resting values. The hemodynamic work performed by the right ventricle increases even more dramatically (more than eightfold) during exercise. This observation has important implications for patients with congenital heart disease, in whom the right ventricle may be absent (as in patients with Fontan) or structurally abnormal (as in postoperative patients with tetralogy of Fallot).

The dramatic increase in ventricular work rate during exercise is supported by a concomitant increase in coronary blood flow during exercise, from values of 60 mL per minute per gram of tissue at rest to as much as 240 mL per minute per gram of tissue at peak exercise. This increase in coronary blood flow results from a decline in coronary vascular resistance and other factors related to the structure of the coronary vascular bed and its unique relationship to the myocardium.[20,21]

The myocardial blood supply during exercise may be compromised by congenital or acquired coronary artery lesions. It is also important to recall that coronary arterial blood flow occurs primarily during diastole.[21] Consequently, aortic regurgitation and diastolic run-off lesions (e.g., aortopulmonary shunting lesions) can compromise coronary perfusion by lowering diastolic blood pressure (and, therefore, coronary perfusion pressure).

CONDUCT OF AN EXERCISE TEST

The protocol chosen for an exercise test should be determined by the clinical questions that the test is to address. Table 16-1 lists some of the more common and important clinical questions that may be encountered in the exercise physiology laboratory. Most of these questions can be addressed with a bicycle or a treadmill ergometer. The relative advantages of these modalities are listed in Table 16-2. The most popular bicycle protocol (Fig. 16-1) is a *ramp* protocol. This protocol requires the subject to pedal at a rate of 60 rpm. After an initial 2- to 3-minute warm-up period during which the subject pedals against

TABLE 16–1. Important Clinical Questions That May Be Addressed in the Exercise Physiology Laboratory

What causes a patient to stop exercising? Is the patient limited by cardiovascular, respiratory, musculoskeletal, hematologic, metabolic, neurologic, emotional, or other factors?
If the patient's ability to exercise is limited by the function of his/her cardiovascular system, which cardiovascular factors are responsible for the limitation?
If the patient's ability to exercise is limited by respiratory or other factors, can the pathophysiologic processes responsible for the poor exercise function be identified more clearly?
How does the patient's condition compare to healthy subjects?
How does the patient's condition compare to his/her past status?
What interventions might improve his/her status?
How might the effectiveness of these interventions be assessed?
Does exercise pose any risk for this patient?
Can anything be done to minimize these risks?
How can the effectiveness of these risk-lowering strategies be assessed?

TABLE 16–2. Relative Advantages of Bicycle and Treadmill Ergometer

Bicycle	Treadmill
Easy to measure external work	Can achieve slightly higher peak VO_2 and peak heart rate and peak myocardial VO_2
External work performed relatively independent of patient size	May more closely simulate a patient's usual physical activities
Ramp protocols → easier to determine ventilatory anaerobic threshold	Can easily accommodate very small patients
Can more easily accommodate extremely fit individuals	
Less noisy → easier to determine blood pressure	
Less motion artifact on electrocardiogram	
Less risk of injury	
Less expensive	
Requires less space	

VO_2, oxygen consumption.

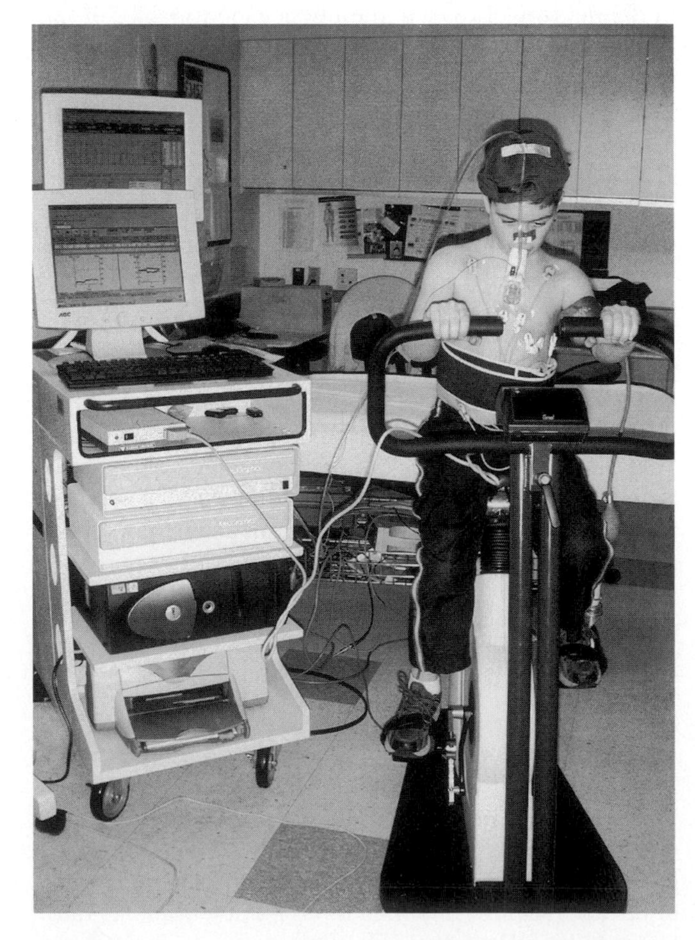

FIGURE 16–1 *A typical patient undergoing a bicycle ergometry stress test.*

TABLE 16–3. The Standard Bruce Protocol

Stage	Speed, mph	Grade, %	Duration, min
1	1.7	10	3
2	2.5	12	3
3	3.4	14	3
4	4.2	16	3
5	5.0	18	3
6	5.5	20	3
7	6.0	22	3

zero resistance, the resistance in the pedals is increased progressively at a constant rate until the 60 rpm pedaling rate can no longer be maintained. The rate at which the resistance is increased is selected so that the subject will reach peak exercise after about 10 minutes.[22] The most popular treadmill protocol is the *Bruce protocol* (Table 16-3). In this protocol, the treadmill speed and elevation are increased by standardized, predetermined amounts every 3 minutes, until the subject can go no further or the desired information has been acquired.[23] The standard Bruce protocol has only seven stages and is therefore not ideal for extremely fit individuals whose exercise capacity exceeds that required to complete the seventh stage. Baseline (and sometimes postexercise) spirometric measurements are also commonly obtained at the time of exercise testing, as these measurements often aid in the interpretation of the exercise physiology data.

In general, for patients with congenital heart disease, the most relevant questions addressed in the exercise physiology laboratory are those related to exercise capacity and the cardiopulmonary response to exercise. At Children's Hospital Boston, we find that the advantages of the bicycle ergometer ramp protocol generally render this modality preferable for these purposes. In cases where issues relating to myocardial perfusion/ischemia are of paramount importance, treadmill protocols are often preferable because of the slightly higher myocardial oxygen consumption that may be achieved with a treadmill ergometer. Treadmill protocols may at times also be preferable when assessing a patient for exercise-related symptoms, as they may more closely simulate the circumstances that produced the symptoms. Other protocols, or modifications of standard protocols, may be desirable in special clinical circumstances.

INTERPRETATION OF EXERCISE PHYSIOLOGY TESTS

Table 16-4 lists the physiologic variables that are directly measured during a noninvasive exercise physiology test and some of the clinically relevant physiologic parameters

TABLE 16–4. Physiologic and Clinical Parameters Determined During Exercise Tests

Measured Variables	Derived Variables	Clinical Parameters
RR	$\dot{V}E$	$\dot{V}O_2$ max
V_T	$\dot{V}CO_2$	Peak work rate
P_ECO_2	$\dot{V}O_2$	VAT
P_EO_2	HR	Peak RER
$P_{ET}CO_2$	Arrhythmias	Peak HR
$P_{ET}O_2$	ST changes	Peak oxygen pulse
Blood pressure	—	Peak $\dot{V}E$
Work rate	—	Breathing Reserve
Oxygen saturation	—	$\Delta\dot{V}E/\Delta\dot{V}CO_2$
Electrocardiogram	—	Peak V_T and RR

HR, heart rate; RER, respiratory exchange ratio; RR, respiratory rate; VAT, ventilatory exchange ratio.

that may be derived from them. The manner in which some of the more important and useful individual parameters may be analyzed, interpreted, and integrated into a coherent picture of a patient's exercise function and cardiopulmonary status will now be discussed. Emphasis will be placed on the application of this analytic approach to the unique clinical and physiologic problems encountered by the pediatric cardiologist.

$\dot{V}_{O_2}$ Max

During a progressive exercise test $\dot{V}_{O_2}$ increases linearly in proportion to work rate. However, near peak exercise, $\dot{V}_{O_2}$ plateaus, and further increases in work rate do not induce additional increases in $\dot{V}_{O_2}$. The level of $\dot{V}_{O_2}$ at this plateau is defined as $\dot{V}_{O_2}$ *max*. The level of motivation and effort required to reach the $\dot{V}_{O_2}$ max plateau is not always achieved during an exercise test, especially when the subject is a young child. In recognition of this fact, many exercise physiologists refer to the highest $\dot{V}_{O_2}$ achieved during an exercise test as the *peak* $\dot{V}_{O_2}$ rather than the $\dot{V}_{O_2}$ *max*. Under ideal circumstances, the peak $\dot{V}_{O_2}$ and $\dot{V}_{O_2}$ max are equal. However, when an exercise test is terminated due to motivational factors or factors other than the cardiopulmonary system's ability to deliver oxygen to the exercising muscles, peak $\dot{V}_{O_2}$ will be less than $\dot{V}_{O_2}$ max.

$\dot{V}_{O_2}$ max is one of the best indicators of exercise capacity and cardiopulmonary fitness. However, defining a *normal* value for $\dot{V}_{O_2}$ max is a complicated matter. $\dot{V}_{O_2}$ max, when expressed as milliliter of oxygen per minute, increases as body mass increases. $\dot{V}_{O_2}$ max is therefore commonly normalized for weight. However, the relationship between $\dot{V}_{O_2}$ max and body weight is not linear. Moreover, $\dot{V}_{O_2}$ max is also affected by other factors such as body habitus and composition, and since adipose tissue consumes almost no oxygen during exercise, normalizing $\dot{V}_{O_2}$ max for weight alone may be misleading and predispose to erroneous conclusions concerning an individual subject's cardiopulmonary status. For instance, suppose that a 50-kg individual who had a $\dot{V}_{O_2}$ max of 2000 mL O_2/minute (40 mL O_2/kg/minute) went on an eating binge, increased his weight to 100 kg and once again achieved a $\dot{V}_{O_2}$ max of 2000 mL O_2/kg/minute (now 20 mL/kg/minute). Although the weight-normalized $\dot{V}_{O_2}$ max has declined by 50%, it would be inappropriate to conclude, based on the data, that there has been a decline in the subject's cardiopulmonary system's ability to deliver oxygen per se.

In recognition of these problems, and based on theoretical considerations regarding the relationship between body size and $\dot{V}_{O_2}$ max, some physiologists have suggested methods of normalizing $\dot{V}_{O_2}$ max using an exponent of body length or weight.[24,25] There is no conformity of opinion concerning the optimal method and these approaches invariably result in rather unwieldy and unfamiliar units (e.g., mL $O_2/kg^{2/3}$/minute). Although each approach has its advantages and disadvantages, as a practical matter, at Children's Hospital (and most pediatric exercise physiology laboratories) estimates of a subject's $\dot{V}_{O_2}$ max are generated using a regression equation that takes into account age, gender, height and/or weight. Ideally each laboratory should generate its own regression equations based upon a local population of normal subjects. Alternatively, predicted values may be calculated using one of the published regression equations.[26–28] It is important to use a regression equation that was generated with an appropriate study population, and account must be taken of the protocol used to generate the regression equation. In addition, one must bear in mind that regression equations can produce unrealistic results when a subject's age and/or size are near or beyond the limits of the patient population from which the equation was derived. Some of the more commonly used regression equations are listed in Table 16-5.

$\dot{V}_{O_2}$ max may be compromised by deficiencies in any of the cardiovascular adaptations that contribute to the normal exercise-related increase in oxygen delivery. Among patients with congenital heart disease the most common factors responsible for a low $\dot{V}_{O_2}$ max are (a) an inability to increase stroke volume during exercise (e.g., patients with ventricular dysfunction, valvular disease, left-to-right shunts, elevated systemic afterload, or pulmonary vascular disease); (b) an inability to increase heart rate to appropriate levels at peak exercise (e.g., patients with sinus or atrioventricular node dysfunction); and (c) systemic hypoxemia (e.g., patients with right-to-left shunts).

TABLE 16–5. Some Useful Prediction Equations for $\dot{V}_{O_2}$ Max*

Predicted $\dot{V}_{O_2}$ max (l/min)	Comments
For males: 4.36 ht – 4.55 For females: 2.25 ht – 1.84	These equations, derived from normal subjects aged 6–17 years, are the ones used most frequently for pediatric patients.[27] They tend to generate unrealistically high estimates for extremely tall, thin subjects, and for extremely short subjects (< 130 cm tall) paradoxically predict lower values for boys than for girls.
For males: 0.053 wt – 0.30 For females: 0.029 wt – 0.29	These equations, derived from healthy subjects aged 6–17 years,[28] yield unrealistically high values for overweight subjects, but may provide superior estimates for tall, thin subjects.
For males: 3.45 ht – 0.028A + 0.022 wt – 3.76 For females: 2.49 ht – 0.018A + 0.010 wt – 2.26	These equations are for subjects > 17 years.[26]
For males: 0.67 $ht^{2.7}$ For females: 0.48 $ht^{2.7}$	These equations are appropriate for subjects < 20 years old.[26] Because wt is not taken into account, they may produce unrealistically high values for tall, thin subjects.
For males: 5.14 $ht^{1.88}/A^{0.49}$ For females: 3.55 $ht^{1.88}/A^{0.49}$	These equations are appropriate for subjects > 20 years old.[26] Because wt is not taken into account, they may produce unrealistically high values for tall, thin subjects.

Ht, height in meters; wt, weight in kilograms; A, age in years.
*Predicted values are for bicycle ergometry. Treadmill values are 5% to 10% higher.

Peak Work Rate

The peak work rate achieved during a progressive exercise test is another useful index of exercise function. This parameter is not readily determined during treadmill exercise testing, because the external work performed on a treadmill is a function not only of the speed and elevation of the treadmill, but also of the weight borne by the subject's feet. This last variable is a function of the subject's body weight and the difficult-to-quantify degree to which he/she leans on the handrails. On account of these complexities, the endurance time on a standard protocol (e.g., the Bruce protocol) is used as a surrogate for the peak work rate. Nomograms and tables are available for the prediction of an individual's expected endurance time on the basis of age and gender (Table 16-6).[23] The normal ranges tend to be quite broad and it must be emphasized that, for the reasons alluded to in prior sections, endurance time on a treadmill does not provide quantitative information regarding the amount of external work that an individual's cardiopulmonary system may support. It is therefore often inappropriate and misleading to compare the endurance

TABLE 16–6. Endurance Time on Bruce Protocol for Healthy Children with Innocent Murmurs

	Percentiles						
Age Group (yr)	**10**	**25**	**50**	**75**	**90**	**Mean**	**SD**
				Boys			
4–5	8.1	9.0	10.0	12.0	13.3	10.4	1.9
6–7	9.7	10.0	12.0	12.3	13.5	11.8	1.6
8–9	9.6	10.5	12.4	13.7	16.2	12.6	2.3
10–12	9.9	12.0	12.5	14.0	15.4	12.7	1.9
13–15	11.2	13.0	14.3	16.0	16.1	14.1	1.7
16–18	11.3	12.1	13.8	14.5	15.8	13.5	1.4
				Girls			
4–5	7.0	8.0	9.0	11.2	12.3	9.5	1.8
6–7	9.5	9.6	11.4	13.0	13.0	11.2	1.5
8–9	9.9	10.5	11.0	13.0	14.2	11.8	1.6
10–12	10.5	11.3	12.0	13.0	14.6	12.3	1.4
13–15	9.4	10.0	11.5	12.0	13.0	11.1	1.3
16–18	8.1	10.0	10.5	12.0	12.4	10.7	1.4

times of different subjects. Comparisons of the endurance times from exercise tests performed on different occasions by the same subject are frequently worthwhile, but the potential influence of changes in a subject's age, size, and exercise technique must be taken into account when interpreting the results of these comparisons.

The external work performed on a bicycle ergometer derives primarily from the work required to overcome the resistance in the pedals. This quantity is readily measured during a progressive exercise test. It is generally expressed in the units of watts or kilopond-meters per minute (1 watt = 6.12 kilopond-meters meters). Identifying a *normal value* for the peak work rate is complicated by many of the same considerations that applied to peak $\dot{V}_{O_2}$. Consequently, as a practical matter, regression equations are generally used to calculate predicted values for peak work rate, and results are expressed as a percentage of this predicted value.

Because the amount of work performed during an exercise test is dependent, to a large extent, on the amount of oxygen that can be delivered to the exercising muscles, the peak work rate is influenced by the same factors that influence peak $\dot{V}_{O_2}$. The peak work rate may also be influenced by orthopedic, neurologic, and other issues that can affect the efficiency of exercise.

Ventilatory Anaerobic Threshold

During a progressive exercise test, the anaerobic threshold occurs when aerobic metabolism, limited as it is by the amount of oxygen delivered by the cardiovascular system, is insufficient to meet the energy requirements of the exercising muscles. The anaerobic threshold is a physiologic phenomenon that is not affected by patient effort or motivation, and may be determined on a submaximal exercise test. Consequently, it is an excellent index of the cardiovascular system's capacity to adapt to the hemodynamic demands of exercise. Because anaerobic metabolism produces carbon dioxide (through the buffering of lactic acid by bicarbonate) but does not consume oxygen, during a progressive exercise test the ventilatory anaerobic threshold (VAT) is marked by an increase in $\dot{V}_{CO_2}$ out of proportion to the associated increase in $\dot{V}_{O_2}$. This phenomenon is manifested by a change in the slope of the $\dot{V}_{CO_2}$ versus $\dot{V}_{O_2}$ curve or the $\dot{V}_E$ versus $\dot{V}_{O_2}$ curve. The VAT may also be determined by detecting the point where the $\dot{V}_E/\dot{V}_{O_2}$ reaches a minimum and begins to increase while the $\dot{V}_E/\dot{V}_{CO_2}$ is flat or decreasing. End-tidal P_{O_2} also reaches a minimum at the VAT (Fig. 16-2).[12,14] Computer algorithms are available for detecting the VAT.[29] These algorithms are sometimes confounded by erratic breathing patterns near the start of an exercise test (a not uncommon problem among anxious young patients) and it is important to assure that the computer-determined VAT corresponds with the value determined by visual inspection of the appropriate graphs.

The VAT is usually expressed in the units *mL O_2/kg/minute*. Prediction equations exist for the calculation of normal values for the VAT on the basis of age, size and gender.[30] VAT is also commonly expressed as a percentage of predicted $\dot{V}_{O_2}$ max. In the absence of cardiovascular disease, VAT rarely falls below 40% of predicted $\dot{V}_{O_2}$ max. However, VAT is typically depressed below this value in patients with conditions that significantly impair the ability to increase cardiac output or oxygen delivery appropriately during exercise.[15,31,32] VAT is also dramatically depressed in patients with coarctation of the aorta,[33] peripheral vascular disease (e.g., patients with

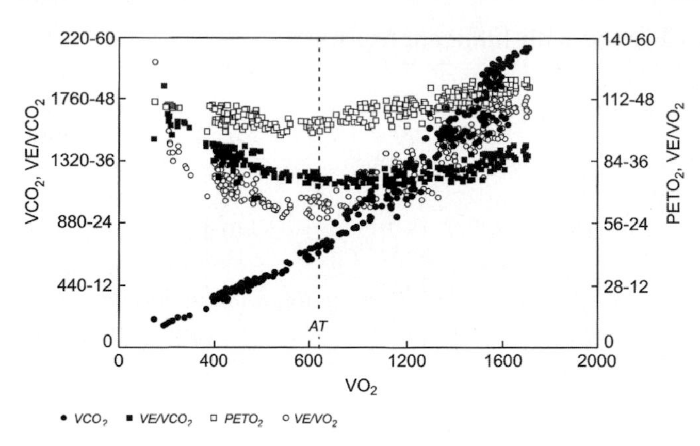

FIGURE 16–2 *Noninvasive detection of the ventilatory anaerobic threshold. At the anaerobic threshold the VE/VO$_2$ reaches a minimum and begins to rise while the VE/VCO$_2$ is flat or declining, the PETO$_2$ reaches a minimum and begins to rise, and the slope of the VCO$_2$ vs. VO$_2$ relationship increases. VE, minute ventilation; VO$_2$, oxygen consumption; PETO$_2$, end-tidal oxygen; AT, ventilatory anaerobic threshold.*

Takayasu arteritis), and other conditions that limit blood flow to the legs during lower extremity exercise.[31,32]

The Respiratory Exchange Ratio

During a progressive exercise test, the respiratory exchange ratio (RER) ($\dot{V}_{CO_2}/\dot{V}_{O_2}$) rises progressively after the VAT has been passed and the exercising muscles must rely on anaerobic metabolism to provide an ever-increasing proportion of their energy requirements. Hence, the RER at peak exercise is a good, objective physiologic index of the degree to which the oxygen delivery capacity of the cardiovascular system has been stressed (and the degree to which the exercising muscles have been forced to rely upon anaerobic metabolism) at peak exercise.[12,13] For adults and older children, a peak RER below 1.09 implies that exercise was not terminated on account of a cardiovascular limitation.[15] (Young children tend to have less anaerobic capacity and their peak-exercise RER therefore tends to be slightly lower.[34]) Conversely, a peak-exercise RER above 1.09 strongly suggests that a cardiovascular limitation (i.e., an inability to provide sufficient oxygen to the muscles to support ongoing exercise) was a major, if not the major, factor responsible for the termination of exercise. These considerations are of particular importance in patients with a compromised chronotropic response to exercise, a condition commonly encountered among patients who have had surgery for congenital heart disease.[35] These patients will typically have a low heart rate at peak exercise. In these cases, an elevated peak-exercise RER would indicate that the low peak heart rate is not due to a suboptimal effort. On the contrary, these data would indicate that the patient cannot increase his heart rate to normal levels, despite expending an excellent effort and pushing his/her cardiovascular system close to its limit. Determination of the peak-exercise RER is also very helpful in the interpretation of exercise tests of patients receiving beta blockers or other anti-arrhythmic agents that may depress the chronotropic response to exercise.

Heart Rate

The maximum heart rate achievable at peak exercise tends to decline with age. For treadmill exercise, the normal peak heart rate is commonly estimated from the equation:

$$\text{Peak HR} = 220 - \text{age (in years)}$$ [36]

Peak heart rate on a bicycle tends to be about 5% to 10% less than on a treadmill.[37]

Normally, during a progressive exercise test, heart rate rises linearly in proportion to $\dot{V}_{O_2}$, from resting to peak values. In patients with isolated chronotropic defects, the slope of the heart rate versus $\dot{V}_{O_2}$ curve is depressed and a normal peak heart rate is not achieved. Patients with a depressed stroke volume response to exercise rely excessively on a rise in heart rate to increase their cardiac output during exercise, and the slope of the heart rate versus $\dot{V}_{O_2}$ curve tends to be abnormally steep. This abnormal heart rate response may be seen even in patients with coexisting chronotropic defects. In these individuals the stimulus to increase heart rate in compensation for the depressed stroke volume response partially overwhelms the chronotropic defect and causes the heart rate rise to be abnormally steep relative to the rise in $\dot{V}_{O_2}$, even though the peak exercise heart rate remains abnormally low. In contrast, athletes tend to have larger than normal stroke volumes and therefore, at submaximal levels of exercise tend to have a below-normal heart rate for any given $\dot{V}_{O_2}$. The athlete's peak-exercise heart rate, however, is normal (Fig. 16-3).

The Oxygen Pulse

The oxygen pulse at peak exercise is related to the stroke volume at peak exercise and is therefore, for the clinician, one of the most useful indices available from the exercise physiology laboratory. The relationship between the oxygen pulse and stroke volume is best understood by dividing both sides of the Fick equation by heart rate:

$$\dot{V}_{O_2}/\text{HR} = \text{oxygen pulse} = \text{C.O./HR} \times \text{oxygen extraction}$$
$$= \text{SV} \times \text{oxygen extraction.}$$

At peak exercise, oxygen extraction is maximized and may be assumed to be the same value in most patients. Therefore, at peak exercise, the oxygen pulse is proportional to stroke volume, provided the assumption regarding the oxygen

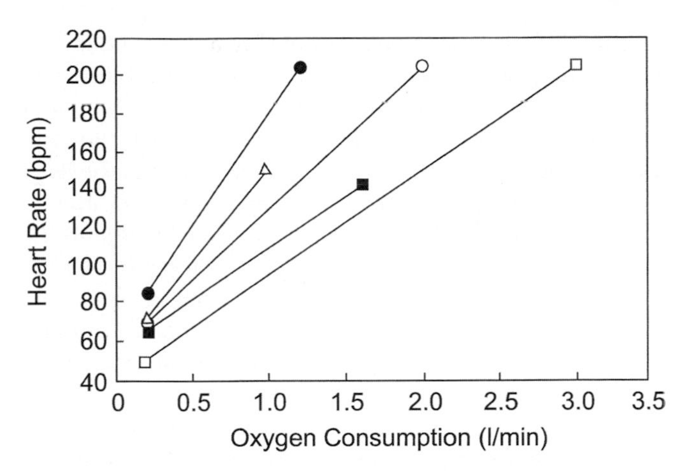

FIGURE 16–3 *Influence of various clinical conditions upon the relationship between heart rate and oxygen consumption during exercise. Variation of heart rate with respect to oxygen consumption during a progressive exercise test for a hypothetical 50-kg 15-year-old healthy subject (solid triangle), athlete (diamond), patient with a depressed chronotropic response (circle), patient with a depressed stroke volume response (square), and a patient with both a depressed chronotropic and stroke volume response (open triangles). Note that the athlete's peak oxygen pulse (peak oxygen consumption divided by peak heart rate) is above normal. The patient with a depressed stroke volume response has a below-normal peak oxygen pulse and partially compensates for this condition by increasing heart rate more rapidly than normal, causing the slope of the heart rate–oxygen consumption curve to be abnormally steep. In contrast, the patient with a depressed chronotropic response has an abnormally flattened curve and cannot achieve a normal peak heart rate, although a partial compensation for the chronotropic deficiency is achieved by increasing the peak oxygen pulse (i.e., stroke volume) to above-normal levels. The patient with the depressed chronotropic and stroke volume response still has a steeper-than-normal slope, but cannot achieve a normal peak heart rate and cannot compensate for this chronotropic deficiency by increasing stroke volume. This individual's peak oxygen consumption is therefore more depressed than any of the other subjects'.*

extraction at peak exercise is valid.[38] Normal values for oxygen pulse at peak exercise may be calculated by dividing the predicted peak $\dot{V}_{O_2}$ by the predicted peak heart rate. Peak-exercise oxygen pulse is best expressed as an absolute value (mL O_2/beat) and as a percentage of the predicted peak-exercise oxygen pulse.

When using the oxygen pulse to draw conclusions concerning a subject's stroke volume at peak exercise, it is important to recall that oxygen extraction is equal to the arterial oxygen content minus the mixed venous oxygen content. Consequently, in patients with depressed arterial oxygen content at peak exercise (e.g., patients with anemia or patients with significant arterial desaturation at peak exercise), oxygen extraction at peak exercise would be less than normal and the oxygen pulse would therefore underestimate stroke volume. In contrast, polycythemia increases arterial oxygen content and would therefore cause the oxygen pulse to overestimate the stroke volume. Similarly, among athletes the peak oxygen pulse tends to overestimate stroke volume because their oxygen extraction at peak exercise is slightly higher than that of normal subjects (i.e., their mixed venous oxygen saturation at peak exercise is slightly lower than normal subjects'). If these potential confounding factors are borne in mind, calculation of the oxygen pulse can permit clinicians to make valid and valuable inferences regarding a subject's cardiovascular response to exercise.

It is important to note that, for the purposes of this discussion, the term *stroke volume* refers to the forward, or physiologic stroke volume (i.e., the amount of blood that goes to the body with each heart beat). It is therefore not equivalent to the anatomic stroke volume (i.e., end diastolic volume minus end systolic volume) when valvular regurgitation or shunt lesions are present.

The oxygen pulse tends to be depressed in patients with conditions that impair their ability to increase forward stroke volume to appropriate levels at peak exercise. Patients with depressed ventricular function, severe valvular disease, systemic hypertension, coronary artery disease,[36] and pulmonary vascular obstructive disease[39] often have a low peak-exercise oxygen pulse. The peak-exercise oxygen pulse is often depressed in patients who have undergone a Fontan procedure, even in the absence of ventricular or valvular dysfunction.[40,41] In these patients, the low oxygen pulse probably reflects the absence of a pulmonary ventricle and the consequent inability of the passively perfused pulmonary vascular bed to accommodate the high rate of blood flow normally present at peak exercise.

Young patients with chronic aortic regurgitation usually have well-preserved exercise function and peak-exercise oxygen pulse.[42] In these patients, the fall in systemic vascular resistance that normally accompanies exercise tends to lessen the severity of the regurgitation during exercise. In addition, the left ventricular dilation typically present in chronic aortic regurgitation helps to maintain forward stroke volume and usually compensates effectively for the hemodynamic burden imposed by the leaky valve. Similar factors may also help to preserve the exercise function of patients with other valvular insufficiency lesions.

Minute Ventilation and Breathing Reserve

The exercise capacity of healthy subjects and patients with isolated cardiovascular disease is limited by the body's ability to deliver blood (i.e., oxygen) to the exercising muscles. Hence, at peak exercise, minute ventilation is usually less than the maximum voluntary ventilation (MVV, the maximum amount of air that a subject can breathe in and out in 1 minute). The MVV is usually estimated by measuring the maximum amount of air a subject can breathe out during 12 seconds of maximal hyperventilation, and multiplying this quantity by 5. This maneuver requires a degree of patient cooperation that is often beyond the capacity of most young subjects (and many older subjects as well). Alternatively, the MVV may be estimated by multiplying the FEV_1 ([forced expiratory volume in 1 second] from baseline spirometry) by 40.[43] The breathing reserve is the percentage of a subject's MVV that is not used at peak exercise, i.e.,

$$\text{Breathing reserve} = 100(\text{MVV} - \text{peak } \dot{V}_E)/\text{MVV}$$

The normal breathing reserve at peak exercise is 20% to 45%.[15] Patients with isolated cardiovascular disease tend to have normal MVVs, but their peak $\dot{V}_E$ tends to be low because their exercise capacity is depressed because of their cardiovascular disease. Consequently, these patients have higher than normal breathing reserves. In contrast, patients with severe lung disease, especially those with obstructive lung disease, are often *respiratorily limited.* They will typically have a lower than normal MVV and will have little or no breathing reserve at peak exercise. For instance, a healthy subject might have an MVV of 100 L/minute, a peak $\dot{V}_E$ of 65 L/minute and a breathing reserve of 35%. A patient with severe obstructive lung disease who is respiratorily limited might have an MVV of only 50 L/minute, a peak $\dot{V}_E$ of 50 L/minute and a breathing reserve of 0%.

$\Delta\dot{V}_E/\Delta\dot{V}CO_2$

Normally, during a progressive exercise test, $\dot{V}_E$ rises linearly in proportion to $\dot{V}_{CO2}$ until above the anaerobic threshold, when the accumulating lactic acidosis causes a compensatory increase in $\dot{V}_E$ out of proportion to the increase in $\dot{V}_{CO2}$. The slope of the linear (subanaerobic threshold) portion of the $\dot{V}_E$ vs. $\dot{V}_{CO2}$ curve ($\Delta\dot{V}_E/\Delta\dot{V}_{CO2}$, i.e., the number of liters of air that must be breathed to eliminate 1 L of carbon dioxide; normal value < 28) is a useful index of pulmonary function that reflects the efficiency of gas exchange during exercise. For gas exchange to proceed optimally, ventilation and perfusion must be optimally matched. Consequently, conditions that cause maldistribution of pulmonary blood flow are associated with an elevated $\Delta\dot{V}_E/\Delta\dot{V}_{CO2}$.[44,45] This phenomenon is commonly encountered among patients with residual pulmonary artery stenoses following repair of tetralogy of Fallot. In these subjects there is a positive correlation between the $\Delta\dot{V}_E/\Delta\dot{V}_{CO2}$ and the degree of pulmonary blood flow maldistribution present on radionuclide lung perfusion scans.[45] The $\Delta\dot{V}_E/\Delta\dot{V}_{CO2}$ has also been found to be one of the best predictors of postoperative peak $\dot{V}_{O2}$ in patients who have undergone surgical repair of tetralogy of Fallot.[44,45] This observation probably reflects the critical impact that pulmonary artery stenoses, when combined with the pulmonary regurgitation that is almost invariably present postoperatively in these patients, may have upon the right ventricle's ability to increase cardiac output during exercise.[45]

The $\Delta\dot{V}_E/\Delta\dot{V}_{CO2}$ is also almost invariably elevated in Fontan patients.[46] This observation is probably due to the absence of a pulmonary ventricle. The consequent loss of the normal pulmonary artery pulsatility results in ventilation/perfusion mismatch secondary to a suboptimal distribution of pulmonary blood flow.[47] Elevations of the $\Delta\dot{V}_E/\Delta\dot{V}_{CO2}$ may also be seen in patients in whom the transport of gases across the alveolar-capillary membrane is impaired (e.g., patients with elevated pulmonary capillary wedge pressures), in patients with right-to-left intracardiac shunts,[48] and in patients with pulmonary vascular disease.[39]

Tidal Volume and Respiratory Rate

The tidal volume at peak exercise typically increases to about 60% of the baseline forced vital capacity (FVC).[15] The FVC of patients who have undergone multiple cardiothoracic surgical procedures is often reduced, however, and their tidal volume at peak exercise often comprises an abnormally large percentage of their baseline FVC. Patients with reactive airway disease may develop bronchoconstriction and air trapping during exercise and have abnormally small tidal volumes at peak exercise.[49] In these patients post-exercise spirometric measurements would typically demonstrate an obstructive pattern more severe than that present on baseline spirometry. In contrast, upper airway obstruction (e.g., tracheal compression secondary to a vascular ring) tends to take unusually large, slow breaths during exercise. The peak respiratory rate usually does not exceed 60 breaths per minute in healthy subjects (70 breaths per minute in young children).[15] More rapid respiratory rates are often seen in patients with restrictive or interstitial lung disease.[49]

End-Tidal P_{CO_2}

Normally, end-tidal P_{CO_2} approximates arterial P_{CO_2}. (In fact, at rest end-tidal P_{CO_2} slightly underestimates arterial P_{CO_2}, and during heavy exercise it slightly overestimates arterial P_{CO_2}.[50]) However, in the presence of ventilation/perfusion mismatch, the close relationship between end-tidal and arterial P_{CO_2} is disrupted. Under these circumstances, end-tidal air is disproportionately derived from alveoli with high ventilation/perfusion ratios (and consequently low CO_2 concentrations) and end-tidal P_{CO_2} would therefore be less than arterial P_{CO_2}. Hence a persistently low end-tidal P_{CO_2} throughout an exercise test is most often encountered in patients with ventilation/perfusion mismatch. Low end-tidal P_{CO_2} is also seen in patients with chronic metabolic acidosis (because of an associated compensatory respiratory alkalosis) and in patients with right-to-left intracardiac shunts. In these latter individuals, the P_{CO_2} of the blood returning from the lungs in the pulmonary veins (and hence equal to the end-tidal P_{CO_2}) must be reduced to below normal values so that the blood ultimately entering the systemic circulation, composed of a mixture of pulmonary venous and right-to-left shunting blood, contains a normal P_{CO_2}.[50] In patients with right-to-left intracardiac shunts following a fenestrated Fontan procedure, the end-tidal P_{CO_2} (and the $\Delta\acute{v}_E/\Delta\acute{v}_{CO2}$) during exercise trend toward normal values following transcatheter closure of the Fontan fenestration.[51]

Rarely, a persistently low end-tidal P_{CO_2} may be due to hyperventilation secondary to emotional or psychological factors. However, in these situations, it is unusual for one to continue to hyperventilate throughout an exercise test. Arterial blood sampling is helpful in circumstances where doubt exists concerning the factors responsible for a low end-tidal P_{CO_2}. An elevated end-tidal P_{CO_2} almost invariably reflects CO_2 retention, usually secondary to respiratory disease.[50]

Blood Pressure

Peak systolic blood pressure rarely exceeds 200 mm Hg in healthy adolescents.[37,52] In pediatric patients, an excessive rise in right upper extremity blood pressure during exercise is most commonly encountered in patients with coarctation of the aorta. This abnormality may be encountered even after a successful repair.[53] An excessive rise in blood pressure may also be seen in patients with renal vascular disease, essential hypertension, and diffuse vascular disease secondary to Takayasu arteritis. At peak exercise, systolic blood pressure should exceed resting values by at least 25%.[52,54] A depressed blood pressure response may be seen in patients with cardiomyopathies, ventricular outflow tract obstruction, severe atrioventricular valve insufficiency, severe pulmonary insufficiency, pulmonary vascular obstructive disease and coronary artery disease. Systolic blood pressure should never fall during exercise (a fall in systolic blood pressure is an indication for termination of an exercise test). Abrupt, dramatic declines in blood pressure following exercise are sometimes seen in patients with vasodepressor syncope.

The Exercise Electrocardiogram

Analysis of exercise electrocardiogram (ECG) data is an integral component of an exercise test. The influence of exercise on the incidence and nature of rhythm disturbances should be assessed. In structurally normal hearts, ectopy that is suppressed by exercise is thought to be benign.[55] In contrast, myocardial ischemia, cardiomyopathies, and conditions such as the prolonged QT syndrome and catecholamine sensitive ventricular tachycardia are often characterized by an increase in the frequency and complexity of ectopy during exercise.[56] Rhythm disturbances are also commonly encountered in patients who have had surgery for congenital heart disease. In these patients the absence or suppression of an arrhythmia during an exercise test may have little predictive value. However, patients whose arrhythmias develop or worsen with exercise appear to be at greater risk for future serious arrhythmic events, and exercise testing therefore plays an important role in the assessment and management of this difficult clinical issue.[56]

The influence of exercise on conduction abnormalities should also be assessed. Patients with significant atrioventricular (AV) nodal disease may develop progressively higher grade AV block during exercise. In contrast, patients with AV block secondary to elevated resting vagal tone (e.g., many athletes) typically develop normal AV conduction during exercise.[57] In patients with Wolff-Parkinson-White syndrome, the sudden loss of pre-excitation during exercise is thought to indicate that the bypass tract has a relatively long anterograde effective refractory period and that the subject is therefore at low risk for sudden cardiac death.[58] Patients with the prolonged QT syndrome may have normal QT intervals at rest but may be unable to shorten their QT interval appropriately during exercise.[59,60] In patients with pacemakers, analysis of the exercise ECG findings may help assess whether the pacemaker is functioning properly and whether the pacemaker settings are optimal.[61]

The influence of exercise on the ST segment and T wave morphology should also be analyzed. It must be emphasized, however, that the incidence of coronary artery disease in the pediatric population is quite low, and the sensitivity and specificity of ST-T wave changes for the detection of coronary artery anomalies in pediatric subjects is unknown.[52,62,63] Exercise-induced ST-T wave changes are more commonly encountered in pediatric patients with cardiomyopathies and/or myocardial ischemia secondary to excessively high myocardial oxygen demand during exercise (e.g., patients with aortic stenosis). More severe ST changes are certainly more suggestive of myocardial ischemia, especially when associated with chest pain and other abnormalities.[52,64,65] However, the correlation between ST changes and myocardial ischemia in pediatric patients, although not precisely known, is probably no more than moderate. Radionuclide-based myocardial perfusion imaging is often used to help in the assessment of patients thought to be at increased risk for myocardial ischemia, and has been found to be helpful in patients with Kawasaki disease[66] and hypertrophic cardiomyopathy.[67] However, perfusion abnormalities of questionable clinical significance, unassociated with significant detectable coronary artery pathology, are commonly found in patients following the arterial switch operation.[62] The value of myocardial perfusion studies in patients with congenital coronary artery malformations has also not been established.

REFERENCES

1. Franciosa J, Park M, Levine T. Lack of correlation between exercise capacity and indices of resting left ventricular performance in heart failure. Am J Cardiol 47:33–39, 1981.
2. Rogers R, Reybrouck T, Weymans M, Dumoulin M, Van der HL, Gewillig M. Reliability of subjective estimates of exercise capacity after total repair of tetralogy of Fallot. Act Paediatr 83:866–869, 1994.
3. Cooper KH, Purdy J, White S, Pollock M, Linerud AC. Age-fitness adjusted maximal heart rates. Med Sci Sports 10: 78–86, 1977.
4. Cooper DM, Weiler-Ravell D, Whipp BJ, Wasserman K. Growth-related changes in oxygen uptake and heart rate during progressive exercise in children. Pediatr Res 18: 845–851, 1984.
5. McElroy PA, Janicki JS, Weber KT. Physiologic correlates of the heart rate response to upright isotonic exercise: relevance to rate-responsive pacemakers. J Am Coll Cardiol 11:94–99, 1988.
6. Loeppky JA, Greene ER, Hoekenga DE, Caprihan A, Luft UC. Beat-by-beat stroke volume assessment by pulsed Doppler in upright and supine exercise. J Appl Physiol 50:1173–1182, 1981.
7. Braunwald E, Sonnenblick EH, Ross JJr, Glick G, Epstein SE. An analysis of the cardiac response to exercise. Circ Res XXII (Suppl 1):I, 1967.
8. Udelson JE, Bacharach SL, Cannon RO, III, Bonow RO. Minimum left ventricular pressure during beta-adrenergic stimulation in human subjects. Evidence for elastic recoil and diastolic "suction" in the normal heart. Circulation 82:1174–1182, 1990.
9. Casaburi R, Daly J, Hansen JE, Effros RM. Abrupt changes in mixed venous blood gas composition after the onset of exercise. J Appl Physiol 67:1106–1112, 1989.
10. Yeh MP, Gardner RM, Adams TD, Yanowitz FG, Crapo RO. "Anaerobic threshold": problems of determination and validation. J Appl Physiol 55:1178–1186, 1983.
11. Hagberg JM, Coyle EF, Carroll JE, Miller JM, Martin WH, Brooke MH. Exercise hyperventilation in patients with McArdle's disease. J Appl Physiol 52:991–994, 1982.
12. Wasserman K. Determinants and detection of anaerobic threshold and consequences of exercise above it. Circulation 76(Supp VI):VI29–VI39, 1987.
13. Wasserman K. The Dickinson W. Richards lecture. New concepts in assessing cardiovascular function. Circulation 78: 1060–1071, 1988.
14. Washington RL. Cardiorespiratory testing: anaerobic threshold/respiratory threshold. Pediatr Cardiol 20:12–15, 1999.
15. Hansen JE, Sue DY, Wasserman K. Predicted values for clinical exercise testing. Amer Rev Respir Dis 129:S49–S55, 1984.
16. Jones NL, McHardy GJ, Naimark A, Campbell EJ. Physiological dead space and alveolar-arterial gas pressure differences during exercise. Clin Sci 31:19–29, 1966.
17. Whipp BJ, Wasserman K. Alveolar-arterial gas tension differences during graded exercise. J Appl Physiol 27:361–365, 1969.
18. Ekelund LG, Holmgren A. Central hemodynamics during exercise. Circ Res XX and XXI:I, 1967.
19. Linehan JH, Dawson CA. Pulmonary vascular resistance. In Fishman AP (ed). The Pulmonary Circulation, Philadelphia, 1990, pp 41–55.
20. Braunwald E. Control of myocardial oxygen consumption: physiologic and clinical considerations. Am J Cardiol 27: 416–432, 1971.
21. Tsujioka K, Goto M, Hiramatsu O, Wada Y, Ogasawara Y, Kajiya F. Functional characteristics of intramyocardial capacitance vessels and their effects on coronary arterial inflow and arterial outflow. In Kajiya F, Klassen GA, Hoffman JIE (eds). Coronary Circulation: Basic Mechanism and Clinical Relevance. Tokyo, 1990, pp 89–97.
22. Whipp BJ, Davis JA, Torres F, Wasserman K. A test to determine parameters of aerobic function during exercise. J Appl Physiol 50:217–221, 1981.
23. Cumming GR, Everatt D, Hastman L. Bruce treadmill test in children: normal values in a clinic population. Am J Cardiol 41:69–75, 1978.
24. Rogers DM, Olson BL, Wilmore JH. Scaling for the V_{O2}-to-body size relationship among children and adults. J Appl Physiol 79:958–967, 1995.
25. Jones NL. In Clinical Exercise Testing, Philadelphia, 1997, pp 131–134.
26. Jones NL. In Clinical Exercise Testing, Philadelphia, 1997, pp 243.
27. Cooper DM, Weiler-Ravell D. Gas exchange response to exercise in children. Amer Rev Respir Dis 129:S47–S48, 1984.
28. Cooper DM, Weiler-Ravell D, Whipp BJ, Wasserman K. Aerobic parameters of exercise as a function of body size during growth in children. J Appl Physiol 56:628–634, 1984.
29. Beaver WL, Wasserman K, Whipp BJ. A new method for detecting anaerobic threshold by gas exchange. J Appl Physiol 60:2020–2027, 1986.
30. Reybrouck T, Weymans M, Stijns H, Knops J, Van der HL. Ventilatory anaerobic threshold in healthy children. Age and sex differences. Eur J Appl Physiol 54:278–284, 1985.
31. Wasserman K. The anaerobic threshold measurement to evaluate exercise performance. Amer Rev Respir Dis 129: S35–S40, 1984.
32. Hansen JE, Sue DY, Oren A, Wasserman K. Relation of oxygen uptake to work rate in normal men and men with circulatory disorders. Am J Cardiol 59:669–674, 1987.
33. Rhodes J, Geggel RL, Marx GR, Bevilacqua L, Dambach YB, Hijazi ZM. Excessive anaerobic metabolism during exercise after repair of aortic coarctation. J Pediatr 131:210–214, 1997.
34. Hansen HS, Froberg K, Nielsen JR, Hyldebrandt N. A new approach to assessing maximal aerobic power in children: the Odense School Child Study. Eur J Appl Physiol 58:618–624, 1989.
35. Reybrouck T, Weymans M, Stijns H, Van der Hauwaert LG. Exercise testing after correction of tetralogy of Fallot: the

fallacy of a reduced heart rate response. Am Heart J 112: 998–1003, 1986.
36. Wasserman K, Hansen JE, Sue DY, et al. Principles of Exercise Testing and Interpretation (ed Third). Philadelphia, Lippincott, 1999, pp 150–151.
37. Braden DS, Carroll JF. Normative cardiovascular responses to exercise in children. Pediatr Cardiol 20:4–10, 1999.
38. Jones NL. Clinical Exercise Testing, 4th ed. Philadelphia: WB Saunders, 1997, p 135.
39. Garofano RP, Barst RJ. Exercise testing in children with primary pulmonary hypertension. Pediatr Cardiol 20:61–64, 1999.
40. Nir A, Driscoll DJ, Mottram CD, Offord KP, Puga FJ, Schaff HV, Danielson GK. Cardiorespiratory response to exercise after the Fontan operation: a serial study.[erratum appears in J Am Coll Cardiol 1993 Oct;22(4):1272]. J Am Coll Cardiol 22:216–220, 1993.
41. Harrison DA, Liu P, Walters JE, Goodman JM, Siu SC, Webb GD, Williams WG, McLaughlin PR. Cardiopulmonary function in adult patients late after Fontan repair. J Am Coll Cardiol 26:1016–1021, 1995.
42. Rhodes J, Fischbach PS, Patel H, Hijazi ZM. Factors affecting the exercise capacity of pediatric patients with aortic regurgitation. Pediatr Cardiol 21:328–333, 2000.
43. Campbell SC. A comparison of the maximum voluntary ventilation with the forced expiratory volume in one second: an assessment of subject cooperation. J Occupat Med 24: 531–533, 1982.
44. Clark AL, Gatzoulis MA, Redington AN. Ventilatory responses to exercise in adults after repair of tetralogy of Fallot. Br Heart J 73:445–449, 1995.
45. Rhodes J, Dave A, Pulling MC, Geggel RL, Marx GR, Fulton DR, Hijazi ZM. Effect of pulmonary artery stenoses on the cardiopulmonary response to exercise following repair of tetralogy of Fallot. Am J Cardiol 81:1217–1219, 1998.
46. Troutman WB, Barstow TJ, Galindo AJ, Cooper DM. Abnormal dynamic cardiorespiratory responses to exercise in pediatric patients after Fontan procedure. J Am Coll Cardiol 31:668–673, 1998.
47. Rhodes J. Concerning the Fontan patient's excessive minute ventilation during exercise. J Am Coll Cardiol 32:1132, 1998.
48. Wasserman K, Hansen JE, Sue DY, Casaburi R, Whipp BJ. Principles of Exercise Testing and Interpretation. Philadelphia, 1999, pp 173–174.
49. Wasserman K, Hansen JE, Sue DY, Casaburi R, Whipp BJ. Principles of Exercise Testing and Interpretation. Philadelphia, 1999, pp 104–109.
50. Wasserman K, Hansen JE, Sue DY, Casaburi R, Whipp BJ. Principles of Exercise Testing and Interpretation. Philadelphia, 1999, p 82.
51. Rhodes, J. Personal observation.
52. James FW, Kaplan S, Glueck CJ, Tsay JY, Knight MJ, Sarwar CJ. Responses of normal children and young adults to controlled bicycle exercise. Circulation 61:902–912, 1980.
53. Ruttenberg HD. Pre- and postoperative exercise testing of the child with coarctation of the aorta. Pediatr Cardiol 20: 33–37, 1999.
54. Alpert BS. Exercise in hypertensive children and adolescents: any harm done? Pediatr Cardiol 20:66–69, 1999.
55. Jacobsen J, Garson A, Jr., Gillette PC, McNamara DG. Premature ventricular contractions in normal children. J Pediatr 92:36–38, 1978.
56. Wiles H. Exercise testing for arrhythmia: Children and adolescents. Prog Pediatr Cardiol 2:51–60, 1993.
57. Jones NL. Clinical Exercise Testing, 4th ed. Philadelphia: WB Saunders, 1997, p 119.
58. Bricker JT, Porter CJ, Garson A, Jr., Gillette PC, McVey P, Traweek M, McNamara DG. Exercise testing in children with Wolff-Parkinson-White syndrome. Am J Cardiol 55: 1001–1004, 1985.
59. Vincent GM, Jaiswal D, Timothy KW. Effects of exercise on heart rate, QT, QTc and QT/QS2 in the Romano-Ward inherited long QT syndrome. Am J Cardiol 68:498–503, 1991.
60. Weintraub RG, Gow RM, Wilkinson JL. The congenital long QT syndromes in childhood. J Am Coll Cardiol 16: 674–680, 1990.
61. Bricker JT, Garson A, Jr., Traweek MS, Smith RT, Ward KA, Vargo TA, Gillette PC. The use of exercise testing in children to evaluate abnormalities of pacemaker function not apparent at rest. Pacing Clin Electrophysiol 8:656–660, 1985.
62. Mahle WT, McBride MG, Paridon SM. Exercise performance after the arterial switch operation for D-transposition of the great arteries. Am J Cardiol 87:753–758, 2001.
63. Weindling SN, Wernovsky G, Colan SD, Parker JA, Boutin C, Mone SM, Costello J, Castaneda AR, Treves ST. Myocardial perfusion, function and exercise tolerance after the arterial switch operation. J Am Coll Cardiol 23:424–433, 1994.
64. Shimizu M, Ino H, Okeie K, Emoto Y, Yamaguchi M, Yasuda T, Fujino N, Fujii H, Fujita S, Mabuchi T, Taki J, Mabuchi H. Exercise-induced ST-segment depression and systolic dysfunction in patients with nonobstructive hypertrophic cardiomyopathy. Am Heart J 140:52–60, 2000.
65. Yetman AT, Hamilton RM, Benson LN, McCrindle BW. Long-term outcome and prognostic determinants in children with hypertrophic cardiomyopathy. J Am Coll Cardiol 32: 1943–1950, 1998.
66. Hijazi ZM, Udelson JE, Snapper H, Rhodes J, Marx GR, Schwartz SL, Fulton DR. Physiologic significance of chronic coronary aneurysms in patients with Kawasaki disease. J Am Coll Cardiol 24:1633–1638, 1994.
67. Dilsizian V, Bonow RO, Epstein SE, Fananapazir L. Myocardial ischemia detected by thallium scintigraphy is frequently related to cardiac arrest and syncope in young patients with hypertrophic cardiomyopathy. J Am Coll Cardiol 22:796–804, 1993.

VII

Allied Disciplines

17

Sedation and Anesthesia in Cardiac Procedures

PETER C. LAUSSEN, MBBS

The development and expansion of pediatric cardiac anesthesia has occurred in parallel with the advances made in the diagnosis and treatment of congenital heart defects. The cardiac anesthesia service, a division of the Department of Anesthesia, Pain and Perioperative Medicine, at Children's Hospital Boston, provides anesthesia for procedures in the cardiac operating rooms, cardiac catheterization laboratories, cardiac magnetic resonance imaging suite and the cardiac intensive care unit, and also provides a consultative service for patients with cardiac disease undergoing noncardiac procedures in the general operating rooms and interventional radiology.

OVERVIEW

A unique feature of managing patients with congenital heart defects is the knowledge, expertise, and technical skills required to manage a heterogeneous population of patients with a wide variety of diagnoses and pathophysiology. An illustration of our experience and procedures performed in the cardiac operating room at Children's Hospital, Boston, over the past 5 years is shown in Figure 17-1; 69% of procedures were performed on cardiopulmonary bypass (*open* procedures), and 31% were *closed* procedures that did not require cardiotomy or cardiopulmonary bypass. Because of the diversity of congenital heart disease (CHD) lesions and the variations of severity and pathophysiology of each lesion, individualized anesthetic management is critical and should be based on the known effects of anesthetics and other drugs in patients with variable hemodynamic reserve.

New challenges over recent years for anesthesia management are the extremes of patient size and age presenting for surgical and catheterization procedures. Improvements in surgical techniques and cardiopulmonary bypass management have resulted in extension of successful reparative procedures to premature and very low–birth-weight neonates. These patients pose additional considerations of organ immaturity along with technical considerations for surgical repair. At the other end of this spectrum, adults with long-standing congenital heart disease and pathophysiologic derangements often have limited reserve and may have significant end-organ dysfunction that compromises postoperative recovery. Because of the unique and complex nature of their underlying defects and pathophysiology, these adults are often best managed within pediatric cardiovascular centers where the expertise to manage specific congenital heart defects is readily available.

Despite the change in patient demographics over the past two decades, the mortality associated with congenital heart surgery has continued to decline. The mortality for patients following cardiac surgical procedures managed in the cardiac intensive care unit at Children's Hospital Boston has declined from 5% in 1992 to 1.3% in 2004, regardless of diagnosis or surgical technique. This decline in mortality has occurred despite the increase in the case-mix index, a marker of the complexity of diagnoses and surgical procedures. However, along with the substantial decrease in mortality has been a steady increase in the costs related to management of these patients. Therefore, an important focus is the provision of efficient and cost-effective care, and anesthesia practices such as early tracheal extubation

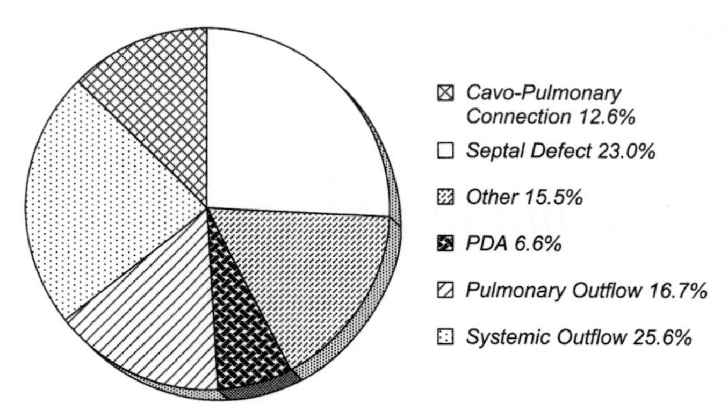

FIGURE 17–1 *Procedures performed in the cardiac operating room at Children's Hospital 2000 through 2003. Septal defects include atrial septal defect, ventricular septal defect, and complete atrioventricular canal. Cavopulmonary connection includes bidirectional Glenn and Fontan procedures. Systemic outflow procedures include the arterial switch operation, stage 1 Norwood procedure, coarctation and interrupted aortic arch repair, subaortic membrane resection, and aortic and mitral valve replacement or valvuloplasty. Pulmonary outflow procedures include repair of pulmonary atresia and tetralogy of Fallot variants, right ventricle–to–pulmonary artery conduit placement and tricuspid valve replacement or valvuloplasty, PDA (patent ductus arteriosus). Others include all other closed and open procedures performed in the cardiac operating rooms.*

may have a bearing on costs by impacting the length of intensive care stay as well as total hospital stay.

STRUCTURE OF THE CARDIAC ANESTHESIA SERVICE

For many years, the care of children with cardiac disease at Children's Hospital has been undertaken using a collaborative programmatic model that includes cardiology, cardiac surgery, cardiac anesthesia, and nursing actively participating in management plans, teaching and education, and research efforts. Our success has served as a model for the development of similar cardiac or heart centers throughout the United States and world wide. An operating committee oversees the activities, resources, and planning within the cardiovascular program (CVP). The chief of the cardiac anesthesia division is a participating member of the operating committee, and for the most part anesthesia-related resources and equipment for the cardiac operating rooms and the catheterization laboratories are approved through the CVP operating committee capital budgets.

The cardiac anesthesia service at Children's Hospital Boston has nine attending staff, all of whom have additional training and experience in a wide range of areas such as pediatrics, internal medicine, pediatric anesthesia, cardiac anesthesia, and critical care medicine. To meet clinical commitments each weekday, two attending physicians are assigned to the cardiac operating rooms, two attending physicians are assigned to provide coverage for the cardiac catheterization laboratory and cardiac magnetic resonance imaging (MRI) suite, and one attending provides a consultative service for patients with cardiac disease undergoing noncardiac surgery or patients who need review in the preoperative clinics.

Each month, the cardiac anesthesia service provides an active training program for five rotating fellows who are completing their pediatric or cardiac anesthesia fellowship programs. In addition, there is one senior clinical fellow position each year to provide concentrated training in pediatric cardiac anesthesia. Teaching is primarily by direct case-by-case teaching with weekly tutorials and regular didactic lectures for anesthesia fellows. The cardiac anesthesia service participates in CVP case conferences, mortality and morbidity meetings, and clinical research protocols.

RISK FOR CARDIAC ARREST DURING CONGENITAL CARDIAC SURGERY

The incidence of cardiac arrests in children during general anesthesia has been reported by Pediatric Perioperative Cardiac Arrest (POCA) registry as 1.4 per 10,000 anesthetics, with a mortality of 26%.[1] The cardiac anesthesia service at Children's Hospital Boston maintains a database of patients undergoing an open or closed procedure in the cardiac operating room, and over the past 5 years, our incidence of cardiac arrests classified as possibly anesthesia-related as defined by the POCA registry, is 24 per 10,000 anesthetics or 0.24%, but with no mortality. This is 17 times higher than the incidence of anesthesia-related cardiac arrests reported to the POCA registry and confirms the increased risk during anesthesia for congenital cardiac surgery. This is perhaps not surprising given the underlying pathophysiology and surgical procedures in patients with congenital cardiac disease, but it supports our contention that these patients ought to be managed by an experienced and dedicated cardiac anesthesia team who work closely with the cardiac surgical and operating room staff, and who can anticipate and manage at-risk patients and situations.

ANESTHESIA FOR CARDIAC SURGERY

Preoperative Assessment and Preparation

Complete and accurate preoperative assessment is essential for the successful anesthetic management of patients with CHD. It is often difficult to determine the management for a particular patient based solely on the specific and often complex anatomic defects. Rather, the appropriate organization of preoperative patient data, preparation of the patient, and decisions about monitoring, anesthetic agents, and postoperative care are best accomplished by focusing on major pathophysiologic problems. Together with a careful patient history and examination for cardiac failure, low cardiac output state, or pulmonary hypertension, the anesthesiologist will know the acceptable arterial oxygen saturation range for a particular patient during a procedure and will have formed an assessment of the cardiorespiratory reserve, which in turn will determine the amount of vasoactive support and likely postoperative course.

The introduction of Clinical Practice Guidelines (CPG) for the management of specific surgical procedures at Children's Hospital leads to a number of significant changes aimed at reducing hospital length of stay. Two important initiatives that had a direct impact on anesthetic preparation and management included the admission of elective patients on the day of surgery and catheterization (same day admission, SDA) and early tracheal extubation (qv). To facilitate SDA, a dedicated cardiology and cardiac surgery preoperative clinic, staffed by nurse practitioners, enables all preoperative tests and examinations to be performed, data from relevant studies such as echocardiography and cardiac catheterization to be reviewed, and important patient and family discussions and signing of consent forms to take place. This is particularly important before procedures and allows a complete discussion of sedation and anesthesia techniques, expectations of patient and families, and postoperative management considerations. It is also useful to provide an indication as to the anticipated length of stay, which we can readily do based on our CPG practices. Fasting guidelines established by the cardiac anesthesia service at Children's Hospital are shown in Table 17-1. For children who have undergone multiple procedures and who are anxious about subsequent interventions or examinations, it is useful to establish a specific relationship with one anesthesiologist so that consistent plans are maintained, and confidence developed.

TABLE 17–1. Nothing by Mouth (NPO) Guidelines

	Solids/Milk/ Formula, hr	Clear Liquids, hr	Breast Milk, hr
Adults	NPO after midnight		
Children > 36 mo	6	2	NA
Children 6-36 mo	6	2	3
Children < 6 mo	4	2	3

Clears: water, clear juice drinks, popsicles, Pedialyte, noncarbonated beverages; solids: food, candy, chewing gum, juice with pulp, milk and milk products including formula, carbonated beverages

Note: Medical necessity may dictate modification of the NPO guidelines as determined by cardiologist/cardiac anesthesiologist. Special consideration must be taken with complex congenital heart disease such as severe congestive heart failure, significant ventricular dysfunction, cyanosis, failing Fontan circulation, ascites, and severe gastrointestinal reflux. This should also include evaluation of the infant/child who has been NPO more than 6 hours and who may require intravenous hydration.

Although more than 90% of elective patients are suitable for SDA for cardiac surgical and catheterization procedures, admission to the hospital before the procedure is recommended when hydration with intravenous (IV) fluids is necessary because of polycythemia (hematocrit level above 55%), to initiate vasoactive or inotropic support if the patient has a significant low cardiac output state, for monitoring of heart rate and rhythm after discontinuing antiarrhythmic drugs prior to electrophysiology studies, and in certain anxious and frightened patients to facilitate overnight sedation and premedication.

Premedication

The immediate preoperative period is an anxious time for patients and parents. Many patients may have undergone prior surgery or investigational procedures, and separation from parents may be difficult. Oral midazolam is often an effective anxiolytic, and although it may not produce hypnosis, will enable separation from parents. In young children up to 5 years old who are particularly anxious and those who have undergone previous procedures, we commonly add oral ketamine 5 to 7.5 mg/kg to midazolam to provide a reliable state of hypnosis and dissociation. In circumstances where premedication is deemed important because of the extreme separation anxiety and limited hemodynamic reserve, an intramuscular premedication with ketamine 4 to 5 mg/kg, glycopyrolate 10 to 20 μg/kg, and midazolam 0.1 mg/kg is effective.

Midazolam is a short-acting, water-soluble benzodiazepine that can be administered intravenously, intramuscularly, orally, and rectally. While it is a commonly prescribed premedicant before anesthesia and surgical procedures and is an effective sedative, if the cardiac output and splanchnic perfusion is reduced, hepatic metabolism of midazolam will be reduced and drug accumulation is likely. The onset time is between 15 and 30 minutes with a duration of action of 2 to 4 hours. While IV midazolam is well tolerated for the most part, significant hypotension may occur in patients with poorly compensated cardiac failure who are dependent on endogenous catecholamines to maintain vascular resistance and blood pressure.

Chloral hydrate is commonly used for sedating children prior to medical procedures and imaging studies, and can be used as a premedication prior to surgery. It can be administered orally or rectally in a dose ranging from 50 to 80 mg/kg (maximum dose 1 gm). Onset of action is within 15 to 30 minutes with a duration of action between 2 to 4 hours. Between 10 to 20% of children will have a dysphoric reaction to chloral hydrate frequently being excitable and uncooperative. Alternatively, some children may become excessively sedated with respiratory depression and potential inability to protect their airway.

Monitoring

Because of the potential for rapid and dramatic hemodynamic changes in young patients with CHD, especially infants, complete preparation of anesthetic and monitoring equipment and resuscitation drugs is essential. Assistance should be immediately available during the induction of anesthesia in case problems develop.

Standard Monitoring

Routine monitoring for any pediatric patient undergoing anesthesia includes pulse oximetry, electrocardiogram (ECG), noninvasive blood pressure, and end-tidal CO_2. Pulse oximetry may reflect the adequacy of gas exchange, cardiac output, pulmonary blood flow, and intracardiac shunting, although its accuracy at low oxygen saturations (<75%–80%) is limited.[2] Direct arterial pressure monitoring yields important beat-to-beat information in cardiac patients. In general, radial arterial lines are preferred, but caution is required in flushing radial artery catheters because volumes as small as 0.3 mL force microbubbles and small thrombi retrograde into the carotid arteries.[3] Although femoral arterial lines are an excellent alternative to radial artery lines, they may be associated with a higher complication rate in neonates. Femoral artery catheters should be removed as soon as practical after surgery to reduce the risk for nosocomial infection and to prevent occlusion from thrombus, which will affect access for cardiac catheterization if later studies are necessary. Peripheral arterial lines, particularly those in the foot, may not accurately reflect the central aortic pressure of hypothermic children, especially during CPB and deep hypothermia.

Systemic air emboli are a constant risk in patients with CHD, regardless of their usual shunting pattern, because of the dynamic nature of shunts during anesthesia and surgery. Air traps are advisable for all IV lines but are not a substitute for meticulous attention and constant vigilance concerning the purging of air bubbles.

End-tidal CO_2 monitoring should be used for all patients who are intubated to monitor for misplacement or obstruction of the endotracheal tube and as guide to the effectiveness of mechanical ventilation and the amount of pulmonary blood flow. The gradient between the Pa_{CO_2} and end-tidal CO_2 should be established soon after intubation and once arterial access has been established; the normal Pa_{CO_2} minus end-tidal CO_2 difference being 5 to 10 mm Hg. An increase in the arterial to end-tidal CO_2 difference may occur with altered ventilation/perfusion matching in the lung. Conversely, a sudden decrease in pulmonary blood flow will cause a sudden fall in end-tidal CO_2; specific clinical circumstances include a fall in cardiac output, an increase in right to left intracardiac shunt, air embolism, occlusion to a systemic to pulmonary artery shunt or restriction of pulmonary blood flow such as from a vessel loop or during balloon dilation.

Intracardiac Pressure Measurement

Placement of a percutaneous central venous catheter is not necessary for all patients undergoing cardiac surgery. They are indicated in situations where large blood loss may be anticipated and when inotrope support is necessary before bypass. Measurement of the superior vena cava (SVC) O_2 saturation and the arterial minus SVC O_2 saturation difference (normally less than 20%–30%) may provide information as to the adequacy of the cardiac output. During surgery and bypass, the central venous pressure may be a useful monitor for adequate cerebral venous drainage after placement of the SVC venous cannula. Postoperative complications of transvenous central lines include venous thrombus and infection, particularly in neonates and infants, which may cause SVC syndrome and persistent pleural effusions and will significantly affect the success of later surgical procedures in patients undergoing staged repairs. The central venous line should therefore be removed as soon as practical following the procedure.

Transthoracic atrial and pulmonary artery catheters, placed by the surgeon before discontinuing bypass can be used for volume replacement and drug infusions and can generally remain for a longer period of time after surgery.[4] Left atrial pressure gives useful information about the adequacy of circulating blood volume and of ventricular and atrioventricular valve function. Oxygen saturation data and pressure recording from pulmonary arterial and atrial catheters provides reliable clues about the presence of residual shunts. Changes in pressure recorded when the pulmonary artery catheter is pulled back from the pulmonary artery to the right ventricle provide useful information about the adequacy of the right ventricular outflow tract repair.[5] Transcutaneous pulmonary artery balloon catheters may be difficult to place, and measurement of the thermodilution cardiac output is inaccurate in patients with intracardiac shunting.

Intraoperative Echocardiography

Intraoperative echocardiography has an established role in intraoperative monitoring of patients undergoing repair of CHD, although is not necessary for all procedures.[6] Placement of a transesophageal probe after the induction of anesthesia in the operating room affords the opportunity to reevaluate the anatomy before surgical intervention but, more important, the adequacy of surgical repair can be evaluated as soon as the patient is weaned from CPB. Interference of the airway by the probe and the effect on unstable hemodynamics before and after CPB must be carefully evaluated to avoid complications.

INDUCTION OF ANESTHESIA

Whatever the method of anesthesia or sedation, it is essential the procedure is discussed with staff prior to starting, and that the potential complications during the procedure are appreciated. At Children's Hospital, a *time-out* is mandatory before starting every procedure in the operating room or catheterization laboratory to ensure the correct procedure is about to be performed on the correct patient, and that all resources and equipment have been checked and are immediately available.

The choice of induction technique is influenced by the response to premedication and the anesthetic management plan. IV induction is simple and rapid; however, establishing IV access may be difficult in some cases. As a general rule, a patient with limited cardiorespiratory reserve should have an IV line placed for safe induction, and in some circumstances a fluid bolus or starting an inotropic or vasoactive infusion may be necessary before induction to prevent possible hemodynamic compromise. To facilitate IV access, a heavy premedication may be necessary, but the use of a topical local anesthetic cream or the combination with inhaled nitrous oxide may simplify placement of an IV catheter.

Intravenous Induction

Fentanyl, 15 to 25 μg/kg, in combination with pancuronium 0.2 mg/kg provides hemodynamic stability and prompt airway control.[7,8] Etomidate 0.3 mg/kg and ketamine 2 to 3 mg/kg IV are alternative IV induction agents that provide loss of consciousness with hemodynamic stability and minimal increases in pulmonary vascular resistance. They are particularly useful in patients with severe congestive heart failure (CHF) and ventricular outflow obstructions. Atropine 20 μg/kg or glycopyrrolate 10 μg/kg is traditionally given concurrently due to increased secretions. If IV access is difficult and stressful in infants, a combination ketamine 4 mg/kg, glycopyrrolate 10 μg/kg, and suxamethonium 2 mg/kg intramuscularly (IM) allows prompt induction and airway control.

Ketamine is a phencyclidine derivative, classified as a dissociative anesthetic agent. It effectively dissociates the thalamic and limbic systems and provides intense analgesia. An IV dose of 2 to 3 mg/kg has a rapid onset, short duration of action between 10 and 15 minutes, and elimination half-life between 2 and 3 hours. It produces a type of catalepsy whereby the eyes remain open, usually with nystagmus and intact corneal reflexes. Occasionally, nonpurposeful myoclonic movements may occur. It will dilate cerebral blood vessels and should be avoided in patients with intracranial hypertension. Ketamine usually provides hemodynamic stability because both heart rate and blood pressure usually increase through sympathomimetic actions resulting from central stimulation and diminished postganglionic catecholamine uptake. However, it does have direct myocardial depressant effects and should be used with caution in patients with limited myocardial reserve. There are conflicting reports about the effect of ketamine on pulmonary vascular resistance.[9] Although patients predisposed to pulmonary hypertension may demonstrate an increase in pulmonary artery pressure after ketamine administration, the response is usually minimal. On balance, therefore, ketamine can be used in patients with pulmonary hypertension, provided events such as hypoventilation and airway obstruction are avoided. Airway secretions are increased, and even though airway reflexes seem intact, aspiration may occur. Therefore, it is essential that patients are fasting prior to administration of ketamine and that complete airway management equipment is available. The increase in airway secretions can result in laryngospasm during airway manipulation and an antisialagogue agent such as atropine or glycopyrrolate should be administered concurrently. The major side effects during emergence are delirium, hallucinations, and nightmares. These may be ameliorated with the concurrent use of benzodiazepines.

Etomidate is an anesthetic induction agent with the advantage of minimal cardiovascular and respiratory depression.[10] An IV dose of 0.3 mg/kg induces a rapid loss of consciousness with a duration of 3 to 5 minutes. It may cause pain on injection and is associated with spontaneous movements, hiccupping, and myoclonus. Etomidate may be used as an alternative to the synthetic opioids for induction of patients with limited myocardial reserve. It is not approved for continuous infusion because of depression to adrenal steroidogenesis.[11]

The induction agents thiopental (3–5 mg/kg) and propofol (2–3 mg/kg) cause direct myocardial depression and venodilation and are suited only for patients with preserved ventricular function. They must be used with caution in patients who have undergone a previous cavopulmonary connection. The resting venous tone may be increased in this patient group, and the fall in preload could result in significant hypotension during induction. Propofol is a phenol derivative supplied in a soy emulsion and egg phospholipid to make an injectable emulsion. Because propofol has a short duration of action and rapid clearance, it has been used by infusion or repeated bolus doses with patients awakening rapidly when it is discontinued. A major disadvantage is pain on injection, although this can be overcome by the addition of lidocaine. Titrated dose of propofol 1 to 2 mg/kg is suitable to induce loss of consciousness for short procedures such as cardioversion and transesophageal echocardiography.

Inhalation Induction

An inhalation induction with sevoflurane is suitable for most infants and children if they have stable ventricular function and adequate hemodynamic reserve. This emphasizes the importance of preoperative evaluation when planning the induction technique. Inhalational induction can be used safely in patients with cyanotic heart disease, although uptake may be slower due to the right-to-left shunt.[12] Peripheral oxygen saturations will generally increase, provided cardiac output is maintained and airway obstruction avoided.

For many younger children, the presence of a parent during inhalation induction may be preferable for both the patient and parent.[13] This is a common technique for normal children undergoing induction of anesthesia for noncardiac surgery; however careful preoperative preparation and explanation are necessary before this is undertaken in the cardiac operating room.

TABLE 17–2. Factors Determining the Technique for Maintenance of Anesthesia

Patient factors	Patient age and size Timing of surgery and preoperative management Pathophysiology of specific congenital heart defects Cardiorespiratory reserve
Anesthetic factors	Depth of premedication Drug distribution and maintenance of anesthesia on CPB Postoperative analgesia requirements
Surgical factors	Extent and complexity of surgery Residual cardiac defects Risks for bleeding and protection of high-pressure suture lines
Conduct of CPB	Degree of hypothermia Myocardial protection Modulation of the inflammatory response and reperfusion injury
Postoperative management	Myocardial function Cardiorespiratory interactions Neurologic recovery Analgesia management

CPB, cardiopulmonary bypass.

MAINTENANCE OF ANESTHESIA

There are no specific *recipes* to maintain anesthesia during pediatric cardiac surgery and catheterization procedures, and the technique should be individualized for each patient. Table 17-2 shows the factors to consider when planning the anesthetic technique for a particular patient and surgical procedure.

Inhalational Anesthetic Agents

A balanced anesthetic technique, using a lower dose of opioid to provide analgesia and maintaining anesthesia with an inhalational agent such as isoflurane throughout the procedure, is a useful strategy for patients with stable cardiac reserve who are suitable for early tracheal extubation after surgery. This approach can be used for patients undergoing simple atrial and ventricular septal defect repair, conduit revision or replacement, and uncomplicated systemic outflow tract surgery such as subaortic membrane resection and aortic valve replacement.[14]

The volatile agents most commonly used during pediatric anesthesia are isoflurane and sevoflurane. Increased sensitivity of the immature cardiovascular system and decreased cardiovascular reserves reduce the margin of safety in infants and younger children with severe CHD. Volatile anesthetics cause dose-dependent direct myocardial depression primarily by limiting calcium availability within the myocyte, and given the immaturity of the neonatal and infant myocardium, the potential for systolic dysfunction in these patients may be increased when volatile agents are used. They also have a direct vasodilating effect on arteriole smooth muscle. These agents must therefore be titrated with caution because of their ability to cause hypotension. They have minimal direct effect on intracardiac conduction.[15,16]

Historically, halothane was used successfully during pediatric cardiac anesthesia for many years, both as an induction agent and to maintain anesthesia. However, it is rarely used nowadays because of the increased risk for significant myocardial depression and bradycardia during induction, along with an increased sensitization of the myocardium to endogenous and exogenous catecholamines, which may cause ventricular tachycardia.

Isoflurane causes less direct myocardial depression, has a faster uptake and emergence, has no effect on intracardiac conduction, and causes much less sensitization of the myocardium to catecholamines compared with halothane. It is a very useful agent to maintain anesthesia throughout cardiac surgery and CPB. It may be used as a sole agent for patients in whom extubation in the immediate postoperative period is planned. Because of peripheral vasodilating properties, isoflurane is a useful adjunct during high-dose opioid anesthesia, particularly if the patient is hypertensive. During bypass, isoflurane 0.5% to 1.0% can be delivered into the fresh gas flow of the bypass circuit and titrated to hemodynamic response.

Sevoflurane is a popular agent for induction of anesthesia in children and can be safely used for most patients with congenital heart disease.[17] Its low solubility contributes to faster onset of action and subsequent emergence from anesthesia. As with isoflurane, it causes less myocardial depression and has a low risk for arrhythmias in children compared to halothane. However, because of cost and rapid emergence, there appears little advantage to continue sevoflurane during maintenance of anesthesia.

The use of nitrous oxide in children with CHD and shunts is limited because of its potential for enlarging systemic air emboli and for potentially increasing pulmonary vascular resistance.

Opioid-Based Anesthesia

A high-dose opioid anesthetic technique is generally preferred for patients with limited cardiorespiratory reserve; when the surgical procedure is extensive and complex; when the cardiopulmonary technique includes a long duration or deep hypothermia with circulatory arrest; when there are anticipated postcardiotomy complications such as bleeding from high-pressure suture lines, dysrhythmias, or residual lesions such as atrioventricular valve insufficiency; and when the anticipated postoperative course in the intensive care unit is prolonged.[14,18]

High-dose narcotic anesthesia provides excellent cardiovascular stability in children with CHD. Morphine (1 mg/kg or more) given slowly over a prolonged period provides reasonable cardiovascular stability in children; however, as in adults, histamine release can occur and cause hypotension. The more potent synthetic opioids, fentanyl (25–75 μg/kg) and sufentanil (5–15 μg/kg), provide better stability of the cardiovascular system on induction of anesthesia when used with pancuronium in very sick infants with CHD.[19]

In our practice, fentanyl is commonly used to maintain anesthesia, with a usual dosing strategy of 50 μg/kg administered prior CPB, a further 25 μg/kg at the onset of rewarming on CPB, and a further 25 μg/kg after bypass depending upon hemodynamic stability. Additional doses or a continuous infusion of potent narcotics may be necessary for surgery involving cardiopulmonary bypass because narcotic concentrations may decrease during CPB. Drug pharmacokinetics may be substantially altered by hypothermia, hemodilution, reduced protein binding, binding of drugs to the bypass circuit and oxygenator membrane, sequestration of drugs within the pulmonary vascular bed, and reduced hepatic and renal clearance. Drug pharmacodynamics may be altered due to CPB variables such as flow rate and perfusion pressure and the use of vasoactive drugs.

Remifentanil is a new synthetic ultra–short-acting opioid, rapidly metabolized by nonspecific tissue esterases.[20] It is unique among the currently available opioids because of its extremely short context-sensitive half time (3–5 minutes), which is largely independent of the duration of infusion. Administered only as a continuous infusion 0.25 to 1.0 μg/kg per minute, remifentanil may cause significant respiratory depression and is usually administered to patients who are mechanically ventilated. It may be useful for patients with limited cardiorespiratory reserve undergoing procedures such as cardiac catheterization or pacemaker placement because intense analgesia is provided without significant hemodynamic complications. It may also be used to maintain anesthesia during mild hypothermic CPB for patients who are extubated immediately after surgery in the operating room, such as after atrial septal defect repair.[14] Patients usually emerge quickly once the infusion has been stopped, and opioid side effects are reduced because of the short duration of action.

STRESS RESPONSE TO SURGERY AND CARDIOPULMONARY BYPASS

The link between stress and adverse postoperative outcome in critically ill newborns and infants undergoing surgery is not surprising given their precarious balance of limited metabolic reserve and increased resting metabolic rate.[21] In the early experience of CPB in neonates and infants, the use of high-dose opioid techniques as the basis for anesthesia, with continuance of this strategy into the immediate postoperative period to modulate the stress response, was perceived to be one of the few clinical strategies associated with a measurable reduction in morbidity and mortality.[22,23] To a large extent, this experience formed the basis of anesthesia management for neonates, infants, and older children undergoing congenital cardiac surgery.

It is now recognized, however, that the activation and magnitude of the stress response to cardiac surgery is related not only to the surgical procedure and tissue trauma directly, but also by exposure of blood to the nonendothelial surfaces of the cardiopulmonary bypass circuit and the systemic inflammatory response. More recent studies in neonates, infants, and children undergoing cardiac surgery have demonstrated that high-dose opioid anesthesia (specifically fentanyl 30–50 μg/kg) attenuates the *prebypass* endocrine and hemodynamic response to surgical stimulation, but does not have a consistent or substantial impact on modifying activation of this response on CPB.[24,25] Based on these data, it is possible to conclude that high-dose opioid anesthesia followed by continuation into the immediate postoperative period specifically to attenuate the stress response has a less critical role in determining outcome than was reported in early studies. Opioids have an important role during anesthesia for cardiac surgery because of the hemodynamic stability they provide, but high doses are not necessary for all patients.

Muscle Relaxants

Pancuronium is a slow-onset, long-acting, nondepolarizing aminosteroid muscle relaxant. A bolus dose of 0.1 to 0.2 mg/kg can produce tachycardia and hypertension in children through its sympathomimetic effect, but with a duration of action up to 60 minutes, it is the agent of choice for most patients during long cardiac surgical and catheterization procedures. For patients in whom a short-acting, nondepolarizing muscle relaxant is desirable (i.e., duration of action 30 minutes), *cis*-atracurium 0.2 mg/kg and vecuronium 0.1 mg/kg are ideal agents with few cardiovascular side effects.

Succinylcholine 1 to 2 mg/kg is a rapid-onset, short-duration, depolarizing muscle relaxant that is used primarily during a rapid sequence induction in patients with a full stomach to facilitate intubation and control of the airway. Succinylcholine acts on nicotinic and muscurinic parasympathetic receptors, and atropine or glycopyrrolate 10 to 20 μg/kg should also be given to avoid associated bradycardia or even sinus arrest.

Rocuronium is a newer, rapid-onset, intermediate-duration of action, aminosteroid nondepolarizing muscle relaxant. Time to complete neuromuscular blockade for an intubating dose of 0.6 mg/kg ranges from 30 to 180 seconds, although adequate intubating conditions are usually achieved within 60 seconds. It is therefore a suitable alternative to succinylcholine during rapid-sequence induction. The duration of action averages 25 minutes although recovery is slower in infants. It is a safe drug to administer to patients with limited hemodynamic reserve and does not cause histamine release.

EARLY TRACHEAL EXTUBATION

The early tracheal extubation of children after congenital heart surgery has received renewed attention with the development of clinical practice guidelines and the evolution of *fast track* management for cardiac surgical patients. Early extubation refers to tracheal extubation within a few hours (4–8 hours) after surgery, although functionally it means the avoidance of routine, overnight mechanical ventilation. A number of reports have described successful tracheal extubation in neonates and older children following congenital heart surgery, either in the operating room (OR) or soon after in the cardiac intensive care unit.[26–29] We have reviewed our experience of early tracheal extubation as a component of the clinical practice guideline following atrial septal defect surgery and demonstrated this strategy was cost-effective without compromising patient management.[30]

The surgical approach and techniques for many cardiac procedures have also substantially changed over recent years, particularly with the development of minimally invasive techniques in adults and children. Although it may be thought that a minimally invasive incision could be associated with a more rapid postoperative recovery because of less pain or analgesic requirements, this has not been demonstrated. In a controlled study of children undergoing atrial septal defect repair using either a minimally invasive incision or full sternotomy, we concluded that the primary advantage of the minimally invasive approach was cosmetic, and we were unable to demonstrate any difference in pain scores and other markers of postoperative recovery.[31]

MANAGEMENT DURING CARDIOPULMONARY BYPASS

Once the patient is on CPB, systemic perfusion and gas exchange are maintained directly from the bypass pump and membrane oxygenator. The adequacy of systemic perfusion is regularly checked during bypass by following the mixed venous oxygen saturation and lactate levels. Ventilation is discontinued when full flow has been established during the cooling phase of CPB.

Anesthesia can be maintained using different strategies, including bolus dosing or continuous infusions of opioids and/or benzodiazepines and intermittent use of isoflurane via a vaporizer connected to the sweep gas to the bypass circuit. The depth of hypothermia is an important variable affecting anesthesia level, and in general as the core and brain temperature decreases and reaches deep hypothermic levels (i.e., $< 22°C$), the electroencephalogram (EEG) in effect becomes isoelectric and anesthetic agents or drugs are generally not necessary during this phase. However, at mild to moderate hypothermic levels (i.e., $> 28°C$), cerebral metabolic rate and EEG activity increase and loss of consciousness can not be guaranteed. This is particularly a concern for patients undergoing surgical repair at mild hypothermic levels ($> 32°C$) and also during the rewarming phase of CPB.

Anesthesia during CPB is associated with an increased risk of patient awareness.[32] Although these studies have been performed in adults, there is no reason to suspect that infants and children do not have the same potential risk. Monitoring the adequacy of anesthetic depth during CPB is difficult, but possible indices include changes in autonomic responses such as an increase in perfusion pressure for a given flow rate, tearing and diaphoresis, and metabolic responses such as a fall in mixed venous oxygen saturation and a rise in lactate level. Monitoring the depth of anesthesia during a procedure is critically important to ensure patients are adequately anesthetized, and devices such as the Bispectral Index (Aspect Medical, Newton, MA), which monitor a processed EEG signal, have been developed. We have evaluated this form of monitoring in pediatric patients undergoing cardiac and noncardiac surgery, but at this time, their role in routine monitoring of anesthetic depth remains debated.[33–37]

MANAGEMENT AFTER CARDIOPULMONARY BYPASS

Chest closure is a time of particular instability after operations for CHD. If there are concerns for ventricular dysfunction or inadequate hemostasis, it is common for the chest to be left open and covered with a scialastic membrane after surgery. Delayed closure of the sternum can be undertaken in the CICU once the patient is in a stable condition, and we have previously demonstrated that this approach is associated with improved outcome and low risk for morbidity and infection.[38]

Transfer from the operating table and to the intensive care unit from the OR can be associated with substantial hemodynamic instability. All monitoring must be continued uninterrupted. A full oxygen cylinder must be used and the breathing circuit checked for leaks. Equipment for reintubation and resuscitation drugs must be taken with the patient in case of inadvertent problems during transport. The endotracheal tube should be secure and suctioned to remove secretions to reduce the risk for obstruction. Additional anesthesia and muscle relaxants may be necessary if the patient becomes hypertensive or tachycardic when moved. If there is unexpected hypotension or dysrhythmia before the patient leaves the OR, further evaluation is essential immediately to determine the cause and establish stability.

ANESTHESIA FOR CARDIAC CATHETERIZATION

Adequate sedation and anesthesia during cardiac catheterization are essential to facilitate acquisition of meaningful hemodynamic data and to assist during interventional procedures. For the most part, hemodynamic or diagnostic catheterization procedures can be performed under sedation in all age groups. For many interventional procedures sedation may be appropriate; however for procedures that are associated with significant hemodynamic compromise, or are prolonged, general anesthesia is preferable.

Whatever technique is used, it is essential that hemodynamic data be attained in conditions as close to normal as possible. When using sedation, full monitoring is essential to ensure that respiratory depression is avoided. During anesthesia, the effects of inspired oxygen concentration, mechanical ventilation and hemodynamic side effects of various anesthesia agents must also be appreciated. Postprocedure monitoring either in a recovery room or intensive care unit is mandatory.

CATHETERIZATION LABORATORY ENVIRONMENT

Cardiac catheterization laboratories are usually remote from the operating room and rarely configured to accommodate anesthetic personnel. Relative to patient size, the lateral and anteroposterior cameras used for imaging are in close proximity to the patients' head and neck, limiting access to the airway. An anesthetic machine and monitors around the patient will further confine the space in which the anesthesiologist may work and limit access to the patient. In addition, the environment is darkened to facilitate viewing of images, and monitoring with capnography and pulse oximetry is mandatory.

The large surface area to body mass ratio of infants and neonates predisposes them to hypothermia, which may significantly increase metabolic rate and delay recovery from sedation and anesthesia. Hypothermia is a particular concern in the catheterization laboratory because of radiant and convective heat loss; prolonged exposure of the patient after sedation or general anesthesia and during preparation for catheterization may result in significant heat loss. In addition, the use of cold flush solutions and damp towels in contact with the patient will also contribute to hypothermia.

Care must be taken when positioning a patient on the catheterization table because of the risk for pressure areas and nerve traction injury. In particular, brachial plexus injury may occur when patients have their arms positioned above their heads for a prolonged period of time to make room for the lateral cameras. To facilitate femoral vein and arterial access, the pelvis is commonly elevated from the catheterization table. This may displace abdominal contents cephalad, restricting diaphragm excursion and increasing the risk for respiratory depression in a sedated patient: It is thus most important to eliminate this pelvic elevation once vessel access is attained.

Although the underlying cardiac status or physiologic status of a patient may increase the risk for adverse events during catheterization, in many circumstances complications are sudden, occurring without warning, and reflect the inherent risk for specific procedures. The frequency of critical events requiring cardiopulmonary resuscitation in patients in the CVP at Children's Hospital is continually tracked and evaluated by our Resuscitation Review Committee. The current frequency of an unexpected event requiring resuscitation with chest compressions during cardiac catheterization is 7.0 (0.7%) per 1000 procedures. Further, from 1996 through 2004 following the establishment of a rapid response extracorporeal membrane oxygenation (ECMO) system, 22 patients (0.2% of all catheterizations over this period) have been emergently cannulated for ECMO support in the catheterization laboratory because of extreme hemodynamic instability or as part of cardiopulmonary resuscitation; of these patients 67% survived to discharge. These figures emphasize the inherent risk for a sudden adverse event during catheterization even in the most optimal of settings, and all staff, including catheterizers, anesthesiologists, nurses, and technicians, must be vigilant and prepared for immediate intervention.

Complications of various interventional procedures are related in part to the type of procedure, but all share the risks associated with percutaneous vascular access with large catheters that course through the heart and vessels. Although limited cardiac reserve of the patient may increase his or her risk for adverse events during catheterization, in many circumstances complications are sudden, occurring without warning, and reflect the inherent risk for specific procedure. Placement of catheters in and through the heart increases the risk for dysrhythmias, perforation of the myocardium, damage to valve leaflets and chordae, cerebral vascular accidents, and air embolism. The use of radiopaque contrast material may cause an acute allergic reaction (although this is rare in children with nonionic contrast media), pulmonary hypertension, and myocardial depression. Blood loss may be sudden and unexpected when using large-bore catheters, vessels are ruptured, or vessel entry sites are inadvertently beyond the pubic ramus in the pelvis and cannot be compressed following catheter removal. More insidious blood loss may occur over several hours in heparinized small children or neonates owing to bleeding around the catheter site or multiple aspirations and flushes of catheters. Transfusion requirements and appropriate vascular access should be continually assessed. Arrhythmias, albeit transient, may be recurrent and fatal if not promptly treated. On most occasions, removal of the wire or catheter is sufficient for the arrhythmia to resolve, but when this does not happen, it is important that full resuscitation and cardioversion equipment be available.

SEDATION FOR CARDIAC CATHETERIZATION

Most diagnostic, noninterventional hemodynamic catheterization studies can be performed with the patient sedated and breathing room air. This allows meaningful hemodynamic data and oxygen saturations to be measured, together with accurate calculations of cardiac output, shunt fraction, and vascular resistances. It is important that adequate local anesthetic be used at vascular access sites to limit the amount of sedation. Interventional procedures that cause minimal or transient hemodynamic perturbations can be performed using sedation techniques, including patent ductus arteriosus and atrial septal defect device occlusion, balloon dilation of stenotic aortic and pulmonary semilunar valves, balloon dilation of recoarctation of the aorta and of main or branch pulmonary artery stenosis, and coil embolization of vessels.

Well-prepared intermittent sedation protocols can be managed by nurses trained in pediatric sedation and the cardiac catheterization environment. At Children's Hospital, nurses administering sedation must undergo a specific training and accreditation program. Procedural sedation orders and limits for dose range of specific sedative drugs are shown in Figure 17-2. Cardiac anesthesia staff are available to manage respiratory depression and airway obstruction and to intervene if the limits of the sedation protocol have been reached and the patient remains unsettled on the catheterization table.

In select cases, a continuous IV sedation technique can be used by an anesthesiologist who is immediately available to

CHILDREN'S HOSPITAL BOSTON ☐ NAME ______________

If STAT – check box above

CARDIAC CATHETERIZATION LABORATORY
PROCEDURAL SEDATION ORDERS CH MRN ______________

Page 1 of 1 DOB ______________
Template Revision Date: 8-13-03
Approval by Pharmacy and Therapeutics Committee: 3-8-04

☐ NKDA Allergies / Adverse Reaction: ______________
Dose Basis: **Weight:** _____ kg **Age:** _____

PRE-MEDICATIONS:
☐ <9 kg: Consult with Anesthesia
☐ 9 - 20 kg: **Demerol Compound** (Meperidine 25 mg/mL, Chlorpromazine 6.25 mg/mL, Promethazine 6.25 mg/mL)
☐ acyanotic: 0.11 mL/kg x _____ kg = _____ mL (MAX 2 mL) IM x1
☐ cyanotic (SaO_2 ≥70): 0.078 mL/kg x _____ kg = _____ mL (MAX 1.4 mL) IM x1
☐ markedly cyanotic (SaO_2 <70): Consult with Anesthesia
☐ >20 kg: **Midazolam 20 mg PO x1**

IV ACCESS
☐ Establish intravenous access if necessary
☐ Infuse IV Fluids (choose one) ☐ Lactated Ringers Solution / ☐ Other _____ Run at: ☐ TKO *or* ☐ ____ mL/hr

SEDATION - For procedures lasting longer than 4 hours, consult anesthesia for further sedation.
☐ ≤20 kg
☐ **Midazolam** 0.025 mg/kg x _____ kg = _____ mg (MAX 0.5 mg) **IV Q10min PRN procedural sedation.**
MAX cumulative dose 0.3 mg/kg or 6 mg (whichever is less) over 4 hours
☐ **Morphine** 0.025 mg/kg x _____ kg = _____ mg (MAX 0.5 mg) **IV Q10min PRN procedural sedation.**
MAX cumulative dose 0.3 mg/kg or 6 mg (whichever is less) over 4 hours
☐ >20 kg
☐ **Midazolam 0.5 mg IV Q10min PRN procedural sedation.**
MAX cumulative dose 0.3 mg/kg or 12 mg (whichever is less) over 4 hours.
☐ **Morphine 0.5 mg IV Q10min PRN procedural sedation.**
MAX cumulative dose 0.3 mg/kg or 12 mg (whichever is less) over 4 hours.

REVERSAL AGENTS
☐ **Naloxone** 1 mcg/kg x _____ kg = _____ **mcg IV x1 PRN respiratory depression.**
Wait 90 secs. If no response, give **Naloxone** 2 mcg/kg x _____ kg = _____ **mcg IV x1 PRN respiratory depression.**
Wait 90 more secs. If no response, give **Naloxone** 4 mcg/kg x _____ kg = _____ **mcg IV x1 PRN respiratory depression.**
MAX cumulative dose for all 3 doses is 400 mcg or 1 ampule.
If still no response after this sequence. Anesthesia STAT (x5-5555) must be activated if this hasn't already been done.
☐ **Flumazenil** 0.01 mg/kg x _____ kg = _____ mg (MAX 0.2 mg) **IV Q1min PRN respiratory depression unresponsive to naloxone.** MAX cumulative dose of 0.05 mg/kg or 1 mg, whichever is less.

MONITORING: Continuous Pulse Oximetry, Heart Rate and Respiratory Rate Monitoring per protocol.

DISCHARGE: to PACU after procedure.

DATE TIME Physician/Nurse Practitioner signature PRINTED NAME PAGER #

DATE TIME RN #1 SIGNATURE RN #2 SIGNATURE DATE TIME
ORDERS MAY NOT BE MODIFIED ONCE SIGNED BY PRESCRIBER

FIGURE 17–2 *Sedation template used for cardiac catheterization.*

manage the airway. A combination of ketamine and midazolam infused at 2 to 5 mg/kg/hr and 0.05 to 0.1 mg/kg/hr, respectively, is often successful in maintaining sedation without respiratory depression or airway compromise. Alternative sedation techniques include propofol 50 to 150 μg/kg/min and remifentanil 0.25 to 0.5 μg/kg/min.

GENERAL ANESTHESIA FOR CARDIAC CATHETERIZATION

Patient and procedural factors are considerations when planning general anesthesia. Patients who have a limited cardiorespiratory reserve may not tolerate prolonged procedures under IV sedation, particularly if respiratory depression or airway obstruction occurs concurrently. Respiratory distress may occur in some patients when positioned supine, particularly if they have significant congestive cardiac failure, pulmonary hypertension, or limited diaphragm excursion secondary to an enlarged liver or ascites. Certain anesthetic agents may cause significant hemodynamic changes secondary to direct myocardial depression or to their effects on the peripheral circulation, which can alter the interpretation of catheterization data.

General anesthesia may be indicated because of the risks and possible complications associated with certain procedures. At critical phases during some interventions such as device and stent placement, it is essential patients remain absolutely still because sudden patient movement may dislodge the device or alter stent position. In addition, if hemodynamic compromise may occur during an intervention, such as placement of ventral septal defect occlusion devices, dilation of multiple peripheral pulmonary artery stenoses or balloon dilation of a stenotic mitral valve, general anesthesia is usually recommended.

Patients may breathe spontaneously or have assisted ventilation during general anesthesia. Spontaneous ventilation techniques can be achieved with IV anesthesia agents such as ketamine and propofol or with inhalation anesthetic agents and airway protection using a laryngeal mask. For the most part, however, general anesthesia will require assisted ventilation following paralysis with a neuromuscular blocking drug and endotracheal intubation.

MAGNETIC RESONANCE IMAGING AND ANGIOGRAPHY

The claustrophobic small bore of the MRI machine and noise during imaging means that sedation is necessary for most children undergoing cardiac MRI and magnetic resonance angiography procedures. To allow three-dimensional magnetic resonance angiography and gradient echo sequences for images of blood flow, breath-holding is necessary during image acquisition, and therefore general anesthesia is frequently required for neonates, infants, and young children. As in the catheterization laboratory, administering general anesthesia amid the MRI equipment is often difficult and hemodynamic monitoring may be limited.[40]

REFERENCES

1. Morray J. Anesthesia-related cardiac arrests in children: an update. Anesthesiol Clin North America 20(1):1, 2002.
2. Schmitt HJ, Schuetz WH, Proeschel PA, et al. Accuracy of pulse oximetry in children with cyanotic congenital heart disease. J Cardiothorac Vasc Anesth 7:61, 1993.
3. Butt WW, Gow R, Whyte H. Complications resulting from use of arterial catheters: retrograde flow and rapid elevation in blood pressure. Pediatrics 76:250, 1985.
4. Gold JP, Jonas RA, Lang P, et al. Transthoracic intracardiac monitoring lines in pediatric surgical patients: a ten-year experience. Ann Thorac Surg 42:185, 1986.
5. Lang P, Chipman CW, Siden H. Early assessment of hemodynamic status after 24 hours (intensive care unit) and one year postoperative data in 98 patients. Am J Cardiol 49:1733, 1982.
6. McGowan FX, Laussen PC.Con: Transesophageal echocardiography should be used routinely for pediatric open heart surgery. J Cardiothorac Vasc Anesth 13:632, 1999.
7. Hickey PR, Hansen DD, Wessel DL, et al. Pulmonary and systemic hemodynamic responses to fentanyl in infants. Anesth Analg 64:483, 1985.
8. Yaster M.The dose response of fentanyl in neonatal anesthesia. Anesth 66:433, 1987.
9. Hickey PR, Hansen DD, Cramolini GM. Pulmonary and systemic hemodynamic responses to ketamine in infants with normal and elevated pulmonary vascular resistance. Anesth 62:287, 1985.
10. Sarkar M, Laussen PC, Zurakowski D, et al. Hemodynamic responses to an induction dose of etomidate in pediatric patients. Anesthesiology 95:A1263, 2001.
11. Ostwald P, Doenicke AW. Etomidate revisited. Anesth 11:391, 1998.
12. Tanner GE, Angers DG, Barash PG. Effect of left-to-right, mixed left-to-right, and right-to-left shunts on inhalational anesthetic induction in children. Anesth Analg 64:101, 1985.
13. Odegard KC, Modest S, Laussen PC. Parental presence during induction of anaesthesia for children undergoing cardiac surgery. Paediatr Anaesth 12:261, 2002.
14. Laussen PC, Roth PJ. Fast tracking: efficiently and safely moving patients through the intensive care unit. Prog Ped Cardiol 18;149, 2003.
15. Lovoie J, Walsh EP, Laussen PC, et al. Effects of propofol or isoflurane anesthesia on cardiac conduction in children undergoing radiofrequency ablation for tachydysrhythmias. Anesthesiology 82:884, 1995.
16. Zimmerman AA, Ibrahim AE, Epstein MR, et al. The effects of halothane and sevoflurane on cardiac electrophysiology in

children undergoing radiofrequency catheter ablation. Anesth 87:A1066, 1997.
17. Holzman RS, van der Velde ME, Kaus SJ, et al. Sevoflurane depresses myocardial contractility less than halothane during induction of anesthesia in children. Anesth 85:1260, 1996.
18. Hansen DD, Hickey PR. Anesthesia for hypoplastic left heart syndrome: high dose fentanyl in 30 neonates. Anesth Analg 65:127, 1986.
19. Hickey PR, Hansen DD. Fentanyl- and sufentanil-oxygen-pancuronium anesthesia for cardiac surgery in infants. Anesth Analg 63:117, 1984.
20. Lynn AM. Editorial. Remifentanil. The paediatric anaesthetist's opiate? Paediatr Anaesth 6:433, 1996.
21. Shew SB, Jaksic T. The metabolic needs of critically ill children and neonates. Sem Ped Surg 8:131, 1999.
22. Anand KJS, Hansen DD, Hickey PR. Hormonal-metabolic stress responses in neonates undergoing cardiac surgery. Anesthesiology 73:661, 1990.
23. Anand KJS, Hickey, PR. Halothane-morphine compared with high-dose sufentanil for anesthesia and postoperative analgesia in neonatal cardiac surgery. N Eng J Med 326:1, 1992.
24. Gruber EM, Laussen PC, Casta A, et al. Stress response in infants undergoing cardiac surgery: a randomized study of fentanyl bolus, fentanyl infusion, and fentanyl-midazolam infusion. Anesth Analg 92:882, 2001.
25. Duncan HP, Clotte A, Weir PM, et al. Reducing stress responses in the pre-bypass phase of open heart surgery in infants and young children: a comparison of different fentanyl doses. Br J Anaesth 84:556, 2000.
26. Barash PJ, Lescovich F, Katz JD, et al. Early extubation following pediatric cardiothoracic operations: a viable alternative. Ann Thorac Surg 29:228, 1990.
27. Hinle JS, Diaz LK, Fox LS. Early extubation after cardiac operations in neonates and young infants. J Thorac Cardio Surg 114:413, 1997.
28. Vricells LA, Dearani JA, Grundy SR, et al. Ultra-fast track in elective congenital heart surgery. Ann Thorac Surg 69: 865, 2000.
29. Burrows FA, Taylor RH, Hillier SC. Early extubation of the trachea after repair of secundum-type atrial septal defects in children. Can Anaesth Soc J 39:1041, 1992.
30. Laussen PC, Reid W, Stene RA, et al. Tracheal extubation of children in the operating room after atrial septal defect repair as part of a clinical practice guideline. Anesth Analg 82: 988, 1996.
31. Laussen PC, Bichell DP, McGowan FX, et al. An evaluation of patient recovery after minimally invasive surgery and full length sternotomy for repair of atrial septal defects in children. Ann Thoracic Surg 69:591, 2000.
32. Dowd NP, Cheng DCH, Karski JM, et al. Intraoperative awareness in fast-track cardiac anesthesia. Anesth 89: 1068, 1998.
33. Davidson AJ, McCann ME, Devavaram P, et al. Differences in the Bispectral index between infants and children during emergence from anesthesia after circumcision surgery. Anesth Analg 93:326, 2001.
34. McCann ME, Brustowicz RM, Bacsik JA, et al. The Bispectral index and explicit recall during the intraoperative wake-up test for scoliosis surgery. Anesth Analg 94: 1474, 2002.
35. McCann ME, Bacsik JA, Davidson A, et al. The correlation of Bispectral index with end-tidal sevoflurane concentration and hemodynamic parameters in preschoolers. Paediatr Anaesth 12:519, 2002.
36. Laussen PC, Murphy JA, Zurakowski D, et al. Bispectral index monitoring in children undergoing mild hypothermic cardiopulmonary bypass. Paediatr Anaesth 11:567, 2001.
37. Kussman BD, Gruber EM, Zurakowski D, et al. Bispectral index monitoring during infant cardiac surgery: relationship of BIS to the stress response and plasma fentanyl levels. Paediatr Anaesth 11:663, 2001.
38. Tabbatt S, Duncan BW, McLaughlin D, et al. Delayed sternal closure following cardiac surgery in a pediatric population. J Thorac Cardiovasc Surg 113:886, 1997.
39. O'Hare B, Laussen PC. Anesthesia for pediatric cardiac interventional catheterization procedures. In Bissonnette B, and Dalens B. (eds). Pediatric Anesthesia, Principles and Practice. New York: McGraw Hill, 2001, pp 1372–1386.
40. Odegard KO, DiNardo JA, Tsai-Goodman B, et al. Anaesthesia considerations for cardiac MRI in infants and small children. Paediatr Anaesth 14:1339, 2003.

18

Intensive Care Unit

David L. Wessel, MD and
Peter C. Laussen, MBBS

In the past three decades, the development of surgical and catheter techniques for the diagnosis and treatment of critical heart disease in children has been paralleled by major advances in the field of intensive care. Increasingly, children with congenital heart disease (CHD) are now managed in units specifically dedicated to pediatric intensive care or, in particular, pediatric *cardiac* intensive care, rather than in surgical units caring primarily for adults following surgical management of acquired heart disease.[1] Optimal care of these neonates, infants, and children requires an understanding of the subtleties of complex congenital cardiac anomalies, respiratory mechanics and physiology, the transitional circulation of the neonate, pharmacologic and mechanical support of the circulation, the effects of cardiopulmonary bypass (CPB) on the heart, lungs, brain, and abdominal organs; airway management; mechanical ventilation; and treatment of multiorgan system failure. A pediatric cardiology knowledge base assumes a central role in the intensive care management of these patients as more complex therapeutic options become available.

HISTORY

The concepts and value of a hospital ward dedicated to patients requiring intensive care were appreciated during the polio epidemic of the 1950s. The need to mechanically ventilate dozens of patients simultaneously demanded a reorganization of hospital-based care. The modern era of continuous invasive monitoring, pharmacologic manipulation of blood pressure and cardiac output, and resuscitation of critically ill patients of all types arose in large part because of the advent of CPB techniques in the 1950s, the ability to conduct open heart surgery and therefore the need for specialized postoperative care. By 1966 there were also reports of *pediatric* cardiac surgery intensive care units (Minneapolis, Toronto, Boston, etc.) devoted to the specialty. However there was also serious morbidity and mortality associated with critical care of children with heart disease, with one 1966 publication reporting 50% mortality for postoperative children with CHD who required overnight mechanical ventilation.[2] The hazards and implications of requiring cardiac intensive care were staggering.

During the early 1970s, CPB techniques improved substantially and younger children and infants became appropriate candidates for cardiac catheterization and interventions (septostomy) along with cardiac surgical repairs. At the same time, pediatric critical care emerged as a specialized discipline in North America, Australia, parts of Europe, and later in the United Kingdom, attracting subspecialists primarily from pediatric cardiology and pediatric anesthesia.

In some institutions like Children's Hospital Boston, pediatric cardiac critical care evolved in parallel with noncardiac intensive care. In other centers, pediatric cardiac intensive care flourished under the umbrella of multidisciplinary pediatric intensive care. But in nearly all examples it expanded to encompass more than just postoperative patients alone. Pediatric cardiac intensivists were gradually embraced by cardiac surgeons, intensivists, neonatologists, anesthesiologists, and cardiologists as important and necessary specialists with roots in many disciplines. The specialized cardiac nursing component was soon also considered to be indispensable to optimal care of children with heart disease.

STAFF AND PATIENTS, CHILDREN'S HOSPITAL BOSTON

The cardiac intensive care unit at Children's Hospital Boston has evolved to encompass a 23,000–square foot floor for 24 patients with critical heart disease, spanning an age range from the very-low–birth-weight premature infant to the adult with CHD. The physician staff includes eight full-time intensive care physicians who are trained in critical care and usually in pediatric cardiology or cardiac anesthesia. Two experienced senior clinical fellows concentrating in pediatric cardiac intensive care for 1 or more years beyond regular fellowship training provide clinical support and obtain research experience during their period of specialized training. A full complement of clinical trainees derived from cardiology and/or critical care training programs are assigned to the intensive care unit in 1-month rotations. They join cardiac surgical residents in advanced years of training who rotate through the cardiac intensive care unit in 6-month, or longer, blocks. Because of the complexity of illness and required skills, pediatric residents are not routinely part of the physician clinical group until they have entered their fellowship training. More than 80 cardiac intensive care nurses comprise the nursing roster along with respiratory therapists, a cardiac intensive care clinical pharmacist, a cardiovascular social worker, and other hospital-based support staff.

Nearly 1200 admissions to the cardiac intensive care unit (CICU) are encountered each year (Fig. 18-1). Expanding the scope of reparative operations to the newborn and premature newborn has altered the demographic makeup of cardiac patients scheduled for surgery and admitted to the intensive care unit. Typically half of the admissions are among patients younger than 1 year and in 2004, 23% of admissions were newborns. However, because of the complexity of illness among newborns, added diagnostic time preoperatively, and longer postoperative lengths of stay, the newborn population comprises nearly 50% of patient days. Thus nearly every other bed space is occupied by a newborn patient with heart disease. Our clinical focus during the past two decades of cardiac intensive care has been on primary corrective surgery early in life.[3]

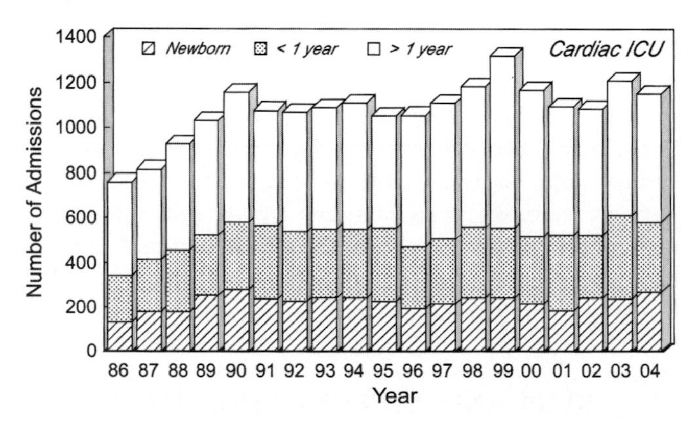

FIGURE 18–1 *Annual admissions to the cardiac intensive care unit at Children's Hospital Boston are nearly 1200. Almost one fourth of admissions are newborns; half are younger than 1 year. Newborns account for 40% to 50% of patient days.*

MULTIDISCIPLINARY CARE

In addition to the important role of the surgeon in postoperative management, care is provided by those with special expertise in critical care, including anesthetic principles, as well as cardiac anatomy and physiology. But the variety of patients with congenital heart disease requiring critical care services requires that clinicians be versed not only in care of the neonate and premature neonate but also in the adult patient with CHD whose care is often referred by adult cardiologists back to a pediatric cardiac intensive care–based program. Few individuals can expect to have such broad training (ranging from newborn medicine through internal medicine), so the challenge has been to develop truly multidisciplinary teams with leadership that can draw upon the expertise of many.

NEWBORN CONSIDERATIONS

Care of the critically ill neonate requires an appreciation of the special structural and functional features of immature organs, the interactions of the *transitional* neonatal circulation and the secondary effects of the congenital heart lesion on other organ systems.[4–8] The neonate appears to respond more quickly and profoundly to physiologically stressful circumstances, which may be expressed in terms of rapid changes in pH, lactic acid, glucose, and temperature. Neonates have diminished fat and carbohydrate reserves. The higher metabolic rate and oxygen consumption of the neonate accounts for the rapid appearance of hypoxia when these patients become apneic. Immaturity of the liver and kidney may be associated with reduced protein synthesis and glomerular filtration such that drug metabolism is altered and hepatic synthetic function is reduced. These issues may be compounded by the normal increased total body water of the neonate compared with that of the older patient, along with the propensity of capillary system of the neonate to leak fluid from the intravascular space. This is especially prominent in the lung of the neonate where the pulmonary vascular bed is nearly fully recruited at rest and lymphatic recruitment required to handle increased mean capillary pressures associated with increases in pulmonary blood flow may be unavailable.[7,8] The neonatal myocardium is less compliant than in the older child, less tolerant of increases in afterload, and less responsive to increases in preload. Younger age also predisposes the myocardium to the adverse effects of CPB and hypothermic ischemia implicit in surgical support techniques used for reparative operations. These factors do not preclude intervention in the neonate but simply dictate that extraordinary vigilance be applied to the care of these children, and that intensive care management plans emerge to account for the immature physiology.

The observed benefits of neonatal reparative operations discussed in Chapter 57 will continue to dictate that care of the newborn with complex congenital heart disease after CPB is a central feature of cardiac intensive care. At Children's Hospital Boston our approach to neonates with CHD has been toward complete surgical correction rather than palliation in order to avoid the pathophysiologic consequences and limits on neonatal growth.[3] This concept has been extended to include the premature newborns who now as a group are admitted to the CICU before surgical correction. One in 10 newborns is premature. Palliative medical or surgical interventions were often preferred management options in premature infants with CHD, however, current experience supports the notion that early biventricular repair can be achieved with low mortality.[9]

PREOPERATIVE CARE

Optimal preoperative care involves (a) initial stabilization, airway management, and establishment of vascular access; (b) a complete and thorough noninvasive delineation of the anatomic defect(s); (c) resuscitation with evaluation and treatment of secondary organ dysfunction, particularly the brain, kidneys, and liver; (d) cardiac catheterization if necessary—typically for (1) physiologic assessment, (2) interventional procedures such as balloon atrial septostomy or valvotomy, or (3) anatomic definition not visible by echocardiography (e.g., coronary artery distribution in pulmonary atresia with intact ventricular septum or delineation of aorticopulmonary collaterals in tetralogy of Fallot with pulmonary atresia); and (e) surgical management when cardiac, pulmonary, renal and central nervous systems are optimized. Crucial in this process is the continued communication among medical, surgical and nursing disciplines.

POSTOPERATIVE CARE

Assessment

When the clinical course of patients after cardiac surgery deviates from the usual expectation of uncomplicated recovery, our first responsibility is to verify the accuracy of the preoperative diagnosis and the adequacy of the surgical repair. For example, a young infant who is acidotic, hypotensive, and cyanotic after surgical repair of tetralogy of Fallot may tempt us to ascribe the findings to the vagaries of ischemia–reperfusion injury of CPB or transient, postoperative stiffness of the right ventricle. However, the real culprit may be an additional ventricular septal defect undetected preoperatively and therefore not closed, a residual ventricular septal defect around the surgical patch, or residual right ventricular outflow obstruction. Any of these anatomic issues—and more—can produce serious adverse outcomes. Getting the right postoperative assessment is therefore imperative and treatment follows accordingly. Evaluation of the postoperative patient relies on examination, monitoring, and interpretation of vital signs or other bedside data and imaging (Table 18-1). When the accuracy of the diagnosis and adequacy of the repair are established, then a low cardiac output state can be presumed and treatment optimized. Treating low cardiac output states and preventing cardiovascular collapse are often the central features of pediatric cardiac intensive care. This topic will be the focus of this chapter, without detailing the specific considerations for each lesion, which instead are presented in their respective chapters.

Optimizing preload involves more than just giving volume to a hypotensive patient. There are numerous considerations to fluid balance involving types of isotonic fluid, ultrafiltration in the operating room, optimal hematocrit, use of furosemide, thiazides, and newer drugs like fenoldapam or nesiritide. Fluid itself can be detrimental if excess extravascular water results in interstitial edema and end-organ dysfunction of vital organs like the heart, lungs, and brain. Perhaps permitting a right-to-left shunt at atrial level would optimize preload to the left ventricle in some conditions (see below). Maintaining aortic perfusion after CPB and improving the contractile state of the heart with higher doses of catecholamines is a reasonable goal but may have particularly deleterious consequences in the newborn myocardium after hypothermic CPB. The benefits of afterload reduction are well known but in excess there is hypotension and cardiovascular collapse or renal or cerebral insufficiency. Pacing the heart can stabilize the rhythm and hemodynamics but may also contribute to dysynchronous, inefficient contraction of the heart or

TABLE 18–1. Intensive Care Strategies to Diagnose and Support Low Cardiac Output States

Know the cardiac anatomy in detail and its physiologic consequences
Understand the specialized considerations of the newborn and implications of reparative rather than palliative surgery
Diversify personnel to include expertise in neonatal and adult congenital heart disease
Monitor, measure, and image the heart to rule out residual disease as a cause of postoperative hemodynamic instability or low cardiac output, then maintain aortic perfusion and improve the contractile state
Optimize preload (including atrial shunting)
Reduce afterload
Control heart rate, rhythm and synchrony
Optimize heart lung interactions
Provide mechanical support when needed

induce other arrhythmias. And finally, mechanical support of the failing myocardium in the form of extracorporeal membrane oxygenation (ECMO) or ventricular assist devices, while life-saving in many instances, presents their own set of time limitations and morbid complications. One must recognize that almost every treatment approach has its own set of adverse effects that may be damaging. Supporting cardiac output in the postoperative patient is a balance between the promise and poison of therapy.

The initial assessment following cardiac surgery begins with review of the operative findings. This includes details of the operative repair and CPB, particularly total CPB or myocardial ischemia (aortic cross clamp) times, concerns about myocardial protection, recovery of myocardial contractility, typical postoperative systemic arterial and central venous pressures, findings from intraoperative transesophageal echocardiogram, if performed, and vasoactive medication requirement. This information will guide subsequent examination, which should focus on the quality of the repair or palliation plus a clinical assessment of cardiac output (Table 18-2). In addition to a complete cardiovascular examination, a routine set of laboratory tests should be obtained, including a chest radiograph, 12- or 15-lead electrocardiogram, blood gas analysis, serum electrolytes and glucose, an ionized calcium level, complete blood count, and coagulation profile.

Monitoring

The level of bedside monitoring that is appropriate for each patient depends upon his or her cardiac diagnosis, the type of repair or palliation, and anticipated requirements for hemodynamic and respiratory data. All patients should have continuous monitoring of their heart rate and rhythm by electrocardiogram, systemic arterial blood pressure (invasive or noninvasive), oxygen saturation by pulse oximetry, and respiratory rate. Breath-to-breath end-tidal CO_2 monitoring is routine in mechanically ventilated patients to monitor for possible disconnection, misplacement, or obstruction of the endotracheal tube. It is also a useful indicator for acute changes in pulmonary blood flow.

Monitoring central venous pressure is routine for many patients following cardiac surgery, except those who undergo the least complex procedures. For example, we do not routinely place a central venous catheter in patients undergoing thoracic procedures, such as coarctation of the aorta or vascular ring and patent ductus arteriosus (PDA) ligation, nor in patients undergoing cardiotomy with a short period of mildly hypothermic CPB, such as an atrial septal defect repair. Intracardiac or transthoracic left atrial (LA) catheters are often used to monitor patients after complex reparative procedures. Pulmonary artery (PA) catheters are now seldom used but may be particularly useful if the postoperative management anticipates a problem such as (a) a residual lesion producing an intracardiac left-to-right shunt (e.g., multiple ventral septal defects [VSDs]); (b) residual right ventricle (RV) outflow tract obstruction, since a catheter *pull-back* can be performed to measure the RV-to-PA pressure gradient; and (c) pulmonary hypertension, thereby allowing rapid detection of pressure changes and assessment of the response to interventions.

LA catheters are especially helpful in the management of patients with ventricular dysfunction, coronary artery perfusion abnormalities, and mitral valve disease. The mean LA pressure is typically 1 to 2 mm Hg greater than mean RA pressure, which generally varies between 1 and 6 mm Hg in nonpostoperative pediatric patients undergoing cardiac catheterization. In postoperative patients, mean LA and RA pressures are both often greater than 6 to 8 mm Hg. However, they should generally be less than 15 mm Hg. The compliance of the RA is greater than that of the LA except in the newborn, so pressure elevations in the RA of older patients with two ventricles are typically less pronounced.

Table 18-3 shows possible causes of abnormally elevated LA pressure. In addition to pressure data, intracardiac catheters in the RA (or a percutaneously placed central venous catheter), LA, and PA can be used to monitor the oxygen saturation of systemic venous or pulmonary venous blood.

Table 18-4 lists the causes of abnormally high or low RA, LA, and PA oxygen saturations, which can be measured at the bedside in the ICU. Following reparative surgery, patients with no intracardiac shunts and an adequate cardiac output may have a mild reduction in RA oxygen saturation to approximately 60%. Lower RA oxygen saturation does not

TABLE 18–2. Signs of Heart Failure or Low Cardiac Output States

Signs:
Cool extremities/poor perfusion
Oliguria and other end organ failure
Tachycardia
Hypotension
Acidosis
Cardiomegaly
Pleural effusions
Monitor and measure:
Heart rate, blood pressure, intracardiac pressure
Extremity temperature, central temperature
Urine output
Mixed venous oxygen saturation
Arterial blood gas pH and lactate
Laboratory measures of end organ function
Echocardiography

TABLE 18–3. Common Causes of Elevated Left Atrial Pressure After Cardiotomy

Decreased ventricular systolic or diastolic function
Myocardial ischemia
Dilated cardiomyopathy
Systemic ventricular hypertrophy
Left atrioventricular valve disease
Large left-to-right intracardiac shunt
Chamber hypoplasia
Intravascular or ventricular volume overload
Cardiac tamponade
Arrhythmia:
Tachyarrhythmia, junctional rhythm
Complete heart block

necessarily indicate low cardiac output; if a patient has arterial desaturation (common mixing lessons, lung diseases, etc.) an arteriovenous oxygen difference of 25% is normal, and there may be appropriate oxygen delivery and extraction. Elevated RA oxygen saturation is often due to left-to-right shunting at the atrial level (e.g., from the LA, from an anomalous pulmonary vein, or from an LV-to-RA shunt). Blood in the LA is normally fully saturated with oxygen (i.e., approximately 100%). The two chief causes of reduced LA oxygen saturation are an atrial level right-to-left shunt and pulmonary venous desaturation from abnormal gas exchange.

In the absence of left-to-right shunts, the PA oxygen saturation is the best representation of the *true* mixed venous oxygen saturation, because all sources of systemic venous blood should be thoroughly combined as they are ejected from the RV. When elevated, this saturation is useful in the identification of residual left-to-right shunts following repair of VSD. The absolute valve of the PA oxygen saturation is a predictor of significant postoperative residual shunt. In patients following tetralogy of Fallot (TOF) or VSD repair, a PA oxygen saturation above 80% within 48 hours of surgery with supplemental oxygen (O_2) at a fractional inspired oxygen concentration (F_IO_2) below 0.5 has been shown to be a sensitive indicator of a significant left-to-right shunt (Qp/Qs > 1.5) 1 year after surgery.[10] Determination of the PA oxygen saturation can also be useful in patients with systemic-to–pulmonary artery collaterals, because flow from these vessels into the pulmonary arteries can increase the oxygen saturation.

Low Cardiac Output Syndrome

Although some causes of low cardiac output after cardiopulmonary bypass are attributable to residual or undiagnosed structural lesions, progressive low cardiac output states do occur. A number of factors have been implicated in the development of myocardial dysfunction following cardiopulmonary bypass including (a) the inflammatory response associated with cardiopulmonary bypass; (b) the effects of myocardial ischemia from aortic cross clamping; (c) hypothermia; (d) reperfusion injury; (e) inadequate myocardial protection; and (f) ventriculotomy (when performed). The expression and prevention of reperfusion injury after aortic cross clamping on cardiopulmonary bypass is currently the subject of intense investigation. We have previously shown the typical decrease in cardiac index in newborns following an arterial switch operation (Fig. 18-2).[11] In this group of 122 newborns, the median maximal decrease in cardiac index, which occurred typically 6 to 12 hours after separation from cardiopulmonary bypass, was 32%. A fourth of all of these newborns reached a nadir of cardiac index that was less than 2 L/min/m^2 on the first postoperative night.

TABLE 18–4. Causes of Abnormal Right Atrial, Left Atrial, or Pulmonary Artery Oxygen Saturation

Location	Elevated	Reduced
RA	Atrial level left-to-right shunt	↑ VO_2 (e.g., low CO, fever)
	Anomalous pulmonary venous return	↓ SaO_2 saturation with a normal A-V O_2 difference
	Left ventricular-to-right atrial shunt	Anemia
	↑ dissolved O_2 content	Catheter tip position (e.g., near CS)
	↓ O_2 extraction	
	Catheter tip position (e.g., near renal veins)	
LA	Does not occur	Atrial level right-to-left shunt
		↓ PvO_2 (e.g., parenchymal lung disease)
PA	Significant left-to-right shunt	↑ O_2 extraction (e.g., low CO, fever)
	Small left-to-right shunt with incomplete mixing of blood	↓ SaO_2 saturation with a normal A-V O_2 difference
	Catheter tip position (e.g., PA "wedge")	Anemia

RA, right atrium; LA, left atrium; CO, cardiac output; PA, pulmonary artery; A-V, arterio-venous; VO_2, oxygentation consumption; CS, coronary sinus; PvO_2, pulmonary vein oxygen tension; SaO_2, arterial oxygen saturation.

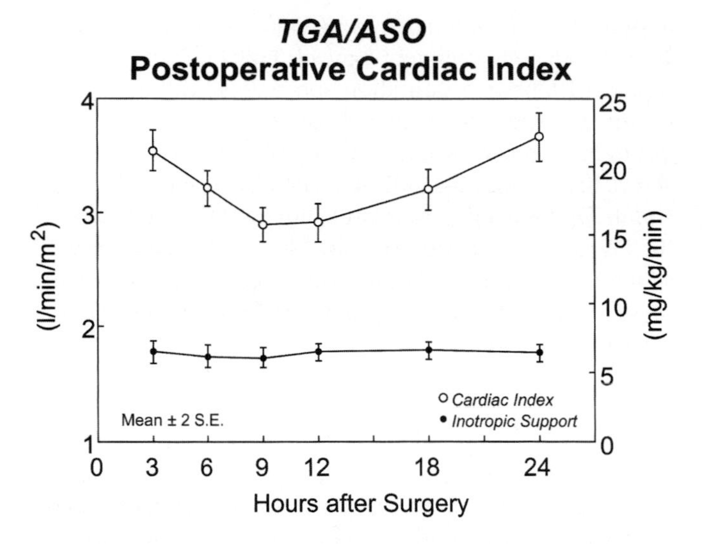

FIGURE 18–2 *Cardiac index measured in infants following the arterial switch operation declines during the first 12 hours. A fourth of the patients reach a value less than 2.0 L/min/m². The median reduction in cardiac index the first night is 33%. See Wernovsky G, Wypij D, Jonas RA, et al. Postoperative course and hemodynamic profile after the arterial switch operation in neonates and infants. A comparison of low-flow cardiopulmonary bypass and circulatory arrest. Circulation 92(8):2226, 1995, with permission.*

Low cardiac output syndrome (LCOS) does occur in the postoperative patient, but appropriate anticipation and intervention can do much to avert morbidity or the need for mechanical support. Signs of low cardiac output are listed in Table 18-2. Mixed venous oxygen saturation, whole-blood pH, and lactate are laboratory measures commonly used to evaluate the adequacy of tissue perfusion and hence, cardiac output.

Volume Adjustments

After CPB, the factors that influence cardiac output such as preload, afterload, myocardial contractility, heart rate, and rhythm must be assessed and manipulated. Volume therapy (increased preload) is commonly necessary, followed by appropriate use of inotropic and afterload-reducing agents.[4] Atrial pressure and the ventricular response to changes in atrial pressure must be evaluated. Ventricular response is judged by observing systemic arterial pressure and waveform, heart rate, skin color and peripheral extremity temperature, peripheral pulse magnitude, urine flow, core body temperature, and acid-base balance.

Preserving and Creating Right-to-Left Shunts

Selected children with low cardiac output may benefit from strategies that allow right-to-left shunting at the atrial level in the face of postoperative right ventricular dysfunction. A typical example is early repair of TOF, when the moderately hypertrophied, noncompliant right ventricle has undergone a ventriculotomy and may be further compromised by an increased volume load from pulmonary regurgitation secondary to a transannular patch on the right ventricular outflow tract. In these children, it is very useful to leave the foramen ovale patent to permit right-to-left shunting of blood, thus preserving cardiac output and oxygen delivery despite the attendant transient cyanosis. If the foramen is not patent or is surgically closed, right ventricular dysfunction can lead to reduced left ventricular filling, low cardiac output, and ultimately, left ventricular dysfunction. In infants and neonates with repaired truncus arteriosus, the same concerns apply and may even be exaggerated if right ventricular afterload is elevated because of pulmonary artery hypertension. This concept has been extended to older patients with single-ventricle physiology who are at high risk for Fontan operations.[12] The Fontan circulation relies on passive flow of blood through the pulmonary circulation without benefit of a pulmonary ventricle. If an atrial septal communication or fenestration is left at the time of the Fontan procedure, the resulting right-to-left shunt helps to preserve cardiac output. These children have fewer postoperative complications.[13] It is better to shunt blood right to left, accept some decrement in oxygen saturation, but maintain ventricular filling and cardiac output, than to have high oxygen saturation but low blood pressure and cardiac output.

Pharmacologic Support

Catecholamines

Preload adjustments often do not suffice to provide adequate cardiac output. Use of pharmacologic agents to support cardiac output is common.[14,15] Table 18-5 lists common vasoactive drugs used in the ICU and their actions. Many prefer to use dopamine first in doses of 3 to 10 μg/kg per minute. One rarely uses more than 15 μg/kg/minute because of the known vasoconstrictor and chronotropic properties of dopamine at very high doses. However, extreme biologic variability in pharmacokinetics and pharmacodynamics defies placing narrow limits on recommended dosages. Dobutamine's chronotropic and vasodilatory advantages recognized in adults with coronary artery disease have not always proved equally efficacious in clinical studies in children. In fact, dobutamine has fewer, or no, dopaminergic advantages for the kidney.[16] This may be an especially important limitation in infants with excess total body water and interstitial edema. The significant chronotropic effect and increased oxygen consumption induced by isoproterenol have also increasingly limited its use in neonates and infants. Epinephrine is occasionally useful for short-term therapy when high systemic pressures are sought, provided that the temporary increase in

TABLE 18–5. Summary of Selected Vasoactive Agents

Noncatecholamines

Agent	Doses (IV)	Peripheral Vascular Effect	Cardiac Effect	Conduction System Effect
Digoxin	20 µg/kg premature	Increases peripheral vascular resistance 1–2+;	Inotropic effect 3–4+; acts	Slows sinus node
(Total digitalizing	30 µg/kg neonate	acts directly on vascular smooth muscle.	directly on myocardium.	slightly; decreases
dose)	(0–1 mo)	Variable; age dependent. Vasoconstrictor.	Inotropic effect 3+; depends	atrioventricular
Calcium:	40 µg/kg infant (< 2 yr)	Donates nitric oxide group to relax smooth	on ionized Ca^{++}.	conduction more.
Chloride	30 µg/kg child (2–5 yr)	muscle and dilate pulmonary and systemic	Indirectly increases cardiac	Slows sinus node;
Gluconate	20 µg/kg child (> 5 yr)	vessels.	output by decreasing afterload.	decreases atrioven-
Nitroprusside	10–20 mg/kg/dose (slowly)	Primarily venodilator. As a nitric oxide donor	Decreases preload, may decrease	tricular conduction.
Nitroglycerin	50–100 mg/kg/dose (slowly)	may cause pulmonary vasodilation, and	afterload. Reduces myocardial	Reflex tachycardia
Amrinone	0.5–5 µg/kg/min	enhance coronary vasoreactivity after aortic	work related to change in wall	Minimal
Milrinone	0.5–10 µ/kg/min	cross-clamping.	stress.	Minimal tachycardia
Vasopressin	1–3 mg/kg loading dose	Systemic and pulmonary vasodilator.	Diastolic relaxation (lusiotropy)	As above
Thyroid Hormone	5–20 mcg/kg/min	Thrombocytopenia.	As above	None known
Tri-iodothyronine	maintenance	As above	No direct effect	Tachycardia
(T3)	50 µg/kg loading dose	Shorter half-life	Positive inotropy	
Natriuretic peptide	0.25–1.0 µ/kg/min	Potent vasoconstrictior	Positive inotropy	
(Nesiritide)	maintenance	Mild vasodilator	Diastolic relaxation	
	.002–.003 U/kg/min	Vasodilation		
	0.05–0.10 µ/kg/min	Natriuresis		
	0.01–0.03 µ/kg/min	Little experience in children. Diuretic effects controversial		

(Continued)

TABLE 18–5. Summary of Selected Vasoactive Agents—cont'd

Catecholamines								
				Peripheral Vascular Effect			Cardiac Effect
Agent	Dose Range	Alpha	$Beta_2$	Delta	$Beta_1$	$Beta_2$	Comment
Phenylephrine	0.1–0.5 μg/kg/min	4+	0	0	0	0	Increases systemic resistance, no inotropy; may cause renal
Isoproterenol	0.05–0.5 μg/kg/min	0	4+	0	4+	4+	ischemia; useful for treatment of tetralogy of
Norepinephrine	0.1–0.5 μg/kg/min	4+	0	0	2+	0	Fallot spells
Epinephrine	0.03–0.1 μg/kg/min	2+	1–2+	0	2–3+	2+	Strong inotropic and chronotropic agent; peripheral vasodilator;
Dopamine	0.2–0.5 μg/kg/min	4+	0	0	4+	3+	reduces preload; pulmonary vasodilator. Limited by tachycardia
Dobutamine	2–4 μg/kg/min	0	0	2+	0	0	and oxygen consumption
Fenoldapam	4–8 μg/kg/min	0	2+	2+	1–2+	1+	Increases systemic resistance; moderately inotropic; may cause
	>10 μg/kg/min	2–4+	0	0	1–2+	2+	renal ischemia $beta_2$ effect with lower doses; best for blood
	2–10 μg/kg/min	1+	2+	0	3–4+	1–2+	pressure in anaphylaxis and drug toxicity
	0.05–1 μg/kg/min						Splanchnic and renal vasodilator; may be used with isoproterenol;
	See text						increasing doses produce increasing alpha effect
	Little experience in children						Less chronotropy and arrhythmias at lower doses; effects vary with
							dose similar to dopamine; chronotropic advantage compared
							with dopamine may not be apparent in neonates
							Powerful D_1 agonist. Little chronotropic or inotropic effect but
							may redistribute flow to renal bed and improve urine output

peripheral vascular resistance can be tolerated. High doses of epinephrine are occasionally necessary to increase pulmonary blood flow across significantly narrowed systemic-to-pulmonary artery shunts when oxygen saturations are low and falling. Arginine vasopressin has been advocated for states of refractory vasodilation associated with low circulating vasopressin levels as may rarely occur after CPB in children.[17]

In the past, the side effects of inotropic support of the heart with catecholamines seemed a lesser concern in children than in adults with an ischemic, noncompliant heart. Tachycardia, an increased end-diastolic pressure and afterload, or increased myocardial oxygen consumption, in spite of their undesirable side effects, were tolerated by most children in need of inotropic support after CPB. However, with increasing perioperative experience in neonates and young infants, the adverse effects of vasoactive drugs have become more evident. The less compliant neonatal myocardium, like the ischemic adult heart, may raise its end-diastolic pressure during higher doses of dopamine infusion or may develop even more extreme noncompliance. Actual myocardial necrosis caused by high doses of epinephrine infusions has been identified in neonatal animal models after CPB.[18,19] Although these agents do increase the cardiac output, the concomitant increase in ventricular filling pressure is less well tolerated by the immature myocardium than it is in older children. Many of the complex corrective procedures performed in neonates and small infants are accompanied by transient postoperative arrhythmias that are either induced or exacerbated by catecholamines, which can have a profound adverse effect on the patient's recovery after surgery. Diastolic function is crucial in older patients with single ventricles and can be adversely affected by catecholamines. Nevertheless, the predictable and often significant decrease in cardiac output documented by many investigators after CPB in infants and older children continues to justify the practice of judiciously using catecholamines to support the heart and circulation while weaning them from CPB and during the immediate postoperative period.

Phosphodiesterase III Inhibitors

Milrinone has emerged as an important inotropic agent for use in children after open heart surgery.[20–22] It is a nonglycosidic, noncatecholamine inotropic agent with additional vasodilatory and lusitropic properties. Used extensively in adults for treatment of heart failure, and more recently introduced to pediatric practice, this class of drugs exerts their principle effects by inhibiting phosphodiesterase III, the enzyme that metabolizes cyclic adenosine monophosphate (cAMP). By increasing intracellular cAMP, calcium transport into the cell is favored, and the increased intracellular calcium stores enhance the contractile state of the myocyte. In addition, the re-uptake of calcium is a cAMP-dependent process, and these agents may therefore enhance diastolic relaxation of the myocardium by increasing the rate of calcium re-uptake after systole (lusitropy). The drug also appears to work synergistically with low doses of β-agonists and has fewer side effects than other catecholamine vasodilators, such as isoproterenol. In critically ill postoperative newborns, milrinone increased cardiac output, lowered filling pressures, and reduced pulmonary artery pressures.[21]

The PRIMACORP trial investigated the efficacy and safety of prophylactic milrinone use to prevent LCOS after cardiac surgery in high-risk pediatric patients.[22] The study was a multicenter, randomized, double-blind, placebo-controlled trial using three parallel treatment groups (low-dose: 25-μg/kg bolus over 60 minutes followed by a 0.25-μg/kg per minute infusion for 35 hours; high-dose: 75-μg/kg bolus followed by 0.75 μg/kg per minute, or placebo). The composite end point of death or the development of LCOS was evaluated at 36 hours and at the follow-up visit. Among 238 treated patients, the prophylactic use of high-dose milrinone significantly reduced the risk of death or the development of LCOS relative to placebo with a relative risk reduction of 55% ($P = 0.023$) in the treated patients. Patients who developed LCOS had a significantly longer cumulative duration of mechanical ventilation and hospital stay in comparison with those who did not develop LCOS. The authors concluded that the prophylactic use of high-dose milrinone following pediatric congenital heart surgery reduces the risk of LCOS. Dopamine and milrinone have emerged as our most commonly used inotropic agents, often used in combination to achieve increased cardiac output, maintain arterial perfusion pressure, and improve diastolic relaxation.

Thyroid Hormone

LCOS typically overlaps with the time that free and total tri-iodothyronine (T3) levels are significantly suppressed following surgical reconstruction, namely during the first 24 to 48 hours postoperatively. This is a significant observation, as T3 is the predominant form of biologically active thyroid hormone and is known to improve cardiac output by improving the inotropic state of animal and human hearts, while decreasing systemic vascular resistance. Limited studies of T3 supplementation after cardiac surgery have been performed in children. Mainwaring et al.[23] gave 2 bolus doses of T3 after the Fontan procedure to 10 children aged 19 to 42 months. Compared with a historical control group, the T3 patients had a significantly shorter period of mechanical ventilation. Bettendorf et al.[24] randomized 40 children undergoing a wide variety of cardiac procedures to receive bolus dosing of T3 or placebo. Cardiac output was reported to be higher in the treatment group, estimated by echocardiography. Chowdhury et al.[25] randomized 28 children aged 0 to 18 years to a 5-day continuous infusion of

T3 (0.05–0.15 μg/kg/hr) or placebo. Among neonates, the T3 group had lower severity of illness scores and lower inotrope requirements. The T3 group also had a trend toward higher mixed venous oxygen saturations, fewer days of mechanical ventilation, and a shorter postoperative length of stay. No adverse effects of T3 administration were recorded in any of these small series.

Thus the current literature demonstrates that infants undergoing cardiac surgery experience significant depression of T3 levels and that supplementation of T3 may have an impact on physiologic variables and perhaps other measures of improved outcomes. Larger trials with more rigorous trial design are under way and may address whether certain subgroups at particular risk for LCOS may benefit from T3 administration. Preliminary analysis of a blinded trial of T3 administration to patients after reconstructive surgery for hypoplastic left heart syndrome at Children's Hospital Boston was disappointing.

Other Afterload-Reducing Agents

When systemic blood pressure is elevated and cardiac output appears low or normal, a primary vasodilator is indicated to normalize blood pressure and to decrease the afterload on the left ventricle. This is especially true for the newborn myocardium, which is especially sensitive to changes in afterload and tolerates elevated systemic resistances poorly. Although nitroprusside has no known direct inotropic effects, this potent vasodilator has the advantage of being readily titratable and possessing a short biologic half-life. Use of nitroglycerin avoids the toxic metabolites, cyanide and thiocyanate, associated with nitroprusside use (especially in hepatic and renal insufficiency), but its potency as a vasodilator is less than that of nitroprusside. Inhibitors of angiotensin-converting enzyme have proven to be important adjuvants to chronic anticongestive therapy in pediatric patients. Intravenous forms are available and may be useful in treatment of systemic hypertension immediately after coarctation repair or when afterload reduction with these inhibitors would benefit patients unable to receive oral medications. Sudden hypotension with the intravenous forms may limit use among infants.

The natriuretic hormone system is an important regulator of neurohumoral activation, vascular tone, diastolic function, and fluid balance. Preliminary data suggest that the endogenous biologic activity of the natriuretic hormone system is decreased following pediatric cardiopulmonary bypass. In theory, infusions of brain natriuretic peptide could oppose the neurohumoral mechanism associated with vasoconstriction and fluid retention after pediatric CPB. In randomized adult studies following cardiopulmonary bypass, natriuretic hormone infusions suppress the renin-angiotensin-aldosterone axis and improve cardiac loading conditions, cardiac index, and urine output.[26–29] We have increasing experience with nesiritide infusions in children.

Fenoldapam is a new dopaminergic agent useful in the treatment of systemic hypertension and may have salutary effects on renal blood flow. It has no known chronotropic or inotropic effects on the heart but reduces afterload and may augment urine output in critically ill newborns after cardiac surgery.

Levosimendan is a calcium sensitizer that enhances the contractile state of the ventricle by increasing myocyte sensitivity to calcium and induces vasodilation. Levosimendan increases cardiac output by increasing stroke volume. It is independent of cAMP pathways that characterize the mechanism of action of both the catecholamines and the type III phosphodiesterase inhibitors. With its positive inotropic effects, levosimendan may be of value as adjunctive therapy to other inotropic drugs in patients who are refractory or tachyphylactic to other forms of inotropic support. Its hemodynamic effect in children is uncertain, but its pharmacokinetic profile seems similar to adults.[30]

Other Strategies

Newer strategies to support low cardiac output associated with cardiac surgery in children include use of atrio-biventricular pacing for patients with complete heart block or prolonged interventricular conduction delays and asynchronous contraction.[31] Appreciation of the hemodynamic effects of positive and negative pressure ventilation may facilitate cardiac output. Avoidance of hyperthermia and even induced hypothermia may provide end-organ protection during periods of low cardiac output. Anti-inflammatory agents including monoclonal antibodies, competitive receptor blockers, inhibitors of compliment activation, and preoperative preparation with steroids are being actively investigated in an effort to prevent and protect major organs from ischemic injury imposed by cardiopulmonary bypass and the reperfusion injury associated with the recovery period.

DIASTOLIC DYSFUNCTION

Occasionally there is an alteration of ventricular relaxation, an active energy-dependent process, which reduces ventricular compliance. This is particularly problematic in patients with a hypertrophied ventricle undergoing surgical repair (e.g., tetralogy of Fallot or Fontan surgery) and following CPB in some neonates when myocardial edema may significantly restrict diastolic function (i.e., *restrictive physiology*).[32,33] The ventricular cavity size is small and the stroke volume is decreased. β-Adrenergic antagonists and calcium channel blockers add little to the treatment of this condition. In fact, hypotension or myocardial depression produced by these agents frequently outweighs any gain from slowing the heart rate. Calcium channel blockers are relatively contraindicated in neonates and small infants because of their dependence on transsarcolemmal flux of calcium to both initiate and sustain contraction.

A gradual increase in intravascular volume to augment ventricular capacity, in addition to the use of low doses of inotropic agents, has proven to provide modest benefit in patients with diastolic dysfunction. Tachycardia must be avoided to optimize diastolic filling time and to decrease myocardial oxygen demands. If low cardiac output continues despite the above-outlined treatment, therapy with vasodilators can be carefully attempted to alter systolic wall tension (afterload) and thus decrease the impediment to ventricular ejection. Because the capacity of the vascular bed increases after vasodilation, simultaneous volume replacement is often indicated. Milrinone or enoximone is useful under these circumstances since these agents are noncatecholamine so-called inodilators with vasodilating and lusitropic (improved diastolic state) properties, in contrast to other inotropic agents. Nesiritide also may have a particularly important role to play in lowering left ventricular filling pressures in patients with heart failure.

MANAGING ACUTE PULMONARY HYPERTENSION IN THE INTENSIVE CARE UNIT

Children with many forms of CHD are prone to develop perioperative elevations in pulmonary vascular resistance (PVR). This may complicate the postoperative course, when transient myocardial dysfunction requires optimal control of right ventricular afterload.[34]

Although one often presumes that postoperative patients with pulmonary hypertension have active and reversible pulmonary vasoconstriction as the source of their pathophysiology, the critical care physician is obligated to explore anatomic causes of mechanical obstruction that impose a barrier to pulmonary blood flow. Elevated LA pressure, pulmonary venous obstruction, branch pulmonary artery stenosis, or surgically induced loss of the vascular tree all will raise right ventricular pressure and impose an unnecessary burden on the right heart. Similarly a residual or undiagnosed left-to-right shunt will raise pulmonary artery pressure postoperatively and must be addressed. Extended use of pulmonary vasodilator strategies will only augment residual or undiagnosed shunts and increase the volume load on the heart.

Several factors peculiar to CPB may raise PVR: Pulmonary vascular endothelial dysfunction, microemboli, pulmonary leukosequestration, excess thromboxane production, atelectasis, hypoxic pulmonary vasoconstriction, and adrenergic events have all been suggested to play a role in postoperative pulmonary hypertension. Postoperative pulmonary vascular reactivity has been related not only to the presence of preoperative pulmonary hypertension and left-to-right shunts, but also to the duration of total CPB. Treatment of postoperative pulmonary hypertensive crises has been partially addressed by surgery at earlier ages, pharmacologic intervention, and other postoperative management strategies (Table 18-6).

Pulmonary Vasodilators

Many intravenous vasodilators have been used with variable success in patients with pulmonary hypertensive disorders requiring critical care. Older style vasodilators such as tolazaline, phenoxybenzamine, nitroprusside, or isoproterenol had little biologic basis for selectivity or enhanced activity in the pulmonary vascular bed.[35] However, if myocardial function is depressed and the afterload-reducing effect on the left ventricle is beneficial to myocardial function and cardiac output, there may be some value to these drugs. However, in addition to drug-specific side effects, they all have the limitation of potentially profound systemic hypotension, critically lowering right (and left) coronary perfusion pressure and simultaneously increasing intrapulmonary shunt. Even with selective infusions of rapidly metabolized intravenously administered vasoactive drugs into the pulmonary circulation, systemic drug concentrations and systemic hemodynamic effects can be appreciable.

Prostacyclin appears to have somewhat more selectivity for the pulmonary circulation but at high doses can precipitate a hypotensive crisis in unstable postoperative patients with refractory pulmonary hypertension. It is best suited for chronic outpatient therapy in severe forms of primary pulmonary hypertension.[36–39] Agents that improve ventricular

TABLE 18–6. Critical Care Strategies for Postoperative Treatment of Pulmonary Hypertension

Encourage	Avoid
1. Anatomic investigation	1. Residual anatomic disease
2. Opportunities for right-to-left shunt as "pop off"	2. Intact atrial septum in right heart failure
3. Sedation/anesthesia	3. Agitation/pain
4. Moderate hyperventilation	4. Respiratory acidosis
5. Moderate alkalosis	5. Metabolic acidosis
6. Adequate inspired oxygen	6. Alveolar hypoxia
7. Normal lung volumes	7. Atelectasis or overdistention
8. Optimal hematocrit	8. Excessive hematocrit
9. Inotropic support	9. Low output and coronary perfusion
10. Vasodilators	10. Vasoconstrictors/increased afterload

function in addition to reducing afterload (e.g., type III phosphodiesterase inhibitors) are more appealing when cardiac output is low.

As an alternative approach to nonspecific vasodilators, it seems logical to target vasoconstrictors known to be associated with pathologic states or critical events. In this regard, endothelin, a potent vasoconstrictor, elevated in newborns with persistent pulmonary hypertension, children with congenital heart disease, and patients after cardiopulmonary bypass seems a likely candidate for investigation of specific receptor blockers. Petrossian and colleagues[40] have shown promising amelioration of postoperative pulmonary hypertension associated with cardiopulmonary bypass in animal models of increased pulmonary blood flow (from intracardiac shunts) when pretreated with endothelin-A receptor blockers. Undoubtedly, since the causes of pulmonary hypertension in the intensive care setting are frequently multifactorial, our *best* therapy will be multiply targeted. Adding phosphodiesterase inhibitors to prostacyclin infusions, endothelin blockers, thromboxane inhibitors, and inhaled nitric oxide (NO) may all have individual and combined merit with synergism enhancing efficacy.

NO is a selective pulmonary vasodilator that can be breathed as a gas and distributed across the alveoli to the pulmonary vascular smooth muscle.[41,42] It is formed by the endothelium from L-arginine and molecular oxygen in a reaction catalyzed by NO synthase. It then diffuses to the adjacent vascular smooth muscle cells where it induces vasodilation through a cyclic guanosine monophosphate–dependent pathway.[43] Since NO exists as a gas, it can be delivered by inhalation to the alveoli and then to the blood vessels that lie in close proximity to ventilated lung. Because of its rapid inactivation by hemoglobin, inhaled NO may achieve selective pulmonary vasodilation when pulmonary vasoconstriction exists. It has advantages over intravenously administered vasodilators that cause systemic hypotension and increase intrapulmonary shunting. Inhaled NO lowers pulmonary artery pressure in a number of diseases without the unwanted effect of systemic hypotension. This is especially dramatic in children with cardiovascular disorders and postoperative patients with pulmonary hypertensive crises.[34,44–46]

Therapeutic uses of inhaled NO in children with congenital heart disease abound in the ICU. For example, newborns with total anomalous pulmonary venous connection (TAPVC) frequently have obstruction of the pulmonary venous pathway as it connects anomalously to the systemic venous circulation. When pulmonary venous return is obstructed preoperatively, pulmonary hypertension is severe and demands urgent surgical relief. Increased neonatal pulmonary vasoreactivity, endothelial injury induced by cardiopulmonary bypass, and intrauterine anatomic changes in the pulmonary vascular bed in this disease contribute to postoperative pulmonary hypertension. Inhaled nitric oxide dramatically reduces pulmonary hypertension without change in heart rate, systemic blood pressure or vascular resistance.

Patients with TAPVC, congenital mitral stenosis, and other pulmonary venous hypertensive disorders associated with low cardiac output appear to be among the most responsive to NO. These children are born with significantly increased amounts of smooth muscle in their pulmonary arterioles and veins. Histologic evidence of muscularized pulmonary veins as well as pulmonary arteries suggests the presence of vascular tone and capacity for change in resistance at both the arterial and venous sites. The increased responsiveness seen in younger patients with pulmonary venous hypertension to NO may result from pulmonary vasorelaxation at a combination of pre- and postcapillary vessels.

Successful use of inhaled NO in a variety of other congenital heart defects following cardiac surgery has been reported by several groups. It may be especially helpful when administered during a pulmonary hypertensive crisis.[46] Descriptions of use after Fontan procedures[47] and following VSD repair have been described along with a variety of other anatomic lesions. Prophylactic use of inhaled NO in patients at risk of developing postoperative pulmonary hypertensive crises is thought by some to reduce the duration of mechanical ventilation.[48] Very young infants who are excessively cyanotic after a bidirectional Glenn anastomosis do not generally improve oxygen saturation in response to inhaled NO. Increasing cardiac output and cerebral blood flow may have much greater impact on arterial oxygenation. Elevated pulmonary vascular tone is seldom the limiting factor in the hypoxemic patient after the bidirectional Glenn operation.[49]

Inhaled NO can also be used diagnostically in neonates with right ventricular hypertension after cardiac surgery to discern those with reversible vasoconstriction. Failure of the postoperative neonate with pulmonary hypertension to respond to NO successfully discriminated anatomical obstruction to pulmonary blood flow from pulmonary vasoconstriction. Failure of the postoperative neonate to respond to NO should be regarded as strong evidence of anatomic and possibly surgically remediable obstruction.[50]

If withdrawal of NO is necessary before resolution of the pathologic process, hemodynamic instability may be expected. We have previously suggested that the withdrawal response to inhaled NO can be attenuated by pretreatment with the type V phosphodiesterase inhibitor, sildenafil (Viagra).[51] Sildenafil inhibits the inactivation of cGMP within the vascular smooth muscle cell and has the potential to augment the effects of endogenous or exogenously administered nitric oxide to effect vascular smooth muscle relaxation. Sildenafil can be administered in oral or intravenous forms and has been shown to have somewhat selective pulmonary vasodilating capacity while lowering the left atrial pressure and providing a modest degree of afterload reduction in some postoperative children. Chronic oral administration of sildenafil to adults with primary pulmonary hypertension improves the exercise capacity and this may suggest an important therapeutic application of the intravenous preparation in postoperative congenital heart surgery.

In summary, aggressive identification and treatment of low cardiac output conditions after cardiac surgery is central to the critical care of children with congenital heart disease. Successful application of these strategies and thoughtful use of pharmacologic intervention has undoubtedly contributed to the remarkable decline in mortality associated with congenital heart surgery in the past two decades. However, despite these interventions, additional (mechanical) support is sometimes necessary as a bridge to recovery.

Mechanical Support of the Circulation

Despite the expanding options for pharmacologic support, the circulation cannot be adequately supported in some patients in both preoperative and postoperative situations. Mechanical assist devices have an important role providing short-term circulatory support to enable myocardial recovery and the potential for longer-term support while awaiting cardiac transplantation. Although a variety of assist devices are available for adult-sized patients, ECMO is the predominant mode of support for children (see Chapter 59).

Currently, more than 300 children per year receive ECMO for cardiac support, according to reports to the Extracorporeal Life Support Registry, with most patients placed on ECMO following cardiotomy.[52–54] While over 50% of these patients are decannulated from ECMO, the overall survival to discharge has only been between 35% and 40% of reported cases over the past decade.

At Children's Hospital Boston, we have used ECMO to support the circulation in more than 200 patients. Neonates comprise 41% of all our cardiac ECMO, with a survival rate to discharge of 50%. The pediatric group (infants through to 16 years of age) comprises 55% of our total experience, with an improved survival rate to discharge of 59%.

Substantial institutional variability in patient selection for ECMO makes comparison of published experience difficult. Centers with an efficient and well-established ECMO service are more likely to use this form of support in patients with low cardiac output. Furthermore, surgical technique and bypass management are additional confounding factors that make comparisons of the use and indications for ECMO between institutions difficult to interpret. Nevertheless, this form of mechanical support can be demonstrated to be lifesaving, and it can be argued that it should be available when needed for selected patients following congenital heart surgery. ECMO for pediatric resuscitation (rapid deployment during active cardiopulmonary resuscitation [CPR]) in a pulseless circulation remains a controversial issue. A rapid-response ECMO system was started at Children's Hospital Boston in 1996.[55] Of more than 200 cardiac ECMO patients, 50% were cannulated during active CPR (rapid-response system), and 55% of these patients have been successfully discharged from hospital. General indications and contraindications for ECMO support of the circulation in patients with CHD are summarized in Tables 18-7 and 18-8.

CARDIOVASCULAR INTERACTIONS WITH OTHER ORGANS

Respiratory Function and Heart–Lung Interaction

Altered respiratory mechanics and positive pressure ventilation may have significant influence on hemodynamics after congenital heart surgery. Therefore, the approach to mechanical ventilation should not only be directed at achieving a desired gas exchange, but also influenced by the potential cardiorespiratory interactions of mechanical ventilation and method of weaning. The mode of ventilation must be matched to the hemodynamic status of each patient to

TABLE 18–7. Typical Indications for ECMO

I. Inadequate oxygen delivery
  A. *Low cardiac output:*
    1. Chronic (cardiomyopathy)
    2. Acute (myocarditis)
    3. Weaning from cardiopulmonary bypass
    4. Preoperative stabilization
    5. Progressive postoperative failure
    6. Pulmonary hypertension
    7. Refractory arrhythmias
    8. Cardiac arrest
  B. *Profound cyanosis:*
    1. Intracardiac shunting and cardiovascular collapse
    2. Acute shunt thrombosis
    3. Acute respiratory failure exaggerated by underlying heart disease
    4. Congenital heart defect, complicated by other newborn indications for ECMO such as meconium aspiration syndrome, PPHN, pneumonia, sepsis, respiratory distress syndrome
II. Support for intervention during cardiac catheterization

ECMO, extracorporeal membrane oxygenation.

TABLE 18–8. Relative Contraindications for ECMO

End-stage, irreversible or inoperable disease
Family, patient directives to limit resuscitation
Significant neurologic or end organ impairment
Uncontrolled bleeding within major organs
Extremes of size and weight
Inaccessible vessels during resuscitation

ECMO, extracorporeal membrane oxygenation.

achieve adequate cardiac output and gas exchange. Frequent modifications to the mode and pattern of ventilation may be necessary during recovery after surgery, with attention to changes in lung volume and airway pressure. Changes in lung volume have a major effect on PVR, which is lowest at the lung's functional residual capacity (FRC), while both hypo- or hyperinflation may result in a significant increase in PVR because of altered traction on alveolar septae and extra-alveolar vessels.

Positive pressure ventilation influences preload and afterload on the heart (Table 18-9).[56–58] An increase in lung volume and intrathoracic pressure decreases preload to the right and left atria. The afterload on the pulmonary ventricle is increased during a positive pressure breath secondary to the changes in lung volume and increase in mean intrathoracic pressure. If this is significant, or there is limited functional reserve, RV stroke volume may be reduced and end-diastolic pressure increased. This in turn may contribute to a LCOS and signs of RV dysfunction including tricuspid regurgitation, hepatomegaly, ascites, and pleural effusions. In contrast to the RV, the afterload on the systemic ventricle is decreased during a positive pressure breath secondary to a fall in the ventricle transmural pressure. The systemic arteries are under higher pressure and not exposed to radial traction effects during inflation or deflation of the lungs. Therefore, changes in lung volume will affect LV preload, but the effect on afterload is dependent on changes in intrathoracic pressure alone rather than changes in lung volume. Positive pressure ventilation and PEEP therefore may have significant beneficial effect in patients with left ventricular failure.

TABLE 18–9. The Cardiorespiratory Interactions of a Positive Pressure Mechanical Breath

	Afterload	Preload
Pulmonary ventricle	Elevated Effect: ↑ RVEDp ↑ RVp ↓ Antegrade PBF ↑ PR and/or TR	Reduced Effect: ↓ RVEDV ↓ RAp
Systemic ventricle	Reduced Effect: ↓ LVEDp ↓ LAp ↓ Pulmonary edema ↑ Increase cardiac output	Reduced Effect: ↓ LVEDV ↓ LAp

RVEDp, right ventricle end diastolic pressure; RVp, right ventricle pressure; RVEDV, right ventricle end diastolic volume; PBF, pulmonary blood flow; PR, pulmonary regurgitation; TR, tricuspid regurgitation; LVEDp, left ventricle end diastolic pressure; LVEDV, left ventricle end diastolic volume; LAp, left atrial pressure; RAp, right atrial pressure.

Patients with LV dysfunction and increased end-diastolic volume and pressure can have impaired pulmonary mechanics secondary to increased lung water, decreased lung compliance and increased airway resistance. The work of breathing is increased and neonates can fatigue early because of limited respiratory reserve. A significant proportion of total body oxygen consumption is directed at the increased work of breathing in neonates and infants with LV dysfunction, contributing to poor feeding and failure to thrive. Therefore, positive pressure ventilation has an additional benefit in patients with significant volume overload and systemic ventricular dysfunction by reducing the work of breathing and oxygen demand.

The use of positive end expiratory pressure (PEEP) in patients with congenital heart disease has been controversial. It was initially perceived not to have a significant positive impact on gas exchange, and there was concern that the increased airway pressure could have a detrimental effect on hemodynamics and contribute to lung injury and air leak. Nevertheless, PEEP increases FRC, enabling lung recruitment, and redistributes lung water from alveolar septal regions to the more compliant perihilar regions. Both of these actions will improve gas exchange and reduce PVR. PEEP should, therefore, be used in mechanically ventilated patients following congenital heart surgery. However, excessive levels of PEEP can be detrimental by increasing afterload on the right side of the circulation. This may be especially true in the Fontan circulation. Usually 3 to 5 cm H_2O of PEEP will help maintain FRC and redistribute lung water without causing hemodynamic compromise. Of course the optimal condition for the Fontan circulation occurs when the patient can breathe spontaneously, generating negative pleural and intrathoracic pressures, which facilitate systemic venous return. If lung volume can be maintained and work of breathing minimized without any positive pressure ventilation, then the Fontan circulation is best served. Early transition to a pressure-support mode of breathing and aim to extubation during the first few postoperative hours is our goal.

Diaphragmatic paresis (reduced motion) or paralysis (paradoxical movement) may precipitate and promote respiratory failure, particularly in the neonate or young infant who relies on diaphragmatic function for breathing more than older infants and children (who can recruit accessory and intercostal muscles if diaphragmatic function proves inadequate). Injury to the phrenic nerve, usually the left, may occur during operations that require dissection of the branch pulmonary arteries well out to the hilum (e.g., tetralogy of Fallot, arterial switch operation), arch reconstruction from the midline (e.g., Norwood operation), manipulation of the superior vena cava (Glenn shunts), takedown of previous systemic-to-pulmonary shunts, or after percutaneous central venous access. Phrenic injury may occur more frequently at reoperation, when adhesions and scarring may obscure landmarks. Topical cooling with ice during deep hypothermia may also cause transient phrenic palsy. Increased work of breathing on low ventilator settings, increased P_{CO_2}, and a chest radiograph revealing an elevated hemidiaphragm are suggestive of diaphragmatic dysfunction. The chest radiograph may be misleading, however, if taken during peak positive pressure ventilation. Ultrasonography or fluoroscopy is useful for identifying diaphragmatic motion or paradoxical excursion. Recovery of diaphragmatic contraction usually occurs; however, if a patient fails to tolerate repeated extubations despite optimizing cardiovascular and nutritional status, and diaphragmatic dysfunction persists with volume loss in the affected lung, then the diaphragm may need to be surgically plicated. Although only a temporary effect is gained the avoidance of collapse and volume loss in the affected lung may provide the critical advantage.

Increased airway resistance arises from several pathologic changes alone or in combination: secretions, either excessive in quantity or viscosity; swelling of the mucosa due to hyperemia or edema, most often resulting from trauma or infection; hyperactive bronchial smooth muscle; or extrinsic compression by neighboring structures or diminished forces pulling the conducting passages open. Patients who have secretions from the tracheal aspirate that has many visible organisms and polymorphonuclear cells on microscopy, together with fever, an elevated white blood cell count, and consolidation on the chest radiograph require treatment with appropriate antibiotics.

Postextubation stridor may be due to mucosal swelling of the large airway; a nebulized, inhaled (alpha) agonist (e.g., racemic epinephrine) promotes vasoconstriction and decreases hyperemia and, possibly, edema. If re-intubation is necessary, a smaller endotracheal tube should be used if possible along with diuresis and often a short term administration of steroids, prior to a subsequent attempt at extubation in 24-36 hours. An evaluation for vocal cord dysfunction should be considered, especially in patients with surgery near the recurrent laryngeal nerve.

Bronchospasm may be treated by inhaled or systemically administered bronchodilators, but must be used with caution in light of their chronotropic and tachyarrhythmic potential. If all of these maneuvers fail to improve the patient's condition, the minimum tidal volume and frequency that provide sufficient mechanical minute ventilation to satisfactorily supplement spontaneous ventilation and minimize overinflation of the lungs are determined and used during the recovery phase.

Pulmonary edema, *pneumonia*, and *atelectasis* are the most common causes of lower airway and alveolar abnormalities that interfere with gas exchange. If a bacterial pathogen is identified, therapy includes antibiotics and pulmonary toilet. If the cause is pulmonary edema, therapy is aimed toward lowering the left atrial pressure through diuresis and pharmacologic means to reduce afterload and improve the lusitropic state of the heart. For infants, fluid restriction is frequently incompatible with adequate nutrition and, therefore, an aggressive diuretic regimen is preferable to restriction of caloric intake. Adjustment of end expiratory pressure and mechanical ventilation serve as supportive therapies until the alveoli and pulmonary interstitium are cleared of the fluid that interferes with gas entry.

Pleural effusions, and less often *ascites*, may occur in patients after a Fontan operation or reparative procedures requiring a right ventriculotomy (e.g., tetralogy of Fallot, truncus arteriosus) with transient right ventricular dysfunction. Especially in young patients, pleural effusions and increased interstitial lung water may be a manifestation of right heart failure. This seems logically related to raised systemic venous pressure impeding lymphatic return to the venous circulation. The lymphatic circuit is often functioning at full capacity in these children. Fluid in the pleural space or peritoneum and intestinal distention compete with intrapulmonary gas for thoracic space. Evacuation of the pleural space or drainage of ascites and decompression of the intestinal lumen allow the intrapulmonary gas volume to increase.

Central Nervous System

The dramatic reduction in surgical mortality in recent decades has been accompanied by a growing recognition of adverse neurologic sequelae in some survivors. Central nervous system (CNS) abnormalities may be a function of coexisting brain abnormalities or acquired events unrelated to surgical management (e.g., paradoxical embolus, brain infection, effects of chronic cyanosis), but CNS insults appear to occur most frequently during or immediately after surgery. In particular, support techniques used during neonatal and infant cardiac surgery—CPB, profound hypothermia and circulatory arrest—have been implicated as important causes of brain injury.[59]

During hypothermic CPB, there are multiple perfusion variables that might influence the risk of brain injury. These include (but are probably not limited to) (a) the total duration of CPB and the duration and rate of core cooling; (b) pH management during core cooling; (c) duration of circulatory arrest; (d) type of oxygenator; (e) presence of arterial filtration; and (f) depth of hypothermia. Undoubtedly, there is interaction between these various elements, and CNS injury following CPB is most likely multifactorial. Early postoperative studies (in the ICU) revealed a higher incidence of neurologic perturbation in patients undergoing circulatory arrest including a higher incidence of clinical and electroencephalographic (EEG) seizures, a longer recovery time to the first reappearance of EEG activity, and greater release of the brain isoenzyme of creatine kinase (see Chapter 9).

Seizures are the most frequently observed neurologic consequence of cardiac surgery using CPB with an incidence in older studies of 4% to 25%. Although the incidence of seizures in the ICU has dramatically declined in recent years, we treat seizures aggressively using benzodiazepines, phenobarbital, or phenytoin. Importantly, we have reduced or eliminated, where possible, practices that may have been associated with brain injury after CPB: rapid cooling on cardiopulmonary bypass and use of prolonged hypothermic circulatory arrest, extreme alpha stat strategy of intraoperative pH management, extreme hemodilution to hematocrit less than 20, applying heat lamps to infants on arrival in ICU, hypocapnic hyperventilation, prolonged muscle relaxation (masking seizure observations), and so forth. We are especially loath to permit hyperthermia to any degree in the early postoperative period.

Intraventricular hemorrhage may occur as a consequence of perinatal events or circulatory collapse in the first few days of life. It is commonly associated with prematurity. Our approach has been to screen all premature infants or asphyxiated babies with a head ultrasound prior to cardiopulmonary bypass, which of course involves extensive anticoagulation, hemodynamic perturbation, and risk that bleeding will extend. Surgical intervention is delayed for several days if intraventricular bleeding is documented. Our strategy of deferring operations in very premature newborns for several days after birth is associated with a low incidence of intraventricular hemorrhage in these high risk patients despite use of cardiopulmonary bypass.[9]

Renal Function and Postoperative Fluid Management

Risk factors for postoperative renal failure include preoperative renal dysfunction, prolonged bypass time, low cardiac output, and cardiac arrest. In addition to relative ischemia and nonpulsatile flow on CPB, an angiotensin II–mediated renal vasoconstriction and delayed healing of renal tubular epithelium has been proposed as one mechanism for renal failure. Postoperative sepsis and nephrotoxic drugs may cause further damage to the kidneys.

Because of the inflammatory response to bypass and significant increase in total body water, fluid management in the immediate postoperative period is critical. Capillary leak and interstitial fluid accumulation may continue for the first 24 to 48 hours after surgery, necessitating ongoing volume replacement with colloid or blood products. A fall in cardiac output and increased antidiuretic hormone secretion contribute to delayed water clearance and potential prerenal dysfunction, which could progress to acute tubular necrosis and renal failure if a low cardiac output state persists.

During CPB, optimizing the circuit prime, hematocrit, and oncotic pressure, attenuating the inflammatory response with steroids and protease inhibitors such as aprotinin,[60] and the use of modified ultrafiltration techniques have all been recommended to limit interstitial fluid accumulation.[61] During the first 24 hours after surgery, maintenance fluids should be restricted to 50% of full maintenance, and volume replacement titrated to appropriate filling pressures and hemodynamic response.

Oliguria in the first 24 hours after complex surgery and CPB is common in neonates and infants until cardiac output recovers and neurohumoral mechanisms abate. Although diuretics are commonly prescribed in the immediate postoperative period, the neurohumoral influence on urine output is powerful. Time after CPB and enhancement of cardiac output through volume and pharmacologic adjustments are the most important factors that will promote diuresis.

Peritoneal dialysis, *hemodialysis*, and continuous *veno-venous hemofiltration* (CVVH) provide alternate renal support in patients with severe oliguria and renal failure.[62] Besides enabling water and solute clearance, maintenance fluids can be increased to ensure adequate nutrition. The indications for renal support vary, but include blood urea nitrogen (BUN) level above 100 mg/dL, life-threatening electrolyte imbalance such as severe hyperkalemia, ongoing metabolic acidosis, fluid restrictions limiting nutrition, and increased mechanical ventilation requirements secondary to persistent pulmonary edema or ascites.

A peritoneal dialysis catheter may be placed into the peritoneal cavity at the completion of surgery or later in the ICU. Indications in the ICU include the need for renal support or to reduce intra-abdominal pressure from ascites that may be compromising mechanical ventilation. Drainage may be significant in the immediate postoperative period as third-space fluid losses continue, and replacement with albumin and/or fresh frozen plasma may be necessary to treat hypovolemia and hypoproteinemia.

Gastrointestinal Issues

Following cardiac surgery in neonates and children, adequate nutrition is exceedingly important. These critically ill children often have decreased caloric intake and increased energy demand after surgery; the neonate in particular has limited metabolic and fat reserves. Total parenteral nutrition can provide adequate nutrition in the early hypercatabolic phases of the early postoperative period.

Upper gastrointestinal bleeding and ulcer formation may occur following the stress of cardiac surgery in children and adults. There are limited reports of the efficacy of histamine H_2 antireceptors, sucralfate, or oral antacids in pediatric cardiac patients, although their use is common in many intensive care units. Hepatic failure may occur after cardiac surgery (particularly after the Fontan operation and is typically characterized by elevated liver enzymes and coagulopathy).

Necrotizing enterocolitis, although typically a disease of premature infants, is seen with considerable frequency in neonates with CHD. Risk factors include (a) left-sided obstructive lesions, (b) umbilical or femoral arterial catheterization/angiography, (c) hypoxemia, and (d) lesions with wide pulse pressures (e.g., systemic to pulmonary shunts, patent ductus arteriosus, especially in transposition of the great arteries and severe aortic regurgitation) producing retrograde flow in the mesenteric vessels during diastole. Frequently, multiple risk factors exist in the same patient, making a specific etiology difficult to establish. Treatment includes continuous nasogastric suction, parenteral nutrition, and broad-spectrum antibiotics. Bowel exploration or resection may be necessary in severe cases.

Infection

Low-grade (< 38.5°C) fever during the immediate postoperative period is common and may be present for 3 to 4 days, even without a demonstrable infectious etiology. However, there are several reports of increased susceptibility to infection after CPB. CPB may activate compliment and other mediators of inflammation, but can also lead to derangements of the immune system and increase the likelihood of infection. A centrally mediated etiology of fever following CPB has been postulated.

Sepsis and nosocomial infection after cardiac surgery contribute substantially to overall morbidity. Despite the recent increased use of broad coverage, third-generation cephalosporins, these agents did not seem to be more effective in decreasing postoperative infections. Meticulous catheter insertion and daily care routines along with early removal of indwelling catheters in the postoperative patient may potentially reduce the incidence of sepsis.

Mediastinitis occurs in up to 2% of patients undergoing cardiac surgery; risk factors may include delayed sternal closure, early re-exploration for bleeding, or reoperation. Mediastinitis is characterized by persistent fever, purulent drainage from the sternotomy wound, instability of the sternum, and leukocytosis. *Staphylococcus* is the most common offending organism. Treatment usually involves

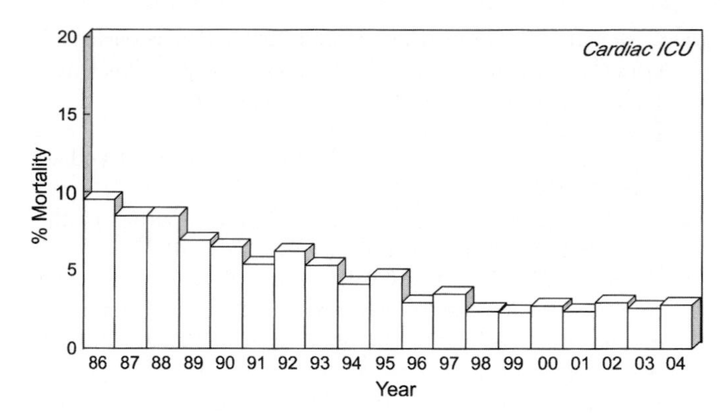

FIGURE 18–3 *Mortality for all patients in the cardiac intensive care unit at Children's Hospital Boston declined dramatically through the 1990s and is now 2.5%.*

débridement and irrigation with parenteral antibiotic therapy. Duration of therapy seldom exceeds 2 weeks.

SUMMARY

The cardiac intensive care unit has become the epicenter of activity in large cardiovascular programs. Nowhere are collaborative practices and multidisciplinary skills more valued or necessary. A curriculum in cardiac intensive care is now formally incorporated into cardiology training; pediatric intensive care training programs have a mandate to include curricula and experience in management of postoperative cardiac patients. Specialists in this field must have in-depth training in cardiology but be well versed in diagnosis and management of multiorgan system dysfunction, which is so vital to the discipline of intensive care. Increased complexity of disease, advances in technology and applied research, shortened lengths of stay, and improved survival all describe the fast-paced specialized environment that has accompanied the development of this new specialty of pediatric cardiac intensive care. Although the dramatic reduction in mortality has been gratifying in cardiac intensive care (Fig. 18-3) and is attributable to many factors, achieving 100% survival with minimal morbidity remains our elusive goal. It will challenge the next generation of practitioners.

REFERENCES

1. Chang AC. How to start and sustain a successful pediatric cardiac intensive care program: A combined clinical and administrative strategy. Pediatr Crit Care Med 3:107, 2002.
2. Brown K, Johnston AE, Conn AW. Respiratory insufficiency and its treatment following paediatric cardiovascular surgery. Can Anaesth Soc J 13:342, 1966.

3. Castaneda AR, Mayer JE, Jr., Jonas RA, et al. The neonate with critical congenital heart disease: repair: a surgical challenge. J Thorac Cardiovasc Surg 98(5 Pt 2):869, 1989.
4. Friedman WF, George BL. Treatment of congestive heart failure by altering loading conditions of the heart. J Pediatr 106:697, 1985.
5. Friedman WF. The intrinsic physiologic properties of the developing heart. Prog Cardiovasc Dis 15:87, 1972.
6. Romero TE, Friedman WF. Limited left ventricular response to volume overload in the neonatal period: a comparative study with the adult animal. Pediatr Res 13: 910, 1979.
7. Mills AN, Haworth SG. Greater permeability of the neonatal lung. Postnatal changes in surface charge and biochemistry of porcine pulmonary capillary endothelium. J Thorac Cardiovasc Surg 101:909, 1991.
8. Feltes TF, Hansen TN. Effects of an aorticopulmonary shunt on lung fluid balance in the young lamb. Pediatr Res 26: 94, 1989.
9. Reddy VM, McElhinney DB, Sagrado T, et al. Results of 102 cases of complete repair of congenital heart defects in patients weighing 700 to 2500 grams. J Thorac Cardiovasc Surg 117:324, 1999.
10. Lang P, Chipman CW, Siden M. Early assessment of hemodynamic status after repair of tetralogy of Fallot: a comparison of 24 hour and one year postoperative data in 98 patients. Am J Cardiol 58:795, 1982.
11. Wernovsky G, Wypij D, Jonas RA, et al. Postoperative course and hemodynamic profile after the arterial switch operation in neonates and infants: a comparison of low-flow cardiopulmonary bypass and circulatory arrest. Circulation 92: 2226, 1995.
12. Bridges ND, Mayer JE, Jr., Lock JE, et al. Effect of baffle fenestration on outcome of the modified Fontan operation. Circulation 86:1762, 1992.
13. Lemler MS, Scott WA, Leonard SR, et al. Fenestration improves clinical outcome of the Fontan procedure: a prospective, randomized study. Circulation 105:207, 2002.
14. Bohn DJ, Poirer CS, Demonds JF. Efficacy of dopamine, dobutamine, and epinephrine during emergence from cardiopulmonary bypass in children. Crit Care Med 8: 367, 1980.
15. Wessel DL. Managing low cardiac output syndrome after congenital heart surgery. [Review]. Critical Care Medicine 29(Suppl):S220, 2001.
16. Habib DM, Padbury JF, Anas NG, et al. Dobutamine pharmacokinetics and pharmacodynamics in pediatric intensive care patients. Crit Care Med 20:601, 1992.
17. Rosenzweig EB, Starc TJ, Chen JM, et al. Intravenous arginine-vasopressin in children with vasodilatory shock after cardiac surgery. Circulation 100:182, 1999.
18. Caspi J, Coles JG, Benson LN, et al. Age-related response to epinephrine-induced myocardial stress: a functional and ulstrastructural study. Circulation 84(Suppl):III-394, 1991.
19. Caspi J, Coles JG, Benson LN, et al. Effects of high plasma epinephrine and Ca2+ concentrations on neonatal myocardial function after ischemia. J Thorac Cardiovasc Surg 105:59, 1993.
20. Bailey JM, Miller BE, Lu W, et al. The pharmacokinetics of milrinone in pediatric patients after cardiac surgery. Anesth 90:1012, 1999.
21. Chang AC, Atz AM, Wernovsky G, et al. Milrinone: systemic and pulmonary hemodynamic effects in neonates after cardiac surgery. Crit Care Med 23:1907, 1995.
22. Hoffman TM, Wernovsky G, Atz AM, et al. Efficacy and safety of milrinone in preventing low cardiac output syndrome in infants and children after corrective surgery for congenital heart disease. Circulation 107:996, 2003.
23. Mainwaring R, Lamberti J, Nelson J, et al. Effects of tri-iodothyronine supplementation following modified Fontan procedure. Cardiol Young 7:194, 1997.
24. Bettendorf M, Schmidt KG, Grulich-Henn J, et al. Tri-iodothyronine treatment in children after cardiac surgery: a double-blind, randomised, placebo-controlled study. Lancet 356:529, 2000.
25. Chowdhury D, Parnell VA, Ojamaa K, et al. Usefulness of triiodothyronine (T3) treatment after surgery for complex congenital heart disease in infants and children. Am J Cardiol 84:1107, 1999.
26. Colucci WS, Elkayam U, Horton DP, et al. Intravenous nesiritide, a natriuretic peptide, in the treatment of decompensated congestive heart failure. Nesiritide Study Group. [erratum appears in N Engl J Med 2000;343:1504]. New England Journal of Medicine 343:246, 2000.
27. Mills RM, LeJemtel TH, Horton DP, et al. Sustained hemodynamic effects of an infusion of nesiritide (human b-type natriuretic peptide) in heart failure: a randomized, double-blind, placebo-controlled clinical trial. Natrecor Study Group. J Am Coll Cardiol 34:155, 1999.
28. Publication Committee for the VMAC Investigators (Vasodilatation in the Management of Acute CHF): Intravenous nesiritide vs nitroglycerin for treatment of decompensated congestive heart failure: a randomized controlled trial.[see comment][erratum appears in JAMA;288:577, 2002.] JAMA 287:1531, 2002.
29. Yancy CW, Saltzberg MT, Berkowitz RL, et al. Safety and feasibility of using serial infusions of nesiritide for heart failure in an outpatient setting (from the FUSION I trial). Am J Cardiol 94:595, 2004.
30. Turanlahti M, Boldt T, Palkama T, et al. Pharmacokinetics of levosimendan in pediatric patients evaluated for cardiac surgery. Pediatr Crit Care Med 5:457, 2004.
31. Janousek J, Vojtovic P, Hucin B, et al. Resynchronization pacing is a useful adjunct to the management of acute heart failure after surgery for congenital heart defects. Am J Cardiol 88: 145, 2001.
32. Cullen S, Shore D, Redington A. Characterization of right ventricular diastolic performance after complete repair of tetralogy of Fallot. Restrictive physiology predicts slow postoperative recovery. Circulation 91:1782, 1995.
33. Redington AN, Penny D, Rigby ML. Antegrade diastolic pulmonary arterial flow as a marker of right ventricular restriction after complete repair of pulmonary atresia with intact ventricular septum and critical pulmonary valve stenosis. Cardiol Young 2:382, 1992.

34. Wessel DL. Current and future strategies in the treatment of childhood pulmonary hypertension. Prog Ped Cardiol 12:289, 2001.
35. Drummond WH, Gregory GA, Heymann MA, et al. The independent effects of hyperventilation, tolazoline, and dopamine on infants with persistent pulmonary hypertension. J Pediatr 98:603, 1981.
36. Barst RJ, Rubin LJ, Long WA, et al. A comparison of continuous intravenous epoprostenol (prostacyclin) with conventional therapy for primary pulmonary hypertension. The Primary Pulmonary Hypertension Study Group. [see comment]. N Engl J Med 334:296, 1996.
37. Palevsky HI, Long W, Crow J, et al. Prostacyclin and acetylcholine as screening agents for acute pulmonary vasodilator responsiveness in primary pulmonary hypertension. Circulation 82:2018, 1990.
38. Rosenzweig EB, Kerstein D, Barst RJ. Long-term prostacyclin for pulmonary hypertension with associated congenital heart defects. Circulation 99:1858, 1999.
39. Zobel G, Dacar D, Rodl S, et al. Inhaled nitric oxide versus inhaled prostacyclin and intravenous versus inhaled prostacyclin in acute respiratory failure with pulmonary hypertension in piglets. Pediatr Res 38:198, 1995.
40. Petrossian E, Parry AJ, Reddy VM, et al. Endothelin receptor blockade prevents the rise in pulmonary vascular resistance after cardiopulmonary bypass in lambs with increased pulmonary blood flow. J Thorac Cardiovasc Surg 117:314, 1999.
41. Frostell CG, Fratacci MD, Wain JC, et al. Inhaled nitric oxide: A selective pulmonary vasodilator reversing hypoxic pulmonary vasoconstriction. Circulation 83:2038, 1991.
42. Furchgott RF, Zawadzki JV. The obligatory role of endothelial cells in the relaxation of arterial smooth muscle by acetylcholine. Nature 288:373, 1980.
43. Ignarro LJ, Buga GM, Wood KS, et al. Endothelium-derived relaxing factor produced and released from artery and vein is nitric oxide. Proc Natl Acad Sci U S A 84:9265, 1987.
44. Atz AM, Wessel DL. Inhaled nitric oxide in the neonate with cardiac disease. Semin Perinatol 21:441, 1997.
45. Wessel DL, Adatia I, Giglia TM, et al. Use of inhaled nitric oxide and acetylcholine in the evaluation of pulmonary hypertension and endothelial function after cardiopulmonary bypass. Circulation 88(5 Pt 1):2128, 1993.
46. Journois D, Pouard P, Mauriat P, et al. Inhaled nitric oxide as a therapy for pulmonary hypertension after operations for congenital heart defects. J Thorac Cardiovasc Surg 107:1129, 1994.
47. Goldman AP, Delius RE, Deanfield JE, et al. Pharmacological control of pulmonary blood flow with inhaled nitric oxide after the fenestrated Fontan operation. Circulation 94(Suppl): II44, 1996.
48. Miller OI, Tang SF, Keech A, et al. Inhaled nitric oxide and prevention of pulmonary hypertension after congenital heart surgery: a randomised double-blind study. Lancet 356:1464, 2000.
49. Adatia I, Atz AM, Wessel DL. Inhaled nitric oxide does not improve systemic oxygenation after bidirectional superior cavopulmonary anastomosis. J Thorac Cardiovasc Surg 129:217, 2005.
50. Adatia I, Atz AM, Jonas RA, et al. Diagnostic use of inhaled nitric oxide after neonatal cardiac operations. J Thorac Cardiovasc Surg 112:1403, 1996.
51. Atz AM, Wessel DL. Sildenafil ameliorates effects of inhaled nitric oxide withdrawal. Anesthesiology 91:307, 1999.
52. Duncan BW, Hraska V, Jonas RA, et al. Mechanical circulatory support in children with cardiac disease. J Thorac Cardiovasc Surg 117:529, 1999.
53. Extracorporeal Life Support Organization. ECLS Registry Report: International Summary. 2002. Ann Arbor, MI, Extracorporeal Life Support Organization.
54. Wessel D, Almodovar M, Laussen P. Intensive care management of cardiac patients on extracorporeal membrane oxygenation. In Duncan B (ed). Mechanical Support for Cardiac and Respiratory Failure. 2000, pp 75–111.
55. Duncan BW, Ibrahim AE, Hraska V, et al. Use of rapid-deployment extracorporeal membrane oxygenation for the resuscitation of pediatric patients with heart disease after cardiac arrest. J Thorac Cardiovasc Surg 116:305, 1998.
56. Jenkins J, Lynn A, Edmonds J, et al. Effects of mechanical ventilation on cardiopulmonary function in children after open-heart surgery. Crit Care Med 13:77, 1985.
57. Robotham JL, Lixfeld W, Holland L, et al. The effects of positive end-expiratory pressure on right and left ventricular performance. Am Rev Respir Dis 121:677, 1980.
58. Pinsky MR, Summer WR, Wise RA, et al. Augmentation of cardiac function by elevation of intrathoracic pressure. J Appl Physiol 54:950, 1983.
59. Newburger JW, Jonas RA, Wernovsky G, et al. Perioperative neurologic effects of hypothermic arrest during infant heart surgery. The Boston Circulatory Arrest Study. N Engl J Med 329:1057, 1993.
60. Costello JM, Backer CL, de Hoyos A, et al. Aprotinin reduces operative closure time and blood product use after pediatric bypass. Ann Thorac Surg 75:1261, 2003.
61. Elliott M. Modified ultrafiltration and open heart surgery in children. Paediatr Anaesth 9:1, 1999.
62. Paret G, Cohen AJ, Bohn DJ, et al. Continuous arteriovenous hemofiltration after cardiac operations in infants and children. J Thorac Cardiovasc Surg 104:1225, 1992.

19

Methodologic Issues for Database Development: Trends

John K. Triedman, MD

The value of computers for the collection, accounting, and administration of medical data has been appreciated for many years. However, over the last decade, the advent of high-speed networked communication between computers, in concert with the ongoing decrease in the size and cost of computer processors, has revolutionized the role of information technology in pediatric cardiology, as it has in health care generally. As recently as 1990, electronic computing in cardiology was the province of administrators running business systems and a small number of clinical and academic practitioners with interest and expertise in these devices. Now, digital systems mediate the entire range of medical practice. In addition to business functions of schedule and billing, current uses of digital devices include the performance, analysis, and reporting of diagnostic studies and the transmission and storage of clinical images in digital form. Perhaps the most important change has been effected by the capacity for nearly immediate transmission of large amounts of digital information at very low cost, anywhere within institutions or around the world. This has resulted in a massive proliferation of information exchange and presentation among physicians and scientists, and simultaneously has revealed the need for a common but secure digital language that protects the privacy of individuals while facilitating information transmission for the purposes of clinical care and research.

Within the cardiovascular program at Children's Hospital Boston, paper-based systems for research and administration are rapidly becoming extinct. Several hundred personal computers are used by clinicians, researchers, administrators, and technologists to facilitate virtually all departmental processes. These computers are networked locally as a cardiovascular information systems network, served by specialized applications specific to the needs of the cardiovascular program, communications and Web servers, and storage and backup facilities to manage the enormous amount of information generated by the systems users. In 2004, the volume of digital imaging data generated by over 15,000 catheterization and echocardiographic studies in this program exceeded 8,000 GB! This departmental information system is integrated with the hospital-wide information systems, which provide the hardware infrastructure for the system and many more general administrative and clinical functions that are not specific to the needs of the cardiovascular program. The development of these information systems has been the result of decades of investment and represents the contributions of hundreds of individuals. As with all large, organic endeavors, it has responded to changing demands with some false starts and mistakes, but it has, over time, developed a strong internal logic and organization based on its many successes.

The emergence of digital computing as the information backbone of current health practice should not obscure the fact that computers were initially useful primarily as rapid, highly organized and searchable managers of simple numbers and text. The purpose of this chapter is to explore the role of computing in cardiology as it has related to the historical development of clinical practice in the cardiovascular program over the prior three decades. This will necessarily involve comparison and analysis of data that have been available in our systems both then and now, limiting us to the analysis of patient records. The myriad advanced and emerging applications of health care computers in imaging, monitoring, and networked communications are discussed only at this superficial level, and the interested reader is directed to a number of excellent references on these topics.[1–4]

PURPOSE

The principle purpose of a health care information system is the storage and retrieval of patient information. This patient information database constitutes an archive of all clinical activities and a resource for data mining—the search for new knowledge in the complex associations that may be identified by careful examination of the data. Facilitated information retrieval is the desired capability; the physician using the information system would ideally be able to ask a variety of structured questions of the patient database, which is comprehensive in scope and complex in structure, and obtain an accurate and complete response that is not dependent on an individual's memory.

Modern computer systems will accept almost unlimited quantities of digital data. Although this scalable capacity is a great asset, careful planning is necessary to store these data in a manner that is useful for the specific, intended purpose of data retrieval. In fact, it is relatively common that, although all apparently relevant data on the patient are collected and stored, limitations imposed by the design of clinical databases and the software tools available to query them in turn limit the types and scope of questions that can be successfully asked of them. To exploit these resources, clinicians who wish to learn from database research must understand the structure of the database and the nature of the software algorithms used to query them.

DATA COLLECTION AND CODING

Currently, all our reports are created using software and digital equipment. After having demographic data and procedural and diagnostic codes attached, they are sent directly to a central cardiovascular database. The resulting data are then archived on magnetic and optical media, where they serve as a resource for online patient care and review, a source of copies of reports and a basis for research and study. An increasing volume of image data, including echocardiographic and cineangiographic images, is also now being stored in digital format and available online for review. The infrastructure of high-speed networked communications now available in this and most modern hospitals means that such information can be accessed for continuous, real-time review at many locations.

To ensure that the database responds in a useful way to queries, it is important that the description of diagnoses and procedures be as unambiguous as possible. This defines the science of coding, the goal of which is to ensure the accurate, consistent and complete description of clinical events and processes, both for clinical and business information systems. The use of a defined set of codes, which among them can be used to describe all recorded events, diminishes the amount of vague and confusing language retained in the database. Given the complexities of congenital and acquired heart defects and their treatment, this is a formidable task.

All coding systems are structured by the requirement for precision in digital computing. Any recorded event must correspond to precisely one code—no more and no less. Additionally, coding systems are more robust and useful when all individuals assigning a code to an event come up with the same answer. Codes that are based on esoteric physiologic or embryologic principles, while perhaps intellectually elegant and appropriate for certain applications, generally require significant interpretative judgment in the coding assignment, which may negate the value of the entire process unless all of the coding is done by the same individual. Like most health information systems, our system depends on the data input of many physicians and others from different disciplines. For this reason, it is necessary to make the principle diagnostic codes as unambiguous and as easy to assign as possible. In particular, fuzzy, qualitative modifiers of diagnoses (e.g., *virtually intact septum, tiny patent foramen ovale, possible …, mild mitral valve prolapse*) must be carefully isolated from the primary diagnosis itself in the coding system, lest an infinite number of idiosyncratic versions of the same disease populate the data fields. Important data must be identified clearly and with precision, while less important qualifiers and subsidiary diagnoses, which are useful principally to the originator of the data, may also be recorded, but kept separate.

Our principle coding system was developed here several decades ago and has been denoted as the *Fyler System*. This system assigns a six-digit code to each diagnosis and condition: the initial four digits identify and specify certain aspects of the diagnosis, while the fifth and sixth digits are used as modifiers to identify the etiology, severity, and/or conditional presence of that condition. This system has evolved along with our clinical and computing experience, and has been modified several times to accommodate new information, broader clinical experience, and changing concepts as they have arisen, while preserving historical information.

In coding, the balance between too much and too little information must be confronted with respect to the intended use of the data. For example, for the purposes of billing, all patients with a diagnosis of isolated ventricular septal defect may be reasonably lumped together, whereas for the purpose of surgical research, the distinction between anatomic subtypes of the malformation may be critical. It is reasonable to assume that use of a single, comprehensive coding system would allow better communication between physicians by providing a common coding language. However, this form of restriction is unnecessary, and not in every case is it even desirable. In our institution, we have found it useful to use multiple coding schemes that may be mapped to one another, allowing the databases to be searched using different approaches to queries. As long as coding systems are designed in a manner that allows every case to be classified, it is generally possible for any coding system to be readily translated into any other by simple algorithm when the need arises. The intended function of a database (clinical research, billing, quality of care review) will dictate its structure, as will the specific needs of its audience of users. In addition to the Fyler codes, other systems are used in parallel in our hospital, including the ICD-9 and CPT coding systems[5] for billing and hospital administration; the Society for Thoracic Surgeons codes[6,7] for congenital heart surgeries; the Pediatric Cardiac Care Consortium codes[8] for multicenter outcomes analysis; and a variety of project-specific systems for narrowly specified clinical research databases. Although the proliferation of many coding systems may result in a *Tower of Babel*, attempts to limit the coding system to a single uniform classification may also be counterproductive, because limitations of language lead to limitations in thought that are not always apparent.

```
                        Patient Number: XXXXXXX
                        Name: XXXXXXXXX
                        Sex: M
                        Birth Date: XX/XX/200X
Event     Date    Age at Event  DXCode  Diagnosis
CATH      XX/XX/200X  1 Yr 2 Mo 15 Days     Xxxx Xxxx, M.D.
                  DIAG 101000  PULMONARY ATRESIA WITH INTACT VENTRICULAR SEPTUM
                  DIAG 223100  RIGHT VENTRICULAR SINUSOIDS
                  DIAG 309900  RIGHT VENTRICULAR DEPENDENT CORONARY CIRCULATION
                  DIAG 592100  S/P RIGHT BLALOCK SHUNT
                  DIAG 600100  S/P PATENT DUCTUS ARTERIOSUS LIGATION
                  DIAG 242000  PULMONARY HYPERTENSION, RIGHT LUNG
                  DIAG 390800  LPA STENOSIS
                  PROC 642750  DILATION LEFT PULMONARY ARTERY
                  COMP 730500  COMPLETE HEART BLOCK
SURG      XX/XX/200X  1 Yr 2 Mo 17 Days     Xxxx Xxxx, M.D.
                  DIAG 101000  PULMONARY ATRESIA WITH INTACT VENTRICULAR SEPTUM
                  PROC 691300  ECMO DECANNULATION
SURG      XX/XX/200X  1 Yr 3 Mo 1 Day       Xxxx Xxxx, M.D.
                  DIAG 101000  PULMONARY ATRESIA WITH INTACT VENTRICULAR SEPTUM
                  DIAG 592100  S/P RIGHT BLALOCK SHUNT
                  PROC 670000  BANDING PROCEDURE, ANY VESSEL
CATH      XX/XX/200X  1 Yr 6 Mo 25 Days     Xxxx Xxxx, M.D..
                  DIAG 101000  PULMONARY ATRESIA WITH INTACT VENTRICULAR SEPTUM
                  DIAG 223100  RIGHT VENTRICULAR SINUSOIDS
                  DIAG 592100  S/P RIGHT BLALOCK SHUNT
                  DIAG 240000  PULMONARY HYPERTENSION
                  DIAG 642750  S/P DILATION OF LEFT PULMONARY ARTERY
                  DIAG 280200  RIGHT FEMORAL VEIN OCCLUSION
SURG      XX/XX/200X  1 Yr 6 Mo 27 Days     Xxxx Xxxx, M.D..
                  DIAG 101000  PULMONARY ATRESIA WITH INTACT VENTRICULAR SEPTUM
```

FIGURE 19–1 *Example of cardiology patient summary.*

PATIENT SUMMARY FILE

In our institution, a patient summary file was established as a clinical tool for output of database information, allowing the most relevant information for patient care to be readily retrieved in concise form, without nonessential detail. This file is organized in a manner similar to a hospital medical record, with procedures and events organized chronologically, and can be described as an extract of cardiac information about each patient (Fig. 19-1). It is *created on demand* from the larger patient information database, whenever the request is made for information on a given patient.

The value of the patient summary file is dependent on what data are considered to be essential for inclusion in the cardiac medical history. Not all physicians would be in agreement of the key facts to be retrieved from the database to create this file. However, the tendency to store and retrieve excessive amounts of information in response to a desire to be flexible and complete must be balanced against the limited intellectual abilities of human beings to process large amounts of data. Importantly, the cost and human resources needed to enter and maintain the accuracy of information placed in the database increases according to its size and complexity.

The theory behind the patient summary file is that carefully selected information can be reliably collected prospectively, and used as core data or for retrospective searches later. Thus, the first order of business in designing a database and patient summary tool is to obtain a consensus regarding the principle uses of the database, and the specific factual material necessary to accomplish those ends. Then, less relevant and more ambiguous information can be winnowed out of the clinical reports that are produced. When necessary, the format of these reports can be expanded to include additional topical areas, or specific reports can be *drilled down* to provide detailed data from that clinical event.

An example of the value of concise data presentation is the occurrence of clinic visits. These are recorded in the patient information database, but in our experience coded diagnoses from clinic are often erroneous, and rarely if ever produce new clinical facts that supersede the information produced and more effectively documented in simultaneously ordered tests. In fact, the most important information obtained from most clinic visits may be the fact that the patient was alive on that date. Similarly, chest radiographs are not included in the patient summary file; although a radiograph may help diagnose a pulmonary artery sling, the subsequent diagnostic evaluation, including echocardiography, magnetic resonance imaging (MRI), and surgery, identifies that patient's diagnosis with certainty. With the exception of certain arrhythmia diagnoses (e.g., heart block, ventricular and supraventricular tachycardia), electrocardiogram (ECG) diagnoses are also of little marginal value to the summary file. In contrast, catheterizations, echocardiograms, surgeries and, more recently, magnetic resonance imaging all reliably generate detailed and comprehensive and correct diagnostic summaries. Although these occasionally conflict with one another, they are invariably of value in refining the patient's clinical diagnosis, and thus are included *in toto* in the summary file presentation.

MANAGEMENT OF NEGATIVE INFORMATION AND OTHER DIFFICULTIES

Coding of negative information—diagnoses that have been proposed by one modality and subsequently ruled out by a second, surgical modifications that have been taken down or otherwise rendered nonfunctional or diagnoses that have resolved spontaneously over time—is an important and difficult problem in these systems. We have adopted change in a single digit in the six-digit diagnostic code as the marker of *diagnosis ruled-out*. Although this may appear to be an efficient solution to this type of problem, it means that every search for a given diagnosis must take this into account, lest the patients of interest become mixed together with those that are to be excluded. Similar problems exist with the management of semiquantitative grading applied to certain physiologic observations (e.g., trivial, mild, moderate, and severe valvular regurgitation). The difficulties in managing the concept of absence or grade of a diagnosis cannot be overstated, and some effects of this problem on determining the prevalence of certain common lesions will be covered below.

In addition to problems coding severity and absence with regard to diagnostic categories, other problems relate to issues of patient history and identification. As in other major congenital heart centers, we see a large number of patients referred with a known diagnosis and often with a history of prior procedures. Inclusion of relevant cardiologic data acquired elsewhere thus becomes crucial in ensuring that individual records are sufficiently complete to fulfill their role as a working patient summary capable of guiding clinical management. If detailed information about prior surgical and diagnostic events is available, this may be entered in the patient database and identified by location. Often, however, critical information such as procedure date, location, or codable diagnosis is not reliably available, in which case prior procedures are entered as diagnostic codes. These codes indicate a prior procedure—equivalent to the common notation *s/p* or status post. Unfortunately, the quality and origin of outside data are diverse, and systematic entry is difficult.

A more novel problem relates to the identification and classification of diagnoses made during fetal echocardiography. Retroactive management of patient identification is often necessary in patients followed postnatally, as the fetal echocardiogram is performed under the mother's name. Additionally, several diagnostic findings that are physiologic in the fetus are classified as abnormal, making the process of retrospective census of these lesions more difficult.

SOURCES OF ERROR

The presence of a sufficient number of errors in data entry can degrade or even completely cripple the ability of a computer-based system to perform its desired functions. Although it is impossible to eliminate data entry errors altogether, it is critical to view the prevention, detection, and correction of data entry errors as an integral piece of cardiovascular information system management.

To ascertain that each patient record contains all of the requisite information and no more, patient record numbers must be unique, precise, and reliable. Linking the patient record numbers to the hospital-wide medical records system is useful in this respect. In recent years, implementation of systems that check demographics online to ensure that information on each patient remains identical from encounter to encounter has reduced problems with single-digit errors in record numbers and patient names. However, problems still arise with patients who have changed their names or who, for some other reason, have been issued multiple medical record numbers. Additionally, patients not yet registered in the hospital system (e.g., fetal patients, outside studies sent in advance from other institutions) require identification by a proxy while awaiting the patient's arrival.

A second major source of error occurs with the generation of the diagnostic and procedural codes themselves. These errors can be very complex—not only can they be propagated by clerical and keystroke error, but they may reflect lack of knowledge or even legitimate difference of opinion on the part of the individuals assigning the codes or inconsistencies and design flaws of the coding system itself. In general, there are fewer coding errors produced if the physician responsible for the procedure does the coding at the time the procedure is completed.

Scrubbing the database of errors is an ongoing and labor-intensive process. Regular comparison of the patient files against those maintained by the hospital uncovers most errors in patient identifiers and updates demographics. Programs that regularly search files for patients with nearly identical names, birthdates, and/or medical record numbers are also helpful. However, the single most valuable method to maintenance of an error-free database is continuous, day-to-day use of patient information files by physicians and others who will recognize and correct any errors that are entered into the database. The more useful and more used the database, the lower will be the tolerance for errors, and fewer that will be allowed.

PRESENT SIZE AND COST OF CARDIOVASCULAR PATIENT DATABASE

As of January 2004, our database contained more than 131,000 patient records and nearly 731,000 encounters and diagnostic or procedural events. Given the progressive increase in the power, bandwidth, and storage capacity of networked computers, as well as the decline in the cost per computational unit of the hardware, it may seem surprising that the cost of computing continues to rise. A variety of influences contribute to this, representing demand for simple, reliable, and secure computing systems for an ever-increasing number of data storage, retrieval, and communications functions. Also underlying the expense of computing in any organization is a simple fact: The accuracy of the data is ultimately determined by the humans overseeing its entry into the database. As the flow of data increases, more trained personnel are necessary each year to organize and maintain these systems and ensure the accuracy of each datum entered. These information technology professionals represent the major ongoing expense of database computing. Within the cardiovascular program, expenses for information technology are increasing steadily and in recent years have ranged from 5% to 7% of operating budgets.

DATA ANALYSIS FOR THIS TEXTBOOK: CASE SELECTION

In the penultimate edition of this textbook, we reviewed our clinical experience of those seen between January 1, 1973 and December 31, 1987, and in the current edition those seen between January 1, 1988 and January 1, 2002. These will be referred to below as the historic and recent periods, respectively. A minimum of 1-year follow-up time was selected to ensure the precision afforded by multiple observations and to provide the possibility of 1-year follow-up of survivors. The number of patients seen in the historic period (15 years) was 23,612. This number has increased to 59,832 in the recent period (14 years).

DIAGNOSTIC CATEGORIZATION OF PATIENTS: THE HIERARCHICAL SYSTEM

Ignoring administrative entries such as *diagnosis unchanged*, the diagnoses listed for any event were generalized to a single diagnosis for that event, using a hierarchical system of assigning the label (Tables 19-1 and 19-2). The hierarchical order of categoric diagnoses was designed, as much as possible, to mimic our general usage of these terms. The system ranks most highly those diagnoses that are most complex, distinctive, and unambiguous. For example, a diagnosis of hypoplastic left heart syndrome appearing even once on a patient record is likely to describe in accurate and clinically useful terms a consensus diagnosis for a patient regardless of most associated lesions that might also be used to describe the specifics of that patient's cardiovascular status: This categoric diagnosis is ranked highly in the hierarchical scheme. In contrast, the diagnosis of patent ductus arteriosus (PDA) is considerably less likely to be the single descriptor of a patient's anatomy because it is commonly associated and commented in association with a wide variety of more clinically significant anatomic lesions. Only when these other lesions are not present is this likely to be a principle diagnosis, and accordingly, PDA is ranked low in the hierarchical system.

Using the hierarchical system, the diagnoses recorded for all events for each patient were used to assign a preliminary, overall categoric diagnosis for that patient, in the following manner. All the collected diagnoses recorded for a given patient in the patient summary file were reviewed. From these diagnoses, the patient was then assigned to the highest-ranking diagnostic category identified. Clearly, the benefits of this approach are that it allows researchers to take advantage of the use of computerized analysis of a large database. In the present case, the use of a uniform approach to categorization of patients in this manner also allows a direct comparison to patient categories cited in the prior edition of this textbook. At the same time, the simplicity of the hierarchical system and the complexities of congenital anatomy, coupled with the inevitable occurrence over the years of error and variability in the data collection, interpretation, and coding result in miscategorization of some patients. If there was discordance among the event diagnoses, the combination of data from echocardiography, catheterization, surgery, and/or autopsy was used to determine the best possible diagnosis, biased toward the more recent findings. Unusual and unexpected output was further sight-checked through examination of the detailed reports available via the computer, and in some cases samples of various diagnoses were chosen to determine the prevalence of systematic errors in diagnostic category due to changes in coding procedures. Rarely, hospital charts were consulted to confirm apparent results that might influence generalizations about a particular topic. The entire patient file was then divided into groups based on the assigned categoric diagnoses. Subsequently, each diagnostic group was reviewed in detail.

PREVALENCE OF PEDIATRIC HEART DISEASE

Heart disease in children continues to be a major public health problem worldwide. This remains largely due to rheumatic heart disease, the incidence of which seems to

TABLE 19–1. Hierarchical Diagnostic Categories

- Malposition
  - Dextrocardia with situs solitus
  - Visceral heterotaxy
  - Polysplenia
  - Cantrell's syndrome
  - Ectopia cordis
- Hypoplastic left heart syndrome (HLHS)
  - Left atrioventricular (AV) valve atresia
  - Aortic atresia
- Tricuspid atresia (TA)
  - Right AV valve atresia
- Single ventricle
- Truncus arteriosus
  - Truncus
  - Hemitruncus
  - Aortopulmonary window
- Double-outlet right ventricle (DORV)
- d-Transposition of the great arteries (d-TGA)
- L-Transposition of the great arteries (L-TGA)
- Total anomalous pulmonary venous return (TAPVC)
- Pulmonary atresia with intact ventricular septum (PA/IVS)
- Tetralogy of Fallot (TOF)
  - Pulmonary atresia
  - Tetralogy of Fallot with endocardial cushion defect
- Endocardial cushion defects (ECD)
  - Atrial septal defect primum
  - Atrioventricular canal
  - Common atrium
- Coarctation of the aorta (Coarc)
  - Intact ventricular septum
  - Ventricular septal defect
- Ventricular septal defect (VSD)
  - With pulmonary vascular disease
  - With aortic regurgitation
  - With aortic stenosis
  - With mitral valve abnormality
  - With pulmonary stenosis
  - With pulmonary regurgitation
- Aortic valve abnormality (AoV)
  - Valvar aortic stenosis
  - Subaortic stenosis
  - Supravalvar aortic stenosis
  - Aortic regurgitation
- Pulmonary valve (PV) abnormalities
  - Valvar pulmonic strenosis
  - Subvalvar stenosis
  - Double chamber right ventricle
  - Supravalvar stenosis
  - Peripheral pulmonic stenosis
  - Pulmonary regurgitation
- Tricuspid valve (TV) abnormalities
  - Tricuspid regurgitation
  - Tricuspid stenosis
  - Ebstein anomaly
- Mitral valve (MV) abnormalities
  - Mitral stenosis
  - Mitral regurgitation
- Myocardial disease
  - Myocarditis
  - Dilated cardiomyopathy
  - Inborn errors of metabolism
  - Hypertrophic cardiomyopathy
  - Muscular dystrophy
  - Friedrich's ataxia
- Pericardial disease
- Atrial septal defect secundum (ASD2)
  - Partially anomalous pulmonary venous connection
- Patent ductus arteriosus (PDA)
- Aneurysms
- Fistulas
  - Systemic
  - Pulmonary
- Pulmonary hypertension
- Systemic hypertension
- Miscellaneous

be directly related to poverty and social circumstances. In the United States, rheumatic heart disease has become quite rare, and congenital heart disease accounts for almost all heart disease in children. The incidence of congenital heart disease has been remarkably constant throughout the world and over the years, with most estimates ranging between 5 and 10 cases per 1000 live births (Fig. 19-2).[9] This is concordant with a recent careful study of heart defects in a large metropolitan population, showing the prevalence of significant congenital diagnoses increasing from 6.2 to 9.0 cases per 1000 live births over the last 30 years.[9a]

The relative frequencies of the various specific congenital cardiac defects are also quite predictable. The worldwide literature on this topic has recently been reviewed by Hoffman and Kaplan,[9] who surveyed findings from 44 published studies with significant numbers of patients. Their findings are summarized in Table 19-3, together with comparable data drawn from the findings of the New England Regional Infant Cardiac Program (NERICP), a hospital consortium that comprehensively reported the prevalence of more serious cardiac lesions over a 2-year period in the 1970s.[10] Both the common features and differences in these data are worthy of consideration. A major contributor to variation in estimates of prevalence of congenital heart disease in general and the frequency of certain lesions of low clinical severity, such as small ventral septal defects (VSDs), atrial septal defects (ASDs), and PDAs, depends very much on the practice setting from which the patients have been drawn (inpatient vs. outpatient) and the diagnostic and therapeutic technologies available to the practitioner—particularly echocardiography. This will be further analyzed below. What variation is encountered in cardiac lesions that are more rare and severe is more difficult to interpret, but may be attributable to the vagaries of classification or inadequate enumeration.

TABLE 19–2. Frequency of Hierarchical Diagnoses Recorded in the Cardiovascular Program of Children's Hospital Boston during Historical and Recent Periods

Lesion	1973–1987		1988–2002	
Ventricular septal defect	3,322	14.5%	5,117	8.6%
Pulmonary valve abnormality	1,500	6.6%	3,370	5.7%
Tetralogy of Fallot	1,403	6.1%	1,538	2.6%
Aortic valve abnormality	1,060	4.6%	3,299	5.5%
Atrial septal defect	891	3.9%	3,554	6.0%
Patent ductus arteriosus	866	3.8%	544	0.9%
Coarctation	826	3.6%	1,238	2.1%
d-Transposition of great arteries	755	3.3%	991	1.7%
Endocardial cushion defect	717	3.1%	1,188	2.0%
Ventricular dysfunction	369	1.6%	1,160	1.9%
Malposition	335	1.5%	724	1.2%
Mitral valve abnormality	663	2.9%	4,814	8.1%
Hypoplastic left heart syndrome	287	1.3%	518	0.9%
Double-outlet right ventricle	224	1.0%	303	0.5%
Single ventricle	192	0.8%	275	0.5%
Tricuspid atresia	154	0.7%	223	0.4%
Pulmonary hypertension	135	0.6%	124	0.2%
Total anom pulmonary venous connection	118	0.5%	142	0.2%
Pericardial abnormality	111	0.5%	309	0.5%
Truncus arteriosus	107	0.5%	171	0.3%
Rheumatic heart disease	102	0.4%	153	0.3%
l-Transposition of the great arteries	90	0.4%	83	0.1%
Pulmonary atresia/intact ventric septum	83	0.4%	161	0.3%
Hypertension	76	0.3%	92	0.2%
Tricuspid valve abnormality	151	0.7%	3,177	5.3%
Systemic arterial abnormality	70	0.3%	188	0.3%
Atrioventricular fistula	34	0.1%	92	0.2%
Tumor	32	0.1%	91	0.2%
Anomalous left coronary from pulmonary artery	29	0.1%	51	0.1%
Aortopulmonary window	19	0.1%	34	0.1%
Aneurysm	13	0.1%	58	0.1%
RPA from aorta	10	0.0%	19	0.0%
Arrhythmia	883	3.9%	9,168	15.4%
Fetal studies	0	0.0%	1,147	1.9%
No significant heart disease	6,743	29.5%	15,395	25.8%
Missing data	466	2.0%	113	0.2%
Total	23,612	100.0%	59,832	100.0%

Perhaps of more interest than the number of children born with heart disease is the number of babies who will require special medical facilities because of heart disease. The NERICP reported that, excluding premature infants with patent ductus arteriosus, 3 infants of every 1000 live births needed cardiac catheterization and surgery and/or will die with congenital heart disease in early infancy. Although mortality figures have decreased since the time of this study, it is reasonable to assume that the rate of need for cardiac intervention early in infancy has not. Approximately 5 per 1000 live births will require specialized facilities at some time during their lives.[10] The personnel and facilities needed to diagnose and document less hemodynamically serious forms of heart disease, to follow up patients who have undergone surgical repair procedures, and to manage such problems as Kawasaki disease or the dyslipidemias will vary with local interest and resources. All together, about 10 per 1000 live births, or about 1% of children born each year make up the patient material of pediatric cardiology in the United States.

CODING AND CARDIAC LESIONS

For the 59,832 patients seen in the recent period, 1,375,701 diagnostic codes were generated, an average of 23 codes per patient. Looking at these codes from the perspective of the hierarchical system put forward in Table 19-1, nearly half (43%) are accounted for by over 6000 patients with complex cardiovascular disease who fall within the first 11 diagnostic categories (malposition through tetralogy of Fallot). Comparing historic and recent periods,

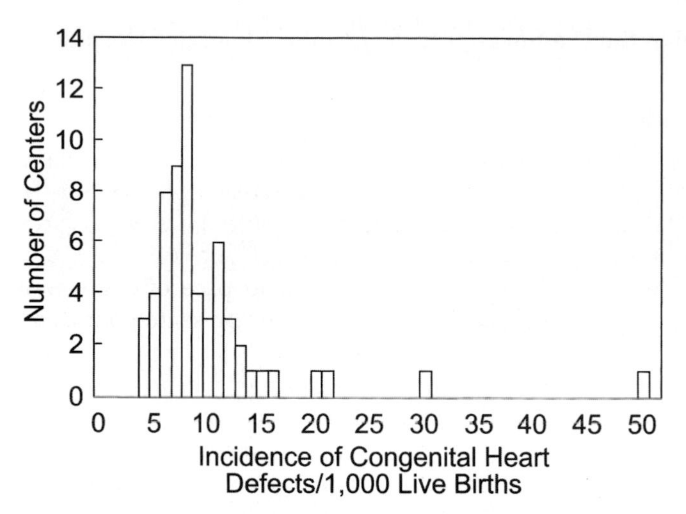

FIGURE 19–2 *Prevalence of congenital heart disease in the general population.*
Adapted from Hoffman JIE, Kaplan S. The incidence of congenital heart disease. J Am Coll Cardiol 39:1890, 2002, with permission.

it is clear that the prevalence and, in some cases, the rank orders of cardiac defects seen at the Children's Hospital Boston have changed (Tables 19-2 and 19-4). If we make the reasonable assumption that the biologic incidence of structural congenital heart disease itself is probably relatively stable in this region over this short period, such changes must reflect changes in the practice of the department. Factors that appear to have affected this practice include changes in patterns of patient referral and reimbursement; adoption and expansion in use of new diagnostic and therapeutic tools; the development of specific areas of interest, specialization, and expertise; institution of broadly based research protocols and outpatient services that increase the scope of the patient population; and changes in the application of the coding system itself. For example, the increase in atrial septal defects is almost certainly related to local interests in closing these defects with devices introduced during cardiac catheterization, to referrals of patients to this center for that purpose, and to the increased utilization and sensitivity of diagnostic echocardiographic techniques. The increase in the number of patients with cardiac malposition/heterotaxy is caused not only by an absolute increase in numbers but also by the fact that these patients now survive and return. The increase in the number of patients with ventricular dysfunction, in many cases an acquired condition, may reflect changes in the population itself. However, it has almost certainly also been affected by the development and wide application of noninvasive, quantitative echocardiographic techniques for measurement of myocardial function and their wide application in this program to large populations of children at risk for myocardial disease due to chemotherapy, HIV infection, and Kawasaki disease and enrolled in research protocols that provided intensive diagnostic follow-up.

Certain changes deserve careful consideration. As mentioned above, rheumatic heart disease has declined in prevalence to the point of becoming a rarity, a phenomenon probably attributable to improvements in public health in the United States. Also decreasing is the category of patients

TABLE 19–3. Studies of Congenital Heart Disease Epidemiology

Lesion	Hoffman and Kaplan Studies	Incidence		Lesion	NERICP Frequency	
VSD	43	3,570	38.8%	VSD	345	18.9%
ASD2	43	941	10.2%	d-TGA	218	12.0%
PDA	40	799	8.7%	TOF	196	10.8%
Pulmonary stenosis	39	729	7.9%	Coarctation	165	9.1%
TOF	41	421	4.6%	HLHS	163	8.9%
Coarctation	39	409	4.4%	PDA	135	7.4%
Aortic stenosis	37	401	4.4%	ECD	110	6.0%
ECD	40	348	3.8%	Pulmonary stenosis	73	4.0%
d-TGA	41	315	3.4%	PA/IVS	69	3.8%
HLHS	36	266	2.9%	ASD2	65	3.6%
DORV	16	157	1.7%	TAPVC	58	3.2%
PA/IVS	11	132	1.4%	Tricuspid atresia	56	3.1%
Truncus arteriosus	30	107	1.2%	Single ventricle	54	3.0%
Single ventricle	23	106	1.2%	Aortic stenosis	41	2.3%
TAPVC	25	94	1.0%	DORV	32	1.8%
Tricuspid atresia	11	79	0.9%	Truncus arteriosus	30	1.6%

ASD2, atrial septal defect secundum; ECD, endocardial cushion defect; d-TGA, d-transposition of the great vessels; DORV, double-outlet right ventricle; HLHS, hypoplastic left heart syndrome; NERICP, New England Regional Infant Cardiac Program; PA/IVS, pulmonary atresia with intact ventricular septum; PDA, patent ductus arteriosus; TAPVC, total anomalous pulmonary venous return; TOF, tetralogy of Fallot; VSD, ventral septal defect.

TABLE 19–4. Relative Incidence of Most Common Cardiac Problems in Historical and Recent Periods

1973–1988		1988–2002	
VSD	14.2%	VSD	8.6%
PV abnormality	6.4%	MV abnormality	8.1%
TOF	6.0%	ASD2	6.0%
AoV abnormality	4.5%	PV abnormality	5.7%
ASD2	3.8%	AoV abnormality	5.5%
PDA	3.7%	TV abnormality	5.3%
COARC	3.5%	TOF	2.6%
DTGA	3.2%	COARC	2.1%
ECD	3.1%	ECD	2.0%
Ventricular dysfunction	1.6%	Ventricular dysfunction	1.9%
Malposition	1.4%	DTGA	1.7%
MV abnormality	1.3%	Malposition	1.2%
Arrhythmia*	3.8%	Arrhythmia	15.4%
No heart disease	28.7%	No heart disease	25.8%

*Diagnosis of "arrhythmia" in historic period does not exclude other, concomitant cardiac diagnosis. See other tables for abbreviations.

with pulmonary hypertension. It seems likely that widespread delivery of cardiac services to infants has reduced the number of patients with pulmonary vascular disease secondary to unrepaired congenital heart disease, and many patients in this category now represent the sporadic occurrence of primary pulmonary hypertension.

A second important change, and one that is perhaps more difficult to understand, is the apparent remarkable increases in the prevalence of valve abnormalities of all types, but especially patients with mitral and tricuspid valve diagnoses. To investigate this finding, a sample of ~360 patients from these categories was examined to determine the meaning of this finding. What was revealed was that these changes in fact show the evolution of our coding and reporting practice in echocardiography, which reflects the comprehensive, anatomic survey approach used in the examination itself. It is now common practice to generate diagnostic codes to indicate the presence of clinically trivial abnormalities or physiologic findings of the valves. This has resulted in spuriously large counts, particularly in the cases of tricuspid and mitral regurgitation. Additionally, approximately 15% to 20% of these patients underwent echocardiography without clinical indication, but instead as part of a clinical research protocol. In combination with the expansion of echocardiographic diagnostic services to large numbers of clinic and protocol patients, this has resulted in a large number of patients with normal cardiac anatomy and function classified as having a valvular abnormality. The exact numbers by which such lesions are overcounted in the recent period are unknown, so caution must be used in interpretation of direct comparison between recent and historic periods.

EFFECTS OF CHANGING TECHNOLOGY ON THE PRACTICE OF PEDIATRIC CARDIOLOGY

Patient volume and utilization of diagnostic and therapeutic resources are presented in Tables 19-5 and 19-6. In contrast to the epidemiology of congenital heart disease, the technology and institutions associated with its management have been evolving at a rapid pace over the past 30 years, and for this reason we have presented our experience in four 7-year epochs to better illustrate trends over that period. An increasing number of patients are being seen each year, with both the number of patients and the number with significant heart disease increasing by ~9% per year over this period. Much of this increase can be accounted for by expansion of outpatient services and referral of patients, especially for specialized techniques not widely available, such as electrophysiologic studies, fetal echocardiography, magnetic resonance imaging, minimally invasive surgical techniques, and interventional cardiac catheterizations.

It was anticipated that the increasing number of echocardiograms would result in decreased numbers of diagnostic cardiac catheterizations. When considering only the patients who are ultimately proved to have heart disease, there is a trend compatible with this theory. Less constrained by requirements for dedicated facilities and personnel, the number of echocardiograms performed has increased by 11% per year and has far outstripped the growth in both the catheterization and surgical procedures, which have increasing by 2% to 3% per year. This increase in echocardiographic volume is due to increases both in the number of patients echoed and the number of echoes performed per patient.

For the average patient, the likelihood that cardiac catheterization will be needed has decreased from 0.94 to 0.35, even though the absolute number of cardiac catheterizations is rising and the number of cardiac catheterizations per patient requiring catheterization has remained relatively constant at ~1.6 (Table 19-6). Similarly, it was thought that the increasing number of interventional cardiac catheterizations would result in fewer cardiac operations. This may also be the case, because the proportion of patients undergoing cardiac surgery has decreased from 0.75 to 0.29 of patients with nontrivial heart disease. Again, despite this drop, the average number of surgeries needed by patients who require at least one surgical procedure has remained quite constant, at ~1.3.

It seems that many patients with congenital heart disease who survive will require medical supervision indefinitely. As more patients survive to adult life, the average number and age of patients being followed will increase over the years. This is reflected in the increase in the percentage of

TABLE 19–5. Annual Number of Procedures in Patients

Categories	1974–1981	1981–1988	1988–1995	1995–2002	Growth Rate
All patients					
Number/yr	1,538	2,612	4,936	8,577	9%/yr
Number with nontrivial heart disease/yr*	624	1,081	2,432	3,490	9%/yr
Surgeries					
Patients/yr	374	533	696	741	3%/yr
Procedures/yr	467	687	893	1,003	4%/yr
Patients ≤30 d	16%	24%	26%	28%	—
Patients ≥18 yr	15%	9%	6%	8%	—
Catheterizations					
Patients/yr	442	526	697	708	2%/yr
Procedures/yr	586	784	1,165	1,208	4%/yr
Patients ≤30 days	16%	23%	17%	13%	—
Patients ≥18 yr	16%	17%	15%	23%	—
Echocardiograms					
Patients/yr	3	1,269	2,586	4,636	10%/yr
Procedures/yr	6	2,425	5,918	10,834	11%/yr
Fetal procedures	—	2%	5%	10%	—
Arrhythmia	61	97	211	496	11%/yr
Deaths					
Number/yr	89	127	161	131	2%/yr
Death as % of all patients	5.8%	4.9%	3.3%	1.5%	−6%/yr

*"Patients with nontrivial heart disease" is estimated from "All patient" by exclusion of patients coded as having no heart disease, or findings such as trivial valvular regurgitation, bicuspid aortic valve, peripheral pulmonary stenosis, murmur, or patent foramen ovale.

both catheterization and surgical patients older than 18 years in the most recent time period (Table 19-5). Who will take care of surviving adult patients with congenital heart disease is a matter of practical concern, now very well recognized. As has been the case at many major academic pediatric cardiac centers, an adult congenital heart program to care for the medical and surgical needs for this unique and rapidly growing group of patients has been established (see Chapter 56). This service is based in both Children's Hospital Boston and the adjacent Brigham and Women's Hospital. We anticipate that this clinical activity will continue to expand rapidly, and that training of practitioners in this field will soon establish a distinct area of specialization drawing on both pediatric cardiology and adult internal medicine.

Echocardiography and Magnetic Resonance Imaging

Echocardiography can be performed with mobile equipment, without exposure to X-radiation, and can be repeated as often as needed. The role of echo in the current era as the core diagnostic technology for children with heart disease is well established. Over the last 15 years, new

TABLE 19–6. Number of Procedures per Cardiac Patient

Procedures	1974–1981	1981–1988	1988–1995	1995–2002
Procedures/patients with nontrivial heart disease	1.70	3.61	3.28	3.74
Procedures/all patients	0.69	1.49	1.62	1.52
Surgeries/patients having at least one surgery	1.25	1.29	1.28	1.35
Surgeries/patients with nontrivial heart disease	0.75	0.64	0.37	0.29
Surgeries/all patients	0.30	0.26	0.18	0.12
Caths/patients having at least one cath	1.57	1.47	1.67	1.63
Caths/patients with nontrivial heart disease	0.94	0.73	0.48	0.35
Caths/all patients	0.38	0.30	0.24	0.14
Echos/patients having at least one echo	—	1.91	2.29	2.34
Echos/patients with nontrivial heart disease	—	2.24	2.43	3.10
Echos/all patients	—	0.93	1.20	1.26

Caths, catheterizations; echo, echocardiograms.

applications of echocardiography and additional techniques for noninvasive anatomic and functional imaging have begun to establish their roles in pediatric cardiology (Fig. 19-3).

Fetal echocardiograms are performed with increasing frequency at the request of ultrasonographers when there is concern about the anatomy of the fetal heart on routine obstetric screening or when a prior child has been born with congenital heart disease. A surprising but certainly predictable outcome of this has been a shift to more proactive prenatal and perinatal management of mothers carrying children with major congenital heart disease. In many practice settings, early diagnosis of major congenital heart disease may influence a decision to terminate pregnancy, with measurable effects on the incidence of major congenital lesions.[11,12] Conversely, deliveries of affected infants are now often planned in a tertiary care center, with immediate transfer of the infant to inpatient cardiac services and a decrease in the number of infants first diagnosed during physiologic crises occurring in the first weeks of life. Indeed, many parents now have visited the cardiac intensive care unit and met with their child's cardiologist and cardiac surgeon before the child is born.

The utilization of transesophageal echocardiography has experienced similar growth. In addition to providing excellent visualization of cardiac structures in adults and large children with complex heart disease and poor echocardiographic windows, transesophageal echocardiography is also now used to evaluate ongoing progress during cardiac surgery and to guide intracardiac intervention in the catheterization laboratory and in the intensive care unit.

Magnetic resonance imaging (MRI) is now also experiencing the rapid growth seen in imaging technologies, which contribute novel and valuable information to clinical appreciation of anatomic structure and function. Although it is more expensive and less flexible in its application than echocardiography, due to the requirement for a large, specialized facility for installation, the need for patient immobility for long periods and incompatibility with implanted metal devices, it provides unparalleled three-dimensional visualization of the structure and function of all anatomic structures in the chest. A variety of innovative approaches have already been developed to increase the range of clinical situations to which MRI might be applied, and the feasibility of measuring vascular flow rates,[13] characterizing tissue injury,[14] and guiding catheter manipulation and cardiovascular intervention[15] has been demonstrated. The expansion of the clinical utility of this modality will be an interesting topic for the next edition of this textbook.

Cardiac Catheterization

The steady improvement in diagnosis by echocardiography results in the need for fewer diagnostic cardiac catheterizations. Yet, because of the increasing frequency of interventional procedures and numbers of patients who have undergone cardiac transplantation to then subsequently require recurrent biopsy, the number of cardiac catheterizations has reached an all-time high (Fig. 19-4). The numbers and types of interventional catheterization procedures continue to expand. Patent ductus arteriosus, atrial and ventricular defects of suitable anatomy, surgically created shunts, and vascular connections are now routinely closed at cardiac catheterization, and stents are used to reinforce dilated vascular and cardiac structures. In developmental stages is the catheter-deployed heart valve, which may be of value in the therapy of pulmonary regurgitation.[16] Administration of local therapy using radioactive isotopes, topical drugs, and genetic agents also seem likely to have some application in the future.

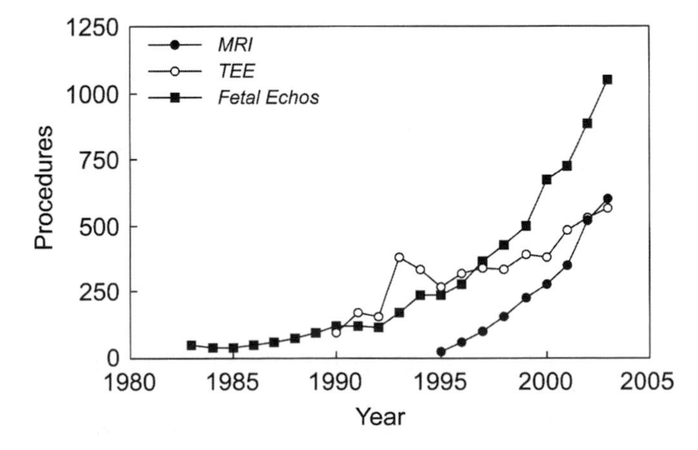

FIGURE 19–3 *Trends in utilization of newer noninvasive imaging modalities at Children's Hospital Boston. MRI, magnetic resonance imaging; TEE, transesophageal echocardiogram.*

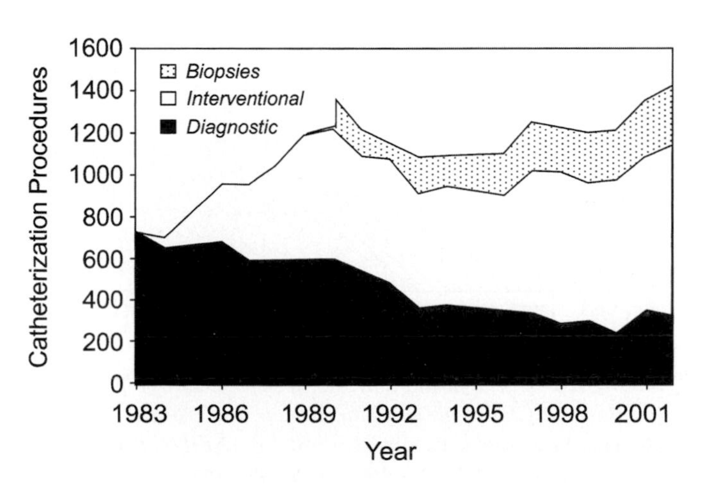

FIGURE 19–4 *Trends in cardiac catheterization.*

Arrhythmia and Electrophysiologic Studies

Over the past 15 years, the technique of radiofrequency catheter ablation has been firmly established as a curative procedure for a wide variety of tachyarrhythmias, most notably those causing supraventricular tachycardia in children with otherwise normal hearts.[17] Additionally, it has become very clear that among patients with congenital heart disease, rhythm problems are a major cause of morbidity and mortality over the long term. Steady improvement and miniaturization has also been seen in technology and implantation techniques used for permanent cardiac pacing and AICDs (automatic implantable cardioverter defibrillators), resulting in less reservation about the use of pacemakers, with ~700 patients having undergone placement of a pacemaker or AICD. The number of patients with an electrocardiographic diagnosis of tachy- or bradyarrhythmia recorded in our database has been growing at a rate of 11% per year, as is noted in Table 19-5. Similar growth has been seen in the number of patients requiring procedures, primarily radiofrequency catheter ablation, for evaluation and/or therapy of arrhythmia, as outlined in Figure 19-5.

Surgery

Even though many patients with conditions formerly corrected by surgical operations are now being treated with interventional catheter techniques, the number of surgical operations being performed at our institution continues to increase (Table 19-5). Some of the less complicated cardiac defects are being managed by catheter techniques or in some cases by the use of less invasive, thoracoscopic surgical approaches.[18] A variety of advances in surgical technique and perioperative management continue to improve surgical survival of patients with complex defects, with concomitant reductions of surgical morbidity and length of stay.

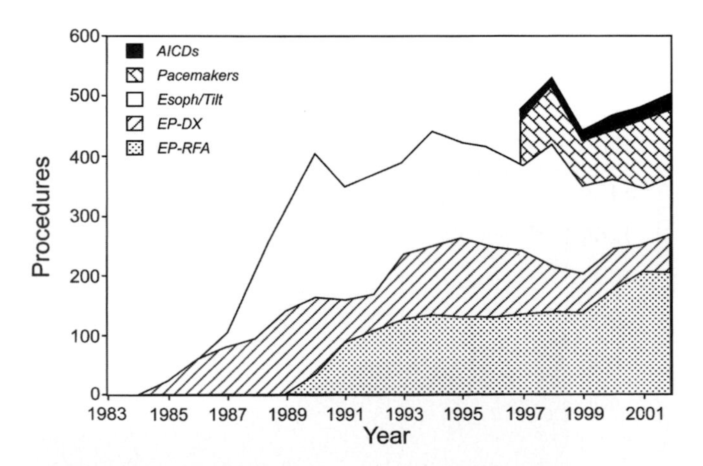

FIGURE 19–5 *Diagnostic and therapeutic electrophysiological procedures at Children's Hospital, Boston, 1983 to 2002. AICDs, automatic implantable cardiac defibrillators; EP-Dx, electrophysiologic diagnosis; RFA, radiofrequency ablation.*

For some years it has been our belief that the earliest discovery, diagnosis, and surgical treatment produce the best long-term results for patients with congenital heart disease. A trend toward increasing use of surgery in neonates continues, with patients younger than 30 days constituting 28% of the surgical population in the most recent 7-year period (Table 19-5). Of note, in this same period there was a slight increase in the number of surgical patients older than 18 years, the first such increase in 15 years. It seems likely that this also represents the emergence of the adult congenital patient population, now returning to surgery for revisions of their prior surgical repairs.

Improved understanding of the hemodynamics involved in the Fontan principle has led to newer surgical methods that achieve better results. Cavopulmonary connections, single or multiple, between the superior vena cava and the right and left pulmonary arteries are favored, with connection of the inferior vena cava effected by intracardiac baffle or extracardiac conduit. A small right-to-left shunt in the form of a fenestration is intentionally created to support the cardiac output. Despite the attendant systemic arterial oxygen desaturation, an upper limit to the right atrial pressure appears to reduce the likelihood of postoperative pleural effusion. The resulting hemodynamics are better than might be expected. This improved understanding of the implications of single ventricle physiology has led to a larger number of patients who are candidates for Fontan surgery and an improved overall survival rate.[19] Recent surgical mortality in patients undergoing a fenestrated Fontan or bidirectional Glenn operation has been less than 2%.

Other recent trends in cardiovascular surgery and perioperative management have also contributed significantly to survival of the sickest children. These include the increasing availability of and experience with extracorporeal membrane oxygenation (ECMO; see Chapter 59) and other forms of long-term cardiorespiratory support, and the establishment of cardiac transplantation as a reasonable option for children with end-stage cardiac disease of both acquired and congenital etiology. To date, we have performed 152 transplantation procedures. About half of the transplant recipients had an original diagnosis of congenital heart disease (see Chapter 60). Pretransplant evaluations and follow-up visits of more than 110 surviving recipients account for ~640 outpatient visits per year.

SURVIVAL AND ANALYSIS OF OUTCOMES

Survival in patients with congenital heart disease is dependent on the anatomic diagnosis and its associated natural history, the possibility of and perioperative risks attached to surgical correction or palliation, and the long-term sequelae of those surgeries experienced by operated patients. Overall survival has clearly improved remarkably in the past 30 years. For example, whereas mortality among infants with transposition of the great arteries was formerly nearly 100%, today it is minimal.[20,21] At the other end of the spectrum, remarkable growth has been observed in adult populations with major congenital heart diagnoses, testifying to increases in longevity as well as decreases in perioperative mortality, and presenting clinical practitioners with a novel spectrum of difficult management problems.[22]

The frequencies of known deaths reported in our database are noted in Table 19-5. Although these are suggestive of decreased mortality rates in more recent periods, these raw numbers are of limited value in assessing survival and outcomes in our patient population because of the many factors that may influence them. On the basis of the trends we have noted in imaging and interventional catheterization, we have speculated in this chapter that cardiac surgery will increasingly be applied to children with increasingly complex and difficult anatomies and physiologies. One would typically expect a greater percentage of loss with such complex surgeries, offsetting to some degree improvements in other areas of care.

Refined tools for assessing outcomes of surgery and interventional procedures are now being developed to allow us to measure the effects of clinical innovation and institutional improvement with greater precision. Most important is the development of the concept of risk adjustment of populations of patients, to account for the overall severity of illness that they present. This approach has been applied with great success in recent years to demonstrate the relations between institutional procedural volume and mortality in congenital heart surgery.[23] It is likely that application of such risk-adjustment methodologies to our historical database will demonstrate an overall increase in the complexity of our patient population undergoing both catheterization and surgery, which complements the increases in volume that are more easily seen and validating some of the interpretations that we have put forward above. The topic of clinical research design is an important one, which will be taken up in detail in the following chapter.

REFERENCES

1. Hersh WR. Information Retrieval: A Health and Biomedical Perspective, 2nd ed. New York: Springer-Verlag, 2003.
2. van de Velde R, Degoulet P. Clinical Information Systems: A Component-Based Approach. New York: Springer Verlag, 2003.
3. Shortliffe EH. Medical Informatics: Computer Applications in Health Care and Biomedicine, 2nd ed. New York: Springer Verlag, 2000.
4. Coiera E. Guide to Medical Informatics, the Internet and Telemedicine. London: Chapman & Hall Medical, 1977.
5. Franklin RC, Anderson RH, Daniels O, et al. Report of the Coding Committee of the Association for European Paediatric Cardiology. Cardiology in the Young 12:611, 2002
6. Gaynor JW, Jacobs JP, Jacobs ML, et al. Congenital Heart Surgery Nomenclature and Database Project: update and proposed data harvest. Ann Thor Surg 73:1016, 2002.
7. Mavroudis C, Jacobs JP. Congenital heart disease outcome analysis: methodology and rationale. J Thor Cardiovasc Surg 123: 6, 2002.
8. Caldarone CA, Raghuveer G, Hills CB, et al. Long-term survival after mitral valve replacement in children aged <5 years: a multi-institutional study. Circulation 104 (Suppl 1): I143, 2001.
9. Hoffman JIE, Kaplan S. The incidence of congenital heart disease. J Am Coll Cardiol 39:1890, 2002.

9a. Botto LD, Correa A, Erickson JD. Racial and temporal variations in the prevalence of heart defects. Pediatrics 107:E32, 2001

10. Fyler DC, Buckley LP, Hellenbrand WE, et al. Report of the New England Regional Infant Cardiac Program. Pediatrics 65(Suppl):376, 1980.
11. Bull C. Current and potential impact of fetal diagnosis on prevalence and spectrum of serious congenital heart disease at term in the UK. Lancet 354: 1242, 1999.
12. Stumpflen I, Stumpflen A, Wimmer M, et al. Effect of detailed fetal echocardiography as part of routine prenatal ultrasonographic screening on detection of congenital heart disease. Lancet 348: 854, 1996.
13. Petersen SE, Voigtlander T, Kreitner KF, et al. Quantification of shunt volumes in congenital heart diseases using a breath-hold MR phase contrast technique: comparison with oximetry. Intl J Cardiovasc Imag 18:53, 2002.
14. Lardo AC, McVeigh ER, Jumrussirikul P, et al. Visualization and temporal/spatial characterization of cardiac radiofrequency ablation lesions using magnetic resonance imaging. Circulation 102:698, 2000.
15. Razavi R, Hill DL, Keevil SF, et al. Cardiac catheterisation guided by MRI in children and adults with congenital heart disease. Lancet 362:1877, 2003.
16. Bonhoeffer P, Boudjemline Y, Qureshi SA, et al. Percutaneous insertion of the pulmonary valve. J Am Coll Cardiol 39:1664, 2002.
17. Kugler JD, Danford DA, Houston KA, et al. Pediatric radiofrequency catheter ablation registry success, fluoroscopy time, and complication rate for supraventricular tachycardia: comparison of early and recent eras. J Cardiovasc Electrophysiol. 13:336, 2002.
18. Cannon JW, Howe RD, Dupont PE, et al. Application of robotics in congenital cardiac surgery. Semin Thorac Cardiovasc Surg 6:72, 2003.
19. Stamm C, Friehs I, Mayer JE Jr, et al. Long-term results of the lateral tunnel Fontan operation. J Thorac Cardiovasc Surg. 121:28, 2001.

20. Williams WG, McCrindle BW, Ashburn DA, et al. Outcomes of 829 neonates with complete transposition of the great arteries 12-17 years after repair. Eur J Cardiothorac Surg 24:1, 2003.
21. Gutgesell HP, Garson A, McNamara DG. Prognosis for the newborn with transposition of the great arteries. Am J Cardiol 44:96, 1979.
22. Somerville J. Management of adults with congenital heart disease: an increasing problem. Ann Rev Med 48:283, 1997.
23. Jenkins KJ, Gauvreau K, Newburger JW, et al. Consensus-based method for risk adjustment for surgery for congenital heart disease. J Thorac Cardiovasc Surg. 123:110, 2002.

20

Methodological Issues in Clinical Research

KATHY J. JENKINS, KIMBERLEE GAUVREAU,
AND STEVEN D. COLAN

CLINICAL RESEARCH IN PEDIATRIC CARDIOLOGY

Although fruitful information can be obtained from simple descriptions of patient outcomes, determination of best practices often requires the formal rigor of clinical study design and analysis. Clinical research techniques are increasingly being applied to create "evidence-based practice" in pediatric cardiac medicine, and modern era researchers often obtain advanced degrees in research methodology. Many texts discuss fundamental principles of study design and analysis; this chapter addresses several issues that are especially important to clinical research in pediatric cardiology. Even though large-scale, multicenter, randomized clinical trials have become a mainstay in the development of evidence-based practice for adult cardiac conditions, this is not the case in pediatrics. Because pediatric cardiac conditions, especially congenital heart defects, are both rare and diverse, simple principles of study design—such as homogeneous study populations and robust sample sizes—are often much harder to achieve. Methodological strategies to overcome problems associated with small sample size are discussed in the first section, with representative examples. Similarly, many issues must be considered when performing cardiac measurements in patients across a broad range of ages and sizes, and linear growth must be taken into account when patients are followed longitudinally. Strategies to appropriately address such age- and size-based differences are presented in the second section. Lastly, tools are increasingly being developed to allow meaningful study across a diverse array of pediatric cardiac conditions. Some of these tools are discussed in the last section.

METHODOLOGICAL ISSUES RELATED TO SMALL STUDY POPULATIONS

Hypothesis-Driven Analytical Studies

Although much of the literature in pediatric cardiology has been generated from descriptive studies in a single institution, hypothesis-driven studies with a predetermined analytical plan and sample size will generally, by design, give a much clearer answer to questions about best practice with the smallest possible sample size. Even though the actual mechanism by which a study will be performed (e.g., a chart review of cases over a 10-year period) may be very similar whether a study is done to "describe outcomes for tetralogy of Fallot at our institution between 1990 and 1999" or to "determine predictors of poor outcome after tetralogy of Fallot repair performed between 1990 and 1999," more specific information about how to change practice is likely possible from the second study than from the first. Patient characteristics, such as age at surgery or prior Blalock-Taussig shunt placement, will be simple descriptive information in the first design, but will serve as potential predictors of a specific outcome in the second. For example, study investigators may hypothesize that early age at surgery is a risk factor for poor outcome among patients with tetralogy of Fallot (TOF).

Studying Informative Patients

The improved information obtained from a study with a specific hypothesis comes from a variety of sources, the most important of which is limiting the study to patients

can be difficult to derive and are computationally intensive. The principle behind these techniques is that the data collected in a particular study represent but one of the many outcomes that could have occurred. The observed data are permuted in all possible ways, and what actually occurred (in the sample) is compared with what might have occurred (the permutations) to calculate a *P* value. For large data sets, it makes little difference which method is used because a *P* value based on the approximations made by traditional techniques and one based on an exact test will be very similar. This is not the case for small samples. Fortunately, a growing number of statistical packages now implement the more commonly used exact tests, allowing computation of valid *P* values even for rare outcomes.

Bayesian inference is another analytical strategy that could be useful when sample sizes are small.[6] When interpreting the results of a clinical research study analyzed using standard techniques, an investigator looks at more than just statistical significance as determined by a *P* value; he or she also considers the context of the research and any previous data that might exist. Bayesian methods allow such previously existing data to be formally integrated into the current research. Prior knowledge—which may be derived from studies on adults, or on a population of children with similar characteristics—is expressed in terms of the probability of a certain outcome. Data from the current study are then used to revise this probability. Existing beliefs about a relationship are modified by the new information, synthesizing evidence from multiple sources. Because inference does not rely solely on a single research study, estimated sample sizes tend to be smaller.

METHODOLOGICAL ISSUES RELATED TO AGE AND SIZE

The diagnostic evaluation of children is invariably subject to the need to differentiate between the effects of disease or treatment and those due to age and somatic growth. For example, the presence or absence of ventricular dilation cannot be assessed without knowledge of both a patient's body size and the normal relationship between the size of the ventricle and the size of the body. Because all cardiovascular structures increase in size as a child grows, comparisons of subjects whose body sizes are not identical require some method of standardization or adjustment. In addition to differences in size, comparisons of children with varying ages could also be affected by differences in body composition, organ maturation, and maturation-induced changes in enzyme activity or hormone levels.

Differences in age and body size are important potential confounders in pediatric research and often dictate study design in terms of the selection of an appropriate control group with which to compare the cases. However, there are many circumstances in which selection of a proper control group alone is simply not sufficient to overcome this problem, particularly when the disease or treatment can affect growth. For example, a study undertaken to determine whether angiotensin-converting enzyme (ACE) inhibitor therapy can favorably alter the severity of left ventricular dilation in infants with dilated cardiomyopathy might include treated and untreated cohorts of patients matched for age and body surface area (BSA) at the time of study enrollment, allowing a direct comparison of ventricular size without the need to account for differences in body size. If growth during the study period were similar in the two groups of children, this simple analysis would address the study question. However, if the treated group had greater somatic growth (a likely outcome), the change in left ventricular size would be expected to be larger in this group simply because of the effects of growth, even if there was no direct impact of use of ACE inhibition on left ventricular dilation. Confounding of this sort could be either counterbalancing (as in this example), masking a treatment effect, or synergistic, mimicking a treatment effect. A method of adjusting for growth-related change is needed to separate the potentially confounded effects of treatment and growth. Three general approaches to this problem are described next.

Indexing or Normalization

Historically, the most common approach to adjusting the size of a cardiovascular structure for overall body size has been to calculate the ratio of structure size to body surface area, often referred to as "indexing" or the "per-BSA method." For example, cardiac index is calculated as cardiac output divided by BSA, and ventricular mass index is ventricular mass divided by BSA. The continued reliance on such "per-surface area standards"[7] justifies a critical discussion of the deficiencies in this method,[8–10] as well as an exploration of alternative approaches to the problem.

Simply stated, the purpose of "indexing" or "normalizing" a variable such as cardiac output is to permit valid comparisons between individuals of differing BSA by eliminating the dependence of the indexed variable on body size. From a practical point of view, this implies that the values of the indexed variable should have the same distribution regardless of BSA, with both the same mean and the same amount of variability (as measured by the standard deviation or variance). Based on numerous intraspecies and interspecies studies, cardiac output has been recognized to be linearly related to BSA over a broad range of body sizes. Consequently, calculation of cardiac index—cardiac output divided by BSA—was adopted as a method of normalization that yielded a mean value of output relatively independent of BSA, thereby allowing comparisons of patients of differing sizes. The extrapolation of this method to other cardiac and vascular structures was predicated on two observations: (1) there is a direct, mostly linear relationship between average cardiac output and the size of most cardiovascular structures; and (2) numerous studies have reported a direct, mostly linear relationship between these structures and BSA.

Unfortunately, although the relationship between two variables can often be described as fairly linear, this does not mean that a straight line is the *best* descriptor of their relationship. There is a generally linear relationship between left ventricular volume and BSA, and also between left ventricular dimension and BSA, even though volume and dimension are related by a cubic function that is most certainly not linear; it is not mathematically possible for both volume and dimension to have a truly linear relationship with BSA. In general, the shortcoming of the indexing technique has been its reliance on simple linear regression analysis without an evaluation of whether the assumptions required to use this method have been fulfilled.[11] It is easy to be misled by a high correlation coefficient. Figure 20-1 illustrates the strong linear relationship between aortic valve annulus (AVA) diameter and BSA in more than 500 normal children varying in age from newborn to 18 years. The correlation coefficient associated with this linear regression analysis is 0.92. Without ever determining whether this is the *best* possible model, such observations have led to the common per-BSA approach of normalization. In fact, looking at the data more closely, there appears to be some curvature, with the AVA measurements of children with the smallest and largest BSAs being more likely to fall below the regression line, whereas the measurements for children in the middle range of BSA are more likely to fall above the line. Figure 20-2 shows the AVA/BSA ratio ("indexed aortic valve annulus diameter") plotted against BSA.

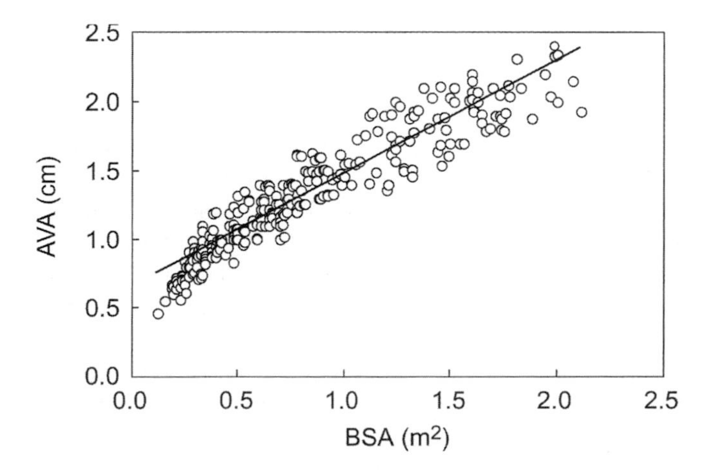

FIGURE 20–1 *Aortic valve annulus (AVA) versus body surface area (BSA) for a sample of normal children, ages 0 to 18 years.*

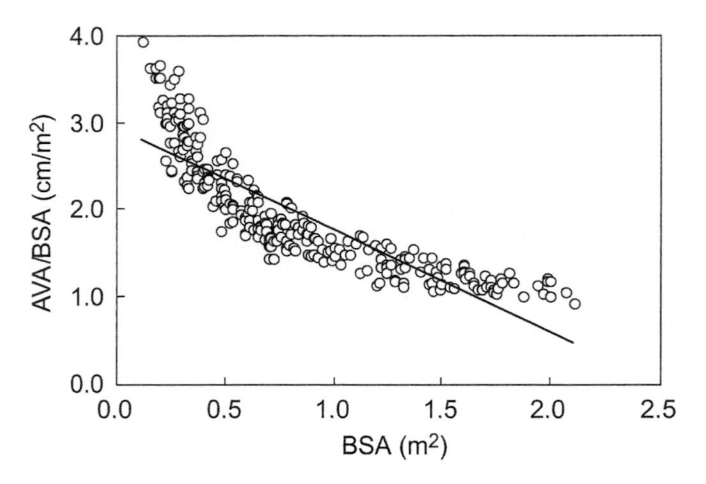

FIGURE 20–2 *Aortic valve annulus (AVA) divided by body surface area (BSA) versus BSA for a sample of normal children, ages 0 to 18 years.*

This relationship is clearly curvilinear; the mean AVA/BSA ratio for a child with BSA 2.0 m^2 is 1.1, whereas the mean for a child with BSA 0.2 m^2 is 3.6. Clearly, the indexing technique does not come close to meeting the requirements for an adequate method of normalization if the simple linear regression model is not appropriate.

In order for the per-BSA method of indexing to work, three assumptions underlying the simple linear regression model must be met. First, the relationship between structure size and BSA must be linear, meaning that size = m × BSA + b must be the best mathematical relationship between the measured structure size and BSA, where *m* is the slope of the line and *b* is its intercept. Second, the intercept of the regression line must be zero (b = 0), meaning that structure size is equal to 0 when BSA is equal to 0. Third, the amount of variability in structure size (as measured by the standard deviation or variance) must be constant over the entire range of BSA values. If we look back at Figure 20-1, the regression line does not appear to have an intercept of 0, and although the correlation is high, the data points do not fall on a straight line. In fact, a significantly better fit (r = 0.96) can be achieved with a nonlinear regression curve of the form size = m × (BSA)(a) + b. The failure to meet the third assumption (constant variability) is also evident in Figure 20-1, where the spread of AVA measurements around the regression line increases as BSA increases. Virtually all cardiovascular structure measurements display this pattern of increasing variance as BSA gets larger[11–15]; this can be explained by the age-related increase in variation for other factors that influence the size of these structures, such as blood pressure, adiposity, and habitual activity level. In general, the per-BSA method of adjusting for the effect of BSA does not work for cardiac structures other than cardiac output and certainly cannot be assumed to do so without specific proof.

Transformation

Two other common approaches to adjusting the size of a cardiovascular structure for body size do not begin by assuming that the relationship between structure size and BSA is necessarily linear. The first and simpler method involves transforming the measurements of either structure size or BSA before indexing, so that the new relationship becomes linear and can be used for normalization. One example of a transformation would be to take the square root of each BSA value ($BSA^{0.5}$); another is to square each value ($BSA^{2.0}$). Several authors have noted that the areas of cardiovascular structures tend to have a linear relationship with BSA, whereas their diameters have a linear relationship with the square root of BSA. To illustrate this, if we examine the graph of AVA versus $BSA^{0.5}$ in Figure 20-3, we see that the relationship does appear to be linear; AVA is not more likely to be either above or below the regression line depending on the value of BSA. Furthermore, when AVA/ $BSA^{0.5}$ is plotted against BSA (Fig. 20-4), the mean ratio is constant across the entire range of BSA values. In general, normalized variables are dimensionless, and this example does yield a dimensionless value; looking at the units, $cm/[(m^2)^{0.5}]$ or cm/m is a constant. It has been suggested that this approach can be generalized such that linear measurements are normalized to $BSA^{0.5}$, area measurements to BSA, and volume measurements to $BSA^{1.5}$. Unfortunately, this approach has not been uniformly successful because certain structures such as left ventricular dimension and left ventricular volume do not have the expected relationship to BSA.[16] Also, even if the mean value of an indexed variable is constant across BSA, this does not ensure that the variability or standard deviation of values around the mean is constant as well, which is required if linear regression is to be used.[17,18] In Figure 20-4, there is more variability of AVA/$BSA^{0.5}$ measurements for subjects with lower BSA than for those with higher BSA.

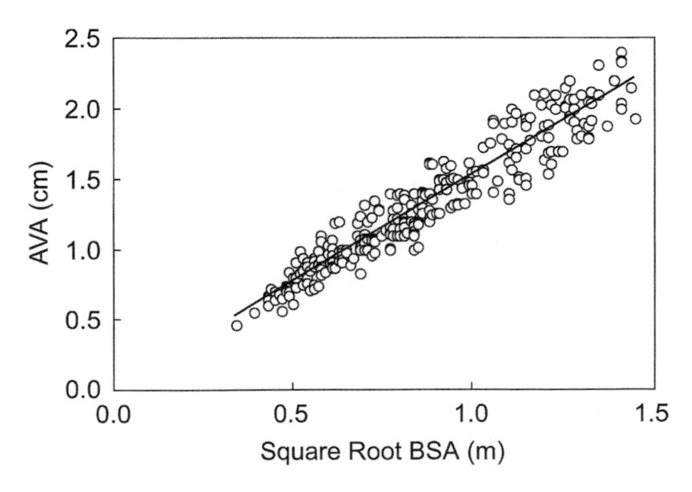

FIGURE 20–3 *Aortic valve annulus (AVA) versus the square root of body surface area (BSA) for a sample of normal children, ages 0 to 18 years.*

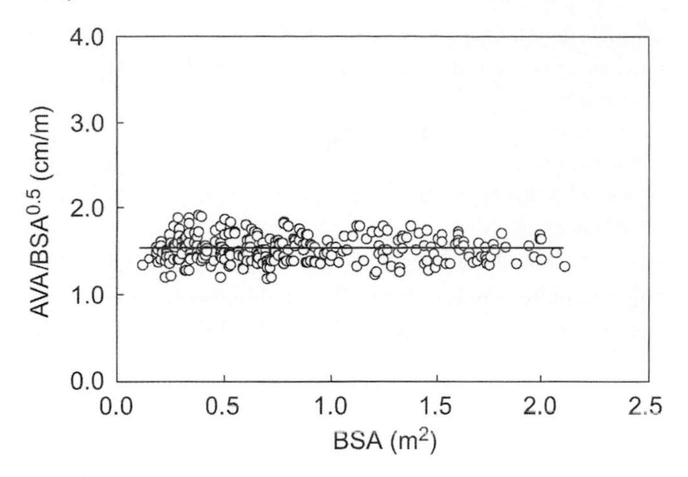

FIGURE 20–4 *Aortic valve annulus (AVA) divided by the square root of body surface area (BSA) versus BSA for a sample of normal children, ages 0 to 18 years.*

Z Scores

A third method of adjusting the size of a cardiovascular structure for either age or body size that has become increasingly popular in pediatric cardiology relies on the calculation of *z* scores, also known as *normal deviates*.[19] The *z* score of a measurement is the distance of this measurement from the mean of the population, expressed in units of the standard deviation. For example, a *z* score of 2.5 indicates that a measurement lies 2.5 standard deviations above the population mean, whereas a *z* score of −1.4 means that the measurement lies 1.4 standard deviations below the mean. For a cardiovascular structure, the calculation of *z* scores is performed relative to the distribution of that structure in the normal, healthy population. This distribution is determined across a range of values for age or body size; *z* scores can then be calculated for subjects of any size within that range. As an example, the relationship between AVA and BSA could be determined in a large population of normal subjects (whether linear or nonlinear); for each possible value of BSA, the expected mean and standard deviation of AVA measurements could then be estimated. For any new subject with a measured value of AVA, a *z* score could be determined by noting the new subject's BSA, estimating the normal mean and standard deviation of AVA values for that particular BSA, calculating the difference between the subject's AVA measurement and the estimated mean, and dividing by the estimated standard deviation of AVA. In the normal population, the mean *z* score is equal to 0, and the standard deviation is equal to 1 by definition. Z scores of 2.0 and –2.0, representing values that are 2 standard deviations above or below the normal mean, respectively, are commonly considered to be the upper and lower limits of normal.

The *z* score is quite similar to the more familiar percentile, used clinically to express age-adjusted height and weight with respect to the normal population. In the case of height and weight, the calculation of percentiles adjusts for the normally expected age-related changes in these measurements, permitting comparisons of subjects with varying ages. Percentiles for height and weight therefore serve the same purpose as *z* scores. In fact, *z* scores can be easily converted to percentiles, but have the advantage of avoiding compression in the higher and lower ranges. A *z* score of 4 (indicating a measurement 4 standard deviations above the normal population mean) corresponds to a percentile of 99.8, whereas a *z* score of 10 corresponds to a percentile of 99.9; it is easier to appreciate the magnitude of abnormality of a structure when its measurement is expressed as a *z* score on a linear scale.

There are distinct advantages of the *z* score approach over the previously described transformed and untransformed methods of indexing. The calculation of a *z* score does not assume any particular predetermined relationship between the cardiovascular structure size and BSA (linear or otherwise) and does not presume that the variability among the measurements is constant over the range of BSA. Z scores are truly a "normalized" variable, in that they are dimensionless and have mean 0 and standard deviation 1 in the normal population. Finally, although the example presented here examines the relationship of AVA to BSA, *z* scores could also be calculated relative to age, or to the combination of age and BSA, or to other variables alone or in combination. The *z* score approach represents the most powerful and flexible technique for normalizing cardiovascular parameters for the effects of age and BSA and has therefore become the standard approach in pediatric cardiology.[18]

Given the widespread use of *z* scores, there are several caveats concerning their application that are worthy of mention.[20,21] The population in whom the "normal" values are determined must be appropriate. This includes an appropriate range of BSA and age, as well as consideration of other potential confounders such as gender and race. The method of measurement must also be the same for the normal population and the population with heart disease. For example, one cannot assume that values for parameters measured by echocardiography will be the same as those measured by magnetic resonance imaging. Perhaps the most subtle and most often ignored issue is the method of calculating BSA. There are a number of published methods for calculating BSA from height and weight data, and the formulas do not yield the same results, particularly at lower values. Unfortunately, many publications do not indicate which of the several formulas has been applied, making it impossible to compare results. Several of the older formulas continue to be used, despite their poor methodology. For example, the 1916 formula published by DuBois and DuBois[22] continues to be applied by some authors despite the fact that the equation was derived from the measurements of only five subjects, no children were included, and the subjects were certainly not normal because the smallest individual in the study was a 34-year-old cretin. The formula with the soundest experimental basis is that of Haycock and colleagues.[23] In a systematic analysis of the normative data at Children's Hospital Boston, this formula was found to provide the highest correlation between BSA and cardiovascular measurements in normal subjects, and is the one currently used. For purposes of reference, the published formulas in most common use are shown in Table 20-1.[22–27]

METHODOLOGICAL ISSUES RELATED TO ANATOMIC DIVERSITY

Pediatric cardiac diseases, especially congenital heart defects, are characterized by substantial anatomic diversity. Although obvious patterns are encountered frequently, variations on the "typical" anatomy of even common lesions are as much the norm as the exception. Although diverse anatomy may make the practice of pediatric cardiology interesting, such diversity presents an interesting dilemma for pediatric cardiac research; studying reasonable-size samples of homogeneous patients becomes nearly impossible. Methods of enhancing statistical power in the face of

TABLE 20–1. Methods of Calculating Body Surface Area

Investigators	Formula for Body Surface Area
Du Bois & Du Bois, 1916 (22)	$0.007184\ \text{height}^{0.725}\ \text{weight}^{0.425}$
Haycock et al., 1978 (23)	$0.024265\ \text{height}^{0.3964}\ \text{weight}^{0.5378}$
Dreyer & Rey, 1912 (24)	$0.1\ \text{weight}^{0.6666}$
Boyd, 1935 (25)	$0.0004688\ (1000\ \text{weight})^{0.8168 - 0.0154 \log(1000\ \text{weight})}$
	$0.0003207\ (1000\ \text{weight})^{0.7285 - 0.0188 \log(1000\ \text{weight})}\ \text{height}^{0.3}$
Gehan & George, 1970, based on Boyd's data (26)	$0.02350\ \text{height}^{0.42246}\ \text{weight}^{0.51456}$
Mosteller, 1987 (27)	$[(\text{height weight})/3600]^{0.5}$

limited sample size were discussed earlier in this chapter. Some additional issues related to the extreme anatomic diversity encountered in pediatric cardiology are also worthy of mention.

Choice of Study Groups

First, as mentioned in the section entitled "Studying Informative Patients," careful thought must be given to the types of anatomic variation that will be included or excluded to answer a particular research question. Decisions to include or exclude patients, based on anatomy or other factors, should not be arbitrary. A consistent application of well-formulated inclusion and exclusion criteria will result in a well-defined study population. An individual subject will either meet the entry criteria or not; as a litmus test, criteria should be sufficiently specific to ensure that multiple investigators will classify subjects identically as either eligible or not eligible.

The extent to which a study population should be homogeneous or diverse depends on the study question. In some cases, a research question may be applicable across a range of defects; in these instances, anatomic diversity can be incorporated and will improve sample size and enhance generalizability of any study finding to a broader population. In other instances, particularly comparison studies of alternative treatment pathways, it may be important to compare "apples to apples" to protect validity. In such cases, only minor anatomic variants that have little possibility of influencing a particular outcome should be included. As an example, a recent study compared 1-year mortality for alternative strategies as initial treatment for hypoplastic left heart syndrome (HLHS): a staged surgical approach (i.e., Norwood operation) versus neonatal transplantation.[28] Because the primary goal of the study was to compare outcomes for infants with classic HLHS, anatomic variants such as malaligned common atrioventricular canal with hypoplastic left ventricle and aorta were not included, even though such infants are often palliated with a Norwood-type procedure. This restriction was imposed because outcomes for infants with complex anatomic variation were not assumed to be similar to those for more straightforward HLHS patients. Minor anatomic variants, such as tiny ventricular septal defects, were allowed.

Useful Analytical Techniques

Selected analytical techniques can be used to ensure that validity is preserved when patients with diverse anatomy are studied together. Such techniques are often included in a comprehensive analytical plan, especially if the influence of anatomy on the outcome of interest is not known for certain. It is usually best to begin with a stratified analysis, whereby patients in different anatomic subgroups are analyzed separately and are only "pooled" together if it is appropriate to do so. Appropriateness is judged by determining whether the effect of the predictor variable on the outcome is similar in each of the homogeneous anatomic subgroups. Similarity can be assessed formally, using statistical techniques such as the Mantel-Haenszel test.[2] If the effect of the predictor variable on the outcome (such as the effect of early age at surgery on mortality) differs among the anatomic subgroups, known as *effect modification*, the groups cannot be combined. Instead, relationships between the predictor variable and the outcome should be reported separately within each subgroup. Although fairly easy to carry out and often quite useful, stratified analyses have the disadvantage that the study sample is split into a number of smaller samples, thereby reducing statistical power.

Another analytical strategy that can be used to address the problem of patient diversity is multivariate modeling. By including terms representing the various anatomic subgroups in mathematical models, this technique can be used to evaluate the relationship between a predictor variable and an outcome, controlling or adjusting for confounding by inherent anatomic differences. Effect modification can be accounted for by incorporating appropriate interaction terms in the models. Although they can be more difficult to interpret than stratified analyses, and the choice of an appropriate model can be complex, multivariate models have the advantage of greater statistical power because the size of the original sample is preserved.

Useful Research Tools

Increasingly, formal research tools are being developed to address the issue of anatomic diversity, allowing patients with a diverse array of defects to be studied together. For example, the Risk Adjustment for Congenital Heart Surgery (RACHS-1) method allows comparisons of short-term mortality for a large fraction of pediatric cardiac surgical cases.[29] When applying RACHS-1, more than 200 types of surgical procedures are grouped into one of six risk categories based on a similar risk for postoperative in-hospital death, where category 1 has the lowest risk for death and category 6 the highest. This grouping together of cardiac surgical procedures is a data reduction technique and simplifies analyses among anatomically diverse cases.

Clinical research tools such as RACHS-1 must be validated before use; Figure 20-5 displays the actual mortality rates in each of the risk categories in the two original validation data sets.[29] To preserve this validity, the RACHS-1 method must be applied in a fashion similar to the way in which it was originally developed and tested. For example, some cardiac surgical procedures were not categorized when RACHS-1 was created. Although it is tempting for

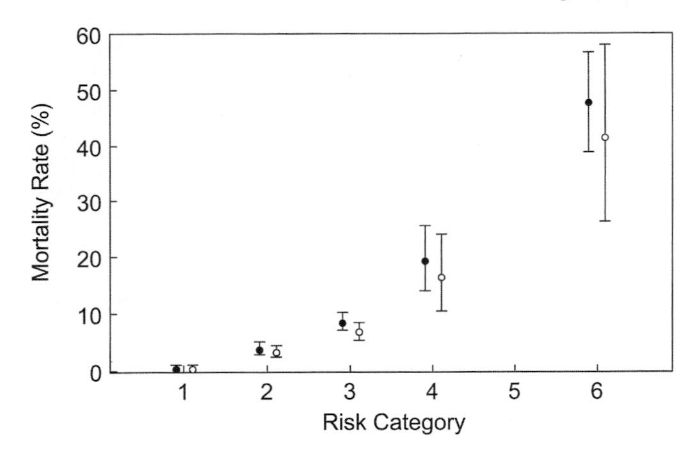

FIGURE 20–5 *Estimated mortality rates (points) and 95% confidence intervals (bars) by RACHS-1 risk category for pediatric patients undergoing single cardiac surgical procedures in two validation data sets (represented by filled and open circles).*

an individual researcher to "add them in" to a seemingly appropriate category, this should not be done without additional validation; the ability of the RACHS-1 method to discriminate between patients who live and those who die, its intended purpose, must be shown to have been preserved. Similarly, RACHS-1 can only be assumed to be valid for the outcome variable for which is was originally designed, postoperative in-hospital mortality. It cannot be presumed to be a valid method of adjusting for case mix for other outcomes, such as morbidity or length of stay in the hospital, without formal testing. Because research tools such as RACHS-1 simultaneously address issues related to both small sample size and anatomic diversity, they are a welcome addition to pediatric cardiology research; the development and validation of additional similar research tools should be encouraged.

REFERENCES

1. Hulley SB, Cummings SR, Browner WS, et al. Designing Clinical Research, 2nd ed Philadelphia: Lippincott Williams & Wilkins, 2001.
2. Hennekens CH, Buring JE. Epidemiology in Medicine. Boston: Little, Brown, 1987.
3. O'Brien PC. Data and safety monitoring. In Armitage P, Colton T (eds). Encyclopedia of Biostatistics, vol 2. New York: John Wiley & Sons, 1998:1058–1066.
4. Pagano M, Gauvreau K. Principles of Biostatistics, 2nd ed. Pacific Grove, CA: Duxbury, 2000.
5. Mehta CR, Patel NR. Exact inference for categorical data. In Armitage P, Colton T (eds). Encyclopedia of Biostatistics, vol 2. New York: John Wiley & Sons, 1998:1411–1422.
6. Press SJ. Bayesian Statistics: Principles, Models, and Applications. New York: John Wiley & Sons, 1989.
7. Tanner JM. Fallacy of per-weight and per-surface area standards, and their relation to spurious correlation. J Appl Physiol 2:1, 1949.
8. Graham TP Jr, Jarmakani JM, Canent RV Jr, et al. Left heart volume estimation in infancy and childhood: Reevaluation of methodology and normal values. Circulation 43:895, 1971.
9. Gutgesell HP, Rembold CM. Growth of the human heart relative to body surface area. Am J Cardiol 65:662, 1990.
10. Henry WL, Ware J, Gardin JM, et al. Echocardiographic measurements in normal subjects: Growth-related changes that occur between infancy and early adulthood. Circulation 57:278, 1978.
11. Abbott RD, Gutgesell HP. Effects of heteroscedasticity and skewness on prediction in regression: modeling growth of the human heart. Methods Enzymol 240:37, 1994.
12. El Habbal M, Somerville J. Size of the normal aortic root in normal subjects and in those with left ventricular outflow obstruction. Am J Cardiol 63:322, 1989.
13. King DH, Smith EO, Huhta JC, et al. Mitral and tricuspid valve annular diameter in normal children determined by two-dimensional echocardiography. Am J Cardiol 55:787, 1985.
14. Gutgesell HP, French M. Echocardiographic determination of aortic and pulmonary valve areas in subjects with normal hearts. Am J Cardiol 68:773, 1991.
15. Lester LA, Sodt PC, Hutcheon N, et al. M-mode echocardiography in normal children and adolescents: Some new perspectives. Pediatr Cardiol 8:27, 1987.
16. Colan SD, Parness IA, Spevak PJ, et al. Developmental modulation of myocardial mechanics: age- and growth-related alterations in afterload and contractility. J Am Coll Cardiol 19:619, 1992.
17. Bates DM, Watts DG. Nonlinear Regression Analysis and Its Applications. New York: John Wiley & Sons, 1988.
18. Kirklin JW, Blackstone EH, Jonas RA, et al. Anatomy, dimensions, and terminology. In: Kirklin JW, Barrat-Boyes BG (eds). Cardiac Surgery. New York: Churchill Livingstone, 1993:21–60.
19. Zar JH. Biostatistical Analysis, 2nd ed. Englewood Cliffs, NJ: Prentice-Hall, 1974.
20. Montgomery DC, Peck EA. Introduction to Linear Regression Analysis, 2nd ed. New York: John Wiley & Sons, 1992.
21. Theil H. Principles of Econometrics. New York: John Wiley & Sons, 1971.
22. DuBois D, DuBois EF. A formula to estimate the approximate surface area if height and weight be known. Arch Intern Med 17:863, 1916.
23. Haycock GB, Schwartz GJ, Wisotsky DH: Geometric method for measuring body surface area: a height-weight formula validated in infants, children, and adults. J Pediatr 93:62, 1978.
24. Dreyer G, Rey W. Further experiments upon the blood volume of mammals and its relation to the surface area of the body: Philosophical transactions of the Royal Society of London 202:191, 1912.

25. Boyd E. The Growth of the Surface Area of the Human Body, reprinted 1975 ed. Westport, CT: Greenwood Press, 1935.
26. Gehan EA, George SL. Estimation of human body surface area from height and weight. Cancer Chemother Rep 54:(4)25, 1970.
27. Mosteller RD. Simplified calculation of body-surface area [letter]. N Engl J Med 317:(17)098, 1987.
28. Jenkins PC, Flanagan MF, Sargent JD, et al. A comparison of treatment strategies for hypoplastic left heart syndrome using decision analysis. J Am Coll Cardiol 38:(4)181, 2001.
29. Jenkins KJ, Gauvreau K, Newburger JW, et al. Consensus-based method for risk adjustment for surgery for congenital heart disease. J Thorac Cardiovasc Surg 123:110, 2002.

21

Contemporary Pediatric Cardiovascular Nursing

PATRICIA O'BRIEN, MARTHA A. Q. CURLEY, AND PATRICIA A. HICKEY

Remarkable progress has been made in the field of pediatric cardiovascular nursing over the past 20 years. Today, nurses titrate multiple intravenous pharmacologic agents, perform complex procedures, educate patients and families, and conduct clinical research to better understand their unique contributions to patient outcomes. The commitment to knowledge dissemination through publications and presentations has never been greater. In the words of Florence Nightingale, "Unless we are making progress in our nursing every year, every month, every week, take my word for it, we are going back."[1] As we enter the 21st century, pediatric cardiovascular nursing is moving steadily forward.

A strong collaborative relationship between physicians and nurses is a key factor in successful patient outcomes. The American Association of Critical Care Nurses' demonstration project[2] linked nurse–physician collaboration, a positive organizational climate, and nurse job satisfaction to lower mortality rates, lower complication rates, and higher levels of patient satisfaction. The Institute of Medicine[3] emphasized that effective collaboration among team members was critical to patient safety. Successful programs understand the unique contribution of each discipline and how the collective intelligence and talent of the entire team is greater than any single individual or discipline. Nurse and physician leaders actively assume the responsibility for creating and supporting a professional practice milieu that fosters interdisciplinary collaboration.

All disciplines require a scientific foundation for their practice. This chapter highlights the major phenomena of concern to pediatric cardiovascular nurses and aspects of professional nursing practice that are considered essential in caring for vulnerable patients and their families. Essential elements include leadership and organization, the nurse–patient relationship, and knowledge and skills fundamental to cardiovascular nursing practice.

LEADERSHIP AND ORGANIZATIONAL STRUCTURE

It is incumbent on the leaders to design systems that integrate multiple patient care services to optimize the patient's and family's experience. To be successful, clinical leaders influence and execute system-wide decisions at the pivotal juncture of cost and quality. The breadth and depth of their responsibility is reflected in making difficult decisions regarding the allocation of scarce resources, managing simultaneous systems of care delivery, and responding to the perceptions of patients and families at the point of service.

At Children's Hospital Boston, the departments of Cardiovascular Surgery, Cardiology, Cardiac Anesthesia, and Cardiovascular Nursing are merged under a common administrative structure called the Cardiovascular Program. For the past decade, this structure has served to provide seamless care to children with cardiovascular disease across the inpatient, diagnostic, interventional, and ambulatory continuum.

The Cardiovascular Operating Committee meets at least monthly and is responsible for program strategy and clinical and fiscal operations. The membership includes the Cardiovascular-Surgeon-in-Chief, Cardiologist-in-Chief, Associate Cardiologist-in-Chief, Vice President for Cardiovascular and Critical Care Services, three senior cardiovascular physicians, and the administrators for the Departments of Cardiology and Cardiovascular Surgery.

The Vice President for Cardiovascular Services oversees nursing and patient services within the five patient care areas: (1) the cardiovascular intensive care unit, (2) cardiology ward, (3) cardiac catheterization laboratories with recovery rooms, (4) cardiac operating rooms, and (5) cardiovascular ambulatory clinics and graphics laboratory, including echocardiography, electrophysiology, and cardiac magnetic resonance imaging (MRI). Nurse Managers are responsible for the daily operations of each patient care area with the respective medical directors.

The Cardiovascular Program is staffed with more than 150 specialized cardiovascular nurses. Most are prepared with a bachelor's degree and receive an extensive orientation program to prepare them to work in the specialty (Table 21-1). Clinical assistants have been successfully added in all patient care areas to perform nonprofessional tasks such as setting up equipment and transporting patients. The cardiac operating room is staffed with a specialized team of cardiac surgical nurses and perfusionists. Other members of the interdisciplinary team include social workers, respiratory therapists, child life specialists, clinical pharmacists, clinical nutritionists, patient care coordinators, patient resource specialists, interpreters, and pastoral care staff.

The contiguous location of the cardiac intensive care unit and the cardiology ward enhances patient safety by having critical care personnel readily available to all patients during emergencies. It also fosters teamwork among the staff in both areas that is important to the successful transition of patients between units. To provide staffing flexibility, a cadre of nurses is cross-trained to other patient care areas within the program.

Nurses care for the spectrum of patients with congenital heart disease, from newly diagnosed premature infants to older adults. The nursing hour standard in the cardiac intensive care unit allows for a nurse-to-patient ratio of 1:1 to 1:2. Nurses on the cardiology floor care for two to four patients at a time. Nurse staffing is determined by the individual needs of the patients. Process efficiencies and economies of scale are achieved because of the large volume of patients in this program. Nurses are promoted within the department as they demonstrate advancement in their clinical skills and expertise. Level I staff nurses are entry-level competent nurses. Level II staff nurses are members of the leadership group with responsibility to support unit operations such as orientation of new staff and special projects. Level III, attained by a small number of staff nurses, requires clinical expertise.

TABLE 21–1. Children's Hospital Boston Cardiovascular Intensive Care Unit Orientation Program

Week	Class Schedule	Clinical Orientation
1	Hospital/nursing orientation (5 days)	**Weeks 1–3** Main focus:
2	**Class Day 1** Introduction to CVP/CICU CVP tour Documentation Preorientation knowledge evaluation	Complete/thorough physical assessment, assessing changes Documentation of assessments Review complete
3	**Class Day 2** Computerized documentation Clinical documentation **Class Day 3** Fetal circulation Cardiac anatomy & assessment Nutrition management Respiratory therapy Arterial blood gas analysis	patient assessment with CNS **Weeks 3–4** Focus on pieces of care: Bedside setup Safety check Drips Computer Documentation Calculations Dressings
4	**Class Day 4** Lesions decreasing PBF Pain management Lesions increasing PBF	**Weeks 4–5** Clinical skills day
5	**Class Day 5** Lesions obstructing SBF Embryology Electrolytes	Focus on applying classroom learning to clinical practice Clinical orientation
6	**Class Day 6** Cardiopulmonary bypass Postoperative management External pacing Hemodynamic monitoring	**Weeks 6-8** More integration of knowledge and bedside practice Beginning independence
7	**Class Day 7** Arrhythmias Cardiac registry Cardiac pharmacology Clinical inquiry/QI	**Weeks 8–11** Mastery of two-patient assignment Taking cases Observation in OR,
8	**Class Day 8** Care of the adult Care of the premature infant Mechanical ventilation Care of CICU patient in cath lab	cath lab, clinic Surgical conference, QI meetings, etc. Increasing independence Separate lunches
9	**Class Day 9** Immunology/acquired heart disease Cardiac transplantation Research in the CVP Emergency situations Professional responsibilities	
10	**Class Day 10** Management of the surgical patient Management of the neurosurgical patient Bereavement Advance directives Chain of command Patient/family teaching	

The number of advanced practice nurses, those with a Master's degree in Nursing, has dramatically increased in the past 20 years. This group of nurses brings advanced clinical skills, knowledge of the research process, and an understanding of organizational systems to the clinical arena and has moved the profession forward with evidenced-based clinical projects. In response to increasing patient volume and complexity (Fig. 21-1), nurse practitioners provide direct patient care in both inpatient and outpatient settings. Clinical nurse specialists focus on the support and development of the nursing staff. A growing group of doctorally prepared nurses are now practicing within the clinical arena and conducting programs of nursing research to help build the science of nursing practice. The role of nurse researcher was recently added to the cardiovascular program to foster nursing research initiatives within the program.

In response to the dramatic increase in cardiac catheterization volume and complexity, nurse and technician staffing has increased to provide for one nurse and two technicians in each of three laboratories plus one nurse for every two patients in the recovery room. The recovery area cares for patients after catheterization procedures and, increasingly, after MRI. The expansion of the recovery area was also driven by the need to perform specialized outpatient procedures with sedation such as transesophageal echocardiograms and cardioversions.

As the clinic population grew and specialized clinics were added, the care delivery system in the clinics (hospital based and satellite) was reorganized into physician and nurse teams. This model has resulted in improved patient flow through the clinics, better utilization of resources, improved continuity and follow-up care, and greater patient satisfaction.

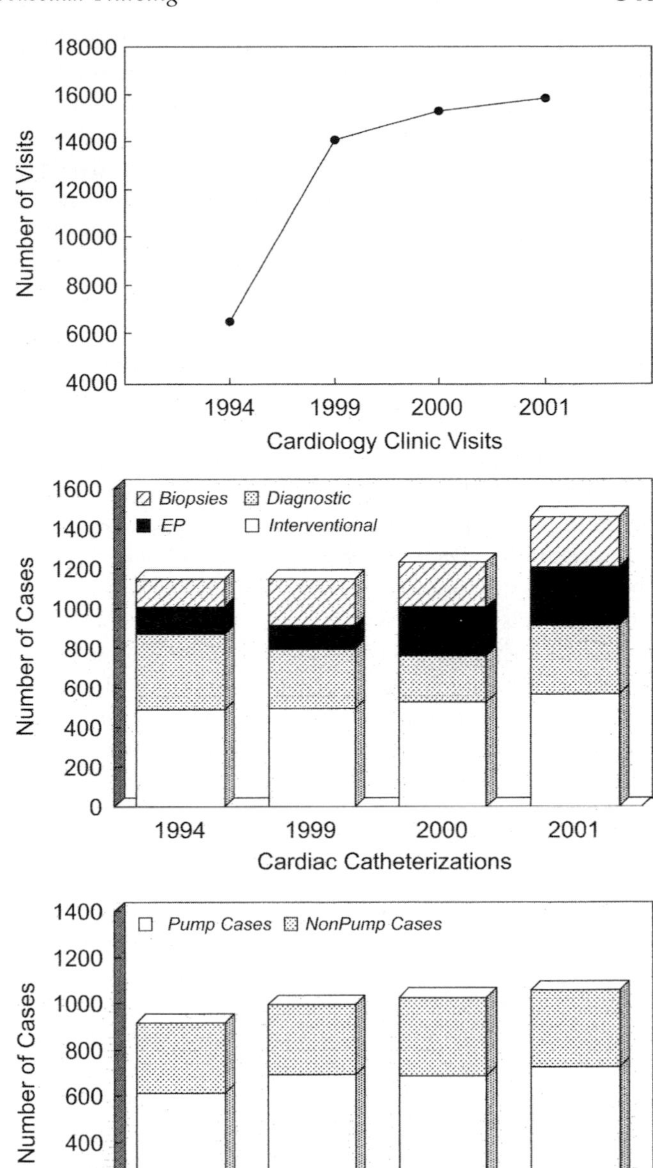

FIGURE 21–1 *Children's Hospital Boston experience, 1994–2002. Clinic visits and catheterization numbers continue to increase significantly. Cardiac surgical numbers also are increasing, albeit at a slower rate, largely because many former surgically managed lesions such as pulmonary and aortic stenosis, atrial septal defects, and patent ductus arteriosus are now repaired by catheterization.*

NURSE–PATIENT RELATIONSHIP

Because of the pivotal role of the family in the life of a developing child, parents are their child's greatest resource and source of support and comfort. It is clear that optimal care of children requires supporting the family. Pediatric nurses have a unique role in collaborating with parents and supporting them in the care of their child.

Family-Centered Care

Parents are not visitors at the bedside but equal partners in providing care to their children. Because most patients with serious congenital heart disease are now diagnosed prenatally or in the newborn period and undergo their first interventions soon after diagnosis, most families new to the cardiovascular care system are the families of newborns and infants. Understandably, these families are highly stressed. One of their worst fears, that is, a serious, possibly life-threatening illness, has happened to their infant. Many nursing research studies have identified the needs of parents during a critical illness. These include the need for information, assurance that their child is receiving the best care, the need for hope, proximity to their child, helping with physical care, being recognized as important to their child's recovery, talking with other parents, prayer, and concrete resources (e.g., transportation and food).[4–6]

Nurses are in an ideal position to meet parents' needs by providing frequent information and flexible visiting, and by working with parents in the care of their child. Parents have described nurses' most significant role in the care of their child as "interpreter" of their critically ill child's responses and the intensive care unit environment. Outlining the trajectory of illness so that parents can anticipate events and teaching parents the skills they need to care for their child at home are important nursing interventions.

To provide holistic care to patients and families, nurses collaborate with their colleagues in the psychosocial disciplines to offer support services to families, such as prenatal support and bereavement programs, educational resources about heart disease, and parent cardiopulmonary resuscitation classes. Internet services help to reduce feelings of isolation during hospitalization and enable families to maintain contact with their extended family and friends at home. Ongoing parent feedback is obtained through a follow-up phone call program. Hearing from families about their hospital experience after discharge provides clinicians and program leaders with suggestions for system changes and improves departmental services for patients and families.

Developmentally Appropriate Care

Nurses, along with child life therapists, are instrumental in normalizing the hospital environment, making it "child friendly," and encouraging children and their families to carry on their normal routines as much as possible. Nurses are sensitive to the unique stressors at each developmental stage, such as separation from parents, stranger anxiety, fear of pain, fear of the unknown, loss of control, and limited attention spans. Because many pediatric cardiovascular patients undergo multiple invasive procedures such as catheterizations and operations during childhood, efforts to minimize stress and enhance coping are especially important. The American Heart Association[7] recently published "Recommendations for Preparing Children and Adolescents for Invasive Cardiac Procedures,"[7] written by an expert panel of cardiovascular nurses, that describes evidence-based interventions to reduce procedural stress in children.

After heart surgery, children are at increased risk for developmental delays, especially in the areas of motor development, speech and language, and cognitive development. Nurses are involved in developmental screening, family counseling, and referral to appropriate resources for early intervention or educational services.

FUNDAMENTALS OF CARDIOVASCULAR NURSING PRACTICE

The nursing management plan for a child after cardiac surgery emphasizes both physiologic alterations and psychosocial issues of concern to nursing (Table 21-2).

Providing Comfort

Relief of pain and suffering is central to the caring practices of nurses. In the past 20 years, a significant body of research on neonatal and pediatric pain has been generated. We now know that even the smallest neonates experience pain and that routine pain assessment and management strategies can provide effective pain relief. In the pediatric cardiovascular population, hospitalized patients must cope with uncomfortable monitoring devices and invasive procedures; thus, effective pain management is a nursing priority. Physiologic consequences of pain, such as decreased respiratory function and atelectasis, increased heart rate, tissue ischemia, and impaired mobility, can slow postoperative recovery. Effective pain management results in earlier mobilization, shorter hospital stays, and decreased costs.[8] Indeed, the Joint Commission on Accreditation of Hospitals[9] considers pain management so important that it designated pain assessment as the fifth vital sign. An institution-wide, interdisciplinary pain initiative established evidence-based standards for the assessment and management of pediatric pain. Standards help decrease random variation and assure a minimal level of care for all patients.

A number of options are available to manage pediatric pain. The administration of narcotics, both intravenous and oral, for severe pain and acetaminophen for minor pain has been employed for many years. In the past decade, patient-controlled analgesia (PCA) and epidural analgesia have become more common in pediatrics. Nonsteroidal anti-inflammatory medications, both intravenous and oral, are especially effective in the management of postoperative pain. Topical anesthetics such as EMLA are used to decrease the experience of pain during procedures such as venipuncture. Widely practiced is "pain prevention," in which around-the-clock scheduled (rather than "as needed") pain medication is administered during known periods of pain and discomfort, such as in the early postoperative period after heart surgery. Increasing attention has appropriately been given to nonpharmacologic methods of providing patient comfort. Parent presence, the use of pacifiers or favorite objects, containment in a quiet environment, and the therapeutic use of music or videos are all easily done in the hospital environment. Many distraction techniques, such as visual distraction, breathing techniques, diversional talk, or guided imagery, are very useful during stressful events and episodic painful procedures, such as

TABLE 21–2. Children's Hospital Boston Sample Postoperative Management Plans for Two Nursing Problems

#/Date	Problem/Need	Outcome Criteria	Process Criteria		D/C Date
			Practice Guidelines	**Individualized Care**	
	Alteration in Cardiac Output				
	Etiology: Decreased pre-load Increased after-load Arrhythmias Ventricular dysfunction	Patient will maintain adequate cardiac output. Patient will remain in normal sinus rhythm.	**Repair:** ________ ________ Assess CO Assess for arrhythmias Inotropic support BP range: Labs: ABG, electrolytes, CBC **Upon transfer from ICU:**	Cardiologist: ________ Surgeon: ________ TPT: ____ CAT: ____ XCT: Date and Time to P6: __/__/__;__:__ Dopamine	
	Defining Characteristics: Signs of poor perfusion Signs of CHF Low urine output Cyanosis		Monitor VS q4h and PRN Monitor cardiac rhythm Assess peripheral perfusion and pulses Assess accurate fluid balance Encourage ambulation Daily weight	Milrinone ECG Postop Pacing wires: ________ Temporary pacing:	
	Alteration in Parenting/Family Dynamics				
	Etiology: Stress and anxiety Learning needs Altered coping responses Availability of support systems Powerlessness Disruption of parental role Delayed parent–infant bonding	A trusting, collaborative relationship will develop between patient's caregiver/significant other and health care team. Effective coping responses and support systems will be developed and maintained. Parent/family participation in care and involvement in decision making will be encouraged and supported.	Assess knowledge and learning needs of patient's caregiver/significant other and develop a plan for meeting those needs. Assess current support systems and coping mechanisms of family. Identify and assess spiritual and cultural needs and practices that may be affected by hospitalization. Utilize chaplain services for further support as needed. Encourage verbalization of concerns, hopes, fears; support emotional well-being. Assess psychosocial and economic situation for eligibility for meal tickets (breast-feeding moms are eligible for two meals per day), transportation assistance, and housing assistance. Utilize social work services for assistance as needed.	Encourage family visitation and participation in care. If appropriate, develop a schedule for care. Provide consistency in nursing care through development of a primary team. Support patient caregiver/significant others in self-care (i.e., encouraging breaks, healthy meals, sleep and rest time). Encourage caring interactions between caregiver/significant other and patient, including physical touch (e.g., stroking, kissing, holding), positive communication, and bringing familiar items from home (e.g., pictures, phone messages, special comfort items).	

during dressing changes. More alternative modalities, such as acupuncture, massage therapy, and Reiki, are also gaining momentum.

Managing procedural sedation is often the responsibility of pediatric cardiovascular nurses. Successful cardiac imaging, such as echocardiograms, MRI, and cardiac catheterization and interventional procedures all require an immobile, comfortable, yet cooperative patient. For infants and small children, this state generally requires sedation. Nurse staffing in the outpatient areas and catheterization laboratory has increased substantially in the past decade to meet the increased need for nursing vigilance of sedated patients. Nurse-managed procedural sedation, usually with narcotics and benzodiazepines, is used for many diagnostic and interventional catheterization procedures and for other painful procedures. Oral chloral hydrate is routinely used for echocardiograms in young children. Lipschitz and others[10] completed an early study demonstrating the safe and effective use of this drug in the pediatric cardiovascular population. An interdisciplinary sedation task force oversees sedation practices within the institution.

Optimizing Nutrition

Poor nutrition is a well-known problem in patients with congenital heart disease. These patients have the dual problem of increased metabolic rates, resulting in increased caloric demands and a hampered ability to ingest adequate nutrients because of fatigue, poor oral-motor skills, and other problems. Feeding issues slow recovery and increase hospital stays.

The expertise of an interdisciplinary team, with nurses playing a prominent role, is often needed to address nutrition problems. Breast-feeding is encouraged, and several studies have demonstrated breast-feeding success in infants with congenital heart defects.[11,12] Nurses manage a variety of nutrition modalities, including enteral and intravenous nutrition. Some infants are unable to meet their nutritional goals safely with oral feeds and require supplemental nutrition with gastric or jejunal tubes. In two nursing studies of infants after cardiac surgery, 10% to 28% of infants were not orally feeding at the time of hospital discharge.[13,14] Nurses have primary responsibility for teaching parents to manage feeding tubes at home.

Managing Complex Therapies

Nurses practice at the patient–technology interface. They master a growing array of monitors, pumps, and machines deployed to benefit the most critically ill and guard against harm from the same technology. With their continuous presence at the bedside, nurses integrate a tremendous volume of data, vigilantly watch for signs of trouble, and assess nuances in the patient's condition. Anticipating problems and intervening to prevent them is a core competency for proficient cardiovascular nurses. Nurses also have a special responsibility to humanize the environment and reassure and comfort parents as they watch their child with fear and anxiety, beneath all the lines, tubes, and technology. In the past decade, nurses have added care of patients requiring extracorporeal membrane oxygenation, continuous venovenous hemofiltration, inhaled nitric oxide, and high-frequency oscillatory ventilation to their repertoire.

Care Coordination

In the complicated world of the hospital, nurses who have a consistent presence with the patient and family assume the responsibility for coordinating the care of the entire interdisciplinary team. As the father of a patient put it, "Nursing is where the rubber meets the road. It's also where improvisation and humanizing of an ill-conceived healthcare system takes place."[15] Nurses collaborate closely with the health care team and family in assessing patient needs and routinely marshal an array of resources to address patient problems. For a child with multisystem problems, the number of specialists and services involved can be overwhelming for the patient and family and challenge the organizational skills of the nurse. As care becomes more complex, the nurses' ability to "keep everyone on the same page" becomes vital.

Complex patients and innovative technologies no longer reside solely in the intensive care unit—they have moved into the home. Nurses teach patients and their families to self-manage complex therapies, and their success is critical in today's health care environment, in which length of stay is often unrelated to reimbursement. With shortened hospital stays, cost-containment pressures, and the use of complex therapies at home, the role of the patient care coordinator has evolved to facilitate continuity in care. The patient care coordinator collaborates with the primary care team and the family to assess home care needs, identifies community resources and initiates referrals, and coordinates activities with payers.

Clinical Practice Guidelines

The development and implementation of clinical practice guidelines (CPGs) has been a successful strategy to provide cost-effective care without compromising quality. A diagnosis-based daily management plan, the CPG involves all disciplines and all aspects of care and is used as a guide for patient care while maintaining continuity and cost effectiveness. Program goals increase the clinical autonomy of each discipline, decrease practice variations, contribute to efficient allocation of resources, decrease costs, and promote interdisciplinary care.[16] The program has produced a wealth of outcome data and information on patient variances and trends in care, which lead to practice improvements. Examples of practice changes since the implementation of the CPG process include the same-day admission program, more effective utilization of ancillary services, and an early endotracheal extubation initiative.

CONCLUSION

In 2001, the Institute of Medicine's Committee on the Quality of Health Care in America issued a landmark report, "Crossing the Quality Chasm: A New Health System for the 21st Century."[3] Many have called this report a mandate for creating new environments of care and a fundamental redesign of the United Sates health care system. Emphatically woven throughout this report is the importance of interdisciplinary teams and effective collaboration among team members. This chapter has presented interdisciplinary collaboration as a central theme in our pediatric cardiovascular program. Nurses uniquely contribute to this goal by providing patients and families with care that creates both a safe environment and safe passage through complex systems.[17]

REFERENCES

1. Nightingale F. Notes on Nursing: What It Is, and What It Is Not. New York: D. Appleton, 1860.
2. Mitchell PH, Armstrong S, Simpson TF, et al. American Association of Critical Care Nurses Demonstration Project: Profile of excellence in critical care nursing. Heart Lung 18:219, 1989.
3. IOM (Institute of Medicine). Crossing the Quality Chasm: A New Health System for the 21st Century. Washington, DC: National Academy Press, 2001.
4. Lewandowski LA. Stressors and coping styles of parents of children undergoing open heart surgery. Crit Care Q 3:75, 1980.
5. Miles MS, Carter ML. Sources of parental stress in the pediatric intensive care unit. Child Health Care 11:65, 1982.
6. Farrel MJ, Frost C. The most important needs of parents of critically ill children: Parents' perceptions. Intens Crit Care Nurs 8:1, 1993.
7. LeRoy S, Elixson EM, O'Brien P, et al. Recommendations for preparing children and adolescents for invasive cardiac procedures. Circulation 108:2550, 2003.
8. U.S. Department of Health and Human Services, Public Health Service, Agency for Health Care Policy and Research. Acute Pain Management: Operative or Medical Procedures and Trauma. Clinical Practice Guidelines. DHHS Pub. No. (AHCPR) 92-1132, Silver Springs, MD: AHCPR Clearinghouse, 1992.
9. Joint Commission on Accreditation of Health Care Organizations. CAMH Update 3. Standard for Pain: PE1.4, August 1999.
10. Lipschitz M, Marino BL, Sanders SP. Chloral hydrate side effects in young children: Causes and management. Heart Lung 22:408, 1993.
11. Coombs VL, Marino BL. A comparison of growth patterns in bottle and breast fed infants with congenital heart disease. Pediatr Nurs 19:175, 1993.
12. Barbas KH, Kelleher DK. Breastfeeding success among infants with congenital heart disease. Pediatr Nurs (in press).
13. O'Brien P, Pelletier M, Reidy S, et al. Determinants of oral feeding in infants following cardiac surgery. Proceedings of the 2nd World Congress of Pediatric Cardiology and Cardiac Surgery, 1997:300.
14. Einarson KD, Arthur HM. Predictors of oral feeding difficulty in cardiac surgical infants. Pediatr Nurs 29:315, 2003.
15. Beckham JD. Andrew's not-so-excellent adventure. Health Care Forum J 36:90, 1993.
16. Poppleton VK, Moynihan PJ, Hickey PA. Clinical practice guidelines: The Boston experience. Prog Pediatr Cardiol 18: 75, 2003.
17. Curley MAQ. Patient-nurse synergy, optimizing patient outcomes. Am J Crit Care 7:64, 1998.

VIII

Acquired Heart Disease

22

Innocent Murmurs, Syncope, and Chest Pain

JANE W. NEWBURGER,
MARK E. ALEXANDER, AND
DAVID R. FULTON

INNOCENT HEART MURMURS

Innocent heart murmurs occur in about half of all children.[1,2] They occur in the absence of either anatomic or physiologic abnormalities of the heart and are not associated with subsequent cardiovascular disease.[3–5] The differentiation of innocent from organic murmurs for purposes of therapy, prognosis, and insurability is a leading cause for referral to a pediatric cardiologist (Exhibit 22-1). Discrimination of innocent from organic murmurs requires knowledge of the auscultatory findings in structural cardiac abnormalities, as well as of the characteristic findings of innocent murmurs. Innocent murmurs generally can be recognized using history, skilled physical examination including auscultation, and electrocardiography.[6–13]

Prevalence

The reported prevalence of murmurs in the neonatal period varies widely, from 0.6% to 77.4%, with differing estimates probably attributable to differences in the frequency and timing of examinations, examining conditions, auscultatory skill, and the threshold for the inclusion of very soft murmurs.[14–18] The estimated likelihood of congenital heart disease among neonates with heart murmurs varies from about 1:2 to 1:12, with higher estimates occurring, not surprisingly, in studies in which residents or senior house officers detect murmurs under uncontrolled conditions. Echocardiography performed in newborn infants thought to have innocent heart murmurs reveals benign (physiologic) pulmonary branch stenosis in half, patent ductus arteriosus in 60%, and patent foramen ovale in all.[19] A heart murmur heard first at 6 months has been estimated to carry a 1:7 risk for structural heart disease, and one heard first at 12 months, only a 1:50 risk.[15]

After infancy, the reported prevalence of innocent heart murmurs ranges between 17% and 66%, with most authors reporting between 40% and 60%.[1,2,20–23] With exercise or with the use of phonocardiography, about 90% of children have murmurs.[22,24,25] Even in reviews from cardiology referral centers, most children with newly referred murmurs have no significant heart disease.[13,22,26]

Clinical Manifestations

General Characteristics

Innocent heart murmurs are always associated with normal heart sounds. The murmurs occur in systole, with the exception of the venous hum, which is continuous. Whereas organic murmurs may be of any length, innocent murmurs are usually brief, peaking in the first half of systole. Organic murmurs often have widespread transmission, with a pattern determined by the lesion, whereas innocent murmurs are often well localized, usually along the left sternal border. It is unusual for the grade of an innocent murmur to be greater than 3 (on a scale of 1 to 6).

EXHIBIT 22–1. Children's Hospital Boston Experience 1988-2002

Age First Seen (years)*	Congenital Heart Disease (n = 52,721)	No Significant Heart Disease (n = 6,902)	Mitral Valve Prolapse (n = 1,567)	Bicuspid Aortic Valve (n = 1,123)
	(%)	(%)	(%)	(%)
0–1	34	21	8	22
1–5	18	25	12	22
5–10	15	22	21	20
10–15	14	19	28	18
15–20	9	11	21	12
20+	10	2	10	6
% Male	50	56	42	71
% Female	50	44	58	39

*Age when patients were first seen by a cardiologist.

The murmur's intensity often changes with position and, occasionally, from examination to examination. With the exception of venous hums, there are no innocent thrills. Cyanosis should never accompany an innocent murmur. The quality of the innocent murmur is often vibratory and musical, or sometimes blowing, in contrast to the harsh quality of many organic murmurs. Independent predictors of structural heart disease during the first evaluation of children with heart murmurs at a tertiary pediatric cardiology center included specific features of the murmur (pansystolic timing, harsh quality, murmur intensity at least grade 3, and location at the left upper sternal border), as well as the presence of a click or abnormal second heart sound.[13] In the future, screening of heart murmurs in children may be accomplished using artificial neural networks or automated spectral analysis.[27,28]

The most common innocent heart murmurs are described below.

Still's Murmur

Still's murmur[3,29] is most commonly heard in patients between the ages of 2 and 7 years. Characteristically, it is a grade 1 to 3, vibratory, buzzing, or twanging systolic ejection murmur, the quality of which is similar to that of a tuning fork. It is usually maximal between the third intercostal space, left lower sternal border, and apex; is much louder in the supine position than in the sitting position; and is characteristically louder with exercise, excitement, or fever. The intensity of ejection murmurs has been demonstrated by invasive phonocardiography to be greater above the aortic valve than above the pulmonary valve.[30] The association of Still's murmur with false chordae tendineae in the left ventricle is controversial, with some authors finding a strong relationship[31,32] and others finding a high prevalence of both Still's murmurs and false tendons in healthy hearts, but no association.[33] The cardiac index of children with Still's murmur is similar to that of children without murmurs.[34] However, individuals with Still's murmurs have been reported to have a significantly smaller mean ascending aortic diameter relative to body surface area, with higher average peak velocities in the ascending and descending aorta than are found in children and young adults without murmurs. These observations suggest that the origin of Still's murmur is in many cases related to a small aortic root and ascending aortic diameter with concomitant high-velocity flow across the left ventricular outflow tract and ascending aorta.[35–38]

Physiologic Ejection Murmur

The physiologic ejection murmur, also called the *innocent pulmonic systolic murmur*, is identical in quality to the murmur of an atrial septal defect, comprising a murmur caused by flow through the normal pulmonic valve but associated with a normal second sound. Using phonocardiography, this murmur may be detected in most normal subjects.[39] It is a grade 1 to 3, blowing, rather high-pitched, diamond-shaped murmur that always peaks in the first half of systole and is maximal in intensity in the second left intercostal space, without wide transmission. Like the Still's murmur, it is louder when the patient is in the supine position and is accentuated by exercise, fever, or excitement. The physiologic ejection murmur may be heard in children of any age and frequently occurs in children with asthenic builds who have narrow anteroposterior diameters or who have pectus excavatum. Studies with intracardiac phonocatheters have demonstrated that the physiologic ejection murmur is located in the main pulmonary artery and is associated with the ejection of blood into the pulmonary artery.[40,41] The physiologic ejection murmur was the type of murmur most likely to be misdiagnosed by pediatric residents.[42]

Cervical Venous Hum

The cervical venous hum[4] is a continuous murmur with diastolic accentuation that may be elicited almost universally in normal children. It is located in the low anterior part of the neck, more often on the right than the left.

The murmur is loudest with the patient in the sitting position and disappears or diminishes in the supine position. Usually the venous hum is accentuated by turning the patient's head away from the side of the murmur and elevating the chin. The murmur may be obliterated by pressing lightly over the jugular vein with the stethoscope or a finger. The mechanism of the venous hum has not been definitively delineated, although it has been postulated to be secondary to turbulence of venous flow in the internal jugular veins and, occasionally, in the external jugular veins.[26,40,43–48]

Physiologic Pulmonary Artery Branch Stenosis of the Newborn

Physiologic pulmonary artery branch stenosis or peripheral pulmonary artery stenosis is heard in the newborn period as a low-frequency systolic ejection murmur maximal in the lateral chest, axillae, and occasionally the back, but is heard less well over the precordium itself. This murmur generally wanes by age 3 months and is believed to be caused by turbulence from the relative discordance in size between the larger main pulmonary artery and smaller branch pulmonary arteries.

Supraclavicular Arterial Bruit

The supraclavicular arterial bruit is a crescendo–decrescendo systolic murmur heard best just above the clavicles, usually on the right side more than on the left. It radiates better to the neck than below the clavicles and, very occasionally, can generate a faint carotid thrill. The bruit may be accentuated by exercise but is not affected by posture and respiration. It can be distinguished from the murmur of aortic stenosis by the disappearance of the supraclavicular murmur with the maneuver of hyperextension of the shoulders[5] or compression of the subclavian artery against the first rib. Supraclavicular systolic murmurs have been postulated to arise from the major brachiocephalic arteries near their aortic origins.[40,49–51]

Laboratory Findings

Diagnostic testing should be tailored to the clinical situation. Most children older than 1 year of age can be evaluated with history, physical examination, and an electrocardiogram (ECG) alone. The qualifications of the examiner have been shown to have a major bearing on the ability to distinguish innocent from organic murmurs in children.[42,52,53] In patients newly referred for evaluation of a heart murmur, the results of echocardiography are unlikely to change the clinical diagnosis of no significant heart disease when a pediatric cardiologist is certain of this diagnosis before echocardiography.[7,12,13] Perhaps for this reason, it is more cost-effective for pediatricians to refer patients with newly diagnosed heart murmurs to pediatric cardiologists than to order two-dimensional echocardiograms.[54] Heart disease is seldom diagnosed when a pediatric cardiologist orders an echocardiogram because of a family's or referring physician's anxiety if patients are older than age 6 weeks with innocent-sounding murmurs and have no worrisome signs or symptoms.[12] Conversely, the threshold for performing a two-dimensional echocardiogram should be low in patients with innocent-sounding heart murmurs on skilled auscultation when structural heart disease is suspected by a pediatric cardiologist because of young age or worrisome history, signs, symptoms, or abnormalities on electrocardiography or chest radiography.[12] In general, echocardiography for evaluation of heart murmurs after infancy in the outpatient setting should be performed if, after skilled clinical assessment, the pediatric cardiologist believes echocardiography is useful because of uncertainty in the diagnosis or to delineate the nature of suspected heart disease.

Management

For children younger than 2 years old in whom the diagnosis of innocent murmur is first made, the authors recommend reevaluation after 2 or 3 years if the murmur persists. Children older than age 2 years do not require reevaluation unless some uncertainty exists (e.g., because of suboptimal patient cooperation or a possible abnormality on a diagnostic test).

It is of the utmost importance to reassure the family of a child with an innocent murmur. The label of heart disease may have adverse effects on the child and the family.[55,56] Even temporary mislabeling may increase the morbidity from cardiac nondisease.[57]

Prognosis

The reliability of the diagnosis of "innocent" heart murmur on initial evaluation by a pediatric cardiologist is supported by published follow-up and actuarial studies. Follow-up studies of series of patients diagnosed as having innocent murmurs have confirmed the original diagnosis in 97% to 100% of the patients.[58,59] Furthermore, actuarial data on people with systolic murmurs thought to be innocent show no deviation from the expected mortality—a discovery that led to a decision to remove restrictions on insurance and employment for those with innocent murmurs.[60]

SYNCOPE

Definition

Syncope is the transient and abrupt loss of consciousness resulting from a decrease in cerebral blood flow, resulting in collapse and relatively prompt recovery over a period of seconds. Syncope should be distinguished from cardiac arrest in which the collapse requires intervention or results in significant end-organ damage. *Presyncope* or *near syncope* has symptoms including dizziness and visual changes that suggest an impending faint, but that do not progress sufficiently to result in collapse. Although these definitions are clear in the abstract, frequently the history is sufficiently vague that the primary question is how to classify a spell.

Incidence

Syncope is common, with a peak incidence in adolescent girls and a lower but increased incidence in toddlers. Many faints, appropriately, are managed without seeking medical care and if those are included, as many as 25% of adults will have had at least a single episode of fainting during childhood and adolescence, and 10% to 40% of adolescents will either faint or have significant presyncopal symptoms with provocative testing.[61,62] About 1 in 1000 seek care for syncope each year.[63] In toddlers with pallid breath-holding spells, boys and girls are equally affected, with the incidence of at least some symptoms being as high as 5%.[64] By school age and adolescence, there is a marked female predominance, which extends well into adult life. The incidence of syncope remains relatively steady in early adult life, before gradually and steadily increasing in older age.[65] Syncope represents a common cause of referral for patients seen in the cardiology outpatient setting at Children's Hospital Boston, with 3820 clinic visits in 1923 patients over 13 years, or 5% of all new patients.

This high incidence of syncope contrasts with the exceptionally low incidence of sudden death and aborted sudden death (1 per 100,000 patient-years) in the pediatric and young adult population.[66,67] The incidence of sudden cardiac death remains low (about 1 per 100 patient-years), even in most patients with significant heart disease. Nonetheless, *syncope with heart disease or syncope closely associated with exercise represents clear risk factors for sudden death and serious heart disease.*[63,68] Resolving the *overall low incidence of serious outcomes and the high incidence of potentially serious symptoms* represents the primary challenge of evaluating these patients.

Physiology

The core physiology of any true syncopal event is abruptly ineffective cerebral blood flow resulting from ineffective cardiac output or cardiovascular control.

Cardiac syncope occurs secondary to combinations of obstruction to left ventricular filling (pulmonary hypertension, tachycardia), left ventricular ejection (aortic stenosis or hypertrophic cardiomyopathy), or ineffective contraction (profound bradycardia, dilated cardiomyopathy, pathologic tachyarrhythmia) with an underlying substrate of either structural, functional, or electrical heart disease. By definition, these episodes are transient.

Common fainting, or *neurally mediated syncope*, goes by many names, some of them emphasizing the dominant line of disordered cardiac and vascular regulation that results in symptoms. These include *vasovagal syncope, cardioinhibitory syncope, pallid breath-holding spells (or reflex anoxic seizures), vasodepressor syncope, postural orthostatic tachycardia syndrome*, and many others. Although there are clear distinctions between both the clinical manifestations and the patients who demonstrate each subtype of physiology, the summary terminology of neurally mediated or neuro cardiogenic syncope emphasizes the inter-relationships between each kind of syncope.

The most classic form of syncope, often called *vasodepressor* or *vasovagal syncope*, is initiated by blood pooling in the extremities, typically with standing. That results in decreased right ventricular and, several heart beats later, left ventricular filling, which in turn triggers combinations of left ventricular sensory activation to the brain stem, combined with carotid body and carotid sinus activation. Each of these initially results in decreased vagal and parasympathetic activation and increased sympathetic and catecholamine activation to raise heart rate, increase venous and arteriolar tone, and enhance left ventricular contractility. When these are sufficient, there is a modest increase in heart rate and narrowing of pulse pressure with an effective transition to upright posture. When the initial homeostatic responses are either inadequate or exaggerated, the homeostatic control mechanisms increase their efforts to maintain adequate blood flow; however, these same mechanisms can produce paradoxical parasympathetic (vagal) stimulation, resulting in heart rate slowing, with or without sympathetic withdrawal resulting in decreased vascular tone and lower blood pressure. External influences, including anxiety and hyperventilation, can exacerbate these responses. Active use of the skeletal muscle pump (jogging, isometrics) can enhance venous return and raise systemic blood pressure, blunting the initial responses. Medications or concomitant medical disorders can also exacerbate or blunt the cyclic swings in cardiac and vascular control. Implicit in this summary is the view of cardiac physiology as a series of inter-related sensors and amplifiers, so that the specific clinical manifestations are the result of dynamic control, including but not limited to the baroreflex, not of simple action–reaction reflexes.[69]

Clinical Manifestations

Overview

Cardiac syncope is characterized by an abrupt onset of collapse with few premonitory symptoms. The typical history is one of acute collapse, often with activity or exercise, with nearly immediate recovery. Palpitations are sometimes noted, but are not diagnostic in any clear fashion. When there is significant residual of confusion, disorientation, or need for CPR the event is best classified as aborted sudden cardiac death. For transient events, recovery is similarly rapid. While symptoms of palpitations, occurrence with exercise, injury, urinary incontinence and an onset while sitting or supine all increase suspicions of a serious arrhythmia, none are diagnostic (Table 22-1). Indeed the responses to arrhythmias, and other transient impairments in cardiac output, are in part determined by the effectiveness of baroreflex controls. Hence the most critical distinction is whether there is historical or exam evidence of heart disease.

Neurally Mediated Syncope

Typical adolescent syncope has a history that is almost pathognomonic. An adolescent girl, having been standing upright on a hot day, possibly at chorus or band practice, has pre-monitory symptoms of feeling warm, constriction of visual fields with the "world going dark" and nausea with a sense that her heart is pounding hard. She may attempt to move away from where she is standing and walk to the nurse's office but turns pale and falls, with only a brief period of unconsciousness. When she recovers, she continues to feel somewhat dizzy, remains pale for minutes and is typically exhausted, often is diaphoretic and clammy, sometimes with a headache. While she has occasional "head rushes" when she stands, she generally feels terrific, is active in school, and has minimal additional medical concerns. With that history, sufficient evaluation is comprised of a normal detailed physical examination, including orthostatic heart rate and blood pressure, dynamic cardiac auscultation, a normal ECG, a reassuring family history focusing on a sibling and parental history of adolescent syncope[70] (common), and of sudden cardiac death (a worrisome finding). For single episodes, the only important reason for referral is parental or patient anxiety.

Convulsive Syncope

Acute pain, anxiety, or other less clear provocation can trigger acute vagal activation resulting in cardiac slowing and sometimes dramatic cardiac pauses captured on event monitoring or during head-up tilt (see Fig. 22-1). When induced during head-up tilt, there are often presyncopal findings of relative hypotension and cyclic heart rate accelerations. These dramatic events can result in opisthotonos that mimics a seizure, often triggering the rescue squad and emergency room evaluation. While these spells can be highly suggestive of cardiac syncope and deserve thoughtful consultation, many children will have no heart disease and

TABLE 22–1. Relative Frequency of Premonitory Symptoms and Residual Findings in Patients with Common Neurally Mediated Syncope and those with More Serious Cardiac Syncope

	Neurally Mediated	Cardiac Syncope
Symptoms		
Premonitory Symptoms	+++	±
Lightheadedness	+++	+/±
Palpitations	+	++
Occurs while upright	+++	+
Occurs while sitting	+/±	+
Emotional Trigger	++	++
Exercise Trigger	+	++
Residual Findings		
Pallor	+++	+/±
Incontinence	–	+
Disorientation	–	+
Fatigue	++	±
Diaphoresis	++	±
Injury	+	++

+++, Very common (> ~50%); ++ common (> ~ 20%); + not rare (>~ 5%); ± uncommon (< 5%); – rare (< ~1%).

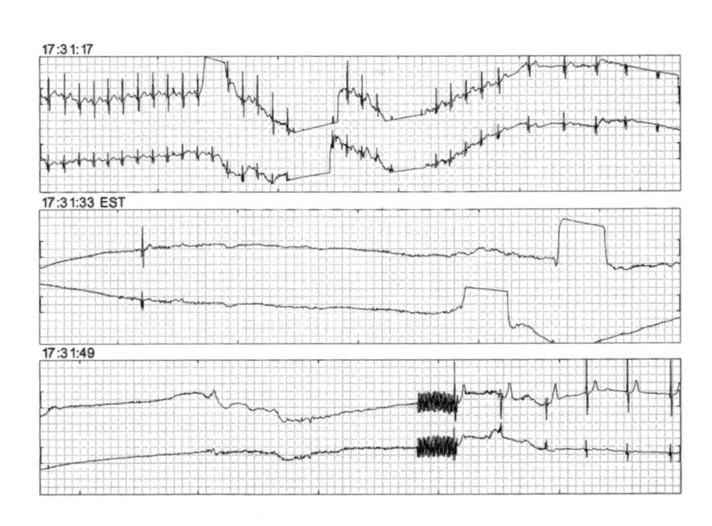

FIGURE 22–1 *Recording from a memory looping event monitor of a toddler with recurrent spells with negative neurology evaluation. There is brief sinus acceleration before dramatic sinus slowing with associated motion artifact. The second panel demonstrates a 2-second pause, a single escape beat, and a second 23-second pause before gradual recovery that includes continued sinus bradycardia with a junctional escape rhythm. This pattern is repeated on subsequent spells, confirming the diagnosis of pallid breath-holding spells.*

a favorable prognosis. While prolonged pauses can be seen in as many as 5% of head-up tilts,[71] but this finding is neither reliably reproduced nor predictive of clinical course in children and adolescents. The precise mechanisms of this dramatic response are complex, as patients have been observed with both sinus tachycardia and profound AV block. This variable rhythm, combined with the failure of pacemakers to completely eliminate symptoms in syncope,[72–74] emphasizes both the dynamic nature of the physiology and the importance for careful symptom/rhythm correlation.

Postural Orthostatic Tachycardia and Recurrent Symptoms

A syndrome of recurrent postural orthostatic tachycardia, characterized by a greater than a 30 to 40 beat/minute heart rate increase with a 6-minute stand test, similar findings on head-up tilt, and multiple symptoms, is well described in young adults[75] and has been observed in adolescents, some of whom are quite disabled by their symptoms and may be determined to have chronic fatigue syndrome.[76,77] Although many of these patients have minimal actual syncope, they have recurrent presyncopal symptoms that may be manifest as palpitations or exercise intolerance. Like other syncope patients, they have an adolescent female dominance. Typically, the referring physicians already have excluded thyroid disease, anemia, and the other obvious causes of this chronic disorder. Recognition can allow some focus to subsequent diagnostic and therapy choices.

Exercise-Induced or Exercise-Associated Syncope

The rare deaths that have been reported in adolescents with syncope invariably highlight that *syncope with exercise is a worrisome finding.*[63,68] Hypertrophic, dilated, and electrical myopathies all can present with exercise-associated syncope with no prior symptoms. All patients with syncope associated with exercise deserve prompt cardiac referral and additional testing with at least an echocardiogram if no diagnosis is apparent on initial evaluation.

Exercise also represents an almost optimal trigger for neurally mediated syncope. Particularly with highly dynamic sports like distance running, the cardiovascular response to exercise is to vasodilate, increase sympathetic output, and shift blood flow to the legs. During running, the skeletal muscle pump action of the leg muscles enhances venous return, facilitating increased cardiac output. Immediately after exertion, that pump function is decreased or absent and can permit the same reflex responses seen in any other example of venous pooling. When an initial evaluation does not identify clear heart disease, most cases of exercise-induced syncope can eventually be demonstrated to be some form of neurally mediated syncope.[68,78,79]

Psychogenic Syncope and Situational Syncope

The relationship between fainting and "nerves" is not always as obvious as it eventually becomes. There are numerous examples of convulsive events and faints triggered by acute anxiety and resulting in prolonged cardiac pauses. In those cases, the emotional trigger (e.g., the sight of blood) results in the physiologic event of profound bradycardia.

More problematic are patients in whom some of the events seem to be typical neurally mediated syncope, but over time, there is acceleration and potential embellishment of the symptoms, so that some events seem to result from panic or anxiety. The history in this setting does not make sense; physical examination, laboratory testing, and monitoring are neither consistent nor diagnostic of clear pathology. In young adults, measures of anxiety are a better predictor of future faints than syncope during head-up tilt.[80] In practice, this interaction is often easy to recognize, but may be difficult to prove.

Toddler Syncope

Variously called *pallid breath-holding spells, white syncope, reflex anoxic seizures*, and *toddler syncope*, there is a well-recognized, generally stereotypical syndrome of paroxysmal collapse in toddlers.[64,81] Repeated spells are often referred to cardiologists or neurologists for further evaluation. In the typical spell, a trivial physical or emotional trauma triggers an aborted cry, opisthotonic stiffening, and pallor that resolves over about a minute and is often followed by sleep. Rarely, such spells trigger true seizures. They contrast and overlap with classic breath-holding spells, with ongoing crying with cyanosis, breath-holding, and then symptoms. Onset is typically between age 6 months and 3 years, with termination in more than 65% of cases by age 5 years and in the vast majority by age 8 years, after which they would generally be classified as convulsive syncope. Nearly 20% of toddlers with breath-holding spells have some syncope as adolescents.

When isolated and typical, toddler syncope is generally managed by the primary care physician with little formal investigation. When recurrent, evaluation for anemia,[82,83] arrhythmia, and epilepsy is appropriate. Iron therapy may be useful, but efficacy has been more impressive in developing countries than in recent U.S. experience. Although the level of bradycardia can be quite impressive, most toddlers have infrequent episodes that resolve without specific therapy.

Diagnostic Evaluation

Similar to the experience in evaluating heart murmurs in the minimally symptomatic child, the diagnosis of neurally mediated syncope can be confidently made in most children with a detailed history, physical examination, and ECG. In 480 patients referred to a pediatric cardiology practice for syncope, 22 (5%) had cardiac syncope. Of those, 21 were identified either by the historical linkage to exercise (10 of 153, 6%), abnormal ECG,[16,68] a concerning family history of arrhythmia, or abnormal physical examination.

The history is the critical test and focuses on triggers, presyncopal symptoms that can serve as both clues to the physiology and a proxy for therapy efforts, and some assessment of the severity of symptoms. A 10-point visual analogue scale (0, no symptoms, 10 constant dizziness and recurrent syncope) allows rapid self-assessment and a quick way to track symptoms over time. Family history focuses on a history of sudden unexpected death before age 40, congenital deafness, or cardiomyopathy, all of which are worrisome, and the common history of recurrent adolescent or toddler syncope that was outgrown.

Physical examination should include orthostatic vital signs, repeating heart rate and blood pressure supine, then having the patient move directly to standing and repeating the heart rate and blood pressure at 1 and 3 minutes. A brief neurologic examination is appropriate, as is a detailed cardiac examination in several positions, examining for transient murmurs from dynamic subaortic stenosis and mitral valve prolapse. Focused history and examination should explore signs and symptoms of systemic disease, connective tissue disorders like Marfan syndrome, and underlying eating disorders.

Electrocardiography

The ECG is examined for left ventricular hypertrophy, Wolff-Parkinson-White syndrome, atrioventricular and interventricular conduction defects, and electrical myopathies, most notably long QT syndrome. The ECG is an imperfect screen for hypertrophic cardiomyopathy and has no value in screening for most coronary anomalies that present after the first year of life. It is not surprising to see somewhat prominent respiratory sinus arrhythmia. For patients with combinations of borderline ECGs or worrisome family histories, ECGs on siblings and parents are useful tools. Ambulatory ECG monitoring, including 24-hour Holter monitors, portable event monitoring,[84] and rarely implantable loop recorders,[85] can each be useful in correlating clinical symptoms with arrhythmias, although, like echocardiograms, the primary yield is demonstrating the absence of serious disease.

Echocardiography

Routine echo screening with syncope referred to pediatric cardiology has a low yield, 5% in those with normal screening examinations, with most of those findings representing minor valvular findings that are unrelated to the syncope.[68] A careful echocardiographic examination, including examination of the coronary origins,[86] is indicated when the history, physical, ECG, or family history is suggestive of cardiac disease or cardiac syncope, or when the frequency of the episodes is becoming worrisome.

Cardiac Catheterization

For patients with structurally and functionally normal hearts by echocardiogram, nondiagnostic or normal ECGs, and unrevealing ambulatory monitoring, there is little to no yield in cardiac catheterization, even if it includes programmed electrical stimulation. Most pediatric echo laboratories can adequately image the coronaries to exclude anomalous coronaries. Other diagnoses are effectively excluded by echo or may require drug challenges.

For patients with congenital heart disease, particularly those with combinations of syncope, palpitations, nonsustained ventricular tachycardia, or other arrhythmias, cardiac catheterization, including programmed atrial and ventricular stimulation and appropriate hemodynamic evaluation, is indicated.[87] The role of catheterization in evaluating arrhythmia risk in patients with cardiomyopathy remains poorly defined.

Other Studies

Head-up tilt testing is an effective way to recreate neurally mediated syncope and can be effectively performed in adolescents.[88] Unfortunately, these same maneuvers can induce syncope in completely asymptomatic adolescent volunteers,[61,62] of whom up to 40% will have presyncopal symptoms with a 70-degree tilt.

Because of the high incidence of false-positive results, head-up tilt testing cannot be viewed as a diagnostic test. Rather, it should be used as confirmatory test or a physiologic probe. At Children's Hospital Boston, the test has evolved as a way of exploring challenging and recurrent symptoms.

Treadmill exercise testing has a poorly defined role in evaluating patients with syncope. It has advantages of being relatively nonthreatening, easy to obtain, and a reasonable screen for a number of occult arrhythmias. In some series, as many as 15% to 20% of syncope patients recreated their symptoms during or immediately after exercise. At Children's Hospital Boston, exercise testing is obtained more frequently than head-up tilt testing in patients with problematic syncope, although it is still performed in less than 5% of syncope patients.

Management

For cardiac syncope, therapy is directed at the underlying disorder. For neurally mediated syncope, the episodic, self-resolving nature of the disorder contributes to inadequate double-blind, placebo-controlled data regarding therapeutic choices in adults and even fewer data in children. Therapy recommendations are based on limited series, more limited trials, and rational planning based on the clinical physiology.

Nonpharmacologic, Nondevice Therapy

Education regarding the nature of syncopal events and ways to either prevent or abort spells represents the cornerstone of therapy. Most patients will have significant relief with a combination of *overhydration*, including increased fluid, decreased caffeine, and increased sodium intake, and *antigravity maneuvers*, including isometric leg or arm contractions, staged shifts from supine to upright, squatting or lying down with onset of presyncopal symptoms, and possibly use of compression stockings. In difficult cases, "tilt training" with supervised upright time leaning against a wall[89] can be beneficial. Upright, weight-bearing aerobic exercise may also be beneficial.[90] Education on these techniques can also be diagnostic because symptoms caused by arrhythmia will not be reliably eliminated by these maneuvers.

For many cases of situational syncope and certainly for hysterical or psychogenic fits, behavioral therapy is critical. When patients will not accept a purely behavioral approach, many accept a combined approach of modest medical therapy along with a cognitive-behavioral approach through psychiatry.

Drug Therapy

Pharmacologic management focuses on volume enhancement, limiting excessive catecholamine drive, blood pressure augmentation, and rarely anticholinergic therapy. In refractory cases, the effects of these agents appear at least additive, and many have been used in combination.[91]

Volume enhancement using fludrocortisone represents a mainstay in therapy.[92] An essentially pure mineralocorticoid, fludrocortisone appears to work by increasing blood volume by enhancing sodium renal reabsorption. Advantages include rare side effects, once-daily dosing, and low cost. Disadvantages include slow onset of action and, particularly with higher doses, the potential for chronic hypokalemia or chronic hypertension, although the incidence of those side effects is low.[93] Low doses, by themselves, are ineffective for severe postural tachycardia symptoms.[94]

Use of β blockers has a long history of apparent success in pediatric syncope,[95] and atenolol is neither superior nor inferior to fludrocortisone in a small pediatric series.[92] The use of β blockers for syncope aims at decreasing excessive catecholamine stimulation and hence blunting catecholamine-mediated vasodilation and potentially cardiac sensory triggers associated with a hyperdynamic, underfilled left ventricle. Several recent randomized trials in adults have shown no benefit[96,97] to nonselective β blockers. Pindolol, a unique agent with intrinsic sympathomimetic activity, may have some clinical advantages.

Midodrine hydrochloride is a unique prodrug that is metabolized into a peripherally active direct α_1 agonist. It has been useful in repeated trials of adults with neurally mediated hypotension.[98,99] Side effects are related to its direct drug effects and include piloerection, scalp itching, and rarely urinary symptoms. Advantages of midodrine include its direct and rapid action, allowing titration when required, and the very narrow therapeutic effect. Disadvantages include a short duration of action (3 to 5 hours) and high cost, limiting its use to highly symptomatic and highly motivated patients.

Limited case series, almost always in highly symptomatic patients, have used selective serotonin reuptake inhibitors, erythropoietin, and disopyramide.

For highly refractory syncope with documented, clinical pauses, both ventricular and dual-chamber pacing have been effective at decreasing, but not eliminating, symptoms. The published pediatric experience is very limited, and at Children's Hospital Boston, this indication for pacing was present in 12 of 497 patients treated with permanent pacemakers. When focusing on the specific indication for pacing of toddlers with pallid breath-holding spells, either ventricular or dual-chamber pacemakers can eliminate the seizure-like events in most severe cases, limiting them in the remainder.[74,100] Although highly effective in the most difficult cases, it is critical to note that the Mayo clinic implants about one pacemaker a year for this indication.[101]

Course

Neurally mediated syncope is not associated with increased risk for mortality. Toddlers with breath-holding spells are more likely to have neurally mediated syncope than adolescents, but symptoms resolve in most by age 4.[64] Most adolescents, even those most disabled, appear to outgrow their episodes over several years. For teens, improvement may result from effective use of behavioral and physical approaches to their symptoms. The episodic nature of syncope, its benign natural history, and the lack of perfect drug therapy lead to an initial nonpharmacologic approach. When drug therapy is needed, therapy is typically continued for about 1 year, followed by trials of decreasing therapy.

CHEST PAIN

After murmurs, chest pain in children and adolescents is the most frequent complaint leading to referral to a pediatric cardiologist.[102] In most cases, the pain is not related to a serious underlying cause, and cardiac origins of chest pain are infrequent[103]; however, accurate assessment of the clinical presentation is essential so that pathology is not overlooked.

By the time a patient reaches the cardiologist, the anxiety level of the family is high, reinforced by knowledge that cardiac causes of chest pain in older individuals can be life threatening. Therefore, appropriate care for this group of patients must address not only the etiology but also reassurance about the nature of what is often a self-limited condition.

Epidemiology

Depending on the point of entry to the medical system, the epidemiology of chest pain varies in children. Estimates suggest that chest pain is the primary complaint in 650,000 pediatric encounters yearly,[104,105] with such complaints accounting for 5% to 15% of patients referred to a pediatric cardiology clinic.[106,107] Cardiac causes of chest pain in younger patients presenting to emergency rooms are sparse, constituting only 1% of patients evaluated in one review with idiopathic (21%) or musculoskeletal (5%) etiologies far more common.[108–110]

Etiology

Noncardiac Causes of Chest Pain

Chest Wall. Pain attributable to the chest wall is the most common explanation in the pediatric age range, seen in as many as 31% of patients,[109,111] and may involve connective, bony, or muscular tissue. The underlying cause can be traumatic or atraumatic. Costochondritis related to inflammation at the costochondral junction is a common explanation for chest pain, particularly in adolescents, and can be traced to traumatic strain in athletes or lifting of relatively heavy objects.[112–114] Precordial catch syndrome is generally sharp pain of short duration and unclear etiology isolated to the left lower sternal border or apex that is sometimes exercise induced and may recur.[115–117] Some patients are able to relieve the pain with deep inspiration. Slipping rib syndrome is pain caused by trauma or tension on the fibrous connections to the 8th, 9th, or 10th ribs. These ribs are not attached to the sternum but to each other, and with unrestrained motion of a rib, pain is produced by irritation of the intercostal nerves.[118–120] The pain can be sharp or dull and is sometimes reproducible. The sternum itself can be the source of chest pain with a uncommon condition known as *hypersensitive xiphoid* that improves spontaneously.[121] Pectus deformities of the chest wall can be associated with occasional pain that may be accentuated by exercise.[122,123] Sickle cell disease is associated with acute chest syndrome, an important cause of death in this group of patients and frequently responsible for hospital admissions.[124,125] The etiology of the pain remains unclear, with episodes attributed to fat embolism, infection, or bony infarction.[126] Aggressive therapy with prophylactic transfusion and hydroxyurea has been used successfully to reduce frequency of these episodes.[127,128] Breast conditions may produce pain in both males and females, although far more commonly in the latter. Causes include infection, pubertal or menstrual change, and pregnancy. Traumatic chest pain is very common in adolescents related to muscular strain or tears, rib fractures, or spasm. Such pain is almost always self-limited.

Pulmonary. Underlying pulmonary pathology leads to chest pain in a variety of settings. Reactive airway disease causes pain related to strain from persistent cough, dyspnea, or pneumothorax. In particular, exercise-induced bronchospasm is present in many children and adolescents, limiting their ability to participate in sports. Pretreatment with bronchodilator therapy may avert recurrent episodes.[129,130] Pneumonia is associated with chest pain in many patients in the setting of acute febrile illness. Chest pain is a frequent presenting symptom after a pulmonary embolus. Although uncommon, a family history of hypercoagulability may provide insight into the diagnosis. Pleural disease is associated with chest pain that may be acute in onset, accentuated by inspiration and prolonged in duration. Pleural effusion is most frequently of infectious origin but can also be produced by systemic inflammatory conditions or malignancy. Pleural irritation can also result from pneumothorax producing inspiratory pain; however, the pain can also be referred to the shoulder from diaphragmatic irritation. Pneumothorax can present spontaneously in Marfan syndrome[131] and cystic fibrosis,[132] or it may follow trauma.

Gastrointestinal. Chest pain may derive from a number of common gastrointestinal conditions. Gastroesophageal reflux with esophagitis produces a burning sensation in the retrosternal area, sometimes exacerbated by supine positioning.[133,134] Signs of reflux in infants include arching of the back with feeding, spitting or recurrent vomiting, and respiratory changes related to aspiration, including wheezing and rhonchi. Peptic ulcer disease most frequently associated with *Helicobacter pylori* infection can be an important source of pain localized to the epigastric region or lower chest.[135] Spasm of the esophagus can produce marked chest pain.[133] When a possible gastrointestinal source of pain is suspected, evaluation of both motility and tissue involvement is warranted using manometry and endoscopy with biopsy.

Psychogenic. Among pediatric patients presenting to a cardiology clinic with chest pain, a substantial number have symptoms that are psychogenic in origin.[108,109] The history can pinpoint a preceding event that can act as a trigger for the pain, including death of a friend or family member, divorce or separation, illness or trauma in a family member, or depression.[136,137] Chest pain can present as a symptom in hyperventilation syndrome. Despite the inclination to ascribe the complaint to a nonorganic cause, the provider must consider the social setting. Family members are generally very anxious about the possibility of underlying organ pathology and may not be ready to accept an alternate explanation. Often, reassurance about the anticipated benign outcome is helpful. Adolescents with chest pain frequently believe they have heart disease and tend to change their lifestyle as a result.[138] In some cases, it may be necessary to obtain some noninvasive testing to provide support for the absence of underlying disease. Several encounters may allow the development of trust and rapport, so that the family is more amenable to a diagnosis of psychogenic origin and likely to seek further counseling if necessary.[139]

Cardiac Causes of Chest Pain

Myocardial. Cardiomyopathy, either hypertrophic or dilated, is associated with chest pain. The pain is the result of imbalance between myocardial demand and cardiac output. In the former case, marked increase in myocardial oxygen demand exceeds coronary flow during exercise, resulting in angina. Mid-cavitary obstruction exacerbates the imbalance, leading to increased myocardial work and myocardial oxygen consumption. In addition, coronary artery compression produced by myocardial bridging may cause myocardial ischemia and angina.[140] In dilated cardiomyopathy, the muscle mass is decreased, but the capacity of the heart to deliver adequate coronary blood flow is impaired by diminished stroke volume. Acute myocarditis generally of viral origin may present with chest pain, usually the result of concomitant pericarditis.

Valvular. Severe aortic valve or subaortic obstruction produces chest pain due to limitation of cardiac output during exercise in the setting of left ventricular hypertrophy. The supply–demand mismatch is similar to that of hypertrophic cardiomyopathy. Mitral regurgitation can be the source of chest pain when severe, related to volume overload of the left ventricle producing increased myocardial work with output limited by the large regurgitant fraction of blood. Although more likely to occur as a chronic condition, the onset of mitral regurgitation can be acute after ruptured chordae tendineae in individuals with mitral valve prolapse or connective tissue disease. Less acute and poorly understood is the pain that has been associated in a small percentage of patients with mitral valve prolapse, which may in fact be unrelated to this condition.[141,142]

Pericardial. Acute inflammation of the pericardium is frequently accompanied by chest pain thought to result from opposition of the inflamed parietal and visceral pericardial surfaces. The underlying cause can be viral, bacterial, autoimmune, or related to operative procedures in which the pericardium is entered. In the presence of effusion, the pericardial surfaces are separated, so that the pain is diminished or absent.

Coronary. Kawasaki disease results in the formation of coronary abnormalities in 20% to 25% of those not treated early in the course with intravenous γ-globulin and in 2% to 4% of those receiving treatment before 10 days from the onset of fever. Giant aneurysm (> 8 mm diameter) formation puts patients at risk for late progressive stenosis at the distal or proximal ends of the aneurysm. Exercise produces chest pain in those with critical narrowing.[143] Uncommonly, coronary artery abnormalities of congenital origin produce chest pain during exercise, which is thought related to compression of an artery between the aortic and pulmonic roots or insufficient coronary flow through a kinked acute-angle takeoff of the artery or spasm of the artery.[144] Rarely, the left coronary artery may arise from the pulmonary artery, a condition that presents in infancy with heart failure after left ventricular infarction, but it can remain silent until later in childhood when symptoms of pain with exercise may prevail.

Aortic. Dissection of the aorta in Marfan syndrome, other connective tissue disorders, Turner's syndrome, and familial aneurysmal diseases causes acute severe chest pain that may radiate to the back. A sinus of Valsalva aneurysm can rupture unexpectedly into the right atrium or ventricle.

Rhythm Abnormalities. Children with supraventricular tachycardia may complain of chest pain during acute events. The pain may be the result of coronary ischemia related to diminished ventricular diastolic filling and low cardiac output. Some patients describe chest discomfort rather than pain. Ventricular tachycardia producing chest pain is most commonly seen in patients who have undergone repair or palliation of congenital lesions, as well as individuals with cardiomyopathy, long QTc syndrome, or severe electrolyte disturbances.

Clinical Evaluation

History

More than any other component of the clinical assessment, the history is most critical because careful exploration of the present illness can often identify the cause of chest pain. If possible, the history should be obtained from the patient rather than the parents, who may be prone to overinterpretation, exaggeration, or inaccuracy related to their personal experiences or anxiety. The patient should establish total duration of the symptom from the first episode. In most circumstances, chest pain is present for many months if not years before parents seek input, supporting a noncardiac cause. The manner of onset, whether acute or chronic, gradual or sudden, may suggest an etiology, with cardiac causes more acute in nature. Precipitating and predisposing factors provide insight, such as pain occurring with physical exertion (cardiac or musculoskeletal), injury or strain (musculoskeletal), response to rest or analgesics (musculoskeletal), emotional circumstances related to family disruption, school difficulties, illness of a friend or relative, or depression (psychogenic). The characteristics of the symptom should be detailed first with a subjective description of the pain (i.e., squeezing, sharp, dull, aching, cramping), and the patient should locate the pain by pointing directly to the site of greatest intensity and then areas of possible radiation. Cardiac chest pain is generally mid-precordial and can radiate to the left arm. Severe crushing pain radiating to the back is experienced with aortic tears. Subcostal pain is generally chest wall related. The intensity of the pain should be estimated using a scale of 1 to 10, with the lower and upper ranges defined for reference. The temporal nature of the episode should be identified as continuous, constant, intermittent, or recurrent. Aggravating and relieving factors may provide insight about the nature of the cause with respect to exertion, position, meals, or breathing. The course of the symptoms since initial presentation may indicate that the process is improving or progressing. It is often helpful to ask patients if they are worried about the pain, and if so, why—a line of questioning that can help to disclose emotional factors influencing the symptoms. Associated symptoms may be helpful clues, including palpitations, dizziness, syncope, epigastric pain, nausea, vomiting, fatigue, fever, cough, coryza, shortness of breath, and orthopnea or dyspnea on exertion. The family history can identify other individuals with possible connective tissue disease.

Physical Examination

The appearance of the patient may suggest a connective tissue disorder in a tall individual with dolichocephaly and pectus excavatum or carinatum. The costochondral junctions should be palpated to elicit tenderness. Auscultation may identify wheezing associated with reactive airway disease or rales found with pneumonia or congestive failure. The cardiac assessment may suggest underlying heart disease by its hyperdynamic quality and displacement of the point of maximal intensity in patients with volume-overloaded lesions. A palpable thrill along the left sternal border, at the base bilaterally, and the suprasternal notch supports left ventricular outflow tract obstruction. An apical or parasternal heave is associated with right or left ventricular hypertrophy, respectively. On auscultation, underlying cardiac disease may be heralded by the presence of a loud S_2 associated with pulmonary hypertension, whereas muffled heart sounds are found in moderate to large pericardial effusions. Systolic clicks are noted with bicuspid aortic valves or mitral valve prolapse. The harsh systolic ejection murmur of valvar or subvalvar aortic stenosis is heard along the left sternal border with radiation to the base and neck. Mitral regurgitation is heard at the apex with radiation to the left axilla, although murmurs associated with posterior mitral leaflet abnormalities may be heard at the left mid to upper sternal border, related to a more anteriorly and superiorly directed regurgitant jet. Aortic regurgitation of at least mild to moderate degree produces a regurgitant murmur radiating from the right base, down the left lower sternal border toward the apex. S_3 gallops are heard in the presence of at least moderate mitral regurgitation or dilated cardiomyopathy, whereas S_4 gallops, although far less common, are noted in hypertrophic cardiomyopathy or severe aortic stenosis. A friction rub is present with acute pericarditis.

Electrocardiogram

The ECG is of occasional benefit in the assessment of the patient with chest pain. A short PR interval and delta wave on ECG identifies the presence of an accessory bypass tract that can support supraventricular tachycardia in the patient who complains of chest pain with fast heart rate. Left ventricular hypertrophy is sometimes seen in patients with hypertrophic cardiomyopathy, moderate to severe aortic valve stenosis, subaortic stenosis, or aortic regurgitation and dilated cardiomyopathy. Long QTc interval may suggest the possibility of ventricular tachyarrhythmia. An infarct pattern can be present in anomalous left coronary artery from the pulmonary artery or rarely in Kawasaki disease. In pericarditis, diffuse T-wave abnormalities are common.

Chest X-ray

As with the ECG, chest x-rays are helpful in a limited number of those presenting with chest pain and therefore can be used selectively. In the patient with myocarditis, pericarditis, dilated cardiomyopathy, or aortic regurgitation of at least moderate degree, the x-ray may show cardiac chamber enlargement. A dilated ascending aorta can be present in those with Marfan syndrome. Reactive airway disease produces air trapping with hyperexpansion of the lung fields and flattened diaphragms. Pleural effusions or infiltrates are noted in infectious processes, and peripheral lung field abnormalities may be suggestive of pulmonary embolus. Spontaneous pneumothorax producing chest pain is readily recognized by radiograph.

Echocardiography

The echocardiogram is a useful modality if applied prudently in the assessment of the patient with chest pain because most patients do not have underlying heart disease. Echo can make the diagnosis of hypertrophic cardiomyopathy with or without left ventricular outflow tract obstruction. The left ventricular function is reduced in dilated cardiomyopathy or myocarditis with reduced ventricular function. Pericardial fluid is easily identified, and in the setting of large effusions, tamponade physiology is marked by atrial wall collapse and variability of the Doppler flow velocity across the mitral valve or in the descending thoracic aorta. In Marfan syndrome, the aortic dimensions can be markedly increased; associated findings include mitral valve prolapse with or without mitral regurgitation and aortic regurgitation related to a dilated aortic root. Coronary artery dilation or aneurysm formation is virtually pathognomonic for Kawasaki disease in a patient with a history of a prolonged febrile illness. Patients with giant aneurysms are at particular risk for stenotic lesions. Although echo identification of these stenoses is difficult, chest pain in the presence of giant aneurysms should prompt further workup for coronary ischemia. The course and distribution of rare coronary abnormalities predisposing to chest pain can be visualized by echo including single right or left coronary arteries.

Exercise Testing

In most patients with chest pain, exercise testing is not necessary. In some cases, rhythm abnormalities such as supraventricular tachycardia are unmasked during exercise testing. Ventricular arrhythmias can either suppress with exercise (generally thought to have benign implications) or degenerate during testing, potentially correlating with the patient's symptoms. When ischemia is suggested by history, upright treadmill exercise testing is a useful first step. Sesta-MIBI stress testing provides additional sensitivity by identifying regions of abnormal coronary perfusion. Such evaluation is helpful in patients with large aneurysms after Kawasaki disease and in those with congenital coronary artery anomalies identified by echo. In some cases, although the clinician is convinced that chest pain is unrelated to underlying heart disease or exercise-induced bronchospasm, exercise testing may be necessary to reassure an anxious family about the benign nature of the pain.

REFERENCES

1. Epstein N. The heart in normal infants and children. J Pediatr 32:39, 1948.
2. Sampson JJ, Hahman PT, Halverson WL, et al. Incidence of heart disease and rheumatic fever in school children in their climatically different California communities. Am Heart J 29:178, 1945.
3. Caceres CA, Perry LW. The innocent murmur: A problem in clinical practice. Boston: Little, Brown, 1967.
4. The cervical venous hum. In Caceres CA, Perry LW (eds). The Innocent Murmur. Boston: Little, Brown, 1967:181–192.
5. Perloff JK. Normal or innocent murmurs. In The Clinical Recognition of Congenital Heart Disease. Philadelphia: WB Saunders, 1987:8–18.
6. Lembo NJ, Dell'Italia LJ, Crawford MH, et al. Bedside diagnosis of systolic murmurs. N Engl J Med 318:1572, 1988.
7. Newburger JW, Rosenthal A, Williams RG, et al. Noninvasive tests in the initial evaluation of heart murmurs in children. N Engl J Med 308:61, 1983.
8. Smythe JF, Teixeira OH, Vlad P, et al. Initial evaluation of heart murmurs: Are laboratory tests necessary? Pediatrics 86(4):497, 1990.
9. Geva T, Hegesh J, Frand M. Reappraisal of the approach to the child with heart murmurs: Is echocardiography mandatory? Int J Cardiol 19(1):107, 1988.
10. Advani N, Menahem S, Wilkinson JL. The diagnosis of innocent murmurs in childhood. Cardiol Young 10:340, 2000.
11. Zufelt K, Rosenberg HC, Li MD, et al. The electrocardiogram and the secundum atrial septal defect: A reexamination in the era of echocardiography. Can J Cardiol 14(2): 227, 1998.
12. Danford DA, Martin AB, Fletcher SE, et al. Echocardiographic yield in children when innocent murmur seems likely but doubts linger. Pediatr Cardiol 23(4):410, 2002.
13. McCrindle BW, Shaffer KM, Kan JS, et al. Cardinal clinical signs in the differentiation of heart murmurs in children. Arch Pediatr Adolesc Med 150(2):169, 1996.
14. Braudo M, et al. Auscultation of the heart. Early neonatal period. Am J Dis Child 101:575, 1961.
15. Richards MR, Merritt KK, Samuels MH, et al. Frequency and significance of systolic cardiac murmurs in infants. Pediatrics 15:196, 1955.
16. Farrer KF, Rennie JM. Neonatal murmurs: Are senior house officers good enough? Arch Dis Child Fetal Neonatal Ed 88(2):F147, 2003.
17. Ainsworth S, Wyllie JP, Wren C. Prevalence and clinical significance of cardiac murmurs in neonates. Arch Dis Child Fetal Neonatal Ed 80(1):F43, 1999.
18. Van Oort A, Blanc-Botden M, De Boo T, et al. The vibratory innocent heart murmur in schoolchildren: Difference in auscultatory findings between school medical officers and a pediatric cardiologist. Pediatr Cardiol 15(6):282, 1994.
19. Arlettaz R, Archer N, Wilkinson AR. Natural history of innocent heart murmurs in newborn babies: Controlled echocardiographic study. Arch Dis Child Fetal Neonatal Ed 78(3):F166, 1998.
20. Friedman S, Robie WA, Harris TN. Occurrence of innocent-adventitious cardiac sounds in childhood. Pediatrics 4:782, 1949.
21. Rauh LW. Cardiac murmurs in children. Ohio State Med J 36:973, 1970.
22. Schwartzman J. Cardiac status of adolescents. Arch Pediatr 58:443, 1941.
23. Thayer WS. Reflections on the interpretation of systolic cardiac murmurs. Am J Med Sci 169:313, 1925.
24. Lessof M, Brigden W. Systolic murmurs in healthy children and in children with rheumatic fever. Lancet 2:673, 1957.
25. McKee MH. Heart sounds in normal children. Am Heart J 16:79, 1938.
26. Fogel DH. The innocent systolic murmur in children: A clinical study of its incidence and characteristics. Am Heart J 59:844, 1960.
27. DeGroff CG, Bhatikar S, Hertzberg J, et al. Artificial neural network-based method of screening heart murmurs in children. Circulation 103(22):2711, 2001.

28. Thompson WR, Hayek CS, Tuchinda C, et al. Automated cardiac auscultation for detection of pathologic heart murmurs. Pediatr Cardiol 22(5):373, 2001.
29. Still GF. Common Disorders and Diseases of Childhood. London: Frowde, Hodder & Stoughton, 1909.
30. Stein PD, Sabbah HN. Aortic origin of innocent murmurs. Am J Cardiol 39:655, 1977.
31. Perry LW, Ruckman RN, Shapiro SR, et al. Left ventricular false tendons in children. Am J Cardiol 52:1264, 1983.
32. Wessel A, Beyer C, Pulss W, et al. False chordae tendineae in the left ventricle: Echo and phonocardiographic findings. Z Kardiol 74(5):303, 1985.
33. Van Oort A, Van-Dam I, Heringa A, et al. The vibratory innocent heart murmur studied by echo-Doppler. Acta Paediatr Scand 329(Suppl):103, 1986.
34. Sholler GF, Celermajer JM, Whight CM. Doppler echocardiographic assessment of cardiac output in normal children with and without innocent precordial murmurs. Am J Cardiol 59(5):487, 1987.
35. Kato H, Sugimura T, Akagi T, et al. Long-term consequences of Kawasaki disease: A 10- to 21-year follow-up study of 594 patients. Circulation 94:1379, 1996.
36. Klewer SE, Donnerstein RL, Goldberg SJ. Still's-like innocent murmur can be produced by increasing aortic velocity to a threshold value. Am J Cardiol 68(8):810, 1991.
37. Donnerstein RL, Thomsen VS. Hemodynamic and anatomic factors affecting the frequency content of Still's innocent murmur. Am J Cardiol 74(5):508, 1994.
38. Van Oort A, Blanc-Botden M, De Boo T, et al. The vibratory innocent heart murmur in schoolchildren: Difference in auscultatory findings between school medical officers and a pediatric cardiologist. Pediatr Cardiol 15(6):282, 1994.
39. Groom D, Sihvonen YT. A high sensitivity pick up for cardiovascular sounds. Am Heart J 54:592, 1957.
40. Castle RF. Clinical recognition of innocent cardiac murmurs in infants and children. JAMA 177:71, 1961.
41. Segal BL, Novack P, Kasparian H. Intracardiac phonocardiography. Am J Cardiol 13:188, 1964.
42. Gaskin PR, Owens SE, Talner NS, et al. Clinical auscultation skills in pediatric residents. Pediatr 105(6):1184, 2000.
43. Cutforth R, Wiseman J, Sutherland RD. The genesis of the cervical venous hum. Am Heart J 80:488, 1970.
44. Edwards EA, Levine HD. Peripheral vascular murmurs: Mechanism of production and diagnostic significance. Arch Intern Med 90:284, 1952.
45. Levine SA, Harvey WP. Clinical Auscultation of the Heart, 2nd ed. Philadelphia: WB Saunders, 1959.
46. Mannheimer E. Phonocardiography in children. In Advances in Pediatrics. Chicago: Year Book, 1955.
47. Moscovitz HL. The venous hum. Am Heart J 62:141, 1961.
48. Segal BL. Innocent murmurs. In The Theory and Practice of Auscultation. Philadelphia: FA Davis, 1964:168–179.
49. Cassels DE. Cardiovascular murmurs in infants and children. Med Clin North Am 1957;41:75.
50. Fowler NO. The innocent murmur. In Physical Diagnosis of Heart Disease. New York: MacMillan, 1962:49–61.
51. Kawabori I, Stevenson JG, Dooley TK, et al. The significance of carotid bruits in children: Transmitted murmur of vascular origin, studied by pulsed Doppler ultrasound. Am Heart J 98:160, 1979.
52. Miller RA, Stamler J, Smith JM, et al. The detection of heart disease in children: Results of mass field trials with use of tape recorded heart sounds. Circulation 32:956,1965.
53. Haney I, Ipp M, Feldman W, et al. Accuracy of clinical assessment of heart murmurs by office based (general practice) paediatricians. Arch Dis Child 81(5):409, 1999.
54. Danford DA, Nasir A, Gumbiner C. Cost assessment of the evaluation of heart murmurs in children. Pediatrics 91(2): 365, 1993.
55. Glaser HH, Harrison GS, Lynn DB. Emotional implications of congenital heart disease in children. Pediatrics 33:367, 1964.
56. Linde LM, Rasof B, Dunn OJ, et al. Attitudinal factors in congenital heart disease. Pediatrics 38:92, 1966.
57. Bergman AB, Stamm SJ. The morbidity of cardiac nondisease in schoolchildren. N Engl J Med 276:1008, 1967.
58. Lynxwiler CP, Donahoe JC. Evaluation of innocent heart murmurs. South Med J 48:164, 1955.
59. Marienfeld CJ, Telles N, Silvera J, et al. A 20 year follow-up study of "innocent" murmurs. Pediatrics 30:42, 1962.
60. Engle MA. Insurability and employability: Congenital heart disease and innocent murmurs. Circulation 56:143, 1977.
61. Lewis DA, Zlotocha J, Henke L, et al. Specificity of head-up tilt testing in adolescents: Effect of various degrees of tilt challenge in normal control subjects. J Am Coll Cardiol 30(4):1057, 1997.
62. de Jong-de Vos van Steenwijk CC, Wieling W, et al. Incidence and hemodynamic characteristics of near-fainting in healthy 6- to 16-year old subjects. J Am Coll Cardiol 25(7):1615, 1995.
63. Driscoll DJ, Jacobsen SJ, Porter CJ, et al. Syncope in children and adolescents. J Am Coll Cardiol 29(5):1039, 1997.
64. DiMario FJ Jr. Prospective study of children with cyanotic and pallid breath-holding spells. Pediatr 107(2):265, 2001.
65. Soteriades ES, Evans JC, Larson MG, et al. Incidence and prognosis of syncope. N Engl J Med 347(12):878, 2002.
66. Neuspiel DR, Kuller LH. Sudden and unexpected natural death in childhood and adolescence. JAMA 254(10):1321, 1985.
67. Driscoll DJ, Edwards WD. Sudden unexpected death in children and adolescents. J Am Coll Cardiol 5(6 Suppl):118B, 1985.
68. Ritter S, Tani LY, Etheridge SP, et al. What is the yield of screening echocardiography in pediatric syncope? Pediatrics 105(5):E58, 2000.
69. Saul JP, Alexander ME. Reflex and mechanical aspects of cardiovascular development: Techniques for assessment and implications. J Electrocardiol 30(Suppl):57, 1998.
70. Camfield PR, Camfield CS. Syncope in childhood: A case control clinical study of the familial tendency to faint. Le Journal Canadien Des Sciences Neurologiques 17:306, 1990.

23

Preventive Heart Disease: Dyslipidemia and Hypertension (Systemic)

JANE W. NEWBURGER

Atherosclerotic cardiovascular disease is the leading cause of death and disability in the United States. In 2001, 38.5% of all deaths were caused by cardiovascular diseases, and coronary heart disease was the leading killer, accounting for about one in five deaths. Major risk factors for coronary heart disease include elevated low-density lipoprotein (LDL) cholesterol, low high-density lipoprotein cholesterol (HDL), diabetes mellitus (for adults, diabetes mellitus is regarded as a coronary heart disease equivalent), cigarette smoking, hypertension, and family history of premature coronary heart disease. In large part, atherosclerotic heart disease is preventable with modification of risk factors. This chapter focuses on two of the major risk factors for adult cardiovascular disease managed by the pediatric cardiologist, namely hyperlipidemia and hypertension. Internet sites providing useful information related to these risk factors are provided in Table 23-1.

Autopsy studies have shown that atherosclerosis begins early in life. A seminal study demonstrated advanced coronary lesions in young American soldiers killed in the Korean war.[1] The Pathobiological Determinants of Atherosclerosis in Youth (PDAY) Study, a multi-institutional study of atherosclerosis, reported frequent fibrous plaques in the aortas and coronary arteries in postmortem examinations of subjects aged 15 to 19 years.[2] Furthermore, in young people dying primarily as a result of trauma, Berenson and colleagues[3] demonstrated that the severity of asymptomatic coronary and aortic atherosclerosis was directly related to the severity and numbers of proven cardiovascular risk factors in adults.

Epidemiologic studies have also highlighted the importance of risk factors in childhood. Children and adolescents with severe dyslipidemia are more likely than the general population to have abnormal lipid profiles as they grow older.[4,5] Furthermore, long-term prospective studies have shown a strong association between cholesterol levels in young adult life and later risk for cardiovascular disease.[6] Children whose adult relatives have coronary artery disease have a higher likelihood of elevated levels of total and LDL cholesterol than those without such a family history. About half of children whose parents have premature coronary artery disease will be hyperlipidemic.[7] Similarly, hypertension in childhood has a high correlation with adult hypertension,[8] and children with higher blood pressure are more likely to have first-degree relatives with a history of hypertension.[9,10] Similarly, the racial and ethnic distribution of the metabolic syndrome—including hypertriglyceridemia, low high-density lipoprotein (HDL), high fasting glucose, excessive waist circumference, and hypertension—in American adolescents is similar to that in American adults.[11]

Recently, advances in imaging have facilitated the assessment of preclinical vascular disease. Brachial artery reactivity, a surrogate for coronary artery function, is abnormal in adolescents with hyperlipidemia.[12] High-risk adolescents have been shown to have carotid and coronary artery atherosclerosis, as indicated by increased carotid intima-media thickness[13–15] and coronary artery calcification on electron beam computed tomography,[16] respectively. Finally, modification of risk factors in childhood may improve markers of preclinical disease; a recent randomized controlled trial of statin therapy for 2 years demonstrated significant regression of carotid atherosclerosis in children with familial hyperlipidemia.[15]

TABLE 23–1. Useful Internet Sites

Third Report of the NCEP Expert Panel on Detection, Evaluation, and Treatment of High Blood Cholesterol in Adults (Adult Treatment Panel III, or ATP III): http://www.nhlbi.nih.gov/guidelines/cholesterol/atp3full.pdf

Third National Health and Nutrition Examination Survey (NHANES III): http://www.cdc.gov/nchs/about/major/nhanes/datatblelink.htm)

Normative data for height, weight, and body size by BMI percentiles: http://www.cdc.gov/growthcharts/

Blood pressure percentiles: http://www.nhlbi.nih.gov/guidelines/hypertension/child_tbl.htm

The Seventh Report of the Joint National Committee on Prevention, Detection, Evaluation, and Treatment of High Blood Pressure (JNC 7): http://www.nhlbi.nih.gov/guidelines/hypertension/index.htm

The Fourth Report on the Diagnosis, Evaluation, and Treatment of High Blood Pressure in Children and Adolescents: http://pediatrics.aappublications.org/cgi/reprint/114/2/S2/555

Because decades of follow-up would be required, no published investigations have yet demonstrated that risk factor reduction in childhood will reduce the incidence of coronary artery disease and stroke in adulthood. However, postmortem, epidemiologic, and clinical data have demonstrated that the precursors of atherosclerosis begin in childhood. Recent studies have shown that risk factor modification can improve preclinical vascular abnormalities in childhood and adolescence. Based on these data, it is overwhelmingly likely that risk factor modification early in life and extending into adulthood will reduce the adult burden of atherosclerosis.

HYPERLIPIDEMIA

Description of Lipids and Lipoproteins

Cholesterol is a fatlike substance (lipid) that travels in the blood in particles called *lipoproteins,* which are molecules containing both fats and proteins.[17] Lipids plays an important role in normal biologic processes, including the formation of bile salts and steroid hormones and composition of cell membranes. Cholesterol is transported in serum by lipoproteins, containing a core of nonpolar lipids, including esterified cholesterol and triglycerides, and a surface monolayer that is composed of phospholipids, unesterified cholesterol, and apoproteins.

The major classes of lipoproteins found in the serum in fasting individuals are as follows:

Low-density lipoproteins constitute 60% to 70% of total serum cholesterol. The major apolipoprotein for LDL is apo B-100 (apo B). Higher levels of LDL cholesterol are associated with greater risk for cardiovascular disease, and lowering of LDL reduces the risk for coronary heart disease. LDL cholesterol is the primary target of lipid-lowering therapy.

High-density lipoproteins constitute 20% to 30% of total serum cholesterol and are carried by apo A-1 and apo A-II. Low HDL is a risk factor for atherosclerotic cardiovascular disease.

Very-low-density lipoproteins (VLDLs) are triglyceride-rich lipoproteins, produced by the liver, constituting 10% to 15% of total serum cholesterol and involving apo B-100; apo C-I, C-II, and C-III; and apo E. VLDLs are precursors of LDLs. VLDL remnants, consisting of partially degraded VLDLs, are atherogenic.

Intermediate-density lipoprotein (IDL) is a remnant lipoprotein that is usually included in the measured LDL fraction.

Chylomicrons are triglyceride-rich lipoproteins formed in the intestine from dietary fat. The apolipoproteins of chylomicrons include apo B-48; apo C-I, C-II, and C-III; and apo E. Chylomicron remnants may be mildly atherogenic.

Screening for Dyslipidemias

The optimal strategy in childhood for hyperlipidemia screening (i.e., selective versus universal) has been controversial. In the *selective screening strategy*, advocated by the National Cholesterol Education Program,[18] screening is performed only in children older than age 2 years deemed to be at high risk as follows: those whose parents or grandparents, at 55 years of age or less, underwent diagnostic coronary arteriography and were found to have coronary atherosclerosis or suffered a documented myocardial infarction, angina pectoris, peripheral vascular disease, cerebrovascular disease, or sudden cardiac death; those whose parent has a total cholesterol level of 240 mg/dL or higher; and those for whom the health history of a parent or grandparent is unknown. Screening should also be performed in children whose personal health includes risk factors, such as diabetes, hypertension, obesity, sedentary lifestyle, history of Kawasaki disease, or disease states associated with increased risk, such as diabetes mellitus or nephrotic syndrome.[19]

Advocates for universal screening note that almost half of children with elevated cholesterol levels do not have a positive family history.[20–22] Furthermore, the most severely affected hyperlipidemic children are not selectively identified by positive family history.[22] The Bogalusa Heart Study found that only 40% of white children and 21% of black children with elevated levels of LDL cholesterol had a parent with a history of vascular diseases.[20]

Measurement of Lipids and Lipoproteins

Levels of total cholesterol and HDL cholesterol can be measured in the nonfasting state any time of day. Both measurements should always be obtained because measurement of total cholesterol alone may miss those at risk from low HDL cholesterol.

More information is obtained when measuring a lipid profile after fasting, except for water intake, for 12 hours. Fasting profiles are the ideal way to screen children at high risk. Total cholesterol is equal to the sum of LDL, HDL, and VLDL. When chylomicrons are eliminated by fasting for 12 hours, VLDL can be calculated by dividing the triglyceride level by 5. LDL can be calculated in fasting patients as follows:

$$\text{LDL} = \text{total cholesterol} - \text{HDL} - (\text{triglycerides}/5).$$

If triglyceride levels are greater than 400 mg/dL, either a lipoprotein electrophoresis or direct measurement of LDL cholesterol should be performed.

Because lipid values may vary, it is useful to repeat a fasting lipid profile if the first profile reveals abnormalities in the range that require alterations in management.

Normative Lipid Values

"Normal" lipid values in childhood were first established in the 1970s by the Lipid Research Clinics. The distribution of fasting lipid and lipoprotein levels in children and adolescents, displayed in Table 23-2 ,were used to establish cutoff points for classification and intervention in the 1991 National Cholesterol Education Program recommendations for management of hypercholesterolemia in children.[18] More recent data were established in the Third National Health and Nutrition Examination Survey.[23]

The American Heart Association sets the following definitions of acceptable, borderline, and high total and LDL cholesterol in individuals between 2 and 19 years of age[19]:

Total Cholesterol (mg/dL)	LDL Cholesterol (mg/dL)
Acceptable	
<170	<110
Borderline	
170–199	110–129
High	
≥200	≥130

Because LDL cholesterol is the major atherogenic lipoprotein, all children with LDL cholesterols greater than 130 mg/dL should receive targeted intervention and follow-up (see later discussion).

HDL cholesterol values below 40 mg/dL are considered a risk factor for coronary heart disease, whereas those above 60 mg/dL are considered protective. Factors associated with low HDL cholesterol include genetic or metabolic causes, obesity, smoking, and use of certain medications. HDL cholesterol may be raised by weight

TABLE 23–2. Fasting Lipids and Lipoprotein Levels (mg/dL) in Children by Age

	Males			Females		
Age (yr)	**5%**	**50%**	**95%**	**5%**	**50%**	**95%**
Cholesterol						
0 – 4	114	155	203	112	156	200
5 – 9	121	160	203	126	164	205
10 – 14	119	158	202	124	160	201
15 – 19	113	150	197	120	158	203
Triglycerides						
0 – 4	29	56	98	34	64	112
5 – 9	30	56	101	32	60	105
10 – 14	32	66	125	37	75	131
15 – 19	37	78	148	39	75	132
HDL cholesterol						
5 – 9	38	56	74	36	53	73
10 – 14	37	55	74	37	52	70
15 – 19	30	46	63	35	52	74
LDL cholesterol						
5 – 9	63	93	129	68	100	140
10 – 14	64	100	140	68	97	132
15 – 19	62	94	130	59	96	137

HDL, high-density lipoprotein; LDL, low-density lipoprotein.

Data from Lipid Research Clinic. Population Studies Data Book, vol 1: The Prevalence Study. Bethesda, MD: Department of Health and Human Services, Publication (NIH) 80-1527.

reduction, exercise, and increased consumption of dietary fat, ideally monounsaturated and omega-3 fatty acids.

High triglyceride levels, greater than 150 mg/dL, can be related to genetic or metabolic causes, obesity, or use of medications. For obese patients, weight reduction is likely to decrease triglyceride levels. Triglyceride levels greater than 500 mg/dL are associated with a risk for pancreatitis and must be treated urgently, with stringent dietary management, medication, or both. Such patients should be evaluated for genetic metabolic disorders.

Children with the most severe forms of dyslipidemia often have familial or genetic causes. Familial hyperlipidemia (FH) is one of the most common genetic disorders, transmitted by an autosomal codominant inheritance pattern. Phenotypic FH may be caused by more than 60 different allelic mutations affecting the quantity or functions of the LDL receptor (see http://www.ncbi.nlm.nih.gov/Omim/allresources.html). In heterozygous FH, affecting 1 in every 500 people, LDL receptor function in the liver is reduced by about half, and total cholesterol and LDL levels are about doubled from normal levels. Risk is compounded in some FH patients by low HDL cholesterol. Without treatment, about half of FH patients have premature coronary heart disease (before age 50 in men or age 60 in women). In childhood and adolescence, however, few patients have the cardinal manifestations seen in adults, such as cutaneous or tendinous xanthomas or arcus corneae. In FH families, LDL cholesterol levels allow accurate diagnosis of FH in childhood. Of note, increased LDL cholesterol and lipoprotein (a) and decreased HDL cholesterol levels in children identify FH kindred at highest risk for coronary heart disease.[24]

Homozygous FH, occurring in about 1 in every 1 million people, is associated with total cholesterol levels between 600 and 1200 mg/dL. Typical cutaneous and tendon stigmata are evident by school age, and untreated patients can have symptomatic coronary heart disease in childhood and adolescence. Patients with homozygous FH are usually treated with lipid apheresis every 2 weeks, sometimes together with high-dose statins and ezetimibe.[25]

Descriptions of other genetic forms of dyslipidemia, including familial combined hyperlipidemia and elevated lipoprotein (a), a subclass of the LDL particle with shared gene sequence and structural homology with plasminogen, appear elsewhere.[26,27]

Secondary Causes of Dyslipidemia

Although lipid abnormalities in childhood most often result from inherited metabolic disorders and suboptimal lifestyle (e.g., obesity, poor diet, sedentary lifestyle), dyslipidemia can also be secondary to systemic disorders. Most secondary causes of dyslipidemia can be discerned from a careful history and physical examination. Common secondary causes include use of medications, endocrine and metabolic disorders, obstructive liver disease, and renal disease. Profound perturbations of serum lipids occur after significant infections; thus, lipids should be measured no sooner than three weeks 3 a viral or bacterial infection associated with fever. The most common secondary cause of dyslipidemia occurring in the first year of life is obstructive liver disease. Later in childhood, endocrine disorders, especially hypothyroidism, diabetes mellitus, and renal diseases, are the leading secondary causes of dyslipidemia. In adolescence, factors such as medications and smoking play an increased role. For children without a positive family history of hyperlipidemia or obvious secondary causes, measurement of thyroid-stimulating hormone, liver function tests, renal function tests, and urinalysis may be considered.

Management

The first step in management of normal children with LDL cholesterol of 130 mg/dL or higher, or diabetics with LDL cholesterol of at least 100 mg/dL, is counseling for therapeutic lifestyle changes. The Dietary Intervention Study in Children[28] showed that lower-fat diets are safe, effective, and acceptable in high-risk pubertal children. Children and their families should meet with a nutritionist with expertise in lipids, with goals of consuming less than 7% of calories from saturated fat and less than 200 mg cholesterol per day, and increasing dietary fiber. A practical example for families is that each plate of food should be filled by half with salads or vegetables, one fourth with a starch (ideally brown rather than white), and one fourth with protein, such as chicken or fish. In addition, children and adolescents should be counseled to increase their physical activity, ideally to more than 30 minutes of vigorous activity at least 5 days a week. For children who are not involved in team sports, an exercise bicycle or treadmill by the television can motivate exercise. Hyperlipidemic children and their families should be counseled as early as possible, ideally in grade school, regarding the risks of smoking.

Children with elevated triglycerides (≥150 mg/dL) or low HDL cholesterol (<40 mg/dL) are often overweight (body mass index > 85th percentile) or obese (body mass index > 95th percentile). Weight management should be addressed by dietary changes, including smaller portion sizes, lower calorie snacks, and removal of high-calorie foods from the home. Children with elevated triglycerides are advised to decrease intake of simple sugars and refined carbohydrate. Increased physical activity is critical to the success of weight management. Behavior modification programs for weight loss in obese children also may produce long-term success. Isolated elevation of fasting triglyceride is not treated pharmacologically unless fasting levels are greater than 400 mg/dL, when risk for pancreatitis increases.

Children with familial or genetic hyperlipidemia rarely decrease their LDL by more than 15% with diet management alone.[29] If elevation of LDL cholesterol persists and secondary causes of hyperlipidemia are excluded, pharmacologic management may be initiated. Medication is recommended for children older than age 10 years who, despite diet modification, have LDL cholesterol levels of 190 mg/dL or greater without other risk factors, or have LDL levels greater than 160 mg/dL together with at least two other risk factors, such as hypertension, low HDL cholesterol, diabetes, obesity, physical inactivity, or strong family history of premature coronary heart disease.[18]

First-line agents for hyperlipidemia in children and adolescents include both bile acid resin binders, such as cholestyramine, and statins. Cholestyramine has a long track record of safety, with minor gastrointestinal side effects, and reduces LDL cholesterol by 10% to 30%. However, its inconvenience and unpalatability limit patient compliance and hence its utility in later childhood and adolescence.[30–33]

HMG-CoA reductase inhibitors (statins) are the first-line agents for lowering cholesterol in adults, for whom they have been proven to reduce mortality and morbidity from coronary heart disease in both primary and secondary prevention trials.[34,35] In childhood, statins are prescribed primarily to individuals with severe forms of dyslipidemia, such as heterozygous familial hyperlipidemia, or to those with other systemic disorders that put them at high risk, such as diabetes mellitus or cardiac transplantation. Safety and efficacy of statin use in childhood and adolescence have been reported in observational studies[31,36] and short-term clinical trials.[15,33,37–40] Furthermore, statin therapy over a 2-year period decreases carotid atherosclerosis in adolescents with familial hyperlipidemia.[15] Most statins have been approved by the Food and Drug Administration for use in boys older than age 10 years and in girls after menarche. Serious adverse effects include elevation of liver transaminases and, very rarely, rhabdomyolysis, which can lead to renal failure. Because statins are teratogenic, they cannot be used during pregnancy. For this reason, they should be prescribed with caution in sexually active adolescent girls, for whom concomitant use of oral contraceptives may be advisable.

Ezetimibe is a selective inhibitor of cholesterol absorption that lowers LDL cholesterol by preventing the intestinal uptake of dietary and biliary cholesterol.[41–44] When combined with a statin, ezetimibe produces further LDL reduction of about 25%, sometimes accompanied by small increases in HDL cholesterol and modest reductions in triglycerides. Ezetimibe has been approved by the Food and Drug Administration for boys older than age 10 years and adolescent girls after menarche.

Other lipid-lowering agents are seldom used in childhood and adolescence. Nicotinic acid (niacin) is highly effective in increasing HDL cholesterol but is poorly tolerated in children,[45] and fibric acid derivatives have been associated with significant transaminase elevations.[32,46,47]

HYPERTENSION

Hypertension is a leading risk factor for atherosclerotic cardiovascular disease, including coronary heart disease, stroke, and renal failure. In adults, the risk for cardiovascular disease doubles for every increment of 20 mm Hg in systolic blood pressure and 10 mm Hg in diastolic blood pressure starting at 115/75 mm Hg.[48] Because blood pressure tends to track along similar percentiles with increasing age, children with high blood pressure are likely to become hypertensive adults. Furthermore, hypertension is an important component of the metabolic syndrome, which has become increasingly common in children as the U.S. obesity epidemic strikes even the young.

Updated normative values for systolic and diastolic blood pressure in children and adolescents based on age, gender, and height percentile are summarized in Tables 23-3 and 23-4. Hypertension is defined as average systolic or diastolic blood pressure greater than the 95th percentile for age, gender, and height percentile measured on at least three separate occasions.[49] Those with systolic or diastolic blood pressures between the 90th and 95th percentiles are classified as having prehypertension. As in adults, children and adolescents whose blood pressures are between 120 mm Hg (systolic) or 80 mm Hg (diastolic), respectively, and the 95th percentiles for systolic or diastolic blood pressure are now classified as prehypertensive. "White-coat hypertension" refers to the patient whose blood pressure is greater than the 95th percentile in the physician's office but less than the 90th percentile outside a clinical setting. Because end-organ damage from hypertension can occur even in young people, well children should undergo regular measurement of blood pressure during well-child visits to the pediatrician beginning at age 3 years.

Decisions regarding evaluation and management of children and adolescents with hypertension depend on the degree of elevation of blood pressure.[49] Stage 1 hypertension is defined as blood pressure levels ranging from the 95th percentile to 5 mm Hg above the 99th percentile. Stage 2 hypertension is defined as blood pressure levels greater than 5 mm Hg above the 99th percentile. Asymptomatic patients with stage 1 hypertension may undergo a diagnostic evaluation before initiation of treatment. Those with stage 2 hypertension should undergo more timely evaluation and initiation of

TABLE 23–3. Blood Pressure Levels for Boys by Age and Height Percentile

		SBP (mm Hg)							DBP (mm Hg)						
		Percentile of Height							Percentile of Height						
Age (y)	BP Percentile	*5th*	*10th*	*25th*	*50th*	*75th*	*90th*	*95th*	*5th*	*10th*	*25th*	*50th*	*75th*	*90th*	*95th*
1	50th	80	81	83	85	87	88	89	34	35	36	37	38	39	39
	90th	94	95	97	99	100	102	103	49	50	51	52	53	53	54
	95th	98	99	101	103	104	106	106	54	54	55	56	57	58	58
	99th	105	106	108	110	112	113	114	61	62	63	64	65	66	66
2	50th	84	85	87	88	90	92	92	39	40	41	42	43	44	44
	90th	97	99	100	102	104	105	106	54	55	56	57	58	58	59
	95th	101	102	104	106	108	109	110	59	59	60	61	62	63	63
	99th	109	110	111	113	115	117	117	66	67	68	69	70	71	71
3	50th	86	87	89	91	93	94	95	44	44	45	46	47	48	48
	90th	100	101	103	105	107	108	109	59	59	60	61	62	63	63
	95th	104	105	107	109	110	112	113	63	63	64	65	66	67	67
	99th	111	112	114	116	118	119	120	71	71	72	73	74	75	75
4	50th	88	89	91	93	95	96	97	47	48	49	50	51	51	52
	90th	102	103	105	107	109	110	111	62	63	64	65	66	66	67
	95th	106	107	109	111	112	114	115	66	67	68	69	70	71	71
	99th	113	114	116	118	120	121	122	74	75	76	77	78	78	79
5	50th	90	91	93	95	96	98	98	50	51	52	53	54	55	55
	90th	104	105	106	108	110	111	112	65	66	67	68	69	69	70
	95th	108	109	110	112	114	115	116	69	70	71	725	73	74	74
	99th	115	116	118	120	121	123	123	77	78	79	80	81	81	82
6	50th	91	92	94	96	98	99	100	53	53	54	55	56	57	57
	90th	105	106	108	110	111	113	113	68	68	69	70	71	72	72
	95th	109	110	112	114	115	117	117	72	72	73	74	75	76	76
	99th	116	117	119	121	123	124	125	80	80	81	82	83	84	84
7	50th	92	94	95	97	99	100	101	55	55	56	57	58	59	59
	90th	106	107	109	111	113	114	115	70	70	71	72	73	74	74
	95th	110	111	113	115	117	118	119	74	74	75	76	77	78	78
	99th	117	118	120	122	124	125	126	82	82	83	84	85	86	86
8	50th	94	95	97	99	100	102	102	56	57	58	59	60	60	61
	90th	107	109	110	112	114	115	116	71	72	72	73	74	75	76
	95th	111	112	114	116	118	119	120	75	76	77	78	79	79	80
	99th	119	120	122	123	125	127	127	83	84	85	86	87	87	88
9	50th	95	96	98	100	102	103	104	57	58	59	60	61	61	62
	90th	109	110	112	114	115	117	118	72	73	74	75	76	76	77
	95th	113	114	116	118	119	121	121	76	77	78	79	80	81	81
	99th	120	121	123	125	127	128	129	84	85	86	87	88	88	89
10	50th	97	98	100	102	103	105	106	58	59	60	61	61	62	63
	90th	111	112	114	115	117	119	119	73	73	74	75	76	77	78
	95th	115	116	117	119	121	122	123	77	78	79	80	81	81	82
	99th	122	123	15	127	128	130	130	85	86	86	88	88	89	90
11	50th	99	100	102	104	105	107	107	59	59	60	61	62	63	63
	90th	113	114	115	117	119	120	121	74	74	75	76	77	78	78
	95th	117	118	119	121	123	124	125	78	78	79	80	81	82	82
	99th	124	125	127	129	130	132	132	86	86	87	88	89	90	90
12	50th	101	102	104	106	108	109	110	59	60	61	62	63	63	64
	90th	115	116	118	120	121	123	123	74	75	75	76	77	78	79
	95th	119	120	122	123	125	127	127	78	79	80	81	82	82	83
	99th	126	127	129	131	133	134	135	86	87	88	89	90	90	91
13	50th	104	105	106	108	110	111	112	60	60	61	62	63	64	64
	90th	117	118	120	122	124	125	126	75	75	76	77	78	79	79
	95th	121	122	124	126	128	129	130	79	79	80	81	82	83	83
	99th	128	130	131	133	135	136	137	98	98	88	89	90	91	91

TABLE 23–3. Blood Pressure Levels for Boys by Age and Height Percentile—cont'd

		SBP (mm Hg)							DBP (mm Hg)						
		Percentile of Height							Percentile of Height						
Age (y)	BP Percentile	*5th*	*10th*	*25th*	*50th*	*75th*	*90th*	*95th*	*5th*	*10th*	*25th*	*50th*	*75th*	*90th*	*95th*
14	50th	106	107	109	111	113	114	115	60	61	62	63	64	65	65
	90th	120	121	123	125	126	128	128	75	76	77	78	79	79	80
	95th	124	125	127	128	130	132	132	80	80	81	82	83	84	84
	99th	131	132	134	136	138	139	140	87	88	89	90	91	92	92
15	50th	109	110	112	113	115	117	117	61	62	63	64	65	66	66
	90th	122	124	125	127	129	130	131	76	77	78	79	80	80	81
	95th	126	127	129	131	133	134	135	81	81	82	83	84	85	85
	99th	134	135	136	138	140	142	142	88	89	90	91	92	93	93
16	50th	111	112	114	116	118	119	120	63	63	64	65	66	67	67
	90th	125	126	128	130	131	133	134	78	78	79	80	8	82	82
	95th	129	130	132	134	135	137	137	82	83	83	84	85	86	87
	99th	136	137	139	141	143	144	145	90	90	91	92	93	94	94
17	50th	114	115	116	118	120	121	122	65	66	66	67	68	69	70
	90th	127	128	130	132	134	135	136	80	80	81	82	83	84	84
	95th	131	132	134	136	138	139	140	84	85	86	87	87	88	89
	99th	139	140	141	143	145	146	147	92	93	93	94	95	96	97

The 90th percentile is 1.28 SD, the 95th percentile is 1.645 SD, and the 9th percentile is 2.326 SD over the mean.
For research purposes, the SDs in Table B1 allow one to compute BP *z* scores and percentiles for boys with height percentiles given in Table 3 (ie, the 5th, 10th, 20th, 25th, 50th, 75th, 90th, and 95th percentiles). These height percentiles must be converted to height z scores given by: 5% = −1.645; 10% = −1.28; 25% = −0.68; 50% = 0; 75% = 0.68; 90% = 1.28; and 95% = 1.645, and then computed according to the methodology in steps 2 through 4 described in Appendix B. For children with height percentiles other than these, follow steps 1 through 4 as described in Appendix B.
From National High Blood Pressure Education Program Working Group on High Blood Pressure in Children and Adolescents. The fourth report on the diagnosis, evaluation, and treatment of high blood pressure in children and adolescents. Pediatrics, 114:555, 2004.

TABLE 23–4. Blood Pressure Levels for Girls by Age and Height Percentile

		SBP (mm Hg)							DBP (mm Hg)						
		Percentile of Height							Percentile of Height						
Age (y)	BP Percentile	*5th*	*10th*	*25th*	*50th*	*75th*	*90th*	*95th*	*5th*	*10th*	*25th*	*50th*	*75th*	*90th*	*95th*
1	50th	83	84	85	86	88	89	90	38	39	39	40	41	41	42
	90th	97	97	98	100	101	102	103	52	53	53	54	55	55	56
	95th	100	101	102	104	105	106	107	56	57	57	58	59	59	60
	99th	108	108	109	111	112	113	114	64	64	65	65	66	67	67
2	50th	85	85	87	88	89	91	91	43	44	44	45	46	46	47
	90th	98	99	100	101	103	104	105	57	58	58	59	60	61	61
	95th	102	103	104	105	107	108	109	61	62	62	63	64	65	65
	99th	109	110	111	112	114	115	116	69	69	70	70	71	72	72
3	50th	86	87	88	89	91	92	93	47	48	48	49	50	50	51
	90th	100	100	102	103	104	106	106	61	62	62	63	64	64	65
	95th	104	104	105	107	108	109	110	65	66	66	67	68	68	69
	99th	111	111	113	114	115	116	117	73	73	74	74	75	76	76
4	50th	88	88	90	91	92	94	94	50	50	51	52	52	53	54
	90th	101	102	103	104	106	107	108	64	64	65	66	67	67	68
	95th	105	106	107	108	110	111	112	68	68	69	70	71	71	72
	99th	112	113	114	115	117	118	119	76	76	76	77	78	79	79
5	50th	89	90	91	93	94	95	96	52	53	53	54	55	55	56
	90th	103	103	105	106	107	109	109	66	67	67	68	69	69	70
	95th	107	107	108	110	111	112	113	70	71	71	72	73	73	74
	99th	114	114	116	117	118	120	120	78	78	79	79	80	81	81

(Continued)

TABLE 23–4. Blood Pressure Levels for Girls by Age and Height Percentile—cont'd

		SBP (mm Hg)							DBP (mm Hg)						
		Percentile of Height							Percentile of Height						
Age (y)	BP Percentile	*5th*	*10th*	*25th*	*50th*	*75th*	*90th*	*95th*	*5th*	*10th*	*25th*	*50th*	*75th*	*90th*	*95th*
6	50th	91	92	93	94	96	97	98	54	54	55	56	56	57	58
	90th	104	105	106	108	109	110	111	68	68	69	70	70	71	72
	95th	108	109	110	111	113	114	115	72	72	73	74	74	75	76
	99th	115	116	117	119	120	121	122	80	80	80	81	82	83	83
7	50th	93	93	95	96	97	99	99	55	56	56	57	58	58	59
	90th	106	107	108	109	111	112	113	69	70	70	71	72	72	73
	95th	110	111	112	113	115	116	116	73	74	74	75	76	76	77
	99th	117	118	119	120	122	123	124	81	81	82	82	83	84	84
8	50th	95	95	96	98	99	100	101	57	57	57	58	59	60	60
	90th	108	109	110	111	113	114	114	71	71	71	72	73	74	74
	95th	112	112	114	115	116	118	118	75	75	75	76	77	78	78
	99th	119	120	121	122	123	125	125	82	82	83	83	84	85	85
9	50th	96	97	98	100	101	102	103	58	58	58	59	60	61	61
	90th	110	110	112	113	114	116	116	72	72	72	73	74	75	75
	95th	114	114	115	117	118	119	120	76	76	76	77	78	79	79
	99th	121	121	123	124	125	127	127	83	83	84	84	85	86	87
10	50th	98	99	100	102	103	104	105	59	59	59	60	61	62	62
	90th	112	112	114	115	116	118	118	73	73	73	74	75	76	76
	95th	116	116	117	119	120	121	122	77	77	77	78	79	80	80
	99th	123	123	125	126	127	129	129	84	84	85	86	86	87	88
11	50th	100	101	102	103	105	106	107	60	60	60	61	62	63	63
	90th	114	114	116	117	118	119	120	74	74	74	75	76	77	77
	95th	118	118	119	121	122	123	124	78	78	78	79	80	81	81
	99th	125	125	126	128	129	130	131	85	85	86	87	87	88	89
12	50th	102	103	104	105	107	108	109	61	61	61	62	63	64	64
	90th	116	116	117	119	120	121	122	75	75	75	76	77	78	78
	95th	119	120	121	123	124	125	126	79	79	79	80	81	82	82
	99th	127	127	128	130	131	132	133	86	86	87	88	88	89	90
13	50th	104	105	106	107	109	110	110	62	62	62	63	64	65	65
	90th	117	118	119	121	122	123	124	76	76	76	77	78	79	79
	95th	121	122	123	124	126	127	128	80	80	80	81	82	83	83
	99th	128	129	130	132	133	134	135	87	87	88	89	89	90	91
14	50th	106	106	107	109	110	111	112	63	63	63	64	65	66	66
	90th	119	120	121	122	124	125	125	77	77	77	78	79	80	80
	95th	123	123	125	126	127	129	129	81	81	81	82	83	84	84
	99th	130	131	132	133	135	136	136	88	88	89	90	90	91	92
15	50th	107	108	109	110	111	113	113	4	64	64	65	66	67	67
	90th	120	121	122	123	125	126	127	78	78	78	79	80	81	81
	95th	124	125	126	127	129	130	131	82	82	82	83	84	85	85
	99th	131	132	133	134	136	137	138	89	89	90	91	91	92	93
16	50th	108	108	110	111	112	114	114	64	64	65	66	66	67	68
	90th	121	122	123	124	126	127	128	78	78	79	80	81	81	82
	95th	125	126	127	128	130	131	132	82	82	83	84	85	85	86
	99th	132	133	134	135	137	138	139	90	90	90	91	92	93	93
17	50th	108	109	110	111	113	114	115	64	65	65	66	67	67	68
	90th	122	122	123	125	126	127	128	78	79	79	80	81	81	82
	95th	125	126	127	129	130	131	132	82	83	83	84	85	85	86
	99th	133	133	134	136	137	138	139	90	90	91	91	92	93	93

The 90th percentile is 1.28 SD, the 95th percentile is 1.645 SD, and the 9th percentile is 2.326 SD over the mean.

For research purposes, the SDs in Table B1 allow one to compute BP z scores and percentiles for girls with height percentiles given in Table 4 (ie, the 5th, 10th, 20th, 25th, 50th, 75th, 90th, and 95th opercentiles). These height percentiles must be converted to height z scores given by: 5% = −1.645; 10% = −1.28; 25% = −0.68; 50% = 0; 75% = 0.68; 90% = 1.28; and 95% = 1.645, and then computed according to the methodology in steps 2 through 4 described in Appendix B. For children with height percentiles other than these, follow steps 1 through 4 as described in Appendix B.

From National High Blood Pressure Education Program Working Group on High Blood Pressure in Children and Adolescents. The fourth report on the diagnosis, evaluation, and treatment of high blood pressure in children and adolescents. Pediatrics, 114:555, 2004.

antihypertensive therapy. When symptomatic, patients with stage 2 hypertension require immediate pharmacologic treatment and consultation with an expert.

Measurement

Systolic blood pressure occurs at the moment of ventricular systole, whereas diastolic pressure occurs in ventricular diastole immediately preceding systole. Although these definitions were originally based on studies using indwelling catheters, an array of noninvasive methods are available for blood pressure assessment. Traditionally, blood pressure has been taken by auscultation with a mercury sphygmomanometer or a calibrated aneroid device in a patient at rest in the sitting position for at least 5 minutes with feet on the floor and arm supported at the heart level. The cuff bladder should cover 80% to 100% of the arm circumference and two thirds of the length of the upper arm; smaller cuff sizes result in erroneous elevation of blood pressure. The cuff should be inflated to a pressure 20 to 30 mm Hg higher than the patient's systolic pressure, and then deflated at 2- to 3-mm Hg each second. Systolic pressure occurs when the first sound is heard during cuff deflation (i.e., the first Korotkoff sound, or K_1), and diastolic pressure occurs at the point before disappearance of sounds (K_5). Many centers now use automated oscillometric devices, which are easy to use and eliminate inter observer variation, but for which measurements may vary from those obtained by auscultation.[50] If blood pressure is greater than the 90th percentile by oscillometric device, the measurement should be repeated by auscultation.[49] Some patients have home measurement devices; these should be calibrated at regular intervals for accuracy. Ambulatory 24-hour blood pressure monitoring, obtained with oscillometric devices, identifies patients with white-coat hypertension and nocturnal hypertension and is useful for management of patients with known hypertension.[51,52] The results of 24-hour blood pressure monitoring correlate better with end-organ damage than does the office blood pressure[52] and may be useful in differentiating primary and secondary hypertension.[53]

Diagnostic Evaluation

Figure 23-1 summarizes the management algorithm for evaluation and treatment of children and adolescents with stage 1 and 2 hypertension. Similar to evaluation of hypertensive adults, evaluation of the child and adolescent with hypertension aims to (1) assess lifestyle and identify other cardiovascular risk factors or concomitant diseases that could affect prognosis and guide treatment; (2) detect secondary causes of hypertension; and (3) assess end-organ damage (e.g., left ventricular hypertrophy).[48] Most children

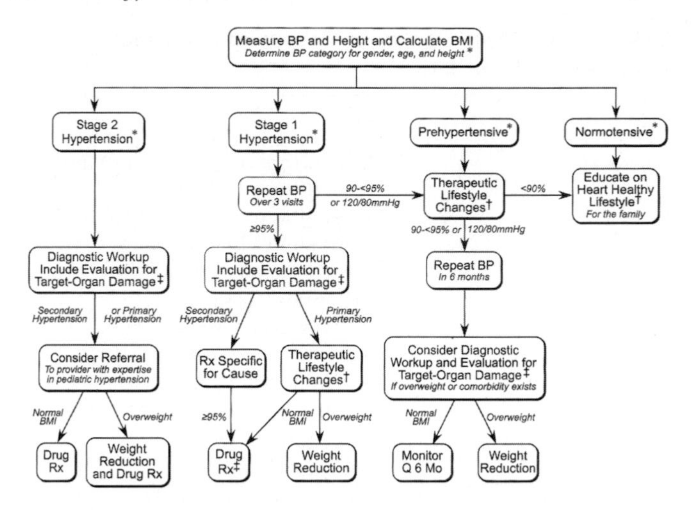

FIGURE 23–1 *Management algorithm. Rx, prescription; Q, every; *, see text; ‡, especially if younger, very high blood pressure, little or no family history, diabetic, or other risk factors.*

have no symptoms. Medical history should inquire about medical conditions; use of medications; family history of hypertension, premature atherosclerotic cardiovascular disease, diabetes, and renal disease; and, in adolescents, substance abuse. In addition to the routine cardiovascular exam, physical examination should include calculation of body mass index, examination of the optic fundi, palpation of the thyroid gland, and auscultation for carotid and abdominal bruits.

Most children older than age 6 years and adolescents with blood pressure at the 95th percentile have primary hypertension, with positive family histories or with obesity.[19] Obese patients with prehypertension and all patients with hypertension should undergo a fasting lipid profile and fasting glucose to better assess risk for future atherosclerotic cardiovascular disease.[48,49] A hemoglobin A1c test should be performed in those with obesity and a strong family history of type 2 diabetes. Children, especially those who are obese, with a history of loud, frequent snoring should undergo polysomnography to exclude hypertension on the basis of a sleep disorder.

Diagnostic tests that are recommended in the initial evaluation of all patients with hypertension include a complete blood count, urinalysis, urine culture, serum electrolytes, blood urea nitrogen, and creatinine.[49] In addition, a renal Doppler ultrasound is recommended to screen for hydronephrosis, renovascular hypertension, or renal parenchymal abnormalities.[49] When substance abuse is suspected, laboratory testing should include a drug screen. Finally, prehypertensive patients with comorbid risk factors, as well as all hypertensive patients, should undergo two-dimensional echocardiography to identify left ventricular hypertrophy.[49]

TABLE 23–5. Most Common Causes of Secondary Hypertension, by Age

Age Group	Cause
Newborn	Renal artery or venous thrombosis Renal artery stenosis Congenital renal abnormalities Coarctation of the aorta Bronchopulmonary dysplasia
First year	Coarctation of the aorta Renovascular disease Renal parenchymal disease Iatrogenic (medication, volume) Tumor
Infancy to 6 yr	Renal parenchymal disease Renovascular disease Coarctation of the aorta Endocrine causes* Iatrogenic Essential hypertension* Renal parenchymal disease
6-10 yr	Renovascular disease Essential hypertension Coarctation of the aorta Endocrine causes* Iatrogenic* Essential hypertension
12-18 yr	Iatrogenic Renal parenchymal disease* Endocrine causes* Coarctation of the aorta*

*Uncommon for category.
From Swinford RD, Ingelfinger JR. Evaluation of hypertension in childhood diseases. In Barratt TM, Avner ED, Harmon WD (eds). Pediatric Nephrology, 4th ed. Baltimore: Lippincott Williams & Wilkins, 1999:1007.

Secondary causes of hypertension are much more likely in young children with stage 1 hypertension, children or adolescents with stage 2 hypertension, and those with a history or findings on screening tests suggestive of underlying medical conditions (Table 23-5). By far the most common cause of secondary hypertension is renal disease, usually renal parenchymal disease secondary to reflux nephropathy, pyelonephritis, or obstructive uropathy.[54] Other renal causes of hypertension include glomerulonephritis, nephrotic syndrome, hemolytic-uremic syndrome, polycystic kidney disease, or congenital renal dysplasia. Studies to image renal parenchymal disease include the renal ultrasound, voiding cystourethrogram, or renal scintiscan.

In 8% to 10% of children, secondary hypertension is caused by renovascular abnormalities, including unilateral or bilateral renal artery stenosis, occurring in the main renal artery or in segmental branch arteries.[54,55] A variety of noninvasive diagnostic tests are used for evaluation of renovascular hypertension, including renal scintiscan with angiotensin-converting enzyme (ACE) inhibition and noninvasive angiography using digital subtraction, computed tomography, or magnetic resonance imaging. The gold standard for diagnosis remains conventional angiography, sometimes with intra-arterial digital subtraction, and this test should be performed in children with severe hypertension, especially when it occurs together with very high plasma renin activity, an abdominal bruit, or a solitary kidney.[54]

Coarctation of the aorta is one of the most common causes of hypertension cared for by the pediatric cardiologist. The diagnosis of coarctation is made easily on the physical examination by finding diminished or delayed femoral pulses and higher blood pressure in the arms than the legs (see Chapter 36). Coarctation of the aorta accounts for one third of cases of secondary hypertension in infancy, but only 2% of cases first detected in childhood and adolescence.[54,56,57] Even after repair, many children continue to have systemic hypertension with a mild residual gradient from upper to lower extremities at rest or sometimes only evident with exercise. For this reason, patients often require chronic antihypertensive medication after coarctation repair, together with stenting of the aorta in those with persistent gradients.[58]

Endocrine disorders may also cause secondary hypertension.[59] Pheochromocytoma, accounting for 0.5% to 2.0% of childhood secondary hypertension, may cause sustained or, much less commonly, episodic hypertension.[54,60,61] The diagnosis is suggested by elevated urinary catecholamines on 24-hour urine collection or elevation of plasma catecholamines. Imaging tests for pheochromocytoma include the T2-weighted or gadolinium-DPTA enhanced magnetic resonance imaging or meta-iodo-benzyl guanidine (MIBG) scanning.[54,62,63] Other endocrine causes of secondary hypertension, such as excess glucocorticoids or mineralocorticoids, or hyperthyroidism, should be excluded as appropriate based on initial screening.

Hypertension of central nervous system origin is rare but may have a fulminant presentation.[54,64] Central nervous system causes may be primary (e.g., brain tumor) or secondary to the biochemical milieu (e.g., hypercalcemia, lead poisoning).

Management

Initial management of mild hypertension or prehypertension includes counseling regarding healthy lifestyles. Lifestyle modifications that have been proven in adults to lower blood pressure include weight reduction in those who are overweight or obese[65]; adoption of the Dietary Approaches to Stop Hypertension (DASH) diet, which is rich in fruits, vegetables, and low-fat dairy products, with reduced saturated fat[66]; reduction in intake of sodium chloride[67]; and increase in physical activity.[68] Indeed, uncomplicated hypertension should not lead to restriction of physical activity because regular exercise may actually lower blood pressure, especially in obese subjects.[69] Those who smoke should be vigorously encouraged to quit, and use of anabolic steroids should be strongly discouraged. Although few adolescents will admit to excessive alcohol intake, they should nonetheless be instructed about the role of alcohol in hypertension.[70] Whenever possible, these lifestyle modifications should be combined and adopted by the entire family.

Indications for use of antihypertensive medication in children and adolescents include symptomatic hypertension, secondary hypertension, high risk for future atherosclerotic cardiovascular disease based on presence of additional risk factors (e.g., diabetes mellitus or multiple other cardiovascular risk factors), or evidence of end-organ effects, such as increased left ventricular mass on two-dimensional echocardiography or cardiac magnetic resonance imaging.[49] Medication also should be initiated when nonpharmacologic measures fail to control hypertension.[49] The goal of pharmacologic management in children and adolescents should be to reduce blood pressure to below the 95th percentile, or lower in patients with diabetes, renal disease, or other major risk factors.

Excellent data in adults suggest that complications of hypertension can be reduced by lowering blood pressure with many classes of agents, including thiazide-type diuretics, ACE inhibitors, β blockers, angiotensin receptor blockers (ARBs), and calcium channel blockers.[48] Each of these classes of antihypertensive agent has been shown to lower blood pressure in children.[49] Of note, because ACE inhibitors and ARBs are teratogenic, they should not be used in adolescent girls who may become pregnant.

The long-term risks and benefits of specific antihypertensive medications in children and adolescents are not known. Therefore, the choice of an optimal antihypertensive regimen must derive, in part, from studies in adults. The recently published trial in adults, Antihypertensive and Lipid Lowering Treatment to Prevent Heart Attack Trial (ALLHAT), recommended that thiazide-type diuretics be used as initial therapy for most adults with hypertension, either alone or in combination with other classes of medication.[71] The Second Australian National Blood Pressure Study found that males treated with ACE inhibitors as initial therapy had a slightly lower incidence of cardiovascular events or all-cause mortality than those treated with thiazides.[72] There is consensus that ACE inhibitors are a better choice for first-line therapy in those with ventricular dysfunction or heart failure.[48,73] For patients with hyperlipidemia, chronic renal disease, or diabetes, initial antihypertensive management should include an ACE inhibitor or ARB.[48] ACE inhibitors and ARBs have been shown to have a favorable effect on the progression of diabetic and nondiabetic renal disease.[48] For patients with mild renal disease, these can be used as long as serum creatinine does not rise more than 35% above baseline and there is no hyperkalemia. For patients with hypertension and stable coronary artery disease, a rarity in pediatrics except for FH homozygotes and Kawasaki disease patients, β blockers are the drug of first choice.[48,73] African American patients with hypertension often respond better to monotherapy with diuretics and calcium channel blockers than to ACE inhibitors, β blockers, or ARBs.[48] Of note, patients with severe hypertension often require management with more than one therapy, and many drugs are available in convenient combination products.[73]

REFERENCES

1. Enos WF, Holmes RH, Beyer J. Coronary disease among United States soldiers killed in action in Korea. JAMA 152:1090, 1953.
2. Strong JP, Malcom GT, McMahan CA, et al. Prevalence and extent of atherosclerosis in adolescents and young adults: Implications for prevention from the Pathobiological Determinants of Atherosclerosis in Youth Study. JAMA 281:727, 1999.
3. Berenson GS, Srinivasan SR, Bao W et al. Association between multiple cardiovascular risk factors and atherosclerosis in children and young adults. N Engl J Med 338:1650, 1998.
4. Nicklas TA, von Duvillard SP, Berenson GS. Tracking of serum lipids and lipoproteins from childhood to dyslipidemia in adults: The Bogalusa Heart Study. Int J Sports Med 23(Suppl 1):S39, 2002.
5. Fuentes RM, Notkola IL, Shemeikka S, et al. Tracking of serum total cholesterol during childhood: An 8-year follow-up population-based family study in eastern Finland. Acta Paediatr 92:420, 2003.
6. Klag MJ, Ford DE, Mead LA, et al. Serum cholesterol in young men and subsequent cardiovascular disease. N Engl J Med 328:313, 1993.
7. Lee J, Lauer RM, Clarke WR. Lipoproteins in the progeny of young men with coronary artery disease: Children with increased risk. Pediatrics 78:330, 1986.
8. Lauer RM, Clarke WR. Childhood risk factors for high adult blood pressure: The Muscatine Study. Pediatrics 84:633, 1984.
9. Shear CL, Burke GL, Freedman DS, et al. Value of childhood blood pressure measurements and family history in predicting future blood pressure status: Results from 8 years of follow-up in the Bogalusa. Pediatrics 77:862, 1986.
10. Prineas RJ, Gomez-Marin O, Gillum RF. Tracking of blood pressure in children and nonpharmacological approaches to the prevention of hypertension. Ann Behav Med 7:25, 1985.
11. de Ferranti SD, Gauvreau K, Ludwig DS, et al. Prevalence of the metabolic syndrome in American adolescents:

Findings from the Third National Health and Nutrition Examination Survey. Circulation 2004 (in press).
12. Mietus-Snyder M, Malloy MJ. Endothelial dysfunction occurs in children with two genetic hyperlipidemias: Improvement with antioxidant vitamin therapy. J Pediatr 133:35, 1998.
13. Pauciullo P, Arcangelo I, Renata S, et al. Increased intima-media thickness of the common carotid artery in hypercholesterolemic children. Arterioscler Thromb 7:1075, 1994.
14. Tonstad S, Joakimsen O, Stensland-Bugge E, et al. Risk factors related to carotid intima-media thickness and plaque in children with familial hypercholesterolemia and control subjects. Arterioscler Thromb Vasc Biol 16:984, 1996.
15. Wiegman A, de Groot E, Hutten BA, et al. Arterial intima-media thickness in children heterozygous for familial hypercholesterolaemia. Lancet 363:369, 2004.
16. Mahoney LT, Burns TL, Stanford W, et al. Coronary risk factors measured in childhood and young adult life are associated with coronary artery calcification in young adults: The Muscatine Study. J Am Coll Cardiol 27:277, 1996.
17. Third Report of the National Cholesterol Education Program (NCEP) Expert Panel on Detection, Evaluation, and Treatment of High Blood Cholesterol in Adults (Adult Treatment Panel III). NIH Publication No. 02-5215. Bethesda, MD: National Heart, Lung, and Blood Institute, National Institutes of Health, 2002
18. National Cholesterol Education Program. Report of the Expert Panel on Blood Cholesterol Levels in Children and Adolescents. NIH Publication 91-2732. Bethesda, MD: National Heart, Lung, and Blood Institute, 1991.
19. Williams CL, Hayman LL, Daniels SR, et al. Cardiovascular health in childhood: A statement for health professionals from the Committee on Atherosclerosis, Hypertension, and Obesity in the Young (AHOY) of the Council on Cardiovascular Disease in the Young, American Heart Association. Circulation 106:143, 2002.
20. Dennison BA, Kikuchi DA, Srinivasan SR, et al. Parental history of cardiovascular disease as an indication for screening for lipoprotein abnormalities in children. J Pediatr 115:186, 1989.
21. Garcia RE, Moodie DS. Routine cholesterol surveillance in childhood. Pediatrics 84:751, 1989.
22. Griffin TC, Christoffel KK, Binns HJ, et al. Family history evaluation as a predictive screen for childhood hypercholesterolemia. Pediatrics 84:365, 1989.
23. Hickman TB, Briefel RR, Carroll MD, et al. Distributions and trends of serum lipid levels among United States children and adolescents ages 4–19 years: Data from the Third National Health and Nutrition Examination Survey. Prev Med 27:879, 1998.
24. Wiegman A, Rodenburg J, de Jongh S, et al. Family history and cardiovascular risk in familial hypercholesterolemia: Data in more than 1000 children. Circulation 107:1473, 2003.
25. Marais AD, Firth JC, Blom DJ. Homozygous familial hypercholesterolemia and its management. Semin Vasc Med 4:43, 2004.
26. Wilcken DE. Overview of inherited metabolic disorders causing cardiovascular disease. J Inherit Metab Dis 26:245, 2003.
27. Belay B, Belamarich P, Racine AD. Pediatric precursors of adult atherosclerosis. Pediatr Rev 25:4, 2004.
28. The Writing Group for the DISC Collaborative Research Group. Efficacy and Safety of Lowering Dietary Intake of Fat and Cholesterol in Children with Elevated Low-Density Lipoprotein Cholesterol: The Dietary Intervention Study in Children (DISC). JAMA 18:1429, 1995.
29. Glueck CJ, Mellies MJ, Dine M, et al. Safety and efficacy of long-term diet and diet plus bile acid-binding resin cholesterol-lowering therapy in 73 children heterozygous for familial hypercholesterolemia. Pediatrics 78:338, 1986.
30. West RJ, Lloyd JK, Leonard JV. Long-term follow-up of children with familial hypercholesterolemia tested with cholestyramine. Lancet 2:873, 1980.
31. Stein EA. Treatment of familial hypercholesterolemia with drugs in children. Arteriosclerosis Suppl I:I-145, 1989.
32. Tonstad S, Knudtzon J, Siversten M, et al. Efficacy and safety of cholestyramine therapy in peripubertal and prepubertal children with familial hypercholesterolemia. J Pediatr 129:42, 1996.
33. McCrindle BW, Helden E, Cullen-Dean G, et al. A randomized crossover trial of combination pharmacologic therapy in children with familial hyperlipidemia. Pediatr Res 51:715, 2002.
34. Scandinavian Simvastatin Survival Study Group. Randomized trial of cholesterol-lowering in 4444 patients with coronary heart disease: The Scandinavian Simvastatin Survival Study. Lancet 344:1383, 1994.
35. Shepherd J, Cobbe SM, Ford I, et al. Prevention of coronary heart disease with pravastatin in men with hypercholesterolemia. N Engl J Med 333:1301, 1995.
36. Ducobu J, Brasseur D, Chaudron JM, et al. Simvastatin use in children. Lancet 339:1488, 1992.
37. Knipscheer HC, Boelen CC, Kastelein JJP, et al. Short-term efficacy and safety of pravastatin in 72 children with familial hypercholesterolemia. Pediatr Res 39:867, 1996.
38. Lambert M, Lupien PJ, Gagne C, et al. Treatment of familial hypercholesterolemia in children and adolescents: Effect of lovastatin. Pediatrics 97:619, 1996.
39. Summary of Recommendations of the Conference on Blood Lipids in Children: Optimal levels for early prevention of coronary artery disease. Prev Med 12:728, 1983.
40. McCrindle BW, Ose L, Marais AD. Efficacy and safety of atorvastatin in children and adolescents with familial hypercholesterolemia or severe hyperlipidemia: A multicenter, randomized, placebo-controlled trial. J Pediatr 143:74, 2003.
41. Gagne C, Bays HE, Weiss SR, et al. Efficacy and safety of ezetimibe added to ongoing statin therapy for treatment of patients with primary hypercholesterolemia. Am J Cardiol 90:1084, 2002.
42. Harris M, Davis W, Brown WV. Ezetimibe. Drugs Today (Barc) 39:229, 2003.
43. Hopkins PN. Familial hypercholesterolemia: Improving treatment and meeting guidelines. Int J Cardiol 89:13, 2003.
44. Rudel LL. Preclinical and clinical pharmacology of a new class of lipid management agents. Am J Manag Care 8:S33, 2002.

45. Colletti RB, Neufeld EJ, Roff NK, et al. Niacin treatment of hypercholesterolemia in children. Pediatrics 92:78, 1993.
46. Steinmetz J, Morin C, Panek E, et al. Biological variations in hyperlipidemic children and adolescents treated with fenofibrate. Clin Chim Acta 112:43, 1981.
47. Wheeler KA, West RJ, Lloyd JK, et al. Double-blind trial of bezafibrate in familial hypercholesterolemia. Arch Dis Child 60:34, 1985.
48. Chobanian AV, Bakris GL, Black HR, et al. Seventh report of the Joint National Committee on Prevention, Detection, Evaluation, and Treatment of High Blood Pressure. Hypertension 42:1206, 2003.
49. National High Blood Pressure Education Program Working Group on High Blood Pressure in Children and Adolescents. The Fourth Report on the Diagnosis, Evaluation, and Treatment of High Blood Pressure in Children and Adolescents. Pediatrics 114:555, 2004.
50. Park MK, Menard SW, Yuan C. Comparison of auscultatory and oscillometric blood pressures. Arch Pediatr Adolesc Med 155:50, 2001.
51. Morgenstern B. Blood pressure, hypertension, and ambulatory blood pressure monitoring in children and adolescents. Am J Hypertens 15:64S, 2002.
52. Lurbe E, Redon J. Reproducibility and validity of ambulatory blood pressure monitoring in children. Am J Hypertens 15: 69S, 2002.
53. Flynn JT. Differentiation between primary and secondary hypertension in children using ambulatory blood pressure monitoring. Pediatrics 110:89, 2002.
54. Swinford RD, Ingelfinger JR. Evaluation of hypertension in childhood diseases. In Barratt TM AEHW (ed). Pediatric Nephrology. Baltimore: Lippincott Williams & Wilkins, 1999: 1007–1030.
55. Sinaiko AR. Childhood hypertension. In Hypertension: Pathophysiology, Diagnosis, and Management. New York: Raven Press, 1995:209–225.
56. Londe S. Causes of hypertension in the young. Pediatr Clin North Am 25:55, 1978.
57. Alpert BS, Bain HH, Balfe JW. Role of the renin-angiotensin-aldosterone system in hypertensive children with coarctation of the aorta. Am J Cardiol 43:828, 1979.
58. Hornung TS, Benson LN, McLaughlin PR. Interventions for aortic coarctation. Cardiol Rev 10:139, 2002.
59. Rodd CJ, Sockalosky JJ. Endocrine causes of hypertension in children. Pediatr Clin North Am 40:149, 1993.
60. Deal JE, Sever PS, Barratt TM, et al. Phaeochromocytoma: Investigation and management of 10 cases. Arch Dis Child 65:269, 1990.
61. Stackpole RH, Melicow MM, Uson AC. Pheochromocytoma in children. J Pediatr 63:315, 1963.
62. Schmedtje JF, Sax S, Poole JL et al. Imaging methods in diagnosis of pheochromocytoma. Bildgeb Chir 122:438, 1997.
63. Boraschi P, Braccini G, Grassi L, et al. Incidentally discovered adrenal masses: Evaluation with gadolinium enhancement and fat-suppressed MR imaging at 0.5. Eur J Radiol 24:245, 1997.
64. Phillips SJ, Whisnant JP. Hypertension and the brain. National High Blood Pressure Education Program. Arch Intern Med 152:938, 1992.
65. He J, Whelton PK, Appel LJ, et al. Long-term effects of weight loss and dietary sodium reduction on incidence of hypertension. Hypertension 35:544, 2000.
66. Sacks FM, Svetkey LP, Vollmer WM, et al. Effects on blood pressure of reduced dietary sodium and the Dietary Approaches to Stop Hypertension (DASH) diet. DASH-Sodium Collaborative Research Group. N Engl J Med 344:3, 2001.
67. Chobanian AV, Hill M. National Heart, Lung, and Blood Institute Workshop on Sodium and Blood Pressure: A critical review of current scientific evidence. Hypertension 35:858, 2000.
68. Whelton SP, Chin A, Xin X, et al. Effect of aerobic exercise on blood pressure: A meta-analysis of randomized, controlled trials. Ann Intern Med 136:493, 2002.
69. Barlow SE, Dietz WH. Obesity evaluation and treatment: Expert Committee recommendations. Maternal and Child Health Bureau, Health Resources and Services Administration and the Department of Health and Human Services. Pediatrics 102:E29, 1998.
70. Xin X, He J, Frontini MG, et al. Effects of alcohol reduction on blood pressure: A meta-analysis of randomized controlled trials. Hypertension 38:1112, 2001.
71. Major outcomes in high-risk hypertensive patients randomized to angiotensin-converting enzyme inhibitor or calcium channel blocker vs diuretic. The Antihypertensive and Lipid-Lowering Treatment to Prevent Heart Attack Trial (ALLHAT). JAMA 288:2981, 2002.
72. Wing LM, Reid CM, Ryan P, et al. A comparison of outcomes with angiotensin-converting–enzyme inhibitors and diuretics for hypertension in the elderly. N Engl J Med 348:583, 2003.
73. Initial therapy of hypertension. Med Lett 46:53, 2004.

24

Rheumatic Fever

DONALD C. FYLER

DEFINITION

Rheumatic fever, although still without precise pathogenesis, is considered to be a delayed autoimmune reaction in genetically predisposed individuals to group A, β-hemolytic, streptococcal pharyngitis. It is a self-limited disease that may involve joints, skin, brain, serous surfaces, and the heart. Were it not for cardiac valve damage, the disease would be of little practical consequence.

PREVALENCE

"In the 1920's rheumatic fever was the leading cause of death in individuals between 5 and 20 years of age ... in 1938 there were more than a thousand deaths in New York City alone ... In New England, childhood rheumatism accounted for nearly half of adult heart disease and in Boston's crowded North End hardly a family was spared"[1] (Fig. 24-1).

In developed countries, rheumatic fever and rheumatic heart disease had almost disappeared by the early 1980s. Some localized resurgences, peaking in 1985, then occurred[2] related to reappearance of streptococci with virulent M-protein serotypes once prevalent in epidemics[3] some of which have again decreased[4–7] (Table 24-1). In stark contrast, rheumatic fever and rheumatic heart disease remain a major problem in developing countries, where it is estimated that rheumatic fever affects some 10 to 20 million people each year.[4–8] Rheumatic heart disease remains the primary cause of death from heart disease in those younger than age 50 years,[5] with valve operations accounting for some 30% of all cardiac operations in some countries.[9] The incidence of rheumatic fever in developing countries has been estimated to be at least 150 per 100,000 population, with mortality rates as high as 8.2 per 100,000 from heart involvement, compared with less than 1 per 100,000 and less than or equal to 1.8 per 100,000 respectively, in developed countries.[6]

Several terms, including *developing, Third World, disadvantaged, semitropical*, and *tropical*, are accurate generalized descriptions of the countries in which rheumatic fever is common. It is a disease of the socially disadvantaged; it is associated with poverty. Still, it must be remembered that these are only generalizations. Pockets of rheumatic fever have been reported in developed, First World, advantaged, countries with cool climates (e.g., the Navajos in the United States[10] and the Maoris in New Zealand,[11] as well as in Polynesia,[12] Hawaii,[13] and Utah[2]). To those familiar with the era when patients were sent to warm climates ("safely free of rheumatic fever") to recover,[14] the irony of the situation is sobering. It is apparent that the prevalence data from that period were seriously flawed and may still be. The figures for the precise prevalence of rheumatic fever and rheumatic heart disease probably vary, in part because there is no specific test for rheumatic fever and in part because an attack may cause so few symptoms that an episode of active disease may be overlooked. Indeed, there was so much confusion about the diagnosis of rheumatic fever among military personnel during World War II that criteria were invented to provide a rational basis for management of patients.[15,16] Those labeled as having rheumatic fever who did not meet Jones criteria often exceeded those who did. In the past, before modern knowledge of mitral valve prolapse as a cause of mitral valve regurgitation or a bicuspid aortic valve as a cause of aortic regurgitation, surveys counted many of these patients as having rheumatic heart disease. Still, admitting the obvious confusion, if the main features of rheumatic disease are considered, rheumatic fever

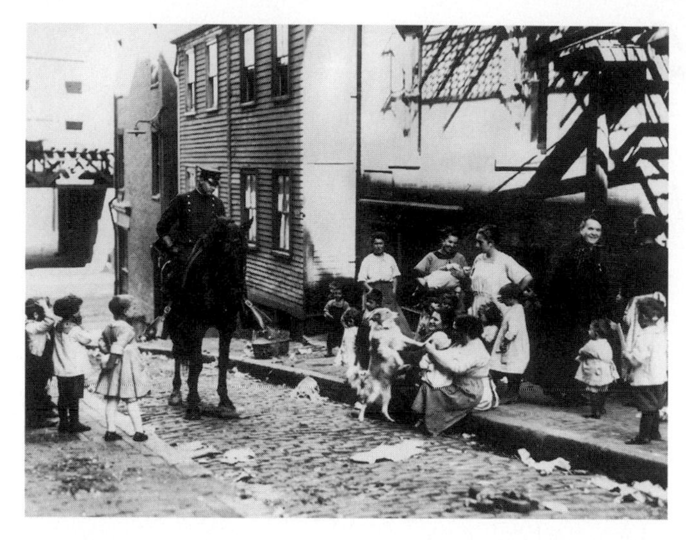

FIGURE 24–1 *Foster Street, North End, Boston, 1905. Courtesy of Gates and Tripp.*

has once again nearly disappeared from the United States in a lifetime (see Table 24-1). To emphasize this situation, one needs only to go to a disadvantaged country in which rheumatic fever and rheumatic heart disease are common to get a sense of déjà vu.

PATHOGENESIS

A "Social Disease"

Rheumatic fever is found mainly in poverty-stricken populations. In the past, in the United States, it seemed to be predominantly a disease of the Caucasian ghettos (see Fig. 24-1) and later a disease of blacks.[17] Whether this is because of poor nutrition, crowding, or unavailability of medical services is not known. There is good reason to believe that prevalence decreased due to the availability of penicillin,[5,18] during which rheumatogenic strains also declined.[3]

TABLE 24–1. Children's Hospital Boston Experience: Rheumatic Fever and Rheumatic Heart Disease*

	1973-1987	1988-2002
Total patient number	102	153
Acute rheumatic fever	12	15
Older than age 20 years	11	34
Interventional procedure	0	24
Electrophysiologic study	1	5

*Compared with 1973-1987, a modest increase in total patient numbers was seen in the recent 1988-2002 era. However, only 15 patients with acute rheumatic fever were encountered, 9 of whom had valvar involvement. There has been an increase in older patients, some of whom underwent interventional catheterization procedures such as device closure of perivalvar prosthetic mitral leaks; arrhythmia ablations were undertaken in 5 others.

Group A Streptococcal Pharyngitis

Since Cheadle's[19] Harveian lectures 100 years ago, physicians have noted that pharyngitis often occurs a week or so before the onset of rheumatic fever and that, at least in temperate climates, there is a seasonal incidence of rheumatic fever. Throat cultures often grew β-hemolytic streptococci. Still, it was not generally accepted until some 45 years ago that group A, β-hemolytic streptococcal infection invariably preceded an attack of acute rheumatic fever.[16] The convincing evidence was the high rising levels of streptococcal antibodies (antistreptolysin O) in the sera of children with active rheumatic fever. With the acceptance of group A, β-hemolytic streptococcal pharyngitis as being inextricably involved in the pathogenesis of rheumatic fever, research focused sharply on the streptococcus as a causative agent.

The following observations must be reconciled in any theory of the causation of rheumatic fever:

1. From the clinical point of view it, is established that infants with β-hemolytic streptococcal infections do not get rheumatic fever. The youngest age at which rheumatic fever occurs is about 2 years, with the disease being rare in the third year. The age range at which a child has a first attack of acute rheumatic fever is 5 to 15 years, the average being 8 years.
2. There is a latent period from the onset of streptococcal pharyngitis to the onset of rheumatic fever (average, 18 days).[20]
3. At most, during an epidemic of β-hemolytic streptococcal pharyngitis, rheumatic fever occurs in 3% of untreated patients.[21]
4. Chorea may manifest without evidence of preceding streptococcal infection; yet it may be followed some years later by mitral stenosis.
5. The dramatic inflammatory suppression by adrenocorticotropic hormone or cortisone suggests that an immunologic mechanism is involved in the pathogenesis.[22,23]
6. Rheumatic fever damages primarily the mitral valve, to a lesser extent the aortic valve, rarely the tricuspid valve, and extremely rarely the pulmonary valve. Why one valve is more prone to rheumatic damage than another is unknown. At the worst, 50% to 60% of patients with acute rheumatic fever develop damaged valves.
7. Group A, β-hemolytic streptococcal pharyngitis in a child who has recovered from rheumatic fever is likely to reactivate the disease; indeed, the second attack is likely

to mimic the first in its manifestations.[24,25] Whether recurrent streptococcal infection with the original M type will produce a second attack is unknown.

8. Group A, β-hemolytic streptococcal impetigo is *not* followed by rheumatic fever.[26] Why the patient must have pharyngitis to stimulate rheumatic fever is unknown. Perhaps the weak antibody response to streptococcal skin infection compared with pharyngeal infection is a clue to understanding this difference.[27] The difference in recognizable "rheumatic antigens" on blood cells versus cells from the tonsils of patients with rheumatic heart disease compared with controls may provide further understanding.[28] Equally mysterious is that impetigo may trigger glomerulonephritis but not rheumatic fever. A limited number of specific group A streptococcal M types cause glomerulonephritis; only rarely do both acute rheumatic fever and acute glomerulonephritis occur together. In contrast, no M-type specificity for rheumatic fever has been found.[29] There are at least 130 M types of group A, β-hemolytic streptococci, many of which have been associated with epidemics of rheumatic fever.

Genetic Factors

The familial incidence of rheumatic fever has been mentioned in literature for about 100 years. Numerous studies of siblings and relatives have been carried out, largely confirming the impression that a familial factor plays a role.[30] An alloantigen has been demonstrated on B cells in 75% of patients with rheumatic fever, whereas it is noted in only about 16% of nonrheumatic patients.[31] Others have suggested that the HLA-DR antigen is a marker for patients known to have rheumatic heart disease.[32] These observations tend to confirm the idea that there is a genetic background for rheumatic fever, but laboratory demonstration of a host factor in rheumatic fever is still less than completely overwhelming.

Pathogenetic Hypothesis

Thus, it is apparent that despite extensive experience with and investigation of rheumatic fever, questions remain about its exact pathogenesis. What is known is that of the streptococcal subgroups, group A is the most pathogenic to humans. In this group, the virulence of the organism is related to its M protein,[33] of which there are at least 130 varieties.[6] Some are found to be associated with rheumatic fever (also called class I) after pharyngitis, and others are associated with skin infections (also called class II), which may be followed by glomerulonephritis. The M-protein type varies both over time and in location. It is postulated that the group A, ß-hemolytic streptococcus with the appropriate M protein (which resembles myosin) adheres to the pharyngeal mucosa of the genetically susceptible host. Antigens and superantigens are then produced that activate T-cell and B-cell lymphocytes, which produce cytokines and antibodies directed against myosin, leading to carditis.[6] Streptococcal antibodies have been described in the caudate nucleus of patients who have had chorea.[34]

From a clinical standpoint, the following scenario seems reasonable. In a genetically susceptible individual, repeated, untreated, streptococcal infections in early life sensitize the child to the possibility of rheumatic fever. Sometime after the age of 2 years, a group A, β-hemolytic streptococcal pharyngitis sets off an unusually high antibody response. After recovery from the pharyngitis, there is a 10-day latent period of relative well-being, following which an autoimmune response involving the excess streptococcal antibodies begins, lasts many weeks, and gradually damages the left heart valves. Later, a recurrent streptococcal infection may reactivate the disease. There is continuing valve damage after clinical evidence of rheumatic activity has subsided. How much of this is caused by recurrent rheumatic fever, by smoldering activity, or by hemodynamic factors causing scarring is unknown. It is known that Aschoff nodules (accepted by most as a sign of rheumatic activity) are found in the heart structures at cardiac biopsy years after the known attack.[35]

PATHOLOGY

There are inflammatory lesions in the heart, blood vessels, brain, and serous surfaces of the joints and pleura. The pathologic picture is characterized by a distinctive and pathognomonic granuloma, consisting of perivascular infiltration of cells and fibrinoid protoplasm (Aschoff bodies). Aschoff bodies (Fig. 24-2) are found in all patients with clinical rheumatic activity, in those who have died after rheumatic fever, and in many with chronic rheumatic valvar abnormalities as well,[35] suggesting that many patients with this disease have subclinical, active, rheumatic fever smoldering for years.

As many as half of patients with a first attack of rheumatic fever have valve involvement. The mitral vale is most commonly involved, being at first incompetent and, later, in some patients, becoming stenotic. When first involved, the aortic valve becomes incompetent, but unlike the mitral valve, almost never becomes stenotic. Aortic regurgitation does occur as a solitary lesion (5% of patients) but is more often seen in combination with mitral regurgitation. Mitral regurgitation alone or associated with aortic regurgitation is by far the most common lesion, so much so that the diagnosis of rheumatic heart disease without mitral disease is suspect. Incompetent and even stenotic tricuspid valves

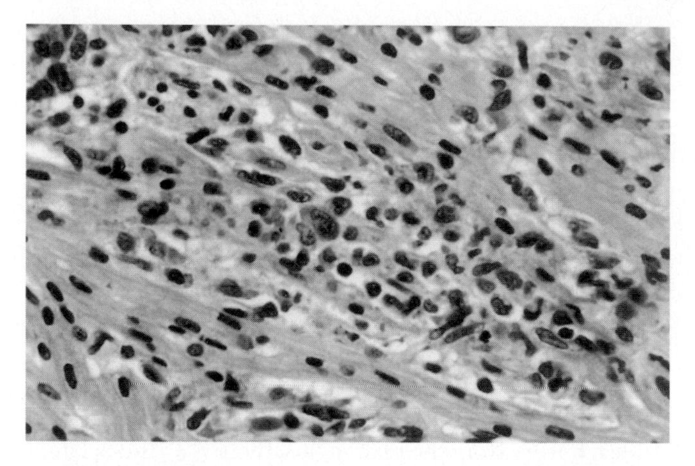

FIGURE 24–2 *Granulomatous stage of an Aschoff nodule showing central necrosis with fibrinoid degeneration and a mixed inflammatory infiltrate of lymphocytes, plasma cells, and large histiocytic cells (Anitschkow cells).*
Courtesy of Antonio Perez, MD, Children's Hospital Boston.

are seen (Fig. 24-3), and rarely an incompetent pulmonary valve is reported.

CLINICAL MANIFESTATIONS

A history of pharyngitis is reported by about half of patients with acute rheumatic fever. Pharyngitis ranges from typical symptoms of streptococcal pharyngeal infection to vague symptoms of upper respiratory illness. With spontaneous subsidence of the sore throat, there is a latent period when the child is afebrile and seems well. About 10 days later, the child becomes ill again. At this point, elevation of the antistreptolysin-O titer is demonstrable, and throat culture may produce β-hemolytic streptococci, which prove to be group A.

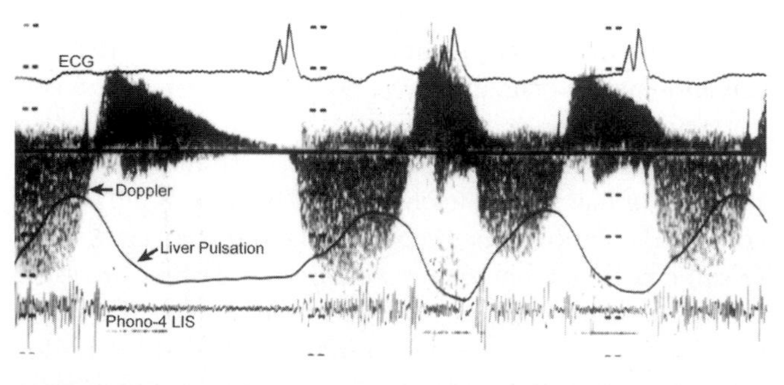

FIGURE 24–3 *These tracings were obtained from a 16-year-old Grenadian girl who had severe rheumatic mitral and tricuspid disease. Tricuspid regurgitation is demonstrated by the Doppler tracing and coincident pulsation of a grossly enlarged liver.*
From Fyler DC [ed]. Nadas' Pediatric Cardiology. Philadelphia: Hanley & Belfus, 1992.

The fever associated with acute rheumatic fever is not high, rarely over 103°F. It may be so low as to be recognized only with systematic recording on a temperature chart. Much has been made of tachycardia being out of proportion to fever as a sign of rheumatic fever. In my experience, this has not been a prominent feature in the usual case of active disease except when there is a congestive heart failure, a more adequate explanation for tachycardia. A child with active rheumatic fever who is febrile is rarely flushed and is more often pale.

Polyarthritis

Most patients have some joint symptoms[36,37] (Table 24-2). Several joints may be intermittently involved (polyarthritis), ranging from vague arthralgia to florid swelling, heat, redness, and demonstrable joint fluid. Occasionally, it is difficult to elicit objective evidence of arthritis; intermittent limping and other limitations of function to guard painful joints may be the only historical data. When there is active involvement (swollen, red, or tender joints), there is fever. The joints most involved are the knees, hips, ankles, elbows, wrists, and shoulders; characteristically the joint symptoms are migratory, rarely involving a single joint for more than 2 days. Unlike joint involvement in rheumatoid arthritis, the small joints of the hands and feet, the temporomandibular joints, and sternoclavicular joints are not commonly involved. The pain can be exquisite, the child reacting to any contact with the inflamed joint, including the weight of bed sheets. A swollen joint that is not tender results from some disease

TABLE 24–2. Principal Manifestations of Rheumatic Fever in 457 Initial Attacks, Exclusive of Cases of Pure Chorea

Manifestations	Cases	%
Significant murmurs	240	53
Pericarditis	29	6
Congestive heart failure	36	8
Prolonged P-R interval	115	25
Subcutaneous nodules	54	12
Erythema marginatum	48	11
Chorea (exclusive of pure chorea)	61	13
Fever	405	89
Elevated sedimentation rate	421	92
Fever and/or elevated sedimentation rate	442	97
Antistreptolysin-O titer of 400 units or more	376	82
Joint pain	412	90
Syndrome of joint pain, fever, and/or elevated sedimentation rate, and elevated antistreptolysin-O titer	338	74
Total cases	457	

From Massell BF, Flyer DC, Roy SB: Am J Cardiol 1:436, 1958,[38] with permission.

other than rheumatic fever. The stage of acute arthritis associated with obvious fever is self-limited, commonly subsiding within a few days and rarely lasting longer than a month. It is a striking clinical observation that chorea and acute polyarthritis never occur together. This is readily believable because the combination of these two problems would produce memorable difficulties.

Carditis

Although roughly half of patients with rheumatic fever have evidence of carditis on first examination, symptoms of congestive heart failure are relatively uncommon. When there is congestive failure, the patients are sometimes very ill with dyspnea, hepatomegaly, vomiting, tachycardia, and fever, as well as florid joint involvement.

When there is pericardial effusion, there may be a cough and often precordial or left shoulder pain that varies with position.

Carditis is mainly manifested by the appearance of murmurs. By far the most common cardiac observation is the presence of an apical systolic murmur. The murmur of mitral regurgitation is characteristically blowing, of high frequency, and transmits to the axilla. It extends through most of systole, beginning with the first sound. Often, there is a short, apical, mid-diastolic rumble (Carey-Coombs murmur) that does not signify mitral stenosis. The presystolic crescendo of mitral stenosis is not encountered in a first attack of acute rheumatic fever. A repeated, careful search for an early diastolic blowing murmur is required because there may be aortic insufficiency. Occasional irregularity can be documented with a variable 2:1 block. A friction rub indicates pericarditis. With pancarditis, there may be gross congestive heart failure, enlarged liver, visible pulsating neck veins when the patient is in the sitting position, shortness of breath, and pulmonary rales.

Erythema Marginatum

In a small percentage of patients with active rheumatic fever, a distinctive rash, erythema marginatum, may be observed. When present, it is virtually a certain sign of rheumatic fever (Fig. 24-4). It is an irregular, geometric, circinate, marginate, red rash over the torso that is evanescent. This rash may be brought out by hot baths and does not itch.

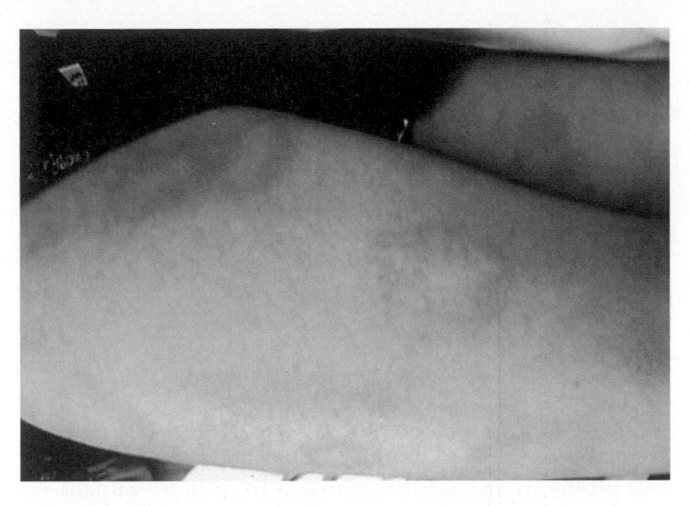

FIGURE 24–4 *Erythema marginatum of the thighs in an 8-year-old boy.*
Courtesy of John K. Triedman, MD.

Subcutaneous Nodules

Firm nodules over hard bony surfaces such as the elbows, wrists, shins, knees, ankles, vertebral column, and occiput are seen occasionally in patients with active rheumatic fever. On microscopy, these structures resemble Aschoff nodules and almost invariably signify rheumatic activity. This phenomenon is uncommon in first attacks, generally being seen in patients who already have well-established heart disease. Nodules are best detected under side-lighting when the skin is slowly moved over the bony surfaces such as the elbows or knees. Nodules are more often seen than palpated and are small, nontender lumps attached to the underlying bone. It is interesting that injections of small amounts of the patient's own blood into these bony surfaces will often produce nodules similar in appearance and on histologic examination. Production of nodules by Massell's method has been used as a test of rheumatic activity.[38] These observations support the suggestion that nodules are the result of trauma to the hard bony areas in patients who have active disease.

Chorea

Sydenham's chorea (St. Vitus' dance) is a distinctive clinical entity with virtually no differential diagnosis. There are purposeless, choreiform movements, aggravated by stress, in an emotionally labile child or young adolescent (usually female). Chorea is less common in older adolescents and is not seen in adults. There may be slurred speech, grotesque facial grimacing, and illegible penmanship. The outstretched hands assume a characteristic "spooning" position; asked to show the tongue, it flicks out and in like a snake's tongue; a fine tremor is palpable in the outstretched hands. In a severe attack, the child may be unable to feed, and the thrashing movements of the extremities may result in bruises. The more the parents chastise the child about spilling food, nervousness, and dropping things, the more the child's equanimity and coordination disintegrate.

Often the onset of chorea is reported to have followed some major trauma such as a bad automobile accident.

Chorea may exist in two circumstances. It simply may be part of an otherwise active rheumatic process (almost never with simultaneous arthritis), in which case there is an elevated sedimentation rate, fever, and evidence of a preceding streptococcal infection; or it may be an isolated phenomenon, pure chorea, without evidence of rheumatic activity.

Pure Chorea

The number of patients with pure chorea is variable. As many as 10% of rheumatic patients may have pure chorea. The choreiform movements, labile mood, and coordination problems are indistinguishable from those in patients who have chorea associated with active rheumatic fever. However, with pure chorea, all other manifestations of rheumatic fever are absent. There is no fever, and there may be no evidence of a preceding streptococcal infection by history, throat culture, or antistreptolysin titer. There is no evidence of cardiac involvement and no elevation of the sedimentation rate.

Occasionally, a patient will have unilateral chorea (hemichorea), all features being characteristic except that abnormal movements are confined to one side. It is probably pure chance that my experience with hemichorea has been of the pure form, without evidence of rheumatic activity. With observation, hemichorea often extends to involve the other side; indeed, with careful observation, many patients with bilateral chorea have more pronounced signs on one side.

Whether a child has chorea or not can usually be determined in the first minutes of the physical examination because the disease is readily recognized if it is has ever been seen before. If a question remains, the performance of the child should be observed under varying circumstances. The outstretched hands, the movements of the tongue, the ability to pronounce Methodist-Episcopal or some other equally difficult phrase, the response to irritation (usually the examination alone is irritating enough), and the inability to write may resolve the question.

Abdominal Pain

At intervals in the past, children were hospitalized for abdominal pain with fever and ended up with abdominal exploration for appendicitis, after which it was discovered that the child had acute rheumatic fever. Whether this abdominal pain is a consequence of pericardial effusion or inflammation of the abdominal serous surfaces is not clear. However, it has occurred often enough to be reasonably well documented in my experience. Nevertheless, if the patient fulfills the criteria for abdominal exploration, it is safer to go ahead with surgery than to assume that the pain results from rheumatic fever.

ANCILLARY STUDIES

Minor Laboratory Tests

A throat culture from an untreated patient often grows hemolytic streptococci. The antistreptolysin-O titer is elevated and may continue to rise, sometimes to remarkably high levels, as the period of observation continues. Other indirect tests of infection, such as rapid antigen diagnostic tests, may be positive but do not provide strain virulence information.[39,40]

The sedimentation rate is almost invariably elevated, as is the C-reactive protein. The possibility of finding a normal sedimentation rate in a child with a severely congested liver should be kept in mind but is rarely seen in practice. The sedimentation rate must be corrected for anemia because anemia is common in these patients. A number of nuclear imaging techniques, using gallium, radiolabeled leukocytes, and antimyosin antibody, which identify myocardial inflammation are currently being studied and may be of value.

Electrocardiogram

The electrocardiogram is not particularly useful in the diagnosis of acute rheumatic fever. Roughly 20% of patients have a prolonged PR interval, particularly if repeated electrocardiograms are taken. Atropine shortens the prolonged PR interval to normal. Occasionally, patients have intermittent 2:1 block, and rarely complete heart block has been reported. Nonspecific changes in the T wave and ST segments are seen, but are neither common nor specific to this diagnosis.

Chest X-Ray

The heart size may be variably enlarged if there is carditis (Fig. 24-5).

Echocardiogram

Where rheumatic fever is common, echocardiographers report that many patients with acute rheumatic fever, including some patients with pure chorea, have mitral regurgitation.[2] A high incidence of mitral valve prolapse in patients with rheumatic heart disease has been noted.[41] In the acute attack, there may be evidence of myocardial depression with reduced shortening fraction and dilation

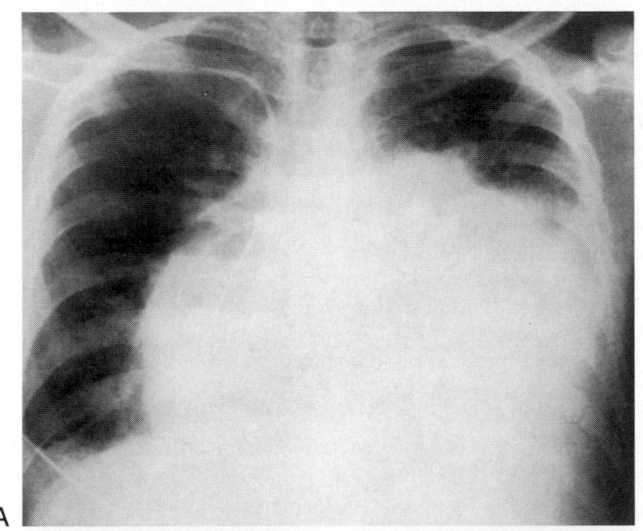

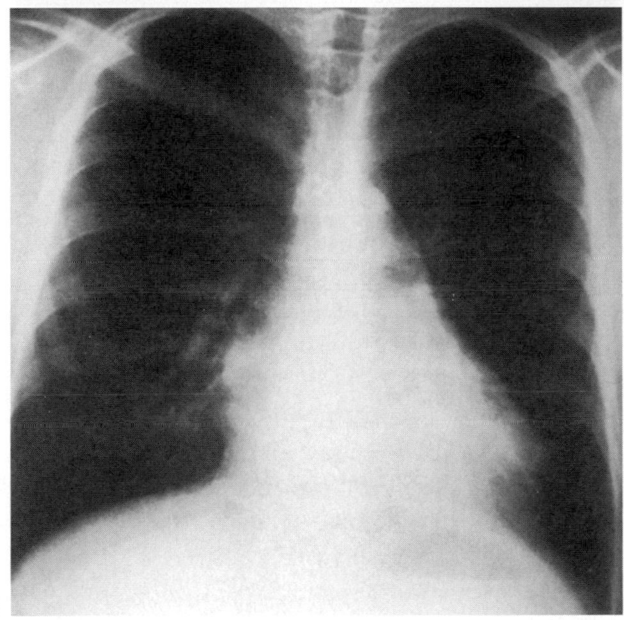

FIGURE 24–5 *Chest x-rays from a 14-year-old with active rheumatic fever for 8 months despite steroid and salicylate therapy.* ***A****, Preoperative, without significant pericardial fluid.* ***B****, Postoperative, following replacement of the mitral and aortic valves for gross congestive heart failure.*
From Fyler DC [ed]. Nadas' Pediatric Cardiology. Philadelphia: Hanley & Belfus, 1992.

of the left ventricle. Clearly, echocardiography has become of considerable value in both identifying and following mitral or aortic regurgitation.[42,43] However, echocardiographic Doppler incidence of regurgitation should be interpreted with caution because at least 45% of normal people have minor degrees of mitral regurgitation.[44] Some 80% of mitral regurgitation murmurs detected echocardiographically are audible, and thus echocardiography is felt not necessary for diagnosis by experienced physicians.[39] Echocardiograms are, however, the method of choice in evaluating the presence and amount of pericardial fluid.

Cardiac Catheterization

There is no need for cardiac catheterization for physiologic or anatomic reasons and cardiac biopsy because of a very low yield[45] is unnecessary, except perhaps in cases of unexplained congestive heart failure.[39]

DIAGNOSIS

There being no specific tests for rheumatic fever, T. Duckett Jones, in 1944,[15] published clinical criteria for the diagnosis of rheumatic fever that have had widespread use with slight modifications over the years (Table 24-3). In Jones' scheme, two major or one major and two minor criteria are required to make the diagnosis of rheumatic fever. The use of the Jones criteria in the diagnosis of acute rheumatic fever is straightforward for most patients. There are, however, two groups who cause some confusion.

1. **Chorea.** For practical purposes, the presence of chorea alone proves the diagnosis of acute rheumatic fever. Confusion often arises when there is hemichorea or when the physician has not seen this disease. Usually, the diagnosis is self-evident.
2. **Probable Rheumatic Fever.** There is a sizeable group of patients who have arthritis, fever, and evidence of a preceding streptococcal infection who are labeled as having probable rheumatic fever. For some of these patients, the diagnosis is ultimately shown to be erroneous, but the group as whole tends to develop valvar damage in significant numbers over the years.

Arthralgia alone is not sufficient to suggest the diagnosis of acute rheumatic fever, regardless of positive ancillary laboratory results. Obviously, such patients are encountered. However, if all such patients were labeled as being prone to rheumatic fever (and all that designation implies), the large number of mistaken diagnoses could scarcely be justified.

Similarly, although in theory a patient with acute rheumatic fever might have monoarticular arthritis, this entity is sufficiently rare, and other forms of monoarticular arthritis are sufficiently common that a diagnosis of acute rheumatic fever based on involvement of one joint is most often an error.

TABLE 24–3. 2002-2003 WHO Revision of Jones Criteria for the Diagnosis of Rheumatic Fever and Rheumatic Heart Disease

Diagnostic Categories	Criteria
Primary episode of RF.[a]	Two major* or one major and two minor** manifestations **plus** evidence of a preceding group A streptococcal infection***.
Recurrent attack of RF in a patient **without** established rheumatic heart disease.	Two major or one major and two minor manifestations **plus** evidence of a preceding group A streptococcal infection.
Recurrent attack of RF in a patient **with** established rheumatic heart disease.	Two minor manifestations **plus** evidence of a preceding group A streptococcal infection.[c]
Rheumatic chorea.	Other major manifestations or evidence of group A streptococcal infection not required.
Insidious onset rheumatic carditis.[b]	
Chronic valve lesions of RHD (patients presenting for the first time with pure mitral stenosis or mixed mitral valve disease and/or aortic valve disease).[d]	Do not require any other criteria to be diagnosed as having rheumatic heart disease.
*Major manifestations	— Carditis — Polyarthritis — Chorea — Erythema marginatum — Subcutaneous nodules
**Minor manifestations	— Clinical: fever, polyarthralgia — Laboratory: elevated acute phase reactants (erythrocyte sedimentation rate or leukocyte count) — Electrocardiogram: prolonged P-R interval
***Supporting evidence of a preceding streptococcal infection within the last 45 days	— Elevated or rising antistreptolysin-O or other streptococcal antibody, or — A positive throat culture, or — Rapid antigen test for group A streptococci, or — Recent scarlet fever

[a]Patients may present with polyarthritis (or with only polyarthralgia or monoarthritis) and with several (3 or more) other minor manifestations, together with evidence of recent group A streptococcal infection. Some of these cases may later turn out to be rheumatic fever. It is prudent to consider them as cases of "probable rheumatic fever" (once other diagnoses are excluded) and advise regular secondary prophylaxis. Such patients require close follow up and regular examination of the heart. This approach is particularly suitable for patients in vulnerable age groups in high incidence settings.
[b]Infective endocarditis should be excluded.
[c]Some patients with recurrent attacks may not fulfill these criteria.
[d]Congential heart disease should be excluded.
From Rheumatic fever and rheumatic heart disease: report of a WHO expert consultation. World Health Organization, Geneva 2004. Technical Report Series No. 923, with permission.

I believe that the minimal joint involvement needed to label a patient *rheumatic*, with its lifelong implication, is a single "objective" joint and at least one other joint with arthralgia. Anything observed by someone other that the patient is taken as an objective sign (i.e., limping, swelling, redness, or inability to use an arm to lift objects). Arthritis without tenderness is not acceptable. Using this as the minimal acceptable evidence of joint involvement, there are a number of patients with joint involvement, evidence of recent streptococcal infection, and an elevated sedimentation rate. I believe these children should be considered to have rheumatic fever and observed for the late development of valvar disease. With follow-up, only a small percentage of these patients have turned out to have other diseases, most commonly rheumatoid arthritis or lupus erythematosus.

Differential Diagnosis

Myocardial Disease

The differential diagnosis between rheumatic fever and acute myocardial disease is a common clinical problem. Often, there is good evidence for a myocardial or pericardial disorder but no evidence of valvar disease. It is an important principle that *there is no rheumatic heart disease without valvar involvement. There must be a murmur to diagnose rheumatic heart disease*. An obvious difficulty arises in the patient with no murmur and echocardiographic evidence of mitral regurgitation. Over the years, it has become accepted that a murmur is required to diagnose rheumatic carditis. Echo-Doppler demonstration of pathologic mitral regurgitation in the absence of a murmur does not change this dictum. On the other hand, inability to demonstrate mitral regurgitation by echo-Doppler, in the presence of a murmur, is taken as virtual proof of the absence of mitral regurgitation, and some other explanation of the murmur should be sought. It is evident that some years of observation will be required to learn the full value of echocardiography in the diagnosis and management of rheumatic fever.

Rheumatoid Arthritis

Rheumatoid arthritis can be confused with acute rheumatic fever in two ways. With continued follow-up, the syndrome of arthritis, elevated antistreptolysin titer, and elevated sedimentation rate may turn out to be rheumatoid arthritis. One should be wary of this possibility, particularly if the joints involved are the small joints of the hands and feet. In any case, follow-up usually solves this problem.

A more pressing differential difficulty occurs when the patient has pericardial effusion, fever, evidence of a prior streptococcal infection, and an elevated sedimentation rate. Without murmurs typical of rheumatic heart disease, these patients have most often turned out to have rheumatoid arthritis or, rarely, lupus erythematosus.

Other Joint Diseases

Rarely, there may be more than one joint involved with septic arthritis. This differential resolves itself in days with observation. Trauma and aseptic forms of arthritis are almost invariably monoarticular and are usually readily recognized. For practical purposes, monoarticular arthritis is not rheumatic fever.

Sickle Cell Disease

Sickle cell disease may mimic acute rheumatic fever in many respects, including cardiomegaly, systolic and diastolic murmurs, and joint pain. A family history may provide a clue, and a sickle cell preparation and electrophoresis of the hemoglobin will confirm the diagnosis. All black patients in whom the diagnosis of acute rheumatic fever or rheumatic heart disease is under consideration should be studied for sickle cell anemia before treatment of rheumatic fever is begun.

Infective Endocarditis

Infective endocarditis may be the cause of fever in a child who has murmurs compatible with rheumatic heart disease. Differentiation between infective endocarditis and active rheumatic fever may be difficult because both diseases cause murmurs and may be associated with elevated sedimentation rates and arthritis or arthralgia. Observation over a few days generally makes it possible to distinguish between the two possibilities. Any question of infective endocarditis is a mandatory indication for multiple blood cultures. It is said that active rheumatic fever and bacterial endocarditis do not occur together; I cannot deny this from my own experience.

MANAGEMENT

Acute Attack

After throat cultures have been obtained, *penicillin therapy is begun*. The doses used are therapeutic (600,000 to 900,000 U of benzathine penicillin intramuscularly for children, and 1,200,000 U for adolescents [or penicillin, 200,000 U orally, four times daily and continued until the patient has been treated 10 days]).[30] At that time, a preventive maintenance dose of penicillin is begun (200,000 U orally, twice daily, every day). Management of a patient with clearly active rheumatic fever or suspected rheumatic fever without the use of antibiotics is an unconscionable error because continued streptococcal infection can be expected to aggravate the disease. Despite the absence of demonstrable streptococci or an elevated antistreptolysin titer, patients with chorea are given penicillin just like all others with acute rheumatic fever.

The hoary recommendation that all physical activity for patients with active rheumatic fever should be rigidly limited has dwindled into obscurity. No longer do we limit activity as a means to prevent further heart damage. The idea that rheumatic cardiac involvement is different from other types of myocardial disease, or that exercise is more likely to cause scarring, simply has no basis in fact. Limitation of activity is managed as it is in everyone else with a febrile illness, congestive heart failure, or both. Avoidance of vigorous activity is ordinarily left to the patient who, when sick, scarcely feels like moving around anyway. Rigorous attention to eradication and prevention of streptococcal infection is a much more rewarding enterprise.

Salicylates are used for control of pain and suppression of rheumatic activity in patients who do not have carditis or have only questionable evidence of cardiac involvement (Table 24-4). In those who cannot tolerate salicylates, a nonsteroidal anti-inflammatory drug such as naproxen (10 to 20 mg/kg/day) may be used.[46] On the other end of the spectrum, it is mandatory that the child with pancarditis and congestive heart failure receive prednisone as a lifesaving measure. There is room for debate about the use of prednisone for the child with valvulitis that is not life threatening because unassailable evidence that further valve damage can be prevented is lacking. One can find data to support whatever course of treatment is proposed.[24,47,48] In my view, the risks of prednisone therapy are outweighed, even in this intermediate group, by the possibility that valve damage may be reduced. Consequently, for all children with acute active disease and unequivocal valve involvement,

TABLE 24–4. Treatment of Acute Rheumatic Fever

Treatment and prophylaxis of group A, hemolytic, streptococcal infection:
- Benzathine penicillin, 1.2 million units intramuscularly every month
- Suppressive therapy

With no heart involvement:
- Aspirin 100 mg/kg/day in four divided doses.
- Reduce dose if salicylate level exceeds 25 mg/100 ml
- Reduce dose if symptoms of salicylism (tinnitus)
- Reduce dose by 25% after 1 week if good clinical response and continue for 6-8 weeks, tapering the dose in last 2 weeks.

With valvar involvement:
- Prednisone, 2.0 mg/kg/day for 2 weeks, then taper for 2 weeks
- With good response begin aspirin 75 mg/kg/day in the 3rd week and continue until the 8th week , tapering in the final 2 weeks.
- Increase suppressive dose if symptoms return or sedimentation rate rises.

From Markowitz M, Gordis L: Rheumatic Fever, 2nd ed. Philadelphia, W.B. Saunders, 1972, with permission.

I use steroid therapy initially and later switch to salicylates (see Table 24-4). As mentioned, the discovery of mitral regurgitation by echocardiography, without a murmur, is considered equivocal evidence.

How long treatment should be continued is, perhaps, even more controversial. There is an initial response of joint symptoms, fever, and sedimentation rate to treatment with prednisone or salicylates. Demonstrable response, often dramatic, occurs in 48 to 72 hours, and complete suppression in 7 to 10 days. The sedimentation rate returns to normal sooner when prednisone is used. After 2 to 3 weeks without clinical or laboratory evidence of activity, the dose of prednisone can be tapered and aspirin added while observing the response. Sometimes there is a reappearance of symptoms or laboratory findings (rebound phenomenon) despite this weaning process. The dose then should be increased until suppression is again attained. In any case, treatment is rarely needed beyond 12 to 16 weeks.

Management of congestive heart failure is usually best accomplished with diuretics. Digoxin is also used but requires caution because digoxin in the presence of an inflamed myocardium is known to precipitate dangerous rhythm problems, fortunately rarely.

Rheumatic pericardial effusion tends to accumulate slowly and rarely causes tamponade even with a large accumulation.

Although chorea is a self-limited disease, the emotional distress can be alleviated with phenobarbital or valium. With an improved mood, the choreiform movements are less marked. If chorea is associated with other manifestations of rheumatic activity, particularly if there is valvar involvement, corticosteroids may provide measurable improvement, although I do not use prednisone for pure chorea. In severe cases, hospitalization may be needed, if for no other reason than to assist the child in eating and to prevent injury from flailing movements.

Course

Untreated active rheumatic fever lasts from a few weeks to several months, averaging between 8 and 16 weeks for rheumatic activity as measured by the presence of an elevated sedimentation rate, congestive failure, nodules, erythema marginatum, or continued chorea. In those younger than age 5 years, carditis is more severe and chronic heart disease more common than in older patients.[49] Rheumatic activity persists longer in patients who have carditis.

At the time of initial presentation, as many as half of children with rheumatic fever already have a significant murmur. As the days and weeks go by, under appropriate therapy, some children lose the murmur, whereas others develop murmurs for the first time (Table 24-5). These changes are less frequent the longer the disease lasts, but the cardiac status never completely stabilizes; some individuals first develop new cardiac murmurs 20 years later. Young women who had pure chorea as children tend to develop pure mitral stenosis; there is only a presystolic crescendo murmur and no murmur of mitral regurgitation.

Individuals with mitral or aortic regurgitation or both may experience worsening of the existing valvar damage as the years go by. Although this may be the result of recurrent rheumatic fever, it also may simply be a result of the hemodynamics (*mitral regurgitation begets mitral regurgitation*). Mitral stenosis (Fig. 24-6) usually requires years to develop, sometimes as many as 20 years, although it has occurred as early as 2 to 3 years after the apparent onset of rheumatic fever. In countries in which rheumatic fever is common, mitral stenosis develops more rapidly, being seen in small children. Biopsy specimens of the atrial appendages in patients undergoing mitral valve surgery show Aschoff nodules in high frequency the nearer the surgery is to the attack of active rheumatic fever, but they are still present in some patients many years later. The presence of Aschoff nodules is taken as evidence of smoldering, low-grade rheumatic activity.

When chorea is associated with other signs of activity, the incidence of ultimate valve damage is comparable to that caused by active rheumatic fever without chorea. When there is chorea with no other signs of rheumatic activity (pure chorea), ultimate heart damage is less frequent, appears late, and is most often pure mitral stenosis without preceding mitral regurgitation.

Recurrent Rheumatic Fever

A second attack of rheumatic fever represents a failure of secondary prevention. Most often there has been a lapse

TABLE 24–5. Incidence of Development of Significant Murmurs at Various Intervals after the Onset of 206 Initial Attacks of Rheumatic Fever*

Duration of Illness (days)	Number	Patients Developing Murmurs During Interval: *Percent of Patients with Carditis*	*Percent of Total Patients*
1-7	78	76	38
8-14	7	6.8	3.4
15-28	4	3.9	1.9
29-42	3	2.9	1.4
43-91	4	3.9	1.9
More than 91	7	6.8	3.4
Total	103	100	50

From Massell BF, Flyer DC, Roy SB,[38] with permission.
*Data for patients observed between 1941 and 1951.

of penicillin prophylaxis; less often, oral penicillin has been ineffective. It is usually possible to document the intervening streptococcal infection by throat culture and by a rise in antibodies. The first order of business is to eliminate oral streptococci and reestablish adequate prevention. If the recurrence appeared while the patient was receiving oral penicillin, a switch to monthly injection is required. In all other respects, the treatment of a recurrent attack of acute rheumatic fever is the same as for a first attack. The question of adequate prophylaxis must be examined. Perhaps a switch to intramuscular benzathine penicillin is needed. Perhaps the interval between doses of intramuscular penicillin should be shortened to 3 weeks instead of 4 weeks.

A recurrent attack usually resembles the earlier attack, although valvar involvement may be extended. The appearance of congestive heart failure in a rheumatic child is always interpreted as evidence of active disease and, by implication, involvement of the myocardium as well as the valves. Although this is a useful working hypothesis, some patients develop sufficient valvar deformity within months of the apparent first onset of the disease to be the main cause of congestive heart failure (see Fig. 24-5). The problem may necessitate a decision between treating active myocardial involvement or advanced valvar disease as the cause of congestive heart failure. Echocardiography usually solves this question. Cardiac catheterization is usually unnecessary, except if the dominant lesion is significant mitral stenosis for which balloon dilation has become very effective (Fig. 24-7), although restenosis may occur in some.[50] When there is valvar regurgitation sufficient to cause

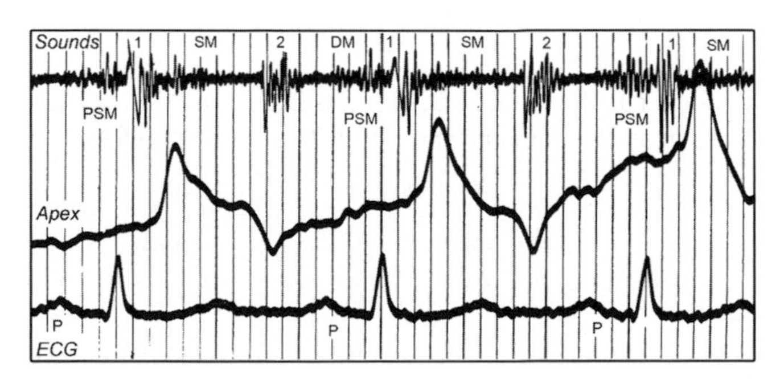

FIGURE 24–6 *Typical presystolic crescendo murmur in a patient with rheumatic heart disease and mitral valve involvement. Tracing recorded at cardiac apex. 1, Prominent first heart sound; 2, moderately split second heart sound; SM, decrescendo medium-frequency moderate-intensity systolic murmur; DM, mid-diastolic murmur; PSM, presystolic crescendo murmur From Fyler DC [ed]. Nadas' Pediatric Cardiology. Philadelphia: Hanley & Belfus, 1992.*

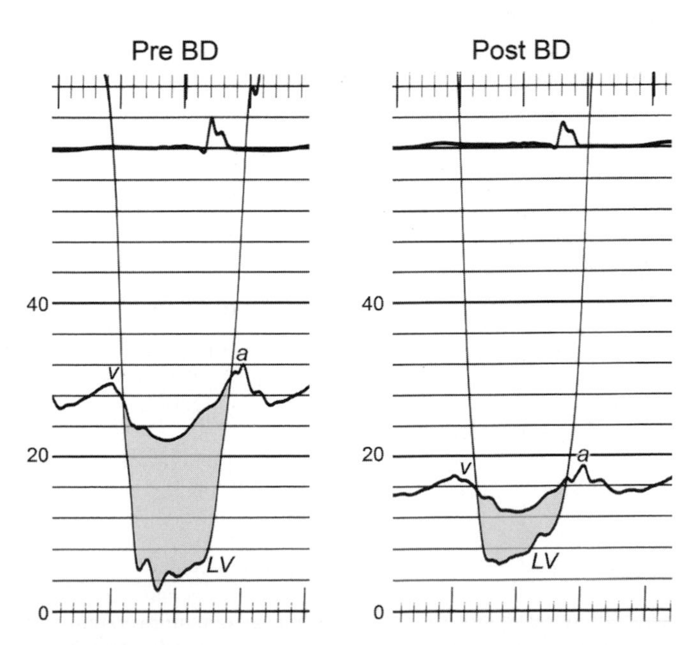

FIGURE 24–7 *Pressure tracings obtained at catheterization in a 14-year-old boy with severe mitral stenosis of rheumatic origin showing marked reduction of the gradient (shaded area) across the mitral valve following balloon dilation (BD).*

congestive heart failure, surgery may be needed and may be life-saving, despite associated myocardial damage. When in doubt, surgery is probably the best choice because any myocardial problem is only aggravated by the valvar abnormality. The idea that cardiac surgery is specifically prohibited in the face of active rheumatic disease is no longer tenable.[51]

Primary Prevention

The idea that rheumatic fever could be prevented through control of streptococcal infection was proposed as early as 1937,[52] but sulfanilamide was ineffective. During World War II, it was possible to document the spread of streptococcal infection through military camps and to establish that adequate and timely treatment of streptococcal pharyngitis prevents rheumatic fever.[53] Based on these studies, it was determined that treatment of streptococcal pharyngitis begun as late as 9 days after onset will prevent rheumatic fever. It was recommended that group A streptococcal infection be treated for a full 10 days (Table 24-6).

The practical question is the management of pharyngitis in modern-day pediatric practice. Surely, children with febrile sore throats should have throat cultures, which continue to be the most accurate diagnostic test but require up to 48 hours for results. If these are positive for hemolytic streptococci, antibiotic therapy should be continued for 10 days, even in this era of declining rheumatic fever in the United States.[54,55] Rapid detection of group A streptococci on throat swabs, by which specific antigens are identified, although comparing favorably with blood agar cultures,[40] varies considerably with equipment used.[6]

Where there is organized throat culturing and central reporting of β-hemolytic streptococcal recovery, community physicians respond to this information, resulting in a reduction in the spread of streptococcal infection and elimination of rheumatic fever.[56]

There has been considerable interest for many years in developing a vaccine to prevent rheumatic fever, without success to date. Initial attempts included injection of streptococcal toxins and killed organisms. Subsequent vaccine development attempts followed identification of the M protein of the organism's capsule as the virulent factor. However, these attempts have been complicated by the identification of more than 130 M-protein serotypes and by evidence of cross-reactions occurring between some of these with human heart tissue and synovium. Multivalent M-protein recombinant vaccines aimed at preventing group A streptococcal pharyngitis and whose antibodies do not cross-react with human tissue have been made and are being evaluated,[57] and they may be available for use in several years. These attempts may be complicated by findings suggesting that acute rheumatic fever may follow skin infections in Australian aboriginal populations.[58]

Secondary Prevention

A patient who has had acute rheumatic fever is susceptible to recurrent rheumatic fever for the rest of his life. *Once a rheumatic, always a rheumatic*. The likelihood of recurrence is greater the shorter the time interval since rheumatic activity, and when there has been valve damage. Recurrences are more common among children than adults, especially when there has already been a preceding recurrence.[59]

Although oral penicillin V (250 mg administered twice each day) will prevent secondary attacks of rheumatic fever, compliance with this routine is often less than optimum.

TABLE 24–6. Primary Prevention of Rheumatic Fever (Treatment of Streptococcal Tonsillopharyngitis)

Agent	Dose	Mode	Duration
Benzathine penicillin G	600,000 units of patients 60 lb 1,200,000 units of patients >60 lb	Intramuscular	Once
Penicillin V (phenoxymethylpenicillin)	250 mg 3 times daily	Oral	10 days
	For individuals allergic to penicillin:		
Erythromycin estolate	20-40 mg/kg/day 2-4 times daily (maximum 1 g/day) or	Oral	10 days
Ethylsuccinate	40 mg/kg/day 2-4 times daily (maximum 1 g/day)	Oral	10 days

The following agents are acceptable but usually not recommended: amoxicillin, dicloxacillin, oral cephalosporins, and clindamycin.
The following are not acceptable: sulfonamides, trimethoprim, tetracyclines, and chloramphenicol.

From Dajani AS, Bisno AL, Chung KJ, et al: Prevention of rheumatic fever. Circulation 78:1082-1086, 1988, by permission of the American Heart Association, Inc.

TABLE 24–7. Secondary Prevention of Rheumatic Fever (Prevention of Recurrent Attacks)

Agent	Dose	Mode
Benzathine penicillin G	1,200,000 units	Intramuscularly Every 4 weeks*
	or	
Penicillin V	250 mg twice daily	Oral
	or	
Sulfadiazine	0.5 g once daily for patients <60 lb 1.0 g once daily for patients >60 lb	Oral
For individuals allergic to penicillin or sulfadiazine:		
Erythromycin	250 mg twice daily	Oral

From Dajani AS, Bisno AL, Chung KJ, et al: Prevention of rheumatic fever. Circulation 78:1082-1086, 1988, by permission of the American Heart Association, Inc.

*In high-risk situations, administration every 3 weeks is advised.

For more reliable coverage the use of benzathine penicillin G (120,000 units intramuscularly every 4 weeks) is more dependable, although more painful (Table 24-7). Some problems with oral penicillin have been traced to mouth organisms that produce penicillinase, but most are a result of forgetfulness or active rebellion.

Any patient who has had a known attack of rheumatic fever should be followed for at least 5 years (the time of greatest recurrence), and those with valvar damage should be followed indefinitely. When following these patients, it is useful to record the antistreptolysin-O titer, as well as the sedimentation rate, to serve as a baseline if subsequent concern about rheumatic activity arises.

REFERENCES

1. Bland EF. The way it was. Circulation 76:1190, 1987.
2. Veasy LG, Wiedmeier SE, Orsmond GS, et al. Resurgence of acute rheumatic fever in the intermountain area of the United States. N Engl J Med 316:421, 1987.
3. Stollerman GH. Rheumatic fever. Lancet 349:935, 1997.
4. Derry FW Jr. A 45-year perspective on the streptococcus and rheumatic fever: The Edward H Kass lecture in infectious disease history. Clin Infect Dis 19:110, 1994.
5. Veasy LG, Hill HR. Immunologic and clinical correlations in rheumatic fever and rheumatic heart disease. Pediatr Infect Dis J 16:400, 1997.
6. Rheumatic fever and rheumatic heart disease: Report of WHO Expert Consultation. Geneva: World Health Organization, 2004 (Technical Report Series No. 923).
7. Kaplan EL. Global assessment of rheumatic fever and rheumatic heart disease at the close of the century. Circulation 88:1964, 1993.
8. McLaren MJ, Markowitz M, Gerber MA. Rheumatic heart disease in developing countries: The consequence of inadequate prevention. Ann Intern Med 120:243, 1994.
9. Snitcowsky R. Rheumatic fever prevention in industrializing countries: Problems and approaches. Pediatrics (Suppl) 996, 1996.
10. Coulehan J, Grant S, Reisinger K, et al. Acute rheumatic fever and rheumatic heart disease on the Navajo reservation, 1962–1977. Pub Health Rep 95:62, 1980.
11. Stanhope JM. New Zealand trends in rheumatic fever, 1885–1971. N Z Med J 82:297, 1975.
12. Neutze JM. The third international conference on rheumatic fever and rheumatic heart disease: Rheumatic fever and rheumatic heart disease in the western Pacific region. N Z Med J 101:202, 1988.
13. Chun LT, Reddy V, Yamamoto LG. Rheumatic fever in children and adolescents in Hawaii. Pediatrics 79:549, 1987.
14. Jones TD, White PD, Roche CF, et al. The transportation of rheumatic fever patients to a subtropical climate. JAMA 109:1308, 1937.
15. Jones TD. The diagnosis of rheumatic fever. JAMA 126:481, 1944.
16. Stollerman GH, Markowitz M, Taranta A, et al. Jones criteria (revised) for guidance in diagnosis of rheumatic fever. Circulation 32:664, 1965.
17. Gordis L. The virtual disappearance of rheumatic fever in the United States: Lessons in the rise and fall of disease. Circulation 72:1155, 1985.
18. Massell BF, Chute CG, Walker AM, et al. Penicillin and the marked decrease in morbidity and mortality from rheumatic fever in the United States. N Engl J Med 318: 280, 1988.
19. Cheadle WB. Harveian Lectures on the various manifestation of the rheumatic state as exemplified in childhood and early life. Lancet 1:821, 871, 921, 1889.
20. Rammelkamp CH Jr, Strolzer BL. The latent period before the onset of acute rheumatic fever. Yale J Biol Med 34:386, 1961.
21. Rammelkamp CH, Wannamaker LW, Denny FW. The epidemiology and prevention of rheumatic fever. Bull N Y Acad Med 28:321, 1952.
22. Tomaru T, Uchida Y, Mohri N, et al. Post inflammatory mitral and aortic valve prolapse: A clinical and pathological study. Circulation 76:68, 1987.
23. United Kingdom and U.S. Joint Report on Rheumatic Heart Disease. The natural history of rheumatic fever and rheumatic heart disease: Ten-year report of cooperative clinical trial of ACTH, cortisone and aspirin. Circulation 32: 457, 1965.
24. DiSciasco G and Taranta A: Rheumatic fever in children. Am Heart J 99:635, 1980.
25. Sanyal SK, Berry AM, Duggal S, et al. Sequelae of the initial attack of acute rheumatic fever in children from North India: A prospective 5-year follow-up study. Circulation 65:375, 1982.
26. Wannamaker LW. The chain that links the heart to the throat. Circulation 48:9, 1973.

27. Kaplan EL, Anthony BF, Chapman SS, et al. The influence of the site of infection on the immune response to group A streptococci. J Clin Invest 49:1405–1414, 1970.
28. Gray ED, Regelmann WE, Abdin Z, et al. Compartmentalization of cells bearing "rheumatic" cell surface antigens in peripheral blood and tonsils in rheumatic heart disease. J Infect Dis 155:247, 1987.
29. Zabriskie JB. Rheumatic fever: A streptococcal-induced autoimmune disease? Pediatr Annu 11:383, 1982.
30. Markowitz M, Gordis L. Rheumatic fever, 2nd ed. Philadelphia: WB Saunders, 1972.
31. Pattarroyo ME, Winchester RJ, Vejerano A, et al. Association of B-cell alloantigen with susceptibility to rheumatic fever. Nature 278:173, 1979.
32. Rajapakse CAN, Halim K, Al-Orainey I, et al. A genetic marker for rheumatic heart disease. Br Heart J 58:659, 1987.
33. Lancefield RC. Current knowledge of the type specific M antigens of group A streptococci. J Immunol 89:307, 1962.
34. Husby G, van de Rijn I, Zabriskie JB, et al. Antibodies reacting with cytoplasm of subthalamic and caudate nuclei neurons in chorea and acute rheumatic fever. J Exp Med 144:1094, 1944.
35. Thomas WA, Averill JH, Castleman B, et al. The significance of Aschoff bodies in the left atrial appendage: A comparison of 40 biopsies removed during mitral commissurotomy with autopsy material from 40 patients dying from rheumatic fever. N Engl J Med 249:761, 1983.
36. Lahiri K, Rane HS, Desai AG. Clinical profile of rheumatic fever: A study of 168 cases. J Trop Pediatr 31:273, 1985.
37. Bhattacharya S, Reddy KS, Sundaram KR, et al. Differentiation of patients with rheumatic fever from those with inactive rheumatic heart disease using the artificial subcutaneous nodule test, myocardial reactive antibodies, serum immunoglobin and serum complement levels. Int J Cardiol 14:71, 1987.
38. Massell BF, Fyler DC, Roy SB. The clinical picture of rheumatic fever: Diagnosis, immediate prognosis, course and therapeutic implications. Am J Cardiol 1:436, 1958.
39. Stollerman GH. Rheumatic Fever in the 21st Century. Clin Infect Dis 33:806, 2001.
40. Bisno AL. Treatment of group A streptococcal pharyngitis. N Engl J Med 344:205, 2001.
41. Lembo NJ, Dellitalia LJ, Crawford MH, et al. Mitral valve prolapse in patients with prior rheumatic fever. Circulation 77:830, 1988.
42. Narula J, Chandrasekhar Y, Rahimtoola S. Diagnosis of active carditis: The echoes of change. Circulation 100:1576, 1999.
43. Minich LL, Tani LY, Pagotto LT, et al. Doppler echocardiography distinguished between physiologic and pathologic "silent" mitral regurgitation in patients with rheumatic fever. Clin Cardiol 20:924, 1997.
44. Yoshida K, Yoshikawa J, Shakido M, et al. Color Doppler evaluation of valvular regurgitation in normal subjects. Circulation 78:840, 1988.
45. Narula J, Chopra P, Talwar KK, et al. Does endomyocardial biopsy aid in the diagnosis of active rheumatic carditis? Circulation 88:2198, 1993.
46. Uziel Y, et al. The use of naproxen in the treatment of children with rheumatic fever. J Pediatr 137:269, 2000.
47. United Kingsom and U.S. Joint Report on Rheumatic Fever. The treatment of rheumatic fever in children: A cooperative clinical trial of ACTH, cortisone and aspirin. Circulation 11:343, 1955.
48. United Kingdom and U.S. Joint Report on Rheumatic Fever. The evolution of rheumatic heart disease in children: Five-year report of a cooperative clinical trial of ACTH, cortisone and aspirin. Circulation 22:503, 1960.
49. Tani LY, Veasy LG, Minich LL, et al. Rheumatic fever in children younger than 5 years: Is the presentation different? Pediatrics 112(5):1065, 2003.
50. Farhat BF, Ayari M, Maatouk F, et al. Percutaneous balloon versus surgical closed and open mitral commissurotomy: Seven year follow-up results of a randomized trial. Circulation 97:245, 1998.
51. Hellman ND, Tani LY, Veasy G, et al. Current states of surgery for rheumatic carditis in Children. Ann Thorac Surg 78:1403, 2004.
52. Massell BF. Studies on the use of Prontylin in rheumatic fever. N Engl J Med 216:487, 1937.
53. Catanzaro FJ, Stetson CA, Morris AJ, et al. The role of streptococcus in the pathogenesis of rheumatic fever. Am J Med 17:749, 1954.
54. Dajani AS, Bisno AL, Chung KJ, et al. Prevention of rheumatic fever: A statement for health professionals by the committee on rheumatic fever, endocarditis, and Kawasaki disease of the Council on Cardiovascular Disease in the Young, the American Heart Association. Circulation 78: 1082, 1988.
55. Shulman ST (ed). Pharyngitis: Management in an Era of Declining Rheumatic Fever. New York: Praeger, 1984.
56. Phibbs B, Taylor J, Simmerman RA. A community-wide streptococcal control project. The Natrona County Primary Prevention Program, Casper, Wyoming. JAMA 214:2018, 1970.
57. Dale JB. Multivalent group A streptococcal vaccine designed to optimize the immunogenicity of six tandem M protein fragments. Vaccine 17:193, 1999.
58. McDonald M, Currie BJ, Carapetes JR. Acute rheumatic fever: A chink in the chain that links the heart to the throat? Lancet Infect Dis 4:240, 2004.
59. Markowitz M. The decline of rheumatic fever: Role of medical intervention. J Pediatr 106:545, 1985.

25

Kawasaki Disease

DAVID R. FULTON, MD AND
JANE W. NEWBURGER, MD, MPH

DEFINITION

Kawasaki disease is an acute, systemic vasculitis of uncertain etiology, occurring predominantly in infants and young children. It is characterized by fever, bilateral nonexudative conjunctivitis, erythema of the lips and oral mucosa, changes in the extremities, rash, and cervical lymphadenopathy. Coronary artery aneurysms or ectasia develop in 15% to 25% of cases and may lead to myocardial infarction, sudden death, or chronic coronary insufficiency.

PREVALENCE

Though noted initially in Japan in 1967[1] and most prevalent there, Kawasaki disease occurs worldwide in both endemic and community-based epidemic forms in children of all races.[2,3] The most recent Japanese statistics from a nationwide survey in 2000 note 168,394 affected children, with higher rates in males and infants younger than 1 year. In 2000, the incidence rate was 134.2 per 100,000 children younger than 5 years.[2] The absence of a mandatory national reporting system in the United States makes estimates difficult. Administrative data from hospital discharge abstracts indicate that more than 4000 hospitalizations were associated with Kawasaki disease in the United States in 2000.[4] Current data show that among children younger than 5 years, the occurrence is greatest in children of Asian origin (33.3/100,000), somewhat less in African Americans 23.4/100,000), and lowest in whites 12.7/100,000).[5] The pattern of involvement is generally endemic, with occasional epidemics among primarily younger children, with a male-to-female ratio of 1.4/1; however, the illness is being more commonly recognized in older children and adolescents.[6] Outbreaks are more likely in the spring, suggesting an infectious etiology, but a steady background activity of cases is noted throughout the remainder of the year. The disease can recur (approximately 3% in Japan), and person-to-person transmission is unusual.

ETIOLOGY AND PATHOGENESIS

The search for an etiologic agent has been wide-ranging. Features suggesting that the process is infectious include young age at presentation, higher frequency of cases in the spring, and clustering of individuals in near proximity without direct contact. Prior exposure of index cases to freshly cleaned carpets has been noted for many years, although no specific organism or toxin has been identified in the rugs. Some investigators believe that an agent triggers a typical immune response resulting in the clinical manifestations of the disease, whereas others think that the marked immune response is related to exposure of the host to a superantigen.[7] A number of reports have implicated specific superantigens, including TSST-1–secreting strains of *Staphylococcus aureus* and streptococcal pyrogenic exotoxin B– and C–producing streptococci[7] as well as *Lactobacillus casei*, which induce coronary arteritis in mice.[8] Other investigators have found support for a typical antigen immune response by demonstrating oligo-IgA plasma cells and IgA heavy-chain genes in vascular tissue of individuals with fatal Kawasaki disease.[9,10]

Regardless of the initiating event, Kawasaki disease is accompanied by significant derangements in the immunoregulatory system that lead to coronary inflammation and coronary artery abnormalities, dilatation, aneurysm formation, and giant aneurysms in some patients. The presence of T-cell activation has been detailed widely with increased circulating monocytes, activation of helper T cells, and decreased suppressor T cells. B-cell activation has also been shown, with increased secretion of IgG and IgM antibodies.[11] A number of investigators have shown T-cell stimulation bearing specific Vβ T-cell receptors capable of interacting with antigen-presenting cells. The markedly skewed expansion of circulating T cells with Vβ2 and Vβ8 repertoires suggests that superantigens may initiate this interaction.[12–18] Endothelial cell damage appears to occur as a result of this increased immune activity. Leung and colleagues[19] have reported that IgM antibodies from acute sera can damage cultured human vascular endothelial cells when pretreated with gamma interferon, as have IgG and IgM antibodies when cells are stimulated with interleukin-1 or tumor necrosis factor.[20] Cytokines released by stimulated T cells and macrophages could incite damage to endothelial cells in the acute phase of the illness; many reports detail the increased levels of circulating mediators including interleukins,[9,10,21–24] soluble selectins,[25] leukotrienes[26] and tumor necrosis factor in the acute phase of the illness. Thus, the features of an immune reaction induced by a superantigen are supported by documented VB skewing of T-lymphocytes, a polyclonal B-lymphocyte activation, and inflammatory cytokine production.[27]

Vascular endothelial growth factor (VEGF), a glycoprotein that acts on endothelium to increase vascular permeability, is activated to markedly elevated levels in the acute phase of Kawasaki disease,[28] an effect possibly explaining the edema of the distal extremities and hypoalbuminemia. This theory is supported by the presence of microvascular dilation and subendothelial edema[29] on skin biopsy. VEGF stimulates nitric oxide production in endothelial cells through nitric oxide synthase enzyme expression,[30] and it has been reported that nitric oxide production is greater in those patients with Kawasaki disease who develop coronary aneurysms.[31] Although serum VEGF levels remain elevated following intravenous gamma globulin administration (IVIG), VEGF levels in patients with persistent fever after IVIG were higher than in IVIG responders, with serum albumin lower in the IVIG-resistant group.[32] Of those in the latter category, 44% had coronary abnormalities, whereas IVIG responders had no coronary abnormalities, supporting a role for VEGF in the pathogenesis of coronary artery damage.

Matrix metalloproteinases (MMPs) 2 and 9 degrade extracellular matrix, collagen, and elastin and are in balance with their specific tissue inhibitors (TIMPs). Imbalance between the MMPs and TIMPs has been shown to degrade the tissue matrix in abdominal aortic aneurysms.[33] Patients with Kawasaki disease have higher levels of MMPs than afebrile and febrile controls prior to treatment with IVIG. In addition, patients with Kawasaki disease with coronary artery lesions have higher levels of MMPs and MMP/TIMP ratios than those without coronary abnormalities,[34] suggesting that these circulating proteins may play an active role in coronary arterial remodeling.

PATHOLOGY

The mortality in cases of Kawasaki disease approximates 0.1% with virtually all deaths occurring secondary to the cardiac sequelae of this disease.[35] Fujiwara and Hamashima[36] initially described the pathology from autopsy findings of children dying in the acute and subacute phases prior to available treatment with IVIG. They established four categories of the illness based on the time from onset of the disease (stage I, 0–9 days; stage II, 12–25 days; stage III, 28–31 days; and stage IV, 40 days to 4 years). The inflammatory changes in stage I are highlighted by vasculitis of small vessels and microvessels and perivasculitis and endarteritis of the coronary vessels. Pancarditis is present and is also found in stage II, with panvasculitis of the coronary bed sometimes with aneurysm formation and coronary thrombosis. By stage III, the acute inflammation has subsided but myointimal proliferation of the coronary arteries proceeds. In stage IV, stenosis is noted for the first time with scarring. Early in the course, death is the result of arrhythmia and myocarditis, with increasing trends toward ischemia and infarction as time progresses from onset of disease. Of note is the concomitant onset of a hypercoagulable state[37] and thrombocytosis in stages II and III, when the mortality rate is highest. Sudden death from myocardial infarction may occur many years later in those children with aneurysms and stenosis of the coronary arteries. At autopsy in addition to coronary artery abnormalities, aneurysms at other sites involving small- to medium-sized vessels and including femoral, iliac, renal, axillary, and brachial arteries have been reported.

CLINICAL MANIFESTATIONS

Because no diagnostic test is available for Kawasaki disease, the diagnosis must be made on clinical grounds (Exhibit 25-1). Often the illness begins with fever and what appears to be a prodromal gastroenteritis or otitis media in a child between the ages of 1 and 5 years. The persistence of fever with the onset of the other signs may lead the clinician to consider the diagnosis. First described by Kawasaki in Japanese children,[38] the classic criteria have continued to serve as the standard adopted by the American Heart Association (Exhibit 25-1) for arriving at the diagnosis[39] and include fever for 5 days or more and at least four of the five

Exhibit 25–1
Principal Clinical Findings*

Fever persisting at least 5 days‡ or more without other source in association with at least 4 principal features:
Oral changes that may include erythema or cracking of the lips, strawberry tongue, erythema of the oral mucosa
Bilateral, non-exudative conjunctival injection
Polymorphous rash, generally truncal involvement, non-vesicular
Changes of extremities that may include erythema and edema of the hands or feet; desquamation of fingers and toes 1-3 weeks after onset of illness
Cervical lymphadenopathy often unilateral with at least 1 node = 1.5 cm

*Patients with fever and fewer than four criteria can be diagnosed with the presence of coronary artery disease by two-dimensional echocardiography or coronary angiography.
‡Many experts believe that in the presence of classic features, the diagnosis of Kawasaki disease can be made by experienced observers before day 5 of fever.
From Anonymous Diagnostic guidelines for Kawasaki disease. Circulation 103: 335, 2004.

following findings: (a) a nonexudative, bilateral conjunctivitis; (b) oral changes with erythematous or dry fissured lips, strawberry tongue, or pharyngitis; (c) a nonvesicular, morbilliform rash involving the trunk, perineum, and extremities, often sparing the face; (d) erythema of the palmar and plantar surfaces, edema of the hands or feet, or periungual desquamation; and (e) anterior cervical lymphadenopathy of 1.5 cm or greater. Alternatively, the diagnosis can be made with fewer than four of five criteria in the presence of coronary artery abnormalities on echocardiogram.[39] Not all criteria need to be present simultaneously to make the diagnosis; indeed, it is common for some findings to resolve as others appear, making serial evaluation of the patient essential (Exhibit 25-1).

Because a sizeable number of children with coronary artery aneurysms never meet the classic criteria, the American Heart Association is currently considering new criteria for IVIG treatment of Kawasaki disease separate from the classic epidemiologic case definition. Other illnesses that may mimic Kawasaki disease include toxin-mediated disease related to staphylococcal or streptococcal diseases, scarlet fever, enterovirus, adenovirus, measles, parvovirus, Epstein-Barr virus, mycoplasma, and rickettsial disease. Infants younger than 6 months present a particular challenge because they often lack clinical criteria for the diagnosis, yet are at greater risk for development for coronary artery abnormalities.[40] The diagnosis should be considered and echocardiography performed in young infants who have

Exhibit 25–2
Other Significant Clinical and Laboratory Findings

Cardiovascular: On auscultation, gallop rhythm or distant heart sounds; ECG changes (arrhythmias, abnormal Q waves, prolonged PR and/or QT intervals, occasionally low voltage or ST-T wave changes); chest x-ray abnormalities (cardiomegaly); echocardiographic changes (pericardial effusion, coronary aneurysms, or decreased contractility); mitral and/or aortic valvular insufficiency; and rarely, aneurysms or peripheral arteries (eg., axillary), angina pectoris, or myocardial infarction
Gastrointestinal: Diarrhea, vomiting, abdominal pain, hydrops of gallbladder, paralytic ileus, mild jaundice, and mild increase of serum transaminase levels
Blood: Increased erythrocyte sedimentation rate, leukocytosis with left shift, positive C-reactive protein, hypoalbuminemia, and mild anemia in acute phase of illness (thrombocytosis in subacute phase)
Urine: Sterile pyuria of urethral origin and occasional proteinuria
Skin: Perineal rash and desquamation in subacute phase and transverse furrows of fingernails (Beau's lines) during convalescence
Respiratory: Cough, rhinorrhea, and pulmonary infiltrate
Joint: Arthralgia and arthritis
Neurologic: Mononuclear pleocytosis in cerebrospinal fluid, striking irritability, and rarely facial palsy

From Anonymous Diagnostic guidelines for Kawasaki disease. Circulation 103: 335, 2004.

fever of greater than 5 days' duration without documented source and whose laboratory data are consistent with moderate or severe systemic inflammation.[41–43]

Other supportive signs are present in many children with Kawasaki disease (Exhibit 25-2). The rash, when perineal in location, often desquamates by the end of the first week of illness. Anterior uveitis can be identified by slit-lamp examination in 83% of patients early in the course.[44] Arthralgia and arthritis of large and small joints may be severe enough that children refuse to walk or perform tasks with their hands, but the arthritis is virtually never chronic.[44] Abdominal signs including vomiting, diarrhea, or hydrops of the gallbladder[45] are common. Other typical findings include sterile pyuria and aseptic meningitis.[46]

Tachycardia and gallop rhythm are frequently present, often thought to be out of proportion to the degree of anemia or tachycardia and therefore a manifestation of underlying myocarditis. In some cases, overt congestive heart failure occurs; however, the presence of myocarditis does not appear to correlate with risk of coronary artery aneurysm.[47] Pericarditis may present during the acute phase noted by the presence of a rub, but tamponade is very rare and resolution without long-term sequelae is the rule. A blowing systolic murmur can indicate mitral regurgitation resulting from myocarditis and aortic regurgitation, although rarely apparent clinically is identified occasionally on echocardiogram with aortic root dilation.[48] Regurgitation generally resolves with improvement of myocardial inflammation.

Kawasaki disease causes coronary artery abnormalities in 15% to 25% of patients who are not treated in the acute phase of the disease with high-dose IVIG.[49] Lesions may be observed by echocardiography as early as 1 week from the onset of fever, with further progression ensuing in the next 3 to 4 weeks. Given the difficulty in reaching diagnostic confirmation of the illness using the classic criteria, identification of those at higher risk for coronary disease and for whom early treatment could reduce extent of involvement has led investigators to focus on predictive factors for coronary artery abnormalities. The Asai score[50] assigned risk by including age younger than 1 year, male gender, fever for more than 14 days, hemoglobin below 10 g/dL, white blood cell (WBC) count above 30,000/mm^3, erythrocyte sedimentation rate (ESR) above 101 mm/hr, and elevation of C-reactive protein (CRP) or ESR beyond 30 days. Other reports have supported the concept of prolonged fever as a marker for ongoing vasculitis.[51,52] In a multicenter prospective trial of IVIG, risk for coronary involvement was increased by male gender, age under 1 year, elevated CRP, and higher absolute band count.[53,54] For those treated early with IVIG, a risk assignment methodology has been developed that uses higher baseline neutrophil and band counts, lower hemoglobin concentration, lower platelet count and fever on the day after IVIG administration.[55]

Laboratory Data

Laboratory values in the acute phase reflect the systemic vasculitis uniformly present early in the disease. Acute-phase reactants are increased markedly including ESR, CRP. and α_1-antitrypsin measurements.[56] The WBC count is elevated with a leftward shift, and a normochromic, normocytic anemia[57] is noted within the first week of illness. Thrombocytosis is usually present by the second week of the disease, often peaking at counts greater than 1,000,000 mm^3 in association with hypercoagulability. These parameters often persist over the first month of the illness and gradually decline. Hepatocellular inflammation is accompanied by increases in gamma-glutamyltransferase.[58] Sterile pyuria and pleocytosis of cerebrospinal fluid,[46] both with mononuclear cells, are found frequently.

Electrocardiography

The electrocardiogram is generally not helpful in Kawasaki disease, but in the acute phase, nonspecific ST-T wave changes are present and the PR interval may be prolonged. These findings are probably related to myocarditis.

Chest Radiography

Chest radiographs are usually unremarkable, but have been reported rarely to show pulmonary infiltrates, pulmonary effusions, or pulmonary nodules. When chest radiographs show such findings, other potentially explanatory diagnosis should be sought.

Echocardiography

Two-dimensional echocardiography provides excellent visualization of the proximal coronary arteries in young children with measurements correlating closely with those identified by angiography.[59] Measurement of the proximal left main, anterior descending, circumflex, proximal, and middle right and posterior descending branches should be made. Assessment of ventricular function, pericardial fluid, and mitral and aortic regurgitation should be obtained. Coronary artery dilation may be present as early as the end of the first week of illness with *periluminal brightness* preceding dilation, suggesting the presence of inflammatory changes of the endothelium. Dilation can proceed to coronary artery aneurysm formation (Fig. 25-1). Echocardiography should be undertaken as soon as the diagnosis is entertained, particularly because an incomplete clinical picture with coronary

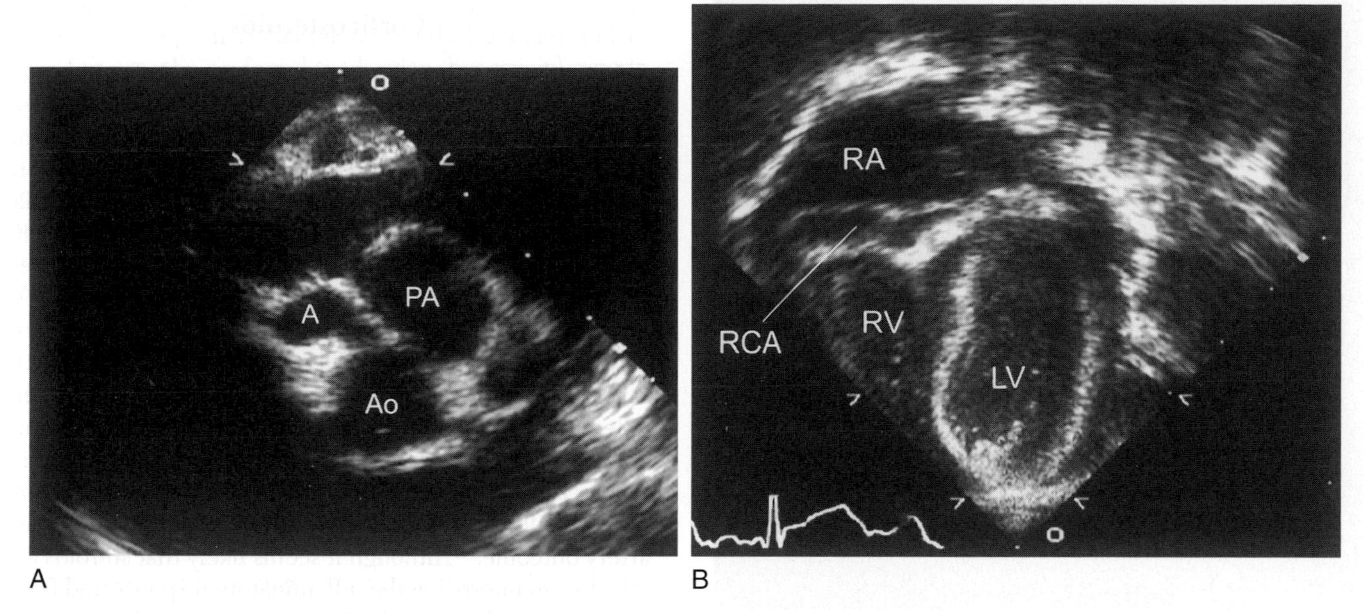

FIGURE 25–1 *A, Echocardiogram showing an aneurysm (A) of the proximal right coronary artery obtained from a short axis parasternal view. B, Ectasia of the right distal coronary artery seen from a foreshortened apical four-chamber image. Ao, aortic root; LV, left ventricle; PA, pulmonary artery; RA, right atrium; RCA, right coronary artery; RV, right ventricle.*

artery abnormalities is sufficient to make the diagnosis and initiate therapy.[60] Serial studies are obtained 10 to 14 days from onset of illness and at the end of the subacute phase (6–8 weeks).

In 1984, the Japanese Ministry of Health defined as abnormal those coronary arteries with lumen diameter larger than 3 mm in children younger than 5 years, larger than 4 mm in those older than 5 years and lumen diameter 1.5 times the size of an adjacent segment or an irregular lumen.[61] Others have shown that coronary artery size in healthy children correlates linearly with increasing body size.[62] In patients with Kawasaki disease whose coronary arteries are classified as normal by Japanese Ministry of Health criteria, the dimensions are larger than expected when adjusted for body surface area (BSA) in all phases of the disease.[62–64] This observation suggests that the prevalence of coronary artery abnormalities may be underestimated.

Cardiac Catheterization

Historically, selective coronary arteriography has been used for diagnostic assessment of coronary abnormalities,[49,65] but given the current technical quality of echocardiographic imaging, invasive studies are generally reserved for the child with large aneurysms or those with symptoms suggestive of angina. Aneurysms are described as localized or extensive,[66] the former being further subclassified as fusiform or saccular. Extensive aneurysms, those that involve more than one segment, are ectatic (dilated uniformly) or segmented (multiple dilated segments joined by normal or stenotic segments) (Fig. 25-2). Aneurysms may also involve other medium to large extraparenchymal arteries, particularly the subclavian, axillary, femoral, iliac, renal, and mesenteric arteries.[67] Occasionally, aneurysms of the aorta may occur.

MANAGEMENT

Salicylates

Aspirin is a standard therapy for Kawasaki disease, both for its anti-inflammatory and antithrombotic effects. At diagnosis, most clinicians begin high-dose aspirin, 80 to 100 mg/kg/day divided into four daily doses, until defervescence and then reduce the dose to 3 to 5 mg/kg/day, administered once daily until the end of the sub-acute phase 6-8 weeks), to reduce the likelihood for Reye syndrome[68] or gastrointestinal bleeding.[69] Meta-analysis has shown that low-dose or high-dose aspirin regimens in conjunction with IVIG have a similar incidence of coronary abnormalities at 30 and 60 days from onset of illness.[70] In patients with aneurysms, low-dose aspirin therapy is continued, sometimes in combination with anticoagulants or other antiplatelet agents.

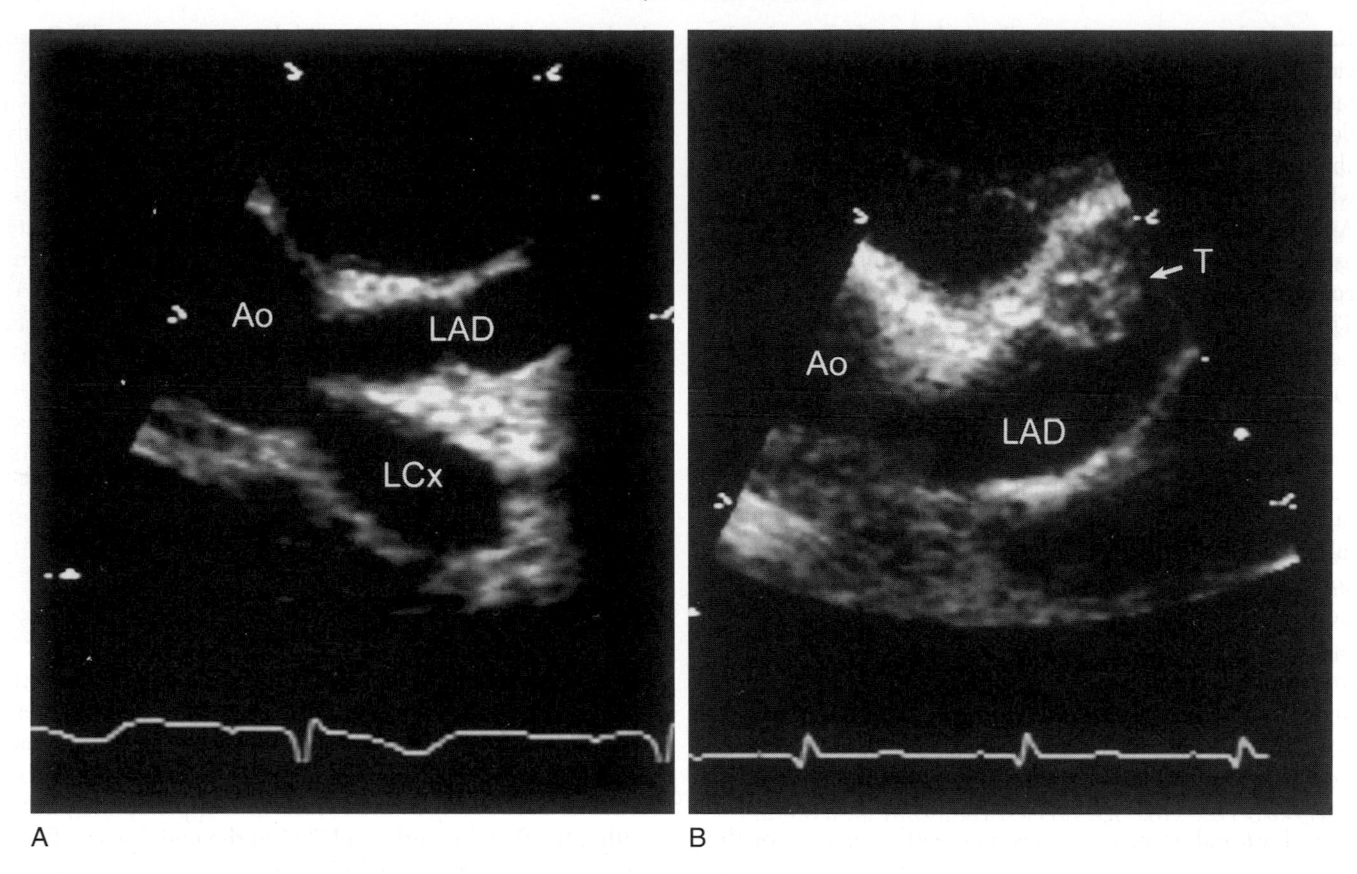

FIGURE 25–3 *A, Giant aneurysm formation of the left anterior descending (LAD) and circumflex (LCX) coronary arteries. B, Thrombus formation (T) adherent to the wall of the left anterior coronary artery.*

abnormal ventricular function in response to dobutamine infusion.[112] Abnormalities of coronary flow velocity and reserve in patients with at least moderate aneurysms or stenosis have been demonstrated using intracoronary Doppler flow guide wires.[113] Transthoracic Doppler assessment of coronary flow reserve in the right and left anterior descending coronary arteries have correlated well with invasive measurements,[114,115] providing a useful method in younger children who cannot undergo stress testing. Adenosine stress testing in combination with cardiac magnetic resonance imaging has been introduced recently.

Patients with Spontaneous Regression of Aneurysm

Regression of aneurysms occurs as a result of myointimal proliferation,[116–118] has been identified at postmortem examination and with use of transluminal ultrasound.[119] Histologic examination of regressed aneurysms show pathologic findings similar to those seen in atherosclerosis,[120] raising the concern that individuals with Kawasaki disease may be predisposed to early onset of coronary disease.[66,118]

Abnormal coronary artery function in regressed aneurysms has been demonstrated during invasive studies, with decreased vascular diastolic reactivity,[121] in addition to decreased response to intravenous dipyridamole[122] and nitroglycerine.[123] In patients receiving isosorbide dinitrate at catheterization, segments with regressed aneurysms as well as regions with persistent aneurysms had diminished reactivity relative to coronary arteries that had never been enlarged in Kawasaki disease patients or to coronary arteries of control patients.[124] Further, the decreased reactivity in abnormal areas progressed as duration from illness increased.

Course without Detectable Lesions

Children without coronary aneurysms comprise the largest subset of patients following Kawasaki disease, so that data regarding long-term outcome are essential, yet pathologic evaluation is limited. Four children who died early in the acute phase of disease (9–22 days) had inflammatory changes of the coronary arteries without dilatation,[117] but it was not possible to determine if these arteries might have dilated with prolonged survival. In another series, five children who died of incidental causes following Kawasaki disease underwent postmortem examination of the coronary arteries that showed intimal thickening and fibrosis indistinguishable from those of arteriosclerosis.[118] No correlation with clinical status was available.

Given the diffuse nature of the vasculitis seen in the acute phase of Kawasaki disease, the long-term endothelial function remains unknown. The absence of plasma 6-keto-prostaglandin F-1a, a metabolite of prostacyclin during the acute and sub-acute phase of the illness, suggests abnormal endothelial cell function[125] as well as the presence of altered lipid metabolism.[126] More recently, investigators have found decreased fibrinolytic activity in long-term survivors of Kawasaki disease both with and without coronary abnormalities.[127] Children with a history of Kawasaki disease and normal-appearing epicardial arteries were compared with normal controls with regard to myocardial blood flow and flow reserve measured using positron emission tomography.[128] Those with Kawasaki disease had lower myocardial reserve and higher total coronary resistance without regional perfusion abnormalities suggestive of damage to the coronary microcirculation. Invasive studies in children with apparently normal epicardial arteries after Kawasaki disease showed abnormal constriction with acetylcholine, an endothelium-dependent vasodilator, whereas response to nitroglycerin, an endothelium-independent vasodilator, was preserved.[129] These findings suggest abnormal endothelial function after Kawasaki disease even in those children in whom coronary dilation was never detected. Coronary artery resistance responses to acetylcholine were well preserved, suggesting normal endothelial and smooth muscle function in these arteries. However, data regarding endothelial function in normal coronary segments remain controversial.[130] High-resolution ultrasound of the brachial artery shows marked impairment of flow-mediated dilation in patients with Kawasaki disease without coronary abnormalities, compared with controls, many years after the onset of disease.[131] Endothelial independent responses were intact in both groups. These observations were supported by a similar study that showed abnormal hyperemia in brachial artery response among those with Kawasaki disease compared with controls. Interestingly, there was marked improvement in endothelial function following infusion of intravenous vitamin C in the Kawasaki patients.[132] Following Kawasaki disease, children have shown a proatherogenic lipid profile compared with age-matched healthy subjects.[133] Those with coronary aneurysms had low high-density lipoprotein cholesterol and apoA-I levels, high apoB levels, and increased peripheral conduit arterial stiffness, while even those without coronary abnormalities had increased apoB levels and brachioradial arterial stiffness. Other investigators have shown preserved endothelial function in those with normal coronary arteries following Kawasaki disease compared with those with persistent or regressed aneurysms.

Overall, patients who have not had demonstrable coronary artery abnormalities have continued to do well clinically.[65,133] The long-term management of this group should include follow-up assessment every 3 to 5 years after the first year of illness. Particular attention should be paid to minimizing coronary risk factors by maintaining normal blood pressure and healthy dietary habits, assessing lipid profile every 5 to 10 years, and encouraging routine exercise.

REFERENCES

1. Kawasaki T. [Acute febrile mucocutaneous syndrome with lymphoid involvement with specific desquamation of the fingers and toes in children]. Arerugi 16:178, 1967.
2. Hayasaka S, Nakamura Y, Yashiro M, et al. Analyses of fatal cases of Kawasaki disease in Japan using vital statistical data over 27 years. J Epidemiol 13:246, 2003.
3. Morens D, Anderson L, Hurwitz E. National surveillance of Kawasaki disease. Pediatrics 65:21, 1980.
4. Holman R, Curns A, Belay E, et al. Kawasaki syndrome hospitalizations in the United States, 1997 and 2000. Pediatrics 112:495, 2003.
5. Davis R, Waller P, Mueller BA, et al. Race-specific incidence rates and residential proximity to water. Arch Pediatr Adolesc Med 149:66, 1995.
6. Stockheim J, Innocentini N, Shulman S. Kawasaki disease in children and older adolescents. Pediatrics 137:250, 2000.
7. Meissner H, Leung D. Pediatr Infect Dis 19:91, 2000.
8. Duong T, Silverman E, Bissessar MV, et al. Superantigenic activity is responsible for induction of coronary arteritis in mice: an animal model of Kawasaki disease. Int Immunol 15: 79, 2003.
9. Rowley A, Shulman ST, Mask C, et al. IgA plasma cell infiltration of proximal respiratory tract, pancreas, kidney, coronary artery in acute Kawasaki disease. J Infect Dis 182:1183, 2000.
10. Rowley A, Shulman S, Spike B, et al. Oligoclonal IgA response in the vascular wall in acute Kawasaki disease. J Immunol 166:1334, 2001.
11. Furukawa S, Matubara T, Yabuta K. Mononuclear cell subsets and coronary artery lesions in Kawasaki disease. Arch Dis Child 67:706, 1992.
12. Abe J, Kotzin BL, Jujo K, et al. Selective expansion of T cells expressing T-cell receptor variable regions V beta 2 and V beta 8 in Kawasaki disease. Proc Natl Acad Sci USA 89: 4066, 1992.
13. Abe J, Kotzin B, Meissner H, et al. Characterization of T cell repertoire changes in acute Kawasaki disease. J Exp Med 177:791, 1993.
14. Yamashiro Y, Nagata, Oguchi S, et al. Selective increase of Vβ2+ cells in the small intestinal mucosa in Kawasaki disease. Omission, 1999.
15. Yoshioka T, Matsutani T, Iwagami S, et al. Polyclonal expansion of TCRβV2 and TCRβV6-bearing T cells in patients with Kawasaki disease. Immunol 96:465, 1999.

16. Curtis N, Zheng R, Lamb J. Evidence for a superantigen mediated process in Kawasaki Disease. Arch Dis Child 72:308, 2004.
17. Leung D, Giorno R, Kazemi LV, et al. Evidence for superantigen involvement in cardiovascular injury due to Kawasaki syndrome. J Immunol 155:5018, 1995.
18. Brogan P, Shah V, Klein N, et al. T cell Vß repertoires in childhood vasculitides. Clin Exp Immunol 131:517, 2003.
19. Leung D, Collins T, Lapierre LA, et al. Immunoglobulin M antibodies present in the acute phase of Kawasaki syndrome lyse cultured vascular endothelial cells stimulated by gamma interferon. J Clin Invest 77:1428, 1986.
20. Leung D, Geha R, Newburger J, et al. Two monokines, interleukin 1 and tumor necrosis factor, render cultured vascular endothelial cells susceptible to lysis by antibodies circulating during Kawasaki syndrome. J Exp Med 164:1958, 2004.
21. Fujieda M, Oishi N, Kurashige T, et al. Antibodies to endothelial cells in Kawasaki disease lyse endothelial cells without cytokine pretreatment. Clin Exp Immunol 107:120, 1997.
22. Hashimoto H, Igarashi N, Yachie A, et al. The relationship between serum levels of interleukin-6 and thyroid hormone during the follow-up study in children with nonthyroidal illness: Marked inverse correlation in Kawasaki and infectious disease. Endocrine 43:31, 1996.
23. Hirao J, Hibi S, Andoh T, et al. High levels of circulating interleukin-4 and interleukin-10 in Kawasaki disease. Int Arch Allerg Immun 112:152, 1997.
24. Suzuki H, Uemura S, Tone S. Effects of immunoglobulin and gamma-interferon on the production of tumour necrosis factor-alpha and interleukin-1-β by peripheral blood monocytes in the acute phase of Kawasaki disease. Eur J Pediatr 155:291, 1996.
25. Kim D, Lee KY. Serum Soluble E-selectin levels in Kawasaki Disease. Scand J Rheum 23:283, 1994.
26. Mayatepek E, Lehmann WD. Increased generation of cysteinyl leukotrienes in Kawasaki disease. Arch Dis Child 72:526, 1995.
27. Leung D, Meissner H, Shulman S. Prevalence of superantigen-secreting bacteria in patients with Kawasaki disease. J Pediatr 140:742, 2002.
28. Terai M, Yaukawa K, Narumoto S, et al. Vascular endothelial growth factor in acute Kawasaki disease. Am J Cardiol 83: 337, 1999.
29. Hirose S, Hamashima Y. Morphological observations on the vasculitis in the mucocutaneous lymph node syndrome: a skin biopsy study of 27 patients. Eur J Pediatr 129:215, 1978.
30. Fukumura D, Gohongi T, Kadambi A, et al. Predominant role of endothelial nitric oxide synthase in vascular endothelial growth factor-induced angiogenesis and vascular permeability. Proc Natl Acad Sci U S A 98:2604, 2001.
31. Iizuka T, Oishi K, Sasaki M, et al. Nitric oxide and aneurysm formation in Kawasaki disease. Acta Paediatr 86:470, 1997.
32. Terai M, Honda T, Yasukawa K, et al. Prognostic impact of vascular leakage in acute Kawasaki disease. Circulation 108: 325, 2003.
33. Longo G, Xiong W, Greiner T, et al. Matrix metalloproteinases 2 and 9 work in concert to produce aortic aneurysms. J Clin Invest 96:318, 2002.
34. Gavin P, Crawford SE, Shulman S, et al. Systemic arterial expression of matrix metalloproteinases 2 and 9 in acute Kawasaki disease. Arterioscler Thromb Vasc Biol 23:576, 2003.
35. Yanagawa H, Nakamura Y, Yashiro K, et al. Results of the nationwide epidemiologic survey of Kawsaki disease in 1995 and 1996 in Japan. Pediatrics 102:E65, 1998.
36. Fujiwara H, Kosaki F, Okawa S. Pathology of the heart in Kawasaki disease. Pediatrics 54:271, 1974.
37. Burns J, Glode M, Clarke S, et al. Coagulopathy and platelet activation in Kawasaki syndrome: identification of patients at high risk for development of artery aneurysms. J Pediatr 105:206, 1986.
38. Kawasaki T, Kosaki F, Okawa S, et al. A new infantile acute febrile mucocutaneous lymph node syndrome (MLNS) prevailing in Japan. Pediatrics 54:271, 1974.
39. Anonymous. Diagnostic guidelines for Kawasaki disease. Circulation 103:335, 2004.
40. Burns J, Wiggins J, Toews W, et al. Clinical spectrum of Kawasaki disease in infants younger than 6 months of age. J Pediatr 109:759, 1986.
41. Schuh S, Laxer R, Smallhorn J, et al. Kawasaki disease with atypical presentation. Pediatr Infect Dis 7:208, 1991.
42. Rowley A, Gonzalez Crussi F, Gidding SS. Incomplete Kawasaki disease with coronary artery involvement. J Pediatr 109:759, 1987.
43. Fukushige N, Takahashi N, Ueda K, et al. Incidence and clinical features of incomplete Kawasaki disease. Acta Pediatr 83:1057, 1994.
44. Burns J, Joffe L, Sargent RA. Anterior uveitis associated with Kawasaki syndrome. Pediatr Infect Dis 4:285, 1985.
45. Sty J, Starshak R, Gorenstein L. Gallbladder perforation in a case of Kawasaki disease: image correlation. J Clin Ultrasound 11:381, 1983.
46. Dengler L, Capparelli E, Bastian J, et al. Cerebrospinal fluid profile in patients with acute Kawasaki disease. J Ped Infect Dis 17:478, 1998.
47. Hiraishi S, Yashiro K, Oguchi K, et al. Clinical course of cardiovascular involvement in the mucocutaneous lymph node syndrome: Relation between clinical signs of carditis and development of coronary arterial aneurysm. Am J Cardiol 47:323, 1981.
48. Ravekes W, Colan SD, Gauvreau K, et al. Aortic root dilation in Kawasaki disease. Am J Cardiol 87:919, 2001.
49. Kato H, Ichinose E, Yoshioka F, et al. Fate of coronary aneurysms in Kawasaki disease: serial coronary angiography and long-term follow-up study. Am J Cardiol 49:1758, 1982.
50. Asai T. [Diagnosis and prognosis of coronary artery lesions in Kawasaki disease. Coronary angiography and the conditions for its application a score chart]. Nippon Rinsho 41:2080, 1983.
51. Koren G, Lavi S, Rose V, et al. Kawasaki disease: review of risk factors for coronary aneurysms. Pediatrics 108: 386, 1986.

52. Daniels S, Specker B, CT, et al. Correlates of coronary artery aneurysm formation in patients with Kawasaki disease. Am J Dis Child 141:205, 1987.
53. Nakano M. Predictive factors of coronary aneurysm in Kawasaki disease: correlation between coronary arterial lesions and serum albumin, cholinesterase activity, prealbumin, retinal-binding protein and immature neutrophils. Prog Clin Biol Res 250:535, 1987.
54. Newburger J, Takahashi M, Burns J, et al. The treatment of Kawasaki syndrome with intravenous gamma globulin. N Engl J Med 315:341, 1986.
55. Beiser A, Takahashi M, Baker A, et al. A predictive instrument for coronary artery aneurysms in Kawasaki disease. Am J Cardiol 81:1116, 1998.
56. Burns J, Mason W, Glode MP, et al. Clinical and epidemiologic characteristics of patients referred for evaluation of possible Kawasaki disease. J Pediatr 118:680, 1991.
57. Melish ME. Kawasaki Syndrome: a 1986 perspective. Rheum Dis Clin North Am 13:7, 1987.
58. Ting E, Capparelli E, Billman G, et al. Elevated gamma-glutaryltransferase concentrations in patients with acute Kawasaki disease. Pediatr Infect Dis 17:431, 1998.
59. Capannari T, Daniels S, Meyer R, et al. Sensitivity, specificity and predictive value of two-dimensional echocardiography in detecting coronary artery aneurysms in patients with Kawasaki disease. J Am Coll Cardiol 7:355, 1986.
60. Anonymous. Diagnostic guidelines for Kawasaki disease. Circulation 103:335, 2001.
61. Research Committee on Kawasaki Disease. Report of subcommittee on standardization of diagnostic criteria and reporting coronary artery lesions in Kawasaki disease. Tokyo, Japan: Ministry of Health and Welfare, 1984.
62. de Zorzi A, Colan S, Gauvreau K, et al. Coronary dimensions may be misclassified as normal in Kawasaki disease. J Pediatr 133:254, 1998.
63. Arjunan K, Daniels S, Meyer R, et al. Coronary artery caliber in normal children and patients with Kawasaki disease but without aneurysm: An echocardiographic and angiographic study. J Am Coll Cardiol 8:1119, 1986.
64. Kurotobi S, NT, Kawakami N, et al. Coronary diameter in normal infants, children and patients with Kawasaki disease. Pediatr Inter 44:1, 2002.
65. Kato H, Sugimura T, Akagi T. Long-term consequences of Kawasaki Disease. A 10 to 21 year follow-up study of 594 patients. Circulation 94:1379, 1996.
66. Takahashi M, Mason W, Lewis A. Regression of coronary aneurysms in patients with Kawasaki syndrome. Circulation 75:387, 1987.
67. Suzuki A, Kamiya T, Kuwahara N, et al. Coronary arterial lesion of Kawasaki disease: cardiac catheterization: findings of 1100 cases. Pediatr Cardiol 7:3, 1986.
68. Takahashi M, Mason W, Thomas D, et al. Reye syndrome following Kawasaki syndrome confirmed by liver histopathology. In Kato H (ed). Kawasaki Disease Proceedings of the 5th International Kawasaki Disease Symposium, Fukuoka, Japan, May 22–25, 1995. Amsterdam, Elsevier Science BV, 1995, p 436.
69. Matsubara T, Mason W, Kashani IA, et al. Gastrointestinal hemorrhage complicating aspirin therapy in acute Kawasaki disease. J Pediatr 128:701, 1996.
70. Durongpisitkul K, Guruaj V, Park J. The prevention of coronary artery aneurysm in Kawasaki disease: a meta-analysis on the efficacy of aspirin and immunoglobulin treatment. Pediatrics 96:1057, 1995.
71. Furusho K, Kamiya T, Nakano H. High-dose intravenous gammaglobulin for Kawasaki disease. Lancet ii:1055, 1984.
72. Barron K, Murphy D, Silverman E, et al. Treatment of Kawasaki syndrome: a comparison of two dosage regimens of intravenously administered immune globulin. J Pediatr 117:638, 1990.
73. Morikawa Y, Ohashi Y, Harada K, et al. A multicenter, randomized, controlled trial of intravenous gamma globulin therapy in children with acute Kawasaki Disease. Acta Paediatr Jpn 36:347, 1994.
74. Nagashima M, Matsushima M, Matsuoka H. High-dose gammaglobulin therapy for Kawasaki disease. J Pediatr 110: 710, 1987.
75. Newburger JW, Takahashi M, Beiser AS. A single intravenous infusion of gamma globulin as compared with four infusions in the treatment of acute Kawasaki syndrome. N Engl J Med 324:1663, 1991.
76. Report of the Committee on Infectious Disease. Kawasaki disease. In Pickering L (ed). Red Book: Report of the Committee on Infectious Disease. Elk Grove Village, IL: American Academy of Pediatrics, 2003, p 394.
77. Burns J, Glode M, Capparelli E. Intravenous gammaglobulin treatment in Kawasaki syndrome: are all brands equal? In Kato H (ed). Kawasaki Disease Proceedings of the 5th International Kawasaki Disease Symposium, Fukuoka, Japan. Amsterdam: Elsevier Science BV, 1995.
78. Silverman E, Huang C, Rose V, et al. IVGG treatment of Kawasaki disease: are all brands equal? In Kato H (ed). Kawasaki Disease Proceedings of the 5th International Kawasaki Disease Symposium, Fukuoka, Japan. Amsterdam: Elsevier Science BV, 1995.
79. Rosenfeld EA, SS, Corydon KE. Comparative safety and efficacy of two immune globulin products in Kawasaki disease. In Kato H (ed). Kawasaki Disease Proceedings of the 5th International Kawasaki Disease Symposium, Fukuoka, Japan. Amsterdam: Elsevier Science BV, 1995, p 291.
80. Schneider L, Geha R,, et al. Outbreak of hepatitis C associated with IVGG administration: US, October 1993–June 1994. Morbidity and Mortality Weekly Report 43:505, 1994.
81. Dajani A, Taubert K, Takahashi M, et al. Guidelines for long-term management of patients with Kawasaki disease. Report from the committee on Rheumatic Fever, Endocarditis, and Kawasaki Disease, Council on Cardiovascular Disease in the Young, American Heart Association. Circulation 89:916, 1994.
82. Tse S, Silverman E, McCrindle B, et al. Early treatment with intravenous immunoglobulin in patients with Kawasaki disease. J Pediatr 140:450, 2002.
83. Marasini M, Pongiglione G, Gazzolo D. Late intravenous gamma globulin treatment in infants and children with

Kawasaki Disease and coronary artery abnormalities. Am J Cardiol 68:796, 1991.
84. Kato H, Koike S, Yokoyama T. Kawasaki disease: effect of treatment on coronary artery involvement. Pediatrics 63:175, 1979.
85. Shinohara M, Sone K, Tomomasa T. Corticosteroids in the treatment of the acute phase of Kawasaki disease. J Pediatr 135:465, 1999.
86. Sundel R, Baker A, Fulton D, et al. Corticosteroids in the initial treatment of Kawasaki disease: Report of a randomized trial. J Pediatr 142:611, 2003.
87. Hashino K, Ishii M, Iemura M. Re-treatment for immune globulin-resistant Kawasaki disease: A comparative study of additional immune globulin and steroid pulse therapy. Pediatrics Inter 43:211, 2001.
88. Fujiwara R, Fujiwara H, Hamashima Y. Size of coronary aneurysm as a determinant factor of the prognosis in Kawasaki disease: clinicopathologic study of coronary aneurysms. Prog Clin Biol Res 250:519, 1987.
89. Nakano H, Saito A, Ueda K. Clinical characteristics of myocardial infarction following Kawasaki disease: report of 11 cases. J Pediatr 108:198, 1986.
90. Cheatham JP, Kugler JD, Gumbiner CH. Intracoronary streptokinase in Kawasaki disease; acute and thrombolysis. Prog Clin Biol Res 250:517, 1987.
91. Kato H, Ichinose E, Inoue O, et al. Intracoronary thrombolytic therapy in Kawasaki disease: treatment and prevention of acute myocardial infarction. Prog Clin Biol Res 250:445, 1987.
92. Levy M, Benson L, Burrows P. Tissue plasminogen activator for the treatment of thromboembolism in infants and children. Pediatrics 118:467, 1991.
93. Terai M, Ogata M, Sugimoto K. Coronary arterial thrombi in Kawasaki disease. J Pediatr 106:76, 1985.
94. Hirose S, Kawashima Y, Nakano S, et al. Long-term results in surgical treatment of children 4 years old or younger with coronary involvement due to Kawasaki disease. Circulation 74, 1986.
95. Ino T, Iwahara M, Boku H. Aortocoronary bypass surgery for Kawasaki disease. Pediatr Cardiol 8:195, 2004.
96. Kitamura S, Kawachi K, Oyama C, et al. Kawasaki heart disease treated with an internal mammary artery graft in pediatric patients: a first successful report. J Thor Cardiovasc Surg 89:860, 1985.
97. Kitamura S. Surgical treatment for coronary arterial lesions in Kawasaki disease. Prog Clin Biol Res 250:455, 1987.
98. Suzuki A, Kamiya T, Ono Y. Indication for aortocoronary bypass for coronary arterial obstruction due to Kawasaki disease. Heart Vessels 1:94, 1985.
99. Takeuchi Y, Suma K, Shiroma K, et al. Surgical experience with coronary arterial sequelae of Kawasaki disease in children. J Cardiovasc Surg 22:231, 1981.
100. Kitamura S, Kameda Y, Seki T, et al. Long-term outcome of myocardial revascularization in patients with Kawasaki coronary artery disease. A multi-center cooperative study. J Thorac Cardiovasc Surg 107:663, 1994.
101. Kamiya T, Suzuki A, Ono Y,, et al. Angiographic follow-up study of coronary artery lesions in the cases with a history of Kawasaki disease: with a focus on the follow-up more than ten years after the onset of disease. In Kato H (ed). Kawasaki Disease Proceedings of the 5th International Kawasaki Disease Symposium, Fukuoka, Japan. Amsterdam: Elsevier Science BV, 1995, p 569.
102. Kato H, Sugimura T, Akagi T,, et al. Long-term consequences of Kawasaki Disease. Circulation 94:1379, 1996.
103. Tatara K, Kusakawa S. Long term prognosis of giant coronary aneurysms in Kawasaki disease. Prog Clin Biol Res 250:579, 1987.
104. Suzuki A, Kamiya T, Arakaki Y. Fate of coronary arterial lesions in Kawasaki disease. Am J Cardiol 74:822, 1994.
105. Kato H, Ichinose E, Kawasaki T. Myocardial infarction in Kawasaki disease: clinical analyses in 195 cases. J Pediatr 108:123, 1986.
106. Suzuki A, Kamiya T, Ono Y, et al. Myocardial ischemia in Kawasaki disease: follow-up study by cardiac catheterization and coronary angiography. Pediatr Cardiol 9:1, 1988.
107. Fukuda T, Akagi T, Ishibashi M, et al. Non-invasive evaluation of myocardial ischemia in Kawasaki disease: comparison between dipyridamole stress thallium and exercise stress testing. Am Heart J 135:482, 1998.
108. Kimball T, Witt S, Daniels S. Dobutamine stress echocardiography in the assessment of suspected myocardial ischemia in children and young adults. Am J Cardiol 79:380, 1997.
109. Pahl E, Seghal R, Chrystof D, et al. Feasibility of exercise stress echocardiography for follow-up of children with coronary involvement secondary to Kawasaki disease. Circulation 91:122, 1996.
110. Hijazi Z, Udelson J, Snapper H, et al. Physiologic significance of chronic coronary aneurysms in patients with Kawasaki disease. J Am Coll Cardiol 24:1633, 1994.
111. Furuyama H, Odagawa Y, Katoh C, et al. Altered myocardial flow reserve and endothelial function late after Kawasaki disease. J Pediatr 142:149, 2003.
112. Harada K, Tamura M, Toyono M, et al. Effect of dobutamine on a Doppler echocardiographic index of combined systolic and diastolic performance. Pediatr Cardiol 23:613, 2002.
113. Hamaoka K, Onouchi Z, Kamiya Y, et al. Evaluation of coronary arterial flow-velocity dynamics and flow reserve in patients with Kawasaki disease by means of a Doppler guide wire. J Am Coll Cardiol 31:833, 1998.
114. Hiraishi S, Hirota H, Horiguchi Y, et al. Transthoracic Doppler assessment of coronary flow velocity reserve in children with Kawasaki disease: comparison with coronary angiography and thallium-201 imaging. J Am Coll Cardiol 40:1816, 2002.
115. Noto N, Karasawa K, Kanamaru H, et al. Non-invasive measurement of coronary flow reserve in children with Kawasaki disease. Brit Heart J 87:559, 2002.
116. Fujiwara H, Hamashima Y. Pathology of the heart in Kawasaki disease. Pediatrics 61:100, 1978.
117. Fujiwara T, Fujiwara H, Nakano H. Pathological features of coronary arteries in children with Kawasaki Disease in which coronary arterial aneurysm was absent at autopsy. Circulation 78:345, 1988.

118. Tanaka N, Naoe S, Masuda H, et al. Pathological study of sequelae of Kawasaki disease MCLS. With special reference to the heart and coronary arterial lesions. Acta Pathol Jpn 36:1513, 1986.
119. Sugimura T, Kato H, Inoue O, et al. Intravascular ultrasound of coronary arteries in children. Assessment of the wall morphology and the lumen after Kawasaki disease. Circulation 89:258, 1994.
120. Sasaguri Y, Kato H. Regression of aneurysms in Kawasaki disease: a pathological study? J Pediatr 100:225, 1982.
121. Kurisu Y, Azumi T, Sughara T. Variation in coronary artery dimensions distensible abnormality after disappearing aneurysm in Kawasaki disease. Am Heart J 114:532, 1987.
122. Matsumura K, Okuda Y, Ito T. Coronary angiography of Kawasaki disease with the coronary vasodilator dipyridamole: assessment of distensibility of affected coronary arterial wall. Angiology 39:141, 1988.
123. Spevak P, Newburger J, Keane J, et al. Reactivity of coronary arteries in Kawasaki syndrome: an analysis of function. Am J Cardiol 60:640, 1987.
124. Sugimura T, Kato H, Inoue O. Vasodilatory response of the coronary arteries after Kawasaki disease: evaluation by intracoronary injection of ofisosorbide dintrate. J Pediatr 121: 684, 1992.
125. Fulton D, Meissner H, Peterson M. Effects of current therapy of Kawasaki disease on eicosanoid metabolism. Am J Cardiol 61:1323, 1988.
126. Newburger JW, Burns JC, Beiser A. Altered lipid metabolism following Kawasaki disease. Circulation 84:625, 1991.
127. Albisetti M, Chan A, McCrindle B, et al. Fibrinolytic response to venous occlusion is decreased in patients after Kawasaki disease. Blood Coagul Fibrinolysis 14:181, 2003.
128. Muzik O, Paridon S, Singh T, et al. Quantification of myocardial blood flow and flow reserve in children with a history of Kawasaki Disease and normal coronary arteries using positron emission tomography. J Am Coll Cardiol 28:757, 1996.
129. Mitani Y, Okuda Y, Shimpo H, et al. Impaired endothelial function in epicardial coronary arteries after Kawasaki disease. Circulation 96:454, 1997.
130. Yamakawa R, Ishii M, Sugimara T, et al. Coronary endothelial dysfunction after Kawasaki disease: evaluation by intracoronary injection of acetylcholine. J Am Coll Cardiol 31:1074, 1998.
131. Dhillon R, Clarkson P, Donald A, et al. Endothelial dysfunction late after Kawasaki disease. Circulation 94:2103, 1996.
132. Deng YB, Li TL, Xiang HJ, et al. Impaired endothelial function in the brachial artery after Kawasaki disease and the effects of intravenous administration of vitamin C. Pediatr Infect Dis 22:34, 2003.
133. Nakamura Y, Yanagawa H, Harada K, et al. Mortality among persons with a history of Kawasaki disease in Japan: the fifth look. Arch Pediatr Adolesc Med 156:162, 2002.

26

Cardiomyopathies

STEVEN D. COLAN

This diverse group of disorders has historically been understood to represent *heart muscle diseases of unknown etiology*, clearly excluding secondary processes such as hypertension, ischemic heart disease, and valvar and congenital heart disease. However, in 1995 this classification was changed to conform to clinical practice, defining cardiomyopathies as diseases of the myocardium associated with cardiac dysfunction, including primary and secondary forms.[1] The defined secondary forms are generally categorized by etiology, such as anthracycline, hypertensive, inflammatory, metabolic, and ischemic cardiomyopathy. The concept of a *cardiomyopathy of overload* is included under this umbrella and refers to the clinically familiar concept of load-induced myocyte dysfunction. The cardiomyopathies are also classified according to phenotype as (I) dilated, (II) hypertrophic, (III) restrictive, (IV) arrhythmogenic right ventricular, and (V) unclassified. The phenotypic classification is primarily based on morphology but generally has implications as to the underlying physiology. The mixture of morphology and physiology inherent within this classification is clearly problematic, and many overlapping cases are encountered. It is now clear that the etiology is not a reliable predictor of the phenotype insofar as the same etiology can manifest as dilated cardiomyopathy in some patients and as hypertrophic cardiomyopathy in others, and furthermore that individual patients can transition between the two over time. This chapter is organized according to the phenotypic classification primarily because of its utility for management decisions, its implications as to physiology and outcome, and its representation of the standard clinical framework; presented in the following sequence:

I. Dilated cardiomyopathy
   Definition and epidemiology
   Clinical presentation and diagnostic evaluation
   Treatment
   Predictors of outcome in dilated cardiomyopathy
   Outcome
   Infective myocarditis
   Endocardial fibroelastosis
   Dystrophinopathies
   Duchenne muscular dystrophy
   Becker muscular dystrophy
   X-linked dilated cardiomyopathy
   Doxorubicin cardiomyopathy
   Mechanism of anthracycline-mediated cardiac injury
   Clinical characteristics of anthracycline cardiotoxicity
   Risk factors for doxorubicin cardiotoxicity
   Prevention of doxorubicin cardiomyopathy
   Management
   HIV-Associated cardiac disease
   Myotonic dystrophy
   Iron overload cardiomyopathy
   Thalassemia

II. Hypertrophic cardiomyopathy
   Familial hypertrophic cardiomyopathy
   Genetics
   Pathology
   Pathophysiology
   Diastolic dysfunction
   Exercise intolerance
   Ischemia
   Myocardial bridging
   Arrhythmias
   Sudden death
   Clinical description
   Physical
   Electrocardiogram

Echocardiogram
Exercise testing
Magnetic resonance imaging (MRI)
Catheterization
Differential diagnosis
Management
Beta-blockers
Calcium channel blockers
Vasodilators
SBE prophylaxis
Pacemaker therapy
Alcohol septal ablation
Surgical myectomy
Antiarrhythmics
Exercise restriction
Risk stratification
Clinical course
Friedreich ataxia
Heart disease in Friedreich ataxia
III. Restrictive cardiomyopathy
IV. Right ventricular cardiomyopathies
Uhl anomaly
Arrhythmogenic right ventricular cardiomyopathy
V. Noncompaction of the ventricular myocardium

DILATED CARDIOMYOPATHY

Definition and Epidemiology

Dilated cardiomyopathy (DCM) is characterized by dilation and impaired systolic function of the left or both ventricles. Although the term *congestive cardiomyopathy* was formerly used as a synonym, DCM is now preferred because the earliest manifestation is usually ventricular enlargement and dysfunction. Congestive heart failure is not a constant feature and, of course, does not differentiate this from other forms of cardiomyopathy. It is the most common form of cardiomyopathy in children, accounting for at least 50% of cases, and has a population incidence of 0.58 per 100,000 children.[2] DCM has numerous etiologies, clinical manifestations, and outcomes that vary depending on the pathogenesis and host response. The described associations in children include infectious,[3] familial,[4,5] mitochondrial,[6,7] metabolic,[8] arrhythmic,[9] toxic,[10] and inflammatory diseases,[11] but most cases remain idiopathic. Although the true frequency of the various causes of DCM is currently unknown, improved methods of diagnosis have enabled determination of the cause for a progressively larger proportion of the previously idiopathic cases. Between one third and one half of cases are thought to be familial {Crispell, 1999 55679 /id}. Inflammatory heart disease due to viral myocarditis or an abnormal immunologic response to viral infection[13] is believed to account for 30% to 40% of cases.

The variety of causes that can eventuate in DCM suggests that the disorder is the final common pathway for any of the mechanisms that produce myocardial damage, including cytotoxic, metabolic, immunological, and infectious mechanisms. Although generally treated as a distinct entity, the so-called *cardiomyopathy of overload*, representing the clinically indistinguishable cardiomyopathy seen as the end-stage manifestation of untreated pressure or volume overload, almost certainly represents the same final common pathway. The molecular event or events that account for myocardial failure remain elusive, although numerous metabolic abnormalities have been described.[14–16] Many abnormalities often coexist and their relative importance remains unclear. Although most investigators have sought a single final pathway to contractile dysfunction, this may not be correct. Because dilated cardiomyopathy appears as the end result of many quite different processes, it is likely that numerous metabolic disturbances may have ventricular dysfunction as the primary clinical manifestation. Clarification of the disease-specific pathogenesis of contractile failure has no doubt been hampered by our very limited ability to determine etiology. For example, the potential relationship between viral myocarditis and DCM has been a particular focus of speculation and investigation. The proposed scenario is that clinical or subclinical viral myocarditis initiates an autoimmune reaction that ultimately leads to DCM. This topic is discussed in the section on myocarditis, but it is clear that one of the factors impeding clarification of this mechanism is the limited ability to diagnose viral myocarditis.

It is worth noting that although there is a general clinical assumption that the primary functional change at the myofiber level in DCM is depression of contractile function, several groups have shown that isolated cardiac muscle harvested from patients with end-stage heart failure is capable of normal force-generating capacity under ideal conditions and low stimulation frequencies,[17] even when force generation deteriorates at higher stimulation frequencies.[18] In contrast, diastolic abnormalities are a constant property of failing heart muscle.[19] It is likely that in many forms of DCM, the process evolves over time, with depressed contractility present at certain phases of the disease particularly during the early or inciting phase, but that intrinsic failure of the contractile function of individual myocytes is an inconstant feature of the disease.

Clinical Presentation and Diagnostic Evaluation

Regardless of the underlying cause of the ventricular dysfunction, the dilated cardiomyopathies have similar modes of presentation. Older children present with exercise intolerance, dyspnea on exertion, tachycardia, palpitations, chest pain, abdominal distention, syncope or near-syncope, and occasionally with cardiovascular collapse and sudden death. Although many symptoms parallel those seen in adults, primary complaints of peripheral edema and paroxysmal nocturnal dyspnea are uncommon in younger children. Infants are generally recognized on the basis of respiratory distress, abdominal distention, and poor feeding but occasionally the process is subacute and failure to thrive is present at the time of diagnosis. Secondary cardiomyopathies can manifest a broad spectrum of noncardiac abnormalities, depending on the nature of the primary disorder.

Physical findings depend on the severity of clinical compromise. Patients with mild ventricular dysfunction can present with reduced exercise capacity but no abnormal physical findings. Congestive heart failure is nearly always accompanied by tachypnea and tachycardia. Peripheral cyanosis is noted only in the presence of severe compromise. Peripheral pulses are often weak and can be difficult to palpate, reflecting a narrow pulse pressure and hypotension. Cool extremities and poor capillary refill can be noted, particularly in infants. Intercostal retractions are a common finding in infants and young children, but in contrast to adults, pulmonary auscultation rarely reveals rales, even when frank pulmonary edema is present on chest radiograph. Wheezing can be heard at all ages because of attenuated airway relaxation, a process that appears to result from the generalized desensitization of the beta-adrenergic receptors that is characteristic of congestive heart failure.[20] Hepatomegaly is a seminal finding and can be massive in infants, changing rapidly in response to therapy. Neck vein distention and peripheral edema are almost never detected in infants, but become more common with age. The cardiac impulse is often displaced laterally and is diffuse. Gallop rhythm with a third heart sound is common, as is a murmur of mitral regurgitation.

Cardiomegaly, pulmonary venous congestion, pulmonary edema, atelectasis, and pleural effusions are the key radiographic findings, depending on severity. Cardiomegaly on chest radiograph may be the only finding in asymptomatic left ventricular dysfunction, but the sensitivity and specificity of this finding is quite poor in children. The electrocardiogram shows sinus tachycardia in most patients. Nonspecific ST-T wave changes and left ventricular hypertrophy are noted in about half of patients, with atrial and right ventricular hypertrophy in 25%. Nearly 50% of patients have arrhythmias detectable by Holter monitoring at the time of presentation, including atrial fibrillation and flutter, ventricular ectopic beats, and nonsustained ventricular tachycardia. Dilated cardiomyopathy must be differentiated from tachycardia-induced cardiomyopathy, a process that can have a similar presentation but responds to arrhythmia control with complete recovery.[9]

The diagnostic findings on echocardiogram are a dilated left ventricle with diminished systolic performance (Fig. 26-1). Dysfunction is global although moderate regional variation in wall motion is usually present.[21] Quantitative assessment of systolic and diastolic functional parameters and ventricular morphology is diagnostically and prognostically useful.[22] Pericardial effusions are frequent. Intracardiac thrombi have been reported in as many as 23% of children, although rarely in infants.[23] Color flow and spectral Doppler are useful for assessment of mitral regurgitation and diastolic function.[22] The echocardiogram is equally critical for excluding valvar and structural cardiac disease. Anomalous origin of the left main coronary artery from the pulmonary artery can be reliably recognized through the combined use of imaging and color flow Doppler.[24]

Radionuclide studies are not usually helpful for diagnosis or management of dilated cardiomyopathy in children, although some older children with poor echocardiographic windows can require an alternative imaging modality for assessment of ventricular function. Myocardial perfusion scans are often used in adults to differentiate ischemic cardiomyopathy but this differential rarely arises in pediatrics. Gallium-67 citrate has been suggested as a means of detecting inflammatory heart disease,[25] but is not generally believed to be as accurate as biopsy.

Cardiac magnetic resonance imaging has assumed an increasingly important role in the imaging of congenital and acquired heart disease in children. The technique provides an accurate method of measuring left and right ventricular volumes, masses, and ejection fractions. Intracardiac thrombi are readily documented. The method is particularly useful in patients with poor echocardiographic images. The primary limitations relate to exclusion of patients with pacemakers, the safety of which is not established, and the need for anesthesia is young children.

Cardiac catheterization is performed primarily for endomyocardial biopsy. Occasionally the possibility of a coronary anomaly remains in doubt, in which case coronary arteriography is mandatory. Assessment of hemodynamics is rarely useful for patient management unless the clinical presentation is discrepant from the echocardiographic findings, but has important prognostic implications and is needed if transplantation is considered, particularly measurement of pulmonary artery pressure and vascular resistance. Biopsy results in idiopathic dilated cardiomyopathy are nonspecific, demonstrating myocyte hypertrophy and variable amounts of fibrosis without evidence of inflammatory infiltrates. The primary importance of biopsy is detection of known causes of dilated cardiomyopathy,[26] including histologic or polymerase chain reaction evidence of myocarditis,

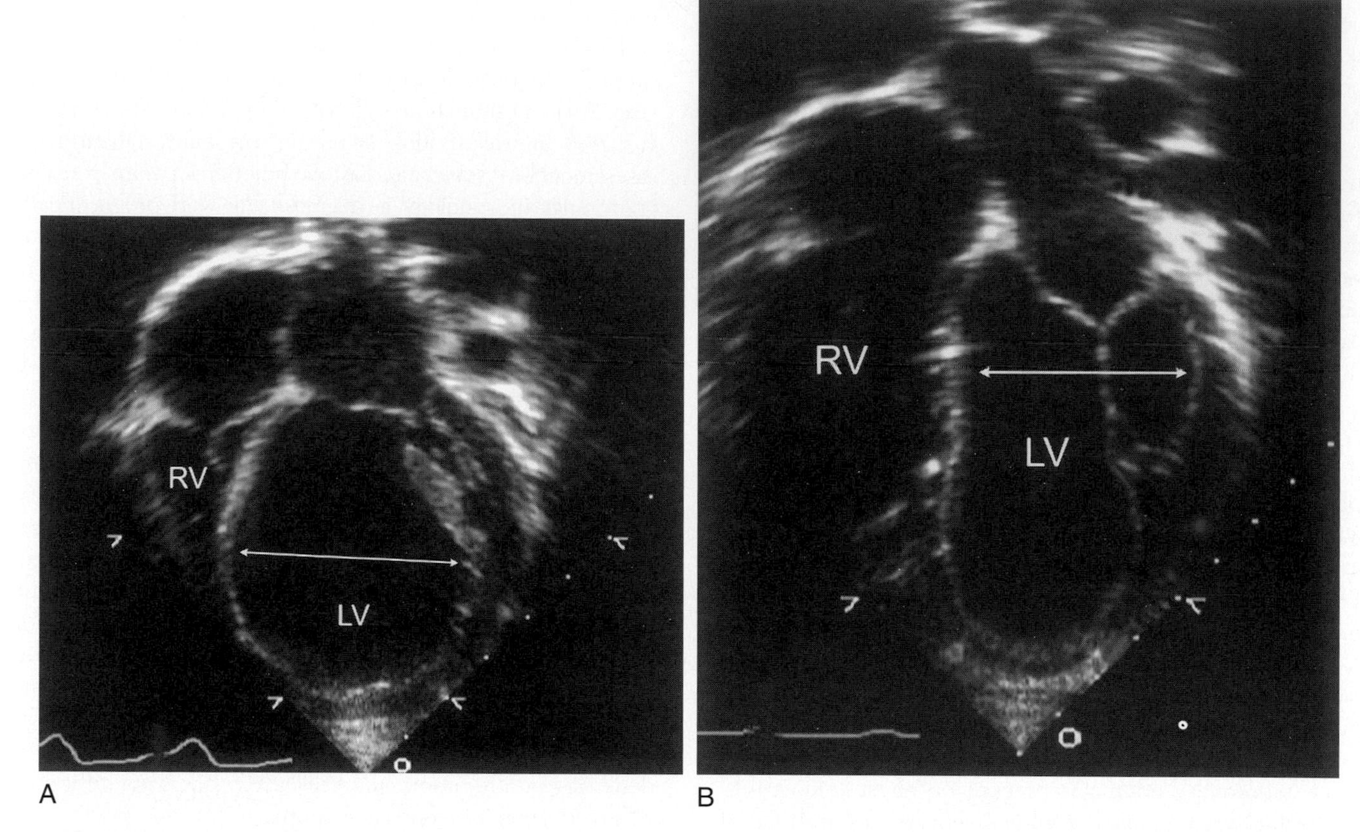

FIGURE 26–1 *Comparison of ventricular configuration in the normal left ventricle (A) and dilated cardiomyopathy (B) in apical, transverse echocardiographic imaging. In the normal heart, the size of the right ventricle (RV) is similar to that of the left ventricle (LV), and the transverse width of the LV (arrow) is about two-thirds the long axis dimension. In patients with dilated cardiomyopathy, the LV dilates more than the RV, and the ventricle is more spherical with a transverse dimension (arrow) that is nearly as great as the long axis dimension.*

infiltrative or mitochondrial disorders, cytoskeletal protein defects and endocardial fibroelastosis.[23] Numerous disorders such as histiocytoid cardiomyopathy of infancy,[27] although rare, can only be diagnosed by tissue analysis. A finding of inflammatory heart disease justifies delay in consideration of transplantation because myocarditis in children is generally associated with a more favorable prognosis,[23] including the potential for complete recovery. The safety of transvenous biopsy has been amply demonstrated,[28] and extensive experience in its use has been gained through routine application in cardiac transplant recipients. The highest risk is noted in infants, where perforation by the stiff biopsy catheters is a recognized complication. However, this is exactly the patient group in whom the results can be most helpful, shifting the risk-benefit ratio in favor of the test even in this age group.

The differential diagnosis of DCM in children and in infants in particular is complex due to the imposing array of possible rare disorders (Table 26-1). An ordered and logical algorithm for diagnostic evaluation has been published,[29] based on standard and widely available laboratory screening tests, leading to targeted specific testing for particular disorders of metabolism. This is a rapidly evolving field as new enzymatic disorders are recognized and must be incorporated within this algorithm. Certain disorders, such as the mitochondrial disorders,[6] can be particularly difficult to diagnose due to tissue-selective and heterogeneous tissue expression, related to tissue-specific isoenzyme or unbalanced segregation of mutated and wild-type mitochondrial DNA. This leads to the biochemical manifestation of the defect when a certain threshold of mutated mitochondrial DNA is reached. The situation is rendered even more complex by the age dependent accumulation of mitochondrial DNA deletions that appear to have no causal relation to DCM.

Treatment

In the absence of an identifiable cause, treatment is supportive and nonspecific, targeted at controlling the symptoms of congestive heart failure. Therapy for congestive

TABLE 26–1. Secondary Forms of Dilated Cardiomyopathy

Familial Cardiomyopathy	Neuromuscular Disorders
Barth syndrome	Duchenne, Becker muscular dystrophy
Endocardial fibroelastosis	Emery-Dreifuss muscular dystrophy
Familial dilated cardiomyopathy (autosomal dominant and recessive, X-linked)	Myotonic dystrophy
	Myotubular myopathy
Infectious myocarditis	Nemaline myopathy
Bacterial (*Brucella*, diphtheria, gonococcus, *Haemophilus influenzae*, meningococcal, mycobacterium, mycoplasma, pneumococcal, salmonella, *Serratia marcescens*, *Staphylococcus aureous, Treponema pallidum*)	Roussey-Levy polyneuropathy
	Scapulohumeral muscular dystrophy
Fungal (actinomyces, aspergillus, blastomyces, candidiasis, coccidiodes, cryptococcus, histoplasma, mucomycosis, nocardia)	Spinal muscular atrophy
Parasitic (ascaris, schistosoma, trichinella)	Systemic disorders
Protozoal (toxoplasma, trypanosoma)	Hemochromatosis (primary, secondary)
Rickettsial (*Rickettsia rickettsii, Coxiella burnetii*)	Hemolytic uremic syndrome
Spirochetal (borrelia, leptospira)	Histiocytosis X
Viral (adenovirus, coxsackie A and B, cytomegalovirus, echoviruses, HIV, hepatitis C, herpes simplex, influenza A and B, measles, mumps, parvovirus, polio, respiratory syncytial virus, rubella, varicella)	Juvenile rheumatoid arthritis
Metabolic and nutritional disorders	Kawasaki disease
Beta-ketothiolase deficiency	Lupus erythematosus
Electrolyte disturbances (hypocalcemia, hypokalemia, hypomagnesemia, hypophosphatemia)	Osteogenesis imperfecta
	Peripartum cardiomyopathy
Endocrine (thyrotoxicosis, hypothyroidism, diabetes, pheochromocytoma, neuroblastoma, catecholamine)	Polyarteritis nodosa
	Polymyositis
Fatty acid oxidation (carnitine deficiency, VLCAD, LCAD, and LCHAD deficiency; MCAD deficiency)	Reye syndrome
	Sarcoidosis
Hypertaurinuria	Systemic sclerosis
Glycogenosis (types IV and V)	Toxic cardiomyopathy
Mitochondrial (Kearns-Sayre, MELAS, MERRF, NADH-Coenzyme Q reductase deficiency, cytochrome C oxidase deficiency)	Alcoholic cardiomyopathy
	Anabolic steroids
	Anthracyclines
Mucopolysaccharidoses (type III, IV, VI)	Arsenic
Selenium deficiency (Keshan disease)	Chloramphenicol
Sphingolipidoses (Gaucher, Farber, gangliosidosis, Niemann-Pick, Refsum, Sandhoff, Tay-Sachs)	Cobalt
	Cocaine
Thiamine deficiency (Beri-beri)	Lead
	Lithium

LCAD, long chain acyl-coa dehydrogenase deficiency; LCHAD, long chain 3-hydroxyacyl coenzyme A dehydrogenase deficiency; MCAD, medium chain acyl-coenzyme A-dehydrogenase deficiency; MELAS, mitochondrial myopathy, encephalopathy lactacidosis, stroke; MERRF, myoclonic epilepsy associated with ragged-red fibers; VLCAD, very long chain acyl-coa- dehydrogenase deficiency.

heart failure and ventricular dysfunction is discussed in detail in Chapters 7, 59, and 60 and will not be considered here. There are, however, several observations that are pertinent to DCM in particular. The severity of clinical compromise determines the level of support that is required. Management at centers that have extracorporeal membrane oxygenator and ventricular assist device support available is advised for these patients. Some patients can experience sufficient recovery within a period of days to permit withdrawal of mechanical myocardial support, and the method can at times be used as a bridge to transplantation procedures.[30]

Carnitine deficiency and disorders of carnitine transport can result in dilated and hypertrophic cardiomyopathy and, in some cases, dietary carnitine supplementation can lead to dramatic cardiac and clinical improvement.[31] In an attempt to avoid delays in therapy, it is not uncommon for clinicians to initiate empirical carnitine supplementation before biochemical confirmation of this disorder. In fact, cardiomyopathy is not a prominent early feature of myopathic carnitine deficiency, in which skeletal muscle weakness and recurrent metabolic crises dominate. In addition to potentially obscuring the diagnostic evaluation, other inborn errors of metabolism have been described that manifest as a dilated cardiomyopathy but deteriorate rapidly in response to carnitine supplementation.[32] Plasma carnitine concentrations and fatty acid metabolism by-products should be evaluated in all infants with cardiomyopathy of unknown etiology to exclude familial carnitine transporter defect, but empirical therapy is not advised.

Children with DCM are at risk for intracardiac thrombus formation and systemic embolization. Intracardiac thrombi are seen in 46% to 84% of children at autopsy, but the relationship of this to premorbid findings is unclear since one of these studies[33] documented no intracardiac thrombus during life. Clinical series report the presence of intracardiac thrombus in 0% to 23%. Comparison of these studies indicates an age-related trend toward higher incidence, but none of the series have been large enough to draw firm conclusions. Use of prophylactic antithrombotic therapy is controversial, because no controlled trials of antithrombotic agents in children with heart failure are available. The adult experience indicates that anticoagulation is beneficial in patients with a previous thromboembolic event, atrial fibrillation, or the presence of a new left ventricular thrombus. Warfarin therapy is recommended in children under these circumstances as well, but the vast majority of pediatric DCM patients will meet none of these criteria. Aspirin monotherapy is beneficial in patients with ischemic heart disease, but evidence of efficacy in other forms of cardiomyopathy is lacking. It appears that aspirin and other nonsteroidal anti-inflammatory agents can attenuate the beneficial effects of angiotensin-converting enzyme (ACE) inhibitors.[34] The new appearance of an intracardiac thrombus justifies a trial of thrombolytic therapy because the incidence of embolization under these circumstances is quite high.

Mitral valve regurgitation is common in DCM and in some instances can be moderate or more in severity. There are reports of clinical improvement after mitral valvuloplasty in patients with DCM, with improved symptoms, ventricular function, and survival. The repair represents a form of afterload reduction, with a fall in wall stress consequent to ventricular remodeling.[35] In patients with moderate to severe mitral regurgitation associated with DCM, valve repair should be seriously considered, but valve replacement almost certainly entails excess risk. Regurgitation in this setting is nearly always secondary to annular dilatation and responds well to annuloplasty.

The beneficial symptomatic effects of exercise training in adults with congestive heart failure have been well documented, but the impact on survival is less clear.[36] Although there is no similar reported experience in children, there is ample documentation that exercise performance in patients with congenital heart disease can be improved by training programs.[37] Based on current data, excluding the relatively high-risk situations of acute ischemia and active myocarditis, exercise training appears advisable for all patients.

Predictors of Outcome in Dilated Cardiomyopathy

Predictors of outcome in children with dilated cardiomyopathy have been evaluated in many studies, with variable findings. Severity of dysfunction has been found to be predictive of outcome in some studies,[23] but not in others.[38] Similar to results in adults, the shape of the ventricle is prognostically important, with a more spherical shape associated with a poorer outcome.[23] Patients who have improved shortening fraction over the first 1 to 6 months after presentation have better survival than those who do not.[38] Familial cardiomyopathy has generally been reported to have a poorer prognosis. Marked elevation of end-diastolic pressure,[39] presence of ventricular arrhythmias,[39] tissue diagnosis of endocardial fibroelastosis,[23] persistent cardiomegaly, and persistent congestive heart failure have also been reported to adversely affect survival, whereas tissue diagnosis of myocarditis has been associated with a better outcome. Ventricular size and mass at presentation have not been found predictive of outcome, although persistent elevation in mass and wall stress are negative predictors.[40] Younger age at presentation has been reported to be associated with a better outcome by some groups,[41] with a worse outcome by other groups,[42] and in other series has not been found to be a significant factor.[39] Symptoms appear to provide poor prognostic capability, because even asymptomatic patients with incidental discovery of dilated cardiomyopathy can have a poor prognosis.[43] Coexistence of right ventricular dysfunction appears to portend a particularly poor outcome.[44]

One motivation for defining factors associated with a poor outcome is to enable early recommendation for cardiac transplantation. It is therefore disturbing that some studies have found certain factors to have major predictive value whereas others have found the same factors to have either no significance or the opposite effect. Given the heterogeneity of the disorder itself and the small number of patients that have been included in many series, it is likely that the patient samples are quite dissimilar. Entry criteria have also varied substantially among these studies, with specific inclusion of myocarditis in some but exclusion in others. If the results among studies are tabulated, one observes that negative studies frequently outnumber positive studies with regard to most hemodynamic and echocardiographic parameters. For many of the variables, it is likely that there is a real association with outcome but the relationship is weak. The fact that commonly employed measures of ventricular performance are only weakly predictive of survival severely limits their utility in decisions concerning transplantation.

Outcome

The natural history is quite variable, depending on the etiology and severity of cardiac compromise. Arrhythmias, congestive heart failure, and death can be seen during any stage of the disease. The clinical course can be a rapid and unremitting progression to overwhelming cardiogenic shock and death, transient dysfunction with full recovery and few or no symptoms, or any course in between these extremes. There are also patients who manifest the insidious appearance of ventricular dysfunction without an identifiable acute precipitating illness. Regardless of the initial presentation, patients with persistent dysfunction remain at risk for progressively impaired cardiac function, congestive failure, and death. For pediatric patients with idiopathic dilated cardiomyopathy, 1-, 2-, 5-, and 10-year survival rates of 41% to 94%,[33,38,45–48] 20% to 88%,[33,39,45,47,48] 34% to 86%,[38,39,46,47] and 52% to 84%,[39,47] respectively, have been reported. Most deaths occur within the first 6 months to 2 years after onset.[39,42,45] In those who survive, nearly half have full normalization of ventricular function,[42,45,49] 25% have improved but abnormal function,[45,49] and 25% have persistently severely depressed function.[45,49] Recovery of function is generally complete within the first year but occasional patients experience continued late improvement.[23,50]

Infective Myocarditis

Myocardial inflammatory diseases are an important cause of dilated cardiomyopathy in children. Although myocarditis has previously been speculated to account for most instances of chronic DCM, it is now clear that a large proportion is due to familial forms of DCM. The relationship between myocarditis and DCM remains uncertain, but a large body of human and animal data has led to the construct of a disease characterized by three sequential phases.[3] The first phase is characterized by an initial myocardial insult that is believed to be a viral infection in most cases. Usually clinically silent, the disease is rarely diagnosed during this phase. The onset of the second phase manifests as progressive myocardial damage due to autoimmunity triggered by the initial injury. Overt congestive heart failure is more common during this phase and the inflammatory process is more overt, but evidence of persistent viral infection is unusual. Despite resolution of the inflammatory process, the third phase with the typical clinical picture of chronic DCM may follow. Clearly, the diagnostic and therapeutic implications of each of these phases are quite different.

Nearly all of the organisms that cause common infectious illnesses in children can also cause myocarditis,[3] although fewer have been associated with the manifestations of dilated cardiomyopathy (Table 26-1). In addition, myocarditis can occur as a hypersensitivity or toxic reaction and is associated with a number of important systemic diseases such as rheumatic fever. Epidemics of viral myocarditis have been reported, particularly with Coxsackie B virus, and the enteroviruses as a group are considered to be the most common cause of viral myocarditis. The relative importance of the various organisms that have been identified as potentially capable of infecting the myocardium has been elucidated by molecular techniques, with Coxsackie B and adenovirus most commonly identified. However, identification of a virus does not establish a causal relationship to the inflammatory process, particularly because most of the population will have been exposed to these agents. In fact, identification of virus in the myocardium of patients dying from myocarditis is rare. Nevertheless, the existing body of animal and human data is sufficiently compelling to justify the pursuit of diagnostic and therapeutic strategies based on the understanding of an initial infectious insult that triggers an autoimmune disorder and may eventually be followed by end-stage DCM.

Myocarditis cannot be reliably distinguished from other forms of dilated cardiomyopathy on clinical grounds alone, presenting in both acute and chronic forms with symptoms and functional consequences related to the severity of ventricular dysfunction. A significant number of cases of myocarditis have manifestations that are subclinical, associated with electrocardiographic changes or arrhythmias, and in a significant number can be occult or present with sudden death.[51] Clinical diagnosis of myocarditis has been based on clinical features including echocardiographic evidence of ventricular dysfunction in association with positive peripheral cultures, serology, or histologic evidence of inflammation on biopsy or necropsy. Clinical diagnosis is unreliable due to a high frequency of unrelated infectious illness in children and an absence of evidence of systemic infectious disease in the majority of patients with myocarditis. The diagnostic yield from serology and peripheral viral culture is low and viral culture from the heart is rarely positive. Despite the development of alternative diagnostic modalities, endomyocardial biopsy remains the only method to confirm the presence of an inflammatory process in the myocardium. Measurement of cardiac enzymes is not helpful as they are rarely elevated. Elevation of cardiac troponin I, a marker of myocyte necrosis, is noted in only one-third of patients with myocarditis on biopsy.[52] Viral culture is rarely positive and serology is not helpful in early management. Several newer methods are reportedly helpful in diagnosis of myocarditis, including the presence of contrast enhancement on magnetic resonance imaging[53] and antimyosin scintigraphic imaging,[54] but their role is at present undefined. Ultimately, endomyocardial biopsy remains the final arbiter of the presence of myocardial inflammation. Even this is a less-than-perfect tool, as the process is often focal and can be missed on spot sampling. Histologic examination of tissue obtained at endomyocardial biopsy has a reported sensitivity of only 50% for the diagnosis of myocarditis using standard methods.[55] The arguments for and against endomyocardial biopsy in individual cases have been recently reviewed.[56,57] The procedure carries sufficient risk to limit its use only to those patients at high clinical risk for a treatable disorder in which biopsy may be useful in diagnosis, treatment planning, or establishing prognosis. For example, presence of viral genome within the myocardium is associated with a worse outcome[11] and has been reported to predispose to graft viral infection.[58]

The lack of reliable and definitive diagnosis has historically resulted in marked uncertainty on the role that particular viral infections play in the etiology of myocarditis. Molecular in situ hybridization has demonstrated viral genome in as many as 50% of cases of myocarditis and idiopathic dilated cardiomyopathy. Recently, identification of viral nucleic acid by means of polymerase chain reaction (PCR) amplification has successfully identified viral genome in a variety of tissues, including myocardium. This technique permits the rapid identification of viral nucleic acid in myocardium and provides a sensitive method for the diagnosis of myocarditis. Based on these methods in children with suspected myocarditis, viral genome has been detected for adenovirus in 40%, enterovirus in 20%, herpes simplex virus in 5%, and cytomegalovirus in 3%.[59] Not infrequently, histologic evidence of inflammation is absent despite the presence of viral genome, particularly for adenovirus, creating uncertainty as to the pathophysiology of the virus in the disease process. Therefore, despite these advances in identification of viral genome in myocardial tissue, the relationship between myocarditis and dilated cardiomyopathy remains controversial.[60] The recent addition to the diagnostic armamentarium of the ability to distinguish between latent infection and persistence of viral genome can help settle some of these issues. The pathogenesis of DCM is believed to represent the combination of direct virus-mediated myocyte dysfunction and immune response–mediated tissue injury. A provocative report that a Coxsackie virus protease cleaves the cytoskeletal protein dystrophin, the same protein that is responsible for inherited forms of dilated cardiomyopathy, indicates additional molecular mechanisms by which viral infection can contribute to the pathogenesis of acquired cardiomyopathy independent of an inflammatory response.[61]

Management of dilated cardiomyopathy secondary to myocarditis is similar to other forms of dilated cardiomyopathy, although there is some evidence that myocarditis predisposes to digoxin toxicity and therefore digoxin should be used with caution and rapid loading should be avoided during the acute phase. Because of the considerable body of evidence indicating that the immune response and autoimmunity may play a central role in the acute and chronic myocardial damage,[62,63] immunosuppression has been proposed as a possible therapeutic option. Small, uncontrolled trials of corticosteroid therapy in children with evidence of myocarditis[64] have reported favorable outcome. Similar to trials of these and other immunosuppressive agents in adults, these uncontrolled studies in a disease with a high rate of spontaneous resolution are impossible to interpret. A multicenter trial of immunosuppressive therapy for biopsy proven myocarditis in adults, consisting of prednisone combined with either cyclosporine or azathioprine, found no benefit.[65] The results of this study have been widely interpreted as showing that immunosuppressive therapy must strike a fine balance between preventing the immune-mediated clearance of virus and permitting an excess response with associated autoimmune damage. Duration of therapy, timing of therapy relative to disease stage, specifics of the inciting virus, and potential activation of latent virus are other factors that may have contributed to the absence of benefit in this trial. Of seven other controlled trials of immunosuppressive therapy in adults with myocarditis, only one found a statistically significant reduction in myocardial inflammation and improvement in cardiac function. Overall, despite the evidence for autoimmunity in mediating the cardiac injury in myocarditis, the currently available data do not support the routine use of immunosuppressive therapy in children with myocarditis.[64]

Treatment with intravenous immunoglobulin (IVIG) was initially proposed as a means to suppress the immune response in myocarditis, regardless of cause and to cause more rapid viral clearance in viral myocarditis. A retrospective analysis of IVIG use in children with myocarditis demonstrated improved 1-year survival and recovery of left ventricular function with IVIG therapy, although improved survival did not achieve statistical significance in the small cohort.[66] Animal studies and preliminary studies in adults were similarly promising, although a single randomized study in adults failed to demonstrate a treatment effect. Nevertheless, based on animal studies indicating that IVIG is more effective during the acute phase, the belief that the therapy may be more effective in children, the lack of other more effective specific therapy, and the very low adverse event rate, IVIG continues to be used by most centers in children suspected of being in the acute phase of myocarditis. Doses have been based on the Kawasaki experience (2 g/kg administered over 6–12 hours). Potential benefits of retreatment are unknown.

Endocardial Fibroelastosis

Diffuse thickening of the left ventricular endocardium secondary to proliferation of fibrous and elastic tissue is an uncommon but nonspecific response to a variety of inciting agents. The finding was at one time thought to represent a specific disease, but as emphasized by Lurie,[67] it is now clear that endocardial fibroelastosis (EFE) represents a final common pathway for many different myocardial stressors. An association with mumps virus infection has been suspected for many years, a theory supported by the finding of mumps virus genome in the myocardium of infants and children.[68] This proposed etiology for a significant proportion of cases is further supported by the observed fall in EFE incidence coincident with implementation of widespread vaccination. Despite the reduction in frequency, the histologic finding continues to be reported in association with a wide variety of cardiac diseases, including pre- and postnatal left ventricular outflow tract obstruction, numerous other forms of congenital heart disease, many forms of dilated and hypertrophic cardiomyopathy (myocarditis, familial cardiomyopathies, idiopathic dilated cardiomyopathy, viral myocarditis, mucopolysaccharidosis, carnitine deficiency, and Adriamycin [doxorubicin] cardiomyopathy) and as a focal finding in adults with various cardiac disorders. Among the various associations, no single theme emerges, supporting the interpretation that this represents a nonspecific tissue response. The pathophysiology of the response is of interest inasmuch as it can provide clues to pathways of injury shared by various diseases.

Clinically, more than 80% of cases occur in the first year of life, with a presentation dependent on which form of the disease is manifest. Most cases have a dilated ventricle with increased wall thickness and depressed systolic function. The clinical manifestations of the dilated form are similar to other types of dilated cardiomyopathy. Rarely, patients present with a contracted form characterized by a small left ventricle and the clinical picture of a restrictive cardiomyopathy. The diagnosis of EFE is most commonly made at autopsy. Although EFE is often suspected on echocardiography when the ultrasound signal from the endocardial surface is unusually strong, this has not been found to be a reliable diagnostic technique.[60] EFE can be recognized on endomyocardial biopsy and despite the greater involvement of the left ventricle in many patients, the diagnosis can frequently be confirmed on right ventricular biopsy. An autopsy series found that most patients with EFE had right ventricular involvement, although to a lesser extent than on the left[70] but the diagnostic accuracy of endomyocardial biopsy of the right ventricle has not been systematically tested. The purpose of the diagnosis is primarily for prognosis, since in some clinical situations the finding of EFE has been associated with a poor outcome. For example, in case series of dilated cardiomyopathy EFE is often identified as one of the risk factors for death.[23,71] Nevertheless, in a group of patients with idiopathic EFE the 4-year survival was 77%, which is not worse than the survival that has been reported in other forms of dilated cardiomyopathy.

Dystrophinopathies

Identification of dystrophin as the mutated protein in Duchenne muscular dystrophy (DMD) was the initial stage in the recognition of a wide clinical spectrum of disease associated with dystrophin gene mutations. *Dystrophinopathy* is now commonly used to describe disorders unified by a defect in the dystrophin gene that range from classic DMD to asymptomatic mild elevation of serum creatine kinase. The disorders include Duchenne and Becker muscular dystrophy, congenital muscular dystrophy, various forms of limb-girdle muscular dystrophy, X-linked dilated cardiomyopathy,[72] and carriers of the Duchenne and Becker muscular dystrophy gene.[73,74] The dystrophinopathies are one of the several forms of cardiomyopathy that manifest X-linked inheritance. Although, as described in subsequent sections, the name "X-linked dilated cardiomyopathy" has been used to describe a specific dystrophinopathy, there are in fact numerous described forms of cardiomyopathy that are inherited in an X-linked fashion, including the dystrophinopathies, Barth syndrome secondary to defects in tafazzin (*G4.5*) gene,[75] the emerin gene (the X-linked variant of Emery-Dreifuss muscular dystrophy),[76] Danon disease,[77] and McLeod syndrome (XK membrane transport syndrome).[78] The dystrophin gene is the largest known human gene, accounting for ~1.5% of the X chromosome. Dystrophin is predominantly localized in the plasma membrane of striated muscle cells and is considered to be a component of the membrane cytoskeleton in myogenic cells.[79] The structure of dystrophin is similar to other cytoskeletal proteins, and it is thought to be important in maintaining the structural integrity of the plasma membrane. The proposed mechanism whereby the absence of dystrophin leads to cell injury is through increased susceptibility to mechanical injury to the sarcolemma during the application of the force of contraction[80] or excess cation permeability leading to excess calcium influx and secondary sarcolemma breakdown.[79] This proposed pathoetiology has been bolstered by the observation that a period of reduced myocardial stress provided by use of a ventricular assist device can result in normalization of acquired dystrophin abnormalities.[81] Dystrophin is absent in nearly all patients with the Duchenne phenotype but in Becker dystrophy there can be either reduced quantities of a normal protein or normal quantities of a structurally abnormal protein. Cases with intermediate severity represent variable expression of these same gene defects.

In addition to skeletal muscle, dystrophin is present in neurons, smooth muscle, and cardiac muscle. Not surprisingly, the dystrophinopathies have clinical findings due to the dystrophin deficiency in these other tissues, such as cognitive deficits and cardiomyopathy in DMD. Despite this, involvement in the various tissues is nonuniform. For example, some families with X-linked dilated cardiomyopathy have severe myocardial dysfunction but normal skeletal muscle strength.[82] Becker dystrophy is a milder disease than DMD with similar clinical manifestations and slower progression, but occasional patients have severe myocardial dysfunction that can precede significant skeletal muscle involvement. At present the reason for the tissue-specific disease expression is not fully explained.[83] One reported cause of the differential effect is in X-linked dilated cardiomyopathy where a specific mutation has been identified that prevents gene transcription in cardiac muscle but permits maintenance of dystrophin synthesis in skeletal muscle via exon skipping or alternative splicing mechanisms not present in cardiac tissue.[84]

Duchenne Muscular Dystrophy

With an incidence of about 30 per 100,000 live births, the Duchenne form of muscular dystrophy is the most common and most severe type of childhood progressive muscular dystrophy. Transmission of the genetic defect is by an X-linked recessive gene, with approximately two thirds of mothers of affected boys thought to be carriers. Although serum levels of creatine kinase and other sarcoplasmic enzymes are elevated from birth, the first clinical manifestation is weakness that becomes apparent when the child begins to walk, or between 2 and 6 years of age at the latest. Weakness progresses to an inability to walk by the end of the first decade, with the development of contractures, progressive deformity, and severe kyphoscoliosis in the later stages. Invariably there is an associated cardiomyopathy, although this is usually masked by the consequences of the skeletal myopathy. Average age of death is 18 to 19 years with occasional survival to beyond age 30. Death is related to respiratory insufficiency in approximately 75% and to congestive heart failure or sudden death in the remainder.[85] Although the cardiomyopathy can contribute to the clinical picture, the distinction between cardiac and pulmonary compromise can be difficult. Many of these patients have major orthopedic procedures, including spinal fusion, to assist them in maintaining motor capabilities and to improve ease of care. Long-term assisted ventilation is also undertaken in some patients when ventilatory capacity is inadequate. The ability to determine the degree of cardiac involvement is of importance for defining which patients are less likely to benefit from assisted ventilation and that are high-risk surgical candidates.

Loss of dystrophin from the cell membrane results in a mechanically inadequate membrane that is more easily damaged during muscular contraction. Muscle inflammation and necrosis is followed by both regrowth of muscle fibers and replacement by fibrous tissue. Thus, the typical histologic pattern is widespread degeneration and regeneration of individual muscle fibers in most skeletal muscle groups with extensive connective tissue proliferation (endomysial fibrosis). The muscle fiber number progressively decreases as the connective tissue content of each muscle group increases, suggesting that the endomysial fibrosis impairs the ability of the individual fibers to regenerate. This concept receives further support from the observation that in mice with an X-linked muscular dystrophy muscle fiber degeneration and regeneration without fibrosis accompany the identical genetic defect but progressive deterioration is not seen, suggesting that in the absence of fibrosis the regenerative process can continue indefinitely. Patients are often observed to sustain mild to moderate left ventricular dysfunction for a long period of time, but with the onset of moderate to severe dysfunction, the rate of myocardial deterioration escalates, progressing rapidly to congestive heart failure and death.[85] This sequence of events can reflect a rise in wall tension secondary to cell loss, inducing further cell loss, a cycle that becomes rapidly self-perpetuating once a critical level of afterload is reached.

Electrocardiographic findings in a patient with Duchenne muscular dystrophy is characterized by tall, narrow R waves in the anterior precordial leads and deep, narrow Q waves in the lateral leads. Because these electrocardiographic findings resemble the changes associated with posterior and lateral infarction, selective scarring in the posterobasal myocardium has been suggested as the basis for the Q waves and right axis shift. Abnormalities of rhythm and conduction are also common. Persistent or labile sinus tachycardia is present from early in the disease. On 24-hour electrocardiogram (ECG) recordings, the rate may never fall below 100 beats per minute. The tachycardia persists and can even progress with age, in contrast to the normal age-related fall in heart rate. The cause of the sinus tachycardia is unknown, but an obvious possibility is enhanced sympathetic drive secondary to ventricular dysfunction. However, the elevated heart rate is present from early in the disease, does not appear to be closely related to the coexistence of systolic dysfunction, and is seen both in subjects with abnormal and those with preserved ventricular performance.[86] All portions of the conduction system can be involved in the degenerative process, with frequent bundle branch or occasional complete atrioventricular block. Dystrophin has been identified as an important molecule for membrane function in the Purkinje conduction system of the heart, presumably accounting for these abnormalities. Ventricular arrhythmias with a risk of sudden death are seen more commonly in patients with severe cardiomyopathy, and QT dispersion can be a useful method to define level of risk.[87] Atrial flutter is commonly encountered in the preterminal stages of Duchenne muscular dystrophy.

Cardiac catheterization is rarely indicated in these patients and most cardiac functional data are derived from echocardiographic and radionuclide studies. Left ventricular posterior wall thickness and cavity dimensions are less than in age-matched healthy controls and the left ventricular free wall thickness and short axis dimension decrease inappropriately with age. This pattern of *atrophic heart* is associated with the most emaciated and motor-impaired patients. However, even when compared with a group of wheelchair-bound control individuals, the left ventricular measurements were reduced.[88] The pattern observed consisted of a normal increase in dimension and wall thickness for a period of years with reversal of this trend during the later, nonambulatory years.

Most studies of ventricular function have noted abnormal systolic function with progressive abnormalities over time.[89] Abnormal systolic function is rarely present before age 10, but increases in prevalence thereafter and is virtually universal after age 18 years.[89] Several reports have noted a close relationship between the reduction in vital capacity or other measures of skeletal muscle strength and reduced shortening fraction or abnormal systolic time intervals.[90,91] Although these observations would suggest a significant association between skeletal and cardiac muscle involvement, other observers have felt that the severity of cardiac impairment does not relate to the degree of skeletal muscle weakness. For example, radionuclide ejection fractions in 38 patients with Duchenne muscular dystrophy aged 13 to 42 years ranged from 17% to 70%, with no relation to age, skeletal muscle involvement, or pulmonary function.[92] The probable explanation for this difference of opinion is that parallel but somewhat independent processes are being examined. That is, when individual patients are evaluated in a longitudinal fashion, there is progressive deterioration of striated muscle, be it cardiac or skeletal. However, when patients at an equivalent stage of the disease are compared, the degree of cardiac deterioration is noted to be poorly correlated with the skeletal muscle weakness, implying that although both aspects are progressive, the two do not reliably progress at a similar rate.[93]

Insofar as skeletal and cardiac involvement in Duchenne muscular dystrophy can progress at different rates, the extent of cardiac impairment cannot be deduced from assessment of skeletal muscle weakness and must therefore be independently assessed. A specific means of assessment of cardiac performance must be used, such as echocardiography, radionuclide ventriculography, or cardiac magnetic resonance imaging. At least 25% of these subjects cannot be adequately evaluated by ultrasound once the nonambulatory phase of the disease is reached, a problem that progresses with time. Cardiac magnetic resonance imaging is not subject to these limitations, providing detailed information about ventricular size and function, and is particularly useful in the older patients.

Therapy for the cardiomyopathy associated with Duchenne muscular dystrophy is largely nonspecific. The observation that fibrosis may play a critical role in the progression of the disease has led to the suggestion that therapy aimed at reducing the fibrotic response might be beneficial. Immunosuppressants, including corticosteroid therapy, have been reported to improve strength in patients with Duchenne muscular dystrophy.[94] Other approaches, such as increasing the rate of protein synthesis, decreasing proteolysis, and, more recently, increasing muscle cell proliferation and regeneration have been pursued (see review by Tidball et al[95]). The cardiac effects of these therapies have been evaluated in several animal models, but their potential in preventing cardiomyopathy in humans is largely unexplored. Currently, cardiac therapy is generally initiated for symptoms and for severe ventricular dysfunction, using standard anticongestive medications. ACE inhibitors and beta-blockers effectively decrease neurohumoral activation and result in symptomatic improvement.[96] The more interesting question is whether early initiation of these potentially cardioprotectant agents could prevent or retard the vicious cycle of stress-induced cell loss, a hypothesis that is as yet untested.

Surgery is known to be somewhat risky in patients with Duchenne muscular dystrophy, leading some institutions to advise against it altogether. If the risks are properly defined and appropriate precautions are taken, the true high-risk patients can be excluded and surgery can be performed in the remainder with reasonable success. It should be understood, however, that these patients could never be considered to have a normal risk for surgery. Delivery of anesthesia is notoriously hazardous, with reports of hyperthermia, cardiac arrest, and acute rhabdomyolysis.[97–99] The Duchenne muscular dystrophy heart has been reported to be excessively sensitive to a number of nonanesthetic agents, including the calcium-channel blocking agent verapamil. Thus, pharmacologic interventions must be carefully considered and creative therapy is to be avoided. In general, anesthetic regimens with the least cardiodepressant actions are used in these patients,[86] but in the presence of known cardiac dysfunction, additional intraoperative and postoperative monitoring is used, with arterial and thermodilution pulmonary artery catheter placement to continuously record cardiac output, pulmonary artery wedge pressure, and arterial pressure. Such additional precautions are relatively easy to implement. The more difficult decision arises when one attempts to define criteria by which patients should be excluded from surgery altogether. Certainly, the nature of the contemplated procedure should influence this decision. Spinal fusion is one of the most common operations performed in the late stages of the disease, and represents a significant cardiovascular stress with marked blood loss and fluid shifts, prolonged anesthesia delivery, induced hypotension, and multiple drug delivery. Although severe cardiomyopathy is believed to be a contraindication to spinal fusion in Duchenne muscular dystrophy, moderate levels of dysfunction are well tolerated.[86] Based on the findings at the time of assessment, the procedure is judged to be relatively low risk (normal echocardiogram), moderate risk (mild to moderate ventricular dysfunction), or high risk (severe ventricular dysfunction). In general, only emergency procedures are undertaken in the high-risk patients. In moderate-risk patients, elective procedures such as spinal fusion are still pursued, but additional anesthesia precautions are taken. Using these methods, spinal fusion can be performed even in the presence of fairly marked ventricular dysfunction (shortening fraction <20%) without incident.

Becker Muscular Dystrophy

The dystrophin mutation in Becker muscular dystrophy results in a decreased amount and/or size of the dystrophin molecule. The clinical course is one of later onset and slower progression than in Duchenne muscular dystrophy. Cardiac involvement can be detected during adolescence and eventually affects nearly all patients. Female carriers also have a high incidence of cardiac involvement, although usually less severe.[100] There is a striking absence of correlation between the degree of skeletal muscle weakness and the severity of the cardiomyopathy.[101,102] Systolic dysfunction similar in magnitude to that seen in Duchenne muscular dystrophy can be identified in children with Becker muscular dystrophy prior to the onset of significant skeletal muscle impairment.[89] In teenagers, the clinical picture may be dominated by a severe, symptomatic cardiomyopathy. The primary implication of these diverse patterns of clinical involvement is that the skeletal muscle manifestations of the muscular dystrophy cannot be assumed to predict the magnitude of cardiomyopathy. Evaluation and management are similar to that for Duchenne muscular dystrophy.

X-Linked Dilated Cardiomyopathy

The presentation of X-linked dilated cardiomyopathy is indistinguishable from other dilated cardiomyopathies except for its X-linked transmission. Affected males typically present in the second or third decade of life with congestive heart failure, progressing to death or transplantation within 1 to 2 years. The unrelenting course of the disease could be explained by the same mechanism as that proposed for the cardiomyopathy associated with Duchenne muscular dystrophy, namely a process of escalating damage secondary to elevated myocardial wall force. Female carriers can occasionally manifest a mild and slowly progressive cardiomyopathy with onset after the childbearing years, making it possible for presentation in the mother and child to coincide. The disease was shown to be due to mutations in the dystrophin gene by Towbin et al,[103] and subsequent reports have identified 16 different mutations in dystrophin as the responsible defect, indicating that the disease is genetically heterogeneous. Generally, dystrophin expression is only mildly diminished in skeletal muscle but is absent in cardiac muscle.[77] Dystrophin abnormalities should be considered in the differential for dilated cardiomyopathy in general, with a higher index of suspicion in boys and in families with an X-linked pattern of transmission. Serum level of muscle-derived creatine kinase is a useful screening test, elevation of which warrants detailed neurologic examination and testing of skeletal muscle strength. Myocardial biopsy with identification of dystrophin protein abnormalities is the most sensitive and specific test for dystrophinopathy as a cause of cardiomyopathy.

Doxorubicin Cardiomyopathy

The anthracycline antibiotics include a number of valuable antitumor agents with doxorubicin (Adriamycin) in particular having the broadest spectrum of antitumor activity of available cancer chemotherapeutic agents. Thousands of children have received doxorubicin over the past 30 years for several of the most common pediatric oncologic disorders, including acute lymphocytic leukemia. A dramatic improvement in long-term survival after childhood cancer has occurred during the same time interval. As a result, late residua from therapy often represent the most important clinical problem for these patients. Among these is doxorubicin-associated cardiomyopathy, the consequences of which continue to unfold as the length of follow-up increases.

Mechanism of Anthracycline-Mediated Cardiac Injury. The cardioselective pathogenesis of doxorubicin cardiotoxicity, although not completely understood, is thought to involve the generation of reactive oxygen species[104] resulting from reduction of doxorubicin to its semiquinone free radical form, particularly within mitochondria.[105] Doxorubicin has a high affinity for iron, providing an additional mechanism whereby doxorubicin could stimulate the generation of reactive oxygen radicals. The cardioselectivity of these actions may reflect an enhanced susceptibility of the heart to oxidant stress[106] due to a high rate of oxygen consumption coupled with low levels of superoxide dismutase, catalase, and glutathione peroxidase. The clinical importance of these findings relates to the potential for reduced toxicity if the cardiac injury can be reduced without interference with antitumor activity. Although the mechanism of antitumor activity is also speculative, doxorubicin is known to bind to mammalian DNA, and is believed to exert antitumor activity through DNA fragmentation and inhibition of DNA synthesis,[107] whereas free radical formation does not appear to play a primary role in its antitumor effect. Free radical scavengers such as N-acetylcysteine and vitamin E are ineffective, both clinically and experimentally, in reducing chronic anthracycline cardiotoxicity. However, iron-chelating agents such as dexrazoxane at present comprise the most promising agents for cardioprotection, possibly by depletion of intra- and extracellular iron and prevention of free hydroxyl radical generation.[108]

Clinical Characteristics of Anthracycline Cardiotoxicity. The clinical toxicity of the anthracycline antibiotics can be divided into acute, subacute, chronic, and late phases. Supraventricular arrhythmias and ventricular premature beats are occasionally noted during and shortly after administration of doxorubicin, but are rarely clinically important. There are rare reports of a subacute syndrome of transient left ventricular dysfunction or a pericarditis/myocarditis syndrome. Clinically, the most significant problems relate to a chronic, dose-related cardiomyopathy. Historically, cardiomyopathy presented with left ventricular dysfunction, elevated filling pressure, and reduced cardiac output at 2 to 4 months after completion of therapy. The myocardial insult is often delayed for a period of time after the last dose of the drug because of a time delay in the full cytotoxic effect of the drug, with a mean latency between 3 and 8 weeks.[109] The initial experience indicated that congestive heart failure secondary to doxorubicin was rapidly progressive, irreversible, and almost always fatal, but more recent reports include survival for years after the onset of clinical cardiotoxicity with occasional recovery of function. Based on endomyocardial biopsy data, it is clear that myocardial injury accompanies even relatively low cumulative doses, with histopathologic evidence of injury present after as little as 180 mg/m^2 of body surface area. Although the morphologic damage is proportional to the total cumulative dose, there is considerable variability in the dose at which adverse effects on myocardial function first appear. In fact, functional abnormalities correlate weakly with dose and little or no clinical deterioration is noted until a certain patient-specific threshold dose is surpassed.[110] The incidence of clinical congestive heart failure is related to cumulative dose in a nonlinear fashion,[110] with 2% to 5% of patients experiencing symptomatic cardiotoxicity after 400 to 500 mg/m^2. However, even with cumulative doses in excess of 1000 mg/m^2, no more than 50% of patients develop clinical congestive heart failure.[111]

More recently, new onset of congestive heart failure has been described in some patients years after completion of therapy.[112] As a group, these patients manifest a low incidence of depressed contractility. The dominant abnormality is elevated afterload related to inadequate hypertrophy in the absence of significant dilation.[112,113] Total cumulative dose, age at the time of doxorubicin therapy, and duration since completion of therapy each relate to the incidence of cardiac abnormalities. Excess afterload is most closely related to age at therapy and time since therapy, whereas abnormal contractility is determined predominantly by total cumulative dose and is strongly related to depression of function early after completion of therapy. These differences as well as the histologic findings indicate two distinct mechanisms of injury. Depressed contractility appears to represent the usual form of cardiotoxicity that has been commonly reported in pediatric and adult studies of doxorubicin recipients. This injury appears to be relatively stable after completion of therapy. However, excess afterload is a particular risk for young children, appearing gradually over time, and manifesting as inadequate myocardial growth compared with the rate of somatic growth. This form of doxorubicin-mediated cardiac injury appears to represent impaired growth capacity of the myocardium, a problem of particular importance to the small child.

Risk Factors for Doxorubicin Cardiotoxicity. Numerous clinical studies have identified certain factors that place patients at increased risk for the adverse cardiac effects of doxorubicin. Patients younger than 4 years are at increased risk.[112] Females are at higher risk on a dose-matched basis.[114,115] Mediastinal irradiation probably increases toxicity though the effect is not marked. However, the factor that has been consistently found to bear the strongest relationship to the incidence of cardiotoxicity is the total cumulative dose. The relationship between total cumulative dose of doxorubicin and symptomatic cardiotoxicity is nonlinear with an inflection point somewhere between 400 and 600 mg/m^2. In one study the incidence of cardiomyopathy was 7% in subjects who received less than 550 mg/m^2, increasing to 18% in the group who received 700 mg/m^2.[116] Although there is some variation in the dose at which the incidence of congestive heart failure has been observed to rise, this general pattern has been observed in the numerous studies that have examined it. The importance of the method of dosing has been suggested as an important factor in cardiac injury, with a weekly dosing regimen associated with less cardiotoxicity than dosing every 3 weeks.[117] Although administration by continuous infusion was initially reported to lower toxicity, more recent reports have not confirmed this benefit.[118,119]

Prevention of Doxorubicin Cardiomyopathy. Historically, recognition of the dose-related nature of early-onset congestive heart failure resulted in modification of chemotherapeutic protocols to a nearly universal limitation of cumulative dose of less than 350 to 450 mg/m^2, successfully reducing this complication to 1% or less. Although late toxicity also appears to be dose-related, doses as low as 90 to 220 mg/m^2 still represent a measurable risk,[112,113] with no *safe* dose having been demonstrated. In addition to uniform dose reduction for all patients, the alternative means of toxicity reduction that have been reported include co-administration of agents aimed at providing cardioprotection and programmed dose reduction as dictated by one of several monitoring programs. Numerous agents with the potential to reduce doxorubicin cardiotoxicity have been tried in animal and human trials, but at present the most promising is dexrazoxane (ICRF-187). Dexrazoxane has a plausible mechanism of action (iron chelation),[120] evidence of reduced early and late toxicity in animals,[121] and promising early results in clinical trials in children.[108,122] The use of troponin I release as a biomarker for anthracycline cardiotoxicity appears to provide a means of assessing the acute benefit of cardioprotectant agents,[108,123] but the long-term relationship to late cardiac outcome is not known. Of particular interest is the recent demonstration of an antiapoptotic action associated with the protective effect, supporting observations that doxorubicin-induced apoptosis initiated a week or more after administration may account for the delayed appearance of congestive heart failure in anthracycline cardiomyopathy.[124,125] Pertinent issues that have not been fully addressed include potential reduction of antitumor activity and tolerance for higher anthracycline dose.

The use of cardiac monitoring programs that attempt to detect cardiotoxicity on an individual basis, thereby permitting individual dosing regimens with dose reduction in those patients with evidence of cardiac injury, are widely used *and* highly contentious.[126,127] Doxorubicin-induced myocardial injury can be detected by several different methods, including endomyocardial biopsy, cardiac catheterization, echocardiography, rest and exercise radionuclide angiography, and magnetic resonance imaging. Although the means used to detect myocardial injury have varied from study to study, in other regards the monitoring programs that have been recommended are quite similar. The basic approach of each of these programs is to evaluate patients periodically during doxorubicin therapy and to delay or discontinue the drug in those patients with an abnormal test result.[126] There is general agreement that onset of congestive heart failure justifies cessation of doxorubicin therapy. However, the more typical scenario is a patient who has received some fraction of the intended cumulative dose of doxorubicin, at which time an asymptomatic drop in left ventricular function is detected. For patients on monitoring protocols, if the fall in function exceeds some pre-defined criteria, cessation of anthracycline therapy is advised with the intent of minimizing adverse cardiac outcome.[126] However, opponents of currently published criteria voice concern that the impact of these programs on overall outcome has not been addressed,[127] because administration of anthracyclines is intrinsically a compromise between cancer cure and cardiac injury such that any reduction in total cumulative dose decreases antitumor effect. Even a reduction in cumulative dose from 270 down to 180 mg/m^2 has been shown to have a detectable impact on cancer cure rate.[113] Thus, a cardiac monitoring program that can trigger discontinuation of anthracycline therapy must seek a balance between what severity of cardiac injury is acceptable and what dose is required to achieve the desired antitumor effect. At present, the available data have not confirmed that drug withholding in response to asymptomatic abnormalities on cardiac testing results in a net increase in overall survival.

Management. If congestive heart failure appears during therapy, outcome is generally poor and availability of the option of cardiac transplant is determined primarily by the probability of tumor recurrence. Recognition of asymptomatic ventricular dysfunction after completion of therapy is a more common clinical scenario but there are few data on the efficacy of therapy in these patients. At least 50% of doxorubicin recipients have abnormal elevation of afterload, with or without abnormal contractility, and the excess afterload appears to progress with time.[112,128] Angiotensin converting enzyme inhibitor (ACEI) treatment of asymptomatic left ventricular dysfunction in adults with idiopathic cardiomyopathy results in delayed disease progression. Based on these data, many survivors of childhood cancer are currently treated with ACEI agents. Administration of ACEI has been shown to reduce blood pressure and left ventricular wall stress,[118,129] but long-term benefit has not been documented. There is evidence that anthracycline cardiomyopathy has features of restrictive cardiomyopathy,[130] a disease for which ACEI therapy has little benefit. Although symptomatic patients should be managed in a fashion similar to other forms of dilated cardiomyopathy, the available data do not support institution of ACEI in asymptomatic patients with anthracycline cardiomyopathy.[131]

HIV-Associated Cardiac Disease

The human immunodeficiency virus (HIV) and acquired immune deficiency syndrome (AIDS) pandemic has not spared the pediatric age group. Vertical (mother to infant) perinatal transmission is overwhelmingly the most common cause of pediatric infection and guarantees that pediatric incidence will rise in parallel with global infection rates unless effective means to prevent transmission can be identified. Offspring are placed at disproportionate hazard because the disease primarily affects adults during their reproductive years. The magnitude of this risk is changing over time, since antiretroviral therapy has been reported to reduce vertical transmission rates from as high as 35% down to 8%.[132] Uncertainty in diagnosis, changing maternal incidence rates, and variable transmission rates make it difficult to project the magnitude of the public health problem that pediatric AIDS will represent in the future, but for affected children, cardiovascular involvement can be a primary cause of morbidity and mortality.

The clinical course in perinatally HIV-infected children typically follows one of two courses. About 25% of patients have a rapid course characterized by early onset of AIDS complex, appearance of *Pneumocystis carinii* pneumonia and encephalopathic manifestations by 6 months of life, and high early mortality.[133] In contrast, the slowly progressive group is relatively healthy with few early complications, late onset of the AIDS complex, and a 50% survival to 9 years of age.[134] In both groups, cardiac complications manifest as pericardial effusions,[135] left ventricular dysfunction, and symptomatic congestive heart failure. Left ventricular dysfunction has been described in 5% to 45% of HIV-infected children in various studies.[136] A multicenter longitudinal study of 130 vertically infected children[137] found that 25% had systolic dysfunction and in 42% of these, the systolic dysfunction was secondary to depressed contractility, as assessed using load-independent indices of contractility. Serial evaluations over time revealed progressive dysfunction. Congestive heart failure often occurs with the acute systemic illnesses to which these patients are predisposed, representing the consequences of reduced cardiac reserve. In other patients, chronic congestive heart failure presents as a primary manifestation of the cardiomyopathy. Cardiac dysfunction is associated with a high mortality rate in children with AIDS, even when it is not the direct cause of death.[138]

There are multiple possible explanations for cardiac dysfunction and cardiomyopathy in the setting of HIV infection. Histologic evidence of lymphocytic infiltrates or myocarditis has been described in both adults and children.[139] These infiltrates may relate to direct myocardial infection but drug reaction, autoimmunity,[140] and selenium deficiency have also been suggested.[141] Direct HIV infection of cardiac myocytes has been demonstrated,[142] but evidence of association of myocytic HIV infection with the lymphocytic infiltrates and with cardiac dysfunction has not been uniform.[143] Coinfection with Epstein-Barr virus is common,[144,145] but the virus has not been found in the myocardium. Disseminated cytomegalovirus is commonly seen in HIV-infected patients and can at times involve the heart.[146] Other viral infections such as adenovirus, coxsackie virus, parvovirus, and herpes viruses, as well as a variety of fungal, mycobacterial, and protozoan infections have been associated in individual cases, and presumably represent a consequence of the generalized immunodeficiency and high rate of pulmonary and opportunistic infections in these patients. Although many patients experience gradual cardiac deterioration, the high prevalence of myocarditis indicates that endomyocardial biopsy is indicated in patients with new-onset cardiomyopathy.

In the absence of a specific treatable cause of myocarditis, therapy is not different from other causes of dilated cardiomyopathy. The potential cardiotoxic role of zidovudine (AZT) therapy in patients with HIV is controversial. Based on the finding that AZT-treated children have a higher incidence of ventricular dysfunction and cardiomyopathy, cessation of antiretroviral therapy in patients with evidence of cardiomyopathy has been recommended.[147] However, this finding is confounded by the fact that only patients with more advanced disease are usually treated with AZT. Several other studies have failed to confirm adverse cardiac affects from these drugs.[145,148] At present, the evidence of cardiotoxic effects of AZT does not appear to justify withholding this otherwise beneficial therapy.

Myotonic Dystrophy

Myotonic dystrophy is an autosomal, dominantly inherited disorder with diffuse but inconstant systemic involvement. The molecular defect relates to a variably increased number of CTG trinucleotide repeats in the 3′ untranslated portion of a protein kinase gene located on chromosome 19, the myotonic dystrophy protein kinase.[149] Although the transmission is autosomal, clinical severity is more marked when the mother is the transmitting parent. In affected mothers, although the transmission rate is 50%, up to 61% of fetuses that inherit the gene manifest the congenital form of the disorder.[150] Prenatal diagnosis is possible and advisable when there is a family history.[151] Cardiac involvement includes repolarization abnormalities on electrocardiography, first degree or higher atrioventricular block, left axis deviation, atrial flutter and fibrillation, bundle branch block, and premature ventricular and supraventricular contractions. Sudden death, usually related to the electrophysiologic abnormalities, is a well-recognized risk that is more commonly related to heart block and less frequently to ventricular tachycardia.

Although the classical form of myotonic dystrophy has an onset between 10 and 60 years, congenital, infantile, and early onset cases are also seen. The congenital form of the disorder leads to delivery problems and onset of symptoms at birth, with respiratory and feeding problems, hypotonia of the skeletal musculature, and arthrogryposis associated with a neonatal mortality as high as 25%.[152] Those who survive have a severe form of myotonic dystrophy resulting in neuromuscular and intellectual disabilities. Cardiac symptoms are generally absent during childhood but electrocardiographic abnormalities similar to the adult-onset form of the disorder are generally recognized by adolescence.[153] The magnitude of myocardial involvement is unclear. Symptomatic myocardial involvement is generally absent, but abnormal function has long been suspected. Congestive heart failure is occasionally reported in adults related to bradycardia and mitral regurgitation but rarely to myocardial dysfunction. In contrast to the dystrophinopathies, systolic function is generally normal in the infantile[154] and adult forms of the disease[155] although rare instances of symptomatic systolic dysfunction have been reported. In contrast, diastolic function has been noted to be abnormal in both forms of the disorder[154,156] with primary manifestations in early diastole, suggestive of impaired relaxation. One of the more striking skeletal muscle manifestations of the disorder in older children and adults is impaired relaxation, raising the intriguing possibility that the diastolic abnormalities of cardiac function relate to cardiac myotonia.[157]

Abnormal relaxation could also relate to asynchronous deactivation consequent to the conduction defects so prevalent in this disorder. Although the observed diastolic dysfunction is not associated with symptomatic manifestations of cardiac impairment in most patients, the finding can still be of considerable clinical importance with regard to the risk for heart block. Diastolic dysfunction is associated with reduced preload reserve and secondary intolerance for bradycardia. In this situation acute heart block can lead to a particularly marked fall in cardiac output, potentially explaining the high incidence of sudden death associated with heart block in this disease.

The primary clinical issue with respect to cardiac involvement is progressive conduction system disease with an associated risk of Stokes-Adams attacks and sudden death. Although any section of the conduction system can be affected, it is the His-Purkinje system that is primarily involved.[158] Due to the significant risk of sudden death, timing of pacemaker implantation is the primary issue in cardiac management. Electrocardiographic and electrophysiologic parameters, including PR, QRS, or HV intervals, have not been predictive of progression. A recent study noted that a PR interval >240 ms was a significant risk factor for atrial fibrillation, syncope, and sudden death in patients >40 years old.[159] Patients with congenital myotonic dystrophy are troubled by respiratory and neurologic complications but do not appear to have an early onset of electrophysiologic manifestations. Onset of conduction system disease is at times noted during adolescence, but complete heart block and cardiac-related mortality during childhood is rare.[160] In one study of 367 patients with myotonic dystrophy,[161] 75 died over a 10-year period at a mean age of 53 years, the earliest death occurring at age 24. Periodic ECGs and 24-hour Holter monitor recordings are advised to detect the onset of conduction system disease. Invasive electrophysiology has not been shown to provide additional prognostic data. Although prophylactic pacemaker insertion may be advisable for older patients with asymptomatic first-degree block, the absence of a verified risk of sudden death in children argues against such an approach. However, in patients with higher grades of AV block, pacemaker implantation appears justified.

Iron-Overload Cardiomyopathy

Myocardial injury due to excess iron deposition is associated with hereditary hemochromatosis and also as a consequence of chronic transfusion therapy in a number of disorders including thalassemia, sickle cell anemia, red cell aplasia, and chronic renal failure. Hereditary hemochromatosis has been identified as the most common hereditary disorder in the United States, found in 0.1% to 0.5% of the population with a gene frequency that can be as high as 10%. Symptomatic involvement is rare in childhood but young adults have been described with onset of congestive heart failure in their early 20s.[162] During childhood, iron overload is primarily seen in conjunction with transfusion therapy. Among these disorders, thalassemia is the disease for which the largest childhood experience in management of hemochromatosis has been accumulated.

Thalassemia

Beta-thalassemia is a hereditary anemia with abnormal synthesis of adult hemoglobin and is among the commonest single gene disorders in the world. Prior to the introduction of transfusion protocols, the outcome of patients with thalassemia was extremely poor. Although children who receive adequate transfusion therapy grow and develop normally with substantially improved survival, survival is ultimately limited by the toxicity of the resultant cumulative iron overload. Life-long transfusion therapy, extravascular hemolysis, and increased intestinal absorption of iron result in systemic iron accumulation with secondary multiorgan injury. Ultimately, myocardial dysfunction limits survival with death from congestive heart failure in the latter half of the second decade if iron accumulation is not treated. Treatment of iron overload with chelating agents such as deferoxamine was first introduced in the early 1960s, but was generally abandoned due to disappointing early results. During the 1970s, studies documenting a reduction in hepatic iron deposits and fibrosis spawned a renewed interest in deferoxamine therapy. Subsequent studies established that a slow, continuous infusion of deferoxamine combined with concurrent ascorbate repletion considerably enhances urinary iron excretion. By the mid 1980s, improved survival was documented as well.[163] Proceeding on the presumption that greater benefit would accrue from early childhood initiation of therapy prior to irreversible tissue injury and fibrosis, programs of early and sustained chelation therapy were initiated in many centers. Patients born during the late 1970s when this therapy was introduced are only now reaching adulthood. Consequently, the impact of the early introduction of chelation therapy in these patients is currently being revealed. Chelation therapy is associated with a clear improvement in event-free cardiac survival. Nevertheless, cardiomyopathy still remains the primary determinant of survival in this disease.[164]

The mechanism of the cardiomyopathy associated with thalassemia is controversial. Kremastinos et al[165] noted that cardiac function is usually normal in patients with thalassemia until the time of onset of congestive heart failure, leading these authors to conclude that iron overload was not the etiology. This interpretation was based on the assumption that progressive accumulation of iron should result in progressive myocardial dysfunction. This group subsequently[166] reported a high prevalence of myocarditis in patients with beta-thalassemia and concluded that infectious myocarditis is involved in the pathogenesis of left ventricular systolic dysfunction and is the main cause of death in these patients.

Rivers et al[167] interpreted the reversal of cardiac dysfunction in patients with hereditary hemochromatosis treated by serial venesection as evidence that the ventricular impairment is due to direct local depressant effect rather than irreversible tissue damage or myocardial fibrosis. Observations in nontransfusional hemochromatosis may not be directly applicable to patients with beta-thalassemia who have iron storage disease superimposed on a chronic hemolytic anemia. Nevertheless, the beneficial response to iron-reduction therapy seen in thalassemia also argues against irreversible tissue damage. As a further indication of the important role of iron removal, thalassemic patients showed little improvement in ventricular function after bone marrow transplantation, but experienced normalization in response to iron reduction therapy by chronic phlebotomy.[168] Numerous case reports and small series have similarly noted reversal of cardiac dysfunction in patients treated with chelation therapy,[169] and clinical management is therefore based on the assumption that iron deposition is primarily at fault.

Most reports of cardiac dysfunction in thalassemia have relied on shortening fraction or ejection fraction. The utility of fiber shortening for evaluation of myocardial contractility is limited by a dependence upon heart rate, preload, and afterload in addition to contractility. The limitations of load-dependent measures of cardiac function such as fractional shortening are clinically relevant in this population. For example, in sickle cell anemia, high preload and reduced afterload have been reported to mask depressed left ventricular contractility.[170] Since the presence of anemia and the need for frequent transfusions affect loading conditions, while the risk of intrinsic myocardial dysfunction due to iron overload is high, use of load-independent indices of contractility is requisite for accurate detection of cardiotoxicity.[171]

There have been a number of reports indicating that diastolic abnormalities precede the onset of systolic dysfunction in patients with beta-thalassemia.[172,173] These findings are of interest in part due to the potential for improved early recognition of cardiomyopathy. The observed abnormalities include a mitral inflow pattern with an increased E/A ratio and rapid early deceleration time, findings consistent with impaired compliance, despite normal systolic function and no history of congestive heart failure. These findings are noted early in the natural history of the disease and are difficult to reconcile with the finding of minimal to at most mild fibrosis in patients with severe left ventricular dysfunction secondary to nontransfusional hemochromatosis.[174] In contrast, Kremastinos et al[175] found that young patients had mitral inflow patterns demonstrating elevation of both E and A waves with a normal E/A ratio, with the pattern of reduced E/A only in older patients who also had left ventricular hypertrophy. Similarly, diastolic dysfunction has been reported to be predictive of the development of systolic dysfunction and congestive heart failure only in older subjects.[176]

The available means by which to assess iron accumulation, total body iron content, specific tissue content, and the balance between active and inactive iron stores remain unsatisfactory. Iron excretion has been used to monitor iron balance and response to chelation therapy. The relative balance between fecal and urinary iron loss is highly variable, depending on deferoxamine dose and rate of erythropoiesis, necessitating collection of both feces and urine. Myocardial biopsy with grading of myocardial iron is possible[177] but is impractical for routine monitoring and has not been shown to be predictive of outcome. Serum ferritin level has previously been shown to correlate (on a population basis) with liver iron content but there is marked individual variation. Serum ferritin levels have been found to correlate with hemochromatosis grade in patients with beta-thalassemia[177] as well as with cardiac disease-free survival,[178] but the correlation is relatively weak. Recently, magnetic resonance imaging relaxation parameter (T2*) has been reported to be inversely related to cardiac iron deposition.[179] Although a relationship to cardiac dysfunction in thalassemia has been identified, the ability of this parameter to predict outcome and document response to therapy remains uncertain.

Although there has been ample anecdotal evidence of the efficacy of chelation therapy in preventing and potentially reversing primary and secondary hemochromatosis,[180] significant issues persist about the overall therapeutic efficacy that can be achieved. Several encouraging early reports of longitudinal evaluation in cohorts followed for 4 to 5 years demonstrated improved systolic function in response to chronic chelation therapy.[169] However, numerous cross-sectional studies of late outcome in patients managed on chronic chelation programs have described limited success, with cardiomyopathy remaining a frequent problem.[181–184] Analysis of cohorts with a high incidence (up to 50%) of cardiomyopathy have indicated that older age at onset of therapy and poor therapeutic compliance are significant risk factors for the development of heart disease.[181,182] In these patients, compliance with chelation therapy correlates more closely with myocardial iron deposition than does number of transfusions.[177] Life-long obligation to a 12-hour per day subcutaneous infusion taxes the cooperation of even the most compliant patient, a category that rarely includes adolescents. Periodic monitoring of ventricular function is useful to detect early evidence of myocardial injury, prior to onset of symptoms. Intensification of chelation therapy with a higher daily dose administered intravenously in response to recognition of clinically significant ventricular dysfunction has been noted to be beneficial but full recovery of ventricular function has not been typical.[182,184] This approach is not risk free. In addition to the potential for direct adverse effects of chelation therapy, dose intensification with indwelling venous catheters carries additional risks. Increased susceptibility to thromboembolic complications in subjects with beta-thalassemia has been described, including arterial occlusion and recurrent pulmonary thromboembolism.[185] Several groups have described a high incidence of pulmonary hypertension in beta-thalassemia,[186,187] which in at least some cases was secondary to recurrent pulmonary thromboembolism.[187]

HYPERTROPHIC CARDIOMYOPATHY

Hypertrophic cardiomyopathy (HCM) is defined as the presence of ventricular hypertrophy without an identifiable hemodynamic cause such as hypertension, valvular heart disease, catecholamine-secreting tumors, hyperthyroidism, or other conditions that could secondarily stimulate cardiac hypertrophy. HCM accounts for 42% of childhood cardiomyopathy and has an incidence of 0.47/100,000 children.[2] The various names have been applied to the disorder over the years such as *asymmetric hypertrophy of the heart, functional subaortic stenosis, idiopathic hypertrophic subaortic stenosis, asymmetric septal hypertrophy*, and numerous others, have each reflected a particular clinical or pathologic aspect of the disease. As understanding of the disorder has advanced, it has become apparent that a rather broad spectrum of disease can be encountered and definitions based on the presence of regional differences in wall thickness or the presence of dynamic left ventricular outflow obstruction are inadequate. The current preferred terminology of *hypertrophic cardiomyopathy* takes into account the broader range of findings, regardless of whether the hypertrophy is localized or global. It is clear that HCM represents a heterogeneous group of disorders and this diversity is more apparent in childhood than at any other age. It is possible to further subdivide these diseases based on etiology into primary and secondary forms, where the primary form is a familial disorder (*familial hypertrophic cardiomyopathy*, FHC) typically devoid of findings outside of the heart. The secondary forms include diseases such as Friedreich ataxia[188] where ventricular hypertrophy is common but is not the dominant clinical manifestation and others, such as glycogenosis Type IX,[189] in which a systemic disorder has primarily or exclusively cardiac manifestations. A classification of the various forms of HCM is provided in Table 26-2, recognizing that the continued evolution of our understanding of this disorder implies that any classification will require frequent revision.

Familial Hypertrophic Cardiomyopathy

Genetics

The genetic transmission of FHC is usually autosomal dominant, with about 50% of cases representing new mutations. Maternally inherited mitochondrial pattern of transmission has also been reported,[190,191] adding to the complexity of the disease, although in some cases the histology of this disease does not manifest the typical myocardial disarray of the autosomal dominant forms.[192] There has been a virtual explosion of information since the early 1990s concerning the genetic abnormalities associated with this disorder. One of the most striking findings has been the sheer number of diverse mutations that manifest clinically as HCM. The results of molecular studies so far have

TABLE 26–2. Classification of the Forms of Hypertrophic Cardiomyopathy

Familial hypertrophic cardiomyopathy
Sarcomeric hypertrophic cardiomyopathy
Maternally inherited hypertrophic cardiomyopathy
Syndromes
Beckwith-Wiedemann syndrome
Cardio-facial-cutaneous syndrome
Costello syndrome
Friedreich ataxia
Lentiginosis (LEOPARD syndrome)
Noonan syndrome
Secondary forms
Anabolic steroid therapy and abuse
Infant of diabetic mother
Prenatal and postnatal corticosteroid therapy
Metabolic disorders
Carnitine deficiency (Carnitine palmitoyl transferase II deficiency, carnitine-acylcarnitine translocase deficiency)
Fucosidosis type 1
Glycogenoses (types 2, 3, and 9; Pompe disease, Forbes disease, phosphorylase kinase deficiency)
Glycolipid lipidosis (Fabry disease)
Glycosylation disorders
I-cell disease
Lipodystrophy, total
Lysosomal disorders (Danon disease)
Mannosidosis
Mitochondrial disorders (multiple forms)
Mucopolysaccharidoses (types 1, 2, and 5; Hurler syndrome, Hunter syndrome, Scheie syndrome)
Selenium deficiency

implicated a number of sarcomeric proteins in the etiology, including beta-myosin heavy chain, alpha-myosin heavy chain, myosin essential light chain, myosin regulatory light chain, cardiac troponin T, cardiac troponin I, α-tropomyosin, titin, and myosin binding protein C.[193] These gene mutations also display allelic heterogeneity; that is, multiple distinct mutations of each of these genes can cause the disease. These findings have led to the paradigm of FHC as a disease of the sarcomere (sarcomeric hypertrophic cardiomyopathy, SHC) and provides a rational basis for a mechanism by which diverse mutations could eventuate in similar phenotypes.[194,195] Familial forms of HCM are due to nonsarcomeric genes, such as those due to mitochondrial defects,[190,191] potassium channel,[196] and the gamma subunit of protein kinase A.[192] Although SHC appears to be the most common cause of FHC, it is not the only cause.

Beyond the potential for furthering our understanding of the pathophysiology of the disease,[197] other benefits could derive from genotyping as a screening tool. That certain mutations predict greater or lesser cardiac risk has been well documented,[198] raising expectations that genotyping will improve risk stratification and clinical management. Recent data cast considerable doubt on the utility of genetic diagnosis for risk prediction[199] insofar as there appears to be a very poor correlation between genotype and clinical expression of the disorder. Development of a commercially viable method for screening for the individual mutations has been impeded by the need to screen for the many point mutations. This approach is also limited by the fact that the point mutations that have been identified appear to account for only 50% to 60% of cases. The alternative of detecting mutant protein has typically not been possible because of the subtle nature of most mutations. Furthermore, potentially unifying observations that could simplify the screening process have often not held true over time. For example, mutations in troponin T were initially reported to have a consistent phenotype of mild or absent hypertrophy associated with a high incidence of sudden death,[200] but families have now been described with troponin T defects who have a low risk of early death.[201] Other factors, such as the coexistence of mitochondrial DNA mutations in some families,[202] multiple mutations,[203] or the impact of coexistent genetic polymorphisms on the renin-angiotensin system,[204] account for some of the variability in disease expression.

In addition to the practical obstacles caused by the complexity of the genetic nature of the disease, it has also been argued that detection of gene carriers in FHC may have too little impact on clinical care to justify the cost and the potential for adverse psychological and social consequences.[205] This is a moot issue, because current technology functionally limits screening to families with several affected individuals in whom linkage analysis can help identify the relevant locus. For these patients, the phenotype can be surmised from the family history, limiting the new information gained by knowledge of the genotype. However, in the 50% of cases without an affected first-degree relative, genetic screening would have an enormous impact on clinically ambiguous cases. Infants, children, and young adults would particularly benefit from this capability. The diagnosis of the disease is often confounded in patients in whom a mild to moderate stimulus for hypertrophy is known to be present, thereby in principle excluding the diagnosis of FHC, but the magnitude and pattern of hypertrophy are typical for FHC. In some cases the chance coexistence of two diseases can be confirmed on genetic screening.[206] The differential diagnosis of FHC in infants is frequently difficult, in part related to problems with unequivocally diagnosing other causes such as mitochondrial disorders. There is overlap in the patterns of physiologic and pathologic hypertrophy, and children and young adults are often excluded from athletics based on a presumptive diagnosis of FHC. For some, this is a life and career altering decision that could benefit from the certainty of a genetic diagnosis.

Pathology

Gross pathology characteristically demonstrates increased heart weight, a nondilated left ventricle often with greater maximal thickness of the septum than that of the free wall, a thickened mitral valve with mural endocardial plaque in the outflow portion of the septum in apposition to the anterior leaflet of mitral valve, dilated atria, and in some cases grossly visible areas of scarring without significant narrowing of the epicardial coronary arteries. Age-related differences include absence of a septal endocardial plaque or myocardial scarring in subjects younger than 10 years. Although it is not possible to determine on postmortem examination whether outflow obstruction was present, mural plaques are more common and both free wall and septal hypertrophy tend to be more marked in these cases. Focal myocardial fiber disarray or disorganization within the ventricular septum is a feature of this disease that is observed in most cases. Although not unique to FHC, normal hearts or heart conditions other than FHC rarely have myocardial fiber disarray that involves more than 5% of the septum, whereas 90% of hearts with FHC have this finding in more than 5% of the septum.[207]

Abnormal intramural coronary arteries are also reported in a high percentage of patients with FHC. The abnormalities consist of increased number and size of arteries with thickened walls and narrowed lumens. These abnormal vessels are most common in the ventricular septum but are also present in the left ventricular free wall.[208,209] The significance of these abnormal vessels is uncertain although they may play a role in the reduced coronary reserve of FHC[209] and/or the occurrence of transmural infarction. Similar abnormal coronary vessels have been observed in normal fetuses and in some forms of congenital heart disease. Thus, similar to asymmetric hypertrophy and focal myocardial disarray, the presence of abnormal intramural coronary arteries is not specific for FHC but is more marked and more common than in other diseases.

Pathophysiology

The mechanism whereby sarcomeric mutations lead to cardiac hypertrophy is not known. Given the similar phenotypes that result from diverse genotypes, a common pathogenesis is believed to exist. Although contractile abnormalities have been proposed as a unifying mechanism,[210] the mutant proteins in HCM do not consistently manifest abnormal contractility.[211] Energy compromise, based on inefficient utilization of adenosine triphosphate, is a common feature of the diffuse mutations that has been proposed as potential pathogenesis.[212] Increased cost of force production resulting in excess myocyte stress with local release of trophic factors is proposed as the stimulus to hypertrophy. It is, however, difficult to reconcile the regional variation in hypertrophy including the predilection for septal hypertrophy with this hypothesis. Similarly, the biochemical abnormalities are present even when hypertrophy is absent.

FHC is usually classified as obstructive or nonobstructive, depending on the presence of a pressure gradient between the left ventricle and aorta. The gradient can be present at rest or latent (provokable) and often demonstrates marked spontaneous lability.[213] Often, clinicians attach too much significance to the presence or absence of outflow obstruction, as discussed by Criley.[214] Dynamic subaortic stenosis can be elicited in normal ventricles with provocation and can be seen in a variety of other disease states. Outflow obstruction is present in less than half of patients with FHC and is not predictive of outcome. In fact, symptomatic patients without obstruction fare more poorly than those who have gradients. Although provocation of latent outflow obstruction has been recommended,[215] there are no data indicating that this is clinically useful. The magnitude of outflow obstruction is unrelated to the occurrence of ventricular tachycardia[216] or risk of sudden death. Surgical or pharmacologic reduction in the outflow gradient in symptomatic patients is usually associated with a reduction in symptoms although the incidence of sudden death is not improved. In general, dynamic outflow obstruction is more common in symptomatic patients but is not a negative prognostic factor, and interventions aimed to reduce the gradient are justified only insofar as symptomatic benefit can be anticipated.

Diastolic Dysfunction. Systolic dysfunction is not a primary feature of FHC, although occasional progression to a dilated, dilated cardiomyopathy has been described. However, a large body of evidence has now accumulated indicating that diastolic dysfunction plays a substantial role in the physiologic consequences of FHC. Both relaxation and passive filling are disturbed in FHC. Several mechanisms probably contribute to the abnormalities in relaxation (a) asynchronous activation and inactivation[217,218]; (b) ischemia; and (c) a possible primary defect in cellular calcium handling. Similarly, abnormal passive properties are also multifactorial: (a) increased wall thickness alone decreases chamber compliance, regardless of whether myocardial compliance is impaired, and (b) myocardial fibrosis may also influence chamber stiffness through increased intrinsic myocardial stiffness. In addition to the congestive symptoms that result from the elevation in diastolic pressure, diastolic dysfunction also impairs myocardial blood flow, further predisposing the hypertrophied ventricle to ischemia.

Exercise Intolerance. Limitation of exercise capacity is often the primary and most disabling symptom in FHC, due either to dyspnea or chest pain. In this group, exercise performance is impaired, even when asymptomatic patients are included.[219] Although presumed secondary to diastolic dysfunction, studies of the relation between exercise capacity and diastolic function have yielded conflicting results.[220–223] Current data would indicate that passive diastolic properties are more important than abnormal relaxation.[223] However, the etiology appears to be multifactorial and variable, depending on the presence of obstruction as well as the magnitude of ventricular asynchrony.

Ischemia. Chest pain is extremely common in FHC and can have characteristics of angina but is often atypical, occurring at rest, having a variable threshold of onset, and at times prolonged in duration. Most patients with FHC are free of epicardial coronary artery disease but have numerous other potential causes of ischemia. Intramural small vessel disease has been documented in areas of myocardial fibrosis, suggesting a causal role. Leftward deviation and systolic compression of septal perforators correlate with exercise thallium defects. Patients with FHC have reduced subendocardial arteriolar density and lumen area in association with diminished coronary reserve.[224] Symptomatic patients with FHC with or without obstruction have metabolic evidence of myocardial ischemia (decreased myocardial lactate uptake or net lactate production) during exercise, pacing, or catecholamine infusion.[225–227] Ischemia is absent at rest and patients without a history of chest pain do not manifest the same ischemic response to these stresses. However, young, asymptomatic patients with severe septal hypertrophy have abnormalities in glucose metabolism similar to those found in ischemic myocardium.[228] Unfortunately, electrocardiographic changes with exercise are an unreliable marker of ischemia, occurring with equal frequency in patients with and without inducible ischemia.[229] Chest pain is common in children and teenagers with FHC and is generally assumed to represent ischemia. Although confirmatory metabolic studies are not available, children and young adults with thallium scintigraphy indicative of ischemia are at increased risk of sudden death.[230]

Myocardial Bridging. Muscle bands overlying epicardial coronary arteries have been identified in a number of heart diseases. Myocardial bridges are congenital and sufficiently common that they are considered an anatomic variant rather than a congenital anomaly, having been observed in 20% to 66% of hearts.[231] Despite evidence of systolic compression of the underlying coronary artery visible on angiography, there has been little evidence to support the hypothesis that bridging is responsible for ischemia. Their presence has been detected angiographically in 30% of adults with FHC,[232] with no evidence of adverse impact on outcome. In a recent provocative report of a relationship between sudden death and the presence of myocardial bridging in children with FHC.[233] Yetman et al[233] suggest that surgical unroofing of the coronary can prevent sudden death. These authors describe delayed diastolic filling of the affected coronary as a mechanism for ischemia. However, based on prior data, it is unclear why myocardial bridges would have a greater impact on children than has been described in adults. Perhaps more troubling is the observation in this report[233] that patients with bridges were older than the patients without, and the overall incidence (28%) was identical to the frequency described in adults (30%).[234] If myocardial bridging, a condition present from birth, has a marked negative impact on survival, one would expect the incidence to decrease with age, not increase or stay the same. Thus, although surgical intervention is possible,[235] further confirmation is required before myocardial bridging can be accepted as an adverse risk factor worthy of surgical intervention.

Arrhythmias. Atrial fibrillation develops in approximately 15% of adults with FHC, but is unusual in children. Early reports indicated a markedly negative impact on survival, but more recent studies do not support this.[236] Ventricular arrhythmias including ventricular tachycardia and fibrillation are common, and are the presumed mechanism of sudden death in most cases. There are conflicting data concerning the prognostic implications of ventricular arrhythmias found on Holter monitor recording in patients with FHC. Although syncope is a risk factor for sudden death,[237] the presence of asymptomatic ventricular tachycardia on Holter monitoring is not a risk factor.[238,239] However, symptomatic ventricular tachycardia on Holter monitor or induced at electrophysiology study appears to identify a high-risk subgroup.[239] In children, ventricular arrhythmias on Holter monitoring are less frequent than in adults,[240] despite a higher annual risk of sudden death. Early studies of increased QT dispersion indicated an increased risk of sudden death[241,242] but more recent studies do not support this.[243]

Sudden Death. Numerous potential mechanisms exist for sudden death in FHC. Individual reports have described asystole, complete heart block,[244] myocardial infarction, and supraventricular tachycardia with rapid ventricular response as antecedent events.[245–247] Hypotension with diminished coronary filling and secondary autonomic reflex activation would be expected to be particularly poorly tolerated in this disease and may represent a common initiating event. In adults, symptomatic nonsustained ventricular tachycardia on ambulatory monitoring is a highly specific risk factor for sudden death. However, adolescent patients, who have the highest incidence of sudden death, are rarely found to have arrhythmias.

Clinical Description

In about half of adult patients it is possible to elicit a history of another family member with FHC or a family history of sudden death at a young age, but in children this percentage is only about 20%. Although many young patients are asymptomatic, the full spectrum of symptoms associated with this disease can be present from early in childhood. The chest pain can be angina-like but is more often atypical, often occurring at rest, and can last for hours without enzymatic evidence of myocardial injury. Subjects can have no pain on maximal exercise testing on one occasion and then experience severe pain early in exercise on another. Reduced exercise tolerance due to dyspnea is common, although congestive symptoms are not, at least beyond the age of one year. In contrast, infants with FHC often have a presentation more typical for congestive heart failure, with a history of tachypnea, hepatomegaly, and poor feeding and growth. Palpitations are common in adults but rarely noted by children. Syncope occurs in 15% to 25% of adult subjects. Although syncope is less common in childhood, it is strongly associated with the risk of sudden death.

Physical. Most children and young adults are remarkably healthy with a frequent predilection for athletics. Although many physical findings have been described in this disease, most relate to dynamic ventricular outflow obstruction and are absent in subjects without obstruction. Therefore, completely normal findings at physical examination in a healthy patient who may be quite athletic does not exclude the presence of this potentially fatal disorder, an observation that has led some observers to suggest echocardiographic screening as part of an evaluation prior to sports participation. The apical and parasternal cardiac impulses are often augmented but rarely displaced. Hepatomegaly is common in infants but is generally not seen beyond this age. In the presence of outflow obstruction, a bisferiens carotid pulse can be encountered, corresponding to the *spike-and-dome* aortic pulse contour in patients with dynamic outflow obstruction. Parasternal and carotid systolic thrills are frequent in patients with left or right ventricular outflow obstruction. The murmur of dynamic left ventricular outflow obstruction can be noted, rising in intensity with physiologic maneuvers that lower preload or afterload or increase contractility.[248] Very loud systolic murmurs are usually found in subjects with subpulmonary stenosis, which is more common in infants and children. The murmur of mitral regurgitation is frequent in subjects with subaortic stenosis, though difficult to separate from the outflow murmur. Aortic regurgitation can be heard but is less commonly encountered than in discrete subaortic stenosis.

Electrocardiogram. Although the vast majority of patients with FHC and obstruction to left ventricular outflow have abnormal ECG findings, about 25% of patients without obstruction have normal ECG findings. The most common abnormalities are left ventricular hypertrophy, ST segment and T wave abnormalities, and abnormal Q waves.

Echocardiogram. The echocardiogram permits noninvasive assessment of ventricular size, wall thickness, systolic and diastolic function, outflow obstruction, and valvar insufficiency (Fig. 26-2). Nearly all children can be adequately imaged by transthoracic echocardiography, but transesophageal imaging plays a valuable role in pre- and intraoperative evaluation. Numerous studies have documented the incidence of involvement of the various anatomic regions.[249] Localized hypertrophy of the anterior septum is seen in 10% to 15% of patients, and 20% to 35% of patients have involvement of both anterior and posterior portions of the septum. At least 50% of patients have involvement of the anterolateral free wall in addition to the septum. The incidence of isolated involvement of the posterior and apical portions of the septum or anterolateral free wall without hypertrophy of the anterior septum is as much as 20%. The reported incidence of concentric hypertrophy is quite variable but can be as much as 20%. The anatomic pattern has not proven to be predictive of outcome but is a primary determinant of outflow obstruction and is an important factor in surgical planning.[250]

In addition to defining the location and extent of hypertrophy, the presence of anterior motion of the mitral apparatus can be seen as well as the presence and extent of septal-mitral apposition (Fig. 26-2*B*). Color flow Doppler echocardiography in conjunction with continuous wave Doppler and two-dimensional imaging has proved uniquely useful in defining the site, extent, and mechanism of left and/or right ventricular outflow obstruction.[251,252] Both M-mode and Doppler[253–256] echocardiographic techniques reveal abnormal filling characteristics in many patients. Systolic and diastolic myocardial velocities are typically subnormal on tissue Doppler.

Exercise Testing. Quantitative assessment of functional capacity is useful to document clinical status as well as to objectively assess the response to therapeutic interventions. High grade arrhythmias are elicited in some patients, with a negative prognostic implication. A hypotensive response to

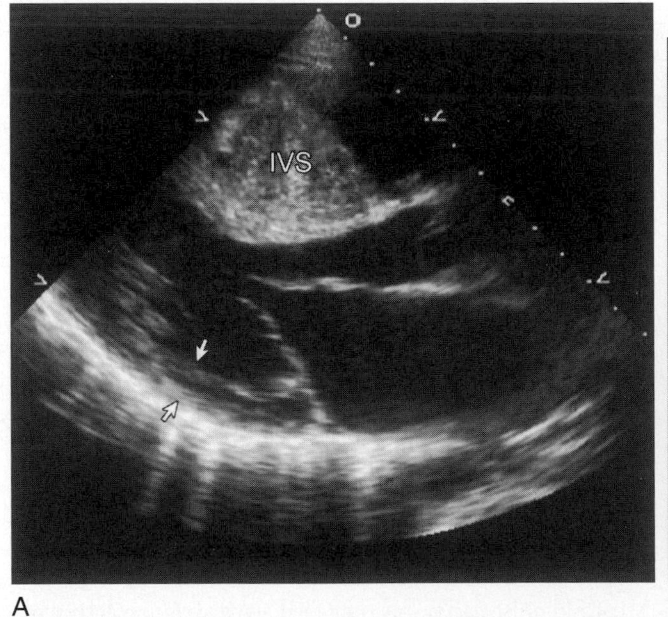

A

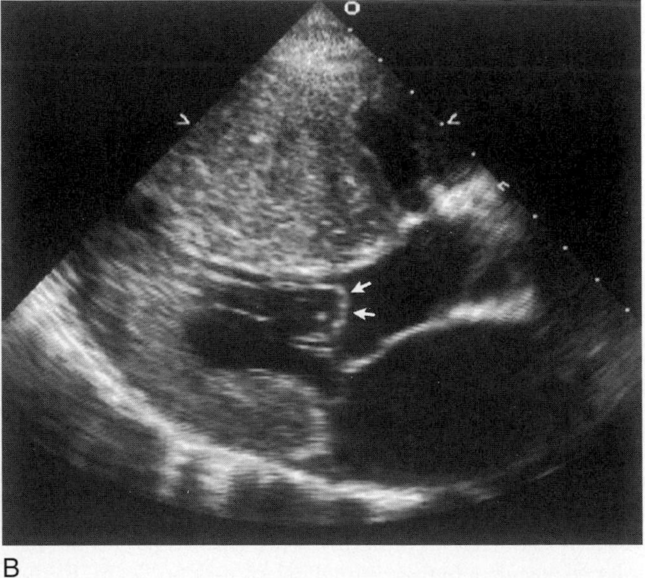

B

FIGURE 26–2 *Parasternal long axis image of a patient with familial sarcomeric hypertrophic cardiomyopathy. A, The marked increase in interventricular septal (IVS) thickness compared with posterior wall thickness (arrows) is seen on this late diastolic frame, and the mitral valve leaflets are in a neutral, nearly closed position. B, Dynamic left ventricular outflow obstruction is illustrated. During ejection, the anterior mitral leaflet moves into apposition with the IVS and buckles anteriorly (arrows), nearly obliterating the left ventricular outflow tract.*

exercise appears to represent a risk for sudden death,[257,258] but more definitively a normal exercise blood pressure response identifies a low-risk cohort.[259,260] In contrast, exercise-associated repolarization changes are seen with and without ischemia, indicating that exercise should be combined with a tracer study if ischemia is suspected.

Magnetic Resonance Imaging (MRI). Cardiac MRI is a useful tool for measurement of myocardial mass and wall thickness,[261,262] particularly for patients in whom echocardiography is inadequate. Three-dimensional reconstruction of MRI data provides improved quantification of the regionally hypertrophied left ventricle in this disorder.[263] Variation in regional and transmural systolic function is uniquely available from myocardial tagging studies that have documented reduced myofiber shortening isolated to areas of increased wall thickness.[264] Recent work using delayed enhancement after gadolinium administration has demonstrated the capacity to identify areas of myocardial fibrosis,[265] a finding that may be of prognostic importance.

Catheterization. The hemodynamic findings in this disorder depend on the presence or absence of obstruction. The pressure gradient can be absent, can be quite labile, varying between 0 and 200 mm Hg, or may be constant. The arterial pulse tracing can have a spike-and-dome configuration, reflecting mid-systolic obstruction to flow. In the obstructive form of the disease, postextrasystolic beats will show a fall in arterial pressure in spite of marked increase in ventricular pressure, reflecting the rise in contractility and secondary increase in dynamic obstruction. Mean atrial and atrial "a" wave pressures are elevated, as is the ventricular end-diastolic pressure. Since cavity size is normal or small, the ventricular diastolic pressure-volume relationship is abnormal, indicating reduced chamber compliance. The right ventricle can be involved, particularly in infants and children, with outflow gradients and elevated diastolic pressure. Left ventriculography shows a hypertrophied ventricle with systolic cavity obliteration. The enlarged papillary muscles can fill the systolic cavity, and anterior motion of the mitral leaflets into the outflow tract can be evident. Simultaneous right and left ventricular angiography in a cranially angulated left anterior oblique projection is useful to display the size and configuration of the interventricular septum. In infants, the septum often impinges on the right ventricular outflow and right ventricular cavity obliteration in systole can be noted.

Differential Diagnosis

Ultimately, diagnosis of FHC depends on molecular identification of the offending gene or the abnormal gene product. Until this test is widely available, reliance on current, less than perfect, diagnostic tools is necessary. Although echocardiographic identification of hypertrophy is the primary diagnostic modality in current clinical use, FHC with an associated risk of sudden death can be present even in the absence of hypertrophy.[266,267] Surprisingly, when a genotyped population is investigated, usual ECG and echocardiographic criteria accurately detect disease in only 83% of adults[268] and only 50% of children.[269] Under these circumstances, the need for alternative diagnostic modalities is apparent. Tissue Doppler has been reported to reliably discriminate between genotypically positive and negative populations, even in patients without hypertrophy.[270–272] The myocardium in FHC has an abnormal pattern of ultrasound integrated backscatter, potentially providing an alternative method of diagnosis.[273] There are no data to suggest that ultrasound tissue characterization will be useful in diagnosing patients without hypertrophy, but it has the potential to differentiate hypertrophy from other causes.[274] The utility of this test is less in children with FHC, in whom myocardial reflectivity has been found to be normal.[275] MRI provides morphologic information similar to that available on echocardiography and improved utility of MRI in diagnosing borderline cases has not been demonstrated. Endomyocardial biopsy is useful for excluding other causes of HCM, including mitochondrial disorders and storage diseases, and is therefore recommended in infants and young children. However, the primary histologic abnormality of focal myocardial disarray is not unique to FHC and cannot be reliably detected on biopsy specimens.

Association of HCM with numerous disorders other than FHC has been described. Although isolated case reports have described HCM in association with many disorders, there are a number of disorders in which HCM is seen with sufficient frequency to indicate that it is an intrinsic element of the disease (Table 26-2). Patients with Friedreich ataxia have a 25% to 50% incidence of HCM, with clinical characteristics quite different from FHC (see below). HCM is seen in up to 20% to 30% of patients with Noonan syndrome[276] with findings similar to FHC. Although the risk of congestive heart failure is more common than in FHC, there is also at least some risk of sudden death.[277] Infants of diabetic mothers and neonates exposed to corticosteroids often have transient biventricular hypertrophy, sometimes with outflow tract obstruction, and occasionally causing symptoms. Finally, there are many genetic disorders that are often accompanied by cardiac hypertrophy. Generally, HCM in infants presents unique problems in differential diagnosis. In various series, diseases other than FHC have accounted for 30% to 70% of HCM cases in patients younger than 2 years.[277] Hypertrophy with depressed function is rare in FHC and highly suggestive of a metabolic or mitochondrial disorder,[278] as is severe concentric hypertrophy in patients younger than 2 years. Myocardial biopsy is often necessary to distinguish among these disorders, is recommended in all patients younger than 2 years, and can be particularly helpful in children with symmetric hypertrophy or depressed function who have no family history of FHC.[278,279] Mitochondrial disorders present a particular problem in diagnosis because of variable and often tissue-specific involvement.

Differentiation between physiologic hypertrophy secondary to athletic participation and pathologic hypertrophy in FHC is a frequent and important problem in children and young adults. The cardiac response to chronic, intense exercise has been well characterized and includes dilation and hypertrophy with preservation of myocardial contractility.[280] The hypertrophic response is most intense in sports that elicit a marked rise in blood pressure during exercise[281] such as rowing, wrestling, and power lifting.[282–284] Wall thicknesses greater than 13 mm are occasionally found in athletes and mild left ventricular hypertrophy is not infrequent in patients with FHC, resulting in a significant incidence of diagnostic ambiguity.

Electrocardiography has not been particularly helpful in differentiation because of the frequent presence of ECG abnormalities in athletes.[285,286] The echocardiographic and clinical features that increase the probability of FHC include (a) a family history of FHC or early sudden death; (b) significant regional differences in hypertrophy; (c) diastolic dysfunction; (d) abnormal tissue Doppler, (e) abnormal ultrasonic myocardial reflectivity; (f) absence of deconditioning-induced regression of hypertrophy, and (g) abnormalities of coronary flow reserve.[272,287–289] Ultimately, there are some subjects in whom differentiation based on available techniques is simply not possible.[290]

Management

The goals of therapy in this disorder are to reduce symptoms and prolong survival. The symptoms of chest pain, dyspnea, and exercise intolerance can often be managed medically, and surgery has been successful in certain patient groups. Digitalis is not helpful and is usually contraindicated unless atrial fibrillation occurs. Although dyspnea is a common symptom, diuretic therapy is usually not beneficial, can increase the outflow gradient due to a reduction in chamber volume, and can reduce cardiac output through inadequate preload on the noncompliant myocardium.

Beta-Blockers. The mainstay of therapy for many years has been beta-adrenergic blockade. Chest pain and dyspnea are often relieved by propranolol, but improved exercise capacity is seen less often. The response appears to be dose dependent, and very high dosage levels have often been used. Unfortunately, side effects such as fatigue and depression are often encountered at these high dosage levels, particularly in children and adolescents, and can be intolerable. Despite early improvement, symptoms often recur and may not respond to dose escalation. Studies of the impact of beta-blocker therapy on survival in adults and children have invariably been uncontrolled but have not identified a measurable effect of propranolol on survival. In a single uncontrolled study in children, comparison of a small number of pediatric patients in each of two geographically distinct areas, one of which treated all HCM patients with high-dose propranolol, found unusually high mortality (52% 10-year survival) in the untreated cohort with no mortality in the treated cohort.[291] It is difficult to reconcile these findings with the many prior, larger studies that have failed to identify a survival benefit from propranolol and large pediatric studies that have found a 10-year survival of 80% in unselected populations.[292] The study design used in this study[291] is potentially highly biased by the potential for genetically similar patients in each geographic region, and the differences in outcome do not exceed those observed between other studies in small groups of pediatric patients with HCM.

Calcium Channel Blockers. Calcium channel blockers in general and verapamil in particular have been used extensively in patients with FHC. Sustained improvement in diastolic relaxation is generally noted in response to verapamil administration with secondary reduction in diastolic pressure and mean left atrial pressure.[293–297] This is believed to be the mechanism for the reduction in dyspnea and increase in exercise capacity that occurs. Improved distribution of subendocardial flow and diminished inducible ischemia have been noted as well.[298] Nearly all patients have a substantial and sustained symptomatic improvement that can be dramatic in some individuals.[277,299] Although older patients with congestive heart failure can be intolerant of these drugs, pediatric tolerance has been excellent, even in neonates.[277,300] Several retrospective studies report a reduced risk of sudden death,[277,301,302] but definitive controlled trials to support this are not available. Early clinical reports suggested that calcium channel blockers could reduce the severity of left ventricular hypertrophy but this observation was never confirmed. Recently, work in mice with a defect in alpha-myosin heavy chain found that administration of diltiazam prior to the appearance of hypertrophy prevented phenotypic expression of the disease,[303] raising the possibility that timing of administration may be critical to achieving an antihypertrophic effect.

Vasodilators. Inhibition of the renin-angiotensin system has a favorable impact on ventricular hypertrophy and diastolic function in hypertension and aortic stenosis, but has rarely been used in FHC, presumably because of concerns that vasodilatation can aggravate subaortic obstruction. Indeed, in patients with dynamic subaortic stenosis, systemically administered angiotensin converting enzyme inhibitors result in reduced preload and afterload with a secondary fall in cavity size and increase in outflow gradient, as well as impaired left ventricular relaxation and compliance.[304] Based on theoretical considerations and data such as these, it is generally believed that these agents as well as other systemic vasodilators are contraindicated in HCM when left ventricular outflow tract obstruction is present. However, there are also recent data indicating a significant role for aldosterone,[204] and the renin-angiotensin system in general[305] in modulating the phenotypic manifestations of HCM, leading to the suggestion that blocking this system might reduce hypertrophy and fibrosis.

Systemic Bacterial Endocarditis (SBE) Prophylaxis. Antibiotic prophylaxis is recommended for patients with outflow tract obstruction, in whom an increased risk of endocarditis has been documented.[306] Patients with nonobstructive FHC who do not have other indications do not require prophylaxis.

Pacemaker Therapy. Asynchronous ventricular pacing has emerged as an effective method of symptomatic treatment in some patients with left ventricular outflow tract obstruction.[307] Although early in the experience with this technique the mechanism of reduced left ventricular outflow tract obstruction was thought secondary to altered septal motion, it has become clear over time that pacing-induced asynchronous activation impairs contractility, thereby reducing the force of contraction.[308,309] The secondary reduction in Venturi forces in the outflow tract and the rise in end systolic volume, changes seen with any negative inotrope, result in a reduction in outflow gradients through the same mechanism as beta-blockers or calcium channel blockers.[310] This explains the observation that the combination of atrioventricular delay and pacing site that induces the greatest magnitude of ventricular asynchrony, as reflected by the longest achievable QRS interval, has the maximum impact on outflow gradient. Results in small cohorts of children with outflow obstruction who were symptomatic despite medical therapy have reported symptomatic improvement, reduced outflow obstruction, reduced left ventricular hypertrophy, and improved exercise tolerance.[311–313] Despite reports of nearly all subjects experiencing benefit in early studies,[314,315] subsequent controlled studies found that only about 60% of subjects improved. Furthermore, in two thirds of these the benefit appeared to reflect placebo effect and an adverse effect on symptoms was seen in 5%.[316] The significant placebo effect has been seen in other studies,[317] perhaps explaining reports of persistent symptom relief after pacing termination.[314] Early reports of persistent reduction of gradient after termination of gradient[314] have not been confirmed in later studies.[318] Dual-chamber pacing in patients without obstruction has not been beneficial.[319] This mode of therapy is not free of theoretical and known adverse consequences. Although intended to reduce the stimulus to myocardial hypertrophy in patients with FHC, asynchronous ventricular activation causes asymmetric hypertrophy in animal models.[320] Asynchronous activation is intimately related to asynchronous deactivation, one of the primary causes of abnormal diastolic filling in FHC. Exacerbation of this asynchrony has a measurable negative impact on diastolic function.[321] Pacemaker implantation is associated with a significant incidence of complications,[322] particularly in growing children. Based on current information, dual-chamber pacing should at best be considered as an alternative to surgical or transcatheter septal reduction in patients with obstructive FHC who are symptomatic despite maximum medical therapy.

Alcohol Septal Ablation. Septal infarction induced by direct, transcatheter septal infusion of absolute alcohol results in reduction of septal thickness and secondary relief of left ventricular outflow tract obstruction, with symptomatic improvement and increased exercise tolerance. Toxicity has included a 50% incidence of transient heart block and a 15% to 20% incidence of permanent complete heart block, periprocedure ventricular arrhythmias that may require cardioversion, unintended distal infarction due to inadvertent alcohol infusion into the anterior descending coronary, and late appearance of complete heart block.[323–327] The technical feasibility in adolescents has been demonstrated, although experience in this age group is limited. Success is highest when obstruction is related to localized basilar hypertrophy. Patients with mitral valve abnormalities or obstruction that is deeper within the ventricular chamber are poor candidates. Late outcome is unknown for this new technique, but current results indicate this may represent a reasonable alternative to surgery for relief of outflow tract obstruction in selected patients.[328]

Surgical Myectomy. In symptomatic subaortic stenosis, septal myotomy–myectomy results in symptomatic improvement in nearly all patients, despite the fact that symptoms are generally not correlated with the presence and degree of obstruction. Numerous recent studies have documented a high success rate, low mortality, and few complications with the procedure.[235,329–331] Results in children have been similar to those reported in adults.[332,333] There has been a striking reduction in complication rates compared with those reported in earlier series. Surgery permits concomitant mitral valve repair in patients with underlying mitral valve abnormalities and significant mitral regurgitation. Mitral valve replacement may be needed in some patients to achieve adequate relief of outflow obstruction, but recent advances in surgical technique have significantly reduced the number of such patients.[334] Recent results indicate no operative mortality and a survival advantage, both of which are significantly different from earlier experience.[335] Consequently, surgery should be considered for relief of symptoms in patients with intractable and debilitating symptoms in spite of maximum medical therapy. However, intervention based on gradient alone cannot be recommended.

Antiarrhythmics. Although most instances of sudden death in FHC are arrhythmic events, antiarrhythmic therapy has not proved highly effective. Amiodarone was initially reported to reduce the incidence of sudden death in certain high-risk subgroups, but subsequent studies indicated that treatment in fact may increase the risk of sudden death.[336] Furthermore, the pediatric experience with amiodarone therapy for FHC is very limited due to the toxicity associated with chronic therapy. The promising early experience with implantable cardioverter defibrillators (ICD) has resulted in a shift to recommending an ICD for patients with syncope, symptomatic ventricular tachycardia on Holter monitor, or resuscitated cardiac arrest.[337–339] The risk-benefit ratio for the use of ICDs in children is skewed compared with that of adults. In a recent review, 28% of children experienced appropriate, potentially life-saving ICD discharges and 25% experienced inappropriate discharges; however, there was a 21% incidence of lead failure.[340] The low rate of device utilization implies that better methods of risk stratification in children are needed. Children are also at high risk for more device-related infections and adverse psychosocial impact than adults. Therefore, although potentially life-saving, pediatric-specific implantation indications must be developed and tested before this technology will achieve its potential in children.

Exercise Restriction. Avoidance of strenuous exercise is generally recommended for patients with FHC. The rational for this restriction is based on the observations that sudden death is the usual cause of death in FHC and has a higher-than-expected association with exercise[341] and that FHC is believed to be the most common cause of sudden death in young, competitive athletes.[342] Nevertheless, the basis for this recommendation has several serious weaknesses.[343] The true incidence of FHC in athletes who experience sudden death is uncertain because genetic confirmation was not available and diagnosis was based on morphologic criteria that cannot unequivocally differentiate FHC from physiologic hypertrophy. Clearly, some patients with FHC tolerate intense, competitive athletic participation without symptoms or sudden death.[344] Population studies have documented the apparent paradox that although there is a transient increase in the risk for sudden death during intense exercise in patients with coronary artery disease who regularly participate in low- and high-level exertion, these individuals experience an overall reduction in the risk for sudden death.[345,346] Additionally, individuals who do not exercise regularly have an exaggerated risk of sudden death during exercise.[347] In fact, it is precisely those individuals with cardiovascular risk factors who derive the largest risk reduction from regular participation in moderate to intense exercise.[347] Several population studies have now documented that exercise and sports participation during childhood are predictive of activity level in adults.[348,349] Detraining and social stigmatization are particularly difficult problems for the adolescent who is excluded from the usual school activities and peer interactions. Competitive team sports elicit an emotional overlay that appears to increase the risk associated with the sport itself, in addition to demanding more intense exercise, and can therefore be justifiably proscribed. Certain activities, such as weight lifting, are associated with high levels of circulating catecholamines that can predispose to arrhythmias and elicit a marked stimulus to eccentric cardiac hypertrophy. However, in patients who do not manifest high-grade arrhythmias or exercise-induced arrhythmias or hypotension, there is little evidence to indicate that moderate aerobic-type exercise represents a significant risk and it does provide measurable hemodynamic and psychological benefits.

Risk Stratification

Many prognostic factors for sudden death have been reported, but few have been confirmed. It is likely that availability of genotyping will improve risk stratification, but four major risk factors have been identified: a family history of sudden death, exercise-induced hypotension, syncope, and symptomatic nonsustained ventricular tachycardia on Holter monitor. Patients free of all risk factors are considered at low risk and interventions (other than for symptoms such as chest pain or exercise intolerance) are not indicated. With two or more risk factors or with syncope alone in children, risk is considered high and aggressive management such as ICD implantation is recommended. There is no consensus on management of intermediate-risk patients. Several recent reports have evaluated the impact of the severity of left ventricular hypertrophy on survival and risk of sudden death. Extreme wall thickness, in particular, has been suggested as an important risk factor[350] and therefore as a potential indication for an implantable cardioverter-defibrillator.[351] Other reports have not confirmed this association.[352–355] In a recent study of 237 patients, patients with a wall thickness less than 15 mm were at lower risk, but risk did not vary by degree of hypertrophy.[356] None of these studies included a large number of children, and none examined the risk associated with the severity of hypertrophy adjusted for body size. Overall, available data do not support inclusion of severity of hypertrophy as a risk factor in children with HCM. Additional negative prognostic factors such as evidence of ischemia on exercise thallium, marked QT dispersion, and myocardial bridging may also be useful in management decisions for these patients.[357]

Clinical Course

The clinical course for FHC is highly age-dependent. Hypertrophic cardiomyopathy presenting in infancy appears to carry a worse prognosis than in older age groups. Symptomatic infants generally manifest congestive heart failure and cyanosis and have been reported to have a particularly poor outlook, with 9 of 11 dying within the first 5 years in one series[358] and 10 of 19 dying in the first year of life in another.[359] However, some series have noted survival not dissimilar to older children, with reported survival of 100% at 6 years[360] and 85% survival at 12 years,[277] likely representing differences related to small series and numerous etiologies of HCM in this age group. Ventricular hypertrophy can develop during childhood or adolescence and ECG abnormalities can precede its appearance,[361] but new appearance in a previously normal adult has not been described. The severity of hypertrophy can progress during periods of accelerated somatic growth, particularly during adolescence.[362] Importantly, the increase in magnitude of hypertrophy that is sometimes seen does not appear to have negative prognostic importance and does not justify an alteration in management.[362] Regression of hypertrophy occurs in older adults[363] but is rarely observed in children.[364] Systolic function is nearly always normal or hyperdynamic and generally does not change over time unless there is a transition to a thin-walled dilated cardiomyopathy,[365] a transformation only occasionally observed during childhood[366,367] and invariably associated with a grim prognosis. In patients with obstruction, the pressure gradient is also generally stable in adult subjects, although progression does occur in children and adolescents.[368] Sudden death in patients referred to tertiary care centers is seen annually in 3% to 5% of adults but more recent population studies find an unbiased rate of 0.1% to 1%.[352,369–372] Although prior small reports in children have described an annual mortality of 6-8% of children,[245,247,373] recent large studies indicate an annual mortality of 1%,[292] similar to results in adult populations. Asymptomatic adults appear to be at even lower risk[374] although a similar relationship to symptoms has not been demonstrated in children. While improved survival has been reported with medical and surgical interventions, the studies are invariably retrospective and usually rely on historical controls.

Friedreich Ataxia

Friedreich ataxia is an autosomal recessive heredofamilial disorder characterized by progressive degeneration of the spinocerebellar tracts. In addition to the neurologic deficit, there is muscular weakness in most patients after the first few years with initial involvement of the lower extremities and later development of weakness in the upper limbs. Diabetes is frequent and cardiomyopathy is present in most patients. The chief clinical expression is ataxia that usually becomes manifest before adolescence. Although the mean age of onset is 9 years, there is a wide range (2 to 25 years and occasionally even later). Affected children frequently become wheelchair bound in the second or third decade of life, and scoliosis is almost universal. Cardiac abnormalities have been reported to be identifiable in nearly all subjects with Friedreich ataxia, and the presence or absence of cardiac involvement is often used to aid diagnosis.

The gene responsible for Friedreich ataxia encodes frataxin, a mitochondrial protein that is highly expressed in the normal heart.[375] Nearly all mutations appear to be secondary to an unstable expansion of a GAA triplet repeat.[76] with longer repeats associated with earlier age of onset, more rapid disease progression, and more severe left ventricular hypertrophy.[188,377] Although the exact function of frataxin is uncertain, current evidence indicates a mitochondrial membrane location serving a role in iron transport.[378] Frataxin deficiency results in mitochondrial iron accumulation, oxidative damage, and reduced cellular respiratory function.[379] Iron chelation with deferoxamine and treatment with apoptosis inhibitors protected fibroblasts harvested from patients with Friedreich ataxia from oxidant-induced death.[380] These findings are similar to anthracycline cardiomyopathy, have been seen in other neurodegenerative disorders, and suggest that the mitochondrial defects result in oxidative-damage induced apoptotic cell death.[381] Although iron chelation therapy has been suggested as a potential form of therapy, serum iron and ferritin concentrations are normal, suggesting that such therapy could be problematic.[382] The proposed mechanism of oxygen radical injury is further supported by preliminary data indicating coenzyme Q10 and the free-radical scavenger idebenone are cardioprotectant in these patients.[383,384]

Heart Disease in Friedreich Ataxia

Depending on the criteria used to define the presence of heart disease, cardiac involvement can be detected during life in 50% to 100% of patients, but on autopsy the heart is abnormal in virtually all. The histopathology of the heart in Friedreich ataxia has been studied by several observers with similar though nonspecific findings.[385] Although many patients have idiopathic cardiac hypertrophy, the marked myocyte disorganization characteristic of sarcomeric hypertrophic cardiomyopathy is not a feature of Friedreich ataxia. With more severely involved cases there are foci of necrosis interspersed with hypertrophied muscle cells and replacement of cardiac muscle by connective tissue. Abnormalities in the small, intramural coronary arteries have been reported, and cardiac ischemia has been suggested as a potential cause of the necrosis.[385]

The clinical manifestations of cardiac abnormalities in Friedreich ataxia are usually noted during the terminal stages of the disease, with symptoms rarely occurring during childhood.[386] The symptoms noted in most series consist of exertional dyspnea, palpitations, chest pain, and pedal edema. Respiratory failure is the usual late outcome in Friedreich ataxia, and although possibly related to cardiac dysfunction it can also be attributed to the combination of severe scoliosis and neuromuscular dysfunction. As a consequence, it is often difficult to know when to attribute dyspnea to the cardiac involvement in these patients. Although palpitations are often reported, the few studies that have included Holter monitors have not found ventricular arrhythmias to be a common finding. Chest pain is usually atypical or nonspecific. Ankle edema is often seen in the most severely disabled patients who are wheelchair bound and relatively immobile, making this sign unreliable as a means to recognize cardiac failure. Thus, the nonspecific nature of the described symptoms and the failure of significant clinical involvement to be manifest prior to the terminal phase of the illness make clinical assessment an unreliable means of detecting cardiac disease in Friedreich ataxia.

Electrocardiographic abnormalities are a sensitive but nonspecific indicator of myocardial involvement in Friedreich ataxia. Some abnormality of the electrocardiogram has been described in 75% to 90% of patients.[387] Repolarization abnormalities, including diffuse T-wave inversion, are the most commonly reported finding, being seen in 40% to 90% of patients. Interestingly, repolarization abnormalities are seen in some patients with echocardiographically normal hearts. Furthermore, the electrocardiogram is quite insensitive to the presence of ventricular hypertrophy, with 80% to 90% of patients with significant hypertrophy on echocardiogram not meeting electrocardiographic criteria for left or right ventricular hypertrophy.[387] Ventricular arrhythmias and conduction disturbances in Friedreich ataxia are rare, but atrial arrhythmias are often noted late in the disease. Atrial tachycardias, particularly atrial flutter or fibrillation, are the most common arrhythmias, and are found in up to 50% of patients before death.

The results of the various imaging modalities have basically revealed the same range of findings. Nearly all patterns and gradations of hypertrophy can be found, with concentric, asymmetric, and no hypertrophy each seen in some percentage of patients. The pattern can evolve over time and the severity correlates with the age of onset, with younger diagnosis manifesting more severe hypertrophy.[388] Hypertrophy has been seen by echocardiography in 20% to 100% of subjects aged 3 years and older. In a large, systematic, prospective study of all patients with Friedreich ataxia followed at one institution,[389] hypertrophy was identified in only 20%, with concentric hypertrophy in 11% and asymmetric hypertrophy in 9%. Dilated cardiomyopathy was seen in 7%. The much smaller incidence of significant echocardiographic abnormalities noted in this study compared with other, less comprehensive studies is probably more representative of the true incidence.

Dilated cardiomyopathy is occasionally seen in Friedreich ataxia. Histopathology in these hearts shows myocyte hypertrophy, degeneration and atrophy of muscle fibers, and myocardial interstitial fibrosis, findings similar to the nonspecific histopathologic findings in hearts with other forms of idiopathic dilated cardiomyopathy.[387] The dilated form of the cardiomyopathy has been speculated to represent an end-stage progression of the HCM of Friedreich ataxia, but the conversion from concentric hypertrophy to dilated cardiomyopathy has not actually been observed. It is unlikely that this is the course in all cases, since there are several reports of dilated cardiomyopathy as the primary cardiac presentation at ages 3 to 6 years of age, even before onset of neurologic symptoms.[390] There are few longitudinal studies of the cardiac disease in Friedreich ataxia. In one study in which 10 patients were followed over a 5-year period, three were found to manifest some dilation with a fall in systolic function, but the changes were not sufficient to warrant the diagnosis of dilated cardiomyopathy.[391] In another study, 17% of patients evolved into a dilated cardiomyopathy pattern over a mean period of 8 years, and almost all had a hypertrophic ventricle on initial evaluation.[392]

The importance of the cardiac disease to the ultimate clinical course in Friedreich ataxia is somewhat difficult to ascertain. Although many authors have stated that cardiac disease is the cause of death in most patients, verification is scant. For example, cardiac symptoms were reported in 46 of 115 patients aged 10 to 72 years with signs of heart failure in only one.[390] The symptoms in this group of patients are difficult to interpret because the most common symptom was exertional dyspnea (46/46), followed by palpitations (13/46), and angina (44/46). Even if cardiac dysfunction contributes to the symptoms of dyspnea and chest pain, only in occasional cases does the cardiac disease present a significant management problem prior to the terminal stages. It is important to note that despite the morphologic similarities between the cardiac findings in Friedreich ataxia and familial hypertrophic cardiomyopathy, the clinical picture in the two diseases differs in many regards. Myocardial disarray, the pathologic hallmark of familial hypertrophic cardiomyopathy, is absent in Friedreich ataxia. Ventricular arrhythmias and sudden death, which are frequent in familial hypertrophic cardiomyopathy, are uncommonly reported in Friedreich ataxia and when they occur, are generally seen in association with respiratory failure, atrial flutter and fibrillation, and congestive heart failure.[393]

RESTRICTIVE CARDIOMYOPATHY

Restrictive cardiomyopathy is defined as a disease of the myocardium characterized by restrictive filling and reduced diastolic volume of either or both ventricles with normal or near normal systolic function. Similar to dilated and hypertrophic forms, restrictive myopathies occur as primary and secondary forms, where the secondary types are related to a multisystem disorder including infiltrative and storage diseases. Restrictive cardiomyopathy is the least common form of cardiomyopathy, and among children is quite rare, accounting for fewer than 3% of pediatric cardiomyopathy cases.[2] As reviewed recently by Denfield,[394] the reported experience in children is comprised of a handful of small case series and occasional case reports. Presentation in children is often with respiratory symptoms similar to asthma or recurrent respiratory infections, with hepatomegaly, ascites, and peripheral edema, or sometimes with syncope or sudden death. The characteristic feature of restrictive cardiomyopathy is a marked increase in the stiffness of the myocardium or endocardium, resulting in a reduced ventricular capacitance. The physiologic consequence is impaired ventricular filling, leading to elevated diastolic filling pressure and marked atrial dilation (Fig. 26-3).[395] Pulmonary hypertension secondary to left atrial hypertension is present from the early stages of this disease. Although numerous secondary causes of restrictive cardiomyopathy have been described in adults (Table 26-3), the pediatric cases are generally idiopathic or related to either anthracycline cardiotoxicity or endocardial fibroelastosis, with up to one third manifesting in families.[396] Differentiation from many of the secondary causes such as myocardial noncompaction relies on morphologic criteria. Tissue analysis is generally undertaken given the dismal prognosis of the disease and the desire to exclude any potentially treatable disorder. Methods of differentiation between restrictive cardiomyopathy and constrictive pericarditis have not been specifically investigated in children, primarily because constrictive pericarditis is extraordinarily rare in children. Recent reports suggest that noninvasive differentiation between restrictive cardiomyopathy and pericardial disease can be achieved in 95% of adult patients using tissue Doppler.[397] The most striking characteristic of the reports in children has been the uniformly poor prognosis, with a 2-year survival of approximately 50%. Death is usually due to congestive heart failure, although 25-30% may have sudden death. Anticoagulation is recommended as a 25% incidence of thromboembolism has been seen in children. Therapy is otherwise nonspecific and usually of very limited benefit. Onset of irreversible elevation of pulmonary vascular resistance can occur within 1 to 4 years in these patients and early cardiac transplantation is therefore recommended to avoid the need for heart and lung transplantation.[398] The survival curve for restrictive cardiomyopathy is significantly worse than the outcome for children who have undergone cardiac transplantation, leading to the recommendation that patients should be listed for transplant at the time of diagnosis.

TABLE 26–3. Causes of Restrictive Cardiomyopathy

Primary restrictive cardiomyopathy
Endomyocardial fibrosis
Hypereosinophilic syndrome (Löffler's disease)
Familial
Idiopathic
Secondary restrictive cardiomyopathy
Infiltrative
Interstitial
Amyloidosis
Anthracycline cardiomyopathy
Radiation toxicity
Sarcoidosis
Scleroderma
Storage
Fabry disease
Gaucher disease
Glycogenosis
Hemochromatosis
Hurler disease
Noninfiltrative
Carcinoid heart disease
Noncompaction of the ventricular myocardium
Pseudoxanthoma elasticum

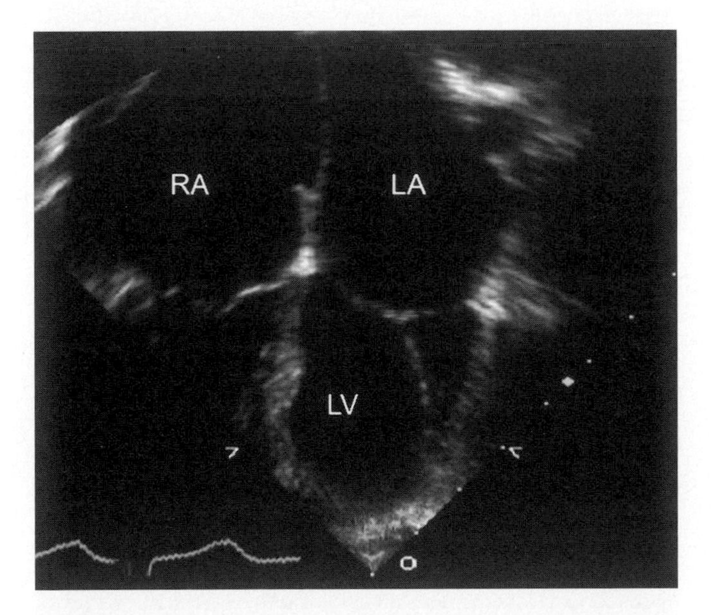

FIGURE 26–3 *Apical transverse end-diastolic echocardiographic image in a patient with restrictive cardiomyopathy. The left (LA) and right atria (RA) are markedly dilated (see Fig. 26-1A for comparison with normal) and often exceed the size of the left ventricle (LV).*

RIGHT VENTRICULAR CARDIOMYOPATHIES

Uhl Anomaly

Uhl anomaly is an exceedingly rare disorder characterized by virtual absence of the myocardial layer of the right ventricular free wall, resulting in a thin wall consisting of endocardium apposed to endocardium, explaining the alternative name of parchment right ventricle. It has been often confused with arrhythmogenic right ventricular cardiomyopathy, which, although rare, is certainly the more common of the two.[399] Occurrence is usually sporadic, but occasional familial cases have been described. Congestive heart failure is the primary mode of presentation, and findings may be dramatic with massive peripheral edema. Arrhythmias are not a prominent feature, in contradistinction to arrhythmogenic right ventricular cardiomyopathy. Palliative treatment with standard anticongestive therapy has limited success. Surgical intervention with either exclusion of the right ventricle and direct cavopulmonary anastomosis[400] or cardiac transplantation has been successful.

Arrhythmogenic Right Ventricular Cardiomyopathy

Arrhythmogenic right ventricular cardiomyopathy (ARVC), also known as *arrhythmogenic right ventricular dysplasia*, is a rare disorder in which the right ventricular myocardium is characterized by progressive noninflammatory loss of myocytes with replacement by fat and fibrous tissue. The process begins locally but progresses to global right and usually modest left ventricular involvement but relative lack of septal changes. ARVC is familial in more than half of cases with generally autosomal dominant inheritance with incomplete penetrance, although recessive forms have also been reported. The genetic basis for the disorder results in marked regional variation in incidence. Although rare in the United States, the disorder accounts for a large percentage of sudden, unexpected deaths in young adults in Italy.[401] Presentation with arrhythmias and sudden death is common, particularly in adolescents and young adults, with presentation having been reported as early as age 10.[402] Biventricular dysfunction is typical,[403] and differentiation from other forms of dilated cardiomyopathy such as myocarditis can be problematic. Although a hyperintense MRI signal typical of fatty tissue has been considered useful in diagnosis, recent reports indicate this finding is unreliable.[404] Clinical, arrhythmic, and MRI findings can be identical in both ARVC and myocarditis.[405] Tissue diagnosis of transmural fibrofatty infiltration requires surgical biopsy. Endomyocardial biopsy may be helpful[406] but focal involvement and sparing of the septum limit the utility of this technique. Although antiarrhythmic drug therapy has not been effective, the use of implantable cardioverter defibrillator therapy appears to improve outcome in ARVC.[407,408] However, similar to the situation with hypertrophic cardiomyopathy, identification of the high-risk patients most likely to benefit from defibrillator implantation remains problematic.

NONCOMPACTION OF THE VENTRICULAR MYOCARDIUM

Numerous synonyms have been used to describe this abnormality of the myocardium, each based on the peculiar appearance most notable in the left ventricle, including spongy myocardium, spongioform cardiomyopathy, noncompaction, hypertrabeculation, and persisting myocardial sinusoids. The fundamental abnormality is a pattern of multiple prominent trabeculations in the left ventricular apex and to a variable extent the apical aspect of the left ventricular free wall with deep intertrabecular recesses (Fig. 26-4). These trabeculae typically overlie a thin rim of compact myocardium and account for more than half of the wall thickness in the affected areas. Although described as early as 1932, the disorder was largely unrecognized until the widespread availability of echocardiography, which has greatly facilitated its recognition. The morphologic pattern of left ventricular noncompaction (LVNC) has been seen both as an isolated finding and also in association with

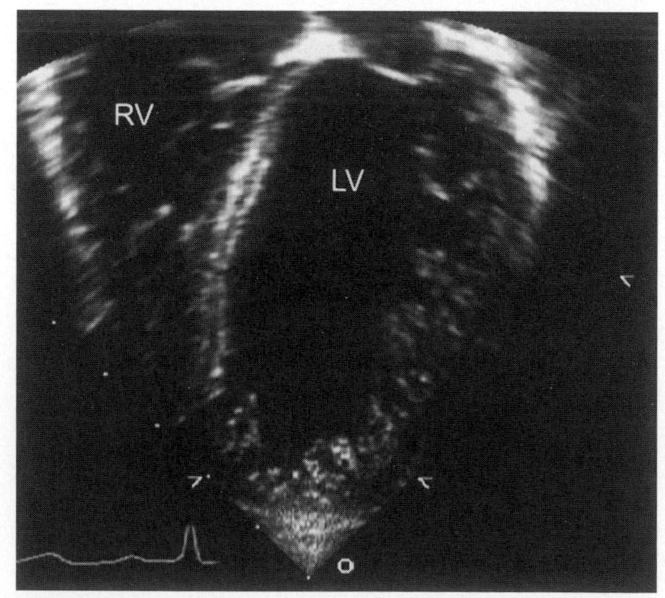

FIGURE 26–4 *Atypical transverse end-diastolic echocardiographic image in a patient with left ventricular noncompaction. The smooth surface of the LV interventricular surface contrasts with the finger-like projections of myocardium from the apical and lateral free wall into the LV cavity. LV, left ventricle; RV, right ventricle.*

congenital heart disease.[409] Similarly, the myocardial abnormality can be seen with and without ventricular dysfunction. On the basis of a morphologic appearance similar to the embryonic myocardium, the disorder has been believed to represent an arrest of normal embryogenesis of the endocardium and myocardium. This understanding has been challenged by the observation that the pattern can also be acquired.[410] Although initially described as a highly fatal disorder of early childhood, it is now frequently seen in adults, indicating that either the prognosis is not as grave as previously believed or that new development of the pattern is common.[411,412] In addition to congenital heart disease, the pattern has been described in conjunction with neuromuscular disorders,[413,414] mitochondrial disorders,[8] Barth syndrome,[415] trisomy 13,[416] Fabry disease,[417] and other systemic disorders.[418] Multiple genetic loci have been described, but none account for a large proportion of cases.[419] Altogether, as information accumulates it has become increasingly apparent that this is a diverse disorder that may not represent a distinct cardiomyopathy but rather a nonspecific myocardial response to a variety of stimuli.[420] The clinical course of the described cases has also not been sufficiently characteristic to permit identification of noncompaction as a unique cardiomyopathy.

Patients with LVNC may have normal ventricular function and hemodynamics. In those with a manifest cardiomyopathy, restrictive or dilated patterns of disease may be present. Clinical findings include heart failure, arrhythmias, and thromboembolic events.[418,421–424] Although most documented cases have had symptoms, there is clearly a significant ascertainment bias with underdiagnosis of asymptomatic cases. Diagnosis is usually based on recognition of the typical findings on cross-sectional echocardiography. In addition to multiple prominent ventricular trabeculations most prominent at the left ventricular apex, blood flow into the deep intertrabecular recesses can be documented by color Doppler. Although specific criteria related to the number of trabeculae or the relative thickness of the compacted and noncompacted layers of the myocardium have been suggested,[418] the validity of these criteria remains unknown because of the poorly defined nature of the underlying disorder. Left ventricular trabeculations can be seen in the normal heart,[425] adding to the diagnostic confusion. Management is symptom based and nonspecific. Although the suggestion has been put forward that these patients may be more susceptible to ventricular thrombi and thromboembolism due to the apical sinusoids, it is not known whether the incidence is higher than in other forms of dilated or restrictive myopathy with similar clinical severity, nor is it clear whether anticoagulation is effective. Prognosis has been strikingly variable, and again it is not clear whether the presence of the noncompaction pattern portends a worse outcome than predicted by the severity of congestive or restrictive physiology. Although subjects with LVNC and normal ventricular function may be at risk for development of systolic or diastolic dysfunction, it is not currently known how frequently or how rapidly this transition takes place.[418,421]

REFERENCES

1. Richardson P, McKenna W, Bristow M, et al. Report of the 1995 World Health Organization International Society and Federation of Cardiology Task Force on the Definition and Classification of Cardiomyopathies. Circulation 93:841, 1996.
2. Lipshultz SE, Sleeper LA, Towbin JA, et al. The incidence of pediatric cardiomyopathy in two regions of the United States. N Engl J Med 348:1647, 2003.
3. Wheeler DS, Kooy NW. A formidable challenge: the diagnosis and treatment of viral myocarditis in children. Crit Care Clin 19:365, 2003.
4. Bowles KR, Bowles NE. Genetics of inherited cardiomyopathies. Expert Rev Cardiovasc Ther 2:683, 2004.
5. Towbin JA, Solaro RJ. Genetics of dilated cardiomyopathy: more genes that kill. J Am Coll Cardiol 44:2041, 2004.
6. Holmgren D, Wahlander H, Eriksson BO, et al. Cardiomyopathy in children with mitochondrial disease; clinical course and cardiological findings. Eur Heart J 24: 280, 2003.
7. Chinnery PF, DiMauro S, Shanske S, et al. Risk of developing a mitochondrial DNA deletion disorder. Lancet 364: 592, 2004.
8. Scaglia F, Towbin JA, Craigen WJ, et al. Clinical spectrum, morbidity, and mortality in 113 pediatric patients with mitochondrial disease. Pediatrics 114:925, 2004.
9. Fishberger SB, Colan SD, Saul JP, et al. Myocardial mechanics before and after ablation of chronic tachycardia. Pacing Clin Electrophysiol 19:42, 1996.
10. Lipshultz SE, Lipsitz SR, Mone SM, et al. Female sex and higher drug dose as risk factors for late cardiotoxic effects of doxorubicin therapy for childhood cancer. N Engl J Med 332:1738, 1995.
11. Calabrese F, Thiene G. Myocarditis and inflammatory cardiomyopathy: microbiological and molecular biological aspects. Cardiovasc Res 60:11, 2003.
12. Crispell KA, Wray A, Ni H, et al. Clinical profiles of four large pedigrees with familial dilated cardiomyopathy: preliminary recommendations for clinical practice. J Am Coll Cardiol 34:837, 1999.
13. Luppi P, Rudert WA, Zanone MM, et al. Idiopathic dilated cardiomyopathy - A superantigen-driven autoimmune disease. Circulation 98:777, 1998.
14. Marks AR. A guide for the perplexed - Towards an understanding of the molecular basis of heart failure. Circulation 107: 1456, 2003.
15. Van Bilsen M, Smeets PJH, Gilde AJ, et al. Metabolic remodelling of the failing heart: the cardiac burn-out syndrome? Cardiovasc Res 61:218, 2004.

16. Ventura-Clapier R, Garnier A, Veksler V. Energy metabolism in heart failure. J Physiol (Lond) 555:1, 2004.
17. Bristow MR, Minobe W, Rasmussen R, et al. Beta-adrenergic neuroeffector abnormalities in the failing human heart are produced by local rather than systemic mechanisms. J Clin Invest 89:803, 1992.
18. Böhm M, La Rosée K, Schmidt U, et al. Force-frequency relationship and inotropic stimulation in the nonfailing and failing human myocardium: Implications for the medical treatment of heart failure. Klin Wochenschr 70:421, 1992.
19. Gwathmey JK, Liao R, Helm PA, et al. Is contractility depressed in the failing human heart. Cardiovasc Drugs Ther 9:581, 1995.
20. Borst MM, Beuthien W, Schwencke C, et al. Desensitization of the pulmonary adenylyl cyclase system: a cause of airway hyperresponsiveness in congestive heart failure? [In Process Citation]. J Am Coll Cardiol 34:848, 1999.
21. Rein AJ, Colan SD, Parness IA, et al. Regional and global left ventricular function in infants with anomalous origin of the left coronary artery from the pulmonary trunk: preoperative and postoperative assessment. Circulation 75:115, 1987.
22. McMahon CJ, Nagueh SF, Eapen RS, et al. Echocardiographic predictors of adverse clinical events in children with dilated cardiomyopathy: a prospective clinical study. Heart 90:908, 2004.
23. Matitiau A, Perez-Atayde A, Sanders SP, et al. Infantile dilated cardiomyopathy: Relation of outcome to left ventricular mechanics, hemodynamics, and histology at the time of presentation. Circulation 90:1310, 1994.
24. Karr SS, Parness IA, Spevak PJ, et al. Diagnosis of anomalous left coronary artery by Doppler color flow mapping: Distinction from other causes of dilated cardiomyopathy. J Am Coll Cardiol 19:1271, 1992.
25. Camargo PR, Mazzieri R, Snitcowsky R, et al. Correlation between gallium-67 imaging and endomyocardial biopsy in children with severe dilated cardiomyopathy. Int J Cardiol 28:293, 1990.
26. Ardehali H, Qasim A, Cappola T, et al. Endomyocardial biopsy plays a role in diagnosing patients with unexplained cardiomyopathy. Am Heart J 147:919, 2004.
27. Malhotra V, Ferrans VJ, Virmani R. Infantile histiocytoid cardiomyopathy: Three cases and literature review. Am Heart J 128:1009, 1994.
28. Cowley CG, Lozier JS, Orsmond GS, et al. Safety of endomyocardial biopsy in children. Cardiol Young 13:404, 2003.
29. Schwartz ML, Cox GF, Lin AE, et al. Clinical approach to genetic cardiomyopathy in children. Circulation 94:2021, 1996.
30. Reddy M, Hanley FL. Mechanical support of the myocardium. *In* Chang AC, Hanley FL, Wernovsky G, Wessel DL, (eds): Pediatric cardiac intensive care. Baltimore: Williams & Wilkins, 1998, pp 345-9.
31. Pierpont ME, Breningstall GN, Stanley CA, et al. Familial carnitine transporter defect: A treatable cause of cardiomyopathy in children. Am Heart J 139:S96, 2000.
32. Östman-Smith I, Brown G, Johnson A, et al. Dilated cardiomyopathy due to type II X-linked 3-methylglutaconic aciduria: Successful treatment with pantothenic acid. Br Heart J 72:349, 1994.
33. Akagi T, Benson LN, Lightfoot NE, et al. Natural history of dilated cardiomyopathy in children. Am Heart J 121:1502, 1991.
34. Teerlink JR, Massie BM. The interaction of ACE inhibitors and aspirin in heart failure: Torn between two lovers. Am Heart J 138:193, 1999.
35. Goldfine H, Aurigemma GP, Zile MR, et al. Left ventricular length-force-shortening relations before and after surgical correction of chronic mitral regurgitation. J Am Coll Cardiol 31:180, 1998.
36. Coats AJS. Exercise training for heart failure - Coming of age. Circulation 99:1138, 1999.
37. Rowland TW. Trainability of the cardiorespiratory system during childhood. [Review]. Canadian Journal of Sport Sciences 17:259, 1992.
38. Lewis AB. Prognostic value of echocardiography in children with idiopathic dilated cardiomyopathy. Am Heart J 128:133, 1994.
39. Lewis AB, Chabot M. Outcome of infants and children with dilated cardiomyopathy. Am J Cardiol 68:365, 1991.
40. Kimball TR, Daniels SR, Meyer RA, et al. Left ventricular mass in childhood dilated cardiomyopathy: A possible predictor for selection of patients for cardiac transplantation. Am Heart J 122:126, 1991.
41. Burch M, Siddiqi SA, Celermajer DS, et al. Dilated cardiomyopathy in children: Determinants of outcome. Br Heart J 72:246, 1994.
42. Pongpanich B, Isaraprasart S. Congestive cardiomyopathy in infants and children. Clinical features and natural history. Jpn Heart J 27:11, 1986.
43. Redfield MM, Gersh BJ, Bailey KR, et al. Natural history of incidentally discovered, asymptomatic idiopathic dilated cardiomyopathy. Am J Cardiol 74:737, 1994.
44. Mendes LA, Dec GW, Picard MH, et al. Right ventricular dysfunction: An independent predictor of adverse outcome in patients with myocarditis. Am Heart J 128:301, 1994.
45. Ciszewski A, Bilinska ZT, Lubiszewska B, et al. Dilated cardiomyopathy in children: clinical course and prognosis. Pediatr Cardiol 15:121, 1994.
46. Taliercio CP, Seward JB, Driscoll DJ, et al. Idiopathic dilated cardiomyopathy in the young: clinical profile and natural history. J Am Coll Cardiol 6:1126, 1985.
47. Friedman RA, Moak JP, Garson A, Jr. Clinical course of idiopathic dilated cardiomyopathy in children. J Am Coll Cardiol 18:152, 1991.
48. Venugopalan P, Agarwal AK, Akinbami FO, et al. Improved prognosis of heart failure due to idiopathic dilated cardiomyopathy in children. Int J Cardiol 65:125, 1998.
49. Van der Hauwaert LG, Denef B, Dumoulin M. Long-term echocardiographic assessment of dilated cardiomyopathy in children. Am J Cardiol 52:1066, 1983.
50. Lewis AB. Late recovery of ventricular function in children with idiopathic dilated cardiomyopathy. Am Heart J 138:334, 1999.
51. Nakagawa M, Sato A, Okagawa H, et al. Detection and evaluation of asymptomatic myocarditis in schoolchildren - Report of four cases. Chest 116:340, 1999.

52. Lauer B, Niederau C, Kühl U, et al. Cardiac troponin T in patients with clinically suspected myocarditis. J Am Coll Cardiol 30:1354, 1997.
53. Mahrholdt H, Goedecke C, Wagner A, et al. Cardiovascular magnetic resonance assessment of human myocarditis - A comparison to histology and molecular pathology. Circulation 109:1250, 2004.
54. Martin MER, Moya-Mur JL, Casanova M, et al. Role of noninvasive antimyosin imaging in infants and children with clinically suspected myocarditis. J Nucl Med 45:429, 2004.
55. Chow LH, Radio SJ, Sears TD, et al. Insensitivity of right ventricular endomyocardial biopsy in the diagnosis of myocarditis. J Am Coll Cardiol 14:915, 1989.
56. Bohn D, Benson L. Diagnosis and management of pediatric myocarditis. Paediatr Drugs 4:171, 2002.
57. Wu LA, Lapeyre AC, III, Cooper LT. Current role of endomyocardial biopsy in the management of dilated cardiomyopathy and myocarditis. Mayo Clin Proc 76:1030, 2001.
58. Calabrese F, Rigo E, Milanesi O, et al. Molecular diagnosis of myocarditis and dilated cardiomyopathy in children: Clinicopathologic features and prognostic implications. Diagn Mol Pathol 11:212, 2002.
59. Martin AB, Webber S, Fricker FJ, et al. Acute myocarditis: Rapid diagnosis by PCR in children. Circulation 90:330, 1994.
60. Kawai C. From myocarditis to cardiomyopathy: Mechanisms of inflammation and cell death - Learning from the past for the future. Circulation 99:1091, 1999.
61. Badorff C, Lee GH, Lamphear BJ, et al. Enteroviral protease 2A cleaves dystrophin: Evidence of cytoskeletal disruption in an acquired cardiomyopathy. Nature Med 5:320, 1999.
62. Mason JW. Myocarditis and dilated cardiomyopathy: An inflammatory link. Cardiovasc Res 60:5, 2003.
63. Staudt A, Staudt Y, Dorr M, et al. Potential role of humoral immunity in cardiac dysfunction of patients suffering from dilated cardiomyopathy. J Am Coll Cardiol 44:829, 2004.
64. Gagliardi MG, Bevilacqua M, Bassano C, et al. Long term follow up of children with myocarditis treated by immunosuppression and of children with dilated cardiomyopathy. Heart 90:1167, 2004.
65. Mason JW, O'Connell JB, Herskowitz A, et al. A clinical trial of immunosuppressive therapy for myocarditis. The Myocarditis Treatment Trial Investigators [see comments]. N Engl J Med 333:269, 1995.
66. Drucker NA, Colan SD, Lewis AB, et al. Gamma-globulin treatment of acute myocarditis in the pediatric population. Circulation 89:252, 1994.
67. Lurie PR. Endocardial fibroelastosis is not a disease. Am J Cardiol 62:468, 1988.
68. Ni JY, Bowles NE, Kim YH, et al. Viral infection of the myocardium in endocardial fibroelastosis - Molecular evidence for the role of mumps virus as an etiologic agent. Circulation 95:133, 1997.
69. Mahle WT, Weinberg PM, Rychik J. Can echocardiography predict the presence or absence of endocardial fibroelastosis in infants <1 year of age with left ventricular outflow obstruction? Am J Cardiol 82:122, 1998.
70. Angelov A, Kulova A, Gurdevsky M. Endocardial fibroelastosis. Clinico-pathological study of 38 cases. Pathol Res Pract 178:384, 1984.
71. Arola A, Tuominen J, Ruuskanen O, et al. Idiopathic dilated cardiomyopathy in children: Prognostic indicators and outcome. Pediatrics 101:369, 1998.
72. Feng J, Yan JY, Buzin CH, et al. Comprehensive mutation scanning of the dystrophin gene in patients with nonsyndromic X-linked dilated cardiomyopathy. J Am Coll Cardiol 40:1120, 2002.
73. Culligan KG, Mackey AJ, Finn DM, et al. Role of dystrophin isoforms and associated proteins in muscular dystrophy (review). Bioorganic & Medicinal Chemistry Letters 2:639, 1998.
74. Hoogerwaard EM, Van der Wouw PA, Wilde AAM, et al. Cardiac involvement in carriers of Duchenne and Becker muscular dystrophy. Neuromusc Disord 9:347, 1999.
75. Vesel S, Stopar-Obreza M, Trebusak-Podkrajsek K, et al. A novel mutation in the G4.5 (TAZ) gene in a kindred with Barth syndrome. Eur J Hum Genet 11:97, 2003.
76. McNally E, Allikian M, Wheeler MT, et al. Cytoskeletal defects in cardiomyopathy. J Mol Cell Cardiol 35:231, 2003.
77. Cohen N, Muntoni F. Multiple pathogenetic mechanisms in X linked dilated cardiomyopathy. Heart 90:835, 2004.
78. Singleton BK, Green CA, Renaud S, et al. McLeod syndrome resulting from a novel XK mutation. Br J Haematol 122:682, 2003.
79. Lapidos KA, Kakkar R, McNally EM. The dystrophin glycoprotein complex: signaling strength and integrity for the sarcolemma. Circ Res 94:1023, 2004.
80. Cziner DG, Levin RI. The cardiomyopathy of Duchenne's muscular dystrophy and the function of dystrophin. Med Hypotheses 40:169, 1993.
81. Vatta M, Stetson SJ, Jimenez S, et al. Molecular normalization of dystrophin in the failing left and right ventricle of patients treated with either pulsatile or continuous flow-type ventricular assist devices. J Am Coll Cardiol 43:811, 2004.
82. Ortiz-Lopez R, Li H, Su J, et al. Evidence for a dystrophin missense mutation as a cause of X-linked dilated cardiomyopathy. Circulation 95:2434, 1997.
83. Beggs AH. Dystrophinopathy, the expanding phenotype-Dystrophin abnormalities in X-linked dilated cardiomyopathy. Circulation 95:2344, 1997.
84. Ferlini A, Sewry C, Melis MA, et al. X-linked dilated cardiomyopathy and the dystrophin gene. Neuromusc Disord 9:339, 1999.
85. Sasaki K, Sakata K, Kachi E, et al. Sequential changes in cardiac structure and function in patients with Duchenne type muscular dystrophy: a two-dimensional echocardiographic study. Am Heart J 135:937, 1998.
86. Shapiro F, Sethna N, Colan S, et al. Spinal fusion in Duchenne muscular dystrophy: A multidisciplinary approach. Muscle Nerve 15:604, 1992.
87. Yotsukura M, Yamamoto A, Kajiwara T, et al. QT dispersion in patients with Duchenne-type progressive muscular dystrophy. Am Heart J 137:672, 1999.

88. Goldberg SJ, Stern LZ, Feldman L, et al. Serial left ventricular wall measurements in Duchenne's muscular dystrophy. J Am Coll Cardiol 2:136, 1983.
89. Brockmeier K, Schmitz L, von Moers A, et al. X-chromosomal (p21) muscular dystrophy and left ventricular diastolic and systolic function. Pediatr Cardiol 19:139, 1998.
90. Matsuoka S, Ii K, Akita H, et al. Clinical features and cardiopulmonary function of patients with atrophic heart in Duchenne muscular dystrophy. Jpn Heart J 28:687, 1987.
91. Chenard AA, Becane HM, Tertrain F, et al. Systolic time intervals in Duchenne muscular dystrophy: evaluation of left ventricular performance. Clin Cardiol 11:407, 1988.
92. Stewart CA, Gilgoff I, Baydur A, et al. Gated radionuclide ventriculography in the evaluation of cardiac function in Duchenne's muscular dystrophy. Chest 94:1245, 1988.
93. Melacini P, Vianello A, Villanova C, et al. Cardiac and respiratory involvement in advanced stage Duchenne muscular dystrophy. Neuromusc Disord 6:367, 1996.
94. Biggar WD, Politano L, Harris VA, et al. Deflazacort in Duchenne muscular dystrophy: a comparison of two different protocols. Neuromuscul Disord 14:476, 2004.
95. Tidball JG, Wehling-Henricks M. Evolving therapeutic strategies for Duchenne muscular dystrophy: targeting downstream events. Pediatr Res 56:831, 2004.
96. Ishikawa Y, Bach JR, Minami R. Cardioprotection for Duchenne's muscular dystrophy. Am Heart J 137:895, 1999.
97. Buzello W, Huttarsch H. Muscle relaxation in patients with Duchenne's muscular dystrophy. Use of vecuronium in two patients. Br J Anaesth 60:228, 1988.
98. Sethna NF, Rockoff MA. Cardiac arrest following inhalation induction of anaesthesia in a child with Duchenne's muscular dystrophy. Can Anaesth Soc J 33:799, 1986.
99. Lang SA, Duncan PG, Dupuis PR. Fatal air embolism in an adolescent with Duchenne muscular dystrophy during Harrington instrumentation. Anesth Analg 69:132, 1989.
100. Politano L, Nigro V, Nigro G, et al. Development of cardiomyopathy in female carriers of Duchenne and Becker muscular dystrophies. J Am Med Assoc 275:1335, 1996.
101. Melacini P, Fanin M, Danieli GA, et al. Myocardial involvement is very frequent among patients affected with subclinical Becker's muscular dystrophy. Circulation 94:3168, 1996.
102. Saito M, Kawai H, Akaike M, et al. Cardiac dysfunction with Becker muscular dystrophy. Am Heart J 132:642, 1996.
103. Towbin JA, Hejtmancik JF, Brink P, et al. X-linked dilated cardiomyopathy: Molecular genetic evidence of linkage to the Duchenne muscular dystrophy (dystrophin) gene at the Xp21 locus. Circulation 87:1854, 1993.
104. Sarvazyan N. Visualization of doxorubicin-induced oxidative stress in isolated cardiac myocytes. Am J Physiol Heart Circ Physiol 271:H2079, 1996.
105. Yen HC, Oberley TD, Gairola CG, et al. Manganese superoxide dismutase protects mitochondrial complex I against adriamycin-induced cardiomyopathy in transgenic mice. Arch Biochem Biophys 362:59, 1999.
106. Papadopoulou LC, Theophilidis G, Thomopoulos GN, et al. Structural and functional impairment of mitochondria in adriamycin-induced cardiomyopathy in mice: Suppression of cytochrome *c* oxidase II gene expression. Biochem Pharmacol 57:481, 1999.
107. Cera C, Palumbo M. Anti-cancer activity of anthracycline antibiotics and DNA condensation. Anticancer Drug Des 5:265, 1990.
108. Lipshultz SE, Rifai N, Dalton VM, et al. The effect of dexrazoxane on myocardial injury in doxorubicin-treated children with acute lymphoblastic leukemia. N Engl J Med 351:145, 2004.
109. Von Hoff DD, Layard M. Risk factors for the development of daunorubicin cardiotoxicity. Cancer Treat Rep 65(suppl 4):19, 1982.
110. Bristow MR, Mason JW, Billingham ME, et al. Dose-effect and structure-function relationships in doxorubicin cardiomyopathy. Am Heart J 102:709, 1981.
111. Von Hoff DD, Layard MW, Basa P, et al. Risk factors for doxorubicin-induced congestive heart failure. Ann Intern Med 91:710, 1979.
112. Lipshultz SE, Colan SD, Gelber RD, et al. Late cardiac effects of Doxorubicin therapy for acute lymphoblastic leukemia in childhood. N Engl J Med 324:808, 1991.
113. Sorensen K, Levitt G, Bull C, et al. Anthracycline dose in childhood acute lymphoblastic leukemia: issues of early survival versus late cardiotoxicity. J Clin Oncol 15:61, 1997.
114. Lipshultz SE, Lipsitz SR, Mone SM, et al. Female sex and drug dose as risk factors for late cardiotoxic effects of doxorubicin therapy for childhood cancer [see comments]. N Engl J Med 332:1738, 1995.
115. Ewer MS, Jaffe N, Ried H, et al. Doxorubicin cardiotoxicity in children: comparison of a consecutive divided daily dose administration schedule with single dose (rapid) infusion administration. Medical & Pediatric Oncology 31:512, 1998.
116. Von Hoff DD, Layard MW, Basa P, et al. Risk factors for doxorubicin-induced congestive heart failure. Ann Intern Med 91:710, 1979.
117. Umsawasdi T, Valdivieso M, Booser DJ, et al. Weekly doxorubicin versus doxorubicin every 3 weeks in cyclophosphamide, doxorubicin, and cisplatin chemotherapy for non-small cell lung cancer. Cancer 64:1995, 1989.
118. Lipshultz SE, Giantris AL, Lipsitz SR, et al. Doxorubicin administration by continuous infusion is not cardioprotective: the Dana-Farber 91-01 Acute Lymphoblastic Leukemia protocol. J Clin Oncol 20:1677, 2002.
119. Levitt GA, Dorup I, Sorensen K, et al. Does anthracycline administration by infusion in children affect late cardiotoxicity? Br J Haematol 124:463, 2004.
120. Wiseman LR, Spencer CM. Dexrazoxane. A review of its use as a cardioprotective agent in patients receiving anthracycline-based chemotherapy. [Review] [75 refs]. Drugs 56:385, 1998.
121. Herman EH, Ferrans VJ, Young RS, et al. Effect of pretreatment with ICRF-187 on the total cumulative dose of doxorubicin tolerated by beagle dogs. Cancer Res 48:6918, 1988.
122. Schiavetti A, Castello MA, Versacci P, et al. Use of ICRF-187 for prevention of anthracycline cardiotoxicity in children: preliminary results. Pediatr Hematol Oncol 14:213, 1997.

123. Cardinale D, Sandri MT, Colombo A, et al. Prognostic value of troponin I in cardiac risk stratification of cancer patients undergoing high-dose chemotherapy. Circulation 109:2749, 2004.
124. Sawyer DB, Fukazawa R, Arstall MA, et al. Daunorubicin-induced apoptosis in rat cardiac myocytes is inhibited by dexrazoxane. Circ Res 84:257, 1999.
125. Delpy E, Hatem SN, Andrieu N, et al. Doxorubicin induces slow ceramide accumulation and late apoptosis in cultured adult rat ventricular myocytes. Cardiovasc Res 43:398, 1999.
126. Steinherz LJ, Graham T, Hurwitz R, et al. Guidelines for cardiac monitoring of children during and after anthracycline therapy: Report of the Cardiology Committee of the Childrens Cancer Study Group. Pediatrics 89:942, 1992.
127. Lipshultz SE, Sanders SP, Goorin AM, et al. Monitoring for anthracycline cardiotoxicity. Pediatrics 93:433, 1994.
128. Makinen L, Makipernaa A, Rautonen J, et al. Long-term cardiac sequelae after treatment of malignant tumors with radiotherapy or cytostatics in childhood. Cancer 65:1913, 1990.
129. Lipshultz SE, Lipsitz SR, Sallan SE, et al. Long-term enalapril therapy for left ventricular dysfunction in doxorubicin-treated survivors of childhood cancer. J Clin Oncol 20:4517, 2002.
130. Dorup I, Levitt G, Sullivan I, et al. Prospective longitudinal assessment of late anthracycline cardiotoxicity after childhood cancer: the role of diastolic function. Heart 90:1214, 2004.
131. Lipshultz SE, Colan SD. Cardiovascular trials in long-term survivors of childhood cancer. J Clin Oncol 22:769, 2004.
132. Connor EM, Sperling R, Gelber R. Reduction of maternal-infant transmission of human immunodeficiency virus type 1 with zidovudine treatment. N Engl J Med 331:1173, 1994.
133. Peckham C, Gibb D. Mother-to-child transmission of the human immunodeficiency virus. N Engl J Med 333:298, 1995.
134. Tovo PA, de Marino M, Gabiano C. Prognostic factors and survival in children with perinatal HIV-1 infection. Lancet 339:1249, 1992.
135. Silva-Cardoso J, Moura B, Martins L, et al. Pericardial involvement in human immunodeficiency virus infection. Chest 115:418, 1999.
136. Lipshultz SE. Dilated cardiomyopathy in HIV-infected patients [editorial; comment] [see comments]. N Engl J Med 339:1153, 1998.
137. Lipshultz SE, Easley KA, Orav EJ, et al. Left ventricular structure and function in children infected with human immunodeficiency virus: the prospective P^2C^2 HIV multicenter study. Circulation 97:1246, 1998.
138. Starc TJ, Lipshultz SE, Kaplan S, et al. Cardiac complications in children with human immunodeficiency virus infection. Pediatrics 104:E141, 1999.
139. Lipshultz SE, Chanock S, Sanders SP, et al. Cardiovascular manifestations of human immunodeficiency virus infection in infants and children. Am J Cardiol 63:1489, 1989.
140. Currie PF, Goldman JH, Caforio AL, et al. Cardiac autoimmunity in HIV related heart muscle disease. Heart 79: 599, 1998.
141. Herskowitz A, Wu T-C, Willoughby SB, et al. Myocarditis and cardiotropic viral infection associated with severe left ventricular dysfunction in late-stage infection with human immunodeficiency virus. J Am Coll Cardiol 24:1025, 1994.
142. Lipshultz SE, Fox CH, Perez-Atayde AR, et al. Identification of human immunodeficiency virus-1 RNA and DNA in the heart of a child with cardiovascular abnormalities and congenital acquired immune deficiency syndrome. Am J Cardiol 66:246, 1990.
143. Rodriguez ER, Nasim S, Hsia J, et al. Cardiac myocytes and dendritic cells harbor human immunodeficiency virus in infected patients with and without cardiac dysfunction: Detection by multiplex, nested, polymerase chain reaction in individually microdissected cells from right ventricular endomyocardial biopsy tissue. Am J Cardiol 68:1511, 1991.
144. Luginbuhl LM, Orav EJ, McIntosh K, et al. Cardiac morbidity and related mortality in children with HIV infection. J Am Med Assoc 269:2869, 1993.
145. Lipshultz SE, Orav EJ, Sanders SP, et al. Cardiac structure and function in children with human immunodeficiency virus infection treated with zidovudine. N Engl J Med 327: 1260, 1992.
146. Mast HL, Haller JO, Schiller MS, et al. Pericardial effusion and its relationship to cardiac disease in children with acquired immunodeficiency syndrome. Pediatr Radiol 22:548, 1992.
147. Domanski MJ, Sloas MM, Follmann DA, et al. Effect of zidovudine and didanosine treatment on heart function in children infected with human immunodeficiency virus. J Pediatr 127:137, 1995.
148. Levi G, Patrizio M, Bernardo A, et al. Human immunodeficiency virus coat protein gp120 inhibits the beta-adrenergic regulation of astroglial and microglial functions. Proc Natl Acad Sci USA 90:1541, 1993.
149. Berul CI, Maguire CT, Aronovitz MJ, et al. DMPK dosage alterations result in atrioventricular conduction abnormalities in a mouse myotonic dystrophy model. J Clin Invest 103:R1, 1999.
150. Rudnik-Schoneborn S, Nicholson GA, Morgan G, et al. Different patterns of obstetric complications in myotonic dystrophy in relation to the disease status of the fetus. Am J Med Genet 80:314, 1998.
151. Geifman-Holtzman O, Fay K. Prenatal diagnosis of congenital myotonic dystrophy and counseling of the pregnant mother: case report and literature review. [Review] [27 refs]. Am J Med Genet 78:250, 1998.
152. Reardon W, Newcombe R, Fenton I, et al. The natural history of congenital myotonic dystrophy and long term clinical aspects. Arch Dis Child 68:177, 1993.
153. Forsberg H, Olofsson B-O, Eriksson A, et al. Cardiac involvement in congenital myotonic dystrophy. Br Heart J 63:119, 1990.
154. Bu'Lock FA, Sood M, De Giovanni JV, et al. Left ventricular diastolic function in congenital myotonic dystrophy. Archives of Disease in Childhood 80:267, 1999.
155. Hayashi Y, Ikeda U, Kojo T, et al. Cardiac abnormalities and cytosine-thymine-guanine trinucleotide repeats in myotonic dystrophy. Am Heart J 134:292, 1997.

156. Fragola PV, Calo L, Luzi M, et al. Doppler echocardiographic assessment of left ventricular diastolic function in myotonic dystrophy. Cardiology 88:498, 1997.
157. Child JS, Perloff JK. Myocardial myotonia in myotonic muscular dystrophy. Am Heart J 129:982, 1995.
158. Lazarus A, Varin J, Ounnoughene Z, et al. Relationships among electrophysiological findings and clinical status, heart function, and extent of DNA mutation in myotonic dystrophy. Circulation 99:1041, 1999.
159. Colleran JA, Hawley RJ, Pinnow EE, et al. Value of the electrocardiogram in determining cardiac events and mortality in myotonic dystrophy. Am J Cardiol 80:1494, 1997.
160. Die-Smulders CE, Howeler CJ, Thijs C, et al. Age and causes of death in adult-onset myotonic dystrophy. Brain 121:1557, 1998.
161. Mathieu J, Allard P, Potvin L, et al. A 10-year study of mortality in a cohort of patients with myotonic dystrophy. Neurology 52:1658, 1999.
162. Porter J, Cary N, Schofield P. Haemochromatosis presenting as congestive cardiac failure. Br Heart J 73:73, 1995.
163. Marcus RE, Huehns ER. Transfusional iron overload. [Review] [100 refs]. Clinical & Laboratory Haematology 7:195, 1985.
164. Economou-Petersen E, Aessopos A, Kladi A, et al. Apolipoprotein E epsilon4 allele as a genetic risk factor for left ventricular failure in homozygous beta-thalassemia. Blood 92:3455, 1998.
165. Kremastinos DT, Toutouzas PK, Vyssoulis GP, et al. Global and segmental left ventricular function in beta-thalassemia. Cardiology 72:129, 1985.
166. Kremastinos DT, Tiniakos G, Theodorakis GN, et al. Myocarditis in b-thalassemia major: A cause of heart failure. Circulation 91:66, 1995.
167. Rivers J, Garrahy P, Robinson W, et al. Reversible cardiac dysfunction in hemochromatosis. Am Heart J 113:216, 1987.
168. Mariotti E, Angelucci E, Agostini A, et al. Evaluation of cardiac status in iron-loaded thalassaemia patients following bone marrow transplantation: improvement in cardiac function during reduction in body iron burden. British Journal of Haematology 103:916, 1998.
169. Freeman AP, Giles RW, Berdoukas VA, et al. Sustained normalization of cardiac function by chelation therapy in thalassaemia major. Clinical & Laboratory Haematology 11:299, 1989.
170. Denenberg BS, Criner G, Jones R, et al. Cardiac function in sickle cell anemia. Am J Cardiol 51:1674, 1983.
171. Colan SD, Borow KM, Neumann A. Left ventricular end-systolic wall stress-velocity of fiber shortening relation: a load-independent index of myocardial contractility. J Am Coll Cardiol 4:715, 1984.
172. Yaprak I, Aksit S, Ozturk C, et al. Left ventricular diastolic abnormalities in children with beta- thalassemia major: a Doppler echocardiographic study. Turkish Journal of Pediatrics 40:201, 1998.
173. Brili SV, Tzonou AI, Castelanos SS, et al. The effect of iron overload in the hearts of patients with beta-thalassemia. Clin Cardiol 20:541, 1997.
174. Olson LJ, Edwards WD, Holmes DR, Jr., et al. Endomyocardial biopsy in hemochromatosis: Clinicopathologic correlates in six cases. J Am Coll Cardiol 13:116, 1989.
175. Kremastinos DT, Tsiapras DP, Tsetsos GA, et al. Left ventricular diastolic Doppler characteristics in b-thalassemia major. Circulation 88:1127, 1993.
176. Hou JW, Wu MH, Lin KH, et al. Prognostic significance of left ventricular diastolic indexes in beta-thalassemia major. Archives of Pediatrics & Adolescent Medicine 148:862, 1994.
177. Lombardo T, Morrone ML, Privitera A, et al. Cardiac iron overload in thalassemic patients: An endomyocardial biopsy study. Ann Hematol 71:135, 1995.
178. Olivieri NF, Liu PP, Sher GD, et al. Brief report: combined liver and heart transplantation for end- stage iron-induced organ failure in an adult with homozygous beta-thalassemia. N Engl J Med 330:1125, 1994.
179. Wood JC, Tyszka JM, Carson S, et al. Myocardial iron loading in transfusion-dependent thalassemia and sickle cell disease. Blood 103:1934, 2004.
180. Politi A, Sticca M, Galli M. Reversal of haemochromatotic cardiomyopathy in b thalassaemia by chelation therapy. Br Heart J 73:486, 1995.
181. Richardson ME, Matthews RN, Alison JF, et al. Prevention of heart disease by subcutaneous desferrioxamine in patients with thalassaemia major. Aust N Z J Med 23: 656, 1993.
182. Lerner N, Blei F, Bierman F, et al. Chelation therapy and cardiac status in older patients with thalassemia major. American Journal of Pediatric Hematology-Oncology 12: 56, 1990.
183. Desideri A, Scattolin G, Gabellini A, et al. Left ventricular function in thalassemia major: protective effect of deferoxamine. Can J Cardiol 10:93, 1994.
184. Aldouri MA, Wonke B, Hoffbrand AV, et al. High incidence of cardiomyopathy in beta-thalassaemia patients receiving regular transfusion and iron chelation: reversal by intensified chelation. Acta Haematologica 84:113, 1990.
185. Michaeli J, Mittelman M, Grisaru D, et al. Thromboembolic complications in beta thalassemia major. Acta Haematologica 87:71, 1992.
186. Koren A, Garty I, Antonelli D, et al. Right ventricular cardiac dysfunction in beta-thalassemia major. Am J Dis Child 141:93, 1987.
187. Jootar P, Fucharoen S. Cardiac involvement in beta-thalassemia/hemoglobin E disease: clinical and hemodynamic findings. Southeast Asian Journal of Tropical Medicine & Public Health 21:269, 1990.
188. Dutka DP, Donnelly JE, Nihoyannopoulos P, et al. Marked variation in the cardiomyopathy associated with Friedreich's ataxia. Heart 81:141, 1999.
189. Regalado JJ, Rodriguez MM, Ferrer PL. Infantile hypertrophic cardiomyopathy of glycogenosis Type IX: isolated cardiac phosphorylase kinase deficiency. Pediatr Cardiol 20:304, 1999.
190. Geier C, Perrot A, Özcelik C, et al. Mutations in the human muscle LIM protein gene in families with hypertrophic cardiomyopathy. Circulation 107:1390, 2003.

191. Taylor RW, Giordano C, Davidson MM, et al. A homoplasmic mitochondrial transfer ribonucleic acid mutation as a cause of maternally inherited hypertrophic cardiomyopathy. J Am Coll Cardiol 41:1786, 2003.
192. Arad M, Benson DW, Perez-Atayde AR, et al. Constitutively active AMP kinase mutations cause glycogen storage disease mimicking hypertrophic cardiomyopathy. J Clin Invest 109:357, 2002.
193. Bonne G, Carrier L, Richard P, et al. Familial hypertrophic cardiomyopathy from mutations to functional defects. Circ Res 83:580, 1998.
194. Marian AJ, Zhao G, Seta Y, et al. Expression of a mutant (Arg92Gln) human cardiac troponin T, known to cause hypertrophic cardiomyopathy, impairs adult cardiac myocyte contractility. Circ Res 81:76, 1997.
195. Nakaura H, Morimoto S, Yanaga F, et al. Functional changes in troponin T by a splice donor site mutation that causes hypertrophic cardiomyopathy. Am J Physiol Cell Physiol 277:C225, 1999.
196. Marian AJ, Roberts R. The molecular genetic basis for hypertrophic cardiomyopathy. J Mol Cell Cardiol 33: 655, 2001.
197. Lombardi R, Betocchi S. Aetiology and pathogenesis of hypertrophic cardiomyopathy. Acta Paediatr 91:10, 2002.
198. Hengstenberg C, Erdmann J, Charron P. Outcome of clinical versus genetic family screening in hypertrophic cardiomyopathy with focus on cardiac beta-myosin gene mutations: Prediction of clinical status: is molecular genetics a new tool for the management of hypertrophic cardiomyopathy in clinical practice? Cardiovasc Res 57:298, 2003.
199. Mogensen J, Murphy RT, Shaw T, et al. Severe disease expression of cardiac troponin C and T mutations in patients with idiopathic dilated cardiomyopathy. J Am Coll Cardiol 44:2033, 2004.
200. Moolman JC, Corfield VA, Posen B, et al. Sudden death due to troponin T mutations. J Am Coll Cardiol 29:549, 1997.
201. Anan R, Shono H, Kisanuki A, et al. Patients with familial hypertrophic cardiomyopathy caused by a Phe110Ile missense mutation in the cardiac troponin T gene have variable cardiac morphologies and a favorable prognosis. Circulation 98:391, 1998.
202. Arbustini E, Fasani R, Morbini P, et al. Coexistence of mitochondrial DNA and b myosin heavy chain mutations in hypertrophic cardiomyopathy with late congestive heart failure. Heart 80:548, 1998.
203. Van Driest SL, Vasile VC, Ommen SR, et al. Myosin binding protein C mutations and compound heterozygosity in hypertrophic cardiomyopathy. J Am Coll Cardiol 44:1903, 2004.
204. Ortlepp JR, Vosberg HP, Reith S, et al. Genetic polymorphisms in the renin-angiotensin-aldosterone system associated with expression of left ventricular hypertrophy in hypertrophic cardiomyopathy: a study of five polymorphic genes in a family with a disease causing mutation in the myosin binding protein C gene. Heart 87:270, 2002.
205. Burn J, Camm J, Davies MJ, et al. The phenotype/genotype relation and the current status of genetic screening in hypertrophic cardiomyopathy, Marfan syndrome, and the long QT syndrome. Heart 78:110, 1997.
206. Tikanoja T, Jääskeläinen P, Laakso M, et al. Simultanous hypertrophic cardiomyopathy and ventricular septal defect in children. Am J Cardiol 84:485, 1999.
207. Maron BJ, Roberts WC. Hypertrophic cardiomyopathy and cardiac muscle cell disorganization revisited: relation between the two and significance. Am Heart J 102:95, 1981.
208. Maron BJ, Wolfson JK, Epstein SE, et al. Intramural ("small vessel") coronary artery disease in hypertrophic cardiomyopathy. J Am Coll Cardiol 8:545, 1986.
209. Tanaka M, Fujiwara H, Onodera T, et al. Quantitative analysis of narrowings of intramyocardial small arteries in normal hearts, hypertensive hearts, and hearts with hypertrophic cardiomyopathy. Circulation 75:1130, 1987.
210. Thierfelder L, Watkins H, MacRae C, et al. a-tropomyosin and cardiac troponin T mutations cause familial hypertrophic cardiomyopathy: A disease of the sarcomere. Cell 77:701, 1994.
211. Redwood CS, Moolman-Smook JC, Watkins H. Properties of mutant contractile proteins that cause hypertrophic cardiomyopathy. Cardiovasc Res 44:20, 1999.
212. Crilley JG, Boehm EA, Blair E, et al. Hypertrophic cardiomyopathy due to sarcomeric gene mutations is characterized by impaired energy metabolism irrespective of the degree of hypertrophy. J Am Coll Cardiol 41:1776, 2003.
213. Kizilbash AM, Heinle SK, Grayburn PA. Spontaneous variability of left ventricular outflow tract gradient in hypertrophic obstructive cardiomyopathy. Circulation 97:461, 1998.
214. Criley JM. Unobstructed thinking (and terminology) is called for in the understanding and management of hypertrophic cardiomyopathy. J Am Coll Cardiol 29:741, 1997.
215. Marwick TH, Nakatani S, Haluska B, et al. Provocation of latent left ventricular outflow tract gradients with amyl nitrite and exercise in hypertrophic cardiomyopathy. Am J Cardiol 75:805, 1995.
216. Dritsas A, Gilligan D, Sbarouni E, et al. Influence of left ventricular hypertrophy and function on the occurrence of ventricular tachycardia in hypertrophic cardiomyopathy. Am J Cardiol 70:913, 1992.
217. Pak PH, Maughan WL, Baughman KL, et al. Marked discordance between dynamic and passive diastolic pressure-volume relations in idiopathic hypertrophic cardiomyopathy. Circulation 94:52, 1996.
218. Betocchi S, Hess OM, Losi MA, et al. Regional left ventricular mechanics in hypertrophic cardiomyopathy. Circulation 88:2206, 1993.
219. Jones S, Elliott PM, Sharma S, et al. Cardiopulmonary responses to exercise in patients with hypertrophic cardiomyopathy. Heart 80:60, 1998.
220. Nihoyannopoulos P, Karatasakis G, Frenneaux M, et al. Diastolic function in hypertrophic cardiomyopathy: Relation to exercise capacity. J Am Coll Cardiol 19:536, 1992.
221. Chikamori T, Counihan PJ, Doi YL, et al. Mechanisms of exercise limitation in hypertrophic cardiomyopathy. J Am Coll Cardiol 19:507, 1992.
222. Lele SS, Thomson HL, Seo H, et al. Exercise capacity in hypertrophic cardiomyopathy - Role of stroke volume

limitation, heart rate, and diastolic filling characteristics. Circulation 92:2886, 1995.

223. Briguori C, Betocchi S, Romano M, et al. Exercise capacity in hypertrophic cardiomyopathy depends on left ventricular diastolic function. Am J Cardiol 84:309, 1999.
224. Schwartzkopff B, Mundhenke M, Strauer BE. Alterations of the architecture of subendocardial arterioles in patients with hypertrophic cardiomyopathy and impaired coronary vasodilator reserve: a possible cause for myocardial ischemia. J Am Coll Cardiol 31:1089, 1998.
225. Cannon RO3d, Schenke WH, Maron BJ, et al. Differences in coronary flow and myocardial metabolism at rest and during pacing between patients with obstructive and patients with nonobstructive hypertrophic cardiomyopathy. J Am Coll Cardiol 10:53, 1987.
226. Ogata Y, Hiyamuta K, Terasawa M, et al. Relationship of exercise or pacing induced ST segment depression and myocardial lactate metabolism in patients with hypertrophic cardiomyopathy. Jpn Heart J 27:145, 1986.
227. Cuccurullo F, Mezzetti A, Lapenna D, et al. Mechanism of isoproterenol-induced angina pectoris in patients with obstructive hypertrophic cardiomyopathy and normal coronary arteries. Am J Cardiol 60:667, 1987.
228. Jung WI, Sieverding L, Breuer J, et al. ^{31}P NMR spectroscopy detects metabolic abnormalities in asymptomatic patients with hypertrophic cardiomyopathy. Circulation 97:2536, 1998.
229. Cannon RO, III, Dilsizian V, O'Gara PT, et al. Myocardial metabolic, hemodynamic, and electrocardiographic significance of reversible thallium-201 abnormalities in hypertrophic cardiomyopathy. Circulation 83:1660, 1991.
230. Dilsizian V, Bonow RO, Epstein SE, et al. Myocardial ischemia detected by thallium scintigraphy is frequently related to cardiac arrest and syncope in young patients with hypertrophic cardiomyopathy. J Am Coll Cardiol 22:796, 1993.
231. Yamaguchi M, Tangkawattana P, Hamlin RL. Myocardial bridging as a factor in heart disorders: Critical review and hypothesis. Acta Anat (Basel) 157:248, 1996.
232. Kitazume H, Kramer JR, Krauthamer D, et al. Myocardial bridges in obstructive hypertrophic cardiomyopathy. Am Heart J 106:131, 1983.
233. Yetman AT, McCrindle BW, MacDonald C, et al. Myocardial bridging in children with hypertrophic cardiomyopathy - a risk factor for sudden death. N Engl J Med 339:1201, 1998.
234. Miller GL. Functional assessment of coronary stenoses. J Am Coll Cardiol 32:1134, 1998.
235. Hillman ND, Mavroudis C, Backer CL, et al. Supraarterial decompression myotomy for myocardial bridging in a child. Ann Thorac Surg 68:244, 1999.
236. Robinson K, Frenneaux MP, Stockins B, et al. Atrial fibrillation in hypertrophic cardiomyopathy: A longitudinal study. J Am Coll Cardiol 15:1279, 1990.
237. Nienaber CA, Hiller S, Spielmann RP, et al. Syncope in hypertrophic cardiomyopathy: Multivariate analysis of prognostic determinants. J Am Coll Cardiol 15:948, 1990.
238. Spirito P, Rapezzi C, Autore C, et al. Prognosis of asymptomatic patients with hypertrophic cardiomyopathy and nonsustained ventricular tachycardia. Circulation 90:2743, 1994.
239. Fananapazir L, Chang AC, Epstein SE, et al. Prognostic determinants in hypertrophic cardiomyopathy: Prospective evaluation of a therapeutic strategy based on clinical, Holter, hemodynamic, and electrophysiological findings. Circulation 86:730, 1992.
240. McKenna WJ, Franklin RCG, Nihoyannopoulos P, et al. Arrhythmia and prognosis in infants, children and adolescents with hypertrophic cardiomyopathy. J Am Coll Cardiol 11:147, 1988.
241. Miorelli M, Buja G, Melacini P, et al. QT-interval variability in hypertrophic cardiomyopathy patients with cardiac arrest. Int J Cardiol 45:121, 1994.
242. Dritsas A, Sbarouni E, Gilligan D, et al. QT-interval abnormalities in hypertrophic cardiomyopathy. Clin Cardiol 15: 739, 1992.
243. Yi G, Elliott P, McKenna WJ, et al. QT dispersion and risk factors for sudden cardiac death in patients with hypertrophic cardiomyopathy. Am J Cardiol 82:1514, 1998.
244. Calderon-Colmenero J, Baltazares M, Buendia A. Complete heart block as a cause of syncope in hypertrophic cardiomyopathy. Cardiol Young 4:79, 1994.
245. McKenna WJ, Goodwin JF. The natural history of hypertrophic cardiomyopathy. Curr Probl Cardiol 6:1, 1981.
246. Maron BJ, Bonow RO, Cannon RO3d, et al. Hypertrophic cardiomyopathy. Interrelations of clinical manifestations, pathophysiology, and therapy (2). N Engl J Med 316:844, 1987.
247. McKenna WJ. The natural history of hypertrophic cardiomyopathy. Cardiovasc Clin 19:135, 1988.
248. Kramer DS, French WJ, Criley JM. The postextrasystolic murmur response to gradient in hypertrophic cardiomyopathy. Ann Intern Med 104:772, 1986.
249. Klues HG, Schiffers A, Maron BJ. Phenotypic spectrum and patterns of left ventricular hypertrophy in hypertrophic cardiomyopathy: Morphologic observations and significance as assessed by two-dimensional echocardiography in 600 patients. J Am Coll Cardiol 26:1699, 1995.
250. Lewis JF, Maron BJ. Hypertrophic cardiomyopathy characterized by marked hypertrophy of the posterior left ventricular free wall: significance and clinical implications. J Am Coll Cardiol 18:421, 1991.
251. Maron BJ, McIntosh CL, Klues HG, et al. Morphologic basis for obstruction to right ventricular outflow in hypertrophic cardiomyopathy. Am J Cardiol 71:1089, 1993.
252. Schwammenthal E, Block M, Schwartzkopff B, et al. Prediction of the site and severity of obstruction in hypertrophic cardiomyopathy by color flow mapping and continuous wave Doppler echocardiography. J Am Coll Cardiol 20:964, 1992.
253. Gidding SS, Snider AR, Rocchini AP, et al. Left ventricular diastolic filling in children with hypertrophic cardiomyopathy: assessment with pulsed Doppler echocardiography. J Am Coll Cardiol 8:310, 1986.
254. Iwase M, Sotobata I, Takagi S, et al. Effects of diltiazem on left ventricular diastolic behavior in patients with hypertrophic

cardiomyopathy: evaluation with exercise pulsed Doppler echocardiography. J Am Coll Cardiol 9:1099, 1987.
255. Maron BJ, Spirito P, Green KJ, et al. Noninvasive assessment of left ventricular diastolic function by pulsed Doppler echocardiography in patients with hypertrophic cardiomyopathy. J Am Coll Cardiol 10:733, 1987.
256. Choong CY, Herrmann HC, Weyman AE, et al. Preload dependence of Doppler-derived indexes of left ventricular diastolic function in humans. J Am Coll Cardiol 10:800, 1987.
257. Frenneaux MP, Counihan PJ, Caforio ALP, et al. Abnormal blood pressure response during exercise in hypertrophic cardiomyopathy. Circulation 82:1995, 1990.
258. Maki S, Ikeda H, Muro A, et al. Predictors of sudden cardiac death in hypertrophic cardiomyopathy. Am J Cardiol 82:774, 1998.
259. Sadoul N, Prasad K, Elliott PM, et al. Prospective prognostic assessment of blood pressure response during exercise in patients with hypertrophic cardiomyopathy. Circulation 96:2987, 1997.
260. Olivotto I, Maron BJ, Montereggi A, et al. Prognostic value of systemic blood pressure response during exercise in a community-based patient population with hypertrophic cardiomyopathy. J Am Coll Cardiol 33:2044, 1999.
261. Posma JL, Blanksma PK, Van der Wall EE, et al. Assessment of quantitative hypertrophy scores in hypertrophic cardiomyopathy: Magnetic resonance imaging versus echocardiography. Am Heart J 132:1020, 1996.
262. Allison JD, Flickinger FW, Wright JC, et al. Measurement of left ventricular mass in hypertrophic cardiomyopathy using MRI: Comparison with echocardiography. Magn Reson Imaging 11:329, 1993.
263. Soler R, Rodríguez E, Marini M. Left ventricular mass in hypertrophic cardiomyopathy: Assessment by three-dimensional and geometric MR methods. J Comput Assist Tomogr 23:577, 1999.
264. Kramer CM, Reichek N, Ferrari VA, et al. Regional heterogeneity of function in hypertrophic cardiomyopathy. Circulation 90:186, 1994.
265. Moon JC, Reed E, Sheppard MN, et al. The histologic basis of late gadolinium enhancement cardiovascular magnetic resonance in hypertrophic cardiomyopathy. J Am Coll Cardiol 43:2260, 2004.
266. McKenna WJ, Stewart JT, Nihoyannopoulos P, et al. Hypertrophic cardiomyopathy without hypertrophy: Two families with myocardial disarray in the absence of increased myocardial mass. Br Heart J 63:287, 1990.
267. Maron BJ, Kragel AH, Roberts WC. Sudden death in hypertrophic cardiomyopathy with normal left ventricular mass. Br Heart J 63:308, 1990.
268. Charron P, Dubourg O, Desnos M, et al. Diagnostic value of electrocardiography and echocardiography for familial hypertrophic cardiomyopathy in a genotyped adult population. Circulation 96:214, 1997.
269. Charron P, Dubourg O, Desnos M, et al. Diagnostic value of electrocardiography and echocardiography for familial hypertrophic cardiomyopathy in genotyped children. Eur Heart J 19:1377, 1998.
270. Nagueh SF, Kopelen HA, Lim DS, et al. Tissue Doppler imaging consistently detects myocardial contraction and relaxation abnormalities, irrespective of cardiac hypertrophy, in a transgenic rabbit model of human hypertrophic cardiomyopathy. Circulation 102:1346, 2000.
271. Nagueh SF, Bachinski LL, Meyer D, et al. Tissue Doppler imaging consistently detects myocardial abnormalities in patients with hypertrophic cardiomyopathy and provides a novel means for an early diagnosis before and independently of hypertrophy. Circulation 104:128, 2001.
272. Nagueh SF, McFalls J, Meyer D, et al. Tissue Doppler imaging predicts the development of hypertrophic cardiomyopathy in subjects with subclinical disease. Circulation 108: 395, 2003.
273. Lattanzi F, Spirito P, Picano E, et al. Quantitative assessment of ultrasonic myocardial reflectivity in hypertrophic cardiomyopathy. J Am Coll Cardiol 17:1085, 1991.
274. Naito J, Masuyama T, Tanouchi J, et al. Analysis of transmural trend of myocardial integrated ultrasound backscatter for differentiation of hypertrophic cardiomyopathy and ventricular hypertrophy due to hypertension. J Am Coll Cardiol 24:517, 1994.
275. Vitale DF, Bonow RO, Calabrò R, et al. Myocardial ultrasonic tissue characterization in pediatric and adult patients with hypertrophic cardiomyopathy. Circulation 94:2826, 1996.
276. Noonan J, O'Connor W. Noonan syndrome: a clinical description emphasizing the cardiac findings. Acta Paediatrica Japonica 38:76, 1996.
277. Moran AM, Colan SD. Verapamil therapy in infants with hypertrophic cardiomyopathy. Cardiol Young 8:310, 1998.
278. Goldstein JD, Shanske S, Bruno C, et al. Maternally inherited mitochondrial cardiomyopathy associated with a C-to-T transition at nucleotide 3303 of mitochondrial DNA in the tRNA(Leu(UUR)) gene. [Review] [14 refs]. Pediatr Dev Pathol 2:78, 1999.
279. Leatherbury L, Chandra RS, Shapiro SR, et al. Value of endomyocardial biopsy in infants, children and adolescents with dilated or hypertrophic cardiomyopathy and myocarditis. J Am Coll Cardiol 12:1547, 1988.
280. Colan SD. Mechanics of left ventricular systolic and diastolic function in physiologic hypertrophy of the athlete heart. Cardiol Clin 15:355, 1997.
281. Karjalainen J, Mäntysaari M, Viitasalo M, et al. Left ventricular mass, geometry, and filling in endurance athletes: Association with exercise blood pressure. J Appl Physiol 82:531, 1997.
282. Spirito P, Pelliccia A, Proschan MA, et al. Morphology of the "athlete's heart" assessed by echocardiography in 947 elite athletes representing 27 sports. Am J Cardiol 74:802, 1994.
283. Colan SD, Sanders SP, Borow KM. Physiologic hypertrophy: effects on left ventricular systolic mechanics in athletes. J Am Coll Cardiol 9:776, 1987.
284. Douglas PS, O'Toole ML, Katz SE, et al. Left ventricular hypertrophy in athletes. Am J Cardiol 80:1384, 1997.
285. Bjornstad H, Storstein L, Meen HD, et al. Electrocardiographic findings of repolarization in athletic students and control subjects. Cardiology 84:51, 1994.

286. Björnstad H, Smith G, Storstein L, et al. Electrocardiographic and echocardiographic findings in top athletes, athletic students and sedentary controls. Cardiology 82:66, 1993.
287. Dickhuth H-H, Röcker K, Hipp A, et al. Echocardiographic findings in endurance athletes with hypertrophic non-obstructive cardiomyopathy (HNCM) compared to non-athletes with HNCM and to physiological hypertrophy (athlete's heart). Int J Sports Med 15:273, 1994.
288. Radvan J, Choudhury L, Sheridan DJ, et al. Comparison of coronary vasodilator reserve in elite rowing athletes versus hypertrophic cardiomyopathy. Am J Cardiol 80:1621, 1997.
289. Manolas J, Kyriakidis M, Anastasakis A, et al. Usefulness of noninvasive detection of left ventricular diastolic abnormalities during isometric stress in hypertrophic cardiomyopathy and in athletes. Am J Cardiol 81:306, 1998.
290. Maron BJ, Pelliccia A, Spirito P. Cardiac disease in young trained athletes: Insights into methods for distinguishing athlete's heart from structural heart disease, with particular emphasis on hypertrophic cardiomyopathy. Circulation 91:1596, 1995.
291. Ostman-Smith I, Wettrell G, Riesenfeld T. A cohort study of childhood hypertrophic cardiomyopathy: improved survival following high-dose beta-adrenoceptor antagonist treatment. J Am Coll Cardiol 34:1813, 1999.
292. Colan SD, Lowe AM, Lipshultz SE, et al. Etiology specific outcome in pediatric hypertrophic cardiomyopathy. Circulation 110:III-516, 2004.
293. Hess OM, Murakami T, Krayenbuehl HP. Does verapamil improve left ventricular relaxation in patients with myocardial hypertrophy. Circulation 74:530, 1986.
294. Posma JL, Blanksma PK, Van der Wall E, et al. Acute intravenous versus chronic oral drug effects of verapamil on left ventricular diastolic function in patients with hypertrophic cardiomyopathy. J Cardiovasc Pharmacol 24:969, 1994.
295. Hartmann A, Schnell J, Hopf R, et al. Persisting effect of Ca(2+)-channel blockers on left ventricular function in hypertrophic cardiomyopathy after 14 years' treatment. Angiology 47:765, 1996.
296. Shaffer EM, Rocchini AP, Spicer RL, et al. Effects of verapamil on left ventricular diastolic filling in children with hypertrophic cardiomyopathy. Am J Cardiol 61:413, 1988.
297. Spicer RL, Rocchini AP, Crowley DC, et al. Hemodynamic effects of verapamil in children and adolescents with hypertrophic cardiomyopathy. Circulation 67:413, 1983.
298. Gistri R, Cecchi F, Choudhury L, et al. Effect of verapamil on absolute myocardial blood flow in hypertrophic cardiomyopathy. Am J Cardiol 74:363, 1994.
299. Spicer RL, Rocchini AP, Crowley DC, et al. Chronic verapamil therapy in pediatric and young adult patients with hypertrophic cardiomyopathy. Am J Cardiol 53:1614, 1984.
300. Dickinson DF, Wilson N, Curry P. Use of nifedipine in hypertrophic cardiomyopathy in infants. A report of two cases. Int J Cardiol 7:159, 1985.
301. Seiler C, Hess OM, Schoenbeck M, et al. Long-term follow-up of medical versus surgical therapy for hypertrophic cardiomyopathy: a retrospective study. J Am Coll Cardiol 17:634, 1991.
302. Pelliccia F, Cianfrocca C, Romeo F, et al. Hypertrophic cardiomyopathy: Long-term effects of propranolol versus verapamil in preventing sudden death in "low-risk" patients. Cardiovasc Drugs Ther 4:1515, 1990.
303. Semsarian C, Ahmad I, Giewat M, et al. The L-type calcium channel inhibitor diltiazem prevents cardiomyopathy in a mouse model. J Clin Invest 109:1013, 2002.
304. Kyriakidis M, Triposkiadis F, Dernellis J, et al. Effects of cardiac versus circulatory angiotensin-converting enzyme inhibition on left ventricular diastolic function and coronary blood flow in hypertrophic obstructive cardiomyopathy. Circulation 97:1342, 1998.
305. Tsybouleva N, Zhang LF, Chen SN, et al. Aldosterone, through novel signaling proteins, is a fundamental molecular bridge between the genetic defect and the cardiac phenotype of hypertrophic cardiomyopathy. Circulation 109:1284, 2004.
306. Spirito P, Rapezzi C, Bellone P, et al. Infective endocarditis in hypertrophic cardiomyopathy - Prevalence, incidence, and indications for antibiotic prophylaxis. Circulation 99:2132, 1999.
307. O'Rourke RA. Cardiac pacing. An alternative treatment for selected patients with hypertrophic cardiomyopathy and adjunctive therapy for certain patients with dilated cardiomyopathy. Circulation 100:786, 1999.
308. Pak PH, Maughan WL, Baughman KL, et al. Mechanism of acute mechanical benefit from VDD pacing in hypertrophied heart - Similarity of responses in hypertrophic cardiomyopathy and hypertensive heart disease. Circulation 98:242, 1998.
309. Prinzen FW, Van Oosterhout MFM, Vanagt WYR, et al. Optimization of ventricular function by improving the activation sequence during ventricular pacing. Pacing Clin Electrophysiol 21:2256, 1998.
310. Sherrid MV, Pearle G, Gunsburg DZ. Mechanism of benefit of negative inotropes in obstructive hypertrophic cardiomyopathy. Circulation 97:41, 1998.
311. Alday LE, Bruno E, Moreyra E, et al. Mid-term results of dual-chamber pacing in children with hypertrophic obstructive cardiomyopathy. Echocardiogr J Cardiovasc Ultrasound Allied Tech 15:289, 1998.
312. Rishi F, Hulse JE, Auld DO, et al. Effects of dual-chamber pacing for pediatric patients with hypertrophic obstructive cardiomyopathy. J Am Coll Cardiol 29:734, 1997.
313. Dimitrow PP, Podolec P, Grodecki J, et al. Comparison of dual-chamber pacing with nonsurgical septal reduction effect in patients with hypertrophic obstructive cardiomyopathy. Int J Cardiol 94:31, 2004.
314. Fananapazir L, Cannon RO, III, Tripodi D, et al. Impact of dual-chamber permanent pacing in patients with obstructive hypertrophic cardiomyopathy with symptoms refractory to verapamil and b-adrenergic blocker therapy. Circulation 85:2149, 1992.
315. Fananapazir L, Epstein ND, Curiel RV, et al. Long-term results of dual-chamber (DDD) pacing in obstructive hypertrophic cardiomyopathy: Evidence for progressive symptomatic and hemodynamic improvement and reduction of left ventricular hypertrophy. Circulation 90:2731, 1994.

316. Nishimura RA, Trusty JM, Hayes DL, et al. Dual-chamber pacing for hypertrophic cardiomyopathy: A randomized, double-blind, crossover trial. J Am Coll Cardiol 29:435, 1997.
317. Linde C, Gadler F, Kappenberger L, et al. Placebo effect of pacemaker implantation in obstructive hypertrophic cardiomyopathy. Am J Cardiol 83:903, 1999.
318. Gadler F, Linde C, Rydén L. Rapid return of left ventricular outflow tract obstruction and symptoms following cessation of long-term atrioventricular synchronous pacing for obstructive hypertrophic cardiomyopathy. Am J Cardiol 83:553, 1999.
319. Cannon RO3d, Tripodi D, Dilsizian V, et al. Results of permanent dual-chamber pacing in symptomatic nonobstructive hypertrophic cardiomyopathy. Am J Cardiol 73:571, 1994.
320. Van Oosterhout MFM, Prinzen FW, Arts T, et al. Asynchronous electrical activation induces asymmetrical hypertrophy of the left ventricular wall. Circulation 98: 588, 1998.
321. Betocchi S, Losi MA, Piscione F, et al. Effects of dual-chamber pacing in hypertrophic cardiomyopathy on left ventricular outflow tract obstruction and on diastolic function. Am J Cardiol 77:498, 1996.
322. Kiviniemi MS, Pirnes MA, Eränen HJK, et al. Complications related to permanent pacemaker therapy. Pacing Clin Electrophysiol 22:711, 1999.
323. Chang SM, Nagueh SF, Spencer WH, III, et al. Complete heart block: Determinants and clinical impact in patients with hypertrophic obstructive cardiomyopathy undergoing nonsurgical septal reduction therapy. J Am Coll Cardiol 42:296, 2003.
324. Chang SM, Lakkis NM, Franklin J, et al. Predictors of outcome after alcohol septal ablation therapy in patients with hypertrophic obstructive cardiomyopathy. Circulation 109:824, 2004.
325. Gietzen FH, Leuner CJ, Obergassel L, et al. Transcoronary ablation of septal hypertrophy for hypertrophic obstructive cardiomyopathy: feasibility, clinical benefit, and short term results in elderly patients. Heart 90:638, 2004.
326. Qin JX, Shiota T, Lever HM, et al. Conduction system abnormalities in patients with obstructive hypertrophic cardiomyopathy following septal reduction interventions. Am J Cardiol 93:171, 2004.
327. Talreja DR, Nishimura RA, Edwards WD, et al. Alcohol septal ablation versus surgical septal myectomy: comparison of effects on atrioventricular conduction tissue. J Am Coll Cardiol 44:2329, 2004.
328. Kimmelstiel CD, Maron BJ. Role of percutaneous septal ablation in hypertrophic obstructive cardiomyopathy. Circulation 109:452, 2004.
329. Robbins RC, Stinson EB. Long-term results of left ventricular myotomy and myectomy for obstructive hypertrophic cardiomyopathy. J Thorac Cardiovasc Surg 111:586, 1996.
330. McCully RB, Nishimura RA, Tajik AJ, et al. Extent of clinical improvement after surgical treatment of hypertrophic obstructive cardiomyopathy. Circulation 94:467, 1996.
331. Schönbeck MH, Rocca HPB, Vogt PR, et al. Long-term follow-up in hypertrophic obstructive cardiomyopathy after septal myectomy. Ann Thorac Surg 65:1207, 1998.
332. Mohr R, Schaff HV, Puga FJ, et al. Results of operation for hypertrophic obstructive cardiomyopathy in children and adults less than 40 years of age. Circulation 80 Suppl.:I191, 1989.
333. Theodoro DA, Danielson GK, Feldt RH, et al. Hypertrophic obstructive cardiomyopathy in pediatric patients: results of surgical treatment. J Thorac Cardiovasc Surg 112:1589, 1996.
334. Minakata K, Dearani JA, Nishimura RA, et al. Extended septal myectomy for hypertrophic obstructive cardiomyopathy with anomalous mitral papillary muscles or chordae. J Thorac Cardiovasc Surg 127:481, 2004.
335. Maron BJ, Dearani JA, Ommen SR, et al. The case for surgery in obstructive hypertrophic cardiomyopathy. J Am Coll Cardiol 44:2044, 2004.
336. Fananapazir L, Leon MB, Bonow RO, et al. Sudden death during empiric amiodarone therapy in symptomatic hypertrophic cardiomyopathy. Am J Cardiol 67:169, 1991.
337. Elliott PM, Sharma S, Varnava A, et al. Survival after cardiac arrest or sustained ventricular tachycardia in patients with hypertrophic cardiomyopathy. J Am Coll Cardiol 33:1596, 1999.
338. Hamilton RM, Dorian P, Gow RM, et al. Five-year experience with implantable defibrillators in children. Am J Cardiol 77: 524, 1996.
339. Wilson WR, Greer GE, Grubb BP. Implantable cardioverter-defibrillators in children: a single-institutional experience. Ann Thorac Surg 65:775, 1998.
340. Alexander ME, Cecchin F, Walsh EP, et al. Implications of implantable cardioverter defibrillator therapy in congenital heart disease and pediatrics. J Cardiovasc Electrophysiol 15:72, 2004.
341. Semsarian C, Richmond DR. Sudden cardiac death in familial hypertrophic cardiomyopathy: an Australian experience. Aust N Z J Med 29:368, 1999.
342. Maron BJ, Shirani J, Poliac LC, et al. Sudden death in young competitive athletes. Clinical, demographic, and pathological profiles. J Am Med Assoc 276:199, 1996.
343. Shephard RJ. The athlete's heart: is big beautiful? British Journal of Sports Medicine 30:5, 1996.
344. Maron BJ, Klues HG. Surviving competitive athletics with hypertrophic cardiomyopathy. Am J Cardiol 73:1098, 1994.
345. Friedewald VE, Jr., Spence DW. Sudden cardiac death associated with exercise: The risk- benefit issue. Am J Cardiol 66:183, 1990.
346. Kohl HW, Powell KE, Gordon NF, et al. Physical activity, physical fitness, and sudden cardiac death. Epidemiologic Reviews 14:37, 1992.
347. Richardson CR, Kriska AM, Lantz PM, et al. Physical activity and mortality across cardiovascular disease risk groups. Med Sci Sports Exerc 36:1923, 2004.
348. Beunen GP, Lefevre J, Philippaerts RM, et al. Adolescent correlates of adult physical activity: a 26-year follow-up. Med Sci Sports Exerc 36:1930, 2004.
349. Kraut A, Melamed S, Gofer D, et al. Effect of school age sports on leisure time physical activity in adults: The CORDIS Study. Med Sci Sports Exerc 35:2038, 2003.
350. Spirito P, Maron BJ. Relation between extent of left ventricular hypertrophy and occurrence of sudden cardiac death in

hypertrophic cardiomyopathy. J Am Coll Cardiol 15:1521, 1990.

351. Spirito P, Bellone P, Harris KM, et al. Magnitude of left ventricular hypertrophy and risk of sudden death in hypertrophic cardiomyopathy. N Engl J Med 342:1778, 2000.
352. Cecchi F, Olivotto I, Montereggi A, et al. Hypertrophic cardiomyopathy in Tuscany: Clinical course and outcome in an unselected regional population. J Am Coll Cardiol 26: 1529, 1995.
353. Maron BJ, Olivotto I, Spirito P, et al. Epidemiology of hypertrophic cardiomyopathy-related death - Revisited in a large non-referral-based patient population. Circulation 102:858, 2000.
354. Maron BJ, Roberts WC, Epstein SE. Sudden death in hypertrophic cardiomyopathy: a profile of 78 patients. Circulation 65:1388, 1982.
355. Elliott PM, Blanes JRG, Mahon NG, et al. Relation between severity of left-ventricular hypertrophy and prognosis in patients with hypertrophic cardiomyopathy. Lancet 357: 420, 2001.
356. Olivotto I, Gistri R, Petrone P, et al. Maximum left ventricular thickness and risk of sudden death in patients with hypertrophic cardiomyopathy. J Am Coll Cardiol 41:315, 2003.
357. Yetman AT, Hamilton RM, Benson LN, et al. Long-term outcome and prognostic determinants in children with hypertrophic cardiomyopathy. J Am Coll Cardiol 32:1943, 1998.
358. Maron BJ, Tajik AJ, Ruttenberg HD, et al. Hypertrophic cardiomyopathy in infants: clinical features and natural history. Circulation 65:7, 1982.
359. Suda K, Kohl T, Kovalchin JP, et al. Echocardiographic predictors of poor outcome in infants with hypertrophic cardiomyopathy. Am J Cardiol 80:595, 1997.
360. Schaffer MS, Freedom RM, Rowe RD. Hypertrophic cardiomyopathy presenting before 2 years of age in 13 patients. Pediatr Cardiol 4:113, 1983.
361. Panza JA, Maron BJ. Relation of electrocardiographic abnormalities to evolving left ventricular hypertrophy in hypertrophic cardiomyopathy during childhood. Am J Cardiol 63:1258, 1989.
362. Maron BJ, Spirito P. Implications of left ventricular remodeling in hypertrophic cardiomyopathy. Am J Cardiol 81: 1339, 1998.
363. Thaman R, Gimeno JR, Reith S, et al. Progressive left ventricular remodeling in patients with hypertrophic cardiomyopathy and severe left ventricular hypertrophy. J Am Coll Cardiol 44:398, 2004.
364. Eidem BW, Lindor NM, Driscoll DJ. Resolution of neonatal hypertrophic cardiomyopathy in an infant with an affected mother. Pediatr Cardiol 20:208, 1999.
365. Seiler C, Jenni R, Vassalli G, et al. Left ventricular chamber dilatation in hypertrophic cardiomyopathy: Related variables and prognosis in patients with medical and surgical therapy. Br Heart J 74:508, 1995.
366. Ino T, Nishimoto K, Okubo M, et al. Apoptosis as a possible cause of wall thinning in end-stage hypertrophic cardiomyopathy. Am J Cardiol 79:1137, 1997.
367. Ino T, Okubo M, Nishimoto K, et al. Clinicopathologic characteristics of hypertrophic cardiomyopathy detected during mass screening for heart disease. Pediatr Cardiol 17:295, 1996.
368. Panza JA, Maris TJ, Maron BJ. Development and determinants of dynamic obstruction to left ventricular outflow in young patients with hypertrophic cardiomyopathy. Circulation 85:1398, 1992.
369. Spirito P, Chiarella F, Carratino L, et al. Clinical course and prognosis of hypertrophic cardiomyopathy in an outpatient population. N Engl J Med 320:749, 1989.
370. Agnarsson UT, Hardarson T, Hallgrimsson J, et al. The prevalence of hypertrophic cardiomyopathy in men: An echocardiographic population screening study with a review of death records. J Intern Med 232:499, 1992.
371. Cannan CR, Reeder GS, Bailey KR, et al. Natural history of hypertrophic cardiomyopathy - A population- based study, 1976 through 1990. Circulation 92:2488, 1995.
372. Maron BJ, Casey SA, Poliac LC, et al. Clinical course of hypertrophic cardiomyopathy in a regional United States cohort. J Am Med Assoc 281:650, 1999.
373. McKenna WJ, Deanfield JE. Hypertrophic cardiomyopathy: an important cause of sudden death. Arch Dis Child 59: 971, 1984.
374. Takagi E, Yamakado T, Nakano T. Prognosis of completely asymptomatic adult patients with hypertrophic cardiomyopathy. J Am Coll Cardiol 33:206, 1999.
375. Campuzano V, Montermini L, Lutz Y, et al. Frataxin is reduced in Friedreich ataxia patients and is associated with mitochondrial membranes. Human Molecular Genetics 6:1771, 1997.
376. Brice A. Unstable mutations and neurodegenerative disorders. [Review] [58 refs]. J Neurol 245:505, 1998.
377. Klockgether T, Ludtke R, Kramer B, et al. The natural history of degenerative ataxia: a retrospective study in 466 patients. Brain 121:589, 1998.
378. Bulteau AL, O'Neill HA, Kennedy MC, et al. Frataxin acts as an iron chaperone protein to modulate mitochondrial aconitase activity. Science 305:242, 2004.
379. Delatycki MB, Camakaris J, Brooks H, et al. Direct evidence that mitochondrial iron accumulation occurs in Friedreich ataxia. Annals of Neurology 45:673, 1999.
380. Wong A, Yang J, Cavadini P, et al. The Friedreich's ataxia mutation confers cellular sensitivity to oxidant stress which is rescued by chelators of iron and calcium and inhibitors of apoptosis. Human Molecular Genetics 8:425, 1999.
381. Schapira AH. Mitochondrial involvement in Parkinson's disease, Huntington's disease, hereditary spastic paraplegia and Friedreich's ataxia [see comments]. [Review] [112 refs]. Biochimica et Biophysica Acta 1410:159, 1999.
382. Wilson RB, Lynch DR, Fischbeck KH. Normal serum iron and ferritin concentrations in patients with Friedreich's ataxia. Annals of Neurology 44:132, 1998.
383. Buyse G, Mertens L, Di SG, et al. Idebenone treatment in Friedreich's ataxia: neurological, cardiac, and biochemical monitoring. Neurology 60:1679, 2003.

384. Mariotti C, Solari A, Torta D, et al. Idebenone treatment in Friedreich patients: one-year-long randomized placebo-controlled trial. Neurology 60:1676, 2003.
385. James TN, Cobbs BW, Coghlan HC, et al. Coronary disease, cardioneuropathy, and conduction system abnormalities in the cardiomyopathy of Friedreich's ataxia. Br Heart J 57: 446, 1987.
386. Ulku A, Arac N, Ozeren A. Friedreich's ataxia: a clinical review of 20 childhood cases. Acta Neurol Scand 77:493, 1988.
387. Alboliras ET, Shub C, Gomez MR, et al. Spectrum of cardiac involvement in Friedreich's ataxia: Clinical, electrocardiographic and echocardiographic observations. Am J Cardiol 58:518, 1986.
388. Maione S, Giunta A, Filla A, et al. May age onset be relevant in the occurrence of left ventricular hypertrophy in Friedreich's ataxia? Clin Cardiol 20:141, 1997.
389. Child JS, Perloff JK, Bach PM, et al. Cardiac involvement in Friedreich's ataxia: a clinical study of 75 patients. J Am Coll Cardiol 7:1370, 1986.
390. Casazza F, Ferrari F, Finocchiaro G, et al. Echocardiographic evaluation of verapamil in Friedreich's ataxia. Br Heart J 55:400, 1986.
391. Hawley RJ, Gottdiener JS. Five-year follow-up of Friedreich's ataxia cardiomyopathy. Arch Intern Med 146:483, 1986.
392. Casazza F, Morpurgo M. The varying evolution of Friedreich's ataxia cardiomyopathy. Am J Cardiol 77:895, 1996.
393. Zimmermann M, Gabathuler J, Adamec R, et al. Unusual manifestations of heart involvement in Friedreich's ataxia. Am Heart J 111:184, 1986.
394. Denfield SW. Sudden death in children with restrictive cardiomyopathy. Card Electrophysiol Rev 6:163, 2002.
395. Guadalajara JF, Vera-Delgado A, Gaspar-Hernandez J, et al. Echocardiographic aspects of restrictive cardiomyopathy: Their relationship with pathophysiology. Echocardiogr J Cardiovasc Ultrasound Allied Tech 15:297, 1998.
396. Schwartz ML, Colan SD. Familial restrictive cardiomyopathy with skeletal abnormalities. Am J Cardiol 92:636, 2003.
397. Ha JW, Ommen SR, Tajik AJ, et al. Differentiation of constrictive pericarditis from restrictive cardiomyopathy using mitral annular velocity by tissue Doppler echocardiography. Am J Cardiol 94:316, 2004.
398. Weller RJ, Weintraub R, Addonizio LJ, et al. Outcome of idiopathic restrictive cardiomyopathy in children. Am J Cardiol 90:501, 2002.
399. Gerlis LM, Schmidt-Ott SC, Ho SY, et al. Dysplastic conditions of the right ventricular myocardium: Uhl's anomaly *v* arrhythmogenic right ventricular dysplasia. Br Heart J 69:142, 1993.
400. Azhari N, Assaqqat M, Bulbul Z. Successful surgical repair of Uhl's anomaly. Cardiol Young 12:192, 2002.
401. Corrado D, Basso C, Nava A, et al. Arrhythmogenic right ventricular cardiomyopathy: current diagnostic and management strategies. Cardiol Rev 9:259, 2001.
402. Hulot JS, Jouven X, Empana JP, et al. Natural history and risk stratification of arrhythmogenic right ventricular dysplasia/cardiomyopathy. Circulation 110:1879, 2004.
403. Hébert JL, Chemla D, Gérard O, et al. Angiographic right and left ventricular function in arrhythmogenic right ventricular dysplasia. Am J Cardiol 93:728, 2004.
404. Bomma C, Rutberg J, Tandri H, et al. Misdiagnosis of Arrhythmogenic right ventricular Dysplasia/Cardiomyopathy. Journal of Cardiovascular Electrophysiology 15:300, 2004.
405. Sen-Chowdhry S, Lowe MD, Sporton SC, et al. Arrhythmogenic right ventricular cardiomyopathy: clinical presentation, diagnosis, and management. Am J Med 117:685, 2004.
406. Chimenti C, Pieroni M, Maseri A, et al. Histologic findings in patients with clinical and instrumental diagnosis of sporadic arrhythmogenic right ventricular dysplasia. J Am Coll Cardiol 43:2305, 2004.
407. Wichter T, Paul M, Wollmann C, et al. Implantable cardioverter/defibrillator therapy in arrhythmogenic right ventricular cardiomyopathy - Single-center experience of long-term follow-up and complications in 60 patients. Circulation 109:1503, 2004.
408. Roguin A, Bomma CS, Nasir K, et al. Implantable cardioverter-defibrillators in patients with arrhythmogenic right ventricular dysplasia/cardiomyopathy. J Am Coll Cardiol 43:1843, 2004.
409. Pignatelli RH, McMahon CJ, Dreyer WJ, et al. Clinical characterization of left ventricular noncompaction in children - A relatively common form of cardiomyopathy. Circulation 108:2672, 2003.
410. Finsterer J, Stollberger C, Schubert B. Acquired left ventricular hypertrabeculation/noncompaction in mitochondriopathy. Cardiology 102:228, 2004.
411. Rigopoulos A, Rizos IK, Aggeli C, et al. Isolated left ventricular noncompaction: An unclassified cardiomyopathy with severe prognosis in adults. Cardiology 98:25, 2002.
412. Oechslin EN, Jost CHA, Rojas JR, et al. Long-term follow-up of 34 adults with isolated left ventricular noncompaction: A distinct cardiomyopathy with poor prognosis. J Am Coll Cardiol 36:493, 2000.
413. Stollberger C, Winkler-Dworak M, Blazek G, et al. Left ventricular hypertrabeculation/noncompaction with and without neuromuscular disorders. Int J Cardiol 97:89, 2004.
414. Finsterer J, Stollberger C, Kopsa W. Familial left ventricular hypertrabeculation in myotonic dystrophy type 1. Herz 28:466, 2003.
415. Chen R, Tsuji T, Ichida F, et al. Mutation analysis of the G4.5 gene in patients with isolated left ventricular noncompaction. Mol Genet Metab 77:319, 2002.
416. McMahon CJ, Chang AC, Pignatelli RH, et al. Left Ventricular Noncompaction Cardiomyopathy in Association with Trisomy 13. Pediatr Cardiol, 2004.
417. Stollberger C, Finsterer J, Voigtlander T, et al. Is left ventricular hypertrabeculation/noncompaction a cardiac manifestation of Fabry's disease? Z Kardiol 92:966, 2003.
418. Stollberger C, Finsterer J. Left ventricular hypertrabeculation/noncompaction. J Am Soc Echocardiogr 17:91, 2004.
419. Kenton AB, Sanchez X, Coveler KJ, et al. Isolated left ventricular noncompaction is rarely caused by mutations in G4.5, alpha-dystrobrevin and FK Binding Protein-12. Mol Genet Metab 82:162, 2004.

420. Varvava AM. Isolated left ventricular non-compaction: a distinct cardiomyopathy? Heart 86:599, 2001.
421. Weiford BC, Subbarao VD, Mulhern KM. Noncompaction of the ventricular myocardium. Circulation 109:2965, 2004.
422. Alehan D. Clinical features of isolated left ventricular noncompaction in children. Int J Cardiol 97:233, 2004.
423. Murphy RT, Thaman R, Blanes JG, et al. Natural history and familial characteristics of isolated left ventricular non-compaction. Eur Heart J 26:187, 2005.
424. Wald R, Veldtman G, Golding F, et al. Determinants of outcome in isolated ventricular noncompaction in childhood. Am J Cardiol 94:1581, 2004.
425. Tamborini G, Pepi M, Celeste F, et al. Incidence and characteristics of left ventricular false tendons and trabeculations in the normal and pathologic heart by second harmonic echocardiography. J Am Soc Echocardiogr 17:367, 2004.

27

Pericardial Diseases

Roger E. Breitbart

DEFINITION

Pericardial diseases are those that involve the pericardial membranes and fluid space surrounding the heart. These diseases include congenital abnormalities, primary inflammatory and infectious processes, secondary reactive processes, and chronic conditions.

The pericardium comprises outer fibrosal and inner serosal layers. The serosa is actually a *collapsed* sac that envelopes the heart and proximal great vessels. The innermost layer forms the visceral pericardium or epicardium. This is continuous via reflections with the outer serosal layer that is adherent to the outermost fibrosa, forming the parietal pericardium. The pericardial sac in the normal adult contains 15 to 35 mL of serous fluid that resides principally in a series of pericardial sinuses, the remainder of the collapsed sac being virtual space.[1]

This chapter presents an overview of pericardial conditions pertinent to pediatric practice but it is, of necessity, not exhaustive. The author has relied heavily on the comprehensive and authoritative work of Spodick[1,2] and other cited references.

ACUTE PERICARDITIS

Acute pericarditis is the most common pericardial disease encountered in routine clinical practice. There are myriad causes, some of which are listed in Table 27-1. Most are idiopathic cases, which, for the most part, are thought to be viral or postviral.[1,2] Whether infectious, postinfectious, or autoimmune, there is inflammatory infiltration of the pericardial membranes, with (effusive) or without (noneffusive) accumulation of excess pericardial fluid. Features common to both effusive and noneffusive pericarditis are presented in this section whereas those related specifically to clinically significant fluid accumulation and tamponade are considered in the next. It is beyond the scope of this chapter to address features unique to each underlying cause.

Chest pain is a prominent symptom in many cases of acute pericarditis, although it is often lacking in the more indolent or insidious etiologies. When present, the pain tends to be sharp and precordial, sometimes radiating, worse with inspiration or cough, and characteristically positional. Patients are particularly uncomfortable when recumbent and typically find some relief sitting up and leaning forward. Fever is common, especially in viral and bacterial pericarditis. On physical examination, patients may appear quite uncomfortable. In cases of bacterial pericarditis the patient may be severely ill with systemic signs of sepsis and shock. There is typically a pericardial friction rub on auscultation; contrary to some teaching, a rub is often audible even when there is a large effusion.[3]

Several tests may aid in the diagnosis of acute pericarditis. Progressive electrocardiographic abnormalities are pathognomonic, and discrete stages in this progression have been described.[1,2] Early in the disease, there is characteristic widespread J-point and ST segment elevation in inferior and anterior leads (Fig. 27-1). PR segments are deflected in a direction opposite the P wave (i.e., downward in leads with upright P waves and upward in those with downgoing P waves).[4] Later in the disease, J-points return to baseline, followed by flattening and eventual inversion of the T waves. It is critical to distinguish pericarditis from acute coronary syndromes in adult patients presenting with chest pain.[2]

TABLE 27–1. Etiologies of Pediatric Acute Pericarditis and Pericardial Effusion

Idiopathic (probably viral)
Infection
Bacterial
Neisseria meningiditis
Hemophilus influenza
Staphylococcus aureus
Mycobacterium tuberculosis
Borrelia burgdorferi
Other bacteria, including obligate intracellular species
Viral
Coxsackie virus
Cytomegalovirus
Human immunodeficiency virus
Other viruses
Fungal
Candida
Other
Parasitic
Toxoplasma gondii
Other
Connective tissue disease and vasculitis
Systemic lupus erythematosus
Rheumatoid arthritis
Rheumatic fever
Inflammatory bowel disease
Kawasaki disease
Other vasculitides and connective tissue syndromes
Other etiologies
Postpericardiotomy syndrome
Renal failure, including uremia and chronic dialysis
Malignancy, especially leukemia and lymphoma
Graft versus host disease
Pneumonia
Myxedema
Drug, especially mesalamine
Trauma, including hemopericardium
Extravasation from indwelling central venous catheters, especially in low-birth-weight neonates
Other

Adapted from Spodick DH. The Pericardium: A Comprehensive Textbook. New York: Marcel Dekker, 1997.

On chest radiograph, the cardiac silhouette may appear normal or, if there is an appreciable pericardial effusion, enlarged. Pleural fluid may be present, more often on the left. Other findings, for example pulmonary infiltrates or a mediastinal mass, may indicate specific etiologies for pericarditis.

The echocardiogram may have normal findings in noneffusive acute pericarditis but more typically shows at least a small collection of pericardial fluid, often localized posteriorly, if not a circumferential effusion (Fig. 27-2).

Screening blood tests are of limited value in most cases of acute pericarditis. A rise in circulating cardiac troponin I has been found in 32% of adult patients with viral or idiopathic acute pericarditis and may be indicative of

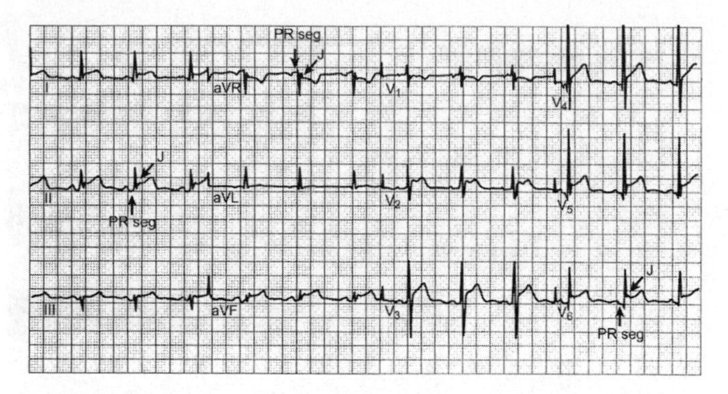

FIGURE 27–1 *Electrocardiogram showing stage I changes pathognomonic of acute pericarditis, including widespread J-point and ST segment elevation and deflection of the PR segments in the direction opposite that of the P wave, generally PR depression with upright P waves.*
Adapted from Spodick DH. Pericardial diseases. In Braunwald E, Zipes D.P, Libby P [eds]. Heart Disease, 6th ed. Philadelphia: WB Saunders, 2001: 1823, with permission.

inflammation of adjacent epicardial myocardium.[5] An elevated white blood cell count may be found in patients with bacterial pericarditis. The erythrocyte sedimentation rate may be elevated, particularly in association with collagen vascular diseases. Other tests related to specific diagnoses (Table 27-1) may be useful when indicated by history and physical findings. Analysis of fluid obtained by pericardiocentesis may be diagnostic in cases of malignant, mycobacterial, and other bacterial pericarditis; pericardial biopsy is rarely informative.[6–8]

The management of acute pericarditis, aside from treatment of the underlying cause where possible, involves anti-inflammatory therapy to relieve symptoms and accelerate resolution. Nonsteroidal drugs such as ibuprofen are often very effective. Refractory cases may respond to corticosteroids. The addition of colchicine has been effective in anecdotal reports.[1,2,9] Therapeutic pericardiocentesis is necessary for tamponade and may also be indicated for otherwise large effusions.

POSTPERICARDIOTOMY SYNDROME

Postpericardiotomy syndrome is a form of acute pericarditis that merits special note because it is frequently encountered in centers with active pediatric cardiac surgery programs. It may occur after any cardiac operation including transplantation.[10] A similar or identical syndrome develops in some patients after chest trauma and rarely as a complication of transvenous pacing.[1,2,11] The precise etiology is unknown and potential immune-mediated pathophysiologic mechanisms are debated.[10,12–14] Patients present 1 week to several months after surgery with low-grade fever and

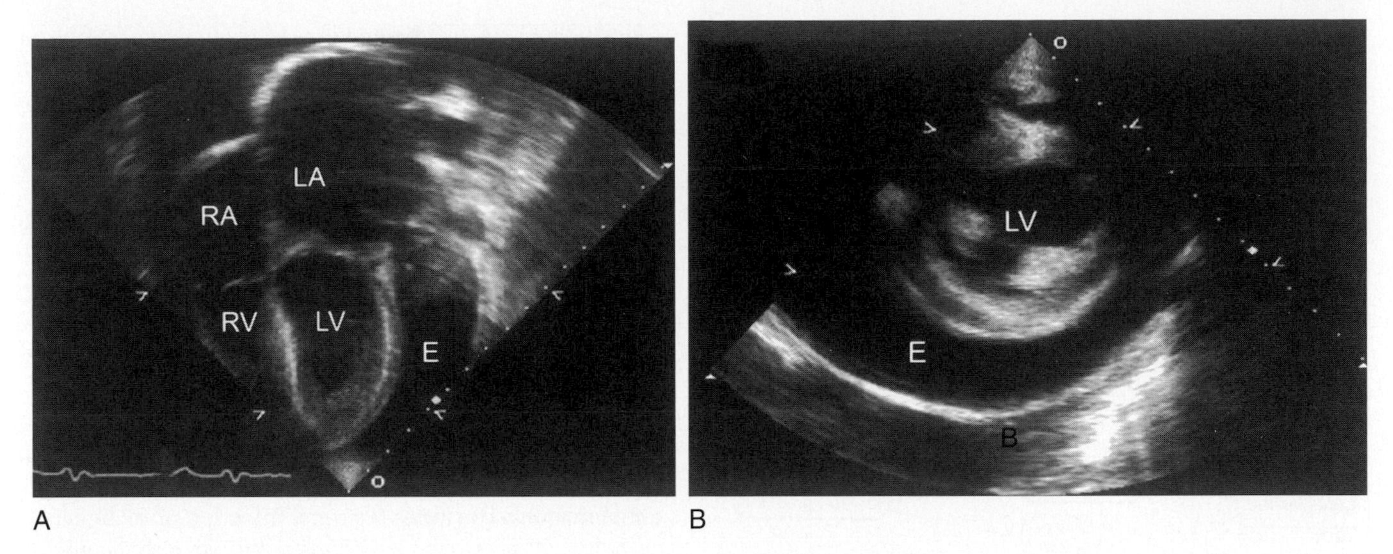

FIGURE 27–2 *Echocardiogram of a patient with a large, circumferential pericardial effusion (E). A, Apical four chamber view including right atrium (RA), left atrium (LA), right ventricle (RV), and left ventricle (LV). B, Parasternal short-axis view.*

the typical signs and symptoms of pericardial inflammation noted in prior sections of this chapter. Cardiac tamponade may develop.[15] Patients may also have findings indicating associated pleuritis and pleural effusion. Strategies for the evaluation and management of postpericardiotomy syndrome are essentially as reviewed above for acute pericarditis, and below when complicated by tamponade. Nonsteroidal anti-inflammatory drugs are the mainstay of therapy. Corticosteroids may hasten recovery but are not effective for prevention when administered prophylactically.[16,17]

PERICARDIAL EFFUSION AND TAMPONADE

Excess pericardial fluid of any volume may accumulate in acute pericarditis, postpericardiotomy syndrome, or in any of a number of more chronic conditions associated with pericardial transudation (see Table 27-1). Pericardial effusion may have little effect on cardiac function in some patients, particularly if it accumulates slowly and the pericardium is sufficiently compliant to avoid the development of high intrapericardial pressure. Importantly, however, cardiac tamponade may occur in the presence of pericardial effusion, whether large or small. Rapid accumulation and tamponade are often the rule in hemopericardium caused by external trauma or iatrogenic cardiac perforation. In tamponade, increased intrapericardial pressure limits venous return to the heart and impairs chamber compliance, resulting in decreased diastolic filling and compromised cardiac output. Cardiogenic shock and death may ensue, often precipitously.

Depending on the degree of tamponade, patients with pericardial effusion may have variable dyspnea, tachypnea, tachycardia, hypotension, poor perfusion, distant heart sounds, friction rub, jugular venous distention, hepatomegaly, and/or altered consciousness.[18–20] Some children may have emesis.[15] Pulsus paradoxus, defined as a decline is systolic blood pressure greater than or equal to 10 mm Hg during inspiration, is a key diagnostic finding indicative of tamponade physiology (Figs. 27-3 and 27-4). Such respiratory variation can be measured conventionally using the Korotkoff sounds and may be evident on the pulse-oximetry waveform.[21]

Electrocardiographic findings may be normal or may show changes typical of acute pericarditis. In addition, there may be electrical alternation of the QRS complex

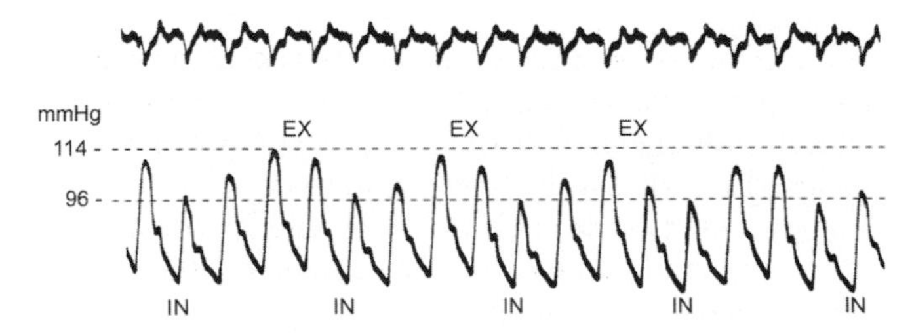

FIGURE 27–3 *Brachial artery pressure tracing demonstrating pulsus paradoxus, with the corresponding electrocardiogram above. The systolic pressures at end inspiration (IN), 96 mm Hg, and peak expiration (EX), 114 mm Hg, differ by 18 mm Hg, which is the size of the pulsus.*
Adapted from Spodick DH. The Pericardium: A Comprehensive Textbook. New York: Marcel Dekker, 1997, with permission.

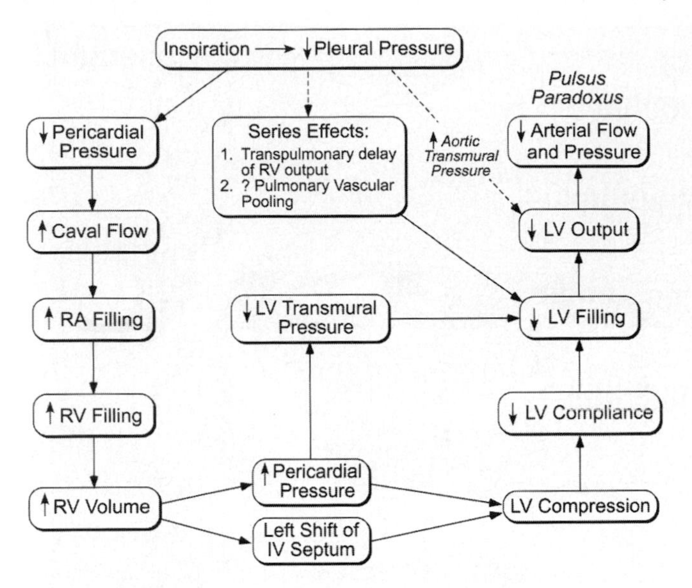

FIGURE 27–4 *Physiology of pulsus paradoxus. Responses to inspiratory reduction of pleural pressure combine to produce the inspiratory fall in left ventricular output and arterial systolic pressure.*
Adapted from Spodick DH. The Pericardium: A Comprehensive Textbook. New York: Marcel Dekker, 1997, with permission.

attributed to oscillation of the heart within the effusion.[18] There may be diffusely low QRS voltages, reported to be indicative of tamponade rather than effusion alone.[22]

On chest radiograph, the cardiac silhouette may appear enlarged. If there is a large pericardial effusion, the normal contours of the right and left heart borders may be obscured, with the heart taking on a more globular or spherical configuration.

On echocardiography there is typically a circumferential pericardial effusion. Exaggerated respiratory variation in transvalvular flows measured by Doppler is a key diagnostic finding in tamponade. Less specific is diastolic invagination or collapse of the right atrial and right ventricular free walls on imaging.[23,24]

At cardiac catheterization, needed occasionally to confirm the diagnosis of tamponade, there is elevation of ventricular pressures throughout diastole and near-equilibration of atrial and ventricular diastolic pressures.[1,2]

Signs of tamponade in a patient with a pericardial effusion represent an indication for urgent or emergent therapeutic pericardial drainage, either percutaneously or occasionally by open surgical drainage. Percutaneous needle aspiration, ideally including insertion of a pericardial catheter over a guide wire, is typically accomplished via a sub-xiphoid approach in infants and children with at least 1 cm of pericardial fluid along the diaphragmatic contour of the heart.[25,26] Ultrasound or fluoroscopic guidance, if available, is often helpful. Medical management is of only limited value in this setting.[1,2] Acute intravascular volume expansion aids cardiac filling and may be temporarily helpful while necessary preparations are made to drain the pericardium. Inotropes and vasoconstrictors are typically ineffective. Positive pressure ventilation may further compromise venous return and is to be avoided if possible.

In the absence of tamponade, there are few indications for therapeutic pericardial drainage.[1,2] Very large pericardial effusions may compress significant portions of lung, with associated dyspnea, and this is relieved with drainage. Chronic, recurring effusions that are refractory to medical therapies may in some cases respond to surgical pericardiotomy[27,28]; percutaneous balloon pericardiotomy has also been reported in children.[29] In acute, effusive pericarditis, diagnostic pericardiocentesis is indicated when the differential diagnosis includes bacterial infection or malignancy.

CONSTRICTIVE PERICARDITIS

Constrictive pericarditis, rarely described in children, occurs when cardiac filling is limited by a scarred, fibrotic, and sometimes calcified pericardium. Typically, the pericardium is thickened and the pericardial space obliterated; however, pericardial thickness may be normal,[30] and pericardial fluid may be present in a syndrome of effusive-constrictive pericarditis.[31] Constriction may develop days to months after acute pericarditis of any cause, whether clinically manifest or silent. It is most often idiopathic and typically becomes chronic, although transient acute constriction soon after effusive pericarditis is described.[1,2,32] Rarely, constrictive pericarditis may develop years after cardiac surgery.

The symptoms and signs of constrictive pericarditis may be very mild or severe and generally resemble those of congestive right heart failure.[1,2] Patients may also have exertional dyspnea to the extent that ventricular filling, stroke volume, and hence cardiac output cannot increase adequately. Dyspnea may be exacerbated in the presence of pleural effusions. On examination, there is typically a relative sinus tachycardia; atrial fibrillation and other atrial tachyarrhythmias may ensue due to atrial dilation. Pulsus paradoxus may be present in effusive-constrictive pericarditis. Jugular venous distention is prominent, and there is often pulsatile hepatomegaly, ascites, and dependent edema. On cardiac auscultation there may be a diastolic S_3 *knock*.

Electrocardiographic findings typically show nonspecific T-wave abnormalities, and there are often low ventricular voltages and wide P waves. The chest radiograph may show a dilated SVC, pleural effusions, and, in more chronic cases, calcium in the pericardium. Computed tomography and magnetic resonance imaging may demonstrate a thickened

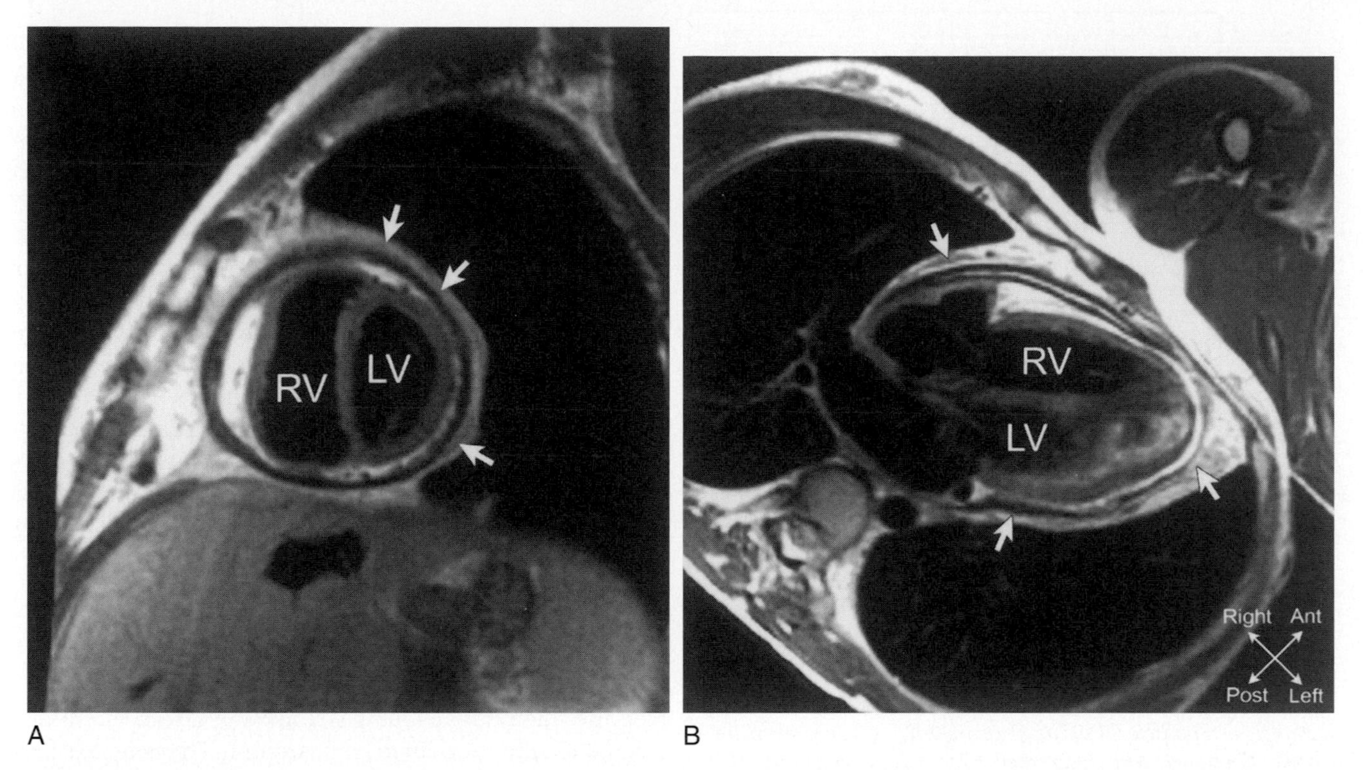

FIGURE 27–5 *Magnetic resonance images of a patient with a constrictive pericardium (arrows) encasing the right (RV) and left (LV) ventricles. A, Parasagittal cut. B, Axial cut.*

pericardium (Fig. 27-5) and enlarged atria and venae cavae.[33] Echocardiography may show pericardial thickening whereas Doppler analysis reveals characteristic abnormalities of mitral and tricuspid inflow and ventricular filling.[1,2,23] Cardiac catheterization is necessary to distinguish constrictive physiology from that associated with restrictive cardiomyopathy. Both exhibit the characteristic *square root sign* in the ventricular pressure tracings, reflecting an acute pressure fall at the onset of diastole and rapid rise in early diastole followed by a plateau (Fig. 27-6). In restrictive disease, however, the left ventricular diastolic pressure exceeds that of the right, accentuated by fluid challenge, whereas in constrictive disease they are nearly equal.

Surgical pericardiectomy is required to treat constrictive pericarditis as medical management is ineffective.[1,2,34]

CONGENITAL PARTIAL OR COMPLETE ABSENCE OF THE PERICARDIUM

Absence of the pericardium is a rare malformation in which the pericardium is incomplete, in part or in total, presumably the result of defective embryonic development. When such defects occur, it is the left side of the pericardium that is most often absent, whereas absence of the right pericardium is less common. Absence of the inferior pericardium is associated with diaphragmatic defects. Complete absence of the pericardium is exceedingly rare.[1,2] A family with absence of the left pericardium has been described.[35]

Absence of the pericardium is most often clinically silent but may become manifest, particularly in partial absence, when there is herniation, incarceration, or torsion of critical cardiovascular structures including the atria, atrial appendages, ventricles, and great vessels, impairing cardiac filling and output.[36] Rupture of tricuspid valve chordae has been reported.[37] Compression of the epicardial coronary vessels can produce atypical angina pectoris and myocardial infarction.[38,39]

The clinical presentation is variable.[40] Some patients may have paroxysmal chest pain but most are asymptomatic. Findings on physical examination and electrocardiogram may be absent or nonspecific.[41] Displacement of cardiac structures, mainly left lateral displacement of the apex, may be recognized on plain chest radiograph (Fig. 27-7A) and particularly exaggerated on decubitus films.[42] Echocardiography may show unusual acoustical windows and abnormal cardiac and septal motion.[43] Magnetic resonance imaging is the definitive modality for delineating the precise anatomy (Fig. 27-7B).[44]

Management of symptomatic patients may involve surgical reconstruction of the defective pericardium using

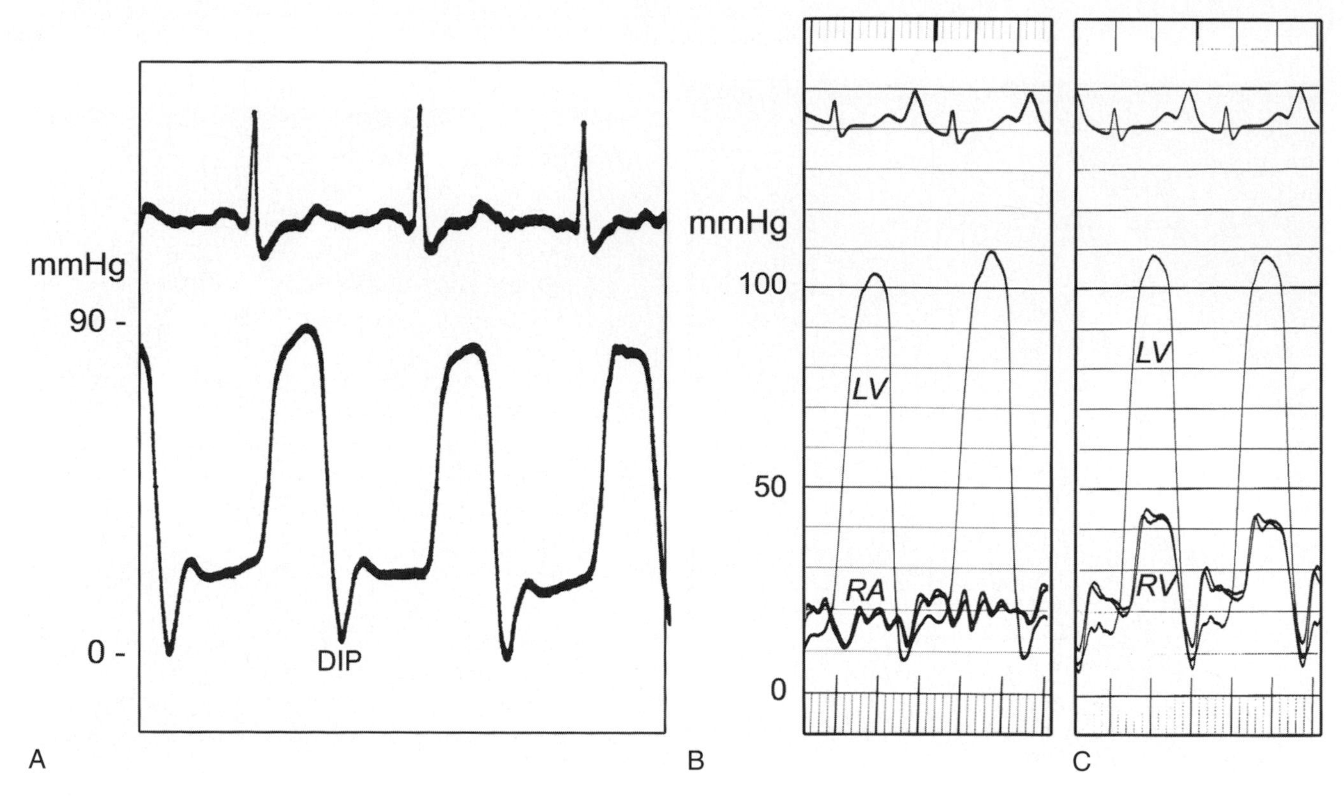

FIGURE 27–6 *Intracardiac pressure recordings in constrictive pericarditis. A, Left ventricular pressure tracing, with corresponding electrocardiogram above, demonstrating the square root sign with dip and rapid rise in early diastole. Reprinted with permission from Spodick DH. The pericardium: A comprehensive textbook. New York Marcel Dekker, 1997. B,C, Simultaneous pressure tracings from a patient with constrictive pericarditis showing equalization of left ventricular (LV), right atrial (RA), and right ventricular (RV) diastolic filling pressures.*

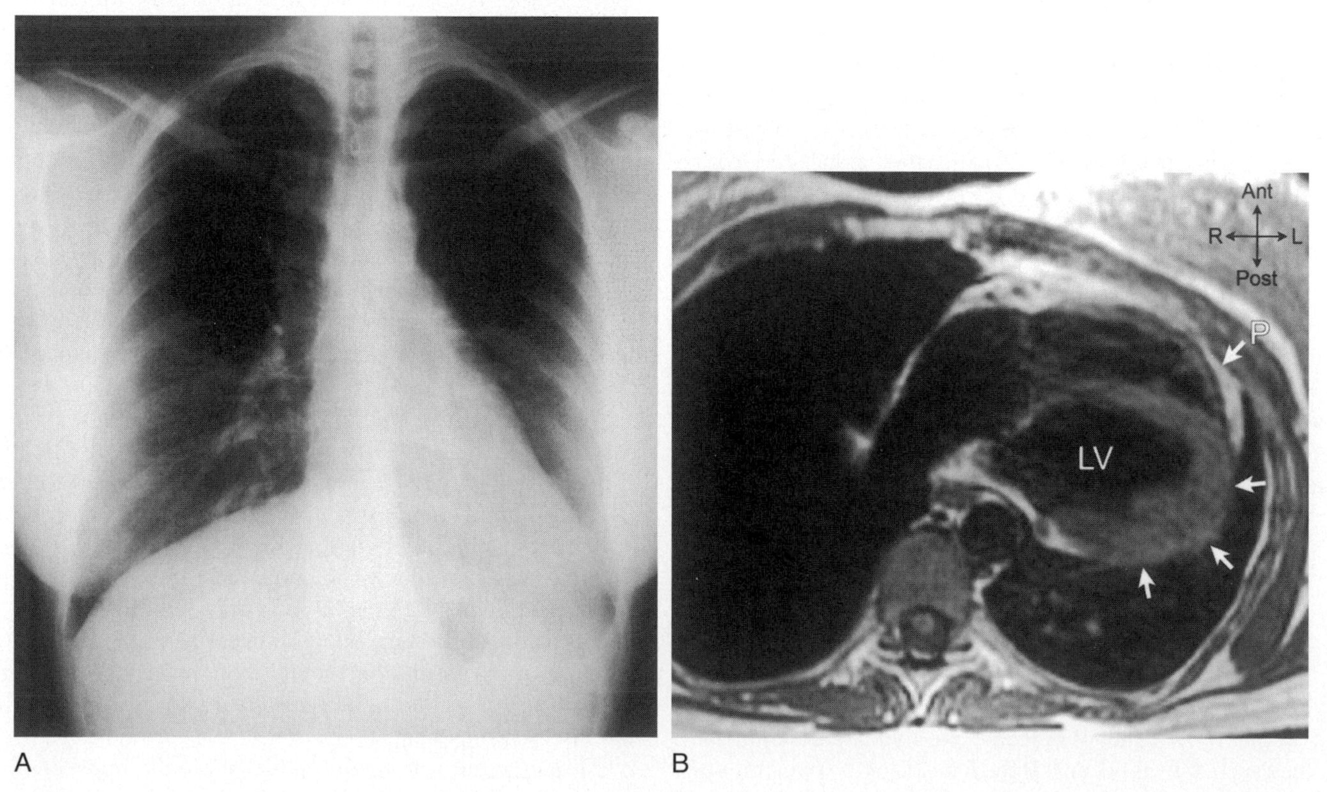

FIGURE 27–7 *Images of a patient with congenital absence of the left pericardium. A, Chest radiograph showing leftward displacement of the cardiac apex. B, Magnetic resonance image showing that the pericardium (P) is absent posterolaterally (arrows) around the left ventricle (LV) in an axial cut.*

synthetic or xenograft membrane or, alternatively, partial pericardiectomy to enlarge small incarcerating defects.[39,40]

PERICARDIAL CYSTS AND TUMORS

Isolated, fluid-filled pericardial cysts of several types may be found at any location on the pericardium, usually incidentally.[1] If large, however, they can produce symptoms by compression of the heart, mimicking tamponade, or of other adjacent structures. They must be differentiated from other cystic mediastinal masses with the aid of computed tomography, echocardiography, or magnetic resonance imaging. Treatment, if necessary, may involve aspiration or excision.[45]

Primary pericardial tumors are exceedingly rare. Teratoma,[46] lipoma, [47] hibernoma,[48] and mesothelioma[49] have been reported.

REFERENCES

1. Spodick DH. The Pericardium: A Comprehensive Textbook. New York: Marcel Dekker, 1997.
2. Spodick DH. Pericardial diseases. In Braunwald E, Zipes DP, Libby P (eds). Heart Disease, 6th ed. Philadelphia: WB Saunders, 2001: 1823.
3. Markiewicz W, Brik A, Brook G, et al. Pericardial rub in pericardial effusion: lack of correlation with amount of fluid. Chest 77:643, 1980.
4. Kudo Y, Yamasaki F, Doi Y, et al. Clinical correlates of PR-segment depression in asymptomatic patients with pericardial effusion. J Am Coll Cardiol 39:2000, 2002.
5. Imazio M, Demichelis B, Cecchi E, et al. Cardiac troponin I in acute pericarditis. J Am Coll Cardiol 42:2144, 2003.
6. Zayas R, Anguita M, Torres F, et al. Incidence of specific etiology and role of methods for specific etiologic diagnosis of primary acute pericarditis. Am J Cardiol 75:378, 1995.
7. Meyers DG, Meyers RE, Prendergast TW. The usefulness of diagnostic tests on pericardial fluid. Chest 111:1213, 1997.
8. Seferovic PM, Ristic AD, Maksimovic R, et al. Diagnostic value of pericardial biopsy: improvement with extensive sampling enabled by pericardioscopy. Circulation 107:978, 2003.
9. Brucato A, Cimaz R, Balla E. Prevention of recurrences of corticosteroid-dependent idiopathic pericarditis by colchicine in an adolescent patient. Pediatr Card 21:395, 2000.
10. Cabalka AK, Rosenblatt HM, Towbin JA, et al. Postpericardiotomy syndrome in pediatric heart transplant recipients: immunologic characteristics. Tex Heart Inst J 22:170, 1995.
11. Bajaj BP, Evans KE, Thomas P. Postpericardiotomy syndrome following temporary and permanent transvenous pacing. Postgrad Med J 75:357, 1999.
12. Hoffman M, Fried M, Jabareen F, et al. Anti-heart antibodies in postpericardiotomy syndrome: cause or epiphenomenon? A prospective, longitudinal pilot study. Autoimmunity 35:241, 2002.
13. Bartels C, Honig R, Burger G, et al. The significance of anticardiolipin antibodies and anti-heart muscle antibodies for the diagnosis of postpericardiotomy syndrome. Eur Heart J 15:1494, 1994.
14. Webber SA, Wilson NJ, Fung MY, et al. Autoantibody production after cardiopulmonary bypass with special reference to postpericardiotomy syndrome. J Pediatr 121(5 Pt 1): 744, 1992.
15. Scarfone RJ, Donoghue AJ, Alessandrini EA. Cardiac tamponade complicating postpericardiotomy syndrome. Pediatr Emerg Care 19:268, 2003.
16. Wilson NJ, Webber SA, Patterson MW, et al. Double-blind placebo-controlled trial of corticosteroids in children with postpericardiotomy syndrome. Pediatr Card 15:62, 1994.
17. Mott AR, Fraser CD, Jr., Kusnoor AV, et al. The effect of short-term prophylactic methylprednisolone on the incidence and severity of postpericardiotomy syndrome in children undergoing cardiac surgery with cardiopulmonary bypass. J Am Coll Cardiol 37:1700, 2001.
18. Spodick DH. Acute cardiac tamponade. N Engl J Med 349:684, 2003.
19. Milner D, Losek JD, Schiff J, et al. Pediatric pericardial tamponade presenting as altered mental status. Pediatr Emerg Care 19:35, 2003.
20. Browne GJ, Hort J, Lau KC. Pericardial effusions in a pediatric emergency department. Pediatr Emerg Care 18:285, 2002.
21. Tamburro RF, Ring JC, Womback K. Detection of pulsus paradoxus associated with large pericardial effusions in pediatric patients by analysis of the pulse-oximetry waveform. Pediatrics 109:673, 2002.
22. Bruch C, Schmermund A, Dagres N, et al. Changes in QRS voltage in cardiac tamponade and pericardial effusion: reversibility after pericardiocentesis and after anti-inflammatory drug treatment. J Am Coll Cardiol 38: 219, 2001.
23. D'Cruz I, Rehman AU, Hancock HI. Quantitative echocardiographic assessment in pericardial disease. Echocardiography 14:207, 1997.
24. Reydel B, Spodick DH. Frequency and significance of chamber collapses during cardiac tamponade. Am Heart J 119:1160, 1990.
25. Lock JE, Bass JL, Kulik TJ, et al. Chronic percutaneous pericardial drainage with modified pigtail catheters in children. Am J Cardiol 53:1179, 1984.
26. Zahn EM, Houde C, Benson L, et al. Percutaneous pericardial catheter drainage in childhood. Am J Cardiol 70: 678, 1992.
27. Sagrista-Sauleda J, Angel J, Permanyer-Miralda G, et al. Long-term follow-up of idiopathic chronic pericardial effusion. N Engl J Med 341:2054, 1999.
28. Mueller XM, Tevaearai HT, Hurni M, et al. Long-term results of surgical subxiphoid pericardial drainage. Thorac Cardiovasc Surg 45:65, 1997.
29. Thanopoulos BD, Georgakopoulos D, Tsaousis GS, et al. Percutaneous balloon pericardiotomy for the treatment of large, nonmalignant pericardial effusions in children: immediate and medium-term results. Cathet Cardiovasc Diagn 40:97, 1997.

30. Talreja DR, Edwards WD, Danielson GK, et al. Constrictive pericarditis in 26 patients with histologically normal pericardial thickness. Circulation 108:1852, 2003.
31. Sagrista-Sauleda J, Angel J, Sanchez A, et al. Effusive-constrictive pericarditis. N Engl J Med 350:469, 2004.
32. Haley JH, Tajik AJ, Danielson GK, et al. Transient constrictive pericarditis: causes and natural history. J Am Coll Cardiol 43:271, 2004.
33. Chen SJ, Li YW, Wu MH, et al. CT and MRI findings in a child with constrictive pericarditis. Pediatr Card 119:259, 1998.
34. Ling LH, Oh JK, Schaff HV, et al. Constrictive pericarditis in the modern era: evolving clinical spectrum and impact on outcome after pericardiectomy. Circulation 100:1380, 1999.
35. Taysi K, Hartmann AF, Shackelford GD, et al. Congenital absence of left pericardium in a family. Am J Med Genet 21:77, 1985.
36. McIlhenny J, Campbell SE, Raible RJ, et al. Pediatric case of the day. Congenital absence of the pericardium. Am J Roentgenol 167:270-274-275, 1996.
37. van Son JA, Danielson GK, Callahan JA. Congenital absence of the pericardium: displacement of the heart associated with tricuspid insufficiency. Ann Thorac Surg 56:1405, 1993.
38. Chapman JE, Jr., Rubin JW, Gross CM, et al. Congenital absence of pericardium: an unusual cause of atypical angina. Ann Thorac Surg 45:91, 1988.
39. Rusk RA, Kenny A. Congenital pericardial defect presenting as chest pain. Heart (British Cardiac Society) 81:327, 1999.
40. Gatzoulis MA, Munk MD, Merchant N, et al. Isolated congenital absence of the pericardium: clinical presentation, diagnosis, and management. Ann Thorac Surg 69:1209, 2000.
41. Di Pasquale G, Ruffini M, Piolanti S, et al. Congenital absence of pericardium as unusual cause of T wave abnormalities in a young athlete. Clin Cardiol 15:859, 1992.
42. Faridah Y, Julsrud PR. Congenital absence of pericardium revisited. Int J Cardiovasc Imaging 18:67, 2002.
43. Connolly HM, Click RL, Schattenberg TT, et al. Congenital absence of the pericardium: echocardiography as a diagnostic tool. J Am Soc Echocardiogr 8:87, 1995.
44. Gassner I, Judmaier W, Fink C, et al. Diagnosis of congenital pericardial defects, including a pathognomic sign for dangerous apical ventricular herniation, on magnetic resonance imaging. Br Heart J 74:60, 1995.
45. Eto A, Arima T, Nagashima A. Pericardial cyst in a child treated with video-assisted thoracoscopic surgery. Eur J Pediatr 159:889, 2000.
46. Garcia CM, Mulet J, Caralps J, et al. Fast-growing pericardial mass as first manifestation of intrapericardial teratoma in a young man. Am J Med 89:818, 1990.
47. Trusen A, Beissert M, Schultz G, et al. Progressively enlarging pericardial lipoma in a child. Br J Radiol 77:68, 2004.
48. Heifetz SA, Parikh SR, Brown JW. Hibernoma of the pericardium presenting as pericardial effusion in a child. Pediatr Pathol 10:575, 1990.
49. Eker R, Cantez T, Dogan O, et al. Pericardial mesothelioma. A pediatric case report. Turk J Pediatr 31:305, 1989.

28

Infective Endocarditis

GERALD R. MARX

Endocarditis, relatively rare in pediatrics, continues to be associated with significant morbidity and mortality. Although the commonly used terminology is *SBE*, or subacute bacterial endocarditis, a more practical terminology would be *infective endocarditis*. This latter reflects the evolving change, over time, in microbial organisms related to infectious-mediated inflammation of the endocardial surface of the heart. Recently, fungal endocarditis has become increasingly prevalent in pediatric centers. Additionally, the demarcation between acute and subacute clinical presentation is less clear in the pediatric age group, with increasing incidence of more acute or toxic episodes of infectious endocarditis in young infants and children.

The diagnosis of endocarditis continues to be vexing to the practicing pediatrician, neonatologist, internist, family practitioner, and pediatric cardiologist. However, all must be aware of this disease to initiate rapid diagnosis and corresponding effective treatment. Due to the insidious nature of the disease, and significant associated illness, the infectious disease laboratory, infectious disease specialist, cardiologist, and cardiovascular surgeon must work together to ensure a successful outcome.

EPIDEMIOLOGY

Infective endocarditis in childhood has unique features that differentiate it from disease in adults. Equally important, these features are evolving over time.[1–7] With the increased survival of pediatric patients with congenital heart disease, and the overall decrease in rheumatic fever, congenital heart disease has become the predominant substrate for infective endocarditis in the pediatric age group. In recent years, 50%, 78%, and 84% of infective endocarditis in the pediatric patient has been associated with congenital heart disease.[2–4] Moreover, the frequency of endocarditis in children seems to be increasing over time. Using pediatric hospital admissions as the denominator, 0.4[4] to 0.8[1] of 1000 hospital admissions was for infective endocarditis. The increase in frequency is due to the increased survival of patients with congenital heart disease and improved care and survival of critically ill and chronically hospitalized newborn infants. Some might argue that the increased frequency also may be due to enhanced detection and diagnosis with the advent of echocardiography.

The incidence of endocarditis in children younger than 2 years has significantly increased.[4] Equally striking is the increased incidence in the premature infant who does not have underlying structural heart disease,[6] particularly among those with indwelling catheters, and may represent 8% to 10% of pediatric infective endocarditis. In one report from a high-risk nursery, the incidence was 4.3%.[6] The microbes associated with endocarditis in this particular pediatric age group have also changed, resulting in the presentation of this disease entity being acute rather than subacute.[6]

Surgery itself may be an important risk factor for the development of endocarditis, with 50% of children having had previous cardiac surgery.[2] Although the incidence for endocarditis increases with time since surgery, with the use of prosthetic valves or conduits the risk is high even in the immediate postoperative period. In a 30-year analysis of postoperative infective endocarditis, 22% of cases occurred immediately postoperatively, with 6% involving patch material.[8]

Postoperative endocarditis occurs most commonly in those with aortic stenosis[8]: 13.3 % at 25 years, and 20.6% at 30 years.[9] The risk is highest after valve replacement. In comparison, the 25-year cumulative incidence is 1.3% after tetralogy of Fallot repair, 2.5% in ventricular septal defect, 2.8% in isolated primum atrial septal defect, and 3.5% in isolated aortic coarctation. The 20-year cumulative rate was reported as 6.4% after repair of tetralogy of Fallot with pulmonary atresia probably related to the right ventricular to pulmonary arterial conduit. On the other hand, endocarditis was not encountered after secundum atrial septal defect, pulmonic stenosis, or patent ductus arteriosus repair during 30 years of follow-up.[9]

Valvar endocarditis has also been encountered in some patients with *normal* aortic or mitral valves, often due to infection with *Staphylococcus aureus*.[2] Among patients with congenital heart disease, this organism has become more common than *Streptococcus viridans*. This shift in microbial organisms has transformed the corresponding clinical course to a more acute presentation. In the pediatric age group, staphylococcal endocarditis has been associated with a more indolent course with higher complication, surgical intervention, and mortality rates than those that occur with other infectious agents.

In almost all reported series, males are more commonly affected, perhaps related to the very high incidence of aortic valve lesions in males.

PATHOPHYSIOLOGY

Nonbacterial thrombotic endocarditic lesions are proposed to be the substrate for the development of endocarditis in patients with congenital heart disease and those with indwelling intravenous catheters.[5] The high-velocity jet streams of some congenital defects create shear forces that are thought to damage or denude endothelium, resulting in deposition of red blood cells, platelets, and fibrin. Similarly, indwelling catheters may injure the endocardial or endothelial layer. These lesions may then become infected during episodes of bacteremia. Once the bacteria adhere to the damaged endothelial layer, further fibrin and platelet deposition trap the bacteria in the evolving vegetation. Hence, the pathophysiology of infective endocarditis involves generalized bacteremia and regional endocardial injury and valvulitis. Peripheral manifestations, in more chronic disease, are mediated by immune-complex reactions, most notably resulting in glomerulonephritis. However, other organs beside the kidneys can be involved. Equally important to the causation of peripheral manifestations of disease are the potential for both infectious and noninfectious embolic phenomena, with the possibility of many organ systems being involved.

DIAGNOSIS

The clinical presentation of infective endocarditis is quite variable and is related to multiple factors including the patient's age; organism; site of endocarditis; presence of prosthetic material such as a conduit, valve, or indwelling catheter; heart defect; and recent surgery. The clinical findings relate to four underlying factors, namely bacteremia (fungemia), valvulitis, immunologic responses, and emboli, and may be difficult to differentiate from immune complex reactions.[5]

For practical purposes, the endocarditis presentation in the child and/or adolescent may be acute or subacute. Some investigators suggest this terminology be replaced by "describing the disease based on the etiologic agent involved."[10] Although this recommendation has merit, it belies the importance of recognition of the acuity of the clinical disease. Prompt recognition and institution of antibiotic therapy is essential for survival because patients may present in extremis and require antibiotics urgently before laboratory recognition of the infective agent and antibiotic susceptibility are known. However, in patients with a less-indolent subacute disease, delay of antibiotic treatment for up to 48 hours may be the more sagacious course.

Subacute endocarditis generally is associated with persistent low-grade fevers, malaise, weight loss, fatigue, arthralgias, myalgias, rigors, and diaphoresis. In addition, older patients often manifest petechiae, hemorrhages, Roth spots, Osler nodes, and splenomegaly. In contrast, these features are often not obvious in the pediatric patient in whom embolic episodes with distal extremity or major organ ischemia and/or infarction may be early presenting features. Such patients may have gastrointestinal, renal, or central nervous symptoms. In some, neurologic symptoms including headache, seizures, altered mental status and coma may be the initial presenting features.

Acute infective endocarditis is a rapidly progressive, fulminating disease. Such individuals usually present with high spiking fevers and are severely ill and toxic. However, the newborn infant may not present with fever. Signs and symptoms of congestive heart failure and/or even low cardiac output may inexorably progress. The causative organism is often *S. aureus,* which may cause rapid destruction of heart valve tissue, abscess formation, embolic phenomena, and a rapidly progressive deterioration in hemodynamic status. Fungal endocarditis may present with a similar clinical scenario, again especially in the newborn.

Such observations may be helpful if one detects a new murmur of valvar regurgitation or a ventricular septal defect from abscess progression. Occasionally, murmur intensity may increase secondary to the patient's high-output state. Alternatively, murmurs may be inaudible even in patients with acute and fulminant valvar destruction. For example, the murmur of aortic regurgitation may diminish as incompetence increases, aortic diastolic pressure decreases, and the left ventricular end-diastolic pressure increases, and may even become inaudible while being easily discerned by two-dimensional Doppler echocardiography.

The newborn infant, in particular the premature infant, may not present with typical signs of either acute or subacute endocarditis. Fever may be absent even in the presence of septicemia, and/or congestive heart failure. A high proportion of infants have no underlying congenital heart defect and many, especially in an intensive care unit, have indwelling catheters. Such premature infants may present with pneumonia, meningitis or with septic emboli to distal extremities, often with osteomyelitis.[6] Vegetations can occur on either side of the heart. A mortality rate of 55% in this patient population has been reported.[6]

Bacterial endocarditis in the neonate is most often associated with *S. aureus*, coagulase-negative staphylococci, and *Candida albicans*. These organisms reflect the use of indwelling catheters. The latter, used for hyperalimentation and infusion of high-glucose concentration solutions, are also associated with fungal endocarditis and large friable vegetations that may embolize.[6]

Nonspecific laboratory tests such as sedimentation rate, C-reactive protein, and/or rheumatoid factor are frequently elevated indicating an inflammatory process. Anemia may result from hemolysis or as a feature of chronic disease. Renal involvement due to emboli or immune complex reaction may occur, manifested by hematuria, red blood cell casts, and, in severe, cases renal failure.

Diagnosis may be made by acquisition of infected tissue at the time of surgery or from biopsy of septic emboli and supported by polymerase chain reactivity of involved tissue.

LABORATORY DIAGNOSIS

Positive blood cultures continue to be the mainstay for the diagnosis of infective endocarditis. The bacteremia is continuous; therefore, blood cultures can be drawn regardless of the fever cycle.[10] Although sometimes difficult to acquire, 1 to 3 mL of blood in infants and 3 to 5 mL in older children are preferable, with samples from three different sites being initially recommended. If there is no growth by day 2, then two more sets are recommended.[10] Since organisms may be fastidious and slow growing, the laboratory should be alerted to culture the media for 2 weeks or longer.

In a collation of several reported series of infective endocarditis in pediatric patients, gram-positive cocci were the most common causative organisms.[5] *S. viridans* (alpha-hemolytic), and *S. aureus* accounted for 59% to 76% of proven cases. In children older than 1 year, the most prevalent organism was *S. viridans*, whereas *S. aureus* was most often found in newborns and infants. Coagulase-negative staphylococcal endocarditis occurred in 3% to 7% of patients, and enterococcal endocarditis in 4% to 7%. The latter organism is less common than that reported in adult endocarditis series. The fastidious coccobacilli HACEK bacteria (*Haemophilus, Actinobacillus, Vardiobacterium, Eikenella*, and *Kingella*) occurred in 4% to 5% and streptococcal pneumonia in 3% to 7% of cases. The latter organism may be resistant to antibiotics and rapid clinical deterioration may result. Culture-negative endocarditis was reported in 5% to 7% of cases. *S. aureus* or coagulase-negative staphylococcal species are often associated with endocarditis related to prosthetic material, prosthetic valves, and indwelling catheters.[5] Endocarditis related to surgery can occur within 60 days, often requiring removal of the infected prosthetic material.

ECHOCARDIOGRAPHY

Echocardiography has become enormously helpful in diagnosis, allowing for visualization of vegetations and/or other evidence of endocarditis detectable in 50%[11,12] to 82%[13] of pediatric patients. These vegetations may be seen as oscillating intracardiac masses on a valve leaflet or supporting chordae, or be visualized in the path of a turbulent jet of blood passing through an incompetent valve or septal defect. The mass should be confirmed in more than one imaging plane and be seen consistently throughout the cardiac cycle (Fig. 28-1). No other alternative anatomic explanation for the mass should be possible.

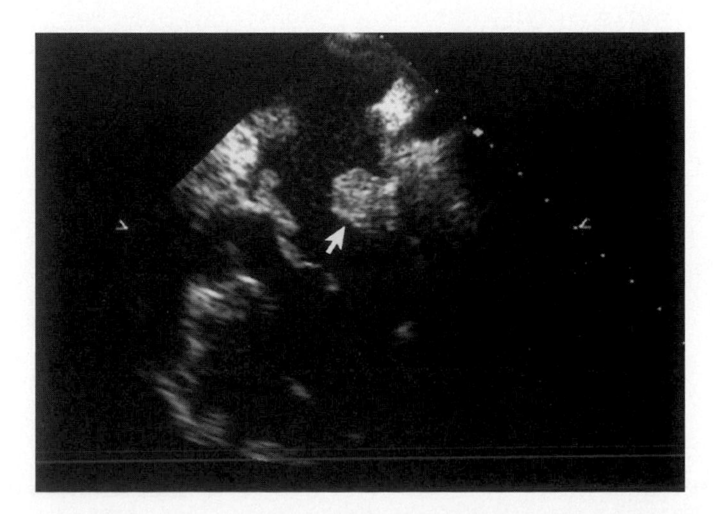

FIGURE 28–1 *Two-dimensional echocardiogram of a mobile echogenic mass on the tricuspid valve leaflet in a neonate with an indwelling line and Candida albicans endocarditis.*

Other abnormalities that may be visualized include an intracardiac abscess (Fig. 28-2) and new dehiscence of a prosthetic valve.

In addition to this important diagnostic role, echocardiography allows for invaluable follow-up for potential complications, including abscess formation, valve destruction and perforation, rupture of chordae, and development or progression of prosthetic paravalvar leaks. Many of these observations have been made in adult patients. Persistence of these vegetations has been reported in some adults even after successful medical treatment.[14] Persistence and morphologic changes in these vegetations have been associated with late complications such as emboli. Severe valvar regurgitation may require valve replacement.[14] Other investigators using transesophageal echocardiography have noted that vegetations larger than 1 cm in diameter were associated with a high incidence of embolization especially if located on the mitral valve.[15]

Thus, although echocardiography has become most important in both diagnosis and follow-up, it is of low yield *as a screening tool* for diagnosis of endocarditis in the pediatric population, especially in those with a low clinical probability of disease, including those with indwelling catheters.[11,16] The yield however is markedly improved when the patient probability is intermediate to high and when blood cultures show positive findings.[16]

In an attempt to improve diagnostic accuracy, scoring systems have been introduced over the years (Tables 28-1 and 28-2). Before echocardiography, Von Reyn and colleagues[17] proposed a classification system in adults that would predict the probability of endocarditis as definite, probable, possible, and absent. The *definite category* mandated a

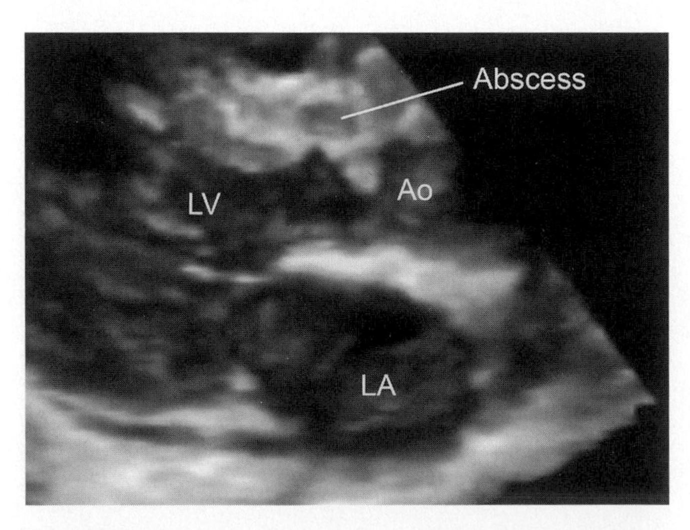

FIGURE 28–2 *Three-dimensional echocardiogram of a retroaortic abscess seen as an echolucent space behind the aortic valve in a teenaged boy with staphylococcal endocarditis.*

TABLE 28–1. Definition of Infective Endocarditis According to the Proposed Modified Duke Criteria*

Definite infective endocarditis
Pathologic criteria
1. Microorganisms demonstrated by culture of histologic examination of vegetation, a vegetation that has embolized, or an intracardiac abscess specimen or
2. Pathologic lesions; vegetation or intracardiac abscess confirmed by histologic examination showing active endocarditis.

Clinical criteria
1. Two major criteria or
2. One major criterion and three minor criteria or
3. Five minor criteria

Possible infective endocarditis
1. One major criterion and one minor criterion or
2. Three minor criteria

Rejected
1. Firm alternate diagnosis explaining evidence of infective endocarditis or
2. Resolution of infective endocarditis syndrome with antibiotic therapy for < 4 d or
3. No pathologic evidence of infective endocarditis at surgery or autopsy, with antibiotic therapy for < 4 d or
4. Does not meet criteria for possible infective endocarditis, as above.

*Modifications shown in bold.
From Li JS, Sexton DJ, Mick N, et al. Proposed modifications to the Duke Criteria for the diagnosis of infective endocarditis. Clin Inf Dis; 30: 633, 2000, with permission.

histologic confirmation and the others were based on physical signs and blood cultures. Because of persistent diagnostic imprecision, the so-called *Duke criteria*[18] were introduced. This revision added echocardiographic observations to the clinical and laboratory findings, while excluding histologic confirmation for the definite category. This system improved diagnostic sensitivity, and in this adult population, transesophageal echocardiography further enhanced diagnostic accuracy. Subsequent studies confirmed these findings.[19,21] However, diagnostic difficulties persisted particularly among those in the *possible group*, those with *S. aureus* bacteremia, and suspected cases of Q fever—even the role of transesophageal echocardiography was questioned.[20,21] These observations led to further revisions such as the addition of specific major and minor criteria. These criteria included a single blood culture or positive IgG antibody titer for *Coxiella burnetii* as a major criterion for diagnosis of Q fever and excluded the echocardiographic minor criteria[21] (Tables 28-1 and 28-2). It was noted by these investigators that transesophageal echocardiography detected evidence of endocarditis in 19% of patients with a negative findings and 21% of patients with intermediate findings. The resulting recommendations included transesophageal echocardiography as an echocardiographic

TABLE 28–2. Definition of Terms Used in the Proposed Modified Duke Criteria for the Diagnosis of Infective Endocarditis (IE)*

Major criteria
Blood culture positive for IE
Typical microorganisms consistent with IE from two separate blood cultures
Viridans streptococci, *Streptococcus bovis*, HACEK group, *Staphylocuccus aureus*; or community-acquired enterococci, in the absence of a primary focus or
Microorganisms consistent with IE from persistently positive blood cultures, defined as follows:
At least two positive cultures of blood samples drawn more than 12 hr apart or
All of three or most of more than four separate cultures of blood (with first and last sample drawn at least 1 hr apart)
Single positive blood culture for *Coxiella burnetii* or antiphase I IgG antibody titer > 1:800
Evidence of endocardial involvement
Echocardiogram positive for IE (**TEE recommended in patients with prosthetic valves, rated at least "possible IE" by clinical criteria, or complicated by IE [paravalvular abscess]; TTE as first test in other patients),** defined as follows:
Oscillating intracardiac mass on valve or supporting structures, in the path of regurgitant jets, or on implanted material in the absence of an alternative anatomic explanation or
Abscess or
New partial dehiscence of prosthetic valve
New valvular regurgitation (worsening or changing of preexisting murmur not sufficient)
Minor criteria
Predisposition, predisposing heart condition or injection drug use
Fever, temperature above 38°C
Vascular phenomena, major arterial emboli, septic pulmonary infarcts, mycotic aneurysm, intracranial hemorrhage, conjunctival hemorrhages, and Janeway lesions
Immunologic phenomena: glomerulonephritis, Osler nodes, Roth spots, and rheumatoid factor
Microbiologic evidence: positive blood culture but does not meet a major criterion as noted above^{+} or serologic evidence of active infection with organism consistent with IE
Echocardiographic minor criteria eliminated

TEE, transesophageal echocardiography; TTE, transthoracic echocardiography.
*Modifications shown in bold.
$^{+}$Excludes single positive culture for coagulase-negative staphylococci and organisms that do not cause endocarditis.
From Li JS, Sexton DJ, Mick N, et al. Proposed modifications to the Duke criteria for the diagnosis of infective endocarditis. Clin Inf Dis; 30:633, 2000. with permission.

first test in patients with prosthetic valves, in those designated as *possible* cases of endocarditis, and in those with complicated infections such as paravalvar abscess. However, transesophageal echocardiography was found to be of limited value in patients with two or fewer minor criteria and in those with definite endocarditis by the standard Duke criteria. In pediatric patients the Duke Criteria sensitivity was better than those with the earlier systems: More cases were classified as definite and fewer were rejected.[22,23] The authors concluded that echocardiographic findings significantly improved diagnostic accuracy and positive blood cultures remained essential for diagnosis.

The superior sensitivity of transesophageal echocardiography among adults compared with that of the transthoracic modality, particularly in those with prosthetic valves, has also been noted by others.[24,25] However, in pediatric patients with positive Duke criteria, transthoracic echocardiography was comparable to the transesophageal approach, although the negative predictive value of transesophageal echocardiography was not studied in the children, none of whom had a prosthetic valve.[26]

TREATMENT

In patients with suspected endocarditis who are not acutely ill, antibiotics may be withheld for up to 48 hours while awaiting blood culture results. However, those presenting with evidence of acute endocarditis or neonates with indwelling lines, sepsis, and hemodynamic instability should receive immediate broad-spectrum coverage. A prolonged course of therapy is necessary because organisms are embedded in a fibrin platelet matrix in high concentrations. The infective organisms' low rates of cell division render them more resistant to antibiotics that affect cellular wall division. Antibiotic sensitivity for the organisms must be determined, including minimal inhibitory concentrations. Blood cultures should be repeated after initiation of therapy to document clearance of bacteremia. All patients are initially treated in the hospital. Later outpatient therapy can be undertaken if the patient is afebrile, has negative blood cultures, and is at negligible risk for complications. Excellent patient and parent compliance is mandatory.

In terms of antibiotic treatment in children, *S. viridans* endocarditis is treated for 4 to 6 weeks with penicillin G or ampicillin intravenously.[5] This assumes penicillin-sensitive streptococci with a minimal inhibitory concentration (MIC) of less than 0.1 μg of penicillin per milliliter. In adults with uncomplicated *S. viridans* endocarditis, a 2-week intravenous course of penicillin, ampicillin, or ceftriaxine combined with gentamicin or a 4-week regimen of ceftriaxine once daily are used. When the streptococci are relatively resistant to penicillin, a 4-week course of penicillin, ampicillin, or ceftriaxine combined with a 2-week course of gentamicin is recommended. Relative resistance implies a MIC above 0.1 μg/mL and below 0.5 μg/m. For children who cannot tolerate a β-lactam antibiotic, the combination of vancomycin and gentamycin has been recommended. However when infection involves a prosthetic valve or patch material, a minimum of 6 weeks of penicillin, ampicillin, or ceftriaxine with 2 weeks of gentamicin is mandatory.

Staphylococcal endocarditis, both coagulase positive and negative, requires a minimum of 6 weeks of intravenous antibiotic therapy with β-lactamase–resistant penicillin, often oxacillin or nafcillin. Again, initial additional synergistic coverage with gentamicin for 3 to 5 days may aid in the destruction of the staphylococcal organisms. For patients that are unable to receive the β-lactamase–resistant penicillin antibiotics, a 6-week course of vancomycin, with or without a 5-day course of gentamicin is recommended. Patients in whom the staphylococcal organism is resistant to the β-lactamase–resistant antibiotics should receive vancomycin. When staphylococcal endocarditis involves prosthetic valve or patch material, surgical intervention is often necessary.

Treatment of culture negative endocarditis should cover staphylococcal, streptococcal (including *S. pneumoniae*), and HACEK organisms. The combination of antibiotic coverage should include ceftriaxine and gentamicin. If staphylococcal endocarditis is suspected, a β-lactamase–resistant penicillin should be added to the regimen. If the organism is not susceptible to a β-lactamase–resistant penicillin, vancomycin should be substituted. Patients with suspected culture-negative endocarditis should be treated for 4 to 6 weeks.

Streptococcal pneumonia endocarditis is relatively rare, accounting for only 3% to 7% of endocarditis in children[5,27] and is accompanied by pneumonia or meningitis in 25%. Although fever occurs in all, vascular- and/or immunologic-related findings are minimal. This is due in part to the acute illness onset and the short interval (4 days) before treatment begins. This infection has been diagnosed at an early age (mean age, 15 months) and is commonly associated with congenital heart disease (91%), and prior heart surgery (50%). In pediatric patients, this organism has been susceptible to penicillin and ceftriaxine. However, despite early treatment, complications requiring cardiovascular surgery have occurred in 36%[11,27] and a mortality rate of 9% has been noted.[27] Fortunately, only 0.4% of pneumococcal bacteremia is associated with endocarditis in children. Considering the pneumococcal serotypes associated with endocarditis in children, polyvalent conjugated vaccine should help to prevent pneumococcal-related disease.

Fungal endocarditis is becoming more prevalent, especially in the newborn infant who is receiving hyperalimentation with a chronic indwelling central venous line. Medical therapy alone is often unsuccessful and surgery may be required. A combination of amphotericin B with 5-fluorocytosine is recommended for candidal fungal endocarditis. Enterococcal endocarditis is rare in pediatrics, and the organism has a high degree of resistance to antibiotics. The recommended treatment is a 6-week course of parenteral ampicillin and gentamicin.

COMPLICATIONS

The cardiovascular complications of endocarditis include abscess formation with para-annular extension and fistulous tract development. The former may be associated with the development of atrioventricular or bundle branch block on the electrocardiogram. Valve leaflet perforation or destruction and chordal rupture may occur as may embolization of vegetations to the central nervous system, kidneys, and other organs. The risk of emboli is more likely with staphylococcal and fungal organisms. Peri-annular extension and abscess formation almost always require surgical intervention, a very difficult undertaking especially when a prosthetic valve is involved or in the presence of paravalvar abscess formation. If feasible, a delay of 1 or more weeks with antibiotic therapy may be beneficial before surgery. However, this is frequently not possible as many of these patients have relentless heart failure and tissue destruction. The Ross procedure has theoretical advantages when acute intervention is necessary in those children whose aortic valve or aortic root are involved. At surgery the infected valve is removed, the root is débrided, and the *pulmonary autograft*, including valve and pulmonary outflow tract, is placed in the native aortic position, with satisfactory short-term results.[28]

PROPHYLAXIS

Endocarditis usually occurs in those with underlying structural cardiac defects who develop bacteremia with organisms likely to cause endocarditis.[29] Using this premise, patients are stratified into high-, moderate-, and negligible-risk groups on the basis of potential outcome if endocarditis develops (Table 28-3). Prophylaxis is recommended for those in the high- and moderate-risk groups. High-risk patients include those with prosthetic valves, a previous history of endocarditis, complex cyanotic heart disease, or surgically created systemic-to-pulmonary artery shunts or conduits. The moderate category includes uncorrected congenital cardiac lesions such as patent ductus arteriosus, ventricular septal defect, primum atrial septal defect, coarctation of the aorta, and bicuspid aortic valve. Other moderate-risk lesions include hypertrophic cardiomyopathy and acquired valve dysfunction from rheumatic heart disease or collagen vascular disorders. The negligible-risk category, for which bacterial endocarditis prophylaxis is not recommended, includes isolated secundum atrial septal defects, atrial and ventricular septal defects, and patent ductus arteriosi 6 months after surgical repair without residual shunts. Although prophylaxis for mitral valve prolapse alone continues to be debatable, it is recommended in those with a mitral regurgitation murmur or echocardiographic

TABLE 28–3. Cardiac Conditions Associated with Endocarditis

Endocarditis prophylaxis recommended
High-risk category
Prosthetic cardiac valves, including bioprosthetic and homograft valves
Previous bacterial endocarditis
Complex cyanotic heart disease (e.g., single-ventricle states, transposition of the great arteries, tetralogy of Fallot)
Surgically constructed systemic pulmonary shunts or conduits
Moderate-risk category
Most other congenital cardiac malformations (other than above and below)
Acquired valvar dysfunction (e.g., rheumatic heart disease)
Hypertrophic cardiomyopathy
Mitral valve prolapse with valvar regurgitation and/or thickened leaflets*
Endocarditis prophylaxis not recommended
Negligible-risk category (no greater risk than the general population)
Isolated secundum atrial septal defect
Surgical repair of atrial septal defect, ventricular septal defect, or patent ductus arteriosus (without residua beyond 6 mo)
Previous coronary artery bypass graft surgery
Mitral valve prolapse without valvar regurgitation*
Physiologic, functional, or innocent heart murmurs*
Previous Kawasaki disease without valvar dysfunction
Previous rheumatic fever without valvar dysfunction
Cardiac pacemakers (intracardiac and epicardial) and implanted defibrillators

*From Dajani AS, Taubert KA, Wilson W. Prevention of bacterial endocarditis, Recommendations by the American Heart Association. JAMA 277:1794, 1997, with permission.

evidence of real regurgitation. Adequate dental hygiene, with antibiotic prophylaxis in those at risk at times of treatment, is most important, albeit still misunderstood by many patients and parents.[30,31]

Thus current recommendations for prophylaxis (Tables 28-4 and 28-5)[29] include coverage for at-risk patients undergoing dental or oral procedures likely to cause bacteremia, these being invariably associated with bleeding. In addition, coverage is also advised for procedures such as tonsillectomy, adenoidectomy, and some respiratory tract manipulations such as rigid bronchoscopy. Coverage is not deemed necessary for flexible bronchoscopy, endotracheal intubation, and tympanostomy tube insertion. Concerning the gastrointestinal tract, prophylaxis is recommended for procedures likely associated with bacteremia, such as sclerotherapy for esophageal varices, dilation of esophageal strictures, and biliary tract procedures and operations that involve the intestinal mucosa. Coverage for transesophageal echocardiography or endoscopy is not considered necessary.

The genitourinary tract is second only to the oral cavity as a portal of entry for organisms that are likely to cause endocarditis. Certain procedures such as prostate surgery, cystoscopy, and urethral dilation are associated with a particularly high rate of bacteremia in the presence of a urinary tract infection, and hence prophylaxis is recommended. It is not considered necessary for certain procedures in uninfected tissues, including urethral catheterization, circumcision, uterine dilation and curettage, therapeutic abortion, sterilization procedures, removal or insertion of intrauterine devices, vaginal hysterectomy, vaginal delivery, and cesarean delivery. Antibiotics effective against the urinary pathogen (e.g., enteric gram-negative bacilli),

TABLE 28–4. Prophylactic Regimens for Dental, Oral, Respiratory Tract, or Esophageal Procedures

Situation	Agents*	Regimen⁺
Standard general prophylaxis	Amoxicillin	Adults; 2 g; children: 50 mg/kg orally 1 hr before procedure
Unable to take oral medication	Ampicillin	Adults: 2 g intramuscularly (IM) or intravenously (IV); children 50 mg/kg IM or IV within 30 min before procedure
Allergic to penicillin	Clindamycin	Adults: 600 mg; children 20 mg/kg or orally 1 hr before procedure
	Cephalexin⁺ or cefadroxil⁺	Adults: 2.0 g; children 50 mg/kg or orally 1 hr before procedure
	Azithromicin or clarithromycin	Adults: 500 mg; children: 15 mg/kg or orally 1 hr before procedure
Allergic to penicillin and unable to take oral medications	Clindamycin or Cefazolin⁺	Adults: 600 mg; children 20 mg/kg IV within 30 min before procedure
		Adults: 1.0 g; children: 25 mg/kg or IV within 30 min before procedure

*Total children's dose should not exceed adult dose.
⁺Cephalosporins should not be used in individuals with immediate-type hypesensitivity reaction (urticaria, angloedema, or anaphylaxis) to penicillins.
From Dajani AS, Taubert KA, Wilson W. Prevention of bacterial endocarditis: recommendations by the American Heart Association. JAMA 277: 1794, 1997, with permission.

TABLE 28–5. Prophylactic Regimens for Genitourinary, Gastrointestinal (Excluding Esophageal) Procedures

Situation	Agents*	Regimen+
High-risk patients	Ampicillin plus Gentamicin	Adults: ampicillin 2 g intramuscularly (IM) or intravenously (IV) plus gentamicin 1.5 mg/kg (not to exceed 120 mg) within 30 min of starting the procedure; 6 hr later, ampicillin 1 g IM/IV or amoxicillin 1 g orally Children: ampicillin 50 mg/kg IM or IV (not to exceed 2.0 g) plus gentamicin 1.5 mg/kg within 30 min of starting the procedure, 6 hr later, ampicillin 25 mg/kg IM/IV or amoxicillin 25 mg/kg orally
High-risk patients allergic to ampicillin/ amoxicillin	Vancomycin plus Gentamicin	Adults: vancomycin 1.0 g IV over 1-2 hr plus gentamicin 1.5 IV/IM (not to exceed 120 mg; complete injection/infusion within 30 min of starting procedure) Children: vancomycin 20 mg/kg IV over 1–2 hr plus gentamicin 1.5 mg/kg IV/IM; complete injection/infusion within 30 min of starting the procedure
Moderate-risk patients	Amoxicillin or Ampicillin	Adults: amoxicillin 2.0 g orally 1 hr before procedure, or ampicillin 2.0 g IM/IV within 30 min of starting the procedure Children: amoxicillin 50 mg/kg orally 1 hr before procedure, or ampicillin 50 mg/kg IM/IV within 30 min of starting the procedure
Moderate-risk patients allergic to ampicillin/ amoxicillin	Vancomycin	Adults: vancomycin 1.0 g IV over 1–2 hr; complete infusion within 30 min of starting the procedure Children: vancomycin 20 mg/kg IV over 1–2 hr; complete infusion within 30 min of starting the procedure

*Total children's dose should not exceed adult dose.

+No second dose of vancomycin or gentamycin is recommended.

From Dajani AS, Taubert KA, Wilson W, et al. Prevention of bacterial endocarditis: recommendations by the American Heart Association. JAMA 277:1794, 1997, with permission.

in addition to the enterococcus, should be administered before invasive genitourinary procedures.

The most common causative organisms of endocarditis after dental, oral, or upper respiratory procedures, rigid bronchoscopy, and surgery involving the upper respiratory tract and esophagus is *S. viridans*. For coverage, a single dose of amoxacillin orally 1 hour before the procedure is the current recommendation, 2 g in adults and 50 mg/kg (not to exceed 2 g) in children. Although ampicillin and penicillin V provide equally adequate coverage, amoxacillin is preferred because of enhanced absorption and higher and more sustained serum levels. A second dose, 4 to 6 hours after the procedure, is no longer recommended. For those patients who cannot receive oral medication, intramuscular or intravenous ampicillin is recommended within 30 minutes of the procedure. Erythromycin is no longer recommended: Significant gastrointestinal disturbance sometimes resulted and, in this author's experience, was often the reason for prophylaxis noncompliance. Clindamycin is recommended as an alternative, orally or intravenously. Orally, the recommended adult dose is 600 mg and in children 20 mg/kg 1 hour before the procedure. Rarely, but importantly, clindamycin has been associated with life-threatening pseudo-membranous colitis. In the absence of penicillin allergy, first-generation cephalosporin antibiotics may be used, including cephalexin or cefadroxil (adult dose, 2 g; pediatric dose, 50 mg/kg) orally 1 hour before the procedure or intravenous cefazolin 1 g in adults and 25 mg/kg in children. Alternatives for oral drugs include azithromycin or clarithromycin.

Prophylaxis for genitourinary procedures should include coverage against enterococci for the high-risk, but not the low-risk, patient. High-risk patients should receive parenteral ampicillin and gentamicin 30 minutes before the procedure, and intravenous ampicillin or oral amoxacillin 6 hours later. The preprocedure dose of ampicillin in adults is 2 g, and 50 mg/kg in children, and for gentamicin the childhood and adult dose is 1.5 mg/kg, not to exceed 120 mg. Six hours after the procedure, the adult can receive either 1 g of intravenous ampicillin, or 1 g of amoxacillin, and the child ampicillin or amoxacillin 25 mg/kg. High-risk patients allergic to penicillin should receive vancomycin and gentamycin. In adults the intravenous dose is 1 g over 1 to 2 hours, and in children the vancomycin dose is 20 mg/kg. Medium-risk patients can receive oral amoxacillin or intravenous ampicillin before the procedure. No post-procedural antibiotic is recommended. Patients allergic to penicillin can receive vancomycin as an alternative.

Patients receiving antibiotics chronically should receive an antibiotic from a different class for prophylaxis. If a patient is undergoing an incision and drainage procedure involving infected material, he or she should receive prophylaxis directed toward the most common pathogen. Antibiotic coverage directed toward *S. aureus* should be used for nonoral soft-tissue infections such as cellulitis, osteomyelitis, and pyogenic arthritis. As the author has seen *S. aureus* acute endocarditis in teenagers and young adults with pustular acne, it is reasonable to refer such patients to a dermatologist for skin care.

The preceding prophylactic recommendations are not universally accepted.[32,33] Some investigators believe that (a) no correlation exists between oral postprocedural bleeding and the risk of endocarditis and (b) that significant bacteremia can occur in the absence of clinically discernible bleeding. In addition, (c) bacteremia intensity in humans after an oral procedure is significantly less than that in an experimental model, and therefore unlikely in children to result in endocarditis and (d) the cumulative exposure to bacteremia is significantly greater from everyday procedures than when compared with that of dental procedures. Nevertheless, although prophylaxis for dental procedures may be controversial, good oral hygiene and a health care system supporting regular dental visits remains vital.

REFERENCES

1. Van Hare GF, Ben-Shachar G, Liebman J, et al. Infective endocarditis in infants and children during the past 10 years: a decade of change. Am Heart J 107:1234; 1984.
2. Saiman L, Prince A, Gersony WM. Pediatric infective endocarditis in the modern era. J Pediatr 122: 847,1993.
3. Martin JM, Neches WH, Wald ER. Infective endocarditis: 35 years of experience at a children's hospital. Clin Inf Dis 24:669, 1997.
4. Ashkenazi S, Leavy O, Bleiden L. Trends of childhood infective endocarditis in Israel with emphasis on children under 2 years of age. Pediatr Cardiol 18:419, 1997.
5. Ferrieri P, Gewitz MH, Gerber MA, et al. Unique features of infective endocarditis in childhood. Circulation 105:2115, 2002.
6. Pearlman SA, Higgins S, Eppes S, et al. Infective endocarditis in the premature infant. Clin Pediatr 37:741,1998.
7. Oelberg DG. Editorial. Neonatal endocarditis: neither rare nor fatal. Clin Pediatr 37:747, 1998.
8. Gersony WM, Hayes CJ, Driscoll DJ, et al. Bacterial endocarditis in patients with aortic stenosis, pulmonary stenosis or ventricular septal defect. Circulation 87(Suppl):1, 1993.
9. Morris CD, Reller MD, Menashe VD.Thirty-year incidence of infective endocarditis after surgery for congenital heart disease. JAMA 279:599, 1998.
10. Dajani AS, Taubert KA.Infective endocarditis. In Allen HD, Gutgesell HP, Clark EB, Driscoll DJ (eds). Heart Disease in Infants, Children, and Adolescents. Philadelphia: Lippincott Williams and Wilkins, 2001, pp 1297–1308.
11. Aly AM, Simpson PM, Humes RA, et al. The role of transthoracic echocardiography in the diagnosis of infective endocarditis in children. Ach Pediatr Adolesc Med 153:950, 1999.
12. McMahon CJ, Ayres N, Pignatelli RH.Echocardiographic presentations of endocarditis, and risk factors for rupture of a sinus of Valsalva in childhood. Cardiol Young 13:168, 2003.
13. Kavey RE, Frank DM, Byrum CJ, et al. Two-dimensional echocardiographic assessment of endocarditis in children. Am J Dis Child 137: 851, 1983.
14. Vuille C, Nidorf M, Weyman AE. Natural history of vegetations during successful medical treatment of endocarditis. Am Heart J 128:1200,1994.
15. Mugge A, Werner GD, Frank G. Echocardiography in infective endocarditis: reassessment of prognostic implications of vegetation size determined by the transthoracic and transesophageal approach. J Am Coll Cardiol 14: 631, 1989.
16. Michelfelder EC, Ochsner JE, Khoury P, et al. Does assessment of pretest probability of disease improve the utility of echocardiography in suspected endocarditis in children? J Pediatr 142: 263, 2003.
17. Von Reyn CF, Levy BS, Arbeit RD, et al. Infective endocarditis: An analysis based on strict case definitions. Ann Int Med 94:505, 1981.
18. Durack DT, Lukes AS, Bright DK. New criteria for diagnosis of infective endocarditis: utilization of specific echocardiographic findings. Am J Med 96:200, 1994.
19. Heiro M, Nikoskelainen J, Hartiala J, et al. Diagnosis of endocarditis: sensitivity of the Duke vs von Reyn criteria. Arc Inter Med 158:18, 1998.
20. Habib G, Derumeaux G, Avierinos JF, et al. Value and limitations of the Duke criteria for the diagnosis of infective endocarditis. J Am Coll Cardiol 22:2023, 1999.
21. Li JS, Sexton DJ, Mick N, et al. Proposed modifications to the Duke criteria for the diagnosis of infective endocarditis. Clin Inf Dis 30:633, 2000.
22. Stockheim, et al. Are the Duke criteria superior to the Beth Israel criteria for the diagnosis of infective endocarditis in children? Clin Inf Dis 27:1451, 1998.
23. Tissieres P, Gervaix A, Beghetti M, et al. Value and limitations of the von Reyn, Duke and modified Duke criteria for the diagnosis of infective endocarditis in children. Pediatrics 112: 467,2003.
24. Roe MT, Abramson MA, Li J, et al. Clinical information determines the impact of transesophageal echocardiography on the diagnosis of infective endocarditis by the Duke criteria. Am Heart J 139:945, 2000.
25. Sochowski R, Kwan-Leung K. Implication of negative results on a monoplane transesophageal echocardiographic study in patients with suspected infective endocarditis. J Am Coll Cardiol 21:216, 1993.
26. Humpl T, McCrindle B, Smallhorn J. The relative roles of transthoracic compared with transesophageal echocardiography in children with suspected infective endocarditis. J Am Coll Cardiol 41: 2068, 2003.
27. Givner LB, Mason EO, Tan TQ, et al; Pneumococcal endocarditis in children. Clin Inf Dis 38:1273, 2004.

28. Birk E, Sharoni E, Dagan O, et al. The Ross procedure as the surgical treatment of active aortic valve endocarditis. J Heart Valve Dis 13:73, 2004.
29. Dajani AS, Taubert KA, Wilson W. Prevention of bacterial endocarditis: recommendations by the American Heart Association. JAMA 277:1794, 1997.
30. Knirsch W, Hassberg D, Beyer A, et al. Knowledge, compliance and practice of antibiotic endocarditis prophylaxis of patients with congenital heart disease. Pediatr Cardiol 24: 344, 2003.
31. Balmer R, Bulock FA. The experiences with oral health and dental prevention of children with congenital heart disease. Cardiol Young 13:439, 2003.
32. Roberts GJ, Holzel HS, Sury MR. Dental bacteremia in children. Pediatr Cardiol 18:24, 1997.
33. Roberts GJ. Dentists are innocent! "Everyday" bacteremia is the real culprit: a review and assessment of the evidence that dental surgical procedures are a principal cause of bacterial endocarditis in children. Pediatr Cardiol 20:317, 1999.

29

Cardiac Arrhythmias

EDWARD P. WALSH, CHARLES I. BERUL,
AND JOHN K. TRIEDMAN

This chapter is intended as a practical overview of the diagnosis and treatment of cardiac arrhythmias in young patients. Although the topic has occupied entire textbooks, the purpose here is to focus on select material that would be of most benefit to residents, fellows, and clinicians working in an acute care setting. For this reason, emphasis has been placed on the surface electrocardiogram (ECG) as the principal tool for diagnosis, with only brief reference to intracardiac electrophysiologic testing and catheter mapping procedures. Readers who are inexperienced or tentative with ECG interpretation may wish to consult Chapters 12 and 61 of this textbook to familiarize themselves with the principals of normal cellular electrophysiology and ECG recording theory before embarking on a discussion of abnormal rhythms. Conversely, those who desire more comprehensive information on arrhythmia management are directed to any of the contemporary textbooks dedicated exclusively to this topic.[1–4]

PATHOPHYSIOLOGY OF ARRHYTHMIAS

Arrhythmias may result from disorders of impulse generation (too fast or too slow), disorders of impulse conduction (block or reentry), or any combination thereof. These abnormalities are best understood by first examining their cellular origin.[5] Admittedly, some of the cellular models used to explain arrhythmias are derived from experimental preparations of isolated heart tissue and cannot always be verified as the exact cause of a clinical rhythm disorder in the intact human heart.[6] Nevertheless, close correlation between these *in vitro* models, and the often stereotypic pattern of rhythm disorders *in vivo*, permits intelligent speculation regarding underlying mechanisms.

Etiology of Premature Beats and Tachycardias

Normally, by virtue of its rapid spontaneous depolarization, the sinoatrial (SA) node can claim priority as the natural pacemaker of the heart. Premature beats and tachycardias may preempt SA node activity owing to disorders of either reentry or automaticity.

Reentry

By far the most common mechanism for tachycardia is the phenomenon of reentry. Reentry implies that a single stimulus or excitation wavefront can return and reactivate the same tissue from whence it came (Fig. 29-1). Because cardiac cells require a refractory period after initial depolarization, the return stimulus cannot simply walk backward in its old footsteps. There must be a second pathway in the circuit (limb B in Fig. 29-1), and the excitation wavefront must be sufficiently delayed at some point in the circuit to allow recovery of the original tissue (limb A in Fig. 29-1). An additional requirement is that the return limb somehow be protected against the initial depolarization, which is to say there must be unidirectional anterograde block of the original stimulus in limb B so that it will not be refractory to retrograde conduction. When all three conditions (dual pathways, conduction delay, and unidirectional block) are satisfied, single echo beats or a sustained reentrant arrhythmia can follow. Reentry will terminate promptly whenever conduction in one limb is sufficiently modified

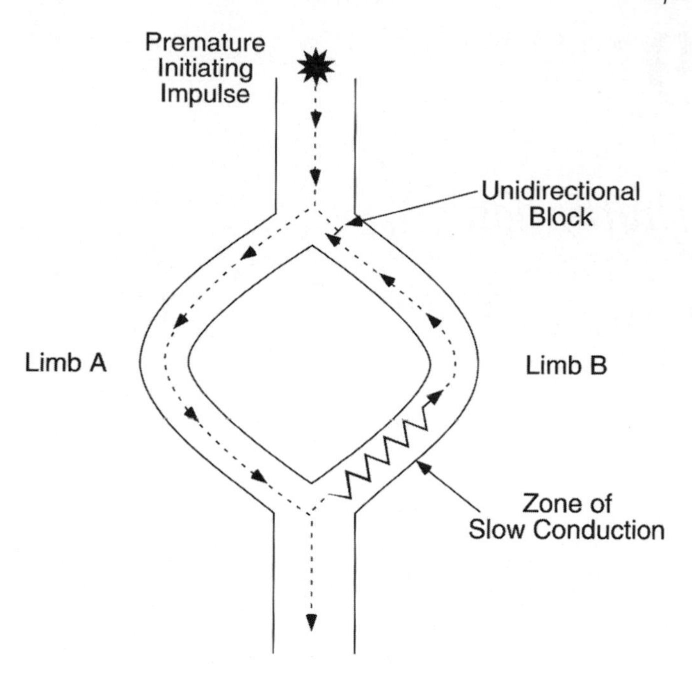

FIGURE 29–1 *Diagram showing the three classic requirements for reentry: (1) dual pathways, (2) unidirectional, anterograde block in limb B, and (3) an area of slow conduction (wavy line in limb B) that allows time for limb A to recover from initial depolarization. The zone of slow conduction can be located anywhere along the circuit.*
From Fyler DC [ed]. Nadas' Pediatric Cardiology. Philadelphia: Hanley & Belfus, 1992.

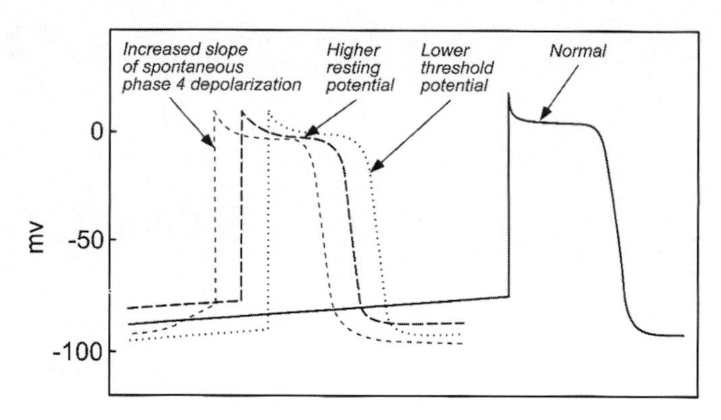

FIGURE 29–2 *Theoretical changes in cellular conditions that can promote abnormal automaticity. The "normal" action potential in this example is a hypothetical Purkinje cell with gradual phase 4 depolarization that will eventually reach threshold potential and generator action potentials at slow rates. Changes in resting potential, threshold potential, or the slope of phase 4 can cause premature depolarization.*
From Fyler DC [ed]. Nadas' Pediatric Cardiology. Philadelphia: Hanley & Belfus, 1992.

or interrupted, using such techniques as overdrive pacing, medications, electrical cardioversion, or catheter ablation.[7]

A classic example of reentry occurs in Wolff-Parkinson White syndrome (WPW), which utilizes the atrioventricular (AV) node and an accessory AV pathway as the two limbs of the circuit. This syndrome represents a natural laboratory for study of the reentry phenomenon to the point of being called the "Rosetta Stone" of electrophysiology.[8] Reentry also appears to be the operative mechanism for atrial flutter (reentry in atrial muscle), atrial fibrillation (multiple atrial reentry circuits), AV node reentry, and probably most forms of ventricular tachycardia. The detailed physiology of these individual disorders is presented later in this chapter.

The general clinical features of reentry include: (1) ability to initiate and terminate tachycardia with appropriately timed premature beats, (2) a narrow range of rates with minimal beat-to-beat variation, (3) paroxysmal onset and termination, (4) predictable pharmacologic response, (5) successful termination with direct-current (DC) shock, and (6) elimination with strategic ablation of one limb of the circuit. Such characteristics can be used to assign a mechanism of reentry to a clinical arrhythmia with reasonable certainty.

Abnormal Automaticity

Enhanced automaticity of a focus outside the SA node can result from any change in cell membrane condition that promotes early achievement of threshold potential (Fig. 29-2). A single abnormal discharge can generate an isolated ectopic beat, whereas repetitive discharge can create a sustained automatic tachycardia.[9] Abnormal automaticity of this type has been implicated as the possible mechanism for a few unusual arrhythmias in children, including ectopic atrial tachycardia,[10] junctional ectopic tachycardia, and some atypical ventricular tachycardias. Clinical characteristics that suggest such a mechanism include (1) inability to initiate or terminate the arrhythmia with pacing maneuvers, (2) resistance to DC cardioversion, (3) wide variation in tachycardia rate proportional to sympathetic tone, (4) very atypical pharmacologic response, and (5) a focal disorder by intracardiac mapping that can be eliminated with a single well-positioned ablation lesion at the epicenter of electrical activation. These characteristics stand in sharp contrast to the behavior of reentrant tachycardia and are easily distinguished in the clinical setting.

Triggered Automaticity

A third possible form of spontaneous cellular depolarization is the phenomenon of triggered automaticity. The electrical triggers in this case are small oscillations that can occur during phase 3 (*early afterdepolarizations*) or phase 4 (*late afterdepolarizations*) of a cellular action potential (Fig. 29-3). If the oscillations are sufficiently high in amplitude, the threshold potential is exceeded, and the cell will be triggered to generate one or more premature beats.[11,12]

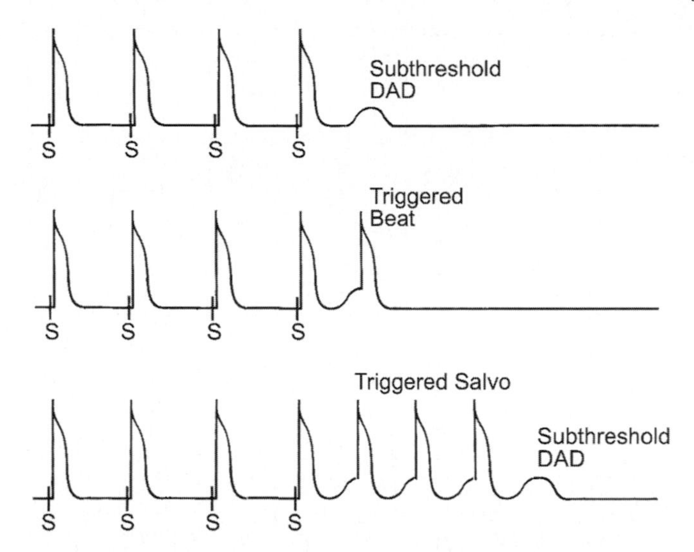

FIGURE 29–3 *Diagrammatic demonstration of delayed afterdepolarization (DAD) and triggered activity. A cell is paced (s) to generate action potentials. At termination of the pacing drive train, there is a delayed oscillation of the cellular potential. If the oscillation is of low amplitude, triggering does not occur (A). If the oscillation exceeds threshold potential, it may trigger single beats (B) or series of beats (C).*
From Fyler DC [ed]. Nadas' Pediatric Cardiology. Philadelphia: Hanley & Belfus, 1992.

In experimental preparations, hypokalemia, high levels of catecholamines, certain antiarrhythmic drugs, and hypoxic injury can produce early afterdepolarizations. Toxic levels of cardiac glycosides, acute hyponatremia, and exposure to norepinephrine can produce the delayed type.

Efforts to define clinical features of triggered tachycardias in the intact heart can be frustrating because there is wide overlap with characteristics of both reentry and abnormal automatic foci. Features in common with reentry include ability to initiate and terminate tachycardia with pacing maneuvers[13] and termination with DC shock. Features in common with abnormal automaticity include wide variation in rate (with *warm-up* at initiation and *cool-down* at termination), as well as sensitivity to catecholamines. Microelectrode studies of human atrial and ventricular tissue have clearly demonstrated early and late afterdepolarizations in vitro,[14] and it is highly likely that triggered activity is operative in some clinical rhythm disorders such as long QT syndrome. However, at present, there is no clinical recording tool that can positively confirm afterdepolarizations in the intact heart.

Bradycardia and Block

Slow heart rates result from depressed depolarization in natural pacemaker cells, block of electrical activation, or both. When SA node automaticity is impaired, one of several latent pacemaker sites in the atrium or AV conducting tissue normally assumes responsibility for generating cardiac rhythm. The escape rate depends on the level of the new pacemaker; foci located in more distal portions of the conducting system have slower phase 4 depolarization and, hence, produce lower rates. Latent pacemakers (particularly those below the AV node) also lack the rich autonomic influence found at the SA node and may exhibit a blunted chronotropic response to exertion and stress.

Block may occur at any stage of the cardiac excitation process. This includes *exit block* (Fig. 29-4) and *entrance block* at a pacemaker focus, or *conduction block* of an established depolarization wavefront at various levels of the heart. Block is a physiologic event if an initiating impulse is premature and arrives at a cardiac site during normal refractoriness, whereas pathologic block occurs in the setting of abnormally long refractory periods, abnormally slow conduction velocity, or complete electrical discontinuity.

There is some merit to a scheme that correlates patterns of block on the surface ECG with the specific type of cardiac cells involved in the event. Generally, slow-response cells of the SA node and AV node (mostly dependent on calcium channel activation) demonstrate a characteristic sequence of gradual and progressive conduction delay in response to an increasingly premature stimulus, culminating in block of an impulse. This pattern is known as *decremental conduction* and creates the familiar Wenckebach periodicity that is a hallmark of conduction delay in these tissues. It is rather unusual to observe this same phenomenon in fast-response cells of the His-Purkinje system, accessory pathways (APs), or working myocardium. With few exceptions, conduction through these areas tends to be all or none,

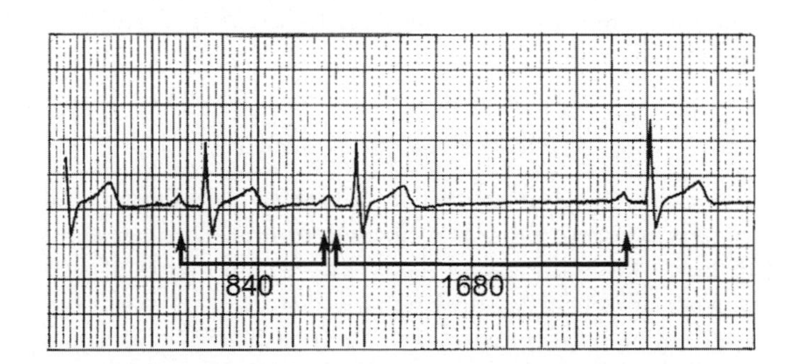

FIGURE 29–4 *An example of probable exit block from the sinoatrial (SA) node. The resting cycle length for sinus node discharge is 840 msec. An abrupt pause in sinus rhythm is then observed, lasting exactly twice that interval. This presumably corresponds to block of conduction between the SA node discharge and atrial muscle.*
From Fyler DC [ed]. Nadas' Pediatric Cardiology. Philadelphia: Hanley & Belfus, 1992.

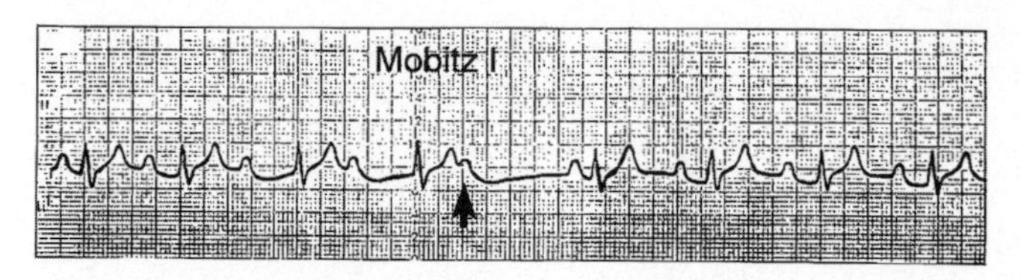

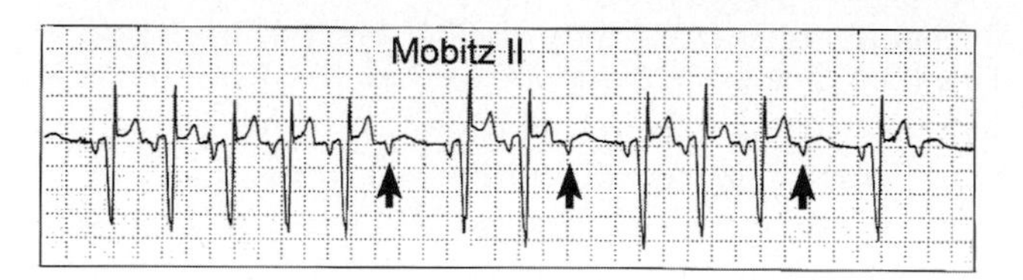

FIGURE 29–5 *Comparison of conduction block in the slow-response cells of the AV node (Mobitz I) and the fast-response cells of the His Purkinje system (Mobitz II).*
From Fyler DC [ed]. Nadas' Pediatric Cardiology. Philadelphia: Hanley & Belfus, 1992.

such that episodic block is an unheralded event. A familiar clinical example of these concepts involves the contrast between AV conduction disturbances due to disease in the AV node (Mobitz I block) and disease in the bundle of His (Mobitz II block). The former shows gradual lengthening of the P-R interval before a blocked P wave, whereas the latter shows only an abrupt nonconducted beat (Fig. 29-5).

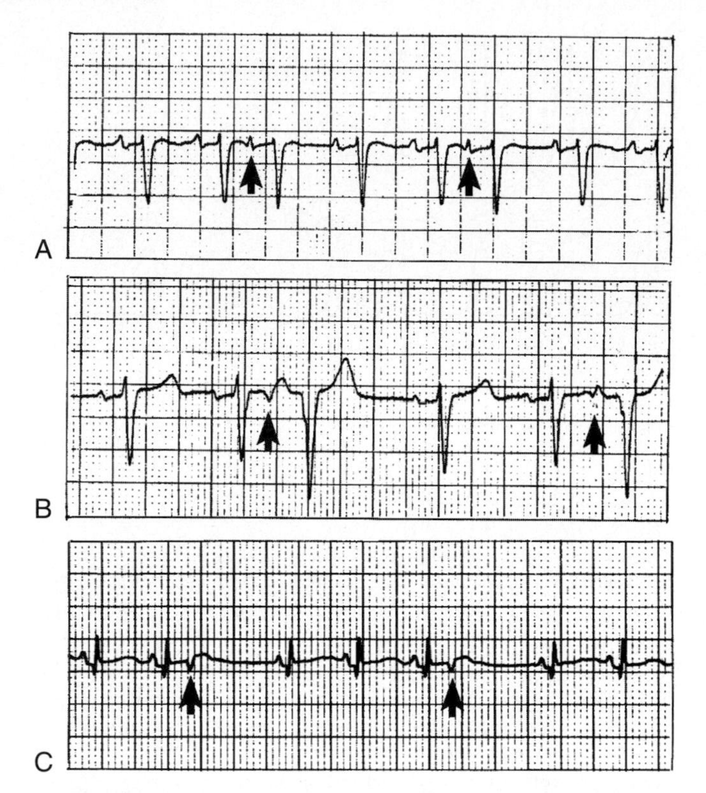

FIGURE 29–6 *Atrial premature beats (marked by arrow) causing (A) normal QRS, (B) conduction with aberration, and (C) block.*
From Fyler DC [ed]. Nadas' Pediatric Cardiology. Philadelphia: Hanley & Belfus, 1992.

PREMATURE BEATS

Premature beats are common in the pediatric age group, with atrial ectopy predominating in infants or young children, and ventricular ectopy during adolescence.[15] Although isolated premature beats are usually benign, they may serve as markers of more serious underlying pathology or as the initiating impulses for reentry tachycardias in susceptible individuals.

Atrial Premature Beats

Atrial ectopy appears on the ECG as an early P wave with an axis and morphology differing from the normal sinus P wave. Atrial premature beats are usually followed by a normal QRS (Fig. 29-6A), but when sufficiently early, can conduct with QRS aberration (see Fig. 29-6B) or become blocked at the AV node (see Fig. 29-6C). If the patient is completely asymptomatic and the physical examination is otherwise normal, occasional atrial premature beats are most always benign and do not necessarily warrant further investigation. However, in any child with symptoms of dizziness or sustained palpitations, atrial premature beats could be a manifestation of an underlying reentry circuit or automatic focus with the potential for supraventricular tachycardia. Surveillance testing with a Holter monitor or event recorder may be indicated for such patients. In asymptomatic individuals, the diagnostic evaluation is expanded only if the beats are very frequent or seem to arise from multiple foci (i.e., variable morphologies for the P wave), in which case hyperthyroidism, structural heart disease, and cardiomyopathy may need to be considered as possible causes.

Junctional Premature Beats

Single ectopic beats arising from the AV node or proximal His-Purkinje system are rather rare. The ECG reveals an early normal QRS but no preceding P wave (Fig. 29-7). Prognostic and diagnostic considerations are generally similar to those for atrial premature beats. Occasionally, junctional premature beats can affect AV conduction if their timing coincides with a normal atrial depolarization. Collision of the premature beat with a normal atrial impulse can mimic abrupt AV block by the mechanism of *concealed conduction* and, thus, junctional premature beats may be considered in the differential diagnosis of some atypical AV conduction abnormalities.

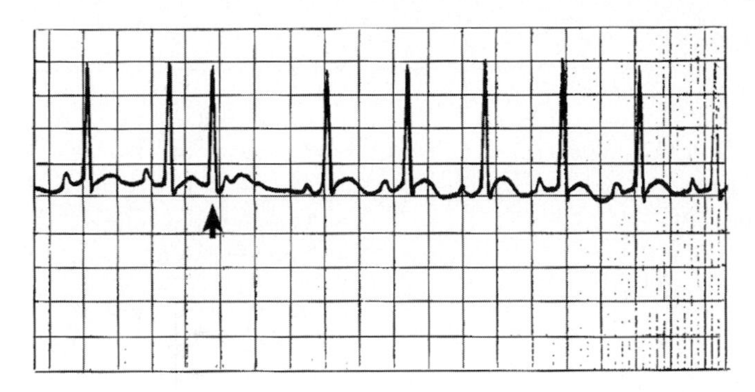

FIGURE 29–7 *Junctional premature beat. Note that the early QRS is identical to a sinus beat, but is not preceded by a P wave. From Fyler DC [ed]. Nadas' Pediatric Cardiology. Philadelphia: Hanley & Belfus, 1992.*

Ventricular Premature Beats

Ventricular ectopy is characterized by an early beat with a wide and abnormal QRS complex, without a preceding P wave (Fig. 29-8). The T-wave axis is usually directed opposite to the QRS. Ventricular ectopy can usually be distinguished from aberrant atrial premature beats by the absence of a premature P wave and the presence of a fully compensatory pause (Fig. 29-9).

Ventricular premature beats are common. They are reported to occur in about 1% to 2% of all pediatric patients with ostensibly normal hearts, and clinical follow-up of such subjects has revealed a generally benign prognosis. However, there does appear to be a definite age predilection for benign ventricular ectopy. From studies of Holter recordings, ventricular ectopy is clearly more common after puberty, occurring in only 1% of normal infants and children[16] compared with 50% to 60% of healthy teenagers and young adults.[17] The physiologic basis for this age distinction is not clear, but it does support the notion that ventricular premature beats may be of less concern during the adolescent years.

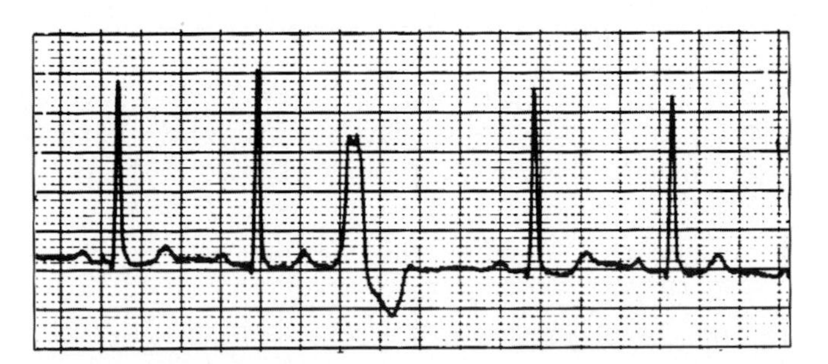

FIGURE 29–8 *Ventricular premature beat showing distortion of the QRS and T wave.*
From Fyler DC [ed]. Nadas' Pediatric Cardiology. Philadelphia: Hanley & Belfus, 1992.

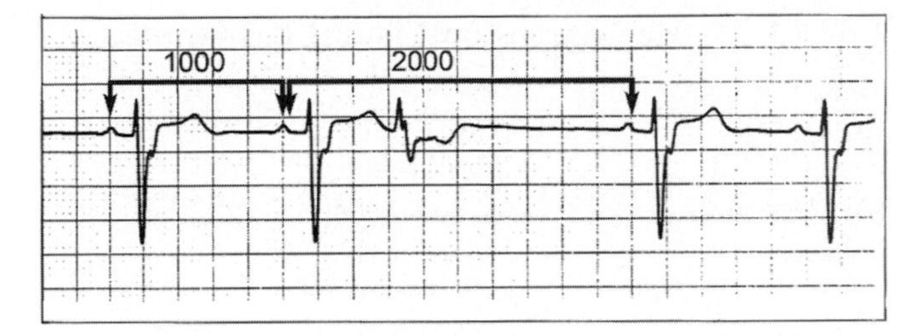

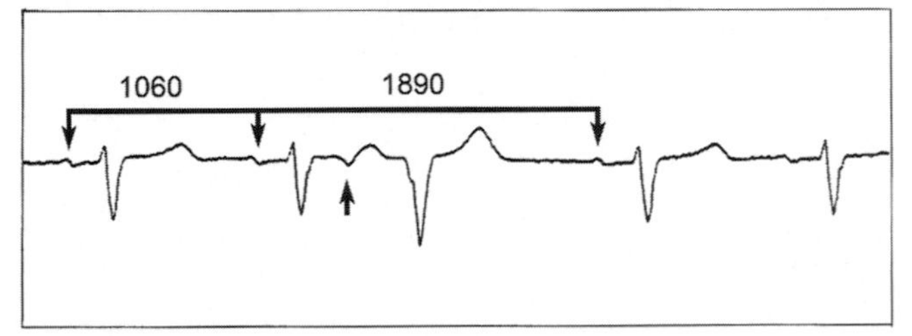

FIGURE 29–9 *Comparison of a ventricular premature beat (A) and an atrial premature beat with aberration (B). Note that the pause following ventricular ectopy is typically "compensatory" (i.e., the interval between P waves for the sinus beats flanking the ectopic beat is exactly twice that for sinus rhythm). The pause following atrial ectopy is "noncompensatory," and the premature P wave (arrow) can be seen.*
From Fyler DC [ed]. Nadas' Pediatric Cardiology. Philadelphia: Hanley & Belfus, 1992.

Unfortunately, ventricular ectopy on a routine ECG cannot always be dismissed out of hand because it may be a manifestation of more serious underlying arrhythmias. For this reason, many patients with ventricular premature beats undergo Holter monitoring. The appearance of higher-grade ectopy on long-term monitoring may indicate the need for an expanded diagnostic evaluation, including such studies as an echocardiogram to rule out myopathy. Some reports suggest that suppression of ventricular premature beats with exercise testing indicate a benign condition, although this is not universally true.

Asymptomatic patients with isolated ventricular premature beats and a normal heart do not require treatment. The management of patients with high-grade ventricular ectopy is discussed later in this chapter.

TACHYCARDIA

The key to effective management of a tachycardia is accurate identification of the underlying mechanism. This must be understood in terms of both site of origin and the electrophysiologic generator (reentry versus automaticity).

TABLE 29–1. Mechanisms for Clinical Tachycardia

Sinoatrial node		Sinus tachycardia	
Atrium	Flutter Fibrillation	Ectopic at tachycardia Multifocal at tachycardia	Some ectopic tachycardia?
AV junction	AV node reentry	Junctional ectopic tachycardia	
Ventricle	Monomorphic VT Polymorphic VT	Focal VT	Torsades de pointes? Some focal VT?
Accessory pathways	ORT (WPW) ORT (URAP) ORT (PJRT) ART (WPW) ART (Mahaim) Preexcited atrial fibrillation		

ART, antidromic reciprocating tachycardia; AV, atrioventricular; ORT, orthodromic reciprocating tachycardia; VT, ventricular tachycardia; WPW, Wolff-Parkinson-White syndrome.

Terminology and Classification

The terms *supraventricular tachycardia* (SVT) and *ventricular tachycardia* (VT) are practical starting points for describing a tachycardia, but they are sorely lacking in specificity. The term SVT is a broad category that includes any rapid rhythm arising from the atrium, the AV junction, or an AP, whereas VT refers to any disorder that arises from cardiac sites below the bifurcation of the bundle of His. Because they convey so little mechanistic information, these terms are often too imprecise for directing therapeutic decisions. By far a more meaningful nomenclature involves a classification scheme similar to the one depicted in Table 29-1. The list is long, but it underscores the diverse nature of clinical tachycardias, each of which requires a fairly unique approach to therapy.

Bedside Diagnosis of Tachycardia Mechanisms

From the 19 different tachycardia mechanisms listed in Table 29-1, it is usually necessary to narrow the differential diagnosis to only one or two choices at the bedside in order to plan therapy and organize further diagnostic testing. Often, careful review of the standard ECG is sufficient to accomplish this goal.

The first step is to examine a full 12- or 15-lead ECG obtained during tachycardia. A single-lead rhythm strip is hopelessly inadequate for this purpose because it lacks definition of the P wave axis and details of QRS morphology. The ECG is initially scrutinized for duration and morphology of the QRS complex. If the QRS is narrow (i.e., identical to a conducted sinus beat in all 12 leads), it can be assumed that the ventricles were activated over the AV node and the His-Purkinje system, a finding that effectively eliminates ventricular tachycardia from the differential diagnosis. If a wide or different QRS is observed, ventricular tachycardia must be the primary consideration, but the differential diagnosis may also include SVT that is distorted by a disturbance of bundle branch conduction or involves anterograde conduction over a preexcitation pathway.

Differential Diagnosis of Narrow QRS Tachycardia

The possible mechanisms for narrow QRS tachycardias are shown in Figure 29-10. Each diagram is accompanied by a sample ECG (hypothetical lead II) that emphasizes the diagnostic clues to be found in the timing and axis of the P wave.

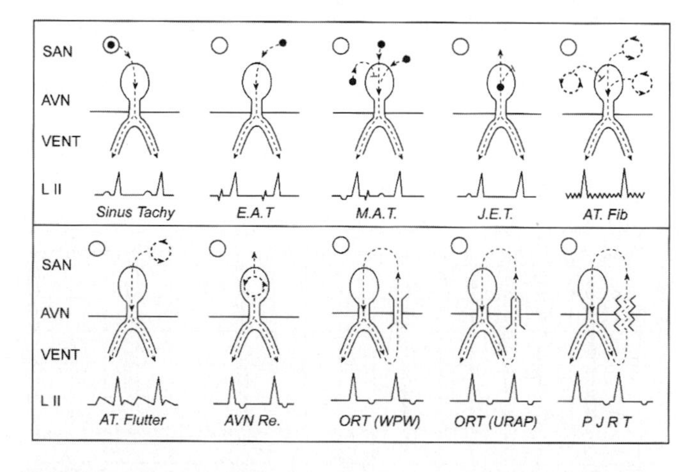

FIGURE 29–10 *Mechanisms for "narrow" QRS tachycardia. Diagrams show the sinoatrial node (SAN; upper left), with the atrioventricular node (AVN) and bundle branches crossing to the ventricle (vent). Surface lead II emphasizes the P-wave timing and morphology.*

The first item is *sinus tachycardia,* which is the prototype automatic arrhythmia. Although not strictly pathologic, it is a good example of the behavior for an automatic focus in that it accelerates and decelerates in a gradual manner and varies in rate with changes in autonomic tone. Note in Figure 29-10 that P waves arising from the SA node register a normal axis of about +60 degrees (i.e., upright in lead II). Because sinus tachycardia usually occurs under conditions of high circulating catecholamines, conduction at the AV node is generally robust, so the A:V ratio is 1:1 in most instances.

In *ectopic atrial tachycardia*, there is an abnormal automatic focus that generates rapid depolarization from an atrial site outside the SA node. Several features distinguish it from sinus tachycardia. First, the P-wave axis is abnormal because of eccentric atrial depolarization. Second, because catecholamine levels are not necessarily elevated and the mechanism does not directly involve the AV node or ventricles, episodic block of AV node conduction can often be observed without interruption of the arrhythmia, especially during vagal stimulation or sleep. *Multifocal atrial tachycardia* presents a similar picture, although in this instance three or more competing P-wave morphologies are observed.

Junctional ectopic tachycardia is a rare condition that is seen almost exclusively in young children following congenital heart surgery but occasionally may occur as a congenital disorder. Note in Figure 29-10 that the focus of rapid discharge is centered in the AV node or the proximal bundle of His. As with other automatic tachycardias, the rate accelerates gradually and exhibits perceptible variation over time. However, the key feature here is potential dissociation of the P and QRS, a consequence of the fact that atrial tissue is not directly linked to the arrhythmia mechanism. In some patients, there may be passive 1:1 retrograde atrial activation with a P axis of −120 degrees, whereas in others, retrograde conduction may be intermittent or even absent altogether. Junctional ectopic tachycardia is the only narrow QRS tachycardia during which the ventricular rate can be faster than the atrial rate.

Automatic tachycardias are sometimes difficult to identify from a surface ECG alone, particularly when P-wave activity is not clearly seen. Perhaps their most notable characteristic is refractoriness to electrical cardioversion, overdrive pacing, and conventional medications. Often, the diagnosis is only considered in retrospect after these remedies have been attempted unsuccessfully.

Reentry mechanisms are the more common cause of a narrow QRS tachycardia. Their most distinctive characteristics are abrupt onset and termination, as well as strictly regular rates. Reentry within atrial muscle produces two very familiar clinical arrhythmias: a single atrial reentry circuit referred to as *atrial flutter*, or multiple, small reentry circuits referred to as *atrial fibrillation*. Atrial fibrillation is readily recognized on the ECG, but atrial flutter is sometimes more difficult. The atrial rate during flutter (classically 300 beats/minute) may vary widely from patient to patient. Rates as fast as 400 beats/minute may be seen in infants, and rates as slow as 130 beats/minute may occur in older patients with congenital heart defects. The hallmark sawtooth pattern in leads II, III, and aV_F may also be difficult to demonstrate at times, particularly during 1:1 AV conduction of slower flutter rates, or during 2:1 conduction when every other flutter wave is buried under a QRS. Careful ECG observation during vagal maneuvers, which can transiently slow AV conduction, may uncover hidden flutter waves.

The final four reentrant circuits for narrow QRS tachycardia include reentry within the AV node, and those tachycardias that reciprocate between the atrium and ventricle through an AP. In all four conditions, a strict 1:1 ratio is generally maintained between the atrium and ventricle, and SVT will terminate immediately when this ratio is disturbed. The atria are depolarized in the retrograde direction to produce a P-wave axis of about −120 degrees. These tachycardias start abruptly, operate at fixed and regular rates, and react to vagal stimulation with either minimal change or abrupt termination. As shown in Figure 29-10, the timing of the retrograde P wave can be used as a marker to differentiate the disorders. In classic *AV node reentry*, retrograde atrial activation occurs nearly simultaneously with ventricular activation, so that the P wave and QRS tend to be superimposed or at least very close in timing. This is reflected in a ventriculoatrial (VA) interval that is less than 70 msec on ECG. By comparison, the reciprocating tachycardias that involve an AP must traverse a physically longer circuit, so that the P wave occurs 70 msec or more after the QRS complex.

Further differentiation among these AV reciprocating circuits is possible by examining the ECG after tachycardia has been terminated. For AV node reentry, the ECG is normal between episodes. For a bidirectional accessory connection (i.e., WPW syndrome), the diagnosis is made by observing the delta wave and short PR interval after sinus rhythm is restored. *Concealed accessory pathways*, which function as unidirectional retrograde conductors, may be harder to diagnose because the ECG in sinus rhythm is completely normal. Differentiation between AV node and concealed pathway reentry may require electrophysiologic study for final resolution. However, one variety of concealed pathway (the *permanent form of junctional reciprocating tachycardia*) can usually be diagnosed with certainty. As the name implies, this form of SVT is very difficult to terminate for more than a few beats and exhibits a dramatically long VA interval during the tachycardia, as depicted in Figure 29-10.

Differential Diagnosis of Wide QRS Tachycardias

A wide QRS tachycardia should always be managed as a VT until proved otherwise. Often, the surface ECG offers no reliable features to eliminate VT from consideration, and proof may come only from invasive electrophysiologic testing. Likewise, patient age and prior medical status should never persuade one to assume that a wide QRS rhythm is a relatively benign SVT. Although rare in the pediatric population, VT may occur at any age, even in previously healthy children.

The possible mechanisms and ECG features of wide QRS tachycardias in pediatric patients are diagrammed in Figure 29-11. One of the most valuable diagnostic observations on an ECG is the presence of dissociation between the rapid QRS and a slower P wave. If the ventricles are seen to beat independently of the atrium, the differential diagnosis is essentially limited to VT. Note, however, that the absence of AV dissociation does not rule out VT because there is frequently passive retrograde 1:1 atrial depolarization in a young patient. One of the potential consequences of AV dissociation is the finding of *fusion beats*, caused by intermittent penetration of atrial impulses. Although fusion is fairly specific for a ventricular tachycardia, it may also occur during some arrhythmias in the WPW syndrome. After resumption of sinus rhythm, the ECG provides

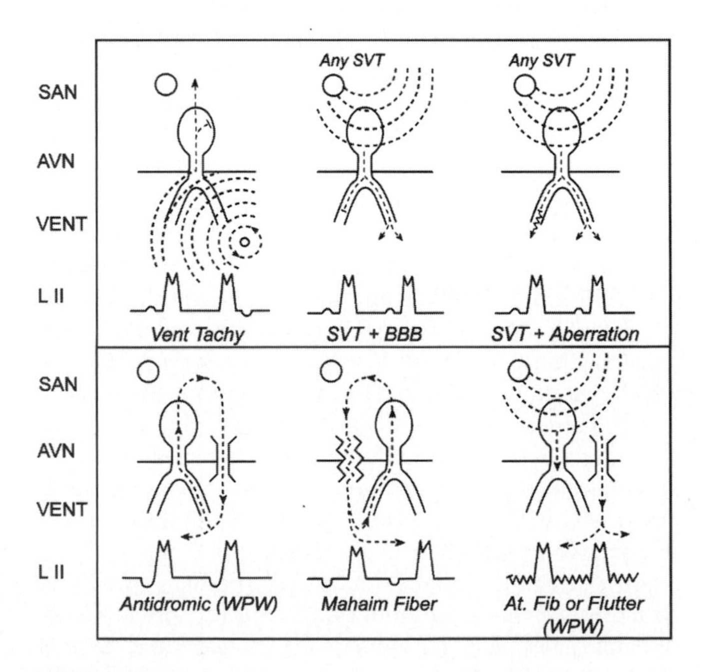

FIGURE 29–11 *Possible mechanisms for "wide" QRS tachycardia.*

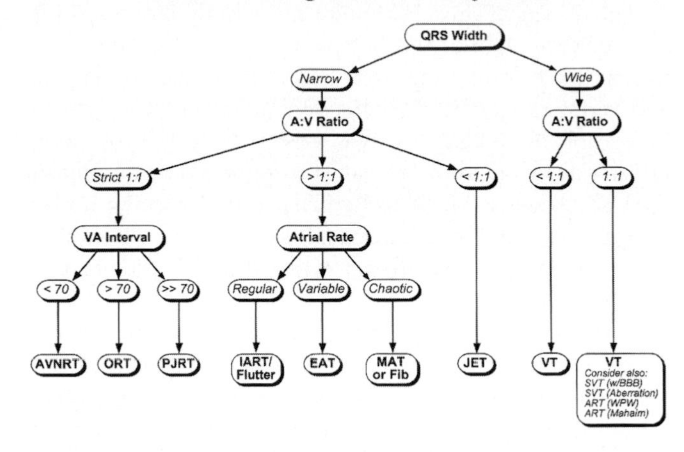

FIGURE 29–12 *Practical scheme for determining the most likely mechanism for a clinical tachycardia based on ECG features. See text for abbreviations.*

additional diagnostic clues. If the patient is noted to have permanent bundle branch block at rest that is identical to the QRS in tachycardia, it is a fairly safe assumption that the primary arrhythmia was SVT. Similarly, if WPW syndrome (short P-R interval and delta wave) or *Mahaim fiber* activity (delta wave with normal P-R) are seen, these pathways are likely to have participated in the tachycardia. The most difficult differential diagnosis involves the choice between VT and SVT with rate-related QRS aberration. In children with SVT, aberration may involve either the right or left bundle branch, often making the ECG indistinguishable from that of VT.

A summary of the diagnostic ECG features for the various tachycardias is provided in Figure 29-12. Note that the degree of diagnostic resolution from the ECG is much less exact for wide QRS compared with narrow QRS tachycardias. A formal electrophysiologic study may be needed when uncertainty exists.

Management of Specific Tachycardias

The preceding section was meant to serve as a rough road map for identification of a tachycardia mechanism at the bedside. Expanded discussion of the physiology and treatment of these individual disorders follows. The tachycardias have been divided into four major groups: (1) automatic SVT, (2) reentrant SVT without APs, (3) reentrant SVT with APs, and (4) ventricular tachycardia.

Automatic Supraventricular Tachycardias

Ectopic Atrial Tachycardia (EAT). EAT is a primary atrial tachycardia resulting from enhanced automaticity of a single nonsinus atrial focus (Fig. 29-13). It accounts for

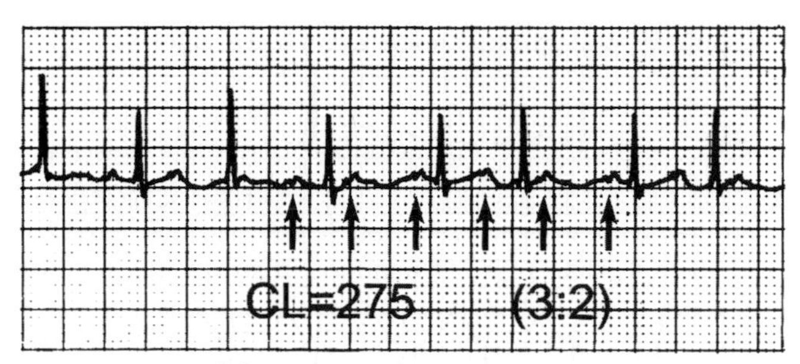

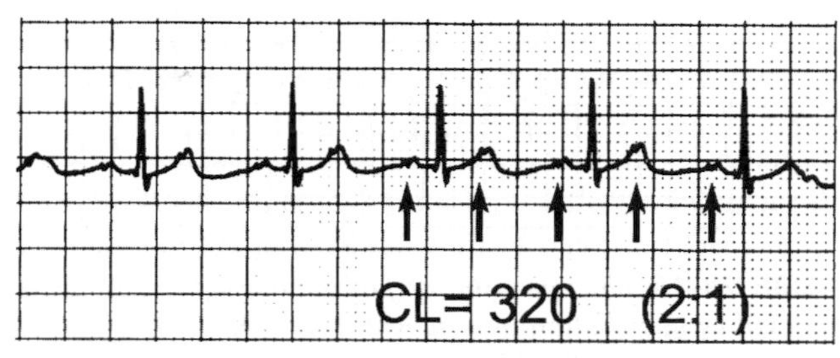

FIGURE 29–13 *Lead II recording from a patient with ectopic atrial tachycardia. The upper strip was obtained after exercise and shows rapid atrial depolarization (arrows) at a cycle length of 275 msec, which conducts with 3:2 ratio. During rest (lower strip), both the atrial rate and A:V ratio are slower.*
From Fyler DC [ed]. Nadas' Pediatric Cardiology. Philadelphia: Hanley & Belfus, 1992.

less than 10% of cases of SVT but may be difficult to treat. This arrhythmia can have a variable presentation, ranging from sporadic episodes that produce only mild symptoms of palpitations and dizziness, all the way to incessant tachycardia with congestive heart failure from tachycardia-induced myopathy.[18] Indeed, it is important not to overlook the possibility of EAT or confuse it with sinus tachycardia when a patient presents with newly diagnosed cardiomyopathy because this type of ventricular dysfunction can be reversed completely in most cases by correcting the rhythm. Ectopic atrial tachycardia can occur at any age. When it is seen in infants and young children, there is a reasonably high likelihood that it could resolve spontaneously after a few months or years, but if it is seen much beyond age 3 years, it is more likely to be a chronic condition.[19] It may also be seen as a transient disorder after cardiac surgery.[20] The precise etiology of EAT is unknown.

On ECG, the hallmark of the arrhythmia is an atrial rate that is inappropriately rapid for age and physiologic state but varies on both a beat-to-beat and a long-term basis to a degree that excludes a reentrant mechanism. The P-wave morphology differs from sinus rhythm and depends on the site of the automatic focus, which may be anywhere in the right or left atrium. Because the arrhythmia mechanism is confined to atrial tissue, the ventricular response rate and the PR interval are determined independently by the AV node. First- and second-degree AV block, as well as episodic bundle branch aberrancy, are common findings (see Fig. 29-13). At electrophysiologic study, earliest atrial activation will map to a point distant from the sinus node (Fig. 29-14). The tachycardia cannot be terminated with pacing or DC cardioversion but may exhibit at least brief overdrive suppression in response to prolonged rapid atrial pacing.

Treatment strategy will depend on the status of ventricular contractility and the patient's age. For patients with depressed function, symptoms may improve somewhat by lowering the ventricular rate, so that acute therapy can be directed toward blocking the AV node. Digoxin can improve ventricular function both through its inotropic effect and through its vagal enhancement of AV node block, but it rarely has any direct effect on the ectopic focus. Although β blockers must be used with care in patients with ventricular dysfunction secondary to EAT, they are sometimes effective in slowing the atrial focus in this disorder and may even be the only necessary therapy for many patients. Amiodarone, sotalol, and flecainide are frequently effective, but an empiric trial is necessary for each agent.

Aggressive efforts at pharmacologic control are usually made in younger children because the condition could eventually resolve. In older children, medical management with a simple agent like a β blocker is usually attempted, but for patients in whom EAT persists despite conservative drug therapy, or who have evidence of tachycardia-induced myopathy, catheter ablation has become the most widely accepted therapy.[21] Ectopic atrial tachycardia in postoperative patients can usually be controlled medically and tends to be transient.

Multifocal Atrial Tachycardia (MAT). MAT (also referred to as chaotic atrial rhythm) is a rare disorder in

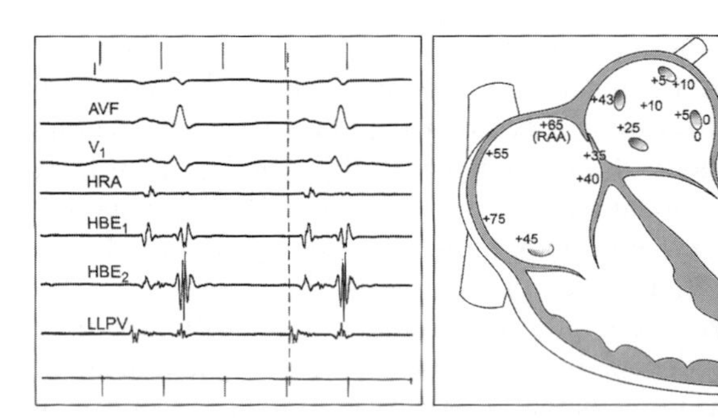

FIGURE 29–14 *Intracardiac mapping of an ectopic atrial focus in the area of the left lower pulmonary vein (LLPV).*
From Fyler DC [ed]. Nadas' Pediatric Cardiology. Philadelphia: Hanley & Belfus, 1992.

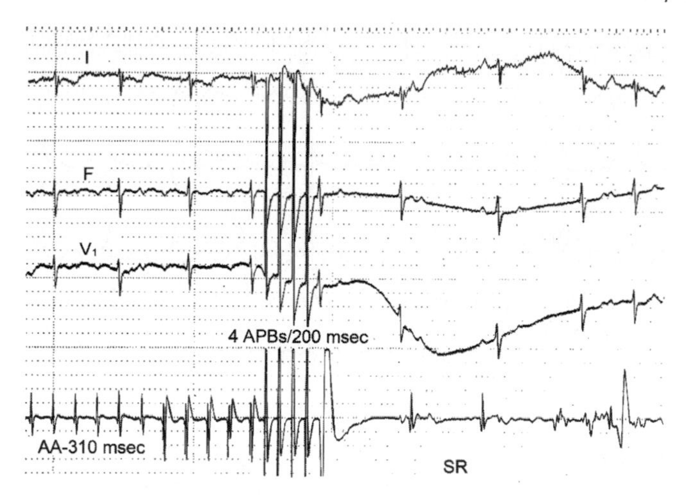

FIGURE 29–19 *Conversion of atrial flutter with esophageal pacing. An atrial esophageal electrogram (bottom trace) confirmed the diagnosis of atrial flutter. A sensing artifact is present in atrial beats 8 to 12, then four pacing artifacts are present, followed by a 200-msec blanking period. After pacing, the first QRS is junctional, and the second beat is sinus.*
From Fyler DC [ed]. Nadas' Pediatric Cardiology. Philadelphia: Hanley & Belfus, 1992.

too severe, it is probably satisfactory to just maintain patients on an AV node blocking drug after conversion of their first episode of atrial flutter, which will help prevent a rapid ventricular response should the arrhythmia recur. If flutter becomes a recurrent issue, management decisions become rather complicated, and consultation with a cardiac electrophysiologist is recommended. The options available for recurrent flutter include catheter ablation,[43–45] chronic drug therapy with potent agents such as sotalol or amiodarone,[46] placement of an atrial antitachycardia pacemaker,[40] and even arrhythmia surgery.[47] None of these can be considered a perfect solution, and all have risks. Final choices for chronic therapy must be made on a case-by-case basis.

Atrial Fibrillation. Atrial fibrillation is thought to arise from multiple small migratory reentry circuits occurring predominately within the left atrium. Although extremely common in elderly patients, atrial fibrillation is rare in children, possibly because of an atrial size that is inadequate to support multiple circuits. The typical clinical settings for atrial fibrillation in the pediatric age group include congenital heart defects involving the mitral and aortic valves,[48] cardiomyopathy, and WPW syndrome. Atrial fibrillation may also be caused by hyperthyroidism in rare cases, and this possibility should be investigated in any new patient without obvious underlying heart disease.

Patients with atrial fibrillation usually experience palpitations, but syncope due to a rapid ventricular response is rare in the absence of the WPW syndrome. Those with compromised ventricular function and particularly slow or fast ventricular response rates may experience weakness or congestive heart failure in addition to palpitations.

The ECG typically reveals low-amplitude irregular atrial activity (Fig. 29-20) that at times may be difficult to differentiate from artifact or rapid atrial flutter. Ventricular response rates are generally between 80 and 150 beats/minute. An ECG highlight is the nearly random variation in length of the RR intervals (irregularly irregular) due to chaotic atrial impulses and variable AV node conduction. Intermittent QRS aberration (*Ashman's phenomenon*) can also be seen (Fig. 29-21).

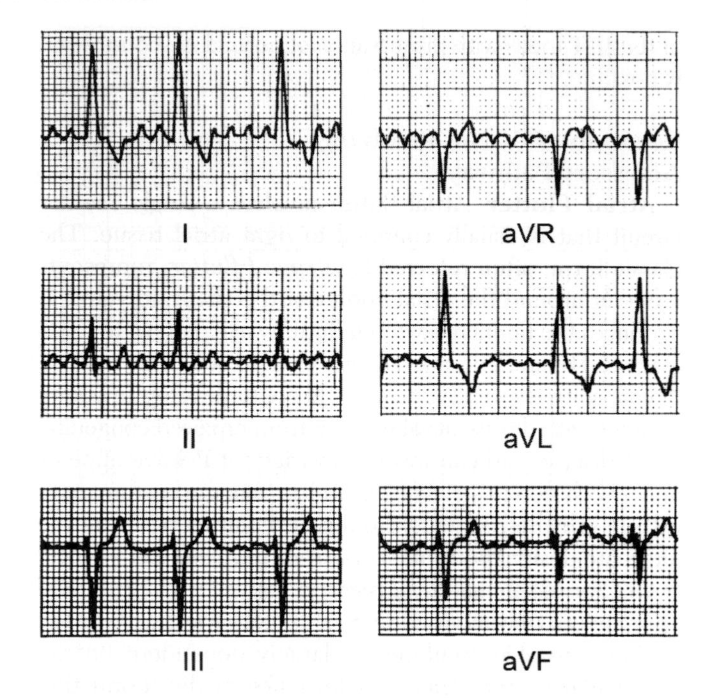

FIGURE 29–20 *Atrial fibrillation that developed in a patient with tricuspid atresia. The ventricular response rate is about 90 beats/min.*
From Fyler DC [ed]. Nadas' Pediatric Cardiology. Philadelphia: Hanley & Belfus, 1992.

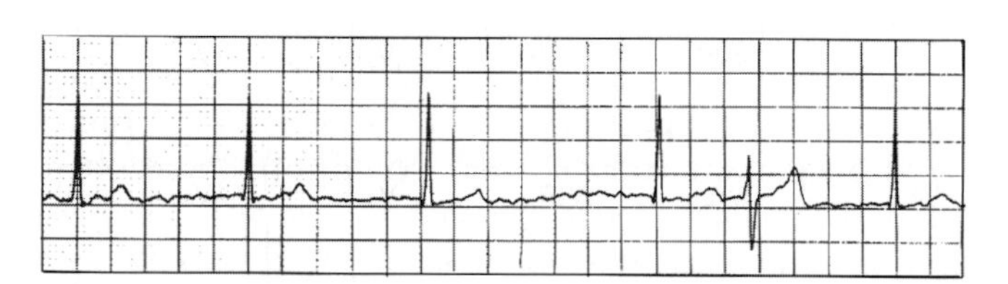

FIGURE 29–21 *Ashman's phenomenon in a patient with atrial fibrillation. There is a relative pause between the 3rd and 4th QRS, followed by closer spacing between the 4th and 5th QRS (which is aberrant). Ashman's typically occurs after such "long–short" intervals.*
From Fyler DC [ed]. Nadas' Pediatric Cardiology. Philadelphia: Hanley & Belfus, 1992.

If the duration of atrial fibrillation is less than about 48 hours, the likelihood of atrial thrombi is minimal; thus, undivided attention can be directed toward converting the rhythm. If initial rate control is required, drugs such as digoxin, esmolol, or verapamil can be used (assuming WPW is not present). Atrial fibrillation can then be terminated reliably with DC cardioversion under appropriate sedation, starting with energies of 1 to 2 joules/kg. Alternatively, pharmacologic conversion can be attempted with intravenous infusion of agents such as procainamide or amiodarone, or with rapid oral loading with sotalol, flecainide, or propafenone.

If the arrhythmia duration is long or uncertain, the risk for atrial thrombi will influence treatment decisions.[49] For a patient with minimal symptoms, it is usually wise to postpone conversion for several weeks while controlling the rate with an AV node blocking agent and providing anticoagulation with warfarin sodium (Coumadin). At the end of this anticoagulation phase, sinus rhythm can be restored by any of the aforementioned techniques. If, on the other hand, the patient has serious symptoms at presentation, the luxury of prolonged anticoagulation may not be available. If no clots are visible on transesophageal echocardiogram, conversion can be performed with reasonably low embolic risk.

Therapy to prevent recurrent atrial fibrillation is similar to that for atrial flutter and may be difficult at times. Catheter ablation techniques for atrial fibrillation are still in the developmental phase but are starting to show some promise.[50]

AV Nodal Reentrant Tachycardia (AVNRT). The reentrant circuit in AVNRT involves two discrete conduction pathways in or around an otherwise normal AV node. One of these pathways, known as the *fast* limb, conducts with a normal PR interval but has a rather long effective refractory period (ERP). If a premature atrial beat arrives at the AV node while the fast pathway is still refractory, conduction can shift to the alternate *slow* limb, which has a short ERP and can therefore handle the impulse but conducts with a very long PR interval. To some extent this is normal physiology, and 30% or more of the general population demonstrate these so-called dual AV nodal pathways.[51] However, when conduction velocity and refractoriness of the two pathways are balanced in just the proper fashion, a reentrant tachycardia can result. There are actually no clear anatomic correlates for the two pathways within the nodal region, but the functional evidence is convincing, including ECG recognition of sudden spontaneous changes in the PR interval (Fig. 29-22) and the demonstration of a discontinuity in the AV nodal conduction time (AH interval) with atrial premature stimuli during electrophysiologic testing (Fig. 29-23). In order for a tachycardia episode to develop in this condition, an appropriately timed premature atrial beat must shift conduction to the slow pathway so that the impulse can then return toward the atrium retrograde in the fast pathway (Fig. 29-24), thereby setting up a *slow–fast* reentry tachycardia.

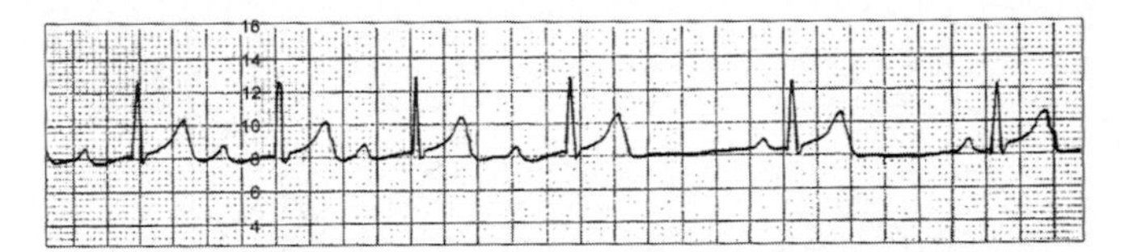

FIGURE 29–22 *Dual AV node pathways on the surface ECG. The P-R interval spontaneously changes from 320 msec to 180 msec when the heart rate slows, indicating a shift from the slow pathway with a shorter refractory period to the fast pathway with a longer refractory period.*
From Fyler DC [ed]. Nadas' Pediatric Cardiology. Philadelphia: Hanley & Belfus, 1992.

AVNRT is rare in very young children. It is probable that the electrophysiologic substrate of dual pathways is present from birth but is simply unmasked with age as both autonomic influences and the refractory characteristics of the AV nodal tissue change with growth. By comparison, AVNRT is the most common mechanism for SVT in patients who first present in adulthood. The tachycardia rate in children with AVNRT is usually between 180 and 250 beats/minute. Severe hemodynamic compromise is rare with AVNRT, but feelings of anxiety, chest pain, and dizziness are frequent. The ECG shows a P wave occurring nearly simultaneously with the QRS complex, and often the P wave

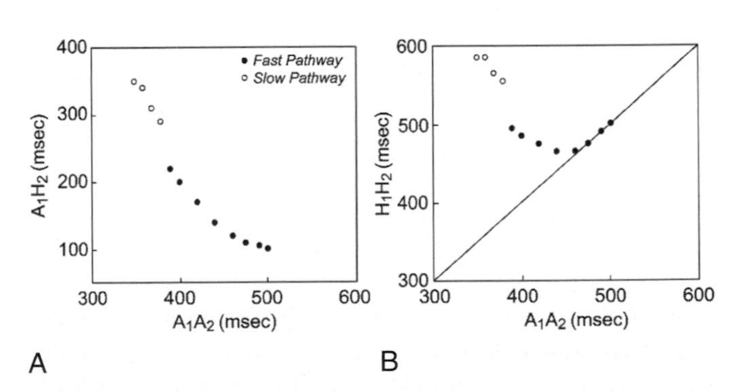

FIGURE 29–23 *Electrophysiologic characteristics of dual AV node pathways. As the A-A interval decreases during atrial extrastimulus testing, the A-H interval increases because of first-degree AV node block (A). The H-H interval decreases, but the change is less than that for the A-A, yielding a slope of less than 1 inch (B). At the effective refractory period of the fast pathway, a 75-msec jump occurs in both the A-H and H-H intervals, with only a 10-msec decrease in A-A, meeting the functional criteria for dual AV node pathways.*
From Fyler DC [ed]. Nadas' Pediatric Cardiology. Philadelphia: Hanley & Belfus, 1992.

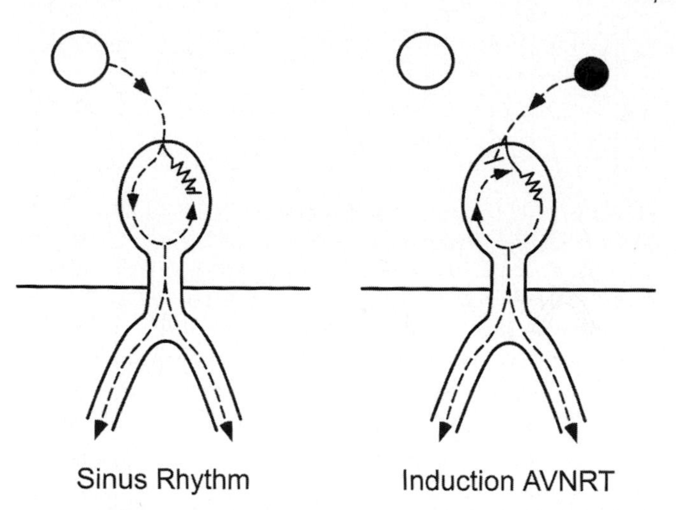

FIGURE 29–24 *Dual AV node pathways. In sinus rhythm (left), antegrade conduction proceeds down both the slow and fast pathways simultaneously, but conduction in the fast pathway usually reaches the point at which they merge again first. The fast pathway then excites the His-Purkinje system, and conduction may proceed retrograde up the slow pathway, blocking its antegrade conduction. Occasionally, slow pathway conduction is so slow that the distal AV node is no longer refractory when its wavefront arrives, giving rise to two ventricular activations from a single atrial stimulus. Tachycardia may be induced (right) when conduction first blocks in the fast pathway because of its short refractory period, then proceeds down the slow pathway, and finally reenters retrograde in the fast pathway.*
From Fyler DC [ed]. Nadas' Pediatric Cardiology. Philadelphia: Hanley & Belfus, 1992.

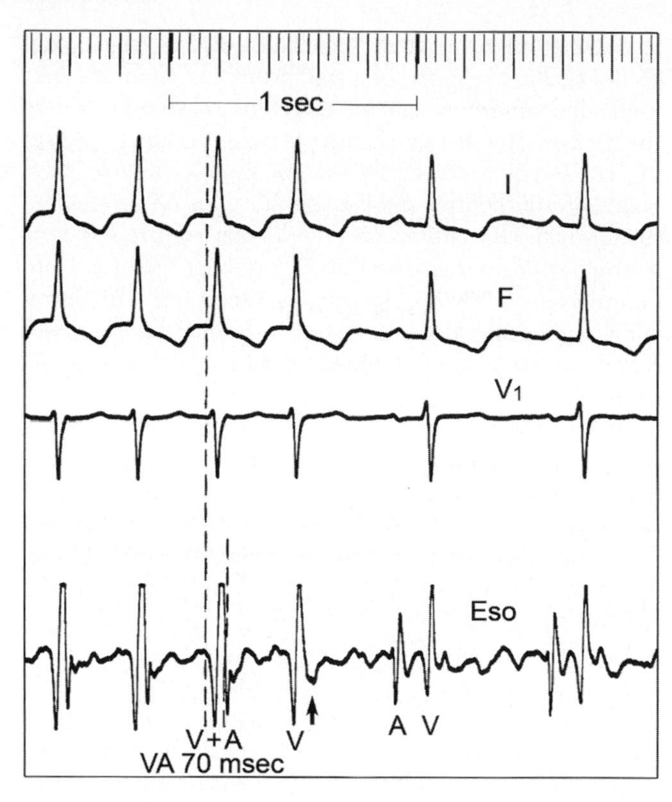

FIGURE 29–25 *ECG (leads I, aV$_F$, and V$_1$), along with an esophageal recording at moment of termination of AV nodal reentry tachycardia. Note that the atrial and ventricular timing are nearly simultaneous during tachycardia, such that discrete P waves are not discernable during the arrhythmia.*
From Fyler DC [ed]. Nadas' Pediatric Cardiology. Philadelphia: Hanley & Belfus, 1992.

will not be clearly discernible because of the superimposed QRS (Fig. 29-25).

In general, any maneuver that enhances vagal tone (Fig. 29-26) to slow AV nodal conduction (e.g., Valsalva maneuver or excitation of the diving reflex with an ice bag applied to the face) may promote termination of AVNRT. If vagal maneuvers fail, pharmacologic therapy is almost universally successful in this disorder. Short-duration AV node blockade with adenosine is very effective, as is administration of a calcium channel blocker like verapamil. Although rarely necessary, AVNRT will also terminate with DC cardioversion using very low energy and can be interrupted promptly with brief bursts of rapid atrial pacing.

Patients with infrequent episodes of AVNRT and minimal symptoms can be managed conservatively with the vagal maneuvers described previously, trading a few minutes of discomfort for the inconvenience and possible side effects of more aggressive treatment options. On the other hand, patients who suffer from frequent bouts of prolonged tachycardia will require either chronic medical therapy or catheter ablation, especially if dizziness is a prominent symptom. The choice between drugs and ablation depends largely on patient age and the attitude of the family. Curative ablation, which modifies or eliminates the slow pathway without damaging the normal fast pathway, is now done on a routine basis in children older than about 4 years, with success rates exceeding 95%.[52] The principal risk during such a procedure is inadvertent fast pathway damage, which could result in high-grade AV block and necessitate pacemaker placement. Although this risk is extremely low, certainly far less than 1% in experienced hands, it is still of sufficient enough concern that some families and physicians may elect to defer ablation in favor of medication trials. The most reasonable agents for preventing or minimizing AVNRT episodes are β blockers and calcium channel blockers, which will be safe and effective in most cases.

SVT Due to Accessory Pathways

In 1930, Wolff, Parkinson, and White described a syndrome that consisted of a short PR interval, bundle

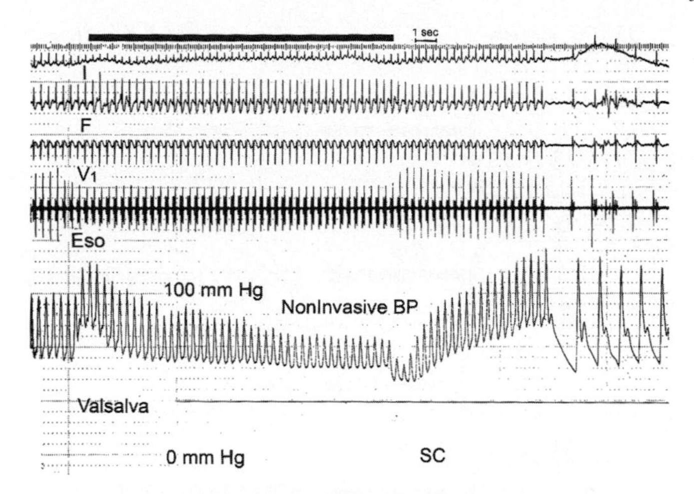

FIGURE 29–26 *In some patients, as in this one with orthodromic reciprocating tachycardia, the Valsalva maneuver is reproducibly effective at terminating tachycardia. Here, tachycardia terminates when the systolic blood pressure reaches 130 mm Hg during phase 4 of the Valsalva maneuver. Although difficult to see on this scale, the tachycardia terminates with an atrial deflection in the esophageal ECG, suggesting block in the AV node.*
From Fyler DC [ed]. Nadas' Pediatric Cardiology. Philadelphia: Hanley & Belfus, 1992.

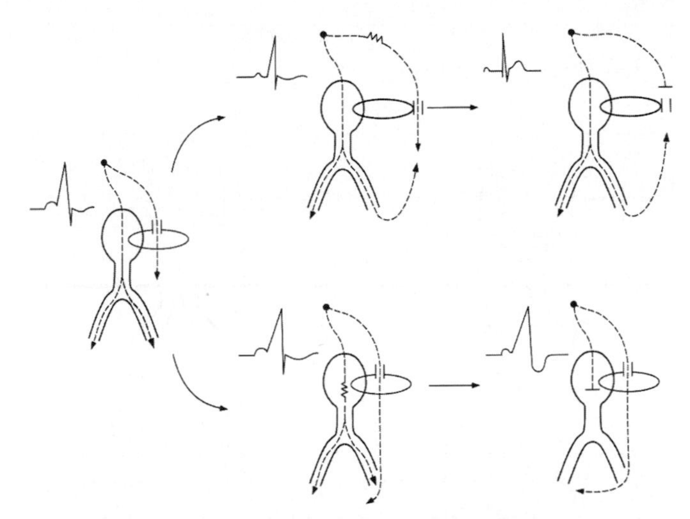

FIGURE 29–27 *Origin of the delta wave in Wolff-Parkinson-White syndrome. During sinus rhythm, the surface ECG appearance is influenced by the balance between ventricular depolarization through the AV node and the accessory pathway (AP), which depends on the relative conduction times from the atria to the ventricles through each pathway. Typically (far left panel), conduction reaches the ventricle first through the AP, yielding a short P-R interval, eccentric depolarization, and a delta wave, but conduction through the AV node also depolarizes a large amount of ventricle. The relative contribution of the accessory pathway may be small (upper panels), yielding relatively normal QRS and P-R intervals. By comparison, if conduction is delayed in the AV node (lower middle panel), more ventricular tissue is depolarized through the AP, yielding a shorter P-R and a more prominent delta wave. Rarely, the AV node may block while the AP remains excitable (lower right panel), yielding fully eccentric ventricular depolarization known as maximal preexcitation.*
From Fyler DC [ed]. Nadas' Pediatric Cardiology. Philadelphia: Hanley & Belfus, 1992.

branch block on the surface ECG, and paroxysmal tachycardia. Although they were unaware of the electrophysiologic or anatomic basis of this disorder, their report sparked further investigation that ultimately confirmed the notion that WPW syndrome was caused by a small AP traversing the AV groove. It is now understood that APs may express themselves through a variety of ECG patterns and arrhythmias dependent on their conduction properties and location.

Several types of APs have been described, including (1) the classic AV pathway of WPW syndrome that is capable of both anterograde and retrograde conduction; (2) concealed APs that conduct only in the retrograde direction; (3) extremely slow conducting concealed APs, which cause the incessant SVT known as PJRT; and (4) Mahaim fibers with very slow anterograde conduction, which arise near the anterolateral tricuspid valve and travel over a long distance to insert near the anterior surface of the right ventricle.

The characteristic appearance of WPW syndrome on the surface ECG during sinus rhythm is that of a short PR interval and a slurred initial QRS deflection, known as a *delta wave*. These findings reflect the fact that conduction from the atrium to the ventricle through the accessory connection is generally faster than conduction in the AV node. Thus, some segment of the ventricle is preexcited by the eccentric spread of activation from the accessory connection. The degree of preexcitation depends on the relative conduction velocities of the AV node and the AP as well as pathway location (Fig. 29-27). Electrophysiologically, preexcitation is characterized by a short or negative HV interval on a His bundle recording (Fig. 29-28).

The axis and morphology of the delta wave can be used to estimate the site of earliest ventricular activation and, hence, the location of the accessory connection. Gallagher and coworkers[53] derived the original algorithm for delta wave mapping based on their pioneering work with surgery for WPW in the 1970s. Subsequently, new algorithms providing more refined localization have arisen in response to the experience and demands of catheter ablation for WPW.[54,55] A simplified version of a modern ECG algorithm for WPW mapping is shown in Figure 29-29.

The most common form of SVT in WPW syndrome, known as *orthodromic reciprocating tachycardia* (ORT),

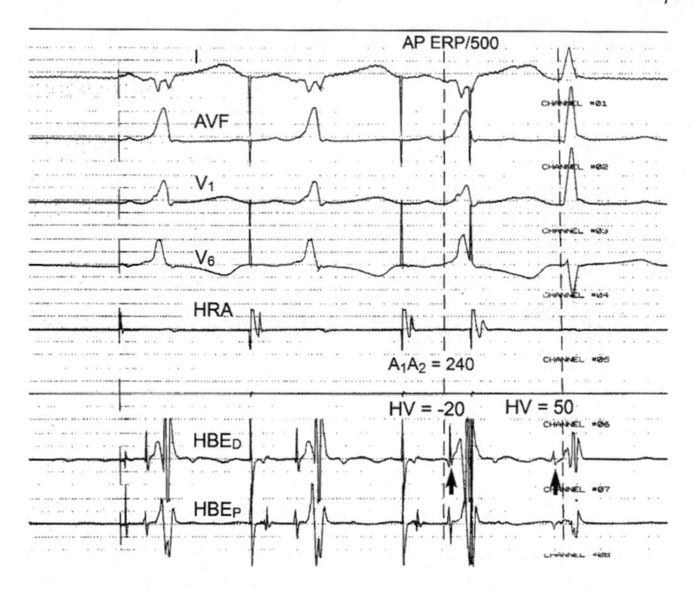

FIGURE 29–28 *Electrophysiologic characteristics of Wolff-Parkinson-White syndrome. During sinus rhythm or atrial pacing, as shown here, ventricular activation occurs first through the accessory pathway (AP), so that the His activation (first arrow) occurs after the beginning of the surface QRS complex. A negative or short H-V interval during an atrial-driven rhythm defines preexcitation. A premature atrial stimulus 240 msec after regular atrial pacing, with a 500-msec interval, causes block in the AP. The result is a long P-R interval, a normal QRS complex, and a positive and normal H-V interval of 50 msec. Because the stimulus was the longest A-A interval that did not produce pre-excitation, it is the AP effective refractory period (ERP), at a drive train of 500 msec.*
From Fyler DC [ed]. Nadas' Pediatric Cardiology. Philadelphia: Hanley & Belfus, 1992.

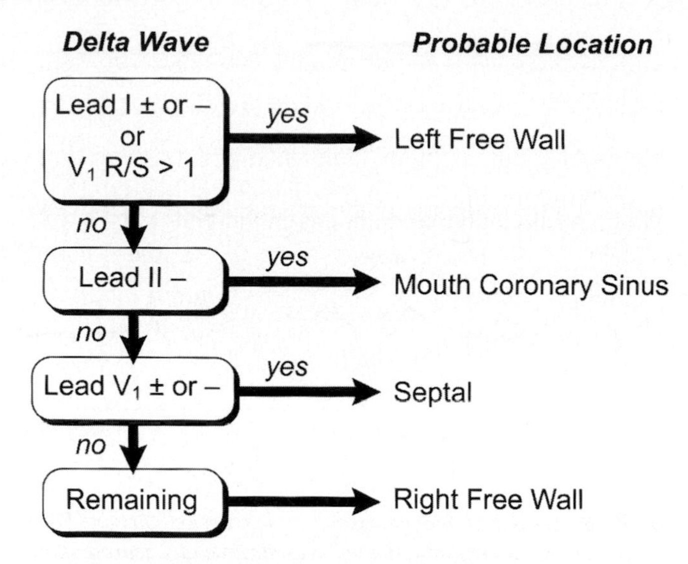

FIGURE 29–29 *Simplified scheme for predicting location of an accessory pathway in Wolff-Parkinson-White syndrome based on the standard 12-lead ECG. The polarity of the delta wave and certain gross features of the preexcited QRS help define the approximate site for the ventricular insertion of the pathway.*[54]

uses the AV node as the anterograde limb, with the AP as the retrograde limb. This circuit generates a narrow QRS complex on ECG because the ventricles are depolarized in the normal fashion over the AV node. Although less common than ORT, other forms of tachycardia can also occur in WPW syndrome, including the opposite reentry circuit using the AP as the anterograde limb and the AV node in the retrograde direction, known as *antidromic reciprocating tachycardia* (ART). The ECG picture of ART will differ markedly from ORT because the ventricles are depolarized by the AP, resulting in a wide QRS that can be hard to distinguish from VT at first glance. Finally, some patients with WPW may experience episodic atrial fibrillation, which actually is the most dangerous tachycardia involving APs. During such episodes, the ventricles can be activated in the anterograde direction by both the AV node and AP. The ECG will therefore contain a mixture of narrow, wide, or intermediate QRS complexes, which may occasionally result in rates that are rapid enough to cause degeneration into ventricular fibrillation (VF).

Concealed pathways, which conduct only in the retrograde direction from ventricle to atrium and do not generate a delta wave on ECG, can participate in ORT but are incapable of supporting antidromic tachycardia or pre-excited conduction of atrial fibrillation. Mahaim fibers are almost exclusively anterograde-only pathways.

ORT in WPW. Tachycardia due to ORT is the most common presentation for WPW in young patients. Episodes may begin as early as intrauterine life, but many patients remain entirely symptomatic until adolescence or adulthood. Severe hemodynamic compromise is rare in ORT. The more common symptoms include palpitations, anxiety, and mild chest discomfort. Some children may experience dizziness and dyspnea during ORT when they attempt to exert themselves. The one scenario in which ORT becomes a serious safety threat is in young infants who may have undetected tachycardia for hours to days, sometimes resulting in congestive heart failure and even cardiovascular collapse at presentation.[56]

The surface ECG during ORT typically displays a narrow QRS morphology with a strictly regular rate. Transient rate-related left or right bundle branch block may occur, particularly at the moment of tachycardia initiation. If the bundle branch block occurs ipsilateral to the side of the AP, the tachycardia cycle length usually increases because of the added conduction time in the ventricular muscle

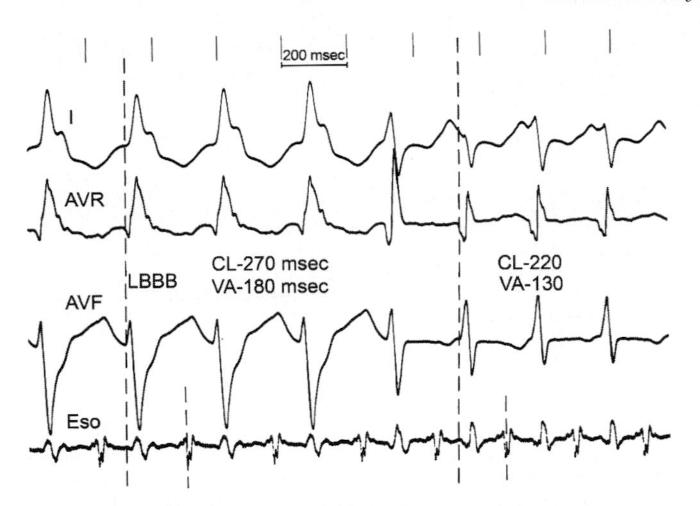

FIGURE 29–30 *A change from left bundle branch block (LBBB) to a normal QRS complex during orthodromic tachycardia led to a 50-msec decrease in the cycle length (CL), and a shortening of the ventriculoatrial (VA) interval from 180 msec to 130 msec, confirming the diagnosis of a left-sided accessory pathway. From Fyler DC [ed]. Nadas' Pediatric Cardiology. Philadelphia: Hanley & Belfus, 1992.*

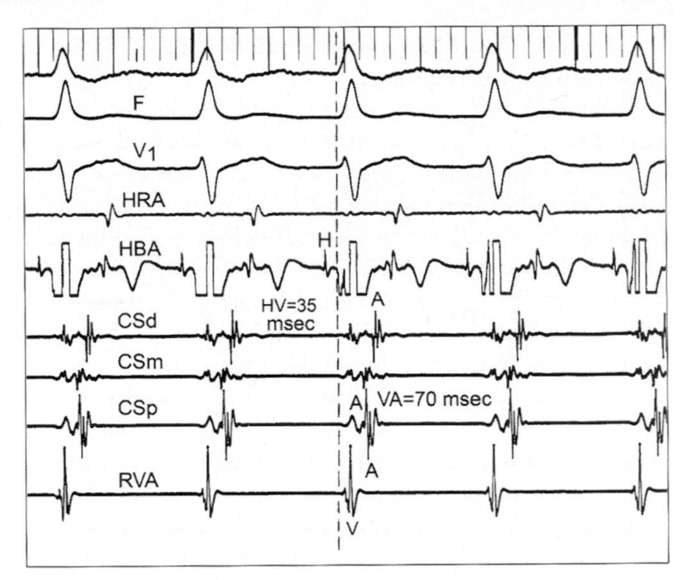

FIGURE 29–31 *Mapping during orthodromic reciprocating tachycardia. The QRS complex is normal on the surface ECG, and the H-V interval is normal, confirming anterograde conduction through the AV node. Retrograde conduction back to the atrium occurs over the accessory pathway. Atrial activation is earliest on the middle coronary sinus electrode (CS), preceding both the HBE lead and the high right atrial (HRA) lead. This corresponds to a left posterior position for the accessory pathway. From Fyler DC [ed]. Nadas' Pediatric Cardiology. Philadelphia: Hanley & Belfus, 1992.*

limb of the tachycardia circuit (Fig. 29-30). When this finding is observed, it helps to identify the location of the AP as either right- or left-sided.[57] The natural initiating events for ORT can include sinus acceleration, atrial premature beats, junctional beats, or ventricular premature beats. The usual requirement for initiation is block of anterograde conduction in the AP plus enough delay in the AV node to allow the AP and atrium to be excitable when the reentrant wavefront reaches them.

During electrophysiologic study, initiation of ORT can usually be achieved with a critically timed atrial premature stimulus that blocks anterograde in the accessory connection and encounters an appropriate delay in the AV node. Thus, the atrial premature stimulus must occur at an interval shorter than the effective refractory period of an accessory connection. Intracardiac recordings during ORT demonstrate an A:V ratio of 1:1 and an interval from the earliest deflection of the QRS to the rapid deflection of the P wave (the VA interval) greater than 70 msec. In addition, to prove that the tachycardia involves an extranodal accessory connection, other conditions must be met. Either the VA interval in tachycardia must increase during transient bundle branch aberration, or it must be possible to preexcite the atrium with a ventricular premature beat placed into tachycardia at a time when the bundle of His is refractory, thus proving that the atrium was not activated through the AV node. Once ORT is confirmed, the location of the accessory connection may be mapped by identifying the site of earliest retrograde atrial activation during ORT (Fig. 29-31). Left-sided pathways can be mapped accurately using a multielectrode catheter in the coronary sinus, whereas right-sided and septal pathways are usually localized during point-by-point mapping along the edge of the tricuspid valve.

Because the AV node is the anterograde limb of the tachycardia circuit in ORT, the therapeutic maneuvers used for conversion of ORT to sinus rhythm parallel those already mentioned for AVNRT. This begins with a Valsalva maneuver or facial application of an ice bag to transiently increase vagal tone. If this proves unsuccessful, an intravenous line can be placed in an antecubital vein, and a rapid dose of adenosine can be given. Intravenous esmolol could also be considered if adenosine fails. If conversion cannot be achieved or maintained by efforts to block the AV nodal limb of the circuit, a medication such as intravenous procainamide, which acts more directly on the AP, can be tried. If at any time during this treatment cascade the patient begins to develop hemodynamic intolerance of ORT, more deliberate therapy with DC cardioversion or transesophageal atrial overdrive pacing can always be instituted. Naturally, if an infant with long-standing ORT has congestive failure and hypotension at first presentation, urgent intervention with DC cardioversion or transesophageal pacing should be considered as initial therapy, rather than squandering time with serial drug trials.

Patient age, severity of presenting symptoms, anterograde conduction properties of the AP, and AP location must all be taken into account when long-term therapy is being planned for ORT in patients with WPW. As many as 30% of infants with ORT from an AP will have spontaneous resolution of the disorder before their first birthday,[58] and this encourages a policy of firm reliance on pharmacologic options throughout the first year or so of life.[59] The drug used most commonly as initial therapy for WPW in young patients is propranolol. Digoxin and verapamil have the potential for enhancing anterograde conduction in the AP, and consequently, most cardiologists view them as contraindicated for long-term therapy of WPW. The only exception may be premature newborns, in whom β blockade can exacerbate hypoglycemia and apnea. Digoxin might still be used cautiously in such cases.[60] If propranolol does not prevent ORT recurrence, therapy can be escalated to a more potent agent, such as flecainide, sotalol, or amiodarone.

For older children, catheter ablation becomes an attractive option for permanently eradicating the AP and avoiding long-term exposure to potentially toxic antiarrhythmic drugs.[61] As will be discussed later in this chapter, the success rate for AP ablation using radiofrequency energy is 92% to 99%, depending on pathway location, and the risks are quite low in experienced hands.[62] Complications seem to be more common in children under 15 kg in body weight; thus, most centers are content to continue medical therapy until children are about 4 years old before recommending elective ablation, assuming no serious symptomatology has occurred.

ART in WPW. This tachycardia, in which the reentry circuit is exactly the opposite of that of ORT, accounts for less than 1% of pediatric SVT cases. Because activation of the ventricle occurs entirely through the AP, the QRS complex is wide and abnormal, demonstrating maximal preexcitation (Fig. 29-32). Retrograde conduction from the ventricles to the atria occurs through the AV node, yielding a retrograde P-wave axis of about −120 degrees.

Initiation of antidromic reentry requires that anterograde conduction blocks in the AV node while it continues in the AP. For this to occur, the anterograde refractory period of the AP must be longer than that of the AV node. Maintenance of the tachycardia then requires that the retrograde refractory period of the AV node be less than the tachycardia cycle length. The relative infrequency of antidromic tachycardia seems to be due to difficulty in meeting all of these conditions. When antidromic tachycardia does occur, the HV interval is markedly negative, with the His bundle deflection occurring near the end of the QRS complex. Retrograde atrial activation, demonstrating

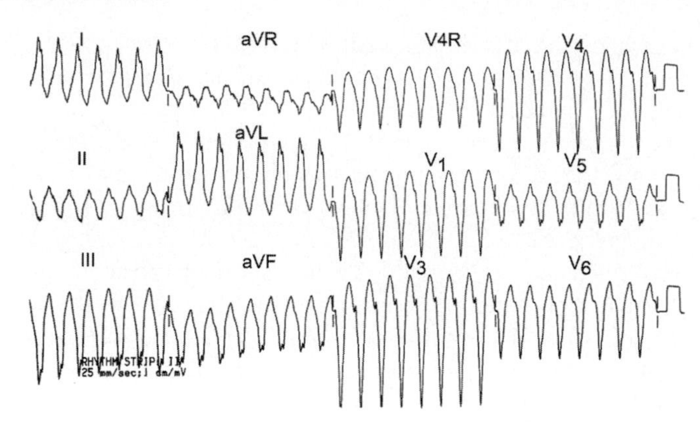

FIGURE 29–32 *Surface ECG showing antidromic tachycardia. This regular, wide-complex tachycardia at a rate of 187 beats/min was induced at electrophysiology study. P waves are not clearly visible. The initial QRS deflections were identical to those in sinus rhythm, strongly suggesting that these complexes represent maximal preexcitation. The electrophysiologic characteristics were those of antidromic reciprocating tachycardia involving a right, posterior accessory pathway.*
From Fyler DC [ed]. Nadas' Pediatric Cardiology. Philadelphia: Hanley & Belfus, 1992.

a pattern of AV nodal origin, occurs after the His deflection and before ventricular activation.

As with ORT, tachycardia maintenance is dependent on conduction through both the AV node and the AP. Consequently, if the diagnosis of antidromic tachycardia is absolutely firm, conversion can be achieved with a protocol identical to that described for ORT. If the episode is the first presentation of a regular wide-complex tachycardia in a patient without a prior ECG in sinus rhythm, the arrhythmia will need to be treated as described for VT until proved otherwise. It is difficult and probably hazardous to make the diagnosis of ART unless a patient already has a well-established diagnosis of WPW. If there is any irregularity whatsoever in the rate or QRS morphology, preexcited atrial fibrillation must be considered and the patient treated accordingly.

Pharmacologic management of ART is similar to that of ORT in patients with WPW syndrome. β Blockers, flecainide, sotalol, and amiodarone are all satisfactory choices for treatment. However, because virtually all patients with antidromic tachycardia have relatively rapidly conducting APs, ablation has now become the preferred option for all but the youngest patient. Not only could ablation be curative, it might also eliminate iatrogenic morbidity that sometimes accompanies treatment of wide QRS tachycardia in a facility unfamiliar with the patient's condition.

Preexcited Atrial Fibrillation in WPW. When an AP is present, every beat of atrial origin may activate the ventricles through the AV node, the APs, both, or neither. Thus, during any rapid atrial tachycardia, the rate and pattern of ventricular activation depend on the conduction times and the refractory period of both the AV node and APs. In such a case, the normal protection of the ventricles from rapid conduction of atrial arrhythmias by the AV node is diminished by the presence of an AP. Thus, a rapid ventricular rate, and possibly VF in response to atrial fibrillation, is a potential cause of syncope and sudden death in patients with WPW.[63] Patients with WPW syndrome are clearly more prone to episodic atrial fibrillation than is the general population. There is little doubt that the AP contributes directly to this tendency because elimination of pathway conduction with medical or ablative therapy effectively prevents recurrence of atrial fibrillation.[64]

A number of factors may be responsible for deterioration of the ventricular rhythm during atrial fibrillation: (1) the presence of multiple APs, (2) shortening of the AP refractory period in response to the sympathetic discharge induced by the initial tachycardia, (3) disorganized ventricular contraction and resultant hypotension due to the extreme irregularity of the rapid ventricular rhythm, and (4) activation of the ventricles on the edge of the refractory period from a prior beat (i.e., effective R-on-T). The presence of a rapid ventricular response to induced atrial fibrillation in the electrophysiology laboratory is reasonably predictive of those who will experience spontaneous syncope or sudden death. Most young patients who have had VF have minimum ventricular cycle lengths during atrial fibrillation of 220 msec or less. Because spontaneous atrial fibrillation is rare in young children with WPW, few pediatric patients present in this fashion. However, the presence of extremely rapidly conducting APs in infants and children makes the potential for disaster high should atrial fibrillation occur.

The surface ECG reveals an irregular rhythm with fluctuating QRS morphology caused by variable fusion between AV node and AP conduction (Fig. 29-33). The presence of two distinct aberrant QRS patterns suggests the possibility of multiple APs. If the purpose of an electrophysiologic procedure is to estimate a patient's risk for future atrial fibrillation episodes, aggressive efforts are made to induce atrial fibrillation with rapid bursts of atrial pacing, and then examine the shortest preexcited RR interval (Fig. 29-34). In practice, atrial fibrillation may be surprisingly difficult to induce in children during electrophysiologic study. The response of the APs to rapid atrial pacing may need to suffice.

The two goals in the acute treatment of atrial fibrillation in WPW are to reduce the ventricular response rate and to terminate the atrial fibrillation. If severe hemodynamic compromise is present, synchronized DC cardioversion will accomplish both goals with the lowest risks and quickest results. If the patient is not severely compromised, medical therapy can be considered. Procainamide administered intravenously is probably the most effective drug because it can slow conduction over the APs and may also terminate atrial fibrillation directly. Although adenosine, digoxin, and calcium channel blockers all lower the rate of impulse conduction in the AV node, they are also known to enhance conduction in an AP, with the net result being an increase

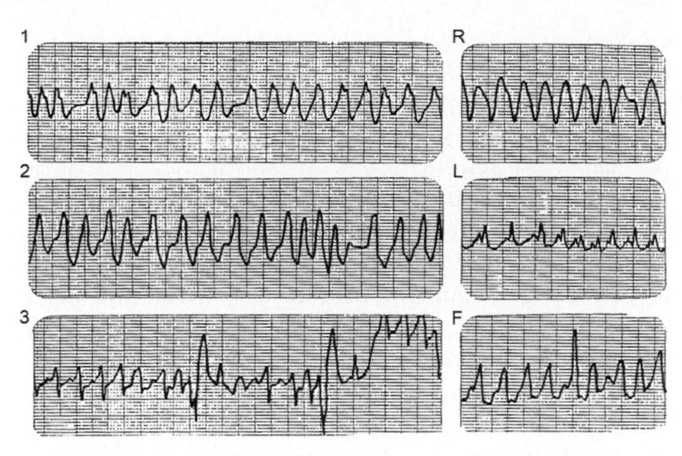

FIGURE 29–33 *Surface ECG showing atrial fibrillation in Wolff-Parkinson-White syndrome. Note the wide-complex, irregular, rapid rhythm. The patient was hypotensive and presyncopal at presentation.*
From Fyler DC [ed]. Nadas' Pediatric Cardiology. Philadelphia: Hanley & Belfus, 1992.

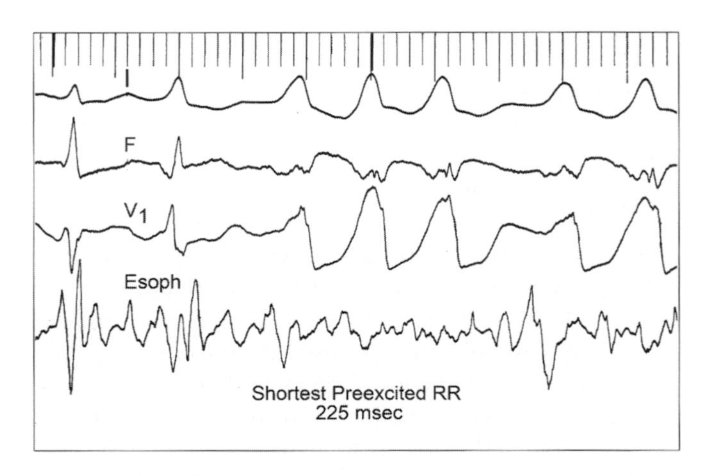

FIGURE 29–34 *Atrial electrogram showing atrial fibrillation in Wolff-Parkinson-White syndrome. The esophageal recording demonstrates continuously irregular atrial activity, whereas surface recordings show an irregular rhythm with variable QRS morphology and a shortest preexcited R-R interval of 225 msec.*
From Fyler DC [ed]. Nadas' Pediatric Cardiology. Philadelphia: Hanley & Belfus, 1992.

in the ventricular rate and potential degeneration to VF. Consequently, adenosine, digoxin, and calcium channel blockers are all absolutely contraindicated in this setting.

If the ventricular response during an episode of atrial fibrillation is documented to be slow, and there are legitimate size issues or other concerns that make catheter ablation an unattractive option, then and only then would one consider medical therapy for chronic management of a patient who experienced an episode of preexcited atrial fibrillation. Agents such as flecainide, amiodarone, or sotalol could be tried, but proof of efficacy based on some sort of follow-up electrophysiologic testing is a prudent precaution. In all other instances, catheter ablation is the treatment of choice for this condition.

ORT Involving a Concealed Accessory Pathway. The syndrome described by Wolff, Parkinson, and White consisted of a delta wave on the ECG and paroxysmal tachycardia. Because the delta wave depends on the ability of an AP to conduct anterograde, only patients with bidirectional conduction in their AP have true WPW syndrome. However, orthodromic tachycardia is not dependent on anterograde conduction. When ORT occurs without evidence of ventricular preexcitation in sinus rhythm, the AP is said to be *concealed* or *unidirectional retrograde*. This has only minimal significance for the presence and management of the ORT but has important implications regarding the risk for sudden death because rapid anterograde conduction of atrial fibrillation is not possible.

The clinical, ECG (Fig. 29-35), and electrophysiologic manifestations of ORT involving a concealed AP are identical to those of ORT in the presence of WPW, except that the PR interval and QRS complex are normal during sinus rhythm on ECG and remain so during changes in atrial rate and various atrial pacing maneuvers. Why some APs are concealed and others have manifest preexcitation is an intriguing question. The site of anterograde block for concealed APs typically occurs at the ventricular insertion and probably relates to dilution of the relatively small current density in the AP relative to the large ventricular muscle mass,[66] leading to a so-called impedance mismatch.

Initial conversion of tachycardia is also identical to that of ORT with WPW. However, the fact that no risk exists for preexcited atrial fibrillation makes the recommendations for long-term management a bit more relaxed. Patients can be safely treated in a fashion similar to AVNRT, including use of verapamil if desired. Young patients who are not yet candidates for ablation can progress through β blockers and calcium channel blockers, all the way to flecainide, sotalol, or amiodarone, until control is achieved. Young patients who fail multiple drug trials, and most all older children, can be considered candidates for catheter ablation.

Permanent Form of Junctional Reciprocating Tachycardia (PJRT). A certain subset of concealed AP is

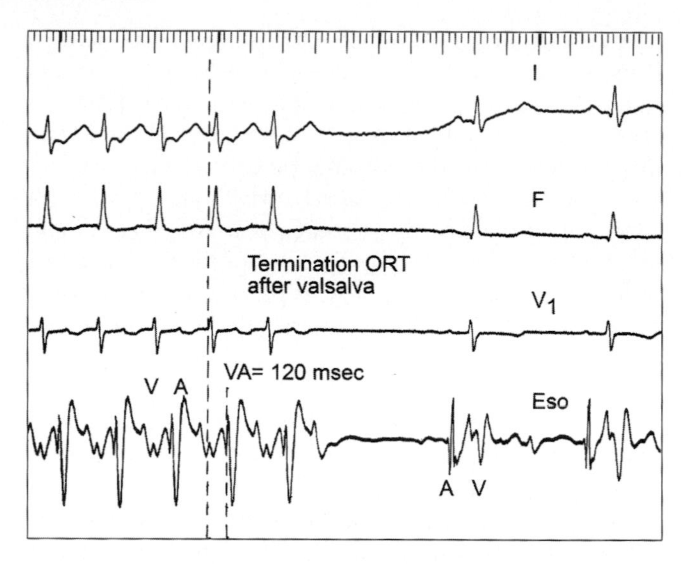

FIGURE 29–35 *Orthodromic tachycardia associated with a concealed accessory pathway. The QRS complex in tachycardia is normal and identical to that in sinus rhythm. The relatively long V-A interval of 120 msec is consistent with an orthodromic mechanism, and there was no evidence of dual AV nodal pathways. From Fyler DC [ed]. Nadas' Pediatric Cardiology. Philadelphia: Hanley & Belfus, 1992.*

characterized by remarkably slow conduction velocity, and this peculiar physiology sets up the conditions for nearly incessant reentry. Because the activation wavefront is so delayed within the AP, atrial muscle and the AV node always have ample time to recover from their refractory period, which eliminates any opportunity for the circuit to extinguish. The end result is an ECG picture of incessant tachycardia at modest rates, with a dramatically long VA interval and a rather normal PR interval. The clinical label attached to this disorder is PJRT. Although uncommon, accounting for only 1% to 3% of SVT cases in children, the striking difficulty in controlling PJRT, coupled with the profound clinical consequences of incessant tachycardia, makes it quite noteworthy.[67]

The relatively slow rates of PJRT rarely cause acute symptoms, but congestive heart failure can eventually arise from the incessant metabolic demand placed on the myocardium by chronically elevated rates. Patients tend to present during infancy or childhood, and only rarely past early adolescence. Similar to EAT, the tachycardia-induced myopathy is reversible once sinus rhythm has been restored.[18]

The AP in PJRT is usually found in the posteroseptal region of the heart. Retrograde conduction into this area will yield an inverted P wave in ECG leads II, III, and aV_F with an axis of about −120 degrees, whereas slow conduction in the AP leads to the very long VA interval (Fig. 29-36).

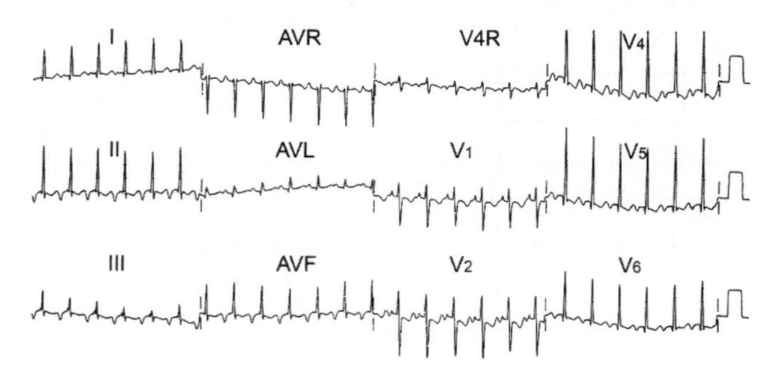

FIGURE 29–36 *Surface ECG showing the permanent form of junctional reciprocating tachycardia. Note the slow tachycardia rate of 150 beats/min, the retrograde P-wave axis of −100 degrees, the extremely long VA interval, and the normal P-R interval. The tachycardia was nearly incessant in this 10-year-old girl.*
From Fyler DC [ed]. Nadas' Pediatric Cardiology. Philadelphia: Hanley & Belfus, 1992.

The tachycardia may stop for a few beats from time to time but promptly reinitiates with either sinus tachycardia or a single premature beat. Subtle variation in conduction velocity through both the AV node and the PJRT pathway in response to changes in sympathetic state can result in tachycardia rates that range on a gradual basis as widely as 120 to 210 beats/minute in the same patient. Anterograde conduction is always through the AV node during tachycardia, resulting in normal QRS morphology. At electrophysiologic study, the atrial excitation pattern during PJRT usually reveals early activation near the mouth of coronary sinus. Often, a discrete potential representing conduction within the AP can be appreciated with careful mapping.[68]

The acute treatment protocol outlined for the more typical forms of ORT is probably a reasonable starting point for PJRT. The caveat to such a protocol is that the tachycardia is likely to recur as soon as the terminating stimulus is removed. Thus, vagal maneuvers, adenosine, atrial pacing, and DC cardioversion may terminate PJRT for as short as one beat. If the diagnosis was not entertained at initial contact, it becomes painfully obvious after frustrating attempts at acute conversion. Effective suppression of PJRT is usually only possible with long-acting medications or catheter ablation.

Many different drugs have been tested for PJRT.[69] Occasionally, control can be achieved with a relatively benign agent such as a β blocker, but more potent drugs are required for most patients. Flecainide stands out as being perhaps the most effective agent for this condition, although sotalol or amiodarone may also be used. Some infants who present with PJRT as newborns can experience spontaneous AP resolution in the first year or so of life similar to WPW; thus, medical management is usually the preferred approach in the very young. However, beyond infancy, PJRT is now treated with catheter ablation at most centers,[68] particularly if there is any evidence of ventricular dysfunction.

Mahaim Fibers. Mahaim fiber is the eponym given to an unusual AP that arises from the anterolateral aspect of the right AV groove and travels a long distance along the free wall of the right ventricle to terminate near the moderator band. Its ventricular end approximates or joins a segment of the right bundle branch, so that it is sometimes described as an *atriofascicular fiber*. Mahaim fibers were misunderstood until very recently. An older model[70] envisioned a connection between the AV node and the right ventricle (*nodoventricular*), and this teaching remained in vogue until detailed mapping data from ablation procedures revealed the true nature of the pathway.[71]

As in WPW syndrome, early ventricular activation results in the ECG appearance of a delta wave with an abnormal QRS. However, Mahaim fibers have very slow conduction, resulting in a fairly normal PR interval (Fig. 29-37). Another feature in common with WPW is a dynamic balance between normal conduction over the His-Purkinje network and abnormal preexcitation over the Mahaim fiber, which varies according to the refractory characteristics and conduction velocity of the two limbs and is also modulated by the timing of the atrial depolarization. This results in a wide array of ECG appearances (Fig. 29-38) and ultimately can predispose to reentry arrhythmias.

Mahaim fibers are rare in both children and adults. The presenting complaint is usually palpitations similar to ORT in an otherwise healthy patient, but Mahaim fibers (like WPW syndrome) seem to occur in a high percentage of patients with Ebstein's anomaly.

The surface ECG in sinus rhythm is variable and at times normal. The preexcitation pattern can wax and wane, depending on sinus rate or the presence of premature beats. Electrophysiologic study may ultimately be necessary to

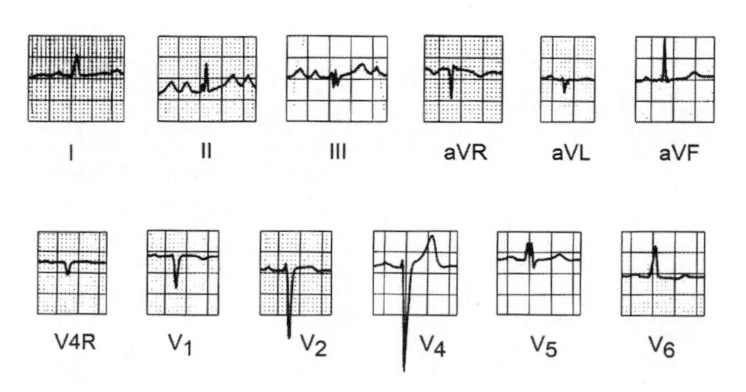

FIGURE 29–37 *Surface ECG from a patient with a Mahaim fiber proven at intracardiac electrophysiologic study. Note the delta waves in many leads but a normal P-R interval.*
From Fyler DC [ed]. Nadas' Pediatric Cardiology. Philadelphia: Hanley & Belfus, 1992.

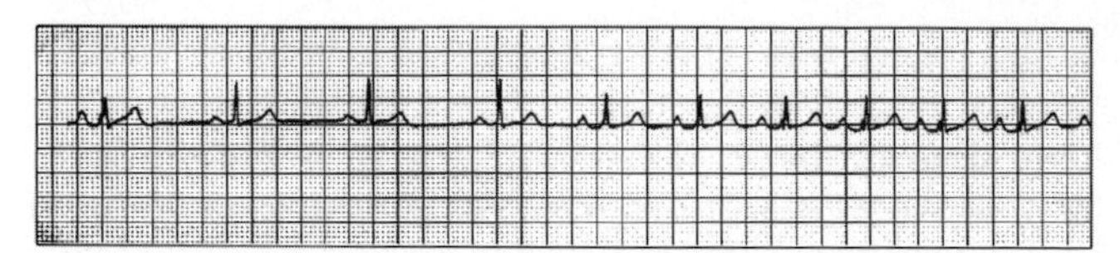

FIGURE 29–38 *Long lead II recording from same patient as in Figure 29-39, showing variability in the degree of preexcitation due to sinus arrhythmia and its effect on the relative contribution of conduction over the Mahaim fiber and normal His-Purkinje pathways.*
From Fyler DC [ed]. Nadas' Pediatric Cardiology. Philadelphia: Hanley & Belfus, 1992.

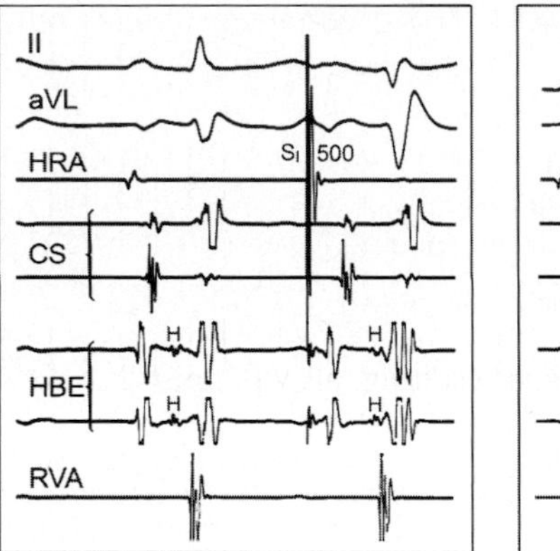

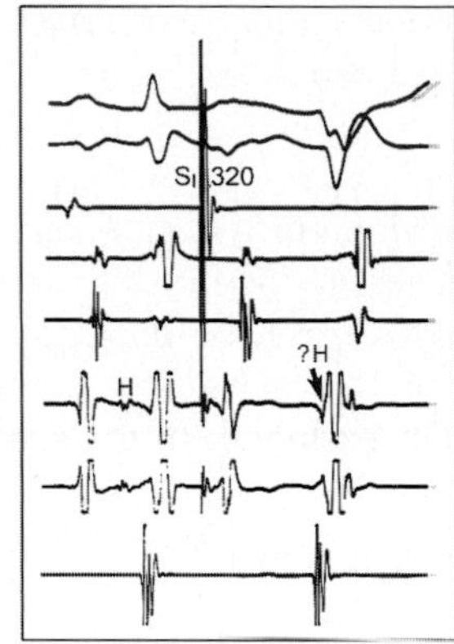

FIGURE 29–40 *Intracardiac recordings during study of a patient with a Mahaim fiber. In the left panel, a sinus beat displays a normal QRS, a normal P-R, and a normal HV. A premature atrial stimulus is then delivered at 500 msec and causes preexcitation with distortion of the QRS and shortening of the HV. In the right panel, an earlier stimulus at 320 msec increases the degree of preexcitation, with further widening of the QRS and a His deflection that is now buried within the QRS. Note, however, that the stimulus-QRS time is increasing progressively, a finding that is not typically seen in conventional Wolff-Parkinson-White syndrome.*
From Fyler DC [ed]. Nadas' Pediatric Cardiology. Philadelphia: Hanley & Belfus, 1992.

unmask Mahaim conduction or to distinguish it from the more conventional AP of WPW syndrome. Because Mahaim fibers preexcite the right ventricle, the delta wave and ventricular activation are directed right to left, sometimes mimicking left bundle branch block.

The typical reentry circuit in this disorder is antidromic, with forward conduction over the Mahaim fiber and return over the normal His-Purkinje system and AV node (Fig. 29-39), resulting in a wide QRS tachycardia with retrograde atrial activation. Atrial fibrillation may also occur, with the Mahaim fiber generating variably preexcited ventricular complexes. Rapidly conducted atrial fibrillation is generally not an issue, owing to the slow conduction potential of these pathways.

The diagnostic keys during electrophysiologic study include demonstration of a short or negative HV interval for a preexcited beat, but with gradual lengthening of the AV time (Fig. 29-40) in response to premature stimuli (unlike WPW, in which the AV time remains fairly constant). During antidromic tachycardia, earliest ventricular activation occurs on the anterior surface of the right ventricle, and earliest retrograde atrial activation occurs near the His bundle catheter. With careful mapping, one can usually record discrete potentials from the Mahaim fiber itself.

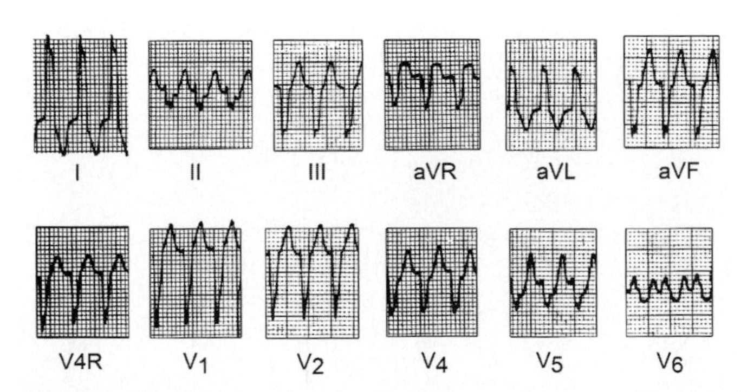

FIGURE 29–39 *Sustained wide QRS tachycardia in a patient with a Mahaim fiber proven at electrophysiologic testing. In an emergency setting, this tracing can be indistinguishable from that of ventricular tachycardia.*
From Fyler DC [ed]. Nadas' Pediatric Cardiology. Philadelphia: Hanley & Belfus, 1992.

In an emergency setting, Mahaim reentry can appear similar to VT or antidromic tachycardia in the WPW syndrome on the surface ECG, so that the diagnosis is often made only after conversion of the initial episode. It may be necessary to employ an emergency treatment strategy similar to that used for ventricular tachycardia at first presentation, using lidocaine, procainamide, esmolol, or DC cardioversion if necessary. If the diagnosis is unquestionably firm in a given patient, simply using a drug that blocks the AV node limb of the circuit, such as adenosine[72] or verapamil, can terminate tachycardia.

Mahaim fiber tachycardia can be prevented with either chronic pharmacologic therapy or catheter ablation.[71,73] Drug choices are essentially the same as for WPW syndrome. Ablation is quite successful for this disorder, although the rate of AP recurrence seems to be higher than for ablation of more conventional WPW pathways, and repeat procedures may be needed.

Ventricular Tachycardia

Tachycardias that originate from myocytes or Purkinje cells below the bifurcation of the bundle of His are grouped under the heading of VT. In general, VT carries a more serious prognosis than SVT. This difference arises not only from the hemodynamic disadvantage of the fast ventricular rate but also, more importantly, from the fact that VT typically occurs in abnormal myocardium with suboptimal function or a channelopathy, which may be vulnerable to degeneration into VF. Some specific forms of VT in young patients can be relatively benign, but this conclusion can only be reached after underlying pathology has been carefully excluded. In the acute setting, all VTs must be taken seriously.

By convention, VT is defined as three or more consecutive ectopic beats of ventricular origin on an ECG. The term *nonsustained* is applied to short self-terminating episodes, whereas the term *sustained* implies an episode lasting longer than 30 seconds or causing hemodynamic instability. The QRS complex during VT appears wide and abnormal, with a P wave that is either dissociated or arises from passive retrograde conduction. There may be competition between the ventricular arrhythmia and episodic anterograde conduction over the AV node such that fusion beats may be noted (Fig. 29-41*A* and *B*). Several varieties of VT can be distinguished by the appearance of the QRS complex during tachycardia. The term *monomorphic* is applied to a uniform QRS morphology, *bidirectional* denotes two alternating QRS types, *polymorphic* indicates a widely varying QRS (see Fig. 29-41*C*), and *torsades de pointes* describes a specific pattern of positive and negative oscillation of the QRS direction, which seems to twist around the isoelectric line of the ECG (see Fig. 29-41*D*).

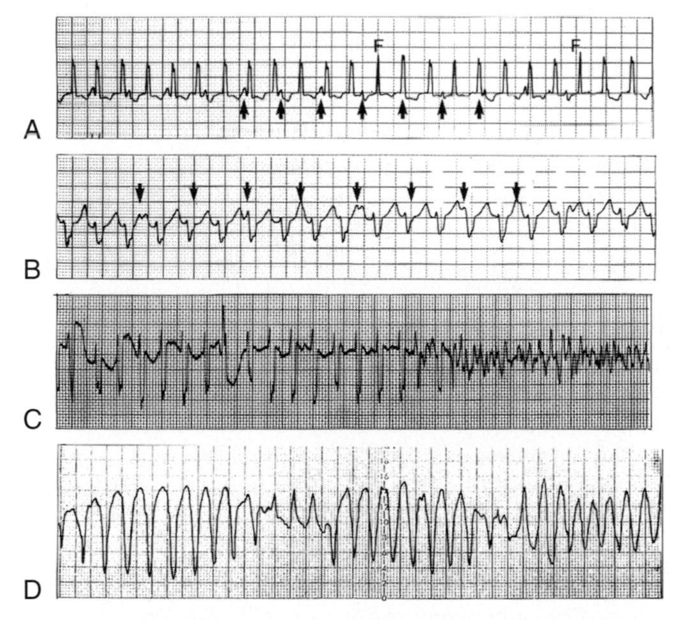

FIGURE 29–41 *Example of ventricular tachycardia.* **A**, *Monomorphic ventricular tachycardia (VT) from an infant with incessant tachycardia, showing dissociated P waves (arrows) and fusion beats (F).* **B**, *Monomorphic VT from a teenager with myocarditis, again showing A-V dissociation.* **C**, *Polymorphic VT from a postoperative patient, degenerating to ventricular fibrillation in the latter portion of the strip.* **D**, *Torsades de pointes from a patient who was being treated with quinidine.*
From Fyler DC [ed]. Nadas' Pediatric Cardiology. Philadelphia: Hanley & Belfus, 1992.

Intracardiac electrophysiologic study is indicated for some VT patients to rule out atypical SVT as the true mechanism for the arrhythmia, or to gain insight into VT mechanism and focus of origin to help plan therapy. In years past, electrophysiologic studies were also performed to evaluate the response to serial antiarrhythmic drug trials, but this role has declined considerably in the era of the implantable cardioverter defibrillator (ICD).

Acute Treatment of VT. Sustained ventricular tachycardia should be treated as an emergency. Arterial blood pressure and perfusion should be assessed immediately and a 12-lead ECG recorded. A history should be obtained with particular attention to medications, possible toxic exposures, and known familial arrhythmias.

Any patient who is unresponsive should be treated with immediate DC shock of 1 to 2 joules/kg. The energy should be synchronized to the QRS if the VT is well organized and has sufficient amplitude, but an unsynchronized discharge is required for VF or rapid polymorphic VT with low-voltage QRS complexes. If an initial shock is unsuccessful, the energy can be doubled and repeated for one or two additional trials.

If the patient is awake and stable, or if electrical conversion is unsuccessful, intravenous drug therapy should be initiated. Lidocaine, administered as a bolus and followed by a continuous infusion, remains the safest first-line agent. Second-line choices depend somewhat on the ECG appearance and the cause of the VT. For monomorphic VT, intravenous procainamide, esmolol, or amiodarone can all be considered. However, if the VT is of the torsades de pointes variety or occurs in the setting of antiarrhythmic drug toxicity, esmolol and magnesium are more appropriate agents. As a general rule, there is no place for adenosine or verapamil in the emergency treatment of a new patient with VT (or any tachycardia with a wide QRS for which the mechanism is uncertain).

Chronic Management of VT. When choosing a long-term treatment plan for VT, the following must be taken into account: (1) the patient's symptoms (or lack thereof), (2) the presence and degree of underlying cardiac pathology, (3) the rate, duration, and morphology of the VT, (4) family history, and (5) the natural history of the specific disorder. Careful evaluation of cardiac structure and function is an important part of the decision process. All patients should undergo echocardiography, and some may require cardiac catheterization or magnetic resonance imaging studies. Subtle pathology such as right ventricular dysplasia, coronary anomalies, and myopathy may be uncovered only with these techniques. If cardiac structure and function are judged to be normal, selected patients with ventricular ectopy who are asymptomatic are often followed closely without therapy, whereas symptomatic patients (whether or not cardiac pathology is demonstrated) are usually treated. Unfortunately this leaves a large and complex gray zone of asymptomatic patients with varied degrees of cardiac pathology who exhibit high-grade ventricular ectopy. The clinician must constantly balance side effects of therapy (including the proarrhythmic potential of some drugs, and the chance of complications with ablation or ICD implant) against the ultimate risk for a malignant arrhythmia. Consultation with a cardiac electrophysiologist is recommended to assist with these difficult decisions.

Specific Forms of VT in Children. VT is a rare arrhythmia in children, and its causes are diverse. Unlike VT related to ischemic heart disease in adult patients, for whom treatment protocols can be driven and refined by enormous clinical experience, no single condition is sufficiently common in children to permit development of authoritative treatment recommendations. The views expressed here reflect our current institutional policy but will certainly be subject to change as new data become available.

Slow Transient VT in Infancy. Relatively slow monomorphic VT can be observed in some neonates or infants with an otherwise normal heart.[74,75] It appears to be due to focal automaticity arising from the right ventricle. The rates (less than 200 beats/min) tend to be just slightly above underlying sinus rhythm, and such mild tachycardia does not result in hemodynamic compromise or symptoms. This benign arrhythmia tends to resolve over the first year of life, although it can persist until age 3 to 5 years in some cases. Treatment is usually unnecessary. β Blockers, which are usually effective in suppressing this disorder, are sometimes prescribed if the VT is present throughout a large percentage of the day.

Rapid Incessant VT in Infancy. This rare condition involves monomorphic VT at rapid rates (more than 200 beats/min) (see Fig. 29-43A, later) and is often so protracted that ventricular function may become compromised or VF may occur. The cellular mechanism is poorly understood, but the VT is usually of left ventricular origin and exhibits many features typical of an automatic focus in that it may fail to respond to DC shock or overdrive pacing. Multiple different VT morphologies may sometimes be seen in the same patient. Some young children have undergone successful surgical excision[76] for uncontrollable VT, and the diseased tissue frequently exhibits pathologic features that suggest epicardial hamartomas of Purkinje cell origin. If the tumor is discrete and solitary, surgery or ablation could be curative, but tumors are sometimes present in a diffuse infiltrative process known as *histiocytoid cardiomyopathy*,[77,78] which is far more difficult to treat. No single antiarrhythmic medication is universally effective in this condition, and potent combinations (e.g., amiodarone plus flecainide plus β blockers) are often required to suppress VT. If the patient has reasonable ventricular function at presentation, chronic pharmacologic treatment[79] can be used for 1 year or so, and this disorder may actually resolve spontaneously over time in some cases.[80] However, in patients with advanced ventricular dysfunction or cardiac arrest, urgent catheter or surgical ablation may need to be considered.

Long QT Syndrome. A prolonged QTc interval on the ECG is a marker for diffuse abnormalities of ventricular repolarization, which in turn may predispose to recurrent VT of the torsades de pointes type.[81] A prolonged QT may be seen as a congenital disorder, or it may be acquired from exposure to certain drugs, toxins, or electrolyte disturbances.

The congenital forms of long QT deserve the most emphasis here. Our understanding of these membrane channelopathies has expanded dramatically over the past decade thanks to identification of specific genetic defects in afflicted families (see Chapter 61). Whereas only two forms of heredity long QT were appreciated in past years (the Romano-Ward type, and the Jervell and Lange-Nielsen type), there are now known to be at least seven distinct gene defects.[82–85] Five of the seven are involved with the function of membrane potassium channels, one involves a sodium channel, and the remaining defect involves a structural protein known as *ankyrin-B*. In simplistic terms, the heterozygous condition for any one of these defects can be viewed as causing the Romano-Ward phenotype of normal hearing and long QT. The homozygous condition for any one defect, or the heterozygous condition for any two defects in combination, can be viewed as causing the Jervell and Lange-Nielsen phenotype of congenital deafness and severe long QT. The individual family mutations or spontaneous mutations that contribute to these seven gene defects are innumerable.[86,87] All blood relatives should have screening ECG performed (regardless of symptom status) whenever an index case of long QT is identified.

The symptoms of long QT syndrome may surface at any age and usually involve episodic dizziness, palpitations, syncope, and even cardiac arrest. These symptoms have been well correlated with episodes of torsades de pointes, and although the VT often stops spontaneously, a prolonged episode can ultimately result in death. The episodes may sometimes be confused with a seizure disorder or benign vasovagal syncope. For this reason, it is recommended that an ECG be obtained as a routine part of the workup for any young patient with unexplained syncope or a first seizure. The long QT syndrome is also thought to be involved in some cases of sudden infant death syndrome.[88]

The diagnosis depends on demonstration of a QT interval that is prolonged beyond the normal range when corrected

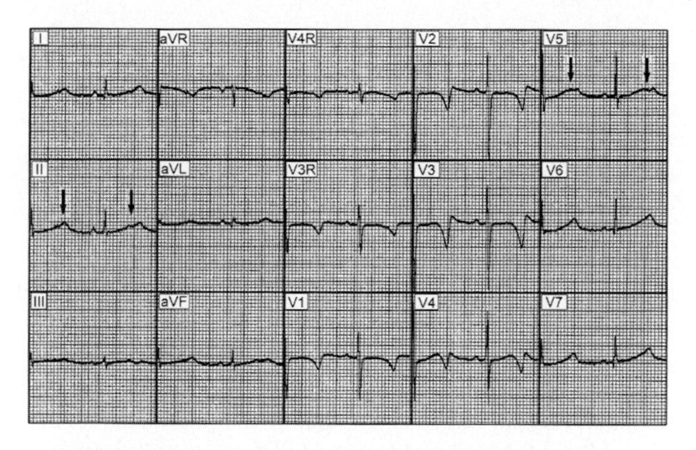

FIGURE 29–42 *Surface ECG from a patient with congenital deafness and long Q-T syndrome who experienced multiple episodes of torsades de pointes with syncope. The T wave is notched and markedly prolonged (arrows). The corrected QT interval at this heart rate exceeded 0.55 msec.*

for heart rate (Fig. 29-42). Certain morphologic features of the T wave (notching or low amplitude), as well as certain clinical features (VT with auditory stimuli or swimming), have been found to correlate with specific gene defects. The ECG findings can be synthesized with the patient's symptoms and family history to generate a clinical risk score,[89] which can be particularly useful when the ECG is borderline or equivocal. Genotyping is also becoming more widely available for this disease.

Programmed ventricular stimulation at electrophysiologic study is not effective for triggering VT or predicting treatment response in the long QT syndromes. Currently, one must still rely on patient symptoms and ambulatory monitoring to gauge effects of therapy. Most often, initial treatment involves high-dose β blockade and activity restriction. Sinus bradycardia and variable AV block may also be seen with this syndrome and may necessitate permanent pacemaker placement[90] both to relieve bradycardia and to reduce VT that may be conditioned by slow ventricular rates. The use of a β blocker, plus pacing when appropriate, has been shown to prevent symptoms in up to 80% of young patients.[91,92] However, cases that remain refractory to these measures could be considered for ICD implantation, surgery, or both to interrupt the left cervical sympathetic ganglion.[93]

Brugada Syndrome. Less common than long QT syndrome is the membrane channelopathy recognized recently as Brugada syndrome.[94] The QT is normal in this condition, but the ECG reveals a right ventricular conduction delay and unusual ST elevation in leads V_1 through V_3 (Fig. 29-43). These findings can fluctuate in some patients to the point that their ECG appears nearly

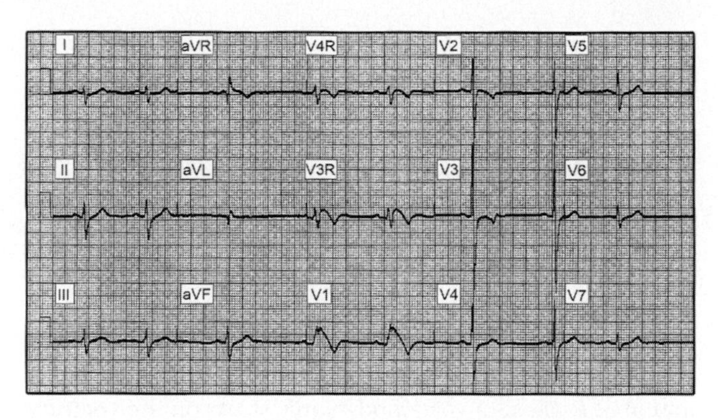

FIGURE 29–43 *ECG from a young patient with Brugada syndrome, showing the right ventricular conduction delay and dramatic ST abnormalities in the right precordial leads.*

normal at times. Provocative challenges with certain antiarrhythmic drugs such as procainamide and flecainide have been used to uncover the abnormalities when the diagnosis is uncertain.[95] Episodic polymorphic VT occurs, which can be fatal. A sodium channel defect has been implicated as the cause of most cases of Brugada syndrome, and the pattern of inheritance suggests an autosomal dominant disorder.[96] Symptoms usually occur in adulthood, but some highly symptomatic children have been observed. Implant of an ICD is recommended in most cases of symptomatic Brugada syndrome. No specific drug has been demonstrated to be effective in preventing sudden death once symptoms begin.[97]

Catecholaminergic VT. As the name implies, this unusual disorder is associated with VT at times of exercise or stress.[98] The tachycardia can be monomorphic but frequently has a distinctive bidirectional appearance with two alternating QRS morphologies.[99] The rates are variable—sometimes just slightly faster than sinus, whereas at other times fast enough to degenerate into VF. Some patients may also demonstrate additional tachycardias of atrial and junctional origin. It has recently become apparent that this disorder is another form of membrane channelopathy, although it appears that the defects responsible are rather diverse. Perhaps the most common of these is a hereditary defect in the cardiac *ryanodine receptor*, which is involved with calcium channels in sarcoplasmic reticulum.[100] An almost identical clinical VT can be seen in *Anderson's syndrome*, which is a defect in membrane potassium channel function whose phenotype can also involve periodic paralysis of skeletal muscle.[101] Regardless of underlying cellular defect, catecholaminergic VT is unpredictable and potentially fatal. Treatment can begin with high-dose β blocker and activity restriction in young patients, but should probably escalate to an ICD if any symptoms persist.

VT in Congenital Heart Disease. Ventricular arrhythmias are often seen as a late complication of congenital heart disease. The lesion most frequently associated with VT is tetralogy of Fallot,[102,103] but it may occur with other defects as well.[104–106] High-grade ventricular arrhythmias may appear even in palliated patients who have not had intracardiac repairs,[107] suggesting that direct surgical scarring is not the lone causative factor. Additionally, there is strong evidence that patients undergoing complete repair of congenital defects early in life are less likely to develop arrhythmias at late follow-up.[108] It may be that early elimination of cyanosis and hemodynamic stress on the ventricle decreases the likelihood of later VT. Other factors correlated with ventricular ectopy and sudden death in the tetralogy population include older age at follow-up, prior large palliative shunts, right ventricular failure, and very wide QRS duration.[109]

Monomorphic VT due to macroreentry appears to be the predominant mechanism for ventricular arrhythmias in these patients. In most instances, patients who experience sustained VT usually demonstrate reproducible initiation of their arrhythmia with programmed stimulation during electrophysiology study.[110] Mapping of VT typically reveals a circuit near areas of scarring, which for the tetralogy group involves the right ventricular outflow tract and the region of the ventricular septal patch.

Although it is universally agreed that patients with sustained VT and symptoms require therapy, decisions are difficult in the absence of symptoms. Firm management guidelines have not been developed for patients who have complex ectopy detected on routine surveillance monitoring, or for tetralogy patients with a dilated right ventricle and a wide QRS who are otherwise doing well. Opinions in such cases range from no therapy all the way to prophylactic ICD. Many centers, including our own, rely on electrophysiologic studies to guide therapy along a middle course in asymptomatic patients. Although no risk stratification scheme is perfect in these cases, a positive ventricular stimulation protocol appears to identify high-risk patients with reasonable accuracy, whereas a negative protocol suggests a low risk for malignant events.[110,111] Aggressive therapy can thus be directed toward those most likely to benefit based on these test results.

Treatment of VT in congenital heart disease may involve correction of residual hemodynamic defects, suppressive drug therapy, ICD implant, catheter ablation, surgical ablation, or some combination of these measures. Surgery to insert a pulmonary valve, coupled with cryoablation of scarred areas in the right ventricular outflow tract, has recently been advocated in older tetralogy patients with severe regurgitation,[112] although data remain limited on long-term outcomes from this intervention. No specific antiarrhythmic drug is likely to be protective in all cases. Experience with mexiletine[113] and β blockers suggests efficacy in suppressing ventricular ectopy by Holter criteria, but parallel data with programmed stimulation are incomplete. Catheter ablation has been used successfully in some patients, but VT recurrences are still too common to support ablation as exclusive therapy in a high-risk patient.[114] In the current era, ICD implant appears to be the safest management strategy for VT in patients with congenital heart defects.[115]

VT in Cardiomyopathies. The management of ventricular arrhythmias in the setting of cardiomyopathy remains a major therapeutic challenge. These conditions are unpredictable, and neither ambulatory monitoring nor electrophysiologic study appears capable of removing the uncertainty surrounding the issue of VT and sudden death. Furthermore, attempts at empiric drug suppression of ectopy may worsen compromised ventricular function through negative inotropic effects, or result in proarrhythmia. Thus, therapeutic emphasis in recent years has shifted steadily toward ICD implant whenever a patient is viewed as at potentially high risk for VT or VF. The true challenge, of course, is generating a reasonably accurate risk-stratification scheme for these conditions.

Hypertrophic cardiomyopathy (HCM) is perhaps the most difficult in this regard because so many patients are entirely asymptomatic until malignant VT occurs. No single drug has been found to be broadly protective against VT for this population.[116] The clinical variables that are currently viewed as predictors of sudden death include (1) a history of syncope, (2) nonsustained VT on Holter, (3) family history of HCM with sudden death, (4) failure to augment blood pressure with exercise, and (5) dramatic septal thickness.[116,117] Data are mixed on the predictive accuracy of some of these items, but when all are viewed in aggregate, the negative predictive value for the absence of all risk factors is probably better than 90%. That is to say, if none of these are present, ICD implant appears unnecessary as a purely prophylactic measure, particularly in young, growing patients, in whom ICD lead complications are so common. How many positive findings are needed to justify an ICD depends somewhat on patient age and size. A single item could perhaps be viewed as sufficient in a fully grown teenager, but not necessarily in a 5-year-old, in whom implantation is still technically demanding. Ventricular stimulation at electrophysiologic study has been used at some centers to help guide decisions in these borderline cases, but this test is not viewed as an absolute predictor of outcome.[118] Multicenter pediatric data are now being gathered to help develop better guidelines for ICD use in young patients with HCM.[119]

Dilated cardiomyopathy (DCM) is likewise associated with unpredictable rhythm status.[120] There is reasonable correlation between ejection fraction (EF) and ventricular arrhythmias,[121] with most data suggesting that an EF much less than 35% places the patient at risk for VT or VF. As with HCM, implantation of an ICD has now become the most generally accepted treatment for VT in this setting, although criteria for patient selection still vary widely from center to center. Use of an ICD as a bridge to transplantation has become increasingly common in children.[122]

A final myopathy that deserves mention is *arrhythmogenic right ventricular dysplasia* (ARVD). This familial disease involves fibrofatty degeneration of the right ventricular free wall and can be associated with recurrent VT. The ECG is one of the most reliable tools for establishing its presence, based on a combination of right ventricular conduction delay, inverted precordial T waves extending out to V_2 and beyond, and a so-called epsilon wave (Fig. 29-44) in the right precordial leads.[123] In advanced cases, abnormalities of right ventricular size, function, and muscle appearance can be appreciated on angiography, magnetic resonance imaging, and echocardiography.[124,125] However, VT may sometimes develop in this condition even before gross structural changes are detectable by these imaging techniques. The VT in this condition usually involves macroreentry within the diseased right ventricular tissue. Electrophysiologic testing is fairly reliable in reproducing these arrhythmias,[126] and the signal-averaged ECG looking for late potentials also appears to be a useful diagnostic tool. As with other the forms of cardiomyopathy, ICD implant has become the most common therapy for ARVD.[127]

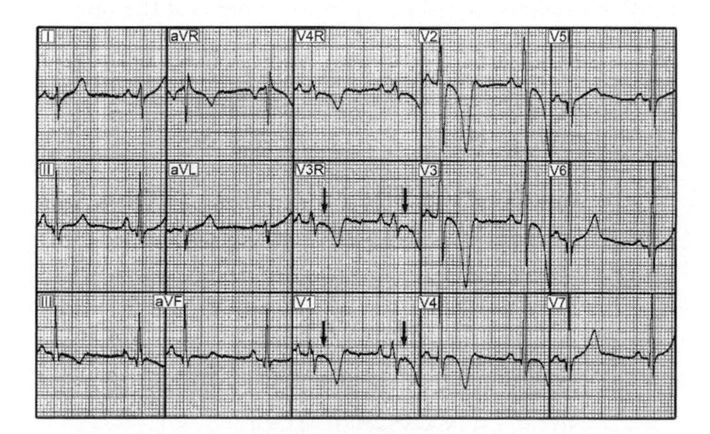

FIGURE 29–44 *ECG from teenager with familial arrhythmogenic right ventricular dysplasia, showing T-wave inversion across the precordium out to lead* V_3*, as well as a sharp epsilon wave in the right precordial leads (arrows).*

Idiopathic VT. Relatively benign forms of VT are seen occasionally in young patients without demonstrable cardiac pathology.[128] Two distinct types are recognized. The first of these is focal automatic VT arising from the right ventricular outflow tract (RVOT). This VT is monomorphic and characterized by relatively slow rates (140 to 190 beats/minute), with a QRS morphology of left bundle branch block and an axis of about +90 degrees on surface ECG. Severe symptoms are uncommon, and some patients are totally unaware of this arrhythmia.[129] However, a few may have nearly incessant VT that can eventually lead to a tachycardia-induced myopathy with congestive symptoms.[18] Furthermore, it is sometimes difficult to distinguish benign RVOT tachycardia from the more concerning VT that may arise in patients with ARVD. Symptoms such as syncope,[130] or very rapid VT rates, would tend to favor the latter diagnosis. Thus, all patients presenting with this morphology of VT should have an echocardiogram performed to evaluate ventricular function, and magnetic resonance imaging along with signal-averaged ECG may be considered if there is ever a concern about ARVD based on family history or ECG findings. Assuming all testing is normal and the patient is asymptomatic, no specific therapy is required for benign RVOT tachycardia. Some cases have been observed to resolve spontaneously with time. If symptoms occur, or the VT is present throughout large portions of the day, treatment with a β blocker can be considered, which suppresses or at least reduces VT in most young patients. Any youngster with depressed ventricular function will usually undergo an attempt at catheter ablation of the RVOT focus. Ablation is highly successful for this disorder as long as the VT remains sufficiently active during the mapping process to permit careful localization.[114,131]

A second form of benign VT is an interesting reentrant circuit along the left ventricular septum that appears to involve the posterior fascicle of the left bundle branch.[132] It goes by many clinical labels, including *Belhassen's tachycardia*[133] and *left posterior fascicular tachycardia*. This VT is abrupt in onset, operates at very regular rates in the range of 130 to 200 beats/minute, and has the ECG appearance of right bundle branch block with a superior QRS axis. It is the only form of VT in children that responds reliably to a calcium channel blocker.[134] In fact, this unanticipated drug sensitivity is responsible for yet another clinical label of *verapamil-sensitive VT* that is often attached to this condition. Assuming underlying cardiac pathology has been removed from consideration, long-term verapamil therapy can be used quite successfully to prevent recurrences of VT. Alternatively, elective catheter ablation can be performed by placing lesions along the left ventricular septal surface, guided by the recording of a sharp potential from a Purkinje fiber.[135] The success rate for ablation of Belhassen's VT approaches 90%, which is the highest for any form of VT encountered in young patients.[114]

SINOATRIAL NODE DYSFUNCTION

Although normal values are well established for resting sinus rates in all age groups, individual variation is so dramatic that it is hazardous to dictate firm cutoff values as indicative of pathologic bradycardia in children. Much depends on the clinical setting. An awake resting sinus rate of 45 beats/minute may be normal for a healthy teenage athlete but would be strictly abnormal for a similar-aged patient with poor cardiac function.

The ECG picture of pathologic sinus node behavior is a slow P-wave rate, usually with marked sinus arrhythmia, allowing a variety of escape rhythms from low atrial and junctional foci (Fig. 29-45). Additionally, the sinus node may display abrupt pauses because of exit block or even complete sinus arrest.

The most common cause of SA node dysfunction in children involves direct injury to the node or its arterial supply as a consequence of surgery for congenital heart disease. No open heart procedure, even simple closure of an atrial septal defect, is without risk for SA node dysfunction, although complex atrial baffling procedures such as the Mustard, Senning, and Fontan operations result in the highest incidence.[42,136,137] Bradycardia is frequently associated with episodic atrial reentry tachycardia (atrial flutter, or fibrillation), in which case the clinical label of *tachy-brady syndrome* is usually applied (Fig. 29-46). The situation may be further complicated by ventricular arrhythmias that can be conditioned by the low rates or arise because of coexistent pathology in ventricular muscle. Occasionally, patients with tachy-brady syndrome experience syncope and even sudden death.[40] The mechanism behind these events may include SVT with rapid ventricular response, abrupt bradycardia (as a primary event or following termination of a prolonged tachycardia), or ventricular tachycardia.

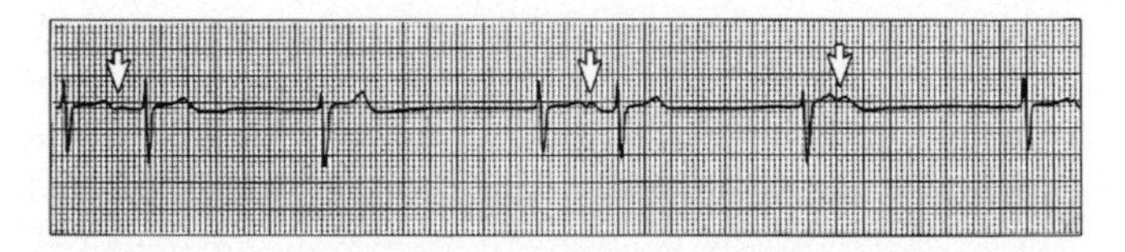

FIGURE 29–45 *Sinus node dysfunction in a patient 10 years after the Mustard operation. The P waves are slow and irregular (arrows), allowing a slow junctional escape rhythm.*
From Fyler DC [ed]. Nadas' Pediatric Cardiology. Philadelphia: Hanley & Belfus, 1992.

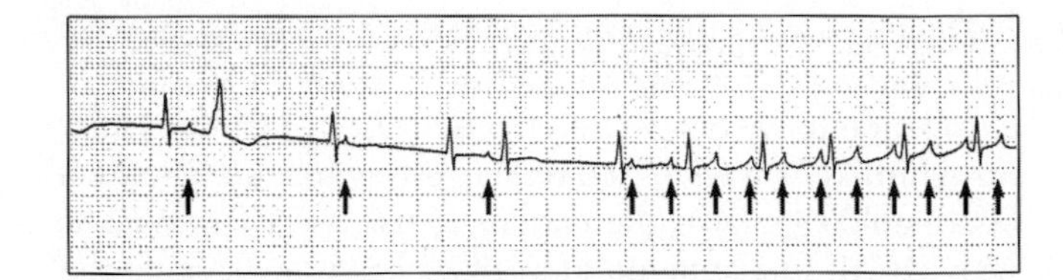

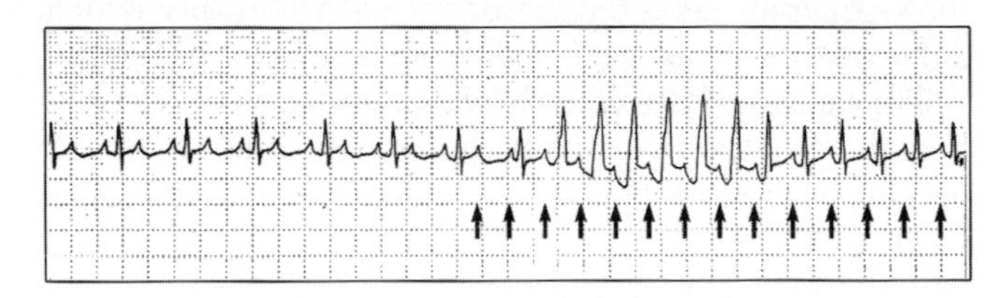

FIGURE 29–46 *Holter recordings from a patient with the "sick sinus syndrome" 5 years after a Senning operation, showing both the "brady" and "tachy" phases. The slow rhythm in the upper strip abruptly changes to a rapid, regular atrial rhythm (arrows), which is atrial muscle reentry or "flutter." This initially conducts 2:1, but on the lower strip changes to 1:1 conduction. There is transient QRS aberration at the onset of the rapid ventricular response.*
From Fyler DC [ed]. Nadas' Pediatric Cardiology. Philadelphia: Hanley & Belfus, 1992.

Asymptomatic patients with isolated sinus bradycardia of mild to moderate degrees may not require therapy unless there are hemodynamic concerns regarding ventricular contractility or valve function. However, any patients with symptoms, profound bradycardia, coexistent tachycardia, or suboptimal hemodynamics should be treated by pacemaker insertion. For those with true tachy-brady syndrome, the simple expedient of correcting bradycardia frequently reduces atrial tachycardia episodes. If atrial tachycardia episodes remain an issue, suppressive medical therapy can be considered once the rate is safely supported. In selected patients, a specialized atrial antitachycardia pacemaker can be inserted as therapy for both the "brady" and "tachy" components of this disorder. Such devices can automatically detect and interrupt atrial flutter with short bursts of rapid pacing in addition to routine antibradycardia function, and may thus eliminate the need for drug therapy in many cases.[138]

DISORDERS OF ATRIOVENTRICULAR CONDUCTION

Abnormalities of AV conduction may involve either the AV node or the proximal His-Purkinje system. They can be subdivided by grades according to the P-QRS relationship on the surface ECG.

First-Degree Atrioventricular Block

In first-degree block, every sinus beat is conducted to the ventricle, but with slow conduction velocity that results in a prolonged PR interval on the ECG (Fig. 29-47). Although delay in the AV node proper is the most common cause of first-degree block, intra-atrial delay or His-Purkinje delay may be operative in some cases.

The causes of first-degree block are numerous and include congenital cardiac malformations (atrial septal defects, AV canal defects, L-transposition), antiarrhythmic medications, myocardial inflammation or myopathy, infection (Lyme disease, viral myocarditis, endocarditis), hypothyroidism, surgical trauma, and high levels of vagal tone. In general, first-degree AV block is a well-tolerated condition. Management is aimed at identifying any reversible underlying cause and following the patient closely to be sure the condition does not progress.

Second-Degree Atrioventricular Block

Second-degree block refers to intermittent failure of conduction for a single sinus impulse. It is subclassified as either the *Mobitz I (Wenckebach)* or *Mobitz II* variety. In the former condition, there is a gradual but progressive increase in the PR interval, culminating in a single nonconducted beat, typically recurring in a sequence that can be described by the ratio of P waves to QRS complexes (2:1 = every other beat blocked, 3:2 = every third beat blocked, etc.). Mobitz I block is usually due to a conduction disorder at the level of the AV node (Fig. 29-48). In Mobitz II block, there is no premonitory conduction delay, but rather an abrupt nonconducted sinus impulse with equal PR intervals for the flanking conducted beats (Fig. 29-49). This disorder usually occurs with disease of the bundle of His and is often associated with a more diffuse disturbance of His-Purkinje conduction, such that it is rare to observe true Mobitz II block in a patient without bundle branch block on their ECG. The distinction between Mobitz I and Mobitz II block is clinically important and can usually be made simply from ECG recordings. When questions remain, intracardiac recordings of the His bundle electrogram by a transvenous catheter will determine the site of the block more precisely.

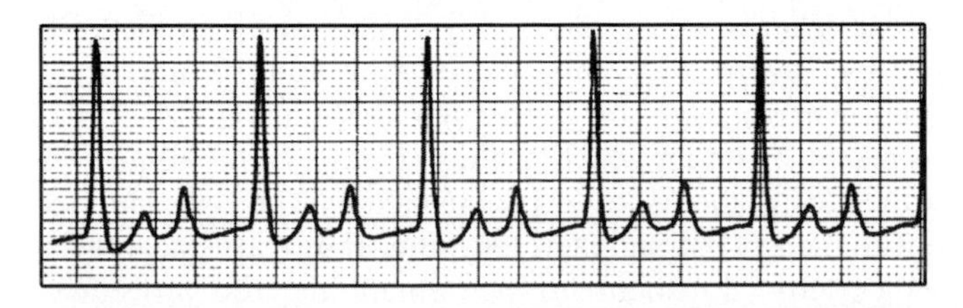

FIGURE 29–47 *First-degree AV block with a P-R interval of 0.39 msec.*
From Fyler DC [ed]. Nadas' Pediatric Cardiology. Philadelphia: Hanley & Belfus, 1992.

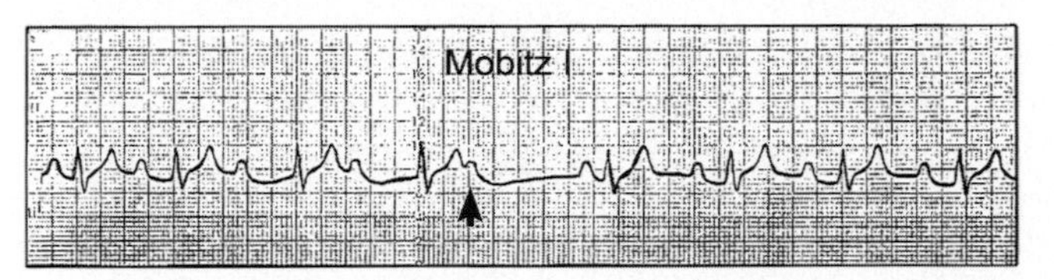

FIGURE 29–48 *Second-degree block of the Mobitz I type, showing gradual and progressive prolongation of the P-R interval before a nonconducted beat (arrow). The subsequent conducted beat has a normal P-R, after which progressive P-R prolongation resumes.*
From Fyler DC [ed]. Nadas' Pediatric Cardiology. Philadelphia: Hanley & Belfus, 1992.

Mobitz I block is well tolerated and does not always require therapy. It may be a normal finding on Holter recordings in many healthy adolescents and young adults during sleep. Etiologies are similar to those associated with first-degree block. Although most patients are asymptomatic, in some there may be progression to higher degrees of block, and in rare instances, symptomatic bradycardia may also occur. For acute symptoms, treatment with intravenous atropine or isoproterenol usually provides temporary improvement in conduction, but a pacemaker is the safest long-term therapy in symptomatic patients if the underlying cause is not reversible.

Mobitz II block due to His-Purkinje disease is a less predictable situation that usually follows inflammatory or traumatic injury below the level of the AV node. Abrupt progression to complete block may occur in this disorder, necessitating a higher level of concern than with Mobitz I block. Mobitz II block is rare in children. When it occurs as the result of surgical trauma, implantation of a pacemaker has been advised.

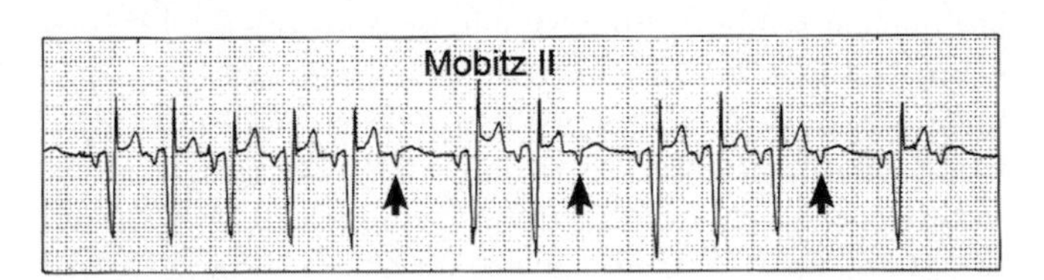

FIGURE 29–49 *Second-degree AV block of the Mobitz II type, which developed in a patient after aortic valve surgery. The P-R intervals are identical for all conducted beats, and the episodic block (arrows) follows no predictable pattern. The QRS is wide because of coexistent bundle branch block.*
From Fyler DC [ed]. Nadas' Pediatric Cardiology. Philadelphia: Hanley & Belfus, 1992.

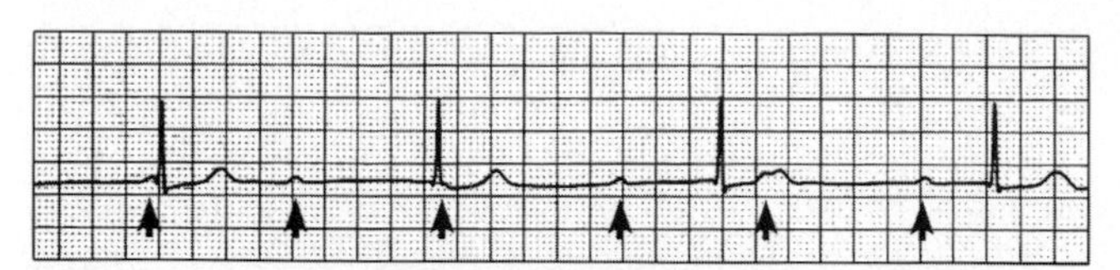

FIGURE 29–50 *Complete heart block showing nonconducted P waves (arrows) and a junctional escape rhythm at 37 beats/min. From Fyler DC [ed]. Nadas' Pediatric Cardiology. Philadelphia: Hanley & Belfus, 1992.*

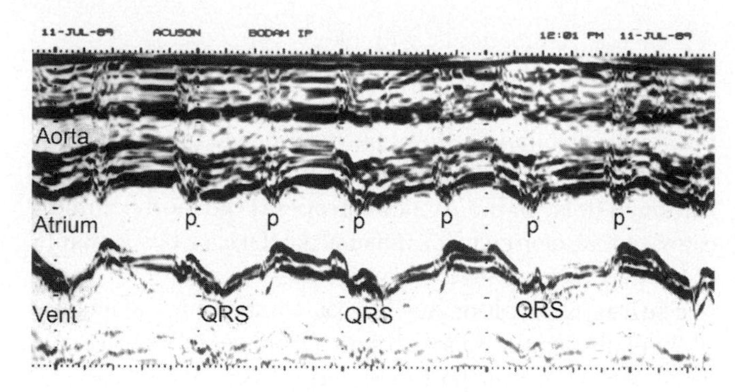

FIGURE 29–51 *M-mode fetal echocardiogram showing complete dissociation of the atrial wall motion (P) and ventricular motion (QRS) in a fetus with congenital heart block. From Fyler DC [ed]. Nadas' Pediatric Cardiology. Philadelphia: Hanley & Belfus, 1992.*

Third-Degree Atrioventricular Block

In third-degree heart block, electrical communication between the atria and ventricles is completely interrupted. The atria continue to beat at their own rate, while the slower ventricular rhythm is supplied by escape foci in the AV node, His-Purkinje system, or ventricular muscle (Fig. 29-50). The QRS complex is narrow when the escape rhythm arises above the bifurcation of the common His bundle, but will be wide if the escape focus arises low in the conducting system or if the patient has concomitant bundle branch block. Third-degree block may be congenital or acquired. The prognosis and therapy vary depending on etiology.

Congenital Complete AV Block

The most common causes of congenital heart block include fetal exposure to maternal antibodies related to connective tissue disease (primarily systemic lupus), and certain congenital cardiac defects (particularly L-transposition or AV canal defects). Often, it is first diagnosed *in utero* when a slow fetal pulse is detected on routine obstetric evaluation.[139] Fetal echocardiography can be performed to rule out structural cardiac defects and to record an M-mode tracing that views simultaneous atrial and ventricular wall motion (Fig. 29-51). Third-degree block is readily diagnosed if the faster atrial motion is completely dissociated from the slow ventricular contraction. If block is seen in the absence of structural defects, maternal testing for antinuclear antibody titers should be performed.[140–142] It is estimated that as many as 80% of mothers will have serologic evidence of connective tissue disease in this setting. Congenital heart block is usually well tolerated *in utero*, but there are well-described instances of fetal hydrops and even fetal death.[141] Unfortunately, treatment of a distressed fetus is difficult because *in utero* pacing techniques have yet to be perfected.[143] At present, the only recourse for a hydropic infant is early delivery and immediate pacing,[144] but this option is frequently limited by fetal lung immaturity.

In most cases, the fetus adapts to slow heart rates and comes to term without difficulty. Delivery should be performed at a high-risk center with pediatric cardiology backup because abrupt extrauterine decompensation may occur even if the fetus did well *in utero*. Emergency pacemaker placement can stabilize such infants promptly. For most newborns with congenital heart block, the transition to extrauterine life is smooth unless complicated by prematurity, lung disease, or anatomic cardiac defects.

Although the short-term prognosis for patients with congenital block is generally good,[145] the long-term outlook is guarded, and most will ultimately require pacemaker insertion. In a review of 30 years of experience with congenital block in patients with normal cardiac anatomy, 32% of unpaced patients eventually developed symptoms, including 5% who had sudden cardiac arrest.[146] A large international review of this condition[147] found the incidence of early death to be 8% for patients with normal cardiac anatomy and 28% for those with structural defects. Certainly, all symptomatic patients should be treated promptly with pacing, but pacemaker implantation should also be considered in advance of symptoms for any patient thought to be at risk for sudden events. Potential risk factors for poor outcome have been sought in multiple studies and include (1) a resting ventricular rate below 55 beats/minute for neonates, (2) a resting ventricular rate below 50 beats/minute for older patients, (3) a prolonged Q-T interval, (4) a wide QRS escape rhythm, (5) ventricular ectopy, and (6) more than mild cardiomegaly or ventricular dysfunction.[146,148–150] It remains uncertain which of these factors is the single best predictor of the need for prophylactic pacer insertion, but given the low risk and high reliability of modern pacer technology, the threshold for recommending the procedure should be low. If none of the above factors are present, it appears reasonable to follow younger patients conservatively if small body size and growth potential could complicate pacemaker implantation and lead maintenance.

Ultimately, all patients will likely receive a permanent pacemaker by the time they are fully grown. Even though the prognosis is generally excellent after pacing, some patients can still develop late-onset ventricular dysfunction.[151] Currently, it is unclear whether this is due to a more generalized cardiac inflammatory process, a result of chronic right ventricular pacing, or some combination of factors.

Acquired Complete AV Block

The most common etiology for acquired AV block in the pediatric age group is direct injury to the conduction tissues during cardiac surgery or catheterization. In about two thirds of cases, traumatic AV block is a transient disturbance that needs only to be treated with temporary pacing until normal conduction returns. If improvement is not observed with 10 days, recovery becomes unlikely.[152]

The prognosis for traumatic AV block is poor unless the patient receives a permanent pacemaker. A fatality rate as high as 50% was observed in follow-up of children with postoperative block in the era before pacemaker therapy was routinely available. At present, there does not appear to be any clinical setting in which pacemaker implant can be safely deferred for persistent third-degree surgical block.

Complete block can also be acquired from inflammatory processes, metabolic disease, neuromuscular disorders, and infectious diseases (e.g., Lyme disease, viral myocarditis) in children.[153] Unless the block can be reversed by treatment of the underlying cause, pacemaker implantation is advisable.

PHARMACOLOGIC THERAPY

The role of antiarrhythmic drugs has decreased dramatically over the past decade, but these agents are still essential tools for rhythm management, especially in the acute setting. Antiarrhythmic drugs are commonly classified according to their effects on cardiac cell action potentials, as initially proposed by Vaughan Williams in 1970. According to this scheme, the drugs are divided into four major groups:

Class I: Local anesthetic agents that reduce upstroke velocity of phase 0 in atrial, ventricular, and Purkinje cells (sodium channel blockers)
Class II: Drugs that inhibit sympathetic activity (β blockers)
Class III: Drugs that prolong action potential duration without changing phase 0
Class IV: Drugs that block the slow inward current (calcium channel blockers)

Class I agents are usually split into subclasses A, B, and C, depending on the degree of modification in the upstroke of phase 0, as well as the effects on repolarization and conduction velocity. This grouping of agents by *in vitro* cellular effect is a useful method for predicting ECG changes during treatment and a reasonable starting point for matching drug effect with arrhythmia mechanism.

A practical formulary of antiarrhythmic agents is reviewed here with emphasis on cellular effects and caveats regarding their use in children. Data regarding pediatric dosages are presented in the Appendix. It is interesting to note that nearly half the antiarrhythmic drugs mentioned in the prior edition of this textbook have now become obsolete or unavailable (including quinidine, disopyramide, tocainide, phenytoin, encainide, moricizine, and bretylium). Better appreciation of proarrhythmic risk[154] and alternate therapy with ablation or an ICD have greatly reduced reliance on chronic pharmacologic treatment. Expanded discussion of all these topics is available from several comprehensive reviews of antiarrhythmic pharmacology for children.[155–157]

Class IA: Procainamide

The actions of a class IA drug involve moderate depression of phase 0 upstroke, a slowing of repolarization, and a prolongation of conduction time in the fast-response cells of atrial muscle, ventricular muscle, His-Purkinje cells, and APs. When these cellular events are translated to the intact heart, the main results are increased duration of the QRS and prolongation of the QT interval in the surface ECG (Fig. 29-52). These agents have minimal direct action on slow-response cells in the SA and AV nodes but may indirectly increase the sinus rate and enhance AV node conduction through anticholinergic side effects. Procainamide is the only IA drug that has remained in active clinical use for children, but it is now largely restricted to short-term intravenous administration. Oral procainamide therapy is complicated by inconsistent absorption, the need for frequent dosing, a potential for proarrhythmia, and the development of a lupus-like syndrome after prolonged use. Procainamide is helpful for acute treatment of reentry tachycardia involving atrial muscle (e.g., atrial fibrillation or flutter), ventricular muscle (monomorphic VT), and APs (e.g., WPW syndrome).

Class IB: Lidocaine and Mexiletine

The cellular effects of IB agents are subtle. In therapeutic concentrations, they cause a trivial decrease in the slope of phase 0 of a normal fast-response action potential, although the effect becomes much more pronounced under conditions of cell damage, acidosis, or hyperkalemia. In both healthy and injured fast-response cells, the duration of the action potential, and to an even greater degree the refractory period, are shortened. This effect appears primarily in

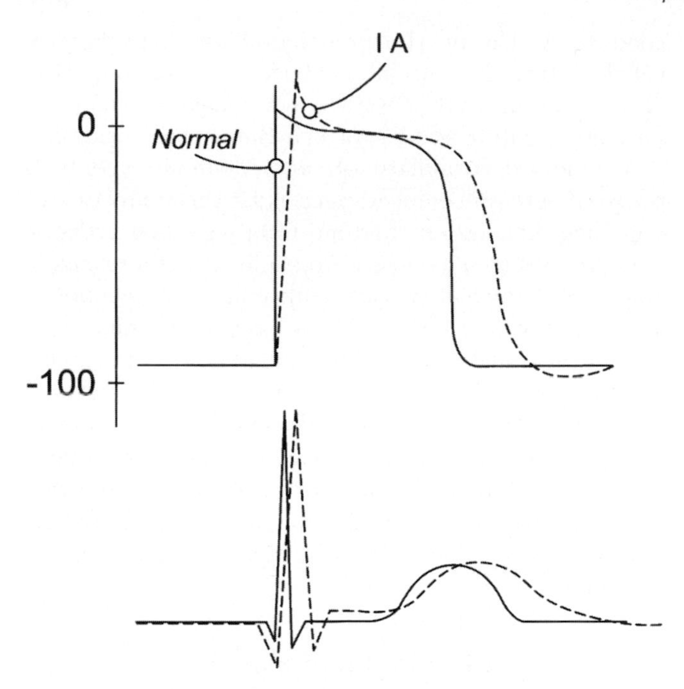

FIGURE 29–52 *Diagrammatic action potential of a fast-response cardiac cell and a corresponding hypothetical ECG stressing the effects of class IA agents.*
From Fyler DC [ed]. Nadas' Pediatric Cardiology. Philadelphia: Hanley & Belfus, 1992.

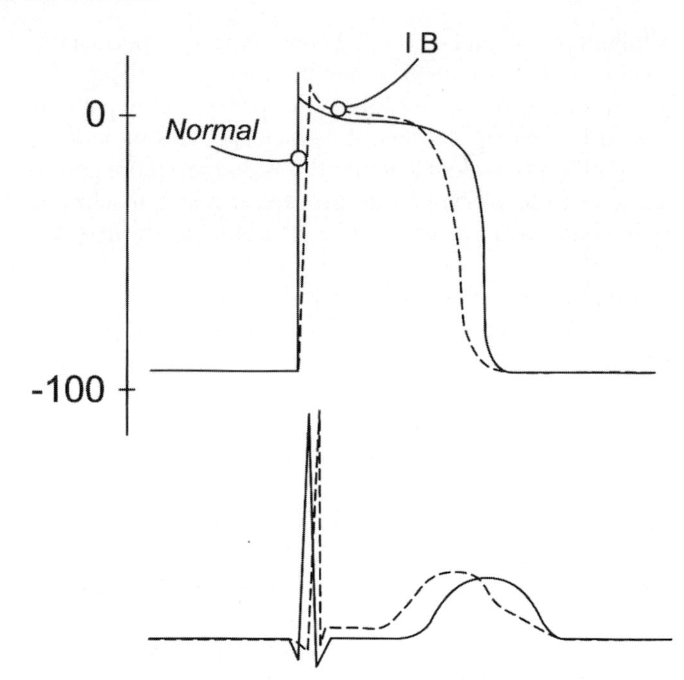

FIGURE 29–53 *Diagrammatic action potential of a fast-response cardiac cell and corresponding hypothetical ECG stressing the effects of class IB agents.*
From Fyler DC [ed]. Nadas' Pediatric Cardiology. Philadelphia: Hanley & Belfus, 1992.

Purkinje fibers and ventricular myocytes and is much less prominent in atrial tissue. Slow-response cells of the normal SA and AV nodes are not affected by IB agents, and the influence on autonomic tone is negligible. These cellular actions all translate to a surface ECG that is largely unchanged from the predrug state, except perhaps for a slight decrease in the QT internal (Fig. 29-53). The IB drugs are used for suppression of ventricular arrhythmias. Having minimal effect on atrial cells, they are usually ineffective for management of supraventricular arrhythmias.

Lidocaine is the prototype IB agent. Owing to rapid hepatic metabolism, it is only available for intravenous use as bolus followed by continuous infusion. Mexiletine is a structural analog of lidocaine with a prolonged elimination half-life that allows oral administration. Proarrhythmia is less common with IB agents than with class IA and IC drugs.

Class IC: Flecainide and Propafenone

The IC agents cause marked depression of phase 0 upstroke and profound slowing of conduction in fast-response cells. The influence on repolarization and action potential duration are minimal, so that the refractory period for an individual cell is not typically prolonged. However, in the intact heart, measured ERPs may be increased, particularly in the His-Purkinje system and APs. Drugs in this class do not appear to affect slow inward calcium currents in vitro nor alter autonomic tone. On the surface ECG, the most notable change is an increase in QRS duration caused by slowing of intraventricular depolarization. The measured QT interval may be prolonged as a consequence of the widened QRS, but the T-wave itself is not significantly modified (Fig. 29-54). Some PR prolongation may be seen.

The IC drugs are potent inhibitors of abnormal automaticity and reentry within atrial muscle, ventricular muscle, and APs, but because of their relatively high proarrhythmic potential,[158] use is reserved for patients with good ventricular function, and initiation of therapy usually requires in-hospital monitoring. Flecainide and propafenone are available for oral use only. No intravenous formulation of a class IC drug is available in the United States.

Class II: Propranolol, Nadolol, Atenolol, Esmolol

The mechanisms by which β blockade modifies cardiac arrhythmias are complex. The predominant effect is competitive inhibition of catecholamine binding at cardiac

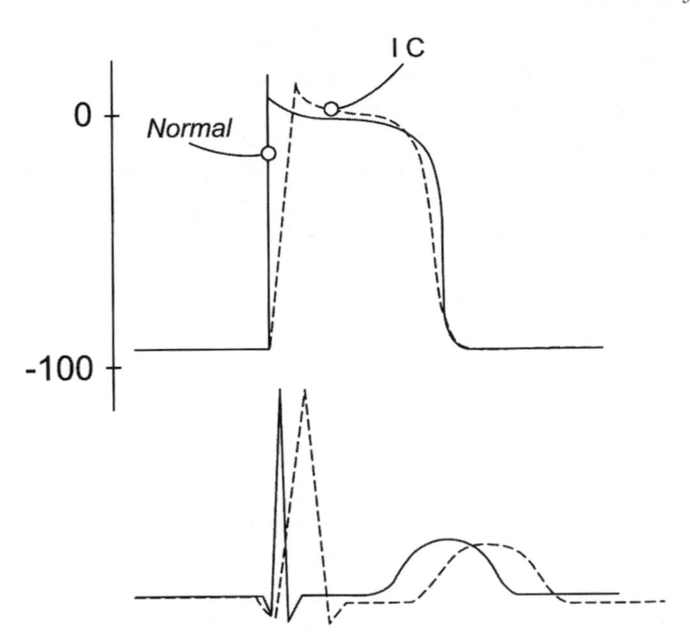

FIGURE 29–54 *Diagrammatic action potential of a fast-response cardiac cell and a corresponding hypothetical ECG stressing the effects of class IC agents.*
From Fyler DC [ed]. Nadas' Pediatric Cardiology. Philadelphia: Hanley & Belfus, 1992.

receptors, which reduces both normal and abnormal automaticity and slows AV node conduction. However, direct membrane effects may also occur, including prolonging the duration of the action potential and ERPs, as well as increasing the threshold for VF. These direct cellular actions are most pronounced during chronic administration of moderate to high doses.

Class II agents are used to treat a diverse spectrum of arrhythmias in children. They are often effective in catecholamine-mediated tachycardias from either abnormal automaticity or triggered activity at both the atrial and ventricular levels. They are less useful for reentry tachycardias but often prove effective if they suppress premature beats that serve as the initiating event for the reentry circuit. Additionally, some forms of reentry SVT may be effectively treated by β blockade if the AV node is a necessary part of the circuit and can be sufficiently slowed to prevent rapid conduction.

Propranolol is the prototype β blocker. It is *nonselective* and affects both B_1 (cardiac) and B_2 (bronchial and blood vessel) receptors. Propranolol is available for oral administration in both solution and tablet form. Important limitations include its B_2 blockade properties, which can aggravate reactive airway disease, and its B_1 blockade, which may further depress ventricular function in patients with poor contractility. Nadolol is likewise a nonselective β blocker that differs from propranolol in requiring less frequent dosing, as well having reduced penetration across the blood–brain barrier.

Atenolol is a *cardioselective* β blocker, although some cross-reactivity with B_2 receptors can still occur at high doses. It has low central nervous system penetration and maintains effectiveness with oral administration only once or twice a day. For most arrhythmias that respond to propranolol, atenolol can be equally effective. There is one report suggesting lower efficacy with atenolol while treating long QT syndrome, although this experience has not been replicated in other studies. Esmolol is an intravenous B_1 selective agent that is unique in its rapid onset and short duration of action, thus lending itself well to emergency management of arrhythmias.

Class III: Amiodarone, Sotalol

Drugs that prolong the action potential plateau without affecting phase 0 (Fig. 29-55) are grouped in class III. All such agents exhibit mixed electrical properties as well as variable effects on the autonomic nervous system.

Amiodarone is the prototype class III agent and is unlike any other antiarrhythmic drug in terms of pharmacokinetics, side effects, and potency.[159] Its electrical effects are felt at

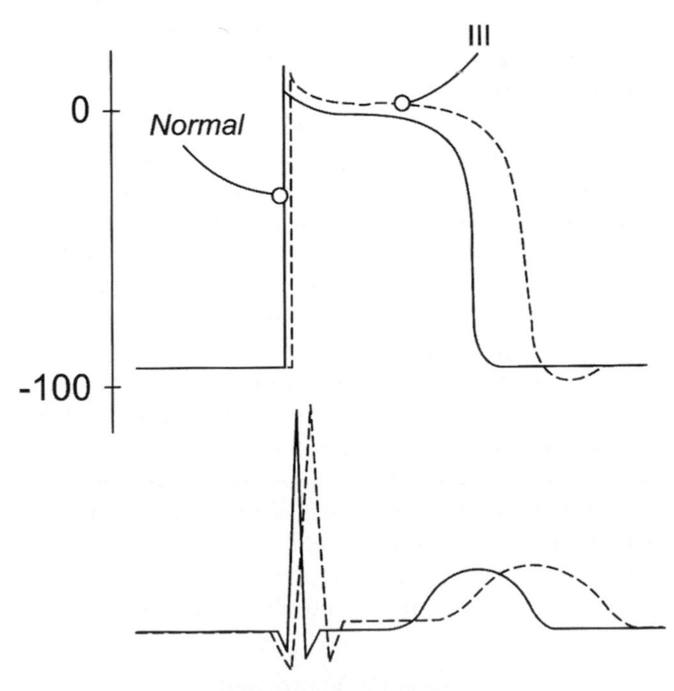

FIGURE 29–55 *Diagrammatic action potential of a fast-response cardiac cell and a corresponding hypothetical ECG stressing the effects of class III agents.*
From Fyler DC [ed]. Nadas' Pediatric Cardiology. Philadelphia: Hanley & Belfus, 1992.

all levels of the heart. Most notable is prolongation of action potential duration (and hence refractory period) in all fast-response cells of atrial muscle, ventricular muscle, Purkinje fibers, and APs. Unlike class I agents, it also has direct effects on the SA and AV nodes, decreasing the rate of automatic discharge in the former and slowing conduction in the latter. Amiodarone also possesses α- and β-blocking properties. Widespread changes occur on the ECG, including sinus slowing, PR prolongation, a slight increase in QRS width, and QT prolongation.

Amiodarone is available for both intravenous and oral administration. Although clinical experience with the intravenous formulation in children is still somewhat limited, it is being used with increasing regularity for acute management of potentially life-threatening conditions such as sustained VT, postoperative JET, and some refractory forms of SVT. Hypotension has been reported while administering intravenous amiodarone, possibly related to an alcohol component of the formulation. Careful hemodynamic monitoring is required when using it intravenously, especially in postoperative infants.

Oral amiodarone is very well tolerated from a hemodynamic point of view. Its α blockade properties are thought to provide afterload reduction through vasodilation, making it one of the few antiarrhythmic drugs that can be tolerated in patients with poor ventricular function. A major disadvantage of oral administration is the protracted loading phase required before significant drug effect is seen (1 to 4 weeks).

Serious side effects are possible with either formulation of amiodarone. This drug should not be used for trivial conditions. Proarrhythmia is a concern, as are the multiple noncardiac toxicities, such as corneal microdeposits, thyroid dysfunction, pulmonary interstitial fibrosis, hepatitis, peripheral neuropathy, photosensitive skin rash, and bluish discoloration of the skin. Amiodarone has an elimination half-life longer than 1 month. Thus, steady serum levels are assured with once-daily administration, but drug elimination is very slow should toxicity develop.

Sotalol is the other class III agent in common clinical use. It acts primarily as a nonselective β blocker at low doses but exhibits class III activity at medium-high levels. It has proved effective[160] in treatment of both supraventricular and ventricular arrhythmias in children, although use must be restricted to those with well-preserved ventricular function because of its negative inotropic properties.

Class IV: Verapamil

Verapamil is the most commonly used calcium channel antagonist in pediatric practice. It acts predominately on the slow inward current in cells of the SA and AV nodes, causing a decrease in the rate of phase 4 automaticity, a slowing of phase 0 depolarization, and a prolongation of refractoriness and conduction time. Except for a slight decrease in plateau amplitude, its effect on the normal fast-response action potential is negligible. These actions all translate to a surface ECG picture of mild sinus slowing and prolongation of the PR interval, but no noticeable change in the QRS or T wave (Fig. 29-56). Under pathologic conditions, however, verapamil can affect injured cells of ventricular or atrial tissue that may deviate from their normal fast-response characteristics. Verapamil is available for both oral and intravenous administration. The most common clinical indication is reentry SVT that requires the AV node as part of the circuit. Thus, AVNRT and ORT involving a concealed AP (but not WPW) are reasonable indications for this agent. Tachycardia arising from atrial muscle (e.g., ectopic atrial tachycardia, atrial flutter) will not respond directly to calcium channel blockade, although AV node conduction can be slowed to control the ventricular response rate in such disorders.

There are several caveats surrounding the use of this agent. Most relevant to the pediatric population is the observation that neonates may develop marked hypotension and bradycardia after intravenous administration.[161] Intravenous verapamil should be avoided in the first 12 months of life, especially now that there are safer alternate techniques for termination of SVT, such as adenosine.

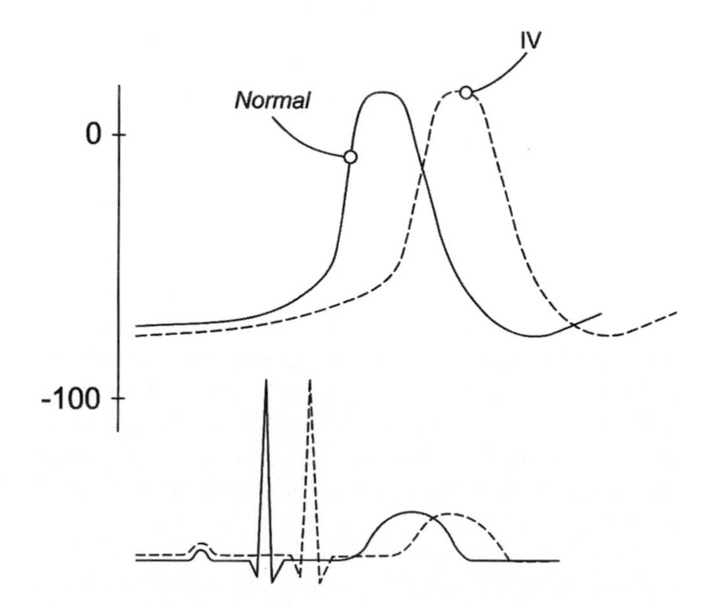

FIGURE 29–56 *Diagrammatic action potential of a slow-response cardiac cell and a corresponding hypothetical ECG stressing the effects of class IV agents.*
From Fyler DC [ed]. Nadas' Pediatric Cardiology. Philadelphia: Hanley & Belfus, 1992.

A second limitation of verapamil relates to its enhancement of anterograde AP conduction in WPW syndrome. In the setting of atrial fibrillation, verapamil could increase the ventricular response rate to dangerous levels, making it contraindicated as long-term treatment in patients with manifest preexcitation. Finally, intravenous verapamil should not be given to patients who are already taking a chronic β blocker, owing to synergistic negative inotropic effects.

Miscellaneous: Adenosine, Digoxin

Adenosine has probably become the most widely used antiarrhythmic agent in pediatric practice. It is an endogenous nucleoside found in all cells of the body, but when administered as a rapid intravenous bolus, it transiently blocks AV node conduction and slows SA node automaticity by a direct cellular effect. Adenosine is promptly removed from the circulation by erythrocytes and endothelial cells, resulting in a half-life of less than 10 seconds. It is extremely effective for interrupting narrow QRS tachycardias such as AVNRT and ORT that involve the AV node as part of the circuit. It can also serve as a useful diagnostic agent to transiently block AV nodal conduction and help elucidate the mechanism of certain tachycardias such as atrial flutter whenever uncertainty exists. It is an extremely well-tolerated drug. There may be mild hypotension and bradycardia lasting several seconds following a dose, but these effects are of little consequence given such rapid drug elimination. Adenosine may aggravate bronchospasm in patients with reactive airway disease and should be used with caution in this setting. It can also enhance anterograde conduction over APs and should thus never be given to a patient with WPW syndrome who is experiencing a wide QRS tachycardia that might possibly be due to preexcited atrial fibrillation.

Digoxin has some direct electrical effects on the cell membrane, but much of its action at standard doses relates to effects on the autonomic nervous system. The predominant clinical response to this agent (SA node slowing and depression of AV node conduction) appears to be due almost exclusively to enhancement of vagal tone. The direct cellular effects on atrial muscle, ventricular muscle, and specialized conduction tissue (including APs) can be best summarized as a mild decrease in the duration of the action potential and shortening of the effective refractory period. The above actions cause predictable changes on the surface ECG that involve sinus slowing, PR prolongation, and a slight shortening of the QT interval. Mild depression of the ST segment and flattening of the T wave may occur also. As an antiarrhythmic agent, digoxin is used primarily to slow AV conduction in patients with a primary atrial SVT such as fibrillation or flutter. With only rare exceptions, it is contraindicated in WPW syndrome.

PACEMAKERS AND IMPLANTABLE DEFIBRILLATORS

Pediatric pacing and defibrillator therapy presents unique challenges because of patient size, growth potential, and the frequent coexistence of congenital structural heart disease.[162] The indications and techniques for implantation differ in many ways from those used for adult patients with more conventional forms of heart disease. In 2002, the American Heart Association, American College of Cardiology, and North American Society of Pacing and Electrophysiology published updated guidelines for pacemaker implantation that included a special section for children.[163] The recommendations were grouped into conditions for which pacing is indicated (class I), conditions for which the consensus is divided or unclear (class II), and conditions for which pacing is not indicated (class III). The current class I indications for pacemakers in children are summarized in Table 29-2. Specific ICD guidelines for pediatric patients have not yet been published but generally follow the criteria used for adult patients.

Of all patients who underwent permanent pacemaker or ICD placement at Children's Hospital Boston from 1980 to 2003, 22% were at least 18 years old. The median age at initial implant was 9.0 years (range, 0 to 54 years), and the patients weighed between 1 and 114 kg. The substantial number of young adult patients reflects the increasing population of survivors of congenital heart disease surgery in whom arrhythmias are a common late complication.

TABLE 29–2. Current Class I Indications for Pacing in Children

1. Advanced second- or third-degree AV block associated with symptomatic bradycardia, ventricular dysfunction, or low cardiac output.
2. Sinus node dysfunction with correlation of symptoms during age-inappropriate bradycardia.
3. Postoperative advanced second- or third-degree AV block that is not expected to resolve or that persists at least 7 days after cardiac surgery.
4. Congenital third-degree AV block with a wide QRS escape rhythm, complex ventricular ectopy, or ventricular dysfunction.
5. Congenital third-degree AV block in the infant with a ventricular rate of less than 50 to 55 beats/min, or with congenital heart disease and a ventricular rate of less than 70 beats/min.
6. Sustained pause-dependent ventricular tachycardia, with or without long QT, in which the efficacy of pacing is thoroughly documented.

See reference 163 for expanded discussion, including Class II and III recommendations.

Pacemakers in Children

There is currently no pacemaker specifically designed for use in children because they make up such a small fraction of the pacemaker market. However, technology has allowed pacemakers to become much smaller in size and weight. Some simple single-chamber generators are now available with a volume of only 6 cc and weight of 12.8 gm, and fully programmable dual chamber devices are now available with a 10-mL volume that can be implanted in a full-term newborn (Fig. 29-57).

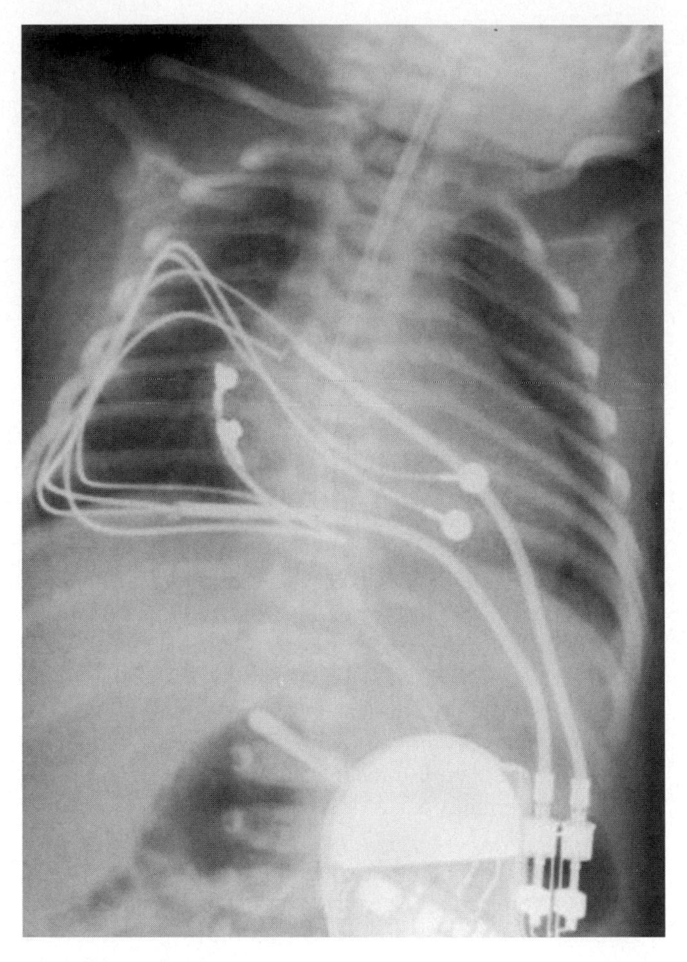

FIGURE 29–57 *Chest x-ray of a 3-kg infant with a DDD pacemaker. Bipolar epicardial leads have been attached to the right atrium and right ventricle. The generator has been placed in a pocket on the abdominal wall.*

Generators and Pacing Modes

The North American Society of Pacing and Electrophysiology (NASPE) and the British Pacing and Electrophysiology Group (BPEG) developed a system of generic codes to describe functionality of pacemakers.[164] This code has been revised several times to incorporate capabilities for programmability, rate modulation, antitachycardia functions, and multisite pacing (Table 29-3). The basic code is a three-letter shorthand description of the chamber paced, chamber sensed, and response to sensing. The fourth and fifth letters are used to describe special features such as rate modulation and multisite pacing (Figs. 29-58 to 29-61).

Atrial-based pacing (including AAI, DDD, and VDD pacing modes) has been shown in adult studies to be superior to simple ventricular-based (VVI) pacing.[165–167] Dual-chamber or atrial pacing may have less morbidity and mortality compared with ventricular pacing in patients with congestive heart failure, valvular heart diseases, and hypertensive heart disease. Although one may still need to resort to VVI pacing in some infants because of size constraints, a pacing system that can ensure AV synchrony is preferred when possible.

There are several types of rate-responsive sensors in modern pacemakers. The most common measure activity, using either a vibration crystal or an accelerometer mounted

TABLE 29–3. Antibradycardia Pacemaker Operation

Standard Three-Letter Code		Special Functions		
I	II	III	IV	V
Chamber Paced	*Chamber Sensed*	*Sensing Response*	*Rate Modulation*	*Multisite Pacing*
O = none A = atrium V = vent D = A & V	O = none A = atrium V = vent D = A & V	O = none T = triggered I = inhibited D = T & I	O = none R = rate	O = none A = two atrial sites responsive V = 2 vent sites D = 2A & 2V sites

From Bernstein AD, Daubert JC, Fletcher RD, et al. The revised NASPE/BPEG generic code for antibradycardia, adaptive-rate, and multisite pacing. North American Society of Pacing and Electrophysiology/British Pacing and Electrophysiology Group. Pacing Clin Electrophysiol 25:260, 2002.

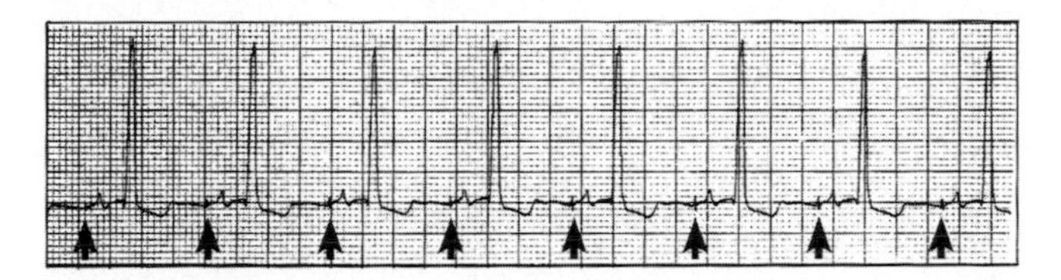

FIGURE 29–58 *Atrial pacing (arrows) in AAI mode for patient with sinus bradycardia and intact AV conduction.*
From Fyler DC [ed]. Nadas' Pediatric Cardiology. Philadelphia: Hanley & Belfus, 1992.

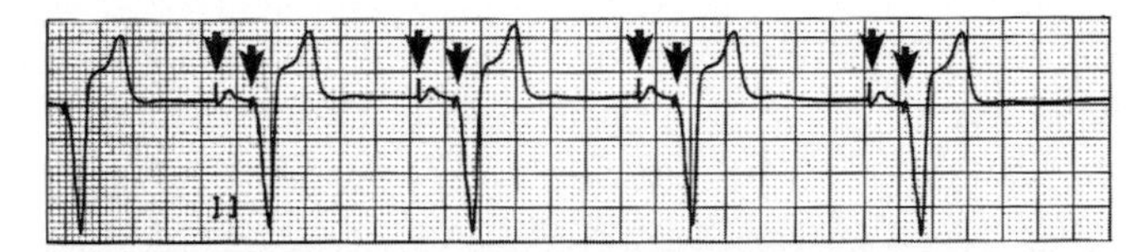

FIGURE 29–60 *Dual-chamber DDD pacing in a patient with sinus bradycardia and complete heart block. Both atrial and ventricular leads pace in this case (arrows).*
From Fyler DC [ed]. Nadas' Pediatric Cardiology. Philadelphia: Hanley & Belfus, 1992.

inside the generator. Minute ventilation rate adaptive sensors are also available and correlate well with physiologic heart rates in children. There are potential pitfalls in using these sensors in pediatric patients, including a more variable pocket location (abdominal or pectoral position) and the type of exercise performed by younger children or patients with congenital heart disease. In patients with normal sinus node function, the intrinsic sinus rate is ordinarily the best physiologic sensor. Exercise testing may be useful for optimizing the sensor response programming.

Biventricular pacing is a new refinement in generator function that activates the right and left ventricles in a nearly simultaneous fashion, thereby eliminating any delay or asynchrony between the two chambers. This feature has proved to be an effective treatment option for adults with congestive heart failure and intraventricular conduction delays.[168,169] The utility of resynchronization therapy in pediatric patients is less well studied; however, the preliminary experience has been promising.[162,170]

Leads and Implant Techniques

The interface between the pacemaker lead and cardiac tissue is the most crucial component of any pacing system. Leads must be positioned such that there is proper recognition of intrinsic electrical activity (*sensing* function), as well as of low energy requirements for pacing (*threshold* or *capture* function).

Although most adult pacemaker recipients have leads placed transvenously, epicardial leads are still required in many children. The primary reasons for epicardial placement include small patient size, significant intracardiac shunting in which thrombus on a transvenous lead might pose an embolic risk, or lack of vascular access (e.g., after a Fontan operation). At Children's Hospital Boston, roughly half of all leads implanted over the past 30 years were epicardial, although the advent of thinner transvenous leads has now overcome size constraints to some extent, and transvenous leads are now preferred whenever possible. The transvenous route has the advantages of avoiding a thoracotomy, lower pacing thresholds, and lower incidence of lead fractures.[171–173] The disadvantages of transvenous leads include a risk for venous occlusion[174] and potential difficulties with lead length as a child grows.

Epicardial leads are available as screw-in, stab-on, or suture-on methods of fixation (Fig. 29-62). Steroid-eluting epicardial leads are now available that suppress the subacute threshold rise secondary to tissue inflammatory response[175] and may contribute to lead longevity and reduced battery drain. Hopefully, improvements in epicardial lead design and the advent of steroid-eluting capability will diminish the historically high rate of epicardial lead failures.

Transvenous leads are attached to the endocardium by either active or passive fixation mechanisms (see Fig. 29-62). Active fixation leads are now used most commonly and operate with a small screw at the tip that anchors into

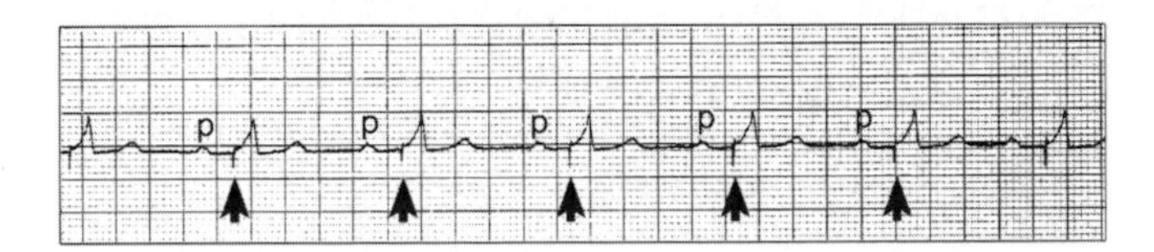

FIGURE 29–59 *Operation of the VDD mode in a patient with heart block but normal sinus node function. One lead senses atrial activity (P); the generator then waits for a 200-msec time delay and paces the ventricle (arrows) through the ventricular lead.*
From Fyler DC [ed]. Nadas' Pediatric Cardiology. Philadelphia: Hanley & Belfus, 1992.

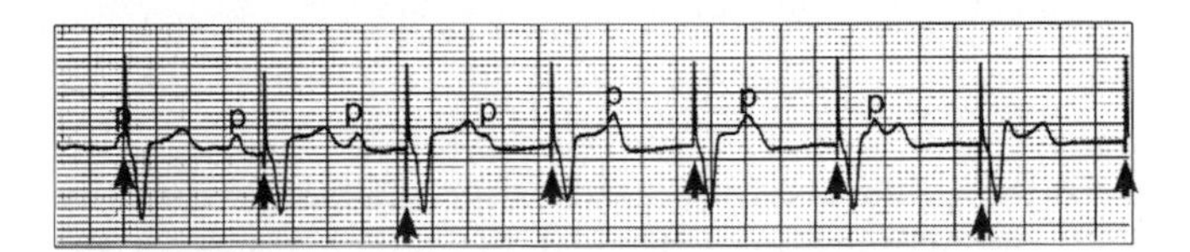

FIGURE 29–61 *Ventricular pacing (arrows) in the VVI mode. Atrial activity (P) is completely dissociated. Absence of AV synchrony caused no difficulties in this patient with congenital heart block and otherwise normal cardiac anatomy and function.*
From Fyler DC [ed]. Nadas' Pediatric Cardiology. Philadelphia: Hanley & Belfus, 1992.

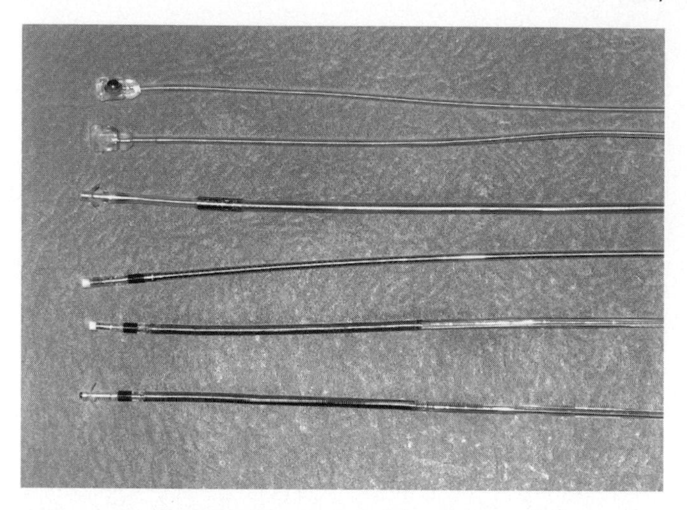

FIGURE 29–62 *Examples of contemporary pacemaker and implantable cardioverter defibrillator (ICD) leads, including (from top to bottom): epicardial sew-on pacing lead (two electrodes from a bipolar lead), bipolar transvenous passive-fixation pacing lead, bipolar transvenous "thin" active-fixation pacing lead, transvenous active-fixation ICD lead, and a transvenous passive-fixation ICD lead.*

the endocardium. Most modern transvenous leads are steroid eluting to minimize inflammation at the site of the lead tip. Although transvenous leads have a generally excellent performance record, a small percentage may still develop high thresholds, poor sensing, insulation breaks, or infection. Malfunctioning or infected leads can be extracted successfully from the vascular space using specialized stylets and sheaths, even in children with complex congenital heart disease.[176]

Implantable Cardioverter Defibrillators

In 1985, only 1300 patients in the United States received an ICD, including 25 children. By 1998, ICD implants had burgeoned to more than 90,000 in the United States, including 600 patients (0.7%) younger than 21 years. Defibrillators have now been demonstrated to be valuable in the treatment of children, particularly those with inheritable channelopathies, cardiomyopathies, or late ventricular arrhythmias after repair of congenital heart disease.

In the Children's Hospital Boston database, more than 150 patients have undergone ICD implantation over the past 10 years, ranging in age from 2 months to adulthood.[177] The indications for ICD implantation included aborted sudden cardiac death (33%), spontaneous sustained VT (24%), syncope with a positive ventricular stimulation study in patients with congenital heart disease (20%), and high-risk patients with hypertrophic cardiomyopathy or congenital long QT syndrome (11%). Overall, 36% of patients have received an appropriate shock, and 16% have received a spurious shock. Lead failure occurred in 20% of patients, with growth over time identified as the variable predicting highest risk for this complication.[115]

ICD Functions

An ICD operates by constantly monitoring cardiac rhythm from a sensing lead that registers ventricular rate, and delivering a shock in the range of 5 to 31 joules whenever a programmed rate limit is violated by an episode of VT or VF (Fig. 29-63). In addition, these devices are capable of providing all standard antibradycardia pacemaker functions, including dual-chamber pacing and even biventricular resynchronization. Some devices are also able to discriminate SVT from VT from VF, and deliver short bursts of atrial or ventricular pacing to interrupt organized episodes of reentrant tachycardia before resorting to shock therapy. The device is obviously larger than a conventional pacemaker because of the added battery requirements for shock energy, but hardware has been reduced to a size that now makes implant quite feasible in children.

ICD Leads and Implant Techniques

Early ICD implants all involved an epicardial approach by sternotomy for placement of epicardial ventricular sensing leads and two large patches through which the shock could be delivered to the epicardial surface of the heart.[178] Early ICD generators were also quite large and

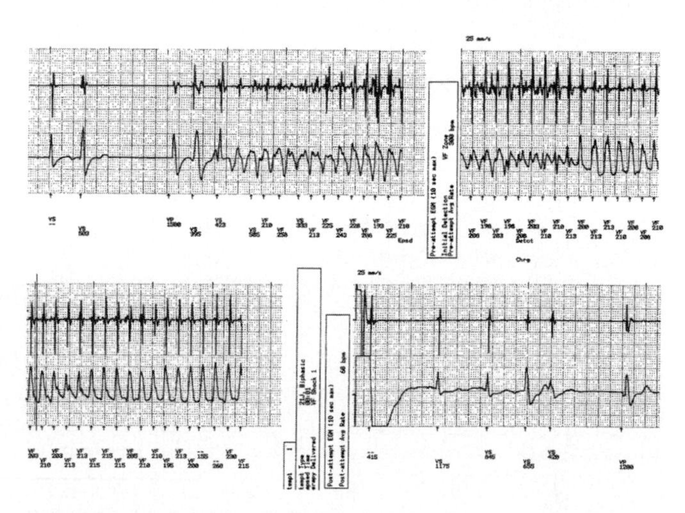

FIGURE 29–63 *Operation of an autonomic implantable cardioverter defibrillator (ICD), as recorded from the ICD lead and stored in the device memory. In the upper panel, the patient develops rapid ventricular arrhythmia that is recognized by the device as ventricular fibrillation (VF). In the lower panel, the device charges and delivers a 21-joule shock to restore normal rhythm.*

had to be placed in an abdominal pocket, even for adult patients. Fortunately, generators quickly became smaller, and the shock function was eventually incorporated into a sophisticated transvenous lead that could combine sensing from the lead tip and shock delivery from coils along the lead shaft.[179] These dramatic technical advances now allow modern ICDs to be placed by a transvenous approach, with the generator positioned in the pectoral area very similar to a standard pacemaker (Fig. 29-64). Modified epicardial or other novel implant techniques are still required in some pediatric cases owing to size constraints and complex cardiac anatomy.[180]

Malfunctions for both epicardial and transvenous ICD leads are relatively common in children.[115,181,182] The increased incidence of lead malfunction in the pediatric population may be due in part to the continued growth of the thorax and the more dynamic activity in young patients.[183] Pediatric ICD recipients also have unique social, developmental, and emotional issues. A recent study identified significant associations between anxiety, depression and quality of life among adolescent ICD recipients.[184] The child's privacy needs to be protected while at the same time reassuring teachers, coaches, and others about the safety of the child's return to school, sports, and recreational activities. Many centers have developed ICD support groups to help young patients and their parents deal with these difficult issues.

CATHETER ABLATION OF ARRHYTHMIAS

When the last edition of this textbook was written in 1991, transcatheter ablation of arrhythmias was still a rather novel procedure. The brief comments devoted to ablation in the earlier text predicted that the technique "... is likely to evolve in this decade as a realistic (and possibly preferred) alternative to drug therapy or surgical therapy for many arrhythmias in childhood." If anything, this prediction has proved to be far too conservative. Catheter ablation has now dramatically altered the standards for clinical management of tachycardias in all age groups.

The earliest transcatheter ablation attempts in the 1980s involved a DC shock to destroy target tissue through a combination of heat and barotraumas.[185] Although effective,

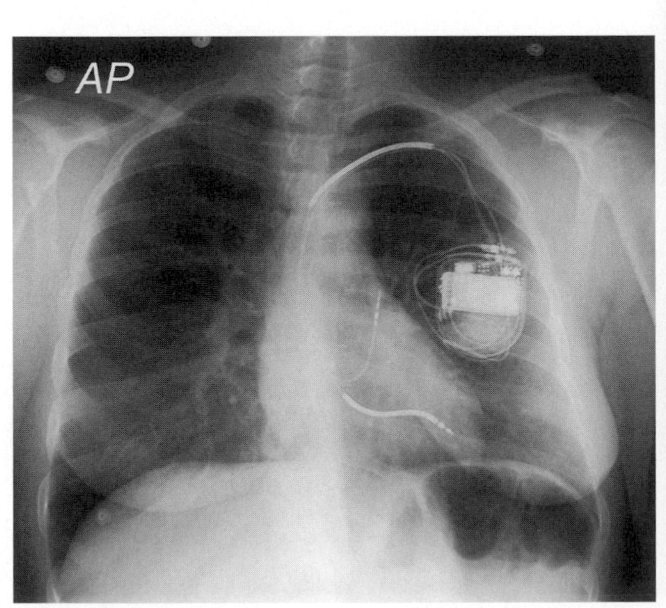

A

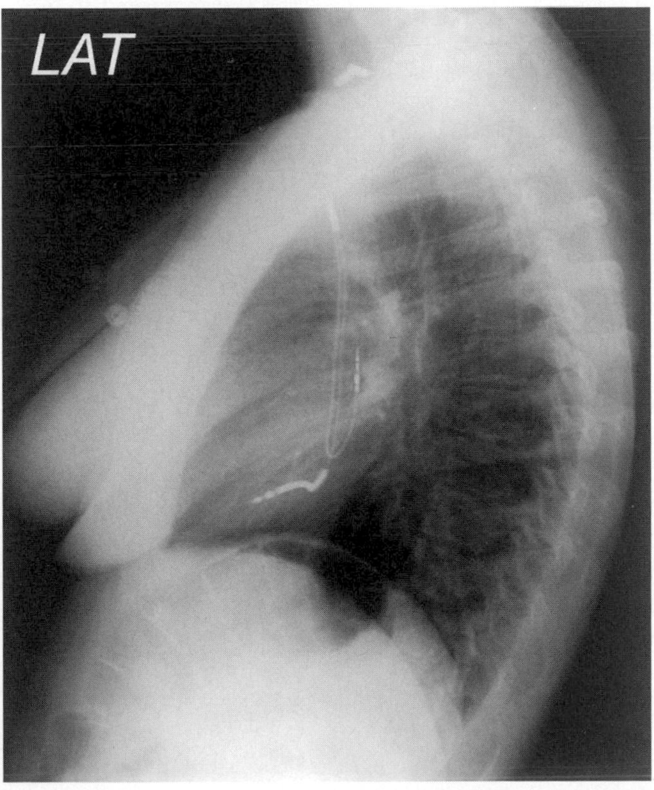

B

FIGURE 29–64 *Chest x-rays (AP, lateral) showing the leads and generator for a dual-chamber transvenous implantable cardioverter defibrillator (ICD) in a patient who has undergone a Mustard operation. A transvenous ICD lead is positioned at the apex of the left ventricle, and a transvenous atrial lead is positioned in the new right atrium. The generator is placed in a pectoral pocket.*

DC ablation was difficult to control and was sometimes complicated by perforation and other major morbidity.[186] In the late 1980s, it was demonstrated that the application of *radiofrequency* (RF) current to the myocardium resulted in more controlled and predictable thermal injury.[187] The effect of RF ablation was both immediate and impressive, leading to rapid adoption of the technique. Alternate energy forms have been investigated for ablation, including microwave heating, ethanol infusion, and tissue freezing with a cryocatheter. Of these, the cryocatheter has now been adopted at many centers as a specialty tool for ablation in the vicinity of critical structures such as the AV node, but RF still remains the most widely used technique.

The mechanism by which RF current ablates tissue is complex (Fig. 29-65). Passage of RF current causes resistive heating in a small zone at the tip of the catheter.[188] Conduction of thermal energy from this zone to the surrounding tissues causes expansion of the thermal lesion, with desiccation of the tissue and tissue death resulting from tissue temperatures above 49° to 50°C. At the same time, heat is carried away from the lesion by convective cooling from circulating blood in the heart, epicardial coronary vessels, and myocardial microcirculation. This convective heat loss ultimately balances the thermal input to the lesion and results in limitation of lesion size at that point. Pathologic studies of RF lesions have shown the formation of pale, macroscopic, well-defined lesions of variable width and depth in the range of 3 to 9 mm.

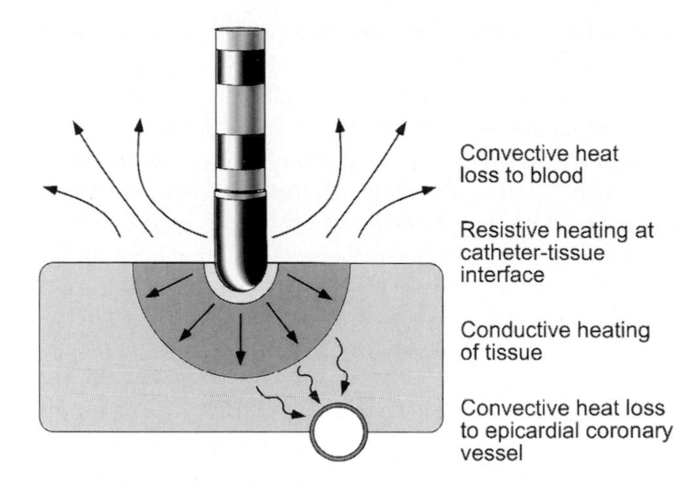

FIGURE 29–65 *Schematic summary of the biophysics for radiofrequency ablation, showing a catheter tip electrode in contact with cardiac tissue. See text for discussion.*

Mapping and Ablation Techniques

Successful application of RF energy for ablation of tachycardias is contingent on a thorough and specific understanding of the anatomy of the heart (Fig. 29-66) and the arrhythmia mechanism, which may be focal or reentrant. Ablation of automatic arrhythmias with a focal origin, such as EAT[21] or certain types of VT,[114] is conceptually simple. Because the electrical activation of the heart spreads radially

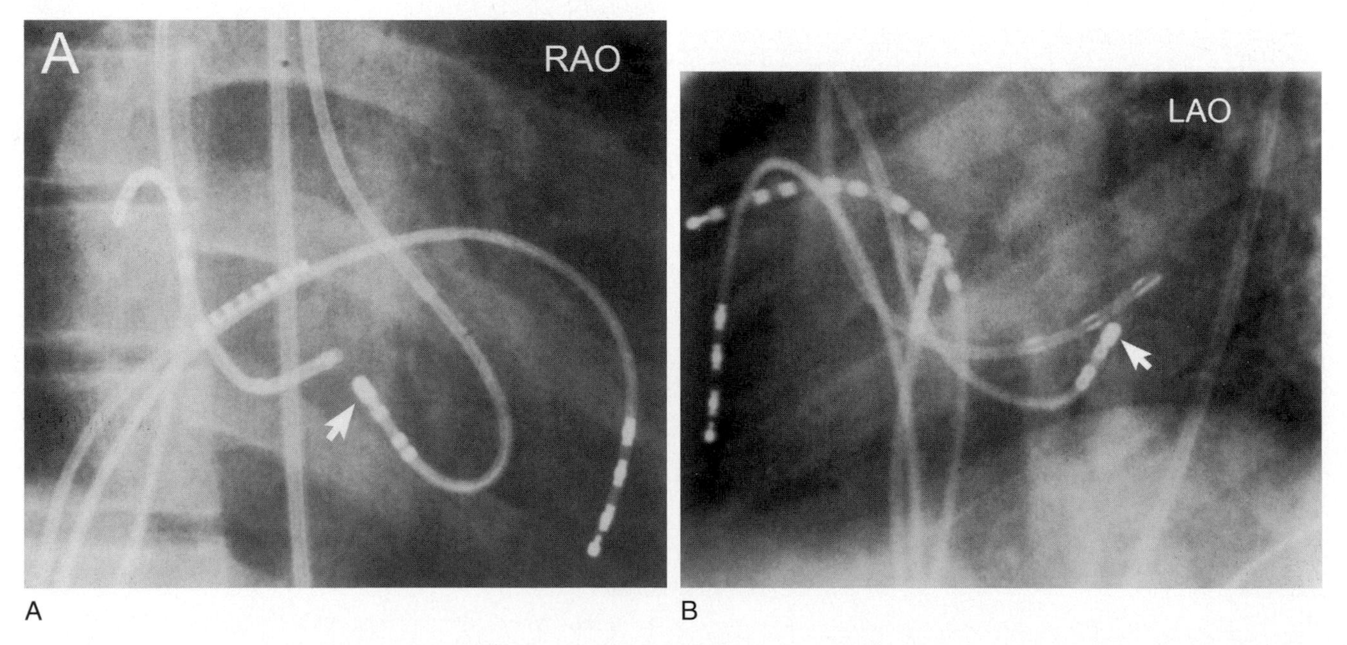

FIGURE 29–66 *Catheter positions (RAO and LAO) during successful radiofrequency ablation of a left-sided accessory pathway. The ablation catheter (arrow) has been inserted into the left ventricle using a retrograde arterial approach, with the tip positioned under the leaflet of the mitral valve at the level of the annulus.*
From Fyler DC [ed]. Nadas' Pediatric Cardiology. Philadelphia: Hanley & Belfus, 1992.

from a focal source, the process of identifying a suitable target for ablation rests simply on the systematic and thorough sampling of endocardial electrical activation of the heart during the rhythm. The earliest site of electrical activation corresponds to the origin of the abnormal rhythm, and ablation at that site typically results in termination of the tachycardia (Fig. 29-67).

Ablation of reentrant arrhythmias is more complex. By definition, the arrhythmia substrate of these tachycardias is a loop, the location of which must be identified within the heart. Fortunately, this process of mapping is considerably simplified for the common types of reentrant SVT caused by the presence of a small discrete AP. These pathways are known to be a relatively safe and susceptible target for ablation and are usually easily accessible from the endocardial surface of the AV groove.[189,190] Thus, for WPW and similar AP-mediated SVT, the process of mapping consists of placing electrode catheters along the mitral or tricuspid annuli and identifying the site of abnormal electrical connection between the atrium and ventricle (Fig. 29-68).

Another form of SVT easily treated by ablation is AV nodal reentrant tachycardia.[52] The arrhythmia substrate in this case is thought to be the tissue interface between atrial muscle and the compact AV node in the perinodal region that can create a pattern of dual conduction pathways. Placement of ablation lesions in a standard location in the posterior AV septum where the slow AV nodal pathway is located has a remarkably high level of efficacy in permanent cure of this arrhythmia.

For reentrant tachycardias other than those mediated by an AP and the AV node (e.g., atrial flutter and atypical atrial and ventricular tachycardias occurring in patients with abnormal hearts), the process of mapping the arrhythmia substrate and identifying an appropriate site for ablation is much more difficult.[44,45,114] In these cases, a variety of advanced techniques must be used, including three-dimensional mapping (Fig. 29-69), sophisticated pacing maneuvers, careful imaging and definition of anatomic detail, and specialized catheters that can ablate larger target areas (Fig. 29-70).

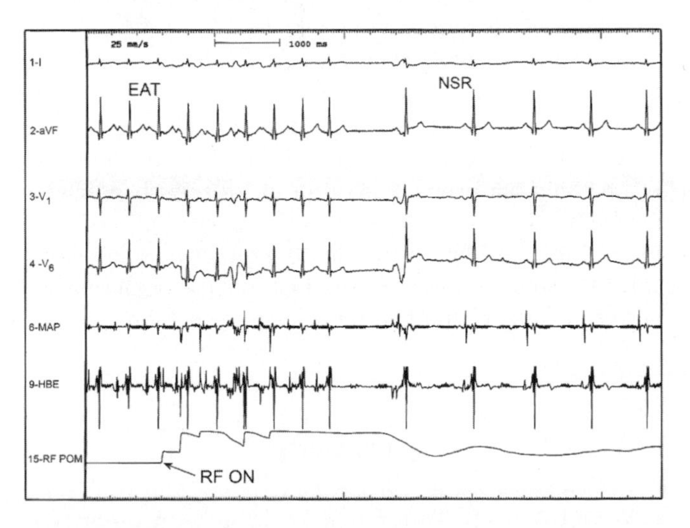

FIGURE 29–67 *Radiofrequency (RF) ablation of ectopic atrial tachycardia (EAT). The focus was extinguished promptly when RF current was applied.*

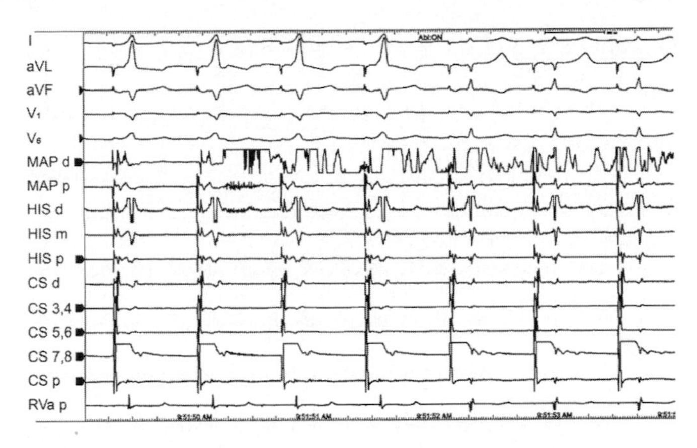

FIGURE 29–68 *Radiofrequency (RF) ablation of Wolff-Parkinson-White syndrome. The delta wave was eliminated promptly when RF current was applied.*

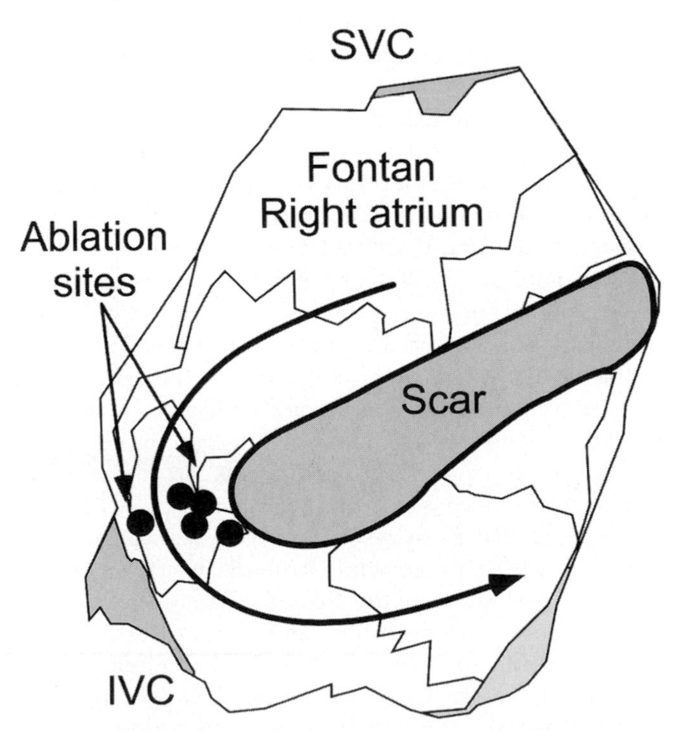

FIGURE 29–69 *Three-dimensional electroanatomic map of intra-atrial reentrant tachycardia. The isochronal time lines delineate the pattern of propagation through the macroreentrant circuit, allowing one to visualize potentially productive sites for ablation. SVC, superior vena cava; IVC, inferior vena cava.*

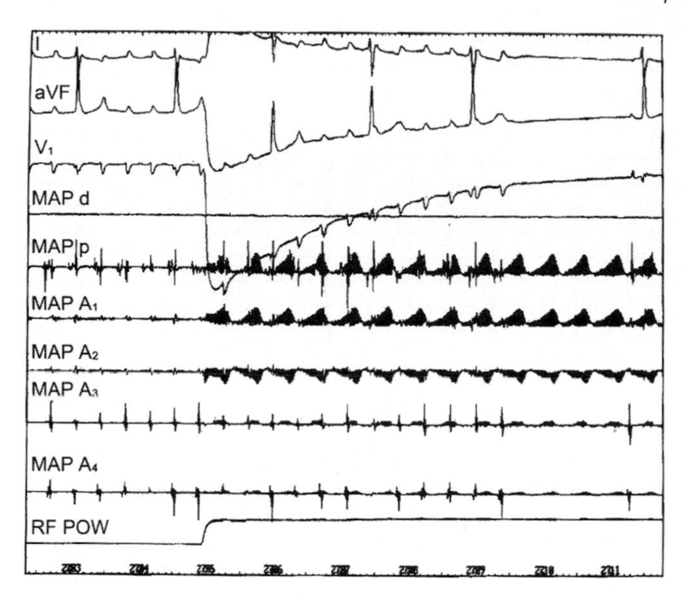

FIGURE 29–70 *Successful radiofrequency ablation of intra-atrial reentrant tachycardia.*

Ablation Outcomes

Initial case reports of RF ablation in pediatrics were published in 1990, and early series were principally notable for demonstrating the feasibility of this procedure in children.[61,62,191] At that time, members of the Pediatric Electrophysiology Society were active in multicenter data collection and were thus prepared to collect the procedural outcomes of this new procedure in a comprehensive manner. The Pediatric RF Ablation Registry has collected the outcomes of nearly 10,000 ablation cases over about a 10-year period and has spawned further prospective studies of pediatric ablation that are currently underway. The results of the Registry studies are impressive in their scope and compare very favorably with studies of ablations performed in adults during the same era. The principal finding of the Registry studies has been that RF ablation is a safe and highly effective means of treating all varieties of SVT in children younger than 21 years with normal cardiac anatomy. The acute efficacy of this procedure in normal hearts varies with the anatomic location of the ablated substrate, with overall efficacy ranging between 90% and 99%. Adverse events, defined broadly to include both major and minor complications, have fallen from 4.2% to less than 3.0% over the years of data collection, with the rate of major adverse events significantly lower. In addition to several subgroup studies of anatomy, age, and specific complication, the Registry database has also been used to assess the outcomes learning curve for participating centers, procedural indications, and fluoroscopy and procedure times, and to track the evolution of all procedural outcomes over time. The most recent assessment of data shows a continued improvement in ablation outcomes, along with a decrease in adverse event rates and fluoroscopy time.[192]

In contrast to children with common forms of SVT occurring in a normal heart, the outcomes of catheter ablation in those with congenital heart disease or unusual tachycardia mechanisms are less favorable. These patients have a variety of features complicating ablation, including their primary anatomic malformations,[193] aberrant location of the normal conduction system,[194] and both macroscopic and microscopic fibrosis. They are prone to both AP-mediated tachycardias (especially patients with Ebstein's disease) and complex atrial and ventricular reentrant tachycardias.[195,196] In addition to constituting difficult problems in arrhythmia substrate mapping, the presence of thickened and fibrotic myocardium may change the biophysics of RF ablation, rendering standard approaches to ablation less effective.[44] Most atypical arrhythmias presenting for catheter ablation can be classified in one of three categories: ventricular tachycardias, atrial reentrant tachycardias (typical and atypical atrial flutter), and AV reciprocating tachycardias occurring in patients with congenital heart defects. Recent reviews of the acute clinical outcomes for ablation in each of these entities have recently been published based on the clinical experience at Children's Hospital Boston.[44,114,197] Acute success rates only range between 60% and 85% for these conditions, but experience and enhanced technology should improve outcomes in the near future.

Looking forward, it is reasonable to predict that our understanding of the natural history of arrhythmia in children and the role of catheter ablation in its management will continue to evolve. Certainly the technical evolution of the field will yield novel approaches to interventional electrophysiology that will allow curative, catheter-based therapy for most varieties of tachycardia, including those currently conceived to be very difficult to ablate.

Note to reader: In the prior edition of this textbook, Dr. J Philip Saul served as coauthor of this chapter with Dr. Walsh.[198] Dr. Saul provided major contributions in the form of text and figures on the topics of AV node reentry and APs. Some of this excellent material has been retained in this updated chapter with his kind permission.

REFERENCES

1. Walsh EP, Saul JP, Triedman JK (eds). Cardiac Arrhythmias in Children and Young Adults With Congenital Heart Disease, Philadelphia: Lippincott Williams & Wilkins, 2001.

2. Deal BJ, Wolff GS, Gelband H (eds). Current Concepts in Diagnosis and Management of Arrhythmias in Infants and Children. Armonk, NY: Futura, 1998.
3. Gillette PC, Garson A (eds). Clinical Pediatric Arrhythmias, 2nd ed. Philadelphia: WB Saunders, 1999.
4. Zipes DP, Jalife J (eds). Cardiac Electrophysiology; From Cell to Bedside, 4th ed. Philadelphia: WB Saunders/Elsevier, 2004.
5. Wit AL, Rosen MR. Pathophysiologic mechanisms of cardiac arrhythmias. Am Heart J 106:798, 1983.
6. Rosen MR. The links between basic and clinical cardiac electrophysiology. Circulation 77:251, 1988.
7. Stevenson WG, Sager PT, Friedman PL. Entrainment techniques for mapping atrial and ventricular tachycardias. J Cardiovasc Electrophysiol 6:201, 1995.
8. Gallagher JJ. Forward. In: Benditt DG, Benson DW (eds). Cardiac Preexcitation Syndromes. Boston: Martinus Nijhoff, 1986:XI-XIII.
9. Hoffman BF, Rosen MR. Cellular mechanisms for cardiac arrhythmias. Circ Res 49:1, 1981.
10. Walsh EP. Transcatheter ablation of ectopic atrial tachycardia using radiofrequency current, In: Huang SK (ed). Catheter Ablation for Cardiac Arrhythmias. Mt. Kisco, NY: Futura, 1994:421–443.
11. Coumel P. Early afterdepolarizations and triggered activity in clinical arrhythmias. In Rosen MR, Janse MJ, Wit AL (eds). Cardiac Electrophysiology: A Textbook. Mount Kisco, NY: Futura, 1990:387–412.
12. Cranefield PF. Action potentials, afterpotentials, and arrhythmias. Circ Res 41:415, 1977.
13. Moak JP, Rosen MR. Induction and termination of triggered activity by pacing in isolated canine Purkinje fibers. Circulation 69:149, 1984.
14. Hiroaka M, Okamoto Y, Sano T. Oscillatory afterpotentials in dog ventricular muscle fibers. Circ Res 48:510, 1981.
15. Dunnigan A, Benditt DG, Benson DW. Modes of onset of paroxysmal atrial tachycardia in infants and children. Am J Cardiol 57:1280, 1986.
16. Southall DP, Johnson F, Shinebourne. The 24 hour electrocardiographic study of heart rate and rhythm in a population of healthy children. Br Heart J 45:281, 1981.
17. Brodsky M, Wu D, Denes P, et al. Arrhythmias documented by 24 hour continuous electrocardiographic monitoring in 50 male medical students without apparent heart disease. Am J Cardiol 39:390, 1977.
18. Fishberger SB, Colan SD, Saul JP, et al. Myocardial mechanics before and after ablation of chronic tachycardia. PACE 19: 42, 1995.
19. Salerno JC, Kertesz NJ, Friedman RA, et al. Clinical course of atrial ectopic tachycardia is age-dependent. J Am Coll Cardiol 43:438, 2004.
20. Rosales AM, Walsh EP, Wessel DL, et al. Postoperative ectopic atrial tachycardia in children with congenital heart disease. Am J Cardiol 88:1169, 2001.
21. Walsh EP, Saul JP, Hulse JE, et al. Transcatheter ablation of ectopic atrial tachycardia in young patients using radiofrequency current. Circulation 86:1138, 1992.
22. Shine KI, Kastor JA, Yurchak PM. Multifocal atrial tachycardia: Clinical and electrocardiographic features in 32 patients. N Engl J Med 279:344, 1968.
23. Liberthson RR, Colan SD. Multifocal or chaotic atrial rhythm: Report of nine infants, delineation of clinical course and management, and review of the literature. Pediatr Cardiol 2:179, 1982.
24. Dodo H, Gow RM, Hamilton RM, et al. Chaotic atrial rhythm in children. Am Heart J 129:990, 1995.
25. Salim MA, Case CL, Gillette PC. Chaotic atrial tachycardia in children. Am Heart J 129:831, 1995.
26. Zeevi B, Berant M, Sclarovsky S, et al. Treatment of multifocal atrial tachycardia with amiodarone in a child with congenital heart disease. Am J Cardiol 57:344, 1986.
27. Levine JH, Michael JR, Guarnieri T. Treatment of multifocal atrial tachycardia with verapamil. N Engl J Med 312:21, 1985.
28. Yeager SB, Hougen TJ, Levy AM. Sudden death in infants with chaotic atrial rhythm. Am J Dis Child 138:689, 1984.
29. Villain E, Vetter VL, Garcia JM, et al. Evolving concepts in the management of congenital junctional ectopic tachycardia: A multicenter study. Circulation 81:1544, 1990.
30. Wren C, Campbell RWF. His bundle tachycardia: Arrhythmogenic and antiarrhythmic effects of therapy. Eur Heart J 8:647, 1987.
31. Grant JW, Serwer GA, Armstrong BE, et al. Junctional tachycardia in infants and children after open heart surgery for congenital heart disease. Am J Cardiol 59:1216, 1987.
32. Till JA, Rowland E. Atrial pacing as an adjunct to the management of post-surgical His bundle tachycardia. Br Heart J 66: 225, 1991.
33. Pfammatter JP, Paul T, Ziemer G, et al. Successful management of junctional tachycardia by hypothermia after cardiac operations in infants. Ann Thorac Surg 60:556, 1995.
34. Walsh EP, Saul JP, Sholler GF, et al. Evaluation of a staged treatment protocol for rapid automatic junctional tachycardia after operation for congenital heart disease. J Am Coll Cardiol 29:1046, 1997.
35. Raja P, Hawker RE, Chaikitpinyo A, et al. Amiodarone management of junctional ectopic tachycardia after cardiac surgery in children. Br Heart J 72:261, 1994.
36. VanHare, Velvis H, Langberg J. Successful transcatheter ablation of congenital junctional ectopic tachycardia in a ten-month old infant using radiofrequency energy. PACE 13: 730, 1990.
37. Fishberger SB, Rossi AF, Messina JJ, et al. Successful radiofrequency catheter ablation of congenital junctional ectopic tachycardia with preservation of atrioventricular conduction in a 9-month old infant. PACE 21:2132, 1998.
38. Ehlert FA, Goldberger JJ, Deal BJ, et al. Successful radiofrequency energy ablation of automatic junctional tachycardia preserving normal atrioventricular nodal conduction. PACE 16:54, 1993.
39. Garson A, Bink-Boelkens MTE, Hesslein PS, et al. Atrial flutter in the young: A collaborative study of 380 cases. J Am Coll Cardiol 6:871, 1985.
40. Rhodes LA, Walsh EP, Gamble WJ, et al. Benefits and potential risks of atrial antitachycardia pacing after repair of

congenital heart disease. Pacing Clin Electrophysiol 18:1005, 1995.
41. Rhodes LA, Walsh EP, Saul JP. Conversion of atrial flutter in pediatric patients using transesophageal atrial pacing: A safe, effective, and minimally invasive technique. Am Heart J 130: 323, 1995.
42. Fishberger SB, Wernovsky G, Gentles TL, et al. Factors that influence the development of atrial flutter after the Fontan operation. J Thorac Cadiovas Surg 113:80, 1997.
43. Collins KK, Love BA, Walsh EP, et al. Location of acutely successful radiofrequency catheter ablation of intraatrial reentrant tachycardia in patients with congenital heart disease. Am J Cardiol 86:969, 2000.
44. Triedman JK, Alexander MA, Love BA, et al. Influence of patient factors and ablative technologies on outcomes of radiofrequency ablation of intra-atrial tachycardia in patients with congenital heart disease. J Am Coll Cardiol 39:1827, 2002.
45. Triedman JK, Alexander ME, Berul CI, et al. Electroanatomic mapping of entrained and exit zones in patients with repaired congenital heart disease and intra-atrial reentrant tachycardia. Circulation 103:2060, 2001.
46. Triedman JK. Atrial reentrant tachycardias. In Walsh EP, Saul JP, Triedman JK (eds). Cardiac Arrhythmias in Children and Young Adults With Congenital Heart Disease. Philadelphia: Lippincott Williams & Wilkins, 2001:137–160.
47. Mavroudis C, Backer CL, Deal BJ, et al. Total cavopulmonary conversion and maze procedure for patients with failure of the Fontan operation. J Thorac Cardiovasc Surg 122:863, 2001.
48. Kirsh JA, Walsh EP, Triedman JK. Prevalence of and risk factors for atrial fibrillation and intraatrial reentrant tachycardia among patients with congenital heart disease. Am J Cardiol 90:338, 2002.
49. ACC/AHA/ESC guidelines for the management of patients with atrial fibrillation: A report of the American College of Cardiology/American Heart Association Task Force on Practice Guidelines and the European Society of Cardiology Committee for Practice Guidelines and Policy Conferences. J Am Coll Cardiol 38:923, 2001.
50. Hsu LF, Jais P, Sanders P, et al. Catheter ablation for atrial fibrillation in congestive heart failure. N Engl J Med 351: 2373, 2004.
51. Casta A, Wolff GS, Mehta AV, et al. Dual atrioventricular nodal pathways: A benign finding in arrhythmia-free children with heart disease. Am J Cardiol 46:1013, 1980.
52. Van Hare GF, Chiesa NA, Campbell RM, et al. Atrioventricular nodal reentrant tachycardia in children: Effect of slow pathway ablation on fast pathway function. J Cardiovasc Electrophysiol 13:203, 2002.
53. Gallagher JJ, Pritchett ELC, Sealy WC. The preexcitation syndrome. Prog Cardiovasc Dis 20:285, 1978.
54. Arruda MS, McClelland JH, Wang X, et al. Development and validation of an ECG algorithm for identifying accessory pathway ablation site in Wolff-Parkinson-White syndrome. J Cardiovasc Electrophysiol 9:2, 1998.
55. Fitzpatrick AP, Gonzales RP, Lesh MD, et al. New algorithm for the localization of accessory atrioventricular connections using a baseline electrocardiogram. J Am Coll Cardiol 23: 107, 1994.
56. Gikonyo BM, Dunnigan A, Benson DW. Cardiovascular collapse in infants: Association with paroxysmal atrial tachycardia. Pediatrics 76:922, 1985.
57. Kerr CR, Gallagher JJ, German LD. Changes in ventriculoatrial intervals with bundle branch block aberration during reciprocating tachycardia in patients with accessory atrioventricular pathways. Circulation 66:196, 1982.
58. Benson DW, Dunnigan A, Benditt DG. Follow-up evaluation of infant paroxysmal atrial tachycardia: Transesophageal study. Circulation 75:542, 1987.
59. Weindling SN, Saul JP, Walsh EP. Risks and efficacy of medical therapy for supraventricular tachycardia in neonates and infants. Am Heart J 131:66, 1996.
60. Deal BJ, Keane JF, Gillette PC, et al. Wolff-Parkinson-White syndrome and supraventricular tachycardia during infancy: management and follow-up. J Am Coll Cardiol 5:130, 1985.
61. Tanel RE, Walsh EP, Triedman JK, et al. A five year experience with radiofrequency catheter ablation: Implications for arrhythmia management in the pediatric and young adult patient. J Pediatr 131:878, 1997.
62. Kugler JD, Danford DA, Deal B, et al. Radiofrequency catheter ablation in children and adolescents: Early results in 572 patients from 24 centers. N Engl J Med 330:1481, 1994.
63. Klein GJ, Bashore TM, Sellers TD, et al. Ventricular fibrillation in the Wolff-Parkinson-White syndrome. N Engl J Med 301: 1080, 1979.
64. Sharma AD, Klein GJ, Guiraudon GM, et al. Atrial fibrillation in patients with Wolff-Parkinson-White syndrome: Incidence after surgical ablation of the accessory pathway. Circulation 72:161, 1985.
65. Bromberg BI, Lindsay BD, Cain ME, et al. Impact of clinical history and electrophysiologic characterization of accessory pathways on management strategies to reduce sudden death among children with Wolff-Parkinson-White syndrome. J Am Coll Cardiol 27:690, 1996.
66. Kuck KH, Jackman WM, Friday KJ, et al. Sites of conduction block in accessory pathways. In Zipes DP, Jalife J (eds). Cardiac Electrophysiology: From Cell to Bedside, 1st ed. Philadelphia: WB Saunders, 1990:503–512.
67. Lindinger A, Heisel A, von Bernuth G, et al. Permanent junctional re-entry tachycardia: A multicentre long-term follow-up study in infants, children and young adults. Eur Heart J 19:936, 1998.
68. Ticho BS, Saul JP, Hulse JE, et al. Variable location of accessory pathway causing the permanent form of junctional reciprocating tachycardia: Confirmation with radiofrequency ablation. Am J Cardiol 70:1559, 1992.
69. van Stuijvenberg M, Beaufort-Krol GC, Haaksma J, et al. Pharmacological treatment of young children with permanent junctional reciprocating tachycardia. Cardiol Young 13: 408, 2003.
70. Gallagher JJ, Smith WM, Kasell JH, et al. Role of Mahaim fibers in cardiac arrhythmias in man. Circulation 64:176, 1981.
71. Klein LS, Hackett FK, Zipes DP, et al. Radiofrequency catheter ablation of Mahaim fibers at the tricuspid annulus. Circulation 87:738, 1993.

72. Ellenbogen KA, Rogers R, Old W. Pharmacological characterization of conduction over a Mahaim fiber: Evidence for adenosine sensitive conduction. Pacing Clin Electrophysiol 12:1396, 1989.
73. Okishige K, Strickberger SA, Walsh EP, et al. Catheter ablation of the atrial origin of a decrementally conducting atriofascicular accessory pathway by radiofrequency current. J Cardiovas Electrophysiol 2:465, 1991.
74. Van Hare GF, Stanger P. Ventricular tachycardia and accelerated ventricular rhythm presenting in the first month of life. Am J Cardiol 67:42, 1991.
75. Davis AM, Gow RM, McCrindle BW, et al. Clinical spectrum, therapeutic management, and follow-up of ventricular tachycardia in infants and young children. Am Heart J 131: 186, 1996.
76. Garson A, Jr., Smith RT, Jr., Moak JP, et al. Incessant ventricular tachycardia in infants: Myocardial hamartomas and surgical cure. J Am Coll Cardiol 10:619, 1987.
77. Otani M, Hoshida H, Saji T, et al. Histiocytoid cardiomyopathy with hypotonia in an infant. Pathol Int 45:774, 1995.
78. Prahlow JA, Teot LA. Histiocytoid cardiomyopathy: Case report and literature review. J Forensic Sci 38:1427, 1993.
79. Gharagozloo F, Porter CJ, Tazelaar HD, et al. Multiple myocardial hamartomas causing ventricular tachycardia in young children: Combined surgical modification and medical treatment. Mayo Clinic Proc 69:262, 1994.
80. Zeigler VL, Gillette PC, Crawford FA Jr, et al. New approaches to treatment of incessant ventricular tachycardia in the very young. J Am Coll Cardiol 16:681, 1990.
81. Jackman WM, Friday KJ, Anderson JL, et al. The long QT syndromes: A critical review, new clinical observations and a unifying hypothesis. Prog Cardiovasc Dis 31:115, 1988.
82. Chiang CE. Congenital and acquired long QT syndrome. Current concepts and management. Cardiol Rev 12:222, 2004.
83. Priori SG. Inherited arrhythmogenic diseases: The complexity beyond monogenic disorders. Circ Res 94:140, 2004.
84. Priori SG, Napolitano C, Vicentini A. Inherited arrhythmia syndromes: Applying the molecular biology and genetic to the clinical management. J Interv Card Electrophysiol 9:93, 2003.
85. Kass RS, Moss AJ. Long QT syndrome: Novel insights into the mechanisms of cardiac arrhythmias. J Clin Invest 112: 810, 2003.
86. Satler CA, Walsh EP, Vesely MR, et al. Novel missense mutation in the cyclic nucleotide-binding domain of HERG causes long QT syndrome. Am J Med Genet 65:27, 1996.
87. Benson DW, MacRea CA, Vesely MR, et al. Missense mutation in the pore region of HERG causes the familial long QT syndrome. Circulation 93:1791, 1996.
88. Schwartz PJ. Stillbirths, sudden infant deaths, and long-QT syndrome: Puzzle or mosaic, the pieces of the jigsaw are being fitted together. Circulation 109:2930, 2004.
89. Schwartz PJ, Moss AJ, Vincent GM, et al. Diagnostic criteria for the long QT syndrome: An update. Circulation 88:782, 1993.
90. Tanel RE, Triedman JK, Walsh EP, et al. High-rate atrial pacing as an innovative therapy in a neonate with congenital long QT syndrome. J Cardiovasc Electrophysiol 8:812, 1997.
91. Dorostkar PC, Eldar M, Belhassen B, et al. Long-term follow-up of patients with long-QT syndrome treated with beta-blockers and continuous pacing. Circulation 100:2431, 1999.
92. Garson A Jr, Dick M 2nd, Fournier A, et al. The long QT syndrome in children: An international study of 287 patients. Circulation 87:1866, 1993.
93. Reardon PR, Matthews BD, Scarborough TK, et al. Left thoracoscopic sympathectomy and stellate ganglionectomy for treatment of the long QT syndrome. Surg Endosc 14:86, 2000.
94. Brugada J, Brugada P. Further characterization of the syndrome of right bundle branch block, ST segment elevation, and sudden cardiac death. J Cardiovasc Electrophysiol 8:325, 1997.
95. Brugada R, Brugada J, Antzelevitch C, et al. Sodium channel blockers identify risk for sudden death in patients with ST-segment elevation and right bundle branch block but structurally normal hearts. Circulation 101:510, 2000.
96. Gussak I, Antzelevitch C, Bjerregaard P, et al. The Brugada syndrome: Clinical, electrophysiologic and genetic aspects. J Am Coll Cardiol 33:5, 1999.
97. Miyazaki T, Mitamura H, Miyoshi S, et al. Autonomic and antiarrhythmic drug modulation of ST segment elevation in patients with Brugada syndrome. J Am Coll Cardiol 27: 1061, 1996.
98. Leenhardt A, Lucet V, Denjoy I, et al. Catecholaminergic polymorphic ventricular tachycardia in children: A 7-year follow-up of 21 patients. Circulation 91:1512, 1995.
99. De Rosa G, Delogu AB, Piastra M, et al. Catecholaminergic polymorphic ventricular tachycardia: Successful emergency treatment with intravenous propranolol. Pediatr Emerg Care 20:175, 2004.
100. Marks AR, Priori S, Memmi M, et al. Involvement of the cardiac ryanodine receptor/calcium release channel in catecholaminergic polymorphic ventricular tachycardia. J Cell Physiol 190:1, 2002.
101. Tawil R, Ptacek LJ, Pavlakis SG, et al. Andersen's syndrome: Potassium-sensitive periodic paralysis, ventricular ectopy, and dysmorphic features. Ann Neurol 35:326, 1994.
102. Nollert G, Fischlein T, Bouterwek S, et al. Long-term survival in patients with repair of tetralogy of Fallot: 36-Year follow-up of 490 survivors of the first year after surgical repair. J Am Coll Cardiol 30:1374, 1997.
103. Murphy JG, Gersh BJ, Mair DD, et al. Long-term outcome in patients undergoing surgical repair of tetralogy of Fallot. N Engl J Med 329:593, 1993.
104. Kirjavainen M, Happonen JM, Louhimo I. Late results of Senning operation. J Thoracic Cardiovasc Surg 117:488, 1999.
105. Keane JF, Driscoll DJ, Gersony WM, et al. Second natural history study of congenital heart defects: Results of treatment of patients with aortic valvar stenosis. Circulation 87: 16, 1993.
106. Houyel L, Vaksmann G, Fournier A, et al. Ventricular arrhythmias after correction of ventricular septal defects: Importance of surgical approach. J Am Coll Cardiol 16:1224, 1990.

107. Deanfield JE, McKenna WJ, Presbitero P, et al. Ventricular arrhythmia in unrepaired and repaired tetralogy of Fallot. Br Heart J 52:77, 1984.
108. Walsh EP, Rockenmacher S, Keane JF, et al. Late results in patients with tetralogy of Fallot repaired during infancy. Circulation 77:1062, 1988.
109. Gatzoulis MA, Till JA, Somerville J, et al. Mechanoelectrical interaction in tetralogy of Fallot: QRS prolongation relates to right ventricular size and predicts malignant ventricular arrhythmias and sudden death. Circulation 92:231, 1995.
110. Khairy P, Landzberg MJ, Gatzoulis MA, et al. Prognostic significance of electrophysiologic testing post tetralogy of Fallot repair: A multicenter study. Circulation 109:1994, 2004.
111. Alexander ME, Walsh EP, Saul JP, et al. Value of programmed ventricular stimulation in patients with congenital heart disease. J Cardiovasc Electrophysiol 10:1033, 1999.
112. Therrien J, Siu SC, Harris L, et al. Impact of pulmonary valve replacement on arrhythmia propensity late after repair of tetralogy of Fallot. Circulation 103:2489, 2001.
113. Moak JP, Smith RT, Garson A Jr. Mexiletine: An effective antiarrhythmic drug for treatment of ventricular arrhythmias in congenital heart disease. J Am Coll Cardiol 10:824, 1987.
114. Morwood JG, Triedman JK, Berul CI, et al. Radiofrequency catheter ablation of ventricular tachycardia in children, and in young adults with congenital heart disease. Heart Rhythm 1:301, 2004.
115. Alexander ME, Cecchin F, Walsh EP, et al. Implications of implantable cardioverter defibrillator therapy in congenital heart disease and pediatrics. J Cardiovasc Electrophysiol 15:72, 2004.
116. Maron BJ, McKenna WJ, Danielson GK, et al. American College of Cardiology/European Society of Cardiology clinical expert consensus document on hypertrophic cardiomyopathy. J Am Coll Cardiol 42:1687, 2003.
117. McKenna WJ, Behr ER. Hypertrophic cardiomyopathy: Management, risk stratification, and prevention of sudden death. Heart 87:169, 2002.
118. Behr ER, Elliott P, McKenna WJ. Role of invasive EP testing in the evaluation and management of hypertrophic cardiomyopathy. Card Electrophysiol Rev 6:482, 2002.
119. Cecchin F, Berul CI, Hamilton RA, et al. Risks and benefits if an ICD for prevention of sudden death in young patients with hypertrophic cardiomyopathy [abstract]. Pace Clin Electrophysiol 26:969, 2003.
120. Friedman RA, Moak JP, Garson A, Jr. Clinical course of idiopathic dilated cardiomyopathy in children. J Am Coll Cardiol 18:152, 1991.
121. Schwartz ML, Cox GF, Lin AE, et al. Clinical approach to genetic cardiomyopathy in children. Circulation 94:2021, 1996.
122. Dubin AM, Berul CI, Bevilacqua LM, et al. The use of implantable cardioverter-defibrillators in pediatric patients awaiting heart transplantation. J Card Fail 9:375, 2003.
123. Fontaine G, Fontaliran F, Hebert JL, et al. Arrhythmogenic right ventricular dysplasia. Annu Rev Med 50:17, 1999.
124. Nasir K, Bomma C, Tandri H, et al. Electrocardiographic features of arrhythmogenic right ventricular dysplasia/cardiomyopathy according to disease severity: A need to broaden diagnostic criteria. Circulation 110:1527, 2004.
125. Dungan WT, Garson A, Jr., Gillette PC. Arrhythmogenic right ventricular dysplasia: A cause of ventricular tachycardia in children with apparently normal hearts. Am Heart J 102:745, 1981.
126. Ellison KE, Friedman PL, Ganz LI, et al. Entrainment mapping and radiofrequency catheter ablation of ventricular tachycardia in right ventricular dysplasia. J Am Coll Cardiol 32:724, 1998.
127. Roguin A, Bomma CS, Nasir K, et al. Implantable cardioverter-defibrillators in patients with arrhythmogenic right ventricular dysplasia/cardiomyopathy. J Am Coll Cardiol 43:1843, 2004.
128. Pfammatter JP, Paul T. Idiopathic ventricular tachycardia in infancy and childhood. J Am Coll Cardiol 33:2067, 1999.
129. Pfammatter JP, Paul T, Kallfelz HC. Recurrent ventricular tachycardia in asymptomatic young children with an apparently normal heart. Eur J Pediatr 154:513, 1995.
130. Tada H, Ohe T, Yutani C, et al. Sudden death in a patient with apparent idiopathic ventricular tachycardia. Japan Circ J 60:133, 1996.
131. O'Connor BK, Case CL, Sokoloski MC, et al. Radiofrequency catheter ablation of right ventricular outflow tachycardia in children and adolescents. J Am Coll Cardiol 27:869, 1996.
132. Ohe T, Aihara N, Kamakura S, et al. Long-term outcome of verapamil-sensitive sustained left ventricular tachycardia in patients without structural heart disease. J Am Coll Cardiol 25:54, 1995.
133. Belhassen B, Shapira I, Pelleg A, et al. Idiopathic recurrent sustained ventricular tachycardia responsive to verapamil: an ECG-electrophysiologic entity. Am Heart J 108:1034, 1984.
134. Kasanuki H, Ohnishi S, Hosoda S. Differentiation and mechanisms of prevention and termination of verapamil-sensitive sustained ventricular tachycardia. Am J Cardiol 64:46, 1989.
135. Nakagawa H, Beckman KJ, McClelland JH, et al. Radiofrequency catheter ablation of idiopathic left ventricular tachycardia guided by a Purkinje potential. Circulation 88:2607, 1993.
136. Manning PB, Mayer JE, Wernovsky G, et al. Staged operation to Fontan increases the incidence of sinoatrial node dysfunction. J Thorac Cardiovasc Surg 111:833, 1996.
137. Walsh EP. Arrhythmias in patients with congenital heart disease. Card Electrophysiol Rev 4:422, 2002.
138. Stevenson EA, Casavant D, Tuzi J, et al. Efficacy of atrial antitachycardia pacing using the Medtronic AT500 pacemaker in patients with congenital heart disease. Am J Cardiol 92:871, 2003.
139. Walsh EP, Sanders SP, Keane JF. Fetal arrhythmias: Detection and management. In Milusky A (ed). Advances in Perinatal Medicine, vol 4. New York: Plenum Medical, 1985:63–94.
140. Chameides L, Truex RC, Vetter V, et al. Association of maternal systemic lupus erythematosus and congenital complete heart block. N Engl J Med 297:1204, 1977.
141. Buyon JP, Hiebert R, Copel J, et al. Autoimmune-associated congenital heart block: Demographics, mortality, and recurrence rates obtained from a national lupus registry. J Am Coll Cardiol 31:1658, 1998.

142. Frohn-Mulder IM, Meilof JF, Szatmari A, et al. Clinical significance of maternal antiRo/SS-A antibodies in children with isolated heart block. J Am Coll Cardiol 23:1677, 1994.
143. Carpenter RJ, Strasburger JF, Garson A, et al. Fetal ventricular pacing for hydrops secondary to complete atrioventricular block. J Am Coll Cardiol 8:1434, 1986.
144. Weindling SN, Saul JP, Triedman JK, et al. Staged pacing therapy for congenital complete heart block in premature infants. Am J Cardiol 74:412, 1994.
145. Esscher E. Congenital complete heart block. Acta Paediatr Scand 70:131, 1981.
146. Scholler GF, Walsh EP. Congenital complete heart block in patients without anatomic cardiac defects. Am Heart J 118:1193, 1998.
147. Michaelson M, Engle MA. Congenital complete heart block: an international study of the natural history. Cardiovasc Clin 4:85, 1972.
148. Dewey RC, Capeless MA, Levy AM. Use of ambulatory electrocardiographic monitoring to identify high-risk patients with congenital complete heart block. N Engl J Med 316:835, 1987.
149. Kertesz NJ, Friedman RA, Colan SD, et al. Left ventricular mechanics and geometry in patients with congenital complete atrioventricular block. Circulation 96:3430, 1997.
150. Esscher E, Michaelsson M. QT interval in congenital complete heart block. Pediatr Cardiol 4:121, 1983.
151. Moak JP, Barron KS, Hougen TJ, et al. Congenital heart block: Development of late-onset cardiomyopathy, a previously underappreciated sequela. J Am Coll Cardiol 37:238, 2001.
152. Weindling SN, Gamble WJ, Mayer JE, et al. Duration of complete atrioventricular block after congenital heart disease surgery. Am J Cardiol 82:525, 1998.
153. Pinto DS. Cardiac manifestations of Lyme disease. Med Clin North Am 86:285, 2002.
154. The Cardiac Arrhythmia Suppression Trial (CAST) Investigators. Preliminary report: Effect of encainide and flecainide on mortality in a randomized trial of arrhythmia suppression after myocardial infarction. N Engl J Med 321:406, 1989.
155. Perry JC. Pharmacologic therapy of arrhythmias. In: Deal BJ, Wolff GS, Gelband H (eds). Current Concepts in Diagnosis and Management of Arrhythmias in Infants and Children. Armonk, NY: Futura, 1998:267–308.
156. Moak JP. Pharmacology and electrophysiology of antiarrhythmic drugs. In Gillette PC, Garson A (eds). Pediatric Arrhythmias: Electrophysiology and Pacing. Philadelphia: WB Saunders, 1990:37–117.
157. Wren C. Practical use of antiarrhythmic drugs. In Wren C, Campbell RWF (eds). Paediatric Cardiac Arrhythmias. Oxford, UK: Oxford Press, 1996:279–289.
158. Fish FA, Gillette PC, Benson DW Jr. Proarrhythmia, cardiac arrest and death in young patients receiving encainide and flecainide. Pediatric Electrophysiology Group. J Am Coll Cardiol 18:356, 1991.
159. Perry JC, Fenrich AL, Hulse JE, et al. Pediatric use of intravenous amiodarone: Efficacy and safety in critically ill patients from a multicenter protocol. J Am Coll Cardiol 27:1246, 1996.
160. Tanel RE, Walsh EP, Lulu JA, et al. Sotalol for refractory arrhythmias in pediatric patients: Initial efficacy and long-term outcome. Am Heart J 130:791, 1995.
161. Epstein, ML, Kiel EA, Victoria BE. Cardiac decompensation following verapamil therapy in infants with supraventricular tachycardia. Pediatrics 75:737, 1985.
162. Walsh EP, Cecchin F. Recent advances in pacemaker and implantable defibrillator therapy for young patients. Curr Opin Cardiol 19:91, 2004.
163. Gregoratos G, Abrams J, Epstein AE, et al. ACC/AHA/NASPE 2002 guideline update for implantation of cardiac pacemakers and antiarrhythmia devices. Circulation 106:2145, 2002.
164. Bernstein AD, Daubert JC, Fletcher RD, et al. The revised NASPE/BPEG generic code for antibradycardia, adaptive-rate, and multisite pacing. North American Society of Pacing and Electrophysiology/British Pacing and Electrophysiology Group. Pacing Clin Electrophysiol 25:260, 2002.
165. Fishberger SB, Wernovsky G, Gentles TL, et al. Long-term outcome in patients with pacemakers following the Fontan operation. Am J Cardiol 77:887, 1996.
166. Connolly SJ, Kerr C, Gent M, et al. Dual-chamber versus ventricular pacing. Circulation 94:578, 1996.
167. Anderson HR, Thuesen L, Bagger JP, et al. Prospective randomized trial of atrial versus ventricular pacing in sick sinus syndrome. Lancet 344:1523, 1994.
168. Auricchio A, Stellbrink C, Sack S, et al. Long-term clinical effect of hemodynamically optimized cardiac resynchronization therapy in patients with heart failure and ventricular conduction delay. J Am Coll Cardiol 39:2026, 2002.
169. Abraham WT, Fisher WG, Smith AL, et al. Cardiac resynchronization in chronic heart failure. N Engl J Med 346:1845, 2002.
170. Janousek J, Vojtovic P, Chaloupecky V, et al. Hemodynamically optimized temporary cardiac pacing after surgery for congenital heart defects. PACE 23:1250, 2000.
171. Fortescue EB, Berul CI, Cecchin F, et al. Patient, procedural, and hardware factors associated with pacemaker lead failures in pediatrics and congenital heart disease. Heart Rhythm 1:150, 2004.
172. Stojanov P, Hrnjak V, Nedeljkovic V, et al. Transvenous permanent pacing in a one-day-old infant. PACE 17:1811, 1994.
173. Molina EJ, Dunnigan AC, Crosson JE. Implantation of transvenous pacemakers in infants and small children. Ann Thorac Surg 59:689, 1995.
174. Figa FH, McCrindle BW, Bigras JL, et al. Risk factors for venous obstruction in children with transvenous pacing leads. PACE 20:1902, 1997.
175. Crossley GH, Brinker JA, Reynolds D, et al. Steroid elution improves the stimulation threshold in an active-fixation atrial permanent pacing lead. Circulation 92:2935, 1995.
176. Friedman RA, Van Zandt H, Collins E, et al. Lead extraction in young patients with and without congenital heart disease using the subclavian approach. PACE 19:778, 1996.
177. Berul CI, Barrett KS, Walsh EP. Implantable cardioverter-defibrillators in pediatric patients. In Walsh EP, Saul JP, Triedman JK (eds). Cardiac Arrhythmias in Children and

Young Adults With Congenital Heart Disease. Philadelphia: Lippincott Williams & Wilkins, 2001:93–111.
178. Silka MJ, Kron J, Dunnigan A, et al. Sudden cardiac death and the use of implantable cardioverter-defibrillators in pediatric patients. Circulation 87:800, 1993.
179. Kron J, Silka MJ, Ohm OJ, et al. Preliminary experience with nonthoracotomy implantable cardioverter-defibrillators in young patients. PACE 17:26, 1994.
180. Berul CI, Triedman JK, Forbess J, et al. Minimally invasive cardioverter defibrillator implantation for children: An animal model and pediatric case report. PACE 24:1789, 2001.
181. Link MS, Hill SL, Cliff DL, et al. Comparison of frequency of complications of implantable cardioverter-defibrillators in children versus adults. Am J Cardiol 83:263, 1999.
182. Stefanelli C, Bradley DJ, Leroy S, et al. Implantable cardioverter defibrillator therapy for life-threatening arrhythmias in young patients. J Intervent Card Electrophys 6:235, 2002.
183. Cooper JM, Stephenson EA, Berul CI, et al. ICD lead complications and laser extraction in children and young adults with congenital heart disease: Implications for implantation and management. J Cardiovasc Electrophysiol 14:344, 2003.
184. DeMaso DR, Lauretti A, Spieth L, et al. Psychosocial Factors and Quality of Life in Children and Adolescents with Implantable Cardioverter Defibrillators. Am J Cardiology 93:582, 2004.
185. Fontaine G, Frank R, Tonet J, et al. Treatment of rhythm disorders by endocardial fulguration. Am J Cardiol 64: 83J, 1989.
186. Boyd EG, Hoet PM. The biophysics of catheter ablation techniques. J Electrophysiol 1:62, 1987.
187. Borggrefe M, Budde T, Podczeck A, et al. High frequency alternating current ablation of an accessory pathway in humans. J Am Coll Cardiol 10:576, 1987.
188. Haines DE, Watson DD. Tissue heating during radiofrequency catheter ablation: A thermodynamic model and observations in perfused and superfused canine right ventricular free wall. PACE 12:962, 1989.
189. Dick M, O'Connor BK, Serwer GA, et al. Use of radiofrequency current to ablate accessory connections in children. Circulation 84:2318, 1991.
190. Saul JP, Hulse JE, De W, et al. Catheter ablation of accessory atrioventricular pathways in young patients: Use of long vascular sheaths, the transseptal approach, and a retrograde left posterior parallel approach. J Am Coll Cardiol 21: 571, 1993.
191. Friedman RA, Walsh EP, Silka MJ, et al. NASPE expert consensus conference: Radiofrequency catheter ablation in children with and without congenital heart disease. Pace Clin Electrophysiol 25:1000, 2002.
192. Van Hare GF, Javitz H, Carmelli D, et al. Prospective assessment after pediatric cardiac ablation: Demographics, medical profiles, and initial outcomes. J Cardiovasc Electrophysiol 15:759, 2004.
193. Levine J, Walsh EP, Saul JP. Catheter ablation of accessory pathways in patients with congenital heart disease including heterotaxy syndrome. Am J Cardiol 72:689, 1993.
194. Epstein MR, Saul JP, Weindling SN, et al. Atrioventricular reciprocating tachycardia involving twin atrioventricular nodes in patients with complex congenital heart disease. J Cardiovasc Electrophysiol 12:671, 2001.
195. Love BA, Collins KK, Walsh EP, et al. Electroanatomic characterization of conduction barriers in sinus/atrial paced rhythm and association with intra-atrial reentrant tachycardia circuits following congenital heart disease surgery. J Cardiovasc Electrophysiol 12:17, 2001.
196. Mandapati R, Walsh EP, Triedman JK. Pericaval and periannular intra-atrial reentrant tachycardias in patients with congenital heart disease. J Cardiovasc Electrophysiol 14:119, 2003.
197. Chetaille P, Walsh EP, Triedman JK. Outcomes of radiofrequency catheter ablation of atrioventricular reciprocating tachycardia in patients with congenital heart disease. Heart Rhythm 1:168, 2004.
198. Walsh EP, Saul JP. Cardiac arrhythmias. In Fyler DC (ed). Nadas' Pediatric Cardiology. Philadelphia: Hanley & Belfus, 1992:377–434.

IX

Congenital Heart Disease

30

Ventricular Septal Defect

JOHN F. KEANE AND DONALD C. FYLER

DEFINITION

The term *ventricular septal defect* describes an opening in the ventricular septum. Ventricular defects may be located anywhere in the ventricular septum, may be single or multiple, and may be of variable size and shape. At Children's Hospital Boston, ventricular septal defect includes patients with isolated or multiple ventricular septal defects and ventricular defects with an associated atrial defect, patent ductus arteriosus, or some valvar abnormalities (Exhibit 30-1).

PREVALENCE

A ventricular septal defect is the most common lesion seen in congenital heart disease. In many, it is part and parcel of a wide range of complicated entities such as tetralogy of Fallot, tricuspid atresia, and transposition. In the past, it has been difficult to determine the precise prevalence of uncomplicated defects for a variety of reasons, including diagnostic imprecision and occurrence of spontaneous closure. In recent years, with improved reporting and diagnosis, particularly using echocardiography, a prevalence rate of 2.5 per 1000 live births has been determined.[1] In an earlier study, 0.35 to 0.50 per 1000 live births had a defect of sufficient size to necessitate catheterization or surgical intervention.[2] Among our patient population with congenital heart disease first seen from 1988 to 2002, 9% had ventricular defects (alone or associated with an atrial defect, patent ductus, or valvar abnormality), and 52% were female (see Exhibit 30-1).

EMBRYOLOGY

A ventricular septal defect results from a delay in closure of the interventricular septum beyond the first 7 weeks of intrauterine life. Although precise reasons for the defect remain unclear, it has been shown that gene mutations result in ventricular septal defects and limb deformities being inherited in the autosomal dominant Holt-Oram syndrome.[3–5] Chromosomal abnormalities[6] and environmental factors[7] also cause ventricular defects. Another risk factor is a parent with a ventricular defect, with 2.9% of offspring having a congenital cardiac lesion, usually a ventricular defect.[8] Ventricular defects are more common among premature and low-birth-weight infants.[9] A subpulmonary defect location is much more common among Asian populations than in Western countries.[10,11]

ANATOMY

Ventricular defects are single or multiple and are classified by their location in the septum (Fig. 30-1).

A wide variety of terms is used to classify the location of ventricular septal defects. A partial list includes membranous, high, subaortic, subarterial, subpulmonary, doubly committed, infundibular, supracristal, intracristal, subcristal, trabecular, muscular, posterior, anterior, mid, apical, Swiss cheese, endocardial cushion type, atrioventricular canal type, malalignment, inlet, outlet, hyphenated combinations of the above, and others[12–17] (see Fig. 30-1). At Children's Hospital Boston, the classifications listed in the following subsections are used.

Exhibit 30–1
Children's Hospital Boston Experience
Ventricular Septal Defect

	1973-1987		1988-2002	
Associated Defects	**All†**	**Hierarchical Listing***	**All†**	**Hierarchical Listing***
Aortic stenosis		117		298
Valvar stenosis	40		27	
Supravalvular stenosis	4		24	
Subvalvar stenosis	69		222	
Stenosis not specified	22		81	
Aortic regurgitation		90		317
Mitral stenosis		22		48
Valvar stenosis	26		83	
Supravalvular stenosis	5		16	
Cor triatriatum	3		6	
Mitral regurgitation		72		527
Pulmonary stenosis		425		428
Valvar stenosis	334		100	
Subvalvar stenosis	61		105	
Double-chambered right ventricle	135		242	
Supravalvar stenosis	37		35	
Peripheral stenosis	98		295	
Pulmonary regurgitation		22		134
Tricuspid valve		83		612
Valvar regurgitation	180		1698	
Ebstein's disease	4		12	
Valvar stenosis	7		20	
Other	20		61	
Atrial septal defect		86		225
Patent ductus arteriosus		70		129
Uncomplicated ventricular septal defect		2235		2399
TOTAL		3322		5117

Note: In the 1988-2002 era, compared with 1973-1987, although the patient number increased by 54%, there was a greater than threefold increase in valve regurgitation (aortic, mitral, pulmonary, tricuspid) and atrial septal defects encountered, reflecting more widespread use of echocardiography.
Of the total 5117 patients seen between 1988 and 2002, 52% were female.
*Arbitrarily records each patient once according to position in the hierarchic list.
†Lists each time a lesion was found; thus, some patients appear several times.

Membranous Defects

Membranous defects, originally considered by far the most common, are now just more common in complicated lesions than muscular defects (Exhibit 30-2). The membranous septum is a small translucent structure located immediately superior to the division of the septal band and adjacent to the commissure between the anterior and septal leaflets of the tricuspid valve. It lies directly under the aortic valve on the left side and overlaps a small segment of the right atrium. Congenital or acquired abnormalities of the aortic valve may be associated with membranous defects. The tricuspid valve may be involved in the formation of a ventricular septal aneurysm and may be damaged by the jet of blood passing through a small membranous defect. Rarely, a defect in the membranous septum opens solely into the right atrium, allowing a left ventricular–right atrial shunt. Because the membranous septum is a small area, most defects extend

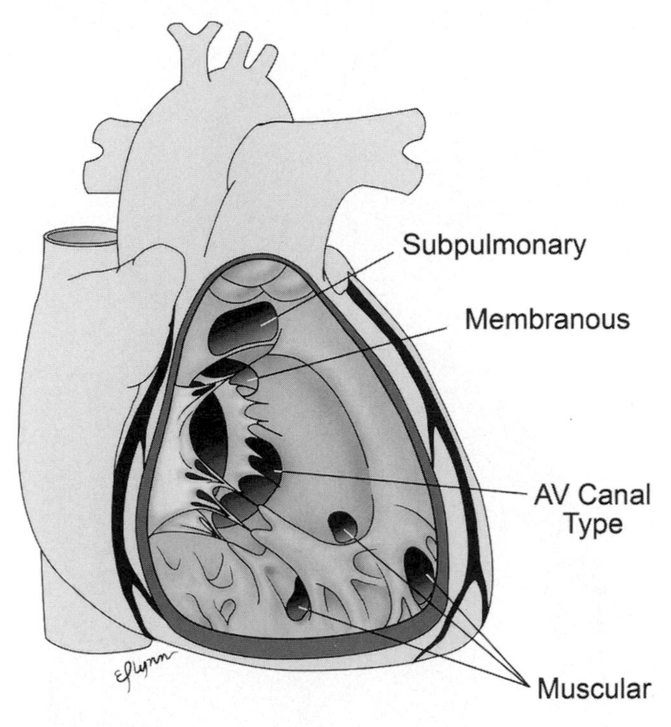

FIGURE 30–1 *Diagram of types of ventricular septal defects as viewed from the right ventricle.*
From Fyler DC [ed]. Nadas' Pediatric Cardiology. Philadelphia: Hanley & Belfus, 1992.

Exhibit 30–2
Childern's Hospital Boston Experience, 1988-2002
Ventricular Septal Defect Location (N = 5177)

Location	*Complicated** *N (%)*	*Non Complicated* *N (%)*
Muscular	858 (34)	781 (59)
Membranous	1021 (41)	360 (27)
Multiple	492 (20)	145 (11)
Malalignment	69 (2.5)	15 (1)
Subpulmonary	48 (2)	9 (1)
Endocardial cushion type	13 (0.5)	8 (1)
LOCATION KNOWN	2501 (100)	1318 (100)
UNKNOWN	217	1081†
TOTAL	2718	2399

*Complicated refers to one or more additional lesions, as in Exhibit 30-1.
-% - % values of known ventricular defect location patients.
-Membranous defects most common in complicated patients.
-Muscular defects most common in complicated patients.
†Of 1081 patients with uncomplicated unknown type defect, 88% had diagnosis of ventricular defect based on physical examination and electrocardiogram; most likely, all were very small.

into the immediately adjacent infundibular region, hence the term *perimembranous*. There may be malalignment of the great arteries and ventricles favoring either the right or left (anterior or posterior) ventricle, often in association with encroachment of either right or left ventricular outflow. Malalignment defects are characteristic of the tetralogy of Fallot syndrome (see Chapter 32).

Muscular Defects

Muscular defects may be located anywhere in the apical, mid, anterior, or posterior muscular septum and are often multiple. With the introduction of echocardiography, these are now more frequently identified and indeed are more common than membranous defects when uncomplicated (see Exhibit 30-2). Sometimes these defects seem multiple when viewed from the right ventricle (the usual surgical approach) because trabeculations overlie a large defect that is discovered to be single when viewed from the left ventricular side (Fig. 30-2).

Infundibular (Subpulmonary) Defects

Infundibular defects are located under the pulmonary valve when viewed from the right ventricle and are immediately beneath the aortic valve when viewed from the left ventricle. The adjacent right coronary aortic valve cusp often prolapses into the ventricular defect with or without aortic regurgitation.

Endocardial Cushion Type of Defects

Endocardial cushion defects are located beneath the tricuspid valve, extending to the tricuspid valve ring, and they occupy the area where an atrioventricularis communis opening would be found. Other stigmata of endocardial cushion defects, such as leftward-superior axis on the electrocardiogram and atrioventricular valve abnormalities, are usually not present.

PHYSIOLOGY

The size of the defect and the pulmonary vascular resistance determine the hemodynamics in these patients. Normally, high fetal pulmonary arteriolar resistance decreases rapidly with the first breath and in the first hours

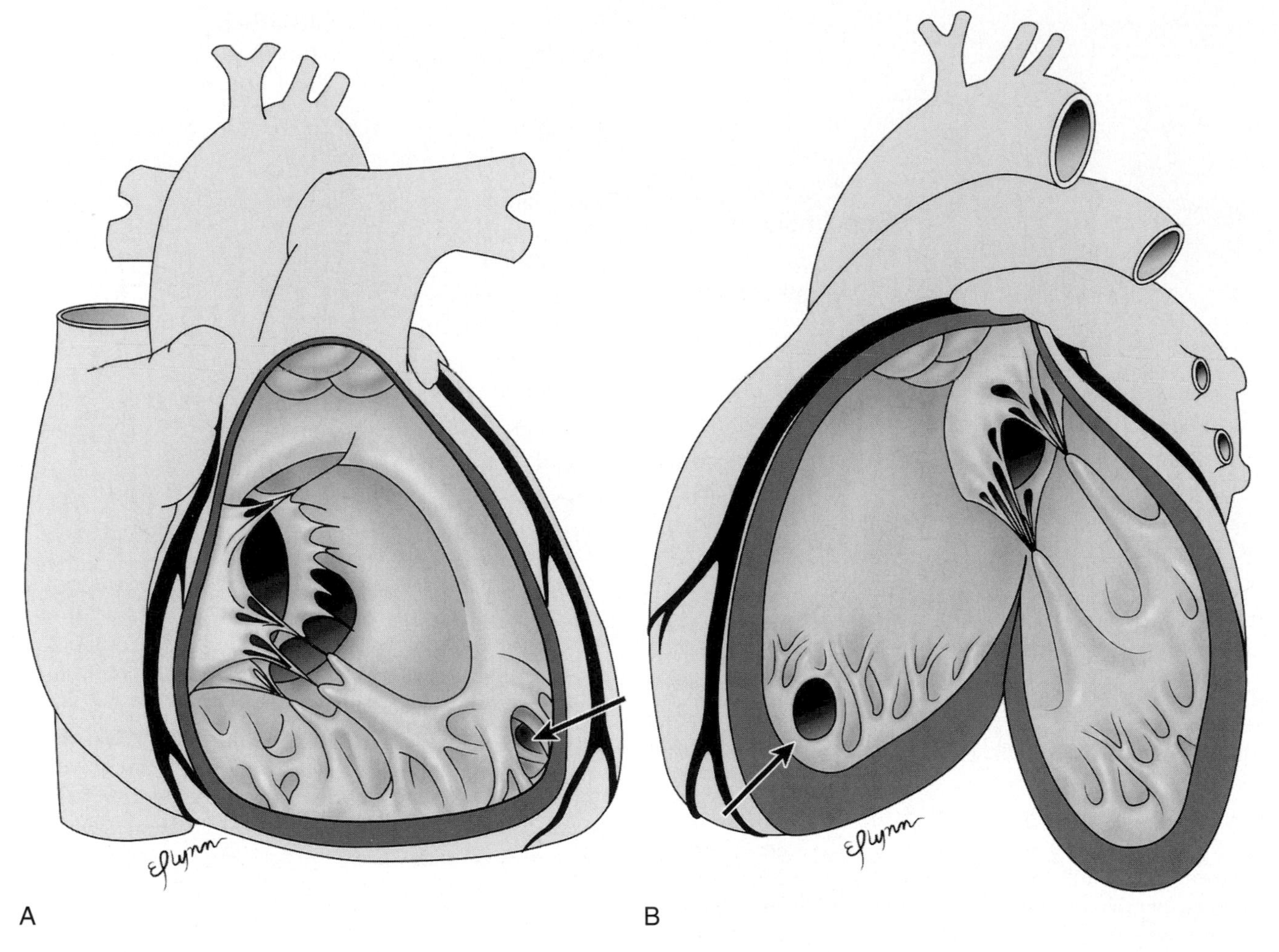

FIGURE 30–2 *Diagram of apical muscular ventricular septal defect as viewed from the right* (**A**) *and left* (**B**) *ventricles. Note that from the right side, shunted blood passes through multiple trabeculations, whereas from the left ventricle, a single defect is present. From Fyler DC [ed]. Nadas' Pediatric Cardiology. Philadelphia: Hanley & Belfus, 1992.*

of life; later the decrease is more gradual (see Chapter 10), and it stabilizes at adult levels about the age of 3 to 6 months. After birth, as pulmonary vascular resistance falls, left-to-right shunting through the ventricular defect begins and increases in the first days and weeks of life. Smaller defects allow the right ventricular and pulmonary arterial pressures to fall proportional to the drop in pulmonary resistance. With large defects (greater than 50% of the aortic diameter), there is obligatory equilibration of pressures between the two ventricles. Fortunately, in these infants, involution of the fetal pulmonary arteriolar structures is variably delayed or reinstated very early[18]; otherwise, the systemic circulation would empty into the pulmonary circulation. The larger the ventricular defect and the lower the pulmonary resistance, the greater the left-to-right shunt. Up to the point of equalization of the right and left ventricular pressures, the size of the shunt is dictated by the size of the hole. When the ventricular pressures are equilibrated, the size of the shunt is determined by the relative levels of the pulmonary arterial and systemic resistances (Fig. 30-3).

The bulk of shunting occurs in systole, with lesser amounts in diastole. Muscular defects may become smaller in systole, allowing less shunting than expected for the size of the defect.

Symptoms are determined by the size of the shunt. If the shunt is small, the infant is asymptomatic; if the shunt is large (pulmonary flow greater than or equal to 2.5 times the systemic blood flow) and the pulmonary artery pressure high, congestive heart failure is common. With a large defect, such heart failure can occur within days of birth, but is usually delayed until the third week of life or, rarely, as late as 6 months after birth with solitary lesions. Other factors that promote the appearance of congestive failure in the first days of life include additional cardiac defects

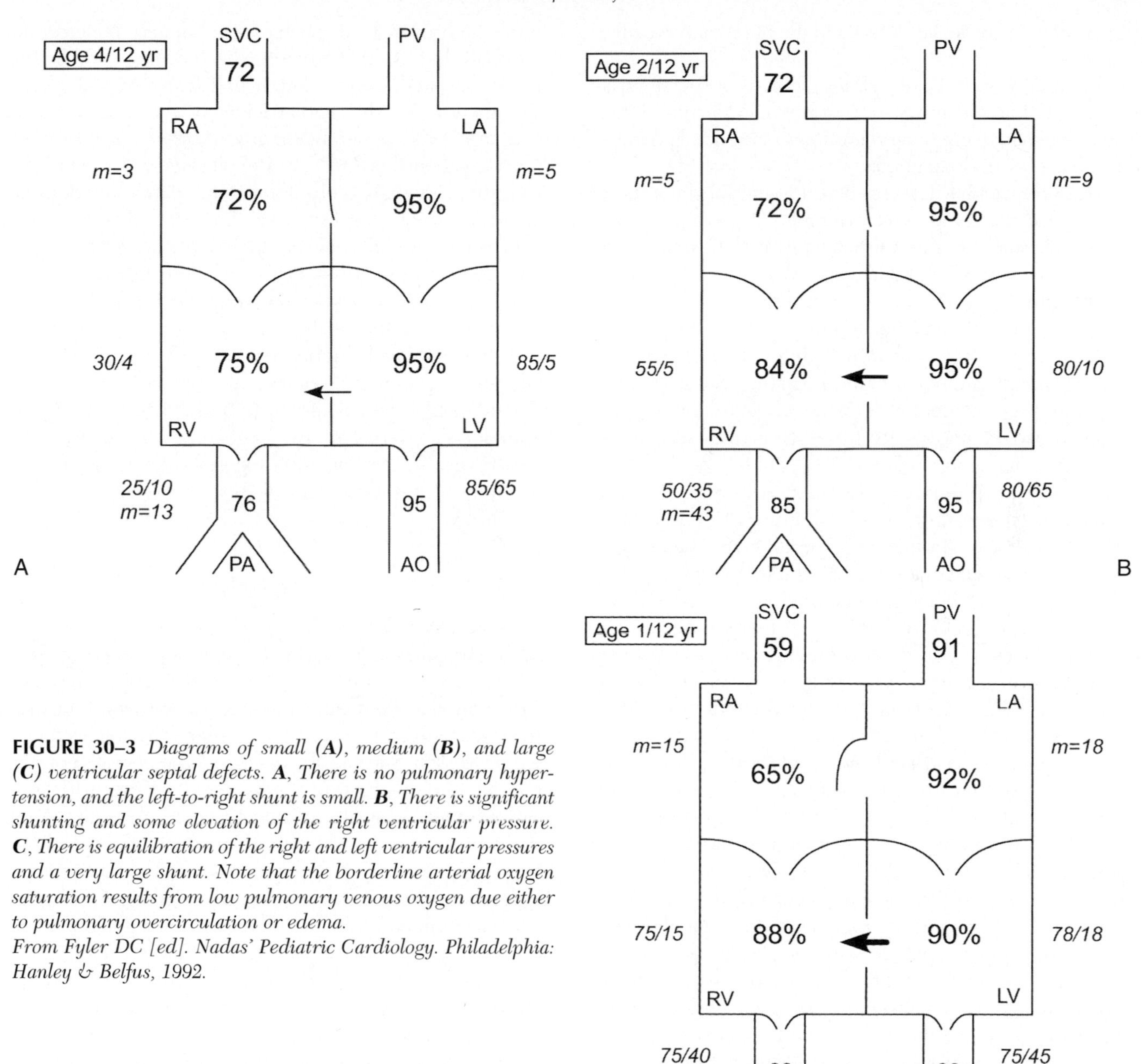

FIGURE 30–3 *Diagrams of small* (**A**), *medium* (**B**), *and large* (**C**) *ventricular septal defects.* **A**, *There is no pulmonary hypertension, and the left-to-right shunt is small.* **B**, *There is significant shunting and some elevation of the right ventricular pressure.* **C**, *There is equilibration of the right and left ventricular pressures and a very large shunt. Note that the borderline arterial oxygen saturation results from low pulmonary venous oxygen due either to pulmonary overcirculation or edema.*
From Fyler DC [ed]. Nadas' Pediatric Cardiology. Philadelphia: Hanley & Belfus, 1992.

(sometimes unsuspected), intercurrent respiratory infection, anemia, noncardiac congenital anomalies, and prematurity.[9]

Left-to-right shunting increases the amount of blood passing through the right ventricle, pulmonary arteries, left atrium, and left ventricle, and if the defect is large enough, there is also hypertension of the pulmonary artery, right ventricle, and left atrium. The abnormalities of chest x-rays, electrocardiograms, angiocardiograms, and echocardiograms are direct functions of these hemodynamic realities.

An additional patent ductus arteriosus increases the amount of left-to-right shunting, but if the combination of a patent ductus arteriosus and a ventricular defect results in equilibration of pressures, the amount shunted depends primarily on the relative pulmonary and systemic resistances, with little relation to the combined size of the defects.

An additional atrial septal defect increases the amount of left-to-right shunting by venting the left atrium, but elevation of right ventricular pressure is still dependent on the size of the ventricular defect and the pulmonary vascular resistance.

Additional valvar abnormalities, such as aortic stenosis or regurgitation and mitral stenosis or regurgitation, influence the hemodynamics in proportion to the added pressure and volume work demanded.

A large ventricular defect is better tolerated when there is counterbalancing pulmonary stenosis. The relation of the systemic resistance to the resistance provided by pulmonary stenosis determines whether there is right-to-left or left-to-right shunting and how much. Some five decades ago when the repair of ventricular septal defects had a high mortality, surgeons successfully reduced the left-to-right shunting though pulmonary artery banding. Subsequently, there was improvement in congestive heart failure and improved growth in infants formerly in critical trouble with ventricular septal defects.

Elevation of pulmonary vascular resistance by any mechanism reduces left-to-right shunting. Hypoxia (high altitude) increases pulmonary vascular resistance and decreases the amount of left-to-right shunt. At high altitudes, children with ventricular defects develop congestive heart failure less commonly than their contemporaries at sea level, and they may develop heart failure on descent to sea level.[19] Similarly, patients with pulmonary arterial hypertension caused by pulmonary venous hypertension have less of a left-to-right shunt. Surgical relief of mitral stenosis in the presence of a large ventricular septal defect can result in a large left-to-right shunt and congestive heart failure even though the patient was cyanotic originally (Fig. 30-4). As patients with large ventricular defects get older (age 12 months or older), irreversible pulmonary vascular obstructive disease may occur.[20–22] The hemodynamic effect is comparable to pulmonary artery banding and may actually help the patient symptomatically by reducing the volume load; however, if the pulmonary vascular disease becomes irreversible, it becomes *the* overriding determinant of the future of the patient.[22,23] Fortunately, normal fetal pulmonary vascular changes usually involute after birth, only rarely persisting and advancing to permanent abnormality after age 12 months. During the window of delayed appearance, the ventricular defect can be repaired safely, but once irreversible pulmonary vascular disease is established, repair of the defect is not helpful and may be fatal.

CLINICAL MANIFESTATIONS

Discovery

Most infants with ventricular septal defect are asymptomatic because most defects are too small to allow sufficient left-to-right shunting to cause symptoms. Murmurs are rarely audible at birth owing to pulmonary hypertension (normal), but as this regresses, they become audible after a few days and are thus often first discovered at routine auscultation by the pediatrician at the first postnatal checkup. Another significant group (20% to 30% of symptomatic patients) is discovered when some other noncardiac congenital anomaly is observed and a search for additional anomalies leads to a discovery of a heart murmur. Larger defects may produce only tachypnea, but among the largest ones, symptoms of gross congestive failure, tachypnea, dyspnea, reduced fluid intake, and poor growth call attention to the underlying abnormality.

Although a small number of infants who are symptomatic because of a ventricular defect are transferred to a cardiac unit in the first week of life, many with heart failure are first seen at some weeks of age. In general, the sickest babies are the youngest. Often, superimposed respiratory infections precipitate hospitalization (respiratory syncytial virus is common).

Symptoms

Infants with large septal defects present with symptoms caused by congestive heart failure and superimposed respiratory infections. Tachypnea, with respiratory rates regularly more than 60 breaths/minute, is a first symptom, often recognized in retrospect by the mother as having been present since birth. Such a baby may grow and develop normally for sometime without other symptoms. Those with more severe dyspnea will be unable to nurse normally, resting frequently and requiring more than 20 minutes to ingest an appropriate feeding. Regurgitation is common, and vomiting occurs when there is severe congestive failure. Growth failure is a common problem,[24–26] sometimes initially seeming satisfactory, only later to slow down. In the worst case, the infant never exceeds birth weight because of poor caloric intake and increased oxygen consumption due to excessive work of the heart and lungs.

Older patients seen for the first time may be referred because of arrhythmia, congestive heart failure, hemoptysis, and bacterial endocarditis.[27]

Physical Examination

The size of the defect and the amount of left-to-right shunting greatly influence the physical findings. Thus, patients of all ages with small or moderate-sized defects have a pressure gradient across the ventricular septum resulting in a pansystolic loud murmur with a thrill (Fig. 30-5). The onset of the murmur diminishes the first heart sound intensity at the left lower sternal border, the second heart sound is normal (splitting interval, pulmonary closure intensity), and patients grow well and are asymptomatic.[28] The very

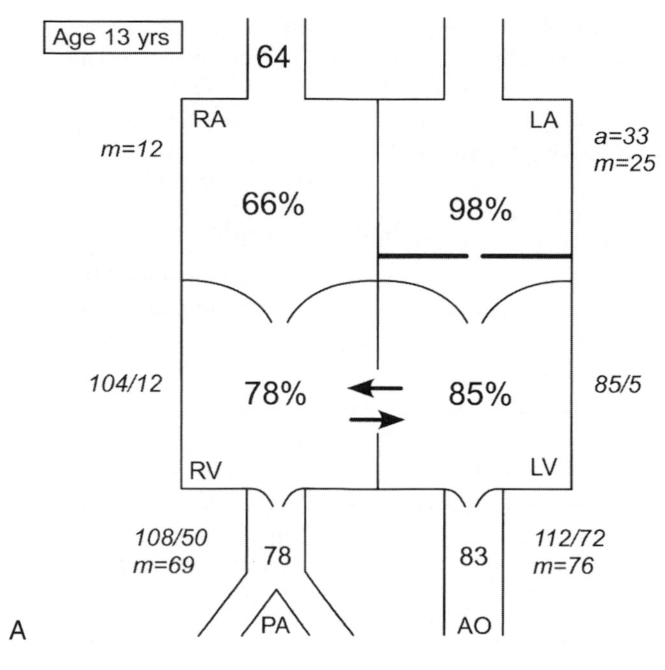

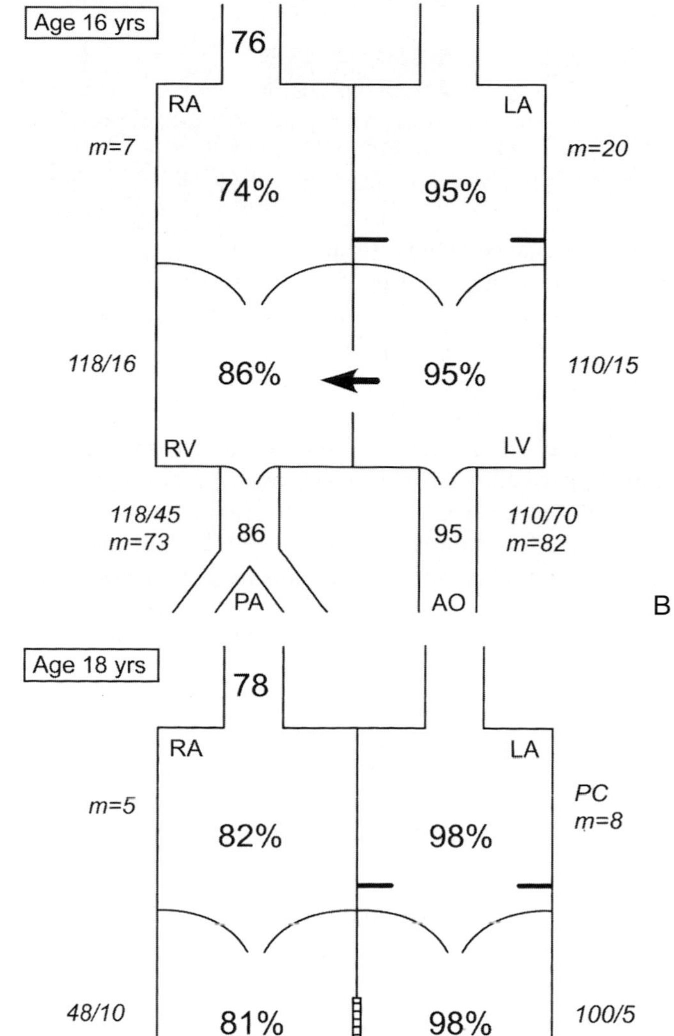

FIGURE 30–4 *Catheterization data from a cyanotic boy who had supravalvar mitral stenosis, a large ventricular septal defect, and elevated pulmonary resistance.* ***A****, Preoperative data at age 13 years.* ***B****, After removal of the supravalvar membrane at age 16 years, showing a decrease in vascular resistance and appearance of a large left-to-right shunt.* ***C****, Data at age 18 years after closure of ventricular septal defect, showing only mild residual pulmonary hypertension.*
From Fyler DC [ed]. Nadas' Pediatric Cardiology. Philadelphia: Hanley & Belfus, 1992.

loud (grade 5) systolic murmur of a small membranous defect (maladie de Roger) is best heard at the third and fourth left intercostal spaces at the sternal border; it is important to remember that a double-chambered right ventricle, a common accompanying lesion, produces a similar murmur. The often equally loud murmur from a subpulmonary defect is best heard at the second intercostal space level. Occasionally, very small muscular defects are associated with a grade 2 or less blowing, high-frequency murmur that ends in mid to late systole.

In contrast, the infant with a large unrestrictive defect is often malnourished and scrawny. The respiratory rate is 80 to 100 breaths/minute with retractions, the liver edge is palpable well below the right costal margin (at least in part owing to hyperexpanded lungs), and the cardiac impulse is hyperdynamic and rapid. Because there is no pressure gradient across the ventricular defect, the systolic murmur is not prominent (thus, thrills are uncommon), but a diastolic flow rumble due to excessive mitral valve flow is often present. Surprisingly, the peripheral pulses are generally

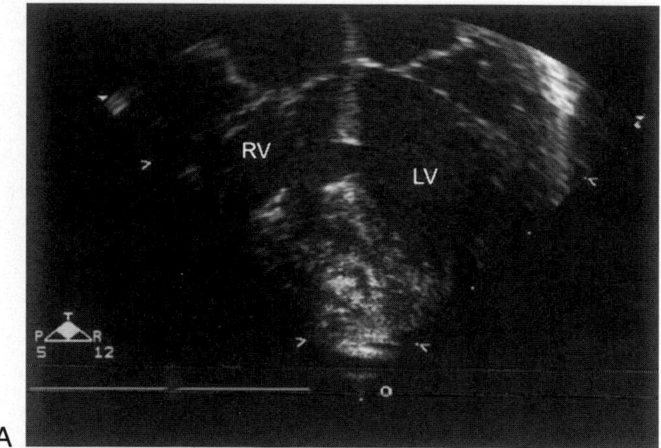

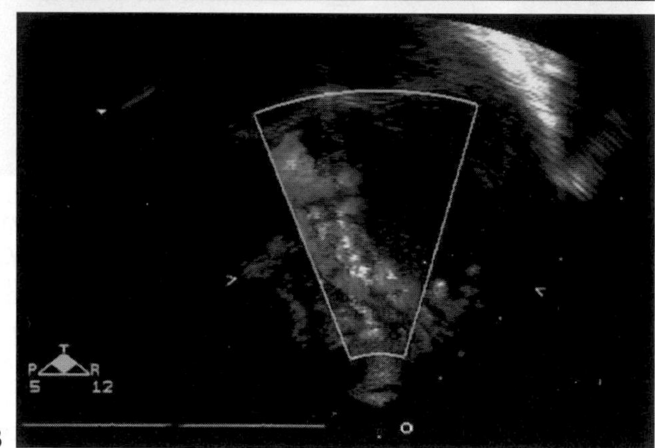

FIGURE 30–9 **A**, *Apical echocardiogram demonstrating a large muscular ventricular septal defect positioned directly between the left ventricular (LV) and right ventricular (RV) labels. There is also a more apical region that could represent an additional defect, but the imaging is ambiguous.* **B**, *Color-flow Doppler of the same image clearly shows the two jets (blue) of flow across the interventricular septum.*

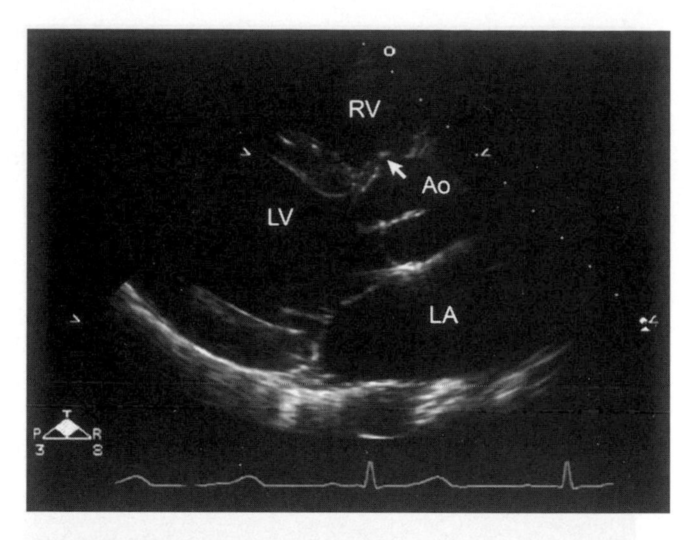

FIGURE 30–10 *Parasternal long-axis echocardiogram of subpulmonary ventricular septal defect with prolapse of the right coronary cusp of the aortic valve. The arrow indicates the position of the aortic annulus. The right coronary cusp below this arrow is dilated and distorted. Ao, aorta; LA, left atrium; LV, left ventricle; RV, right ventricle.*

cardiac positioning views for the different defect locations are used. These were introduced by Bargeron and colleagues in 1988[33] and are also the basis for most views currently used in echocardiography.

1. *Membranous defects* are best seen using the long-axis oblique view in which the contrast is seen to cross the membranous defect directly beneath the aortic valve (Fig. 30-11). On the orthogonal biplane right anterior oblique view, the contrast is also seen to pass beneath the conal septum to the right ventricular outflow tract, and in some patients, the actual defect may be seen as a solid white oval disc because of the contrast jet being viewed "end on" in systole.
2. *Mid-muscular and apical defects* are also best seen using the long axial oblique view (Figs. 30-12, and 30-13),

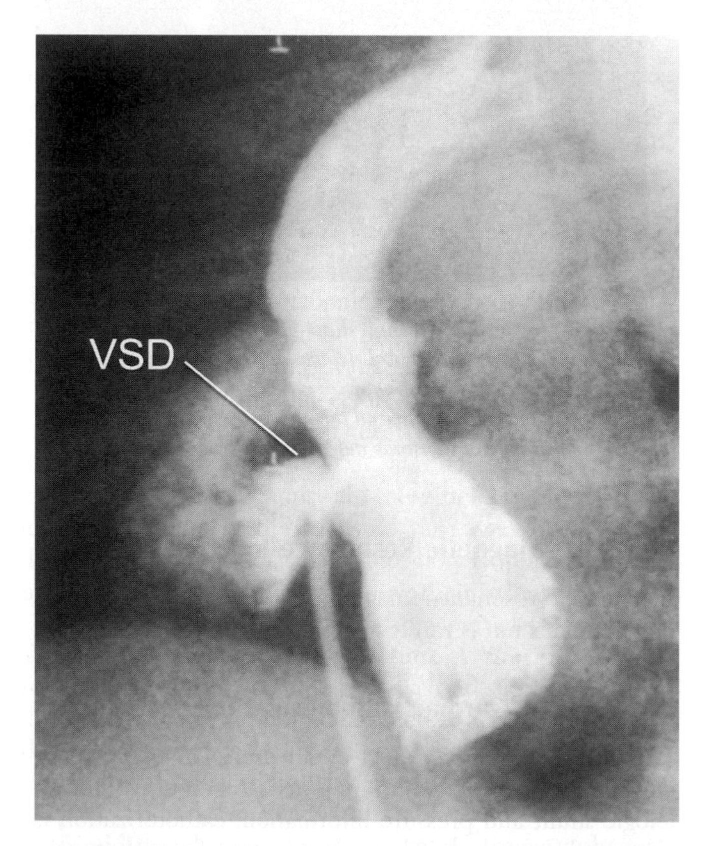

FIGURE 30–11 *Angiogram showing a membranous ventricular septal defect (VSD). The injection is into the left ventricle with the patient in the long axial oblique position. Contrast passes from the left to the right ventricle just beneath the aortic valve.*

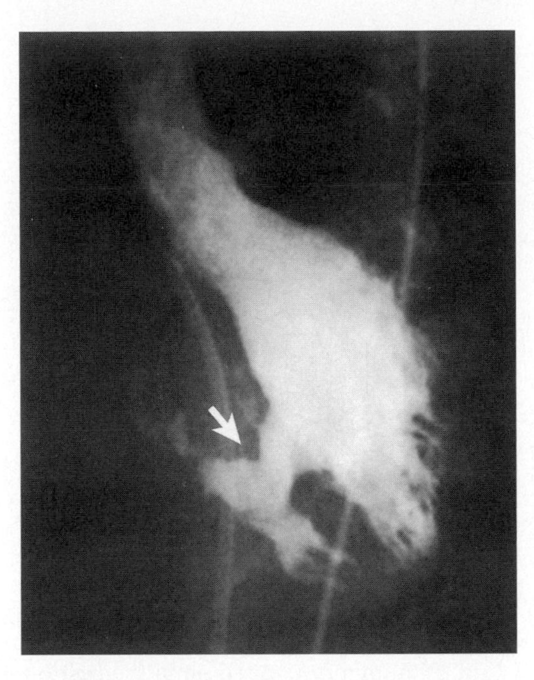

FIGURE 30–12 *Angiogram showing single large muscular defect (arrow) in lower septum, long axial oblique view.*

whereas *anterior muscular defects* are well seen in the right anterior oblique view.

3. *Posterior muscular and inlet type defects* are outlined using the hepatoclavicular (four-chamber) view and an apex-to-base projection, particularly for the former.
4. *Subpulmonary defects* are visualized in the right anterior oblique view, with contrast being seen to pass directly through the conal septum (Fig. 30-14).

Minor Laboratory Tests

Hemoglobin and hematocrit measurements may be important because any degree of anemia aggravates the symptoms produced by a left-to-right shunt. Evidence of a superimposed infection, as demonstrated by fever or an elevated white count, may reveal the aggravating cause of congestive heart failure in infants.

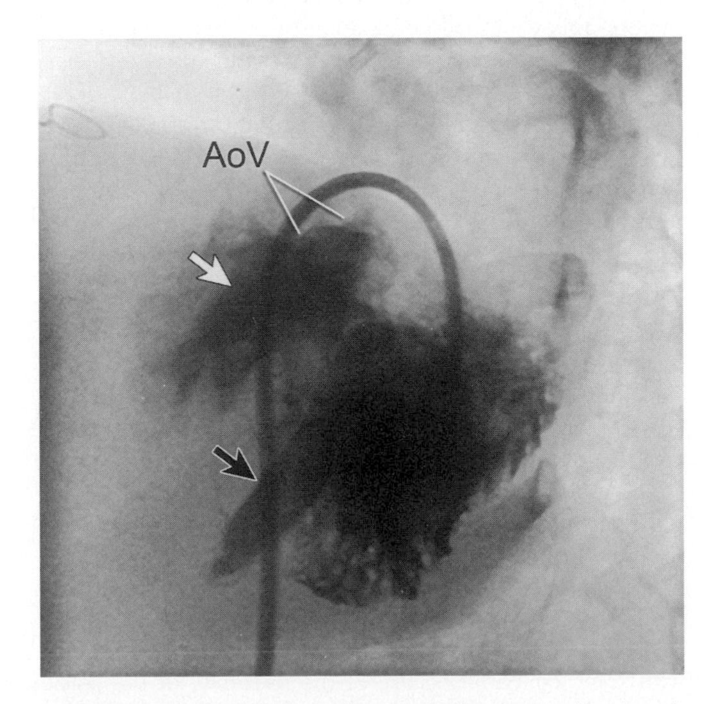

FIGURE 30–13 *Angiogram showing multiple apical and mid-muscular ventricular septal defects (arrows), injecting contrast in the left ventricle with the patient in the left anterior oblique position.*

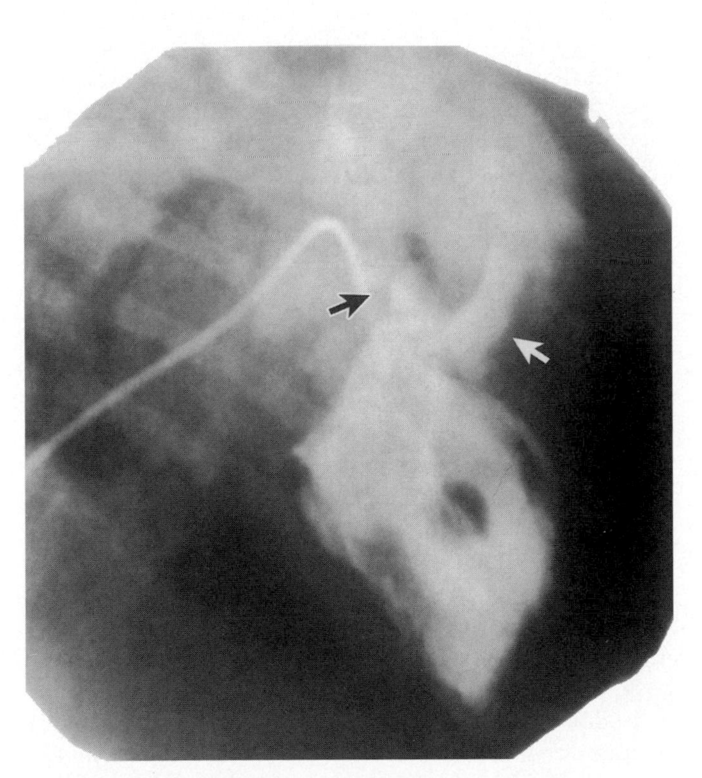

FIGURE 30–14 *Angiogram showing a subpulmonary ventricular septal defect, injection contrast in the left ventricle with the patient in a right anteroposterior oblique position. Dye passes through the conal septum (white arrow) almost directly into the main pulmonary artery (black arrow at noncoronary cusp of aortic valve).*
From Fyler DC [ed]. Nadas' Pediatric Cardiology. Philadelphia: Hanley & Belfus, 1992.

MANAGEMENT

In general, it is reasonable to obtain a two-dimensional echocardiogram soon after detection of a ventricular septal defect murmur because although the initial clinical impression is usually correct, sometimes it is in error. Perhaps one exception to this is the infant with a grade 2 or less high-frequency early mid-systolic murmur and a normal second heart sound and electrocardiogram, which indicate a tiny defect, in whom medical follow-up alone is adequate.

Influence of Size of Defect

Small Ventricular Septal Defects

Most ventricular defects are small.[34–36] The child who has reached the age of 6 months without evidence of congestive heart failure and without evidence of pulmonary hypertension can be managed conservatively. Ventricular defects do not get bigger, only smaller; rarely, left-to-right shunting is increased by the development of additional lesions causing left ventricular hypertension. After the first year of life, asymptomatic infants known to have small, persistently patent defects should be examined every 3 years or so to watch for aortic valve prolapse or regurgitation, document any defect decrease in size, and ensure prophylactic antibiotics are used to prevent the possibility of infective endocarditis whenever oral, dental, or genitourinary surgery is undertaken.

Large Ventricular Septal Defects

The mortality rate with surgical closure has become sufficiently low (less than 1%) that repair even in the first few months of life is now feasible[37,38] (Exhibit 30-3). Thus, in those neonates and infants with poor growth, a single unrestrictive defect, and pulmonary artery pressure at or near systemic level, surgical closure should be undertaken. In addition, those with multiple defects, as long as they are reachable through the tricuspid valve, also should undergo surgical closure. After surgery, improvement in growth is almost universal.[26] On the other hand, babies with restrictive defects (pulmonary artery pressure less than 60% systemic level, and adequate growth) can be followed medically with anticongestive measures and any associated anemia corrected,[39] given that many defects will decrease in size or even close spontaneously with time. In older patients, large defects with significant shunts and left ventricular enlargement should be closed, either surgically or, if muscular septal in location, by catheter-delivered devices.

In terms of surgery, the usual route of closure is through the tricuspid valve (transatrial). With this approach, defects that are membranous, inlet, and muscular proximal to the moderator band, and some that are anteriorly located, can be closed. Subpulmonary defects are usually closed through the pulmonary valve. Apical defects may on occasion be closed through a small apical right ventriculotomy—a left ventriculotomy approach is no longer used because this frequently resulted in left ventricular dysfunction.

In recent years, catheter-delivered devices have been used to close ventricular defects with excellent results[40–47] (see Chapter 14). Most of these have been placed in patients older than 1 year, in muscular defects, often many per patient—a few have been placed in membranous defects, with some concern because of the proximity of the aortic valve to the defect.[45,46] These devices have also been successfully placed intraoperatively.[47–49]

Exhibit 30–3

Childern's Hospital Boston Experience

Ventricular Septal Defect Surgery

	1973-1987		1988-2002	
Age at Repair	*N*	*30-Day Mortality (%)*	*N*	*30-Day Mortality (%)*
0-2 mo	35	20	113	0
3-6 mo	135	4	208	0.5*
7-12 mo	136	3	150	0
1-5 yr	200	1	202	0.5†
6-10 yr	64	0	47	0
11-15 yr	29	0	13	0
16-20 yr	23	4	11	0
21-	15	0	3	33‡
TOTAL	638	3	7460.4	

Note: When compared with the 1973-1987 era, in the 1988-2002 period, (1) 30 day mortality decreased from 3% to 0.4% and (2) number operated on in the first 6 months increased from 27% to 43% with only 1 death in 321 infants, compared with 12 deaths in 170 infants.

*At 4 months, infant with hydrocephalus had closure of membranous ventricular defect, atrial septal defect, and patent ducuts arteriosus, together with tricuspid valve plasty; had small residual anterior muscular defect; died 1 month later at home.

† This 16-month-old infant developed severe mitral regurgitation following balloon dilation for severe stenosis, had valve replacement and defect closure within days, and died three days later.

‡This 17-year-old patient with traumatic ventricular septal defect, initially had two devices placed at two catheterizations while on balloon pump assistance, followed by surgery next day with death within the next 24 hours.

Influence of Type of Defect

In general, the risks of surgery in the current era are sufficiently low and the degree of successful closure high enough to recommend closure of any large defect regardless of location at any age. Pulmonary artery banding is no longer used. In addition, catheter-delivered devices now offer an increasingly satisfactory alternative technique for closure of surgically difficult-to-reach muscular defects in the apical and anterior septal locations.

Membranous Defects

Many defects are located in the membranous septum and often become smaller, with up to 27%, including some large defects, closing spontaneously.[22,36,50] Because of this tendency toward improvement with time, it is reasonable to follow medically many of those with good growth and low pulmonary artery pressure, even though decrease in shunt size is by no means a certainty.

The rare malalignment membranous defect is not thought to close spontaneously or to get smaller. These defects are usually large and associated with pulmonary hypertension; consequently, all should be surgically closed. Most are associated with pulmonary stenosis in the context of cyanotic or acyanotic tetralogy of Fallot and are surgically corrected either electively or because of symptoms.

Muscular Defects

Muscular defects are very common and are often multiple. Small lesions frequently close spontaneously,[36] as may large defects occasionally (Fig. 30-15). Thus, as with membranous defects, it is reasonable to follow infants conservatively for some months as long as they are doing well. If significant shunting persists and pulmonary artery pressure is elevated, then primary closure is indicated. Apical and anterior defects are best managed with catheter-delivered devices (in patients older than 6 months), whereas those proximal to the moderator band are accessible surgically at any age through the tricuspid valve, thus avoiding a ventriculotomy. Although residual shunting persists in some, it is often much less than before the procedure and may disappear with time. Pulmonary artery banding as a palliative procedure is essentially no longer used.

Infundibular (Subpulmonary) Defects

Because subpulmonary defects are rarely small and are not known to get smaller, and because aortic regurgitation develops commonly, all patients with significant anatomic defects are referred to the surgeons after the age of 6 months, or earlier if there is growth failure. It should be remembered that physiologically once a cusp has prolapsed, the shunt size is diminished by the cusp.

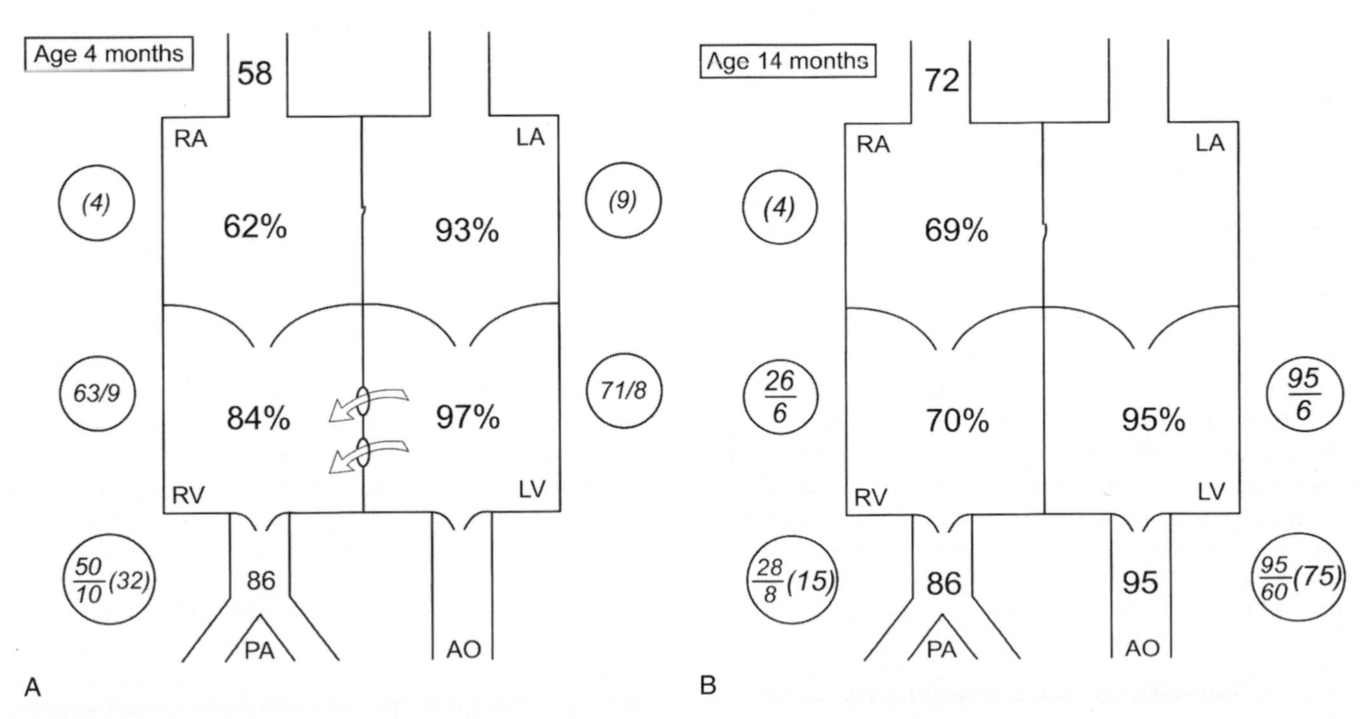

FIGURE 30–15 *Catheterization data in a child.* **A**, *At age 4 months, huge left-to-right shunt (Qp/Qs > 4/1) through multiple muscular ventricular septal defects (arrows).* **B**, *At age 14 months, spontaneous closure of defects with elimination of shunt.*

Endocardial Cushion Type of Defect

Because these defects do not regress spontaneously or get smaller and because small defects are uncommon, surgery is almost invariably needed.

COURSE

Children with smaller defects reach adulthood normally without surgery. Although bacterial endocarditis is uncommon,[50] it is more often seen in those managed medically than in the surgically treated group.[51]

Rarely, the murmur of the small defect becomes so loud that it is distracting to nearby individuals, but more often, it becomes less intense as the chest grows; occasionally, this loud murmur is due to the development of a double-chambered right ventricle. A defect in the membranous area that seems small may be partially occluded by a prolapsed aortic valve, this being visible on echocardiography.

Patients with larger defects that have been surgically closed usually do well, regaining their destined position on the growth chart if surgery is done early enough and if there are no noncardiac anomalies that inhibit growth.[26] Even with late surgical closure, the child is not dwarfed but is smaller than the parent or siblings. There are late deaths: in the Natural History Study,[52] although most occurred in surgically managed patients with Eisenmenger's complex, there were a few sudden deaths even among those managed medically with a small defect. Significant ventricular dysrhythmias were identified in both medical and surgical survivors in that study. Perhaps current management strategies will decrease this risk.

Some surgical survivors have a small residual defect (20%)[26] due to an unrecognized second defect or a leak around the patch, but rarely require a second operation.

Complete right bundle branch block occurs in almost all surgically managed infants younger than 6 months of age. Because the surgical approach is transatrial, this conduction defect is central in origin, but appears to be of no consequence to date. Persistent complete heart block is extremely rare, less than 1%.

When cardiac catheterization was done postoperatively in earlier years, pulmonary artery pressure and resistance had significantly decreased in the very young.[26] Postoperative tricuspid valve deformity related to the patch material and tricuspid regurgitation have not been a problem in the absence of pulmonary hypertension or stenosis.

Spontaneous Diminution in Size

Spontaneous decrease in defect size and even closure has been long recognized. The reported frequencies of such events have varied considerably, related to age, defect location, follow-up duration, and especially methods of detection, particularly echocardiography. Inlet (endocardial cushion), typical malalignment, and subpulmonary defects are usually large and remain so. Although shunting in the former types remains substantial, in the latter, it often decreases as the right coronary cusp of the aortic valve prolapses into the defect, thus functionally reducing the orifice size. Membranous and muscular defects often decrease or close, this often involving the septal leaflet of the tricuspid valve in the membranous variety (often referred to as an "aneurysm of the membranous septum"). In a recent echocardiographic study, although of short duration, 15% of membranous defects closed spontaneously, as did some 57% of muscular defects (often small and multiple).[36] It is of interest that a few large apical defects close by enlargement of muscle bundles near the moderator band such that the right ventricular apex remains in continuity only with the left ventricular cavity[53] (see Figs. 30-12 and 30-15). Other recent spontaneous closure rates include 6%[50] and 15%, the latter over more than 20 years of follow-up.[52]

Development of Pulmonary Vascular Disease

In the past, pulmonary vascular disease (Eisenmenger's complex) appeared with increasing frequency as children survived longer with large ventricular septal defects, occurring in some 15% of patients in the 20-year-old group.[18] Although all patients with large ventricular defects had some pulmonary arteriolar abnormality on biopsy,[26] the development of permanent pulmonary vascular disease is very rare before the first birthday; the numbers increase afterward.[21,54] In general, pulmonary vascular disease is more common when the ventricular septal defect is large, multiple, or associated with a patent ductus arteriosus. With early surgery, the incidence of pulmonary vascular obstructive disease should approach zero, and for practical purposes, it has.

With pulmonary hypertension, the second heart sound is accentuated, often palpable, and usually single. In some patients, the murmur of pulmonary regurgitation is recognizable (Fig. 30-16). The electrocardiogram shows right ventricular hypertrophy. Any degree of left ventricular hypertrophy suggests left-to-right shunting and a potentially operable candidate. Because pulmonary vascular resistance limits the amount of left-to-right shunting, the patient tends to have a smaller heart on the chest x-ray and is much less likely to have congestive heart failure. The pulmonary vasculature is described as "pruned," with prominent central vessels and decreased caliber of the peripheral vessels.

Any suggestion of pulmonary hypertension in patients older than 6 months with ventricular septal defect requires cardiac catheterization for evaluation. Careful estimation of the pressures encountered in the right side of the heart, pulmonary arteries, and left atrium (or as reflected in the

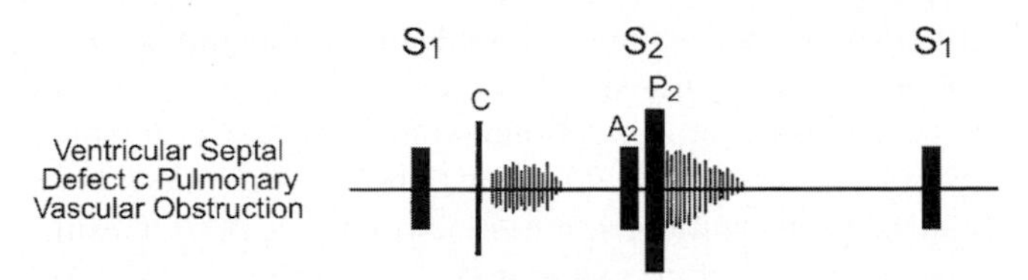

FIGURE 30–16 *Diagram of auscultatory findings in a child with ventricular septal defect and pulmonary vascular obstructive disease. Note the minimal systolic murmur and loud* P_2*. The high-frequency early diastolic murmur following* P_2 *results from pulmonary regurgitation. The diastolic murmur and the click are not invariably present.* S_1*, first heart sound;* S_2*, second heart sound; C, click;* A_2*, aortic valve closure;* P_2*, pulmonary valve closure.*

From Avery ME, First LP [eds]. Pediatric Medicine. Baltimore: Williams & Wilkins, 1989.

pulmonary arterial wedge position) is needed. Measurement of the shunt size should be recorded. The catheterization data should not be confused by general anesthesia or use of agents that might affect the pulmonary circulation. Results suggesting pulmonary vascular disease of any degree should prompt collection of further confirmatory evidence such as the response to pulmonary arterial vasodilators, including oxygen and nitric oxide. Other contributory causes to the pulmonary hypertension, such as living at high altitude or obstructive airway disease, should be carefully evaluated.[55]

Urgent surgical intervention should be undertaken to reverse the process if the pulmonary vascular disease is of recent origin. Virtually all children with ventricular septal defect and any evidence of pulmonary vascular disease undergo surgical correction in the first year of life because it is highly likely that the pulmonary vascular disease must be of recent onset. Beyond the age of 6 months, the decision to operate depends on whether the vascular change is minimal or advanced, is of recent onset, or shows evidence of reversibility. These decisions cannot be readily tabulated and are associated with significant error. In general, all patients with pulmonary resistance estimated at less than 8 units/m^2 and any evidence of developing pulmonary vascular disease are referred for closure, although a perforated patch may offer some safety ("blow-off valve") in borderline cases. Significant left-to-right shunting ($Qp/Qs > 2:1$) is taken as an indication for surgery even in the face of elevated pulmonary vascular resistance. Patients who clearly respond to dilator therapy such as oxygen and nitric oxide are subjected to surgery. Patients with resistance levels higher than 8 units/m^2, particularly those who have no left-to-right shunt, those older than 2 years, and those who show no response to pulmonary arterial vasodilation, are not considered candidates for correction. Some of these patients survive into the fourth or fifth decade. Pregnancy poses a prohibitive risk for women with pulmonary vascular disease secondary to congenital heart problems (50% mortality rate). The tendency to survive pregnancy, even delivery, but then to succumb suddenly within 1 to 2 weeks is well recognized.[56] For this reason, these patients are strongly discouraged from becoming pregnant as a matter of life and death. Contraceptive pills, which might promote pulmonary infarction, and mechanical devices, which promote infection as well as clotting, are also contraindicated. Tubal ligation offers a safe but not always acceptable alternative. Clearly the management of contraception and pregnancy in these young women is a matter of importance.

Acquired Aortic Regurgitation

Prevalence

This discussion concerns those patients who develop regurgitation as a result of prolapse of one or more aortic valve cusps. Audible aortic regurgitation in the United States occurs in some 5% of patients with a ventricular septal defect,[57] in 10% of these due to a bicuspid aortic valve.[58] In the others, the regurgitation follows prolapse of one or more valve cusps into the adjacent ventricular defect, the latter in the United States being perimembranous (also called *subcristal*) in location in most (74%) and subpulmonary in the minority.[58] In Asians, the reverse is quite striking. This combination of ventricular defect and regurgitation is more common in males (64%),[58] whereas the incidence of an uncomplicated ventricular defect is similar in both sexes.[52] Because aortic valve lesions such as stenosis are much more common in males (80%) and because prolapsing leaflets are rarely seen in other diseases with larger unrestrictive ventricular defects similarly located (such as tetralogy of Fallot), the valve in this syndrome may be intrinsically abnormal. This would seem to be supported by the anatomic observation that cusp sizes are unequal in some 84% to 98% of "normal" valves, with the largest cusp being either the right or noncoronary[59–61]; these are the cusps that are adjacent to the ventricular defects. Congenital valve abnormalities other than bicuspid have also been described in surgical series.[62]

The more widespread use of continually improving echocardiographic equipment at Children's Hospital Boston has (1) documented appearance and progression of cusp prolapse in the very young into the defect on serial studies, (2) identified large numbers of patients with a ventricular defect and prolapse of varying degrees (minor to severe), and (3) diagnosed regurgitation (inaudible in most) in about 50% of these. The latter finding would indicate an incidence of prolapse with regurgitation at least twice that of the audible regurgitation in the pre-echocardiography era.

Physiology

The left-to-right shunt tends to be small partly because the ventricular defect is obstructed by the aortic cusp. There is a pressure gradient across the septum and often the right ventricular outflow tract, sometimes due to the prolapsed cusp, but more often the result of mild infundibular obstruction. Pulmonary resistance is rarely elevated.

Clinical Manifestations

A history of congestive heart failure in infancy is rare. Currently, most patients are seen for evaluation of a ventricular septal defect murmur, with the prolapse and regurgitation then being identified on echocardiography. In terms of the septal defect, it is frequently possible to diagnose on physical examination the location of the defect. The perimembranous (subcristal) defect is associated with a thrill and systolic murmur at the third and fourth intercostal spaces at the left sternal border, whereas in a subpulmonary defect, these are distinctly higher, at the second intercostal space level. The second heart sound is normal. The age of audible aortic regurgitation detection is about 5 years[58] and is identifiable as an early diastolic onset murmur often of high frequency ending in mid-diastole. It is separated from the systolic murmur by the second heart sound and is thus not a continuous bruit as in a patent ductus. In the more recent echocardiographic era, among our patients with prolapse, the prolapse has been noted in some 20% of these in the first years of life, associated with minor degrees of regurgitation in about half. The pulse pressure is normal in most cases because the degree of regurgitation is mild at most.

Course

Progression of valve prolapse and regurgitation is well recognized in the young, although many beyond age 15 years have minimal stable hemodynamic disease.[58,62–65] The risk for developing aortic regurgitation in subpulmonary defects is more than twice that in perimembranous (subcristal) defects. On the other hand, in the latter, the development of additional defects such as subpulmonary or subaortic stenosis is much more common.[58,62] The incidence of endocarditis in these cases is very high and occurs even in postoperative patients.

Management

These cases are relatively rare in the United States, being much less common than in Asian countries, where subpulmonary defects are so common. Influenced largely by the latter experience, including current echocardiographic information and surgical results, it is reasonable to recommend surgical closure of any subpulmonary defects (other than rare tiny ones, which do occur) shortly after discovery. If aortic regurgitation is present and mild at most, closure alone is sufficient. If regurgitation is moderate or more, valve plasty, which is quite effective,[62,66–70] is necessary in addition (Fig. 30-17). Valve replacement is rarely needed except in older patients. Beyond age 15 years, if regurgitation is mild at most, shunting minimal, and the patient stable, continued medical observation seems reasonable.[63] With perimembranous (subcristal) defects, obvious prolapse, and a tricuspid valve, similar management indications as for subpulmonary defects are reasonable. Sometimes the additional lesions are the major indication for surgery in these patients. Our recent results with this approach have been satisfactory to date. Strict endocarditis prophylaxis is vital in these patients, before and after surgery.

The diagnosis of aortic regurgitation among those with a ventricular defect, with or without prolapse, has become more common (see Exhibit 30-1), owing to the more widespread use of echocardiography, the exquisite color sensitivity of which identifies inaudible, mostly minute amounts of regurgitation. By and large, this regurgitation in those without prolapse and with a tricuspid valve is viewed largely as being of little significance, requiring only medical management.

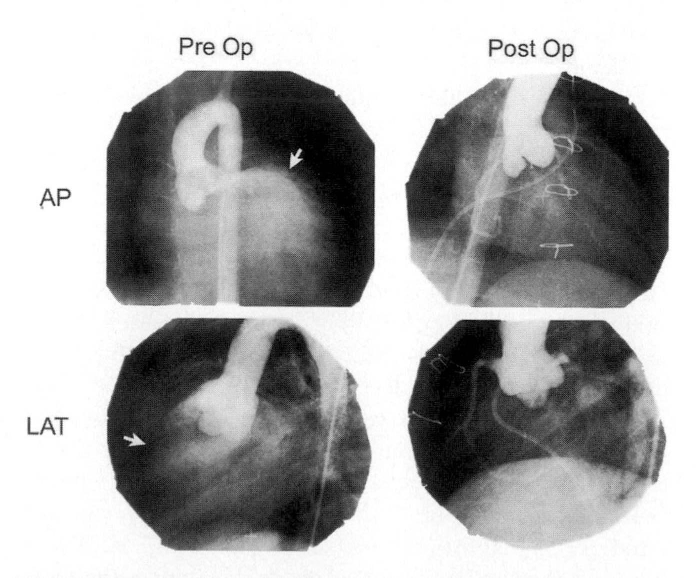

FIGURE 30–17 *Ascending aortograms anteroposterior (AP) and lateral (LAT) projections, preoperatively (Preop) at age 3 years and postoperatively (Postop) at age 4 years after membranous ventricular septal defect closure and aortic valve plasty. Preoperatively, moderate aortic regurgitation is evident (arrows), but is virtually absent on postoperative study. Sixteen years, later only mild aortic regurgitation is present.*

Ventricular Septal Defects and Aortic Stenosis

Valvar or subvalvar stenosis associated with a ventricular septal defect is not rare (see Exhibit 30-1). The subaortic lesion is usually a discrete fibrous or fibromuscular ridge situated at a variable distance beneath the aortic valve, commonly distal to the ventricular defect but occasionally proximal. The ventricular defect may be membranous, muscular, or both in location. These patients are initially seen for evaluation of a systolic murmur. Although a physical examination finding such as a constant apical ejection click may suggest a valvar obstructive aortic lesion in addition to the septal defect, the diagnosis is made echocardiographically in virtually all cases. The degrees of obstruction vary widely at either level, ranging from virtually none at a subaortic membrane or bicuspid valve to severe obstruction at either.

Physiologically, the degree of obstruction may be underestimated and the left-to-right shunt increased when the ventricular defect is proximal to the obstruction. In contrast, subaortic obstruction may be more magnified when the defect is distal (rare) because both the left to right shunt and the systemic output have to cross the obstructing membrane; in this setting, closure of the defect alone may decrease the gradient.

Echocardiography provides (1) the anatomic details of the lesions, together with much physiologic information, including the magnitude of shunting and degree of obstruction by Doppler interrogation; and (2) the ability to follow these parameters by sequential studies.

Defect status changes are common, especially in very young patients. Ventricular defects may decrease in size or close spontaneously, and aortic stenosis lesions may progress, some at an alarming rate (see Chapter 33, Fig. 33-8). Thus, management of these patients varies considerably and is dependent on the current status. Those with stable small defects and mild or less obstruction can be followed medically indefinitely. Stable neonates with moderate septal defects and minimal obstruction can also be followed medically, initially frequently, in the hope the ventricular defect will decrease spontaneously in size. If the defect is large, the infant symptomatic, the pulmonary artery pressure high, and the aortic stenosis mild, then surgical ventricular defect closure alone is necessary. If the ventricular defect is small and the outflow obstruction valvar and significant, then balloon dilation is the treatment of choice. If the subaortic obstruction is moderate or more, then surgical resection is necessary, but better delayed until age 10 years or later because recurrent obstruction is common in those younger. During follow-up of these patients, other lesions, such as infundibular pulmonary stenosis (double-chambered right ventricle), may develop and require treatment. In all, continued endocarditis prophylaxis is essential.

Ventricular Septal Defect and Secundum Atrial Septal Defect

Ventricular and secundum atrial defects are readily recognized on two-dimensional echocardiography and occurred in some 4% of our entire ventricular defect population (see Exhibit 30-1). Although large atrial defects are easily recognized echocardiographically, some are due to a dilated patent foramen ovale because of the left atrial hypertension and atrial left-to-right shunting. This left-to-right shunt disappears after the excess left atrial flow and pressure are relieved by closure of the ventricular septal defect. In those with a true secundum atrial defect, the left atrial overload resulting from the ventricular septal defect is relieved by the atrial defect, and there is no atrial hypertension. From a practical standpoint, the distinction is not important because if the ventricular defect requires surgical closure through the transatrial route, the atrial septal opening is closed at the same time, at no additional risk. The incidence of extracardiac anomalies in these patients is higher than in those with isolated ventricular septal defects.[2]

Ventricular Septal Defect and Patent Ductus Arteriosus

Within the first days of life, all infants have a patent ductus arteriosus, which persists in many with ventricular defects.

Continued patency of the ductus contributes to the equilibration of pressure between the ventricles and may provide additional left-to-right shunting if the pulmonary resistance favors this. When either or both defects are large, the net flow depends on relative pulmonary versus systemic resistance. The differences in ductal versus ventricular shunting because of arterial-to-arterial shunting through the ductus and shunting from ventricle-to-ventricle through the ventricular septal defect, as well as the differences in shunting in systole and diastole, have an almost unfathomable complexity. When both defects are large and the amount of left-to-right shunting is determined by the pulmonary resistance, closing the ductus alone, even if it is large, may not affect the size of the shunt. From a practical standpoint, both defects are closed at surgery in the infant without any additional risk. If the ventricular defect is restrictive, it may be beneficial to close the ductus alone. The diagnosis, particularly in the infant or newborn, is made echocardiographically because the typical continuous murmur is often absent when both defects are large. Peripheral pulses are often bounding. In the older child (now very unusual), if the defects are restrictive and pulmonary artery pressure is less than systemic, then the typical pansystolic ventricular defect and continuous ductal murmurs are evident.

Treatment of significant lesions in very young patients consists of surgical closure of both defects when identified. Clearly restrictive defects in the normally growing infant may be followed medically with the hope for spontaneous closure; if the ductus persists, then it may be coil-occluded at catheterization.

Older patients with significant lesions and low pulmonary resistance should have the defects closed surgically, or by devices if the ventricular defect is in an appropriate location. If significantly elevated pulmonary resistance is suspected, then the patient is catheterized to evaluate pulmonary resistance response to (1) oxygen and nitric oxide and (2) temporary occlusion and device closure of the ductus if indicated.

Ventricular Defects with Pulmonary Stenosis

Ventricular defects associated with pulmonary stenosis occur most commonly in the framework of tetralogy of Fallot. Occasionally, patients with valvar pulmonary stenosis or obstructive muscle bundles in the right ventricle, together with a ventricular defect, do not fit the criteria for diagnosis of tetralogy of Fallot. All types of outflow obstruction may be progressive.[58,70,71] In our population, about 6% of patients with ventricular septal defect will have some degree of peripheral pulmonary stenosis (see Exhibit 30-1).

Those with the anatomy of tetralogy of Fallot most often go on to develop the classic tetralogy of Fallot syndrome (see Chapter 32).

Acyanotic Tetralogy of Fallot

The characteristic physical findings associated with a small ventricular septal defect (loud systolic murmur and thrill) so resemble those of acyanotic tetralogy of Fallot that confusion between the two diagnoses was a common error in pediatric cardiology before more routine echocardiography. Whether there are one or two components of the second heart sound is difficult to recognize, especially in the small infant in whom this differentiation most often is necessary. The heart size and pulmonary vascularity on x-ray may be the same in both conditions. The electrocardiogram may not show evidence of an abnormal degree of right ventricular hypertrophy, particularly in small infants. Any electrocardiographic evidence of an abnormal degree of right ventricular hypertrophy is cause for concern when the tentative diagnosis is isolated ventricular defect; if the electrocardiographic interpretation is correct, there is either pulmonary hypertension or pulmonary stenosis. Echocardiography has essentially eliminated this problem. In the acyanotic tetralogy of Fallot patient, the overriding aorta is seen, as are the large ventricular defect, the infundibular pulmonary stenosis, and any shunting; the systemic level right ventricular pressure is also evident. If the right ventricular pressure is really less than that of the left ventricle, the probability of the development of classic tetralogy of Fallot syndrome is unlikely. Still, occasionally a membranous ventricular septal defect with some outflow gradient and without an overriding aorta is encountered and may develop into tetralogy of Fallot. Therefore, some prognostic reservation is justified because some of these infants develop tetralogy of Fallot, whereas others lose the flow gradient as the ventricular defect becomes smaller.

Cardiac catheterization is seldom necessary and only when anatomic questions of significance persist.

Ventricular Defect and Valvar Pulmonary Stenosis

Valvar pulmonary stenosis occurred in only 2% of our ventricular septal defect population (see Exhibit 30-1) and seemed more common in the infant age group. Spontaneous closure of the ventricular defect, particularly when muscular and small, is not uncommon and may occur even when the valvar stenosis is severe. On physical examination, the point of maximal intensity of the murmur depends on the degree of right ventricular obstruction. With left-to-right shunting, the murmur of a ventricular septal defect may be audible at the fourth left intercostal space, whereas a similarly loud ejection murmur preceded by a variable click may be audible at the second left intercostal space because of the valvar stenosis.

Electrocardiograms show more right ventricular hypertrophy than is expected with simple ventricular septal defects. Chest x-rays may not be very helpful. Two-dimensional echocardiography identifies the anatomic features of the ventricular defect and pulmonary valve and provides reasonable estimates of the degree of valvar stenosis.

Whether treatment is indicated or not depends on the severity of the defects. It may be that neither defect is sufficient to require intervention (catheterization therapy or surgery).

Ventricular Septal Defect with Double-Chambered Right Ventricle

Muscle bundles, usually involving the moderator band from the lower infundibular septal region, traverse and obstruct the right ventricular outflow tract causing a double-chambered right ventricle. This lesion is common and usually progressive. The ventricular defect is usually membranous and may get smaller and even close spontaneously.

Double-chambered right ventricle produces a loud murmur, often louder than that of a small ventricular septal defect. When both lesions coexist, the auscultatory, electrocardiographic, and x-ray features are not sufficiently reliable for a certain diagnosis. The electrocardiographic findings sometimes show significant right ventricular hypertrophy, suggesting right ventricular hypertension;

occasionally, however, because some of the unipolar right ventricular leads are placed over the low-pressure outflow area, this may be absent. The diagnosis is recognized at echocardiography, and the severity is reasonably documented by Doppler techniques. Cardiac catheterization is usually unnecessary. Some of these patients develop membranous subaortic stenosis.[58,72]

Usually, surgical treatment is required because the obstruction is almost invariably progressive. In general, excision of the muscle bundles requires a right ventricular exposure, but occasionally resection is possible through the tricuspid valve.

Ventricular Septal Defect and Mitral Valve Disease

Some patients with ventricular septal defect also have mitral stenosis, regurgitation, or both (see Exhibit 30-1). In those with significant stenosis, increased left atrial pressure or volume may be substantial if the atrial septum is intact. In this case, two possible causes of pulmonary vascular abnormality (left-to-right shunting and elevated pulmonary venous pressure) may coexist. Fortunately, the two are not additive, and for any given level of resistance, the outcome (so far as the pulmonary vascular disease is concerned) is likely to be better than that for a patient with a comparable ventricular defect alone (see Fig. 30-4).

In those with mitral regurgitation, management depends on clinical status, degree of regurgitation, and size of the ventricular defect. Echocardiography provides sufficient hemodynamic and anatomic details such that catheterization is usually unnecessary. When both lesions are mild, medical management is indicated; occasionally, spontaneous ventricular defect closure may occur (see Fig. 30-18). If there is a large left-to-right shunt at the ventricular level and the regurgitation is not severe, then closure of the defect alone may improve the regurgitation. If the latter is severe, then a valvuloplasty is usually effective in the short term.

When there is more than minimal mitral stenosis associated with the ventricular defect, the patient's course usually will be determined by the severity of the mitral stenosis. If the mitral valve is minimally obstructed and there is moderate pulmonary hypertension or less, management is the same as that for the usual ventricular defect. If there is moderate mitral stenosis and the ventricular defect is of some size, there will be systemic levels of pressure in the pulmonary artery. The amount of left-to-right shunting will depend largely on the comparative levels of pulmonary and systemic resistance.

When there is severe mitral stenosis, the level of pulmonary resistance may become so high that ventricular shunting reverses and the patient becomes cyanotic.

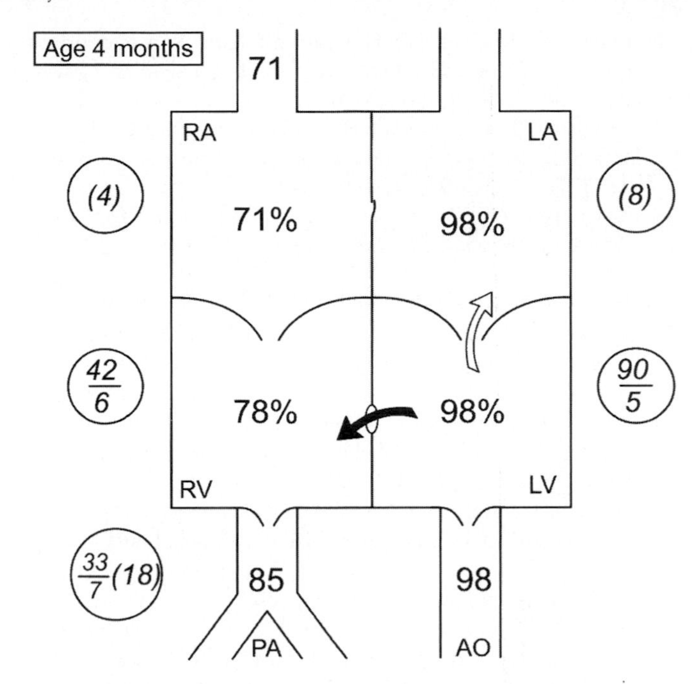

FIGURE 30–18 *Catheterization data in a 4-month-old infant with 2:1 left-to-right shunt, membranous ventricular septal defect (black arrow), and moderate mitral regurgitation through anterior leaflet cleft (open arrow). Four years later, the ventricular defect had spontaneously closed, and at age 10 years, the mitral cleft was successfully closed surgically.*

The ultimate success of management depends on the success in treating the mitral stenosis.

In the infant with severe mitral stenosis and a large ventricular defect, a very difficult problem, echocardiographic assessment preoperatively is usually adequate and is followed by surgical defect closure and valvuloplasty. If the ventricular defect is small, then balloon dilation offers an alternative to surgery in some forms of severe mitral stenosis.[73] If valve replacement is required in those with a small annulus, then a supra-annular prosthesis placement may be effective.[74] In the older patient with a large defect and significant mitral stenosis, catheterization is necessary for hemodynamic reasons. If there is uncertainty concerning resolution of very high pulmonary resistance with surgery, balloon dilation of a suitably anatomically malformed valve may relieve stenosis enough to allow resistance to decrease and left to right shunting to increase sufficiently to safely close the ventricular defect (see Fig. 30-4).

REFERENCES

1. Botto LD, Correa A, Erickson JD. Racial and temporal variations in the prevalence of heart defects. Pediatrics 107(3):1, 2001

2. Fyler DC, Buckley LP, Hellenbrand WE, et al. Report of the New England Regional Infant Cardiac Program. Pediatrics 65(Suppl):376, 1980.
3. Vaughan CJ, Basson CT. Molecular determinants of atrial and ventricular septal defects and patent ductus arteriosus. Am J Med Genet 97(4):304, 2000.
4. Newbury-Ecob RA, Leanage R, Raeburn JA, et al. Holt-Oram syndrome: A clinical genetic study. J Med Genet 33:300, 1996.
5. Basson CT, Bachinsky DR, Lin RC, et al. Mutations in human TBX5 cause limb and cardiac malformation in Holt-Oram syndrome [erratum Nat Genet 15:411, 1997]. Nat Genet 15:30, 1997.
6. Wilkins LE, Brown JA, Nance WE, et al. Clinical heterogeneity in 80 home-reared children with cri du chat syndrome. J Pediatr 102:528, 1983.
7. Ferencz C, Loffredo CA, Correa-Villansenor AC, et al. Genetic and environmental risk factors of major cardiovascular malformations: The Baltimore-Washington Infant Study: 1981–1989. Armonk, NY: Futura, 1997.
8. Driscoll DJ, Michels VV, Gersony WM, et al. Occurrence risk for congenital heart defects in relatives of patients with aortic stenosis, pulmonary stenosis, or ventricular septal defect. Circulation 87(Suppl 1):114, 1993.
9. Moe DG, Guntheroth WG. Spontaneous closure of uncomplicated ventricular septal defect. Am J Cardiol 60:674, 1987.
10. Ando M, Takao A. Racial Differences in the Morphology of Common Cardiac Anomalies. Japan: Bulletin of the Heart Institute, 1979:47.
11. Momma K, Toyama K, Takao A, et al. Natural history of subarterial infundibular ventricular septal defect. Am Heart J 108:1312, 1984.
12. Capelli H, Andrade JL, Somerville J. Classification of the site of ventricular septal defect by 2-dimensional echocardiography. Am J Cardiol 51:1474, 1983.
13. Edwards JE: Congenital malformations of the heart and great vessels. In Gould SE (ed). Pathology of the Heart. Springfield, IL: Charles C. Thomas, 1960.
14. Goor DA, Lillehei CW, Rees R, et al. Isolated ventricular septal defect: Developmental basis for various types and presentation of classification. Chest 58:468, 1970.
15. Hagler DJ. Standardized nomenclature of the ventricular septum and ventricular septal defects, with applications for two-dimensional echocardiography. Mayo Clin Proc 60:741, 1985.
16. Lincoln C, Jamieson S, Joseph M, et al. Transatrial repair of ventricular septal defects with reference to their anatomic classification. J Thorac Cardiovasc Surg 75:183, 1977.
17. Soto B, Becker AE, Moulaert AJ, et al. Classification of ventricular septal defects. Br Heart J 43:332, 1980.
18. Hoffman JIE, Rudolph AM, Heymann MA. Pulmonary vascular disease with congenital heart lesions: Pathologic features and causes. Circulation 64:873, 1981.
19. Vogel JHK, McNamara DG, Blount SG. Role of hypoxia in determining pulmonary vascular resistance in infants with ventricular septal defects. Am J Cardiol 20:346, 1967.
20. Heath D, Edwards JE. The pathology of hypertensive pulmonary vascular disease. Circulation 18:533, 1958.
21. Nadas AS, Ellison RC, Weidman WH. Pulmonary stenosis, aortic stenosis, ventricular septal defect: clinical course and indirect assessment. Circulation 56:(Suppl 1-1), 1977.
22. O'Fallon WM, Weidman WH, Driscoll DJ, et al. Long-term follow up of congenital aortic stenosis, pulmonary stenosis and ventricular septal defect. Circulation 1(Suppl 1): 38, 1993.
23. Rabinovitch M, Keane JF, Norwood WI, et al. Vascular structure in lung tissue obtained at biopsy correlated with pulmonary hemodynamic findings after repair of congenital heart defects. Circulation 69:655, 1984.
24. Levy RJ, Rosenthal A, Miettinen OS, et al. Determinants of growth in patients with ventricular septal defect. Circulation 57:793, 1978.
25. Nadas AS, Fyler DC. Pediatric Cardiology. Philadelphia: WB Saunders, 1981:348–521.
26. Yeager SB, Freed MD, Keane JF, et al. Primary surgical closure of ventricular septal defect in the first year of life: results in 128 infants. J Am Coll Cardiol 3:1269, 1984.
27. Ellis JH, Moodie DS, Sterba R, et al. Ventricular septal defect in the adult: Natural history and unnatural history. Am Heart J 114:115, 1987.
28. Leatham A. Auscultation of the heart. Lancet 2:703, 1958.
29. Partin C. The evolution of Eisenmenger's eponymic enshrinement. Am J Cardiol 92:1187, 2003.
30. Gersony WM, Nugent EW, Weidman WH, et al. Report from the Joint Study on the Natural History of Congenital Heart Disease. Circulation 1(Suppl 1):24, 1977.
31. Vincent RN, Lang P, Elixson EM, et al. Extravascular lung water in children after operative closure of either isolated atrial septal defect or ventricular septal defect. Am J Cardiol 56:536, 1985.
32. Williams RG, Bierman FZ, Sanders SP. Echocardiographic diagnosis of congenital anomalies. Boston: Little, Brown, 1986.
33. Bargeron LM Jr, Elliot LP, Soto B, et al. Axial cineangiography in congenital heart disease. Section 1: Technical and anatomic considerations: Section 2: Specific lesions. Circulation 56: 1075, 1977.
34. Hoffman JIE, Rudolph AM. The natural history of ventricular septal defects in infancy. Am J Cardiol 16:634, 1965.
35. Collins G, Calder L, Rose V, et al. Ventricular septal defect: Clinical and hemodynamic changes in the first five years of life. Am Heart J 84:695, 1972.
36. Eroglu AG, Oztunc F, Saltik L, et al. Evolution of ventricular septal defect with special reference to spontaneous closure rate, subaortic ridge and aortic valve prolapse. Pediatr Cardiol 24(1):31, 2003.
37. Gaynor JW, O'Brien JE, Jr, Rychik J, et al. Outcome following tricuspid valve detachment for ventricular septal defect closure [see comment]. Eur J Cardiothorac Surg 24(1):31, 2003.
38. Bol-Raap G, Weerheim J, Kappetein AP, et al. Follow up after surgical closure of congenital ventricular septal defect. Eur J Cardiothorac Surg 24(4):511, 2003.
39. Lister G, Hellenbrand WE, Kleinman CS, et al. Physiologic effects of increasing hemoglobin concentration in left-to-right shunting in infants with ventricular septal defects. N Engl J Med 306:502, 1982.

40. Bridges ND, Perry SB, Keane JF, et al. Preoperative transcatheter closure of congenital muscular ventricular septal defects. N Engl J Med 324:1312, 1991.
41. Rocchini A, Lock JE. Defect closure: Umbrella devices. In Lock JE, Keane JF, Perry SB (eds). Diagnostic and Interventional Catheterization in Congenital Heart Disease, 2nd ed. Norwell, MA: Kluwer, 2000:199–220.
42. Kalra GS, Verma PK, Dhall A, et al. Transcatheter device closure of ventricular septal defects: Immediate results and intermediate-term follow-up. Am Heart J 138(2 Pt 1):339, 1999.
43. Holzer R, Balzer D, Cao QL, et al. Amplatzer muscular ventricular septal defect. I. Device closure of muscular ventricular septal defects using the Amplatzer muscular ventricular septal defect occluder: Immediate and mid-term results of a U.S. registry. J Am Coll Cardiol 43(7):1257, 2004.
44. Thanopolous BD, Tsaousis GS, Karanasios E, et al. Transcatheter closure of perimembranous ventricular septal defects with the Amplatzer asymmetric ventricular septal defect occluder: Preliminary experience in children. Heart (British Cardiac Society) 89(8):918, 2003.
45. Bass JL, Kalra GS, Arora R, et al. Initial human experience with the Amplatzer perimembranous ventricular septal occluder device. Cath Cardiovasc Intervent 58(2):238, 2003.
46. Ho SY, McCarthy KP, Rigby ML. Morphology of perimembranous ventricular septal defects: Implications for transcatheter device closure. J Intervent Cardiol 17(2):99, 2004.
47. Fishberger SB, Bridges ND, Keane JF, et al. Intraoperative device closure of ventricular septal defects. Circulation 88: 205, 1993.
48. Okubo M, Benson LN, Nykanen D, et al. Outcomes of intraoperative device closure of muscular ventricular septal defects. Ann Thorac Surg 72(2):416, 2001.
49. Konstantinov IE, Coles JG. The role of intraoperative device closure in the management of muscular ventricular septal defects. Semin Thorac Cardiovasc Surg Ped Card Surg Ann 6:84, 2003.
50. Gabriel HM, Heger M, Innerhofer P, et al. Long-term outcome of patients with ventricular septal defect considered not to require surgical closure during childhood. J Am Coll Cardiol 39(6):1066, 2002.
51. Gersony WM, Hayes CJ, Driscoll DJ, et al. Bacterial endocarditis in patients with aortic stenosis, pulmonary stenosis or ventricular septal defect. Circulation 87(Suppl 1):1, 1993
52. Kidd L, Driscoll DJ, Gersony WM, et al. Second natural history study of congenital heart defects: Results of treatment of patients with ventricular septal defects. Circulation 87(Suppl 1):1, 1993.
53. Kumar K, Lock JE, Geva T. Apical muscular ventricular septal defects between the left ventricle and the right ventricular infundibulum. Circulation 95:1207, 1997.
54. Van Hare GF, Soffer LJ, Sivakoff MC, et al. Twenty-five-year experience with ventricular septal defect in infants and children. Am Heart J 114:606, 1987.
55. Levy AM, Tabakin BS, Hanson JS, et al. Hypertrophied adenoids causing pulmonary hypertension and severe congestive heart failure. N Engl J Med 277:506, 1967.
56. Perloff JK. Congenital heart disease and pregnancy. Clin Cardiol 17:578, 1994.
57. Keane JF, Plauth WH, Nadas AS. Ventricular septal defect with aortic regurgitation. Circulation 56(Suppl 1):1, 1977.
58. Rhodes L, Keane JF, Fellows KE, et al. Long follow up (to 43 years) of ventricular septal defect with audible aortic regurgitation. Am J Cardiol 66:340, 1990.
59. Vollerbergh FE, Becker AE. Minor congenital variations of cusp size in tricuspid aortic valves: possible link with isolated aortic stenosis. Br Heart J 39:1006, 1977.
60. Tomita H, Arakaki Y, Ono Y, et al. Imbalance of cusp width and aortic regurgitation associated with aortic cusp prolapse in ventricular septal defect. Jap Circ J 65(6):500, 2001.
61. Silver MA, Roberts WC. Detailed anatomy of the normally functioning aortic valve in hearts of normal and increased weight. Am J Cardiol 55:454, 1985.
62. Trusler GA, Williams WG, Smallhorn JF, et al. Late results after repair of aortic insufficiency associated with ventricular septal defect. J Thorac Cardiovasc Surg 103:276, 1992.
63. Tohyama K, Satomi G, Momma K. Aortic valve prolapse and aortic regurgitation associated with subpulmonic ventricular septal defect. Am J Cardiol 79:1285, 1997.
64. Lun K, Li H, Leung MP, et al. Analysis of indications for surgical closure of subarterial ventricular septal defect without associated aortic cusp prolapse and aortic regurgitation. Am J Cardiol 87(11):1266, 2001.
65. Layangool T, Kirawittaya T, Sangtawesin C. Aortic valve prolapse in subpulmonic ventricular septal defect. J Med Assoc Thai 86(Suppl 3):S549, 2003.
66. Tomita H, Arakaki Y, Yamada O, et al. Severity indices of right coronary cusp prolapse and aortic regurgitation complicating ventricular septal defect in the outlet septum: Which defect should be closed? Circ J 68(2):139, 2004.
67. Hisatomi K, Taira A, Moriyama Y. Is direct closure dangerous for treatment of doubly committed subarterial ventricular septal defect? Ann Thorac Surg 67(3):756, 1999.
68. Cheung YF, Chiu CS, Yung TC, et al. Impact of preoperative aortic cusp prolapse on long-term outcome after surgical closure of subarterial ventricular septal defect. Ann Thorac Surg 73(2):622, 2002.
69. Yacoub MH, Khan H, Stavri, G, et al. Anatomic correction of the syndrome of prolapsing right coronary aortic cusp, dilatation of the sinus of Valsalva, and ventricular septal defect. J Thorac Cardiovasc Surg 113:253, 1997.
70. Gasul BM, Dillon RF, Vrla V, et al. Ventricular septal defects, their natural transformation into those with infundibular stenosis or into the cyanotic or noncyanotic type of tetralogy of Fallot. JAMA 164:847, 1957.
71. Moran AM, Hornberger LK, Jonas RA, et al. Development of double-chambered right ventricle after repair of tetralogy of Fallot. J Am Coll Cardiol 31:1127, 1998.
72. Vogl M, Smallhorn JF, Freedom RM, et al. An echocardiographic study of the association of ventricular septal defect and right ventricular muscle bundles with a fixed subaortic abnormality. Am J Cardiol 61:857, 1988.
73. Moore P, Adatia I, Spevak PJ, et al. Severe congenital mitral stenosis in infants. Circulation 80:2099, 1994.
74. Adatia I, Moore P, Jonas RA, et al. Clinical course and hemodynamic observations after supra annular mitral valve replacement in infants and children. J Am Coll Cardiol 29:1089, 1997.

31

Pulmonary Stenosis

JOHN F. KEANE AND DONALD C. FYLER

DEFINITION

Obstruction to the outflow from the right ventricle, whether within the body of the right ventricle, at the pulmonary valve, or in the pulmonary arteries, is described as pulmonary stenosis. Often these obstructions occur with other major cardiac abnormalities. For the purposes of this discussion, those associated with another cardiac abnormality (except for patent ductus arteriosus, atrial septal defect, and patent foramen ovale) will be excluded; only those with an intact ventricular septum will be considered.

PREVALENCE

Pulmonary stenosis is a common congenital lesion. There were 3370 patients (6%) seen at Children's Hospital Boston between 1988 and 2002 with pulmonary stenosis or regurgitation (Exhibit 31-1), the fifth most common abnormality encountered in that period. The incidence of valvar stenosis has been reported at 0.6 to 0.8 per 1000 live births,[1,2] and when associated with other congenital cardiac lesions, it may occur in as many as 50% of all patients with congenital heart disease. In the Natural History Study, 47% of the 565 patients with valvar stenosis were female.[3]

ANATOMY

Pulmonary valvar stenosis, the most common type of obstruction, is characterized by fused or absent commissures. In most patients, the valve is a mobile, dome-shaped structure with an orifice that may be tiny and sometimes eccentric (Fig. 31-1). The jet of blood through the valve usually causes poststenotic dilation, most often involving the main and left main pulmonary arteries, because that is the direction of the jet (Fig. 31-2). When there is severe valvar stenosis, there is right ventricular hypertrophy, including infundibular muscle, which may contribute to the obstruction.

Dysplastic valves consisting of thickened, irregular, immobile tissue, often with hypoplasia of the valve annulus, and a small, short main pulmonary artery are much less common.[4]

Subvalvar obstruction, also uncommon, is usually muscular and in most cases appears to be caused by displacement of the moderator band. The latter is often associated with a membranous ventricular septal defect, spontaneous closure of which results in isolated outflow obstruction. In very rare instances, the obstruction is ringlike and near the pulmonary valve, resembling subaortic stenosis. In some patients, the subpulmonary obstruction is progressive.[5,6]

Peripheral pulmonary stenosis may take several forms. These include single discrete obstructive lesions at a central pulmonary origin, multiple bilateral stenoses at distal branch origins with poststenotic dilation, and unilateral or bilateral diffuse hypoplasia of long segments of a pulmonary artery (Fig. 31-3). Various combinations of these lesions are encountered in patients with the maternal rubella syndrome,[7] Alagille syndrome,[8] Williams syndrome (often with aortic supravalvar obstruction in addition),[9] and sometimes Noonan's syndrome.[10]

PHYSIOLOGY

To provide adequate cardiac output, the right ventricular pressure must be elevated sufficiently to overcome the

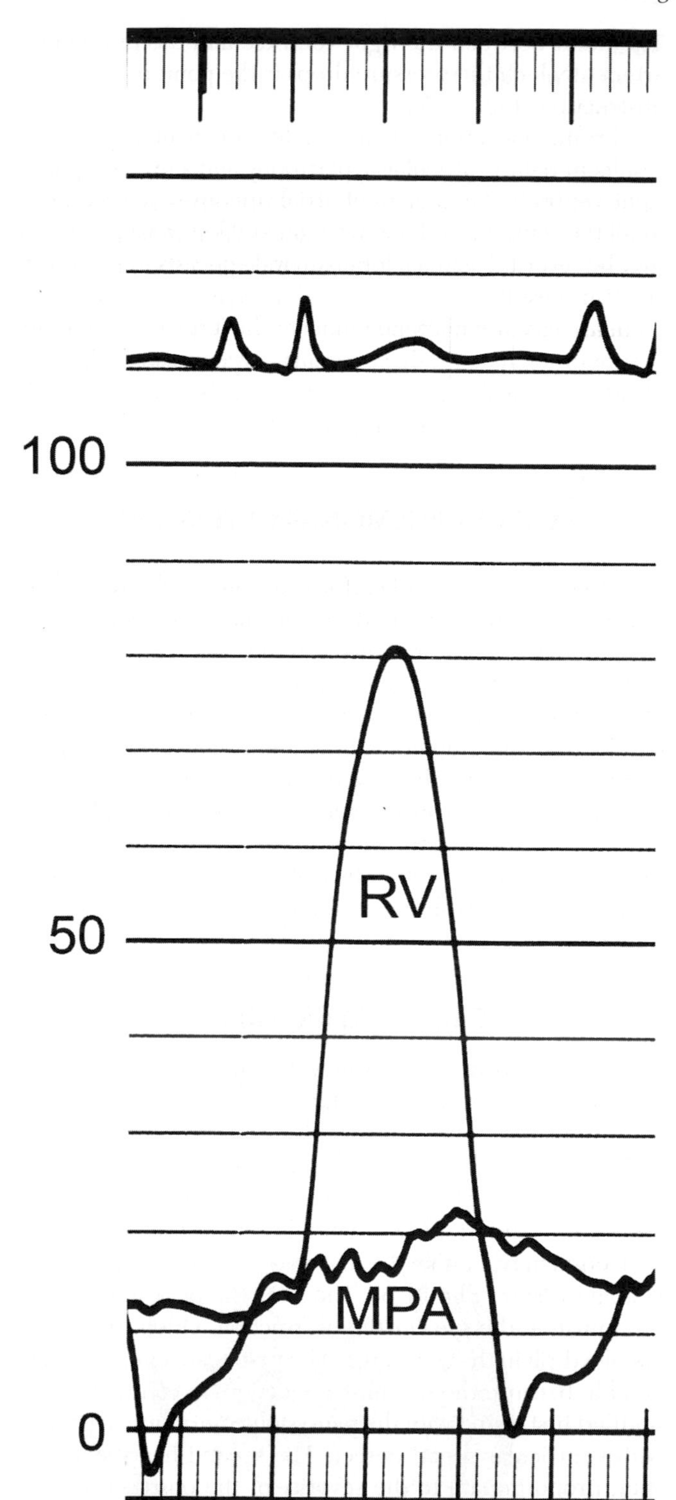

FIGURE 31–5 *Simultaneous right ventricular (RV) and main pulmonary artery (MPA) pressures in a 12-year-old patient with valvar pulmonary stenosis with a peak–peak gradient of 60 mm Hg.*

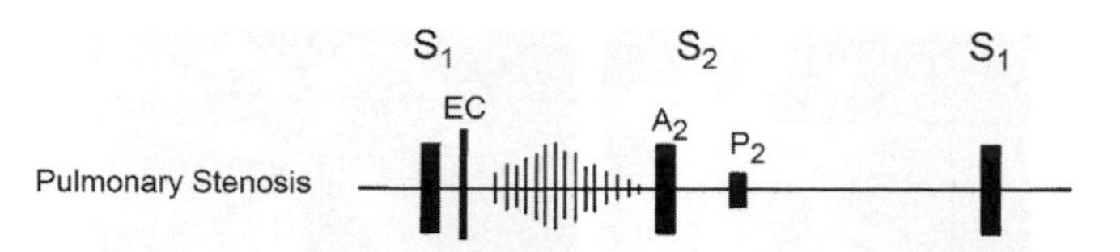

FIGURE 31–6 *Diagrammatic presentation of the murmur in a patient with valvar pulmonary stenosis. S_1, first sound; EC, ejection click; S_2, second sound; A_2, aortic component of the second heart sound.*

From Avery ME, First LP [eds]. Pediatric Medicine. Baltimore: Williams & Wilkins, 1989.

a click, other diagnoses should be considered. The smaller the interval between the first sound and the click, the more severe the stenosis.[13,19] A-wave pulsations in the neck veins are not unusual, but clinical right-sided congestive heart failure is rare. When there are prominent A waves, a fourth heart sound may be audible. A small infant with maximal obstruction may have a minimal murmur, sometimes overlooked, and cyanosis.

Electrocardiography

The electrocardiogram shows right-axis deviation and right ventricular hypertrophy in proportion to the amount of obstruction (Fig. 31-7). The R wave in the right chest leads is commensurate with right ventricular pressure and a superior (negative) T wave in arteriovenous fistula indicates very severe obstruction.[14] There may be P pulmonale.

Chest X-Ray

Except in cases of maximal obstruction in early infancy, the heart size is normal or only slightly enlarged. Poststenotic dilation of the main and left main pulmonary artery is usually visible. In the cyanotic patient, the pulmonary vasculature is decreased. Occasionally, in a patient with maximal obstruction, the right ventricle may be grossly dilated (seen as cardiomegaly on the conventional chest x-ray).

Echocardiography

Measurement of the pressure gradient across the outflow tract by Doppler echocardiography (maximum instantaneous velocity) is quite reliable,[20] being about 10% greater than the peak-to-peak gradient measured at cardiac catheterization.

The size of the pulmonary annulus is readily identifiable, as are the size of structures immediately before and after the obstruction. Poststenotic dilation is well seen, as are the proximal right and left pulmonary arteries.

The mobility, number, and consistency of leaflets are clearly visible, with the valve being noted to dome in

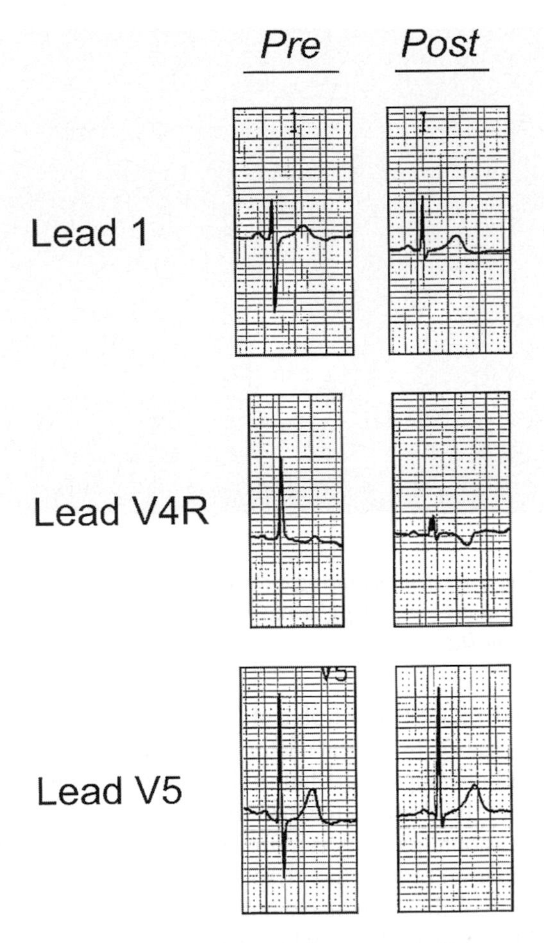

FIGURE 31–7 *Electrocardiogram in patient with severe valvar pulmonary stenosis showing prehypertrophy at age 5 years before dilation and after QRS axis shift, and regression of hypertrophy at age 6 years after gradient reduction of 76 mm to 6 mm by balloon dilation.*

systole (Fig. 31-8). Dysplastic valves are characterized by markedly thickened and immobile leaflets as well as annular hypoplasia. Multiple transducer locations, including parasternal, para-apical, and subxiphoid, should be used to minimize the likelihood of underestimating the gradient.

Cardiac Catheterization

Catheterization for many years has been used only as a therapeutic procedure since the introduction of balloon dilation for management of this lesion.[21] This procedure can be carried out at any age, but elective studies, for safety and technical reasons, are best deferred until age 1 year. At the study, the diameter of the outflow tract at the level of the hinge points of the pulmonary leaflets is measured at end diastole from the lateral projection of a ventricular angiogram. A balloon usually 120% of this value is introduced and inflated across the stenotic valve (see Chapter 14).

Management

When gradient relief is indicated, balloon dilation is the treatment of choice; surgical valvotomy is rarely used (Exhibit 31-2). Although in earlier years, a peak ejection gradient of at least 50 mm Hg across these mobile stenotic valves was used as the indication for dilation (as in valvar aortic stenosis); as experience grew and excellent results were achieved with minimal risk, it became quite reasonable to dilate valves with peak gradients of at least 30 mm Hg. Those with lower gradients require no restrictions or endocarditis prophylaxis.

In the past, among surgical patients with very severe obstruction, some were encountered with so called "suicidal ventricles" due to severe subvalvar obstruction, which was accentuated by acute relief of the valvar stenosis. A few of these patients died. In the dilated population, although residual muscular obstruction is evident to some degree in many, it resolves in time and has been without fatality.

Course

In medically managed patients, mild obstruction in most remains unchanged, whereas moderate or more obstruction does progress in some[17] (Fig. 31-9), more commonly in the young.[18] In those managed surgically, results were excellent, with some 97% being in New York Heart Association class 1 after more than 20 years of follow-up, with only 4% requiring a second procedure, and with endocarditis being a very rare complication.[17,18] In the more recent balloon dilation experience, with shorter follow-up, gradient relief has been excellent, and infundibular obstruction has regressed; residual obstruction due to dysplastic valves or suprapulmonary or subpulmonary stenosis has occurred in a few, and redilation has been necessary in a few others.[16,20–24] Some residual valvar obstruction was probably related to use of an undersized dilating balloon.[25] Pulmonary regurgitation is common after either treatment modality, is usually mild, and has been well tolerated to date.

Critical Pulmonary Stenosis in the Neonate

Maximal pulmonary stenosis in the neonate is a life-threatening problem. Most of these children are blue due to right-to-left atrial shunting, have systemic level or greater right ventricular pressure, are "duct dependent," and require prostaglandin E_1 and intubation. The tricuspid valve and right ventricular size are normal in most, with some degree of hypoplasia in the others. Tricuspid regurgitation is common. The pulmonary valve orifice is severely obstructed and even atretic in a few; occasionally while functionally echocardiographically atretic, it is found at catheterization to

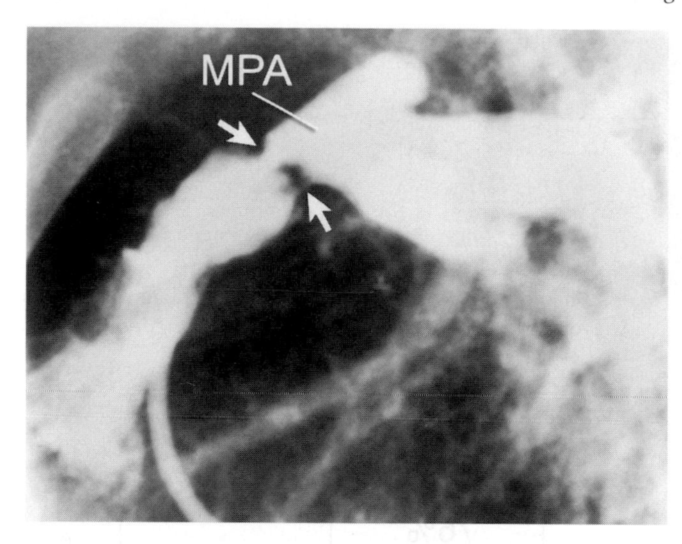

FIGURE 31–10 *Lateral view right ventricular cinegram showing dysplastic pulmonary valve (arrows) and short main pulmonary artery (MPA).*

of minimal intensity heard equally loud in all parts of the chest is virtually diagnostic of peripheral pulmonary stenosis, and if the electrocardiogram is normal, the severity can be said to be mild. Fortunately, these obstructions often regress[48] and thus, for clinical purposes, are largely a curiosity. Most patients with pulmonary stenosis require little or no intervention. These lesions are often seen in patients with Williams and Noonan's syndromes. Currently, the initial treatment in most (see Chapter 14) consists of dilation with conventional high pressure or cutting balloons with or without stent placement[49–54] (see Exhibit 31-2). Surgical management is undertaken in those with central lesions not amenable to catheter-based techniques.

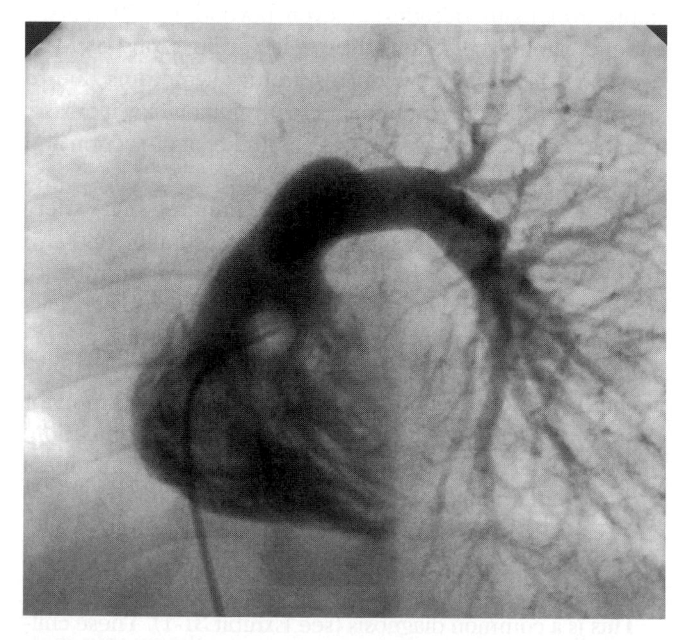

FIGURE 31–11 *Right ventricular angiogram in a 7-month-old infant showing congenital absence of the right pulmonary artery.*

Asymmetric peripheral pulmonary stenosis is occasionally encountered and, rarely, even unilateral congenital absence of a pulmonary artery without any other cardiac abnormality may be identified (Fig. 31-11). When there is unilateral peripheral pulmonary stenosis, it is important to remember that the bulk of pulmonary blood flow goes through the unobstructed lung, often at normal pressure. In this case, the estimation of relative pulmonary blood flow to each lung can be made with radionuclide scans. On occasion, angiography reveals that a mild obstruction to one lung is associated with a predominant blood flow to the opposite lung, and the decision to use surgical or balloon angioplasty is self-evident. A radionuclide scan can be used to assess improvement after angioplasty.

REFERENCES

1. Botto LD, Correa A, Erickson JD. Racial and temporal variations in the prevalence of heart defect. Pediatrics 107(3):1, 2001.
2. Hoffman IE, Kaplan S. The incidence of congenital heart disease. J Am Coll Cardiol 39:1890, 2002.
3. Nugent EW, Freedom RM, Nora JJ, et al. Clinical course in pulmonary stenosis. Report from the Joint Study of the Natural History of Congenital Heart Defects. Circulation (Suppl):1, 1977.
4. Becu L, Somerville J, Gallo A. "Isolated" pulmonary valve stenosis as part of more widespread cardiovascular disease. Br Heart J 38:472, 1976.
5. Pongiglione G, Freedom RM, Cook D, et al. Mechanism of acquired right ventricular outflow tract obstruction in patients with ventricular septal defect: An angiocardiographic study. Am J Cardiol 50:776, 1982.
6. Rowland TW, Rosenthal A, Castaneda AR. Double chamber right ventricle: Experience with 17 cases. Am Heart J 89:455, 1975.
7. Rowe RD. Cardiovascular disease in the rubella syndrome. In Keith JD, Rowe RD, Vlad P (eds). Heart Disease in Infancy and Childhood, 3rd ed. New York: Macmillan, 1979:3–13.
8. Alagille D, Odievre M, Gautier M, et al. Hepatic ductular hypoplasia associated with characteristic facies, vertebral malformations, retarded physical, mental, and skeletal development and cardiac murmur. J Pediatr 86:63, 1975.
9. Williams JCP, Barrett-Boyes BG, Lowe JB. Supravalvar aortic stenosis. Circulation 24:1311, 1961.
10. Noonan JA, Ehmke DA. Associated non-cardiac malformations in children with congenital heart disease. J Pediatr 63: 468, 1963.
11. Steinberger J, Moller JH. Exercise testing in children with pulmonary valvar stenosis. Pediatr Cardiol 20(1):28, 1999.

12. Sholler GF, Colan SD, Sanders SP. Effect of isolated right ventricular outflow obstruction on left ventricular function in infants. Am J Cardiol 62:778, 1988.
13. Gamboa R, Hugenholtz PG, Nadas AS. Accuracy of the phonocardiogram in assessing severity of aortic and pulmonic stenosis. Circulation 30:35, 1964.
14. Ellison RC, Freedom RM, Keane JF, et al. Indirect assessment of severity in pulmonary stenosis. Circulation 56(Suppl 1):1, 1977.
15. Gersony WM, Hayes CJ, Driscoll DJ, et al. Bacterial endocarditis in patients with aortic stenosis, pulmonary stenosis, or ventricular septal defect. Circulation 87(Suppl 1):1, 1993.
16. Jarrar M, Betbout F, Farhat MB, et al. Long-term invasive and noninvasive results of percutaneous balloon pulmonary valvoplasty in children, adolescents, and adults. Am Heart J 138:950, 1999.
17. Hayes CJ, Gersony WM, Driscoll DJ, et al. Second natural history study of congenital heart defects. Results of treatment of patients with pulmonary valvar stenosis. Circulation 87(Suppl 1):1, 1993.
18. Rowland DG, Hammill WW, Allen HD, et al. Natural course of isolated pulmonary valve stenosis in infants and children utilizing Doppler echocardiography. Am J Cardiol 79(3):344, 1997.
19. Driscoll DJ, Wolfe RR, Gersony WM, et al. Cardiorespiratory response to exercise of patients with aortic stenosis, pulmonary stenosis and ventricular septal defect. Circulation 87(Suppl 1):1, 1993.
19. Nadas AS, Fyler DC. Pediatric Cardiology. Philadelphia: WB Saunders, 1972:293–294.
20. Lima CO, Sahn DJ, Valdez-Cruz LM, et al. Noninvasive prediction of transvalvar pressure gradient in patients with pulmonary stenosis by quantitative two-dimensional echocardiographic Doppler studies. Circulation 67:866, 1983.
20. Ray DG, Subramanyan R, Titus T, et al. Balloon pulmonary valvoplasty: Factors determining short- and long-term results. Int J Cardiol 40(1):17, 1993.
21. Kan JS, White RF, Mitchell SE, et al. Percutaneous balloon valvulopasty: A new method for treating congenital pulmonary valve stenosis. N Engl J Med 307:540, 1982.
21. Chen CR, Cheng TO, Huang T, et al. Percutaneous balloon valvuloplasty for pulmonic stenosis in adolescents and adults. N Engl J Med 335(1):21, 1996.
22. Fawzy ME, Awad M, Galal O, et al. Long-term results of pulmonary balloon valvulotomy in adult patients. J Heart Valve Disease 10(6):812, 2001.
23. Rao PS, Galal O, Patnana M, et al. Results of three to 10 years follow up of balloon dilation of the pulmonary valve. Heart 80(6):591, 1998.
24. Radke W, Keane JF, Fellows KE, et al. Percutaneous balloon valvotomy of congenital pulmonary stenosis. J Am Coll Cardiol 8:909, 1986.
25. McCrindle BW. Independent predictors of long-term results after balloon pulmonary valvuloplasty: Valvuloplasty and Angioplasty of Congenital Anomalies (VACA) Registry investigators. Circulation 89(4):1751, 1997.
26. Hanley FL, Sade RM, Freedom RM, et al. Outcomes in critically ill neonates with pulmonary stenosis and intact ventricular septum: A multiinstitutional study. Congenital Heart Surgeons Society. J Am Coll Cardiol 22(1):183, 1993.
27. Colli AM, Perry SB, Lock JE, et al. Balloon dilation of critical valvar pulmonary stenosis in the first month of life. Cath Cardiovasc Diagn 34(1):23, 1995.
28. Gournay V, Piechaud JF, Delogu A, et al. Balloon valvotomy for critical stenosis or atresia of pulmonary valve in newborns. J Am Coll Cardiol 26(7):1725, 1995.
29. Tabatabaei H, Boutin C, Nykanen DG, et al. Morphologic and hemodynamic consequences after percutaneous balloon valvotomy for neonatal pulmonary stenosis: Medium-term follow-up. J Am Coll Cardiol 27(2):473, 1996.
30. Weber HS. Initial and late results after catheter intervention for neonatal critical pulmonary valve stenosis and atresia with intact ventricular septum: A technique in continual evolution. Cath Cardiovasc Intervent 56(3):394, 2002.
31. Kovalchin JP, Forbes TJ, Nihill MR, et al. Echocardiographic determinants of clinical course in infants with critical and severe pulmonary valve stenosis. J Am Coll Cardiol 29(5):1095, 1997.
32. Gildein HP, Kleinhert S, Goh TH, et al. Pulmonary valve annulus grows after balloon dilation of neonatal critical pulmonary valve stenosis. Am Heart J 136(2):276, 1998.
33. Poon LK, Menahem S. Pulmonary regurgitation after percutaneous balloon valvoplasty for isolated pulmonary valvar stenosis in childhood. Cardiol Young 13(5):444, 2003.
34. Berman W Jr, Fripp RR, Raisher BD, et al. Significant pulmonary valve incompetence following oversize balloon pulmonary valvoplasty in small infants: A long-term follow-up study. Cath Cardiovasc Intervent 48(1):61, 1999.
35. Burch M, Sharland M, Shinebourne E, et al. Cardiologic abnormalities in Noonan syndrome: Phenotypic diagnosis and echocardiographic assessment of 118 patients. J Am Coll Cardiol 22(4):1189, 1993.
36. Stamm C, Anderson RH, Ho SY. Clinical anatomy of the normal pulmonary root compared with that in isolated pulmonary valvar stenosis. J Am Coll Cardiol 31(6):1420, 1998.
37. DiSessa TG, Alpert BS, Chase NA, et al. Balloon valvuloplasty in children with dysplastic pulmonary valves. Am J Cardiol 60:405, 1987.
38. Ishizawa A, Oho S, Dodo H, et al. Cardiovascular abnormalities in Noonan syndrome: The clinical findings and treatments. Acta Paediatr Jap 38(1):84, 1996.
39. Stanger P, Cassidy SC, Girod DA, et al. Balloon pulmonary valvuloplasty: Results of the valvuloplasty and angioplasty of congenital anomalies registry. Am J Cardiol 65(11):775, 1990.
40. Ballerini L, Mullins CE, Cifarelli A, et al. Percutaneous balloon valvuloplasty of pulmonary valve stenosis, dysplasia, and residual stenosis after surgical valvotomy for pulmonary atresia with intact ventricular septum: long-term results. Cath Cardiol Diag 19(3):165, 1990.
41. Rose C, Wessel A. Three-decade follow-up in pulmonary artery ectasia: Risk assessment strategy. Ann Thor Surg 73(3):973, 2002.
42. Ring NJ, Marshall AJ. Idiopathic dilation of the pulmonary artery. Br J Radiol 75(894):532, 2002.
43. Shindo T, Kuroda T, Watanabe S, et al. Aneurysmal dilation of the pulmonary trunk with mild pulmonic stenosis. Intern Med 34(3):199, 1995.

44. Veldtman GR, Dearani JA, Warnes CA. Low pressure giant pulmonary artery aneurysms in the adult: Natural history and management strategies. Heart 89(9):1067, 2003.
45. Andrews R, Colloby P, Hubner PJ. Pulmonary artery dissection in a patient with idiopathic dilation of the pulmonary artery: A rare cause of sudden cardiac death. Br Heart J 69(3):268, 1993.
46. Macchi C, Orlandini SZ, Orlandini GE. An anatomical study of the healthy human heart by echocardiography with special reference to physiological valvular regurgitation. Anat Anz 175(1):200, 1994.
47. Van Dijk AP, Van Oort AM, Daniels O. Right-sided valvular regurgitation in normal children determined by combined colour-coded and continuous-wave Doppler echocardiography. Acta Paediatr 83(2):200, 1994.
48. Nomura Y, Nakamura M, Kono Y, et al. Risk factors for persistence of pulmonary arterial branch stenosis in neonates and young infants. Pediatr Int 43(1):36, 2001.
49. Gentles TL, Lock JE, Perry SB. High pressure balloon angioplasty for branch pulmonary artery stenosis: Early experience. J Am Coll Cardiol 22(3):867, 1993.
50. Fogelman R, Nykanen D, Smallhorn JF, et al. Endovascular stents in the pulmonary circulation: Clinical impact on management and medium-term follow-up. Circulation 92(4):881, 1995.
51. Kreutzer J, Landzberg MJ, Preminger TJ, et al. Isolated peripheral pulmonary artery stenosis in the adult. Circulation 93(7):1417, 1996.
52. Ing FF, Grifka RG, Nihill MR, et al. Repeat dilation of intravascular stents in congenital heart defects. Circulation 92(4):893, 1995.
53. Rosales AM, Lock JE, Perry SB, et al. Interventional catheterization management of perioperative peripheral pulmonary stenosis: Balloon angioplasty or endovascular stenting. Cathet Cardiovasc Intervent 56(2):272, 2002.
54. Bergersen LJ, Perry SB, Lock JE. Effect of cutting balloon angioplasty on resistant pulmonary artery stenosis. Am J Cardiol 91(2):272, 2002.

32

Tetralogy of Fallot

ROGER E. BREITBART AND DONALD C. FYLER

DEFINITION

Tetralogy of Fallot is a cyanotic congenital heart malformation comprising infundibular pulmonary stenosis, a conoventricular septal defect, dextroposition of the aorta such that the aortic root overrides the crest of ventricular septum, and right ventricular hypertrophy. This complex of lesions was described in detail by Fallot in 1888,[1] although it had been recognized by others in earlier case reports.[2] In addition to these four defining features, there may be pulmonary valve atresia in a complex known as *tetralogy of Fallot with pulmonary atresia* or alternatively *pulmonary atresia with ventricular septal defect*, previously called truncus arteriosus type IV or pseudotruncus, representing about 20% of all tetralogy of Fallot patients. Rarer variants include *tetralogy of Fallot with absent* (or *dysplastic*) *pulmonary valve* and *tetralogy of Fallot with common atrioventricular canal*. Among a selected group of 1538 tetralogy of Fallot patients seen at Children's Hospital Boston during a 14-year period, 61% had simple tetralogy of Fallot with pulmonary stenosis, 33% had pulmonary atresia, 3% had absent pulmonary valve, and 3% had common atrioventricular canal (Exhibit 32-1).

PREVALENCE

Tetralogy of Fallot is the most common cyanotic cardiac defect, with an incidence of 3.26 per 10,000 live births, or about 1300 new cases per year in the United States.[3–5] Mutations in several human genes have thus far been identified in tetralogy of Fallot: *NKX2.5*, which accounts for 4% of tetralogy of Fallot[6]; *JAG1* in Alagille syndrome. in which the incidence of tetralogy of Fallot is high[7,8]; *TBX5* in Holt-Oram syndrome, in which a few patients have tetralogy of Fallot[9]; and *FOXC2* in hereditary lymphedema-distichiasis, in which rare patients also have tetralogy of Fallot.[10] Deletion of human *TBX1* appears to be the basis for the 15% of tetralogy of Fallot attributable to chromosome 22q11.2 microdeletion, although *TBX1* mutations in nondeleted tetralogy of Fallot patients remain to be identified.[11–13] The gene or genes causing tetralogy of Fallot in trisomy 21, 18, and 13, which together account for 10% of tetralogy of Fallot cases,[14] are as yet unidentified. Thus, in about 70% of tetralogy of Fallot patients, a putative genetic etiology remains to be determined.

PATHOLOGY

Tetralogy of Fallot is one of several cardiac malformations that have defective embryonic neural crest migration and resulting abnormal conotruncal development.[15] Van Praagh and coworkers observed that the severity of subpulmonary stenosis is directly correlated with the degree of aortic override and have proposed that the primary problem in tetralogy of Fallot is underdevelopment of the pulmonary infundibulum, with the other features being secondary.[16]

The surgical anatomy of tetralogy of Fallot has been well described.[17] The ventricular septal defect is typically large, unrestrictive, and subaortic, involving membranous septum (Fig. 32-1). Rarely, it is restrictive or may become so due to partial occlusion by overlying tricuspid valve tissue.[18,19] There is anterior malalignment with anterior deviation of the conal septum and infundibular hypoplasia that constitute the anatomic subpulmonary obstruction. The degree of subpulmonary stenosis is quite variable, ranging from very mild in some patients to critically severe in others; it often increases with age in unrepaired patients.

Exhibit 32–1
Children's Hospital Boston Experience
Tetralogy of Fallot (TOF)
1988-2002

Total* (N = 1538)	**(%) TOF/PS** (N = 937)	**(%) TOF/APV** (N = 50)	**(%) TOF/AVC** (N = 52)	**(%) TOF/PA** (N = 499)
MVSD	5	8	12	5
Abnormal coronary artery	11	8	8	11
PA stenosis/hypoplasia	77	78	79	81
LPA atresia	0.3	0	0	1
RPA atresia	0	2	0	2

*These 1538 (49% female) patients represent all patients seen from January 1988 to January 2002 with tetralogy of Fallot and includes those operated on elsewhere and referred for catheter-based interventional therapies. The incidence of each complicating lesion is similar in all four subgroups.
PS, pulmonary stenosis; APV, absent pulmonary valve; AVC, atrioventricular canal; PA, pulmonary atresia; MVSD, multiple ventricular septal defects; LPA, left pulmonary artery; RPA, right pulmonary artery.

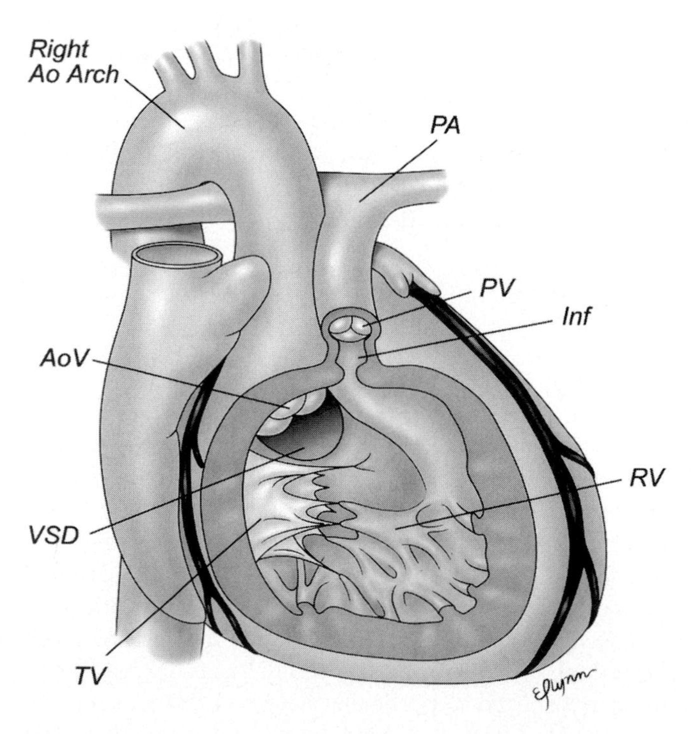

FIGURE 32–1 *Drawing of the cardiac anatomy of tetralogy of Fallot with pulmonary stenosis, viewed through the right ventricle (RV). Features include a conoventricular septal defect (VSD), through which the aortic valve (AoV) is seen; subpulmonary infundibular (Inf) narrowing; hypoplastic pulmonary valve (PV); hypoplastic pulmonary arteries (PA); and normal tricuspid valve (TV). A right aortic (Ao) arch, present in many cases, is also shown.*

Frequently, there are multiple levels of right-sided obstruction in tetralogy of Fallot, consistent with the hypothesis that obstruction to blood flow in the embryonic heart may impair the development of more distal cardiovascular structures.[16] Further, outflow obstruction may become increasingly severe, during both fetal and postnatal development.[20] The pulmonary valve itself is often abnormal, with a variably hypoplastic annulus and thickened, fused, and doming leaflets producing a valvar stenosis. Less commonly, the main and branch pulmonary arteries may be hypoplastic and may have discrete peripheral stenoses, for example, at the origin of the left pulmonary artery at the point of insertion of the ductus arteriosus. This contrasts with isolated valvar pulmonary stenosis and pulmonary atresia with intact ventricular septum, in both of which the pulmonary arteries are well developed (see Chapters 31 and 42). Enlarged bronchial arteries and abnormal aortopulmonary collateral arteries may be present but are most typical of tetralogy of Fallot with pulmonary atresia (see later discussion).

The overriding aortic root is typically enlarged in tetralogy of Fallot; in some cases, there may be aortic valve insufficiency. Further, just as the degree of infundibular hypoplasia varies, so does the extent of aortic override. At the extreme, the aorta is related entirely, or nearly so, to the right ventricle, akin to "tetralogy-like" double-outlet right ventricle with pulmonary stenosis (see Chapter 43). Indeed, the distinction between the two, being subaortic conus with mitral-aortic fibrous discontinuity in double-outlet right ventricle, is clinically unimportant because both malformations exhibit the same physiology and are similarly repaired.

Several other anatomic abnormalities of clinical relevance may be associated with tetralogy of Fallot. Many patients have a patent foramen ovale, but some have a true secundum atrial septal defect meriting closure at surgery. Some may have one or more additional ventricular septal defects involving the muscular septum that may also require surgical or, in selected cases, transcatheter closure if they remain significant. In a small proportion of tetralogy of Fallot cases, infundibular stenosis is complicated by more proximal intracavitary obstruction due to hypertrophied septal and parietal muscle bands akin to double-chamber right ventricle. These must be addressed at the surgical repair. About 25% of patients have a right aortic arch, coursing over the right rather than the left mainstem bronchus, most often with mirror-image branching, that is, left innominate artery first, right common carotid second, and right subclavian third. This anatomy bears on the surgical approach for placement of a systemic-to-pulmonary artery shunt should such palliation be necessary. As many as 5% of patients have an important coronary anomaly in which all or part of the left anterior descending territory is supplied by a large branch of the right coronary artery that crosses over the right ventricular outflow tract. This may complicate and even preclude the infundibulotomy that is part of the standard repair, warranting alternative approaches (see later discussion).

In addition to the previously mentioned features common to all forms of tetralogy of Fallot, there are certain features that are unique to the subgroups of tetralogy with pulmonary atresia, absent pulmonary valve, or common atrioventricular canal. These are considered separately in the following subsections, and similarly in each of the remaining sections of this chapter.

Tetralogy of Fallot with Pulmonary Atresia

A substantial group of patients with tetralogy of Fallot have atresia rather than stenosis of the pulmonary valve, with no physiologic antegrade pulmonary blood flow (Fig. 32-2). In most cases, this is congenital like the other anatomic features, although it may be acquired in rare circumstances.[21] Progression of pulmonary stenosis to atresia in utero has been documented.[20] The atresia may be limited to the pulmonary valve (membranous atresia), or it may additionally involve the subpulmonary infundibulum. Further, there is a spectrum of hypoplasia and atresia of the central pulmonary arteries, arising either directly from the same embryopathy that causes valvar atresia or as a consequence of the lack of blood flow. The main pulmonary artery may be present, supplied retrograde through the ductus arteriosus. In many instances, however, the main pulmonary artery is entirely absent, and the branch pulmonary arteries are diminutive with multiple stenoses. There may be discontinuities of the right and left pulmonary arteries and of individual lobar branches, also either congenital or acquired.

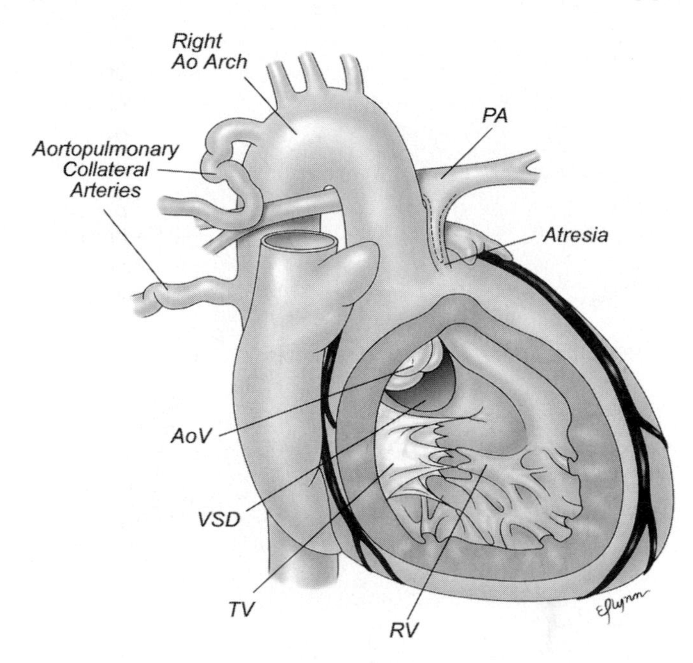

FIGURE 32–2 *Drawing of the cardiac anatomy of tetralogy of Fallot with pulmonary atresia (abbreviations as in Fig. 32-1). There is atresia of the pulmonary outflow tract, and the pulmonary arteries are markedly hypoplastic. The proximal segments of two aortopulmonary collateral arteries are also represented.*

Together with pulmonary artery hypoplasia, aortopulmonary collateral arteries are a hallmark of tetralogy of Fallot with pulmonary atresia.[22,23] These are grossly abnormal vessels that connect the systemic and pulmonary arterial circulations, arising directly from the aorta or its primary or secondary branches, both above and below the diaphragm. They often follow circuitous routes, sometimes crossing the midline, to reach central, lobar, and segmental pulmonary arteries distal to sites of stenosis or discontinuity. The collateral arteries are typically tortuous, variable in caliber, and often stenotic themselves. They clearly appear in association with deficient physiologic pulmonary perfusion and serve a compensatory role, increasing pulmonary blood flow and, hence, systemic arterial oxygenation; however, the vasculogenic mechanisms that underlie their development are as yet unknown.

Right aortic arch, dilation of the ascending aorta, and aortic valve insufficiency are more common in tetralogy of Fallot with pulmonary atresia than other forms of tetralogy.[24]

Tetralogy of Fallot with Absent Pulmonary Valve

In this rare but well described anatomic variant, the pulmonary valve leaflets, rather than being stenotic or atretic, are absent or, more accurately, vestigial (some prefer the term

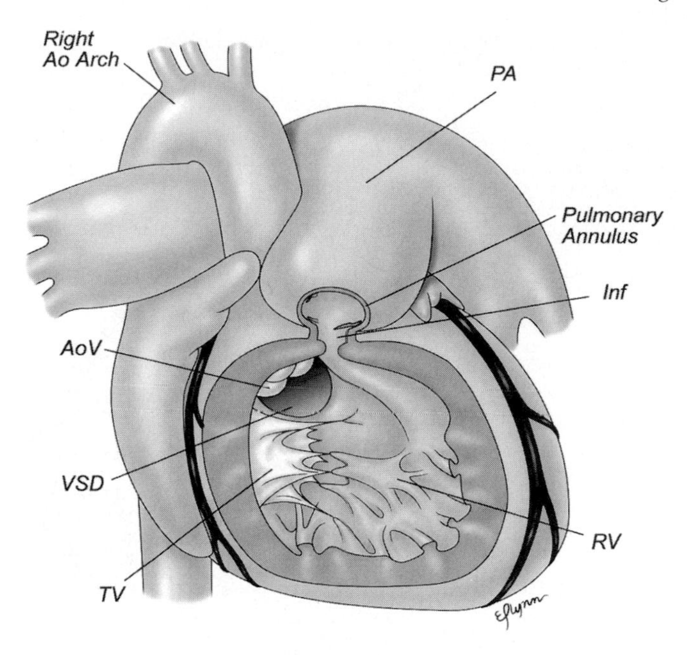

FIGURE 32–3 *Drawing of the cardiac anatomy of tetralogy of Fallot with absent pulmonary valve (abbreviations as in Fig. 32-1). The vestigial pulmonary valve leaflets leave the pulmonary outflow essentially unguarded. The pulmonary annulus is typically small, but there is marked dilation of the main and branch pulmonary arteries.*

dysplastic to *absent*; Fig. 32-3). As a result, the right ventricular outflow is effectively unguarded, with free pulmonary regurgitation and pronounced right ventricular dilation. Associated with this valve malformation is ectasia of the central pulmonary arteries that may be mild or severe; indeed, in many cases, there is massive aneurysmal dilation involving the main and right and left pulmonary arteries. The precise etiology of this vasculopathy is unknown, but it may arise from an inherent abnormality of the pulmonary artery wall, volume overload in utero, or both. The ductus arteriosus is characteristically absent in these patients, a feature that may also contribute to abnormal pulmonary artery flow and development.[25,26] The bronchi are also characteristically obstructed in this syndrome, attributed to external compression by the dilated central pulmonary arteries and abnormally branching segmental pulmonary arteries that appear to intertwine with the intraparenchymal bronchi.[27] There may also be developmental abnormalities intrinsic to the airways themselves. Of note, absent pulmonary valve syndrome also occurs in isolation (i.e., not associated with tetralogy of Fallot).[28]

Tetralogy of Fallot with Common Atrioventricular Canal

A few percentage of tetralogy of Fallot patients have a coexisting common atrioventricular canal. This is truly a combination of the two malformations and may be seen more frequently in trisomy 21 (see Chapter 38). The conoventricular septal defect extends far posterior into the inlet septum, and there is a primum atrial septal defect and a common atrioventricular valve. In addition to requiring more extensive surgical repair, these patients bear other risks associated with the potential for atrioventricular valve regurgitation that affect the timing of repair and the postoperative management (see later discussion).

PHYSIOLOGY

Patients with tetralogy of Fallot are cyanotic because of right-to-left shunting at the ventricular level. This occurs because there is anatomic right ventricular outflow tract obstruction such that the resistance to flow there exceeds the systemic vascular resistance, in the setting of a typically unrestrictive ventricular septal defect. Under these circumstances, oxygen-poor blood in the right ventricle shunts across the defect into the left ventricle and from there into the systemic arterial circulation. When there is a patent foramen ovale or a true atrial septal defect, right-to-left shunting may also occur at the atrial level if the diastolic pressure in the hypertrophic right ventricle and right atrium exceeds the left atrial pressure. In those rare cases in which the ventricular septal defect is restrictive, the right ventricular pressure is suprasystemic and represents a significant added clinical risk.

The volume of the ventricular right-to-left shunt, and hence the degree of cyanosis, is directly proportional to the severity of right ventricular outflow obstruction. When the subpulmonary infundibulum is severely hypoplastic or the pulmonary valve severely stenotic, there is little antegrade pulmonary blood flow, and most of the right ventricular output exits through the ventricular septal defect. Thus, systemic left ventricular output is maintained, albeit with an increasing fraction of oxygen-poor blood. In contrast, when right ventricular outflow obstruction is mild, there is little or no right-to-left shunt at all. Neonates with very mild obstruction may have normal systemic arterial oxygen saturation and are said to have "pink tetralogy." In some of these infants, there may even be left-to-right ventricular shunting with pulmonary overcirculation and heart failure not different from patients with isolated ventricular septal defects (see Chapters 10 and 30). Generally, there is a tendency in tetralogy of Fallot for subpulmonary obstruction, and hence cyanosis, to increase as children grow.

Superimposed on fixed anatomic right ventricular outflow obstruction, dynamic factors may serve to further compromise pulmonary blood flow, increase right-to-left shunting, and worsen cyanosis in tetralogy of Fallot. Dynamic muscular constriction or spasm of the subpulmonary infundibulum will have this effect, as will an increase in pulmonary vascular resistance, for example in a crying infant, or a decrease in systemic vascular resistance, for example during exercise. Catecholamine stimulation of right ventricular mechanoreceptors has also been postulated to increase right-to-left shunting.[29] One or more of these dynamic factors is thought to underlie the physiology of hypercyanotic spells (see later discussion). Conversely, maneuvers that increase systemic vascular impedance limit shunting. Older children with unrepaired tetralogy of Fallot often assume a characteristic squatting position, apparently with this benefit.

Tetralogy of Fallot with Pulmonary Atresia

In the presence of pulmonary atresia, all right ventricular output flows necessarily across the ventricular septal defect. There is no physiologic antegrade pulmonary blood flow. Instead, pulmonary flow derives solely from systemic-to-pulmonary artery communications—patent ductus arteriosus, bronchial arteries, aortopulmonary collaterals, or a combination of these—and comprises mixed arterial and venous blood. These are left-to-right shunts and, therefore, constitute a volume load on the left ventricle. In many instances, these vessels are restrictive, and thus pulmonary artery pressures remain low; however, collateral perfusion may produce excessive flow and pulmonary hypertension in isolated lung segments. Restoration of antegrade pulmonary blood flow by transcatheter or surgical intervention (see later discussion) contributes to improved postnatal growth of the hypoplastic pulmonary arteries.

Tetralogy of Fallot with Absent Pulmonary Valve

In the absence of functional pulmonary valve leaflets, there is free pulmonary regurgitation that represents a volume load both on the right ventricle and on the central pulmonary arteries. Indeed, the stroke volume of the right ventricle may be markedly increased to compensate for a large regurgitant fraction. Ejection of this large stroke volume into the proximal pulmonary arteries may contribute to their characteristically severe dilation. When the accompanying obstructive airway disease is significant, there is segmental air trapping and difficult ventilation that may be severe.

Tetralogy of Fallot with Common Atrioventricular Canal

The physiology in these patients is substantially the same as in tetralogy of Fallot alone, the atrial defect and the more extensive ventricular septal defect notwithstanding. However, there may be insufficiency of the common atrioventricular valve, either congenital or acquired, adding volume load to one or both ventricles. Regurgitation through the tricuspid component after repair can be a difficult problem in the early postoperative period. Right heart failure can ensue if this is superimposed on a right ventricle that is still hypertrophic and stiff, already volume-loaded due to pulmonary regurgitation, or pressure-loaded due to residual outflow tract obstruction.

CLINICAL MANIFESTATIONS

The infant with tetralogy of Fallot may initially come to attention because of a murmur, with or without cyanosis, or increasingly because of fetal echocardiographic diagnosis. The murmur is produced by turbulent flow across a narrowed right ventricular outflow tract, rather than across the unrestrictive ventricular septal defect, and so is present at birth. It is typically a harsh, long, crescendo–decrescendo systolic ejection murmur well heard along the left sternal border and transmitted into the lung fields (Fig. 32-4). The second heart sound is often single, comprising only the aortic component, and accentuated owing to the more anterior dextroposed aorta. There is usually a right ventricular parasternal lift. The degree of cyanosis is a function of the severity of right ventricular outflow obstruction and may be unapparent in the neonate. The remainder of the newborn cardiovascular examination is usually normal.

Before repair, infants with tetralogy of Fallot may be entirely asymptomatic. Alternatively, parents may report variable blueness at rest that is often more apparent with crying. There tends to be increasing cyanosis with growth. However, even with significant cyanosis, many infants may remain otherwise well, without respiratory distress, feeding intolerance, or lethargy. In contrast, in so-called "pink

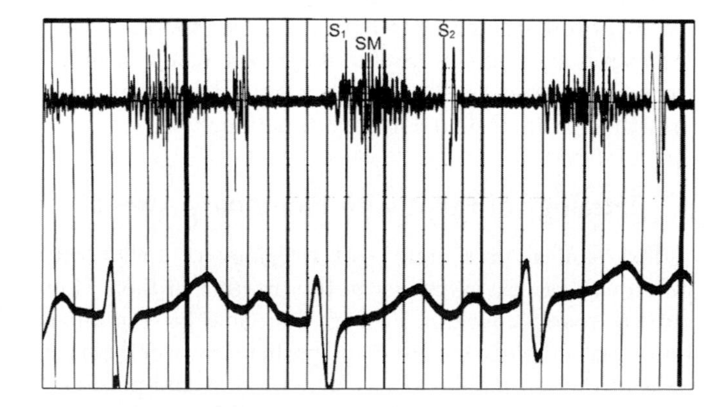

FIGURE 32–4 *Phonocardiogram of a patient with unrepaired tetralogy of Fallot with pulmonary stenosis, with the corresponding electrocardiographic tracing below. Note the long crescendo–decrescendo systolic murmur (SM) between the first (S1) and second (S2) heart sounds, due to turbulent flow across the right ventricular outflow tract. From Tyler DC (ed): Nadas' Pediatric Cardiology. Philadelphia: Harley and Belfus, 1992.*

tetralogy" with little or no outflow obstruction, a substantial ventricular left-to-right shunt, and resulting pulmonary overcirculation may manifest symptoms and signs of heart failure (see Chapters 7 and 30). Parents may report that the baby breathes quickly, feeds poorly, sweats, or is unduly tired, and the baby may not gain weight normally.

Hypercyanotic spells, known colloquially as "tet" spells, are a hallmark of tetralogy of Fallot. In a typical spell, the child becomes distressed and inconsolable, without apparent reason, most often in the morning. Crying is associated with progressively deeper cyanosis and hyperpnea (not tachypnea). Spells are self-aggravating; that is, if unabated, the deepening hypoxemia appears to exacerbate the distress, and more distress brings even more profound cyanosis (again, the physiologic underpinnings of hypercyanotic spells are debated; see previous discussion). Auscultation during the spell reveals a notably diminished or even absent murmur, owing to a significant reduction in flow across the right ventricular outflow tract. Holding the infant with the knees brought up tight to the chest, simulating squatting, has been noted empirically to bring relief in some instances. Not infrequently, the spell terminates with unconsciousness and, rarely, convulsions. If the hypoxemia is extreme, permanent neurologic sequelae and even death may ensue. True hypercyanotic spells are rare in neonates, although cyanosis may increase with crying.

Certain clinical features classically associated with tetralogy of Fallot appear only beyond infancy and, therefore, are rarely seen in contemporary practice in which repair in infants is now the rule. Older children with unrepaired tetralogy of Fallot experience discomfort and air hunger associated with cyanosis, particularly with excitement or exertion, and find that this is relieved when they assume a tight squatting position. Again, this is assumed to increase systemic vascular resistance and, therefore, diminish ventricular right-to-left shunting (see previous discussion). Chronic cyanosis is associated with clubbing of the nail beds of the fingers and toes and may also cause delayed physical growth and diminished cognitive function.[30]

Tetralogy of Fallot with Pulmonary Atresia

The clinical presentation of tetralogy of Fallot with pulmonary atresia is distinct to the extent that there is no outflow systolic murmur. Instead, there may be continuous murmurs audible in the chest and particularly over the back, indicative of aortopulmonary collateral flow and possibly a patent ductus arteriosus. The degree of cyanosis in these infants is a function of the extent of collateralization; that is, they may be very blue if there are few or no collaterals and the ductus arteriosus is closed, or they may be relatively pink, rarely to the point of congestive failure, if there are extensive collaterals with very substantial pulmonary blood flow. To the extent that the collateral murmurs and cyanosis may be relatively subtle, tetralogy of Fallot with pulmonary atresia may not be recognized in the neonate and may come to attention later than with pulmonary stenosis. Also, with pulmonary atresia, hypercyanotic spells are less common, but do occur. Presumably, the physiology in this setting involves shifts in the relative pulmonary and systemic vascular resistances, affecting collateral flow; infundibular spasm would have no effect. Tetralogy of Fallot patients with pulmonary atresia are more likely than those with pulmonary stenosis to have chromosomal abnormalities, particularly chromosome 22q11.2 microdeletion (DiGeorge syndrome) and associated clinical manifestations.[31]

Tetralogy of Fallot with Absent Pulmonary Valve

Additional clinical manifestations of tetralogy of Fallot with absent pulmonary valve are due to the presence of severe pulmonary regurgitation and airways disease. Roughly half of these patients present with severe, even critical, respiratory compromise in the neonatal period, with signs of lower airway obstruction on examination. Ventilation may be worse in the supine, as compared with prone, position because of greater bronchial compression by the aneurysmal pulmonary arteries.[32,33] In other patients, however, respiratory compromise may be quite mild or even absent. Further, the clinical severity appears not to correlate reliably with the degree of pulmonary artery enlargement, suggesting that intrinsic bronchial abnormalities may be a more important determinant. Characteristically, on cardiac auscultation, there is a prominent early to mid-diastolic decrescendo murmur of free pulmonary regurgitation, best heard along the left sternal border, in addition to the typical systolic outflow murmur (i.e., in a "to-and-fro" systolic–diastolic murmur).

Tetralogy of Fallot with Common Atrioventricular Canal

The clinical presentation and auscultatory findings in the setting of common atrioventricular canal are the same as those in simple tetralogy of Fallot, with the possible exception that there may be a pansystolic murmur if there is significant atrioventricular valve regurgitation. Down syndrome with associated features is more common.

ELECTROCARDIOGRAPHY

The electrocardiogram in tetralogy of Fallot characteristically shows evidence of right ventricular hypertrophy that increases with increasing age in the infant, attributable to chronic pressure overload. Right-axis deviation and right atrial enlargement are also present in many cases. If there is a large left-to-right shunt, as in pink tetralogy, or in the presence of a large patent ductus arteriosus or excessive aortopulmonary collateral flow, there may also be left atrial enlargement and biventricular hypertrophy.

Tetralogy of Fallot with Pulmonary Atresia

There are no additional distinctive electrocardiographic features associated with pulmonary atresia.

Tetralogy of Fallot with Absent Pulmonary Valve

There are no additional distinctive electrocardiographic features associated with absent pulmonary valve.

Tetralogy of Fallot with Common Atrioventricular Canal

With common atrioventricular canal, there is a superior QRS axis with counterclockwise loop in the frontal plane, typical of endocardial cushion defects (see Chapter 38).

CHEST RADIOGRAPHY

The chest radiograph of the infant with tetralogy of Fallot typically shows normal visceral situs, levocardia, normal heart size, decreased pulmonary vascularity, and possibly a right aortic arch. If there is a large left-to-right shunt as in pink tetralogy or in the presence of a large patent ductus arteriosus or excessive aortopulmonary collateral flow, the heart may instead be enlarged and pulmonary vascularity increased. The apex of the heart is often elevated owing to right ventricular hypertrophy. This feature, in combination with a relatively concave contour along the left upper heart border due to main pulmonary artery hypoplasia or atresia, gives the cardiac silhouette a so-called boot shape (*coeur en sabot*), although this may not be apparent in the infant with a prominent thymus. Absence of a thymus shadow in the newborn may indicate associated chromosome 22q11.2 microdeletion (DiGeorge syndrome).

Tetralogy of Fallot with Pulmonary Atresia

The pulmonary vascular markings may vary in regions with greater or lesser collateral blood flow. Otherwise, there are no additional distinctive chest radiographic features associated with pulmonary atresia.

Tetralogy of Fallot with Absent Pulmonary Valve

The heart size may be increased due to right ventricular dilation caused by the volume overload of free pulmonary regurgitation. Very large main and branch pulmonary arteries are evident. Signs of bronchial compression may be seen, including segmental or overall hyperinflation.

Tetralogy of Fallot with Common Atrioventricular Canal

There are no additional distinctive chest radiographic features associated with common atrioventricular canal.

ECHOCARDIOGRAPHY

Prenatal diagnosis of tetralogy of Fallot may be made readily by fetal echocardiography.[34] The large malalignment conoventricular septal defect, deviated conal septum, and overriding aorta are seen early in the second trimester on two-dimensional imaging. Later in gestation, the central pulmonary arteries may appear hypoplastic, often progressively so on serial examinations.[20] Doppler interrogation of the ductus arteriosus may show retrograde flow (i.e., from aorta to pulmonary artery) if right ventricular outflow tract obstruction is severe.[35]

Postnatally, echocardiography can identify all the characteristic anatomic features of tetralogy of Fallot in most cases (Fig. 32-5). These include the malaligned conoventricular septal defect, the anterior deviation of the conal septum, the level or levels of right ventricular outflow tract obstruction, and the dextroposed, overriding aorta. The combination of two-dimensional imaging, Doppler interrogation, and color-flow Doppler mapping is usually sufficient to provide all clinically important structural and functional information relevant to planning the surgical repair or, if indicated, palliation, including the following:

- The size and extent of the ventricular septal defect, including the rare restrictive defect
- The location and size of additional muscular ventricular septal defects, if any, that may also require surgical closure
- The levels of right ventricular outflow tract obstruction, including the severity of infundibular stenosis, the presence or absence of more proximal intracavitary muscle bands, and the degree of pulmonary valve abnormality, including annular hypoplasia that may dictate the need for a transannular outflow patch
- The pulmonary artery anatomy, including possible hypoplasia and stenoses of the main or proximal branch pulmonary arteries that may also need to be addressed at operation
- The size and competency of the aortic valve
- The coronary artery anatomy, particularly the presence of a left anterior descending coronary from the right or other important branch of the right coronary crossing the infundibulum that must not be divided and, therefore,

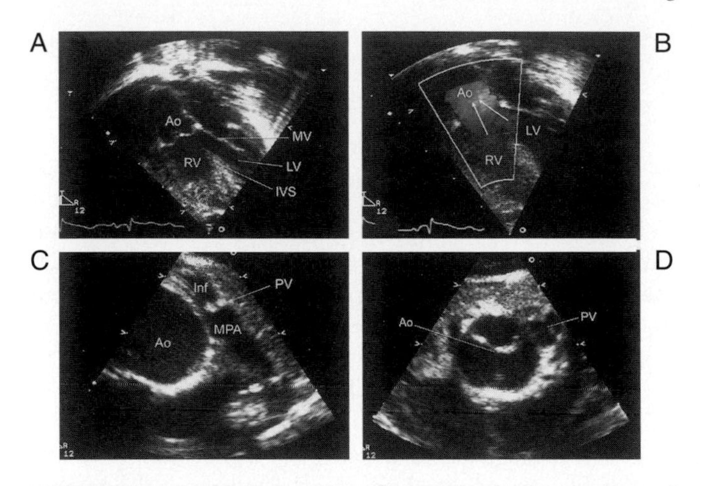

FIGURE 32–5 *Echocardiogram of an infant with tetralogy of Fallot.* ***A****, Modified apical four-chamber view showing the conoventricular septal defect and dextroposed aorta (Ao) overriding the crest of the muscular interventricular septum (IVS) and related substantially to the right ventricle (RV). Note the absence of subaortic conus, with retained fibrous continuity between the aortic valve and mitral valve (MV), distinguishing tetralogy of Fallot, with preserved left ventricle (LV)-to-aorta continuity, from double-outlet right ventricle.* ***B****, Color Doppler mapping corresponding to the image in panel* ***A****, demonstrating systolic flow (blue) from both the left and right ventricles into the aorta (arrows).* ***C****, Parasternal short-axis view demonstrating the hypoplastic subpulmonary infundibulum (Inf) and small, dysplastic pulmonary valve (PV), small main pulmonary artery (MPA), and large aorta.* ***D****, Parasternal short axis view demonstrating the hypoplastic pulmonary valve and large aortic valve.*

may constrain or preclude placement of an outflow patch
- The presence of certain other associated defects that may require surgical attention, such as an atrial septal defect or a patent ductus arteriosus
- The presence of certain other anatomic variants that may impact the surgical approach, such as a right aortic arch or a left superior vena cava to coronary sinus

When acoustical windows are poor, as in some older patients and, rarely, infants, some of these features may not be adequately resolved by echocardiography, and other diagnostic imaging may be necessary before surgery is undertaken.

Echocardiography is also a valuable tool for surveillance and diagnosis after surgical repair of tetralogy of Fallot. In the early postoperative period, it is useful for the identification of atrial right-to-left shunting, residual ventricular septal defects, residual right ventricular outflow tract obstruction, and ventricular systolic dysfunction. In long-term follow-up, it is helpful in the assessment of recurrent right ventricular outflow tract obstruction, pulmonary regurgitation, proximal branch pulmonary artery stenosis, aortic regurgitation, and again ventricular systolic dysfunction. The ongoing utility of echocardiography, however, is often limited by poor acoustical windows in older children and adults. Cardiac magnetic resonance imaging is typically more informative in these patients (discussed later).

Tetralogy of Fallot with Pulmonary Atresia

In addition to the features listed earlier, pulmonary atresia is recognized by two-dimensional imaging and by Doppler analysis demonstrating the absence of right ventricle to pulmonary artery flow. The length of the atretic segment is seen, ranging from very short membranous atresia of the valve alone to longer-segment atresia that also involves part or all of the main pulmonary artery. The branch pulmonary arteries may be visible if good sized; however, they are often severely hypoplastic and not detectable at echocardiography. Aortopulmonary collaterals may be detected by virtue of their characteristic continuous flow pattern on color-flow Doppler mapping. Imaging may show the origins of sizable collaterals, but smaller vessels are not typically resolved, nor are the distal connections to the pulmonary arteries. Thus, in tetralogy of Fallot with pulmonary atresia, echocardiography alone is generally not sufficient to demonstrate key aspects of pulmonary artery anatomy and blood supply, and catheterization is required.

Tetralogy of Fallot with Absent Pulmonary Valve

The key cardiovascular features of the absent pulmonary valve syndrome are readily apparent on the echocardiogram (Fig. 32-6). On two-dimensional imaging, the pulmonary

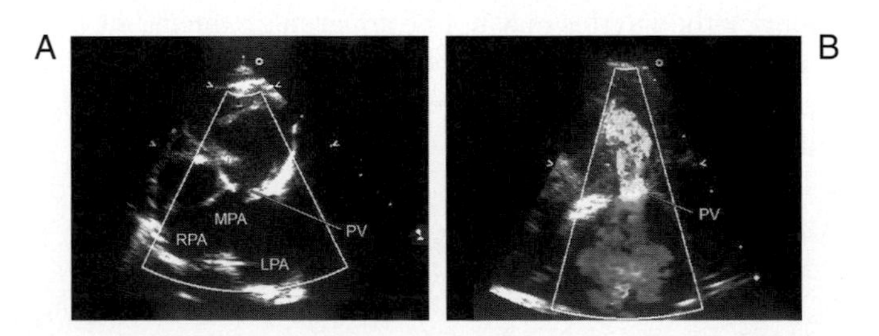

FIGURE 32–6 *Echocardiogram of an infant with tetralogy of Fallot with absent pulmonary valve.* ***A****, Parasternal short-axis view showing the vestigial pulmonary valve leaflets (PV) and markedly dilated main (MPA), right (RPA), and left (LPA) pulmonary arteries.* ***B****, Color Doppler mapping corresponding to the image in panel* ***A****, demonstrating turbulent diastolic flow (multicolor) through the regurgitant pulmonary valve into the right ventricular outflow tract, toward the apex of the scan sector.*

valve leaflets are vestigial, if visible at all, and the main and bilateral branch pulmonary arteries are severely dilated. Doppler analysis shows severe pulmonary regurgitation. The bronchi and their relationship to the pulmonary arteries cannot be demonstrated by echocardiography and other imaging modalities, such as computed tomography or magnetic resonance imaging, may be important in some cases before surgery.

Tetralogy of Fallot with Common Atrioventricular Canal

Imaging shows extension of the ventricular septal defect to involve the inlet septum, the contiguous primum atrial septal defect, and the common atrioventricular valve. Doppler analysis reveals atrioventricular valve regurgitation, if any. As with uncomplicated tetralogy of Fallot, the echocardiographic information is usually sufficient for surgical planning.

CARDIAC CATHETERIZATION

Catheterization was for decades a mandatory part of the diagnostic evaluation of tetralogy of Fallot before surgical repair, principally to document the pulmonary artery anatomy, coronary anatomy, and presence of any additional ventricular septal defects. In recent years, however, with the improvement in the quality of noninvasive evaluation by echocardiography, there has been a steady shift away from catheterization and its attendant risks for patients with tetralogy of Fallot, including those with absent pulmonary valve or common atrioventricular canal (catheterization is still essential for those with pulmonary atresia, discussed later). Most major centers now rely routinely on the echocardiogram to provide all necessary preoperative information, as detailed earlier, reserving diagnostic catheterization for the increasingly rare patient in whom key questions remain unanswered.

In those few cases in which catheterization is undertaken, conventional oximetry and hemodynamic measurements are obtained (see Chapter 14). Angiography is performed with a series of contrast injections in the right ventricle, pulmonary artery, left ventricle, and aortic root, as needed, in projections suited to profile key anatomic features including the right ventricular outflow tract, pulmonary arteries, potential additional ventricular septal defects, and coronary arteries. In addition to the risks inherent in any catheterization (see Chapter 14), unrepaired tetralogy of Fallot patients also incur the risk for hypercyanotic spells during the procedure. Potential precipitating factors include emotional stressors such as restraint and needle puncture, intravascular fluid shifts, and drugs that increase the ratio of pulmonary to systemic vascular resistance.

Aside from diagnostic indications, catheterization may be undertaken for interventional purposes in some cases of tetralogy of Fallot (see Management, later). Large aortopulmonary collateral arteries that may be relatively inaccessible at surgery can be occluded using embolization coils at catheterization before or after the repair. Significant peripheral pulmonary artery stenoses can be dilated using balloon catheters and, if the narrowing is elastic, stented.[36] Balloon dilation of a stenotic pulmonary valve may be useful as a palliative step to increase pulmonary blood flow in certain patients in whom reparative surgery must be delayed[37–41] and to gain access for preoperative pulmonary artery rehabilitation in rare patients with severe pulmonary stenosis and diminutive pulmonary arteries.[36]

Catheterization may also be indicated after surgical repair (see Management). In the early postoperative period, it may be needed to evaluate hemodynamically significant residual lesions, such as right ventricular outflow tract obstruction and residual ventricular septal defects, in patients who are unstable or otherwise unable to wean from support. Catheter interventions may also be indicated in selected postoperative patients for device closure of residual ventricular septal defects, balloon dilation of distal pulmonary artery stenoses, or coil embolization of residual aortopulmonary collaterals.

Tetralogy of Fallot with Pulmonary Atresia

Although catheterization is only rarely required in uncomplicated tetralogy of Fallot, it remains essential in contemporary practice to the complete evaluation and, increasingly, treatment of tetralogy of Fallot with pulmonary atresia (Fig. 32-7). Diagnostic angiography is needed to show the detailed anatomy of the pulmonary arteries, including their arborization within the lungs, and to delineate all sources of pulmonary blood flow—areas in which echocardiography is limited. Key features to be identified include the size and continuity or discontinuity of the central pulmonary arteries, stenosis or atresia involving lobar and segmental branches, and the origins and courses of all aortopulmonary collaterals and their connections to the true pulmonary arteries. Pulmonary vein wedge injections, in addition to contrast injections in the systemic arteries and collaterals, may be required to visualize all lung segments.

Interventional catheterization is a mainstay of therapy, along with surgery, for patients with tetralogy of Fallot with pulmonary atresia (see Management).[42] In selected patients with membranous pulmonary atresia, it may be possible at catheterization to perforate the valve using a guide wire or radiofrequency ablation catheter, followed by balloon dilation of the valve to establish antegrade pulmonary blood flow from the right ventricle.[43,44] Once right ventricle to pulmonary artery continuity has been created, either at catheterization or more commonly surgery, percutaneous

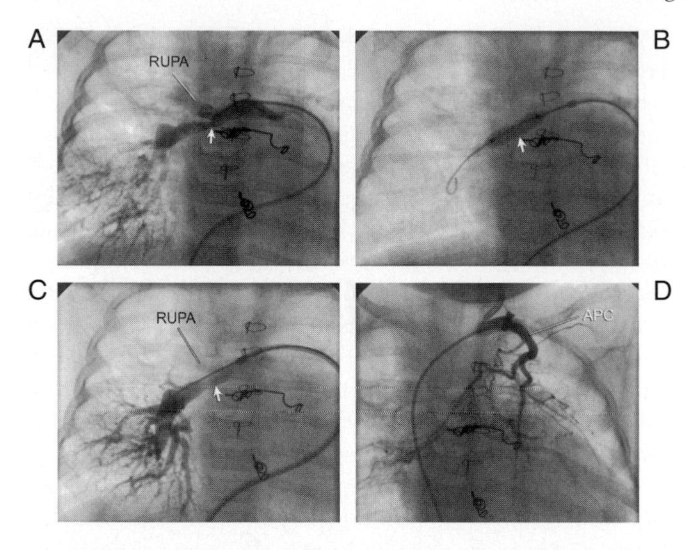

FIGURE 32–7 *Angiograms of a patient with tetralogy of Fallot with pulmonary atresia who had undergone surgery for placement of a right ventricle-to-pulmonary artery conduit, and prior catheterization for vascular coil embolization of aortopulmonary collaterals.* ***A***, *Right pulmonary arteriogram, via a venous catheter (inferior vena cava to right atrium to right ventricle to conduit to pulmonary artery), showing a discrete stenosis (arrow) just distal to the takeoff of the right upper pulmonary artery (RUPA) branch.* ***B***, *Balloon catheter showing a "waist" at the point of narrowing (arrow).* ***C***, *Repeat right pulmonary arteriogram showing increased caliber of the right pulmonary artery stenosis (arrow).* ***D***, *Angiogram demonstrating an aortopulmonary collateral artery (APC) arising from the left innominate artery in this patient with a right aortic arch (note course of retrograde arterial catheter); the collateral was then coil-occluded (not shown).*

balloon angioplasty and stenting are employed for rehabilitation of the hypoplastic and stenotic pulmonary arteries characteristic of this disease. Vascular coils are delivered to occlude aortopulmonary collaterals and palliative surgical systemic-to-pulmonary artery shunts, either when they are in excess or, alternatively, once more effective pulmonary blood flow has been established by catheterization or surgery.

Catheterization is important in the long-term management of repaired tetralogy of Fallot with pulmonary atresia, not only for ongoing pulmonary artery rehabilitation but also for the evaluation and treatment of right ventricle-to-pulmonary artery conduit obstruction. The level of obstruction is documented by appropriate pressure measurements and by angiography. Often, the narrow segment can be dilated and stented, relieving right ventricular hypertension and delaying the need for surgical conduit revision for months or years.

Tetralogy of Fallot with Absent Pulmonary Valve

Pulmonary angiography can provide a more complete picture of the extent and severity of pulmonary artery ectasia than that provided by echocardiography. Before the advent of cardiac magnetic resonance imaging, angiography was sometimes combined with bronchography in the catheterization laboratory to establish the anatomic relationships between the dilated pulmonary arteries and obstructed bronchi.[33] In contemporary practice, however, echocardiography is usually sufficient for surgical planning in tetralogy of Fallot with absent pulmonary valve and angiography is rarely required.

Tetralogy of Fallot with Common Atrioventricular Canal

There are no additional indications for catheterization in patients with tetralogy of Fallot with common atrioventricular canal.

OTHER STUDIES

Cardiac magnetic resonance imaging can provide exquisite anatomic and functional data but is not required in infants with typically excellent echocardiographic images. It is, however, an increasingly important tool for the evaluation of older children and especially adults with repaired tetralogy of Fallot.[45–47] In patients in whom echocardiography is limited by poor acoustical windows, excellent anatomic and functional data can still be obtained noninvasively by magnetic resonance imaging. Moreover, magnetic resonance imaging provides better quantification of ventricular mass, volume, ejection fraction, and regurgitant fraction than can be obtained by echocardiography (Fig. 32-8). This is proving to be particularly important in older repaired patients with right ventricular dysfunction owing to chronic volume overload from free pulmonary regurgitation, with or without pressure overload from residual outflow tract obstruction. Potentially, cardiac magnetic resonance imaging may be useful in the selection of such patients who would benefit from pulmonary valve replacement.[47]

Nuclear lung perfusion scanning (e.g., using technetium-99m–labeled microaggregated albumin) is used in tetralogy of Fallot patients, especially those with pulmonary atresia and hypoplastic pulmonary arteries, for evaluation of pulmonary blood flow distribution to the right and left lungs.[48] This information, typically obtained before and after pulmonary balloon angioplasty, is useful as a measure of the immediate success of the intervention. Followed serially,

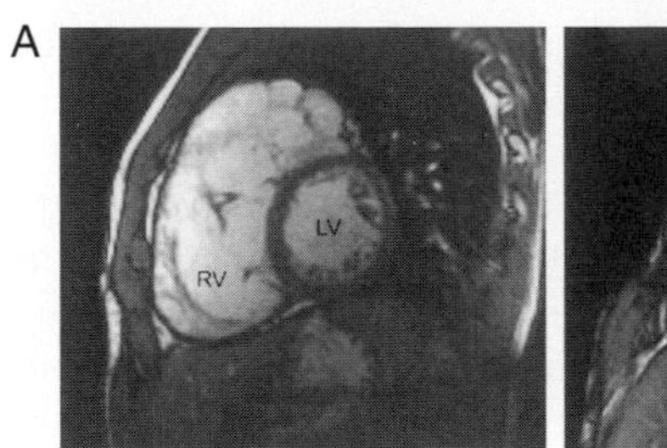

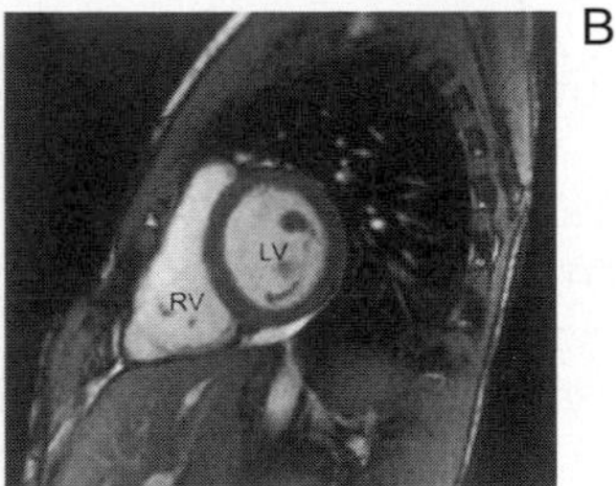

FIGURE 32–8 *Magnetic resonance ventriculography late after repair of tetralogy of Fallot.* ***A****, Parasagittal image showing marked dilation of the right ventricle (RV) with a normal-sized left ventricle (LV).* ***B****, Parasagittal image showing a normal right ventricle for comparison.*

it can also provide evidence of recurrence of stenosis on one side or the other.

Tetralogy of Fallot with Pulmonary Atresia

Magnetic resonance imaging can provide detailed information on sources of pulmonary blood flow, including aortopulmonary collaterals (Fig. 32-9), comparable to that available by x-ray angiography.[49] However, it is not used routinely because most patients require catheterization and angiography for interventional purposes.

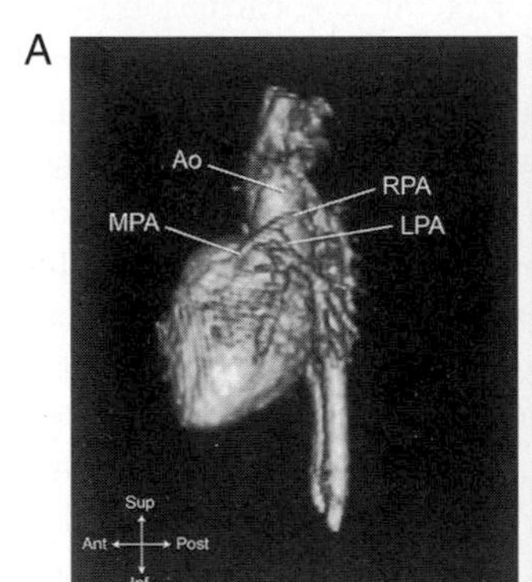

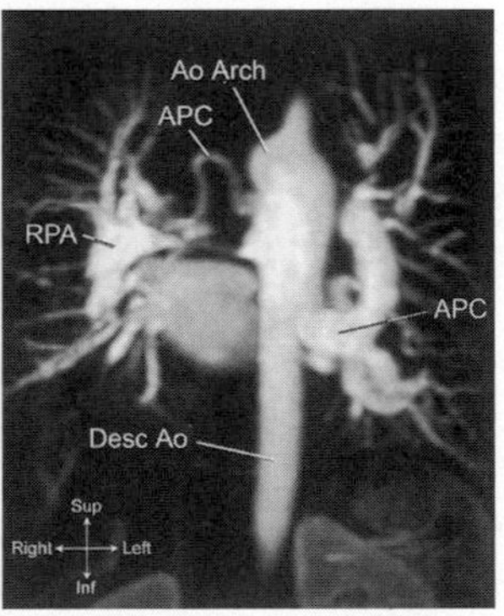

FIGURE 32–9 *Magnetic resonance images of patients with tetralogy of Fallot with pulmonary atresia.* ***A****, Three-dimensional reconstruction of a magnetic resonance angiogram in virtual left lateral projection showing diminutive main (MPA), right (RPA), and left (LPA) mediastinal pulmonary arteries and large rightward ascending aorta (Ao).* ***B****, Magnetic resonance angiogram in coronal projection showing two aortopulmonary collaterals (APC), one very large artery arising from the descending thoracic aorta (Desc Ao) to the left lung, and another smaller artery arising from the aortic arch (Ao Arch) to the right pulmonary artery (RPA) distribution.*

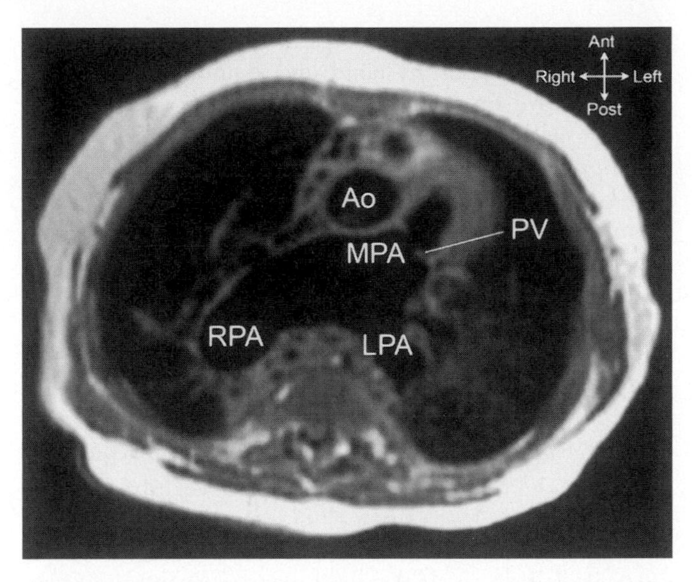

FIGURE 32–10 *Magnetic resonance image of a patient with tetralogy of Fallot with absent pulmonary valve, showing an axial cut through the vestigial pulmonary valve (PV) and markedly dilated main (MPA), right (RPA), and left (LPA) pulmonary arteries, compared with the more normal-caliber aorta (Ao).*

Tetralogy of Fallot with Absent Pulmonary Valve

Magnetic resonance can provide excellent images of the dilated pulmonary arteries (Fig. 32-10), obstructed airways, and their interrelationships. However, in current practice, the echocardiographic images are usually sufficient for diagnosis and surgical planning.

Tetralogy of Fallot with Common Atrioventricular Canal

Magnetic resonance imaging has the same features for common atrioventricular canal as were described previously for absent pulmonary valve.

MANAGEMENT

Most infants with tetralogy of Fallot are only mildly or moderately cyanotic, or even acyanotic, and require no specific medical therapy before surgical repair. Rare newborns with critical right ventricular outflow obstruction and inadequate aortopulmonary collaterals may be ductus arteriosus dependent and require prostaglandin E_1 (alprostadil) infusion to maintain ductal patency pending surgical or catheter intervention. "Pink tetralogy" patients, however, with unobstructed right ventricular outflow tracts, ventricular left-to-right shunting, and pulmonary overcirculation, may develop heart failure and require treatment with anticongestive medicines, including diuretics, digoxin, or angiotensin-converting enzyme inhibitors (see Chapter 7).

Patients who have a hypercyanotic spell are potentially at risk for severe neurologic sequelae and even death and, therefore, merit urgent attention.[50] The spelling patient should be placed in the knee–chest position, if tolerated, to simulate squatting and should be consoled to the extent possible. If outside the hospital, an ambulance should be called. Responding emergency medical personnel, whether in the field or in the hospital, should provide supplemental oxygen and intravenous fluid to expand the intravascular volume and increase pulmonary blood flow. Morphine should be administered immediately to relieve distress and air hunger; this may break the spell in some cases. Propranolol may be infused for β-adrenergic blockade, thought to relax infundibular spasm. If the spell persists, an α-adrenergic agonist such as phenylephrine may be infused to increase the systemic vascular resistance, favoring pulmonary blood flow. Tracheal intubation and mechanical ventilation, extracorporeal membrane oxygenation, or emergency palliative surgery may be necessary to rescue the patient if the spell remains refractory.

Drugs that produce systemic vasodilation can precipitate spells and are to be avoided in tetralogy of Fallot patients. Spells may occur even under sedation, such as for echocardiography or catheterization; therefore, vigilance for the development of signs such as deepening cyanosis, progressive arterial oxygen desaturation, hyperpnea, or metabolic acidosis is important. Patients who have had one or more spells and are awaiting surgery may be maintained on propranolol, which may help to prevent recurrent spells.

Since 1954, when surgical repair of tetralogy of Fallot was first attempted,[51] the recommended age for elective repair of tetralogy of Fallot has declined steadily, now typically about 3 months for infants born at full term with uncomplicated anatomy.[52–55] Repair in early infancy has been made possible by advances in surgical technique and postoperative management (see Chapter 57). Infant repair allows early restoration of normal circulatory physiology, thereby minimizing long-term risks associated with chronic cyanosis and right ventricular hypertension.

Operative repair of tetralogy of Fallot is approached through a median sternotomy, on cardiopulmonary bypass. Both transatrial and transventricular approaches are described; the latter has been favored by surgeons at Children's Hospital Boston in most instances.[56–59] A longitudinal incision is made in the free wall of the infundibulum, with extension proximally to the level of the conal septum. Distally, this incision is extended to just below the pulmonary valve annulus (nontransannular) if the annulus is not hypoplastic, or across the hypoplastic annulus (transannular) and anterior wall of the main pulmonary artery to the bifurcation. The incision may be further extended across one or both origins of the right and left pulmonary arteries if they are also narrowed. Thickened and obstructing pulmonary valve leaflets are resected. Obstructing right ventricular muscle bundles, if any, are also resected. The ventricular septal defect is visualized and repaired through this infundibulotomy, typically with a Dacron patch. Precautions are taken to minimize the risk that the sutures will damage the cardiac conduction system that resides in the margins of the defect. Additional ventricular septal defects, for example, in the anterior muscular septum, are also closed, either with a second patch or sometimes primarily. An outflow patch, comprising glutaraldehyde-treated autologous pericardium, is fashioned to appropriate dimensions and sewn into the infundibulotomy to augment the circumference of the outflow tract. If transannular, the patch continues into the main pulmonary artery and, if narrow, one or both branch pulmonary artery origins. Associated lesions, including patent ductus arteriosus and large atrial septal defects, are also addressed during the operation. Typically, the patent foramen ovale or small atrial septal defect is left open to permit the right atrium to decompress, at the expense of some systemic arterial oxygen desaturation, if the hypertrophic right ventricle remains stiff with a high diastolic filling pressure in the early postoperative period.

Postoperative management in the intensive care unit is typical of that for patients at risk for low cardiac output syndrome after cardiopulmonary bypass.[50] This management includes mechanical ventilation, pleural and mediastinal drainage, intracardiac monitoring, inotropic support, afterload reduction, and diuresis (see Chapter 18). Evaluation for residual outflow obstruction or residual ventricular septal defects with left to right shunting is made by physical examination, pressure and oxygen saturation determinations by means of intracardiac lines, and echocardiography; catheterization may be indicated if these are significant. For the typical tetralogy of Fallot repair, recent statistics from Children's Hospital Boston show a median ventilator time of 29 hours, a median intensive care unit length of stay of 3 days, and a median hospital length of stay of 6 days.[60]

Certain tetralogy of Fallot patients may require different surgical timing or management for a variety of reasons. Infants at any age who are severely cyanotic, or who have had one or more spells, are generally referred immediately for repair. A child who has a severe hypercyanotic spell refractory to medical management may warrant emergent placement of a modified Blalock-Taussig shunt (synthetic tube graft from the innominate or subclavian artery to the ipsilateral pulmonary artery) for immediate, potentially life-saving palliation, deferring elective complete repair.

Repair may also be postponed if certain aspects of the anatomy are unsuitable. There may be significant muscular ventricular defects that would be difficult for the surgeon to close. These may become smaller and even close spontaneously over time, simplifying the ultimate repair. There may be an important coronary artery crossing the infundibulum, precluding infundibulotomy and outflow patch placement. In these cases, a right ventricle-to-pulmonary artery homograft conduit is usually required instead to provide an unobstructed outflow. Because such a fixed conduit will need to be replaced one or more times as the child grows, it may be advantageous to place a palliative shunt and delay definitive repair for 1 year or longer to allow for insertion of the largest possible initial homograft. Also potentially unsuitable for early repair is a severely hypoplastic pulmonary artery tree that may be incapable of conducting a full cardiac output. Again, it may be prudent to delay the repair to allow time for growth of these vessels, often with the aid of interventional catheterization for pulmonary artery rehabilitation in the interim.[36] Finally, surgery may be delayed in premature infants who are still too small at 3 months of age, or in other infants who may have additional noncardiac problems that make the operative risks, particularly associated with cardiopulmonary bypass, unacceptably high.

In all cases in which reparative surgery must be deferred, interim palliation is often necessary because of progressive cyanosis or the onset of tetralogy spells. Usually, such patients require placement of a modified Blalock-Taussig shunt to provide a stable source of pulmonary blood flow. Certain patients with significant valvar pulmonary stenosis may, alternatively, benefit temporarily from transcatheter balloon valvotomy to increase pulmonary blood flow; however, this must be done with caution if the outflow obstruction is predominantly at the valve, lest dilation result in an acute ventricular left to right shunting pulmonary overcirculation.[36–41]

Antibiotic prophylaxis at times of predictable risk for infective endocarditis is indicated in all patients with tetralogy of Fallot, whether unrepaired, palliated, or repaired, according to the recommendations by the American Heart Association current at this writing.[61]

Tetralogy of Fallot with Pulmonary Atresia

The initial medical management of the newborn with tetralogy of Fallot with pulmonary atresia varies according to the sources and amounts of pulmonary blood flow. At one extreme, infants with inadequate aortopulmonary collaterals may be ductus arteriosus dependent and require prostaglandin E_1 (alprostadil) infusion to maintain ductal patency pending surgical or catheter intervention. If, instead, there are adequate collaterals, the ductus may be allowed to close, and many patients will maintain acceptable arterial oxygen saturations in the range of 80% to 90% without treatment. At the other extreme, rare patients may have excessive aortopulmonary collateral flow, and this may increase further as pulmonary arteriolar resistance decreases, even to the extent that anticongestive medicines may be needed.

The definitive management of tetralogy of Fallot with pulmonary atresia includes complementary interventional catheterization and surgical approaches that are orchestrated to establish antegrade pulmonary blood flow from the right ventricle, rehabilitate the pulmonary arteries, and close the ventricular septal defect.[42] Fundamental to this strategy is the understanding that postnatal growth of the hypoplastic pulmonary arterial tree can be promoted by maximizing antegrade flow, minimizing competing collateral flow, and eliminating stenoses. The imperative to achieve antegrade flow has shifted practice at most centers away from formerly routine systemic-to-pulmonary artery shunts, except when urgent palliation is required.

The precise management is dictated by the individual anatomy in each patient, largely the extent of atresia, severity of pulmonary artery hypoplasia, and extent of collateralization. It is possible in some patients to achieve a one-stage surgical repair,[62,63] but many require a staged approach.[64–70] All patients undergo catheterization as a first step to define the pulmonary artery anatomy and all sources of pulmonary blood flow. If there are excessive aortopulmonary collaterals that deliver competing flow, and the arterial oxygen saturation is relatively high, coil embolization of some of these vessels and potentially the patent ductus arteriosus may be undertaken. This is particularly useful for those collaterals that may be relatively inaccessible at surgery.

There are several possibilities for creating continuity between the right ventricle and pulmonary arteries. If there is membranous atresia, limited to the valve, it may be possible at catheterization to perforate and dilate the membrane.[43] Alternatively, a transannular outflow patch may be placed at surgery. If, instead, there is long-segment atresia involving much of the main pulmonary artery, a right ventricle-to-pulmonary artery homograft conduit is placed.[56,57] Additional homograft material may be used at the distal end to augment hypoplastic or even discontinuous branch pulmonary arteries. Occasionally, the mediastinal pulmonary arteries may be so small that a narrow-diameter synthetic tube conduit is used, to be replaced later with a larger homograft.

If the native pulmonary arteries supply only a limited number of bronchopulmonary segments, it is important at operation to recruit additional segments, supplied solely by collateral vessels, into the reconstructed pulmonary arterial tree. This is accomplished in an approach termed *unifocalization*, in which those collateral vessels are detached from the aorta and anastomosed to the central pulmonary artery confluence. In rare cases in which no mediastinal pulmonary arteries of any size can be identified, unifocalization of all major collaterals to the distal conduit may be the only available strategy to establish flow from the right ventricle.

Control of aortopulmonary collaterals and patent ductus arteriosus is a critical issue during cardiopulmonary bypass.[56,57] These must be dissected and looped or ligated to prevent "steal" of systemic flow into the lower-resistance pulmonary circulation, and attendant ischemic injury to end organs, including the brain. Further, because additional smaller collaterals inevitably persist, there is ongoing pulmonary venous return on bypass requiring that a vent be placed to decompress the left ventricle.

Once right ventricle-to-pulmonary artery continuity has been achieved, whether by catheterization or surgery, there is ready antegrade catheter access to the pulmonary arterial tree. More precise delineation of the intrapulmonary vessels is possible. Balloon catheters are used to dilate areas of discrete stenosis. Vascular stents are delivered to segments of elastic narrowing for which dilation alone does not suffice. These interventions serve to decrease right ventricular hypertension, increase flow to distal pulmonary segments, and improve the match between ventilation and perfusion. Further, the advent of more effective pulmonary blood flow from the right ventricle allows remaining aortopulmonary collaterals to be coil-occluded without compromising systemic oxygenation.

The timing of closure of the ventricular septal defect in tetralogy of Fallot with pulmonary atresia also depends on the pulmonary artery anatomy.[67] Once the ventricular defect is closed, the pulmonary arteries must have adequate capacity to receive all systemic venous return (save for that shunting right to left across an atrial septal defect) from the right ventricle. If the total cross-sectional area of the pulmonary arteries is too small, right ventricular failure and low cardiac output will ensue.[71] In some patients born with relatively little pulmonary artery hypoplasia, it may be possible to close the ventricular septal defect at the time of initial right ventricular outflow tract reconstruction.[62,63] More typically, however, ventricular septal defect closure must be deferred until substantial pulmonary artery rehabilitation has been accomplished. The development of left-to-right shunting through the ventricular septal defect is perhaps the most reliable indicator that it can safely be closed. Often, ventricular septal defect closure is scheduled to coincide with surgical revision of the right ventricle-to-pulmonary artery conduit (discussed later). When there is lingering concern about the adequacy of the pulmonary artery tree, a fenestration may intentionally be placed in the ventricular septal defect patch to allow decompression of the right ventricle, to be closed later using a transcatheter occlusion device.[72]

Patients with tetralogy of Fallot with pulmonary atresia typically require one or more additional operations as they grow in size. Right ventricle-to-pulmonary artery conduits are, by their nature, fixed in diameter, and so must be replaced or otherwise enlarged when they become very restrictive. Serial interventional catheterizations are also generally indicated in these patients throughout infancy and childhood, more so than in other tetralogy variants (Exhibit 32-2). New or recurrent pulmonary artery stenoses can be dilated and, if necessary, stented. Existing stents can be redilated up to their maximum diameter. Obstructed right ventricle-to-pulmonary artery homograft conduits can also be dilated and stented, often permitting surgical conduit revision to be postponed for months or years and potentially reducing the total number of such operations that the patient will ultimately have to undergo.

Tetralogy of Fallot with Absent Pulmonary Valve

The initial medical management of tetralogy of Fallot with absent pulmonary valve depends on the degree of the accompanying airway disease.[32,33] Some neonates present with severe bronchial obstruction and require immediate tracheal intubation and mechanical ventilation, followed by early surgical repair. Indeed, in the most severe cases, adequate ventilation may not be achieved even with mechanical support, resulting in death due to respiratory failure. Some of these severely affected infants may benefit from extracorporeal membrane oxygenation as a bridge to surgery. Patients with moderate obstruction may or may not require intubation and may benefit from lying prone rather than supine to help relieve anterior vascular compression of the bronchi. Patients with little or no airway obstruction may require no additional support in the neonatal period and go on to elective repair later in infancy.

The surgical repair of tetralogy of Fallot with absent pulmonary valve, in addition to ventricular septal defect closure and right ventricular outflow reconstruction, involves reduction of the aneurysmal mediastinal pulmonary arteries to relieve bronchial compression.[32,56,57] Approaches include plication or excision of portions of the walls of these vessels, reducing their circumference, or complete removal of dilated segments and replacement with conduit. Some surgeons also place an artificial pulmonary valve in the reconstructed outflow to control pulmonary regurgitation and, thereby, limit the vascular pulsatility, volume load, and ongoing dilation of the vessels that may further compromise the airways.[73]

Exhibit 32–2
Children's Hospital Boston Experience
Tetralogy of Fallot (TOF) Surgery
1988-2002

Total (N = 1059)	TOF/PS (N = 617)	TOF/APV (N = 39)	TOF/AVC (N = 46)	TOF/PA* (N = 357)
Operation/patient	1.1	1.4	1.5	1.9
Catheterization/patient	1.5	1.9	2.1	3.6
	%	%	%	%
Patients catheterized (%)	29	50	22	66
Repair surgery (%)	99	100	83	76
Shunts (%)	5	2	26	27
PA surgical plasty (%)	5	26	4	16
PA balloon dilation (%)	6	18	7	39
Stent placement (%)	3	13	2	26
Coils (%)	1	5	0	15

*The TOF/PA group was the most complicated group to manage, in that, per patient, more operations, catheterizations, pulmonary artery dilations and stents, and vessel occlusions by coils were required, and the proportion who had a repair was the smallest.PS, pulmonary stenosis; APV, absent pulmonary valve; AVC, atrioventricular canal; PA, pulmonary atresia; MVSD, multiple ventricular septal defects; LPA, left pulmonary artery; RPA, right pulmonary artery.

Tetralogy of Fallot with Common Atrioventricular Canal

The medical management of tetralogy of Fallot with common atrioventricular canal is generally no different than that of uncomplicated tetralogy. The surgical repair involves conventional right ventricular outflow tract reconstruction, as described earlier, with closure of the atrioventricular septal defect and division and resuspension of the common atrioventricular valve (see Chapter 38). Division of the common atrioventricular valve may leave the patient with some degree of right-sided (tricuspid) regurgitation, particularly if there is deficient leaflet tissue to fashion two complete valves. Significant tricuspid regurgitation represents a potentially difficult problem early after tetralogy repair because it may further compromise the recently incised right ventricle that is often already doing extra volume work owing to free pulmonary regurgitation and possibly extra pressure work if there is any residual right ventricular outflow tract obstruction or branch pulmonary artery stenoses. Right ventricular failure may seriously complicate the postoperative management of these patients. For this reason, the repair of tetralogy of Fallot with common atrioventricular canal may be postponed until later in infancy when the atrioventricular valve tissue is less friable and technically easier to suture, favoring creation of a more competent tricuspid valve.

Selected statistics regarding the catheterization and surgery of 1059 tetralogy of Fallot patients who underwent operation at Children's Hospital Boston during a 14-year period are shown in Exhibit 32-2.

COURSE

Before repair, infants with tetralogy of Fallot tend to become more cyanotic with time owing primarily to progressive infundibular stenosis and increased ventricular right to left shunting. Beyond the neonatal period, they are also at increasing risk for developing hypercyanotic spells. Chronic hypoxemia is correlated with cognitive impairment in large cohort studies (see Chapter 9). Older children with unrepaired or palliated tetralogy of Fallot may have additional complications associated with chronic cyanosis and polycythemia, including stroke, brain abscess, and pigment gallstones (see Chapter 8). Those patients with large surgical systemic-to-pulmonary artery shunts or persisting large aortopulmonary collaterals may develop pulmonary vascular obstructive disease (see Chapter 10). These problems are increasingly rare in contemporary practice in which infant repair is the rule.

Outcomes after complete repair of tetralogy of Fallot are generally excellent. Actuarial data on patients repaired in the late 1950s and 1960s indicate that nearly 90% were alive 30 years after surgery, excluding early postoperative deaths.[74,75] For patients repaired in more recent decades, the early mortality has been 3% or less.[53–55] Still, even in patients with good initial anatomic results, a number of problems may develop and represent important management issues[76] (see Chapter 56). Some of these may appear in the first few years after repair, but late complications are seen with increasing frequency as increasing numbers of patients are surviving to advanced ages. Many of these patients underwent original repair not in infancy but instead later in childhood. The potential impact of early infant repair on late outcome, positive or negative, will be realized only as larger numbers of patients who underwent repair as infants reach the later decades of life.[77,78]

Clinically important residual ventricular septal defects are often identified and closed early after repair. These are either persistent defects at the patch margin or previously unrecognized or underestimated additional defects in the muscular septum. Rarely, residual defects due to partial patch dehiscence are diagnosed late after repair.

Recurrent right ventricular outflow tract obstruction may develop during childhood at one or more levels and require surgical revision to relieve significant right ventricular hypertension. Muscle bundles may grow to obstruct the os infundibulum in 3% of patients repaired in infancy.[79] In patients with nontransannular outflow patches, the pulmonary valve annulus may be become relatively restrictive as the child grows; this has been a particular concern in patients repaired very early in infancy. Those with transannular patches can develop restriction at the distal insertion of the patch into the branch pulmonary arteries. Patients with significant pulmonary artery hypoplasia at initial presentation may develop additional sites of peripheral pulmonary stenosis over time.

Progressive aortic root dilation and resulting aortic valve insufficiency develop in some tetralogy of Fallot patients. Whether there are tetralogy-associated developmental abnormalities intrinsic to the aortic valve and root that might contribute to this is unknown. In patients with palliative systemic-to-pulmonary artery shunts or significant aortopulmonary collaterals, the obligatory excess flow across the aortic valve, that is, the left-to-right shunt volume, is thought to contribute to aortic dilation. Progression of dilation late after repair has been found to correlate with longer time between palliation and repair and also with pulmonary atresia, right aortic arch, and male gender.[24]

Repaired tetralogy of Fallot patients, as they approach the third decade of life and beyond, are recognized increasingly to have significant right ventricular dilation and systolic and diastolic dysfunction. This is attributed to the accumulated effects, past or ongoing, of excess volume load from pulmonary regurgitation, pressure load from outflow obstruction, hypoxemic coronary perfusion, surgical incision, patch, and scarring, and post–cardiopulmonary bypass ischemia-reperfusion injury—possibly superimposed on tetralogy-associated congenital abnormalities of the myocardium. Transatrial rather than transventricular repair has been advocated to avoid right ventricular incision, but this may be at the expense of residual outflow obstruction in some patients.[80,81] A number of patients with right ventricular dysfunction also have measurable left ventricular dysfunction, an apparent consequence of adverse ventricular interaction.[47,82] Patients with right ventricular dysfunction may remain relatively asymptomatic for years, but many have impaired exercise capacity[83]; ultimately, some, if not most, develop clinical heart failure. Pulmonary valve replacement has been shown to produce short-term improvement in symptoms and exercise tolerance in such patients.[84] However, despite restoration of pulmonary valve competence, the potential for recovery of right ventricular function may be limited, leading some to recommend valve replacement before ventricular function deteriorates.[85,86]

Patients with repaired tetralogy of Fallot are at ongoing risk for rhythm disturbances and sudden cardiac death.[87] Long-term mortality from sudden death is in the range of 3% to 6%. Adverse changes in the ventricular myocardium due to the excess hemodynamic burdens and injuries that cause ventricular dysfunction, enumerated earlier, appear to create the pathologic substrate for arrhythmias. In one prospective study, 45% of repaired patients 3 to 45 years of age had frequent monomorphic ventricular premature beats or higher-grade ventricular ectopy on Holter monitoring, although less such ectopy is found in patients repaired at younger ages. Ventricular ectopy is inducible during treadmill exercise testing in 30% of repaired patients whether or not they manifest ectopy at rest.[88] Sustained ventricular tachycardia can be induced with programmed stimulation in 12% to 28% of patients referred for such studies. However, neither the findings on screening Holter monitoring nor provocative testing have been shown reliably to predict adverse outcomes in tetralogy of Fallot patients, possibly because those with more than low-grade ventricular ectopy are generally treated with antiarrhythmic agents[87] (see Chapter 29). Aside from ventricular arrhythmias, 20% to 30% of repaired patients have sinus node dysfunction and intra-atrial reentrant tachycardia (see Chapter 29).

Like patients with congenital heart disease in general (see Chapter 9), those with tetralogy of Fallot appear as a group to have a lower mean intelligence quotient than control populations, albeit with a large standard deviation, and higher psychosocial morbidity.[89–91] The factors that underlie neurodevelopmental morbidity may include both inborn errors (e.g., genetic syndromes or hypothetical tetralogy-associated central nervous system deficits) and acquired abnormalities that ensue from chronic hypoxemia, hemodynamic instability, and surgery, including cardiopulmonary bypass and circulatory arrest. To date, studies of neurocognitive outcome in tetralogy of Fallot have included substantial numbers of patients repaired in later childhood;

Exhibit 32–3
Boston Children's Hospital Experience
Tetralogy of Fallot Survival
1988-2002

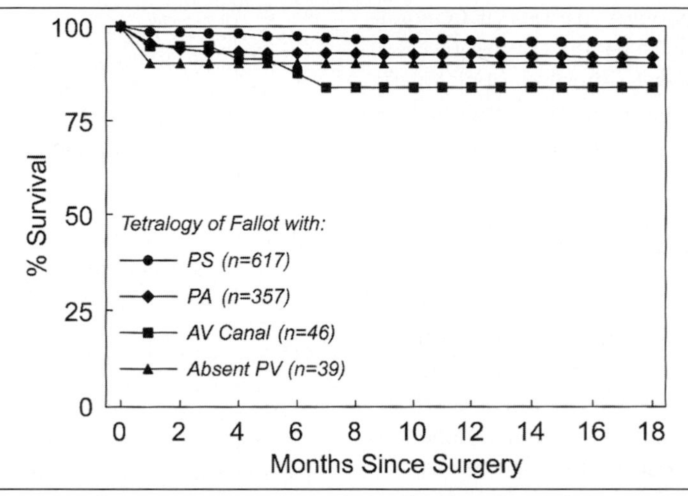

Life table showing survival to 18 months of 1059 patients with tetralogy of Fallot who underwent surgery at Children's Hospital Boston ranging from 84% among those with absent pulmonary valve (APV, the smallest group) to 96% among those with pulmonary stenosis (PS, the largest group).

thus, the potential impact of early infant repair remains to be determined.

Patients with tetralogy of Fallot, whether unrepaired, palliated, or repaired, have a lifelong risk for infective endocarditis and require appropriate antibiotic prophylaxis[61,92] (see Chapter 28). Historically, the most common sites of infection in these patients have been systemic-to-pulmonary artery shunts in palliated patients, or notably the aortic valve, which as noted earlier may be regurgitant.

Tetralogy of Fallot with Pulmonary Atresia

The requirement for a right ventricle-to-pulmonary artery conduit commits patients with tetralogy of Fallot with pulmonary atresia to at least one, often two, and sometimes three reoperations for conduit enlargement or replacement. Typically, this is undertaken when the right ventricular pressure approaches the systemic arterial pressure range. In many instances, reoperation can be postponed, and the number of such procedures minimized, by transcatheter balloon dilation and stenting of an obstructed conduit.[93]

Patients with tetralogy of Fallot with pulmonary atresia are at substantial ongoing risk for recurrent peripheral pulmonary artery stenosis and even acquired atresia of lobar and segmental branches. Serial catheterizations are indicated for ongoing pulmonary artery rehabilitation, often at intervals as short as a few months in young children with severe disease, and less frequently in older children with well-established flow throughout the pulmonary arterial tree.

Some patients with severely hypoplastic pulmonary arteries refractory to rehabilitation may never develop sufficient pulmonary artery cross-sectional area to allow closure of the ventricular septal defect. These patients have a persistent ventricular right to left shunt and are at risk for a range of complications from chronic hypoxemia (see Chapter 8).

Patients with tetralogy of Fallot with pulmonary atresia are at higher risk for progressive aortic root dilation and aortic insufficiency than those with pulmonary stenosis, as noted earlier.[24]

Tetralogy of Fallot with Absent Pulmonary Valve

The outcome for patients with tetralogy of Fallot with absent pulmonary valve depends largely on the severity of airway disease, as noted earlier. Some patients may have little or no clinical evidence of airway narrowing, often despite considerable pulmonary artery dilation. Others present with clinically manifest bronchial obstruction that can be managed if necessary with mechanical ventilation and ultimately relieved at surgery. Still others, however, have such severe airway obstruction that adequate ventilation cannot be achieved even with mechanical support. Even after surgical repair, including reduction of the aneurysmal central pulmonary arteries, some patients continue to have significant bronchial obstruction, owing presumably to residual airway hypoplasia and deformity and to the ongoing impact on intraparenchymal bronchi of abnormally branching segmental pulmonary arteries that cannot be surgically addressed.[27,94] As these patients grow, however, pulmonary function tends generally to improve as pulmonary artery pressures fall and the maturing tracheobronchial tree develops less compressible walls and larger caliber.[28]

Tetralogy of Fallot with Common Atrioventricular Canal

Patients with repaired tetralogy of Fallot with common atrioventricular canal are at risk for any of the long-term complications of either lesion (see Chapter 38). Of particular note is the risk for atrioventricular valve incompetence after canal repair and the extent to which this may compound other residual problems in tetralogy. Right-sided (tricuspid) valve regurgitation adds to the volume overload of the right ventricle, already overloaded by pulmonary regurgitation, accelerating right ventricular dilation, and dysfunction. Similarly, left-sided (mitral) regurgitation adds volume load to the left ventricle that, potentially, may be burdened in the short or long term by aortic insufficiency.

The actuarial survival data of 1059 tetralogy of Fallot patients operated at Children's Hospital Boston, through 18 postoperative months, are shown in Exhibit 32-3.

REFERENCES

1. Fallot A. Contribution a l'anatomie pathologique de la maladie bleue (cyanose cardiaque). Mars Med 25, 1888.
2. Stensen N. Quoted by Goldstein HI. Bull Hist Med 29:526, 1948.
3. Ferencz C, Rubin JD, McCarter RJ, et al. Congenital heart disease: Prevalence at livebirth. The Baltimore-Washington Infant Study. Am J Epidemiol 121:31, 1985.
4. Loffredo CA. Epidemiology of cardiovascular malformations: Prevalence and risk factors. Am J Med Genet 97:319, 2000.
5. National Center for Health Statistics, Birth Data, 2004. Available at: http://www.cdc.gov/nchs/births.htm.
6. Goldmuntz E, Geiger E, Benson DW. NKX2.5 mutations in patients with tetralogy of Fallot. Circulation 104:2565, 2001.
7. Krantz ID, Smith R, Colliton RP, et al. Jagged1 mutations in patients ascertained with isolated congenital heart defects. Am J Med Genet 84:56, 1999.
8. McElhinney DB, Krantz ID, Bason L, et al. Analysis of cardiovascular phenotype and genotype-phenotype correlation in individuals with a JAG1 mutation and/or Alagille syndrome. Circulation 106:2567, 2002.
9. Bruneau BG, Logan M, Davis N, et al. Chamber-specific cardiac expression of Tbx5 and heart defects in Holt-Oram syndrome. Dev Biol 211:100, 1999.
10. Erickson RP, Dagenais SL, Caulder MS, et al. Clinical heterogeneity in lymphoedema-distichiasis with FOXC2 truncating mutations. J Med Genet 38:761, 2001.
11. Merscher S, Funke B, Epstein JA, et al. TBX1 is responsible for cardiovascular defects in velo-cardio-facial/DiGeorge syndrome. Cell 104:619, 2001.
12. Jerome LA, Papaioannou VE. DiGeorge syndrome phenotype in mice mutant for the T-box gene, Tbx1. Nat Genet 27:286, 2001.
13. Gong W, Gottlieb S, Collins J, et al. Mutation analysis of TBX1 in non-deleted patients with features of DGS/VCFS or isolated cardiovascular defects. J Med Genet 38:E45, 2001.
14. Ferencz C, Loffredo CA, Correa-Villasenor A, et al. Genetic and Environmental Risk Factors of Major Cardiovascular Malformations: The Baltimore-Washington Infant Study 1981–1989. Armonk, NY: Futura, 1997.
15. Van Mierop LH, Kutsche LM. Cardiovascular anomalies in DiGeorge syndrome and importance of neural crest as a possible pathogenetic factor. Am J Cardiol 58:133, 1986.
16. Van Praagh R, Van Praagh S, Nebesar RA, et al. Tetralogy of Fallot: Underdevelopment of the pulmonary infundibulum and its sequelae. Am J Cardiol 26:25, 1970.
17. Anderson RH, Allwork SP, Ho SY, et al. Surgical anatomy of tetralogy of Fallot. J Thorac Cardiovasc Surg 81:887, 1981.
18. Flanagan MF, Foran RB, Van Praagh R, et al. Tetralogy of Fallot with obstruction of the ventricular septal defect: Spectrum of echocardiographic findings. J Am Coll Cardiol 11:386, 1988.
19. Musewe NN, Smallhorn JF, Moes CA, et al. Echocardiographic evaluation of obstructive mechanism of tetralogy of Fallot with restrictive ventricular septal defect. Am J Cardiol 61:664, 1988.
20. Hornberger LK, Sanders SP, Sahn DJ, et al. In utero pulmonary artery and aortic growth and potential for progression of pulmonary outflow tract obstruction in tetralogy of Fallot. J Am Coll Cardiol 25:739, 1995.
21. Frater RW, Rudolph AM, Hoffman JI. Acquired pulmonary atresia in tetralogy of Fallot with a functioning Blalock-Taussig shunt. Thorax 21:457, 1966.
22. Haworth SG. Collateral arteries in pulmonary atresia with ventricular septal defect: A precarious blood supply. Br Heart J 44:5, 1980.
23. Liao PK, Edwards WD, Julsrud PR, et al. Pulmonary blood supply in patients with pulmonary atresia and ventricular septal defect. J Am Coll Cardiol 6:1343, 1985.
24. Niwa K, Siu SC, Webb GD, et al. Progressive aortic root dilatation in adults late after repair of tetralogy of Fallot. Circulation 106:1374, 2002.
25. Emmanoulides GC, Thanopoulos B, Siassi B, et al. "Agenesis" of ductus arteriosus associated with the syndrome of tetralogy of Fallot and absent pulmonary valve. Am J Cardiol 37:403, 1976.

26. Fischer DR, Neches WH, Beerman LB, et al. Tetralogy of Fallot with absent pulmonic valve: Analysis of 17 patients. Am J Cardiol 53:1433, 1984.
27. Rabinovitch M, Grady S, David I, et al. Compression of intrapulmonary bronchi by abnormally branching pulmonary arteries associated with absent pulmonary valves. Am J Cardiol 50:804, 1982.
28. Berman W, Jr., Fripp RR, Rowe SA, et al. Congenital isolated pulmonary valve incompetence: Neonatal presentation and early natural history. Am Heart J 124:248, 1992.
29. Kothari SS. Mechanism of cyanotic spells in tetralogy of Fallot—the missing link? Int J Cardiol 37:1, 1992.
30. Newburger JW, Silbert AR, Buckley LP, et al. Cognitive function and age at repair of transposition of the great arteries in children. N Engl J Med 310:1495, 1984.
31. Digilio MC, Marino B, Grazioli S, et al. Comparison of occurrence of genetic syndromes in ventricular septal defect with pulmonic stenosis (classic tetralogy of Fallot) versus ventricular septal defect with pulmonic atresia. Am J Cardiol 77:1375, 1996.
32. Arensman FW, Francis PD, Helmsworth JA, et al. Early medical and surgical intervention for tetralogy of Fallot with absence of pulmonic valve. J Thorac Cardiovasc Surg 84:430, 1982.
33. Heinemann MK, Hanley FL. Preoperative management of neonatal tetralogy of Fallot with absent pulmonary valve syndrome. Ann Thorac Surg 55:172, 1993.
34. Kleinman CS, Weinstein EM, Talner NS, et al. Fetal echocardiography—applications and limitations. Ultrasound Med Biol 10:747, 1984.
35. Berning RA, Silverman NH, Villegas M, et al. Reversed shunting across the ductus arteriosus or atrial septum in utero heralds severe congenital heart disease. J Am Coll Cardiol 27:481, 1996.
36. Kreutzer J, Perry SB, Jonas RA, et al. Tetralogy of Fallot with diminutive pulmonary arteries: Preoperative pulmonary valve dilation and transcatheter rehabilitation of pulmonary arteries. J Am Coll Cardiol 27:1741, 1996.
37. Boucek MM, Webster HE, Orsmond GS, et al. Balloon pulmonary valvotomy: Palliation for cyanotic heart disease. Am Heart J 115:318, 1988.
38. Qureshi SA, Kirk CR, Lamb RK, et al. Balloon dilatation of the pulmonary valve in the first year of life in patients with tetralogy of Fallot: A preliminary study. Br Heart J 60:232, 1988.
39. Sreeram N, Saleem M, Jackson M, et al. Results of balloon pulmonary valvuloplasty as a palliative procedure in tetralogy of Fallot. J Am Coll Cardiol 18:159, 1991.
40. Sluysmans T, Neven B, Rubay J, et al. Early balloon dilatation of the pulmonary valve in infants with tetralogy of Fallot: Risks and benefits. Circulation 91:1506, 1995.
41. Heusch A, Tannous A, Krogmann ON, et al. Balloon valvoplasty in infants with tetralogy of Fallot: effects on oxygen saturation and growth of the pulmonary arteries. Cardiol Young 9:17, 1999.
42. Rome JJ, Mayer JE, Castaneda AR, et al. Tetralogy of Fallot with pulmonary atresia. Rehabilitation of diminutive pulmonary arteries. Circulation 88:1691, 1993.
43. Hausdorf G, Schneider M, Schirmer KR, et al. Interventional high frequency perforation and enlargement of the outflow tract of pulmonary atresia. Z Kardiol 82:123, 1993.
44. Kuhn MA, Mulla NF, Dyar D, et al. Valve perforation and balloon pulmonary valvuloplasty in an infant with tetralogy of Fallot and pulmonary atresia. Cathet Cardiovasc Diagn 40:403, 1997.
45. Niezen RA, Helbing WA, van der Wall EE, et al. Biventricular systolic function and mass studied with MR imaging in children with pulmonary regurgitation after repair for tetralogy of Fallot. Radiology 201:135, 1996.
46. Helbing WA, de Roos A. Clinical applications of cardiac magnetic resonance imaging after repair of tetralogy of Fallot. Pediatr Cardiol 21:70, 2000.
47. Geva T, Sandweiss BM, Gauvreau K, et al. Factors associated with impaired clinical status in long-term survivors of tetralogy of Fallot repair evaluated by magnetic resonance imaging. J Am Coll Cardiol 43:1068, 2004.
48. Oyen WJ, van Oort AM, Tanke RB, et al. Pulmonary perfusion after endovascular stenting of pulmonary artery stenosis. J Nucl Med 36:2006, 1995.
49. Geva T, Greil GF, Marshall AC, et al. Gadolinium-enhanced 3-dimensional magnetic resonance angiography of pulmonary blood supply in patients with complex pulmonary stenosis or atresia: Comparison with x-ray angiography. Circulation 106:473, 2002.
50. Spray TL, Wernovsky G. Right ventricular outflow tract obstruction. In Chang AC, Hanley FL, Wernovsky G, et al (eds). Pediatric Cardiac Intensive Care. Philadelphia: Lippincott Williams & Wilkins, 1998:257.
51. Lillehei CW, Varco RL, Cohen M, et al. The first open heart corrections of tetralogy of Fallot: A 26-31 year follow-up of 106 patients. Ann Surg 204:490, 1986.
52. Di Donato RM, Jonas RA, Lang P, et al. Neonatal repair of tetralogy of Fallot with and without pulmonary atresia. J Thorac Cardiovasc Surg 101:126, 1991.
53. Reddy VM, Liddicoat JR, McElhinney DB, et al. Routine primary repair of tetralogy of Fallot in neonates and infants less than three months of age. Ann Thorac Surg 60:S592, 1995.
54. Pigula FA, Khalil PN, Mayer JE, et al. Repair of tetralogy of Fallot in neonates and young infants. Circulation 100:57, 1999.
55. Parry AJ, McElhinney DB, Kung GC, et al. Elective primary repair of acyanotic tetralogy of Fallot in early infancy: Overall outcome and impact on the pulmonary valve. J Am Coll Cardiol 36:2279, 2000.
56. Castaneda AR, Jonas RA, Mayer JE, et al. Tetralogy of Fallot. In Castaneda AR, Jonas RA, Mayer JE, et al (eds). Cardiac Surgery of the Neonate and Infant. Philadelphia: WB Saunders, 1994:215.
57. Jonas RA. Tetralogy of Fallot with pulmonary stenosis. In Comprehensive Surgical Management of Congenital Heart Disease. New York: Oxford University Press, 2004: 279.
58. Edmunds LH Jr, Saxena NC, Friedman S, et al. Transatrial repair of tetralogy of Fallot. Surgery 80:681, 1976.

59. Pacifico AD, Sand ME, Bargeron LM Jr, et al. Transatrial-transpulmonary repair of tetralogy of Fallot. J Thorac Cardiovasc Surg 93:919, 1987.
60. Laussen PC. Personal communication, 2004.
61. Dajani AS, Taubert KA, Wilson W, et al. Prevention of bacterial endocarditis. Recommendations by the American Heart Association. Circulation 96:358, 1997.
62. Reddy VM, Liddicoat JR, Hanley FL. Midline one-stage complete unifocalization and repair of pulmonary atresia with ventricular septal defect and major aortopulmonary collaterals. J Thorac Cardiovasc Surg 109:832, 1995.
63. Reddy VM, McElhinney DB, Amin Z, et al. Early and intermediate outcomes after repair of pulmonary atresia with ventricular septal defect and major aortopulmonary collateral arteries: Experience with 85 patients. Circulation 101:1826, 2000.
64. Puga FJ, Leoni FE, Julsrud PR, et al. Complete repair of pulmonary atresia, ventricular septal defect, and severe peripheral arborization abnormalities of the central pulmonary arteries: Experience with preliminary unifocalization procedures in 38 patients. J Thorac Cardiovasc Surg 98:1018, 1989.
65. Sawatari K, Imai Y, Kurosawa H, et al. Staged operation for pulmonary atresia and ventricular septal defect with major aortopulmonary collateral arteries: New technique for complete unifocalization. J Thorac Cardiovasc Surg 98:738, 1989.
66. Yagihara T, Yamamoto F, Nishigaki K, et al. Unifocalization for pulmonary atresia with ventricular septal defect and major aortopulmonary collateral arteries. J Thorac Cardiovasc Surg 112:392, 1996.
67. Reddy VM, Petrossian E, McElhinney DB, et al. One-stage complete unifocalization in infants: When should the ventricular septal defect be closed? J Thorac Cardiovasc Surg 113:858, 1997.
68. McElhinney DB, Reddy VM, Hanley FL. Tetralogy of Fallot with major aortopulmonary collaterals: Early total repair. Pediatr Cardiol 19:289, 1998.
69. Duncan BW, Mee RB, Prieto LR, et al. Staged repair of tetralogy of Fallot with pulmonary atresia and major aortopulmonary collateral arteries. J Thorac Cardiovasc Surg 126:694, 2003.
70. Gupta A, Odim J, Levi D, et al. Staged repair of pulmonary atresia with ventricular septal defect and major aortopulmonary collateral arteries: experience with 104 patients. J Thorac Cardiovasc Surg 126:1746, 2003.
71. Nakata S, Imai Y, Takanashi Y, et al. A new method for the quantitative standardization of cross-sectional areas of the pulmonary arteries in congenital heart diseases with decreased pulmonary blood flow. J Thorac Cardiovasc Surg 88:610, 1984.
72. Marshall AC, Love BA, Lang P, et al. Staged repair of tetralogy of Fallot and diminutive pulmonary arteries with a fenestrated ventricular septal defect patch. J Thorac Cardiovasc Surg 126:1427, 2003.
73. Ilbawi MN, Idriss FS, Muster AJ, et al. Tetralogy of Fallot with absent pulmonary valve. Should valve insertion be part of the intracardiac repair? J Thorac Cardiovasc Surg 81:906, 1981.
74. Murphy JG, Gersh BJ, Mair DD, et al. Long-term outcome in patients undergoing surgical repair of tetralogy of Fallot. N Engl J Med 329:593, 1993.
75. Nollert G, Fischlein T, Bouterwek S, et al. Long-term survival in patients with repair of tetralogy of Fallot: 36-Year follow-up of 490 survivors of the first year after surgical repair. J Am Coll Cardiol 30:1374, 1997.
76. Oechslin EN, Harrison DA, Harris L, et al. Reoperation in adults with repair of tetralogy of Fallot: indications and outcomes. J Thorac Cardiovasc Surg 118:245, 1999.
77. Bacha EA, Scheule AM, Zurakowski D, et al. Long-term results after early primary repair of tetralogy of Fallot. J Thorac Cardiovasc Surg 122:154, 2001.
78. Hennein HA, Mosca RS, Urcelay G, et al. Intermediate results after complete repair of tetralogy of Fallot in neonates. J Thorac Cardiovasc Surg 109:332, 1995.
79. Moran AM, Hornberger LK, Jonas RA, et al. Development of a double-chambered right ventricle after repair of tetralogy of Fallot. J Am Coll Cardiol 31:1127, 1998.
80. Karl TR, Sano S, Pornviliwan S, et al. Tetralogy of Fallot: Favorable outcome of nonneonatal transatrial, transpulmonary repair. Ann Thorac Surg 54:903, 1992.
81. Alexiou C, Chen Q, Galogavrou M, et al. Repair of tetralogy of Fallot in infancy with a transventricular or a transatrial approach. Eur J Cardiothorac Surg 22:174, 2002.
82. Davlouros PA, Kilner PJ, Hornung TS, et al. Right ventricular function in adults with repaired tetralogy of Fallot assessed with cardiovascular magnetic resonance imaging: Detrimental role of right ventricular outflow aneurysms or akinesia and adverse right-to-left ventricular interaction. J Am Coll Cardiol 40:2044, 2002.
83. Wessel HU, Paul MH. Exercise studies in tetralogy of Fallot: A review. Pediatr Cardiol 20:39, 1999.
84. Eyskens B, Reybrouck T, Bogaert J, et al. Homograft insertion for pulmonary regurgitation after repair of tetralogy of Fallot improves cardiorespiratory exercise performance. Am J Cardiol 85:221, 2000.
85. Therrien J, Siu SC, McLaughlin PR, et al. Pulmonary valve replacement in adults late after repair of tetralogy of Fallot: Are we operating too late? J Am Coll Cardiol 36:1670, 2000.
86. Vliegen HW, van Straten A, de Roos A, et al. Magnetic resonance imaging to assess the hemodynamic effects of pulmonary valve replacement in adults late after repair of tetralogy of Fallot. Circulation 106:1703, 2002.
87. Alexander ME. Ventricular arrhythmias in children and young adults. In Walsh EP, Saul JP, Triedman JK, eds. Cardiac Arrhythmias in Children and Young Adults with Congenital Heart Disease. Philadelphia: Lippincott Williams & Wilkins, 2001:204.
88. Garson A, Jr., Gillette PC, Gutgesell HP, et al. Stress-induced ventricular arrhythmia after repair of tetralogy of Fallot. Am J Cardiol 46:1006, 1980.
89. Garson A Jr, Williams RB Jr, Reckless J. Long-term follow-up of patients with tetralogy of Fallot: Physical health and psychopathology. J Pediatr 85:429, 1974.

90. Clarkson PM, MacArthur BA, Barratt-Boyes BG, et al. Developmental progress after cardiac surgery in infancy using hypothermia and circulatory arrest. Circulation 62:855, 1980.
91. Shampaine EL, Nadelman L, Rosenthal A, et al. Longitudinal psychological assessment in tetralogy of Fallot. Pediatr Card 10:135, 1989.
92. Morris CD, Reller MD, Menashe VD Thirty-year incidence of infective endocarditis after surgery for congenital heart defect. JAMA 279:599, 1998.
93. Powell AJ, Lock JE, Keane JF, et al. Prolongation of RV-PA conduit life span by percutaneous stent implantation: Intermediate-term results. Circulation 92:3282, 1995.
94. Milanesi O, Talenti E, Pellegrino PA, et al. Abnormal pulmonary artery branching in tetralogy of Fallot with "absent" pulmonary valve. Int J Cardiol 6:375, 1984.

33

Aortic Outflow Abnormalities

John F. Keane and Donald C. Fyler

VALVAR AORTIC STENOSIS

Definition

Obstruction to outflow from the left ventricle by an abnormal aortic valve is described as valvar aortic stenosis.

Prevalence

Reported incidences of valvar aortic stenosis range from 0.04 to 0.38 per 1000 live births.[1–3] It accounted for some 31% of our patients with an aortic outflow abnormality[1] and for some 2% of our total patient population (Exhibit 33-1). This percentage increases with age, becoming by the third decade second only to ventricular septal defect. In most cases, it is associated with a congenitally deformed valve, particularly a bicuspid one, although a few children do have a tricuspid valve. Almost 80% of patients are male.[4]

Pathology

Anatomically, the normal aortic valve has three cusps (tricuspid) and three commissures (tricommissural). Interestingly, cusp sizes are rarely equal (less than 16%), enlargement of the right or noncoronary being the most common observation.[5] In young patients, a congenitally deformed but usually noncalcified mobile valve is almost always present, whereas almost half of elderly patients have very thick calcified immobile tricuspid valves.[6] In children, the most common aortic valve anomaly is a bicuspid (bicommissural) valve, with an incidence in the general population of 0.4% to 2.25%.[3,7,8] In young patients, the right–left commissure is most frequently absent (59%), with absence of the left noncommissure a rarity (less than 2%).[9,10] The two cusps are sometimes unequal in size, such that the valve orifice may be quite eccentric, even in the absence of obstruction; leaflet thickness is also variable, but calcification is very rare. Although stenosis and significant regurgitation are not present in some elderly patients, obstruction in young patients is common and is progressive in about 33% of cases.[4] Progression is likely related to increasing adhesion of remaining commissure margins and leaflet thickening. The more significant degrees of obstruction are seen where the right noncommissure is absent.[9,10] Bicuspid valves are frequently seen in association with other cardiac lesions, particularly left heart anomalies, especially coarctation (55%).[9] Valvar obstruction in neonates is discussed later in this chapter.

Physiology

The degree of obstruction is best expressed in terms of the pressure loss across the valve in systole. This is a mathematical relationship involving the ventricular pressure required to deliver the cardiac output at the required perfusion pressure.[11] With exercise, anemia, hyperthyroidism, or any other cause for increased cardiac output, the left ventricular pressure needed to produce increased output is proportionately higher.

During catheterization, the peak–peak gradient is measured across the aortic valve. This measurement has been considered for several decades the most precise indicator of severity and has been used as the basis for treatment. At catheterization in the sedated patient, this peak–peak ejection gradient is measured preferably from two catheters, one on either side of the aortic valve, or alternatively during withdrawal of a single catheter from ventricle to aorta while

Exhibit 33–1
Children's Hospital Boston Experience, 1988–2002
Aortic Outflow Lesions

Associated Outflow Abnormalities in 3299 Patients

Lesion	*Supravalvar AS (%)*	*Subvalvar AS (%)*		*AR (%)*	*Bicuspid Male Valve (%)*
Valvar AS (N = 1025)	3	9	69	64	72
Supravalvar AS (N = 134)		1041	1	51	
Subvalvar AS (N = 383)			50	5	62
AR (N = 1414)				11	57
Bicuspid valve (N = 310)					63
Root dilation (N = 33+)					76

Note: The total number of patients was (1) identified with left ventricular outflow tract abnormality, using the hierarchical system; (2) then divided into groups by first identifying those with valvar stenosis, followed by searching remainder for supravalvar stenosis, etc. (3) Each patient was counted only once; each group was then searched for associated outflow lesions, these expressed as % values. The large number (N) of patients with aortic regurgitation (AR) reflects sensitivity of echocardiography, 57% of whom had bicuspid valves, and included many others more distant in the hierarchic list with AR. Only 68 patients, almost all with minimal AR and without other cardiac abnormality, were identified, confirming the echocardiographic rarity of AR in normal hearts in contrast to the other cardiac valves.
Those in the bicuspid aortic valve group (N = 310) had neither aortic stenosis nor aortic regurgitation.
All lesions were more common in males.
Thirty-three patients had root dilation (mild in 32) alone, identified by echocardiography, 11 of whom had Kawasaki disease or a syndrome.
Endocarditis occurred in 38 patients: 20 in regurgitation group, 13 in valvar (prior balloon dilation) group, and 5 in subvalvar groups.

simultaneously measuring cardiac output. If the left ventricular pressure is compared with a simultaneous distal arterial pressure (such as a femoral artery), the gradient may be underestimated because the latter systolic value is often higher than the central aortic pressure; this phenomenon is known as the *standing wave effect* (Fig. 33-1).

In recent years, with the remarkable improvements in echocardiographic technology, measurement of obstruction is now done routinely by Doppler techniques. It is important to remember that in using Doppler, it is the maximal instantaneous gradient that is being recorded, usually in an unsedated patient, which is a different measurement than the peak–peak gradient measured in the sedated patient at catheterization. There is a tendency for this Doppler value to be used as the equivalent of the peak–peak gradient, which is an erroneous assumption. Indeed, investigators have shown this comparison to be unreliable, with instances of overestimation and underestimation being common.[12–17] Our own experience, including use of Doppler mean values is similar, although the latter is thought by some investigators to be reliable in adults.[18] Furthermore, instantaneous gradient values may differ in the same patient, depending on the transducer location. Various modifications, such as allowing for pressure recovery, have been studied with some improvement. Nevertheless, the instantaneous gradient measurement is a valuable parameter for use in serial follow-up studies and should be used in conjunction with other variables such as fractional shortening (hyperdynamic function is the usual finding in children), wall stress, and thickness (see Chapter 15).

The systemic arterial pressure is characterized by a smaller than normal pulse pressure. The small pulse of aortic stenosis (pulsus parvus) has stimulated many attempts to determine the severity of the aortic stenosis from the arterial pressure wave. Although this idea is solidly based in science and may be useful to a degree in adults, it is not reliable in children.

Clinical Manifestations

Usually, a child with valvar aortic stenosis is asymptomatic and is growing and developing normally but is discovered to have a heart murmur during a routine physical examination. Discovery of unexpected aortic stenosis in teenagers occurs occasionally, and the required examination of students participating in sports uncovers a few new patients each year.

Less commonly, a child complains of typical angina pectoris with exercise. In toddlers and small children, this symptom is not well articulated, yet sometimes a child is

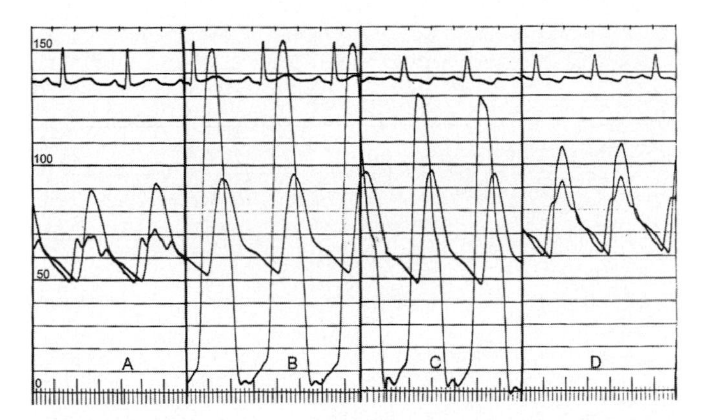

FIGURE 33–1 *Pressure recordings in a patient with valvar aortic stenosis. The numeric scale on the left is in millimeters of mercury (mmHg).* ***A****, Comparison of the pressure recorded from the ascending aorta with that in the femoral artery. Note that the pressure tracing is delayed in the femoral artery and is 20 mmHg higher in the femoral artery than in the ascending aorta ("standing wave"). This is an example of the standing wave effect (see Chapter 14).* ***B****, Comparison of the femoral artery pressure with the left ventricular pressure. Note that the gradient of pressure across the valve measures 60 mmHg but underestimates the true gradient (80 mmHg) by 20 mmHg.* ***C****, Comparison of the femoral artery pressure and the left ventricular pressure after balloon dilation of the aortic valve. Note that the pressure gradient is now smaller, the left ventricular systolic and end-diastolic pressures lower, and the arterial pulse pressure higher. The electrocardiogram now shows bundle branch block, a transitory phenomenon.* ***D****, Comparison of the ascending aorta and femoral artery pressures after dilation. Note that the pulse contour of the ascending aorta has changed: the pulse pressure is greater and the pressures are higher than in panel* ***A****.*
From Fyler DC [ed]. Nadas' Pediatric Cardiology. Philadelphia: Hanley & Belfus, 1992.

observed who suddenly stops and clutches the anterior chest during exercise. Fainting, very rare, is another ominous finding in these children; nevertheless, exercise intolerance is not a common symptom.

On physical examination, the child is well developed and well nourished. The peripheral pulses may be small and the measured pulse pressure less than normal. Often there is a systolic thrill in the suprasternal notch; with more severe stenosis, a thrill may be felt at the second right intercostal space. On auscultation, a constant systolic ejection click usually precedes the crescendo–decrescendo systolic murmur. The murmur is loudest at the second right interspace and is typically stenotic. It transmits well into the neck (Fig. 33-2).

Because ventricular systole is prolonged proportionate to the severity of aortic stenosis, the aortic component at the second heart sound is delayed, producing a narrowly split second heart sound, sometimes with the aortic closure

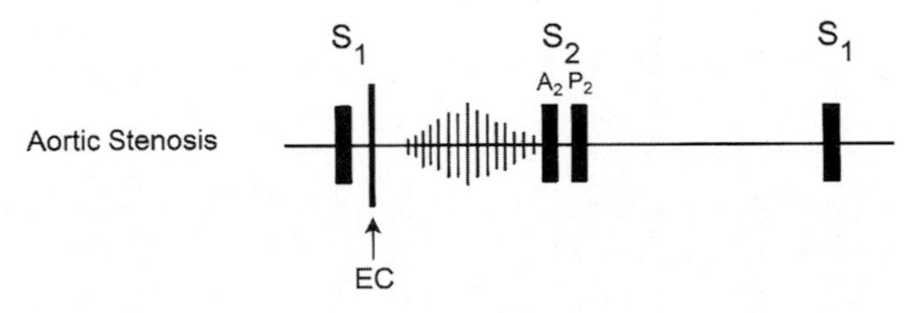

FIGURE 33–2 *Diagram of the ejection murmur of valvar aortic stenosis. Note the early systolic ejection click (EC) characteristic of valvar aortic stenosis. The crescendo–decrescendo murmur reaches peak intensity in mid-systole.*
From Fyler DC [ed]. Nadas' Pediatric Cardiology. Philadelphia: Hanley & Belfus, 1992.

appearing after pulmonary closure (reverse splitting). Similar to left bundle branch block, verification of this phenomenon requires phonocardiography.

Because aortic regurgitation is commonly associated with aortic stenosis, there may be an early diastolic regurgitant murmur as well (Fig. 33-3).

Electrocardiography

The electrocardiogram is not a reliable indicator of obstruction severity other than (1) being almost always normal when the catheterization measured gradient is less than 25 mmHg and (2) abnormalities including increased left ventricular voltages, decreased right anterior forces, and T-wave changes being more likely when the gradient is at least 80 mmHg (Fig. 33-4). In conjunction with physical examination findings, it has some use in identifying small gradients, although the murmur intensity heavily influences the equation.[4]

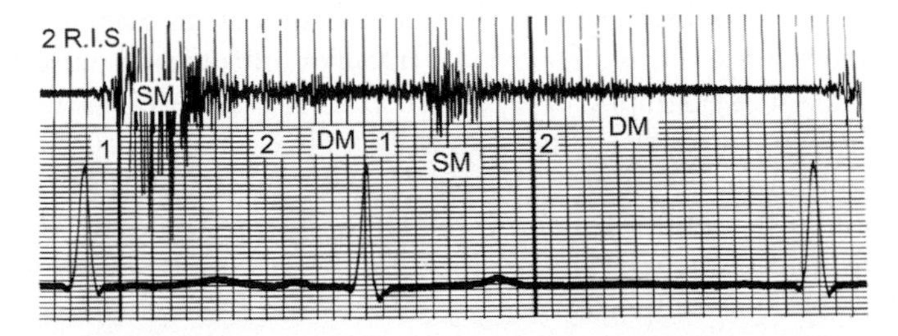

FIGURE 33–3 *Phonocardiogram of the murmurs present in a patient with valvar aortic stenosis and regurgitation. Note the diamond-shaped systolic murmur peaking in early to mid-systole and the high-frequency, lower-intensity murmur throughout diastole. 2RIS, second right intercostal space; SM, systolic murmur; DM, diastolic murmur; 1, first heart sound, 2, second heart sound.*
From Fyler DC [ed]. Nadas' Pediatric Cardiology. Philadelphia: Hanley & Belfus, 1992.

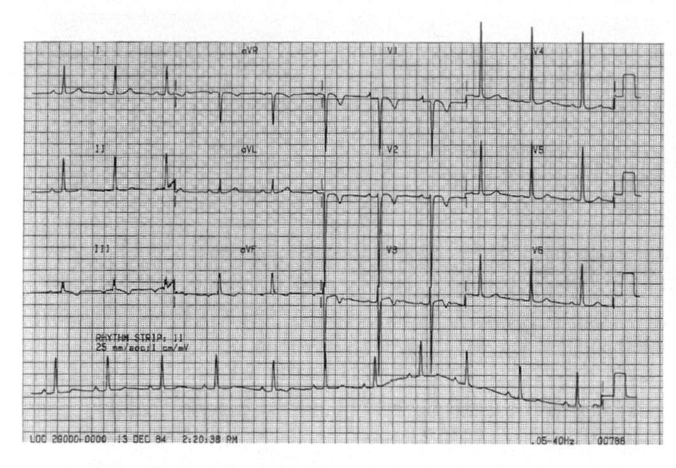

FIGURE 33–4 *Electrocardiogram from a 10-year-old boy, with peak–peak gradient of 107 mm across the aortic valve, showing marked left ventricular hypertrophy by voltage criteria and the significantly diminished anterior forces (V_1, V_2) commonly seen in pressure overload lesions.*

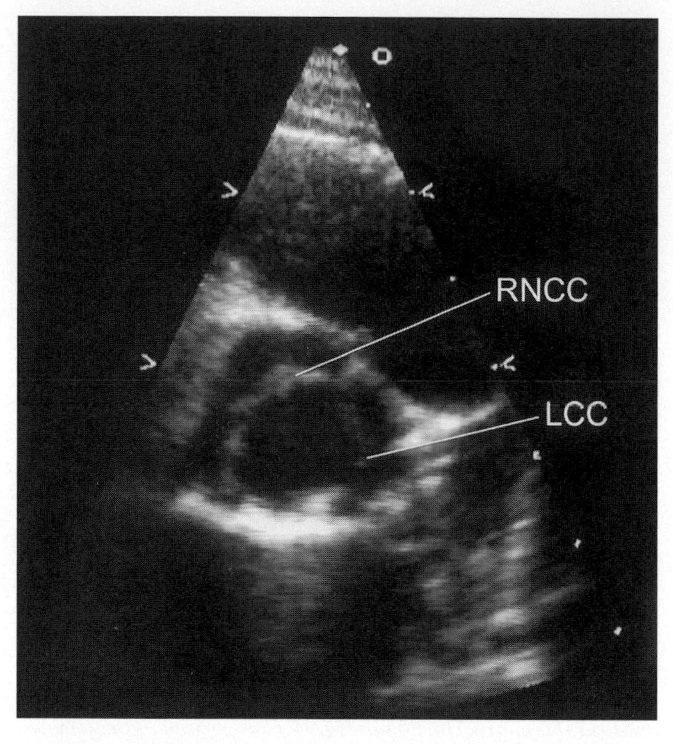

FIGURE 33–5 *Parasternal short-axis echocardiogram of a bicommissural aortic valve with fusion of the right nonaortic commissure. LCC, left coronary cusp; RNCC, right noncoronary cusp; PA, pulmonary artery.*

Chest X-Ray

The heart size (except in small infants in congestive heart failure) is usually normal; because of poststenotic dilation, the ascending aorta is often visible.

Echocardiography

The number, mobility, and thickening of aortic leaflets; size of the ascending aorta; and maximum instantaneous gradient across the valve are all readily achievable. Ventricular function, wall stress, and hypertrophy information is also available (see Chapter 15). Leaflet thickness, mobility, and annular diameter at the hinge points are best evaluated in the long axis view, whereas commissural anatomy is best seen in the short-axis view. In diastole, most aortic valves appear to be trileaflet (or tricuspid), just like on angiography. If a commissure is present, the valve leaflets separate all the way to the valve annulus, but if commissural fusion is present, separation is incomplete, and a raphe can be seen connecting the more peripheral aspects of the adjacent leaflets (Fig. 33-5).

Absence of the right–left commissure is more common than the right coronary–noncoronary commissure, whereas absence of the left coronary–noncoronary commissure is extremely rare.[9]

Regurgitation is seen best in apical or parasternal long-axis views, using color-flow Doppler mapping or pulsed Doppler examination. Quantification of the regurgitation degree is very useful and is based on the diameter of the flow jet at the level of the valve seen by color-flow Doppler mapping, the size of the left ventricle, and the Doppler flow pattern in the descending aorta (see Chapter 13). The instantaneous gradient is evaluated using pulsed or continuous-wave Doppler examination, with the transducer located in the apex, the right sternal border, or the suprasternal notch (recognizing that values may well be different in the same patient), and using sedation in the very young.

Stress Testing

Maximal exercise testing can be a useful procedure. Because the end points of angina, syncope, and changes in the ST segment and T wave are positive outcomes, exercise testing in patients who already have these changes does not add useful information. In asymptomatic patients with normal, borderline, or suspicious findings, especially in those thought to have little obstruction who want to engage in physical activities, a stress test may be very valuable. Significant obstruction may be present if ST-segment and T-wave changes occur.

Cardiac Catheterization

Cardiac catheterization is almost always undertaken to dilate valvar obstruction and only rarely for hemodynamic reasons only. The indications for cardiac catheterization include the following:

1. An echocardiographic maximum instantaneous pressure gradient of 60 mmHg or more is an indication for cardiac catheterization and probable dilation of the valve.
2. Given a lesser echo-Doppler gradient in an asymptomatic child who has no changes in the ST segment and T wave, the decision to catheterize is based on the amount of left ventricular hypertrophy on echocardiography, the intensity of the murmur, and the clinician's estimate of the child's physical activity (a "couch potato" is one type, whereas a weight-lifting, backyard athlete is another).
3. A fainting episode in a patient who has aortic stenosis requires serious consideration of cardiac catheterization. Clearly, if the echo-Doppler evaluation indicates mild obstruction, a search for other causes of syncope is needed; but none being found, fainting, in the presence of aortic stenosis, is a signal for further study and probable therapy. Episodes of feeling dizzy or faint without actual syncope are also encountered and similarly require careful evaluation.
4. Anginal pain that is convincing has the same significance as syncope.
5. Changes in the ST segment and T wave, either on routine follow-up electrocardiograms or during stress tests, requires cardiac catheterization.
6. Because ventricular ectopy further complicates the delivery of cardiac output through an obstructive valve, and may otherwise be a signal of left ventricular impairment, the tendency to intervene is increased when ectopy is present.

The peak–peak pressure gradient across the valve is a precise measure of the degree of obstruction, provided the cardiac output is not depressed. The measured gradient determines whether a balloon angioplasty should be carried out and is usually done if the peak–peak gradient is more than 50 mmHg and aortic regurgitation, if present, is mild at most.

Contrast injected in the mid ascending aorta in the anteroposterior and lateral views outlines the aortic valve, degree of aortic regurgitation if any, and the jet of unopacified blood being ejected through the valve from the left ventricle. Anatomic valve information is also provided; for example, in those with absence of the intercoronary commissure, the most common bicuspid valve anomaly, the conjoined cusp in the lateral view is visible as a continuous band of contrast undivided by a commissure when the valve is open in systole (Fig. 33-6). For measurement of the valve annulus for proposed valve dilation, this is done from a long axial oblique projection with contrast injection in the left ventricle.

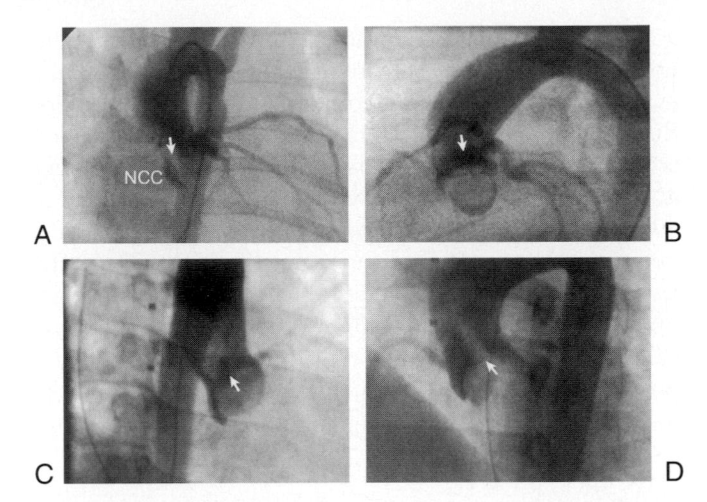

FIGURE 33–6 *Biplane aortic cineangiograms, during ventricular systole, in two children with bicuspid stenotic valves: (1) Absent R-L commissure:* ***A****, Frontal projection showing presence of right noncoronary cusp (NCC) commissure (arrow).* ***B****, Lateral projection showing absence of R-L commissure, identified by solid bar of contrast (arrow) extending the entire width of the common cusp. (2) Absent N-R commissure.* ***C****, Right anterior oblique projection showing solid bar of contrast (arrow) extending across common cusp.* ***D****, Long axial oblique projection showing presence of right–left commissure (arrow); absence of the non–left cusp commissure is extremely rare.*

Management

In marked contrast to pulmonary valvar stenosis, which is easily diagnosed, quantitated, and treated and is essentially free of endocarditis, valvar aortic stenosis is a difficult entity to treat and requires lifelong attention. It is progressive, may be associated with catastrophic incidents such as sudden death, is likely to require repeated interventions, and is a common site of endocarditis. Calcification with age is common, and regurgitation may become a significant problem, as may left ventricular dysfunction, all problems related to its location in the systemic circuit.

Excluding infants in heart failure, it is reasonable to use the severity categories of peak–peak catheterization gradients as outlined in the original Natural History Study as guides to management.[4] These groups consisted of those with gradients of less than 25 mmHg, 25 to 49 mmHg, 50 to 79 mmHg, and greater than 80 mmHg—all require strict endocarditis prophylaxis. For those with a stable gradient of less than 25 mmHg and normal electrocardiogram and stress test, no restriction on physical activities seems reasonable. For those with a 25- to 49-mmHg gradient and normal electrocardiogram and stress test, strenuous competitive level activities should be avoided. Annual evaluations should be done for both groups. For all others, that is with gradients greater than 50 mmHg, intervention is indicated. In earlier years, before balloon valvotomy, a surgical valvotomy was always done for a gradient of 80 mmHg or more, with management strategy varying between institutions for values ranging from 50 to 79 mmHg. In the latter, however, better results at follow-up were evident in those managed surgically.[4] Thus, when balloon valvotomy became available as an alternative to surgery, a peak–peak gradient of 50 mmHg or more, in the absence of more than mild aortic regurgitation, became an indicator for intervention. In many institutions in the United States and other countries, this has replaced surgery as the initial procedure in these patients (Exhibit 33-2). By and large, this approach has been quite effective in that a peak–peak gradient reduction of at least 50% is usual. However, aortic regurgitation has been common, and although mild in most cases, significant incompetence has occurred immediately in some 13%, and in about 38% after 4 years of follow-up. Overall survival rate is 95% at 8 years,[19] comparable to that in some other reports.[20] Results from surgical series of mixed ages, most from earlier years, have been similar.[21–24] In terms of balloon equipment, considerable improvement has continued, such that arterial access

Exhibit 33–2
Children's Hospital Boston Experience
Valvar Aortic Stenosis

Treatment	*1973–1987 N (%)*	*1988–2002 N (%)*
Surgery	126 (65)	7 (3)
Balloon dilation	68 (35)	228 (97)

Balloon Dilation 1988–2002 (228 patients)

	< 1 mo	*1–6 mo*	*6–12 mo*	*1–5 yr*	*5–10 yr*	*>10 yr*
No. of patients	61	50	12	30	26	49
Catheterization-related death (≤48 hr)	2*	0	0	0	0	0

*The only deaths occurred (≤1991) in two neonates (3%): both had critical obstruction, end-diastolic pressures ≥24 mmHg, and severe ventricular dysfunction and were receiving prostaglandins. One of the deaths was related to atrial perforation and tamponade.

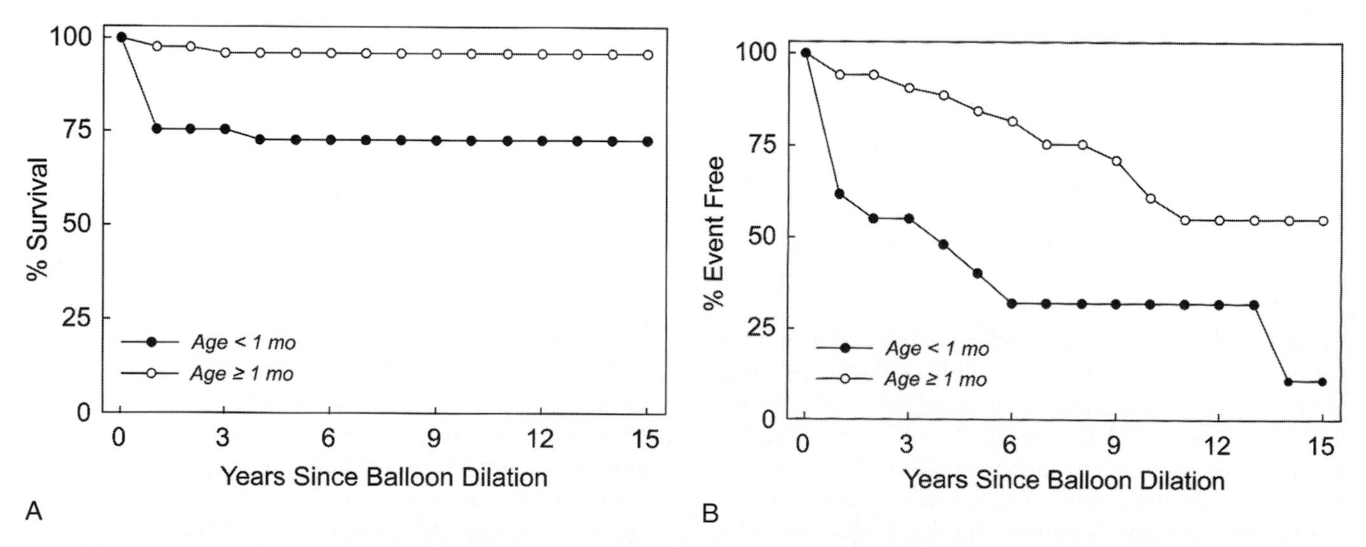

Life tables (A) survival and (B) event-free (surgery, repeat balloon dilation) in those treated initially with balloon dilation by age, showing not unexpectedly better results in those beyond the neonatal period.
Overall, 31 patients have undergone redilation (more than twice in 14); 21 patients (9%) have required surgery (18 of these for regurgitation).

problems are considerably less than they were a decade ago. The effectiveness of balloon dilation is a miracle in itself when one considers that a balloon is being inflated across the usually eccentrically located orifice of a valve whose leaflets vary in both thickness and commissural fusion. Clearly, the weakest site in the orifice "rim" will be the first to tear or separate, whether it be commissure or a leaflet at its free margin edge or its attachment site to the aorta. Indeed, the latter is a frequent observation at later surgery for regurgitation, the detachment frequently being anteriorly located. Nevertheless, balloon dilation will likely remain, at least for the foreseeable future, the initial treatment of choice for significant valvar stenoses given the reasonable results, very short hospital stay, and absence of both a sternotomy scar and cardiopulmonary bypass.

Balloon dilation, however, is largely ineffective in adults,[25] in whom valves are by then often deformed and calcified. Replacement (by prosthesis or Ross procedure) is usually necessary, especially if accompanied by moderate or more regurgitation.

Aortic valvar abnormalities are particularly prone to endocarditis requiring meticulous prophylaxis.[26,27]

Course

The likelihood that progressive obstruction will have occurred by late adult life is very high, even in those with a less than 25-mmHg gradient to begin with. In the pediatric years, significant progression in the Natural History Study occurred in one third of all patients managed medically.[4] The 25-year survival rate for all patients was 85%, 92% for those with initial gradients of less than 50 mmHg, and 80% for those greater. By 25 years, only 60% of medically managed patients remained intervention free, and 60% of the surgically treated patients had undergone reoperation. Sudden death was a rare event, occurring in 25 patients (5%) during the study period. Of these, 75% were postoperative patients, all with significant obstruction, regurgitation, or both; one younger than age 10 years was catheterization related; most were older than 20 years; and one fourth were related to endocarditis. This was, of course, a population studied and operated on between 1958 and 1979, since when surgical and other techniques have improved greatly.

Residual or recurrent obstruction with at most mild regurgitation in pediatric years can be managed by surgical valvotomy[28] or balloon dilation, the latter being both repeatable and effective[29,30] (Fig. 33-7). In later years, valve replacement becomes necessary in many using tissue or prosthetic devices or the patient's transplanted pulmonary valve (Ross procedure). The latter requires replacement of the transplanted pulmonary valve by a homograft from right ventricle to pulmonary artery.

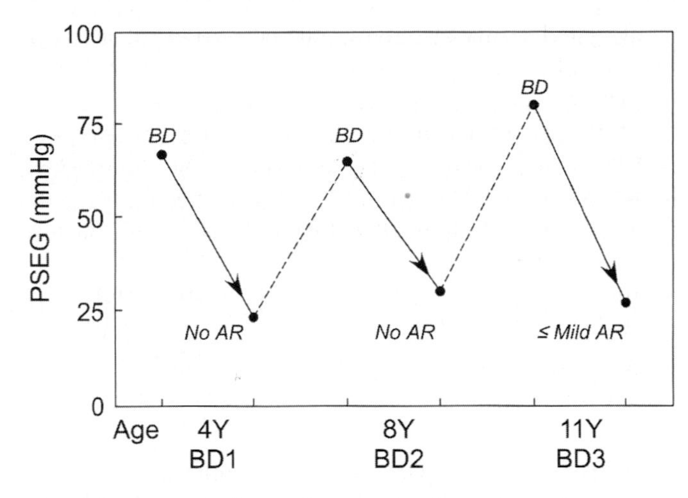

FIGURE 33–7 *Balloon dilation (BD) performed on three occasions in a patient with recurrent obstruction at ages 4, 8, and 11 years for peak–peak gradients of at least 70 mmHg, each followed by reduction to about 25 mmHg with only mild, at most, regurgitation after the final procedure.*

Results have varied from excellent in some series[31,32] to others with problems, as has been our own experience.[33,34] Prosthetic devices requiring anticoagulation are avoided when possible in women of childbearing age. Significant regurgitation usually requires valve replacement, except in those cases related to balloon dilation, in which a valve plasty can be effective for some years.[35]

Exercise intolerance is not a common symptom and is rarely a factor in deciding management questions. In contrast, stress tests do uncover patients who are prone to arrhythmias and changes in the ST segment and T wave during maximal exercise, an observation that should be taken seriously.[36]

Rhythm abnormalities, at rest or on exercise, are encountered[36,37] and are taken as a sign of ventricular dysfunction, and sometimes influence the decision to intervene.

Abnormalities in ventricular function tests, volume measurements, shortening fractions, and other indices (see Chapter 15) should be taken seriously, particularly if a pattern of deterioration is documented in the course of follow-up.

To control the problems associated with aortic stenosis, the following steps should be taken:

1. The average patient with valvar aortic stenosis should be seen at least annually to have an electrocardiogram and echocardiogram. Follow-up is a lifetime commitment and, for most patients, requires visits to the cardiologist when there are, in fact, no symptoms or limitations.
2. In the absence of ST-T changes and with more than minimal obstruction by echocardiography, maximal

exercise tolerance testing should be carried out at 2-year intervals.

3. *Infective endocarditis* is a serious threat, occurring 27.1 times per 10,000 patient-years,[26] and strict prophylaxis is mandatory. Of the 38 instances of endocarditis involving the left heart outflow, 33 occurred in patients with valvar lesions at Children's Hospital Boston (see Exhibit 33-1).
4. Risk for *sudden death* hangs over the head of all patients with aortic stenosis, but it is mainly a threat to those with symptoms, especially those with abnormalities in the S-T segment and T wave and significant valvar disease.[22]

Vigorous exercise, particularly in competitive sports, is associated with sudden death and because of this should be prohibited in those with more than mild obstruction (more than 25 mmHg peak-to-peak), particularly if there is any evidence of changes in the ST segment and T wave, whether or not valvuloplasty has been carried out. This can be a particularly difficult problem because many of these children are well-developed, physically able boys, who sometimes are excellent athletes. For some, in the interest of the child's self-image, some sports, such as baseball and other less violent activities, are permitted. The best outcome results when the parents redesign the child's physical activities and promote a less vigorous type of life while the boy is still prepubertal. This is easier said than done, and when siblings are athletically inclined, especially older siblings, compromises are the only recourse, and sooner or later a rebellious teenager will drop dead.

Avoiding the problem of sudden death while maintaining a healthy psychological outlook is the goal. Obtaining the best compromise with the individual patient is a matter of understanding the family, the child, and the physiology of the cardiac problem.

Infant Aortic Stenosis

Infants with critical valvar aortic stenosis constitute a special group with maximal aortic valve obstruction. A murmur may have been noticed at birth and, indeed, the diagnosis of aortic stenosis may have already been made by fetal echocardiography. Congestive failure develops in the first weeks of life and, very rapidly, a life-threatening situation evolves. It is important to remember that some of these infants initially in the first few days of life look very well and seem to be tolerating some obstruction even with what seems a moderate, at most, instantaneous gradient of less than 30 mmHg. Such gradients may increase greatly within weeks, perhaps related to left ventricular function becoming hyperdynamic and lesions such as patent ductus and muscular ventricular defects spontaneously closing (Fig. 33-8).

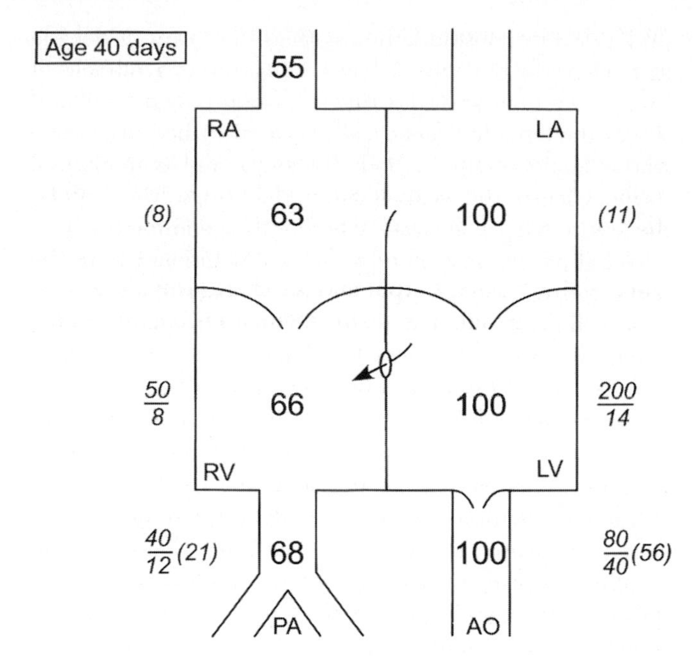

FIGURE 33–8 *Catheterization data in a 40-day-old boy showing a peak–peak ejection gradient of 120 mmHg. An echocardiographic study at age 2 days revealed a maximum instantaneous gradient of 30 mmHg, normal ventricular function, and a moderate muscular ventricular septal defect that had become tiny.*

The valves in these infants are notable, sometimes appearing as gelatinous blobs of tissue unrecognizable as leaflets (Fig. 33-9). The left ventricle may be quite small, and for some infants, it is too small to be compatible with life. A newborn ventricle that can accommodate a maximal volume of 20 mL is borderline in its ability to support life. Because of left ventricular failure, acquired mitral regurgitation,

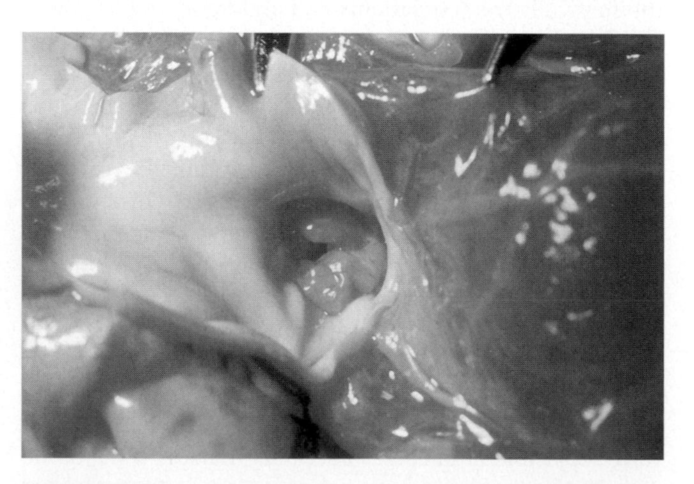

FIGURE 33–9 *Autopsy picture of a nodular primitive-looking critically obstructive valve in a 4-week-old baby who died suddenly at home, undiagnosed. Such valves with survival can mature to become typically bicuspid structures.*

and gross elevation of left atrial pressures, the foramen ovale becomes incompetent, and atrial left-to-right shunting adds to the problems, further aggravating congestive heart failure. Shunting right to left through the ductus arteriosus is helpful in this situation because it supplies some cardiac output that does not have to pass through the aortic valve. Thus, in the most critical situation, administration of prostaglandin E_1 opens the ductus, thereby augmenting cardiac output and stabilizing the infant.

On physical examination, the infant is in congestive heart failure, sometimes in shock, and is ashen and pulseless. Most have an apical ejection click and a systolic murmur. The intensity of the ejection murmur depends on left ventricular function status and indeed may be absent in those with extremely poor function. Many have a murmur of mitral regurgitation due to ventricular dysfunction. The electrocardiogram shows right or left ventricular hypertrophy with changes in the ST segment and T wave (Fig. 33-10). The chest x-ray shows an enlarged heart with pulmonary edema on echocardiography. On echocardiography, the obstructed, usually very thickened aortic valve is well seen, as is any mitral regurgitation, atrial left-to-right shunting, right-to-left shunting at the ductal level, and any aortic arch abnormality. The degree of stenosis can be estimated and related to left ventricular function. Importantly, the adequacy of left ventricular volume can be determined as to whether it is of sufficient size to supply a systemic cardiac output.[38]

Catheterization in these infants, often intubated and being administered prostaglandin E_1, for the past two decades has been carried out as a therapeutic procedure, that is, for balloon dilation. From a historical standpoint, surgical valvotomy was introduced almost four decades ago because medical management had had a universally fatal outcome.[39] Within a decade, it was apparent that only a limited valvotomy, that is, modestly enlarging the orifice, was necessary to achieve excellent early clinical results, including significantly decreasing the incidence of severe aortic regurgitation, often a result of the early extensive valvotomies. It was also noted that at later repeat surgical valvotomy, the originally immature nodular and myxomatous-appearing valves had usually evolved into valves with a more typical bicuspid appearance.[40] Balloon dilation was later introduced as an alternative management strategy,[41] and using the surgical approach of limited valvotomy, smaller balloons with an average balloon-to-annular ratio of 0.8 were used with satisfactory results.[42] Balloon technology has improved considerably over the years, with much lower profiles and sizes becoming available. With balloon dilation, the major immediate changes at catheterization indicating success are significant decreases in left ventricular systolic, diastolic, and atrial pressures and peak–peak gradient (about 50%) (Fig. 33-11). These are followed by rapid extubation, an excellent clinical course, significant improvement in mitral regurgitation, and disappearance of atrial-level shunts.

The survival rate is at least 75% at 8 years, with about one third requiring redilation for obstruction: some 11% have significant regurgitation.[43] In some, initially hypoplastic aortic annuli and left ventricular chambers on echocardiography normalize during follow-up.[43] Occasionally, the annular size measured angiographically in the right anterior oblique view is greater than that in the long-axis view (also the echocardiographic view used for measurement),

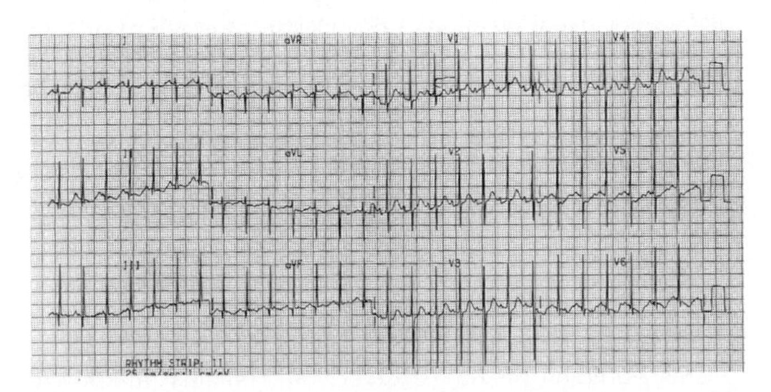

FIGURE 33–10 *Electrocardiogram from 10-day-old boy with critical aortic valvar stenosis with a peak–peak systolic ejection gradient of 90 mmHg showing left ventricular hypertrophy with strain, especially in leads V_5 and V_6.*

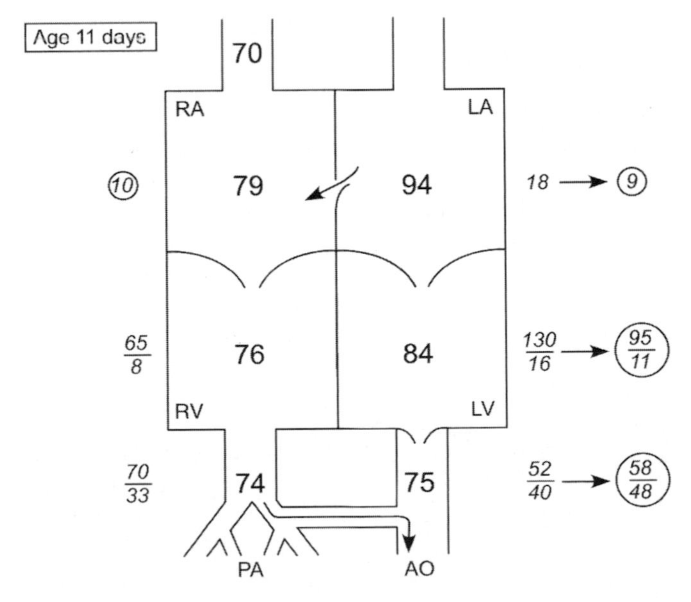

FIGURE 33–11 *Catheterization data in an 11-day-old neonate with critical aortic valvar obstruction who underwent balloon dilation through an umbilical arterial retrograde approach, showing marked immediate reduction (numbers with arrows and circled) in gradient, left ventricular systolic and diastolic, and left atrial pressures.*

suggesting compression of the left heart outflow by the enlarged hypertensive right heart structures. A similar approach has been used by others,[44,45] with results comparable to those of surgical valvotomy in other series.[46] During follow-up in some, membranous progressive subaortic obstruction necessitating surgery occurs.

SUBAORTIC STENOSIS

Definition

Obstruction to outflow from the left ventricle beneath the aortic valve in the presence of two adequate-sized ventricles is called *subaortic stenosis*.

Prevalence

Subaortic stenosis is rarely recognized in the newborn period but is common in infancy and childhood. It is often associated with other lesions, such as ventricular septal defect, coarctation of the aorta, interrupted aortic arch (see Chapter 36), double-chambered right ventricle, and atrioventricular canal. Isolated subaortic stenosis accounted for some 10% of our patients with an aortic outflow abnormality (see Exhibit 33-1).

Pathology

There are four types of subvalvar aortic stenosis (Fig. 33-12).

Discrete Type

The most common form is a discrete, thin, fibromuscular ridge or membrane located at a variable distance beneath the aortic valve, sometimes so close to the valve that the obstructing tissue is difficult to distinguish from the valve itself. Although the term *membranous subaortic stenosis* is occasionally used, this can be misleading because the obstructing tissue usually has some thickness. The opening may be eccentric. Often, there is deformity of the aortic valve (usually tricuspid) caused by the jet of blood passing through the subvalvar obstruction, with resulting aortic regurgitation. The part of the obstruction situated beneath the left coronary cusp, which is frequently attached to the anterior leaflet of the mitral valve, causes the characteristic fluttering and thickening of that leaflet as seen on echocardiography and angiography. The obstruction itself is variable in that a complete circumferential ring is not always present. Indeed, with the advent of echocardiography, small nonobstructive localized protuberances from the region of the membranous septum are frequently identified and are of uncertain significance. Downstream cardiac defects that obstruct blood flow, such as interrupted aortic arch and severe coarctation, are common and sometimes are associated with a membranous ventricular septal defect or a mitral valve deformity. Severe subvalvar obstruction is a great rarity in neonates: however, progression during childhood is well recognized, this also noted decades ago in Newfoundland dogs.[47]

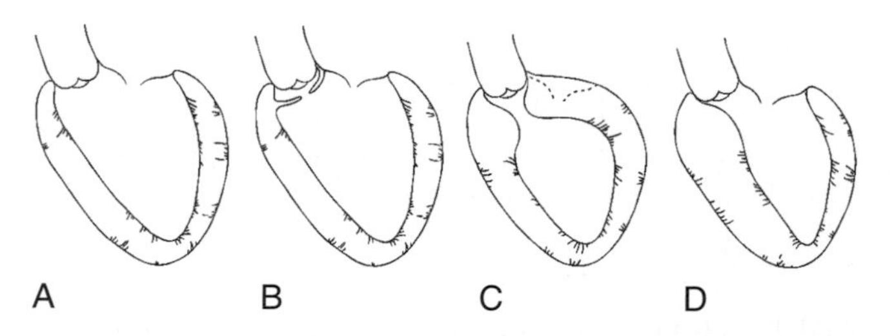

FIGURE 33–12 *Drawings illustrating three types of subaortic stenosis:* ***A****, normal;* ***B****, membranous;* ***C****, fibromuscular tunnel;* ***D****, hypertrophic cardiomyopathy with subaortic obstruction. From Fyler DC [ed]. Nadas' Pediatric Cardiology. Philadelphia: Hanley & Belfus, 1992.*

Tunnel Type

The rarer fibromuscular tunnel has greater length, often affecting 1 cm or more of the outflow tract. Because of its length, or perhaps contributing to it, the anterior leaflet of the mitral valve is often involved, a feature of some significance at the time of surgical correction.

Hypertrophic Subaortic Stenosis

Cardiomyopathy of the idiopathic hypertrophic variety often produces clinically important subaortic obstruction, often solely due to muscle but sometimes involving the anterior leaflet of the mitral valve (see Chapter 24).

Accessory Endocardial Cushion Tissue

Rarely, tissue presumed to be derived from the embryologic endocardial cushions may obstruct the left ventricular outflow tract. It may be attached to a pedicle or act as a sail or sheet across the outflow tract, moving with cardiac contraction and the flow of blood.

Subaortic stenosis is commonly associated with a wide range of other cardiac defects, particularly ventricular septal defect and coarctation (Exhibit 33-3).

Pathogenesis

The etiology of the obstruction remains unknown, but echocardiographic abnormalities of the outflow tract, such as separation of aortic and mitral valve annuli, acute angulation of ventricular septal and ascending aortic axes, and aortic override have been described in these patients.

Exhibit 33–3

Children's Hospital Boston Experience, 1988–2002

Treatment of Supravalvar, Subvalvar Stenosis

Type	*Surgery*	*OP Mortality*	*Reoperation*
Supravalvar (N)	25	0	0
Subvalvar (N)	61	0	3

In the subvalvar group of 61 patients, 3 are known to have been reoperated on for obstruction, representing 8% of those 37 operated on in the first decade of life (N, patient number).

Associated Defects*	
Supravalvar Stenosis (N)	
Pulmonary stenosis	141
Coarctation of aorta	58
Williams syndrome	42
Other	67
Total	308
Subvalvar Stenosis (N)	
Ventricular septal defect	222
Coarctation of aorta	183
Endocardial cushion defect	166
Double-outlet right ventricle	102
D-transposition of great arteries	86
Other	219
Total	1078

*Each patient counted only once and identified by searching entire database.
N, patient number.

These have also been identified before the development of obstruction in some with additional lesions such as coarctation or ventricular septal defect.[48]

Physiology

The physiologic abnormalities are comparable to those seen in valvar aortic stenosis, except that subaortic stenosis is almost never severe enough to cause congestive heart failure in infancy, at least as an isolated lesion. The associated aortic regurgitation is rarely severe in children preoperatively, and indeed significant regurgitation (some 14% of all patients) is largely confined to those who have had surgical or balloon angioplasty procedures.[49] A practical, yet difficult, physiologic problem is the absence of a gradient across the subaortic stenosis when the ductus arteriosus supplies the distal systemic circulation. In this framework, subaortic stenosis may be severe without a significant gradient. Echocardiography has helped greatly in identifying such rare patients, who in the past may have first had interruption of the ductus arteriosus, which then unmasked the subaortic obstruction.

Clinical Manifestations

Isolated subaortic stenosis produces a stenotic systolic murmur that often has a characteristic "shrieking" quality at the mid left sternal border. Usually, there is no systolic click; some patients have an early diastolic blowing murmur of aortic regurgitation. The peripheral pulses are rarely thought of as small, and congestive heart failure resulting from isolated subaortic stenosis is virtually nonexistent.

Electrocardiography

The electrocardiogram usually shows left ventricular hypertrophy in proportion to the degree of obstruction. Mild obstruction produces no abnormality, whereas severe obstruction results in left ventricular hypertrophy with changes in the ST segments and T waves.

Chest X-Ray

The isolated form of subaortic stenosis is not characterized by cardiac enlargement or enlargement of the ascending aorta. Finding an abnormality on the chest x-ray is unusual unless there are associated defects.

Echocardiography

Two-dimensional echocardiography, together with Doppler studies, is the standard diagnostic tool. The anatomy of the lesion is clearly outlined (Fig. 33-13), as is ventricular function. The amount of ventricular muscle hypertrophy is usually proportional to the degree of obstruction, the latter measured as a maximum instantaneous gradient. Fluttering of the left coronary cusp due to the jet across the obstruction is usual, as is leaflet thickening. Aortic regurgitation, present in most and usually mild or less, is evident on color-flow Doppler. Any associated lesions, common, are also outlined.

Cardiac Catheterization

Cardiac catheterization provides a reliable measurement of the peak–peak pressure gradient across the outflow tract of the left ventricle in the sedated patient (Fig. 33-14). This gradient is generally less, sometimes by as much as 50%, than instantaneous gradients of less than 50 mmHg. Because anatomic information is echocardiographically readily available, the only reason for catheterization is for gradient measurement for management decisions. If angiography is carried out, a right anterior oblique with 20 degrees of caudal angulation (Fig. 33-15) and simultaneous long-axis oblique views provide excellent visualization.

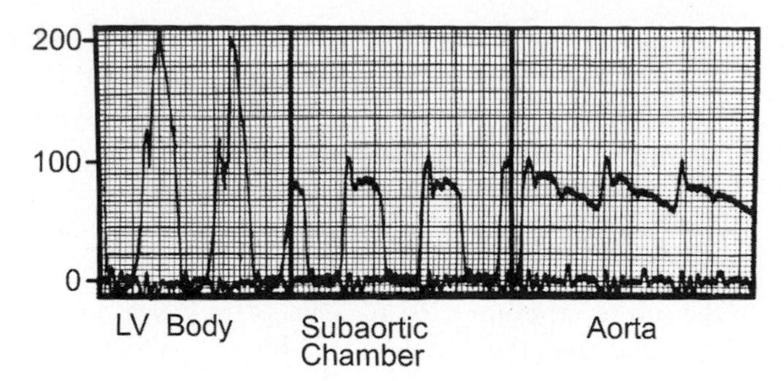

FIGURE 33–14 *Pressure recorded during withdrawal of a catheter from the left ventricle to the aorta in a patient with subaortic stenosis. Note that as the catheter passes the obstructed area, the left ventricular pressure falls; only when it is withdrawn across the aortic valve does a typical arterial pressure contour appear. Sometimes, the space between the subvalvar obstruction and the aortic valve is so small that this type of tracing cannot be recorded.*
From Fyler DC [ed]. Nadas' Pediatric Cardiology. Philadelphia: Hanley & Belfus, 1992.

Management

In the patient with uncomplicated discrete membranous obstruction, surgical treatment is more effective than in the patient with valvar aortic stenosis. Balloon dilation, on the other hand, is ineffective. Thus, because obstruction is progressive in many, and because aortic regurgitation at some point is common, surgical treatment is recommended for a lower peak–peak gradient than for valvar obstruction (30 mmHg versus 50 mmHg).[50] Because the echocardiographically measured instantaneous gradient commonly exceeds the peak–peak value obtained at catheterization (at a different date in a sedated patient), it is reasonable to assume that a catheterization value of 30 mmHg is similar to an instantaneous value of 50 mmHg. Thus, an

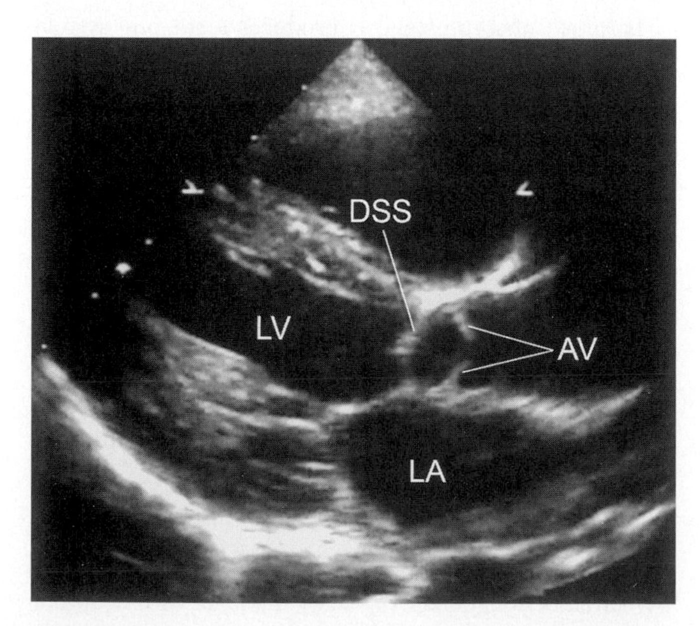

FIGURE 33–13 *Parasternal long-axis echocardiogram of discrete subaortic stenosis (DSS) located just below the aortic valve (AV). LV, left ventricle; LA, left atrium.*

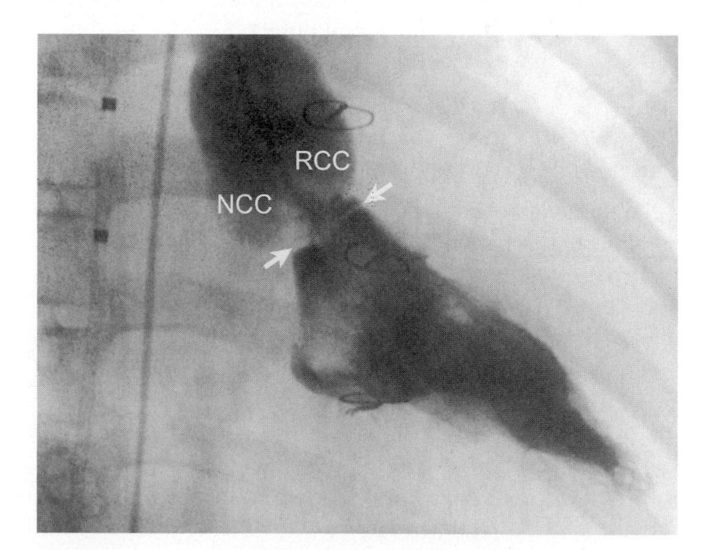

FIGURE 33–15 *Left ventricular cineangiogram in a 9-year-old boy in a right anterior oblique view showing a discrete subaortic membrane (arrows). This had developed since he underwent surgical valve plasty 6 years earlier. RCC, right coronary cusp; NCC,noncoronary cusps.*

instantaneous value exceeding this is used as an indicator for surgery. Because obstruction recurs in some 20% postoperatively,[50–54] patients with instantaneous gradients less than 50 mmHg without other indicators can be followed medically. In one author's (JFK) experience, recurrences are more frequent in those operated on in the first decade of life—perhaps this reflects more significant obstruction initially in these patients. However, some who underwent surgery for peak–peak gradients less than 30 mmHg again had significant obstruction by age 10 years, which was anatomically similar to the preoperative lesion. Although aortic regurgitation commonly develops preoperatively, it is mild in most cases[47,55]; hence, using prevention of regurgitation as the main surgical indicator, especially when the gradient is low, is not warranted.[56]

Echocardiography provides other excellent valuable information, such as muscle thickness and function, all of which should be included in the management decision.

Surgical techniques have changed over the years from simple membrane excision alone to more extensive obstruction removal, including myomectomy. Indeed, the lesion is commonly more than just a thin membrane. Occasionally, in the past, excision of tissue from the anterior leaflet of the mitral valve resulted in perforation of that structure and septal muscle excision resulted in conduction difficulties. In those with more diffuse tunnel-like obstructions, more extensive procedures, such as Ross and Konno or modifications thereof, may be necessary.[57–60]

Subaortic obstruction due to **accessory endocardial tissue** is a very rare entity, encountered by us about once every 2 years. Currently, this entity is identified by echocardiography. Associated cardiac lesions such as tetralogy of Fallot and coarctation occur in some. Echocardiographically, the most common appearance is that of a parachute-like structure appearing in the outflow tract during systole (Fig. 33-16). The degree of obstruction is quite variable. Anatomically, the tissue has a number of attachments to the mitral valve leaflets or papillary muscles. At surgery, the lesion is removed through the aortic valve with elimination of obstruction.[61]

Course

Although discrete obstruction is known to progress in many young patients, a substantial number of patients with mild obstruction remain stable for decades with evidence of slow progression in late life.[55] The number of such patients is likely to increase as echocardiography now identifies many more in childhood with unsuspected nonobstructive membranes. Aortic regurgitation in unoperated patients, although common, is rarely of a significant degree even into adult life; indeed, significant regurgitation almost always occurs only in those who have undergone a procedure (angioplasty or surgery) or who have had endocarditis.[49,56]

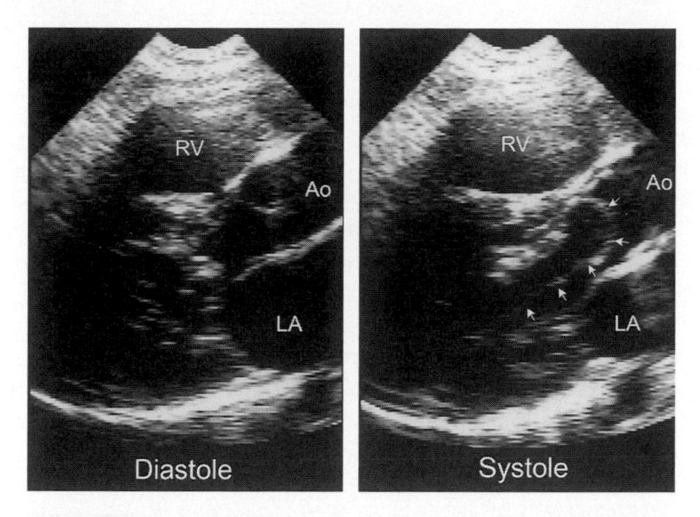

FIGURE 33–16 *Parasternal long-axis echocardiogram of the left ventricular outflow tract at end-diastole (left panel) and mid-systole (right panel) showing atypical subaortic stenosis secondary to accessory atrioventricular valve tissue that billows into the ascending aorta during ejection (arrows). RV, right ventricle; Ao, aorta; LA, left atrium.*

Postoperatively, among series extending over decades, recurrent obstruction occurs in about 20%, often requiring more extensive procedures. Such a scenario is more likely when obstruction is of the tunnel variety.

SUPRAVALVAR AORTIC STENOSIS

Definition

Supravalvar aortic stenosis denotes obstructive constriction of the ascending aorta above the aortic valve. This anomaly is commonly associated with elfin facies (Williams syndrome)[62] and other vascular lesions such as peripheral pulmonary stenosis and coarctation and coronary artery or renal artery stenoses.

Prevalence

Supravalvar aortic stenosis is an uncommon anomaly, with 134 patients with this diagnosis listed in the files of Children's Hospital Boston during the past 14 years. Of these, 42 had Williams syndrome (see Exhibit 33-3). A familial form inherited in an autosomal dominant pattern and without Williams syndrome features has been identified,[63,64] related to an abnormality of chromosome 7q11.23 (see Chapter 5).

The obstructing ring, sometimes asymmetric, is situated above the aortic valve and the sinuses of Valsalva. The edge of the obstructing tissue may impinge on a sinus of Valsalva, compromising flow to the coronary ostia. Occasionally, the coronary occlusion is complete, a leaflet of the distorted aortic valve adhering to the obstructing collar of tissue. When the aortic lumen is compromised, there is proportionate left ventricular hypertension and hypertrophy. The obstruction is commonly localized, but in about 20%, it extends diffusely into the ascending aorta (Fig. 33-17). The aortic cusps are often thickened and distorted, sometimes adherent to the aortic wall, but although aortic regurgitation is common, it is rarely severe.

Some patients have other vascular obstructions. Peripheral pulmonary stenosis with hypoplasia of the pulmonary arteries occurs in 30%, coarctation of the aorta in 15%, renal artery stenosis in 5%; obstructions may also occur in branches of the aorta. In those with Williams syndrome, some 85% have cardiovascular anomalies, with supravalvar aortic stenosis in 71%, peripheral pulmonary stenosis in 38%, and mitral regurgitation in about 20%,[65] sometime progressive.[66] Abdominal coarctation of the aorta has been described and may lead to renal vascular involvement. These obstructions in the aorta can be acquired and are often progressive. Indeed, all these peripheral phenomena may be seen in the absence of supravalvar stenosis and are sometimes readily recognized as part of Williams syndrome.

Physiology

The physiology is comparable to that of valvar aortic stenosis except that coronary blood flow is usually under increased pressure; rarely, the ostia may be obstructed. In any case, the demands of a hypertrophied ventricle, with or without coronary ostial obstruction, are likely to result in a mismatch of myocardial demand and perfusion; indeed, rare sudden death has been reported during exercise in childhood with right cusp fusion (resulting in diminished right coronary flow) to the supravalvar ridge.[67]

Hypercalcemia is seen in patients with Williams syndrome in early infancy.[68]

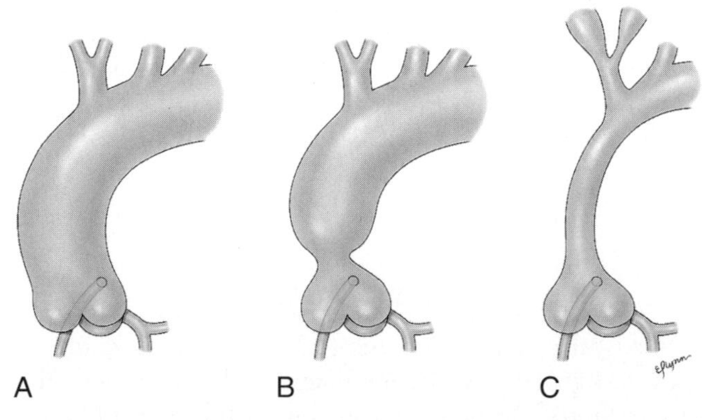

FIGURE 33–17 *The anatomic types of supravalvar aortic stenosis:* ***A****, normal;* ***B*** *and* ***C****, two forms of supravalvar stenosis. The difference between these two forms is in the length of the obstruction, which sometimes involves virtually all the ascending aorta. Note the obstructions in the innominate and common carotid arteries as they arise from the aortic arch. Other obstructions, such as coarctation of the aorta, renal artery stenosis, and pulmonary artery stenosis, are found in some patients.*
From Fyler DC [ed]. Nadas' Pediatric Cardiology. Philadelphia: Hanley & Belfus, 1992.

Clinical Manifestations

Patients with Williams syndrome have typical elfin facies, dental problems, mental retardation, and a very friendly, cheerful personality. Patients in whom this diagnosis is suspected should be evaluated for possible supravalvar aortic stenosis. Otherwise, supravalvar stenosis is discovered in these patients because of a basilar murmur, sometimes associated with a thrill. There may be a family history of supravalvar aortic stenosis. These children tend to grow poorly; they may have exercise intolerance and, occasionally, angina with effort. Syncope has been reported.

On physical examination, other than evidence of Williams syndrome, patients have a systolic murmur over the base of the heart and in the suprasternal notch, the latter often associated with a shudder or thrill. There may be hypertension if coarctation of the aorta or renal artery stenosis is present. Murmurs suggesting peripheral pulmonary stenosis may be audible, as may the murmur of minimal aortic insufficiency.

Electrocardiography

If the obstruction in the ascending aorta is severe, there will be left ventricular hypertrophy.

Chest X-Ray

The heart may be somewhat enlarged, but a chest x-ray is rarely helpful in this diagnosis.

Echocardiography

The diagnosis is identified at echocardiography. The anatomy of the aortic valve leaflets, the sinuses of Valsalva, the coronary arteries, and the supravalvar obstructing collar can be visualized and Doppler estimations of the pressure gradient across the obstructed area made. The supravalvar narrowing is most readily imaged in a parasternal long-axis view (Fig. 33-18), the appearance of the lesion being generally much less impressive than the measured gradient. Wall thickening at the site of obstruction is generally apparent. The aortic valve leaflets may appear thickened and may move abnormally despite absence of commissural fusion. The left ventricular myocardial thickness is generally indicative of the degree of obstruction.

The aortic arch and brachiocephalic vessels should be imaged because coarctation and stenosis of the brachiocephalic arteries commonly accompany supravalvar

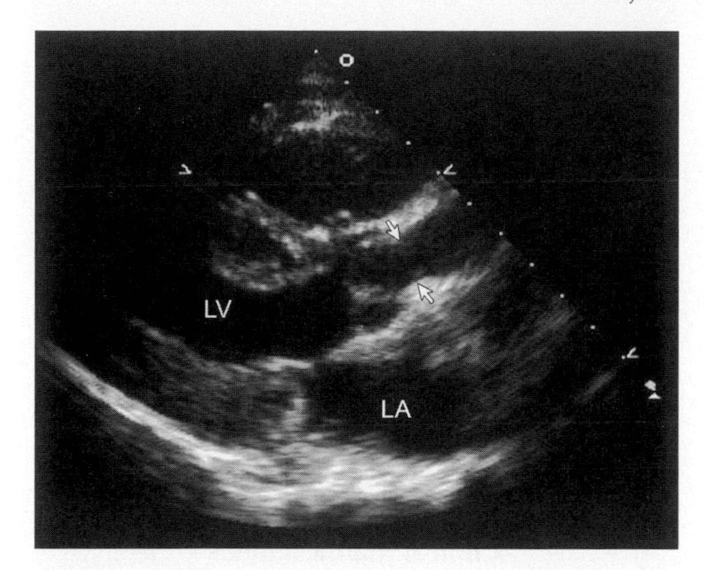

FIGURE 33–18 *Parasternal long-axis echocardiogram of the left ventricle (LV), atrium (LA), and proximal ascending aorta demonstrating typical hourglass-shaped supravalvar aortic stenosis (arrows) just above the sinuses of Valsalva.*

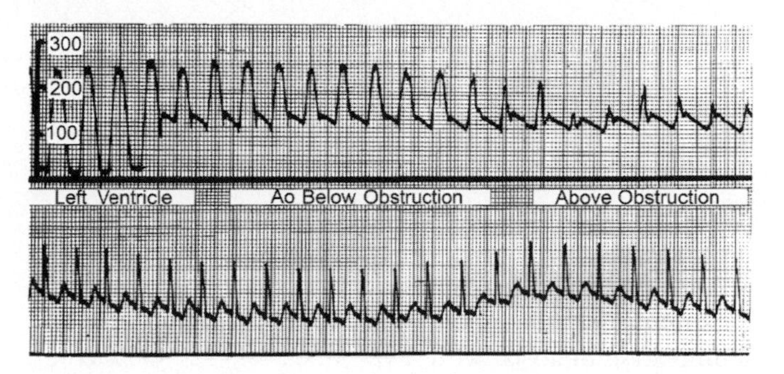

FIGURE 33–19 *Pressure tracing recorded in a patient with supravalvar aortic stenosis during withdrawal of a catheter from the left ventricle to the ascending aorta. Note that there is no change in systemic pressure as the catheter passes the valve and an arterial pressure trace appears. Further withdrawal shows a drop from a higher to a lower arterial pressure.*
From Fyler DC [ed]. Nadas' Pediatric Cardiology. Philadelphia: Hanley & Belfus, 1992.

aortic stenosis. Occasionally, the origin of a coronary artery is stenosed or, rarely, obstructed by a coronary leaflet.[69]

Magnetic Resonance Imaging

This technique provides superior anatomic details but is rarely necessary because of the excellent echocardiographic images.

Cardiac Catheterization

In the uncomplicated patient, in whom all anatomic details are clearly evident on noninvasive studies, cardiac catheterization is unnecessary (Fig. 33-19). If, however, an associated lesion such as significant distal peripheral pulmonary stenosis is suspected, catheterization is undertaken to dilate (with or without stents) these pulmonary lesions because they are generally inaccessible surgically. This combined approach of pulmonary artery dilation and surgical relief of supravalvar aortic stenosis offers better long-term survival than surgery alone in those with the severest elastin arteriopathy.[70] It should be emphasized, however, that catheterization of patients with severe bilateral outflow obstruction may be extremely dangerous. Occasionally, stenoses of individual aortic arch branches can also be managed by dilating and stenting these obstructions.

Management

With symptoms or an instantaneous gradient of more than 30 mmHg, particularly when the lesion is discrete, surgical repair using a variety of techniques is undertaken. These usually decrease the obstruction significantly.[66,71–74]

Course

Further obstructions may develop even though there has been successful surgical relief of the supravalvar obstruction; reoperation has not been necessary to date in our 25 patients operated on in the past 14 years. Coarctation of the aorta, renal artery stenosis, or obstructions of the branches of the aortic arch may develop or recur. Each new problem is evaluated on its own merits and managed independently. Survival and freedom from reintervention rates at 20 years have been reported at 77% and 49%, respectively.[70,72] It is of interest that moderate or lower degrees of peripheral pulmonary stenosis in some of these patients improve spontaneously.[75]

AORTIC REGURGITATION

Definition

The reflux of blood from the ascending aorta into the left ventricle during diastole is described as aortic regurgitation or aortic insufficiency.

Prevalence

Aortic regurgitation is found in association with almost all known pediatric cardiac problems. At Children's Hospital Boston, it was mentioned as a complicating feature

Exhibit 33–4

Children's Hospital Boston Experience

Aortic Regurgitation with Other Congenital Heart Defects

*Defect**	*N*
Aortic stenosis	2271
Tetralogy of Fallot	488
D-transposition of great arteries	461
Ventricular septal defect	418
Coarctation of aorta	278
Malposition	237
Endocardial cushion defect	195
Double-outlet right ventricle	125
Single ventricle	105
Truncus arteriosus	79
Mitral valve disease	2
Other	445
Total	5104

*Categorical diagnoses are mutually exclusive.
N, patient number.

of pediatric heart disease in more than 5000 patients (Exhibit 33-4). It was identified as the sole echocardiographic finding in only 68 patients, mild or less in most cases. From an echocardiographic standpoint, the incidence of aortic regurgitation in a normal heart in childhood has been reported as 0%,[76] increasing to 3% to 8% in adults.[77,78] This is in marked contrast to the frequent identification of regurgitation of other cardiac valves in normal patients, such as less than 77% in tricuspid, less than 88% in pulmonary, and less than 45% in mitral valves.[76–79] There were 61 patients with regurgitation due to rheumatic heart disease.

Pathology

There is no specific pathology for aortic regurgitation because there are multiple causes. There may be dilation of the valve ring, as seen in patients with tetralogy of Fallot (see Chapter 32) or in those with Marfan syndrome. In the latter, there is also commonly great enlargement of all three cusps. The valve may be congenitally abnormal, such as bicuspid, or due to severe underdevelopment of the right coronary cusp. The regurgitation may result from an intervention for stenosis such as balloon angioplasty or surgery. Incompetence of a normal valve may result from the jet effect in patients with subaortic stenosis or because of deformity or adherence of a cusp to a supravalvar obstructing ridge. It may follow prolapse of a cusp into a ventricular septal defect or perforation of a leaflet due to endocarditis. Rheumatic fever remains a major cause in some countries but is rare in the United States.

Physiology

When there is aortic regurgitation, the amount of blood that is refluxed must be pumped forward in addition to that supplying the appropriate cardiac output. The left ventricular volume is thereby enlarged in direct proportion to the amount of regurgitated blood. With increased amounts of regurgitation, the left ventricular volume increases, ultimately resulting in a huge heart. The runoff from the aorta to the left ventricle results in a wide pulse pressure, the systolic pressure becoming higher as the diastolic pressure becomes lower with increasing regurgitation.

Ultimately, over many years, increasing aortic regurgitation leads to congestive heart failure, which presages death, usually within 12 to 24 months.

Clinical Manifestations

A high-frequency, early diastolic blowing murmur, usually best heard along the left sternal border, is virtually diagnostic of aortic regurgitation (Figs. 33-20 and 33-21). The frequency of the murmur (the blowing quality) is higher with aortic regurgitation than it is with pulmonary regurgitation. The murmur is quite difficult to discover, let alone distinguish, when there are continuous murmurs from other causes such as patent ductus arteriosus, collateral circulation, shunt operations, and other lesions. The murmur is heard well in a small child lying down, but among teenagers, it is easier to hear with the patient sitting up and leaning forward. It is best heard with the diaphragm of the stethoscope at the left sternal border, usually at the third interspace. An Austin Flint murmur due to relative mitral stenosis produced by the aortic regurgitant jet may be audible at the apex in mid-diastole when incompetence is significant.

In the past, the discovery of isolated aortic regurgitation was synonymous with the diagnosis of rheumatic heart disease; this is no longer the case. Still, this possibility should be considered for each patient with isolated aortic regurgitation, and any history or family

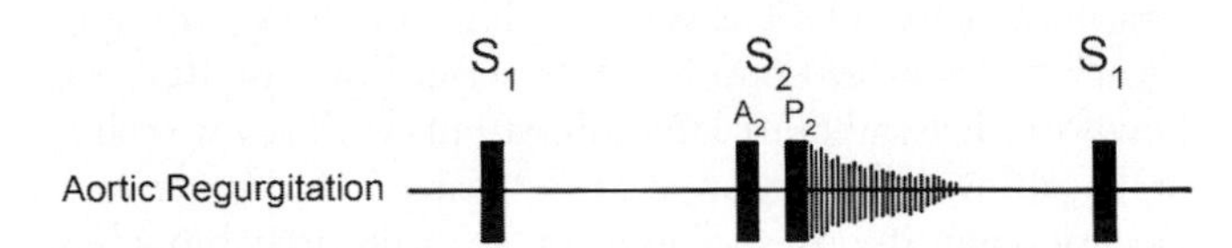

FIGURE 33–20 *Schematic drawing of the murmur of aortic regurgitation. Note the decrescendo, early diastolic murmur that begins after the second heart sound. S1, first heart sound; S2, second heart sound composed of A2 (aortic closure) and P2 (pulmonary closure).*
From Fyler DC [ed]. Nadas' Pediatric Cardiology. Philadelphia: Hanley & Belfus, 1992.

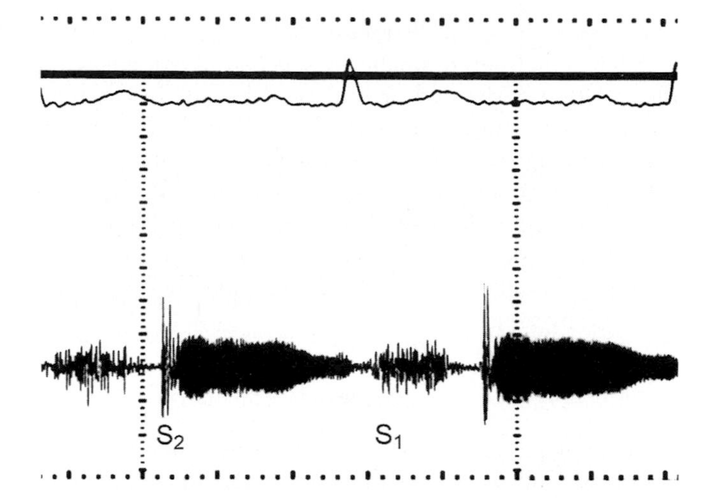

FIGURE 33–21 *Phonocardiogram in a patient who suddenly developed a loud, high-frequency murmur of aortic regurgitation because of a perforation in an aortic valve leaflet.*
From Fyler DC [ed]. Nadas' Pediatric Cardiology. Philadelphia: Hanley & Belfus, 1992.

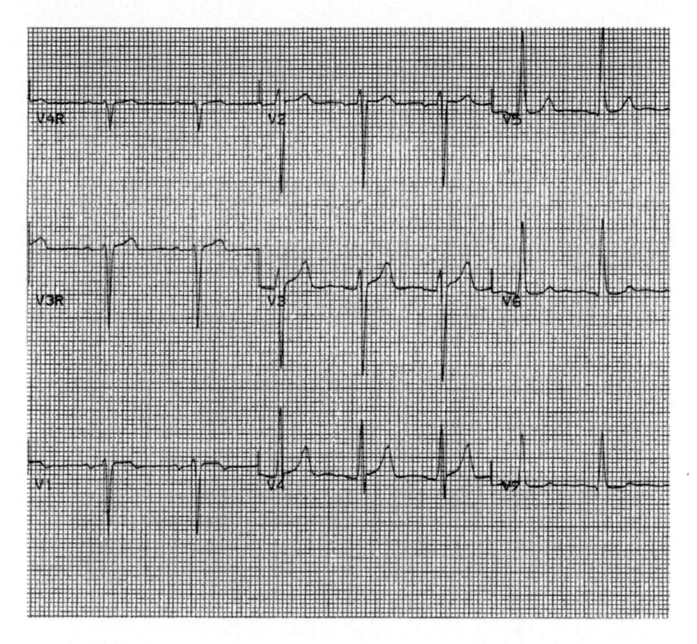

FIGURE 33–22 *Showing left ventricular hypertrophy by voltage criteria (V leads at half standard) in a 19-year-old with bicuspid valve and severe aortic regurgitation.*

history suggesting rheumatic fever should be carefully reviewed.

With increasing degrees of aortic regurgitation, the peripheral pulses become more prominent as the pulse pressure increases. Associated with this wide pulse pressure is a wonderful cacophony of physical findings and signs, including capillary pulsations; de Musset's (head bobbing), Duroziez's, Traube's, Müller's, and Quincke's signs; and Corrigan's (water hammer) pulse.[80] Generally, with routine observation of the carotid pulsations, the pediatrician sees the wide pulse pressure before he or she feels it. Confirmation of the wide pulse pressure by blood pressure measurement documents the somewhat elevated systolic pressure and low diastolic pressure.

The hyperdynamic left ventricular impulse is displaced down and leftward, sometimes reaching the anterior axillary line at the sixth interspace. The hyperactive impulse conveys the impression of forceful ejection of large amounts of blood.

Electrocardiography

With increasing left ventricular volume overload, there is increased left ventricular voltage on the electrocardiogram (Fig. 33-22), and in the extreme form, there may be depression of the ST segment and T-wave inversion.

Chest X-Ray

The heart size is directly proportional to the amount of aortic regurgitation, or it may be grossly enlarged through the dilation of congestive heart failure superimposed on a large regurgitant volume. The dilated ascending aorta is usually visible.

Echocardiography

The regurgitant flow across the aortic valve is readily detected by color Doppler interrogation. Indeed, this sensitive technique frequently identifies aortic regurgitation without an audible murmur. In addition to providing valvar and ascending aorta anatomic information, the former often better delineated on three-dimensional imaging, estimates of the regurgitation severity are possible based on jet dimension and descending aorta runoff information. Very importantly, especially for management guidance, sophisticated ventricular function parameters (end-diastolic and systolic sizes, fractional shortening, wall stress, left ventricular muscle mass) are now readily available (see Chapter 15).

Cardiac Catheterization

Cardiac catheterization is not needed in the evaluation of a patient with aortic regurgitation. However, because most of these children have other defects, cardiac catheterization may be used to provide more physiologic information or to interventionally manage an additional compounding lesion such as a patent ductus arteriosus. Evaluation, if necessary, of the degree of aortic regurgitation during cardiac catheterization is accomplished by the injection of contrast material above the aortic valve (the catheter not in contact with the valve) and observing the amount that enters the ventricle.

Management

Any patient with known aortic regurgitation who has syncope or anginal chest pain or who has developed congestive heart failure is a candidate for surgery. Progressive enlargement and decreasing function, at rest, of the left ventricle on serial echocardiographic studies are surgical indications[81] (Fig. 33-23). The appearance of ventricular dysrhythmias, an event of ominous significance, is another indication for surgery. In asymptomatic patients with significant regurgitation but with stable, modestly increased end-diastolic volumes and normal function, medical management with afterload reduction is a reasonable temporizing measure. Whether levels of B-type natriuretic peptide, secreted by stressed cardiac muscle and known to be elevated in such adult patients,[82] as well as in patients with aortic stenosis[83,84] or heart failure,[85] will be used as a management guide remains to be determined.

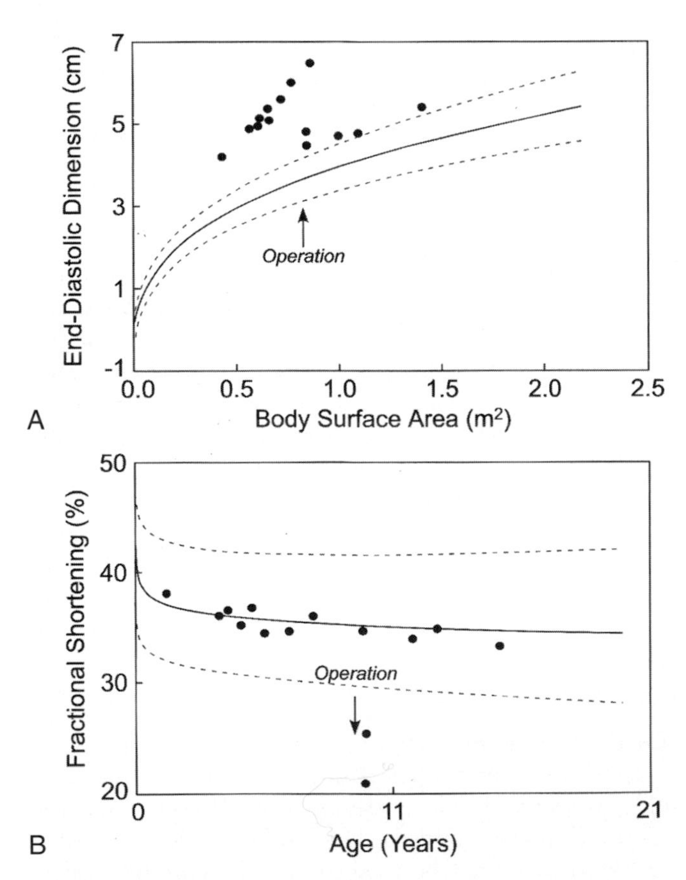

FIGURE 33–23 *Serial echocardiographic measurements showing (**A**) indexed left ventricular end-diastolic volumes and (**B**) fractional shortening before and after surgical valvuloplasty at age 9 years for severe aortic regurgitation after balloon angioplasty for stenosis. Note the dramatic immediate decrease in both parameters postoperatively with recovery of the latter during follow-up. Courtesy of Dr. S. Colan.*

Whenever possible, surgeons undertake valvuloplasty, which is sometimes dramatically successful, particularly in those with a perforated or prolapsed leaflet. In addition, many with a bicuspid valve or a hypoplastic leaflet or torn valve from angioplasty can be satisfactorily palliated by a valve plasty procedure.[35] Some, however, will require a prosthesis and anticoagulation; replacement with a tissue valve has not been effective on a long-term basis in young patients, although success with a Ross operation has been reported by some.

Course

In young patients, relief of severe aortic regurgitation is commonly followed immediately by marked reduction in both end-diastolic volume and shortening fraction, the latter normalizing with time (see Fig. 33-23).

BICUSPID AORTIC VALVE

Definition

Congenital bicuspid aortic valve is characterized by two leaflets and two commissures.

Prevalence

A bicuspid aortic valve is a common anomaly in the general population and frequently occurs without stenosis or regurgitation.[3,7,9] Many are associated with other cardiac defects, such as valvar aortic stenosis, aortic regurgitation, coarctation of the aorta, ventricular septal defect, and endocardial cushion defects.

Clinical Manifestations

A bicuspid aortic valve is more common in males (see Exhibit 33-1).

The diagnosis is suggested by a constant early systolic ejection click at the base or left sternal border or apex. The additional presence of the murmur of aortic regurgitation or aortic stenosis at the second right interspace should raise the question of a bicuspid aortic valve.

Electrocardiography

No specific electrocardiographic changes are associated with bicuspid aortic valve.

Chest X-Ray

There are no specific findings of bicuspid aortic valve on the routine chest x-ray.

Echocardiography

Echocardiographic examination confirms the diagnosis and provides the anatomic details (see Fig. 33-5).

Management

A bicuspid aortic valve is prone to endocarditis, and thus antibiotic prophylaxis is mandatory.

Course

Although many bicuspid aortic valves eventually become stenotic or regurgitant, this is not universal,[86] as evidenced by normal function of such valves in older patients. Among adults, the association of bicuspid aortic valves and dilated aortic roots is well recognized,[87] with progression of dilation occurring in some. Although rare instances of rupture have occurred in adult patients, it does not occur in children.

REFERENCES

1. Fyler DC, Buckley LP, Hellenbrand WE, et al. Report of the New England Regional Infant Cardiac Program. Pediatrics 65(Suppl):376, 1980.
2. Botto LD, Correa A, Erickson JD. Racial and temporal variations in the prevalence of heart defects. Pediatrics 107(3):1, 2001.
3. Hoffman IE, Kaplar S. The incidence of congenital heart disease. J Am Coll Cardiol 39:1890, 2002.
4. Wagner HR, Ellison RC, Keane JF, et al. Clinical course in aortic stenosis. Report from the Joint Study of the Natural History of Congenital Heart Defects. Circulation 56(Suppl 1)1, 1977.
5. Vollebergh FEMG, Becker AB. Minor congenital variations of cusp size in tricuspid aortic valves: Possible link with isolated aortic stenosis. Br Heart J 39:1006, 1977.
6. Roberts WC. The structure of the aortic valve in clinically isolated aortic stenosis: An autopsy study of 162 patients over 15 years of age. Circulation 32:91, 1970.
7. Larsen EW, Edwards WD. Risk factors for aortic dissection: A necropsy study of 161 cases. Am J Cardiol 53:849, 1984.
8. Basso C, Boschello M, Perrone C, et al. An echocardiographic survey of primary school children for bicuspid aortic valve. Am J Cardiol 93:661, 2004.
9. Fernandes SM, Sanders S, Khairy P, et al. Morphology of bicuspid aortic valve in children and adolescents. J Am Coll Cardiol 44:16, 2004.
10. Van Praagh R, Bano-Rodrigo A, Smolinsky A, et al. Anatomic variations in congenital valvar, subvalvar and supravalvar aortic stenosis: A study of 64 post mortem cases. In Takahashi M, Wells WJ, Lindesmith GG (eds). Challenges in the Treatment of Congenital Cardiac Anomalies. New York: Futura, 1986:13–41.
11. Gorlin R, Gorlin SG. Hydraulic formula for calculation of area of stenotic mitral valve, other valves and central circulatory shunts. Am Heart J 41:1, 1951.
12. Lima VC, Zahn E, Houde C, Smallhorn J, et al. Non-invasive determination of the systolic peak-to-peak gradient in children with aortic stenosis: validation of a mathematical model. Cardiol Young 10(2):115, 2000.
13. VanAuker MD, Hla A, Meisner JS, et al. Simultaneous Doppler/catheter measurements of pressure gradients in aortic valve disease: A correction to the Bernoulli equation based on velocity decay in the stenotic jet. J Heart Valve Dis 9(2):291, 2000.
14. Baumgartner H, Stefenelli T, Niederberger J, et al. "Overestimation" of catheter gradients by Doppler ultrasound in patients with aortic stenosis: A predictable manifestation of pressure recovery [see comment]. J Am Coll Cardiol 33(6):1655, 1999.
15. Garcia D, Dumesnil JG, Durand LG, et al. Discrepancies between catheter and Doppler estimates of valve effective orifice area can be predicted from the pressure recovery phenomenon: Practical implications with regard to quantification of aortic stenosis severity [see comment]. J Am Coll Cardiol 41(3):435, 2003.
16. Barker PC, Ensing G, Ludomirsky A, et al. Comparison of simultaneous invasive and noninvasive measurements of pressure gradients in congenital aortic valve stenosis. J Am Society of Echocardiography 15(12):1496, 2002.
17. Villavicencio RE, Forbes TJ, Thomas RL, et al. Pressure recovery in pediatric aortic valve stenosis. Pediatr Cardiol 24(5):457, 2003.
18. Currie PJ, Hagler DJ, Seward JB, et al. Instantaneous pressure gradient: A simultaneous Doppler and dual catheter correlative study. J Am Coll Cardiol 7:800, 1986.
19. Moore P, Egito E, Mowrey H, et al. Midterm results of balloon dilation of congenital aortic stenosis: Predictors of success. J Am Coll Cardiol 27:1257, 1996.
20. Reich O, Tax P, Marek J, et al. Long term results of percutaneous balloon valvuloplasty of congenital aortic stenosis: Independent predictors of outcome. [see comment]. Heart (British Cardiac Society). 90(1):70, 2004.
21. Chartrand CC, Saro-Servando E, Vobecky JS. Long term results of surgical valvuloplasty for congenital valvar aortic stenosis in children. Ann Thorac Surg 68(4):1356, 1999.
22. Keane JF, Driscoll D, Gersony W, et al. Results of treatment of patients with aortic stenosis. The Report of the Second Natural History Study of Congenital Heart Defects. Circulation 87(Suppl 1):1, 1993.
23. Brown JW, Ruzmetov M, Vijay P, et al. Surgery for aortic stenosis in children: A 40 year experience. Ann Thorac Surg 76(5):1398, 2003.
24. Alexiou C, Chen Q, Langley, SM, et al. Is there still a place for open surgical valvotomy in the management of aortic stenosis in children? The view from Southampton. Eur J Cardiothorac Surg 20(2):239, 2001.
25. Rosenfeld HM, Landzberg MJ, Perry SB, et al. Balloon aortic valvuloplasty in the young adult with congenital heart disease. Am J Cardiol 73:112, 1994.

26. Gersony WM, Hayes CJ, Driscoll DJ, et al. Bacterial endocarditis in patients with aortic stenosis, or ventricular septal defect. The Report of the Second Natural History Study of Congenital Heart Defects. Circulation 87(Suppl 1): 1, 1993.
27. Campbell M. The natural history of congenital aortic stenosis. Br Heart J 30:514, 1968.
28. Fulton DR, Hougen TJ, Keane JF, et al. Repeat aortic valvotomy in children. Am Heart J 106:60, 1983.
29. Satou GM, Perry SB, Lock JE, et al. Repeat Balloon Dilation of Congenital Valvar Aortic Stenoses: Immediate Results and Midterm Outcome. Catheter Cardiovasc Intervent 47:47, 1999.
30. Shim D, Lloyd TR, Beekman RH III. Usefulness of repeat balloon aortic valvuloplasty in children. Am J Cardiol 79: 1141, 1997.
31. Elkins RC, Lane MM, McCue C. Ross operation in children: Late results. J Heart Valve Disease 10(6):736, 2001.
32. Rubay JE, Buche M, El Khoury GA, et al. The Ross operation: Mid-term results. Ann Thorac Surg 67(5):1355, 1999.
33. Phillips JR, Daniels CJ, Orsinelli DA, et al. Valvular hemodynamics and arrhythmias with exercise following the Ross procedure. Am J Cardiol 87(5):577, 2001.
34. Solowiejczyk DE, Bourlon F, Apfel HD, et al. Serial echocardiographic measurements of the pulmonary autograft in the aortic valve position after the Ross operation in a pediatric population using normal pulmonary artery dimensions as a reference standard. Am J Cardiol 85(9):1119, 2000.
35. Bacha EA, Satou GM, Moran AM, et al. Valve-sparing surgery for balloon-induced aortic regurgitation in congenital aortic stenosis. J Thorac Cardiovasc Surg 122(1):163, 2001.
36. Driscoll DJ, Wolfe RR, Gersony WM, et al. Cardiorespiratory responses to exercise of patients with aortic stenosis, pulmonary stenosis and ventricular septal defect. Circulation 87(Suppl 1):1, 1993.
37. Wolfe RR, Driscoll DJ, Gersony WM, et al. Arrhythmias in patients with valvar aortic stenosis, valvar pulmonary stenosis, and ventricular septal defect: Results of 24-hour ECG monitoring. Circulation 87(Suppl 1):1, 1993.
38. Rhodes LA, Colan SD, Perry SB, et al. Predictors of survival in neonates with critical aortic stenosis. Circulation 84:2325, 2991.
39. Mody MR, Nadas AS, Bernhard WF. Aortic stenosis in infants. N Engl J Med 276:832, 1967.
40. Keane JF, Bernhard W, Nadas AS. Aortic stenosis surgery in infancy. Circulation 52:1138, 1975.
41. Zeevi B, Keane JF, Castaneda AR, et al. Neonatal critical valvar aortic stenosis: A comparison of surgical and balloon dilation therapy. Circulation 80:831, 1989.
42. Egito EST, Moore P, O'Sullivan J, et al. Transvascular balloon dilation for neonatal critical aortic stenosis: Early and mid-term results. J Am Coll Cardiol 28:442, 1997.
43. McElhinney DB, Lock JE, Keane JF, et al. Left heart growth, function and reintervention after aortic valvuloplasty for neonatal aortic stenosis. Circulation 111:451, 2005.
44. Latiff HA, Sholler GF, Cooper S. Balloon dilation of aortic stenosis in infants younger than 6 months of age: Intermediate outcome. Pediatr Cardiol 24(1):17, 2003.
45. Baram S, McCrindle BW, Han RK, et al. Outcomes of uncomplicated aortic valve stenosis presenting in infants. Am Heart J 145(6):1063, 2003.
46. McCrindle BW, Blackstone EH, Williams WG, et al. Are outcomes of surgical versus transcatheter balloon valvotomy equivalent in neonatal critical aortic stenosis? Circulation 104(12 Suppl 1):I152, 2001.
47. Pyle RL, Patterson DF, Chacko S. The genetics and pathology of discrete subaortic stenosis in the Newfoundland dog. Am Heart J 92:324, 1976.
48. Kleinert S, Geva T. Echocardiographic morphometry and geometry of the left ventricular outflow tract in fixed subaortic stenosis. J Am Coll Cardiol 22:1501, 1993.
49. McMahon C, Gauvreau K, Edwards JC, et al. Risk factors for aortic valve dysfunction in children with discrete subvalvar aortic stenosis. Am J Cardiol 94:459, 2004.
50. Wright GB, Keane JF, Nadas AS, et al. Fixed subaortic stenosis in the young: Medical and surgical course in 83 patients. Am J Cardiol 52:830, 1983.
51. Marasini M, Zannini L, Ussia GP, et al. Discrete subaortic stenosis: Incidence, morphology and surgical impact of associated subaortic anomalies. Ann Thorac Surg 75(6):1763, 2003.
52. Brauner R, Laks H, Drinkwater DC Jr, et al. Benefits of early surgical repair in fixed subaortic stenosis [see comment]. J Am Coll Cardiol 30(7):1835, 1997.
53. de Vries AG, Hess J, Witsenburg M, et al. Management of fixed subaortic stenosis: A retrospective study of 57 cases. [see comment]. J Am Coll Cardiol 19(5):1013, 1992.
54. Frommelt MA, Snider AR, Bove EL, et al. Echocardiographic assessment of subvalvular aortic stenosis before and after operation [see comment]. J Am Coll Cardiol 19(5):1018, 1992.
55. Oliver, JM, Gonzalez A, Allego P, et al. Discrete subaortic stenosis in adults: Increased prevalence and slow rate of progression of the obstruction and aortic regurgitation. J Am Coll Cardiol 38:835, 2001.
56. Gersony WM. Natural history of discrete subvalvar aortic stenosis: Management implications. J Am Coll Cardiol 38:843, 2001.
57. Ohye RG, Gomez CA, Ohye BJ, et al. The Ross/Konno procedure in neonates and infants: Intermediate-term survival and autograft function. Ann Thorac Surg 72(3):823, 2001.
58. Erez E, Kanter KR, Tam VK, et al. Konno aortoventriculoplasty in children and adolescents: From prosthetic valves to the Ross operation. Ann Thorac Surg. 74(1):122, 2002.
59. Jahangiri M, Nicholson IA, del Nido PJ, et al. Surgical management of complex and tunnel-like subaortic stenosis. Eur J Cardiothorac Surg 17(6):637, 2000.
60. Vouhe PR, Ouaknine R, Poulain H, et al. Diffuse subaortic stenosis: Modified Konno procedures with aortic valve preservation. Eur J Cardiothorac Surg 7(3):132, 1993.
61. McElhinney DB, Reddy VM, Silverman NH, et al. Accessory and anomalous atrioventricular valvar tissue causing outflow tract obstruction: Surgical implications of a heterogeneous and complex problem. J Am Coll Cardiol 32(6):1741, 1998.
62. Williams JCP, Barett-Boyes BG, Lowe JB. Supravalvar aortic stenosis. Circulation 24:1311, 1961.

63. Schmidt MA, Ensing GJ, Michels VV, et al. Autosomal dominant supravalvular aortic stenosis: Large three-generation family. Am J Med Genet 32:384, 1989.
64. Kumar A, Stalker HJ, Williams CA. Concurrence of supravalvular aortic stenosis and peripheral pulmonary stenosis in three generations of a family: A form of arterial dysplasia. Am J Med Genet 45:739, 1993.
65. Bruno E, Rossi N, Thuer O, et al. Cardiovascular findings, and clinical course, in patients with Williams syndrome. Cardiol Young 13(6):532, 2003.
66. Keane JF, Fellows KE, LaFarge CG, et al. The surgical management of discrete and diffuse supravalvar aortic stenosis. Circulation 54:112, 1976.
67. Sun CC, Jacot J, Brenner JI. Sudden death in supravalvular aortic stenosis: Fusion of a coronary leaflet to the sinus ridge, dysplasia and stenosis of aortic and pulmonic valves. Pediatr Pathol 12(5):751, 1992.
68. Black JA, Bonham-Carter RE. Association between aortic stenosis and facies of severe infantile hypercalcemia. Lancet 2:745, 1963.
69. Thistlethwaite PA, Madani MM, Kriett JM, et al. Surgical management of congenital obstruction of the left main coronary artery with supravalvular aortic stenosis. J Thorac Cardiovasc Surg 120(6):1040, 2000.
70. Stamm C, Friehs I, Moran AM, et al. Surgery for bilateral outflow tract obstruction in elastin arteriopathy. J Thorac Cardiovasc Surg 120(4):755, 2000.
71. Stamm C, Kreutzer C, Zurakowski D, et al. Forty-one years of surgical experience with congenital supravalvular aortic stenosis. J Thorac Cardiovasc Surg. 118(5):874, 1999.
72. Hazekamp MG, Kappetein AP, Schoof PH, et al. Brom's three-patch technique for repair of supravalvular aortic stenosis. J Thorac Cardiovasc Surg 118(2):252, 1999.
73. McElhinney DB, Petrossian E, Tworetzky W, et al. Issues and outcomes in the management of supravalvar aortic stenosis. Ann Thorac Surg 69(2):562, 2000.
74. Brown JW, Ruzmetov M, Vijay P, et al. Surgical repair of congenital supravalvular aortic stenosis in children. Eur J Cardio Thorac Surg 21(1):50, 2002.
75. Kim YM, Yoo SJ, Choi JY, et al. Natural course of supravalvar aortic stenosis and peripheral pulmonary arterial stenosis in Williams' syndrome. Cardiol Young. 9(1):37, 1999.
76. Yoshida K, Yoshikawa J, Shakudo M, et al. Color Doppler evaluation of valvular regurgitation in normal subjects. Circulation 78:840, 1988.
77. Choong CY, Abascal VM, Weyman J, et al. Prevalence of valvular regurgitation by Doppler echocardiography in patients with structurally normal hearts by two-dimensional echocardiography. Am Heart J 117:636, 1989.
78. Macchi C, Orlandini SZ, Orlandini GE. An anatomical study of the healthy human heart by echocardiography with special reference to physiological valvular regurgitation. Anatomischer Anzeiger 176(1):81, 1994.
79. Van Dijk AP, Van Oort AM, Daniels O. Right-sided valvular regurgitation in normal children determined by combined color-coded and continuous-wave Doppler echocardiography. Acta Paediatr 83(2):200, 1994.
80. Corrigan DJ. Permanent patency of the mouth of the aorta or inadequacy of the aortic valves. Edinburgh Med Surg J 1832.
81. Borer JS, Borow RO. Contemporary approach to aortic and mitral regurgitation. Circulation 108:2432, 2003.
82. Eimer MJ, Ekery DL, Rigolin VH, et al. Elevated B-type natriuretic peptide in asymptomatic men with chronic aortic regurgitation and preserved left ventricular systolic function. Am J Cardiol 94:676, 2004.
83. Weber M, Arnold R, Rau M, et al. Relation of N-terminal pro-b-type natriuretic peptide in severity of valvular aortic stenosis. Am J Cardiol 94:740, 2004.
84. Bergler-Klein J, Klaer U, Heger M, et al. Natriuretic peptides predict symptom-free survival and postoperative outcome in severe aortic stenosis. Circulation 109:2302, 2004.
85. Bettencourt P, Ferriera A, Dias P, et al. Evaluation of brain natriuretic peptide in the diagnosis of heart failure. Cardiology 93:19, 2000.
86. Alegret JM, Duran I, Palagor O, et al. Prevalence of and predictors of bicuspid aortic valves in patients with dilated aortic roots. Am J Cardiol 91:619, 2003.
87. Ferencik M, Pape LA. Changes in size of ascending aorta and aortic valve function with time in patients with congenitally bicuspid aortic valves. Am J Cardiol 92:43, 2003.

34

Atrial Septal Defect

JOHN F. KEANE, TAL GEVA, DONALD C. FYLER

DEFINITION

Any opening in the atrial septum is described as an atrial defect. This definition includes the typical secundum atrial defect, which is most common and usually single (Exhibit 34-1); multiple fenestrations of the septum primum; and sinus venosus defects. The patent foramen ovale is also discussed because of increasing interest in its association with the occurrence of strokes due to emboli from right-to-left atrial shunting in older patients,[1,2] although it has traditionally been considered a normal insignificant finding, especially in infants. Partial anomalous pulmonary venous return to the systemic venous circulation has many of the physiologic characteristics of an atrial defect and in fact is often associated with such a defect. For these reasons, partial anomalous pulmonary veins are also discussed in this chapter.

Large single atrial defects involving the septum primum, which are endocardial in origin, are discussed in the chapter on Endocardial Cushion Defects (see Chapter 38).

PREVALENCE

Because of the absence of symptoms and significant murmurs, many patients with typical significant atrial defects are still seen for the first time in childhood, even adulthood. The incidence of atrial defects in recent studies was 1.0 per 1000 live births,[3,4] far exceeding the 0.073 per 1000 rate in very ill infants reported in earlier years.[5] This large increase is likely due to the more widespread use of echocardiography, which identifies many smaller defects unaccompanied by symptoms or murmurs.

Isolated atrial defects, including those with partial anomalous pulmonary venous return but excluding patent foramina ovale, accounted for 3% of Children's Hospital Boston patients with heart disease and was the eleventh most common lesion. On the other hand, up to 50% of children with congenital heart disease have an atrial defect as part of their cardiac problem.

ANATOMY

Atrial defects may be single or multiple and can be located anywhere in the atrial septum. The defects range from millimeters in diameter to virtual absence of the septum (Fig. 34-1). Atrial septation embryologically involves three structures: the septum primum, septum secundum, and atrioventricular (AV) canal septum. The septum primum is first to appear in the developing atria and consists of a venous valve that grows from the junction between the inferior vena cava and the right atrium toward the septum secundum. The latter is a crescent-shaped muscular ridge that forms in the superior-posterior aspect of the common atrium as an invagination between the developing atria. The AV canal septum is formed, at least in part, by the superior and inferior endocardial cushions and contributes to septation of the outlet portion of the atria and the inlet portion of the ventricles. Normal development of the atrial septum results in formation of the fossa ovalis, which is bounded by septum secundum; the *septum primum*, which attaches to the left atrial aspect of the septum secundum; and a muscular septum between the inferior aspect of the fossa ovalis and the tricuspid and mitral valve annuli—the *AV canal septum*. The tissue that separates the

Exhibit 34–1
Children's Hospital Boston Experience
Atrial Septal Defect

	1973–1987	*1988–2002*
Primary Classification	**N = 956***	**N = 3554***
Atrial septal defect	769	952
Partial anomalous pulmonary veins	78	69
Sinus venosus defect (SVC type)	70	59
Unroofed coronary sinus	3	9
Scimitar syndrome	6	0
Patent foramen ovale	65	2770
TOTAL	991⁺	3859⁺

Note: The huge increase in patent foramen ovale numbers in the more recent 1988–2002 era reflects more widespread use of echocardiography. Listed under other primary diagnoses, and who underwent atrial septal defect closure only, were 25 patients with pulmonary stenosis (17 surgical, 8 device) and 28 with ventricular defects (21 surgical, 7 device). On searching the entire 1988–2002 patient population, there were identified 79 patients with an unroofed coronary sinus and 30 with scimitar syndrome who had other lesions that placed them in other groups as determined by the hierarchic designation. During these same years, in terms of treatment, 238 patients had surgical closure of an isolated atrial secundum defect; atrial defect closure by device was done in 330 patients, many of whom had other lesions.

N, patient number; *, each patient counted only once; ⁺, some had more than one of the lesions under Primary Classification.

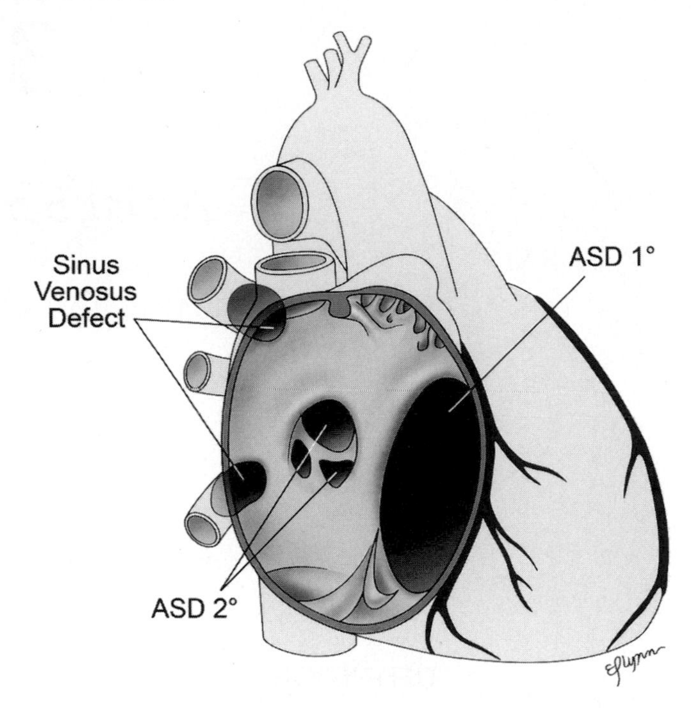

FIGURE 34–1 *Diagram of the atrial septum showing several types of atrial septal defects. An ostium primum defect [ASD1°] is located immediately adjacent to the mitral and tricuspid valves. Ostium secundum defects [ASD2°] are located near the fossa ovalis in the center of the septum. Sinus venosus defects are located in the area derived from the embryologic sinus venosus. From Fyler DC [ed]. Nadas' Pediatric Cardiology. Philadelphia: Hanley & Belfus, 1992.*

right pulmonary veins from the superior vena cava and from the posterior aspect of the right atrium is termed *sinus venosus septum*.[6,7]

A secundum atrial defect in the fossa ovalis is the most common cause of an atrial-level shunt (excluding patent foramen ovale) and is most frequently due to deficiency of septum primum, the valve of the fossa ovalis. Rarely, a secundum defect results in deficiency of septum secundum (the muscular limb of the fossa ovalis).

Patent foramen ovale is a normal interatrial communication during fetal life. It is bordered on the left by septum primum and by the superior limbic band of the fossa ovalis (septum secundum) on the right (Fig. 34-2). During fetal life, right-to-left flow occurs through the foramen because right atrial pressure exceeds that in the left. After birth, the atrial pressures reverse as the lungs aerate, pulmonary vascular resistance decreases, and systemic vascular resistance increases with elimination of placental circulation. As a result, septum primum opposes the superior limbic band of the fossa ovalis, and the foramen ovale narrows. A patent foramen ovale is seen in almost all newborns and with decreasing frequency throughout life.

Sinus venosus defect is a communication between one or more of the right pulmonary veins and the cardiac end of the superior vena cava or the posterior wall of the right atrium[6] (see Fig. 34-1). Anatomically, it is not an atrial septal defect because it does not allow direct communication between the left and right atria, but rather the interatrial communication is through one or more of the pulmonary veins. It is most commonly located between the right upper pulmonary vein and the cardiac end of the superior vena cava (called the *superior vena cava type*), the defect being due to the absence of the anterior wall of the right upper pulmonary vein and the posterolateral wall of the cardiac end of the superior vena cava. The deficiency of the sinus venosus septum can extend peripherally to involve secondary branches of the right pulmonary veins, resulting in the appearance of several pulmonary veins draining into the superior vena cava. The left atrial orifice of the right upper pulmonary vein is usually patent, allowing for an interatrial communication through it. In addition, blood from the right

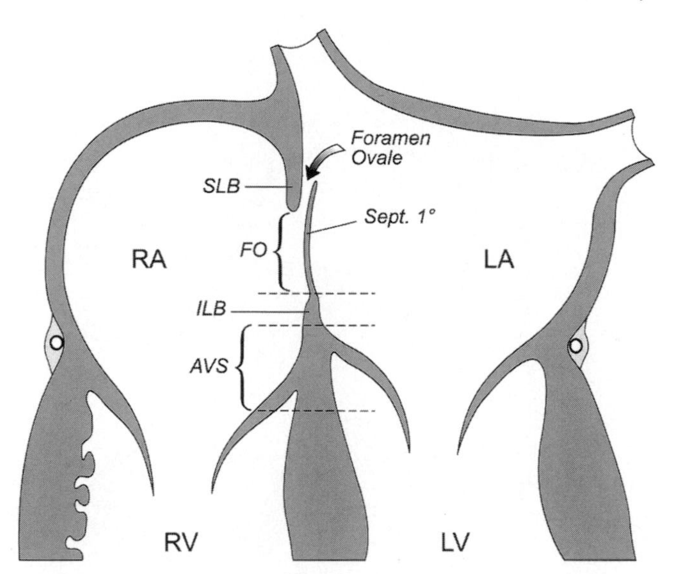

FIGURE 34–2 *Diagram of atrial septal components, showing foramen ovale (arrow), septum primum [Sept 1°], left atrium (LA), left ventricle (LV), fossa ovalis (FO), superior (SLB) and inferior (LMB) limbic bands, atrioventricular septum (AVS), right atrium (RA), and right ventricle (RV).*

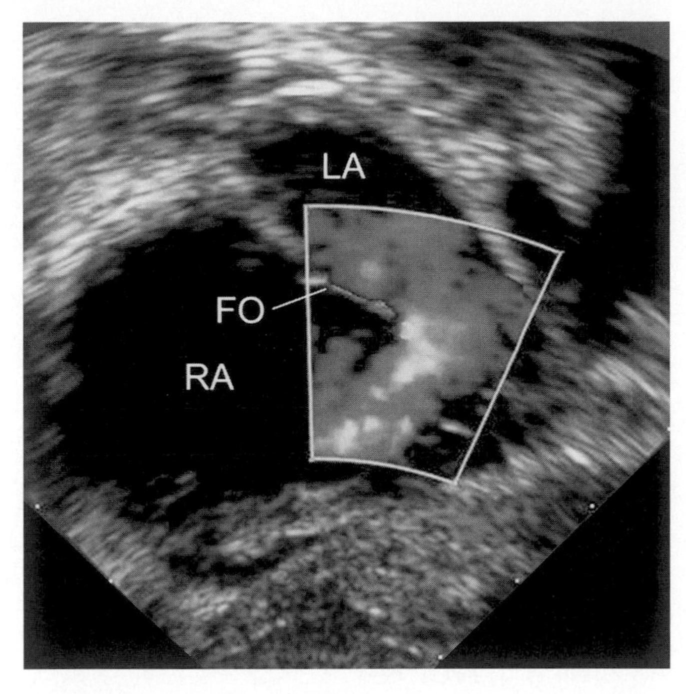

FIGURE 34–3 *Echocardiogram of coronary sinus septal defect outlined by color-flow Doppler. LA, left atrium; FO, foramen ovale; RA, right atrium.*

upper pulmonary vein flows to the right atrium through the defect in the sinus venosus septum. When the left atrial orifice of the right upper pulmonary vein is atretic, there is no interatrial communication, and the anatomic appearance is that of partially anomalous pulmonary venous connection of the right upper pulmonary vein to the superior vena cava. Rarely, the defect involves the right lower or middle pulmonary veins and the middle or superior aspects of the right atrium. This type of sinus venosus defect has been called the *inferior vena cava type*, although direct involvement of the inferior vena cava is either extremely rare or not present. For that reason, the *term sinus venosus of the right atrial type* is preferred.

Coronary sinus septal defect is a rare type of interatrial communication in which the septum between the coronary sinus and the left atrium is either partially or completely unroofed, leading to a left-to-right shunt through the coronary sinus orifice (Fig. 34-3). The orifice of the coronary sinus in this anomaly is usually large as a result of the left-to-right shunt, resulting in a sizeable defect in the inferior aspect of the atrial septum near the entry of the inferior vena cava. The association of a coronary sinus septal defect and persistent left superior vena cava is termed *Raghib syndrome*.[8] When the coronary sinus is completely unroofed, the left superior vena cava enters the left superior corner of the left atrium, anterior to the orifice of the left upper pulmonary vein and posterior to the left atrial appendage.

Common atrium is present when septum primum, septum secundum, and the AV canal septum are absent and is usually associated with heterotaxy syndrome (see Chapter 39).

Partial anomalous pulmonary venous connection is a connection between one or more (but not all) of the pulmonary veins with a systemic vein. An associated interatrial communication is not considered integral to the anomaly. There are several anatomic variations[9] (Fig. 34-4). The most common type is anomalous connection of the left upper pulmonary vein to the left innominate vein. One or more of the left pulmonary veins can connect directly to the right superior vena cava, the coronary sinus, or the hemiazygos vein. Drainage of a right pulmonary vein to the cardiac end of the right superior vena cava or to the right atrium is considered a sinus venosus defect. Anomalous connection of some or all of the right pulmonary veins to the inferior vena cava is termed *scimitar syndrome*.[10] Other elements of the syndrome include hypoplasia of the right lung, secondary dextrocardia, and arterial supply of parts of the right lung by collateral arterial blood vessels, usually from the descending aorta.

Anomalous *drainage* of one or more pulmonary veins to the right atrium results from leftward malposition of septum primum. The normally connecting pulmonary veins drain anomalously.[11] This rare anomaly has been demonstrated in patients with heterotaxy syndrome with polysplenia.

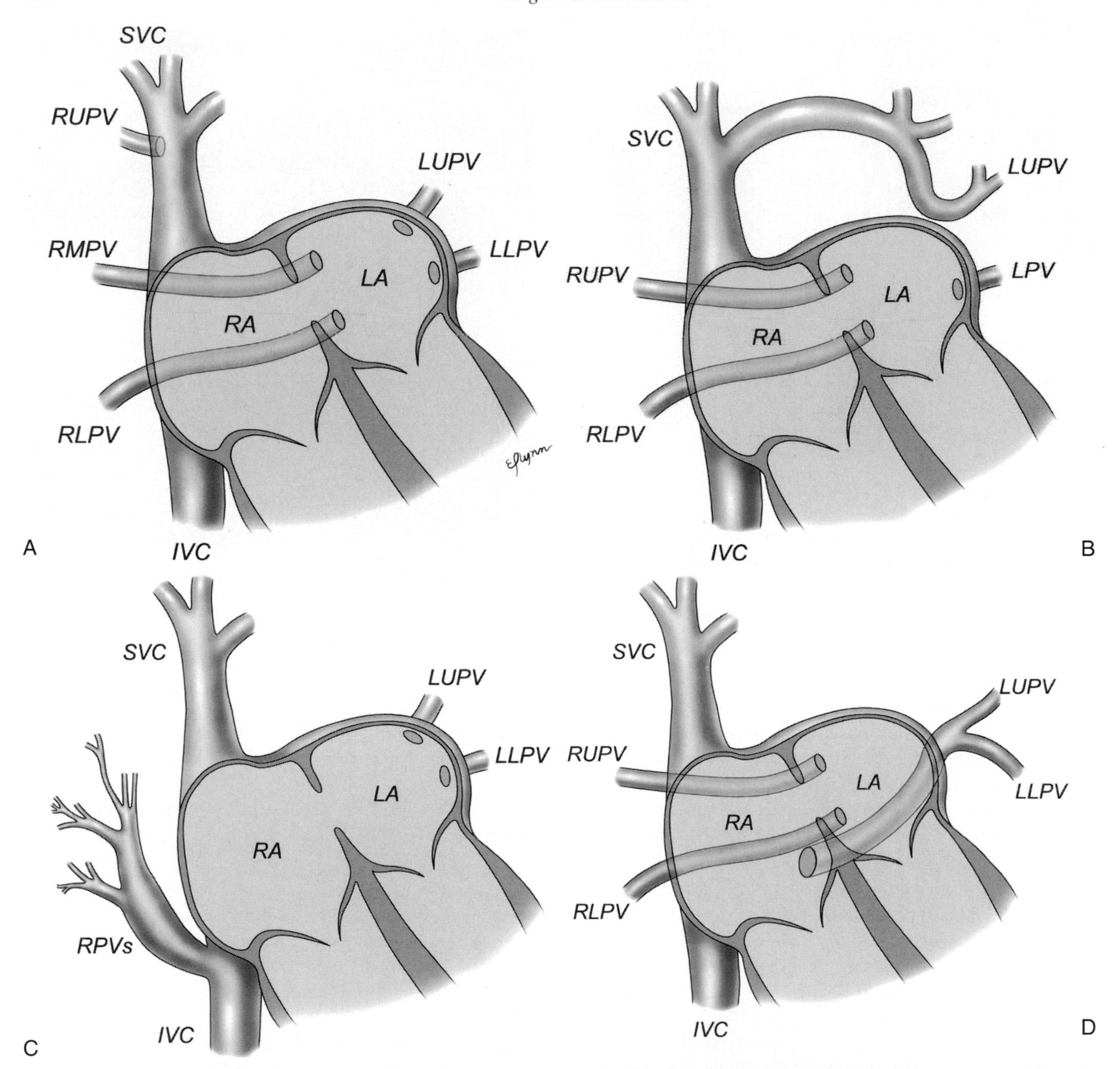

FIGURE 34–4 *Diagram of several connections of anomalous pulmonary veins to the systemic venous circulation. A, Drainage of the right upper veins (RUPV) to the superior vena cava (SVC). B, Drainage of the left upper veins (LUPV) through the left vertical vein to the innominate vein. C, Drainage of lower right-sided veins (RPVs) into the inferior vena cava (IVC; scimitar syndrome). D, Drainage of left pulmonary veins (LPVs) into the coronary sinus.*

PHYSIOLOGY

The amount of shunting through a large atrial defect is determined by the relative right and left ventricular compliance. Early in infancy, the right ventricle is less compliant, and left-to-right shunting is minimal, becoming greater as the right ventricle becomes more compliant with age. Years later, with normally decreasing left ventricular compliance with age and exacerbated by systemic hypertension, which often increases left ventricular end-diastolic pressure, there is a further increase in the left-to-right shunt. Therefore, it is a tenable hypothesis that atrial defects are associated with increasing left-to-right shunting as the patient gets older. Perhaps this hypothesis explains the clinical course of individuals who appear in adulthood with pulmonary vascular obstructive disease or congestive heart failure and an atrial defect but no history of congenital heart disease in childhood.

The left-to-right shunt is phasic, varying with systole and diastole. Often, a small right-to-left shunt can be detected by color-flow Doppler, this accounting for the slightly lower than normal average arterial oxygen saturation found in such patients.[12]

Although most infants with an atrial septal defect are asymptomatic, a few develop congestive heart failure and growth failure. Most often, these atypical infants have large left-to-right shunts in early infancy because there are additional defects, such as ventricular septal defect, patent ductus arteriosus, coarctation, myocardial dysfunction, an anatomically small left ventricle or systemic hypertension. The high incidence of associated extracardiac anomalies[5] accounts for the growth failure in some of these children. Surprisingly, a number of these infants in early difficulty undergo spontaneous closure of the defect,[13–15] suggesting that many of these "defects" are actually dilated patent foramina ovalia that became incompetent because of elevated left atrial pressure for whatever reason. Later, with resolution of the underlying left-sided problem, the foramen ovale closes.

Older patients may develop pulmonary vascular disease. In general, this unfortunate occurrence is rare before the age of 20 years and in the past occurred in 5% to 10% of adults with atrial septal defect who had not undergone surgical repair.[16,17] This incidence is likely to be quite less in the future because most atrial defects are now being closed on discovery, thus preventing the development of pulmonary vascular disease.

CLINICAL MANIFESTATIONS

Children with this congenital anomaly are usually discovered at a few years of age, rarely in the neonatal period. The lack of symptoms and the lack of a readily audible murmur account for the delay in discovering these patients. Generally, the cardiac problem is uncovered during routine examination of an otherwise well child. Discovery at the first preschool examination remains common. Most children with an atrial septal defect of the secundum variety are asymptomatic. A few small infants and many older adults present with congestive heart failure.

Atrial septal defects of the secundum type occur more commonly among females (63%).

Physical Examination

With a large shunt, there is often a left parasternal budge evident, and the underlying enlarged right ventricle is palpable. The first heart sound is characteristically loud at the left lower sternal border (in the presence of a normal or short P-R interval on the electrocardiogram). The second heart sound at the left upper sternal border is widely split, with the splitting interval fixed and unaffected by respiration (Fig. 34-5), owing to the large nonrestrictive atrial defect equalizing the respiratory influence on both right and left ventricular output, with the wide split resulting from delayed emptying of the enlarged right ventricle. The intensity of the pulmonary component is almost always normal, reflecting normal pulmonary pressure and resistance. Murmurs are not loud and may even be absent occasionally. There is usually an ejection systolic murmur (grade 2 at most) at the left upper sternal border due to minor relative pulmonary valve stenosis resulting from the increased flow. There is frequently an early diastolic flow rumble (grade 1 or 2), often of high frequency, at the left lower sternal border due to increased flow-related tricuspid stenosis.

Electrocardiography

On the electrocardiogram, the P-R interval is normal (in contrast to the prolonged interval of the endocardial

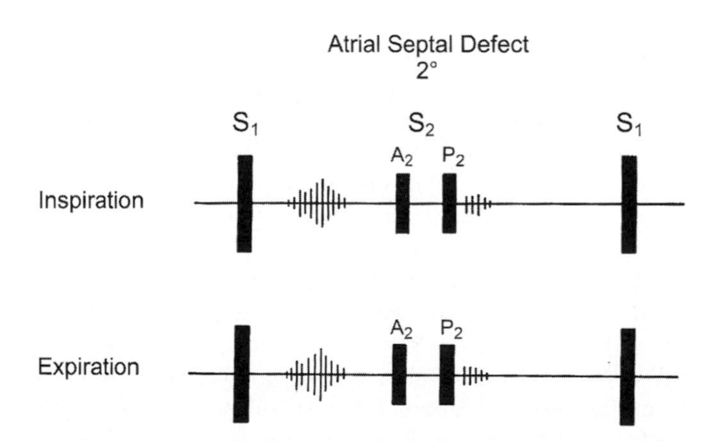

FIGURE 34–5 *Auscultatory findings resulting from an atrial septal defect. The second heart sound (S_2) is widely split and does not vary with respiration. There is a minimal systolic murmur of the ejection type. Often there is an early diastolic rumble that arises from excess flow across the tricuspid valve and seems to occur early in diastole, in part, because of the widely split second heart sound. S_1, first heart sound; A_2, aortic valve closure; P_2; pulmonic valve closure.*
From Fyler DC [ed]. Nadas' Pediatric Cardiology. Philadelphia: Hanley & Belfus, 1992.

cushion ostium primum defect, which decreases the intensity of the first heart closure). Incomplete right bundle branch block is usual (a normal finding in the age group when atrial defects are first discovered). Rarely, there is right ventricular hypertrophy, but later in life in those with pulmonary vascular obstructive disease, right ventricular hypertrophy is common. Right ventricular hypertrophy in the presence of an atrial septal defect may be found also if there is more than minimal pulmonary stenosis, a not unusual concomitant.

Chest X-Ray

On chest x-ray, the heart size is enlarged proportionate to the amount of shunting, and the pulmonary vascularity is increased. The superior vena cava shadow is often absent on the right of the spine on the plain chest film in patients with atrial septal defect, related to right atrial enlargement and clockwise rotation of the heart.

Echocardiography

Echocardiography is the primary imaging modality used for evaluation of atrial septal defects. The atrial septum and the adjacent systemic and pulmonary veins are imaged from several acoustic windows for any abnormal communication. Color-flow Doppler mapping is used to image blood flow direction and velocity. In addition, attention is given to evidence of excess volume load on the right heart structures as a result of the left-to-right shunt.[18] The right atrium, right ventricle, and pulmonary arteries are typically enlarged, and the interventricular septum flattens during diastole as a result of the increased flow.[19] Although echocardiographic measurements of the magnitude of the left-to-right shunt have been reported to correlate with invasive techniques,[20,21] this parameter is not routinely evaluated in clinical practice, in part because of uncertainties about its accuracy and reproducibility.

The atrial septum is best imaged from the subxiphoid window because the ultrasound beam is perpendicular to the atrial septum (Fig. 34-6). Even a thin septum primum is visible from this view, and the likelihood of false dropouts is minimized. In contrast, a false dropout in the mid-portion of the fossa ovalis is common when imaging from the apical view because the ultrasound beam is parallel to the septum. The parasternal short-axis and the right parasternal border (parasagittal) views are also helpful. Particular attention is paid to the location and size of the defect, to its relationship with adjacent structures such as the venae cavae, pulmonary veins, and AV valves, and to the presence of additional defects. In patients who are candidates for transcatheter device closure of the defect, septal rims and total septal length are measured.[22,23]

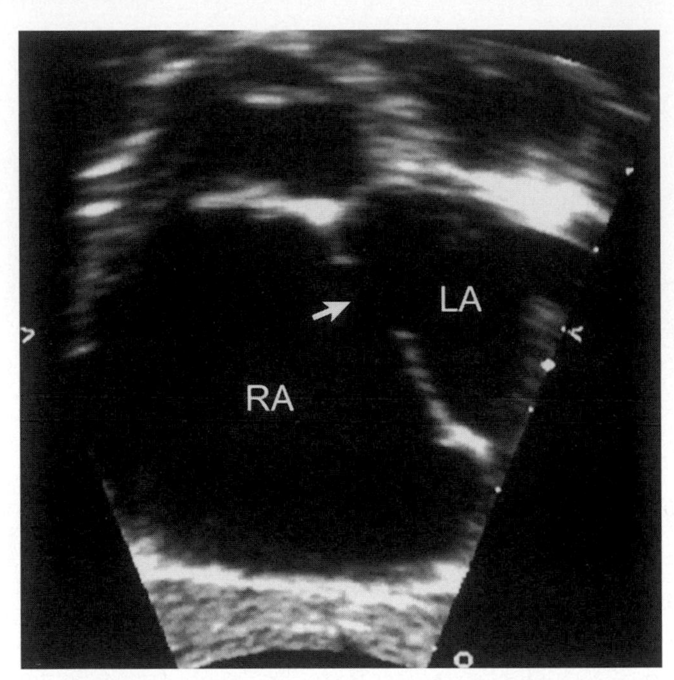

FIGURE 34–6 *Echocardiographic subxiphoid short-axis image of secundum atrial septal defect (arrow). RA, right atrium; LA, left atrium.*

In addition to color-flow Doppler mapping, contrast echo using agitated saline can be helpful in detecting an atrial-level shunt.[24] When a patent foramen ovale is suspected, injection of agitated saline during a Valsalva maneuver (which causes an increase in right atrial pressure) can demonstrate passage of contrast into the left side of the heart, indicating a right-to-left shunt across the foramen. When an unroofed coronary sinus is suspected, injection of agitated saline through an intravenous line placed in the left arm can substantiate the diagnosis by demonstrating appearance of contrast in the left atrium before it appears in the right atrium.

In patients with good acoustic windows and unambiguous delineation of the atrial septal and venous anatomy, transthoracic echocardiography is usually the only diagnostic tool necessary for management planning.[25–27] Transesophageal echocardiography provides an excellent window for imaging of the atrial septum and atrial ends of the systemic and the pulmonary veins[27] and is routinely used for guidance during transcatheter closure of atrial septal defects. Some centers prefer intracardiac echocardiography for the latter. Intraoperative transesophageal echocardiography is seldom used in our center in patients with isolated secundum atrial septal defect, but is frequently used in patients undergoing closure of sinus defects and other complex interatrial communications.

Magnetic Resonance Imaging

Magnetic resonance imaging (MRI) can be helpful in selected patients with a known or suspected atrial septal defect, usually adolescents and adults with inconclusive clinical and echocardiographic findings.[28,29] For example, MRI provides a noninvasive alternative to transesophageal echocardiography and to diagnostic catheterization in patients with right ventricular volume overload in whom transthoracic echo cannot demonstrate the source of the left-to-right shunt. The goals of the MRI examination include delineation of the atrial defect location and size, its relationship to key neighboring structures, and its suitability for transcatheter versus surgical closure, and functional assessment of the hemodynamic burden, including pulmonary-to-systemic flow ratio and right ventricular size and function. The accuracy and reproducibility of these MRI measurements have been demonstrated in several studies.[30,31] MRI is particularly helpful in patients with a sinus venosus defect and anomalous pulmonary venous connection because patient size and acoustic windows do not limit its diagnostic capabilities[32] (Fig. 34-7). In these patients, MRI often provides anatomic and function information that can obviate the need for diagnostic cardiac catheterization.

Cardiac Catheterization

Catheterization is necessary only in those in whom device closure is planned and in whom pulmonary hypertension and vascular obstructive disease are suspected. In the latter rare patients, usually adults, the primary reason for study is to evaluate pressure and resistance responses to vasodilators such as oxygen and nitric oxide to determine whether defect closure is advisable.

If catheterization is undertaken, special care is required when obtaining the right superior vena caval oxygen saturation for shunt calculation purposes. Considerable reflux of left atrial highly saturated blood occurs up the superior vena cava when a large shunt is present. Thus, an uncontaminated venous sample should be obtained high in the vena cava, even from the left innominate vein. We do not use inferior vena caval samples, considering them unreliable because of contamination by both reflux and very high renal vein values. If catheterization data in a patient with pulmonary hypertension suggest a defect might be safely closed, temporary device occlusion may be tested at that study. For defect visualization by angiography, contrast injection in the right upper pulmonary vein in a long-axis oblique projection delineates the defect quite satisfactorily (Fig. 34-8).

MANAGEMENT

Diagnosis of a secundum atrial defect is made or confirmed by echocardiography. For practical purposes, any defect 8 mm or larger with evidence of a significant left-to-right shunt should be closed when identified, even in very young patients, because such a defect will likely never close spontaneously[33,34] and may in fact even get larger.[35,36]

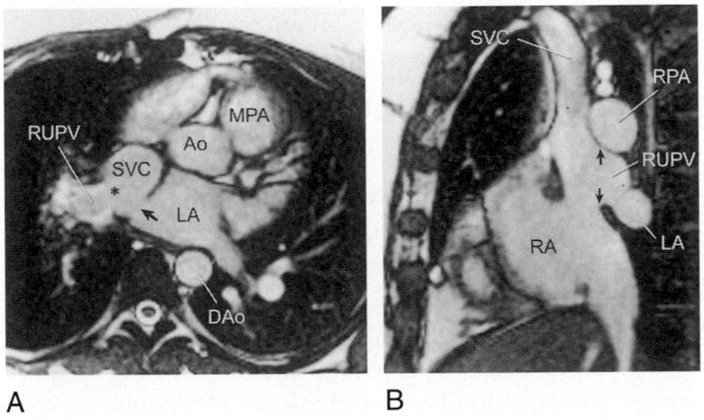

FIGURE 34–7 *Gradient echo cine magnetic resonance images of sinus venosus defect. A, An image in the axial plane showing the sinus venosus defect (*) as an area of unroofing of the wall between the right upper pulmonary vein (RUPV) and the superior vena cava (SVC). The arrow points to the left atrial orifice of the RUPV, which allows communication between the left atrium (LA) and the RUPV and SVC. B, An image in the sagittal plane showing the sinus venosus defect (arrows).*

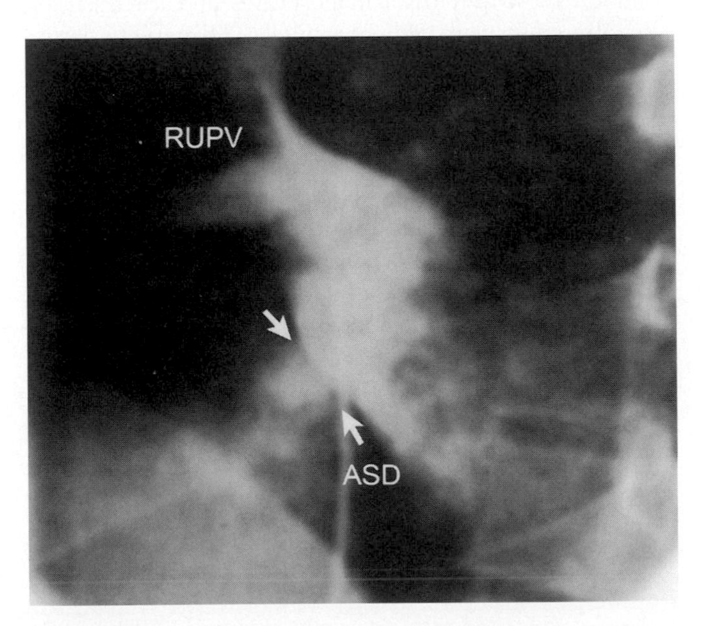

FIGURE 34–8 *Cineangiogram, long-axis oblique view, injecting contrast into right upper pulmonary vein (RUPV), outlining the location of atrial septal defect (ASD; arrows).*

It is reasonable to follow smaller defects in very young patients, which are generally asymptomatic, medically for a few years because many are likely to close spontaneously, particularly those smaller than 3 mm.[33,34,37,38] If, however, after some years of follow-up, echocardiographic evidence of shunting persists and the defect is 5 mm or larger, then it should be closed. The primary reason for closing an atrial defect is to prevent pulmonary vascular disease. Closure also reduces the incidence of supraventricular dysrhythmias (particularly atrial fibrillation), especially when carried out before age 40 years,[39–43] although it does not eliminate this problem even when performed in childhood.[44]

Closure of the secundum defect may be accomplished surgically or by a catheter-delivered device. Although surgery remains the more common approach, use of the latter continues to increase as devices, delivery equipment, and technical skill improve. Surgical techniques have likewise improved such that use of the "ministernotomy" has become widespread, and complete defect closure by suture or patch is almost always accomplished. Mortality is virtually zero, complications are few and mostly minor, and hospital stay has decreased to about 3 days[45–48] (see Chapter 57).

Device closure at catheterization was initially described in 1976,[49] and in those few original patients after 27 years of follow-up, occlusion remained effective, although atrial arrhythmias did occur.[50] During the past two decades, a variety of devices and their modifications have been used, including the clamshell, button, ASDOS, angel wings, and Amplatzer devices.[51] The longest follow-up has been with the clamshell device, and although residual leaks were common, these were trivial in most cases, and arm fractures, albeit frequent, were without sequelae.[52] Complete closure rates with the Amplatzer device in appropriate patients have been very satisfactory, ranging from 94% to 98%, with few severe complications.[53–55]

Clearly, device closure is more appealing than surgery because of absence of a thoracotomy scar and shorter hospital stay. In recent reports comparing surgery and Amplatzer device, defects were often larger in the surgical patients, there were no deaths with either technique, and closure rates were similar (96% to 100%); and although complications occurred in both groups, they were more common in the surgical population.[56–59] In terms of cost in three series, surgery was clearly more expensive in one,[56] slightly more in another,[57] and the same in the third,[58] each report from a different country.

COURSE

The natural course of atrial septal defect, except for the largest openings and those associated with other cardiac defects, is relatively benign.[60] Many patients with significant defects survive for several decades before developing symptoms. It is likely that acquired diseases of adulthood (coronary artery problems, systemic hypertension) often elevate left ventricular end-diastolic pressure, leading to a rise in the left atrial value, which in turn increases the left-to-right shunting. Late problems include congestive heart failure, atrial fibrillation, and rarely pulmonary vascular obstructive disease.

Follow-up of Patients After Closure

Most defects are still closed surgically. Overall, it is remarkable how frequently exercise tolerance improves in patients considered asymptomatic before surgery. It is also quite striking how many patients continue to remain undiagnosed for many decades, with many recent reports containing hundreds of such patients.[39,40,43,46,61] Residual patch leaks are uncommon, and most patients are clinically better. Echocardiographically, right ventricular volumes decrease but do not reach normal values in many, especially in those operated on at older ages.[42,44,61–64] Late appearance of pulmonary vascular obstructive disease or congestive heart failure after repair is virtually unknown, although if some is present preoperatively, it may indeed progress.[65]

Atrial Dysrhythmias

Before closure, atrial dysrhythmias (flutter, fibrillation) are encountered, particularly in older patients. After defect closure, these sometimes improve but are often not eliminated.[39–43] Although their occurrence is age related, supporting repair at a younger age, they have also been seen long after surgical closure in young patients, albeit less frequently.[44] They have also been reported after device closure in those with long follow-up.[50]

Pulmonary Vascular Obstruction

This occurs in about 5% to 10% of patients with unrepaired atrial defects.[17,65] Although most patients exceed age 20 years and are female, rare instances in childhood have occurred[66] (Fig. 34-9). Catheterization with evaluation of response to oxygen and nitric oxide is advisable in all such patients. Any underlying causes such as obstructive airway disease, sleep apnea, high altitude, or drugs require careful investigation because these are reversible.

VARIATIONS

Symptomatic Infants

There are rare infants who fail to thrive, have heart failure or large atrial septal defects, do not respond dramatically to anticongestive drugs, and have no other abnormality.

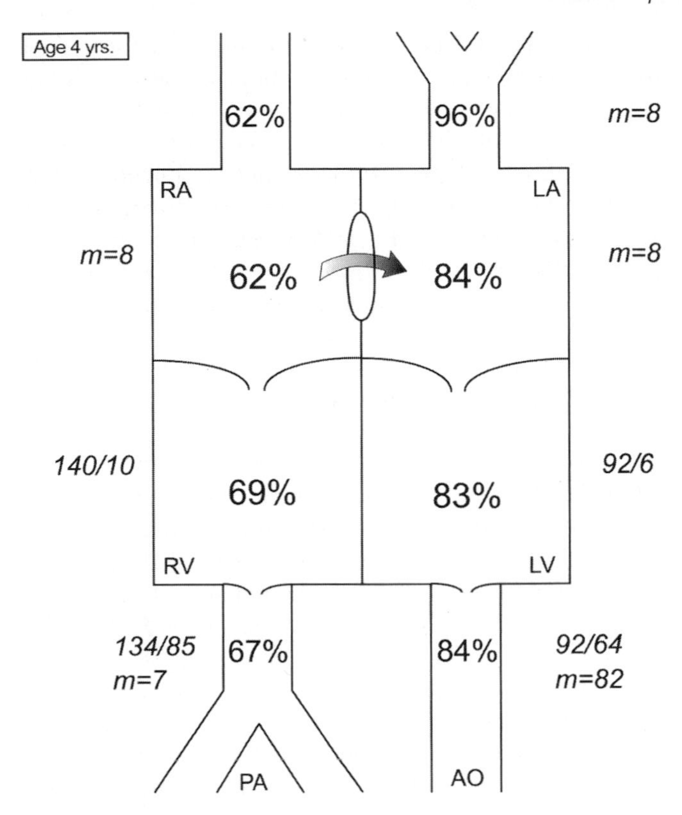

FIGURE 34–9 *Catheterization data in a 4-year-old girl with Down syndrome, a very large atrial defect, right-to-left shunting across this defect (arrows), suprasystemic right ventricle (RV) and pulmonary artery (PA) pressures, and severe pulmonary vascular obstructive disease unresponsive to oxygen and vasodilators. She died 22 months later. RA, right atrium; LA, left atrium; LV, left ventricle; AO, aorta.*

Because spontaneous closure will not occur, surgery, which has minimal risk, is indicated.

Patent Foramen Ovale

Everybody at birth has a patent foramen ovale except in very rare instances such as hypoplastic left heart syndrome. It functionally closes in most within days owing to shifting of the left-sided septum primum against the septum secundum as left atrial pressure rises to exceed that on the right. That it does not anatomically close by fusion for some time has been known to, and appreciated by, catheterization technicians for many years, this foramen providing access to the left heart structures from the right atrium in almost all infants in the first 6 months of life. With increasing use of and technologic improvements in echocardiographic equipment, the patent foramen has become a common observation, especially in young patients (see Exhibit 34-1). Because there is little, if any, shunting and thus no volume overload evidence on the right heart chambers, it has been by and large considered a finding of no significance. Although echocardiographically it has closed in most children by 18 months of age,[38] persistent patency in some 20% of patients older than 90 years has been noted at autopsy.[67]

With the introduction of echocardiographic "bubble studies" and color-flow Doppler, right-to-left atrial shunting, especially with Valsalva maneuvers (which elevate right atrial pressure), became evident. This finding was soon noted to be common in patients with neurologic insults suggestive of an embolic etiology.[68–73] There is thus widespread interest in management of such patients with this combination of lesions. Treatment strategies, including foramen closure surgically or by catheter-delivered devices, are being used that have reduced but not completely eliminated the neurologic events.[73–77]

Sinus Venosus Defects

Superior Vena Caval Sinus Venosus Defect

The superior venal caval sinus venosus defect usually is not large, and shunting usually does not exceed 2:1 Qp/Qs. Clinically, these patients have the physical and electrocardiographic findings of a significant atrial septal secundum defect. Similarly, echocardiographic evaluation demonstrates right heart volume overload characteristics, but with no obvious defect visible in the central atrial septum. Meticulous examination is required to visualize this superior defect (see Fig. 34-6). Although some have real anomalous return of right upper pulmonary veins to the superior vena cava, for the most part, it is the defect location that makes this more apparent than real.[6] All patients are referred to surgery. In older patients, surgery has been very successful using patch defect closure through a transcaval approach.[78] In very young patients, especially when right upper pulmonary venous return is anomalous to the superior vena cava, there is not much room available for a baffle. To circumvent this problem, the superior vena cava is transected superior to the anomalous veins and the distal caval end anastomosed to the right atrial appendage. The atrial defect is then closed in such a way that the proximal vena cava and anomalous veins drain to the left atrium.[79] In older patients, this operation has been quite successful.[79] In our own experience (mean surgical age, 4 years), although dysrhythmias have not been evident, obstruction at the superior vena cava–right atrial anastomosis has occurred in some and has been managed successfully by balloon dilation and stent placement (Fig. 34-10).

Unroofed Coronary Sinus

Diagnosis of unroofed coronary sinus is made by echocardiography (see Fig. 34-3). Surgical repair is tailored to the anatomy present. If a left superior vena cava is present, it is redirected to the right atrial side either through ligation, if an adequate innominate vein is present, or through an intra–left baffle or tunnel to the right atrium.[80] If there is no left superior vena cava and the coronary sinus defect is huge, then the orifice of the coronary sinus is closed. Whether the coronary venous blood flow drains into the left atrium or is redirected to the right is of little practical consequence.

Inferior Vena Caval Sinus Venosus Defect

These rare defects, adjacent to the orifice of the inferior vena cava, often seem to be associated with return of the right lower pulmonary veins. Because the inferior vena caval sinus venosus defect lies between the orifice of the inferior vena cava and the orifices of these veins, this anomalous return is more apparent than real.[81] An appropriate single patch will close the defect with the veins on the correct side, the patch assuming the normal position of the atrial septum.

Partial Anomalous Venous Return

Partial anomalous pulmonary veins are relatively common, usually complicating other cardiac abnormalities. Most often, there is an associated atrial defect, and the hemodynamics are those of an atrial defect. In the absence of an atrial defect, the second sound may be well split but is not fixed relative to respiration. As an isolated defect, partial anomalous pulmonary veins only rarely cause symptoms; pulmonary hypertension is extremely rare, having been reported only in a couple of older patients,[82] and thought due to pulmonary emboli in another.[83]

For the most part, these anomalous veins can be corrected, but the surgical difficulty, the likelihood of success, and the probable benefits should be weighed carefully before proceeding. Abnormal entry of a single small pulmonary vein does not require surgical intervention. The anomalous veins pose the practical problem of what to do when the chest has been opened to repair an atrial defect. Small pulmonary veins entering the left innominate vein may be ligated without a problem or left alone. Pulmonary veins entering the inferior vena cava in older patients can be baffled successfully to the left atrium. In neonates and infants, however, this may be very difficult, and such an attempt in this age group may result in severe obstruction or complete occlusion of the created channel. In those with much or all of the left pulmonary veins returning to the left innominate vein, the connecting vertical vein is usually large and long enough to detach from the innominate vein and anastomose to the left atrium. In each case, tailoring the response to the anatomy is required.

Scimitar Syndrome

Usually, the relatively rare scimitar syndrome is readily recognized on the plain chest x-ray because there is hypoplasia of the right lung, the heart shadow is shifted to the right, and the visible right pulmonary veins (the scimitar) curve toward the inferior vena cava (Fig. 34-11). Sometimes, the physiologic advantage of surgical correction is not obvious in the adult because the amount of blood shunting through the small right lung may be small (less than 1.5/L). In those detected in infancy, symptoms, heart failure, atrial septal defect, pulmonary sequestration, and

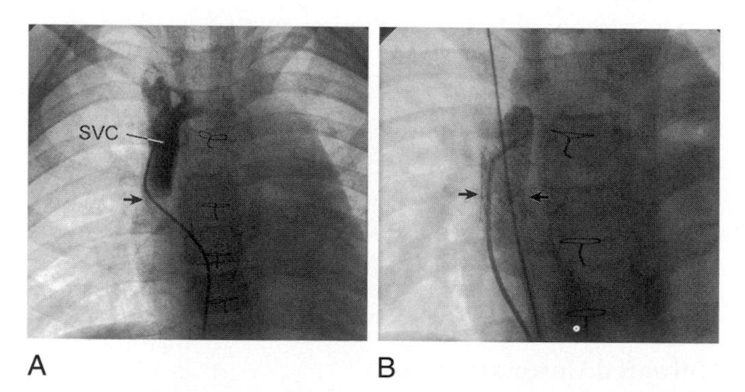

FIGURE 34–10 *Cineangiogram in superior vena cava (SVC) of 7-year-old patient showing (A) virtual occlusion of SVC–right atrial anastomosis (arrow) done as part of repair of sinus venosus atrial defect and (B) now wide-open anastomosis following balloon dilation and stent (arrows) placement.*

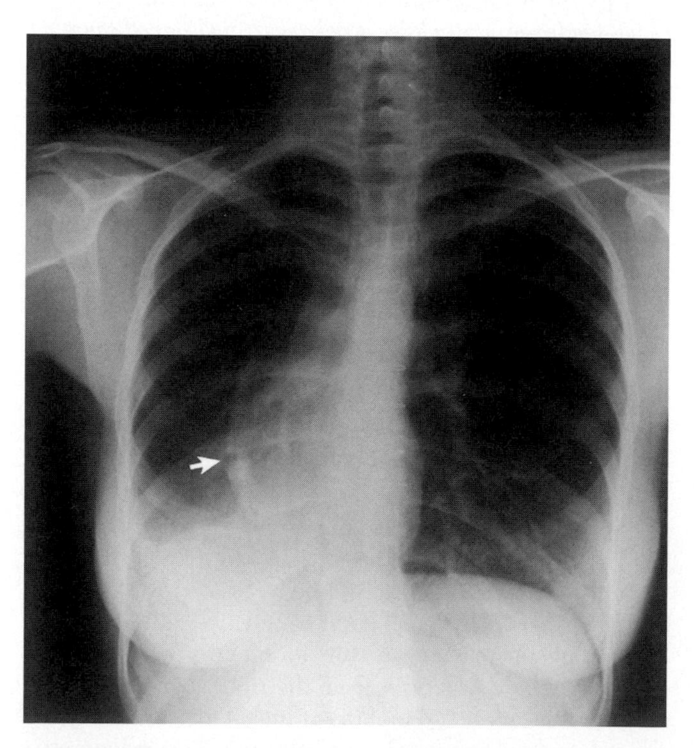

FIGURE 34–11 *X-ray of an asymptomatic 15-year-old patient with scimitar syndrome showing the anomalous pulmonary vein (arrow) draining to the inferior vena cava. Note the dextrocardia because of hypoplasia of the right lung and the corresponding increase in size of the left lung.*

hypertension are common, and some 25% have pulmonary vein stenosis. Postoperative obstruction to pulmonary venous return is very common in infants, and diminished right lung flow is present in almost all.[84]

Uncomplicated Atrial Defect with Cyanosis

Rarely, patients with an atrial septal defect or patent foramen ovale, without other cardiac abnormality, are cyanotic, particularly on exercise.[85,86] This is considered to be an extreme version of the small right-to-left shunt measurable in almost all patients with an atrial septal defect and perhaps is aggravated by an unusually large eustachian valve often found in these people. Closing the defect is curative (Fig. 34-12).

Mitral Valve Prolapse

Mitral valve prolapse (see Chapter 40) is a curious finding seen among some patients with atrial septal defect, without known practical consequence. That mitral valve prolapse is caused by the atrial defect itself is suggested by improvement in the degree of prolapse after repair of the atrial defect.[87]

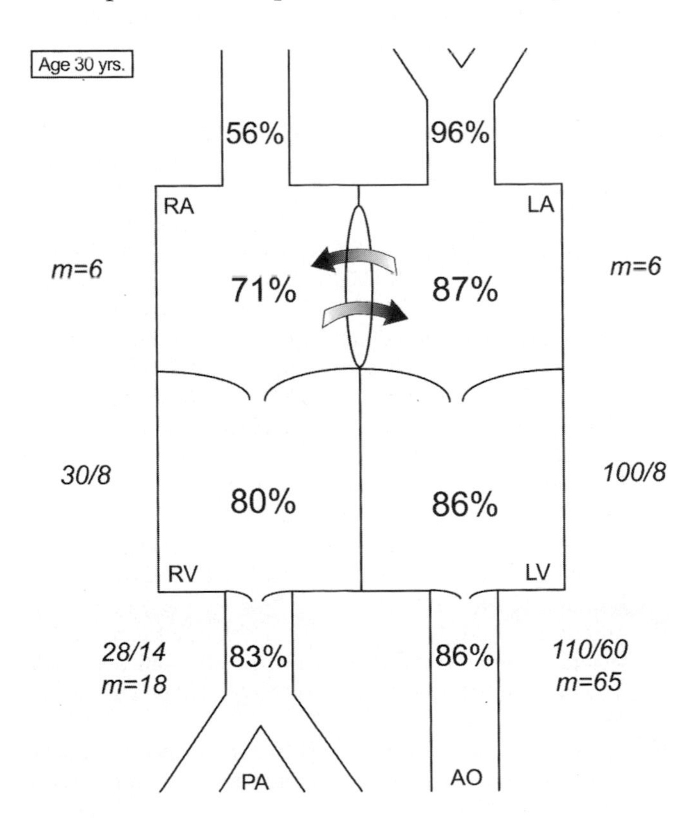

FIGURE 34–12 *Catheterization data in 30-year-old woman with huge atrial secundum septal defect. There is right-to-left shunting at the atrial level and normal pulmonary artery pressure. This atrial defect was surgically closed with a patch, with now normal postoperative physiologic data. RA, right atrium; LA, left atrium; RV, right ventricle; LV, left ventricle; PA, pulmonary artery; AO, aorta; %, oxygen saturation.*

REFERENCES

1. Steiner MM, DiTullio MR, Rundek T, et al. Patent foramen ovale size and embolic brain imaging findings among patients with ischemic stroke. Stroke 29:944, 1998.
2. Mas JL, Arquizan C, Lamy C. Recurrent cerebrovascular events associated with patent foramen ovale, atrial septal aneurysm, or both. N Engl J Med 345:1740, 2001.
3. Botto LD, Correa A, Erickson JD. Racial and temporal variations in the prevalence of heart defects. Pediatrics 107(3), 2001.
4. Hoffman JE, Kaplan S. The incidence of congenital heart disease. J Am Coll Cardiol 39:1890, 2002.
5. Fyler DC, Buckley LP, Hellenbrand WE, et al. Report of the New England Regional Infant Cardiac Program. Pediatrics 65(Suppl):376, 1980.
6. Van Praagh S, Carrera ME, Sanders SP, et al. Sinus venosus defects: Unroofing of the right pulmonary veins—anatomic and echocardiographic findings and surgical treatment. Am Heart J 128:365, 1994.
7. Blom NA, Gittenberger-de Groot AC, Jongeneel TH, et al. Normal development of the pulmonary veins in human embryos and formulation of a morphogenetic concept for sinus venosus defects. Am J Cardiol 87:305, 2001.
8. Raghib G, Ruttenberg HD, Anderson RC, et al. Termination of left superior vena cava in left atrium, atrial septal defect, and absence of coronary sinus: A developmental complex. Circulation 31:906, 1965.
9. Geva T, Van Praagh S. Anomalies of the pulmonary veins. In Allen HD, Gutgessel HP, Clark EB, Driscoll DJ (eds). Moss & Adams' Heart Disease in Infants, Children and Adolescents. Philadelphia: Lippincott Williams & Wilkins, 2001:736.
10. Gao YA, Burrows PE, Benson LN, et al. Scimitar syndrome in infancy. J Am Coll Cardiol 22:873, 1993.
11. Van Praagh S, Carrera ME, Sanders SP, et al. Partial or total direct pulmonary venous drainage to right atrium due to malposition of septum primum. Anatomic and echocardiographic findings and surgical treatment: A study based on 36 cases. Chest 107:1488, 1995.
12. Parisi LF, Nadas AS. Natural history of atrial septal defects. In Kidd BSL, Keith JK (eds). Natural History and Progress in Treatment of Congenital Heart Defects. Springfield, IL: Charles C. Thomas, 1971.
13. Cockerham JT, Martin TC, Gutierrez FR, et al. Spontaneous closure of secundum atrial septal defect in infants and young children. Am J Cardiol 52:1267, 1983.
14. Mahoney LT, Truesdell SC, Krzmarzick TR, et al. Atrial septal defects that present in infancy. Am J Dis Child 140:1115, 1986.
15. Yeager SB, Keane JF. Fate of moderate and large secundum atrial septal defect associated with isolated coarctation in infants. Am J Cardiol 84:362, 1999.

16. Besterman E. Atrial septal defect with pulmonary hypertension. Br Heart J 23:587, 1961.
17. Zaver AG, Nadas AS. Atrial septal defect—secundum type. Circulation 32(Suppl III):24, 1965.
18. Denef B, Dumoulin M, Van der Hauwaert LG. Usefulness of echocardiographic assessment of right ventricular and pulmonary trunk size for estimating magnitude of left-to-right shunt in children with atrial septal defect. Am J Cardiol 55:1571, 1985.
19. Chazal RA, Armstrong WF, Dillon JC, et al. Diastolic ventricular septal motion in atrial septal defect: Analysis of M-mode echocardiograms in 31 patients. Am J Cardiol 52:1088, 1983.
20. Marx GR, Allen HD, Goldberg SJ, et al. Transatrial septal velocity measurement by Doppler echocardiography in atrial septal defect: Correlation with Qp:Qs ratio. Am J Cardiol 55:1162, 1985.
21. Veyrat C, Gourtchiglouian C, Bas S, et al. Quantification of left to right shunt in atrial septal defect using systolic time intervals derived from pulsed Doppler velocimetry. Br Heart J 52:633, 1984.
22. Ishii M, Kato H, Inoue O, et al. Biplane transesophageal echo-Doppler studies of atrial septal defects: Quantitative evaluation and monitoring for transcatheter closure. Am Heart J 125:1363, 1993.
23. Rosenfeld HM, van der Velde ME, Sanders SP, et al. Echocardiographic predictors of candidacy for successful transcatheter atrial septal defect closure. Catheter Cardiovasc Diagn 34:29, 1995.
24. Rosenzweig BP, Nayar AC, Varkay MP, et al. Echo contrast-enhanced diagnosis of atrial septal defect. J Am Soc Echocardiogr 14:155, 2001.
25. Freed MD, Nadas AS, Norwood WI, et al. Is routine preoperative cardiac catheterization necessary before repair of secundum and sinus venosus atrial septal defects? J Am Coll Cardiol 4:333, 1984.
26. Tworetzky W, McElhinney DB, Brook MM, et al. Echocardiographic diagnosis alone for the complete repair of major congenital heart defects. J Am Coll Cardiol 33:228, 1999.
27. van der Velde ME, Sanders SP, Keane JF, et al. Transesophageal echocardiographic guidance of transcatheter ventricular septal defect closure. J Am Coll Cardiol 23:1660, 1994.
28. Taylor AM, Stables RH, Poole-Wilson PA, et al. Definitive clinical assessment of atrial septal defect by magnetic resonance imaging. J Cardiovasc Magn Reson 1:43, 1999.
29. Holmvang G. A magnetic resonance imaging method for evaluating atrial septal defects. J Cardiovasc Magn Reson 1:59, 1999.
30. Powell AJ, Tsai-Goodman B, Prakash A, et al. Comparison between phase-velocity cine magnetic resonance imaging and invasive oximetry for quantification of atrial shunts. Am J Cardiol 91:1523, 2003.
31. Beerbaum P, Korperich H, Barth P, et al. Noninvasive quantification of left-to-right shunt in pediatric patients: Phase-contrast cine magnetic resonance imaging compared with invasive oximetry. Circulation 103:2476, 2001.
32. Ferrari VA, Scott CH, Holland GA, et al. Ultrafast three-dimensional contrast-enhanced magnetic resonance angiography and imaging in the diagnosis of partial anomalous pulmonary venous drainage. J Am Coll Cardiol 37:1120, 2001.
33. Radzik D, Davignon A, van Doesburg N, et al. Predictive factors for spontaneous closure of atrial septal defects diagnosed in the first 3 months of life. J Am Coll Cardiol 22(3):851, 1993.
34. Helgason H, Jonsdottir G. Spontaneous closure of atrial septal defects. Pediatric Cardiol 20(3):195, 1999.
35. McMahon CJ, Feltes TF, Fraley JK, et al. Natural history of growth of secundum atrial septal defects and implications for transcatheter closure. Heart (British Cardiac Society) 87(3):256, 2002.
36. Brassard M, Fouron JC, van Doesburg NH, et al. Outcome of children with atrial septal defect considered too small for surgical closure. Am J Cardiol 83(11):1552, 1999.
37. Riggs T, Sharp SE, Batton D, et al. Spontaneous closure of atrial septal defects in premature vs. full-term neonates. Pediatr Cardiol 21(2):129, 2000.
38. Senocak F, Karademir S, Cabuk F. Spontaneous closure of interatrial septal openings in infants: An echocardiographic study. Int J Cardiol 53(3):221, 1996.
39. Mantovan R, Gatzoulis MA, Pedrocco A, et al. Supraventricular arrhythmia before and after surgical closure of atrial septal defects: spectrum, prognosis and management. Europace 5(2):133, 2003.
40. Oliver JM, Gallego P, Gonzalez A, et al. Predisposing conditions for atrial fibrillation in atrial septal defect with and without operative closure. Am J Cardiol 89(1):39, 2002.
41. Donti A, Bonvicini M, Placci A, et al. Surgical treatment of secundum atrial septal defect in patients older than 50 years. Italian Heart J 2(6):428, 2001.
42. Ghosh S, Chatterjee S, Black E, et al. Surgical closure of atrial septal defect in adults: Effect of age at operation on outcome. Heart (British Cardiac Society) 88(5):485, 2002.
43. Gatzoulis MA, Freeman MA, Siu SC, et al. Atrial arrhythmia after surgical closure of atrial septal defects in adults. N Engl J Med 340(11):839, 1999.
44. Roos-Hesselink JW, Meijboom FJ, Spitaels SE, et al. Excellent survival and low incidence of arrhythmias, stroke and heart failure long-term after surgical ASD closure at young age: A prospective follow-up study of 21-33 years. Eur Heart J 24(2):190, 2003.
45. Attie F, Rosas M, Granados N, et al. Surgical treatment for secundum atrial septal defects in patients > 40 years old: A randomized clinical trial. J Am Coll Cardiol 38(7):2035, 2001.
46. Horvath KA, Burke RP, Collins JJ Jr, et al. Surgical treatment of adult atrial septal defect: early and long-term results. J Am Coll Cardiol 20(5):1156, 1992.
47. Jones DA, Radford DJ, Pohlner PG. Outcome following surgical closure of secundum atrial septal defect. J Paediatr Child Health 37(3):274, 2001.
48. Gessner IH. Atrial septal defect. In Moller JH (ed). Perspectives in Pediatric Cardiology, vol 6. Surgery of Congenital Heart Disease. Pediatric Cardiac Care Consortium 1984–1985. Armonk, NY: Futura, 1998:31.

49. King T, Thompson S, Steiner C, et al. Secundum atrial septal defect: Nonoperative closure during cardiac catheterization. JAMA 235:2506, 1976.
50. Mills NL, King TD. Late follow-up of nonoperative closure of secundum atrial septal defects using the King-Mills double umbrella device. Am J Cardiol 92(3):353, 2003.
51. Rocchini A, Lock JE. Defect closure: Umbrella devices. In Lock JE, Keane JF, Perry SB (eds). Diagnostic and Interventional Catheterization in Congenital Heart Disease. Norwell, MA: Kluwer Academic, 2000:179–198.
52. Prieto L, Foreman C, Cheatham J, et al. Intermediate-term outcome of transcatheter secundum atrial septal defect closure using the Bard Clamshell Septal Umbrella. Am J Cardiol 78(11):1310, 1996.
53. Fischer G, Stieh J, Uebing A, et al. Experience with transcatheter closure of secundum atrial septal defects using the Amplatzer septal occluder: A single centre study in 236 consecutive patients. Heart (British Cardiac Society) 89(2): 199, 2003.
54. Du ZD, Hijazi ZM, Kleinman CS, et al. Comparison between transcatheter and surgical closure of secundum atrial septal defect in children and adults: Results of a multicenter nonrandomized trial. J Am Coll Cardiol 39(11):1836, 2002.
55. Berger F, Ewert P, Bjornstad PG, et al. Transcatheter closure as standard treatment for most interatrial defects: experience in 200 patients treated with the Amplatzer septal occluder [see comment]. Cardiol Young 9(5):468, 1999.
56. Kim JJ, Hijazi ZM. Clinical outcomes and costs of Amplatzer transcatheter closure as compared with surgical closure of ostium secundum atrial septal defects. Med Sci Monitor 8(12):CR787, 2002.
57. Hughes ML, Maskell G, Goh TH, et al. Prospective comparison costs and short term health outcomes of surgical versus device closure of atrial defect in children. Heart (British Cardiac Society) 88(1):67, 2002.
58. Thomson JD, Aburawi EH, Watterson KG, et al. Surgical and transcatheter (Amplatzer) closure of atrial septal defects: A prospective comparison of results and cost. Heart (British Cardiac Society) 87(5):466, 2002.
59. Berger F, Vogel M, Alexi-Meskishvili V, et al. Comparison of results and complications of surgical and Amplatzer device closure of atrial septal defects. J Thorac Cardiovasc Surg 118(4):674, 1999.
60. Campbell M. Natural history of atrial septal defect. Br Heart J 32:820, 1970.
61. Attenhofer Jost CH, Oechslin E, Seifert B, et al. Remodeling after surgical repair of atrial septal defects within the oval fossa. Cardiol Young 12(6):506, 2002.
62. Jemielty M, Dyszkiewicz W, Paluszkiewicz L, et al. Do patients over 40 years of age benefit from surgical closure of atrial septal defects? [see comment]. Heart (British Cardiac Society) 85(3):300, 2001.
63. Celik S, Ozay B, Dagdeviren B, et al. Effect of patient age at surgical intervention on long-term right ventricular performance in atrial septal defect. Jap Heart J 45(2):265, 2004.
64. Veldtman GR, Razack V, Siu S, et al. Right ventricular form and function after percutaneous atrial septal defect device closure. J Am Coll Cardiol 37(8):2108, 2001.
65. Steele PM, Fuster V, Cohen M, et al. Isolated atrial septal defect with pulmonary vascular obstructive disease: Long term follow-up and prediction of outcome after surgical correction. Circulation 76:1037, 1987.
66. Haworth SG. Pulmonary vascular disease in secundum atrial septal defect in childhood. Am J Cardiol 51:265, 1983.
67. Hagen PT, Scholz DG, Edwards WD. Incidence and size of patent foramen ovale during the first 10 decades of life: An autopsy of 965 normal hearts. Mayo Clin Proc 59:17, 1984.
68. DiTullio M, Sacco RL, Gopal A, et al. Patent foramen ovale as a risk factor for cryptogenic stroke. Ann Intern Med 117: 461, 1992
69. Steiner, DiTullio MR, Rundek T, et al. Patent foramen ovale size and embolic brain imaging findings among patients with ischemic stroke. Stroke 29:944, 1998.
70. Serena J, Segura T, Perez-Ayuso J, et al. The need to quantify right-to-left shunt in acute ischemic stroke. Stroke 29:1322, 1998.
71. Mas JL, Arquizan C, Lamy C, et al. Recurrent cerebrovascular events associated with patent foramen ovale, atrial septal aneurysm, or both. N Engl J Med 345:1740, 2001.
72. Schuchlenz HW, Saurer G, Weihs W, et al. Persisting eustachian valve in adults: Relation to patent foramen ovale and cerebrovascular events. J Am Society of Echocardiogr 17(3):231, 2004.
73. Wu LA, Malouf JF, Dearani JA, et al. Patent foramen ovale in cryptogenic stroke: Current understanding and management options. Arch Intern Med 164(9):950, 2004.
74. Dearani JA, Ugurlu BS, Danielson GK, et al. Surgical patent foramen ovale closure for prevention of paradoxical embolism-related cerebrovascular ischemic events. Circulation 100 (19 Suppl II):171, 1999.
75. Bridges ND, Hellenbrand W, Latson L, et al. Transcatheter closure of patent foramen ovale after presumed paradoxical embolism. Circulation 86:1902, 1992.
76. Butera G, Bini MR, Chessa M, et al. Transcatheter closure of patent foramen ovale in patients with cryptogenic stroke [see comment]. Ital Heart J 2(2):115, 2001.
77. Khositseth A, Cabalka AK, Sweeney JP, et al. Transcatheter Amplatzer device closure of atrial septal defect and patent foramen ovale in patients with presumed paradoxical embolism [see comment]. Mayo Clin Proc 79(1):35, 2004.
78. Nicholson IA, Chard RB, Nunn GR, et al. Transcaval repair of the sinus venosus syndrome. J Thorac Cardiovasc Surg 119(4 Pt 1):741, 2000.
79. Gustafson RA, Warden HE, Murray GF. Partial anomalous pulmonary venous connection to the superior vena cava. Ann Thorac Surg 60(6 Suppl):S614, 1995.
80. Sand ME, McGrath LB, Pacifico AD, et al. Repair of left superior vena cava entering the left atrium. Ann Thorac Surg 42:560, 1986.
81. Van Praagh S, Kakou-Guikahue M, Kim H-S, et al. Atrial situs in patients with visceral heterotaxy and congenital heart disease: Conclusions based on findings in 104 postmortem cases. Coeur 19:484, 1988.
82. Babb JD, McGlynn TJ, Pierce WS, et al. Isolated partial anomalous venous connection: A congenital defect with late and serious complications. Ann Thorac Surg 31(6):540, 1981.

83. AboulHosn JA, Criley JM, Stringer WW. Partial anomalous pulmonary venous return: Case report and review of the literature. Catheter Cardiovasc Intervent 58(4):548, 2003.
84. Najm HK, Williams WG, Coles JG, et al. Scimitar syndrome: Twenty years experience and results of repair. J Thorac Cardiovasc Surg 112:1161, 1996.
85. Gallaher ME, Sperling DR, Gwinn JL, et al. Functional drainage of the inferior vena cava into the left atrium—three cases. Am J Cardiol 12:561, 1963.
86. Thomas JD, Tabakin BS, Ittleman FP. Atrial septal defect with right to left shunt despite normal pulmonary artery pressure. J Am Coll Cardiol 9:221, 1987.
87. Schreiber TL, Feigenbaum H, Weyan AE. Effect of atrial septal defect repair on left ventricular geometry and degree of mitral valve prolapse. Circulation 61:888, 1980.

35

Patent Ductus Arteriosus

JOHN F. KEANE AND DONALD C. FYLER

DEFINITION

The ductus is functionally closed in about 90% of full-term infants by 48 hours of age. Persistent, some intermittent, patency for up to 10 days after birth is encountered in patients with circulatory or ventilatory abnormalities and for even longer periods in premature infants. For this chapter, patency of the ductus beyond a few days, and without other significant cardiac lesions, is considered abnormal.

PREVALENCE

The reported incidence of patent ductus in infants ranges from 0.138[1] to 0.8 per 1000 live births,[2] the former value from earlier years among mostly ill infants and the latter in more recent times in the echocardiographic era. At Children's Hospital Boston, the number of patients seen, among all age groups, with a patent ductus during the past 14 years has been smaller than during the preceding 15 years (Exhibit 35-1), related in part to our coding system, continued expansion of neonatology, and the more widespread use of catheter-based closure techniques.

Not only does patency of the ductus arteriosus persist longer among premature infants, but prematurity also accounts for some of the patent ductus arteriosus seen long after infancy. Children born of mothers who have rubella around the time of conception have a high incidence of patent ductus. Maternal rubella is thought to be the cause of its seasonal incidence, which was noted before immunization was widely introduced. Children born at high altitudes more often have a persistently patent ductus than those born at sea level. The number increases as the altitude increases, suggesting that patency is a direct function of ambient oxygen.

ANATOMY

The ductus arteriosus is derived from the left sixth embryologic arch and connects the origin of the left main pulmonary artery to the aorta, just below the left subclavian artery. During fetal life, the ductus is as large or larger than the ascending aorta and carries outflow from the right ventricle to the descending aorta (Fig. 35-1). Within hours of birth, the ductus closes, usually at the pulmonary end, often leaving behind a remnant on the aorta, a ductus diverticulum. Occasionally, a diverticulum persists at the point of origin from the pulmonary artery as well. With a right aortic arch, the ductus is usually left sided, although rarely it arises in a mirror image, entering the right pulmonary artery. Bilateral ductus is rare. In pulmonary atresia, the ductus is small because the left-to-right flow it carries is a small fraction of that normally passing right-to-left to the aorta in the fetus. In patients with tetralogy of Fallot, the ductus is often absent.

The ductus closes through muscular constriction a few hours after birth. Later, there is obliteration of the lumen, initially by a pile up of endothelium and, finally, by complete occlusion through thrombosis, the ductus withering to a fibrous strand. The histopathology of a persistently patent ductus is different from that found in a normal ductus not yet closed, suggesting that persistent patency is usually a primary anomaly and not a secondary effect.[3,4] On histologic

Exhibit 35–1
Children's Hospital Boston Experience
1988–2002
Patent Ductus Arteriosus

There were 544 patients (59% female) with a primary diagnosis of patent ductus arteriosus. Among these were 61 (11%) with a specific syndrome, 12 (2%) with respiratory problems, 1 with endocarditis, and 1 with pulmonary vascular obstructive disease.
Closure of the ductus by surgery (thoracotomy, video-assisted thoracic surgery [VATS]) or by catheter-delivered devices was undertaken in 252 (46%) patients.

Age at Procedure	Thoracotomy	VATS	Device
<1 mo	31	6	0
1–12 mo	21	10	6
1–5 yr	15	27	72
6–10 yr	2	11	26
11+ yr	0	16	49
Total	69	70	153

There were only two deaths, both in the thoracotomy group and both less than 1 month of age, one occurring the following day in a 1.3-kg premature neonate with a large infected intracardiac mass and necrotizing anterocolitis. The other infant died 4 days after surgery, before which a diaphragmatic hernia repair had been carried out and extracorporeal membrane oxygenation had been necessary.

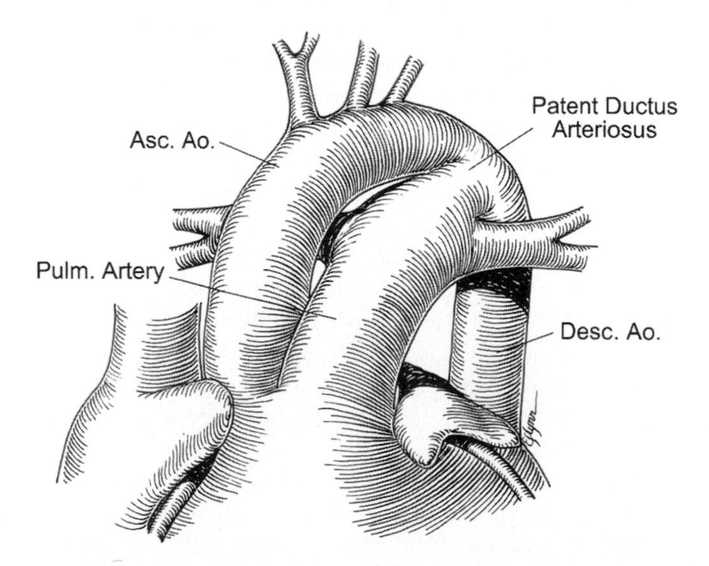

FIGURE 35–1 *Anatomic drawing of a large persistent patent ductus arteriosus.*
From Fyler DC [ed]. Nadas' Pediatric Cardiology. Philadelphia: Hanley & Belfus, 1992.

examination, the ductus is notably edematous, friable, and lacerated after the use of prostaglandins.[5,6]

It is proposed that strands of ductal muscle sometimes snare the descending aorta, causing coarctation,[7,8] or ensnare the proximal pulmonary artery, producing stenosis at the origin of the left pulmonary artery. That constriction of the aorta is associated with a right-to-left shunting duct, whereas constriction of the pulmonary artery is associated with a left-to-right shunt (i.e., in patients with tetralogy of Fallot) remains an intriguing curiosity.

In premature infants, the process of ductal closure is the same but is delayed, sometimes for weeks. The baby is born too soon; ductal closure occurs on schedule. However, not all close. The incidence of persistent patency of the ductus well past infancy in patients who were premature is greater than it is in the normal population.

PHYSIOLOGY

With the first respiratory gasps after birth, pulmonary arteriolar resistance falls abruptly; the ductus arteriosus reverses its flow and begins to shunt from left to right. Normally, the ductus begins to close with the first gasping respiration, and in a matter of hours, the ductus may be functionally closed. If the ductus remains widely patent, there is equilibration of the aortic and pulmonary arterial pressures. In this situation, the pulmonary resistance falls, causing increasing left-to-right shunting and congestive failure. If the ductus is large and there is continued elevation of pulmonary resistance, it may become irreversible, although pulmonary vascular disease is rare before the first birthday.

When there is a persistently large runoff from the aorta to the pulmonary artery, there is excessive blood flow to the lungs, left atrium, left ventricle, and ascending aorta (Fig. 35-2), with enlargement of these structures in proportion to the size of the left-to-right shunt. The volume overload within the thorax is great enough that blood transfusion after ductal ligation is rarely needed. The larger the runoff, the greater is the arterial pulse pressure, and the more striking the peripheral pulsations. When there is a large volume overload, the flap covering the foramen ovale may become incompetent, allowing additional left-to-right shunting and further volume overload.

The mechanism of ductal closure is a complex interaction of the level of arterial oxygen, circulating prostaglandins, genetic predetermination, and unknown factors.[9] Low oxygen tension is a factor in maintaining ductal patency in the fetus, and the sharp increase in arterial oxygen saturation with the first breath is thought to be the initiating step in ductal closure. On the other hand, high ambient oxygen

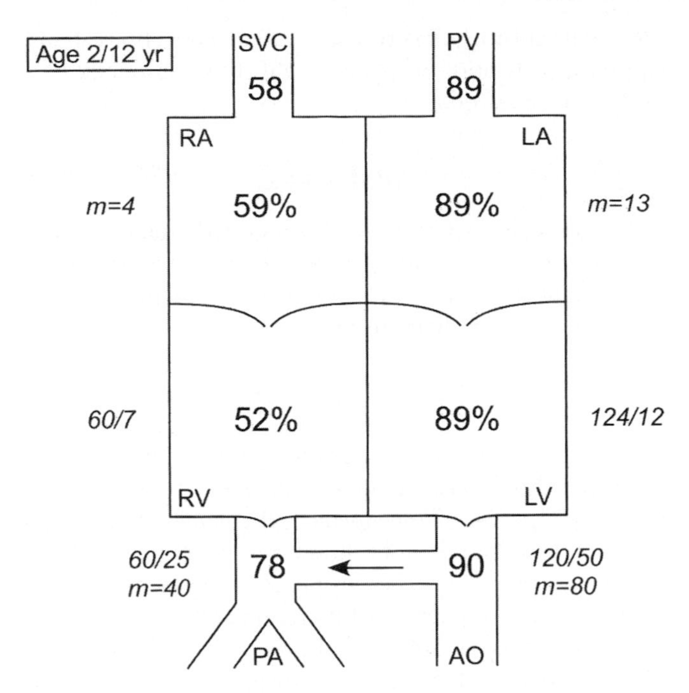

FIGURE 35–2 *Diagram of the hemodynamics in a patient with a patent ductus arteriosus and moderate pulmonary hypertension. Note the low pulmonary venous oxygen that results from a combination of excess pulmonary flow, congestive heart failure, and pulmonary infection. Note also the wide pulmonary arterial and aortic pulses.*
From Fyler DC [ed]. Nadas' Pediatric Cardiology. Philadelphia: Hanley & Belfus, 1992

does not help to close a persistently patent ductus, although the increased incidence of patent ductus in infants born at high altitudes is thought to be the result of low ambient oxygen.[10,11]

Prostaglandin E_1 is a powerful ductal dilator.[12] Prostaglandins may be required to maintain ductal patency *in utero;* in the fetus, their blood levels are high, are found in the wall of the ductus arteriosus, and are also supplied by the placenta. At birth, the levels fall owing to cessation of the placental source and increased pulmonary blood as they are catabolized in the lung; in adults, serum levels are very low.[13–15] The reciprocal relation between the effects of oxygen and prostaglandins varies with maturity. Oxygen is more effective in promoting ductal closure in the mature infant and less in the immature. Prostaglandin E_1 is more effective in promoting ductal patency in the premature infant and less effective in the mature.

Indomethacin given to the baby, or corticosteroids given to the mother,[15] will promote ductal closure. In the natural course of events, the ductus regularly and inappropriately closes in the first days of life even though the baby depends on left-to-right (pulmonary atresia) or right-to-left (interrupted aortic arch) shunting to survive.

CLINICAL MANIFESTATIONS

Patency of the ductus arteriosus in a full-term or older infant or child (female-to-male ration of 2:1) produces symptoms and signs proportionate to the amount of blood passing into the pulmonary circulation. When the ductal shunt is small, the only abnormality may be the presence of a murmur. When the ductus is large, symptoms of congestive heart failure or pulmonary hypertension may be present, and the murmur may not be typical.

Most children are discovered to have a murmur within days or weeks of birth. The murmur is not characteristically continuous in the early weeks of life, but it is recognized as a systolic murmur. If the ductus is large, symptoms of congestive heart failure (tachypnea, dyspnea, intercostal or subcostal retractions, hepatomegaly, or growth failure) may signal the cardiac problem. These children are not cyanotic unless there is pulmonary edema.

Classically, in the older child, there is a crescendo systolic murmur, peaking in intensity at aortic closure and continuing into diastole as a high-frequency, decrescendo diastolic murmur (Fig. 35-3). Usually, though not invariably, the diastolic component of the murmur extends the entire length of diastole. Often, there are coarse sounds (clicks or "shaking dice" noises) during systole, which contribute to the typical machinery sound. The murmur is loudest at the second left intercostal space; maximal intensity anywhere else should raise concern about the diagnosis of a patent ductus arteriosus. In the small infant, it is uncommon to hear the diastolic component of the murmur even if the ductus is large. In older infants with a large ductus and equilibration of aortic and pulmonary pressures, there may be only a systolic murmur, usually recognizable because

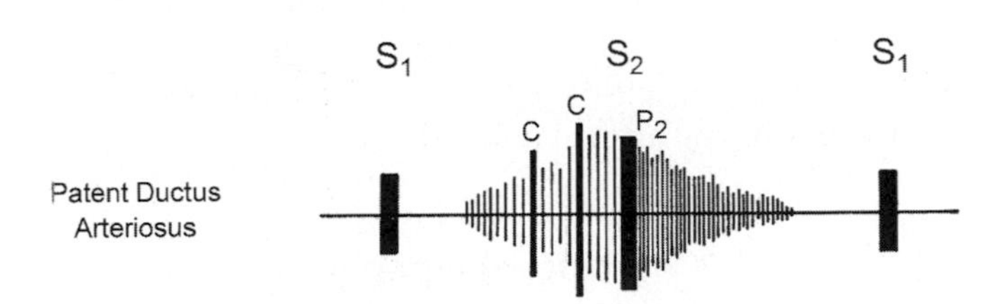

FIGURE 35–3 *Diagram of the machinery murmur of patent ductus arteriosus. Typically, the murmur is maximally loud at the time of the second heart sound (S_2); clicking noises (C) in systole contribute to the machinery sound.*
From Fyler DC [ed]. Nadas' Pediatric Cardiology. Philadelphia: Hanley & Belfus, 1992.

of its location, its crescendo quality, and the clicks. When the ductus is large, there is often an apical diastolic rumble (because of excessive mitral valve flow) that is hard to differentiate from the transmitted sounds of the loud continuous murmur.

The presence of a continuous murmur of crescendo–decrescendo quality, loudest at the time of the second sound, with systolic clicks, and located in the second left intercostal space should be interpreted as resulting from a patent ductus arteriosus. Among other causes of these findings, the most common is an aortopulmonary window; however, even here, the size of the window is usually so big that a continuous murmur is unusual. Other problems that could more or less mimic these findings include the following:

1. A *venous hum* is usually louder when the patient is sitting rather than lying down, and it may be louder to the right of the sternum. Hums have an evanescent quality, changing with respiration as well as position.
2. A *fistula between a coronary artery and a cardiac chamber* may produce a continuous murmur of crescendo–decrescendo quality, which is usually not loudest at the second left intercostal space. The murmur may be louder in systole or diastole, depending on the hemodynamics (see Chapter 52).
3. A *ruptured sinus of Valsalva* also produces a continuous murmur, not previously heard, which most often is also loudest at the second left interspace.
4. *Tetralogy of Fallot with pulmonary atresia and collateral circulation* produces continuous murmurs, which are heard all over the front and back of the chest, and if there are sufficient collaterals, the patient may not be visibly cyanotic.

Usually, all these possibilities are readily eliminated by cardiac auscultation.

In patients with a patent ductus arteriosus, heart failure is a feature of early infancy and is rare after the age of 6 months.

The peripheral arterial pulsations depend on the size of the ductus and the size of the shunt. The larger the ductus and the larger the left-to-right shunt, the more prominent are the peripheral arterial pulsations.

Electrocardiography

The electrocardiogram is normal when there is a small ductus; it shows left ventricular hypertrophy with a somewhat larger ductus and shows combined ventricular hypertrophy with a large ductus and pulmonary hypertension. When pulmonary vascular disease dominates the clinical picture, there may be only right ventricular hypertrophy. Because the presence of a continuous murmur and significant right ventricular hypertrophy are contradictory observations, careful investigation of patients with this combination of findings is required.

Chest X-Ray

The aorta, left ventricle, left atrium, pulmonary vessels, and main pulmonary arteries are enlarged in proportion to the amount of left-to-right shunt and may appropriately affect the cardiac silhouette on the plain chest film.

Echocardiography

On two-dimensional echocardiography, the ductus is easily visualized, and shunting is outlined with color-flow mapping (Fig. 35-4). If the ductal flow is significant, enlargement of the left atrial and ventricular chambers is evident. Estimations of pulmonary artery pressure may be made using the tricuspid regurgitation jet if present and by continuous-wave color Doppler. Although there is usually a gradient of pressure observed between the aorta and pulmonary artery, absence of a gradient may be taken as evidence of pulmonary hypertension at the systemic level. In 60% of patients, incompetence of the foramen ovale allowing left-to-right shunting is evident on color-flow Doppler.[16]

Cardiac Catheterization

Cardiac catheterization for diagnostic purposes has not been used for many decades except in very rare instances of diagnostic uncertainty and to study pulmonary resistance response to vasodilators such as oxygen and nitric oxide when pulmonary hypertension is present (Fig. 35-5). It is, however, very commonly used for interventional closure using a variety of occluding devices.

MANAGEMENT

Interrupting the left-to-right shunt is the goal of management of an uncomplicated patent ductus arteriosus. The reasons for intervention include elimination of congestive heart failure and promotion of growth in the small infant, prevention of infective endocarditis, and pulmonary vascular disease. For practical purposes, every isolated patent ductus arteriosus without associated problems should be closed. Although age and size are not a consideration in surgical management, even in the smallest babies, closure in the catheterization laboratory is generally delayed if feasible until later in the first year of life because of peripheral vessel injury risks. If the patient has failed to thrive or has overt congestive heart failure, the ductus should be interrupted. Legitimate reservations arise when the ductus

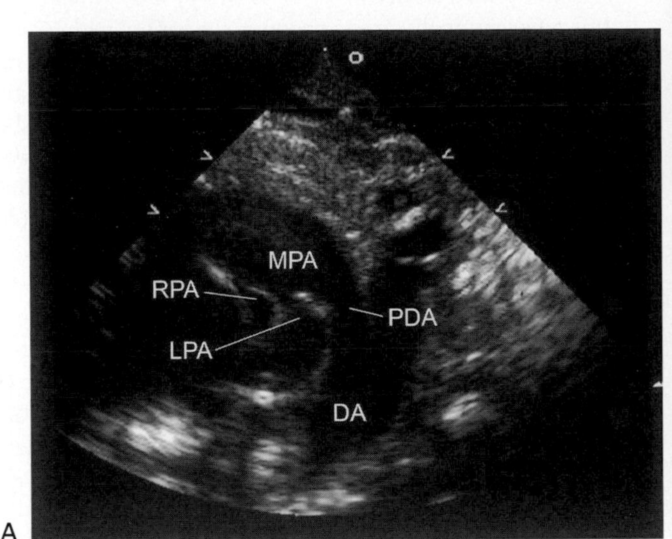

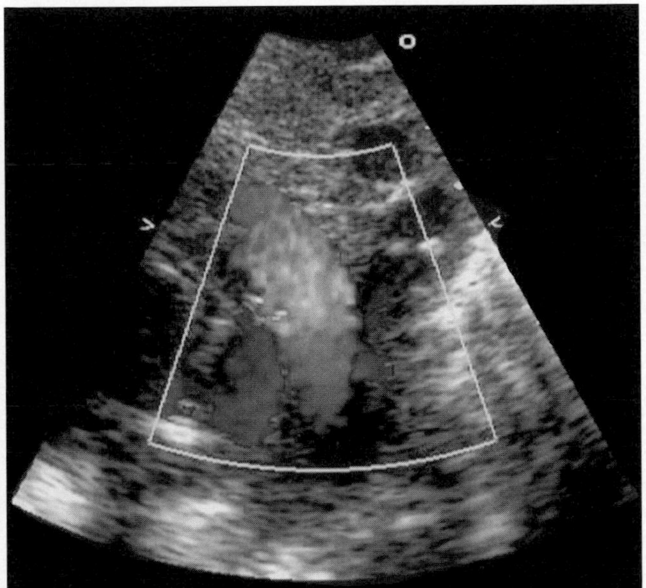

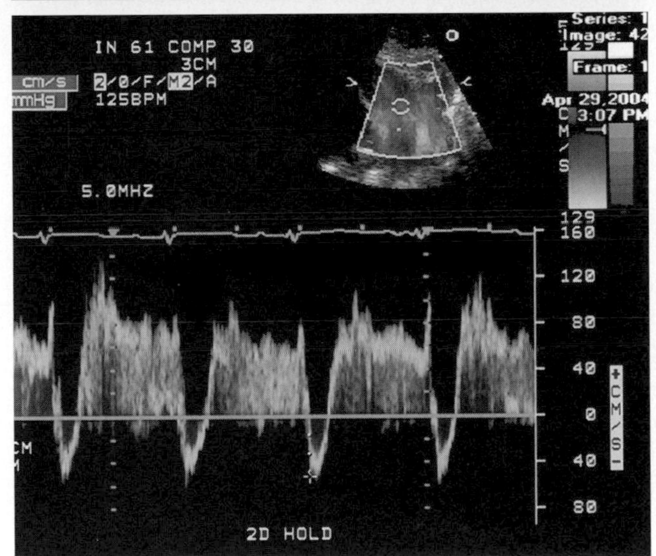

FIGURE 35–4 *A, High left parasternal view of a large patent ductus arteriosus (PDA) between the proximal descending aorta (DA) and the main pulmonary artery (MPA). The anatomic relationship of the PDA arising above left pulmonary artery (LPA), which is superior to the right pulmonary artery (RPA) origin, is shown. B, Color-flow Doppler mapping confirms the presence of flow as the red color jet of the PDA flow is seen to enter the MPA. C, Spectral Doppler is used to show the timing and velocity of flow across the PDA. In this case, there is mostly low-velocity left-to-right flow (signal above the baseline indicates a positive Doppler shift reflecting flow toward the transducer) with transient right-to-left flow in early systole (negative Doppler shift).*

is small and of little physiologic consequence, particularly in those with the so-called silent ductus in whom, in the absence of a murmur, a small ductus is identified echocardiographically; because of the risk for endocarditis[17] and ease and effectiveness of closure techniques, most investigators would recommend closure.

Closure can be accomplished with minimal risk using a variety of techniques (see Exhibit 35-1). Surgical management for many decades involved a thoracotomy with ductal occlusion (preferably by division to prevent recurrence), with excellent results at all ages and sizes. The past decade has seen increasing use of video-assisted thoracoscopic surgery (VATS; see Chapter 59) with remarkable success even in the tiniest of premature babies.[18–22] In the small number of whom this has not been feasible, the traditional thoracotomy approach has been used. Recently, robotic assistance with closure has been introduced[23] (see Chapter 59). Closure using interventional catheterization techniques has been increasingly used over the past two decades. In the current era, it is particularly appealing because it can be done on an outpatient basis[24] and avoids the thoracotomy scar of the traditional surgical approach. It is technically easiest to do when the ductus is quite restrictive, has length, and has an ampulla at the aortic end. As the technique has evolved, a wide variety of devices have been used[25,26] (Fig. 35-6); currently, coils are the most frequently used and are most effective in small lesions,[27] with results comparable to those seen in VATS-treated patients.[28]

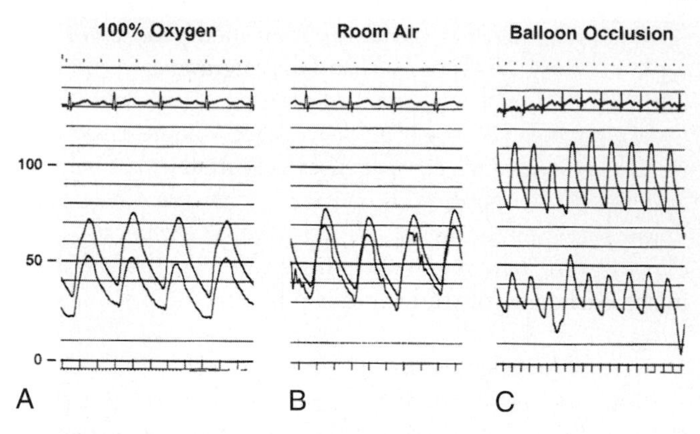

FIGURE 35–5 *Pulmonary and aortic pressure tracings in a 3-year-old child with a large patent ductus arteriosus and elevated pulmonary vascular resistance. A, Breathing 100% oxygen. The pulmonary artery pressure is lower at the time the left-to-right shunt was very large. B, Breathing room air. The pressures are virtually identical at the time the left-to-right shunt was minimal and estimated pulmonary vascular resistance was prohibitively high. C, With the ductus occluded by a balloon. Note the wide separation of pressures. The ductus was later divided, and the child is well without evidence of heart disease.*
From Fyler DC [ed]. Nadas' Pediatric Cardiology. Philadelphia: Hanley & Belfus, 1992.

COURSE

After the first successful closure of a ductus by Gross in 1938,[29] surgery for this lesion became so widespread that a real natural history picture was no longer available. In a retrospective review by Campbell in 1968,[30] high infant mortality, spontaneous closure, endocarditis, heart failure, and pulmonary vascular obstructive disease were described, with a mortality rate of 60% by age 60 years. At present, it is reasonable to suggest, particularly with widespread use of echocardiography, that diagnosis is being made at a younger age, and virtually all cases are being closed either surgically or with devices.

It is now extremely rare to encounter a patient with vascular obstructive disease; this can occur by age 2 years in an untreated large lesion. In such a patient, the characteristic murmur may be absent, the peripheral pulses may not be bounding, and the heart may not be very large. The electrocardiogram may show pure right ventricular hypertrophy. On chest x-ray, a large main pulmonary artery may be visible (Fig. 35-7). If the degree of pulmonary vascular obstruction is uncertain clinically, cardiac catheterization is necessary to measure pulmonary resistance in room air, in oxygen alone, and with a vasodilator such as nitric oxide, with the ductus open and with it temporarily occluded with a balloon. If the resistance value is less than 8.0 Wood units in room air and if there is a significant decrease with the previously mentioned maneuvers, then, especially in the very young, closure by device may be undertaken at that time or by surgery shortly thereafter. Without surgery, survival for several decades with vascular obstructive disease may occur. Differential cyanosis is common in older patients with minimal, if any, cyanosis of the lips and fingers being evident because fully saturated blood comes to these sites from the

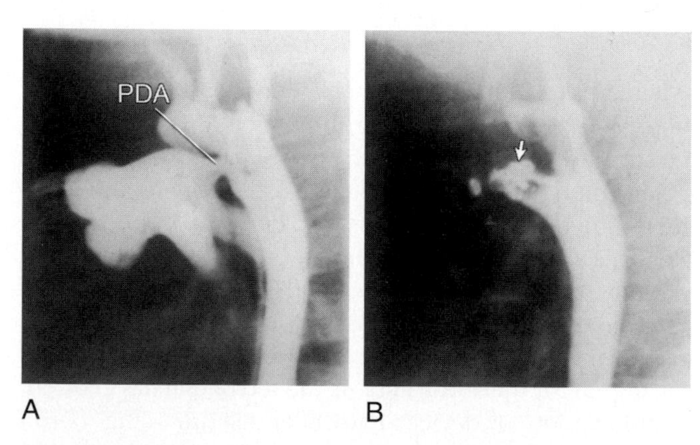

FIGURE 35–6 *Descending aortic cinegrams, lateral view, in a 1-year-old infant with a patent ductus arteriosus (PDA) before (A) and (B) after closure with a Grifka device (arrow).*

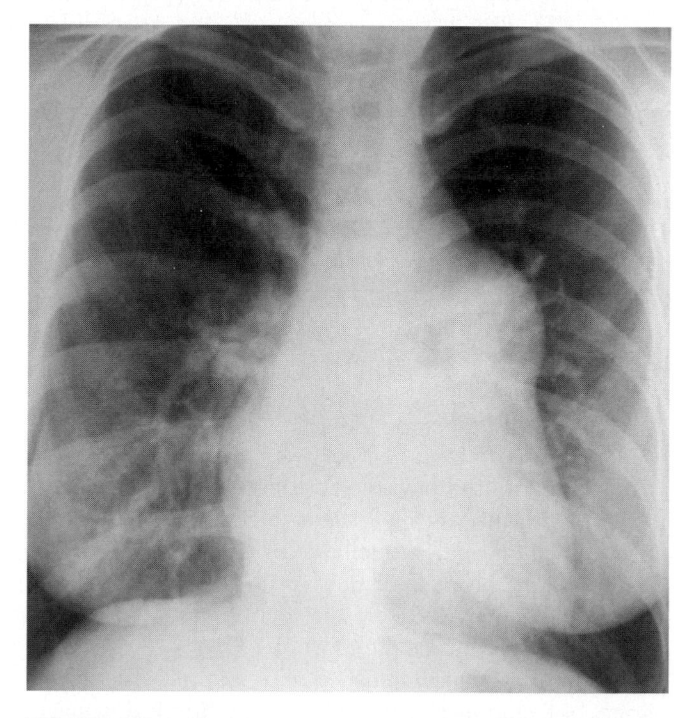

FIGURE 35–7 *Chest x-ray in a young woman with a large patent ductus arteriosus and advanced pulmonary vascular disease. This patient died within a year after this picture was taken. Note the very large main pulmonary artery and the near normal size of the heart.*
From Fyler DC [ed]. Nadas' Pediatric Cardiology. Philadelphia: Hanley & Belfus, 1992.

left ventricle, whereas clubbing and obvious cyanosis of the toes result from the right-to-left shunting through the ductus into the descending aorta. This shunt of desaturated blood also results in increased renal erythropoietin and hemoglobin production, with surprisingly high levels of the latter in the face of minimal upper body desaturation.

An untreated patent ductus arteriosus is a favored site for *infective endocarditis*. The chance of developing endocarditis has been estimated at 0.45% per year.[30] Closure of the ductus eliminates this possibility.[31]

Ductal ligation has been followed by later appearance of a left-to-right shunt because of either incomplete ligation or *recanalization*. Dividing the ductus and oversewing the stumps prevents recanalization. The difficulties and dangers of division, although small, are nonetheless sufficient that some surgeons favor ligation.

In the past, late *spontaneous closure* of a small patent ductus, largely based on auscultation, was noted on a few occasions; since the advent of echocardiography and color flow, this is now rarely encountered.

VARIATIONS

Ductus Arteriosus in Premature Infants

Functional closure of the ductus arteriosus occurs in some 90% of full-term newborns within a couple of days.[32] In premature infants, the ductus persists in many, with those of clinical significance being more common in the smallest babies, many with respiratory distress syndrome, and may add significant morbidity and mortality.[33] Measurement of blood levels of brain natriuretic peptide early may help in predicting such patients.[34]

Prevalence

Of 1700 infants weighing less than 1750 g at birth, 20.5% had a patent ductus arteriosus[15]; 42% of these weighed less than 1000 g, and 7% weighed more than 1500 g.[35] Among 146 older infants with patent ductus arteriosus, 19% weighed less than 2 kg at birth, and 17% were born after less than 34 weeks of gestation.

Anatomy

The gross and histopathologic anatomy of a premature ductus arteriosus is indistinguishable from that of the normal patent ductus arteriosus.[36]

Physiology

The level of pulmonary resistance in premature infants is less than it is in full-term babies. This, coupled with persistent patency of the ductus, favors the early appearance of left-to-right shunt, which may be excessive. The presence of respiratory distress promotes continued patency of the ductus because of hypoxemia, and this aggravates respiratory difficulty either because of congestive heart failure or because of the excessive pulmonary blood volume associated with the shunt, which compromises the intrathoracic volume available for respiration. Pulmonary venous oxygen desaturation and pulmonary hypertension were constant features of premature infants who underwent cardiac catheterization in the early days of studying this problem.

Clinical Manifestations

Although prominence of the peripheral pulses is a good indication that the ductus is large enough to cause problems, the murmur in premature infants is usually atypical, rarely being more than a systolic murmur, and not necessarily crescendo. Indeed, any systolic murmur in a very small premature baby should be considered indicative of a patent ductus arteriosus until proved otherwise.[35] Rarely, a premature infant may have a known patent ductus with no audible murmur.

Electrocardiography

The electrocardiogram shows tachycardia, right-axis deviation, and right ventricular hypertrophy that is rarely in excess of that normally expected for the age.

Chest X-Ray

The chest x-ray is dominated by signs of the respiratory distress syndrome. There is commonly enough gross pulmonary opacity to obscure the cardiac shadow completely.

Echocardiography

Two-dimensional echocardiography with color flow diagnoses the ductus, and serial observations provide information on size and shunt magnitude changes in response to indomethacin therapy.

Cardiac Catheterization

Cardiac catheterization is not used for this condition.

Management

In general, the initial management includes hematocrit level maintenance, ventilatory support, fluid restriction, and diuretic therapy. In those ventilated and weighing less than 1000 g, indomethacin is recommended even in the absence of a significant left-to-right shunt, and in those weighing greater than 1000 g, only when signs relating to a significant shunt appear.[37] If significant patency persists or recurs, another course of indomethacin is given. Using this approach, a 79% closure rate has been achieved.[15] Surgery is recommended for those not responding[37,38]; although ligation has been the traditional approach, in recent years the VATS technique has been very successful[13,18] (see Chapter 59).

The use of prophylactic indomethacin in the absence of a ductus in these babies, although it decreases the ductal and severe periventricular and intraventricular hemorrhage rates, is controversial.[39] It does not decrease the duration of oxygen therapy or ventilatory support, nor the incidence of bronchopulmonary dysplasia,[40–43] nor does it improve survival without neurosensory impairment at 18 months[44]; it is thus not generally recommended.

Course

The overall mortality rate in one large series by the age of 1 year was about 20%,[15] mainly due to pulmonary insufficiency, intracranial hemorrhage, necrotizing enterocolitis, and sepsis. It is unlikely that the ductus played the dominant role in the ultimate outcome for these babies; severe untoward events and death were caused mostly by prematurity and the respiratory distress syndrome. It must be remembered that at 1 year of age, 65% to 70% of the original group were alive without major handicaps.

The mortality associated with surgical closure (VATS or ligation) has improved significantly (see Chapter 59; see Exhibit 35-1).

The surviving small premature babies require continued observation for some months because ductus may remain patent or reopen later, whether they are treated medically or surgically.[32]

Aneurysm of the Ductus Arteriosus

Aneurysm of the closed ductus arteriosus is a variation of the normal ductus diverticulum (the remnant of the ductus at the point of attachment of the aorta). When the diverticulum is large, it is described as an aneurysm. Rarely, the aneurysmal diverticulum may cause obstruction of the aorta,[45] develop clots, obstruct the pulmonary artery,[46,47] be a source of emboli, become infected, or rupture.

Maternal Rubella

The dreadful consequences of maternal rubella about the time of conception are no longer seen because of immunizations. In the past, those affected were often blind, deaf, and retarded, and many had a patent ductus arteriosus. The ductus varied in size. Closure did not improve growth even when the vessel was large. Peripheral pulmonary stenosis was also commonly present.

REFERENCES

1. Fyler DC, Buckley LP, Hellenbrand WE, et al. Report of the New England Regional Infant Cardiac Program. Pediatrics 65(Suppl):398, 1980.
2. Botto LD, Correa A, Erickson JD. Racial and temporal variation in the prevalence of heart defects. Pediatrics 107(3):1, 2001.
3. Gittenberger-de Groot AC. Persistent ductus arteriosus: Most probably a primary congenital malformation. Br Heart J 39:610, 1977.
4. Gittenberger-de Groot AC, Strengers JLM, Mentink LM, et al. Histologic studies on normal and persistent ductus arteriosus in the dog. J Am Coll Cardiol 6:394, 1985.
5. Calder AL, Kirker JA, Neutze JM, et al. Pathology of the ductus arteriosus treated with prostaglandins: Comparison with untreated. Pediatr Cardiol 5:85, 1984.
6. Gittenberger-de Groot AC, Strengers JLM. Histopathology of the arterial duct (ductus arteriosus) with and without treatment with prostaglandin E1. Int J Cardiol 19:153, 1988.
7. Rudolph AM, Heymann MA, Spitznas U. Hemodynamic considerations in the development of narrowing of the aorta. Am J Cardiol 30:514, 1972.
8. Talner NS, Berman MA. Postnatal development of obstruction in coarctation of the aorta, role of the ductus arteriosus. Pediatrics 56:562, 1975.
9. Olley PM, Coceani F. Lipid mediators in the control of the ductus arteriosus. Am Rev Respir Dis 136:218, 1987.
10. Alzamora V, Rotta A, Battilana G, et al. On the possible influence of great altitudes on the determination of certain cardiovascular anomalies. Pediatrics 12:259, 1953.
11. Miao C, Zuberbuhler JA, Zuberbuhler JR. Prevalence of congenital cardiac anomalies at high altitude. J Am Coll Cardiol 12:224, 1988.
12. Olley PM, Coceani F, Bodach E. E type prostaglandins: A new emergency therapy for certain cyanotic congenital heart malformations. Circulation 53:728, 1976.
13. Clyman RI. Ontogeny of the ductus arteriosus response to prostaglandins and inhibitors of their symbols. Semin Perinatol 4:115, 1980.
14. Coceani F, Olley PM. Role of prostaglandins, prostacyclin, and thromboxanes in the control of prenatal patency and postnatal closure of the ductus arteriosus. Semin Perinatol 4:109, 1980.
15. Gersony WM, Peckham GJ, Ellison RC, et al. Effects of indomethacin in premature infants with patent ductus arteriosus: Results of a national collaborative study. J Pediatr 102:895, 1983.
16. Zhou TF, Guntheroth WG. Valve-incompetent foramen ovale in premature infants with ductus arteriosus: Doppler echocardiographic study. J Am Coll Cardiol 10:193, 1987.
17. Sadiq M, Latif F, Ur-Rehman A. Analysis of infective endarteritis in patent ductus arteriosus. Am J Cardio 93(4):513, 2004.
18. Burke RP, Jacobs JP, Cheng W, et al. Video-assisted thoracoscopic surgery for patent ductus arteriosus in low birth weight neonates and infants. Pediatrics 104(2 Pt 1):27, 1999.
19. Hines MH, Raines KH, Payne RM, et al. Video-assisted ductal ligation in premature infants. Ann of Thorac Surg 76(5):1417, 2003.
20. Villa E, Eynden FV, Le Bret E, et al. Paediatric video-assisted thoracoscopic clipping of patent ductus arteriosus: Experience in more than 700 cases. Eur J Cardiothorac Surg 24(3):387, 2004.

21. Nezafati MH. Closure of patent ductus arteriosus by video-assisted thorascopic surgery; minimally invasive, maximally effective: Report of 600 cases. H Surg Forum 6(1), 2003.
22. Odegard KC, Kirse DJ, del Nido PJ, et al. Intraoperative recurrent laryngeal nerve monitoring during video-assisted thoracoscopic surgery for patent ductus arteriosus. J Cardiothorac Vasc Anesth 14(5):562, 2000.
23. Le Bret E, Papadatos S, Folliguet T, et al. Interruption of patent ductus arteriosus in children: robotically assisted versus video-thorascopic surgery. J Thorac Cardiovasc Surg 123(5): 973, 2002.
24. Wessel DL, Keane JF, Parness I, et al. Outpatient closure of the patent ductus arteriosus. Circulation 77:1068, 1988.
25. Rutledge JM. Transcatheter closure of the patent ductus arteriosus. Exp Rev Cardiovasc Ther 1(3):411, 2003.
26. Bilkis AA, Alwi M, Hasri, et al. The Amplatzer duct occluder: Experience in 209 patients. J Am Coll Cardiol 37(1):258, 2001.
27. Wang JK, Laiu CS, Huang JJ, et al. Transcatheter closure of patent ductus arteriosus using Gianturco coils in adolescents and adults. Catheterization and Cardiovascular Interventions 55(4):513, 2002.
28. Jacobs JP, Girous JM, Quintessenza JA, et al. The modern approach to patent ductus arteriosus treatment: Complementary roles of video-assisted thoracoscopic surgery and interventional cardiology coil occlusion. Ann Thorac Surg 76(5):1421, 2003.
29. Gross RE, Hubbard JP. Surgical ligation of a patent ductus arteriosus. Report of the first successful case. JAMA 112:729, 1939.
30. Campbell M. Natural history of persistent ductus arteriosus. Br Heart J 30:4, 1968.
31. Johnson DH, Rosenthal A, Nadas AS. A forty-year review of bacterial endocarditis in infancy and childhood. Circulation 51:581, 1975.
32. Drayton MR, Skidmore R. Ductus arteriosus blood flow during first 48 hours of life. Arch Dis Child 62:1030, 1987.
33. Jones RWA, Pickering D. Persistent ductus arteriosus complicating the respiratory distress syndrome. Arch Dis Child 52:274, 1977.
34. Puddy VF, Amirmansour C, Williams AF, et al. Plasma brain natriuretic peptide as a predictor of haemodynamically significant patent ductus arteriosus in preterm infants. Clin Sci 103(1):75, 2002.
35. Ellison RC, Peckham GJ, Lang P, et al. Evaluation of the preterm infant for patent ductus arteriosus. Pediatrics 71:364, 1983.
36. Gittenberger-de Groot AC, van Ertbruggen I, Moulaert AJMG. The ductus arteriosus in the preterm infant: Histologic and clinical observation. J Pediatr 96:88, 1980.
37. Burns Wechsler S, Wernovsky G. Cardiac disorders. In Cloherty J, Eichenwald EC, Stark AR (eds). Manual of Neonatal Care. Philadelphia: Lippincott Williams & Wilkins, 2004:407–460.
38. Koehne PS, Bein G, Alexi-Meskhishvili V, et al. Patent ductus arteriosus in very low birth weight infants: complications of pharmacological and surgical treatment. J Perinatal Med 29(4):327, 2001.
39. Wyllie J. Treatment of patent ductus arteriosus. Semin Neonatol 8(6):425, 2003.
40. Krueger E, Mellander M, Bratton D, et al. Prevention of symptomatic patent ductus arteriosus with a single dose of indomethacin. J Pediatr 111:749, 1987.
41. Mahoney L, Cladwell RL, Girod DA, et al. Indomethacin therapy on the first day of life in infants with very low birth weight. J Pediatr 106:801, 1985.
42. Rennie JM, Doyle J, Cooke RWL. Early administration indomethacin to preterm infants. Arch Dis Child 61:233, 1986.
43. Mahoney L, Carnero V, Brett C, et al. Prophylactic indomethacin therapy for patent ductus arteriosus in very-low-birth weight infants. N Engl J Med 306:506, 1982.
44. Schmidt B, Davis P, Moddemann D, et al. Trial of indomethacin prophylaxis in preterms investigators: long-term effects of indomethacin prophylaxis in extremely-low-birth-weight infants. N Engl Med 344(26):1966, 2001.
45. McFaul RC, Keane JF, Nowicki ER, et al. Aortic thrombosis in the neonate. J Thorac Cardiovasc Surg 81:334, 1981.
46. Fripp RR, Whitman V, Waldhausen JA, et al. Ductus arteriosus aneurysm presenting as pulmonary artery obstruction: diagnosis and management. J Am Coll Cardiol 6:234, 1985.
47. Jesseph JM, Mahony L, Girod DA, et al. Ductus arteriosus aneurysm in infancy. Ann Thorac Surg 40:620, 1985.

36

Coarctation of the Aorta

JOHN F. KEANE AND DONALD C. FYLER

DEFINITION

Coarctation of the aorta is an obstruction in the descending aorta located almost invariably at the insertion of the ductus arteriosus.

PREVALENCE

Some 4% of all children with congenital cardiac defects have some degree of coarctation of the aorta. When coarctation is the dominant lesion, the incidence has ranged from 0.2/1000 live births among ill infants in New England[1] to 0.3/1000 when all infants are included.[2] At the Children's Hospital Boston, it was the eighth most common cardiac defect and was more common in males (59%) than in females.

This chapter is divided into the following sections:

- Uncomplicated coarctation beyond infancy
- Coarctation of the aorta in neonates/infants without/ with ventricular septal defect
- Coarctation of the aorta with mitral valve abnormalities
- Coarctation of the aorta with aortic stenosis
- Coarctation of the aorta with complex heart disease
- Interrupted aortic arch
- Atypical coarctation of the aorta

EMBRYOLOGY

In the normal fetus, the left fourth arch forms the aortic arch and that on the right regresses. The pulmonary arteries are derived from the sixth arches, the distal part on the left forming the ductus arteriosus while that on the right regresses. The precise cause of coarctation remains unknown but is thought to be due either to an abnormal flow pattern or to extension of the ductal tissue into the wall of the aorta. In the former, lesions which result in decreased flow in the ascending aorta, such as ventricular septal defect, mitral or subaortic obstruction, result in hypoplasia of the transverse arch and aortic isthmic area.[3] In contrast, when ascending aortic flow is increased such as in pulmonary atresia with intact ventricular septum or tetralogy of Fallot, coarctation is extremely rare (Exhibit 36-1). With regard to the ductal tissue theory, it is thought that constriction after birth of aberrant ductal tissue extending into the aortic wall results in obstruction (Fig. 36-1).[4,5] The high incidence of associated intracardiac lesions (Exhibit 36-1), familial recurrence in some and association with syndromes such as Turners[6–8] continue to suggest a genetic substrate (see Chapter 20). Another well-recognized associated anomaly is an intracranial aneurysm, which has been identified in some 10% of adults with coarctation,[9] rupture of which may be the initial presenting feature of a previously unrecognized coarctation.[10]

UNCOMPLICATED COARCTATION BEYOND INFANCY

Anatomy

Almost without exception, the obstructing indentation of the aorta is located opposite the entry of the ductus arteriosus, so called *juxtaductal*. The in-folding of the aortic

Exhibit 36–1

Children's Hospital Boston Experience: 1988-2002–Cardiac Problems Associated with Coarctation of the Aorta

N = 1892* (Males 59%)

Classification	Classified Under Coarctation (1238)			Other
Associated Cardiac Prolems Anomalies	Uncomplicated	Ventricular Defect	Interrupted Aortic Arch	Complicated Cardiac
	(*N* = 806) %	(*N* = 340) %	(*N* = 92) %	(*N* = 654) %
Bicuspid aortic valve	50	48	61	16
Aortic stenosis⁺	29	39	61	44
Aortic regurgitation	28	28	32	24
Mitral stenosis	16	29	3	24
Mitral regurgitation	35	45	59	48
Atrial defect/patent foramen ovale	38	73	77	84
None	17			

Coarctation of the Aorta with Other Complex Cardiac Defects: *N* = 654

	%
Hypoplastic left heart	33
Endocardial cushion defect	21
D-transposition of great arteries	12
Malposition	10
Double-outlet right ventricle	8
Single ventricle	6
Tricuspid atresia	3
Truncus arteriosus	3
Tetralogy of Fallot**	0.3

*Four percent of children with congenital heart disease.
⁺Includes valvar and subvalvar stenosis.
**Consists of two patients (one with pulmonary atresia, the other with virtual pulmonary atresia and extensive aortopulmonary collaterals).

wall is asymmetric and most marked on the posterior and lateral wall opposite the entry of the ductus. Hypoplasia of the aortic arch is common and may be severe, reaching its narrowest point at the coarctation itself (Fig. 36-1). The coarctation may be at, immediately above, or below the origin of the left subclavian artery. An aberrant right subclavian artery arising distal to the coarctation is rare (about 3%), and even rarer still is origin of both subclavian arteries below the obstruction, such that the only vessels above the coarctation are the carotid arteries.

The normal aortic arch tapers, reaching its narrowest diameter at the aortic isthmus just above the ductus arteriosus. In the fetus, the blood supply below this point is supplied by the right ventricle via the ductus arteriosus; the blood above is supplied by flow from the left ventricle via the ascending aorta. For fetal survival, it is not required that blood pass either way through the aorta at the isthmus and, in fact, the blood flow at this point is small enough so that, normally, the aortic diameter here is the narrowest in the thoracic aorta.[11] With growth and increased flow from the left ventricle, this normal narrow point disappears: in those with coarctation the abnormal hypoplasia of the arch may even improve with time but often persists to some degree even after surgical coarctation repair.

Coarctation of the aorta commonly becomes more obstructive as the child grows and is usually accompanied by increasing collateral flow involving the intercostal, internal mammary, and scapular vessels. Thus, because of extensive collateral circulation, it is possible to have severe obstruction of the aorta with only a small difference in blood pressure at

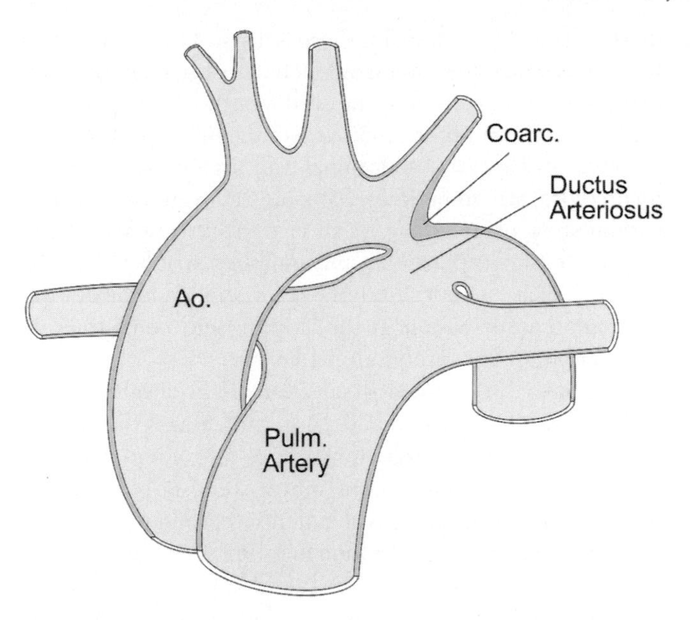

FIGURE 36–1 *Diagram of coarctation of the aorta. From Nadas AS, Fyler DC [eds]. Nadas' Pediatric Cardiology. Philadelphia, PA: Hanley and Belfus, 1992.*

rest between the arms and legs. The collateral vessels become larger and more tortuous with time, the intercostals ultimately eroding the undersurface of the ribs (rib notching). The interconnecting arteries of the collateral circulation are present at birth, enlarging to accommodate the need for increased flow as needed.

Almost any cardiac defect may be associated with coarctation of the aorta. An exception to this rule is the rare association of pulmonary atresia, pulmonary stenosis, or tetralogy of Fallot with coarctation of the aorta (Exhibit 36-1).

Distortion or kinking of the aorta at the usual site of coarctation, without the usual anatomy of coarctation and without demonstrable obstruction, is sometimes called *pseudocoarctation*. This is a misleading term because the aorta is abnormal, not obstructed.

Physiology

The physiologic effects of coarctation of the aorta are a direct function of the difference in blood pressure between the upper and lower body. In theory, this difference could be large but in the average patient is not often more than 30 or 40 mm Hg at rest. This can be accounted for by the fact that collateral blood vessels circumvent the coarctation so that only part of the cardiac output must pass the obstructed area. However, with exercise the upper body pressures and gradient may rise to high levels, even after surgical repair.[12] The mechanisms for the latter are complex, involving baroreceptors, renin-angiotensin system and circulating catecholamines[13–15] but may also be related to some obstruction remaining in the transverse arch or coarctation repair site or older age at repair.

Coarctation affects the heart by causing left ventricular hypertension and hypertrophy, the patient presenting with hypertensive heart disease.

Clinical Manifestations

Patients are usually male (59%), asymptomatic, and older. Some cases are still revealed while searching for the cause of recently identified hypertension: Included in the past a few were first diagnosed because rib notching was observed on a chest radiograph. Most are identified during an evaluation for a heart murmur. Many have other cardiac lesions: indeed only 17% of our *uncomplicated* group had no other cardiac diagnosis (Exhibit 36-1). This is a substantial decrease from the 37% in our earlier (1973–1988) era and likely reflects the more widespread use of echocardiography which detects many items such as inaudible trivial/mild valvar regurgitation and small atrial defects.

Children who have coarctation of the aorta that has not caused symptoms grow normally unless there is some added cardiac or noncardiac anomaly. The femoral pulses are absent or weak and delayed compared with brachial pulses. Because the left subclavian artery may arise above, at, or below the coarctation and the right subclavian artery rarely below, comparisons of brachial and femoral pulses and pressures are important.

Repeated measurements of systolic pressures higher in the arm than in the leg are sufficient to indicate the possibility of coarctation of the aorta. Differences of 20 mm Hg or more usually represent significant obstruction. Normally the systolic pressure in the femoral artery may be up to 20 mm Hg higher than in the arm, so that discovery of a femoral pressure even a few mm Hg lower than that in the arms is suspicious. Generally, the diastolic pressures in the arms and legs are the same, although in some adults and even in older children, diastolic pressure gradients occur. When the pressures are measured directly, there is damping of the lower body pressure curves compared with those for the upper body (Fig. 36-2). Diastolic hypertension in the lower extremities, despite a systolic pressure gradient, suggests hypertension of some other cause (i.e., abdominal coarctation with involvement of the renal arteries).

With direct measurement of the intra-arterial pressures at cardiac catheterization, the pressures differences usually are not as marked as those noted in a clinical situation, although simultaneous measurements of the cuff and intra-arterial pressures compare favorably. The reason for the difference is that many intra-arterial measurements with the patient

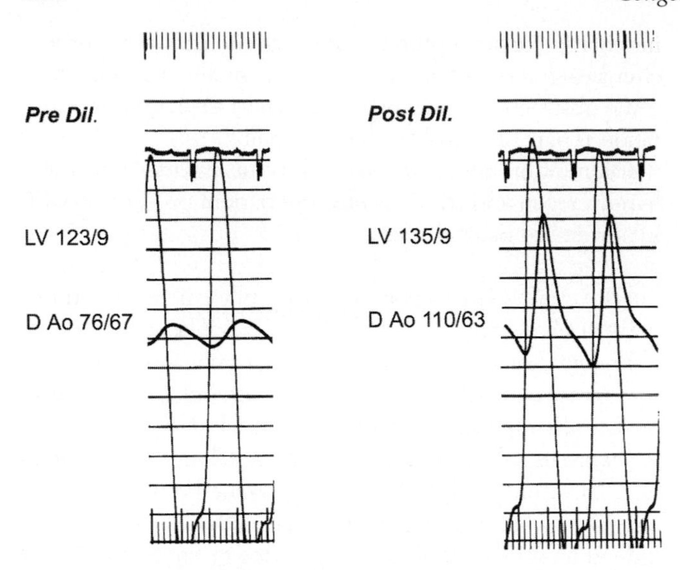

FIGURE 36–2 *A, Simultaneous recording of descending aorta pressure (D Ao) and left ventricular pressure (LV) in a patient with a residual coarctation of the aorta. Note the damped aortic tracing showing a small pulse pressure and a systolic gradient of 47 mm Hg between the left ventricle and the aorta. B, A similar recording following balloon dilatation of the coarctation. Note that a gradient of 15 mm Hg remains. The aortic systolic pressure is now higher and is no longer damped.*
From Nadas AS, Fyler DC [eds]. Nadas' Pediatric Cardiology. Philadelphia, PA: Hanley and Belfus, 1992.

sedated and lying on the catheterization table are being compared with a few cuff measurements in an awake, apprehensive patient who only recently climbed onto the examination table.

A systolic ejection murmur of low intensity from the coarctation is audible over the base of the heart and left interscapular region, usually loudest in the latter area. Because auscultatory identification of systole and diastole is made by listening to the heart sounds and the origin of the murmur is downstream, diastole has begun for the heart before the systolic pulse in the descending aorta has ended. Consequently, the murmur appears to extend into

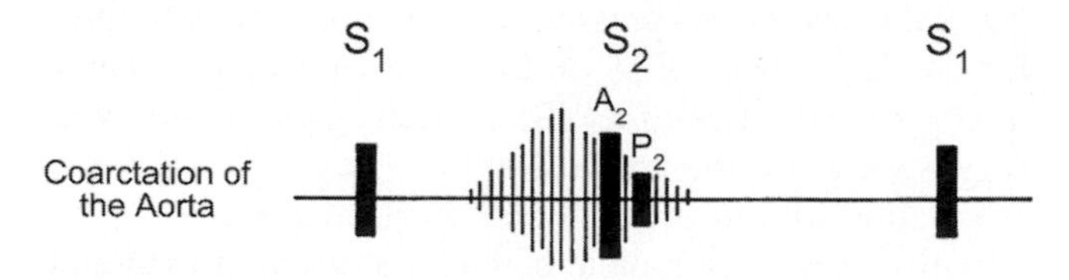

FIGURE 36–3 *Diagram of the murmur of coarctation of the aorta. Usually, the murmur is heard best over the left interscapular area. In relation to the heart sounds, the murmur extends into diastole.*
From Nadas AS, Fyler DC [eds]. Nadas' Pediatric Cardiology. Philadelphia, PA: Hanley and Belfus, 1992.

diastole (Fig. 36-3). Usually, there is a systolic click, due to a bicuspid aortic valve. In the older child, adolescent, or adult, collateral circulation may be sufficiently developed that continuous murmurs are audible over the intercostal arteries, scapulae and anterior abdominal wall. In a more advanced form these are sometimes palpable or even visible. The combination of a systolic ejection murmur loudest at the upper left interscapular area and audible/palpable collaterals in the axillae and/or around the scapulae indicate the obstructed aortic area is at the isthmus and not distally at the diaphragmatic or abdominal levels.

Because of the frequent association of mitral valve abnormalities (Exhibits 36-1 and 36-2), auscultation at the cardiac apex for the apical systolic murmur of mitral regurgitation and the diastolic murmur of mitral stenosis is required. Similarly, as aortic valve involvement is common, murmurs of aortic stenosis or regurgitation may be encountered. Often the question of aortic stenosis is raised because the murmur of coarctation is a stenotic one heard well anteriorly. Generally, however, because the murmur of coarctation is not loudest to the right of the sternum or the suprasternal notch and is at least as loud over the back as it is anteriorly, the distinction is not difficult.

Exhibit 36–2

Children's Hospital Boston Experience: 1973–1987 vs. 1988–2002 Coarctation of the Aorta: Selected Lesions*

Coarctation Interventional Therapy: 1988–2002

Balloon dilation	$N = 164$ (10 < 2 mo age: 61 native)
Stent placement	$N = 69$ (30 native)

There were no deaths associated with these procedures.
*Showing significantly increased incidence (%) in AR (aortic regurgitation), MS (mitral stenosis), MR (mitral regurgitation), and ASD/PFO (atrial septal defect/patent foramen ovale) in recent 1988-2002 period, compared to earlier 1973-1987 era, probably largely due to increasing use of echocardiography.

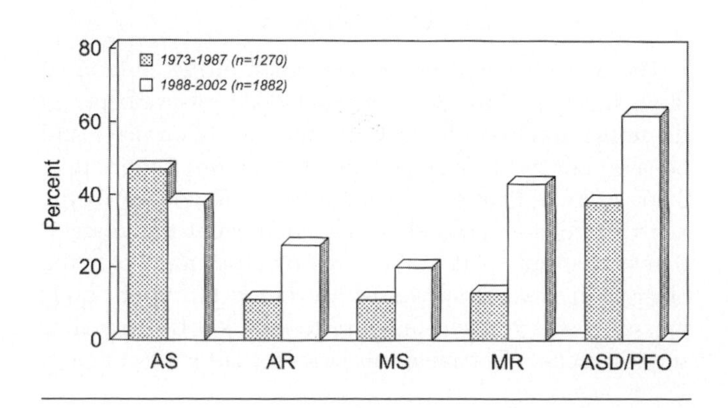

Electrocardiography

The asymptomatic child or adult with coarctation of the aorta may show left ventricular hypertrophy in proportion to the degree of upper body hypertension. Left-sided changes in the S-T segment and T wave in the chest leads are not part of the clinical picture of coarctation of the aorta and raise the possibility of an additional cardiac defect.

Chest Radiography

On chest radiograph, the asymptomatic older child may show a prominent aortic knob, an indentation of the left border of the descending aorta at the usual site of coarctation and, during barium swallow, an opposing indentation on the esophagus. Rib notching is rarely seen before the age of 10 years.

Echocardiography

Simple coarctation almost always occurs just distal to the left subclavian artery, at the site of insertion of the ductus arteriosus (Fig. 36-4). The characteristic feature is indentation of the posterior and lateral aspects of the aorta by a wedge-shaped *shelf* of tissue. The Doppler color flow map gives an estimate of the obstruction width and the continuous wave measurement provides a maximum instantaneous gradient value at that area (often higher than that measured in the sedated patient at catheterization (Fig. 36-5).[16] Distal to the obstruction, the aortic upstroke velocity is reduced and there is continuous flow antegrade throughout the cycle.[17] It is important to carefully evaluate the transverse arch during the study since hypoplasia with some obstruction is a common postoperative finding.[18]

In older patients, the ability to image the aortic isthmus and proximal descending aorta is variable. The flow pattern in the descending aorta may provide evidence that a coarctation is present or absent.

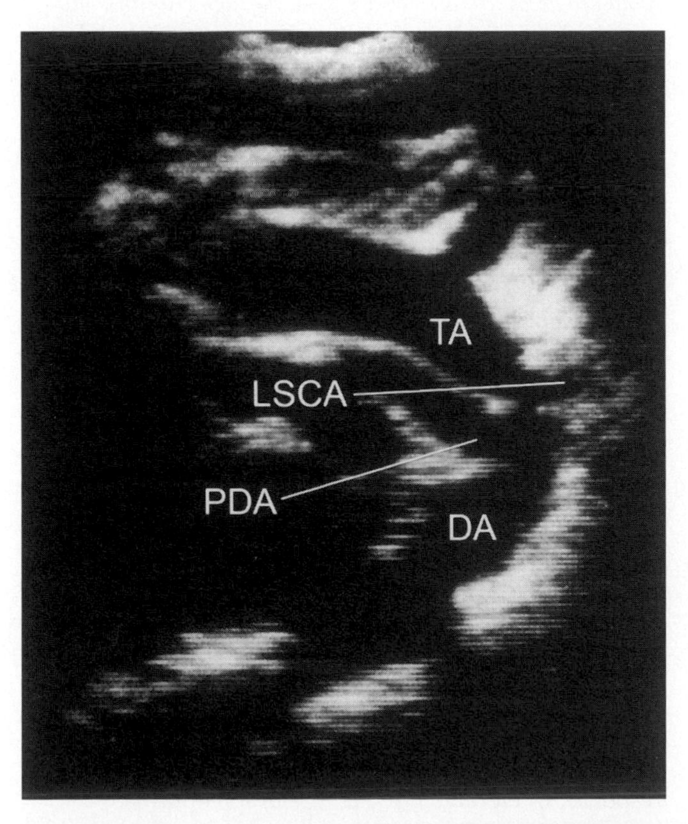

FIGURE 36–4 *Suprasternal notch echocardiogram of the transverse arch (TA), patent ductus arteriosus (PDA), and descending aorta (DA) showing a discrete coarctation between the origin of the left subclavian artery (LSCA) and the PDA.*

Magnetic Resonance Imaging

In older patients, adequate echocardiographic images are often difficult to obtain. In such cases magnetic resonance techniques can provide superb images (Fig. 36-6).

Cardiac Catheterization

There is no need for diagnostic cardiac catheterization in a child with clinically uncomplicated coarctation of the aorta unless there is reason to suspect some additional problem that might be clarified.

MANAGEMENT

Indications for Intervention

An uncomplicated coarctation with a consistent systolic blood pressure gradient between the arms and legs of more than 20 mm Hg is an indication for intervention. This procedure, even in the asymptomatic patient, should be undertaken soon after diagnosis (preferably by age 2 years.) since residual hypertension despite successful relief is very common (24% to 38%) in older patients,[18–20] and ambulatory elevated levels have even been reported after repair at a very young age.[21,22] The intervention performed currently is either surgical (great majority) or balloon angioplasty with or without stent placement.

Surgery

Surgery in most cases consists of resection with end-to-end anastomosis. The mortality rate in uncomplicated patients even at a few months of age is at or near zero (Exhibit 36-3)[20,23,24] with residual obstruction (often at the arch) occurring in some 10% to 14%.[18,20,23,24] Many years ago

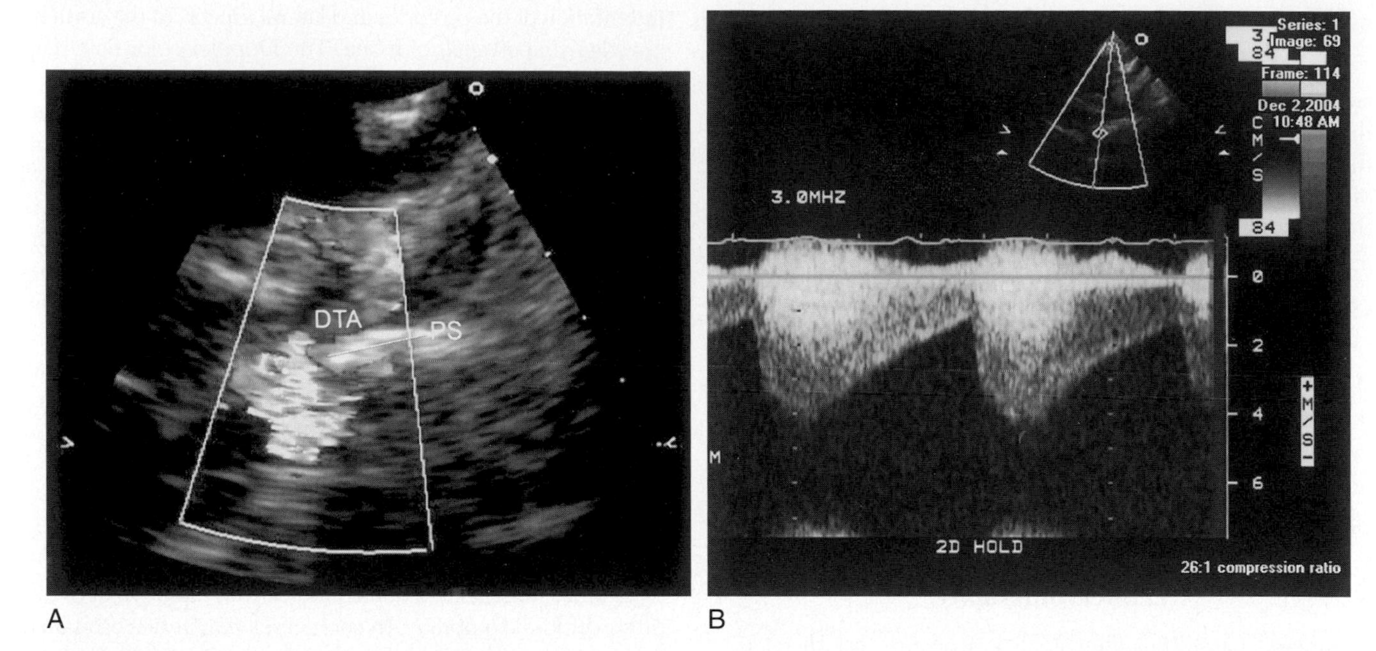

FIGURE 36–5 *A, Color Doppler flow mapping of the narrow and tortuous pathway created by the posterior shelf (PS) at the coarctation site between the distal transverse arch (DTA) and the descending aorta. The laminar flow in the transverse arch is indicated by the uniformly blue color Doppler map, whereas turbulent flow begins at the level of the coarctation, as indicated by the mixture of red and blue signals. B, When a continuous wave Doppler sample is obtained across the arch obstruction, the high velocity continuously antegrade flow signal typical of an arterial obstruction is obtained. Note the double population of Doppler velocities reflecting the fact that the continuous wave Doppler samples velocities along the entire length of the ultrasound beam, detecting the low velocity proximal velocities as well as the high velocity distal velocities.*

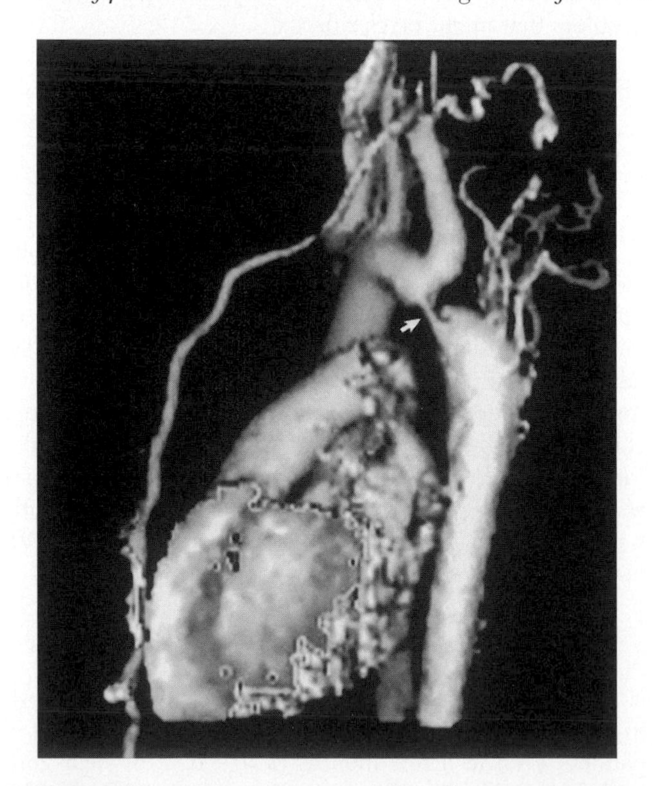

FIGURE 36–6 *Gadolinium-enhanced three-dimensional magnetic resonance angiography of severe aortic coarctation (arrow). Note the collateral vessels to the descending aorta.*

lower limb paralysis due to spinal cord injury resulting from aortic cross clamping in the face of very little collateral flow[25] and mild coarctation occurred in 0.4% of patients.[26] With today's sophisticated imaging modalities and surgical expertise this should no longer occur. Other surgical techniques such as subclavian flap plasty or use of a prosthetic patch are infrequently used, the latter because of aneurysm formation[27,28] and conduit use is very rare. It is important to recognize that reduction of the descending aorta diameter by two thirds is required to produce any systolic pressure gradient: A gradient of 20 mm Hg invariably looks like a severe coarctation.

In the postoperative period there may be significant hypertension and occasionally severe abdominal pain without any residual gradient. These are managed effectively (and even prevented prophylactically) by nitroprusside and esmolol initially, then by captopril and later by enalapril (orally twice daily). These problems are thought related to upper and lower limb vessel resistance differences, disordered renin-angiotensin system, an abnormal baroreceptor response, or elevated circulating norepinephrine.

Balloon Angioplasty

Although in earlier years residual gradients and aneurysms (with some deaths) were not uncommon following balloon

Exhibit 36–3
Children's Hospital Boston Experience: 1988–2002

	Coarctation of Aorta or Interrupted Aortic Arch Surgical Experience							
	Uncomplicated		Ventricular Defect		Interrupted Aortic Arch		Complicated⁺	
Age	*30 day Mortality* N%		*30 day Mortality* N%		*30 day Mortality* N%		*30 day Mortality* N%	
<2 months	116	1*	145	7	62	11	126	7
>2 months	215	0	35	0	11	0	52	4
Total	331	0.3	180	6	73	8	178	6

The initial mortality with surgical management at Children's Hospital Boston of coarctation of the aorta is related to age and associated defects. Compared with 1973 to 1988, the major difference is improvement in the complicated category (21% reduced to 6%).
*This sole mortality in the < 2 months uncomplicated group occurred in a baby with severe untreated valvar aortic stenosis and a left ventricle of marginal size while undergoing stage 1 attempt after successful coarctation repair.
⁺includes some with interrupted aortic arch.
Survival curves for the total 1392 patients seen, many managed in part elsewhere, 806 with *uncomplicated* (simple) coarctation, 340 with coarctation and ventricular septal defect (VSD), 92 with interrupted arch (IAA) and 654 with coarctation and other complicated lesions. Compared to the 1973-1988 era, the most significant improvement occurred in the complicated group with survival at 18 months improving from about 50% to 77%.

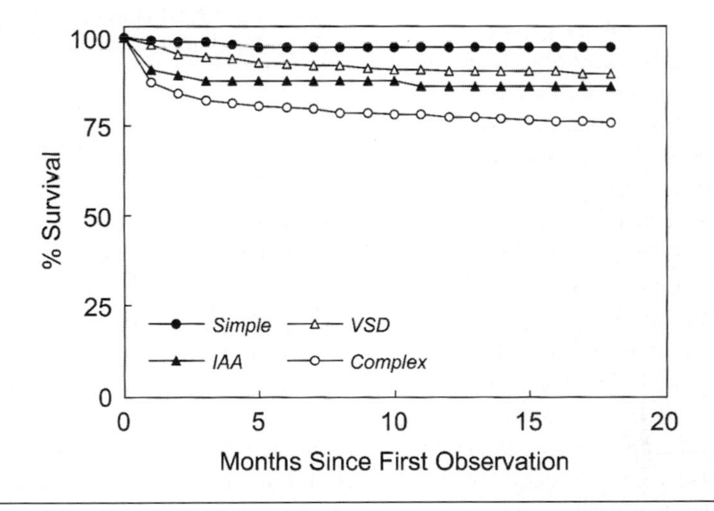

dilation of native coarctation in children and adults, reported results have improved in recent years. In these recent reports the average gradient reduction was 78%, 5% to 13% had significant residual obstruction (some at transverse arch level), aneurysms occurred in 0% to 6%, with one death among 208 patients.[29–32] At Children's Hospital Boston, because of our excellent surgical results, we have limited dilation of native coarctations to (a) those where the coarctation was very discrete and thin, being careful *not* to use balloons greater than three times the coarctation diameter (see Chapter 14) and (b) complex cases such as a patient with a ruptured intracranial aneurysm. In recent reports stents have been placed in native coarctations in some 33 patients with excellent gradient relief, without mortality but with some significant complications.[33,34]

COURSE

Natural History

In the 1970 report of Campbell[35] involving patients beyond infancy, without treatment some 75% of patients died by age 46 years. Heart failure, aortic rupture, endocarditis, and intracranial hemorrhage were common causes of demise. Clearly, at least in this country, the most patients are identified and operated on at an early age. Coarctation of the aorta is a progressive anomaly, and as the collateral circulation increases there may be little change in relative arm and leg blood pressures while the actual point of coarctation becomes more obstructive.

Postoperative Course

Continued follow up indefinitely is necessary in this patient population. Not only is the incidence of associated lesions very high (Exhibit 36-1) but hypertension at rest or with exercise often persists (even in the absence of residual obstruction at rest), early arteriosclerotic heart disease occurs in some[35] and residual obstruction at rest is not uncommon. Although earlier surgery decreases some of these problems, left ventricular echocardiographic abnormalities have been reported in 40% even after a mean surgical age of only 5 years.[36]

Postoperative Balloon Angioplasty

For those with a residual gradient of more than 20 mm Hg, balloon angioplasty has become the primary treatment. Complications in this age group are few and obstruction is alleviated in most, particularly when localized to the repaired isthmic area,[37–39] and is successful regardless of the type of surgical repair.[40] Stent placement in addition in these patients has been a valuable adjunct (see Chapter 14) and can even be later dilated, this being especially necessary in younger patients as they grow.[40,41] Although surgical management can be effective in postoperative obstructions,[42] and is clearly indicated in some for anatomical reasons, interventional techniques in appropriate lesions, given their effectiveness, short hospital stay, absence of thoracotomy incisions and relative safety, are the procedures of choice (Fig. 36-7).

Early surgery and later balloon dilation or reoperation may be double jeopardy but, in our opinion, the dangers of this plan are outweighed by the incidence of late complications with a single, late operation. The fewer years one lives with an obstructed aorta, the fewer problems occur later.

COARCTATION OF THE AORTA IN NEONATES/INFANTS WITHOUT/WITH VENTRICULAR SEPTAL DEFECT

Definition

Because surgery is the initial treatment for severe coarctation and for ventricular septal defect if significant, in this age range, it seemed reasonable to present them together.

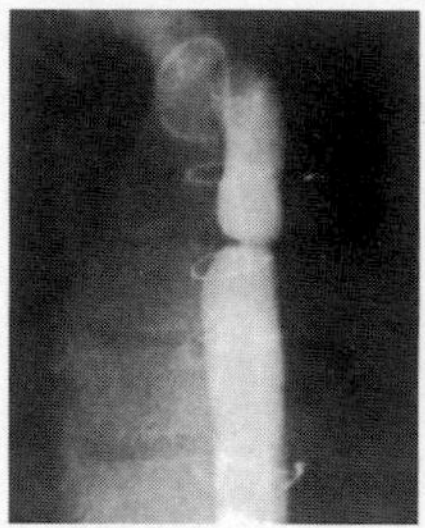
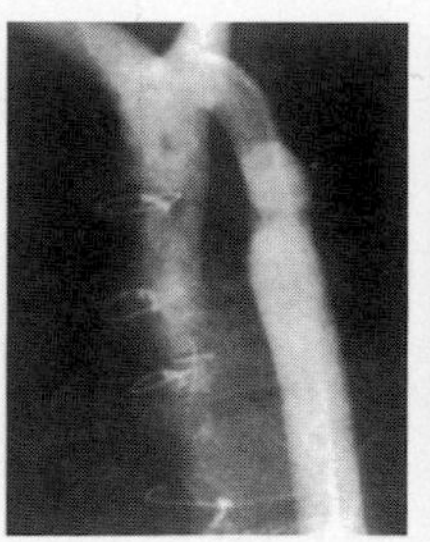
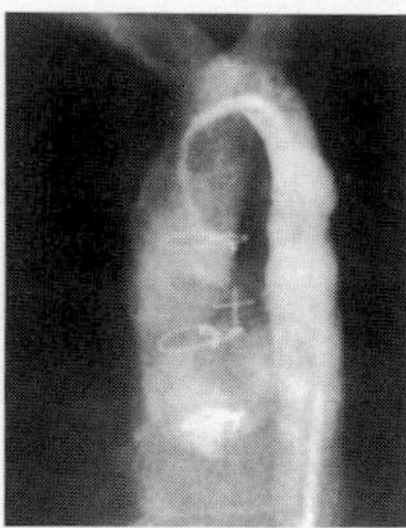
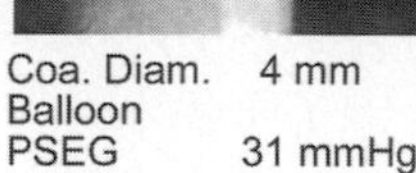

FIGURE 36–7 *Three aortograms of a patient with recurrent coarctation of the aorta. Left, before ballooning. Middle, after using a 10-mm balloon. Right, after using a 12-mm balloon. PSEG, peak systolic gradient; Coa Diam., internal diameter at point of obstruction.*
From Nadas AS, Fyler DC [eds]. Nadas' Pediatric Cardiology. Philadelphia, PA: Hanley and Belfus, 1992.

Anatomy

The anatomy in uncomplicated severe coarctation is similar to that in the older child but if accompanied by a large ventricular septal defect arch hypoplasia is common. The ventricular defects may be single or multiple.

Physiology

Lesser degrees of coarctation with or without a small ventricular septal defect are well tolerated, are without symptoms, are accompanied by a prominent murmur and treatment can be delayed. On the other hand, those with severe aortic obstruction may present very ill with sudden onset of heart failure within weeks of birth whereas those with a large ventricular septal defect often present deathly ill within days of delivery as pulmonary resistance decreases and the ductus closes. Left ventricular failure leads to left atrial hypertension which in turn results in additional left to right shunting at the atrial level (Fig. 36-8).

Clinical Manifestations

An uncomplicated lesser degree of coarctation does not produce symptoms. The patient grows normally and the problem is commonly not diagnosed even for some years as murmurs are not obvious and femoral pulse abnormalities are not detected. On the other hand, patients with an associated small ventricular septal defect are identified much earlier because of the murmur (often loud) produced by this restrictive defect.

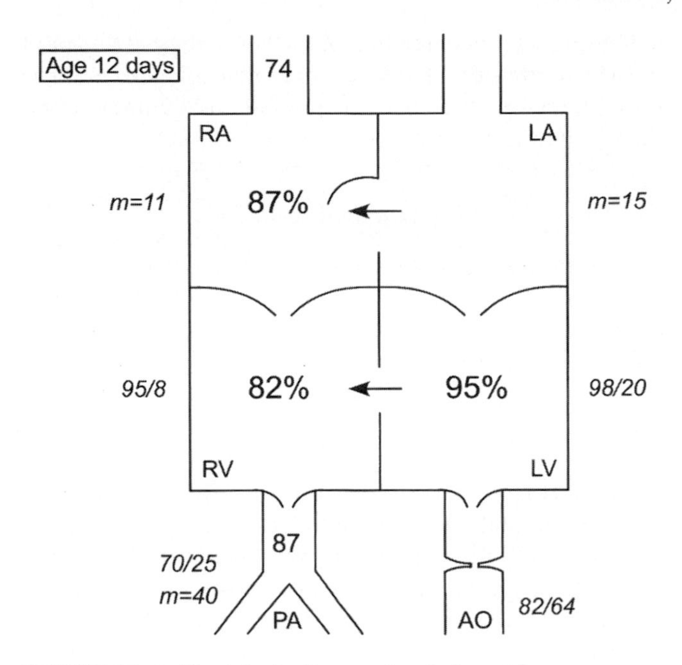

FIGURE 36–8 *Physiologic diagram in a baby with severe coarctation of the aorta and a large ventricular septal defect. This infant was very ill with gross congestive heart failure. Note the elevation of atrial pressures, the incompetent foramen ovale with a large left-to-right shunt, and pulmonary hypertension approaching systemic levels.*
From Nadas AS, Fyler DC [eds]. Nadas' Pediatric Cardiology. Philadelphia, PA: Hanley and Belfus, 1992.

Those with a severe coarctation usually develop heart failure within weeks (60% hospitalized before the fourteenth day of life[1]) and may suddenly become desperately ill. Those with an associated large ventricular defect tend to become critically ill within days of birth as pulmonary resistance falls and the ductus closes spontaneously. Both groups when in this clinical state are ashen, tachypneic, tachycardic, pulseless and acidotic.

Electrocardiography

With significant lesions, electrocardiography reveals that right ventricular hypertrophy dominates in the neonates whereas in uncomplicated lesser obstruction, left ventricular hypertrophy may appear after several months.

Chest Radiography

When the obstruction and ventricular defect are significant, chest radiograph shows cardiomegaly, evidence of congestive failure, and increased pulmonary vascularity.

Echocardiography

With current echocardiographic technology, the anatomic details provided in this age group are superb. The isthmus, transverse arch, ventricular defect(s), patent ductus, left ventricular outflow anatomy and ventricular function, together with shunting details on color flow analysis, are readily identified.

Cardiac Catheterization

Cardiac catheterization for hemodynamic and angiographic data is no longer necessary. Balloon angioplasty has been reported in a few series with high recurrence rates and arterial complications, especially in the first few months of life[43–45] and is used only by us as a palliative procedure if surgical risk is prohibitive.

Management

In the asymptomatic baby with mild obstruction, with or without a small ventricular defect, it is reasonable to follow such a patient medically for several months. During this time a small ventricular defect is likely to spontaneously decrease in size or even close, leaving the coarctation as the only lesion requiring surgery.

At the other end of the spectrum, that is the ill newborn with severe obstruction with a larger ventricular defect, surgery is necessary for both as soon as possible. Preoperative improvement (acidosis and hypotension relief, organ recovery) is often accomplished with prostaglandin E, especially in those just a few days old with a ventricular defect in whom the duct has just closed. This response is much less likely in the older baby with uncomplicated severe obstruction and here a brief preoperative period (hours) of anticongestive measures, afterload reduction, intubation, etc., may make the baby a better surgical candidate. The surgical early mortality is almost zero in uncomplicated neonates, and less than 10% in most series with a ventricular defect (Exhibit 36-3).[46–52] The ventricular defect is primarily closed in the majority, while a pulmonary artery band may be necessary in some with multiple defects.

Course

Postoperative obstruction with current surgical techniques, which also address a hypoplastic arch, occurs in less than 21% of full-term babies.[46–58] In a small series from our hospital of babies weighing less than 2 kg at coarctation repair, 44% had obstruction managed by angioplasty or repeated surgery.[52] Generally, postoperative residual obstruction, especially when located at the suture line, is managed satisfactorily by balloon angioplasty with arterial complications being less frequent in infants as equipment has improved over the years. In those few who had a pulmonary artery band placed, the defects are sometimes found to have become much smaller or even closed spontaneously occasionally such that band removal is all that is necessary, while this is required together with defect closure in others.

COARCTATION OF THE AORTA WITH MITRAL VALVE ABNORMALITIES

Prevalence

Mitral stenosis in association with coarctation is common, occurring in some 20% of our patients. Mitral regurgitation is even more common, 45% (Exhibit 36-1), much more so than 12% in the 1973 to 1988 era. This huge increase probably reflects the widespread use in this era of echocardiography, which identifies minor inaudible regurgitation. In earlier years, significant regurgitation requiring treatment occurred in only about 2% of patients with coarctation.[53]

Anatomy

The structural abnormalities seen in the stenosis group are diverse and include supravalvar mitral ring, hypoplasia of the annulus, parachute deformity and short thick chordae. The regurgitant lesion anatomy is equally variable and includes isolated cleft, leaflet perforation, and abnormal chordae.

Physiology

Because the afterload adversely affects adaptation to mitral regurgitation, otherwise tolerable degrees of mitral regurgitation may be intolerable when there is coarctation of the aorta. The relative severity of the two lesions determines the clinical course.

When there is a ventricular septal defect, the physiologic effect of mitral stenosis is accentuated by left-to-right shunting, the flow across the obstructing mitral valve being greater than normal. Closure of the ventricular defect may reduce the gradient across the mitral valve. When there is severe mitral stenosis and elevated pulmonary venous pressure, there will be pulmonary hypertension which, in the presence of a ventricular defect, may be confusing. Whether the pulmonary vascular disease is caused by pulmonary venous hypertension or by the left-to-right shunt is a critical decision, because the first is reversible with time (see Chapter 30).

Clinical Manifestations

The clinical picture is an amalgam of the clinical features of coarctation of the aorta and the clinical features of mitral regurgitation or mitral stenosis as isolated lesions. In addition to the findings of coarctation of the aorta, there is an apical systolic murmur that transmits well to the axilla when there is mitral regurgitation and an apical diastolic rumble when there is mitral stenosis.

Electrocardiography

With mitral regurgitation and coarctation of the aorta, left ventricular hypertrophy is usual. When there is significant mitral stenosis, right ventricular hypertrophy due to pulmonary hypertension is common.

Chest Radiography

On chest radiograph, the heart is usually very large with severe regurgitation due to both left atrial and ventricular enlargement. With significant mitral stenosis, the left atrium is usually enlarged and pulmonary edema with Kerley B lines may be present, more so when a ventricular defect is present.

Echocardiography

On echocardiogram, with mitral stenosis, the valvar abnormality is evident on two-dimensional examination, a single insertion of the papillary muscles being visible when there is a parachute valve. Hypoplasia of the valve and valve ring are similarly well demonstrated if present. With significant mitral regurgitation, both the left atrium and ventricle seem to be enlarged. The valve anatomy is readily identifiable as is the cause of the regurgitation (e.g., a cleft or prolapse). Assessment of the degree of regurgitation is possible using color flow and the regurgitant orifice dimension may be well seen in systole using three-dimensional echocardiography. Ventricular function assessment is also readily available. Using Doppler techniques, a diastolic gradient across the valve can be measured. The coarctation may be directly visible in smaller children.

Cardiac Catheterization

Cardiac catheterization for diagnostic purposes in these patients is unnecessary because all anatomic and most physiologic details are shown by echocardiography. The only reason for catheterization is if balloon dilation of either mitral stenosis or coarctation or both is planned.

Management

The mitral valve component in this combination of lesions is by far the more difficult of the two to manage. If the mitral valve hemodynamic burden is in the mild range, surgical management of the coarctation is all that is necessary. Indeed, if regurgitation is the primary mitral lesion, coarctation repair alone may improve this.[53] Some types of mitral regurgitation are quite amenable to valve plasty rather than replacement such as an isolated cleft or leaflet perforation. Some forms of congenital mitral stenosis are also surgically repairable such as supravalvar ring, whereas others may require replacement with a prosthesis. The latter is particularly problematic in the very young as most prostheses exceed the annular size—these can be placed in a supraannular position with some success.[54] Balloon dilation can be effective in some stenotic lesions (especially so in those due to rheumatic fever), in some forms of congenital obstruction even in the very young (such as double orifice mitral valve).[55]

Course

Although mitral regurgitation or mitral stenosis is often discovered in early infancy, fortunately mitral valve surgery is rarely required in the first year of life. Either lesion, particularly mitral regurgitation, may become progressively more severe with time.

COARCTATION OF THE AORTA WITH AORTIC STENOSIS

Definition

Aortic stenosis associated with coarctation of the aorta may be valvar, subvalvar, or both and often is associated with ventricular septal defect and/or mitral valve abnormality. This discussion will be confined to those patients with aortic stenosis and coarctation with an intact ventricular septum.

Prevalence

Among critically ill infants with coarctation, 5% have aortic stenosis, of whom some 2% are sufficiently severe to require aortic stenosis surgery.[1] In the current period (1988–2002), 29% of patients with coarctation of all ages had some degree of aortic stenosis (Exhibit 36-1).

Anatomy

The aortic flow obstruction associated with coarctation of the aorta may be valvar, subvalvar, and, in the case of William syndrome, it may be supravalvar. Subvalvar obstruction is more common when there is an interrupted aortic arch.

Physiology

While aortic stenosis and coarctation present the problem of two obstructions in series, the higher coronary perfusion pressure may permit more severe aortic stenosis than might have otherwise been anticipated.

Clinical Manifestations

The problem is diagnosed early in infancy, in some cases because of the development of congestive heart failure and in others because of the discovery of a loud murmur of aortic stenosis. Unlike simple coarctation of the aorta, there is a loud systolic murmur, sometimes with a thrill, at the base of the heart and along the left sternal border. A click is usually audible. The difference in pulse pressure between the arms and legs is sometimes less easily determined because the pulse pressure is generally lower when there is aortic stenosis. Measurements of blood pressures in the arms and legs will establish the presence of coarctation of the aorta.

Electrocardiography

If either of the obstructive lesions or both are severe, electrocardiography will reveal left ventricular hypertrophy. Left ventricular strain pattern is characteristic of the most severe combinations.

Chest Radiography

The chest radiograph will show that the heart is not significantly enlarged unless there is congestive failure or other associated defects.

Echocardiography

The aortic outflow anatomy and degree of obstruction, ventricular function, and the coarctation details are readily visualized on echocardiogram.

Cardiac Catheterization

If the stenosis is mild or less, catheterization is unnecessary before surgical coarctation repair. However, if valvar obstruction is considered severe, balloon dilation at any age is undertaken.

Management

It is uncommon that both lesions are severe. However, in the rare instances of severe obstruction at both valvar and coarctation levels in the neonate or infant, particularly when ventricular function is poor, balloon dilation of both lesions is indicated. In this situation it is recognized that the coarctation dilation is likely temporary but this allows recovery of function with lesser risk at later surgical coarctation repair. When aortic obstruction is mild or less, coarctation surgical repair only is carried out.

Course

In those in whom coarctation reobstruction occurs, balloon dilation is undertaken as it also is in those with progressive valvar stenosis.

COARCTATION OF THE AORTA AND COMPLEX HEART DISEASE

Coarctation of the aorta can be associated with any congenital cardiac defect except pulmonary atresia with intact ventricular septum, and very rarely tetralogy of Fallot (Exhibit 36-1). Infants with coarctation and complex heart disease are usually discovered in early infancy and most are critically ill. The coarctation is sometimes discovered by noting differences in arm and leg pulses or blood pressures, but mostly during echocardiography. Management consists of devising the best plan for the problems identified. With more than trivial obstruction, coarctectomy is undertaken together with repair of other lesions simultaneously. This approach would include for example coarctation repair and a stage 1 procedure simultaneously in hypoplastic left heart syndrome or repair with an arterial switch if d-transposition complicates the coarctation. As might be expected, survival is best among uncomplicated patients but has improved in the complicated cases (Exhibit 36-3).

INTERRUPTED AORTIC ARCH

Definition

Interruption of the aortic arch describes a point of atresia or absence of a segment of the aortic arch.

Prevalence

Of infants with coarctation seen in New England, 12% had complete interruption of the aortic arch. This amounted to 1.3% of all infants critically ill with heart disease with a prevalence of 0.019/1000 live births.[1] At Children's Hospital Boston, interrupted aortic arch accounted for 5% of all patients with aortic obstruction (Exhibit 36-1).

Embryology

The left fourth arch in the embryo forms the transverse aortic arch from the left carotid to the ductal site. Abnormalities in the formation of this area are thought to be responsible for at least two of the types of interrupted arch (type B, the most common; type C, the least common) and perhaps type A (Fig. 36-9). An alternative explanation for type A involves decreased flow across the arch and hence across the isthmus, which leads, in conjunction with right-to-left flow via the ductus to the descending aorta, to absence of the isthmus. From a chromosomal standpoint, deletion of 22q11 is strongly linked to both interrupted aortic arch, especially type B, and the DiGeorge syndrome.[56–58]

Anatomy

Type A (at the isthmus) (Fig. 36-9) occurred in 30% of our 92 patients, type B (interruption between left carotid and subclavian) in 69%, and type C (between innominate and left carotid) in only 1%. A ventricular septal defect of the conoventricular variety is present in the vast majority, being absent in only 5% of our patients (aged 4–20 years when first seen, one of whom had a type B interruption). Aortic stenosis is common (valvar or subvalvar or both) as are bicuspid aortic valves, aberrant subclavian arteries and truncus arteriosus (Exhibit 36-4).

Physiology

Other major defects of the heart commonly associated with interruption of the arch may dominate the physiologic picture. At Children's Hospital Boston we tend to divide the case material: Those with ventricular defect, patent ductus arteriosus, and valve deformity are classified as relatively uncomplicated with all others considered complicated (Exhibits 36-1 and 36-4).

Regardless of associated defects, the ductus arteriosus is required to supply blood to the lower half of the body. In those, spontaneous ductal closure threatens the babies' immediate survival; without circulation to the lower body there is marked metabolic acidosis and circulatory collapse. Average survival is only a matter of days following birth. Presumably, the difference between the infants with coarctation of the aorta who appear in congestive failure in the second week of life and those with interruption of the aorta who appear ill in the first days of life relates to the presence of some antegrade flow in the former through the obstructed isthmus. Clearly, any opening at the point of obstruction makes an appreciable difference, because the ductus arteriosus likely closes at the same time whether there is coarctation or interruption of the aorta. The use of prostaglandins E to open the ductus helps dramatically, more in the interrupted than in the severely coarcted babies (Fig. 36-10).

Clinical Manifestations

These infants become desperately ill in the first days of life whether they have other major cardiac defects or not. Only those with a reliable blood supply to the lower body

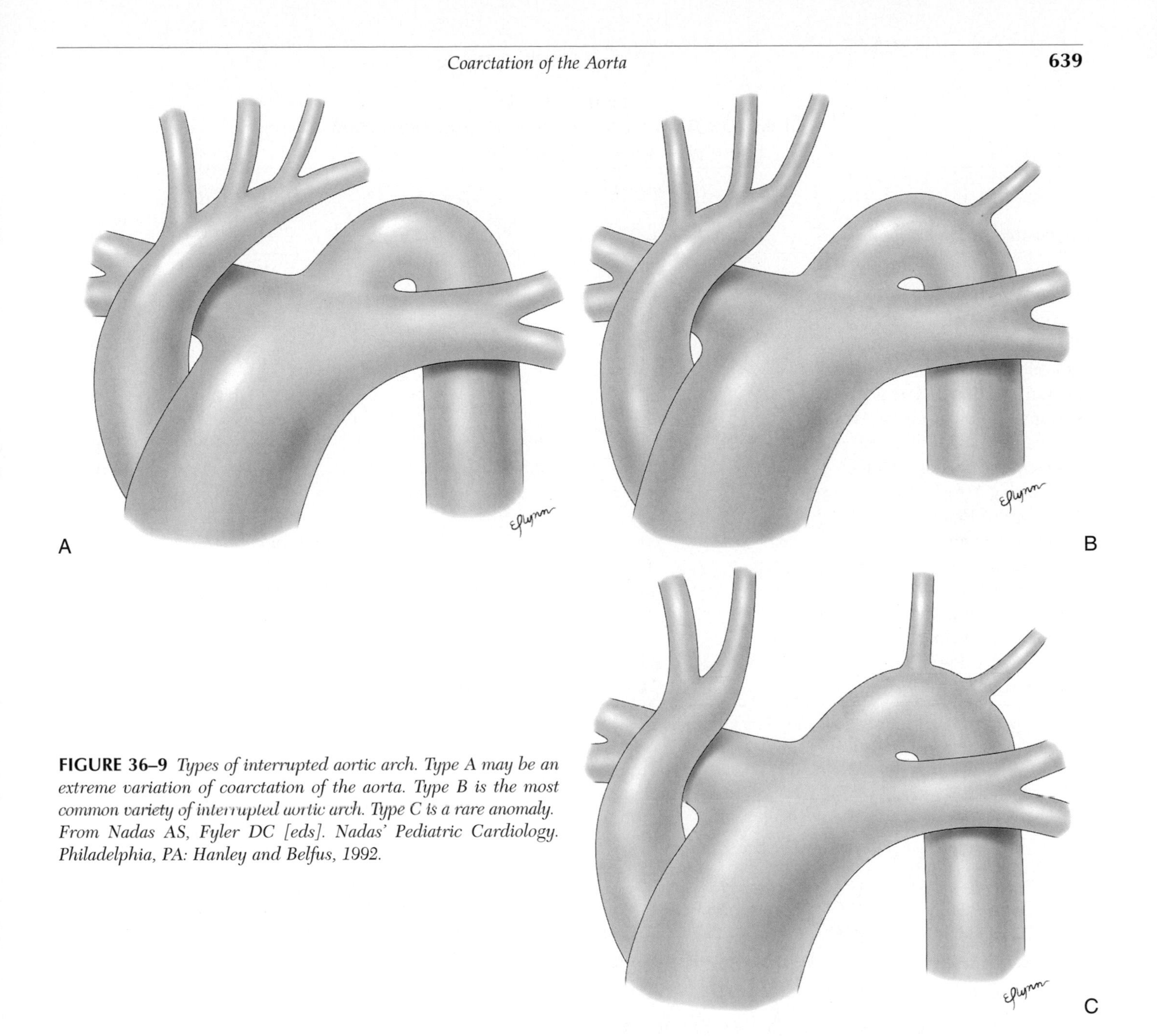

FIGURE 36–9 *Types of interrupted aortic arch. Type A may be an extreme variation of coarctation of the aorta. Type B is the most common variety of interrupted aortic arch. Type C is a rare anomaly. From Nadas AS, Fyler DC [eds]. Nadas' Pediatric Cardiology. Philadelphia, PA: Hanley and Belfus, 1992.*

(i.e., persistent patent ductus arteriosus) survive longer than a few weeks. The infants are *shocky*, tachypneic, and may appear terminally ill. Often, there is a systolic murmur. The peripheral pulses may be weak or absent, sometimes waxing and waning, and only with the improvement following administration of prostaglandins E does the difference between the arm and leg pulses become noticeable. The femoral pulses are usually absent or markedly diminished but may vary in intensity from time to time, depending on whether the ductus is open or closed. The child may be cyanotic or not, depending on the associated cardiac defects.

Electrocardiography

The electrocardiogram shows right ventricular hypertrophy in the uncomplicated cases and reflects the abnormal cardiac pathology in others.

Chest Radiography

The chest radiograph shows cardiomegaly, often marked, and often with increased pulmonary vascularity, although this may not be obvious in the early newborn period.

Exhibit 36–4
Children's Hospital Boston Experience: 1988–2002
Interrupted Aortic Arch: Associated Problems*

	Uncomplicated		*Complicated*	
Associated Problem	*N* = 92	(%)	*N* = 95	(%)
Asplenia	0		5	(5)
Single Ventricle			5	(5)
Hypoplastic Left Heart	0		6	(6)
Tricuspid Atresia	0		6	(6)
Double Outlet Right Ventricle	0		5	(5)
D-transposition of Great Arteries	0		8	(8)
L-transposition of Great Arteries	0		0	
Total anomalous Pulmonary Veins	0			0
Endocardial Cushion Defect	0		9	(9)
Pulmonary Atresia, Intact Septum	0		0	
Tetralogy of Fallot	0		1	(1)
Truncus Arteriosus	0		25	(26)
A-P Window	0		8	(8)
Aortic Stenosis⁺	82	(89)	28	(29)
Aortic Regurgitation	29	(32)	43	(45)
Mitral Valve Anomaly	56	(61)	47	(49)
Pulmonary Valve Anomaly	39	(42)	57	(60)
Tricuspid Valve Anomaly	74	(80)	65	(68)

*Some patients had more than one associated anomaly.
⁺Includes valvar and subvalvar stenosis.

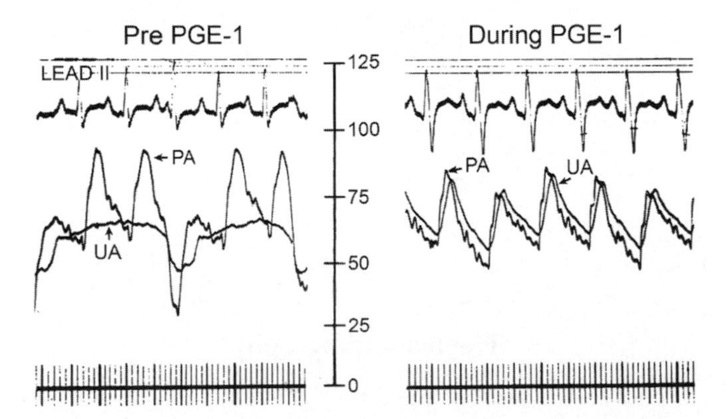

FIGURE 36–10 *Pressure tracings before and after administration of prostaglandins E_1 in a patient with interrupted aortic arch. Note the nonpulsatile tracing from the umbilical artery (UA) (the pressure variation is coincident with mechanical ventilation) and the appearance of pulsatile flow after administration of prostaglandins E_1, PA, pulmonary artery.*
From Nadas AS, Fyler DC [eds]. Nadas' Pediatric Cardiology. Philadelphia, PA: Hanley and Belfus, 1992.

Laboratory Tests

Metabolic acidosis, sometimes quite marked, correlates directly with the state of the patient. The sicker the child appears, the more marked is the acidosis.

Echocardiography

The diagnosis in all its details is made by echocardiography including recognition of ductal dependence, which leads to treatment with prostaglandins E.[59] Later, with a more stable patient, anatomic details may be more precisely outlined. The likely associated cardiac abnormalities should be kept in mind and the patient evaluated for each as the examination proceeds (Exhibits 34-1 and 34-4).[59]

Most infants with interrupted aortic arch have a conoventricular septal defect and deviation of the hypoplastic infundibular septum. Doppler evaluation of the left ventricular outflow tract provides gradient estimates but absence of a detectable gradient does not exclude obstruction. The ascending aorta is seen to end in the brachiocephalic arteries

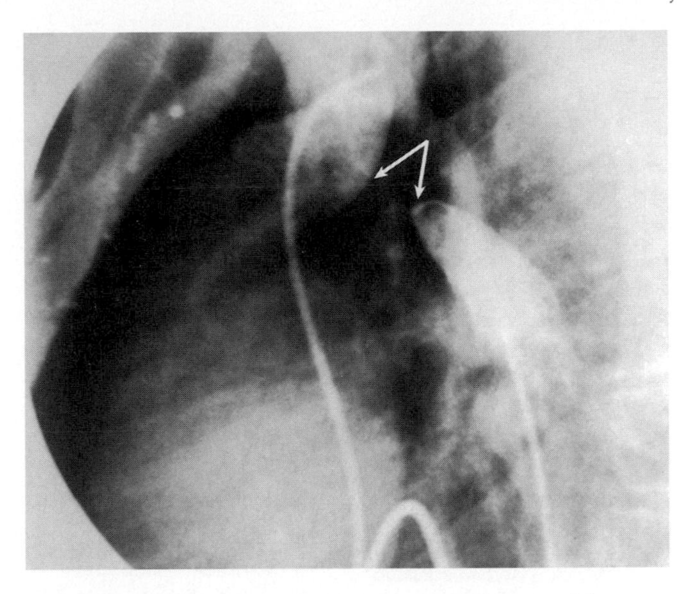

FIGURE 36–11 *Aortogram, lateral view, in 20-year-old patient with long segment type B interruption (arrows) between left carotid and left subclavian arteries*

without a posteriorly coursing transverse arch, and the main pulmonary artery is noted to continue into the descending aorta through the ductus arteriosus. The distance between the distal descending and ascending aorta is also evident in this view.

An aberrant right subclavian artery is a frequent finding in interrupted aortic arch, and is noted to arise from the right side of the proximal descending aorta, adjacent to the origin of the left subclavian artery.

Cardiac Catheterization

Given the precision of anatomic detail by echocardiography together with physiologic information, catheterization is no longer necessary preoperatively in this largely neonatal population, but may be necessary in older patients (Fig. 36-11). In those few older patients with *poor windows*, magnetic resonance imaging provides excellent anatomic details including collateral vessel information.

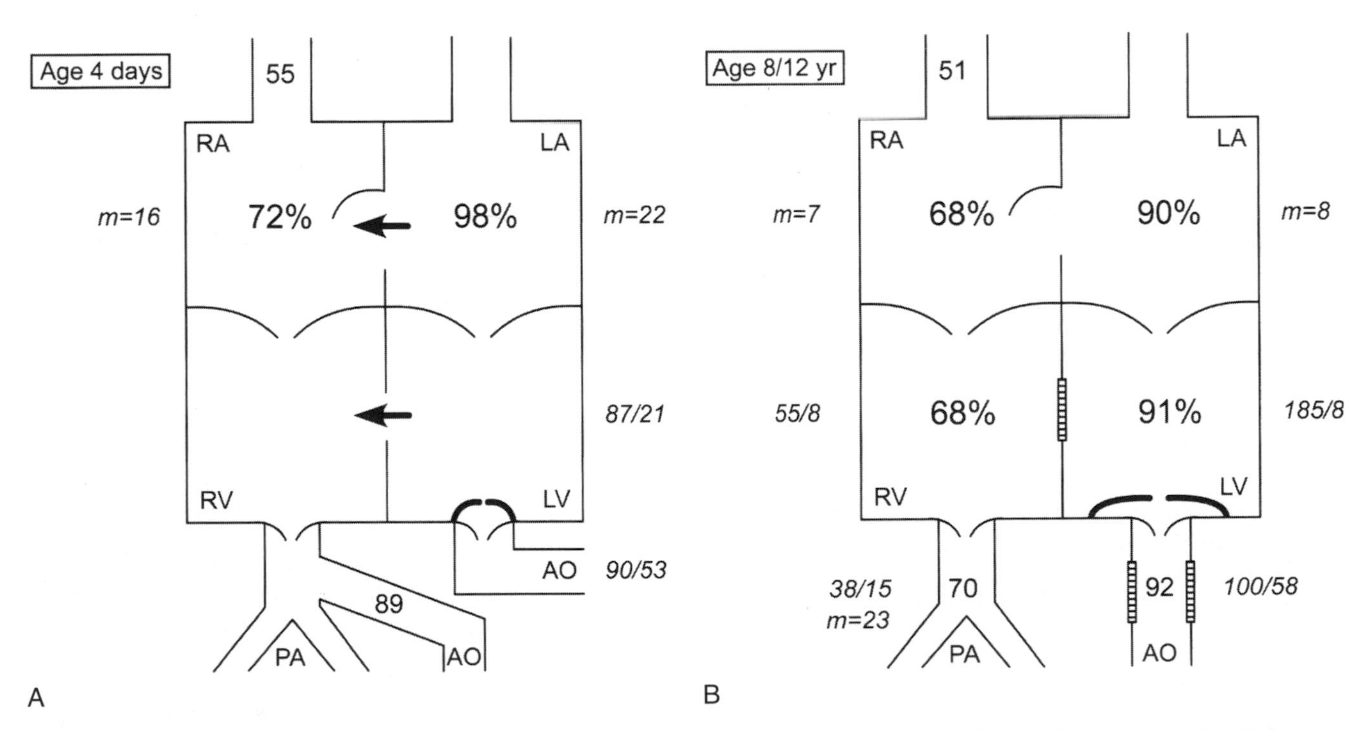

FIGURE 36–12 *This 4-day-old neonate was moribund on arrival and responded to prostaglandins E. A, Catheterization data at age 4 days, using 100% oxygen, showed equal pressures above and below a type B interrupted aortic arch. On angiography, there was a moderately severe subaortic stenosis that became clinically manifest after the ventricular defect was patched and the interruption repaired. B, Same patient 8 months later. Severe subaortic stenosis is evident now that the entire cardiac output passes through the aortic valve. From Nadas AS, Fyler DC [eds]. Nadas' Pediatric Cardiology. Philadelphia, PA: Hanley and Belfus, 1992.*

Management

Infants suspected of having interrupted aortic arch should be treated promptly with prostaglandins E, a response in the patient's condition confirming the impression of ductal dependence (Fig. 36-10). Following echocardiographic evaluation plans for surgery are made. Once the metabolic acidosis has been reasonably controlled, surgical correction should be undertaken as soon as possible.

Generally, in all types, the aortic arch structures can be mobilized and a primary anastomosis of the upper and lower segments of the arch carried out such that artificial conduits or homografts are rarely necessary. In so far as is feasible, all other abnormalities should be repaired at the same operation, although a second operation may be necessary because of intracardiac anatomy. This single-stage approach involves simultaneous correction of such lesions as truncus arteriosus, ventricular septal defect(s), d-transposition and even aortic stenosis. Reported early mortality results range from 0% to 12% (Exhibit 36-3).[60–62] Some investigators have used a two-stage approach but this had been associated with early higher mortality rates (4% to 37%).[60,63,64]

Course

Without surgery, uncomplicated interrupted aortic arch is invariably a fatal illness, with death occurring within days of birth. Additional intracardiac anomalies add to the problem. During follow up, residual problems are common such that freedom from reoperation has been reported as low as 47% at 12 years.[62] A common reason for reoperation is left ventricular outflow tract obstruction, especially if unoperated on at the initial procedure (Fig. 36-12). Preoperative echocardiographic measurements predictive of such future obstruction are now quite useful.[65] In terms of long-term survival, 85% at 12 years represents a most encouraging observation compared to earlier years.[62]

ATYPICAL COARCTATIONS OF THE AORTA

Rarely, coarctation may be atypically located in the thoracic and/or abdominal aorta. It may vary in length from centimeters to the entire descending aorta and may involve major branches such as renal arteries. These obstructions may be associated with William syndrome, neurofibromatosis, Takayasu disease, or rubella syndrome. Treatment depends on severity and location. Among nine patients seen at Children's Hospital Boston between 1988 and 2002, three had a bypass conduit placed and five were treated in the catheterization laboratory using balloon dilation with stent placement in four of these patients (Fig. 36-13).

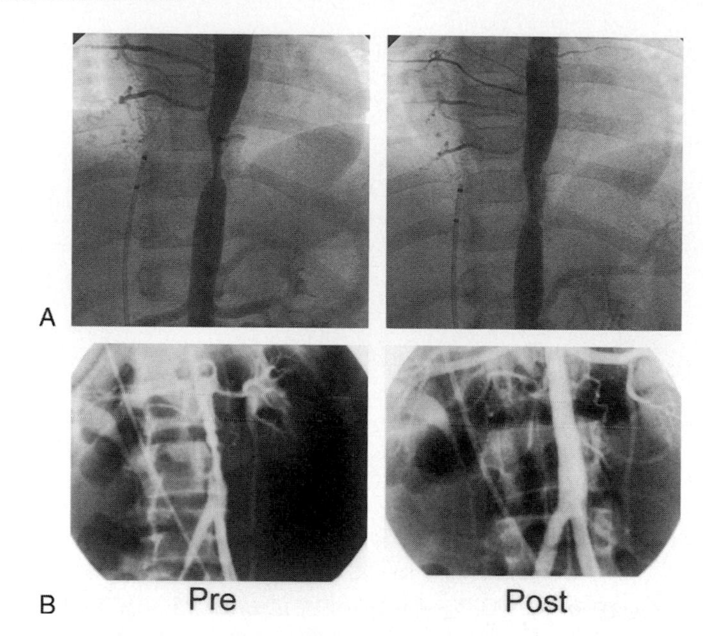

FIGURE 36–13 *Aortic angiograms showing two atypical coarctations and response to interventional therapy. A, Four-year-old child with Takayasu disease with abdominal aorta coarctation pre and post balloon dilation. B, Thirty-year-old patient with Rubella syndrome with diffuse abdominal aorta obstruction pre and post balloon dilation and stent placement.*

REFERENCES

1. Fyler DC, Buckley LP, Hellenbrand WE, et al. Report of the New England Regional Infant Cardiac Program. Pediatrics 65:376, 1980.
2. Botto LD, Correa A, Erickson JD. Racial and temporal variations in prevalence of heart defects. Pediatrics 107(3):1, 2001.
3. Morrow WR, Huhta JC, Murphy DJ, et al. Quantitative morphology of the aortic arch in neonatal circulation. J Am Coll Cardiol 8:616, 1986.
4. Talner NS, Berman MA. Postnatal development of obstruction in coarctation of the aorta: role of the ductus arteriosus. Pediatrics 56:562, 1975.
5. Rudolph A. Aortic arch obstruction. In Rudolph A (ed). Congenital Diseases of the Heart. New York: Futura Publishing, 2001, pp 367–412.
6. Lacro RV, Jones KL, Benirschke K. Coarctation of the aorta in Turner syndrome: a pathologic study of fetuses with nuchal cystic hygromas, hydrops fetalis, and female genitalia. Pediatrics 81:445, 1988.
7. Surerus E, Huggon IC, Allan LD. Turner's syndrome in fetal life. Ultrasound in Obstetrics & Gynecology 22(3):264, 2003.
8. Bordeleau L, Cwinn A, Turek M, et al. Aortic dissection and Turner's syndrome: case report and review of the literature. J Emergency Med. 16(4):593, 1998.

9. Connolly HM, Huston J, 3rd, Brown RD, et al. Intracranial aneurysms in patients with coarctation of the aorta: a prospective magnetic resonance angiographic study of 100 patients. Mayo Clinic Proceedings. 78(12):1491, 2003.
10. Mercado R, Lopez S, Cantu C, et al. Intracranial aneurysms associated with unsuspected aortic coarctation. J Neurosurg. 97(5):1221, 2002.
11. Rudolph AM, Heymann MA, Spitznas U. Hemodynamic considerations in the development of narrowing of the aorta. Am J Cardiol 30:514, 1972.
12. Markel H, Rocchini Ap, Beekman RH, et al. Exercise-induced hypertension after repair of coarctation of the aorta: arm versus leg exercise. J Am Coll Cardiol 8:165, 1986.
13. Beekman RH, Katz BP, Moorehead-Steffens C, et al. Altered baroreceptor function in children with systolic hypertension after coarctation repair. Am J Cardiol 52:112, 1983.
14. Benedict CR, Grahame-Smith DG, Fisher A. Changes in plasma catacholamines and dopamine beta-hydroxylase after corrective surgery for coarctation of the aorta. Circulation 57:598, 1978.
15. Rocchini AP, Rosenthal A, Barger AC, et al. Pathogenesis of paradoxical hypertension after coarctation resection. Circulation 54:382, 1976.
16. Marx GR, Allen HD. Accuracy and pitfalls of Doppler evaluation of the pressure gradient in aortic coarctation. J Am Coll Cardiol 7:1379, 1986.
17. Sanders SP, MacPherson D, Yeager SB. Temporal flow velocity profile in the descending aorta in coarctation. J Am Coll Cardiol 7:603, 1986.
18. Smith Maia MM, CortAs TM, Parga JR, et al. Evolutional aspects of children and adolescents with surgically corrected aortic coarctation: clinical, echocardiographic, and magnetic resonance image analysis of 113 patients. J Thor & Cardiovasc Surg 127(3):712, 2004.
19. Bhat MA, Neelakandhan KS, Unnikrishnan M, et al. Fate of hypertension after repair of coarctation of the aorta in adults. British J Surg 88(4):536, 2001.
20. Roos-Hesselink JW, Scholzel BE, Heijdra RJ, et al. Aortic valve and aortic arch pathology after coarctation repair. Heart (British Cardiac Society) 89(9):1074, 2003.
21. de Divitiis M, Pilla C, Kattenhorn M, et al. Ambulatory blood pressure, left ventricular mass, and conduit artery function late after successful repair of coarctation of the aorta. J Am Coll Cardiol 41(12):2259, 2003.
22. O'Sullivan JJ, Derrick G, Darnell R. Prevalence of hypertension in children after early repair of coarctation of the aorta: a cohort study using casual and 24 hour blood pressure measurement. [see comment]. Heart (British Cardiac Society) 88(2):163, 2002.
23. Dodge-Khatami A, Backer CL, Mavroudis C. Risk factors for recoarctation and results of reoperation: a 40-year review. J Cardiac Surg 15(6):369, 2000.
24. Corno AF, Botta U, Hurni M, et al. Surgery for aortic coarctation: a 30 years experience. Eur J Cardiothorac Surg 20(6): 1202, 2001.
25. Berendes JN, Bredee JJ, Schipperheyn JJ, et al. Mechanism of spinal cord injury after cross-clamping of the descending thoracic aorta. Circulation 66 (Suppl I):112, 1982.
26. Brewer LA, Fosburg RG, Mulder GA, et al. Spinal cord complications following surgery for coarctation of the aorta. J Thorac Cardiovasc Surg 64:368,1972.
27. Napoleone CP, Gabbieri D, Gargiulo G. Coarctation repair with prosthetic material: surgical experience with aneurysm formation. Italian Heart J: Official Journal of the Italian Federation of Cardiology 4(6):404, 2003.
28. von Kodolitsch Y, Aydin MA, Koschyk DH, et al. Predictors of aneurysmal formation after surgical correction of aortic coarctation. J Am Coll Cardiol 39(4):617, 2002.
29. Koerselman J, de Vries H, Jaarsma W, et al. Balloon angioplasty of coarctation of the aorta: a safe alternative for surgery in adults: immediate and mid-term results. Cath & Cardiovasc Interven 50(1):28, 2000.
30. Paddon AJ, Nicholson AA, Ettles DF, et al. Long-term follow-up of percutaneous balloon angioplasty in adult aortic coarctation. Cardiovasc & Interv Radiol 23(5):364, 2000.
31. Ovaert C, McCrindle BW, Nydanen D. Balloon angioplasty of native coarctation: clinical outcomes and predictors of success. J Am Coll Cardiol 35(4):988, 2000.
32. Saba SE, Nimri M, Shamaileh Q, et al. Balloon coarctation angioplasty: follow-up of 103 patients. [see comment]. J Invasive Cardiol 12(8):402, 2000.
33. Harrison DA, McLaughlin PR, Lazzam C, et al. Endovascular stents in the management of coarctation of the aorta in the adolescent and adult: one year follow up. Heart (British Cardiac Society) 85(5):561, 2001.
34. Hamdan MA, Maheshwari S, Fahey JT, et al. Endovascular stents for coarctation of the aorta: initial results and intermediate-term follow-up. [see comment]. J Am Coll Cardiol 38(5):1518, 2001.
35. Maron BJ, Humphries JON, Rowe RD, et al. Prognosis of surgically corrected coarctation of the aorta: a 20-year post-operative appraisal. Circulation 47:119, 1973.
36. Pacileo G, Pisacana C, Russo MG, et al. Left ventricular remodeling and mechanics after successful repair of aortic coarctation. Am J Cardiol 87(6):748, 2001.
37. Hellenbrand WE, Allen HD, Golinko RJ, et al. Balloon angioplasty for aortic recoarctation: results of valvuloplasty and angioplasty of congenital anomalies registry. Am J Cardiol 65:793, 1990.
38. Yetman AT, Nykanen D, McCrindle BW, et al. Balloon angioplasty of recurrent coarctation: a 12-year review. J Am Coll Cardiol 30:811,1997.
39. Siblini G, Rao PS, Nouri S, et al. Long-term follow-up results of balloon angioplasty of postoperative aortic recoarctation. Am J Cardiol 81:61, 1998.
40. Marshall AC, Perry SB, Keane JF, et al. Early results and medium-term follow-up of stent implantation for mild residual or recurrent aortic coarctation. Am Heart J 139(6):1054, 2000.
41. Duke C, Rosenthal E, Quresha SA. The efficacy and safety of stent redilatation in congenital heart disease. Heart (British Cardiac Society). 89(8):905, 2003.

42. Zoghbi J, Serraf A, Mohammadi S, et al. Is surgical intervention still indicated in recurrent arch obstruction: J Thorac & Cardiovasc Surg 127(1):203, 2004.
43. Galal MO, Schmaltz AA, Joufan M, et al. Balloon dilation of native coarctation in infancy. Zeitschrift fur Kardiologie 92(9):735, 2003.
44. Rao PS, Jureidini SB, Balfour IC, et al. Severe aortic coarctation in infants less than 3 months: successful palliation by balloon angioplasty. J Invasive Cardiol 15(4):202, 2003.
45. Koch A, Buheitel G,Gerling S, et al. Balloon dilatation of critical left heart stenoses in low birth weight infants. Acta Paediatrica 89(8):979, 2000.
46. Younoszai AK, Reddy VM, Hanley FL, et al. Intermediate term follow-up of the end-to-side aortic anastomosis for coarctation of the aorta. Ann Thorac Surg 74(5):1631, 2002.
47. Gaynor JW, Wernovsky G, Rychik J, et al. Outcome following single-state repair of coarctation with ventricular septal defect. Eur J Cardiothorac Surg 18(1):62, 2000.
48. Jahangiri M, Shinebourne EA, Zurakowski D, et al. Subclavian flap angioplasty: does the arch look after itself? J Thorac & Cardiovasc Surg 120(2):224, 2000.
49. McElhinney DB, Yang SG, Hogarty AN, et al. Recurrent arch obstruction after repair of isolated coarctation of the aorta in neonates and young infants: is low weight a risk factor? J Thorac & Cardiovasc Surg 122(5):883, 2001.
50. Elgamal MA, McKenzie ED, Fraser CD, Jr. Aortic arch advancement: the optimal one-stage approach for surgical management of neonatal coarctation with arch hypoplasia. Ann Thorac Surg 73(4):1267, 2002.
51. Korbmacher B, Krogmann ON, Rammos S, et al. Repair of critical aortic coarctation in neonatal age. J Cardiovasc Surg 43(1):1, 2002.
52. Bacha EA, Almodovar M, Wessel DL, et al. Surgery for coarctation of the aorta in infants weighing less than 2 kg. Ann Thorac Surg 71(4):1260, 2004.
53. Freed MD, Keane JF, Van Praagh R, et al. Coarctation of the aorta with congenital mitral regurgitation. Circulation 49:1175, 1974.
54. Adatia I, Moore PM, Jonas RA, et al. Clinical course and hemodynamic observations after supraannular mitral valve replacement in infants and children. J Am Coll Cardiol 29:1089, 1997.
55. Moore PM, Adatia I, Spevak PJ, et al. Severe congenital mitral stenosis in infants. Circulation 89:2099, 1994.
56. Botto LD, May K, Fernhoff PM, et al. A population-based study of the 22q11.2 deletion: phenotype, incidence, and contribution to major birth defects in the population. Pediatrics 112(1 pt 1):101, 2003.
57. Loffredo CA, Ferencz C, Wilson PD. Interrupted aortic arch: an epidemiologic study. Tetralogy 61(5):368, 2000.
58. Van Mierop LH, Kutsche LM. Cardiovascular anomalies in DiGeorge syndrome and importance of neural crest as a possible pathogenetic factor. Am J Cardiol 58:133, 1986.
59. Lang P, Freed MD, Rosenthal A, et al. The use of prostaglandin E1 in an infant with interruption of the aortic arch. J Pediatr 91:805, 1977.
60. Schreiber C, Eicken A, Vogt M, et al. Repair of interrupted aortic arch: results after more than 20 years. Ann Thorac Surg 70(6):1896, 2000.
61. Jahangiri M, Zurakowski D, Mayer JE, et al. Repair of the truncal valve and associated interrupted arch in neonates with truncus arteriosus. J Thorac & Cardiovasc Surg 119(3):508, 2000.
62. Fulton JO, Mas C, Brizard CP, et al. Does left ventricular outflow tract obstruction influence outcome of interrupted aortic arch repair? Ann Thorac Surg 67(1):177, 1999.
63. Mainwaring RD, Lamberti JJ. Mid- to long-term results of the two-stage approach for type B interrupted aortic arch and ventricular septal defect. Ann Thorac Surg 64(6): 1782, 1997.
64. Aeba R, Katogi T, Hashizume K, et al. The limitation of staged repair in the surgical management of congenital complex heart anomalies with aortic arch obstruction. Japanese J Thorac & Cardiovasc Surg 51(7):302, 2003.
65. Apfel HD, Levenbraun J, Quaegebeur JM, et al. Usefulness of preoperative echocardiography in predicting left ventricular outflow obstruction after primary repair of interrupted aortic arch with ventricular septal defect. Am J Cardiol 82(4):470, 1998.

37

D-Transposition of the Great Arteries

David R. Fulton and Donald C. Fyler

Definition

D-transposition of the great arteries describes reversal of the anatomic relation of the great arteries. Normally, the aorta is located posterior and rightward and the pulmonary artery anteriorly and leftward; in transposition the aorta is anterior and rightward whereas the pulmonary artery is posterior and leftward. In normally related great arteries, the aorta relates directly to the left ventricle and the pulmonary artery to the right ventricle, while in transposition, the ventricular relationship is reversed. Most patients with transposition are readily characterized using these descriptions. The subject of this chapter is confined to transposition of the great arteries associated with D-looping (see Chapter 4). L-looping and other forms of transposition associated with single ventricle or heterotaxy are found in their respective chapters.

In most infants with D-transposition of the great arteries, there is an intact ventricular septum (Exhibit 37-1). In those with ventricular septal defects, the defects range in size from insignificant to large, sometimes in combination with pulmonic stenosis or pulmonary atresia. Other possible associated cardiac anomalies are coarctation of the aorta, pulmonary stenosis, or mitral valve disease. In a number of instances, classification of transposition is not distinct with the spectrum ranging from double outlet right ventricle (both great arteries arising from the right ventricle) to transposition with ventricular septal defect, and another group having transposition with some ventricular hypoplasia extending to those with single ventricle. Clear demarcation between these groups is not always possible.

Prevalence

D-transposition of the great arteries is the second most common congenital cardiac defect encountered in early infancy and is the leading reason for transfer to a cardiac unit in the first two weeks of life. The number of children born each year with D-transposition (~0.24/1000 live births) is remarkably constant.[1] The constancy of presentation compared to other congenital cardiac defects may be related to ease of clinical recognition in early infancy.

Embryology

The embryologic explanation for transposition remains unknown; however, a widely accepted theory implicates abnormal development of the subarterial conus bilaterally. During normal cardiac formation, both the subaortic conus and subpulmonary conus are present initially with both great arteries situated above the right ventricle. At approximately 30 to 34 days into gestation, the subaortic conus starts to resorb while the aorta migrates inferior and posterior to lie directly over the left ventricle. Simultaneously, the subpulmonary conus persists so that the pulmonary artery remains stationary over the right ventricle. In D-transposition, the subpulmonary conus resorbs, leading to reversal of the normal arterial migration with the pulmonary artery moving inferior and posterior with the pulmonic valve in fibrous continuity with the mitral valve. Because not all forms of D-transposition can be explained simply by this theory, an alternate explanation suggests a failure of the truncus arteriosus to septate normally.

Exhibit 37–1
Boston Children's Hospital Experience
D-Transposition of the Great Arteries

Transposition Associated with	***1973–1987*** *N*	*1988–2002* *N*
*Intact Ventricular Septum	440	565
Ventricular Septal Defect (VSD)	222	376
VSD + ≥moderate Pulmonary Stenosis	93	50
Total	755	991

*Includes those with ≤small VSD: all patients seen at Boston Children's Hospital, including those initially seen elsewhere.

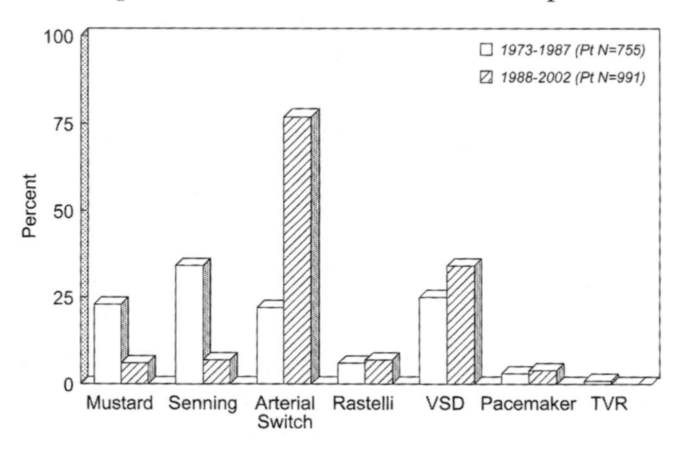

In the 1988-2002 population, (a) there has been a dramatic increase in the number of arterial switch operations, (b) all those with a Mustard or Senning procedure had had that procedure elsewhere before their first visit to Children's Hospital (c) of 41 pacemakers placed, 34 were in Mustard/Senning patients, 4 following arterial switch and VSD closure and 3 after a Rastelli procedure and (d) there were no tricuspid valve replacements (TVR).

To date, no genetic abnormality has been identified to explain the existence of D-transposition. Recurrence in the same family is virtually unrecognized. It is associated with fewer extracardiac anomalies than are most other congenital cardiac defects, perhaps fewer than the general population. Furthermore, transposition of the great arteries is uncommon among premature infants and those with low birth weights.[2] There is evidence of a higher incidence in rural settings,[3] with advanced maternal age and with higher birth order.[4] It does not occur in Down syndrome.

Anatomy

In D-transposition of the great arteries, the aorta arises from the right ventricle, being most often positioned directly in front in a lateral view, and slightly to the right of the pulmonary artery in the antero-posterior view (Fig. 37-1). A small percentage of patients have the aorta positioned somewhat leftward. The pulmonary artery arises behind the aorta from the left ventricle, a position that allows preferential ejection from the left ventricle into the right pulmonary artery and probably accounts for the large right pulmonary artery and the somewhat increased flow to the right lung in these patients.[5] There is a subaortic conus as well as pulmonary and mitral valvar fibrous continuity. Because most of these infants are discovered at birth or shortly afterward, the foramen ovale and ductus arteriosus are often patent at the time of first encounter.

Among infants with an intact ventricular septum, functional obstruction to outflow from the left ventricle (dynamic pulmonary stenosis) is common. This obstruction appears to be caused by bowing of the ventricular septum to the left, because of greater right ventricular pressure; the resulting proximity of the mitral valve and septum causes obstruction.

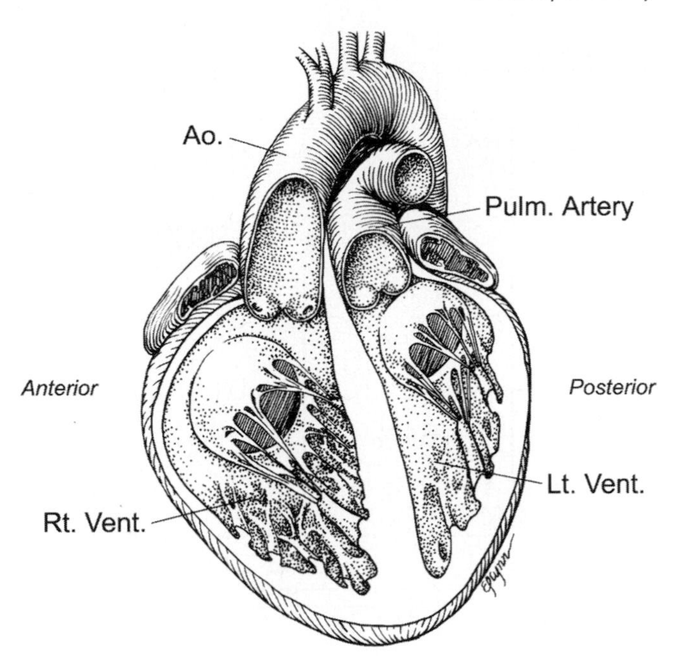

FIGURE 37–1 *Transposition of the great arteries, lateral view. The aorta arises anteriorly from the right ventricle; the pulmonary artery arises posteriorly from the left ventricle. As diagrammed, there is no communication shown between the pulmonary and systemic circulations, a situation not compatible with life. For survival there must be communication between the two circuits, usually as a patent ductus arteriosus, ventricular defect, or atrial opening.*
From Nadas' Pediatric Cardiology, eds: Fyler DC, Hanley & Belfus Inc. Philadelphia 1992

These dynamic gradients disappear with anatomic correction. Rarely, a patient may have anatomic subvalvar stenosis, a challenging management problem,[6] or valvar stenosis. True atrial septal defects are uncommon, but a persistent large ductus arteriosus may be encountered occasionally.

Ventricular defects are present at birth in 50% of the infants with D-transposition of the great arteries, but spontaneous closure in the first year reduces the number of children with ventricular septal defects by one third. Ventricular defects may be located anywhere in the ventricular septum; however, there is some difference of opinion about whether the relative frequency of the different types of ventricular septal defects is similar to that seen in patients who do not have transposition.[7] At Boston Children's Hospital, we have not noticed a distribution convincingly different from that in infants without transposition.[8] The terms *subpulmonary* and *subaortic* ventricular defects are confusing when the great arteries are transposed; the terms *infundibular* and *perimembranous* are preferred. Among the children with transposition of the great arteries and ventricular septal defect, additional cardiac anomalies are more common than among those with transposition of the great arteries and intact ventricular septum. Thus, pulmonary stenosis, pulmonary atresia, an overriding or straddling atrioventricular (AV) valve, coarctation of the aorta, and interruption of the aorta are more likely to be encountered when there is a ventricular septal defect. Right ventricular outflow obstruction is rare.[9]

The coronary anatomy in transposition of the great arteries is important since the location of the coronary arteries influences the outcome of the arterial switch procedure.[10–13] A simple rule that accounts for virtually all variations is that the coronaries arise from the sinuses of Valsalva that face the pulmonary artery and follow the shortest route to their ultimate destination.[14] If the great arteries lie in an anteroposterior position, the right-facing sinus gives rise to the right coronary artery whereas the left coronary artery arises from the left-facing sinus. In side-by-side great arterial relationships, the sinuses face in an anterior and posterior direction. The proximal course of the coronary arteries may follow an intramural path without interposed adventitia, knowledge of which is critical for surgical correction during an arterial switch procedure.

Abnormalities of the tricuspid[15,16] and mitral[17] valves are frequent but are seldom of importance. Infants with a ventricular septal defect of the endocardial cushion type may have an overriding or straddling tricuspid valve. When septal chordal attachments extend into the left ventricle, the valve is said to be *straddling*. When the valve allows direct flow into the left ventricle without straddling chordae, it is described as *overriding*. The implications for surgical correction are vitally important. In either case, with an overriding or straddling tricuspid valve, some right atrial blood is ejected into the left ventricle. When the right ventricle receives less than the usual amount of blood, the result may be ventricular hypoplasia.

Physiology

With transposition of the great arteries, the systemic venous blood passes through the right heart to the aorta, while the pulmonary venous blood passes through the left heart, returning to the lungs. Survival is dependent on the amount of communication between these two parallel circulations. Those with an intact ventricular septum survive because of flow through the ductus arteriosus into the pulmonary circuit, returning from the pulmonary circuit via left atrial to right atrial shunting through a dilated foramen ovale (Fig. 37-2). For the required atrial shunt to occur, the flap of the foramen ovale must become incompetent. At birth the pulmonary circuit is overloaded to the point that elevation of left atrial pressure causes bulging of the atrial septum toward the right, allowing decompression through an incompetent foramen ovale. It is apparent that

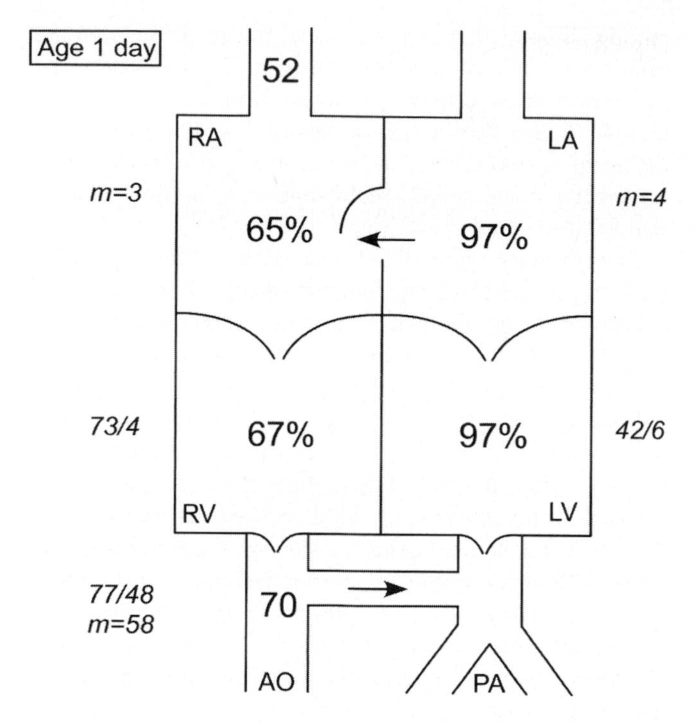

FIGURE 37–2 *Hemodynamic diagram of the circulation with transposition of the great arteries with intact ventricular septum. This infant survives because of flow through the ductus arteriosus to the lungs and return of equal flow from the left atrium to the right through a sprung foramen ovale. It is believed that, at birth, an excess of blood is supplied to the pulmonary circuit by the patent ductus arteriosus, thereby raising the left atrial pressure sufficiently to force open the foramen ovale, and thereby allowing compensatory pulmonary-to-systemic flow. RA, right atrium; RV, right ventricle; Ao, aorta; LA, left atrium; LV, left ventricle; PA, pulmonary artery; italics, pressure in mmHg%; percent oxygen saturation.*
From Nadas' Pediatric Cardiology, eds; Fyler DC, Hanley & Belfus Inc. Philadelphia 1992.

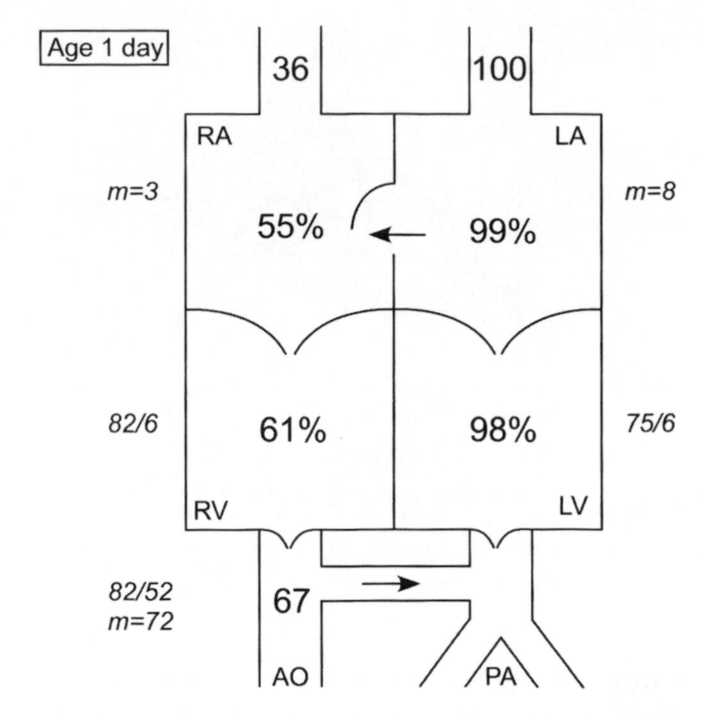

FIGURE 37–3 *Hemodynamic diagram of a newborn infant with transposition of the great vessels and intact ventricular septum who has received prostaglandins E_1. The pulmonary blood flow is excessive, the left atrial pressure is higher than the right, and there is pulmonary hypertension. Compare with Figure 37-4.*
From Nadas AS, Fyler DC [eds]. Nadas' Pediatric Cardiology. Philadelphia, PA: Hanley and Belfus, 1992.

the amount of blood flowing into and out of the pulmonary circulation must be equal, or overloading of blood in one circuit or the other would be rapidly fatal. Increasing the ductal left-to-right shunt, as with infusion of prostaglandin E, increases the flow into the lung,[18,19] which must in turn be compensated for by increased flow toward the right atrium and systemic circuit via the foramen ovale. If the incompetent foramen ovale cannot accommodate the increased blood flow, the pulmonary circuit will be overloaded (Fig. 37-3). At best, a patent foramen ovale and a patent ductus arteriosus allow for marginal survival. Enlarging the atrial opening by balloon atrial septostomy or surgical creation of an atrial defect allows for increased mixing between the two circulations with improved arterial oxygenation. Administering supplemental inspired oxygen has little effect on the systemic arterial oxygen saturation.

Rarely, a patient is born with a *large atrial defect* allowing equal bidirectional shunting with good survival. These patients can be recognized because of the equilibration of atrial pressures and the lack of other shunts.

Infants with *ventricular septal defects* tend to have a larger volume of shunting with higher systemic arterial saturation. The defect allows shunting toward the pulmonary circuit, with return to the systemic circuit via the foramen ovale given the elevated left atrial pressure (Fig. 37-4). Since ventricular defects may close spontaneously over time, survival may be dependent entirely on a shunt at the foramen level since the ductus arteriosus may no longer be patent. On the other hand, a large ventricular defect provides good mixing but the unrestrictive pulmonary blood flow may result in heart failure with minimal cyanosis.

The presence of pulmonary stenosis modifies the balance between resistance to pulmonary and systemic blood flow. In infants with an intact ventricular septum, the outflow of the left ventricle is commonly obstructed by dynamic subpulmonary stenosis. In large part, these obstructions are generally mild and represent a reversible phenomenon that result from the leftward position of the ventricular septum due to right ventricular hypertension.[20]

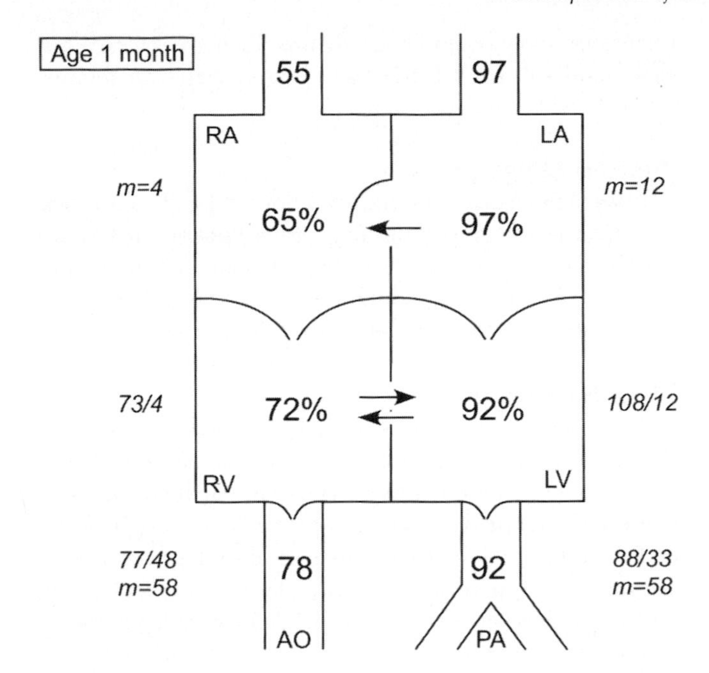

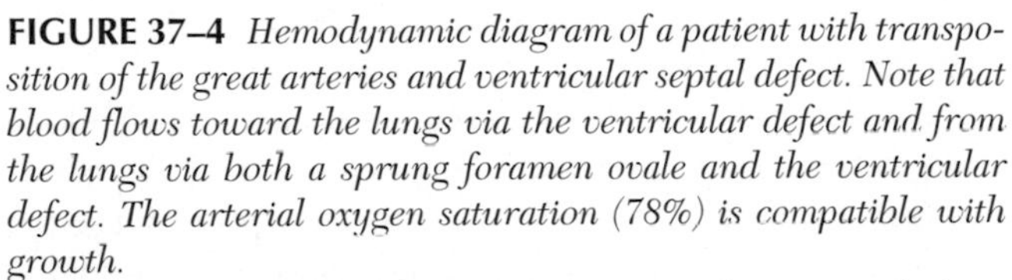

FIGURE 37–4 *Hemodynamic diagram of a patient with transposition of the great arteries and ventricular septal defect. Note that blood flows toward the lungs via the ventricular defect and from the lungs via both a sprung foramen ovale and the ventricular defect. The arterial oxygen saturation (78%) is compatible with growth.*
From Nadas AS, Fyler DC [eds]. Nadas' Pediatric Cardiology. Philadelphia, PA: Hanley and Belfus, 1992.

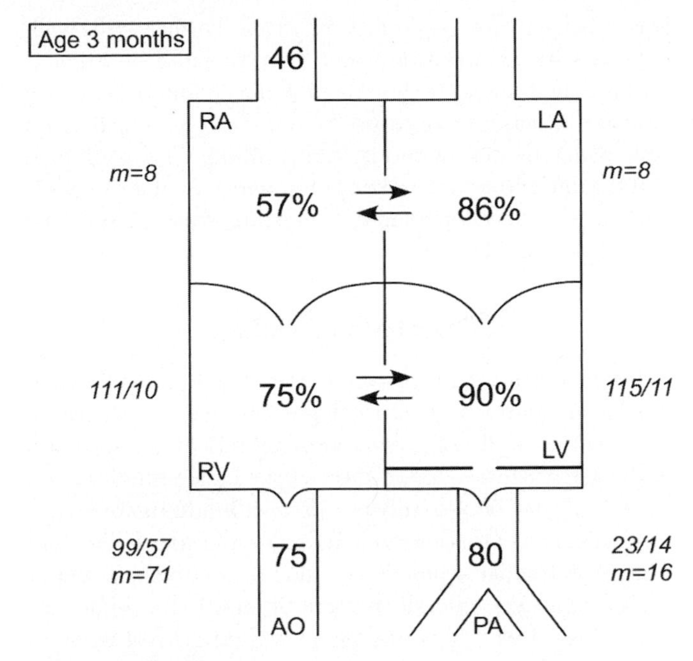

FIGURE 37–5 *Hemodynamic diagram of a patient with transposition of the great arteries, ventricular septal, and subpulmonary stenosis. The balance of the circulation is similar to that shown in Figure 37-4; however, there is normal pulmonary arterial pressure. The pulmonary stenosis prohibits excess pulmonary blood flow; therefore, left atrial pressures are lower.*
From Nadas AS, Fyler DC [eds]. Nadas' Pediatric Cardiology. Philadelphia, PA: Hanley and Belfus, 1992.

Close apposition of the septum to the mitral valve accentuates the obstruction.[21] The obstruction is rarely severe and tends to resolve following the arterial switch procedure. Valvar pulmonic stenosis is rare.

Fixed anatomic pulmonary stenosis, usually subvalvar, is more common in the presence of a ventricular septal defect (Fig. 37-5). The restriction of pulmonary blood flow coupled with a large ventricular defect is likely to result in few symptoms and adequate growth. Consequently, these infants first present to the cardiologist at a somewhat older age than most of the babies with transposition of the great arteries and intact ventricular septum.

Surgical intervention on a single lesion in D-transposition may disturb the precarious balance of circulation between the systemic and pulmonary circuits. Thus the patient with transposition of the great arteries and intact ventricular septum in heart failure related to a large patent ductus arteriosus does poorly with division of the ductus. Similarly, correction of an interrupted aortic arch or coarctation of the aorta may upset the balance between the two circuits particularly if the intercircuit communications are marginal. By contrast, a straddling or overriding AV valve improves mixing. While difficult to repair surgically, these deformities promote higher saturation and therefore a more stable clinical course than those infants without such deformities.

If the ventricular septum is intact, the level of left ventricular pressure required to overcome pulmonary resistance decreases within hours of birth and is less than half of the right ventricular pressure by the end of the first week. Because the arterial switch procedure requires the left ventricle to function at systemic pressure immediately following surgery, most centers operate within the first week of life or as soon as practical. The same approach is undertaken with infants who have a small to moderate sized ventricular defect. The left ventricle of infants with a large ventricular septal defect functions at systemic pressure, making the switch procedure feasible into a prepared left ventricular chamber so that surgical intervention can be planned beyond the first week.

Pulmonary vascular disease is more frequent and occurs earlier in patients with transposition of the great arteries, whether or not a ventricular septal defect is present. Very early pulmonary vascular disease can occur in an infant born with transposition and a large ventricular defect whether or not the defect narrows or closes spontaneously; it is well recognized that infants with an intact ventricular septum from birth can develop pulmonary vascular disease as well. Infants with transposition and an associated ventricular septal defect are at higher risk for developing pulmonary vascular disease than those infants with identical sized ventricular defects without transposition. The additional feature that promotes earlier pulmonary vascular disease is elusive, but may be related to perturbations in systemic Po_2, Pco_2 and pH.[22]

Clinical Manifestations

Infants born with transposition are predominantly male (64%) and often have normal birth weights. Cyanosis in the first day of life suggests the possibility of transposition of the great arteries and, if the ventricular septum is intact, the infant may be severely cyanotic within hours of birth.[2] Cyanosis is less pronounced in infants with transposition and a large ventricular septal defect and may not be apparent at all. Tachypnea is generally present often without prominent retractions. Feeding is prolonged with the infant tiring in the midst of vigorous efforts.

Infants with small ventricular septal defects may get little additional mixing (virtually intact ventricular septum) and may follow a course comparable to that of infants with no ventricular defect. With a somewhat larger defect, recognition of cyanosis may be delayed and tachypnea can vary depending on the degree of pulmonary vascular resistance or pulmonary stenosis. With a large ventricular septal defect, cyanosis may not be present and the respiratory status may progress gradually from mild tachypnea to marked respiratory distress representing heart failure similar to that seen in infants with large ventricular septal defect without transposition. Infants with a straddling tricuspid valve are likely to follow this course. An infant with a ventricular defect and coarctation of the aorta or an interrupted aortic arch may have marked heart failure within days of birth.

Physical Examination

Usually the newborn infant is visibly cyanotic and comfortably tachypneic with a respiratory rate of 60 to 70 beats or more per minute. The cyanosis does not vary with crying or with the administration of oxygen. Systolic murmurs are not a prominent feature in the patients unless there is a pressure gradient across the left ventricular outflow tract. Most observers find that the pulmonic component of the second heart sound is difficult to discern with the posterior position of the pulmonic valve relative to the aorta. After the first 2 weeks of life, growth failure often ensues related to diminished intake and increased caloric requirements from the increased work of breathing.

With a ventricular septal defect, a murmur is present within a few days after birth and, when first examined, the infant may show signs of heart failure. Tachypnea with intercostal and subcostal retractions is frequent with feeding intolerance.

Electrocardiography

In most newborns with transposition of the great arteries, the electrocardiographic findings are within normal limits; later, there is right ventricular hypertrophy. Among infants with an overriding or straddling tricuspid valve, there is left dominance and often a leftward superior axis (Fig. 37-6).

Chest Radiography

The chest radiograph is virtually normal within a few days of birth. In those with a large ventricular defect who present with symptoms of congestion, cardiomegaly and increased pulmonary vascularity are present. A right aortic arch is found in 1% of patients with an intact ventricular septum, 3% of those with a ventricular septal defect and in 10% of patients with ventricular septal defect and pulmonary stenosis or atresia.

Echocardiography

The diagnosis is made by echocardiography particularly using subcostal imaging and a long-axis view, demonstrating that the left ventricle gives rise to a posterior great artery that then branches into a right and left pulmonary artery (Fig. 37-7*A*). The aorta is seen to arise anteriorly from the right ventricle in the short-axis or parasagittal plane with rightward orientation of the transducer (Fig. 37-7*B*). Sweeping leftward from this position demonstrates the posterior pulmonary artery related to the left ventricle. The atrial septum is best visualized from the subcostal four-chamber and sagittal views (Fig. 37-8). Atrial shunting is easily demonstrated using color flow Doppler interrogation. Atrial septal restriction is suggested by deviation of the septum primum into the right atrium as well as a pressure gradient between the atria estimated by Doppler interrogation of the region or by increased velocity of color flow Doppler.

The size, location, and number of ventricular septal defects should be addressed using subxiphoid, apical and parasternal views. The subcostal and parasternal short-axis views are excellent for visualizing peri-membranous and AV canal defects with enhancement using color flow Doppler mapping. Anterior muscular defects are best identified using parasternal short-axis views with color flow Doppler imaging. Posterior and apical muscular defects can be seen best by scanning in the apical four-chamber, short-axis subcostal and short-axis parasternal views.

The left ventricular outflow tract should be examined carefully in parasternal long and short-axis, apical long-axis and subxiphoid long-axis views to exclude obstruction (Fig. 37-9).[23] The morphology of the pulmonary valve should

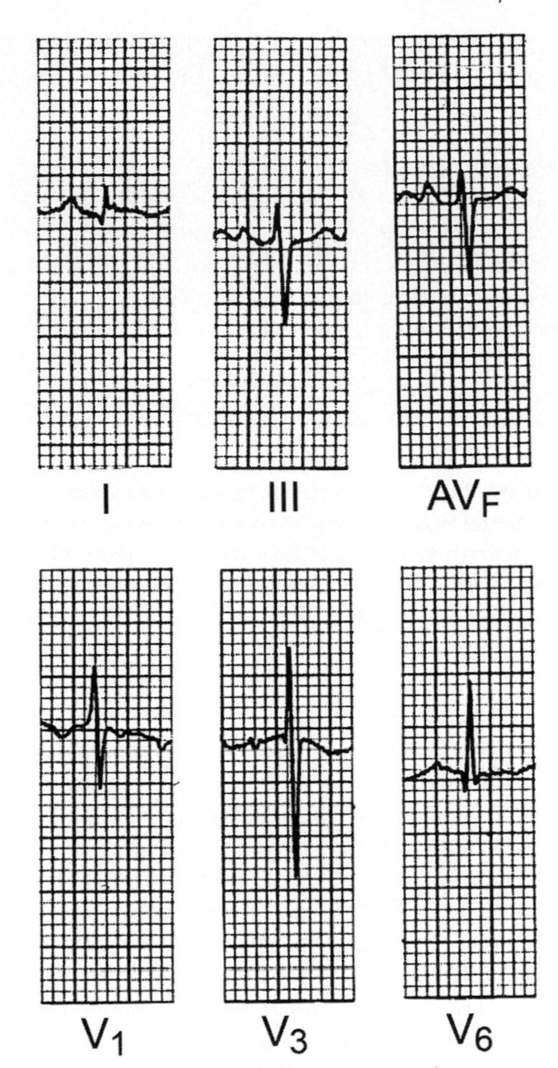

FIGURE 37–6 *Electrocardiogram of a patient with a straddling tricuspid valve. Often when there is an overriding or straddling tricuspid valve, there is hypoplasia of the right ventricle and excessive blood flow through the left ventricle compared with the right. The electrocardiogram may show a leftward-superior axis and left ventricular hypertrophy.*
From Nadas AS, Fyler DC [eds]. Nadas' Pediatric Cardiology. Philadelphia, PA: Hanley and Belfus, 1992.

be determined in a parasternal short-axis view. Causes of left ventricular outflow tract obstruction include posterior malalignment of the infundibular septum, posterior bowing of the interventricular septum (*dynamic* subpulmonary stenosis), valvar stenosis, subvalvar membrane, accessory AV valve tissue and a hypertrophied muscle of Moullaert. The gradient across the outflow tract can be estimated using continuous wave Doppler interrogation from the apical long-axis or subxiphoid short-axis views.

Occasionally in the presence of a basal ventricular septal defect, the AV valve attachments may interfere with repair

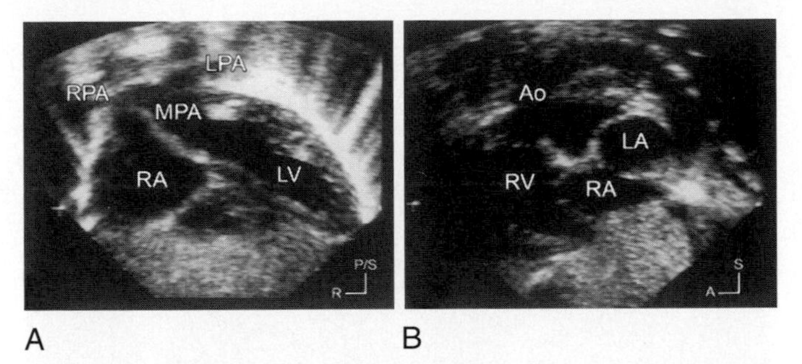

FIGURE 37–7 *D-transposition of the great arteries seen in (A) subxiphoid long-axis view showing the bifurcating pulmonary artery aligned with the left ventricle and (B) Subxiphoid short-axis view demonstrating the aorta, including the arch and brachiocephalic vessels, aligned with the right ventricle. RPA, right pulmonary artery; MPA, main pulmonary artery; RA, right atrium; LV, left ventricle; Ao, aorta.*
From Nadas AS, Fyler DC [eds]. Nadas' Pediatric Cardiology. Philadelphia, PA: Hanley and Belfus, 1992.

of the defect. Usually, abnormal attachment of the tricuspid valve to the infundibular septum can be seen in the subxiphoid short-axis views (Fig. 37-10). Abnormal mitral attachments are best visualized in the parasternal short-axis, subxiphoid short-axis and apical views.

Accurate identification of the coronary artery anatomy is critical in the setting of D-transposition of the great arteries. Multiple views are necessary to provide a composite pattern of the coronary branches.[24] Using the parasternal short-axis view, the left main coronary artery and its bifurcation can be seen with clockwise rotation of the transducer and the proximal right coronary artery is noted best with

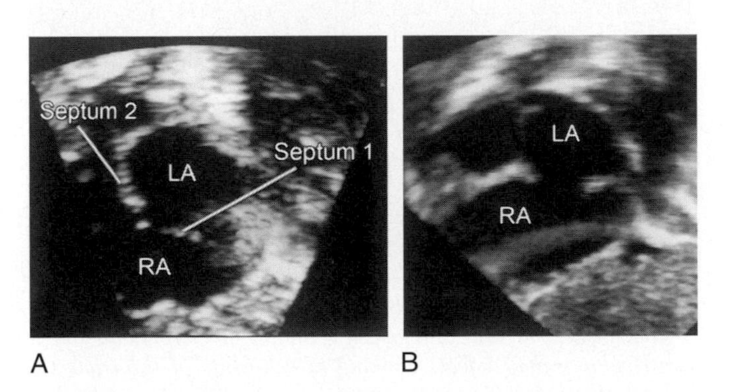

FIGURE 37–8 *Subxiphoid long-axis view of the interarterial septum in an infant with D-transposition of the great arteries. A, Before septostomy. Note the thin septum primum bulging into the right atrium. B, After septostomy. Note the remnants of septum primum around the defect. LA, left atrium; RA, right atrium*
From Nadas AS, Fyler DC [eds]. Nadas' Pediatric Cardiology. Philadelphia, PA: Hanley and Belfus, 1992.

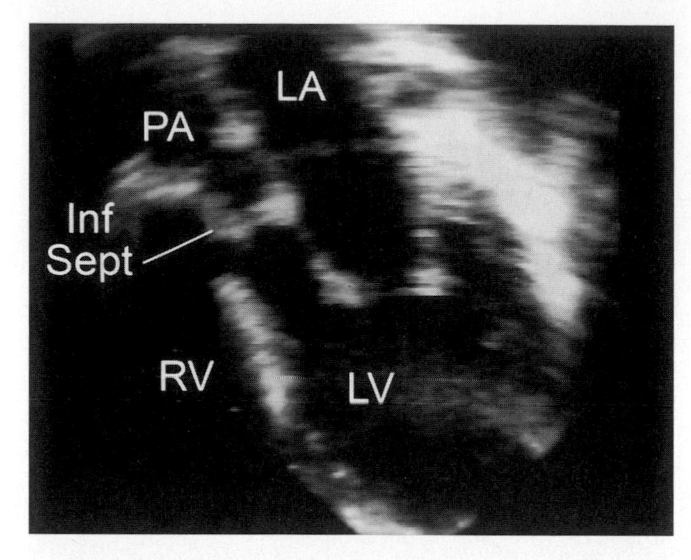

FIGURE 37–9 *Left ventricular outflow tract in a patient with D-transposition of the great arteries, a posterior malalignment ventricular septal defect, and subpulmonary stenosis due to posterior malalignment of the infundibular septum. PA, pulmonary artery; LA, left atrium; LV, left ventricle; RV, right ventricle.*
From Nadas AS, Fyler DC [eds]. Nadas' Pediatric Cardiology. Philadelphia, PA: Hanley and Belfus, 1992.

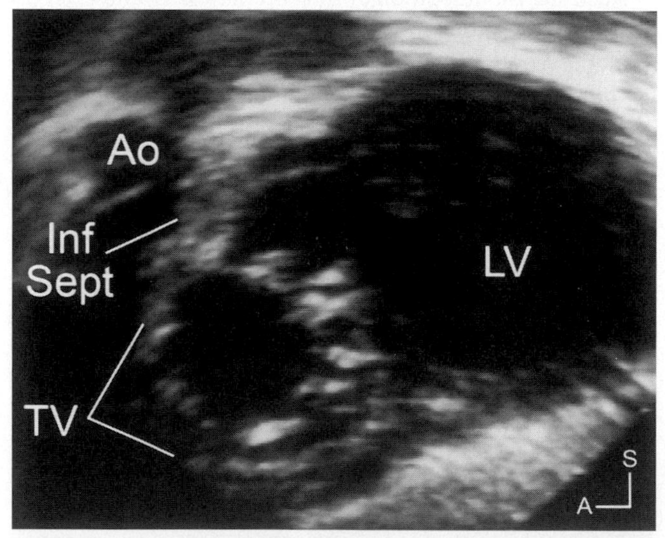

FIGURE 37–10 *Subxiphoid short-axis view in a patient with D-transposition of the great arteries and an anterior malalignment ventricular septal defect, showing attachments of the tricuspid valve to the infundibular septum. Ao, aorta; TV, tricuspid valve; LV, left ventricle.*
From Nadas AS, Fyler DC [eds]. Nadas' Pediatric Cardiology. Philadelphia, PA: Hanley and Belfus, 1992.

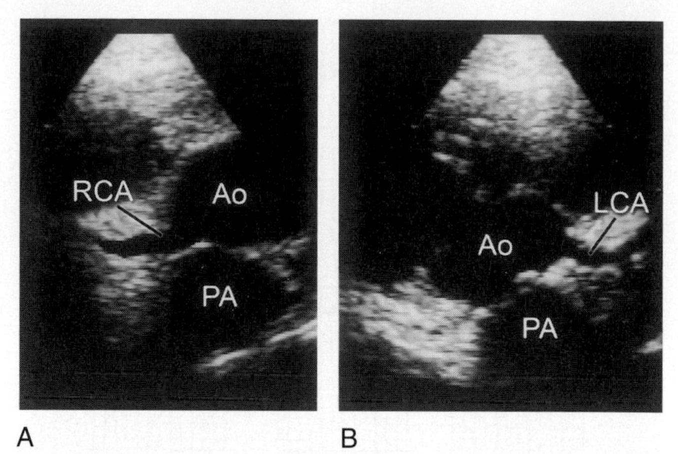

FIGURE 37–11 *Parasternal short-axis views showing the origin on the left and right coronary arteries from the aorta in a patient with D-transposition of the great arteries. Ao, aorta; RCA, right coronary artery; LCA, left coronary artery; PA, pulmonary artery. From Nadas AS, Fyler DC [eds]. Nadas' Pediatric Cardiology. Philadelphia, PA: Hanley and Belfus, 1992.*

counterclockwise rotation (Fig. 37-11). The bifurcation of the left main coronary artery can also be seen well using a parasternal long-axis view with angling toward the left shoulder. Often an apical or subxiphoid four chamber view is useful for demonstrating a coronary artery passing posterior to the pulmonary root in cases of single right coronary artery or origin of the left circumflex coronary artery from the right coronary artery.[25] Intramural coronary arteries, those with proximal segments within the wall of the aorta so that medial layers of the coronary and aorta are not separated by an adventitial layer, are surgically challenging.[10] Careful echocardiographic analysis can detect the presence of intramural coronary arteries with acceptable precision.[26] The variations of coronary anatomy in patients with D-transposition of the great vessels are discussed further in Chapter 57.

Cardiac Catheterization

Little information is needed beyond that furnished by echocardiography. The purpose of cardiac catheterization is to perform balloon atrial septostomy and to confirm the coronary anatomy before an arterial switch procedure. In most cases, the coronary course is well defined by echo (see previous section), obviating the need for coronary angiography but when necessary is best visualized using the *laid back* view (Fig. 37-12).

Balloon Atrial Septostomy, introduced by Rashkind and Miller, remains the standard method of creating an atrial septal defect in the newborn.[27] Although intracardiac complications occurred occasionally in the early years of its implementation, these diminished greatly with the use of biplane fluoroscopy: septostomy may also be performed under echocardiographic guidance.[28,29] The duration of septal

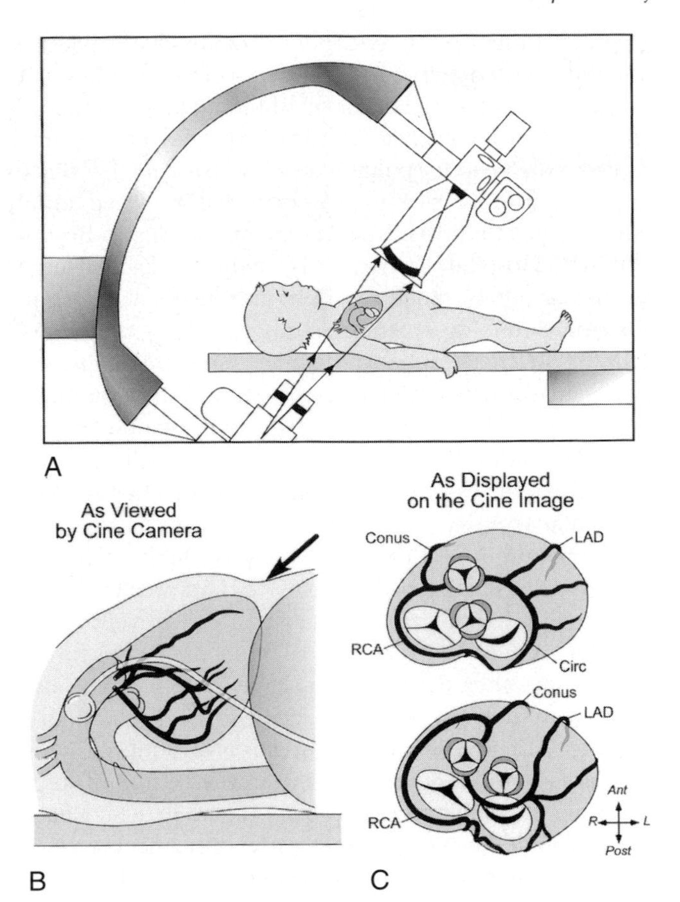

FIGURE 37–12 *The laid-back view to assess the coronary anatomy in transposition of the great arteries. A, Shows the anteroposterior position of the C-arm with maximal caudal angulation. B, A lateral diagram to show the camera's view of the heart and, particularly, the great vessels and the coronary anatomy. C, Shows the cine image of anteroposterior great vessels (upper diagram) and side-by-side vessels (lower diagram).*
From Mandell VS, Lock JE, Mayer JE. Am J Cardiol 65:1379, 1990, with permission.

patency is temporary in some infants, and balloon septostomy is ineffective in most infants older than 2 months. In these circumstances, transseptal needle puncture with balloon dilation, and occasionally stent placement are widely employed to achieve adequate atrial communications. Nonetheless, balloon septostomy remains the procedure of choice in the newborn baby with D-transposition with or without a ventricular septal defect.

Our approach to septostomy at Children's Hospital is to introduce a catheter through a diaphragm via a 7-French sheath, using an umbilical or percutaneous femoral venous entry site. Usually, the balloon is inflated with up to 3 mL of dilute contrast material in the left atrium, provided the cavity is large enough to accommodate this inflated size. Then the balloon is jerked rapidly across the septum and repeated at least once. The size of the defect is then estimated and hemodynamic parameters are measured again.

MANAGEMENT

In the case of known fetal diagnosis of D-transposition of the great arteries, optimal management includes delivery at a center where pediatric cardiologists are present to facilitate care of the infant. At the least, a neonatologist should be present at the delivery so that an early clinical assessment is possible. In the case of the infant without a ventricular septal defect, prostaglandin E_1[18,19] is administered in a starting dose of 0.05 μg/mL per minute. Prostaglandin can induce apnea so the need for intubation should be anticipated. Hypotension from vasodilation is managed with intravascular volume expansion. The infant should be transferred to the neonatal intensive care unit or, when available, a pediatric cardiovascular intensive care unit. Many infants without prior *in utero* diagnosis of D-transposition of the great arteries are born in centers not equipped to provide complete cardiac intervention. These infants present with marked cyanosis and frequently with metabolic acidosis; they require prompt stabilization with prostaglandin infusion and transfer to a cardiac center.

Emergent echocardiography is performed to confirm anatomic impressions from previous fetal ultrasounds. An arterial blood gas is obtained to determine the pH, $P{CO_2}$ and $P{O_2}$. Previously, balloon atrial septostomy was performed routinely in all neonates with transposition of the great arteries; however, with the introduction of the arterial switch procedure and the trend toward performing surgical correction early in infancy, balloon intervention is applied more selectively. In the case of an intact ventricular septum, a balloon atrial septostomy is performed to improve intracardiac mixing and to reduce left atrial pressure. In some institutions, however, balloon atrial septostomy is deferred if surgical repair is imminent, unless the atrial septum is restrictive. When a sizable ventricular septal defect is present, balloon septostomy is less urgent and may be avoided if early surgical repair is planned before the ventricular communication becomes more restrictive. In these cases, infants often require anti-congestive therapy.

Surgery

Creation of an atrial septal defect, by the Blalock-Hanlon technique, provides improved mixing of the pulmonary and systemic circuits and predated the introduction of balloon atrial septostomy. It has been virtually abandoned in the neonate anticipating arterial switch surgery.

Pulmonary artery banding was commonly used in infants with transposition of the great arteries with a large ventricular septal defect. It is now rarely needed because the ventricular septal defects are repaired at the time of the arterial switch procedure unless sizable muscular ventricular defects are present that can be difficult for surgical closure.

Atrial switch procedures represented an important improvement in the management of the infant with transposition culminating in a physiologic repair of the underlying pathophysiology (Exhibit 37-1). In the Mustard procedure (Fig. 37-13),[30] the pulmonary venous blood is baffled to the tricuspid valve and the systemic venous blood to the mitral valve and pulmonary circuit using prosthetic material or pericardium. The Senning procedure became popularized somewhat after the Mustard procedure though its original description predated the Mustard.[31] The Senning procedure accomplishes similar atrial baffling using primarily nonprosthetic material. There is little difference between the results of the two approaches,[32] the mortality for each being less than 5%.[33,34] Timing of surgery is variable depending on the institution but may be delayed for several months if necessary. Both are now rarely used.

The **arterial switch procedure** was performed originally by Jatene[35] and requires transection and reanastomosis of the great arteries to the opposite roots as well as transposing the coronary arteries to the neo-aortic root (Fig. 37-13). Lecompte's modification of this technique is now widely utilized.[36] Initially, the procedure was available for older infants who survived with a ventricular septal defect and systemic pressure in the left ventricle.[37–40] Later, pulmonary artery banding was used to *prepare* the left ventricle for

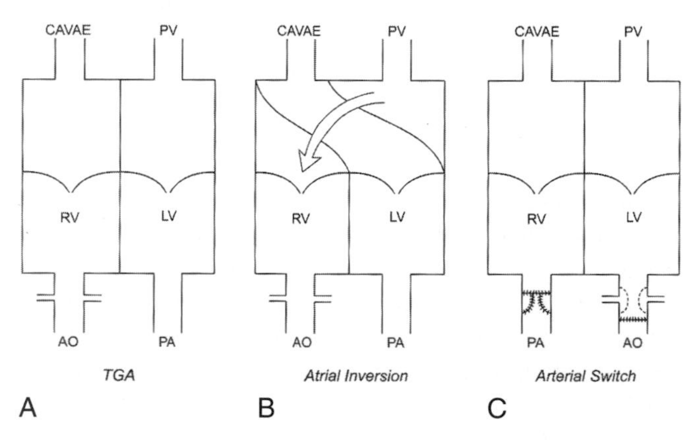

FIGURE 37–13 *Diagrammatic comparison of (A) unrepaired patient with transposition (B) atrial inversion surgery in transposition of the great arteries, and (C) arterial switch surgery. Note that atrial inversion requires long atrial suture lines and results in the right ventricle being the systemic pump. Note the necessity to move the coronary arteries with arterial switching surgery; the left ventricle becomes the systemic pump.*
From Nadas AS, Fyler DC [eds]. Nadas' Pediatric Cardiology. Philadelphia, PA: Hanley and Belfus, 1992.

systemic function at systemic pressure.[41–44] Arterial switching in the newborn can be accomplished in the first 2 weeks of life, taking advantage of the naturally *prepared* left ventricle in the neonate with an intact ventricular septum, obviating the need for pulmonary artery banding.[45–47] Since 1988, the arterial switch procedure has replaced atrial baffle surgery in virtually all patients presenting to Boston Children's Hospital (Exhibit 37-1). In the presence of large ventricular defects, the procedure may be delayed longer. The results for either anatomic subset are very satisfactory (Exhibit 37-2). Potential difficulties using this approach include inadequate coronary perfusion related to anatomic obstruction to flow,[47] stenosis at the anastomotic sites of the great arteries,[48] and aortic regurgitation or left ventricular failure in the case of late repair of the defect with intact ventricular septum.

Ventricular septal defects are closed on the right side of the septum. In atrial baffle repairs, the approach to closure must be through the tricuspid valve since right ventriculotomy can seriously impair ventricular function in this future systemic chamber. Similarly, damage to the tricuspid valve must be avoided because tricuspid regurgitation is poorly tolerated. Tricuspid valve competence is less critical in the arterial switch procedure. Surgery in the setting of large ventricular septal defects, though not urgent in the neonatal period, should be performed as early as practical to avoid the potential complication of pulmonary vascular obstructive disease.[8]

Relief of left ventricular outflow tract obstruction remains a challenge in a modest segment of those infants with transposition of the great arteries. Dynamic obstruction is the most common form of outflow obstruction. It is caused by leftward deviation of the ventricular septum in the setting of higher pressure in the right ventricular chamber relative to the left in those with intact ventricular septum. With arterial switch procedures, the pressure differential is reversed and the obstruction resolves. After atrial baffle procedures, the obstruction may persist but is generally insignificant and rarely requires additional surgery.[6] In those infants with fixed obstruction, the approach is dependent upon the anatomic cause. With discrete fibromuscular obstruction, resection may be possible in some using a transpulmonary approach. In other cases, the obstruction may not be amenable to surgical relief thereby necessitating a Rastelli procedure.

The Rastelli procedure involves closing the ventricular septal defect so that the left ventricular outflow passes through the ventricular defect into the aorta.[49–50] A conduit is placed from the right ventricle to the main pulmonary artery. This approach requires a sizable ventricular septal defect, appropriately located so that a patch can be placed that will redirect the left ventricular flow into the aorta. A restrictive ventricular defect requires enlargement to make the Rastelli procedure feasible.

Exhibit 37–2
Boston Children's Hospital Experience
D-Transposition Surgery
1988-2002

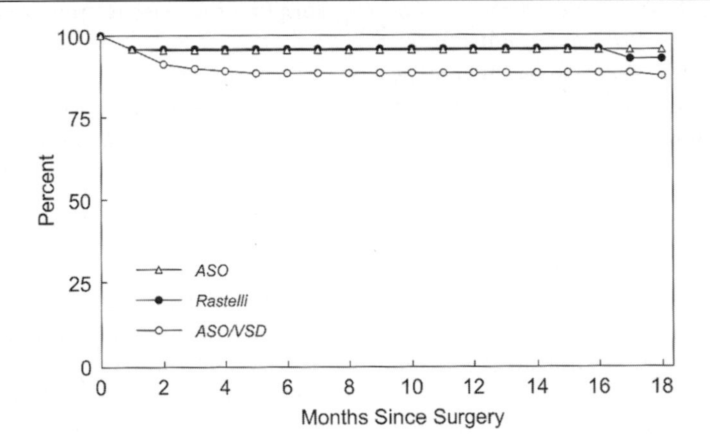

Life Table analysis comparing survival to 18 months following arterial switch alone (469 pts), arterial switch and ventricular septal defect closure (264 pts) and Rastelli procedure (53 pts), all operations done at Boston Childrens Hospital. Survival at 18 months was 96%, 87%, and 92% respectively.

Conversion from an atrial switch to an arterial switch has been used to make the left ventricle the systemic chamber most often in cases of patients with a failing Mustard or Senning procedure.[51–52] The initial step requires banding the main pulmonary artery to prepare the left ventricle for systemic afterload. After a short time, usually several weeks, the patient undergoes an arterial switch procedure with coronary reimplantation and takedown of the atrial baffle.

A staged physiologic repair (Fontan procedure) is the preferred operative approach in the setting of anatomy that is not favorable for standard operative correction. These variants include multiple hemodynamically significant ventricular septal defects, right ventricular hypoplasia or AV valve abnormalities (straddling tricuspid valve).

Palliative atrial (Mustard or Senning) baffle procedures were used in patients with inoperable levels of pulmonary vascular obstructive disease, transposition of the great arteries and a large ventricular septal defect or patent ductus arteriosus.[53–55] Both procedures baffle pulmonary venous, fully saturated blood to the ascending aorta via the right ventricle, thus increasing systemic arterial Po_2. In those with a ventricular defect the increase was evenly distributed throughout all extremities. In those with a patent ductus, preoperatively cyanosis was often more obvious in the upper than in the lower limbs as the ductus perfused the descending aorta with pulmonary arterial fully saturated blood. Postoperatively, the more obvious improvement was in the upper extremities.

COURSE FOLLOWING ATRIAL SWITCH REPAIR

The natural history of D-transposition is marked by limited survival without surgery. Those with an intact ventricular septum do not survive beyond the first year of life with most succumbing early in infancy.[56] Patients with a large ventricular septal defect or patent ductus arteriosus may survive if not operated upon, but pulmonary vascular obstructive disease almost always ensues. In rare cases of balanced physiology, patients with D-transposition of the great arteries, large ventricular septal defect and pulmonic stenosis have survived for a number of years. Even more unusual is late survival of patients with D-transposition and intact ventricular septum with a large atrial septal defect. For the population of those who have undergone physiologic correction with Mustard or Senning procedures, a sizable number have experienced reasonable longevity[57–59] with greater mortality in those with large ventricular septal defects versus those with intact ventricular septum.[57,58] Despite the survival of large numbers of those who have had atrial baffle surgery, a number of late morbidities have been identified.

Rhythm Abnormalities

Supraventricular rhythm disturbances are very commonly encountered in patients following atrial baffle surgery.[60–65] Sinus node dysfunction, manifested by brady-tachyarrhythmias and in some cases overt syncope, is thought to result from injury related to extensive atrial incisions with damage to the sinus node artery.[63–66] Many have required pacemaker implantation to minimize recurrent symptomatic episodes since antiarrhythmic therapy alone may aggravate bradycardia. In addition, atrial arrhythmias are thought to relate to long-standing atrial enlargement in the setting of right ventricular failure or tricuspid regurgitation. Sudden death presumably related to rhythm disorder is a well-recognized phenomenon occurring in up to 1% of patients per year.[57]

Baffle Obstruction and Leak

Obstruction at the right atrial–superior vena caval junction is a well-known sequela associated with the Mustard procedure. The clinical presentation may include chylothorax, edema of the upper extremities or hydrocephalus, although azygous vein decompression may mask the presence of severe obstruction. Catheter intervention or surgical revision of the baffle may be necessary. Inferior vena caval obstruction is uncommon. Pulmonary venous obstruction is noted more frequently following Senning repair. Early manifestations may be pulmonary venous congestion on chest radiograph in the early postoperative period, whereas late survivors with slowly progressive obstruction may have symptoms of reactive airway disease unresponsive to bronchodilator therapy. Baffle leaks are not common but when present are generally noted at the superior aspect of the right atrium. If the predominant shunt is right to left, the patient may show cyanosis, though most often the degree of leak is too small to be clinically apparent. Left-to-right shunts are generally not hemodynamically significant.

Tricuspid Regurgitation

Tricuspid regurgitation is commonly found following surgical repairs that include closure of a membranous ventricular septal defect by a transatrial approach. Although generally of minimal significance in the case of an arterial switch procedure, tricuspid regurgitation is more critical after atrial baffle procedures where the tricuspid valve is the systemic atrioventricular valve. Outcome in this setting is thought to be dependent upon the preservation of tricuspid valve function.[8]

Right Ventricular Function

Failure of the right (systemic) ventricle is widely reported following the Senning or the Mustard procedure,[67–73] although most patients are not symptomatic.[57–74] On the other hand, echocardiographic[74] and stress[75] testing criteria show abnormal ventricular response to stress as well as decreased exercise tolerance that is both chronotropic and inotropic in origin. Cardiac transplantation has been necessary in a small number of patients with severe decompensation of ventricular function.

Central Nervous System Injury

Manifestations of central nervous system injury are not frequent. Causes for such abnormalities have been the subject of extensive study and are addressed in Chapter 9.

COURSE FOLLOWING ARTERIAL SWITCH PROCEDURE

Coronary Insufficiency

Obstruction to coronary arterial flow is most commonly due to kinking of the coronary arteries and often becomes apparent during the perioperative period. Infants with obstruction can show electrocardiographic changes of ischemia or profound low output from myocardial dysfunction.[76] When suspected intraoperatively, inspection and reconfiguration of the proximal coronary segments is mandatory. In some cases, however, infants with important obstruction can show no ill effects and occlusion of a coronary artery may be identified at later catheterization in completely asymptomatic individuals.[77] In such patients arterial collateralization is usually evident.

Supravalvar Obstruction

The presence of supravalvar pulmonary stenosis following the arterial switch procedure was soon noted after this surgical approach was introduced.[47,78] The most frequent types of obstruction are discrete narrowing at the suture line of the anastomosis and long segment obstruction in the pulmonary arteries, especially the right, as they are draped across and anterior to the ascending aorta with the frequency of stenosis above 20 mm Hg noted to be as high as 25%.[79] Balloon dilation angioplasty has met with reasonable success in relieving the gradients with discrete stenosis.[80] For long segment narrowing, balloon dilation is generally inadequate necessitating stent placement or surgical re-intervention. Supravalvar aortic obstruction is far less frequent than supravalvar pulmonary involvement.[81]

Rhythm Abnormalities

In contrast to the atrial switch procedure, rhythm disturbances following the arterial switch procedure have been far less prevalent.[47,79,82] In a review of 390 patients who underwent arterial switch,[82] AV conduction was rarely impaired with 1.7% developing complete AV block all following ventricular septal defect closure and the incidence of late supraventricular tachycardia was 5%. Though ventricular ectopic activity was noted commonly in the postoperative period, late ventricular tachycardia was documented in fewer than 1%.

Left Ventricular Function

Preservation of left ventricular function after the arterial switch procedure is well documented.[47,83,84] Following single-stage arterial switch surgery, including ventricular septal defect closure in some, more than 3 years later by echocardiographic and catheterization assessment quantitative analysis of ventricular function, cardiac index, left ventricular filling pressures, wall dimensions and thickness, systolic function, loading conditions, and contractility were normal.[84] Those undergoing two-stage repair with pulmonary artery banding, showed some mild derangement in function and contractility. Exercise testing in this group of patients shows excellent preservation of cardiopulmonary function.[85]

Neoaortic Regurgitation

By reversing the great arteries in the arterial switch procedure, the native pulmonic valve serves as the neoaortic valve. It is not known how long or how well this valve will be able to function normally in its critical role in the setting of systemic pressure. Reports have shown that the neoaortic annulus and root are larger compared with those of controls several years following surgery[86] and that the size of the aortic root increases over the first several years postoperatively.[87] In addition, mild aortic regurgitation following surgery is present frequently, but progression to a moderate or severe degree is unlikely, and is seen more commonly in patients undergoing arterial switch surgery beyond 1 year of age.[87,88]

VARIATIONS

Transposition of the Great Arteries with Intact Ventricular Septum and Pulmonary Stenosis

Left ventricular outflow tract obstruction with D-transposition of the great arteries and intact ventricular septum occurs in approximately 10% to 30% of patients.[89] The obstruction in most cases is dynamic related to leftward displacement of the ventricular septum, a finding that resolves after the arterial switch procedure.[20] The remainder of cases results from fibrous tissue in the ventricular septum sometimes in association with abnormal mitral valve attachments or rarely valvar pulmonic obstruction. Though early results for surgical intervention were variable, more recent data following the arterial switch procedure indicates a uniformly good outcome for this group.[90]

Transposition and Coarctation of the Aorta

The combination of coarctation of the aorta or interruption of the aortic arch in combination with transposition of the aorta is rare and generally occurs in the setting of a ventricular septal defect.[91] Though survival was uncommon previously, results have improved using a single- or two-stage repair enhanced by intraoperative management and postoperative intensive care.

Transposition of the Great Arteries with Ventricular Defect and Pulmonary Stenosis

Transposition with ventricular defect and pulmonary stenosis is present in approximately 10% of cases. The number, size and location of ventricular defects vary as does left ventricular outflow tract obstruction ranging from mild subvalvar involvement to pulmonary atresia (Fig. 37-14). The clinical presentation is related to the degree of obstruction and size of the ventricular defect. Large ventricular defects with lesser degrees of obstruction present with a murmur or heart failure while those patients with smaller defects or increasing degrees of obstruction will show prominent cyanosis early in the neonatal period.

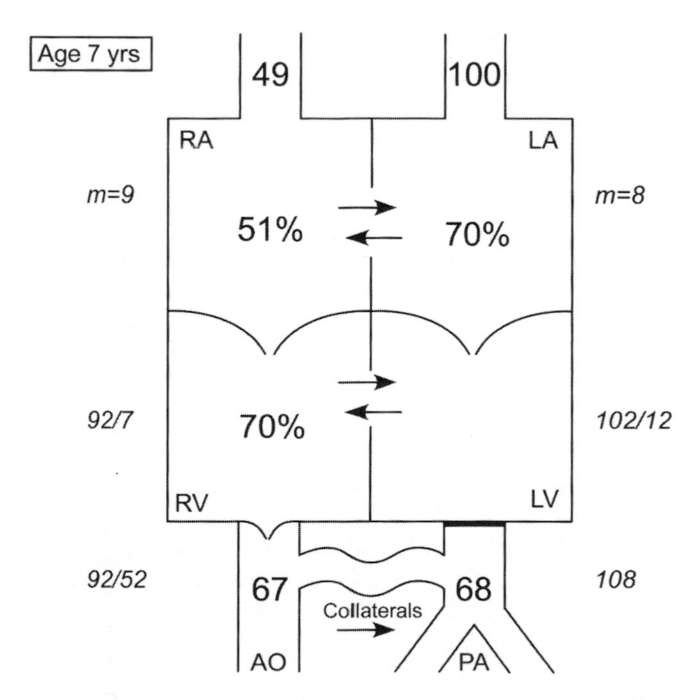

FIGURE 37–14 *A hemodynamic diagram of a patient with transposition of the great arteries, ventricular defect and pulmonary atresia. Note that the only blood supply to the lungs is via major collaterals arising from the descending aorta. Compare with a similar situation encountered in patients with tetralogy of Fallot and pulmonary atresia (see Chapter 32).*
From Nadas AS, Fyler DC [eds]. Nadas' Pediatric Cardiology. Philadelphia, PA: Hanley and Belfus, 1992.

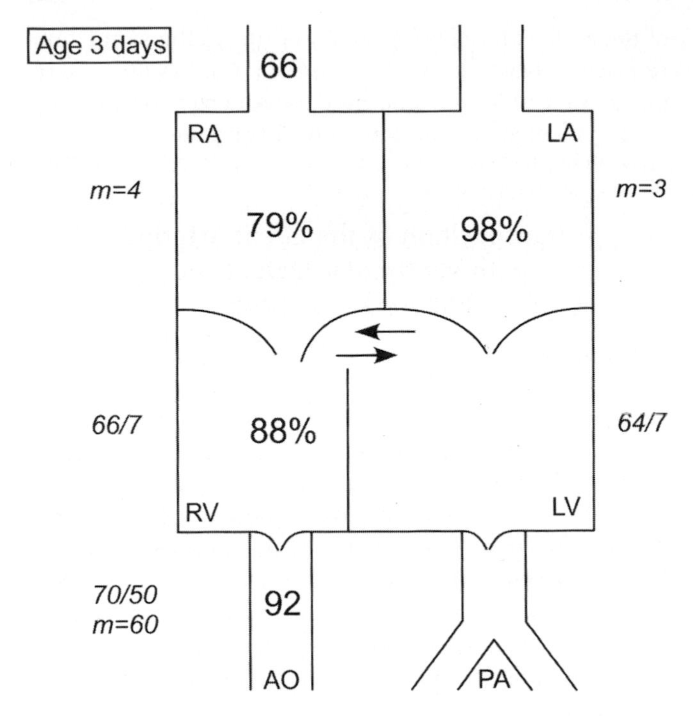

FIGURE 37–15 *Hemodynamic diagram of a patient with transposition of the great arteries, ventricular septal defect, and straddling tricuspid valve. The direct communication of the right atrium to the pulmonary ventricle (anatomic left ventricle) improves mixing of the pulmonary and systemic circulations. The arterial saturation is better than that in the usual patient with transposition of the great arteries despite an added major and surgically uncorrectable problem.*
From Nadas AS, Fyler DC [eds]. Nadas' Pediatric Cardiology. Philadelphia, PA: Hanley and Belfus, 1992.

The surgical approach to this combination of lesions is not straightforward. In cases of severe cyanosis related to marked left ventricular outflow tract obstruction, many centers favor placement of an aortopulmonary shunt in the neonate. This palliative procedure is followed at a later date by a repair that achieves physiologic correction, most often a Rastelli procedure (Exhibit 37-2).[49] If the anatomic size and location of the ventricular defect is acceptable, surgery involves closure of the defect to incorporate continuity between the left ventricle and the aorta in conjunction with placement of a right ventricular to pulmonary artery homograft. Alternatively, the Rastelli procedure can be performed in the neonatal period with anticipated conduit revision at a later time. The Lecompte maneuver utilizes resection of the outlet septum by right ventriculotomy in order to facilitate left ventricular to aortic continuity. This approach requires transection of the pulmonary artery, closure of the native pulmonic valve, and anastomosis of the main pulmonary artery to the right ventricle in order to complete an anatomic and physiologic repair. Alternatively, an arterial switch procedure can be used if left ventricular outflow tract obstruction can be satisfactorily ameliorated.

Overriding Tricuspid Valve and Small Right Ventricle

When the tricuspid valve overrides the ventricular septum in transposition of the great arteries, the right ventricle may be small and arch hypoplasia may co-exist (Fig. 37-15). In the case of a mildly hypoplastic right ventricle, an arterial switch procedure may be sufficient if the right ventricle can provide adequate output. If the right ventricle is diminutive, an arterial switch can be performed and pulmonary flow provided by an aortopulmonary shunt. This initial approach is followed by a bidirectional Glenn shunt within a year, followed eventually by a Fontan procedure. In some cases the aortic arch may be so small as to require augmentation.

REFERENCES

1. Botto LD, Correa A, Erickson DJ. Racial and temporal variations in the prevalence of heart defects. Pediatrics 107:e32, 2001.
2. Fyler DC, Buckley LP, Hellenbrand WE, et al. Report of the New England Regional Infant Cardiac Program. Pediatrics 65(Suppl):376, 1980.
3. Rothman KJ, Fyler DC. Association of congenital heart defects with season and population density. Teratology 13:29, 1976.
4. Rothman KJ, Fyler DC. Sex, birth order and maternal age characteristics of infants with congenital heart defects. Am J Epidemiol 104:527, 1976.
5. Muster AJ, Paul MH, Van Grondelle A, et al. Asymmetric distribution of the pulmonary blood flow between the right and left lungs in d-transposition of the great arteries. Am J Cardiol 38:352, 1976.
6. Idriss FS, DeLeon SY, Nikaidoh H, et al. Resection of left ventricular outflow obstruction in d-transposition of the great arteries. J Thorac Cardiovasc Surg 74:343, 1977.
7. Moene R, Oppenheimer-Dekker A, Weinik A, et al. Morphology of ventricular septal defect in complete transposition of the great arteries. Am J Cardiol 51:1701, 1983.
8. Penskoske P, Westerman G, Marx G, et al. Transposition of the great arteries and ventricular septal defect: results with the Senning operation and closure of the ventricular septal defect in infants. Ann Thorac Surg 36:281, 1983.
9. Moene R, Oppenheimer-Dekker A, Bartelings MM. Anatomic obstruction of the right ventricular outflow tract in transposition of the great arteries. Am J Cardiol 51:1701-1704, 1983.
10. Gittenberger-de Groot AC, Sauer U, Quaegebeur J. Aortic intramural coronary artery in three hearts with transposition of the great arteries. J Thorac Cardiovasc Surg 91:566, 1986.
11. Mayer JE, Jr., Sanders SP, Jonas RA, et al. Coronary artery pattern and outcome of arterial switch operation for transposition of the great arteries. Circulation 82:Suppl IV139, 1990.

12. Smith A, Arnold R, Wilkinson J, et al. An anatomical study of the patterns of coronary arteries and sinus nodal artery in complete transposition. Int J Cardiol 12:295, 1986.
13. Wernovsky G, Sanders SP. Coronary artery anatomy and transposition of the great arteries. Coron Artery Dis 4:148, 1993.
14. Gittenberger-de Groot AC, Sauer U, Oppenheimer-Dekker A, et al. Coronary arterial anatomy in transpostion of the great arteries. Pediatr Cardiol 4(Suppl 1):15, 1983.
15. Deal BJ, Chin AJ, Sanders SP, et al. Subxiphoid two-dimensional echocardiographic identification of tricuspid valve abnormalities in transposition of the great arteries with ventricular septal defect. Am J Cardiol 55:1146, 1985.
16. Huhta JC, Edwards WD, Danielson GK, et al. Abnormalities of the tricuspid valve in complete transposition of the great arteries with ventricular septal defect. J Thorac Cardiovasc Surg 83:569, 1982.
17. Moene RJ, Oppenheimer-Dekker A. Congenital mitral valve anomalies in transposition of the great arteries. Am J Cardiol 49:1972, 1982.
18. Freed MD, Heymann MA, Lewis AB, et al. Prostaglandin E1 infants with ductus arteriosus-dependent congenital heart disease. Circulation 64:899, 1981.
19. Lang P, Freed MD, Bierman FZ, et al. Use of prostaglandin E1 in infants with d-transposition of the great arteries and intact ventricular septum. Am J Cardiol 44:76, 1979.
20. Chiu IS, Anderson RH, Macartney FJ, et al. Morphologic features of an intact ventricular septum susceptible to subpulmonary obstruction in complete transposition. Am J Cardiol 53:1633, 1984.
21. Silove ED, Taylor JF. Angiographic and anatomical features of subvalvar left ventricular outflow obstruction in transposition of the great arteries. The possible role of the anterior mitral valve leaflet. Pediatr Radiol 1:87, 1973.
22. Paul MH. Complete transposition of the great arteries. In Adams FH, Emmanouilides GC, Riemenschneider TA (eds). Moss' Heart Disease in Infants, Children, and Adolescents. Baltimore: Williams and Wilkins, 1968, pp 371–423.
23. Chin AJ, Yeager SB, Sanders SP, et al. Accuracy of prospective two-dimensional echocardiographic evaluation of left ventricular outflow tract in complete transposition of the great arteries. Am J Cardiol 55:759, 1985.
24. Pasquini L, Sanders SP, Parness IA, et al. Diagnosis of coronary artery anatomy by two-dimensional echocardiography in patients with transposition of the great arteries. Circulation 75:557, 1987.
25. Pasquini L, Sanders SP, Parness IA, et al. Coronary echocardiography in 406 patients with d-loop transposition of the great arteries. J Am Coll Cardiol 24:763, 1994.
26. Pasquini L, Parness IA, Colan SD, et al. Diagnosis of intramural coronary artery in transposition of the great arteries using two-dimensional echocardiography. Circulation 88:1136, 1993.
27. Rashkind WJ, Miller WW. Creation of an atrial septal defect without thoracotomy. A palliative approach to complete transposition of the great arteries. JAMA 196:991, 1966.
28. Beitzke A, Stein JI, Suppan C. Balloon atrial septostomy under two-dimensional echocardiographic control. Int J Cardiol 30:33, 1991.
29. Baker EJ, Allan LD, Tynan MJ, et al. Balloon atrial septostomy in the neonatal intensive care unit. Br Heart J 51:377, 1984.
30. Mustard WT. Successful two-stage correction of transposition of the great vessels. Surgery 55:469, 1964.
31. Senning A. Surgical correction of transposition of the great vessels. Surgery 45:966, 1959.
32. Marx GR, Hougen TJ, Norwood WI, et al. Transposition of the great arteries with intact ventricular septum: results of Mustard and Senning operations in 123 consecutive patients. J Am Coll Cardiol 1:476, 1983.
33. deLeon VH, Hougen TJ, Norwood WI, et al. Results of the Senning operation for transposition of the great arteries with intact ventricular septum in neonates. Circulation 70:I21, 1984.
34. Turley K, Hanley FL, Verrier ED, et al. The Mustard procedure in infants (less than 100 days of age). Ten-year follow-up. J Thorac Cardiovasc Surg 96:849, 1988.
35. Jatene AD, Fontes VF, Paulista PP, et al. Anatomic correction of transposition of the great vessels. J Thorac Cardiovasc Surg 72:364, 1976.
36. Lecompte Y, Zannini L, Hazan E, et al. Anatomic correction of transposition of the great arteries. J Thorac Cardiovasc Surg 82:629, 1981.
37. Arensman FW, Sievers HH, Lange P, et al. Assessment of coronary and aortic anastomoses after anatomic correction of transposition of the great arteries. J Thorac Cardiovasc Surg 90:597, 1985.
38. Bical O, Hazan E, Lecompte Y, et al. Anatomic correction of transposition of the great arteries associated with ventricular septal defect: midterm results in 50 patients. Circulation 70:891, 1984.
39. Jatene AD, Fontes VF, Souza LC, et al. Anatomic correction of transposition of the great arteries. J Thorac Cardiovasc Surg 83:20, 1982.
40. Yacoub MH. The case for anatomic correction of transposition of the great arteries. J Thorac Cardiovasc Surg 78:3, 1979.
41. Boutin C, Jonas RA, Sanders SP, et al. Rapid two-stage arterial switch operation. Acquisition of left ventricular mass after pulmonary artery banding in infants with transposition of the great arteries. Circulation 90:1304, 1994.
42. Ilbawi MN, Idriss FS, DeLeon SY, et al. Preparation of the left ventricle for anatomical correction in patients with simple transposition of the great arteries. Surgical guidelines. J Thorac Cardiovasc Surg 94:87, 1987.
43. Sievers HH, Lange PE, Arensman FW, et al. Influence of two-stage anatomic correction on size and distensibility of the anatomic pulmonary/functional aortic root in patients with simple transposition of the great arteries. Circulation 70:202, 1984.
44. Yacoub M, Bernhard A, Lange P, et al. Clinical and hemodynamic results of the two-stage anatomic correction of simple transposition of the great arteries. Circulation 62:I190, 1980.
45. Castaneda AR, Norwood WI, Jonas RA. Transposition of the great arteries and intact ventricular septum: anatomical repair in the neonate. Ann Thorac Surg 5:438, 1984.
46. Mavroudis C. Anatomical repair of transposition of the great arteries with intact ventricular septum in the neonate: guidelines to avoid complications. Ann Thorac Surg 43:495, 1987.

47. Wernovsky G, Hougen TJ, Walsh EP, et al. Midterm results after the arterial switch operation for transposition of the great arteries with intact ventricular septum: clinical, hemodynamic, echocardiographic, and electrophysiologic data. Circulation 77:1333, 1988.
48. Yacoub MH, Bernhard A, Radley-Smith R, et al. Supravalvular pulmonary stenosis after anatomic correction of transposition of the great arteries: causes and prevention. Circulation 66:I193, 1982.
49. Rastelli GC, Wallace RB, Ongley PA. Complete repair of transposition of the great arteries with pulmonary stenosis. A review and report of a case corrected by using a new surgical technique. Circulation 39:83, 1969.
50. Villagra F, Quero-Jimenez M, Maitre-Azcarate MJ, et al. Transposition of the great arteries with ventricular septal defects. Surgical considerations concerning the Rastelli operation. J Thorac Cardiovasc Surg 88:1004, 1984.
51. Cochrane AD, Karl TR, Mee RB. Staged conversion to arterial switch for late failure of the systemic right ventricle. Ann Thorac Surg 56:854, 1993.
52. Mee RB. Severe right ventricular failure after Mustard or Senning operation. Two-stage repair: pulmonary artery banding and switch. J Thorac Cardiovasc Surg 92:385, 1986.
53. Dhasmana JP, Stark J, de Leval M, et al. Long-term results of the "palliative" Mustard operation. J Am Coll Cardiol 6:1138, 1985.
54. Lindesmith GG, Stanton RE, Lurie PR, et al. An assessment of Mustard's operation as a palliative procedure for transposition of the great vessels. Ann Thorac Surg 19:514, 1975.
55. Burkhart HM, Dearani JA, Williams WG, et al. Late results of palliative atrial switch for transposition, ventricular septal defect and pulmonary vascular obstructive disease. Ann Thorac Surg 77:464, 2004.
56. Liebman J, Cullum L, Belloc NB. Natural history of transpositon of the great arteries. Anatomy and birth and death characteristics. Circulation 40:237, 1969.
57. Kirjavainen M, Happonen JM, Louhimo I. Late results of Senning operation. J Thorac Cardiovasc Surg 117:488, 1999.
58. Williams WG, Trusler GA, Kirklin JW, et al. Early and late results of a protocol for simple transposition leading to an atrial switch (Mustard) repair. J Thorac Cardiovasc Surg 95:717, 1988.
59. Williams WG, McCrindle BW, Ashburn DA, et al. Outcomes of 829 neonates with complete transposition of the great arteries 12-17 years after repair. Eur J Cardiothorac Surg 24:1, 2003.
60. Butto F, Dunnigan A, Overholt ED, et al. Transesophageal study of recurrent atrial tachycardia after atrial baffle procedures for complete transposition of the great arteries. Am J Cardiol 57:1356, 1986.
61. Byrum CJ, Bove EL, Sondheimer HM, et al. Hemodynamic and electrophysiologic results of the Senning procedure for transposition of the great arteries. Am J Cardiol 58:138, 1986.
62. Duster MC, Bink-Boelkens MT, Wampler D, et al. Long-term follow-up of dysrhythmias following the Mustard procedure. Am Heart J 109:1323, 1985.
63. Flinn CJ, Wolff GS, Dick M et al. Cardiac rhythm after the Mustard operation for complete transposition of the great arteries. N Engl J Med 310:1635, 1984.
64. Hayes CJ, Gersony WM. Arrhythmias after the Mustard operation for transposition of the great arteries: a long-term study. J Am Coll Cardiol 7:133, 1986.
65. Vetter VL, Tanner CS, Horowitz LN. Electrophysiologic consequences of the Mustard repair of d-transposition of the great arteries. J Am Coll Cardiol 10:1265, 1987.
66. Beerman LB, Neches WH, Fricker FJ, et al. Arrhythmias in transposition of the great arteries after the Mustard operation. Am J Cardiol 51:1530, 1983.
67. Alpert BS, Bloom KR, Olley PM et al. Echocardiographic evaluation of right ventricular function in complete transposition of the great arteries: angiographic correlates. Am J Cardiol 44:270, 1979.
68. Benson LN, Bonet J, McLaughlin P, et al. Assessment of right ventricular function during supine bicycle exercise after Mustard's operation. Circulation 65:1052, 1982.
69. Graham TP, Jr., Atwood GF, Boucek RJ, Jr., et al. Abnormalities of right ventricular function following Mustard's operation for transposition of the great arteries. Circulation 52:678, 1975.
70. Hagler DJ, Ritter DG, Mair DD, et al. Right and left ventricular function after the Mustard procedure in transposition of the great arteries. Am J Cardiol 44:276, 1979.
71. Parrish MD, Graham TP, Jr., Bender HW, et al. Radionuclide angiographic evaluation of right and left ventricular function during exercise after repair of transposition of the great arteries. Comparison with normal subjects and patients with congenitally corrected transposition. Circulation 67:178, 1983.
72. Trowitzsch E, Colan SD, Sanders SP. Global and regional right ventricular function in normal infants and infants with transposition of the great arteries after Senning operation. Circulation 72:1008, 1985.
73. Trowitzsch E, Colan SD, Sanders SP. Two-dimensional echocardiographic estimation of right ventricular area change and ejection fraction in infants with systemic right ventricle (transposition of the great arteries or hypoplastic left heart syndrome). Am J Cardiol 55:1153, 1985.
74. Musewe NN, Reisman J, Benson LN, et al. Cardiopulmonary adaptation at rest and during exercise 10 years after Mustard atrial repair for transposition of the great arteries. Circulation 77:1055, 1988.
75. Paul MH, Wessel HU. Exercise studies in patients with transposition of the great arteries after atrial repair operations (Mustard/Senning): a review. Pediatr Cardiol 20:49, 1999.
76. Tsuda E, Imakita M, Yagihara T, et al. Late death after arterial switch operation for transposition of the great arteries. Am Heart J 124:1551, 1992.
77. Tanel RE, Wernovsky G, Landzberg MJ, et al. Coronary artery abnormalities detected at cardiac catheterization following the arterial switch operation for transposition of the great arteries. Am J Cardiol 76:153, 1995.
78. Yamaguchi M, Hosokawa Y, Imai Y, et al. Early and midterm results of the arterial switch operation for transposition of the great arteries in Japan. J Thorac Cardiovasc Surg 100:261, 1990.
79. Wernovsky G, Mayer JE, Jr., Jonas RA, et al. Factors influencing early and late outcome of the arterial switch operation for transposition of the great arteries. J Thorac Cardiovasc Surg 109:289, 1995.

80. Nakanishi T, Matsumoto Y, Seguchi M, et al. Balloon angioplasty for postoperative pulmonary artery stenosis in transposition of the great arteries. J Am Coll Cardiol 22:859, 1993.
81. Blume ED, Wernovsky G. Long-term results of arterial switch repair of transposition of the great vessels. Semin Thorac Cardiovasc Surg Pediatr Card Surg Annu 1:129, 1998.
82. Rhodes LA, Wernovsky G, Keane JF, et al. Arrhythmias and intracardiac conduction after the arterial switch operation. J Thorac Cardiovasc Surg 109:303, 1995.
83. Colan SD, Trowitzsch E, Wernovsky G, et al. Myocardial performance after arterial switch operation for transposition of the great arteries with intact ventricular septum. Circulation 78:132, 1988.
84. Colan SD, Boutin C, Castaneda AR, et al. Status of the left ventricle after arterial switch operation for transposition of the great arteries. Hemodynamic and echocardiographic evaluation. J Thorac Cardiovasc Surg 109:311, 1995.
85. Mahle WT, McBride MG, Paridon SM. Exercise performance after the arterial switch operation for D-transposition of the great arteries. Am J Cardiol 87:753, 2001.
86. Hourihan M, Colan SD, Wernovsky G, et al. Growth of the aortic anastomosis, annulus, and root after the arterial switch procedure performed in infancy. Circulation 88:615, 1993.
87. Schwartz ML, Gauvreau K, del Nido P, et al. Long-term Predictors of Aortic Root Dilation and Aortic Regugitation Following Arterial Switch Operation. Circulation 110(Suppl 2): 128, 2004.
88. Wernovsky G. Transposition of the great arteries. In Allen HD, Gutgesell HP, Clark EB,, et al. (eds). Moss and Adams' Heart Disease in Infants, Children and Adolescents. New York: Lippincott, Williams and Wilkins, 2000.
89. Sansa M, Tonkin IL, Bargeron LM, Jr., et al. Left ventricular outflow tract obstruction in transposition of the great arteries: an angiographic study of 74 cases. Am J Cardiol 44:88, 1979.
90. Wernovsky G, Jonas RA, Colan SD, et al. Results of the arterial switch operation in patients with transposition of the great arteries and abnormalities of the mitral valve or left ventricular outflow tract. J Am Coll Cardiol 16:1446, 1990.
91. Vogel M, Freedom RM, Smallhorn JF, et al. Complete transposition of the great arteries and coarctation of the aorta. Am J Cardiol 53:1627, 1984.

38

Endocardial Cushion Defects

GERALD R. MARX AND DONALD C. FYLER

DEFINITION

Abnormalities of the structures derived from the embryologic endocardial cushions are called *endocardial cushion defects*. These include a variety of anomalies of the atrial and ventricular septa and the adjacent parts of the mitral and tricuspid valves.

EMBRYOLOGY/GENETICS

The primitive atrioventricular (AV) canal connects the atria to the ventricles. The endocardial cushions make up the circumference of the canal and divide naturally into superior, inferior, right, and left lateral cushions. These ridges of mesenchymal tissue contribute to the adjacent parts of the atrial septum, the ventricular septum, the septal leaflet of the tricuspid valve, and the anterior leaflet of the mitral valve. A flaw in this development results in an endocardial cushion defect.

Molecular studies indicate that the abnormal transformation of epithelial to mesenchymal cells in the development of the endocardial cushions is a result of abnormal coding of protein complexes within the heart jelly. Studies in a mouse model of Down syndrome, the trisomy 16 mouse, have demonstrated a lower density and migration of mesenchymal cells, resulting in an elongated endocardial cushion region.[1] A specific growth factor, found in chick embryos, has been implicated in the transformation of epithelial to mesenchymal cells.[2]

Through molecular mapping, some investigators have reported an *AV canal critical region* at 21q22.1 qter.[3] Others have reported a lack of association of atrioventricular canal defects with a critical region on chromosome 21.[4] Whether or not a specific genetic region has been defined, the relationship of phenotypic expression to genotypic mapping for the wide spectrum of endocardial cushion defects is yet to be defined.

ANATOMY

The anatomic categorization of the endocardial cushion defects has been a controversial topic for some time. To start with, the implication that these defects are derived from the embryologic endocardial cushions is not entirely correct. To discuss the many points of classification that have been raised is beyond the scope of this chapter.

Endocardial cushion defects (also known as *common atrioventricular canals, common atrioventricular orifices*, or *atrioventricular septal defects*) involve the septal portions of the mitral and tricuspid valves and the adjacent ventricular and atrial septa. The degree of abnormality of the septa is variable; at worst, virtually the entire atrial and ventricular septa may be absent. Or there may be a defect confined to one septum or the other. Thus, there may be a very large ventricular defect and no atrial defect (rare), or the reverse (common). Conceptually, the relative size of the atrial or ventricular septal defect is dependent on the position of the AV valves. If the valves attach lower on the AV septum, the primum atrial septal defect is large and the corresponding ventricular septal defect is smaller, and vice versa. When there is deficiency of both the atrial and ventricular septa, the mitral and tricuspid valves cannot attach normally. Their anterior leaflets may form a single saillike structure, which is part of a surprisingly competent valve extending across the septal orifice. When there is dominantly an atrial defect (ostium primum defect), the mitral valve is usually cleft and is often incompetent, sometimes allowing gross regurgitation. Rarely, the atrioventricular valve deformity is the sole abnormality, there being little or no septal defect. The variations in these deformities provide the basis for the many terms used in classification: *complete common, partial; transitional, intermediate; Rastelli type A, B, C; left-sided dominant; right-sided dominant*; and *balanced atrioventricular canal defects*. Many noted pathologists and cardiovascular centers use the term *left versus right-sided AV valve* to denote mitral and corresponding tricuspid valve. This chapter will use the terminology mitral and tricuspid valves and left-sided and right-sided AV valves interchangeably.

The *ventricular defect* can be very large, extending well beyond the part of the septum that is derived from endocardial cushion tissue. Usually, the ventricular opening is large and extends into the adjacent atrial septum as well. (Fig. 38-1), although rarely there may be a large typical ventricular defect with only a minimal atrial opening and, very rarely, no atrial defect at all. An isolated ventricular defect without an atrial opening, usually without atrioventricular valvar deformity, may be located immediately adjacent to the anterior leaflet of the mitral valve and under the septal leaflet of the tricuspid valve, and is described as a ventricular defect of the endocardial cushion type.

The *atrial defects* are equally variable, ranging from a small septal opening to complete absence of the atrial septum (including the entire atrial septum well beyond the territory of the cushions) (i.e., common atrium, single atrium). An isolated atrial defect with little or no ventricular opening is described as an ostium primum defect (Fig. 38-2). The terms *partial, incomplete, transitional*, and *intermediate* describe endocardial cushion defects that range between an ostium primum defect and a persistent, complete common atrioventricular canal.

The *atrioventricular valves* are almost invariably involved in these anomalies. With an ostium primum defect, there is almost always a cleft of the anterior leaflet of the mitral valve (Fig. 38-3), often, but not necessarily, associated with mitral regurgitation. Occasionally a mitral valve has a double orifice (Fig. 38-3), reported in one surgical series to occur in 9% of patients.[5] Although rare, this entity has been associated as a risk factor for poor surgical outcome.[5,6] There may be varying degrees of mitral regurgitation and, occasionally, mitral regurgitation is the dominant lesion, a small associated atrial septal opening being of little

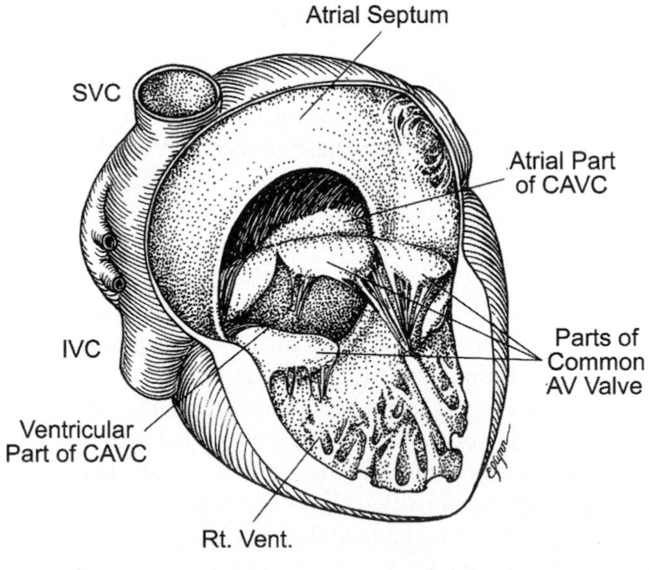

FIGURE 38–1 *Drawing of a common atrioventricular canal. Note the extension of valvar tissue across the defect. Note that the defect extends as one common orifice from the mid-atrial septum to the mid-ventricular septum. There is considerable variation in the size of the orifice and in the relative involvement of the atrial and ventricular septa. IVC, inferior vena cava; SVC, superior vena cava; CAVC, common atrioventricular canal.*
From Nadas AS, Fyler DC [eds]. Nadas' Pediatric Cardiology. Philadelphia, PA: Hanley and Belfus, 1992.

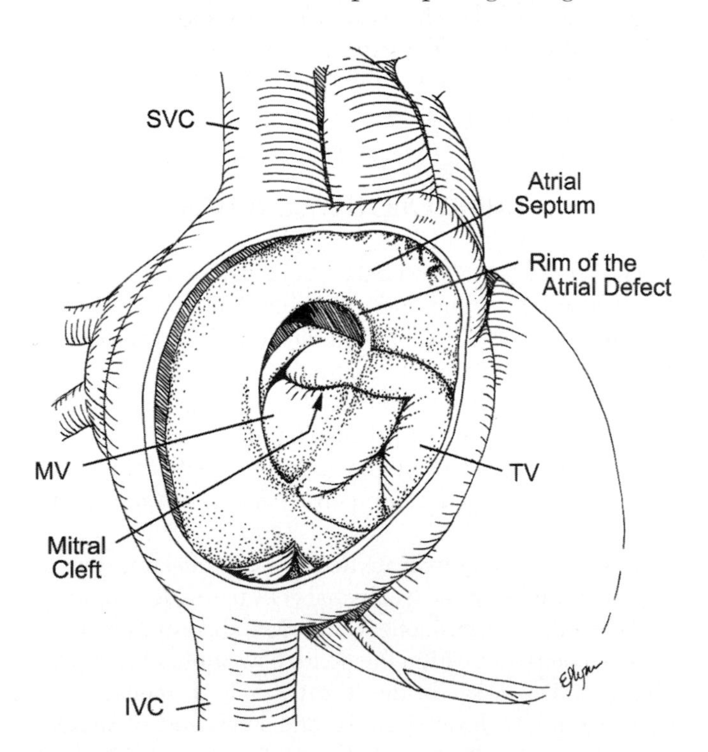

FIGURE 38–2 *Drawing of an atrial septal defect of the ostium primum type. Note that the defect extends to the valve insertions on each side and that there is a cleft in the mitral valve. SVC, superior vena cava; IVC, inferior vena cava; MV, mitral valve; TV tricuspid valve.*
From Nadas AS, Fyler DC [eds]. Nadas' Pediatric Cardiology. Philadelphia, PA: Hanley and Belfus, 1992.

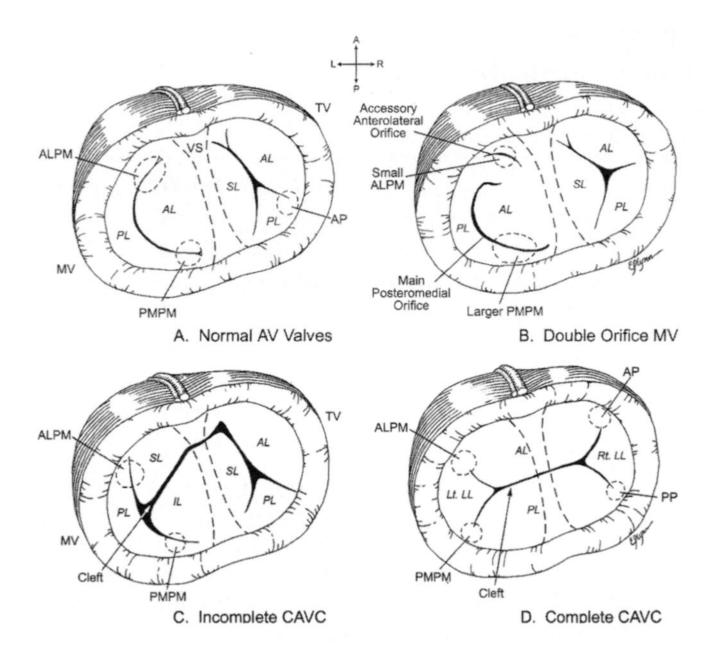

FIGURE 38–3 *Views of the atrioventricular valves from above in patients with endocardial cushion defects compared with those in normal patients. A, Normal. B, Double-orifice mitral valve. Note that there is a papillary muscle associated with each orifice. C, Ostium primum defect (incomplete atrioventricular canal) showing a cleft mitral valve. D, Common atrioventricular canal. Note the valve tissue extending across the defect. PMPM, posterior medial papillary muscle; MV, mitral valve; ALPM, anterolateral papillary muscle; TV, tricuspid valve; AL, anterior leaflet; PL, posterior leaflet; SL. Superior leaflet (mitral side) or septal leaflet (tricuspid side); IL, inferior leaflet; Rt. LL, right lateral leaflet; Lt. LL, Left lateral leaflet; VS, ventricular septum; CAVC, complete atrioventricular canal.*

From Nadas AS, Fyler DC [eds]. Nadas' Pediatric Cardiology. Philadelphia, PA: Hanley and Belfus, 1992.

physiologic consequence. With persistence of the common atrioventricular canal, the anterior leaflet of the atrioventricular valve is shared between the right and left ventricles, forming a saillike structure. This leaflet extends across the septum and poses a significant problem when the atrioventricular canal defect is to be repaired. The relationships of the leaflets to the crest of the ventricular septum have been used as a surgical classification of atrioventricular canal defects.

The tricuspid valve may *override* the ventricular septum or it may *straddle* the septum, with insertion of the chordae in the opposite ventricle. The distinction between overriding and straddling is determined by the insertion of the chordae. If insertion is on the appropriate side of the septum, or on the septal crest the term overriding is used. If insertion is across the septum in the opposing ventricle, the term straddling is used. The implications for surgical repair are obvious. When either the overriding or straddling is significant, the blood from one atrium is distributed to both ventricles, the proportions being dependent on the degree of displacement of the valve. The underlying ventricle will be hypoplastic in proportion to the limitation of blood flow that results from the diversion of flow to the other ventricle. Marked hypoplasia of a ventricle may prohibit any possibility of a two-ventricle repair.

Some patients with a common atrioventricular canal defect have a single left ventricular papillary muscle (or two immediately adjacent papillary muscles), which, when a repair has been undertaken, leaves one papillary muscle in the left ventricle. The functional result amounts to a parachute mitral valve, obstructing left ventricular in-flow.

Equally important, this deformity is a subtle yet important indicator for left ventricular hypoplasia.

Atrioventricular canal defects may be associated with pulmonary stenosis; many of these cases are variants of the tetralogy of Fallot syndrome. In other instances, valvar pulmonary stenosis or peripheral pulmonary stenosis may be associated with the ventricular defect.

However one chooses to think about these questions, it is obvious that the surgeon must be familiar with the anatomy and its variations and must have a philosophy of management that has proved successful, regardless of the nomenclature and the embryologic theories.

Interestingly, the demographics of endocardial cushion defects have changed over time. Before 1973 the ratio of Down to non-Down syndrome for endocardial cushion defects was 10%, which increased to 80% from 1973 to 1987 (Exhibit 38-1). Conjecturally this was related to increased diagnosis, treatment and survival of patients with trisomy 21. As can be seen, from 1988 to 2002 this ratio of Down to non-Down syndrome has shifted downward to 48%. Endocardial cushion defects are an important anatomic substrate of patients with non-Down syndrome and both heterotaxy syndrome and tetralogy of Fallot. Patients with heterotaxy syndrome and endocardial cushion defects often have asplenia with transposition of the great vessels, double outlet right ventricular, and ventricular hypoplasia (Exhibit 38-1). The increased diagnostic acumen of fetal echocardiography, and newborn and infant echocardiography, angiography and magnetic resonance imaging has led to increased detection and treatment of these patients.

Although common AV canal defects are common in patients with Down and non-Down syndrome ostium primum defects are much more common in non-Down syndrome patients (Exhibit 38-1). In patients who do not have Down syndrome, the ventricles are sometimes asymmetric and one of the ventricles is hypoplastic; however, in children with Down syndrome, ventricular hypoplasia is much less common.

Almost any known congenital cardiac defect may be associated with an endocardial cushion defect unless the child has Down syndrome. Except for tetralogy of Fallot,

Exhibit 38–1
Children's Hospital Boston Experience
1988-2002
Endocardial Cushion Defects

Total	*With Down Syndrome*	*Without Down Syndrome*
1188 (F55%)	387 (F53%)	801 (F56%)

In the prior era (1973-1987) the Down/non-Down Syndrome ratio was 1.1, now being 0.3% An additional 724 (40 of whom had Down Syndrome) were categorized under some other heading. (F = female)

Types of Endocardial Cushion Defects

Type	*With Down Syndrome* *N = 387 (%)*	*Without Down Sydnrome* *N = 801 (%)*
Ostium Primum Defect	29 (8)	309 (39)
Common Atrioventricular Canal	337 (87)	376 (47)
Isolated (cleft) Valvar Deformity	21 (5)	116 (14)

While Common Atrioventricular Canal is present in the great majority (87%) of those with Down Syndrome, it is only a little more common than Ostium Primum Defect in those without Down Syndrome (47 vs. 39%).

Primary Diagnoses of Patients with Endocardial Cushion Defects as a Secondary Diagnosis (N = 724)

Total	*With Down Syndrome* *N = 40*	*Without Down Syndrome* *N = 684*
Coarctation of Aorta	0	6
Ventricular Septal Defect	3	5
Aortic Valve Abnormality	0	2
Single Ventricle	0	17
Malposition	1	326
Hypoplastic Left Heart	0	18
Double Outlet Right Ventricle	1	45
D-Transposition of the Great Arteries	0	56
Tetralogy of Fallot	27	57
Atrial Septal Defect	0	4
Other	8	148

other cardiac defects in association with Down syndrome are rare (Exhibit 38-1).

PHYSIOLOGY

The physiologic consequences of endocardial cushion defects are those expected of ventricular or atrial defects or both, with the added possibility of atrioventricular valvar regurgitation. A cleft valve is not necessarily incompetent and a common atrioventricular canal, despite the extensive atrioventricular valve deformity, tends to have little or no regurgitation. However, every possible variation in the size of the defect, the location of the defect, and the degree of atrioventricular valvar incompetence is seen.

When there is mitral regurgitation through a cleft, the presence of an atrial defect may result in the reflux of the blood from the left ventricle to the right atrium. Consequently, the left atrium is not enlarged, despite significant regurgitation and obvious enlargement of the left ventricle.

With valvar overriding there is greater mixing of the pulmonary and systemic venous return, depending on the degree of override, and when one ventricle is very small the degree of mixing is equivalent to that of a single ventricle.

When there is a large ventricular opening, the risk of pulmonary vascular disease is high. In this case there is equilibration of right and left ventricular pressures and, unless there is pulmonary stenosis, there is obligatory pulmonary hypertension from birth. The development of pulmonary vascular disease is age-related and, with a large ventricular component, it occurs at least as early as it does with any other large ventricular defect.

There has been debate about the development of pulmonary vascular disease in patients with persistent atrioventricular canal defects who have Down syndrome. Most agree that the average pulmonary resistance in patients with Down syndrome is higher than it is in comparable children of the same age who do not have the Down syndrome. Some have interpreted this to be irreversible pulmonary vascular obstructive disease of the type seen with large ventricular defects, but appearing earlier because of the genetic abnormality. Histopathologic examination does not bear out this hypothesis. Equally well-established ventilatory problems in children with Down syndrome are a contributing cause for pulmonary hypertension. Respiratory problems such as upper airway obstruction, central hypoventilation, or chronic respiratory disease, in varying combinations, are particularly common in children with Down syndrome and are associated with reversible pulmonary hypertension. The presence of obligatory pulmonary hypertension because of a large ventricular septal defect and a variable left-to-right shunt further impinges on the borderline ventilatory capability. The result is elevation of pulmonary resistance to levels tending to limit left-to-right shunting. This is partly relieved by improved ventilation and oxygenation. However, relaxation of the pulmonary vascularity does not always occur in minutes; sometimes it requires days of improved oxygenation. Whether irreversible pulmonary vascular disease is more common in children who have Down syndrome than in children who do not have Down syndrome remains to be established. One recent published report found no difference in 30-day hospital mortality for patients with Down versus those without Down syndrome for repair of common complete AV canal defects.[6] Despite the inherent pulmonary problems and potential for pulmonary vascular disease in Down syndrome, advances in surgery, operation at younger age, and improvement in postoperative care have culminated in increasingly favorable operative results.

CLINICAL MANIFESTATIONS

Discovery

Fetal Echocardiography

Fetal echocardiography has become a primary tool for the diagnosis of endocardial cushion defects. Seventeen percent of fetuses with congenital heart disease have endocardial cushion defects.[7] This reported high incidence is due in part to mandatory visualization of the four-chamber view on standard level II ultrasound exams. Additionally, 80% of patients with heterotaxy syndrome have endocardial cushion defects, with a significant proportion having complete heart block. *In utero,* the relative bradycardia is readily diagnosed by the obstetrician who will refer the mother to a diagnostic center for more comprehensive evaluation. Furthermore fetal Down syndrome is more readily diagnosed due to elaborate screening based on alpha fetoprotein (AFP) levels, and also ultrasound morphometric characteristics.

Genetic testing and counseling is of paramount importance, once fetal endocardial cushion defects have been diagnosed. In one large study, 50% of such patients with known karyotype had a chromosomal abnormality, of these 39% had trisomy 21. An additional 13% had extracardiac abnormalities and nonkaryotypic syndromes. Furthermore, 33% had a form of heterotaxy syndrome.[8]

Fully 40% of patients with Down syndrome have congenital heart disease, more than half of which are forms of atrioventricular canal abnormality. Common atrium is a characteristic lesion in patients with the Ellis Van Crevald syndrome, and many patients with asplenia (Ivemark syndrome) have common atrioventricular canals. The diagnosis of any one of these syndromes should raise the question of an endocardial cushion defect.

In the absence of a recognizable syndrome, the cardiac lesion is often discovered in early infancy because of a readily audible murmur, although occasionally a baby with Down syndrome has no audible murmur, presumably because of pulmonary hypertension (Fig. 38-4).

One might argue that due to the ever expanding application and omnipresence of echocardiography, and the high prevalence of congenital heart disease, all babies thought to have Down syndrome should undergo a full two-dimensional Doppler echocardiographic evaluation.

Ostium Primum Defects

History

Infants discovered through routine screening methods to have an ostium primum type of atrial septal defect are largely asymptomatic. Rarely, a child with an ostium primum defect will have symptoms of congestive heart failure with tachypnea and growth failure. In such cases, careful attention must be directed to detect important associated hemodynamic abnormalities, such as mitral regurgitation, parachute mitral valve, subaortic stenosis, coarctation of the aorta, and left ventricular hypoplasia.[9]

Physical Examination

Generally, children with atrial septal defects of the ostium primum type grow well and have no signs of congestive heart failure. The cardiac impulse may be hyperactive if the shunt is large and particularly if there is mitral regurgitation. The second heart sound is well split and does not vary with respiration. There is a systolic murmur at the

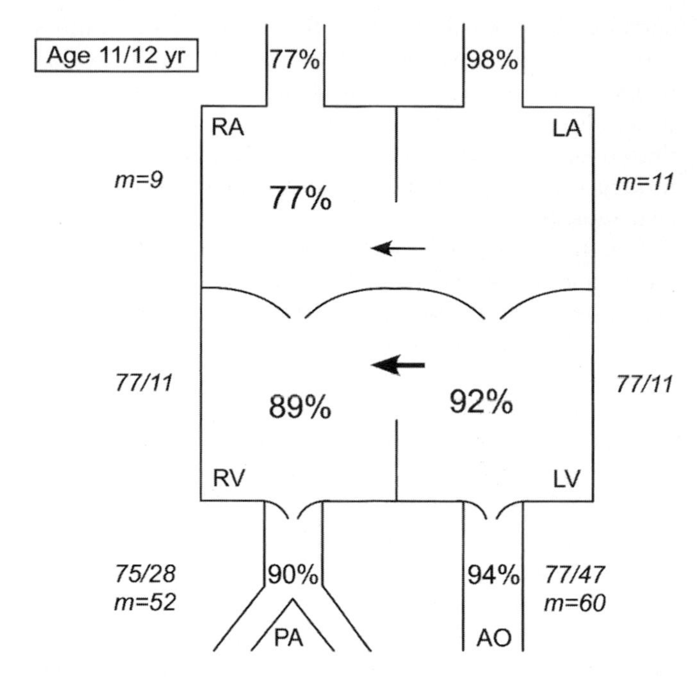

FIGURE 38–4 *This child has Down syndrome. Because there were no abnormal findings on repeated physical examination, she was thought to have no heart disease until an electrocardiogram was taken when she was 11 months old. There was a leftward counterclockwise superior axis (see Fig. 38-5). When examined by a cardiologist there was no abnormality on auscultation. Subsequently, the diagnosis of a very large common atrioventricular canal was made by echocardiography. The infant survived surgery and is now well. Italics, mm Hg; %, percent oxygen saturation; RA, right atrium; RV, right ventricle; LV, left ventricle; LA, left atrium; AO, aorta; PA, pulmonary artery.*
From Nadas AS, Fyler DC [eds]. Nadas' Pediatric Cardiology. Philadelphia, PA: Hanley and Belfus, 1992.

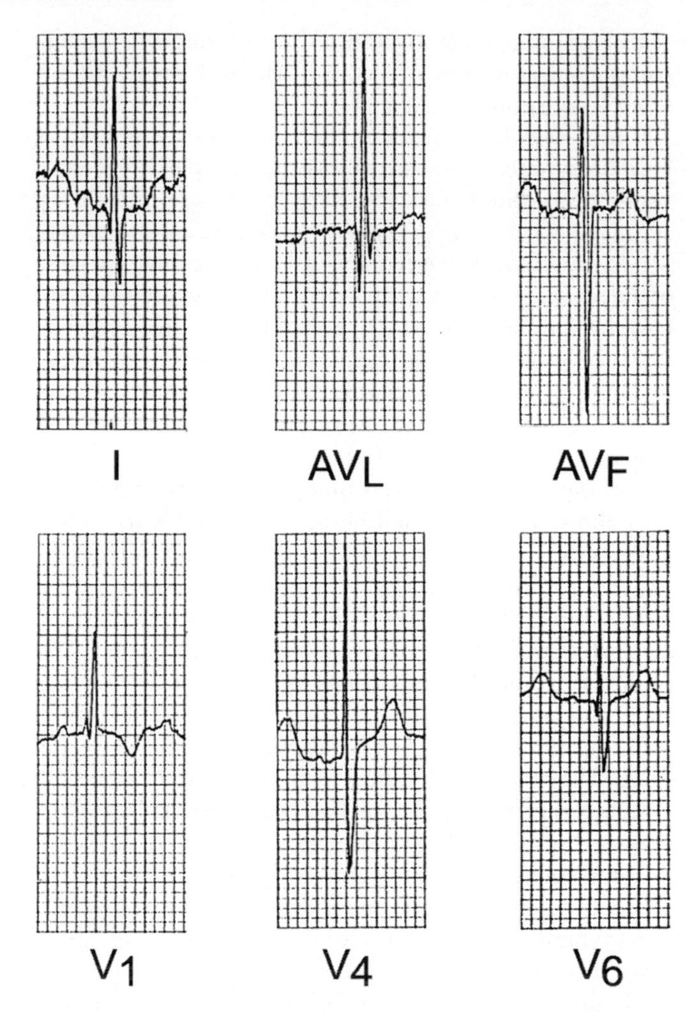

FIGURE 38–5 *This electrocardiogram is typical of the endocardial cushion defects. Note that the QRS axis is leftward counterclockwise and superior.*
From Nadas AS, Fyler DC [eds]. Nadas' Pediatric Cardiology. Philadelphia, PA: Hanley and Belfus, 1992.

upper left sternal border that is stenotic in character and usually is not loud. With a large shunt there may be a rumbling murmur in early to mid diastole at the lower left sternal border. A systolic murmur of mitral regurgitation may be audible at the cardiac apex, although often, in some of these patients, the murmur of mitral regurgitation is heard equally well at the left lower sternal border because the regurgitation is into the right atrium.

Electrocardiography

The electrocardiogram has a leftward, counterclockwise superior axis, usually ranging between –30 degrees and –90 degrees (Fig. 38-5). Incomplete right bundle branch block is usually present and if there is significant mitral regurgitation, there may be left ventricular hypertrophy.

Chest Radiography

Depending on the size of the left-to-right shunt and the amount of mitral regurgitation, the heart may be enlarged and the pulmonary vasculature engorged. The left atrium is not enlarged because it is decompressed by the septal defect; in effect, the left ventricular regurgitant flow passes directly into the right atrium. There may be enlargement of the heart out of proportion to the degree of pulmonary vascular engorgement if mitral regurgitation is a prominent feature.

Echocardiography

The two-dimensional technique demonstrates the atrial defect, and the left-to-right shunt can be recognized with Doppler examination. The presence of a mitral valve cleft and mitral regurgitation are readily appreciated. The diagnostic precision of echocardiography in conjunction with the other clinical findings is accurate enough to avoid the need for diagnostic cardiac catheterization in most of these patients.

The primum atrial septal defect can be imaged using apical, parasternal, and subxiphoid views. The defect is in the atrioventricular canal portion of the atrial septum, adjacent to the atrioventricular valves. The inlet into the atrioventricular valves is common and resembles a complete common atrioventricular canal defect. The attachments of the valve leaflets to the crest of the ventricular septum separate the outlet into the two valve orifices and close the potential ventricular septal defect. The apical four-chamber view shows all of these features (Fig. 38-6*A*). The morphology of the mitral valve is best seen in subcostal and parasternal short axis views (Fig. 38-6*B*). The number and spacing of the left ventricular papillary muscles, the cleft in the anterior mitral leaflet (Fig. 38-6*C*), and the attachments of the valve to the septum can be seen in a short-axis view. Doppler color flow mapping from an apical view is excellent for the detection and quantification of atrioventricular valve regurgitation.

Cardiac Catheterization

With the marked improved diagnostic acumen of echocardiography, catheterization is no longer part of the standard diagnostic evaluation for patients with *uncomplicated* primum atrial septal defects. However, in the child with severe mitral regurgitation it maybe useful to employ cardiac catheterization to assess for other left heart lesions such as subaortic stenosis or aortic coarctation. Importantly, it would be important to assess also for mitral valve stenosis such as in a parachute mitral valve, associated with left ventricular hypoplasia. Determination of the associated

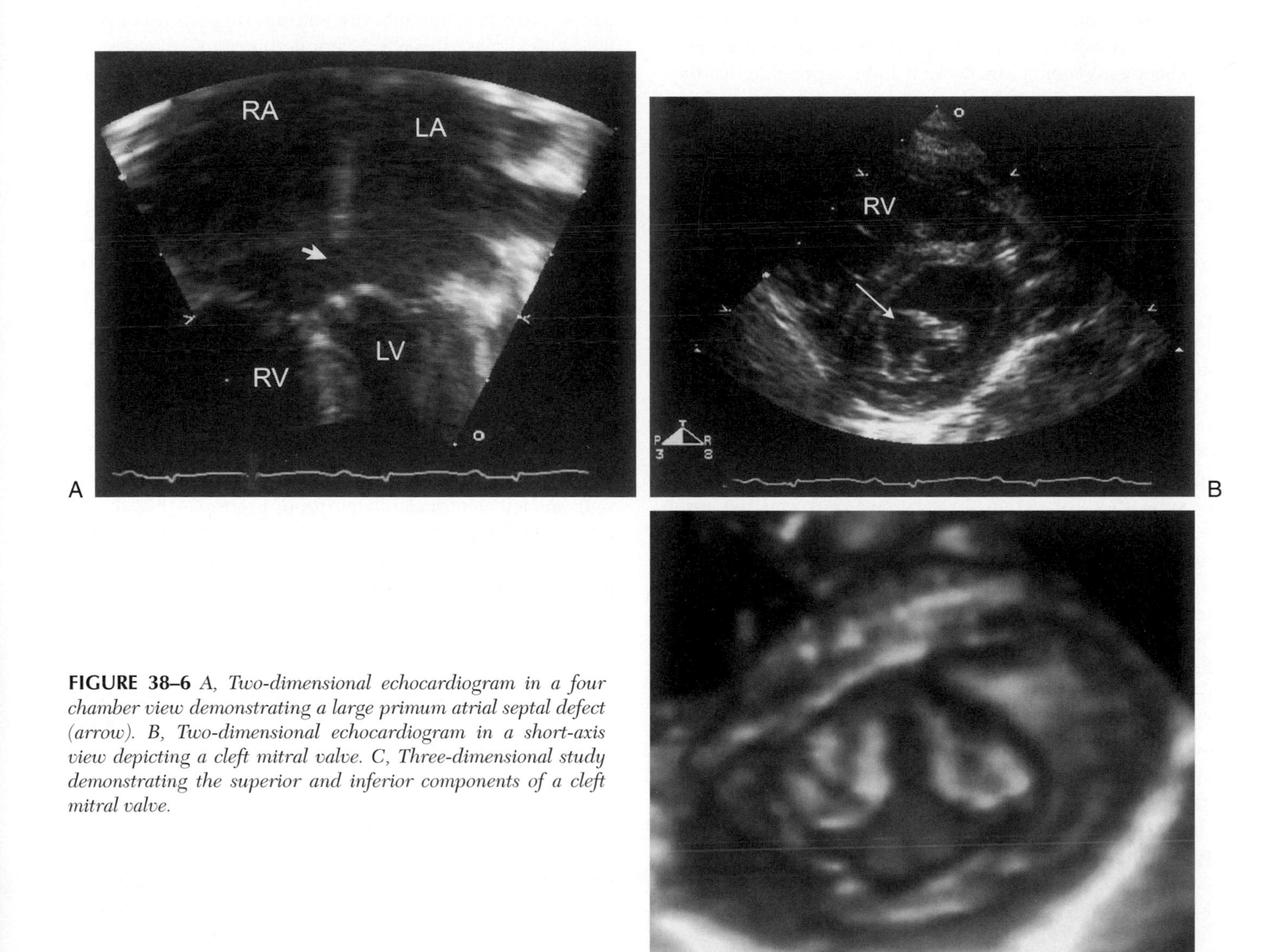

FIGURE 38–6 *A, Two-dimensional echocardiogram in a four chamber view demonstrating a large primum atrial septal defect (arrow). B, Two-dimensional echocardiogram in a short-axis view depicting a cleft mitral valve. C, Three-dimensional study demonstrating the superior and inferior components of a cleft mitral valve.*

hemodynamics may be extremely useful for the patient undergoing extensive left AV valvuloplasty and or replacement. A reliable adage is that patients with atypical echocardiographic findings or observations inconsistent with the other clinical findings should undergo diagnostic catheterization.

Management

In general, in patients with uncomplicated primum atrial septal defects, the accepted age of operation is from 6 to 12 months of age. In the presence of significant left AV valve regurgitation, or associated coarctation, surgical intervention may be undertaken at an earlier age. The results of surgical repair of ostium primum defects are excellent.[19,20,27,28,31,35] Recent centers report an operative mortality rate of 2%, and 10-year survival rate of 91% and 93%, respectively, with late mortality related to reoperations.[10,11] Fortunately, repair of double-orifice mitral valves and most regurgitant valves is possible. As the years go by fewer mitral valve replacements seem to be needed and it is possible that this issue is disappearing. In the meantime, there being little added risk in waiting, it seems wisest to delay surgery until it is possible to replace the valve if it is needed.

Course

It is impossible to close an ostium primum atrial defect, tinker with a regurgitant mitral valve, and leave the patient with a normal heart. Some incompetence of the mitral valve is expected and, therefore, a residual murmur is common. In some situations mitral regurgitation is self-aggravating and becomes more pronounced with the passage of time. The incidence of reoperation for patients with primum atrial septal defects approximates 10%,[10,11] with freedom from reoperation to be 91% at 10 years.[10] Most reoperations are for mitral regurgitation, but some are related to development of subaortic obstruction. In very rare occasions the atrial septal defect patch has undergone dehiscence culminating in residual shunting.

The reoperation for mitral regurgitation seems to best relate to the magnitude of regurgitation immediately following surgery.[12,13] However, one center implied that regurgitation might be progressive with freedom from significant regurgitation to be 89% at 5 years, and 78% at 10 years.[10] Even with marked improvement in surgical techniques, postoperatively arrhythmias do occur. In a 40-year review, 16% of patients developed supraventricular arrhythmias, and 3% complete heart block.[11]

Presently, most patients undergo valvuloplasty rather than replacement as an initial surgery for residual left AV valve regurgitation. Often the cause for regurgitation relates to leaflet dehiscence away from the patch, or the cleft suture line became disrupted, and/or progressive annular dilation culminating in decreased coaptation of the valve leaflets. Surgery may consist of reattachment of the leaflets to the septum, suture of the cleft, and/or annular placement. Present results for reoperation are encouraging.[12]

Atrioventricular Canal

History

In recent years, some 47% of children with common atrioventricular canal defects have Down syndrome (Exhibit 38-1). With recognition that the patient has Down syndrome, the possibility of congenital heart disease must be considered and when heart disease is found, there is a 50% chance that the child has a persistent common atrioventricular canal. While, occasionally, a baby with Down syndrome who has no auscultatory findings has an atrioventricular canal defect, the majority with this defect have easily recognized auscultatory findings suggesting congenital heart disease (usually a systolic murmur). Congestive heart failure and failure to grow adequately are common presenting problems.

Physical Examination

Besides the possible evidences of congestive heart failure, there may be a hyperactive cardiac impulse. Most patients have a systolic murmur that is loudest at the lower left sternal border and sometimes is heard well toward the apex. Third heart sounds, gallop rhythms, and apical diastolic rumbling murmurs are often encountered. The second (pulmonary) component of the second heart sound is usually accentuated.

Electrocardiography

The electrocardiogram has a superior counterclockwise, *northwest* axis, often being between –150 degrees and –90 degrees in the frontal plane. Evidence of right, or both right and left, ventricular hypertrophy is present (Fig. 38-5). Rarely, a patient with severe right ventricular hypertrophy will not have the characteristic leftward-superior axis, but will have right-axis deviation instead.

Chest Radiography

The heart size is enlarged and the pulmonary vascularity is engorged in proportion to the amount of left-to-right shunting. Usually, the left atrium is not enlarged despite evidence of a large shunt.

Echocardiography

Echocardiography has been an invaluable tool in delineating atrioventricular canal defects. Documentation of the size of the ventricular septal defect, the size and shape of the atrial defect, and the relative and absolute sizes of the ventricles, as well as evaluation of the components of the atrioventricular valve, is possible using sophisticated two-dimensional and Doppler echocardiography. The degree of atrioventricular regurgitation, the number and location of the papillary muscles, and the presence of associated defects are recorded.

The subcostal and apical four chamber views demonstrate the primum atrial septal defect, common atrioventricular valve, and the ventricular septal defect component (Fig. 38-7A). The alignment of the common valve vis-à-vis the ventricular septum and left ventricular papillary muscle architecture are well seen in the short axis views (Fig. 38-7*B*). The apical four-chamber view demonstrates the size of the ventricular septal defect and is an excellent view for a Doppler examination of the valves. The apical and parasternal long axis views can demonstrate abnormal valve attachment that produces subaortic stenosis.

Cardiac Catheterization

In the past decade, an important transition has evolved in the preoperative evaluation of patients with complete common AV canal defects. Previously, the recommendation was that all patients with the clinical and echocardiographic diagnosis of a common complete atrioventricular canal defect undergo cardiac catheterization to evaluate the magnitude of pulmonary hypertension and pulmonary resistance. This is no longer necessary. The major factor responsible for this transition is that those patients undergoing two ventricular repairs are operated at 2 to 3 months of age with very good short-term morbidity and mortality results.[14,15] In all patients with a complete common AV canal defect, hence a large nonrestrictive ventricular defect, the pulmonary artery pressure is equal to systemic level. Due to the marked increase in pulmonary blood flow the pulmonary vascular resistance is marginally elevated, if elevated at all. If the surgery is performed before 3 months of age very rarely will the patient have developed *fixed* elevated pulmonary vascular resistance or pulmonary vascular occlusive disease. However, when operated at six months of age the pulmonary arterial resistance can be elevated (Fig. 38-8). In prior surgical eras, when patients were operated at older ages, post-operative pulmonary arterial hypertensive crises were common and difficult to manage. Hence, to optimize post-operative management, cardiac catheterization may be beneficial in the older un-operated patient. During the catheterization the response to various pulmonary vasodilator medications can be tested, such as the response to oxygen, nitroprusside, prostacycline (Fig. 38-8*B*).

Still, certain patients may be considered for cardiac catheterization or other imaging studies such as magnetic resonance imaging or three-dimensional echocardiography. This includes, but is not limited to, patients with parachute left AV valve, left AV valve regurgitation, subaortic stenosis, unbalanced complete common AV canal defects, tetralogy of Fallot, or patients with additional ventricular septal defects. Although not discussed in detail in this chapter,

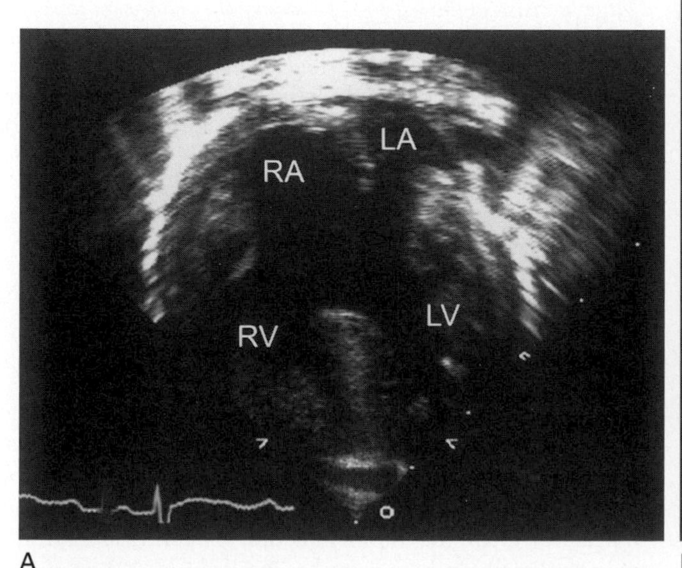

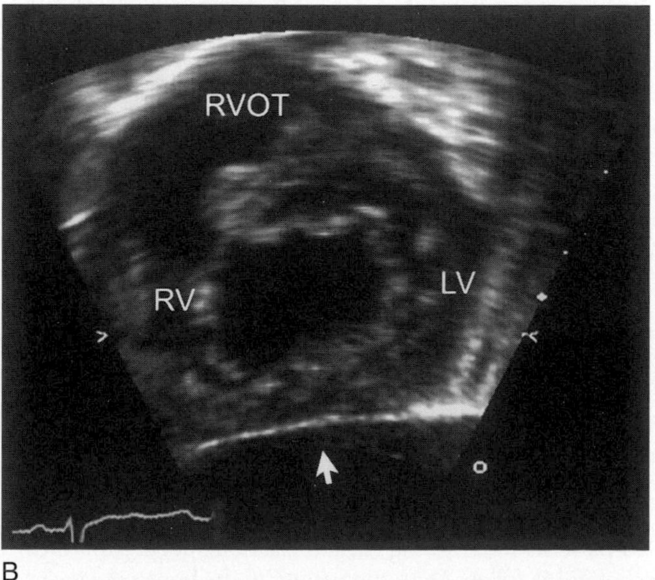

FIGURE 38–7 *A, Two-dimensional echocardiographic four-chamber view incomplete atrioventricular (AV) canal defects showing primum atrial septal defect and common AV valve and large endocardial cushion ventral septal defect. B, Two-dimensional echocardiographic cross sectional view of common AV valve. RA, right atrium; LA, left atrium; RV, right ventricle; RVOT, right ventricular outflow tract; LV, left ventricle.*

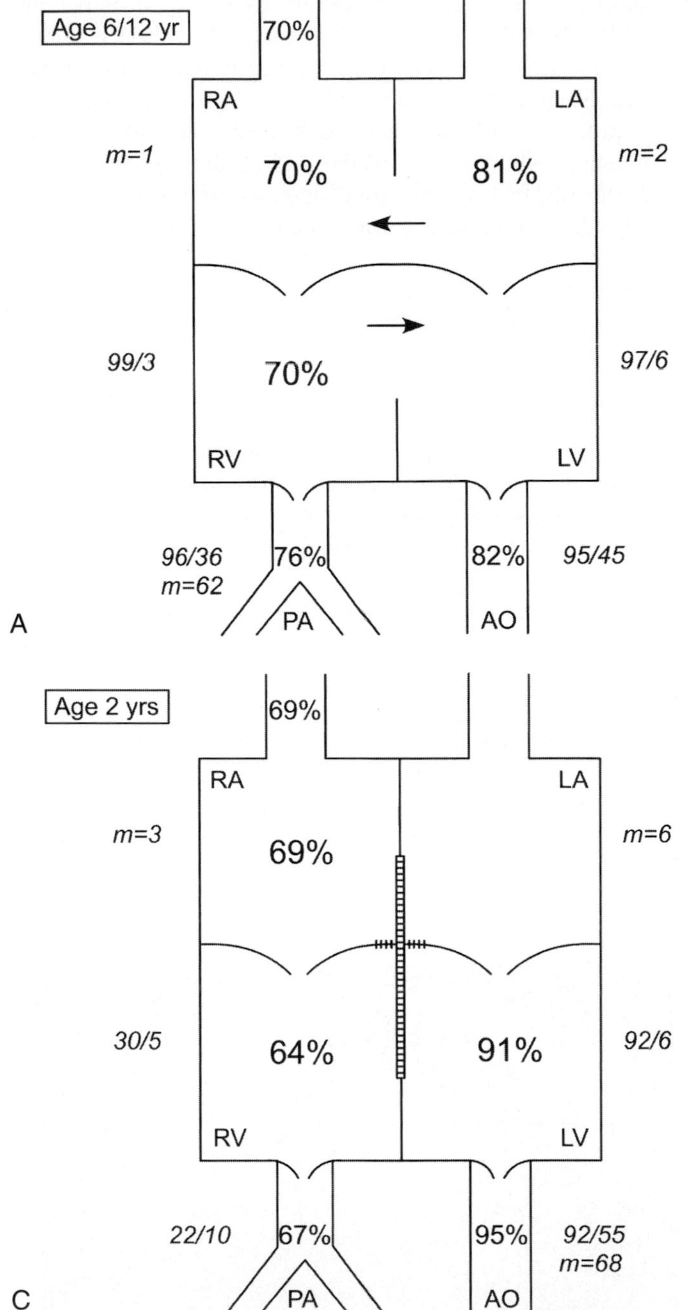

FIGURE 38–8 *A, This infant has Down syndrome and a common atrioventricular canal. At catheterization at age 6 months there was pulmonary hypertension at systemic levels and relatively little left-to-right shunt. As a consequence, the calculated pulmonary resistance was high. B, The child was placed on 100% oxygen and showed a marked increase in the pulmonary blood flow because of a large increase in the left-to-right shunt. He underwent uneventful surgical repair and was brought back for follow-up cardiac catheterization (C) because of a residual murmur. He was found to have a small muscular ventricular septal defect that had been overlooked. There was no evidence of residual elevation of pulmonary resistance. RA, right atrium; RV, right ventricle; LV, left ventricle; LA, left atrium; AO, aorta; PA, pulmonary artery.*
From Nadas AS, Fyler DC [eds]. Nadas' Pediatric Cardiology. Philadelphia, PA: Hanley and Belfus, 1992.

patients with heterotaxy syndrome and AV canal defects should be considered for additional imaging modalities especially to ascertain the pulmonary and systemic venous drainage, especially if considered for Fontan surgery.

In patients undergoing catheterization specific routines are helpful to follow. With the patient in the hepatoclavicular position, a pigtail or balloon angiographic catheter is placed in the left ventricle, across the atrioventricular valve or retrograde across the aortic valve. An angiogram is performed after an injection of contrast of 1.5 mL/kg of body weight. This view will not only outline a complete atrioventricular canal and additional ventricular septal defects, but is as good a view as any for determining the degree of mitral regurgitation. Occasionally, a catheter course across the mitral valve, or the rapid injection of contrast medium, may artificially induce mitral valve leakage. When mitral regurgitation is observed, the angiogram may be repeated with the injection at a lower flow rate (and perhaps with retrograde passage of the catheter) to reduce the chances of catheter-induced valvar regurgitation. The angiogram is used primarily to rule out associated muscular ventricular septal defects to check further on ventricular size, and rule out subaortic stenosis.

An aortogram is recorded to discover a patent ductus arteriosus, a common finding in patients with Down syndrome and a common atrioventricular canal.

Management

Given two ventricles of suitable size, judged adequate to support normal circulation, and no additional defects, surgical correction is undertaken. The defect between the ventricles and atria is patched with one or two patches and the available valve tissue is fashioned into functioning mitral and tricuspid valves. Clearly, the surgeon strives for a functioning mitral valve, because dysfunction on the left side is a major deficit, whereas right-sided atrioventricular valve (tricuspid) dysfunction is much better tolerated. Present standard of care would indicate complete repair of *uncomplicated* complete atrioventricular canal defects between 6 and 12 weeks of age.[14,15] Recent literature reports an early operative mortality (usually indicating death within 1 month of surgery) for complete AV canal defects ranging from 0% to 15% (Exhibit 38-2).[6,14–20] Excluding tetralogy of Fallot or markedly unbalanced AV septal defects, it is generally accepted that the operative mortality for repair of uncomplicated complete atrioventricular canal defects should be less than 4%.

Increased 30-day mortality has been associated with double orifice mitral valve.[6] Interestingly, improved survival has been related to younger age at operation.[15,19] Certainly this seems related to less severe magnitude of elevated pulmonary vascular resistance. The presence of Down syndrome is not related to increased mortality,[6] again related to younger age of operation in these patients. Importantly, the 10-year survival rate of surgery for all patients with common complete AV canal defects ranges from 78% to 93%.[15,16,18,19] The late cardiovascular mortality seems to be related to reoperation.

In following these patients, the major concerns would be for left AV valve regurgitation, subaortic stenosis, and dysrhythmias. The reoperation rate for complete atrioventricular canal defects ranges from 6% to 13%,[15,16,18,30] with most operations for left atrioventricular valve regurgitation. The freedom from reoperation has been variably reported as 73% at 7 years,[18] 79% to 89% at 10 years,[15,16,19] and 89% at 15 years[20] The risk factors for reoperation are early postoperative regurgitation,[12,16] preoperative AV valve regurgitation and presence of parachute mitral valve,[21] surgery at less than 5 kg,[18] surgery at older than 3 months of age[15] and lack of closure of cleft.[17]

The surgery for unbalanced complete AV septal defects, or for complete AV septal defects associated with heterotaxy syndrome is beyond the scope of this chapter. In general, these patients often undergo staging operations for Fontan procedures, with ever improving results.

Exhibit 38–2
Children's Hospital Boston Experience
1988-2002

Endocardial Cushion Defects

Surgical Repair: All procedures at Boston Children's Hospital.

Common Atrioventricular Canal		*N = 332 (%)*
Age at surgery:	< 6 months	208 (63)
	6-12 months	91 (27)
	> 1 year	33 (10)
Reoperation for Mitral Regurgitation		50 (15)
	Valve Plasty	38 (11)
	Valve Replacement	12 (4)

Ostium Primum Defect		*N = 227 (%)*
Age at Surgery:	< 6 months	37 (16)
	6-12 months	30 (13)
	> 1 year	160 (70)
Reoperation for Mitral Regurgitation		8 (4)
	Valve Plasty	4 (2)
	Valve Replacement	4 (2)

Most patients with complete atrioventricular canal were repaired in the first 6 months of life, most with ostium primum defects being greater than age 1 year at repair. Later mitral valve surgery was necessary in 15% of the former compared to 8% of the latter. Survival at 18 months was excellent in both groups.

SUMMARY

Endocardial cushion defects are an important array of congenital heart defects seen in patients with both chromosomal abnormalities and heterotaxy syndrome. Ostium primum defects can be seen in patients without associated problems and most are asymptomatic until surgery. Those patients with primary ostium primum defects that present with symptoms may have important associated abnormalities such as subaortic stenosis, left AV valve disease, and/or aortic arch abnormalities. Over 50% of patients with complete common AV canal defects have Down syndrome. Presently, the preferred age of operation is two to three months of age, to prevent problems with post-operative pulmonary artery hypertension. Early age at operation and improvements in surgical technique and postoperative care have resulted in excellent operative mortality results for complete AV canal defects. In follow-up, the primary concerns for patients operated for endocardial cushion defects are for development of subaortic stenosis and, even more so, left AV valve regurgitation, with good results for repair rather than replacement. Endocarditis prophylaxis is mandatory for all.

REFERENCES

1. Eisenberg LM, Markwald, RR. Molecular regulation of atrioventricular valvuloseptal morphogenesis. Circ Res 77: 1, 1995.
2. Webb S, Anderson RH, Brown NA. Endocardial cushion development and heart loop architecture in the trisomy 16 mouse. Dev Dyn 206:301,1996.
3. Koremburg JR, Bradley C, Disteche CM. Down syndrome: molecular mapping of the congenital heart disease and duodenal atresia. Am J Hum Genet 50:294, 1992.
4. Cousineau J, Lauer RM, Pierpont ME, et al. Linkage analysis of autosomal dominant atrioventricular canal defects: exclusion of chromosome 21. Hum Genet 93: 103, 1994.
5. Nakano T, Kado H, Shiokawa Y, et al. Surgical results of double orifice left atrioventricular valve associated with atrioventricular outcome, risk factors. Ann Thorac Surg 73(1): 695, 2002.
6. Al-Hay AA, MacNeil SJ, Yacoub M, et al. Complete atrioventricular septal defect, Down syndrome, and surgical outcome, risk factors. Ann Thorac Surg 75(2): 412, 2003.
7. Cook AC, All LD, Anderson RH, et al. Atrioventricular septal defect in fetal life: a clinical pathologic correlation. Cardiol Young 1:334, 1991.
8. Huggon IC, Cook AC, Smeeton NC, et al. Atrioventricular septal defects diagnosed in fetal life: associated cardiac and extracardiac abnormalities and outcome. J Am Coll Cardio 36 (2): 593, 2000.
9. Manning PB, Mayer JE, Sanders SP et al. Unique features and prognosis of primum ASD presenting in the first year of life. Circulation 90:1130, 1994.
10. Murashita T, Kubota T, Oba J, et al. Left atrioventricular valve regurgitation after repair of incomplete atrioventricular septal defect. Ann Thor Surg 77 (6): 2157, 2004.
11. El-Najdawi EK, Driscoll DJ, Puga FJ, et al. Operation for partial atrioventricular septal defect: a forty-year review. Thorac & Cardiovasc Surg 119(5): 880, 2000.
12. Moran AM, Daebritz S, Keane JF, et al. Surgical management of mitral regurgitation after repair of endocardial cushion defects: early and midterm results. Circulation 102(19 Suppl 3): III 160, 2000.
13. Rhodes J, Warner KG, Fulton DR, et al. Fate of mitral regurgitation repair of atrioventricular septal defect. Am J Cardio 80(9): 1194, 1997.
14. Jonas RA. Complete Atrioventricular Canal in Comprehensive Surgical Management of Congenital Heart Disease. London: Arnold Publishers of Oxford University Press, 2004.
15. Stellin G, Vida VI, Milanesi O, et al. Surgical treatment of complete A-V canal defects in children before 3 months of age. Eur Cardio-Thorac Surg 23(2): 187, 2003.
16. Bogers AJ, Akkesdijk GP, De Jong PL, et al. Results of primary two-patch repair of complete atrioventricular septal defect. Eur J Cardio-Thorac Surg 18(4): 473, 2000.
17. Nicholson IA, Nunn GR, Sholler GR, et al. Simplified single patch technique for the repair of atrioventricular septal defect. J Thor Cardiovasc Surg 118(4): 642, 1999.
18. Prifti E, Bonacchi M, Bernabei M, et al. Repair of complete atrioventricular septal defects in patients weighing less than 5 kg. Ann Thorac Surg 77(5): 1717, 2004.
19. Boening A, Scheewe J, Heine K, et al. Long-term results after surgical correction of atrioventricular septal defects. Eur J Cardio-Thorac Surg 22(2): 167, 2002.
20. Crawford FA, Jr., Stroud MR. Surgical repair of complete atrioventricular septal defect. Ann Thorac Surg 72(5): 1621, 2001.
21. Fortuna RS, Ashburn DA, Carias De Oliverira N, et al. Atrioventricular septal defects: effect of bridging leaflet division on early valve function. Ann Thorac Surg 277 (3): 895, 2004

39

Cardiac Malpositions and the Heterotaxy Syndromes

STELLA VAN PRAAGH

Abnormal sidedness of the heart, lungs, or abnormal viscera is usually readily recognized and is an important clue for the pediatrician and the cardiologist because this finding is associated with a high incidence of complex cardiac anomalies.

Prior to the introduction of modern two-dimensional echocardiography, accurate diagnosis was difficult and involved multiple cardiac catheterizations and repeated angiocardiograms. At present, detailed diagnosis of all of the cardiac malformations is usually achieved by echocardiography or magnetic resonance imaging.

DEFINITION

The term *cardiac malposition* indicates that the heart is abnormally located within the chest (dextrocardia, mesocardia) or is abnormally located relative to the situs of the abdominal contents (levocardia with abdominal visceral heterotaxy). The heart can also be displaced outside of the thorax (ectopia cordis).

CLASSIFICATION

Dextrocardia indicates that the heart is located in the right chest. Patients with dextrocardia may be divided into those with normally located abdominal viscera (visceroatrial situs solitus), those with inversely located atria and abdominal viscera (visceroatrial situs inversus), and those with visceral heterotaxy (inconsistent visceroatrial situs). Mesocardia indicates that the heart is displaced toward the right though not completely into the right chest. Levocardia describes a heart that is located in the left chest, levocardia with normally located abdominal viscera being normal. The abnormal possibilities include levocardia with visceroatrial situs inversus and levocardia with visceral heterotaxy (isolated levocardia).

It is important to recognize that cardiac malposition does not imply anything specific about the various cardiac segments or the connections and alignments between these segments (see Chapter 4). Segmental analysis of the heart can be achieved with the use of the same criteria in levocardia, mesocardia, or dextrocardia. Accurate diagnosis requires the identification of the situs of the various cardiac segments and the description of the associated defects.

PREVALENCE

In the New England Regional Infant Cardiac report there were 95 infants with malposition (0.103/1000 live births).[1] In the more recent 1988 to 2002 period at Children's Hospital Boston, 724 were patients seen (1% of all patients) with a mortality rate of 19%: In the preceding era among 355 patients the mortality rate was 34% (Exhibit 39-1).

PATHOLOGY

The heart may be misplaced into the right chest because of hypoplasia of the right lung or by virtue of an associated anomaly such as diaphragmatic hernia. Cardiac malposition also occurs with defects or deformities of the anterior chest wall (i.e., the Cantrell syndrome),[2] complete thoracic ectopia cordis, or Siamese twins. In all those cases the cardiac malposition is secondary to noncardiac malformations. Primary cardiac malposition (usually dextrocardia) represents

Exhibit 39–1
Children's Hospital Boston Experience Viscerocardiac Malposition

	1973–1987		1988–2002	
Clinical Diagnosis	*No. Pts.*	*% Mortality*	*No. Pts.*	*% Mortality*
Ectopia cordis	71		22	
Asplenia	52		25	
Polysplenia	37		1	
Dextrocardia*	21		17	
Total	335	34	724	19

*Includes situs inversus totalis, cases of asplenia or polysplenia and cases of secondary dextrocardia: survival has been improved considerably in 1988-2002 era.

a disturbance in the direction of cardiac looping or the lateralization of the thoracic viscera (see Chapter 4).

Any arrangement of cardiac segments and virtually any combination of cardiac defects may be encountered in patients with cardiac malposition.

PHYSIOLOGY

The hemodynamics associated with cardiac malpositions range from normal to those incompatible with life and are a direct consequence of the intracardiac defects.

Clinical Manifestations

The discovery of patients with cardiac malpositions is usually made when a chest x-ray is taken, or because of symptoms of cyanosis or congestive heart failure, or because of the presence of noncardiac anomalies. Dextrocardia or abnormal location of the abdominal viscera is recognized and the patient is referred to a cardiologist. The cardiologist need not be unduly concerned about the malposition, as it has little to do with the ultimate outcome. He or she should concentrate on a systematic segment-by-segment analysis of the heart, using echocardiography and angiocardiography, as the only way to arrive at details needed to plan surgical treatment. Dogged pursuit of the anatomic minutia is the prerequisite to successful management. There are no specific clinical findings and symptoms for cardiac malposition since they depend on the associated cardiac malformations.

SPECIFIC ENTITIES

Visceral Heterotaxy (the Asplenia and Polysplenia Syndromes)

In visceral *heterotaxy*, in addition to the heart several of the abdominal viscera may be malpositioned. This term derives from the Greek words *heteros*, meaning *other*, and *taxis*, meaning *order* or arrangement (i.e., other than normal arrangement.)

Patients with visceral heterotaxy show a high incidence of cardiac malformations. A study of 109 postmortem cases from the Cardiac Registry of the Children's Hospital Boston and of three living patients studied echocardiographically provided important new data that help in the understanding and management of these patients.[3] Hence, this group of patients is presented in detail.

The fundamental characteristics of visceral heterotaxy are an abnormal symmetry of certain viscera and veins (lungs, liver, venae cavae) and situs discordance between various organ systems and between the various segments of the heart.

The spleen is almost always affected in patients with visceral heterotaxy although the reason for this is not understood. The spleen may be absent (asplenia). It may be composed of a cluster of small splenuli, a large spleen and several small ones, or it may be multilobed (polysplenia). It may also be of normal size but abnormally located in the right upper quadrant of the abdomen (single, right-sided spleen), while the heart is left-sided and the lungs are situs inversus or symmetric.[3]

Although the cardiac malformations in heterotaxic individuals show considerable variability, there is also a definite syndromic clustering that often corresponds to the type of splenic malformation present. This association between the cardiac malformations and the status of the spleen, first described by Polhemus in 1952[4] and further elaborated upon by Ivemark in 1955,[5] is responsible for the terms of *asplenia* and *polysplenia syndrome*. Ivemark also observed and emphasized the association between malformations of the conotruncus and the atrioventricular canal in patients with asplenia. Because the atrioventricular canal and the conotruncus undergo division at about the same time that the splenic primordial appear (30–32 days of gestation), he postulated that it was possible for the same teratogenic factor to adversely affect the formation of the spleen and the division of the atrioventricular canal and the conotruncus. The recent identification of the iv locus on chromosome 12 of the *in vitro* and *in vivo* mice,[6] which are known to exhibit a high frequency of visceral heterotaxy with cardiac malformations similar to those observed in humans,[7] and the occurrence of heterotaxy with asplenia or polysplenia in more than one member of the same family[4,8] favors a genetic etiology of the heterotaxy syndromes.

Although the presence of visceral heterotaxy—at least in animals—and the absence or multiplicity of the spleen has been known since the time of Aristotle,[9,10] detailed accounts of abnormalities of the visceral situs began to appear in the German literature in 1745 when Troschel described the existence of partial situs inversus.[11] Eighty-one years later, in 1826, G. Martin[12] (a medical student from L'Ecole-Pratique et des Hopitaux Civils de Paris) described the first known case of asplenia with congenital heart disease and visceral heterotaxy in a human. Since that time, numerous publications have been devoted to this fascinating disturbance in the lateralization of the abdominal and thoracic viscera, which is associated with a wide variety of cardiac malformations, many of them lethal. The realization that, as a rule, patients with asplenia have bilaterally trilobed lungs and bilaterally eparterial bronchi justified the terms *double rightness*[13] and *right pulmonary isomerism*.[10] The observation of bilateral superior venae cavae entering the ipsilateral atrium, bilateral systemic venous connections from below (inferior vena cava and hepatic veins), and totally anomalous pulmonary venous connections to a systemic vein in the majority of patients with asplenia, led to the conclusion that the left atrium was absent; hence the term *right atrial isomerism* appeared appropriate.[14]

The high frequency of bilaterally bilobed lungs and bilateral hyparterial bronchi in patients with polysplenia appeared to justify the term *left lung isomerism*. The frequent absence of the hepatic segment of the inferior vena cava and the *ipsilateral* drainage of the pulmonary veins in several cases of polysplenia, in addition to the tendency of the right atrial appendage to resemble the left atrial appendage, formed the basis of the concept of *bilateral* left-sidedness.[15]

In recent years, new impetus has been given to the concept of right and left atrial isomerism by several investigators who have concluded that the atrial situs in visceral heterotaxy is indeterminate and should be diagnosed as right or left isomerism on the basis of the shape of the atrial appendages.[16–19] Although the proponents of this approach did not really believe that heterotaxic patients have two anatomic right atria or two anatomic left atria,[17,19] the effect of this terminology has been the abandonment of any effort to identify the atrial situs (solitus or inversus) in heterotaxic patients. To clarify this question and to decide if, in fact, it is possible to diagnose the atrial situs in heterotaxic patients with accuracy, the authors undertook the study of 109 heart specimens from patients with visceral heterotaxy and congenital heart disease. This chapter will include the data and conclusions of this study.[3]

Prevalence

Heterotaxy affected 0.8% of patients with congenital heart disease seen at Children's Hospital Boston in a 15-year-period (1973–1987). While, in the past, heterotaxic patients with congenital heart disease were of interest mainly to the pathologist, at present an increasing number of these patients survive, requiring medical and surgical treatment. During a 1-year period (June 1, 1989 to May 31, 1990), 43 patients with visceral heterotaxy underwent echocardiographic examination and cardiac catheterization at this hospital, 14 (38%) of whom were seriously ill infants younger than 6 weeks old.

Pathology

Spleen. The most consistent abnormality involved the spleen. Of the 109 cases of visceral heterotaxy with congenital heart disease seen at autopsy, 58 (53%) had asplenia, 46 (42%) had polysplenia, and 5 (5%) had a single, normal-sized spleen that was abnormally located in the upper right side of the abdomen, while the heart was in the left side of the chest and the situs of the lungs was solitus, inversus or symmetrical. The multiple spleens were right-sided in 29 of 46 patients with polysplenia and left-sided in the remaining 17 patients. It is interesting that right-sided polysplenia was almost twice as frequent as left-sided polysplenia in this postmortem series.

The authors are aware of the existence of living patients who have a normal, left-sided spleen (diagnosed by splenic scan) and cardiac defects similar to those seen in patients with visceral heterotaxy. Those patients were not included in out study, which was limited to postmortem cases.

Lungs. The lungs were abnormally symmetrical. The most common pattern in the asplenia group was bilaterally trilobed lungs with eparterial bronchi; in the polysplenia group, bilaterally bilobed lungs with hyparterial bronchi were most common (Fig. 39-1 and Table 39-1).

Liver. The liver was abnormally symmetric in 76% of the patients with asplenia, 67% of those with polysplenia, and 20% of those with a right-sided, single spleen (Table 39-1). Absence of the gallbladder or extrahepatic biliary atresia has been found in several patients with visceral heterotaxy and polysplenia, usually without significant heart defects.[20]

Mesentery. Mesenteric abnormalities, such as a common mesentery, abnormal mesenteric attachments, and malrotation or malposition of the intestines, are frequent findings with visceral heterotaxy.[21] The mesenteric abnormalities are responsible for the intestinal obstruction observed in heterotaxic patients, usually those with polysplenia.

Systemic Veins. The systemic venous connections are summarized in Table 39-2.

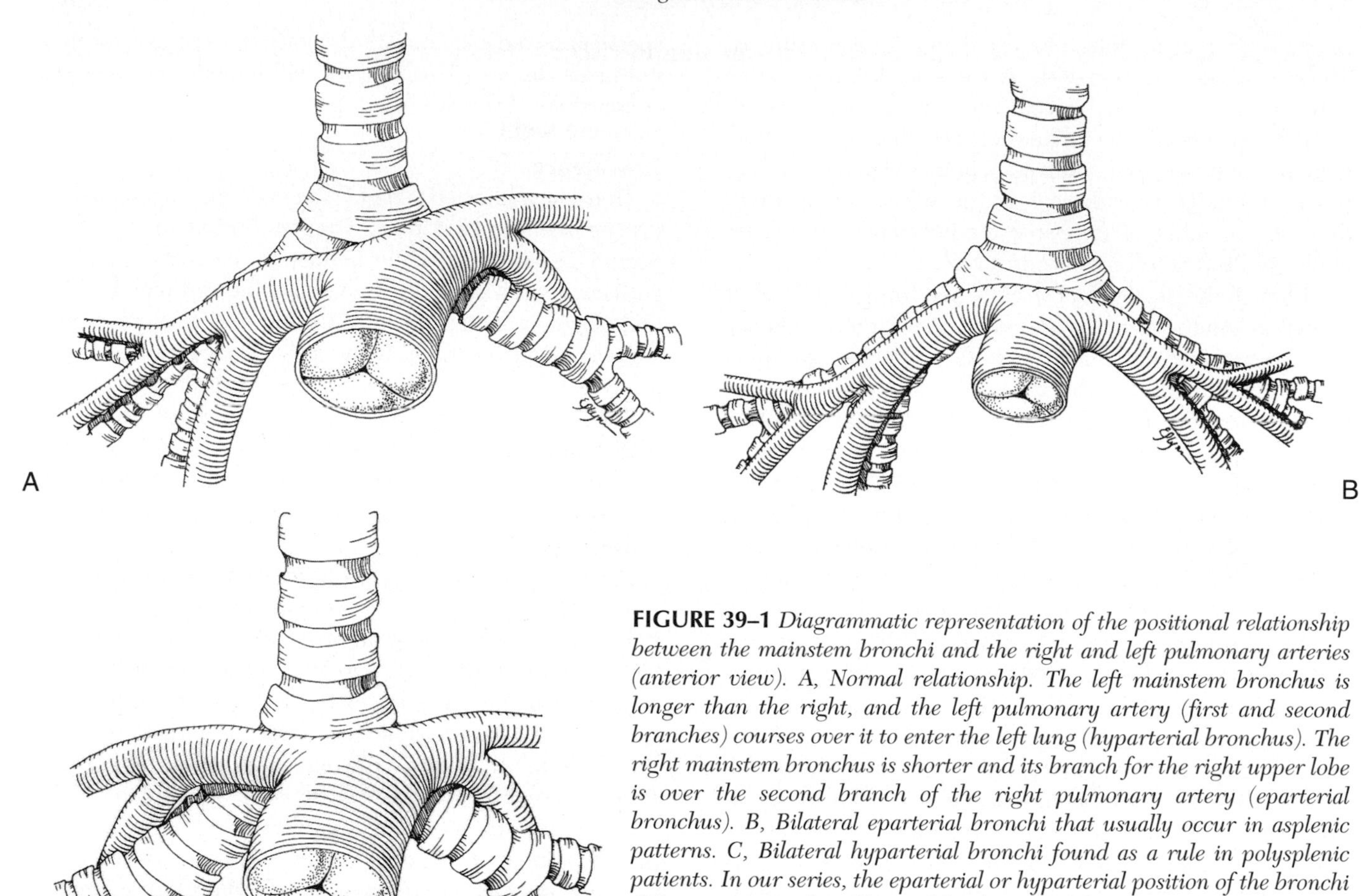

FIGURE 39–1 *Diagrammatic representation of the positional relationship between the mainstem bronchi and the right and left pulmonary arteries (anterior view). A, Normal relationship. The left mainstem bronchus is longer than the right, and the left pulmonary artery (first and second branches) courses over it to enter the left lung (hyparterial bronchus). The right mainstem bronchus is shorter and its branch for the right upper lobe is over the second branch of the right pulmonary artery (eparterial bronchus). B, Bilateral eparterial bronchi that usually occur in asplenic patterns. C, Bilateral hyparterial bronchi found as a rule in polysplenic patients. In our series, the eparterial or hyparterial position of the bronchi did not appear to be influenced by the size of the pulmonary arteries.*

Inferior Vena Cava. The inferior vena cava was intact in all patients with asplenia and in all patients with right-sided, single spleen (Table 39-2) (Fig. 39-2). In one patient with asplenia the inferior vena cava was small and connected with a dilated azygos vein. During cardiac catheterization, the catheter preferentially entered the dilated azygos vein and gave the false impression of an interrupted inferior vena cava. The potential for this venous pattern should be kept in mind if a patient who otherwise has the characteristic features of the asplenia syndrome seems to have interruption of the inferior vena cava and azygos continuation. Since the completion of this study[3] we have described the postmortem findings of a 5-day-old male infant with asplenia who had a left inferior vena cava with azygos entension to a left superior vena cava which entered a left-sided right atrium.[22] Hence an interrupted inferior vena cava may occur rarely in patients with visceral heterotaxy and asplenia.

The inferior vena cava was interrupted (i.e., the renal-to-suprahepatic segment of the inferior vena cava was absent and a dilated azygos vein continued from the renal veins to the superior vena cava) in 80% of the patients with polysplenia (Table 39-2). In one of these, the right-sided, interrupted inferior vena cava had bilateral azygos extensions to the ipsilateral superior vena cava (Fig. 39-3).

Hepatic Veins. All the hepatic veins connected with the inferior vena cava in 72% of the patients with asplenia. In the remaining 28%, the hepatic vein draining the lobe of the liver on the side opposite to the inferior vena cava connected with the atrial segment separately from the inferior vena cava. In one of these latter cases, the hepatic vein connects with an intact coronary sinus, while the coronary sinus was completely unroofed in the others. The point of connection of the hepatic vein was similar externally in both circumstances, suggesting that the apparent connection of a hepatic vein with the left atrium or the left atrial portion of a common atrium is actually a connection with the unroofed coronary sinus. The hepatic veins connected with the inferior vena cava in all five patients with a right-sided, single spleen. In the patients with polysplenia, if the inferior vena cava was intact, both right and left hepatic veins joined the

TABLE 39–1. Lung Lobation, Bronchial Pattern, and Liver Situs in Visceral Heterotaxy with Congenital Heart Disease*

	N = 109 Postmortem Cases					
			Single Right			
	Asplenia (*n* = 58) No.	%	Spleen (*n* = 5) No.	%	Polysplenia (*n* = 46) No.	%
Lung lobation						
Solitus	1	2	2	40	5	12
Inversus	1	2	1	20	4	9
Bilateral trilobed	45	81	2	40	3	7
Bilateral bilobed	1	2			31	72
Bilateral multilobed	6	11				
Bilateral unilobed	1	2				
Unknown	3				3	
Bronchial pattern						
Solitus	1	2	1	20	3	9
Inversus	1	2			3	9
Bilateral eparterial	40	95	4	80	4	12
Bilateral hyparterial					22	68
Unknown	16				14	
Liver situs						
Solitus	7	13			11	26
Inversus	6	11	4	80	3	7
Symmetric	42	76	1	20	29	67
Unknown	3				3	

*All percentages calculated on the basis of known cases; unknowns excluded for the purpose of percentage computations.

inferior vena cava in all except one case. In this case a hepatic vein drained into a normal coronary sinus and, indirectly, into the right atrium. Among patients with interruption of the inferior vena cava, the hepatic veins connected with the anatomically right atrium as a single trunk in all except two cases. In another series of patients, separate connections of the right and left hepatic veins were more common.[19]

Coronary Sinus Septum. The coronary sinus septum (i.e., the anterior wall of the coronary sinus and the adjacent posterior wall of the left atrium) was absent in 95% of patients with asplenia, 80% with a single, right-sided spleen, and 26% with polysplenia (Table 39-2).

Superior Vena Cava. The superior vena cava was present bilaterally in 71% of the patients with asplenia, 40% of patients with a single, right-sided spleen and 50% of patients

TABLE 39–2. Systemic Venous Connections in Visceral Heterotaxy with Congenital Heart Disease

	N = 109 Postmortem Cases					
			Single Right			
Types of Systemic Venous Connections	Asplenia (*n* = 58) No.	%	Spleen (*n* = 5) No.	%	Polysplenia (*n* = 46) No.	%
Continuous (not interrupted) IVC	58	100	5	100	9	20
Continuous IVC and contralateral hepatic vein	16°	28			1*	2
Interrupted IVC					37	80
Interrupted IVC and bilateral hepatic veins					2†	4
Bilateral SVCs	41	71	2	40	23	50
Absent coronary sinus septum	55	95	4	80	12	26

IVC, inferior vena cava; RA, right atrium; SVC, superior vena cava.

°In 1 of the 16 cases of asplenia and in the single case of polysplenia, the hepatic vein contralateral to the IVC drained directly into a normal (not unroofed) coronary sinus and indirectly into the RA.

†In one of these two cases, the coronary sinus septum was partly present, making possible atrial identification. In the other case, the larger of the two hepatic veins was on the same side with the solitus liver and it was interpreted as draining into the anatomic right atrium.

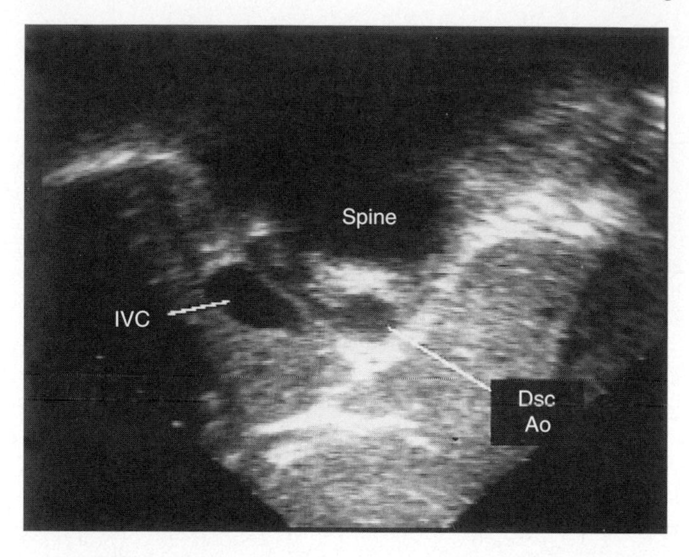

FIGURE 39–2 *Echocardiogram in the subxiphoid transverse view showing the aorta and inferior vena cava on the same side (right) of the spine in a patient with asplenia. IVC, inferior vena cava; Dsc Ao, descending aorta.*

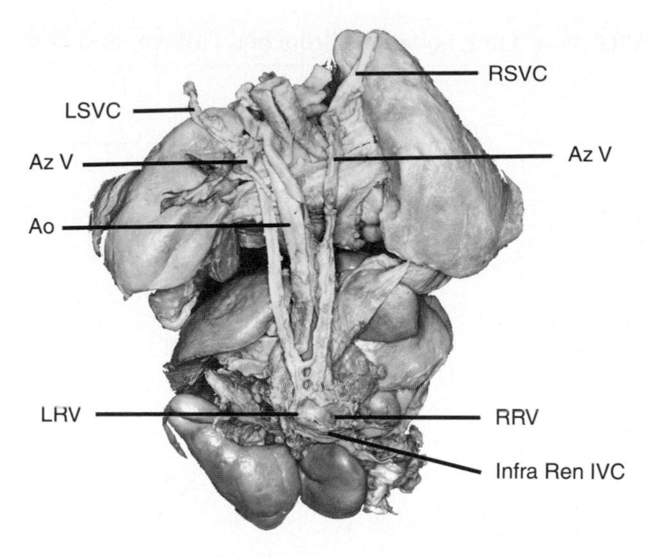

FIGURE 39–3 *Posterior view of the heart, lungs, liver, and kidneys of a 6.5-month-old boy with visceral heterotaxy and left-sided polysplenia. There is interruption of the right-sided inferior vena cava, with bilateral azygos vein (AZV) connecting with bilateral superior venae cavae. The right superior vena cava (RSVC) entered the right atrium directly. The left superior vena cava (LSVC) continued into the coronary sinus, which drained normally into the morphologically right atrium. All the pulmonary veins also drained into the right-sided morphologically right atrium. Multiple fenestrations in the septum primum and a moderate-sized membranous ventricular septal defect allowed blood to enter the morphologically left atrium and left ventricle. There was no deficiency of the atrioventricular canal septum, the atrioventricular valves were normal, and the great arteries were normally related to the ventricles. The segmental combination of this heart was: solitus atria, D-loop ventricles, and normally related great arteries. Ao, aorta; LRV, left renal vein; RRV, right renal vein; Infra Ren IVC, infrarenal inferior vena cava.*

with polysplenia (Table 39-2). The coronary sinus septum was absent in all patients with asplenia who had bilateral superior venae cavae but in only about half of polysplenic patients with bilateral superior venae cavae.

Bilateral Superior Venae Cavae. The high incidence of bilateral superior venae cavae in the patients with absence of the coronary sinus septum indicates that the distal portion of the left horn of the sinus venosus (or the right horn in situs inversus) is present in the majority of these patients. Consequently, the apparent absence of the coronary sinus (the usual derivative of the left horn of the sinus venosus) seems unlikely. It seems more likely that the deep fold that normally develops in embryos older than 25 somites, and separates the left horn of the sinus venosus from the left atrium,[14] failed to form. This makes the coronary sinus inapparent, because it becomes incorporated into the left atrial portion of the common atrium. When, in addition, the common pulmonary vein fails to develop from the back of the common atrium, and the septum primum and secundum are absent, the only component of the left atrium present is its appendage. This type of common atrium is formed primarily from the two horns of the sinus venosus and, in this sense, could be viewed as *bilaterally right atria*. Nonetheless, even this type of common atrium, which occurred in the asplenia cases with totally anomalous pulmonary venous connection to a systemic vein, is not composed of two right atria. It is composed of the right atrium, the unroofed coronary sinus, and the left atrial appendage.

When both atria receive systemic veins (e.g., bilateral superior venae cavae, bilateral hepatic veins, or an inferior vena cava to one atrium and hepatic vein to the other), the true abnormality is not bilaterally right atria but, rather, unroofing of the coronary sinus. Because the coronary sinus is located in the posteroinferior wall of the left atrium, any systemic vein that connects with the coronary sinus will drain into the left atrium when the coronary sinus is unroofed. This is true for all patients with or without visceral heterotaxy, because all the systemic veins connect directly only with the sinus venosus (Fig. 39-4). The proximity of the left atrium to the coronary sinus (the left horn of the sinus venosus) is shown in Fig. 39-4 and is responsible for the apparent *direct* connection of any of the systemic veins with the left atrium when the coronary sinus is unroofed.

Pulmonary Veins. The pulmonary venous connections are summarized in Table 39-3.

Anomalous connections of all the pulmonary veins to a systemic vein occurred in 64% of the patients with asplenia, 60% of those with a right-sided, single spleen, and in only one (2%) with polysplenia.

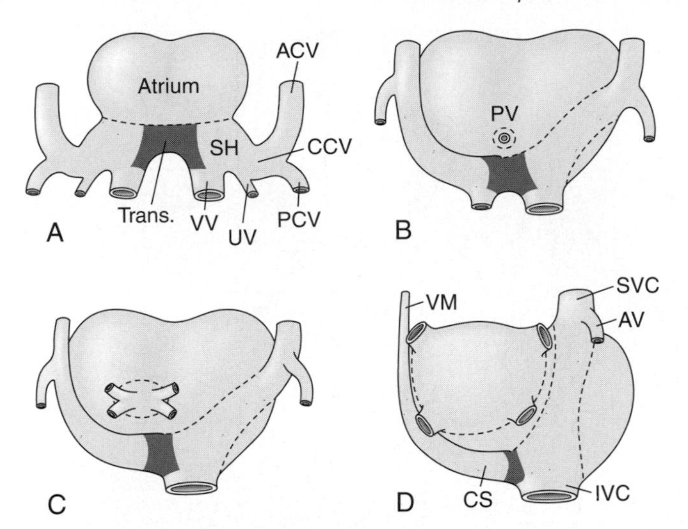

FIGURE 39–4 *Posterior view (diagrammatic) of the sinus venosus in embryos of various ages: A, A 3-mm crown-rump length; B, 5 mm; C, 12 mm; D, newborn. ACV, anterior cardinal vein; AV, azygos vein; CCV, common cardinal vein; CS, coronary sinus; IVC, inferior vena cava; PCV, posterior cardinal vein; PV, pulmonary vein; SH, sinus horn; SVC, superior vena cava; trans., tranverse portion of sinus venosus; UV, umbilical vein; VM, vein of Marshall; VV, vitelline vein.*

From Van Mierop LHS, Wiglesworth FW. Isomerism of the cardiac atria in the asplenia syndrome. Lab Invest 11:1303–1315, 1962, with permission.

In all of the polysplenic patients with partial or total anomalous pulmonary venous return to the right atrium, the connection of the pulmonary veins appeared normal externally. That is, the veins connected with the superior part of the posterior atrial wall between the superior venae cavae when present bilaterally, or to the left of a right superior vena cava in situs solitus, or to the right of a left superior vena cava in situs inversus. The anomalous pulmonary venous return appeared to be due to abnormal *shifting* of the atrial septum toward the anatomically left atrium rather than to an abnormal connection of the pulmonary veins with the right atrium.[15,23,24]

Usually, absence or hypoplasia of the septum secundum appeared to be responsible for the abnormal position and attachments of the septum primum. The abnormal attachments of the superior margin of septum primum to the superoposterior wall of the left atrium allowed in some cases a small or large interatrial communication which, strictly speaking, is not identical with a patent foramen ovale (Figs. 39-5, 39-6, 39-7, and 39-8). For this reason, we refer to this opening as an *interatrial communication*. In postmortem cases the absence of septum secundum made possible the visualization of the upper border of septum primum from the right atrium.

Depending on the extent of displacement of the septum primum, the two right pulmonary veins, or all four pulmonary veins, drained into the anatomically right atrium. In such cases, the anatomically right atrium contained half or all of the common pulmonary vein component that is usually incorporated into the left atrium. The anatomically left atrium was represented by a small chamber that connected with the left atrial appendage and the mitral valve or the mitral component of a common atrioventricular valve, and it received either only the left or none of the pulmonary veins (Figs. 39-6*A*, 39-6*B*, 39-7*A*, 39-7*B*, 39-7*C*, and 39-8). In some rare cases a persistent superior vena cava, associated with an unroofed coronary sinus, drained into the small left atrium.

Therefore, ipsilateral drainage of the pulmonary veins does not indicate bilaterally left atria but, rather, incorporation of part of the left atrium into the right atrium due to malposition of the septum primum.

This realization has significant therapeutic repercussions. Surgical correction of this type of partial or total anomalous pulmonary venous return can be achieved by resecting the malpositioned atrial septum and placing a new atrial septum

TABLE 39–3. Pulmonary Venous Connections in Visceral Heterotaxy with Congenital Heart Disease

	N = 109 Postmortem Cases					
	Asplenia (*n* = 58)		**Spleen (*n* = 5)**		**Polysplenia (*n* = 46)**	
Types of Pulmonary Venous Connections	**No.**	**%**	**No.**	**%**	**No.**	**%**
Normal to LA	6		2	40	15	
Normal to CA	2				13	
To LA with single orifice	12	21				
Total	20	34			28	61
All PVs to RA with abnormal attachments of septum 1°	1	2			10	22
To ipsilateral atrium					7	15
To a systemic vein	37	64	3	60	1	2

CA, common atrium; LA, left atrium; PV, pulmonary vein; RA, right atrium; septum 1°, septum primum.

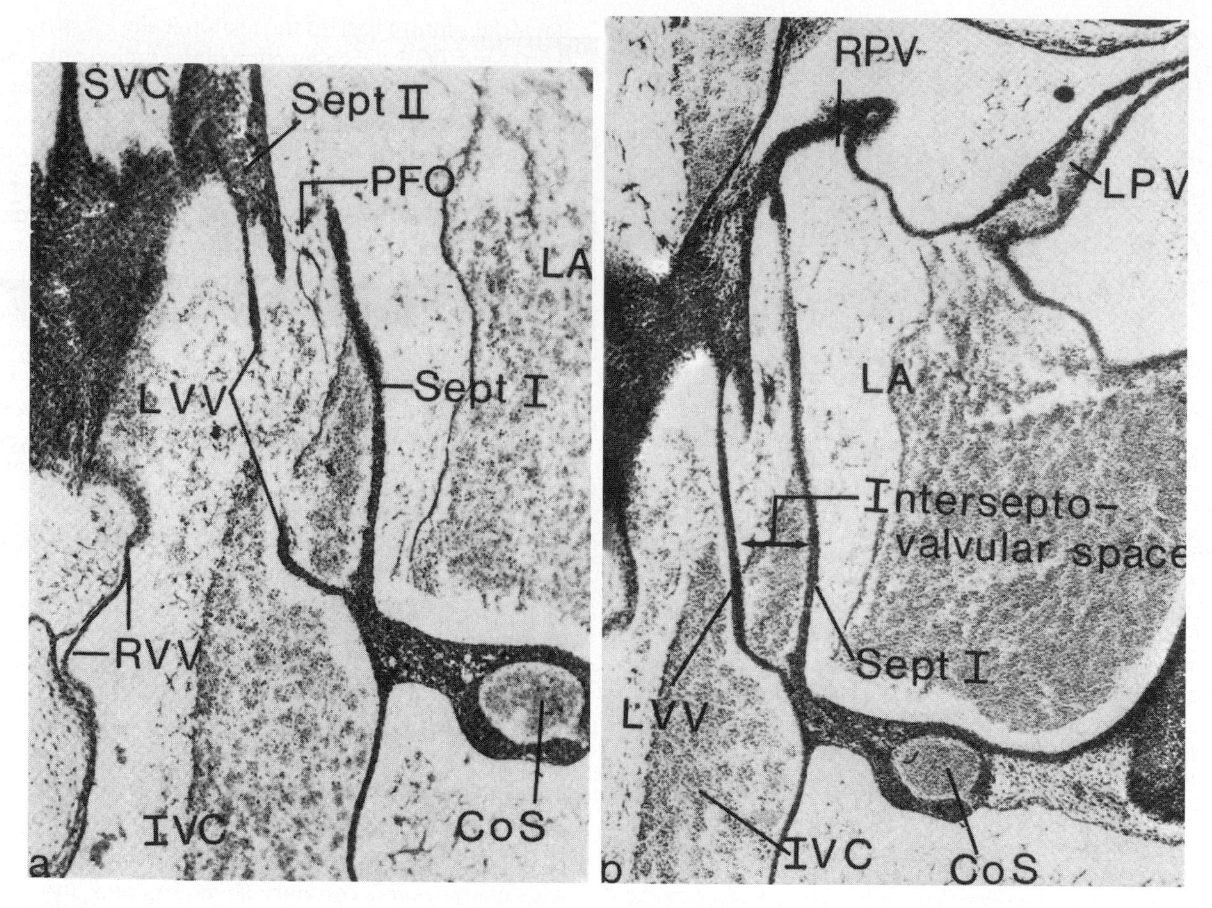

FIGURE 39–5 *A, Septum primum (Sept I) and the left venous valve (LVV) (embryo 914, 29 mm, 56 days of age, from the Minot Embryological Collection, Harvard Medical School). a, frontal section 490; B, frontal section 491, 20 μ dorsal to a. Sept I and the LVV both grow superiorly from sinus venosus fibrous tissue towards the superior limbic band of septum secundum (Sept II). Note that Sept I and the LVV are both directly continuous with the left wall of the inferior vena cava (IVC). Sept II is well developed, and Sept I lies to the left of the Sept II and opens into the left atrium (LA). The patent foramen ovale (PFO) is the space between the top of Sept I to the left, and the inferior rim of Sept II to the right. In B, the space between Sept I to the left and the LVV to the right is the intersepto-valvular space. The right pulmonary veins (RPV) enter the LA just to the left of the attachment of Sept I to Sept II. When the superior limbic band of Sept II is absent, the incoming systemic venous blood from the embryonic right atrium (RA) can displace the unattached upper free margin of Sept I into the LA to the left of the RPVs. Leftward displacement of Sept I into the LA can result in ipsilateral drainage of the pulmonary veins, despite the fact that all of the pulmonary veins are normally connected. Further leftward displacement of the unattached upper free margin of Sept I into the LA to the left of the left pulmonary veins (LPV) will result in totally anomalous pulmonary venous drainage into the RA of the normally connected RPVs and LPVs. See Figures 39-6 and 39-7. (Borax carmine and Lyons blue stain; original magnification ×100). From Van Praagh R, Corsini I. Cor triatriatum: pathologic anatomy and a consideration of morphogenesis based on 13 postmortem cases and a study of normal development of the pulmonary vein and atrial septum in 83 human embryos. Am Heart J 78:379, 1969, with permission.*

in such a position that all the pulmonary veins will be incorporated into the new left atrium. One such patient had only a small additional ventricular septal defect which could be closed easily. Of the 18 patients (17 with polysplenia and 1 with asplenia) with either ipsilateral pulmonary venous drainage or with all the pulmonary veins draining into the anatomically right atrium. 11 had normally related great arteries and anatomy suitable for complete surgical repair.

Atrial Septum and Atrioventricular Canal Septum. The incidence of a deficiency, absence, or malattachment of the septum primum in the various heterotaxic groups is presented in Table 39-4. The same table includes the incidence of deficiency or absence of the atrioventricular canal septum.

Atrial Situs. In patients with visceral heterotaxy the atrial situs is often difficult to determine on the basis of septal

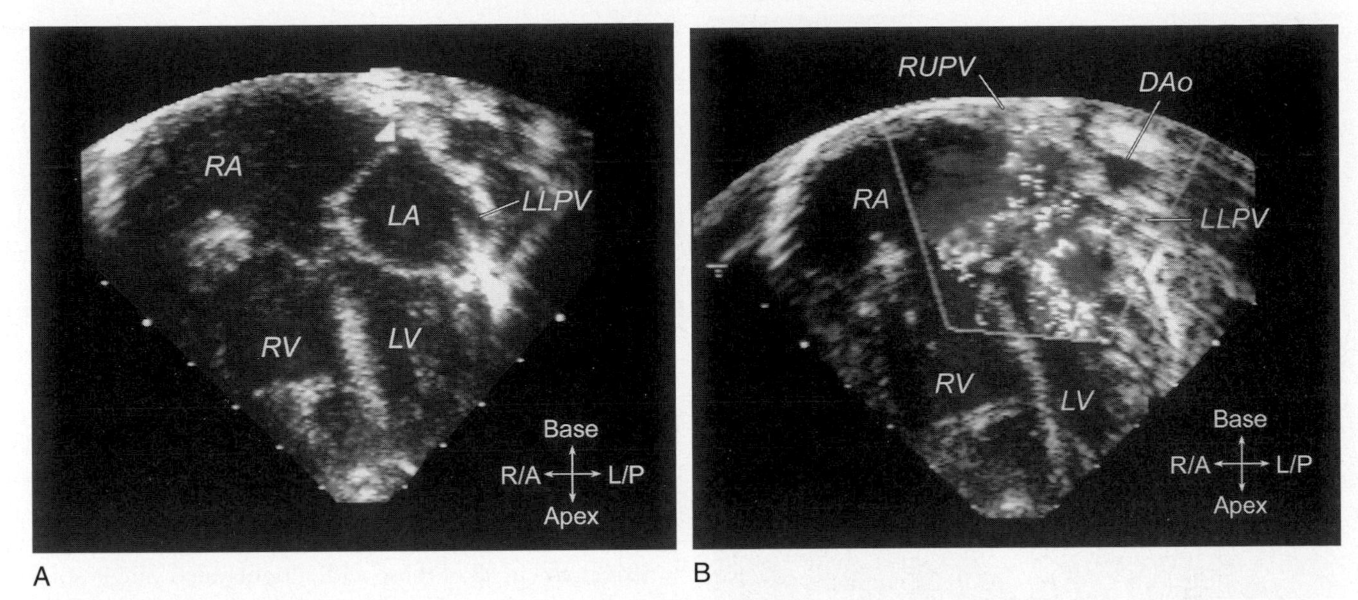

FIGURE 39–6 *A, Apical four-chamber view in a 3-year, 9-month-old child with atrial situs solitus and ventricular D-loop, malposition of septum primum, and drainage of the right pulmonary veins to the right atrium (RA). The left atrium (LA) is smaller than usual due to leftward displacement of the septum primum. The left lower pulmonary vein (LLPV) is seen entering the LA. The RA and right ventricle (RV) are dilated. The interatrial communication, a septum primum malposition defect, is seen between the posterior margin of septum primum and the posterior atrial wall (arrowhead). B, Color flow mapping in the same view confirms flow from the left lower pulmonary vein (LLPV) into the LA and flow from the right upper pulmonary vein (RUPV) into the RA. The descending thoracic aorta (DAo) is indicated as a reference marker to distinguish right and left pulmonary veins.*
From Edwards JE. Pathologic and developmental considerations in anomalous pulmonary venous connection. Mayo Clin Proc 28:411, 1953, with permission.

morphology[25] because the atrial septum is usually very deficient or absent. Consequently, the term *situs ambiguus* was coined to describe patients with unclear situs[26] and should be used when the atrial situs cannot be diagnosed with certainty. The diagnosis of the atrial situs in visceral heterotaxy is considered important for at least two reasons. First, it may lead to enhanced understanding of the etiology of visceral heterotaxy by demonstrating the high incidence of atrial situs inversus in these patients. Second, it makes possible the determination of atrioventricular situs concordance or discordance, which is essential for the more complete understanding of the internal organization of these hearts, and it can be predictive of the course of the conduction system. Review of specimens in this series has shown that atrial situs can be determined in the majority of patients with visceral heterotaxy on the basis of the following considerations.

It is generally accepted that the atrium into which the right horn of the sinus venosus is incorporated is the morphologically right atrium.[14,27] The right horn of the sinus venosus includes the orifices of the inferior and superior venae cavae and the smooth atrial wall between them. The coronary sinus, which represents the reduced left horn of the sinus venosus (Fig. 39-4), normally opens into the sinus venosus component of the morphologically right atrium. Hence, the atrium that receives the superior and inferior venae cavae and the orifice of the coronary sinus is the anatomically right atrium.

It is also well documented that some or all of the pulmonary veins may drain into the right atrium because of malposition of the septum primum. Therefore, when all of the systemic veins and some or all of the pulmonary veins drain into one atrium, which is not a common atrium because another small atrium is present, this large atrium contains the morphologically right atrium.

Until recently, it was thought that the uninterrupted inferior vena cava always connected directly with the right atrium and could be used as a marker for the atrial situs identification. However, the authors are now aware of an angiocardiographically documented case in which a noninterrupted, left-sided, and small inferior vena cava connected with a normally roofed coronary sinus and indirectly with the right atrium.[47] This inferior vena cava received only one hepatic vein. All the other hepatic veins formed a larger confluence that entered the right atrium directly. In such a case, if the coronary sinus were unroofed, it could be possible for the inferior vena cava to drain into the left atrium via the unroofed coronary sinus, leading to an erroneous

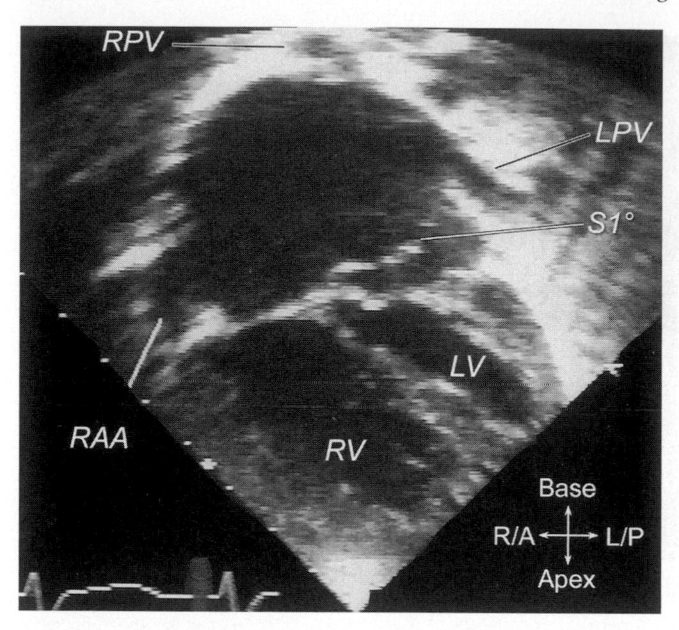

FIGURE 39–7 *An apical four-chamber view in this infant with atrial situs solitus, ventricular D-loop, and tetralogy of Fallot. There is extreme malposition of septum primum (S1°) so that all of the pulmonary veins drain into the right atrium. In this view both a right pulmonary vein (RPV) and a left pulmonary vein (LPV) can be seen entering the right atrium. In addition to the septum primum malposition defect, there are multiple fenestrations in the substance of septum primum. The orifice of the right atrial appendage (RAA) is seen on the right side of the atrium. This is Case 21, Table I, in Van Praagh S, Carrera ME, Sanders SP, et al. Partial or total direct pulmonary venous drainage to the right atrium due to malposition of septum primum. Chest 107:1488, 1995, with permission.*

diagnosis of the atrial situs. In such cases, the size and position of the atrial appendages and the connections of the pulmonary veins could help to determine the atrial situs. The above-mentioned embryologic and pathologic findings were used to identify the atrial situs in the 109 patients in this series.

Anatomically Right Atrium. The anatomically right atrium was considered to be the atrium that received (a) all the systemic veins while a separate atrium received all of the pulmonary veins; (b) all of the systemic veins and some or all of the pulmonary veins without being a common atrium; and (c) the orifice of a normal coronary sinus. A fourth criterion for identifying the right atrium, based on the review of the specimens in this series, was the size and position of the atrial appendages. Although the shape of the atrial appendages may be similar in many cases of visceral heterotaxy, the right atrial appendage is usually the larger and is more anteriorly placed (Fig. 39-9*A* and 39-9*B*).

Anatomically Left Atrium. The anatomically left atrium was the atrium that received (a) half or all of the pulmonary veins and none of the systemic veins (except for a persistent superior vena cava associated with an unroofed coronary sinus in cases with bilateral superior venae cavae); or (b) none of the pulmonary veins and none of the systemic veins. A third, less reliable, criterion for identification of the left atrium, based on review of the specimens of this series, was the size and position of its appendage, which is usually smaller and more posteriorly located than the right atrial appendage (Fig. 39-9*A* and 39-9*B*).

Using criteria 1 through 3 for the right atrium and 1 and 2 for the left atrium (i.e., the systemic and pulmonary venous connections), it was possible to diagnose the atrial situs in all of the patients with polysplenia (100%), in 21 (36%) of those with asplenia, and in 1 (20%) patient with a single, right-sided spleen. When the size and position of the atrial appendages were also taken into consideration, it was possible to diagnose the atrial situs in 47 of those with asplenia (81%) and in all of those with a right-sided, single spleen. In the remaining 11 cases of asplenia (19%), the inferior vena cava was contralateral to the larger and more anterior appendage. In these cases, it could not be ascertained whether the inferior vena cava was connected to the left atrium via an unroofed coronary sinus, or whether the inferior vena cava connected directly with the morphologically right atrium that had the smaller atrial appendage. Consequently, the diagnosis of atrial situs ambiguus seemed to be justified.

The presently used methods of echocardiography do not always allow accurate evaluation of the size and position of the appendages. Hence, the diagnosis of the atrial situs is not always possible during life. For these patients, one should use the term *atrial situs ambiguus*.

In this postmortem series, the incidence of atrial situs inversus, determined with the above-outlined criteria, was highest in patients with a single, right-sided spleen (60%). Next in frequency of situs inversus were the asplenias (31%), and last, the polysplenias (22%) (Table 39-5). There was no significant difference in the distribution of atrial situs between the right and left polysplenic groups. This high incidence of atrial situs inversus in all the heterotaxic patients is noteworthy, and it may provide an important clue in the understanding of the etiology of abnormal visceral lateralization.

Atrioventricular Valves. A common atrioventricular valve (Fig. 39-10) was present in 69% of the patients with asplenia. The single atrioventricular valve that was present in each of the eight cases of asplenia with a single right ventricle (14%) could represent either a common atrioventricular valve entering the single right ventricle or a tricuspid valve with atresia and absence of the mitral valve (Fig. 39-11). Both atrioventricular valves were normal in 7% of asplenic patients. The distribution of atrioventricular valve abnormalities (Table 39-4) was similar in the patients with a single, right-sided spleen.

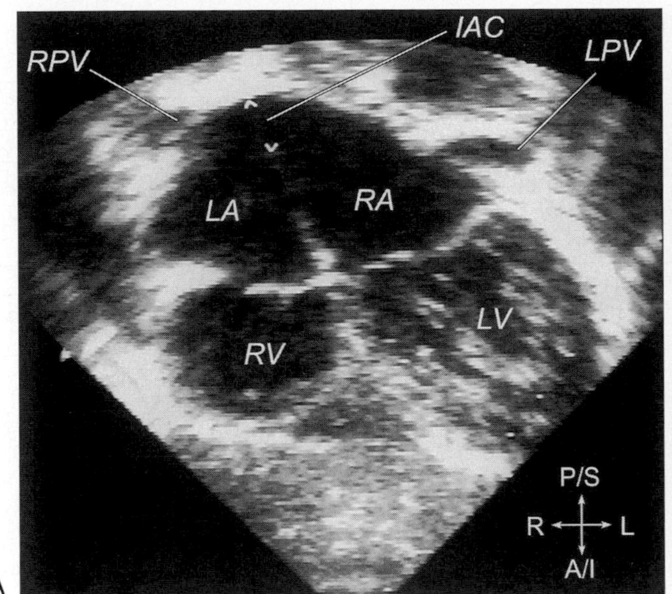

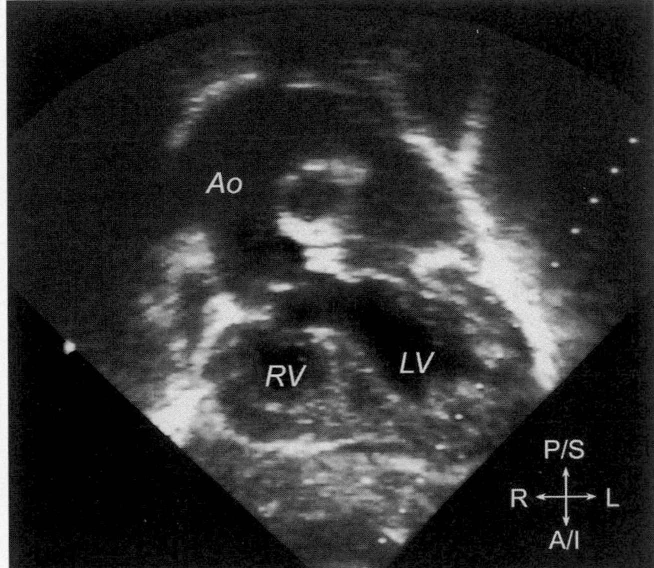

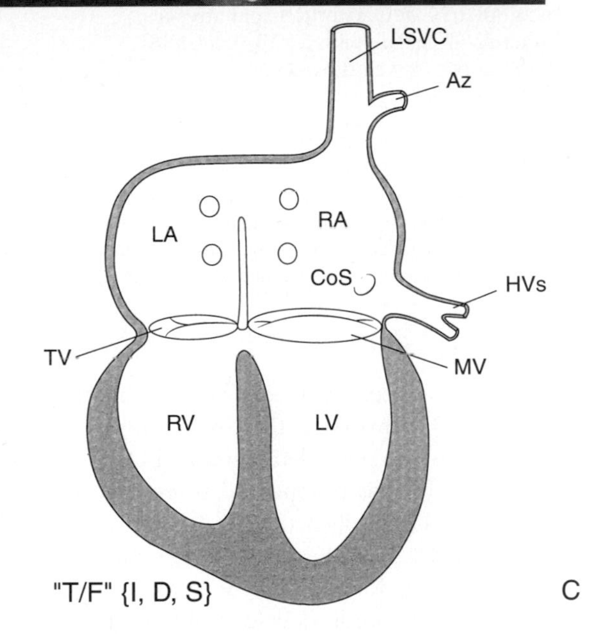

FIGURE 39–8 *A, Posterior subxiphoid long-axis view in a patient with atrial situs inversus, ventricular D-loop, a tetralogy of Fallot type conus, and levocardia. There is a large interatrial communication of the septum primum malposition type (arrowheads) between the rightwardly malposed septum primum and the posterior atrial wall. A right pulmonary vein (RPV) is seen connecting with the right-sided left atrium (LA). A left pulmonary vein (LPV) drains into the left-sided right atrium (RA). B, A more anterior subxiphoid long-axis view in the same patient demonstrates the large conal septal malalignment ventricular septal defect and the overriding aorta (Ao) typical of tetralogy of Fallot. The right ventricle (RV) is mildly hypoplastic. C, Diaphragmatic presentation of the systemic and pulmonary venous connections of the same case. Despite the atrioventricular discordance the ventriculoarterial relationships were normal. The left-sided inferior vena cava was interrupted and extended with a left azygos to the left superior vena cava (LSVC) which entered the left-sided RA. This infant exhibited complete congenital atrioventricular block possibly due to the atrioventricular discordance. Atrioventricular discordance with normally related great arteries occurred frequently in cases of visceral heterotaxy with polysplenia.*

Atrioventricular valve anomalies were present in 65% of patients with polysplenia. A common atrioventricular valve was also the most common anomaly in polysplenia, occurring in 33% of patients. Next most common was a cleft mitral valve with an intact ventricular septum, which occurred in 22%. Two separate and patent atrioventricular valves were present in 35% of patients with polysplenia (Table 39-4).

The frequent occurrence of partial or complete common atrioventricular canal was noted previously by Ivemark.[5] In his series of heterotaxic patients there appeared to be a linkage between atrioventricular canal defects and malformations of the conotruncus. This linkage was also present in our asplenic patients and in our patients with a single, right-sided spleen. A similar linkage did not appear to exist in polysplenic patients. Despite the high incidence of atrioventricular canal defects, conal development was normal in all except five polysplenic patients (Table 39-5).

Ventricles. Ventricular looping did not differ as strikingly between patients with asplenia and polysplenia as did other aspects of cardiac development. A ventricular D-loop was present in 62% of patients with asplenia and 70% of patients with polysplenia, whereas in the remainder a ventricular L-loop was present. A ventricular D-loop was present in all five patients (100%) with a single, right-sided spleen (Table 39-5).

The incidence of ventricular inversion (L-loop ventricles) was almost identical to the incidence of dextrocardia in both the asplenias and the polysplenias. The presence of

TABLE 39–4. Atrial Septa, Atrioventricular Canal, and Ventricular Size in Visceral Heterotaxy with Congenital Heart Disease

	N = 109 Postmortem Cases					
			Single Right			
	Asplenia (n = 58)		Spleen (n = 5)		Polysplenia (n = 46)	
Types of Pulmonary Venous Connections	No.	%	No.	%	No.	%
Atrial septa						
Septum primum present with normal attachments	10	19	3	60	8	19
Septum primum displaced toward the morphologically LA	1	2			15	35
Septum primum resected or artifacted	4°				3*	
Absent septum primum, septum secundum and AVC septum	31	57			13	30
Septum primum present with uncommitted attachments	12	22	2	40	7	16
Atrioventricular Canal						
Complete CAVC with CAVV	40	69	2	40	15	33
Incomplete CAVC (ASD primum or common atrium with cleft MV)					10	22
Incomplete CAVC with MAt	2	3	1	20	2	4
Incomplete CAVC with straddling TV and MS					1	2
CAVC with single RV	8	14				
Incomplete CAVC with tricuspid atresia	4	7	1	20	2	4
Intact AVC septum with 2 AVV Ventricles	4	7	1	20	16	35
Both ventricles well developed	26	45	2	40	29	63
LV hypoplasia	16	28	2	40	11	24
RV hypoplasia	6	10	1	20	5	11
LV absent	8	14				
RV absent	2	3			1	2

°Surgically or postmortem artificiated cases excluded for the purpose of percentage computations.

ASD, atrial septal defect; AVC, atrioventricular canal; AVV, atrioventricular valve; CAVC, common atrioventricular canal; CAVV, common atrioventricular valve; LA, left atrium; LV, left ventricle; MAt, mitral atresia; MS, mitral stenosis; MV, mitral valve; RV, right ventricle; TV, tricuspid valve.

dextrocardia appeared to correlate better with the presence of ventricular inversion than with the presence of atrial inversion in the polysplenic group. Both dextrocardia and ventricular inversion appeared to occur often in patients with visceral heterotaxy (Table 39-5).

The ventricular development in all three groups is summarized in Table 39-4. There was a high incidence of left ventricular underdevelopment in all the heterotaxic patients (Table 39-4). In eight (14%) cases of asplenia, only the right ventricle could be identified (Fig. 39-11). The authors suspect that the right ventricular predominance in many of the heterotaxic patients is related to the hemodynamic effect of the cardiac malformations present prenatally and postnatally.

Ventricular Outflow Tract Obstruction. The pulmonary outflow tract was obstructed in all patients with a single, right-sided spleen and in all except two patients with asplenia. One of the two patients without pulmonary outflow obstruction had aortic atresia, which is very rare, and the other had a double-outlet right ventricle.[28–31] The pulmonary obstruction was subvalvar in 96% of the patients with asplenia and was often associated with valvar stenosis or atresia (Table 39-5). The high incidence of pulmonary outflow tract obstruction has been reported in several series of patients with asplenia.[32]

The picture was much less uniform among polysplenic patients. Both outflow tracts were unobstructed in 35% of patients. Subpulmonary stenosis was seen in 43%, and subaortic stenosis in 22% (Table 39-5 and Fig. 39-9*B*).

Ventriculoarterial Alignment. The ventriculoarterial alignments are detailed in Table 39-5. Asplenic and polysplenic patients diverged widely with respect to ventriculoarterial alignment. In nearly all of the patients with asplenia, the alignment was double-outlet right ventricle (82%) or transposition (9%). Normally related great arteries were present in only 9% of patients. In contrast, the great arteries were normally related in 61% of polysplenic patients. Double-outlet right ventricle was present in 17 (37%) patients with polysplenia, but all except four of these patients had only subpulmonary conus without subaortic conus (Fig. 39-9). Consequently, as a rule, in most of the patients who had polysplenia with a double-outlet right ventricle, the conotruncus was reminiscent of normally related great arteries (subpulmonary conus without subaortic conus). The absence of subaortic conus in cases of double-outlet right ventricle appeared to be responsible for the subaortic

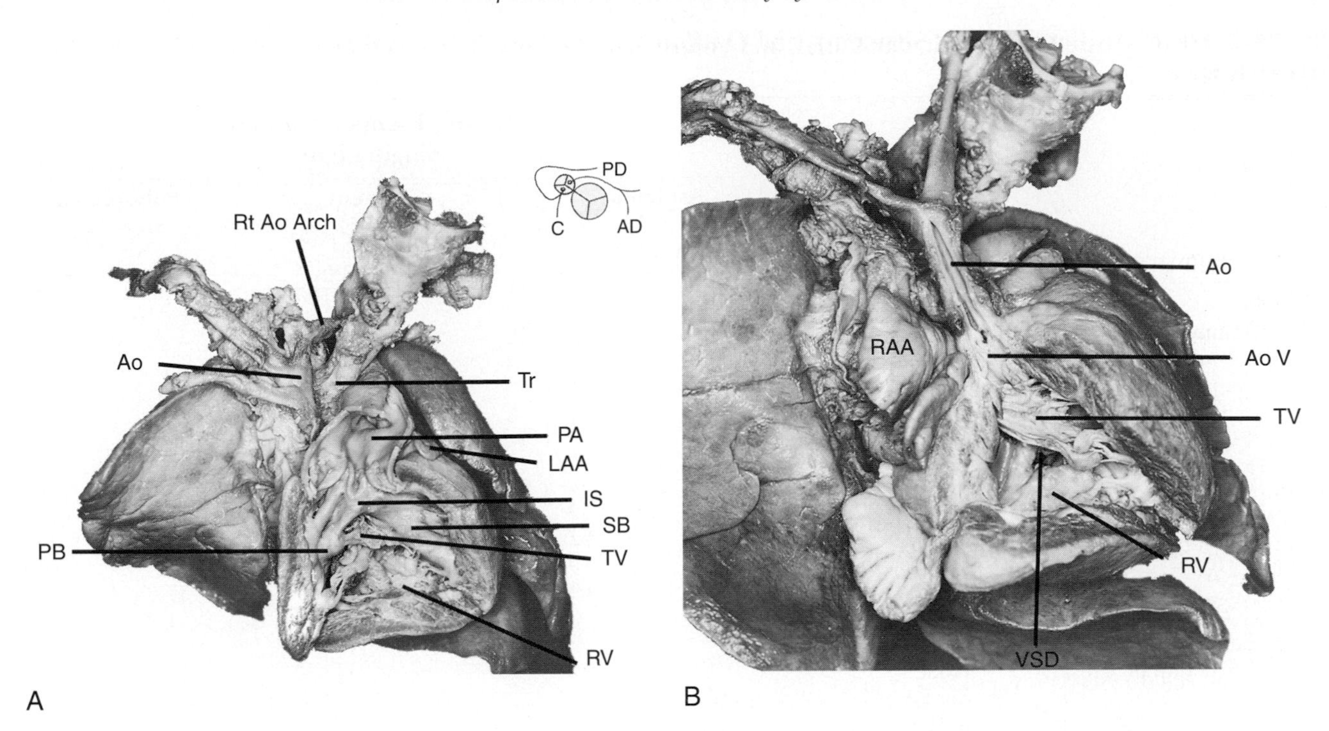

FIGURE 39–9 *The heart and lungs of a 3-day-old girl with visceral heterotaxy and multiple, right-sided spleens. There was a right aortic arch with a left ductus arteriosus and an aberrant left subclavian. A right superior vena cava and the hepatic venous confluence entered the morphologically right atrium. The inferior vena cava was interrupted and continued into a left azygos, which joined the left superior vena cava and entered the morphologically left atrium (unroofed coronary sinus). All the pulmonary veins entered the morphologically right atrium. A, Opened right ventricle (RV) showing the well-developed subpulmonary conus under a normal pulmonary artery (PA). The infundibular septum (IS) and the septal band (SB) are well developed and normally positioned. The small left atrial appendage (LAA) is seen to the left of the PA. PB, parietal band; Tr, trachea. B, Opened RV showing the severe subaortic stenosis caused by the position of the aortic valve (AoV) between the redundant tricuspid valve component (TV) of the common atrioventricular valve and the infundibular septum (not seen in this view). The AoV and the ascending aorta (Ao) are very underdeveloped. The large right atrial appendage (RAA) is seen to the right of the Ao. The ventricular component of the atrioventricular septal defect is partly seen (VSD). This case is an example of double-outlet right ventricle with solitus atria, normally positioned ventricles (D-loop), and normal conus (i.e., only subpulmonary conus). The normalcy of the ventricular loop and the conus are reflected in the normal origin and distribution of the coronary arteries (see insert A). AD, anterior descending coronary; C, conus coronary; PD, posterior descending coronary.*
From Van Praagh S, Antoniadis S, Otero-Coto E, et al. Common atrioventricular canal with and without conotruncal malformations: an anatomic study of 251 postmortem cases. In Nora JJ, Takao A (eds). Congenital Heart Disease: Causes and Processes. Mount Kisco, NY: Futura, 1984, pp 599–639, with permission.

stenosis which was present. The aortic valve had descended to the level of the tricuspid valve and was *squeezed* between the tricuspid valve and the conal septum (Fig. 39-9B). Transposition of the great arteries was present in only one case (2%) of polysplenia. In this single case of polysplenia and transposition of the great arteries, the conus was absent bilaterally, resulting in direct fibrous continuity between both semilunar valves and the anterior leaflet of the common atrioventricular valve.

Segmental Combinations. There was a great diversity of segmental combinations in patients with asplenia and polysplenia, reflecting the inconsistency of the situs of the various cardiac segments, which is the hallmark of visceral heterotaxy. The presence of atrioventricular discordance without transposition of the great arteries in 11% of the patients with polysplenia is noteworthy and reflects one of the most specific characteristics of this group (i.e., absence of subaortic conus) (Table 39-5). Atrioventricular discordance with normally related great arteries results in transposition physiology and can be repaired with the left ventricle as the systemic ventricle by performing an atrial switch operation.[33]

Linkages Between Anomalies. Despite the considerable variation of the situs of the different cardiac segments and the variability of the segmental combinations seen in heterotaxic individuals, several definite linkages between the heart defects were observed.

TABLE 39–5. Heart Position, Cardiac Segments, and Outflow Obstructions in Visceral Heterotaxy with Congenital Heart Disease

		N = 109 Postmortem Cases					
		Asplenia (*n* = 58)		Single Right Spleen (*n* = 5)		Polysplenia (*n* = 46)	
		No.	%	No.	%	No.	%
Levocardia		37	64	5	100	31	67
Dextrocardia		21	36			15	33
Atrial situs	Solitus	29	50	2	40	36	78
	Inversus	18	31	3	60	10	22
	Ambiguus	11	19				
Ventricular loop	D-	36	62	5	100	32	70
	L-	22	38			14	30
Type of conus	SubPA	5	9	1	20	41	89
	SubAo	5	9				
	Bilat	48	82	4	80	5[*]	11
Ventriculo-arterial relationship	Normal	5	9			28	61
	DORV	48	82	5	100	17	37
	TGA	5	9			1	2
AV discordance with NRGA						5	11
Outflow obstruction or atresia	None	1	2			16	35
	SubPA	56[†]	96	5[†]	100	20[†]	43
	SubAo	1[‡]	2			10	22

AV, atrioventricular; Bilat, bilateral; DORV, double-outlet right ventricle; NRGA, normally related great arteries; SubAo, subaortic; SubPA, subpulmonary; TGA, transposition of the great arteries.

[*]In one case there was TGA with bilaterally absent conus, resulting in fibrous continuity of the aortic and pulmonary valves with the anterior leaflet of the common AV valve. The other four patients had DORV.

[†]In 21 cases of asplenia (36%), three cases of right-sided single spleen (60%), and two cases of polysplenia (4%) there was pulmonary atresia.

[‡]A very rare case of aortic atresia.

1. All patients with an unroofed coronary sinus, regardless of the status of the spleen, also had complete or partial common atrioventricular canal. The reverse was true in the groups with asplenia and right-sided, single spleen, but not in patients with polysplenia.
2. All patients who had asplenia or a single, right-sided spleen with an abnormal atrioventricular canal also had an abnormal conus (bilateral or subaortic). The reverse was not always true, and the polysplenic patients did not show this linkage at all.
3. All patients with asplenia, single, right-sided spleen, and polysplenia with totally anomalous pulmonary venous connection to a systemic vein had an abnormal conus (bilateral or subaortic). The reverse was not always true.
4. Polysplenia was characterized by the absence of subaortic conus even in cases of transposition, double-outlet right ventricle or atrioventricular discordance. Only 4 of the 46 polysplenic patients with double-outlet right ventricle had bilateral conus. The single patient with transposition of the great arteries had bilaterally deficient conus.

In patients with visceral heterotaxy, the association of heart defects makes it possible to suspect asplenia or polysplenia.

Associated Anatomic Findings in Asplenia

Asplenia should be suspected when the following defects coexist: (a) an intact inferior vena cava, (b) an unroofed coronary sinus, (c) totally anomalous pulmonary venous connection to a systemic vein, (d) a common atrioventricular canal, (e) double-outlet right ventricle or transposition with bilateral or subaortic conus, and (f) pulmonary stenosis or atresia.

In a few instances, the same defects may exist in patients with a right-sided, single spleen.

Associated Anatomic Finding in Polysplenia

Polysplenia (right- or left-sided) should be suspected when the following defects coexist: (a) an interrupted inferior vena cava, (b) totally or partially anomalous pulmonary venous drainage to the right atrium, (c) complete or partial common atrioventricular canal, and (d) normally related great arteries or double outlet right ventricle without subaortic conus even in cases with atrioventricular discordance (Fig. 39-8).

Clinical Manifestations

Physical Examination. Because nearly all patients with asplenia or a single, right-sided spleen also have pulmonary

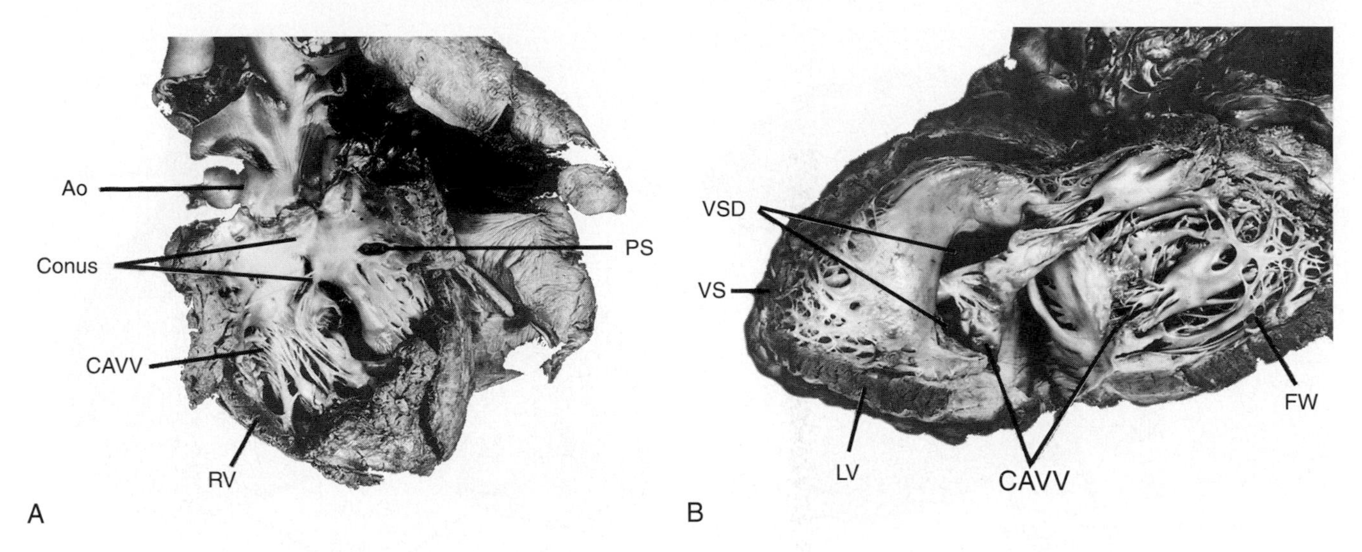

FIGURE 39–10 *The heart and lung of a young girl (4-year, 9 months) with visceral heterotaxy and asplenia. The heart was in the left chest. The inferior vena cava was left-sided below the liver but switched to the right at the level of the liver and entered the right-sided atrium, which had the larger and more anterior appendage. All the pulmonary veins entered the common atrium to the left of the subdividing atrial strand (inferior limbic band) through a common orifice. The ventricles were normally located (D-loop) and both great arteries emerged from the morphologically right ventricle (double-outlet right ventricle). Hence, the segmental combination was: solitus atria (S), D-loop ventricles (D), and D-malposed aorta. A, Opened right ventricle (RV) showing a well-developed subaortic conus (conus) and a defect within the conal septum representing the site of the severe subpulmonary stenosis (PS). The tricuspid component of the common atrioventricular valve (CAVV) and the right ventricular aorta (Ao) are well seen. B, Opened left ventricle (LV) showing the characteristic left ventricular septal surface (VS), the fine trabeculation of the free wall (FW), and the mitral component of the CAVV. VSD, ventricular septal defect.*
Van Praagh S, Antoniadis S, Otero-Coto E, et al. Common atrioventricular canal with and without conotruncal malformations: an anatomic study of 251 postmortem cases. In Nora JJ, Takao A (eds). Congenital Heart Disease: Causes and Processes. Mount Kisco, NY: Futura, 1984, pp 599–639, with permission.

stenosis or atresia with a large ventricular septal defect or single ventricle, cyanosis is almost universal. Large aortopulmonary collateral vessels are rare in heterotaxic patients with pulmonary atresia. Therefore, if the ductus is allowed to constrict, profound cyanosis will develop, with metabolic acidosis and circulatory collapse. A harsh systolic murmur is usually indicative of pulmonary stenosis, whereas the absence of murmur, or a continuous murmur, is more consistent with pulmonary atresia. If atrioventricular valve regurgitation is present it may be difficult to distinguish this murmur from that due to pulmonary stenosis. The liver may be palpable across the abdomen if the two lobes are symmetrical. As previously reported,[31] there was a predominance of males in the group with asplenia and in those with a single, right-sided spleen (Table 39-6).

In contrast, the clinical findings in polysplenia are highly variable because of the variability of the associated heart defects. In general, infants with polysplenia tend to be less seriously ill than infants with asplenia because of the rarity of pulmonary atresia and totally anomalous pulmonary venous connections to a systemic vein in the former patients. This is reflected in the age range and median death (Table 39-6).

Electrocardiography. The electrocardiogram was often helpful in determining atrial situs on the basis of the frontal plane axis of the P wave. In 42 of the patients with asplenia, one or more 12-lead electrocardiograms were examined for atrial situs (Fig. 39-12). In 13 (92%) of 14 patients with the anatomic diagnosis of situs inversus, the P wave axis was greater than 90 degrees, indicating atrial inversion. Also, the P wave axis correctly indicated atrial situs solitus in 24 (86%) of 28 patients who had atrial situs solitus at necropsy.

The P-wave axis of the patients with polysplenia was unreliable for determining atrial situs because ectopic rhythms were common. The atrial pacemaker appeared to vary from one examination to the next in many patients.

As noted by other investigators,[34] conduction disturbances and other rhythm disorders occurred frequently in patients with polysplenia. Complete heart block was present in 22%, nodal rhythm in 9%, and coronary sinus rhythm in 7% of our patients for whom an electrocardiogram was available. In some patients the rhythm disorders followed cardiac catheterization or noncardiac surgery (gastrostomy). In at least 2 of the 19 patients with rhythm disorders, fetal

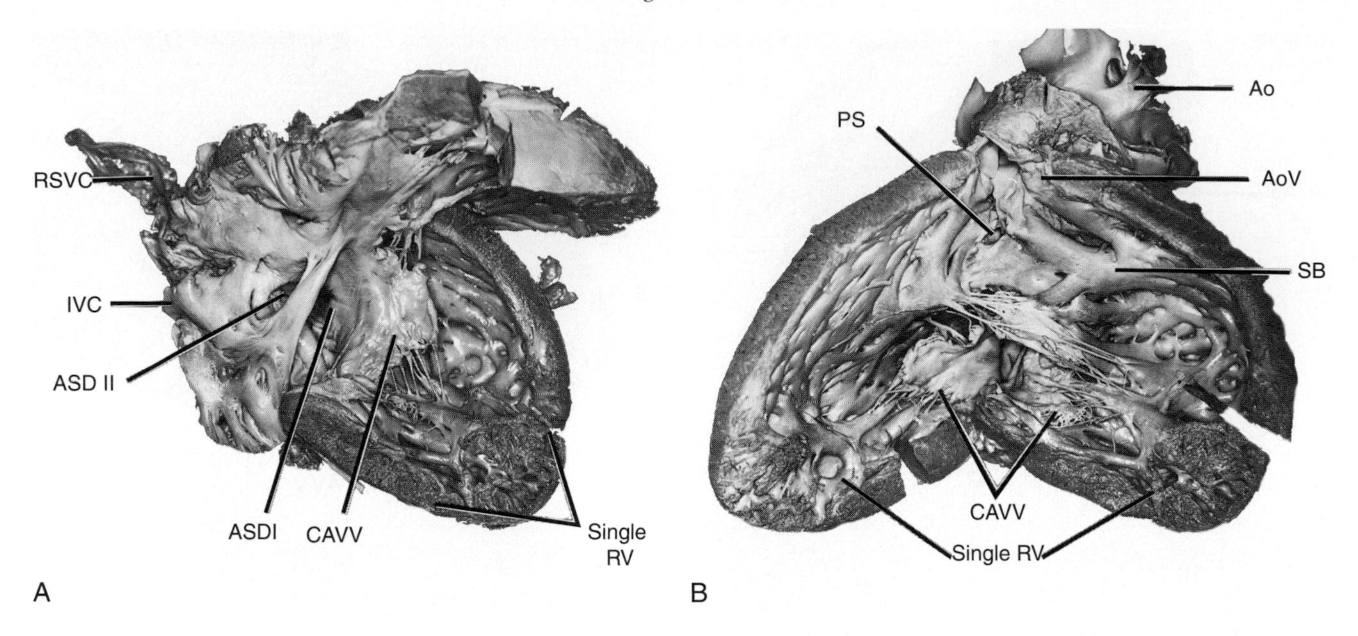

FIGURE 39–11 *The heart of a young boy (3 years, 3 months) with visceral heterotaxy and asplenia. A, Inferior view of the right-sided morphologically right atrium and the inflow of the morphologically single right ventricle (RV). The RA receives the right superior vena cava (RSVC) and the inferior vena cava (IVC). There is a large secundum type of atrial septal defect (ASD II) superior and posterior to the inferior limbic band; a primum type of atrial septal defect (ASD I) is located in front of and below the inferior limbic band. There was totally anomalous pulmonary venous connection to the junction of the RSVC with the RA. The coronary sinus septum was absent and the left superior vena cava appeared to join the left atrium directly. The common atrioventricular valve (CAVV) underlies both the right- and left-sided atrium. B, Anterior view of the opened single RV. The septal band (SB), moderator band, and anterior papillary muscle group are left-sided, indicating that this is a right-handed (D-loop) RV. Double-outlet right ventricle is present with a bilateral conus (subaortic and subpulmonary) separating both semilunar valves from the CAVV. The aortic valve (AoV) lies anteriorly, superiorly, and somewhat to the left of the stenotic pulmonary valve. The subvalvar pulmonary stenosis (PS) mimics a defect within the conal septum. A left ventricular cavity could not be identified, although its microscopic existence cannot be precluded. Ao, aorta.*
Modified from Van Praagh S, Davidoff A, Chin A, et al. Double outlet right ventricle: anatomic types and developmental implications based on a study of 101 autopsied cases. Coeur 13:389, 1982, with permission.

bradycardia was observed. This was subsequently determined to be an inherent atrial bradycardia rather than a sign of fetal distress. The diagnosis of the heterotaxy syndrome by fetal echocardiogram in such circumstances should suggest a rhythm disturbance (heart block or atrial bradycardia) as the cause of the bradycardia rather than fetal distress and, thus, prevent an unnecessary cesarean section.

All the patients with asplenia or a single, right-sided spleen had normal sinus rhythm.

Chest Radiography. In the asplenia syndrome the heart size is usually normal or small and the lungs, oligemic. Cardiac enlargement usually indicates atrioventricular valve regurgitation. Symmetry of the liver and ectopic location of the stomach bubble may be noted as well. An over penetrated frontal view is useful for determining the bronchial anatomy, usually bilaterally eparterial bronchi. Pulmonary venous congestion with hazy lung fields and indistinct vessel outlines may develop in infants with obstructed totally anomalous pulmonary venous connection, especially after the ductus is opened with prostaglandin E_1.

Radiographic findings in patients with polysplenia depend on the heart defect(s) present. On the lateral chest radiograph, the inferior vena cava shadow is absent in patients with an interrupted inferior vena cava and azygos extension. An over penetrated frontal view is useful for determining the bronchial anatomy, usually bilaterally hyparterial bronchi.

Echocardiography.* Discovering the variable, and often complex, anatomy seen in the heterotaxy syndrome is a major undertaking. An organized, segmental approach is essential in such patients. The examiner must develop and consciously go through a checklist of anatomic structures to be sure that all have been examined. Given a compulsive echocardiographer and a comprehensive checklist, most, if not all, pertinent anatomy can be determined using echocardiography.

---

*The section Echocardiography was contributed by Dr. Steven P. Saunders

TABLE 39–6. Age at Death and Male/Female Ratio in Patients with Heterotaxy and Congenital Heart Disease

	Single Right Spleen $n = 5$	Asplenia $n = 58$	Polysplenia* $n = 46$
Age range	1 d to 22 m	5′ to 14 2/12 yr	10 h to 25 yr
Median age at death	6 d	14 d	11.5 m
Male/female ratio	4	1.5	0.9

*Sex and age known in 44 of the 46 patients.
Accent (′), minutes; h, hours; d, days; m, months; yr, years.

The inferior vena cava, hepatic veins and their atrial connection(s), as well as the abdominal aorta, are best seen using subxiphoid views.[35] The superior vena cava on either side can be imaged using suprasternal notch or high, left or right parasternal views.[18,36] The superior vena cava termination of an azygos vein can also be seen using a right or left, high parasternal, parasagittal view. The coronary sinus is seen well in an apical four-chamber view, angled posteriorly.[37] When dilated, the coronary sinus can also be seen from subxiphoid and parasternal long axis views.

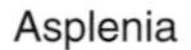

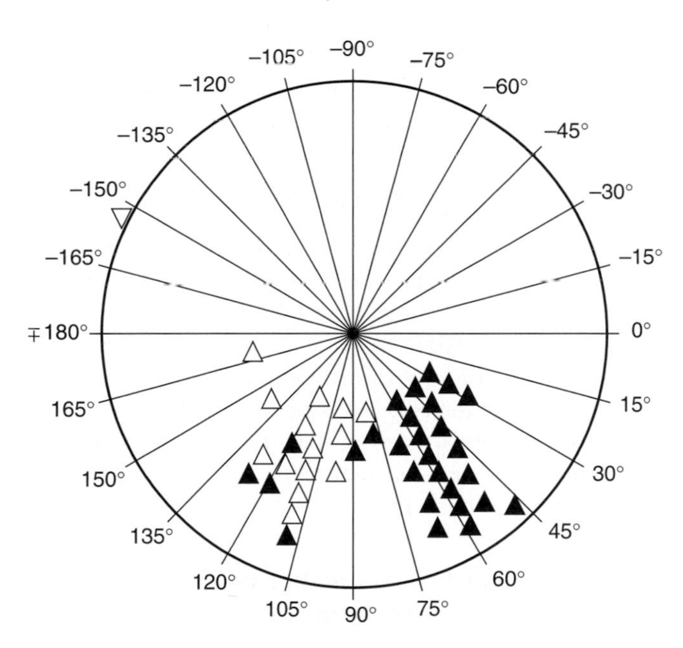

FIGURE 39–12 *The P-wave axis in the electrocardiogram in 42 patients with asplenia compared with the anatomic diagnosis of atrial situs solitus (closed triangles) or atrial situs inversus (open triangles). Of the 28 patients with atrial situs solitus, 24 (86%) had the expected P axis between 30 degrees and 90 degrees. Of the 14 patients with atrial situs inversus, 13 (92%) had the expected P axis between 90 and 150 degrees.*
From Van Praagh S, Kreutzer J, Alday L, et al. Systemic and pulmonary venous connections in visceral heterotaxy, with emphasis on the diagnosis of atrial situs: a study of 109 postmortem cases. In Clark E, Takao A (eds). Developmental Cardiology: Morphogenesis and Function. Mt. Kisco, NY: Futura, 1990, pp. 671–721, with permission.

Normally, connecting pulmonary veins can be seen from a number of views, including apical four-chamber, subxiphoid long- and short-axis, and suprasternal short-axis views. Subxiphoid views are especially good for pulmonary veins connecting below the diaphragm.[38] Pulmonary veins connecting anomalously to the innominate vein or the superior vena cava can usually be imaged using suprasternal notch or high parasternal views.[36] Whatever the connection, the individual pulmonary veins can be seen best from suprasternal or high sternal border views. Doppler color flow mapping is extremely useful for detecting flow in the pulmonary veins and for identifying individual veins.

The atria and atrial septum are best examined using the subxiphoid and apical views.[39,40] The malpositioned septum primum which shifted towards the anatomically left atrium and the resulting drainage of the right or all the pulmonary veins to the right atrium, is well seen in the four chamber apical view (Figs. 39-6*A*, 39-6*B*, 39-7, and 39-8*A*, and 39-8*B*). The atrial appendages can be seen in subxiphoid and parasternal short-axis views. The extent of deficiency of the atrial septum can be determined using apical views.

The atrioventricular valves are best examined from the subxiphoid long- and short-axis and apical four-chamber views. Doppler color flow mapping and pulsed Doppler mapping are useful for detecting and grading regurgitation. Straddling and abnormal attachments of the valves are best appreciated in subxiphoid or parasternal short-axis and apical four-chamber views.[22]

Ventricular size and morphology should be evaluated in at least two orthogonal views, including one sort-axis view. Ventricular volume can be measured using one of the algorithms described elsewhere (see Chapter 15). The method for determining the identity of the ventricles and the direction of looping has been described elsewhere (see Chapter 4). The ventricular septum should also be examined in at least two views, including subxiphoid or parasternal short-axis and apical four-chamber views.[41] Doppler color flow mapping has proved to be reliable for detecting ventricular septal defects if the septum is scanned in several ways.[42]

Outflow tract obstruction should be evaluated using two-dimensional imaging and Doppler flow velocity measurement. Usually subxiphoid or apical views provide a suitable window for Doppler interrogation of the outflow tracts.

The main pulmonary artery and its branches can usually be seen using high parasternal or suprasternal notch views. They should all be measured. Stenosis of the proximal left pulmonary artery at its junction with the ductus arteriosus is common. The side to which the aorta arches can be determined from the orientation of the transducer when the arch is imaged and from the branching pattern. If aortic outflow tract obstruction is present, coarctation should be suspected. A ductus arteriosus can usually be imaged from a high, left parasternal, parasagittal view.

Cardiac Catheterization. Cardiac catheterization may not be necessary for selected, sick infants with critical pulmonary outflow obstruction, with or without anomalous pulmonary venous connection. If the echocardiogram clearly delineates the pulmonary venous anatomy, atrioventricular valve function, pulmonary artery anatomy source(s) of pulmonary blood flow and the anatomy of the aortic arch, creation of an aortopulmonary shunt and repair of totally anomalous venous connection may be safely undertaken on the basis of the echocardiographic diagnosis.

Because many of these patients who survive beyond the first year of life are candidates for a modified Fontan procedure,[43] it is essential that the pulmonary artery pressure be measured and that the pulmonary vascular resistance be calculated. When possible, the pulmonary artery pressure should be measured directly. In exceptional cases where the pulmonary artery cannot be entered for technical reasons or because the source of pulmonary blood flow might be compromised by placing a catheter across it, pulmonary venous wedge pressure may be substituted. Pulmonary blood flow and vascular resistance should be calculated using measured oxygen consumption.

The ventricular end-diastolic pressure has been considered an important factor in predicting the outcome of a Fontan type of repair.[44] This can be measured easily at catheterization.

Angiographic assessment of the pulmonary artery anatomy is essential. Stenosis of one or more branches of the pulmonary artery appears to be a significant risk factor for morbidity and mortality after a Fontan type of operation.

Ventricular angiography provides additional information about atrioventricular valve function, ventricular size and function, and about the size, location, and number of ventricular septal defects.

In patients with severe pulmonary stenosis or atresia, a descending aortogram is useful to detect and define aortopulmonary collaterals. A characteristic angiocardiographic finding indicative of asplenia is the juxtaposition of the inferior vena cava and the descending aorta.[45] This is due to the more medial position of the liver which shifts the position of the inferior vena cava closer to the descending aorta.

Laboratory Tests. The presence of Howell-Jolly bodies in the blood smear is indicative of asplenia or a very small hypofunctioning spleen. A splenic scan is very helpful in diagnosing the presence and position of the spleen. It can also demonstrate the presence of multiple spleens. A small, hypofunctioning spleen may not be detected by a splenic scan. Because patients with a small, hypofunctioning spleen need antibiotic prophylaxis as much as asplenic patients do, this misdiagnosis does not create any therapeutic disadvantage.

Diagnosis of Asplenia

The diagnosis of visceral heterotaxy with asplenia can be established during life on the basis of (a) Howell-Jolly bodies in the blood smear; (b) bilateral eparterial bronchi in the air bronchogram of the chest x-ray; (c) the juxtaposition of the inferior vena cava and the descending aorta; (d) the constellation of the congenital heart defects described above; and (e) the absence of normal uptake on the splenic scan (using heat-damaged red blood cells).

Diagnosis of Polysplenia

The diagnosis of polysplenia can be established during life on the basis of (a) an interrupted inferior vena cava with unilateral (left or right) or bilateral azygos extension to the ipsilateral superior vena cava; (b) bilateral by parterial bronchi in the air bronchogram of the chest x-ray; (c) some or all of the characteristic heart defects described above; (d) ectopic atrial pacemakers in the electrocardiogram; and (e) the presence of multiple spleens or a multilobe spleen on the splenic scan.

Noncardiac Anomalies in Visceral Heterotaxy

In reviewing the medical records and the autopsy reports of the 109 patients in this series, the following additional noncardiac anomalies were found.

Five patients (four with asplenia and one with polysplenia) had multiple, severe, or lethal anomalies involving many organ systems. These included tracheal agenesis with bronchoesophageal fistula (two patients), facial dysmorphism (all five), microphthalmia (three patients), microcephaly (two patients), low-set ears and a short or webbed neck (three patients), cleft palate (three patients), and micrognathia (one patient). All five had central nervous system anomalies, including hydrocephalus (one patient), encephalocele or meningocele (two patients), syringomyelia (one patient), and intraventricular or subarachnoid hemorrhage (one patient). Similarly, all five had skeletal malformations and abnormal kidneys. Three of the five were male and all had cryptorchidism. All five patients died in the first week of life (age range: 42 hours to 7 days).

These five patients appear to represent the result of a more extensive teratogenic mechanism than the one resulting in visceral heterotaxy and congenital heart disease alone. Of interest, three of the five infants had tetralogy of Fallot instead of the rather complex malformations usually seen in heterotaxy with asplenia.

The remaining 104 (95%) patients seldom had malformations other than the ones expected for heterotaxic individuals. Cryptorchidism was an exception. Six of the 35 males with asplenia (17%) had cryptorchidism, which was bilateral in 4. Five of the 20 polysplenic males (25%) had cryptorchidism, and in all 5 it was bilateral. This frequency of cryptorchidism greatly exceeds the incidence of this anomaly in otherwise normal newborns (3.4%).[46] Also the incidence of bilateral cryptorchidism in the affected male with visceral heterotaxy was much higher (66%–100%) than the incidence reported in male infants with cryptorchidism alone (30%).[46]

Management

The presence of a symmetrical liver or a right-sided stomach and dextrocardia in the chest x-ray should alert the clinician to the presence of visceral heterotaxy. When the diagnosis of asplenia is established on the basis of the findings in the blood smear, the air bronchogram, the liver and spleen scan, and the characteristic constellation of the cardiac defects, antibiotic prophylaxis should be given. The recommended regimen for infants and young children is amoxicillin, 125 mg twice daily; for older children and adults, penicillin G, 200,000 units twice daily. Penicillin prophylaxis should continue for life, since fatal septicemia may develop in these patients following a mild upper respiratory infection.[47]

Surgical treatment of the congenital heart defects depends on the nature of the defects. In the asplenic patients with pulmonary atresia, an aortopulmonary or cavopulmonary shunt should not be performed if the pulmonary venous return is abnormal and obstructed. In those cases, the establishment of a normal and nonobstructed pulmonary venous connection should precede the shunt procedure. In some rare cases of asplenia with pulmonary atresia, there may be adequate aortopulmonary collaterals, making survival into adulthood possible without any surgical treatment. When the common atrioventricular valve becomes severely regurgitant, cardiac transplantation is a possible, but not an easily achieved, therapeutic option.[48]

Thoracophagus Twins

Siamese twins joined at the thorax may share vascular and cardiac structures; this usually creates an insurmountable surgical problem. If separation of the heart, liver, and bowel seems possible, surgical separation, often with the view of producing one survivor, can be undertaken.

Ectopia Cordis

Rarely, an infant is born with the heart outside of the thorax, usually through a cleft in the sternum (complete thoracis ectopia cordis). The most frequent cardiac malformation is tetralogy of Fallot. The chest cavity is disproportionately small, a feature that may pose great difficulties in surgical repair.

Cantrell Syndrome

This condition is thoracoabdominal ectopia cordis. It is characterized by midline defects involving the lower part of the sternum and the abdominal epigastrium, with a deficiency in the diaphragm and the diaphragmatic pericardium and, possibly, an omphalocele. Curiously, there is sometimes a peculiar diverticulum from the left ventricle projecting into the epigastric region.

Complete Situs Inversus

When all of the viscera are inverted, situs inversus totalis is said to be present. Although some of these children may have congenital heart disease, there also may be no cardiac anomaly. Situs inversus totalis without heart disease is seldom seen in a hospital population. Hence its prevalence is not known.

Kartagener Syndrome

A syndrome of situs inversus totalis with sinusitis and bronchiectasis has been described.[49] These patients have disordered cilia, which account for the bronchiectasis and the male infertility seen in this syndrome. Similar cilial abnormality is reputed to be present in some patients without complete situs inversus.

Dextrocardia with Visceroatrial Situs Solitus

Extrinsic Causes

The heart may be displaced into the right chest because of hypoplasia of the right lung (for example, in the scimitar syndrome, see Chapter 32), or because of a congenital diaphragmatic hernia, allowing abdominal contents to enter the left side of the chest. In this situation the heart may be normal, although cardiac anomalies are common.

Intrinsic Causes

The heart may occupy the right chest cavity or assume a mesocardial position because of intrinsic reasons related to the process of ventricular looping or the presence of atrial situs inversus. Dextrocardia was frequently present in the heterotaxic patients of this study and appeared to be related to the presence of ventricular L-loop more often than to the presence of atrial situs inversus (Table 39-5).

Because these patients can have almost any cardiac anomaly or combination of anomalies, detailed discussion of the clinical features is scarcely fruitful. As indicated earlier, once malposition has been recognized, the cardiologist begins a systematic evaluation of the segmental relationships and connections of the chambers. That having been done, superimposed anatomic abnormalities can be identified and quantified and a treatment plan outlined.

REFERENCES

1. Fyler DC, Buckley LP, Hellenbrand WE, et al. Report of the New England Regional Infant Cardiac Program. Pediatrics 65:375, 1980.
2. Cantrell JR, Haller JA, Ravitch MM. A syndrome of congenital defects involving the abdominal wall, sternum, diaphragm, pericardium and heart. Surg Gynecol Obstet 197:602, 1958.
3. Van Praagh S, Kreutzer J, Alday L, et al. Systemic and pulmonary venous connections in visceral heterotaxy, with emphasis on the diagnosis of atrial situs: a study of 109 postmortem cases. In Clark E, Takao A (eds). Developmental Cardiology: Morphogenesis and Function. Mt. Kisco, NY: Futura, 1990, pp. 671–721.
4. Polhemus D, Schaefer WB. Congenital absence of the spleen: syndrome with atrioventricularis communes and situs inversus. Pediatrics 9:696, 1952.
5. Ivemark BI. Implications of agenesis of the spleen on the pathogenesis of conotruncus anomalies in childhood. Acta Paediatr Scand [Suppl] 44:1, 1955.
6. Bruekner M, D'Eustachio P, Horwich AL. Linkage mapping of mouse gene, iv, that controls left-right symmetry of the heart and viscera. Proc Natl Acad Sci U S A 86:5035, 1989.
7. Layton WM. Heart malformations in mice homozygous for a gene causing situs inversus. In Rosenquist G, Bersma D (eds). Morphogenesis and Malformations of the Cardiovascular System. New York: Alan R. Liss, 1978, pp. 277–293.
8. Arnold GL, Bixler D, Girod D. Probable autosomal recessive inheritance of polysplenia, situs inversus and cardiac defects in an Amish family. Am J Med Genet 16:35, 1983.
9. Aristotle. Historia Animalium. Book II. Translated by A.L. Peck, Loeb Classical Library, Cambridge, MA, Harvard University Press, 1965, p. 132 (507a, 20).
10. Brandt HM, Liebow AA. Right pulmonary isomerism associated with venous, splenic, and other anomalies. Lab Invest 7:469, 1958.
11. Troschel. quoted by Schelenz K. Ein neuer Beitrag zur Kenntnis des Situs viscerum inversus partialis. Berl Klin Wchnshr 461:188, 840, 1909.
12. Martin G. Observations d'une deviation organique de l'estomac, d'une anomalie dans la situation, dans la configuration du coeur et des vaisseaux qui en partent or qui s'y rendent. Bulletin de la Societe Anatomique de Paris 3:39, 1826.
13. Putschar WGJ, Manion WC. Congenital absence of the spleen and associated anomalies. Am J Clin Pathol 26:429, 1956.
14. Van Mierop LHS, Wiglesworth FW. Isomerism of the cardiac atria in the asplenia syndrome. Lab Invest 11:1303, 1962.
15. Moller JH, Hakib A, Anderson RC. Congenital cardiac disease associated with polysplenia. Circulation 36:789, 1967.
16. Caruso G, Becker AE. How to determine atrial situs? Considerations initiated by 3 cases of absent spleen with a discordant anatomy between bronchi and atria. Br Heart J 41:559, 1979.
17. Freedom RM, Culham JAG, Moes CAF. Asplenia and polysplenia (a consideration of syndromes characterized by right and left atrial isomerism). In Angiocardiography of Congenital Heart Disease. New York, Macmillan 1984, pp. 643–654.
18. Huhta JC, Smallhorn JF, Macartney FJ, et al. Cross-sectional echocardiographic diagnosis of systemic venous return. Br Heart J 48:388, 1982.
19. Macartney FJ, Zuberbuhler JR, Anderson RH. Morphological considerations pertaining to recognition of atrial isomerism. Br Heart J 44:657, 1980.
20. Chandra RS. Biliary atresia and other structural anomalies in the congenital polysplenia syndrome. J Pediatr 85:649, 1974.
21. Van Mierop LHS, Gessner IH, Schiebler GL. Asplenia and polysplenia syndromes. Birth Defects 8:36, 1972.
22. Ruscazio M, Van Praagh S, Marrass AR, et al. Interrupted inferior vena cava in asplenia syndrome and a review of the hereditary patterns of visceral situs abnormalities. Am J Cardiol 81:111, 1998.
23. Edwards JE. Pathologic and developmental considerations in anomalous pulmonary venous connection. Mayo Clin Proc 28:411, 1953.
24. Van Praagh S, Carrera ME, Sanders SP, et al. Partial or total direct pulmonary venous drainage to the right atrium due to malposition of septum primum. Chest 107:1488, 1995.
25. Lev M. Pathologic diagnosis of positional variations in cardiac chambers in congenital heart disease. Lab Invest 3:71, 1954.
26. Van Mierop LHS, Eisen S, Schiebler GL. The radiographic appearance of the tracheobronchial tree as indicator of visceral situs. Am J Cardiol 26:432, 1970.
27. Langman J. Medical Embryology, Human Development: Normal and Abnormal. Baltimore: Williams & Wilkins, 1963, p 180.
28. Freedom RM. Aortic valve and arch anomalies in the congenital asplenia syndrome. Case report, literature review and re-examination of the embryology of the congenital asplenia syndrome. John Hopkins Med J 135:124, 1974.

29. Van Praagh S, Antoniadis S, Otero-Coto E, et al. Common atrioventricular canal with and without conotruncal malformations: an anatomic study of 251 postmortem cases. In Nora JJ, Takao A (eds). Congenital Heart Disease: Causes and Processes. Mount Kisco, NY: Futura, 1984, pp 599–639.
30. Van Praagh S, Davidoff A, Chin A, et al. Double outlet right ventricle: anatomic types and developmental implications based on a study of 101 autopsied cases. Coeur 13:389-439, 1982.
31. Van Praagh S, Geva T, Friedberg DZ, et al. Aortic outflow obstruction in visceral heterotaxy: A study based on twenty postmortem cases. Am Heart J 133:558, 1997.
32. Rose V, Izukawa T, Moes CAF. Syndromes of asplenia and polysplenia. Br Heart J 37:840, 1975.
33. Pasquini L, Sanders SP, Parness I, et al. Echocardiographic and anatomic findings in atrioventricular discordance with ventriculoarterial concordance. Am J Cardiol 62:1256, 1988.
34. Wren C, Macartney FJ, Deanfield JE. Cardiac Rhythm in atrial isomerism. Am J Cardiol 59:1156, 1987.
35. Huhta JC, Smallhorn JF, Macartney FJ. Two-dimensional echocardiographic diagnosis of situs. Br Heart J 48:97, 1982.
36. Snider AR, Silberman NH. Suprasternal notch echocardiography: a two-dimensional technique for evaluating congenital heart disease. Circulation 63:165, 1981.
37. Silverman NH, Schiller NB. Apex echocardiography: a two-dimensional technique for evaluating congenital heart disease. Circulation 57:503, 1978.
38. Cooper MJ, Teitel DF, Silverman NH, et al. Study of the infradiaphragmatic total anomalous pulmonary venous connection with cross-sectional and pulsed Doppler echocardiography. Circulation 70:412, 1984.
39. Bierman FZ, Williams RG. Subxiphoid two-dimensional imaging of the interatrial septum in infants and neonates with congenital heart disease. Circulation 60:80, 1979.
40. Shub C, Dimopoulos In, Seward JB, et al. Sensitivity of two-dimensional echocardiography in the direct visualization of atrial septal defect utilizing the subcostal approach: experience with 154 patients. J Am Coll Cardiol 2:127, 1983.
41. Bierman FZ, Fellows K, Williams RG. Prospective identification of the ventricular septal defects in infancy using subxiphoid two-dimensional echocardiography. Circulation 62: 807, 1980.
42. Ortiz E, Robinson PJ, Deanfield JE, et al. Localization of ventricular septal defects by simultaneous display of superimposed color Doppler and cross-sectional echocardiographic images. Br Heart J 54:53, 1985.
43. Jonas RA, Castaneda AR. Modified Fontan procedure: atrial baffle and systemic venous-to-pulmonary artery anastomotic techniques. J Cardiac Surg 3:91, 1988.
44. Fontan F, De Ville C, Quagebeur J, et al. Repair of tricuspid atresia in 100 patients. J Thorac Cardiovasc Surg 85:647, 1983.
45. Elliot LP, Cramer GG, Ampaltz K. The anomalous relationship of the inferior vena cava and abdominal aorta as a specific angiocardiographic sign in asplenia. Radiology 87:859, 1966.
46. Gonzales R, Michael A. Disorders and anomalies of the scrotal content. In Berhman RE, Vaughn VC, Nelson WL (eds). Nelson's Textbook of Pediatrics, 13th ed. Philadelphia: WB Saunders, 1987, pp 1163–1165.
47. Waldman JD, Rosenthal A, Smith AL, et al. Sepsis and congenital asplenia. J Pediatr 90:555, 1977.
48. Mayer JE, Perry S, O'Brien P, et al. Orthotopic heart transplantation for complex congenital heart disease. J Thorac Cardiovasc Surg 99:484, 1990.
49. Kartagener M. Zur pathogenese der bronchiektasien, bronchietagien bei situs viscerum inversus. Beitr Klin Tuberk 83:489, 1933.
50. Van Praagh R, Corsini I. Cor triatriatum: pathologic anatomy and a consideration of morphogenesis based on 13 postmortem cases and a study of normal development of the pulmonary vein and atrial septum in 83 human embryos. Am Heart J 78:379, 1969.

40

Mitral Valve and Left Atrial Lesions

ROBERT L. GEGGEL AND DONALD C. FYLER

MITRAL VALVE DISEASE

Mitral Regurgitation

Prevalence

Most mitral valve lesions are more commonly associated with other congenital cardiac defects (Exhibit 40-1). Rheumatic mitral disease, the most important cardiac problem in children worldwide, is rare in the United States (see Chapters 19 and 24). Other acquired conditions associated with mitral regurgitation include cardiomyopathy, myocarditis, Kawasaki disease, collagen vascular disease, infective endocarditis, trauma, and ischemic heart disease. Genetic disorders include connective tissue disease (Marfan syndrome, Ehlers-Danlos syndrome), mucopolysaccharidosis (Hurler disease), and homocystinuria.[1,2]

Pathology

Abnormalities of any portion of the mitral valve apparatus can be associated with mitral regurgitation. A forme fruste of endocardial cushion defect involves isolated cleft of the anterior leaflet of the mitral valve with intact septa.[3,4] This condition can be associated with chordal attachments from the anterior mitral leaflet to the interventricular septum that create subaortic obstruction that increases the degree of mitral regurgitation.[1] Incomplete valve coaptation can be produced by a variety of conditions. Redundant mitral valve tissue or lengthened chordae tendineae are present in mitral valve prolapse. The valve leaflets can be hypoplastic[5] or thickened and associated with shortened chordae so that an anomalous mitral arcade with predominant mitral regurgitation is produced.[6,7] Rupture of a chordal attachment produces a flail leaflet; this can occur spontaneously, with connective tissue disorders, with rheumatic fever or endocarditis, or with trauma.[2] Papillary muscle ischemia and dysfunction can be present in anomalous origin of the left coronary artery from the main pulmonary artery (see Chapter 53) or myocarditis. Infective endocarditis can perforate a leaflet. Atrial tumors may prevent valve closure. Conditions associated with dilation of the left ventricle (cardiomyopathy, left-to-right shunts) can lead to mitral annular enlargement. Chronic rheumatic mitral valve disease produces thickened, rigid, and shortened leaflets[2] that histologically contain Aschoff nodules.[8]

Physiology

The degree of mitral regurgitation depends on several factors[2,9]: size of the regurgitant orifice, left ventricular–left atrial pressure gradient, left atrial compliance, duration of systole, and resistance of forward flow to the aorta (left ventricular outlet obstruction and systemic vascular resistance). These features are variable and affected by preload, afterload, and ventricular contractility.

The physiology of mitral regurgitation changes in the acute, chronic compensated, and chronic deompensated stages (Fig. 40-1). Mitral regurgitation can be progressive not only because chronic backflow produces thickening of the valve leaflets and poorer coaptation, but also because increasing degrees of regurgitation produce annular enlargement. With severe mitral regurgitation, pulmonary hypertension can develop both in the acute stage because of low left atrial compliance and in the chronic phase, even if the left atrium is markedly dilated, with the onset of left ventricular dysfunction. Chronic left atrial enlargement is also associated with the development of atrial tachyarrhythmias.

Left ventricular ejection fraction includes forward stroke volume and regurgitant flow. As a result, the ejection fraction

Exhibit 40–1
Boston Children's Hospital Experience
LEFT ATRIAL AND MITRAL VALVE PROBLEMS

Congenital Lesion	*1973–1987* *N*	*1988–2002* *N*
Mitral regurgitation	221	4137
Mitral stenosis	31	68
Supravalvar ring	4	6
Cor triatriatum	10	16
Pulmonary Venous Stenosis	13	9
Mitral Valve Prolapse	367	1148

When comparing the individual lesion numbers between the 2 time periods, most of the 1988-2002 era increases reflect the almost tripled number of patients seen except for the huge nearly 20-fold increase in those with regurgitation. This latter increase, using this hierarchical classification system, is influenced considerably by the more widespread use of echocardiography-among these were 345 patients without any structural heart disease and mostly trivial degrees of regurgitation and 36 other similar patients with Kawasaki disease or a malignancy on chemotherapy.

1988–2002
DISTRIBUTION AMONG OTHER PRIMARY CARDIAC DEFECTS

Primary Diagnosis	***Mitral Stenosis N = 869**	***Supravalvar Stenosis N = 74**	***Cor Triatriatum N = 49**	***Mitral Regurgitation N = 5242**
Coarctation of the Aorta	207	29	0	407
Endocardial Cushion	175	9	5	771
Hypoplastic Left Heart	153	5	3	112
Aortic Outflow Problems	114	8	5	1453
Ventricular Defect	81	14	6	780
Double-outlet right Ventricle	34	5	2	136
Tetralogy of Fallot	29	1	1	375
Malposition	27	3	1	246
Rheumatic Heart Disease	17	0	0	53
Single Ventricle	11	0	0	105
D-Transposition of the Great Arteries	5	0	0	370
L-Transposition of the Great Arteries	1	0	0	39
Tricuspid Atresia	1	0	2	160
Other	14	0	24	230

*These are the patients (6234) in the database with these lesions listed as secondary diagnoses. Counting each patient once the 6234 are then searched for the lesions under "Primary Diagnosis."

is usually increased early in the disease course. A normal ejection fraction in the presence of severe mitral regurgitation represents myocardial dysfunction. Patients with severe mitral regurgitation have clinically significant myocardial dysfunction when the left ventricular ejection fraction is less than 10% greater than the lower limit of normal, which for adults is 50% as assessed by echocardiography.[10]

Clinical Manifestations

Symptoms are related to the degree of regurgitation, the rate of progression, age, and the presence of coexisting cardiac conditions.[2] Mild regurgitation is associated with no symptoms. As regurgitation progresses, fatigue and exercise limitations occur because of limitations in forward stroke volume. Infants with moderate-to-severe regurgitation have

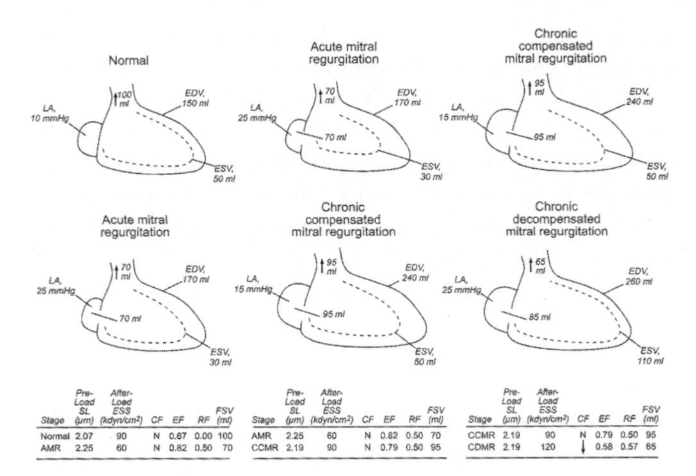

FIGURE 40–1 *Different physiologic stages of mitral regurgitation. A, Changes that occur with acute mitral regurgitation. Left ventricular end-diastolic volume (EDV) and left atrial pressure increase while the contractile function (CF) remains normal (N). The reduction in ventricular afterload created by the regurgitation reduces end-systolic stress (ESS) and left ventricular end-systolic volume (ESV). The ejection fraction (EF) increases but the forward stroke volume (FSV) decreases because of the size of the regurgitant fraction (RF). B, Subsequent transition to chronic compensated mitral regurgitation (CCMR). Left ventricular end-diastolic volume increases and the larger ventricular radius produces a higher end-systolic stress. The increased afterload augments the end-systolic volume. The larger ventricle is able to increase forward stroke volume because of maintenance of normal contractile function and increased ejection fraction. The development of left atrial enlargement enables left atrial pressure to be reduced. C, Subsequent transition to chronic decompensated mitral regurgitation (CDMR). The development of decreased contractile function reduces ejection fraction and forward stoke volume, increases left ventricular end-diastolic and end-systolic volumes. Cardiac dilation increases mitral annular diameter and produces an increased regurgitant fraction.*
From Carabello BA, Crawford FA Jr: Valvular heart disease. N Engl J Med 337:32, 1997, with permission.

poor weight gain, frequent respiratory infections, and tachypnea. Patients with severe mitral regurgitation can develop cardiac *asthma,* which is caused by pulmonary edema and compression of airways by a dilated left atrium and in patients with pulmonary hypertension, by dilated pulmonary arteries.[1,11]

The cardiac examination also varies with the severity of regurgitation. With severe mitral regurgitation, the apical impulse is hyperactive and S_1 is soft because of poor mitral valve coaptation and therefore decreased mitral contribution to this heart sound. In patients with pulmonary hypertension, the pulmonic component of S_2 is increased in intensity. There may be an S_3 due to increased volume flowing across the mitral valve in the rapid-filling phase of ventricular diastole. The systolic murmur has maximal intensity at the apex and radiates to the axilla; this murmur is rarely associated with a thrill so the intensity is lower than grade 3. The intensity of the systolic murmur does not correlate with the degree of regurgitation; *silent* regurgitation can occur with left ventricular dysfunction, elevated left atrial pressure, extrinsic noise from ventilators or prosthetic valves, and noncardiac factors of obesity, chest-wall deformity, or obstructive lung disease.[2,12] The systolic murmur typically is holosytolic, beginning after S_1 and continuing to S_2, and has a blowing quality. In patients with mitral valve prolapse, the murmur may be mid or late systolic. When diastolic flow is greater than twice normal, there can be a diastolic murmur of relative mitral stenosis (see Chapter 11).

Electrocardiography. Moderate and severe mitral regurgitation usually produce the finding of left atrial enlargement and left ventricular hypertrophy. If there is long-standing pulmonary hypertension, right ventricular hypertrophy is present. Chronic severe mitral regurgitation can be complicated by supraventricular tachyarrhythmias, notably atrial flutter and atrial fibrillation.

Chest Radiography. Cardiomegaly is proportionate to the degree of chronic regurgitation. Acute mitral regurgitation or chronic decompensated mitral regurgitation is associated with Kerley's B lines and pulmonary edema.[2] Chronic left atrial enlargement increases the angle of bifurcation of the trachea.[11]

Echocardiography. The mechanism of mitral regurgitation can be determined with the use of two-dimensional echocardiography, Doppler echocardiography, and color flow mapping.[13] Multiple views are required to fully inspect the valve leaflets, chordal attachments, and papillary muscles. These modalities also aid in evaluation of chamber sizes and function. Transesophageal echocardiography may be necessary if transthoracic imaging is limited because of poor acoustic windows and the information obtained can be important in assessing the likelihood of surgical repair.[14] In older patients capable of exercising, stress echocardiography can reveal important pathophysiologic information including exercise-induced pulmonary or systemic hypertension, changes in mitral valve gradient, and exercise tolerance.[15–17]

The various modalities of two-dimensional echocardiography are useful also in assessing the severity of regurgitation. Severe mitral regurgitation is associated with dilation of the left atrium and left ventricle, and often with Doppler echocardiographic evidence for pulmonary venous flow reversal[18] and increased mitral-inflow velocity.[19] Quantitation of the regurgitation can be performed by measuring regurgitant fraction, regurgitant volume, regurgitant orifice area, and vena contracta jet width (Fig. 40-2).[20–23] The vena contracta is defined as the narrowest diameter of the jet as imaged by color Doppler echocardiography. In adult patients, severe mitral regurgitation is associated with more than 50%, more than 60 mL, more than .5 cm^2, and more

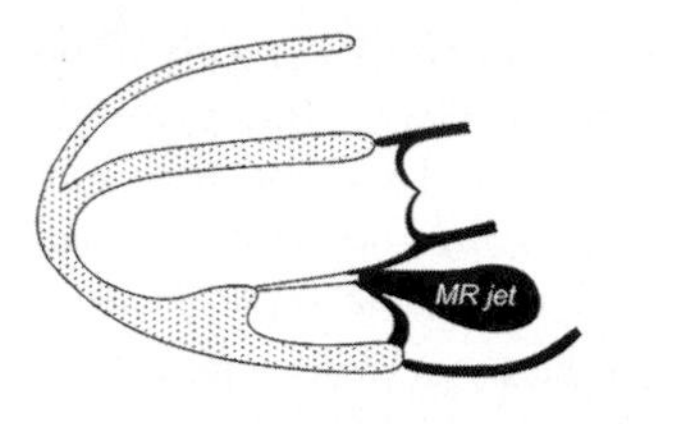

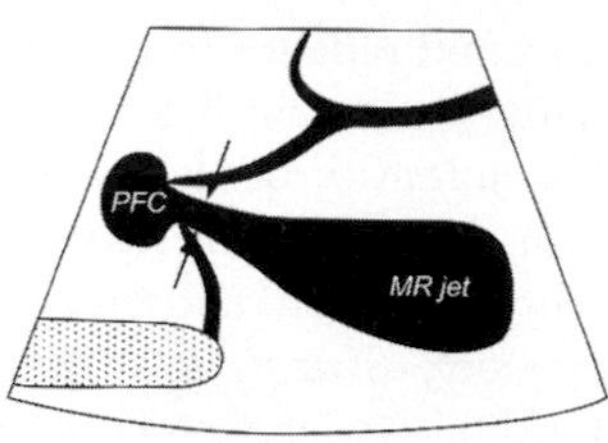

FIGURE 40–2 *Vena contracta jet width. Left panel, Parasternal long-axis view of mitral regurgitation jet. Right panel, zoom mode for measurement of the vena contracta (arrows) just downstream from the orifice. PFC-proximal flow convergence.*
From Hall SA, Brickner E, Willett DL, et al. Assessment of mitral regurgitation severity by Doppler color flow mapping of the vena contracta. Circulation 95:636, 1997, with permission.

than regurgitant fraction, regurgitant volume, orifice area, and vena contracta width, respectively.[21,23] Three-dimensional echocardiography can provide additional information about valve anatomy.[24]

Cardiac Catheterization. Isolated mitral regurgitation usually can be managed without cardiac catheterization[8]: indeed when severe, catheterization may be dangerous. Hemodynamic findings vary with the severity of regurgitation. Severe mitral regurgitation usually has elevated pulmonary capillary wedge or left atrial pressures; tracings from these sites often have a prominent *v* wave that is greater than twice the mean pressure.[9] However, some patients with chronic mitral regurgitation have a markedly dilated, compliant left atrium and normal left atrial pressure.[2,25] Left ventricular diastolic pressure can be elevated with chronic volume overload. In patients with severe regurgitation that is either acute or chronic, pulmonary artery (a) pressure can be elevated, and (b) saturation level may be quite low.

Left ventricular angiography is performed in the right anterior oblique and left anterior oblique views so that the left atrium and left ventricle are not superimposed. Catheter-induced regurgitation is minimized by entering the left ventricle from a retrograde approach via the aorta rather than anterograde across the mitral valve and selecting an injection rate to reduce the occurrence of ventricular premature beats.[2] Some catheter designs are associated with reduced incidence of ectopy.[26] The degree of regurgitation is graded on a qualitative scale of 1 to 4 that rates the degree of left atrial opacification and speed of clearing of contrast.[9] In grade 1 (mild), the left atrium is partially and faintly opacified, and contrast clears with one beat. In grade 2 (moderate), the left atrium is fully opacified but to a lesser degree than the left ventricle, and the contrast takes several beats to clear. In grade 3 (moderately severe), the left atrium is fully opacified to the same degree as the left ventricle. In grade 4 (severe), the left atrium is fully opacified in one beat, becomes progressively opacified with subsequent beats, and contrast fills the pulmonary veins. The degree of regurgitation can be quantified by calculating the regurgitant fraction.[9] Total left ventricular stroke volume (TSV) is determined from the difference between end-diastolic and end-systolic ventricular volumes[27]; the forward stroke volume (FSV) is determined by the Fick method or thermodilution technique. The regurgitant stroke volume (RSV) is calculated as TSV – FSV, whereas the regurgitant fraction is calculated as RSV/TSV.

Management

Mild mitral regurgitation requires observance of endocarditis precautions, but no daily medication or activity restrictions. Periodic re-evaluations are needed to monitor possible progression in the severity of backflow.

Medical management of chronic moderate or severe mitral regurgitation includes the use of diuretics and treatment of systemic hypertension if present. If ventricular dysfunction develops, digoxin can be helpful, especially if there is coexisting atrial fibrillation.[2] Other antiarrhythmic medication may be needed as well. Anticoagulation is required for patients with atrial fibrillation. Afterload reduction agents are beneficial in patients with acute or chronically decompensated mitral regurgitation.[2,28] The use of these agents in patients with chronic compensated mitral regurgitation and normal left ventricular function has not been assessed in large, placebo-controlled trials[28,29]; although acute administration of these agents in this patient group can have dramatic effect,[9,30,31] the long-term effects have been variable and occasionally deleterious, and the reduction in regurgitant volume often small.[10,28,32]

Most patients with mitral regurgitation have mild-to-moderate disease and do not require surgical intervention. In the adult population, approximately 18,000 patients undergo mitral valve surgery annually.[33] Symptomatic patients who do not respond to medical therapy require surgical treatment. The decision to intervene surgically in a patient with compensated hemodynamics is difficult. Surgery exposes the patient to risks that include mortality, need for reoperation,[10,34] complications of anticoagulation if a prosthetic valve is inserted,[35] pacemaker implantation, endocarditis, and cerebrovascular accident.[36] However, in adults, delaying surgery until left or right ventricular dysfunction occurs increases morbidity and mortality.[10,37,38] In pediatric patients postoperative left ventricular function usually normalizes after repair of symptomatic patients but the incidence of atrial arrhythmias is higher the longer severe regurgitation is present.[39]

Criteria for surgical management in asymptomatic adult patients with severe mitral regurgitation require evidence for ventricular dysfunction that includes either left ventricular ejection fraction below 60%, left ventricular end-systolic dimension above 45 mm, subnormal right ventricular ejection fraction at rest, or atrial fibrillation persistent for more than 3 months.[2,10,29,33] In some patients, exercise studies can demonstrate ventricular dysfunction that is not obvious on resting studies.[15,16] Surgery can be offered for patients who do not meet these criteria if there is evidence for progressive loss of ventricular function or if there is a high likelihood of valve repair rather than replacement.[2] Strict criteria for pediatric patients have not been established.

Surgical management includes annuloplasty to prevent progressive annular enlargement, valve reconstruction, or valve replacement. In adolescent or adult patients, annuloplasty can be performed by placement of a prosthetic ring. In younger patients, modified techniques are available to accommodate somatic growth.[40] Valve reconstruction includes repair of anomalies of the chordae tendineae, papillary muscles, or valve leaflets, including closure of clefts, chordal shortening, triangular leaflet resection, chordal substitution, and valve extension with a pericardial patch.[1,40,41] If repair is not possible, the choice of which type of prosthetic valve to place depends on the patient's age. Bioprosthetic valves are preferable in female patients of childbearing age to avoid the teratogenic effects of coumadin.[29] In infants and children, these valves function well for only a limited period so that mechanical valves are preferable despite the challenges involved with maintaining adequate anticoagulation. The need for placement of a second mechanical valve is related to age at initial operation (younger than 2 years) and size of the initial prosthesis (smaller than 20 mm); a larger valve often can be placed at a subsequent operation, suggesting continued annular growth.[42]

Animal studies have demonstrated the feasibility of endovascular repair of mitral regurgitation.[43] Additional investigations will determine the clinical application of such techniques.

Mitral Valve Prolapse

Mitral valve prolapse was initially visualized in the 1960s[44] and subsequently has been the subject of countless reports with contradictory findings varying from innocent variant to structural basis for multiple complications. This variability in apparent significance has led to confusion for clinicians.[45]

Definition

Diagnostic criteria include both auscultatory and echocardiographic features, either or both of which may be present in a patient.[2,46] On physical examination, there can be a constant mid-to-late systolic ejection click with or without a murmur of mitral regurgitation. Some reports suggest that the presence of these features indicate the presence of mitral valve prolapse regardless of the echocardiographic examination,[47] while others require echocardiographic abnormalities.[8] Two- and three-dimensional echocardiography studies have documented that the mitral valve annulus is nonplanar and has a saddle-shaped configuration.[48,49] Systolic displacement of the anterior mitral valve leaflet superior to the mitral annulus that is identified only in the apical four chamber view is a normal finding and not sufficient by itself for the diagnosis of mitral valve prolapse. Although there is no consensus on two-dimensional echocardiographic criteria,[31] recent publications have required superior systolic displacement greater than 2 mm in the parasternal long-axis view and mitral valve thickening greater than 5 mm for the diagnosis of classic mitral valve prolapse. Criteria for nonclassic prolapse include a similar level of displacement but maximal valve thickness less than 5 mm.[50] The thickness is measured in the midportion of the valve leaflet during diastole and excludes areas of focal thickening or chordal insertion (Fig. 40-3). Because the lateral scallop of the posterior leaflet is best imaged in the apical four-chamber view, superior displacement of this portion of the leaflet in this view suggests the diagnosis.[31,51] Occasionally, a definite mid-systolic click is present but the supine echocardiogram is normal; in these patients, obtaining echocardiographic images with the patient sitting, squatting, or standing may document prolapse.

Prevalence

Early reports indicated that up to 35% of patients aged 10 to 18 years of age have superior displacement of the mitral valve in the apical four chamber two-dimensional echocardiographic view.[52] Such a value contradicted the concept that most children have normal cardiac structure, raised the issue of iatrogenic diagnosis, and made it difficult to assess clinical significance since as noted by others, "a disease is particularly benign if you are a false-positive."[53] Some studies have been limited to a hospital-based patient population rather than evaluating a community-based population.

Using strict two-dimensional echocardiographic criteria outlined above, evaluation of 3,736 subjects in the Framingham Heart Study with mean [+ SD] age of 54.7 + 10.0 years, and age range 26 to 84 years, documented a prevalence of 2.4% (1.3% for classic and 1.1% for nonclassic mitral valve prolapse).[50] In this study there was no age or gender predilection. In a study of 193 children aged 5 days to 18 years, superior systolic motion was noted in the parasternal long-axis view in 2.6%.[52]

Mitral valve prolapse occurs both as a primary lesion, and in association with a variety of other conditions (Exhibit 40-2). Mitral valve prolapse is rare in the first decade of life in the absence of an identifiable cause. Principal among these are connective tissue disorders that include Marfan syndrome, Ehlers-Danlos syndrome, osteogenesis imperfecta, pseudoxanthoma elasticum, and Stickler syndrome.[2,51] Skeletal abnormalities include scoliosis, pectus excavatum,[54] asthenic body

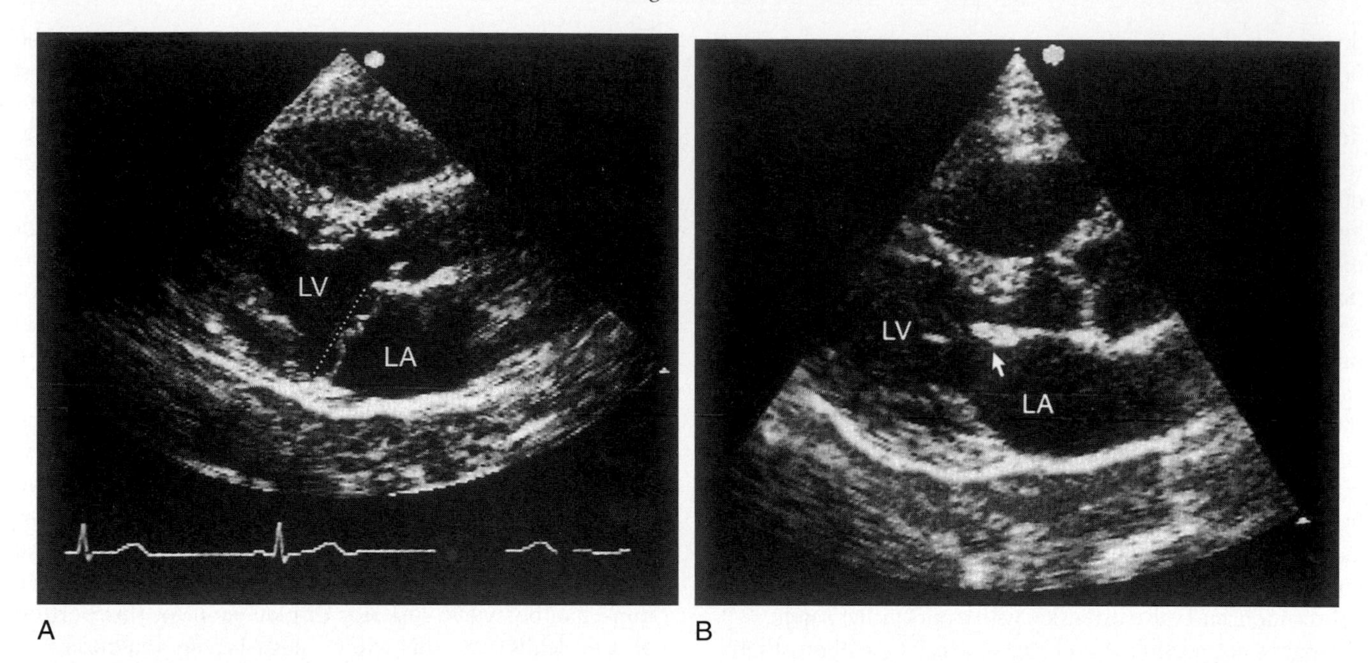

FIGURE 40–3 *Parasternal long-axis view of classic mitral valve prolapse in systole (A) and diastole (B). A, The mitral valve is displaced more than 2 mm superior to the plane of the mitral annulus (dotted line connecting the hinge points of the anterior and posterior valve leaflets) into the left atrium. B, The mitral valve leaflet (arrow) has a thickness more than 5 mm. LA, left atrium; LV, left ventricle.*
From Freed LA, Levy D, Levine RA, et al. Prevalence and clinical outcome of mitral-valve prolapse. N Engl J Med 341:1, 1999, with permission.

habitus,[55] and straight back syndrome.[2] Mitral valve prolapse occurs in 17% to 70% of adult patients with secundum atrial septal defect due to abnormal left ventricular geometric pattern created by right ventricular volume overload[56] or reduction in left ventricular cavity size[55]; the prolapse resolves postoperatively in many patients.[57] Other reported associations include hyperthyroidism, sickle cell disease, muscular dystrophy, hypomastia, and von Willebrand disease.[2,51]

Pathology

Mitral valve prolapse can involve abnormalities of any portion of the mitral valve apparatus including the mitral annulus, valve leaflets, chordae tendineae, and papillary muscles. Primary mitral valve prolapse may involve abnormalities of collagen that produce redundant valve tissue, elongated chordae tendineae, or a dilated annulus. This explanation proposes that mitral valve prolapse is a forme fruste of connective tissue disease.[55,58] Alternatively, the condition may arise as a response to injury that produces collagen disruption and weaker valve components.[55] All components of the valve apparatus can undergo myxomatous changes.[2] The degree of mitral regurgitation is directly proportional to the amount of prolapse and degree of annular dilation. Acute increases in severity of regurgitation occur with rupture of chordae tendineae.[59]

Physiology

Principles reviewed in the discussion of mitral regurgitation apply to patients with mitral valve prolapse. The systolic click moves closer to S_1 when left ventricular volume is reduced (standing position, Valsalva) and occurs later in systole when left ventricular volume is increased (squatting).[8]

Clinical Manifestations

Symptoms are based on the severity of mitral regurgitation. A variety of symptoms have been ascribed to mitral valve prolapse including atypical chest pain, palpitations, fatigue, dizziness, syncope, dyspnea, and anxiety attacks. However, these symptoms are common in the general population and the associations with mitral valve prolapse are weak or nonexistent.[50,55,60,61]

On physical examination, patients often have an asthenic habitus. Skeletal features including a thin anteroposterior diameter, pectus excavatum, or scoliosis are common.[8] Auscultatory findings can be variable. The hallmark feature is a constant, mid-systolic click that is produced by tensing of the valve leaflet or chordae tendineae.[2] The murmur of mitral regurgitation may be absent, limited to late systole, or present throughout systole. A variety of maneuvers have been described to augment the intensity of the click or murmur.[2] The easiest maneuver to perform in children

Exhibit 40–2
Children's Hospital Boston Experience
Cardiac Diagnoses Associated with Mitral Valve Prolapse

Diagnosis	*1973–1987* *N*	*1988–2002* *N*
Mitral valve prolapse	367	340
Mitral regurgitation	68	565
Aortic valve problems	36	274
Atrial septal defect	44	158
Pulmonary stenosis	18	83
Ventricular septal defect	22	73
Endocardial cushion defect	9	53
Cardiomyopathy	5	43
Tetralogy of Fallot	12	22
Transposition of the great arteries	5	4
Arrhythmia	24	4
Other	77	65
TOTAL	704	1684

The total number (*N*) of patients with mitral valve prolapse in the 1988 to 2002 period compared with the 1973 to 1987 era had increased in proportion to the number of patients seen. It was associated with most forms of congenital heart disease. It is likely that echocardiography accounted for the marked increase in some associated lesions such as mitral regurgitation, aortic valve problems, and cardiomyopathy. There were 712 patients with Marfan syndrome in the entire database, 286 (40%) of whom had mitral valve prolapse.

and adolescents is to ask the patient to stand. In this position, left ventricular volume is reduced, the click moves closer to S_1 and is more prominent; mitral regurgitation that is absent or late systolic in the supine position can either develop or become more holosystolic, respectively, because of an increased degree of prolapse.

Cerebral ischemia including stroke and transient ischemic attack has been associated with mitral valve prolapse in studies predating the strict definition of the condition.[62] However, a recent study of 213 patients less than 45 years of age showed no increased risk of this complication in patients with superior displacement of the mitral valve in the two-dimensional echocardiographic long-axis view.[63]

Sudden death occurs rarely in patients with mitral valve prolapse[31] but is uncommon in the absence of a history of syncope caused by an arrhythmia, family history of sudden death associated with mitral valve prolapse, documented supraventricular or ventricular tachyarrhythmia, moderate or severe mitral regurgitation, or a prior embolic event.[64,65]

Electrocardiography. Electrocardiographic findings are usually normal in patients without significant mitral regurgitation. Early reports of T wave inversions in the inferior limb leads or lateral precordial leads have been found to be nonspecific findings that occur also in patients without this condition.[46,55] There is an increased incidence of atrial and ventricular arrhythmias, including atrial or ventricular premature beats, and supraventricular or ventricular tachycardia.[2,66] The mechanism of these arrhythmias is unclear.

Chest Radiography. A chest radiograph (usually not performed for isolated mitral regurgitation) demonstrates normal cardiac findings in patients with less than a moderate degree of mitral regurgitation. Skeletal abnormalities mentioned above can be seen.

Echocardiography. Echocardiography is the main tool used for the diagnosis of mitral valve prolapse. M-mode echocardiography is imprecise and has been supplanted by two-dimensional techniques. As noted in the definition section, the parasternal long-axis view is predominantly used for diagnosis. This view permits visualization of the medial aspect of the anterior leaflet and the middle scallop of the posterior leaflet. The lateral scallop of the posterior leaflet is best imaged in the apical four-chamber view.[31] In addition to noting superior displacement of the valve or coaptation point, chordal lengthening, valve redundancy or thickening, and annular dilation are also evaluated. The degree of mitral regurgitation can be assessed with the use of pulsed or color Doppler echocardiography.

Cardiac Catheterization. In the absence of a significant additional cardiac defect, patients with isolated mitral valve prolapse do not require cardiac catheterization.

Management

Most patients with mitral valve prolapse have a benign course and this natural history should be emphasized to the patient and family.[31,50,67] Mitral regurgitation, if present, is usually trivial or mild. Mitral regurgitation can slowly progress in some patients so that infrequent but regular reevaluation is helpful. Mitral valve prolapse is the most frequent basis for severe mitral regurgitation requiring surgery in adult patients[68]; the need for mitral valve surgery is related to age and gender, being more common after the age of 50 years and in males,[59,69] in patients with thickened valve leaflets or redundancy (classic prolapse), and in those with systolic murmurs.[70–72]

There is an increased risk of endocarditis if the valve leaflets are thickened or there is mitral regurgitation. Endocarditis precautions are recommended for patients with these features but are not necessary for patients without them.[45,71,73,74] Mitral regurgitation should be audible or more than the trivial degree frequently detected by color Doppler echocardiography across normal mitral valves in order for endocarditis precautions to be applied.

Patients with symptomatic arrhythmias are treated by standard regimens (see Chapter 29). Patients in sinus rhythm are treated with aspirin if they have transient ischemic events without other identifiable cause and with warfarin if they have recurrent transient ischemic episodes despite aspirin therapy or if they present initially with a stroke.[2,31] Patients with severe mitral regurgitation usually can have mitral valve reconstruction rather than valve replacement.[68]

Mitral Stenosis

Prevalence

Congenital mitral valve stenosis is a rare condition that occurs in approximately 0.4% of patients with congenital heart disease.[75] Worldwide, most cases represent acquired disease from rheumatic fever but in developed nations, congenital lesions are more common. Congenital mitral stenosis can occur with other left-sided obstructive lesions at the pulmonary vein, supramitral, subaortic, aortic valve, supraaortic valve, or aortic arch level. Shone syndrome encompasses patients with multiple areas of left-sided cardiac obstruction; mitral stenosis by limiting forward flow during development can lead to stenosis or hypoplasia of distal sites.[76] Rarely mitral stenosis can be associated with malignant carcinoid, systemic lupus erythematosus, mucopolysaccharidosis, or Fabry disease.[2]

Pathology

One or more components of the mitral valve apparatus can be affected including the annulus, leaflets, chordae tendineae, and papillary muscles.[31] In typical congenital mitral stenosis, the chordae are short and thickened with obliteration of interchordal spaces, the leaflet margins are thickened and rolled, the papillary muscles are underdeveloped, and the distance between the anterolateral and posteromedial papillary muscles is mildly reduced.[77] Occasionally the chordae may be extremely deficient or absent so that the valve attaches directly onto the papillary muscles and there can be an arcade-like thickening connecting the apices of the papillary muscles along the line of closure of the anterior leaflet.[77–80] The chordae may also attach to a single papillary muscle forming a parachute mitral valve; in this condition, the anterolateral papillary muscle is often absent.[77] A variation of this condition, termed *parachute-like asymmetric mitral valve*, occurs when there are two papillary muscles, one of which is normal and the other, which is elongated toward the annular region with unequal distribution of chordal attachments.[81] An abnormal tensor apparatus can produce a double-orifice mitral valve that can be associated with normal function, stenosis or regurgitation.[82] All components of the mitral valve are small in patients with hypoplastic left heart syndrome.

Physiology

The degree of obstruction depends on the valve area, cardiac output, and heart rate. The valve area can be calculated by applying the Gorlin formula (see Chapter 14). This formula states that for a given valve area, the mean transvalvar pressure gradient varies by the square of the flow rate. The flow rate depends both on cardiac output and heart rate. During tachycardia, diastole is shortened more than systole so that for a given cardiac output, the flow rate increases.[2] The relationship of valve gradient, mitral valve flow, and valve area is depicted in Figure 40-4. A greater pressure gradient is required to maintain cardiac output as the degree of stenosis increases. For a given valve area, increased flow rates are associated with higher valve gradients. With severe stenosis, small increases in flow rate require large increases in pressure gradient. In adults, the normal mitral valve area is 4.0 to 5.0 cm^2; symptoms occur with exertion when the valve area is less than 2.5 cm^2 and are present at rest when the valve area is <1.5 cm^2.[31]

Cardiac output is also reduced by atrial fibrillation. Atrial contraction contributes 15% to 20% of mitral flow so that the development of this arrhythmia can be associated with the development of symptoms.[2,8]

Elevated left atrial pressure is transmitted to the pulmonary circulation. When pulmonary venous pressure exceeds 30 to 40 mm Hg, pulmonary edema develops. Patients with left ventricular dysfunction and elevated left ventricular end-diastolic pressure will therefore develop dyspnea at lower degrees of mitral valve obstruction. Because mitral stenosis is often associated with other left-sided obstructive lesions, some patients do develop left ventricular dysfunction.[8] Moderate-to-severe mitral stenosis can lead to pulmonary artery hypertension due to passive transmission of pressure, reactive vasoconstriction, and structural changes in the vessel wall.[83,84] If pulmonary hypertension is severe, right ventricular dysfunction and tricuspid regurgitation develop.[8]

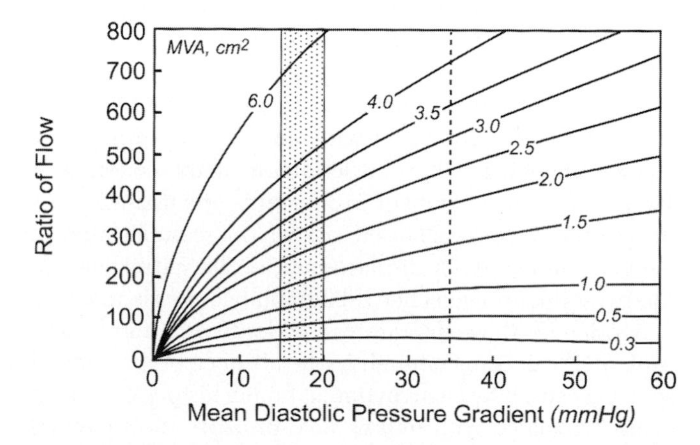

FIGURE 40–4 *Relationship of mitral valve area (MVA) and mitral valve flow to the degree of mitral stenosis.*
From Rahimtoola SH, Durairaj A, Mehra A, et al. Current evaluation and management of patients with mitral stenosis. Circulation 106:1183, 2002, with permission.

Once mitral stenosis is relieved, the pulmonary hypertension often improves but may not become normal if morphologic pulmonary arterial changes are present or if significant stenosis persists.[85,86]

Clinical Manifestations

Mild mitral stenosis is not associated with symptoms. With moderate obstruction patients develop dyspnea or tachypnea with exertion and with severe obstruction symptoms develop at rest. Symptoms depend on the level of cardiac output and level of pulmonary vascular resistance. For patients with moderate or severe obstruction, if cardiac output is maintained with exertion, the left atrial, pulmonary venous, and pulmonary arterial pressures rise significantly and produce pulmonary congestion with cough, wheezing, and occasionally hemoptysis. If cardiac output is limited at rest and increases minimally with exertion, fatigue, orthopnea, and exertional limitation dominate the clinical picture. Infants additionally can have poor oral intake, slow growth, diaphoresis, and recurrent pneumonia. Systemic embolism occurs more commonly in patients with low cardiac output or atrial fibrillation than in patients with mild obstruction or sinus rhythm. Rarely, a markedly dilated left atrium can compress the recurrent laryngeal nerve and produce hoarseness.[2,75,87,88]

The hallmark of the cardiac examination is an apical, low-pitched, rumbling diastolic murmur. The length of the murmur correlates with the severity of stenosis. There usually is presystolic accentuation. The murmur is easier to hear when the patient is in the left lateral decubitus position and during expiration.[2] The intensity of the murmur depends directly on cardiac output, and inversely with chest wall thickness, and severity of associated pulmonary disease. An opening snap created by sudden tensing of the opened valve leaflets is common in rheumatic disease, but often is absent in congenital mitral stenosis.[8] The intensity of S_1 depends on the excursion of the valve leaflets during closing; patients with mild or moderate obstruction have a loud S_1, whereas those with severe obstruction have a soft S_1 (see Chapter 11). Patients with pulmonary hypertension have a prominent right ventricular heave, increased intensity of S_2, and occasionally a murmur of tricuspid regurgitation or pulmonary regurgitation (Graham Steell murmur).

Electrocardiography. The electrocardiogram is normal in patients with mild stenosis. With advancing degrees of obstruction, P-mitrale develops with broad notched P waves in lead II and biphasic P waves in V_1. If pulmonary hypertension develops, right ventricular hypertrophy and right atrial enlargement can also be present. Chronic moderate or severe stenosis can produce atrial tachyarrhythmias, most notably atrial fibrillation.

Chest Radiography. The degree of left atrial enlargement correlates with the severity of stenosis. In the frontal plane, left atrial enlargement creates a double density and splaying of the tracheal bifurcation due to displacement of the left main bronchus superiorly. Enlargement of the left atrium is often easier to appreciate on the lateral projection. Marked left atrial enlargement is unusual in isolated mitral stenosis and its presence implies the coexistence of mitral regurgitation.[2] In severe stenosis, the lung fields demonstrate pulmonary venous congestion, Kerley B lines typically at the costophrenic angle, and redistribution of blood flow to the apical regions.[2,8,87] The pulmonary findings correlate with left atrial pressure: A left atrial pressure above 18 mm Hg produces pulmonary congestion, above 25 mm Hg produces interstitial edema, and above 35 mm Hg produces alveolar edema.[89]

Echocardiography. Two-dimensional, Doppler, and color echocardiography provide information on valve morphology, valve area, pressure gradient, level of pulmonary pressure, presence of left atrial thrombus, and presence of mitral regurgitation or other associated congenital cardiac defects.[89–92] In patients with poor acoustic windows, transesophageal echocardiography provides this information.[93] Multiple views from the parasternal, apical, and subcostal plane are required to identify all components of the valve apparatus and to identify the anatomic contributions to obstruction. The degree of stenosis can be underestimated if there is an associated atrial communication permitting unloading of the left atrium or additional left-sided obstructive lesions that limit cardiac output.[90] The calculation of mitral valve area using the Doppler pressure half-time method correlates well with catheterization-derived measurements in adult patients but not in infants and children possibly due to differences in heart rate, valve size, and atrial and ventricular compliance.[90]

Cardiac Catheterization. A thorough echocardiographic examination generally provides necessary information to determine patient management. Cardiac catheterization is performed if there is discrepancy between echocardiographic findings and clinical features, in older patients with indication for coronary angiography, or if patients fulfill criteria for balloon valvuloplasty.[2,89]

Simultaneous left ventricular and left atrial pressure recordings permit measurement of a direct transmitral pressure gradient (Fig. 40-5). In the absence of an atrial communication, a Brockenbrough transseptal procedure needs to be performed. Pulmonary capillary wedge pressures tend to overestimate left atrial pressure by approximately 2 mm Hg. If a wedge pressure is used care must be taken to ensure that the catheter is not partially wedged, which would yield a higher false gradient; the mean wedge pressure should be lower than the mean pulmonary artery pressure and the oxygen saturation of blood withdrawn from the wedged catheter should exceed 95%.[94] A pulmonary capillary wedge pressure also has delayed transmission compared with

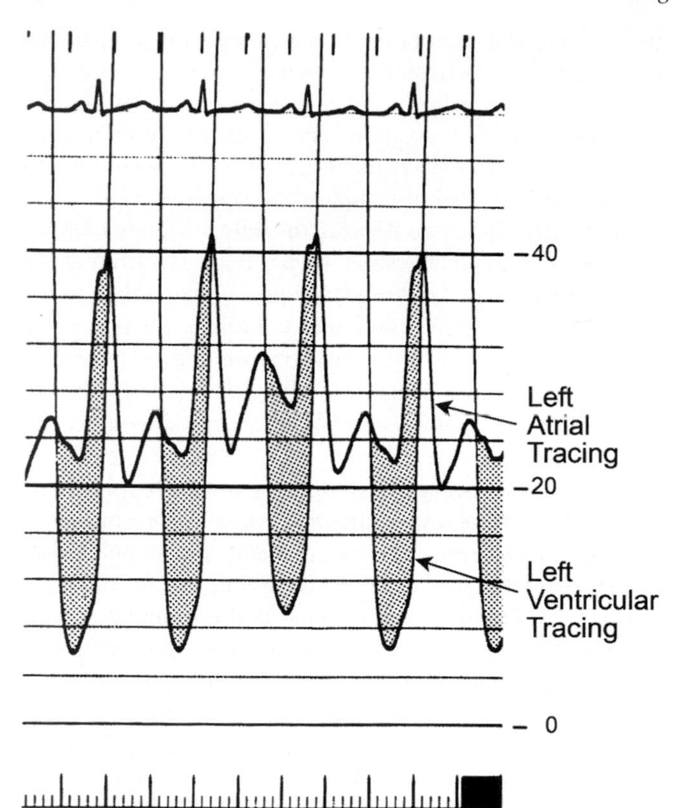

FIGURE 40–5 *Pressure tracings from the left atrium and left ventricle in a 3-month-old infant with severe mitral stenosis. There is a diastolic pressure gradient depicted by the stippled area. From Fyler DC: Mitral valve and left atrial lesions. In Fyler DC (ed). Nadas' Pediatric Cardiology. Philadelphia: Hanley & Belfus, 1992, pp 609–621, with permission.*

a direct left atrial measurement and needs to be realigned by 50 to 70 milliseconds for accurate measurement of mean gradient.[94] Pressure measurements should be obtained close in time to determination of cardiac output. The valve orifice area is determined using the Gorlin formula after calculation of mean diastolic gradient, diastolic filling period, heart rate, and cardiac output[94] (see Chapter 14). Left ventricular angiography permits assessment of the degree of mitral regurgitation and left ventricular function.

Percutaneous balloon valvuloplasty is effective for patients with severe mitral stenosis associated with rheumatic fever.[95,96] Results in patients with severe congenital mitral stenosis are varied and depend on the anatomic basis for obstruction; the best results occur in patients with typical mitral stenosis and symmetric papillary muscles.[97,98] Dilation can reduce the transvalvar gradient in the majority of patients permitting postponement of surgery, but symptomatic improvement at a mean follow-up of 14 months persists in only 44%.[97] This procedure is relatively contraindicated if there is more than mild mitral regurgitation.[99]

Management

The degree of mitral stenosis in many patients is mild and generally does not progress with somatic growth.[8,97] Medical management includes the use of penicillin prophylaxis in patients with rheumatic disease and observance of endocarditis precautions. Symptomatic patients can benefit from the use of beta-blockers or calcium channel blockers by limiting the level of tachycardia associated with exertion. Diuretics and salt restriction are useful in patients with pulmonary venous congestion. Patients with atrial fibrillation require antiarrhythmic medication (see Chapter 29) and anticoagulation. Anticoagulation is also indicated in patients with previous pulmonary or systemic embolic events even if they have sinus rhythm.[2,31,89]

Patients with poor growth, respiratory symptoms, hemoptysis, or severe pulmonary hypertension require intervention. Balloon valvuloplasty can be attempted to delay the time of surgical intervention. Every effort is made to postpone mitral valve surgery as long as possible in infants and children since the results of valve repair are variable and there may be a need for valve replacement. Because of the high incidence of associated heart disease, the surgical approach must be individualized for each patient. The repair of coexisting cardiac conditions that increase left atrial volume, such as ventricular septal defect or patent ductus arteriosus, may be sufficient to significantly reduce the mitral valve gradient.[8] Valvuloplasty techniques vary by the anatomy and include commissurotomy, splitting of papillary muscles, separation of fused chordae tendineae, muscular resection, and annular dilation.[100–105] Many patients require subsequent surgical procedures, including valve replacement, but initial valvuloplasty permits additional growth and avoids the need for anticoagulation.[75] The mitral annulus continues to grow despite the presence of a prosthetic valve ring so that a larger valve can be placed at a subsequent operation to accommodate for growth in a child.[106] Placement of a prosthetic valve in a supraannular position in infants whose annular diameter is too small to accommodate the smallest valve has been associated with poor hemodynamic results.[107] Perioperative pulmonary hypertension can be reduced with inhaled nitric oxide.[108]

LEFT ATRIAL PROBLEMS

Supravalvar Mitral Membrane

A supravalvar mitral membrane consists of a ring of connective tissue that is adherent to the atrial surface of the mitral valve leaflets or slightly superior to the valve annulus. This fibrous tissue is distal to the left atrial appendage, which distinguishes it from the membrane of cor triatriatum.[109,110] This condition can be an isolated finding but usually is associated with other congenital cardiac defects, notably mitral valve stenosis, subaortic stenosis, coarctation, ventricular septal defect, and persistent left superior vena cava draining to the coronary sinus.[8,76,77,88,90,91,97,102,109,111,112] The clinical manifestations depend on the severity of obstruction. Symptoms associated with accompanying defects often dominate the presentation.[110]

The membrane can be identified with the use of two-dimensional echocardiography (Fig. 40-6). Multiple views, including parasternal long-axis, subxiphoid four-chamber, and apical four-chamber, and stop frame diastolic images are often needed to distinguish the membrane from the mitral valve.[90,109] This structure should be carefully searched for in any patient with mitral stenosis since the timing of surgical intervention is earlier when the membrane rather than a valve abnormality primarily causes significant obstruction.[109,113]

Experience of balloon dilation of supravalvar mitral membrane associated with mitral valve abnormality is limited but is associated with the development of significant mitral regurgitation and need for mitral valve replacement.[97] Surgical therapy includes resection of the membrane and repair of associated defects.[102,103,105] Surgical outcome is better in patients with normal mitral valves.[113] While resection usually provides definitive therapy,[102] there is one report that describes the development of recurrent supravalvar mitral membranes, more commonly in infants less than 18 months of age at the time of the initial procedure, so that postoperative follow-up is important.[111]

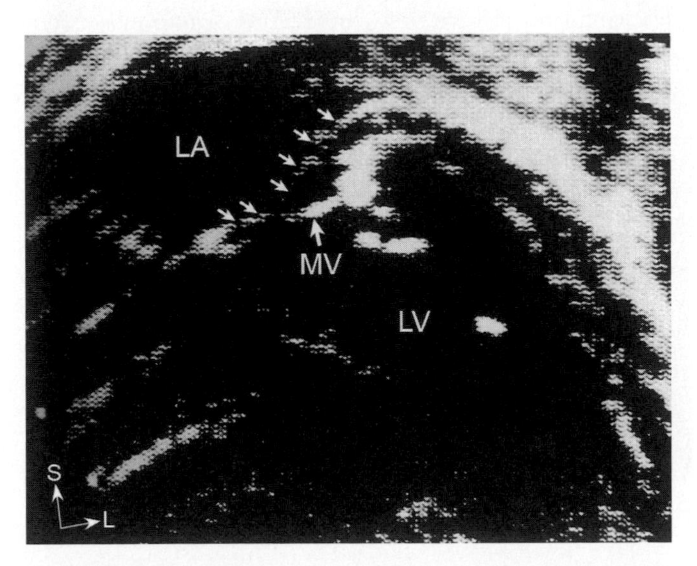

FIGURE 40–6 *Modified subcostal four-chamber echocardiographic views showing supravalvar mitral membrane in diastole (small arrows). L, left; LA, left atrium; LV, left ventricle; MV, mitral valve; S, superior.*
From Sullivan ID, Robinson PJ, de Leval M, et al. Membranous supravalvular mitral stenosis: a treatable form of congenital heart disease. J Am Coll Cardiol 8:159, 1986, with permission.

Cor Triatriatum

Definition

Cor triatriatum consists of an oblique fibromuscular membrane that subdivides the left atrium into a proximal posterior-superior chamber (also termed *accessory chamber*), which typically receives the pulmonary veins, and a distal anterior-inferior chamber communicating with the left atrial appendage and mitral valve.[8,114,115]

Prevalence

Cor triatriatum is very rare and is estimated to comprise 0.1% to 0.4% of congenital heart disease.[114,116,117]

Pathology

Several developmental theories for cor triatriatum have been proposed with incomplete incorporation of the common pulmonary vein to the posterior portion of the primitive left atrium being most accepted.[114–116,118,119] There usually is a single opening in the membrane of variable size and an atrial communication or patent foramen ovale connecting the right atrium and distal chamber. Many variations have been described including no or multiple openings in the membrane,[114,119] an atrial communication connecting the right atrium and proximal chamber,[114–116,119,120] drainage of some pulmonary veins to the distal left atrial chamber,[116,119] presence of other complex cardiac defects,[120,121] or partial or total anomalous pulmonary venous connection to the right side of the circulation.[122,123]

Physiology

The effects on the cardiovascular system are similar to those seen in patients with mitral stenosis, being minimal or absent if the membrane opening is large, and associated with pulmonary venous obstruction, pulmonary edema, pulmonary hypertension, and decreased cardiac output when the opening is small. The degree of obstruction can increase over time arising from calcification, fibrosis, or hypertrophy of muscle fibers in the membrane associated with chronic flow disturbance.[114,124,125] Symptoms of pulmonary venous obstruction are ameliorated not only by the presence of a large opening in the membrane, but also by a large atrial communication between the proximal chamber and right atrium, other cardiac conditions that limit pulmonary flow, or partial anomalous pulmonary venous connection.[110,126] Patients with partial anomalous pulmonary venous connection have variation in pulmonary findings with congestion in lobes draining proximal to an obstructed membrane and increased perfusion in lobes draining to the systemic venous circulation.[8,127]

Clinical Manifestations

Symptoms correlate directly with the diameter of the opening in the membrane as well as with the presence of associated cardiac defects.[121] In a review of 37 reported cases in 1960, patients with an ostial diameter less than 3 mm had a mean age of death of 3.3 months, whereas those with a larger opening had a mean age of death of 16.1 year.[114] With severe obstruction, patients develop respiratory symptoms including tachypnea, cough, dyspnea, wheezing, and frequent pulmonary infections in infancy.[8,121] Older patients can have embolic phenomenon arising from thrombus formation in the proximal chamber.[128] If the membrane opening is large, no symptoms develop and the diagnosis may be made incidentally even occasionally in adults.[129,130] Cor triatriatum should be suspected in patients with unexplained pulmonary edema.[8]

The physical examination differs from patients with mitral stenosis in having no apical diastolic murmur. Patients with pulmonary hypertension have a parasternal right ventricular lift and loud second heart sound. Symptomatic patients frequently have pulmonary rales.

Electrocardiography. Patients with severe obstruction have right axis deviation and right ventricular hypertrophy.[8,121] Right or left atrial hypertrophy is variable.[121]

Chest Radiography. Severe obstruction produces pulmonary venous obstruction, pulmonary edema, and Kerley B lines. In patients with pulmonary hypertension, the main pulmonary artery and right ventricle are dilated.

Echocardiography. Two-dimensional echocardiography is effective for diagnosis of cor triatriatum.[117] Multiple views including parasternal, subxiphoid, and apical, are useful for detecting the left atrial membrane that often curves anteroinferiorly, the number of openings in the membrane, the location of atrial communications, and presence of other congenital cardiac defects (Fig. 40-7). The left atrial appendage is distal to the membrane, a characteristic that distinguishes this condition from supramitral membrane. The entry site of each pulmonary vein should be determined since partial anomalous pulmonary venous connection is present in 9% to 25% of patients with cor triatriatum.[129,131] Color and Doppler echocardiography are useful in assessing the degree of obstruction created by the membrane, level of

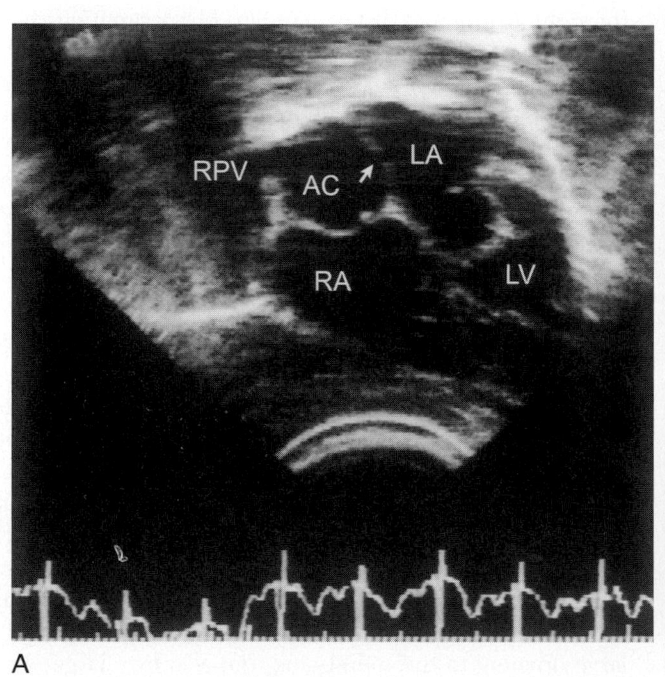

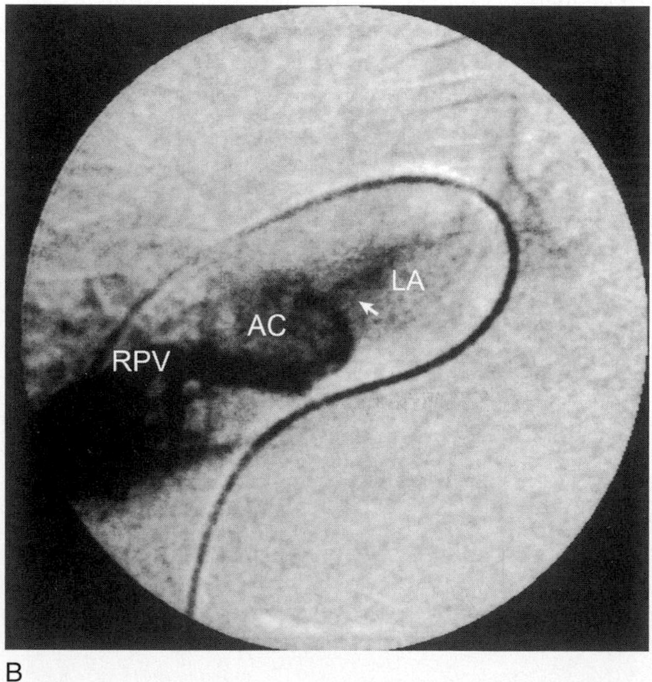

FIGURE 40–7 *Cor triatriatum.*
A, Echocardiogram from the subxiphoid long-axis view (left panel) demonstrating the obstructive left atrial membrane containing a single orifice (arrow) that subdivides the left atrium into a proximal accessory chamber (AC) receiving the right pulmonary vein (RPV) and distal left atrial chamber (LA). LV left ventricle, RA right atrium. B, Levophase of right lower pulmonary artery angiogram demonstrating drainage of the the right pulmonary vein (RPV) to the accessory chamber (AC) and subsequent filling of the distal left atrial chamber (LA) via stenotic opening in the intraatrial membrane (arrow).
From Geggel RL, Fulton DR, Chernoff HL, et al. Cor triatriatum associated with partial anomalous pulmonary venous connection to the coronary sinus: echocardiographic and angiocardiographic features. Pediatr Cardiol 8:279, 1987, with permission.

pulmonary artery pressure, and valve function. In patients with limited transthoracic imaging or for intraoperative assessment, transesophageal echocardiography[132–134] provides diagnostic imaging.

Magnetic resonance imaging and computed tomography: These imaging modalities also effectively detect the presence of a left atrial membrane.[135–137]

Cardiac Catheterization. Cardiac catheterization is generally not needed for management of patients with cor triatriatum. Patients with severe obstruction typically have pulmonary artery hypertension, elevated pulmonary capillary wedge pressure, normal pressure in the distal left atrial chamber, and normal left ventricular end diastolic pressure. The wedge pressure can be normal if there is anomalous pulmonary venous connection to the right heart or an atrial communication between the proximal left atrial chamber and right atrium. In patients in whom this portion of the atrial septum is intact, transseptal catheterization permits direct pressure recording in the accessory chamber.[138] Angiography in this chamber enables visualization of the membrane, which may not be detected on the levophase of a pulmonary arteriogram.[110,121]

Management

The left atrial membrane is resected surgically for patients who are symptomatic or have pulmonary hypertension, or those undergoing repair of other cardiac defects. The diaphragm can be resected from a left atrial or right atrial approach depending on surgical preference, patient size, and coexisting disease.[126,139] In patients with no other significant cardiac disease, surgery is curative.[8,120,121,126]

Pulmonary Vein Stenosis

Pulmonary vein stenosis is a rare condition that represents approximately 0.4% of congenital heart disease.[140] This condition occurs as a congenital and acquired form. Congenital stenosis typically involves the pulmonary vein-left atrial junction and extends a variable distance to the lung parenchyma. This form of the condition often is progressive not only in the degree and length of stenosis but in the number of pulmonary veins affected. Neoproliferation of myofibroblasts is the basis for obstruction in some patients.[141] Acquired pulmonary vein stenosis can occur after surgical repair of anomalous pulmonary venous connection[142] or Mustard procedure for transposition of the great arteries,[143] after cardiac transplantation,[144] as a complication of mediastinal fibrosis,[145] and after treatment of atrial arrhythmias by catheter ablation in or near the pulmonary vein ostia.[146] Compression of a pulmonary vein can occur between the spine and dilated right atrium[147,148] and between the descending aorta and heart in patients with single-ventricle or two-ventricle physiology.[149]

Clinical Manifestations

Pulmonary venous hypertension usually produces respiratory symptoms of tachypnea, cough, frequent respiratory infections, and hemoptysis. Occasional patients with unilateral involvement can be symptom-free,[143] The cardiac examination often has findings of pulmonary hypertension with a prominent right ventricular heave and single S_2 of increased intensity. An electrocardiogram usually demonstrates right ventricular hypertrophy. A chest radiograph typically shows pulmonary edema and Kerley B lines that may be asymmetric if there is differential involvement of the pulmonary veins. An echocardiogram can demonstrate stenosis and increased Doppler turbulence at the left atrial junction and estimate the level of pulmonary hypertension. A pulmonary perfusion scan shows decreased perfusion of affected lobes. Magnetic resonance imaging and computer tomography scans provide excellent imaging[148] (Fig. 40-8) and are useful for serial monitoring of a patient's status. Magnetic resonance imaging of pulmonary veins in adults before catheter ablation of atrial fibrillation has demonstrated that normal pulmonary vein ostia are oval, especially on the left side; the minimal diameter is in the anteroposterior plane and may not be identified on angiograms obtained in that view.[150]

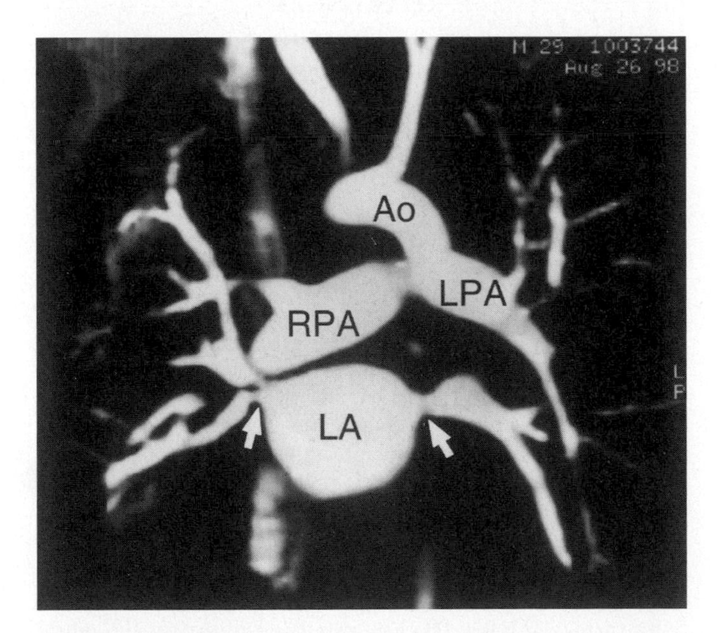

FIGURE 40–8 *Gadolinium-enhanced three-dimensional magnetic resonance angiogram in a young adult with severe bilateral pulmonary vein stenoses (arrows). Ao aorta; LA, left atrium; LPA, left pulmonary artery; RPA, right pulmonary artery.*
From Geva T, Van Praagh S: Anomalies of the pulmonary veins. In Allen HD, Gutgesell HP, Clark EB, Driscoll DJ (eds). Moss and Adams' Heart disease in Infants, Children, And Adolescents, 6th ed. Philadelphia: Lippincott Williams & Wilkins, 2001, pp 736–772, with permission.

Cardiac catheterization demonstrates pulmonary hypertension and usually elevated pulmonary artery wedge pressure, although rarely this value can be normal.[151] The pulmonary artery oxygen saturation in the segment drained by the obstructed vein is elevated because of relative increased contribution of systemic arterial supply to this region.[143] Pulmonary angiography demonstrates slow passage of contrast in the affected lobe and stenosis or atresia of the pulmonary vein. Pulmonary flow is often retrograde in the affected lobe; the pulmonary vein–left atrial junction is imaged more clearly by pulmonary wedge angiography.[152]

Current treatment for congenital pulmonary vein stenosis is challenging and usually unsuccessful. Therapy, including surgery,[153] balloon dilation,[154] or stent placement,[155] despite acute benefit, often is associated with restenosis. Patients with unilateral disease have had occasional long-term improvement by surgery and in some instances by pneumonectomy.[156] Some patients can be considered for lung transplantation.[153] Pulmonary vein compression associated with a giant right atrium after a modified Fontan procedure has been relieved after conversion to a lateral tunnel cavopulmonary anastomosis.[147]

REFERENCES

1. Baylen BG. Congenital mitral insufficiency. In Allen HD, Gutgesell HP, Clark EB, Driscoll DJ (eds). Moss and Adams' Heart Disease in Infants, Children, and Adolescents, 6th ed. Philadelphia: Lippincott Williams & Wilkins, 2001, pp 938–946.
2. Braunwald E. Valvular heart disease. In Braunwald E, Zipes DP, Libby P (eds). Heart Disease: A Textbook of Cardiovascular Medicine, 6th ed. Philadelphia: WB Saunders, 2001, pp 1643–1722.
3. DiSegni E, Edwards J. Cleft anterior leaflet of the mitral valve with intact septa: a study of 20 cases. Am J Cardiol 51:919, 1983.
4. DiSegni E, Bass JL, Lucas RV, et al. Isolated cleft mitral valve: a variety of congenital mitral regurgitation identified by 2-dimensional echocardiography. Am J Cardiol 51:927, 1983.
5. Kalangos A, Oberhansli I, Baldovinos A, et al. Hypoplasia of the posterior leaflet as a rare cause of congenital mitral insufficiency. J Card Surg 12:339, 1997.
6. Layman TE, Edwards JE. Anomalous mitral arcade: a type of congenital mitral insufficiency. Circulation 35:389, 1967.
7. Davachi R, Moller JH, Edwards JE. Diseases of the mitral valve in infancy: anatomic analysis of 55 cases. Circulation 43:565, 1971.
8. Fyler DC. Mitral valve and left atrial lesions. In Fyler DC (ed). Nadas' Pediatric Cardiology. Philadelphia: Hanley & Belfus, 1992, pp 609–621.
9. Grossman W. Profiles in valvular heart disease. In Baim DS, Grossman W (eds). Grossman's Cardiac Catheterization, Angiography, and Intervention, 6th ed. Philadelphia: Lippincott Williams & Wilkins, 2000, pp 759–783.
10. Borer JS, Bonow RO. Contemporary approach to aortic and mitral regurgitation. Circulation 108:2432, 2003.
11. Stanger P, Lucas RV Jr, Edwards JE. Anatomic factors causing respiratory distress in acyanotic congenital heart disease. Pediatrics 43:760, 1969.
12. Schreiber TL, Fisher J, Mangla A, et al. Severe "silent" mitral regurgitation: a potentially reversible cause of refractory heart failure. Chest 96:242, 1989.
13. Banerjee A, Kohl T, Silverman N. Echocardiographic evaluation of congenital mitral valve anomalies in children. Am J Cardiol 76:1284, 1995.
14. Enriquez-Sarano M, Freeman WK, Tribouilloy CM, et al. Functional anatomy of mitral regurgitation: accuracy and outcome implications of transesophageal echocardiography. J Am Coll Cardiol 34:1129, 1999.
15. Feinberg MS, Schwammenthal E, Vered Z. Valvular heart disease (letter to editor). N Engl J Med 337:1474, 1997.
16. Tunick PA, Freedberg RS, Gargiulo A, et al. Exercise Doppler echocardiography as an aid to clinical decision making in mitral valve disease. J Am Soc Echocardiogr 5:225, 1992.
17. Enriquez-Sarano M, Dujardin KS, Tribouilloy CM, et al. Determinants of pulmonary venous flow reversal in mitral regurgitation and its usefulness in determining the severity of regurgitation. Am J Cardiol 83:535, 1999.
18. Leung DY, Griffin BP, Stewart WJ, et al. Left ventricular function after valve repair for chronic mitral regurgitation: predictive value of preoperative assessment of contractile reserve by exercise echocardiography. J Am Coll Cardiol 28: 1198, 1996.
19. Thomas L, Foster E, Schiller NB. Peak mitral inflow velocity predicts mitral regurgitation severity. J Am Coll Cardiol 31:174-9, 1998.
20. Rokey R, Sterling LL, Zoghi WA, et al. Determination of regurgitant fraction in isolated mitral or aortic regurgitation by pulsed Doppler two-dimensional echocardiography. J Am Coll Cardiol 7:1273, 1986.
21. Dujardin KS, Enriquez-Sarano M, Bailey KR, et al. Grading of mitral regurgitation by quantitative Doppler echocardiography: calibration by left ventricular angiography in routine clinical practice. Circulation 96:3409, 1997.
22. Thomas JD. How leaky is that mitral valve? Simplified Doppler methods to measure regurgitant orifice area [editorial comment]. Circulation 95:548, 1997.
23. Hall SA, Brickner E, Willett DL, et al. Assessment of mitral regurgitation severity by Doppler color flow mapping of the vena contracta. Circulation 95:636, 1997.
24. Acar P, Laskari C, Rhodes J, et al. Three-dimensional echocardiographic analysis of valve anatomy as a determinant of mitral regurgitation after surgery for atrioventricular septal defects. Am J Cardiol 83:745, 1999.
25. Braunwald E, Awe WC. The syndrome of severe mitral regurgitation with normal left atrial pressure. Circulation 27:29, 1963.
26. Geggel RL, Hijazi ZM. Reduced incidence of ventricular ectopy with a 4F Halo catheter during pediatric cardiac catheterization. Cathet Cardiovasc Diagn 43:55, 1998.
27. Fifer MA, Grossman W. Measurement of ventricular volumes, ejection fraction, mass, wall stress, and regional wall motion.

In Baim DS, Grossman W (eds). Grossman's Cardiac Catheterization, Angiography, and Intervention, 6th ed. Philadelphia: Lippincott Williams & Wilkins, 2000, pp 353–366.
28. Gaasch WH, Aurigemma GP. Inhibition of the rennin-angiotensin system and the left ventricular adaptation to mitral regurgitation [editorial comment]. J Am Coll Cardiol 39:1380, 2002.
29. ACC/AHA guidelines for the management of patients with valvular heart disease: a report of the American College of Cardiology/American Heart Association Task Force on Practice Guidelines (Committee on Management of Patients with Valvular Heart Disease). J Am Coll Cardiol 32:1486, 1998.
30. Calabrò R, Pisacane C, Pacileo G, et al. Hemodynamic effects of a single oral dose of enalopril among children with asymptomatic chronic mitral regurgitation. Am Heart J 138:955, 1999.
31. Nakano H, Ueda K, Saito A. Acute hemodynamic effects of nitroprusside in children with isolated mitral regurgitation. Am J Cardiol 56:351, 1985.
32. Mori Y, Nakazawa M, Tomimatsu H, et al. Long-term effect of angiotensin-converting enzyme inhibitor in volume overloaded heart during growth: a controlled pilot study. J Am Coll Cardiol 36:270, 2000.
33. Otto CM. Evaluation and management of chronic mitral regurgitation. N Engl J Med 345:740, 2001.
34. Friedman S, Edmunds LH Jr, Cuaso CC. Long-term mitral valve replacement in young children: influence of somatic growth on prosthetic valve adequacy. Circulation 57:981, 1978.
35. Bradley LM, Midgley FM, Watson DC, et al. Anticoagulation therapy in children with mechanical prosthetic cardiac valves. Am J Cardiol 56:533, 1985.
36. Caldarone CA, Raghuveer G, Hills CB, et al. Long-term survival after mitral valve replacement in children aged less than 5 years: a multi-institutional study. Circulation 104[suppl I]:I-143, 2001.
37. Carabello BA, Crawford FA Jr. Valvular heart disease. N Engl J Med 337:32, 1997.
38. Tribouilloy CM, Enriquez-Sarano M, Schaff HV, et al. Impact of preoperative symptoms on survival after surgical correction of organic mitral regurgitation. Circulation 99:400, 1999.
39. Krishnan US, Gersony WM, Berman-Rosenzweig E, et al. Late left ventricular function after surgery for children with chronic symptomatic mitral regurgitation. Circulation 96:4280, 1997.
40. Aharon AS, Laks H, Drinkwater DC, et al. Early and late results of mitral valve repair in children. J Thor Cardiovasc Surg 107:1262, 1994.
41. Chavaud S, Fuzellier JF, Houel R, et al. Reconstruction surgery in congenital mitral valve insufficiency (Carpentier's techniques): long-term results. J Thorac Cardiovasc Surg 115:84, 1998.
42. Raghuveer G, Caldarone CA, Hills CB, et al. Predictors of prosthesis survival, growth, and functional status following mechanical mitral valve replacement in children aged <5 years, a multi-institutional study. Circulation 108[suppl II]:II-174, 2003.
43. St. Goar FG, Fann JI, Komtebedde J, et al. Endovascular edge-to-edge mitral valve repair. Circulation 108:1990, 2003.
44. Barlow JB, Pocock WA, Marchand P, et al. The significance of late systolic murmurs. Am Heart J 66:443, 1963.
45. Nishimura RA, McGoon MD. Perspectives on mitral-valve prolapse [editorial]. N Engl J Med 341:48, 1999.
46. Perloff JK, Child JS, Edwards JE. New guidelines for the clinical diagnosis of mitral valve prolapse. Am J Cardiol 57: 1124, 1986.
47. Krivokapich J, Child JS, Dadourian BJ, et al. Reassessment of echocardiographic criteria for diagnosis of mitral valve prolapse. Am J Cardiol 61:131, 1988.
48. Levine RA, Stathogiannis E, Newell JB, et al. Reconsideration of echocardiographic standards for mitral valve prolapse: lack of association between leaflet displacement isolated to the apical four chamber view and independent echocardiographic evidence of abnormality. J Am Coll Cardiol 11:1010, 1988.
49. Levine RA, Handschumacher MD, Sanfilippo AJ, et al. Three-dimensional echocardiographic reconstruction of the mitral valve, with implications for the diagnosis of mitral valve prolapse. Circulation 80:589, 1989.
50. Freed LA, Levy D, Levine RA, et al. Prevalence and clinical outcome of mitral-valve prolapse. N Engl J Med 341:1, 1999.
51. Warth DC, King ME, Cohen JM, et al. Prevalence of mitral valve prolapse in normal children. J Am Coll Cardiol 5:1173-7, 1985.
52. St. John Sutton M, Weyman AE. Mitral valve prolapse prevalence and complications [editorial]. Circulation 106:1305-7, 2002
53. Boudoulas H, Wooley CF. The floppy mitral valve, mitral valve prolapse, and mitral valvular regurgitation. In Allen HD, Gutgesell HP, Clark EB, Driscoll DJ (eds). Moss and Adams' Heart Disease in Infants, Children, and Adolescents, 6th ed. Philadelphia: Lippincott Williams & Wilkins, 2001, pp 947–969.
54. Shamberger RC, Welch KJ, Sanders SP. Mitral valve prolapse associated with pectus excavatum. J Pediatr 111:404, 1987.
55. Perloff JK, Child JS. Clinical and epidemiologic issues in mitral valve prolapse: Overview and perspective. Am Heart J 113:1324, 1987.
56. Liberthson RR, Boucher CA, Fallon JT, et al. Severe mitral regurgitation: a common occurrence in the aging patient with secundum atrial septal defect. Clin Cardiol 4:229, 1981.
57. Schreiber TL, Feigenbaum H, Weyman AE. Effect of atrial septal defect repair on left ventricular geometry and degree of mitral valve prolapse. Circulation 61:888, 1980.
58. Glesby MJ, Pyeritz RE. Association of mitral valve prolapse and systemic abnormalities of connective tissue: a phenotypic continuum. JAMA 262:523, 1989.
59. Roberts WC, McIntosh CL, Wallace RB. Mechanisms of severe mitral regurgitation in mitral valve prolapse determined from analysis of operatively excised valves. Am Heart J 113: 1316, 1987.
60. Levy D, Savage D. Prevalence and clinical features of mitral valve prolapse. Am Heart J 113:1281, 1987.
61. Arfken CL, Lachman AS, McLaren MJ, et al. Mitral valve prolapse: associations with symptoms and anxiety. Pediatrics 85:311, 1990.
62. Wolf PA, Sila CA. Cerebral ischemia with mitral valve prolapse. Am Heart J 113:1308, 1987.

63. Gilon D, Buonanno FS, Joffe MM, et al. Lack of evidence of an association between mitral-valve prolapse and stroke in young patients. N Engl J Med 341:8, 1999.
64. Maron BJ, Isner JM, McKenna WJ. 26th Bethesda Conference: Recommendations for determining eligibility for competition in athletes with cardiovascular abnormalities. Task Force 3: Hypertrophic cardiomyopathy, myocarditis and other myocardial diseases and mitral valve prolapse. J Am Coll Cardiol 24:880, 1994.
65. Kligfield P, Hochreiter C, Niles N, et al. Relation of sudden death in pure mitral regurgitation, with and without mitral valve prolapse, to repetitive ventricular arrhythmias and right and left ventricular ejection fractions. Am J Cardiol 60:397, 1987.
66. Kavey RW, Sondheimer HM, Blackman MS. Detection of dysrhythmia in pediatric patients with mitral valve prolapse. Circulation 62:582, 1980.
67. Avierinos J, Gersh BJ, Melton LJ II, et al. Natural history of asymptomatic mitral valve prolapse in the community. Circulation 106:1355, 2002.
68. Cohn LH, Couper GS, Aranki SF. Long-term results of mitral valve reconstruction for regurgitation of the myxomatous mitral valve. J Thorac Cardiovasc Surg 107:143, 1994.
69. Wilcken DEL, Hickey AJ. Lifetime risk for patients with mitral valve prolapse of developing severe mitral valve regurgitation requiring surgery. Circulation 78:10, 1988.
70. Fukuda N, Oki T, Iuchi A, et al. Predisposing factors for severe mitral regurgitation in idiopathic mitral valve prolapse. Am J Cardiol 76:503, 1995.
71. Marks AR, Choong CY, Sanfilippo AJ, et al. Identification of high-risk and low-risk subgroups of patients with mitral-valve prolapse. N Engl J Med 320:1031, 1989.
72. Mills P, Rose J, Hollingswoth J, et al. Long-term prognosis of mitral-valve prolapse. N Engl J Med 297:13, 1977.
73. Dajani AD, Taubert KA, Wilson W, et al. Prevention of bacterial endocarditis- recommendations by the American Heart Association. JAMA 277:1794, 1997.
74. Ferrieri P, Gewitz MH, Gerber MA, et al. Unique features of infective endocarditis in childhood- AHA Scientific Statement. Circulation 105:2115, 2002.
75. Baylen BG. Mitral inflow obstruction. In Allen HD, Gutgesell HP, Clark EB, Driscoll DJ (eds). Moss and Adams' Heart Disease in Infants, Children, and Adolescents, 6th ed. Philadelphia: Lippincott Williams & Wilkins, 2001, pp 924–937.
76. Shone JD, Sellers RD, Anderson RC, et al. The developmental complex of "parachute mitral valve," supravalvular ring of left atrium, subaortic stenosis and coarctation of the aorta. Am J Cardiol 11:714, 1963.
77. Ruckman RN, Van Praagh R. Anatomic types of congenital mitral stenosis: report of 49 autopsy cases with consideration of diagnosis and surgical implications. Am J Cardiol 42:592, 1978.
78. Castaneda AR, Anderson RC, Edwards JE. Congenital mitral stenosis resulting from anomalous arcade and obstructing papillary muscles. Report of corrections by use of ball valve prosthesis. Am J Cardiol 24:237, 1969.
79. Pacileo G, Russo MG, Calabro R. Anomalous mitral arcade: echocardiographic and color flow findings. Echocardiography 8:657, 1991.
80. Davachi F, Moller JH, Edwards JE. Diseases of the mitral valve in infancy. Circulation 43:565, 1971.
81. Oosthoek PW, Wenink ACG, Macedo AJ, et al. The parachute-like asymmetric mitral valve and its two papillary muscles. J Thorac Cardiovasc Surg 114:9, 1997.
82. Baño-Rodrigo A, Van Praagh S, Trowitzsch E, et al. Double-orifice mitral valve: a study of 27 postmortem cases with developmental, diagnostic and surgical considerations. Am J Cardiol 61:152, 1988.
83. Otto CM, Davis KB, Reid CL, et al. Relation between pulmonary artery pressure and mitral stenosis severity in patients undergoing balloon mitral commissurotomy. Am J Cardiol 71:874, 1993.
84. Haworth SG, Hall SM, Patel M. Peripheral pulmonary vascular and airway abnormalities in adolescents with rheumatic mitral stenosis. Int J Cardiol 18:405, 1988.
85. Gamra H, Zhang HP, Allen JW, et al. Factors determining normalization of pulmonary vascular resistance following successful balloon mitral valvotomy. Am J Cardiol 83:392, 1999.
86. Fawzy ME, Mimish L, Sivanandam V, et al. Immediate and long-term effect of mitral balloon valvotomy on severe pulmonary hypertension in patients with mitral stenosis. Am Heart J 131:89, 1996.
87. Daoud G, Kaplan S, Perrin EV, et al. Congenital mitral stenosis. Circulation 27:185, 1963.
88. Collins-Nakai RL, Rosenthal A, Castaneda AR, et al. Congenital mitral stenosis-a review of 20 years' experience. Circulation 56:1039, 1977.
89. Rahimtoola SH, Durairaj A, Mehra A, et al. Current evaluation and management of patients with mitral stenosis. Circulation 106:1183, 2002.
90. Banerjee A, Kohl T, Silverman NH. Echocardiographic evaluation of congenital mitral valve anomalies in children. Am J Cardiol 76:1284, 1995.
91. Celano V, Pieroni DR, Morera JA, et al. Two-dimensional echocardiographic examination of mitral valve abnormalities associated with coarctation of the aorta. Circulation 69:924, 1984.
92. Grenadier E, Sahn DJ, Valdes-Cruz LM, et al. Two-dimensional echo Doppler study of congenital disorders of the mitral valve. Am Heart J 107:319, 1984.
93. Ritter SB. Transesophageal real-time echocardiography in infants and children with congenital heart disease. J Am Coll Cardiol 18;569, 1991.
94. Carabello BA, Grossman W. Calculation of stenotic valve orifice area. In Baim DS, Grossman W (eds). Grossman's cardiac catheterization, angiography, and intervention 6th edition. Philadelphia, Lippincott Williams & Wilkins, 2000, pp 193-207.
95. Reyes VP, Raju S, Wynne J, et al. Percutaneous balloon valvuloplasty compared with open surgical commissurotomy for mitral stenosis. N Engl J Med 331:961, 1994.
96. Lock JE, Khalilullah M, Shrivastava S, et al. Percutaneous catheter commissurotomy in rheumatic mitral stenosis. N Engl J Med 313:1515, 1985.
97. Moore P, Adatia I, Spevak PJ, et al. Severe congenital mitral stenosis in infants. Circulation 89:2099, 1994.
98. Spevak PJ, Bass JL, Ben-Shachar G, et al. Balloon angioplasty for congenital mitral stenosis. Am J Cardiol 66:472, 1990.

99. Yeager SB, Flanagan MF, Keane JF. Catheter intervention: balloon valvotomy. In Lock JE, Keane JF, Perry SB, (eds). Diagnostic and interventional catheterization in congenital heart disease, 2nd edition. Boston, Kluwer Academic Publishers, 2000, pp 151-178.
100. Carpentier A. Mitral valve reconstruction in operative surgery. In Jamieson SW, Shumway NE, (eds). Operative surgery 4th ed. Stoneham, MA, Butterworth-Heinemann 1986, pp 405-14.
101. Uva MS, Galletti L, Gayet FL, et al. Surgery for congenital mitral valve disease in the first year of life. J Thorac Cardiovasc Surg 109:164, 1995.
102. Brauner RA, Laks H, Drinkwater DC, et al. Multiple left heart obstructions (Shone's anomaly) with mitral valve involvement: long-term surgical outcome. Ann Thorac Surg 64:721, 1997.
103. Coles JG, Williams WG, Watanabe T, et al. Surgical experience with reparative techniques in patients with congenital mitral valvular anomalies. Circulation 76(suppl III):III-117, 1987.
104. Barbero-Marcial M, Riso A, De Albuquerque AT, et al. Left ventricular apical approach for the surgical treatment of congenital mitral stenosis. J Thorac Cardiovasc Surg 106: 105, 1993.
105. Serraf A, Zoghbi J, Belli E, et al. Congenital mitral stenosis with or without associated defects. Circulation 102[suppl III]: III-166, 2000.
106. Zweng TN, Bluett MK, Mosca R, et al. Mitral valve replacement in the first 5 years of life. Ann Thorac Surg 47:720, 1989.
107. Adatia I, Moore PM, Jonas RA, et al. Clinical course and hemodynamic observations after supraannular mitral valve replacement in infants and children. J Am Coll Cardiol 29:1089, 1997.
108. Atz AM, Adatia I, Jonas RA, et al. Inhaled nitric oxide in children with pulmonary hypertension and congenital mitral stenosis. Am J Cardiol 77:316, 1996.
109. Sullivan ID, Robinson PJ, de Leval M, et al. Membranous supravalvular mitral stenosis: a treatable form of congenital heart disease. J Am Coll Cardiol 8:159, 1986.
110. Jacobstein MD, Hirschfeld SS. Concealed left atrial membrane: pitfalls in the diagnosis of cor triatriatum and supravalve mitral ring. Am J Cardiol 49:780, 1982.
111. Tulloh RMR, Bull C, Elliott MJ, et al. Supravalvar mitral stenosis: risk factors for recurrence or death after resection. Br Heart J 73:164, 1995.
112. Cassano GB. Congenital annular stenosis of the left atrioventricular canal. Am J Cardiol 13:708, 1964.
113. Sethia B, Sullivan ID, Elliott MJ, et al. Congenital left ventricular inflow obstruction: is the outcome related to the site of obstruction? Eur J Cardiothorac Surg 2:312, 1988.
114. Niwayama G. Cor triatriatum. Am Heart J 59:291, 1960.
115. Van Praagh R, Corsini I. Cor triatriatum: pathologic anatomy and a consideration of morphogenesis based on 13 postmortem cases and a study of normal development on the pulmonary vein and atrial septum in 83 human embryos. Am Heart J 78:379, 1969.
116. Lucas RV Jr. Anomalous venous connections, pulmonary and systemic. In Adams FH, Emmanouilides GC (eds). Heart disease in infants, children, and adolescents, 3rd edition. Baltimore, Williams & Wilkins, 1983, pp 458-90.
117. Ostman-Smith I, Silverman NH, Oldershaw P, et al. Cor triatriatum sinistrum: diagnostic features on cross sectional echocardiography. Br Heart J 51:211, 1984.
118. Gharagozloo F, Bulkley BH, Hutchins GM. A proposed pathogenesis of cor triatriatum: impingement of the left superior vena cava on the developing left atrium. Am Heart J 94:618, 1977.
119. Thilenius OG, Bharati S, Lev M. Subdivided left atrium: an expanded concept of cor triatriatum sinistrum. Am J Cardiol 37:743, 1976.
120. Oglietti J, Cooley DA, Izquierdo JP, et al. Cor triatriatum: operative results in 25 patients. Ann Thorac Surg 35:415, 1983.
121. Marin-Garcia J, Tandon R, Lucas RV Jr, et al. Cor triatriatum: study of 20 cases. Am J Cardiol 35:59, 1975.
122. Geggel RL, Fulton DR, Chernoff HL, et al. Cor triatriatum associated with partial anomalous pulmonary venous connection to the coronary sinus: echocardiographic and angiocardiographic features. Pediatr Cardiol 8:279, 1987.
123. Kirk AJB, Pollock JCS. Concomitant cor triatriatum and coronary sinus total anomalous pulmonary venous connection. Ann Thorac Surg 44:203, 1987.
124. McGuire LB, Nolan TB, Reeve R, et al. Cor triatriatum as a problem of adult heart disease. Circulation 31:263, 1965.
125. Feld H, Shani J, Rudansky HW, et al. Initial presentation of cor triatriatum in a 55-year-old woman. Am Heart J 124: 788, 1992.
126. van Son JAM, Danielson GK, Schaff HV, et al. Cor triatriatum: diagnosis, operative approach, and late results. Mayo Clin Proc 68:854, 1993.
127. Somerville J. Masked cor triatriatum. Br Heart J 28:55, 1966.
128. Darbar D, Bridges AB, Roberts R, et al. Cor triatriatum: unusual cause of transient ischemic attacks in a 67-year-old man. Br J Clin Pract 49:166, 1995.
129. Geggel RL, Fulton DR, Rockenmacher S. Nonobstructive cor triatriatum in infancy. Clin Pediatr 38:489, 1999.
130. O'Murchu B, Seward JB. Adult congenital heart disease-obstructive and nonobstructive cor triatriatum. Circulation 92:3574, 1995.
131. Wolf WJ. Diagnostic features and pitfalls in the two-dimensional echocardiographic evaluation of a child with cor triatriatum. Pediatr Cardiol 6:211, 1986.
132. Schlüter M, Langenstein BA, Their W, et al. Transesophageal two-dimensional echocardiography in the diagnosis of cor triatriatum in the adult. J Am Coll Cardiol 2:1011, 1983.
133. Vuocolo LM, Stoddard MF, Longaker RA. Transesophageal two-dimensional and Doppler echocardiographic diagnosis of cor traitriatum in the adult. Am Heart J 124:791, 1992.
134. Shuler CO, Fyfe DA, Sade R, et al. Transesophageal echocardiographic evaluation of cor triatriatum in children. Am Heart J 129:507, 1995.
135. Bissett GS III, Kirks DR, Schwartz DC. Cor triatriatum: diagnosis by MR imaging. AJR 149:567, 1987.
136. Masui T, Seelos KC, Kersting-Sommerhoff BA, et al. Abnormalities of the pulmonary veins: evaluation with

MR imaging and comparison with cardiac angiography and echocardiography. Radiology 181:645, 1991.
137. Tanaka F, Itoh M, Esaki H, et al. Asymptomatic cor triatriatum incidentally revealed by computed tomography. Chest 100:272, 1991.
138. Shaffer EM, Rocchini AP, Dick M II, et al. Transseptal left heart catheterization as an aid in the diagnosis of cor triatriatum. Pediatr Cardiol 8:123, 1987.
139. Richardson JV, Doty DB, Siewers RD, et al. Cor triatriatum (subdivided left atrium). J Thorac Cardiovasc Surg 81: 232, 1981.
140. Edwards J. Congenital stenosis of pulmonary veins. Lab Invest 9:46, 1960.
141. Sadr IM, Tan PE, Kieran MW, et al. Mechanism of pulmonary vein stenosis in infants with normally connected veins. Am J Cardiol 86:577, 2000.
142. van Son JAM, Danielson GK, Puga FJ, et al. Repair of congenital and acquired pulmonary vein stenosis. Ann Thorac Surg 60:144, 1995.
143. Lock JE, Lucas RV Jr, Amplatz K, et al. Silent unilateral pulmonary venous obstruction-occurrence after surgical repair of transposition of the great arteries. Chest 73:224, 1978.
144. Fortuna RS, Chinnock RE, Bailey LL. Heart transplantation among 233 infants during the first six months of life: the Loma Linda experience. Loma Linda pediatric heart transplant group. Clin Transpl 263, 1999.
145. Doyle TP, Loyd JE, Robbins IM. Percutaneous pulmonary artery and vein stenting-a novel treatment for mediastinal fibrosis. Am J Respir Crit Care Med 164:657, 2001.
146. Qureshi AM, Prieto LR, Latson LA, et al. Transcatheter angioplasty for acquired pulmonary vein stenosis after radiofrequency ablation. Circulation 108:1336, 2003.
147. Kreutzer J, Keane JF, Lock JE, et al. Conversion of modified Fontan procedure to lateral atrial tunnel cavopulmonary anastomosis. J Thorac Cardiovasc Surg 111:1169-76, 1996.
148. Valsangiacomo ER, Levasseur S, McCrindle BW, et al. Contrast-enhanced MR angiography of pulmonary venous abnormalities in children. Pediatr Radiol 33:92, 2003.
149. O'Donnell CP, Lock JE, Powell AJ, et al. Compression of pulmonary veins between the left atrium and the descending aorta. Am J Cardiol 91:248, 2003.
150. Wittkampf FHM, Vonken EJ, Derksen R, et al. Pulmonary vein ostium geometry-analysis by magnetic resonance angiography. Circulation 107:21, 2003
151. Geggel RL, Fried R, Tuuri DT, et al. Congenital pulmonary vein stenosis: structural changes in a patient with normal pulmonary artery wedge pressure. J Am Coll Cardiol 3:193, 1984.
152. Kingston HM, Patel RG, Watson GH. Unilateral absence or extreme hypoplasia of pulmonary veins. Br Heart J 49:148, 1983.
153. Spray TL, Bridges ND. Surgical management of congenital and acquired pulmonary vein stenosis. Semin Thorac Cardiovasc Surg Pediatr Card Surg Annu 2:177, 1999.
154. Driscoll DJ, Hesslein PS, Mullins CE. Congenital stenosis of individual pulmonary veins: clinical spectrum and unsuccessful treatment by transvenous balloon dilation. Am J Cardiol 49:1767, 1982.
155. Tomita H, Watanabe K, Yazaki S, et al. Stent implantation and subsequent dilatation for pulmonary vein stenosis in pediatric patients. Circ J 67:187, 2003.
156. Nasrallah AT, Mullins CE, Singer D, et al. Unilateral pulmonary vein atresia: diagnosis and treatment. Am J Cardiol 36:969, 1975.

41

Hypoplastic Left Heart Syndrome, Mitral Atresia, and Aortic Atresia

PETER LANG AND DONALD C. FYLER

HYPOPLASTIC LEFT HEART SYNDROME

Definition

The term *hypoplastic left heart syndrome* describes a diminutive left ventricle with underdevelopment of the mitral and aortic valves.[1] Because of its small size, the left ventricle is incapable of supporting the systemic circulation.

Some patients have mitral or aortic stenosis, or both, but most have aortic or mitral atresia and rarely, some with aortic atresia have a nearly normal-sized left ventricle. These cases are not properly examples of the hypoplastic left heart syndrome. Similarly, cases of mitral atresia with a double-outlet right ventricle are not examples of the hypoplastic left heart syndrome, nor are those rare instances of mitral atresia with inverse ventricles.

Prevalence

The recently reported prevalence of hypoplastic left heart syndrome varies between 0.21 and 0.28 per 1000 live births.[2,3] It is the fifteenth most common defect in the Children's Hospital Boston series, accounting for approximately 1% of patients of all ages with heart disease.

Anatomy

The left ventricle is small, often tiny (Fig. 41-1). Usually the aortic valve is atretic and hypoplastic, although some babies have severe stenosis. Similarly, the mitral valve may be hypoplastic, severely stenotic, or atretic. The ascending aorta is hypoplastic; above an atretic aortic valve, the diameter of the aorta may be 2 mm or less, very small but sufficient to supply adequate coronary circulation in a retrograde fashion. Untreated infants rarely show coarctation of the aorta at autopsy, but coarctation is a common problem among surgically managed survivors, suggesting that the tendency to develop coarctation is inherent in this anomaly.[4,5] The left atrium is small reflecting the limited blood flow in utero. The atrial septum is thickened; the foramen ovale may be small and, occasionally, may be closed. A patent ductus arteriosus is required for survival.

Anomalies of the brain have associated with the hypoplastic left heart syndrome.[6]

Physiology

Overview

With an atretic aortic valve, survival beyond birth is dependent on persistent patency of the ductus arteriosus to maintain the systemic circulation. There have been occasional reports of *long-term* survival of children with hypoplastic left heart syndrome because of prolonged patency of the ductus arteriosus. Survival to 7 years has been reported.[7]

Of necessity, the right ventricle supplies both the pulmonary and the systemic circulations via the ductus arteriosus, the coronary arteries and brachiocephalic vessels are supplied in retrograde fashion. The relative flow to the pulmonary and systemic circuits depends on the relative resistances of the two vascular beds. One of the major influences on total pulmonary resistance is the size of the interatrial orifice. A restrictive atrial defect tends to raise left atrial pressure and total pulmonary resistance, limiting

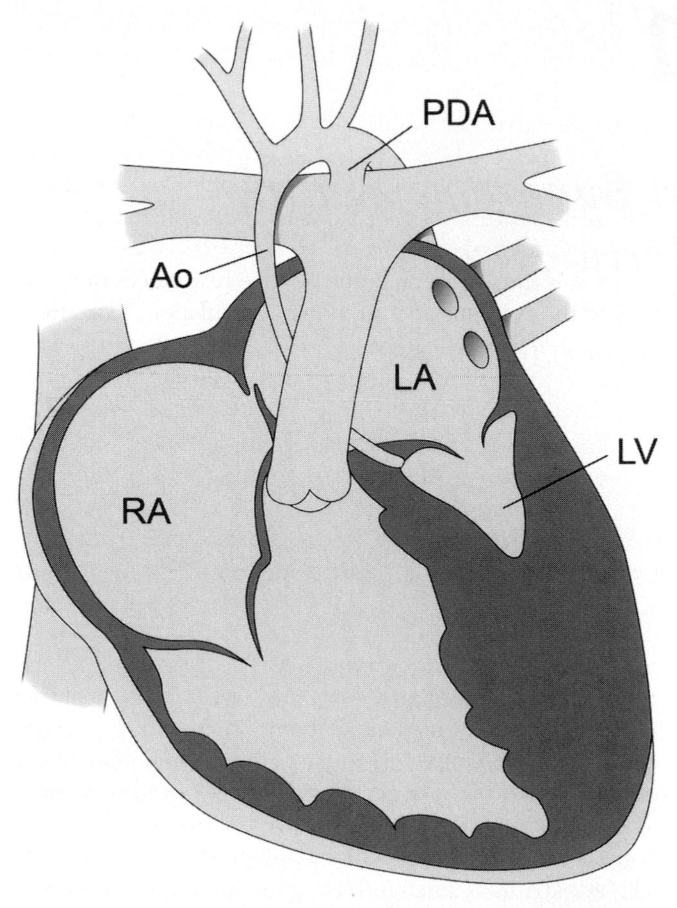

FIGURE 41–1 *Drawing of the anatomy of the hypoplastic left heart syndrome. Note the tiny ascending aorta (Ao) that supplies the coronary circulation in a retrograde direction. No blood passes through the diminutive left ventricle (LV). The left atrium (LA) empties through an incompetent foramen ovale into the right atrium (RA), where all systemic and pulmonary venous blood becomes mixed. The ductus arteriosus (PDA) supplies the entire circulation to the body.*
From Nadas AS, Fyler DC [eds]. Nadas' Pediatric Cardiology. Philadelphia, PA: Hanley and Belfus, 1992.

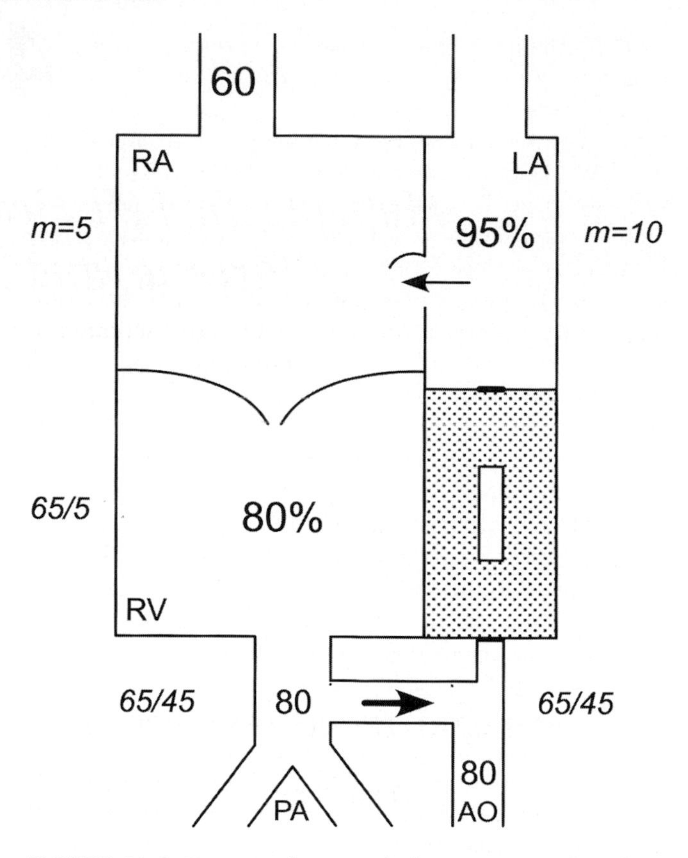

FIGURE 41–2 *Diagram showing ideal preoperative physiology. Low systemic vascular resistance and high pulmonary vascular resistance result in a Q_p/Q_s of approximately 1.*
From Nadas AS, Fyler DC [eds]. Nadas' Pediatric Cardiology. Philadelphia, PA: Hanley and Belfus, 1992.

pulmonary blood flow, whereas a nonrestrictive opening does not.

There is a nearly direct relationship between the amount of pulmonary blood flow and the systemic arterial oxygen saturation. The greater the pulmonary blood flow, the greater the quantity of oxygenated pulmonary venous blood that will return to the heart and mix with the systemic venous return (Fig. 41-2).

It is interesting to speculate that patients with completely unrestricted pulmonary blood flow are likely to succumb to severe congestive heart failure secondary to right ventricular volume overload whereas those individuals with some resistance to pulmonary blood flow may survive. Nonetheless, life for more than a few weeks is precluded.

Transitional Circulation

In the hypoplastic left heart syndrome, as in most forms of congenital heart disease, the intrauterine circulation is adequate to meet the needs of the developing fetus. It is noteworthy that this most lethal congenital heart defect supports normal intrauterine growth.

In utero, all circulation, with the exception of the small amount of pulmonary venous return, passes through the right side of the heart. Streams of superior and inferior vena caval blood return to the right atrium and join the pulmonary venous return (5% to 10% of the cardiac output). The complete admixture of all venous return (that from the placenta as well as the fetus) results in blood flow with identical oxygen saturation to all parts of the fetus. The right atrial return then crosses the tricuspid valve to the right ventricle. The lack of a left ventricular contribution to cardiac output results in a modest right ventricular volume overload.

At this point in the circulation, certain physiological questions emerge, even *in utero*. The relative flow to the pulmonary or systemic circulation is largely dependent on the relative resistance of the pulmonary and systemic vascular beds. Of equal importance is the status of the pulmonary venous return. There is growing evidence that the development of the interatrial septum is abnormal[8] (and of possible primary etiologic significance) in hypoplastic left heart syndrome. In the face of mitral valve atresia, or even severe mitral valve stenosis, an obstructive interatrial septum can result in left atrial hypertension. Even though pulmonary blood flow is low *in utero*, altered intrauterine pulmonary venous pressure might be the best explanation for the abnormal muscularization of the pulmonary veins in these patients. Similarly, the abnormal atrial septal thickness may be caused by left atrial hypertension *in utero*.

There is less speculation about the circulation beyond the ductus arteriosus. It is common to see a posterior aortic ridge of tissue opposite the site of the ductus; systemic blood flow bifurcates at this point. In cases of aortic valve atresia, in which the sole source of systemic blood flow is from the ductus arteriosus, the aortic arch becomes progressively smaller between the ductus and the coronary arteries. Sometimes the origin of the left subclavian artery is involved with ductal tissue and it may become stenotic with time. The ascending aorta, carrying retrograde flow, is an end artery (a common coronary artery) and is frequently 2 mm or less in diameter. This small size is appropriate for the coronary flow required by the newborn heart. However, it must be remembered that coronary blood flow is dependent on a long unobstructed path from the right ventricle to the ascending aorta via the ductus arteriosus. Shortly after birth, coronary flow, as well as cerebral flow, can be compromised, because the aortic isthmus may include ductal tissue that can constrict and obstruct the aorta.

At birth, when the ductus arteriosus is widely patent and the pulmonary arteriolar resistance is relatively high, a brief *honeymoon* begins. The widely patent ductus arteriosus does not restrict systemic blood flow at a *normal* right ventricular systolic pressure. In the absence of ductal constriction, there is no narrowing of the aortic arch, ensuring good coronary and renal perfusion.

A modestly restrictive foramen ovale limits pulmonary blood flow to some extent. More important, in newborns the elevation in pulmonary arteriolar resistance keeps pulmonary blood flow at manageable levels. The moderate limitation in pulmonary blood flow caused by the relatively high resistance is not enough to produce dangerously low systemic arterial oxygen saturation (Fig. 41-2).

Unfortunately, this *ideal* state of physiologic palliation is short lived. Although infants diagnosed *in utero* by two-dimensional echocardiography are seen in this state, most children with the hypoplastic left heart syndrome pass through this honeymoon period without recognition. They behave normally and, unless their *duskiness* is questioned, are often thought to be well.

Two normal physiologic events conspire to bring children with a hypoplastic left heart to medical attention: The ductus arteriosus begins to close and pulmonary vascular resistance decreases. Partial closure of the ductus arteriosus has several profound effects. The first, and the most obvious, is the alteration in the relative resistances of blood flow to the systemic and pulmonary circulation. The effect on the systemic circuit can be either subtle or dramatic. A decrease in systemic output in a newborn has many manifestations. The child's color may be *poor* despite a rise in the systemic oxygen saturation (see below); the peripheral pulses are weak with a narrow pulse pressure; peripheral perfusion can deteriorate; and the child may become lethargic. Concomitant with these changes is an absolute and relative increase in pulmonary blood flow. The major manifestation of this change is tachypnea, with the inevitable inability to breathe and suck at the same time. The *force feeding* of the pulmonary circulation by the closure of the ductus arteriosus is abetted by the normal fall in pulmonary resistance. The relaxation of the pulmonary bed, which may be seen even in the first day of life,[9] may be tempered by the development of acidosis secondary to poor cardiac output.

Usually the end result of progressive ductal closure and falling pulmonary vascular resistance is profound cardiogenic shock. The decreased systemic blood flow is accompanied by poor coronary perfusion. Thus, the right ventricle may have an increased pressure load (secondary to ductal constriction), an increased volume load (secondary to increased pulmonary blood flow), and, because of poor coronary flow, has less wherewithal to do the work. Right ventricular dysfunction and dilation with tricuspid regurgitation only exacerbate the volume overload. Finally, the increased pulmonary blood flow, with obstructed outflow from the left atrium, increases pulmonary venous pressure, contributing to the difficulty in breathing. It is no surprise that children with hypoplastic left heart syndrome often present to medical attention gasping for breath, in a profound low-output state, acidotic, and in renal failure (Fig. 41-3).

Before the introduction of prostaglandin E_1, a child in profound cardiogenic shock secondary to hypoplastic left heart syndrome died quickly, often before surgical intervention could be organized. Although some children did survive to undergo palliative surgery, they were a select few whose systemic circulation was maintained by persistent patency of the ductus arteriosus. With the use of prostaglandin E_1, the ductus arteriosus almost invariably reopens. Once an unobstructed pathway from the right ventricle to the aortic arch has been secured, support for the right ventricle is needed. Usually, the ventricle has

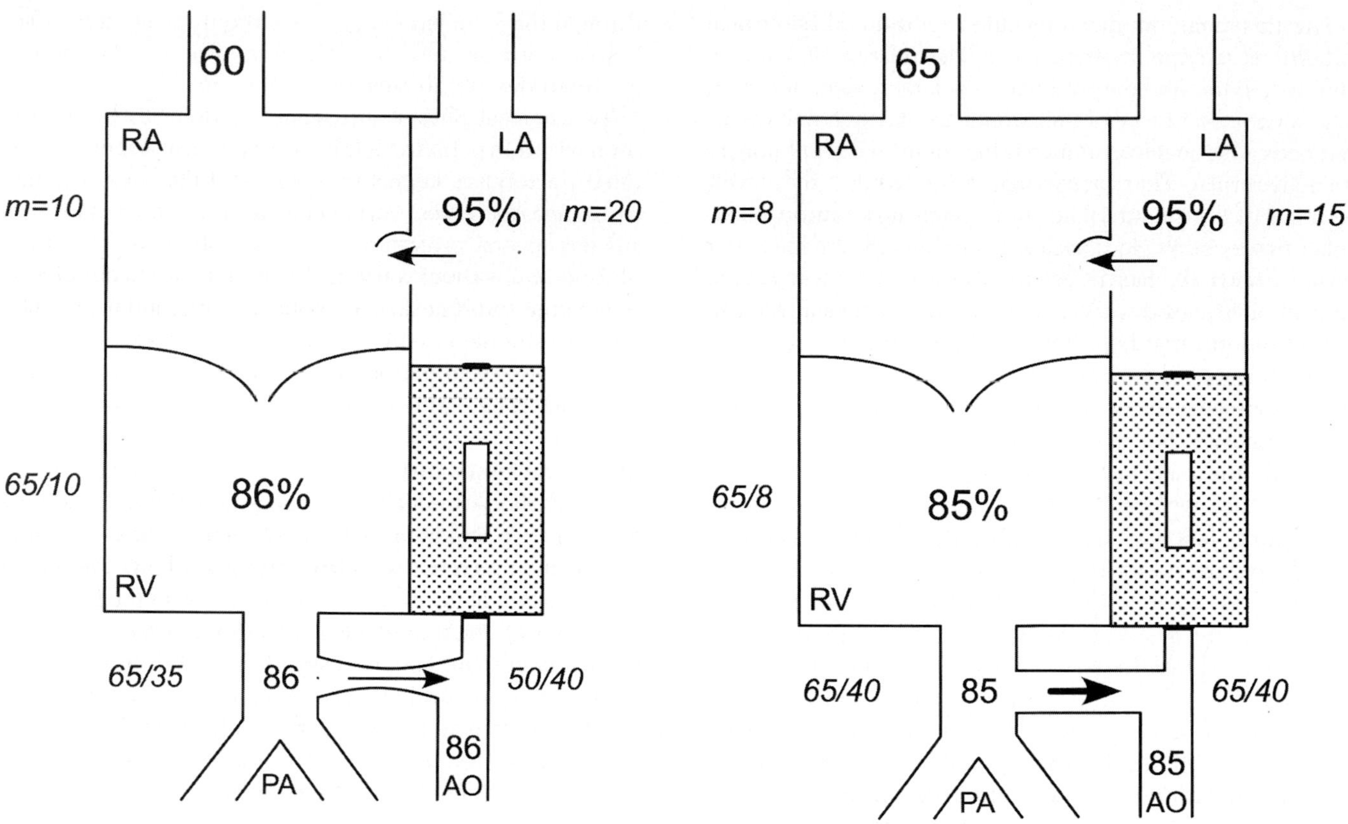

FIGURE 41–3 *Diagram showing closing ductus physiology: decreased systemic blood flow, poor coronary perfusion, increased pulmonary blood flow, and the Q_p/Q_s is approximately 3. There is an increase in right ventricular volume overloading, right ventricular end-diastolic pressure, and left atrial pressure. There is right ventricular dysfunction.*
From Nadas AS, Fyler DC [eds]. Nadas' Pediatric Cardiology. Philadelphia, PA: Hanley and Belfus, 1992.

FIGURE 41–4 *Diagram showing acceptable physiology. The Q_p/Q_s is approximately 2. There is mild right ventricular volume overloading (approximately three times that of normal), a mild increase in right ventricular end-diastolic pressure, and a mild increase in left atrial pressure.*
From Nadas AS, Fyler DC [eds]. Nadas' Pediatric Cardiology. Philadelphia, PA: Hanley and Belfus, 1992.

suffered from a period of relative ischemia secondary to poor coronary perfusion; indeed, right ventricular infarctions have been seen occasionally. In addition, the ventricle has had both a pressure and a volume overload and may have been deprived of adequate metabolic substrate because of hypoglycemia and hypocalcemia. Renal failure may result in an additional fluid overload and hyperkalemia. Finally, hepatic insufficiency, a frequent finding in the setting of low systemic output, may exacerbate the problems of hypoglycemia and acidosis. Inotropic support of the right ventricle must be given gingerly so that whatever metabolic aberrations are present do not contribute to toxic drug reactions.

The physiologic state following resuscitation is never quite as *ideal* as that seen shortly after birth (Fig. 40-4). The relative resistance of the pulmonary and systemic circuits will have changed in the days following birth and that change may have been influenced by the infusion of prostaglandin E_1. The overall pulmonary-to-systemic flow ratio is likely to be at least 2, with resulting systemic arterial oxygen saturation in the range of 85%. Consequently, the right ventricle is volume loaded to the extent that it is pumping three times the normal volume in order to maintain an adequate systemic cardiac output. An increase in right ventricular end-diastolic pressure is a usual finding. The excessive pulmonary blood flow results once again in a volume load to the left atrium. The obstruction to atrial outflow results in pulmonary venous hypertension.

All of this is relatively acceptable. Unfortunately, the transitional circulation is not stable. With the passage of hours, and with, ironically, metabolic improvement, there is a continued decrease in pulmonary vascular resistance. Because the relative resistance of the pulmonary and systemic circulations determines the relative flows to the two circuits, when the maximum volume capacity of the right ventricle is reached (perhaps between four and five times normal, a Qp/Qs of 4), there is a decrease in systemic output. This time, the low output state is not a function of ductal obstruction, but simply a product of the inability of the right ventricle to meet the ever increasing volume demand caused by a decreasing pulmonary vascular resistance. The result of all of this is a continuation of the earlier evolution of the transitional circulatory changes. There is severe right ventricular volume overloading, the right ventricular end-diastolic pressure rises, and there may be right ventricular dilation with tricuspid regurgitation, making matters worse. Once again, the poor systolic perfusion may result in renal failure and acidosis. Left atrial hypertension will impair gas exchange and, in all probability, necessitate intubation and assisted ventilation (Fig. 41-5).

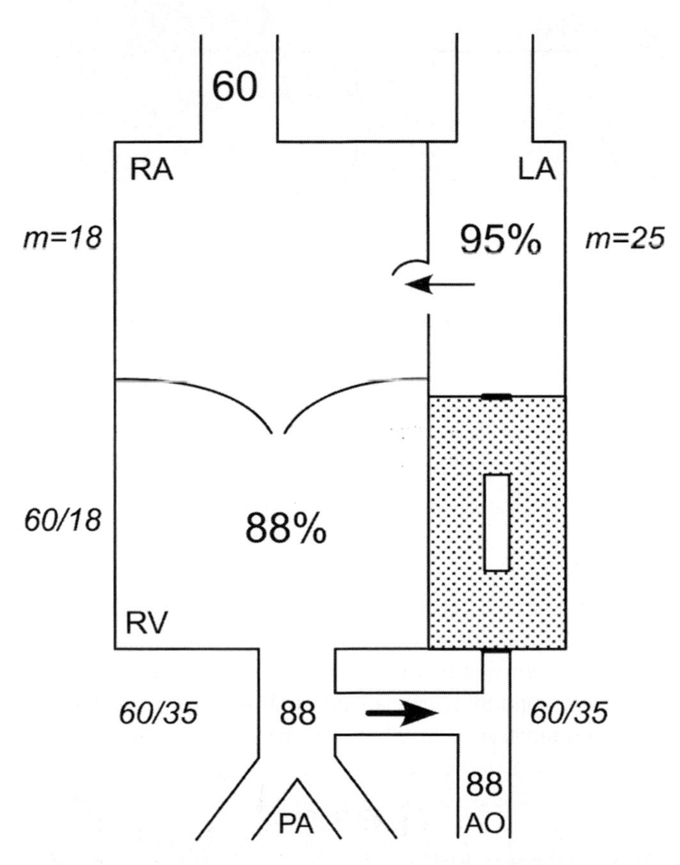

FIGURE 41–5 *Diagram of the low pulmonary resistance physiology. The Q_p/Q_s is approximately 4. There is severe right ventricular volume overloading (approximately five times that of normal), an increase in right ventricular end-diastolic pressure, an increase in left atrial pressure, poor systemic perfusion, low urine output, acidosis, poor right ventricular performance, right ventricular dilation, and tricuspid regurgitation.*
From Nadas AS, Fyler DC [eds]. Nadas' Pediatric Cardiology. Philadelphia, PA: Hanley and Belfus, 1992.

Clinical Manifestations

The infant, usually male (67%), seems healthy at birth. The incidence of prematurity and associated extracardiac anomalies is low. No murmur is heard. Within hours, or a day or so, the nursery nurse may notice that the baby, at times, has poor color, is pale, or somehow just "doesn't seem right." These observations are an exception rather than the rule. More often, without warning, the infant suffers circulatory collapse, becoming ashen, cyanotic, gasping, and near death. There are no palpable pulses. The infant is resuscitated, infusion of prostaglandin E_1 is begun, and the baby is transferred immediately to the nearest pediatric cardiac center.

Electrocardiography

Although, statistically, electrocardiograms in infants with hypoplastic left heart syndrome tend to show less than the usual left ventricular voltages for a newborn infant, this feature is not helpful because many normal newborns also have this pattern. Suffice it to say that the electrocardiogram of an infant with hypoplastic left heart syndrome is rarely interpreted as showing left ventricular hypertrophy and usually shows a little more right ventricular hypertrophy than normal.

Chest Radiography

There is little about the chest radiograph that is specific. The size of the heart and the amount of pulmonary vasculature are variable; the heart may be very large and the pulmonary vasculature increased.

Echocardiography

The hypoplastic left heart syndrome is recognized in detail at echocardiography (Fig. 41-6). Indeed nowadays increasing numbers of affected babies are being recognized by fetal echocardiography long before delivery. The abnormal mitral and aortic valves, the diminutive left ventricle, and the hypoplastic ascending aorta, as well as the flow of blood from the left atrium to the right, are readily identified and confirm the diagnosis. The coronary arteries are supplied from a tiny ascending aorta, often only a few millimeters in diameter. Doppler imaging may reveal retrograde flow in the ascending aorta. The left atrium is small and the atrial septum bulges toward the right. An absent or hypoplastic mitral valve is recognized and the diminutive left ventricle is often visualized. The ductus arteriosus is large and carries blood from the pulmonary artery to the aorta.

The atretic or hypoplastic mitral valve and the hypoplastic left ventricle can be seen in subxiphoid or apical views. Doppler examination of the mitral valve is useful to determine if it is atretic. A potential pitfall in evaluating left ventricular size results from the tendency for the left

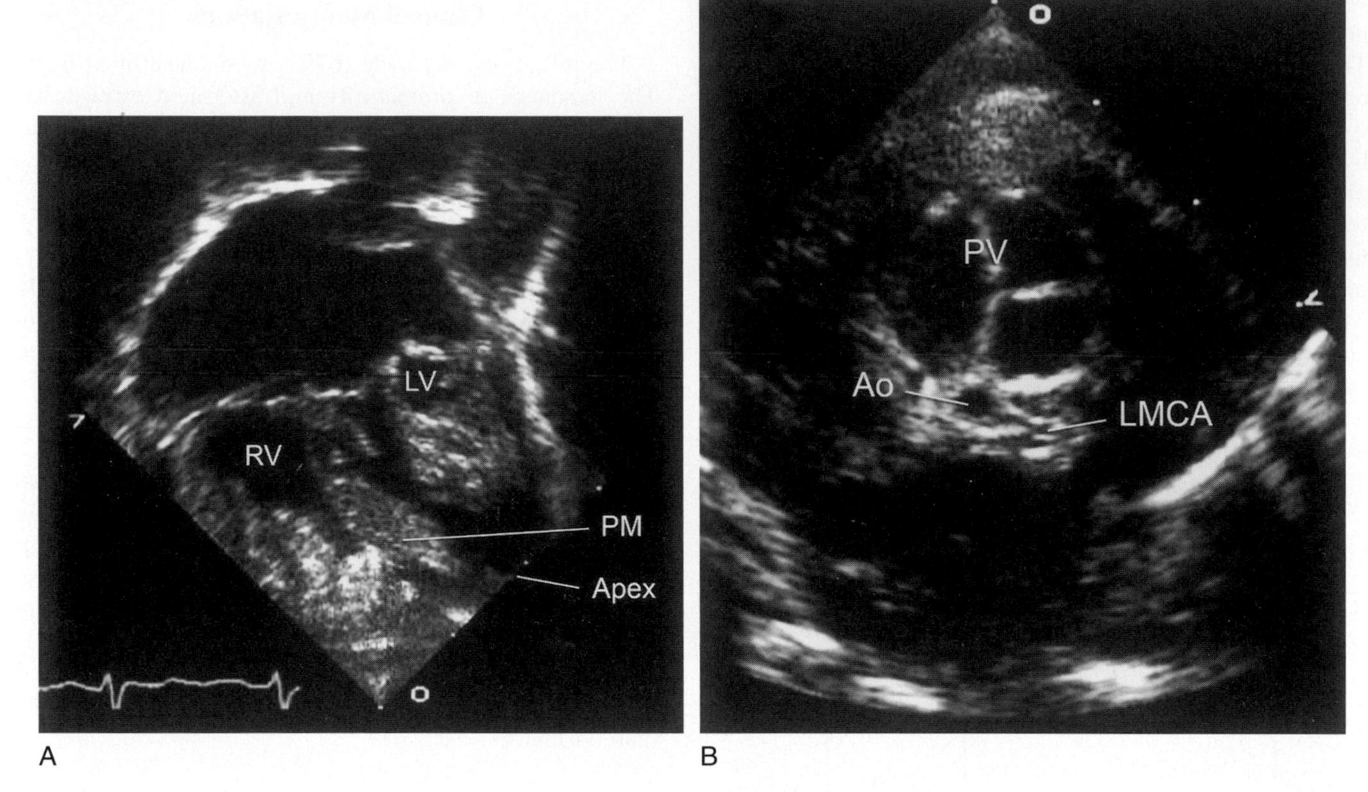

FIGURE 41–6 *Echocardiographic images in newborn with hypoplastic left heart syndrome.*
A, The apical four-chamber view shows the large, apex-forming right ventricle (RV) containing hypertrophied papillary muscles (PM). The diminutive chamber of the left ventricle (LV) extends only a fraction of the heart length. B, In parasternal short axis views, the tiny ascending aorta (Ao) giving rise to the left main coronary artery (LMCA) is seen to lie directly posterior to the very large pulmonary valve (PV).

ventricle long-axis dimension to be reduced before the short-axis dimension. If the left ventricle is evaluated using either two-dimensional or M-mode echocardiography in short-axis projection only, the severity of hypoplasia can be underestimated.

Parasternal and suprasternal views are best for imaging the hypoplastic ascending aorta and aortic arch. The point of juncture of the ductus arteriosus and the arch is often narrow, with a discrete coarctation being present.

The atrial septum can be imaged using subxiphoid views. Tricuspid valve function should be evaluated with Doppler technique from apical and parasternal views, in that tricuspid regurgitation occurs in a significant proportion of patients. Right ventricular function can be evaluated using subxiphoid views.

Cardiac Catheterization

Cardiac catheterization nowadays is rarely necessary in the newborn period, except in those with a virtually intact atrial septum. In those cases, it is undertaken to create a septal defect to relieve left atrial hypertension and pulmonary edema before the stage I surgical procedure. Although most patients require catheterization at age 6 months before the bidirectional Glenn or hemi-Fontan operations, it is likely that it will be replaced by magnetic resonance imaging (MRI) studies in uncomplicated survivors. It is, however, a standard procedure before the Fontan operation.

Management

Medical Treatment

Most infants arrive at the cardiac center intubated and receiving prostaglandin E_1. An attempt must be made to *turn back the clock* and return to the *acceptable* level of pulmonary and systemic blood flow that existed before the patient's collapse. Factors that tend to increase pulmonary vascular resistance (within limits) are needed. The most direct and controllable means of meeting this end is with *controlled hypoventilation*. The FiO_2 should be reduced to as close to 0.21 as possible to maintain an arterial Po_2 of 30 mm Hg. The Pco_2 should be allowed to rise to 40 mm Hg in an attempt to maintain a pH of 7.35 to 7.40. Positive end-expiratory pressure may also be *beneficial* in increasing total pulmonary resistance. Because the intrinsic respiratory drive leads to a lower than desired Pco_2, heavy sedation is often required.

The desired result is reduction of the Qp/Qs from 4 to 2 and reduction of the right ventricular volume load from five to three times normal. This benefit may exceed the potential benefit of intropic medications and vasodilator agents. The judicious use of dopamine and milrinone will aid right ventricular contractibility and reduce systemic vascular resistance, a combination of effects particularly beneficial to this group of patients.

A small subgroup of patients requires separate consideration. Rarely, the interatrial communication can be so obstructive that left atrial hypertension limits pulmonary blood flow to levels that do not permit adequate oxygenation for prolonged survival. In this instance, the Po_2 is below 20 mm Hg despite the reverse of the manipulations described in the preceding paragraphs (i.e., high Fio_2, hyperventilation to the point of hypocarbia, and alkalosis). In this setting, rapid relief of the pulmonary venous obstruction by an atrial septostomy with or without stent placement at catheterization is the only alternative.[10]

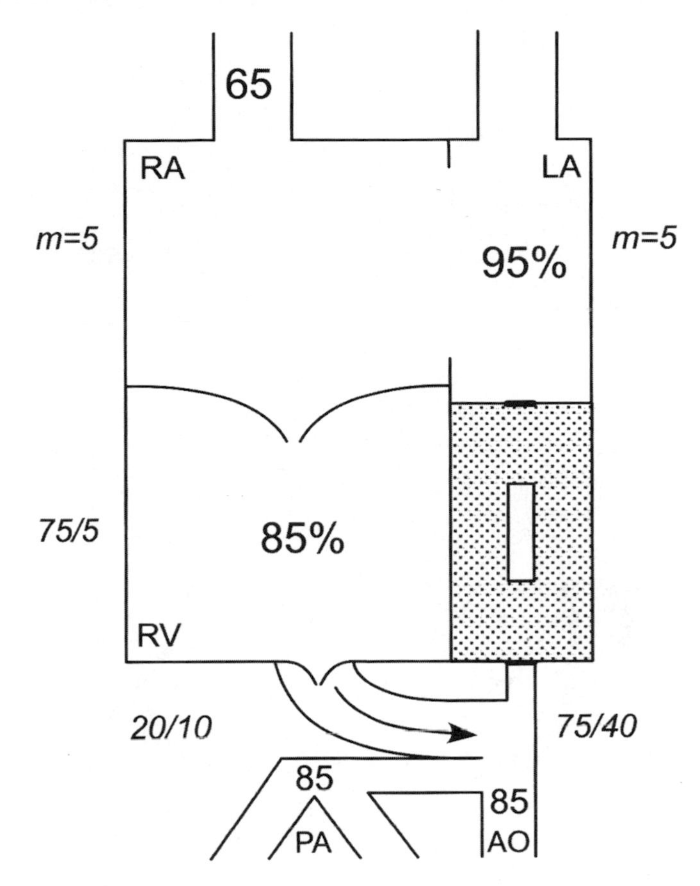

FIGURE 41–7 *Diagram showing ideal postoperative physiology. Widely patent pathway from the right ventricle to the aorta, limitation of pulmonary blood flow without distortion to the pulmonary arteries, unrestricted pulmonary venous return, normal-sized right ventricle, and normal tricuspid valve.*
From Nadas AS, Fyler DC [eds]. Nadas' Pediatric Cardiology. Philadelphia, PA: Hanley and Belfus, 1992.

Surgical Treatment

Based on the initial attempts to manage the hypoplastic left heart syndrome, the following goals for successful palliation were established. *First* is the need to establish a permanent unobstructed communication between the right ventricle and the aorta with preservation of the right ventricular function. *Second* is the necessity of limiting pulmonary blood flow with preservation of pulmonary artery architecture. The *third* goal is to relieve pulmonary venous obstruction (Fig. 41-7).

The surgical procedure developed by Norwood most nearly satisfies the goals for initial palliation and subsequent repair of children with hypoplastic left heart syndrome.[11] Minimal prosthetic material is used in both the systemic and pulmonary circulations, allowing for maximal potential growth. The prosthetic aortopulmonary shunt placed at the time of initial palliation is, of course, removed at the time of reparative surgery. The first-stage operation consists of transection of the distal main pulmonary artery. The aorta, from the takeoff of the left subclavian artery to the ascending aorta, is incised, and an anastomosis is established between the proximal main pulmonary artery and the ascending aorta and the aortic arch. This connection is almost always augmented with homograft tissue in order to avoid arch obstruction. Pulmonary blood flow can be established by a modified Blalock-Taussig shunt, a central shunt, or a right ventricle to distal main pulmonary artery shunt (Fig. 41-8). The latter modification, popularized by Sano[12] has the disadvantage of a small systemic ventriculotomy but the advantage of avoiding diastolic pulmonary artery *run-off*, which can compete with flow to the small ascending aorta and the coronary arteries. This stage of the operation is completed by ligating the ductus arteriosus and opening the atrial septum, unless there is an atrial septal defect.

Surgical Complications

There are numerous potential problems after surgery.[4] Some relate primarily to the underlying anatomic defect, some to the physiologic derangements associated with the circulatory collapse that first signaled the presence of heart disease, and some to the surgery.

Atrial Septum. This structure is thicker and more leftward in orientation than it is in healthy individuals. It is

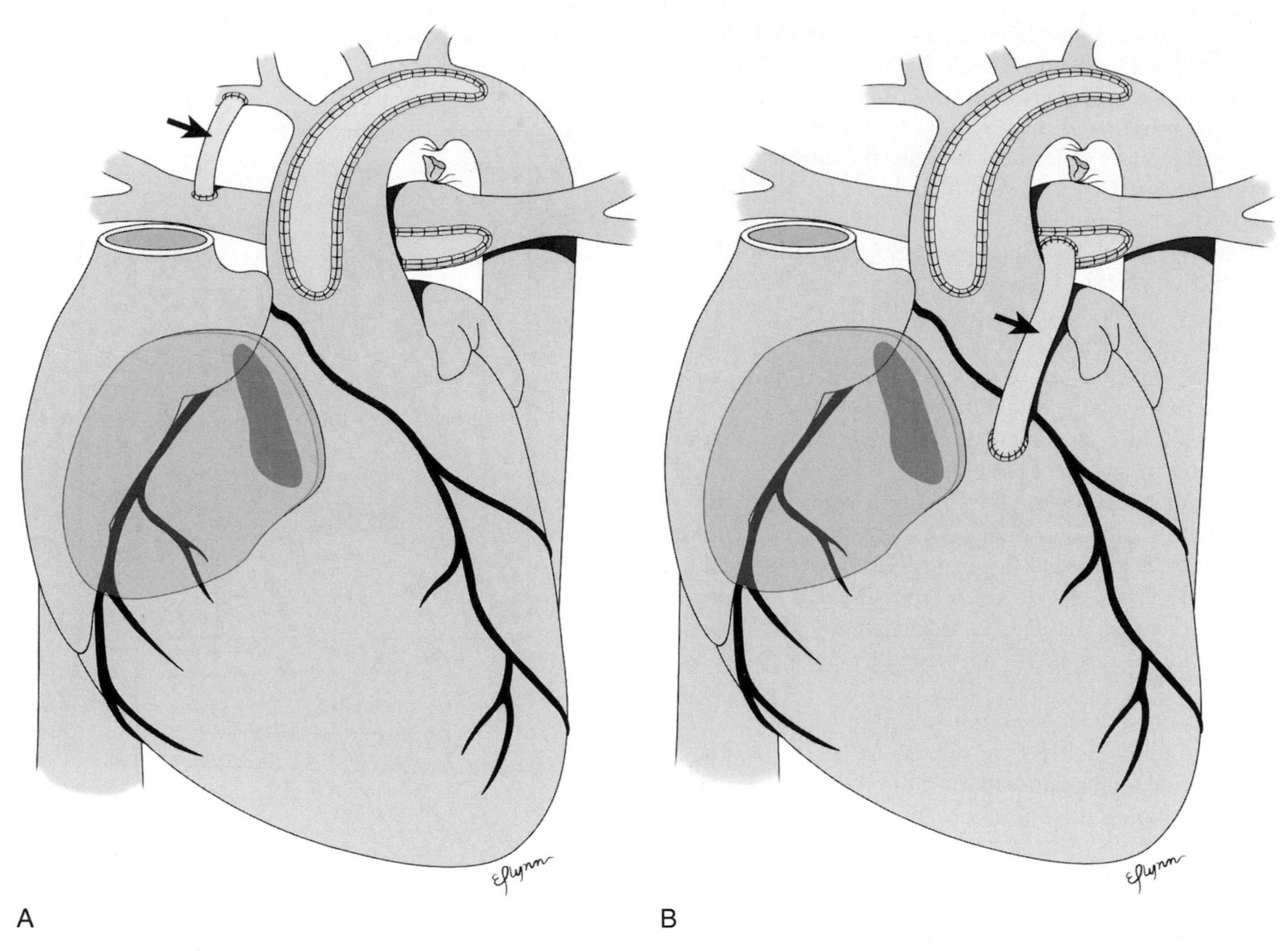

FIGURE 41–8 *Drawing showing pulmonary blood supplied by (A) modified (arrow) Blalock-Taussig shunt (arrow) and (B) right ventricle to pulmonary artery shunt (arrow).*

not readily amenable to balloon septostomy. If obstructive, catheter-directed septostomy, often using a stent, is performed preoperatively to achieve left atrial acute decompression for stabilization before surgery. At surgery, septectomy is an integral part of the initial palliative operation in all. Even with purported wide excision of atrial septal tissue, obstruction to flow has developed (Fig. 40-9). As opposed to initial palliation, subsequent management with stent placement or blade atrial septostomy can be achieved,[10,13] beneficial, although likely temporary, maneuvers. Because pulmonary venous hypertension can adversely affect the development of the pulmonary vascular bed, a restrictive atrial septal defect should be treated aggressively.

Postoperative development of obstruction to flow across the interatrial septum may be subtle. Increasing cyanosis before the time when the child should be *outgrowing* the systemic-to-pulmonary shunt might be the first indication that there is a problem. The intensity of the shunt murmur may decrease as pulmonary artery pressure increases subsequent to pulmonary venous hypertension. Fortunately, two-dimensional echocardiography usually provides a definitive diagnosis of the problem.

Stenosis of the Pulmonary Veins. Progressive stenosis of the pulmonary veins may be associated with extreme left atrial hypoplasia. Whether this occurs because of ongoing underdevelopment of the left heart structures, progressive mediastinal fibrosis, or inflammatory difficulties based on the initial surgery remains unclear.

Tricuspid Regurgitation. The next level of concern following palliative surgery is the status of the tricuspid valve. As mentioned earlier, the right ventricle carries an excess volume and may have been subjected to metabolic and ischemic injury prior to palliation. Thus, some degree of tricuspid regurgitation may be expected. The effect of

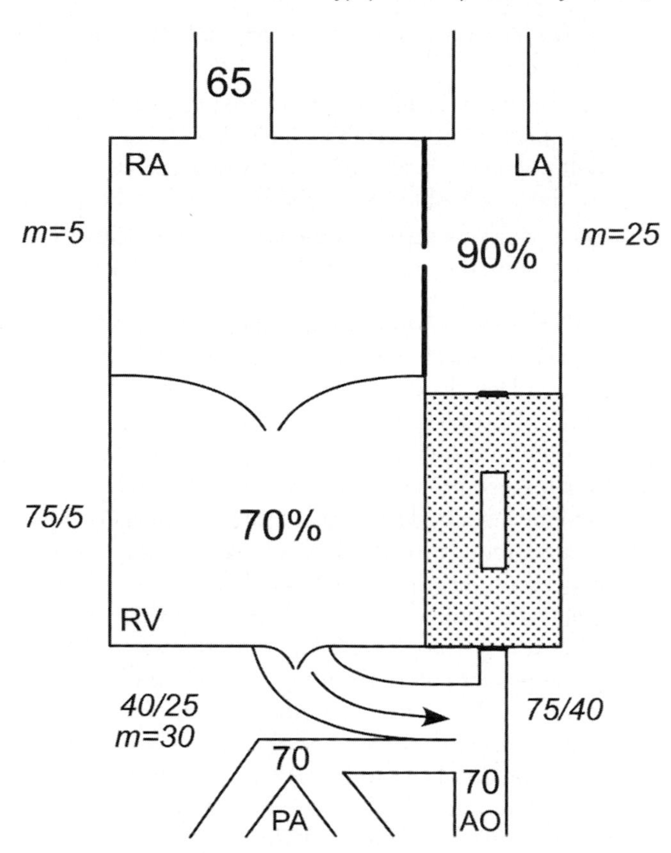

FIGURE 41–9 *Diagram showing restrictive atrial septal defect physiology. The Q_p/Q_s is approximately 1. There is pulmonary artery hypertension due to high left atrial pressure and decreased oxygen saturation caused by low Q_p/Q_s and pulmonary venous desaturation.*
From Nadas AS, Fyler DC [eds]. Nadas' Pediatric Cardiology. Philadelphia, PA: Hanley and Belfus, 1992.

tricuspid regurgitation on early and late mortality is not clear.[14,15] How much tricuspid regurgitation can occur before it is necessary to recommend annuloplasty or valve replacement or simply to refer these children for allotransplantation, remains under discussion.

Right Ventricular Myocardial Problems. The right ventricle may fare poorly regardless of the status of the tricuspid valve. Right ventricular dysfunction secondary to a period of ischemia, acidosis, or severe volume loading may preclude normal (or even adequate) functional status. Ventriculocoronary connections may play a role in poor right ventricular function in the hypoplastic left heart syndrome.[14–19] Thick-walled coronary arteries and myocardial fibrillar disarray have been demonstrated in a subset of these patients, particularly those with a patent left ventricular inflow and obstructed left ventricular outflow tract. If these were to have a major effect on survival following palliative surgery, one would think that overall survival would be significantly better for patients with mitral atresia than for those with mitral stenosis. A study comparing those two groups failed to demonstrate a significant difference. Right ventricular dysfunction after palliative surgery has not been a prominent finding.[4,14] The potentially deleterious effect of the ventriculotomy if the right ventricular to pulmonary artery shunt is used to supply pulmonary blood flow is an important consideration.

Coarctation of the Reconstructed Aorta. Until patients began to survive with palliative surgery, it was not recognized that coarctation of the aorta is a common component of the hypoplastic left heart syndrome (Fig. 41-10).[4,5] How much of this is caused by constricting ductal tissue and how much is the result of surgical manipulation is not always clear. After testing a variety of ways to avoid this problem, our current practice is to bypass the area of potential coarctation with an extensive homograph patch augmented aortic arch reconstruction at the time of initial palliation.[9] If coarctation develops, the resulting increase in right ventricular pressure and the increased pulmonary blood

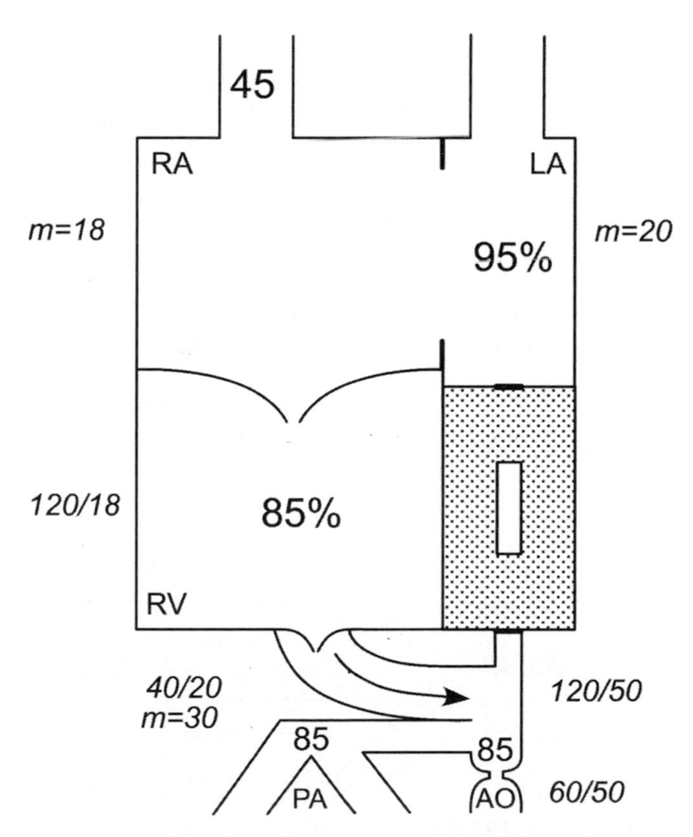

FIGURE 41–10 *Diagram showing coarctation physiology. The Q_p/Q_s is approximately 4. There is increased right ventricular end-diastolic pressure because of decreased ventricular function and tricuspid regurgitation, pulmonary artery hypertension due to increased pulmonary flow, and increased left atrial pressure.*
From Nadas AS, Fyler DC [eds]. Nadas' Pediatric Cardiology. Philadelphia, PA: Hanley and Belfus, 1992.

flow will produce symptoms; the diminished femoral pulses may provide diagnosis. Management with balloon dilation has been successful.[20,21]

Pulmonary Vascular Disease. The pulmonary vascular bed must evolve normally if a successful Fontan operation is to be performed later. The excess of blood volume and pressure to which the pulmonary vasculature is exposed must be kept in mind. Pulmonary vascular disease may be as devastating as right ventricular dysfunction in terms of the subsequent suitability of a patient for a modified Fontan operation.

Peripheral Pulmonary Stenosis. If a later Fontan operation is to be successful, undistorted pulmonary arteries are required (Fig. 41-11). Three features conspire to deform the pulmonary arteries:

1. If the surgeon uses a long segment of the proximal main pulmonary artery in reconstructing the ascending aorta, central pulmonary artery deformity may be the result.[15,22,23]
2. Constricting ductal tissue may produce obstruction at the point of insertion of the ductus into the origin of the left pulmonary artery. Severe narrowing at the takeoff of the proximal left pulmonary artery may be seen.
3. The point of insertion of the arterial-pulmonary shunt may cause distortion of the pulmonary artery.

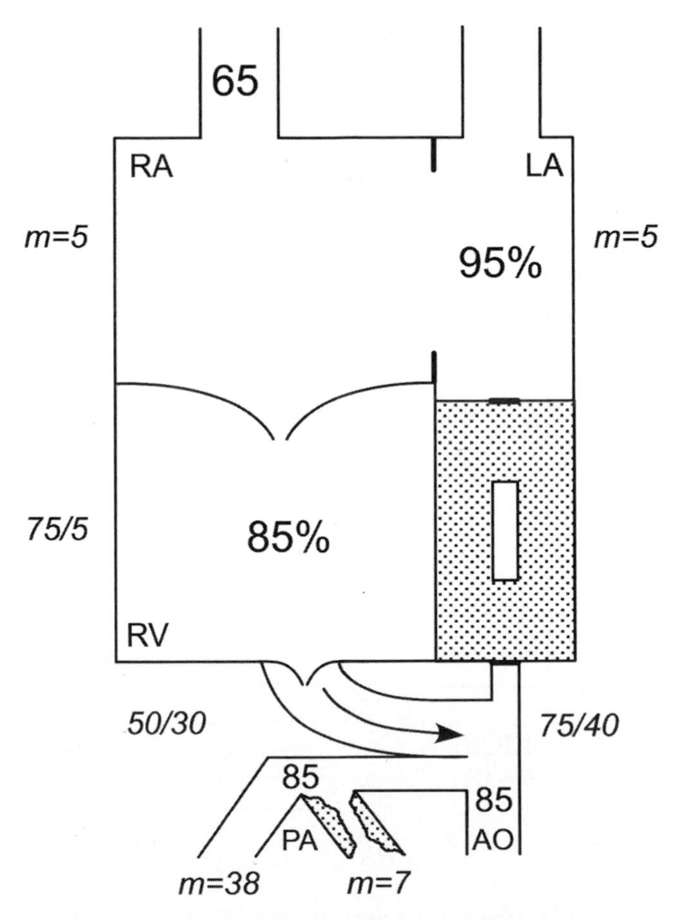

FIGURE 41–11 *Diagram showing distorted pulmonary artery physiology. The Q_p/Q_s is approximately 2. There is right pulmonary artery hypertension and left pulmonary artery hypoplasia because of low flow.*
From Nadas AS, Fyler DC [eds]. Nadas' Pediatric Cardiology. Philadelphia, PA: Hanley and Belfus, 1992.

Arterial-Pulmonary Shunts. A modified right Blalock-Taussig shunt may be the preferred method to supply pulmonary blood flow.[9] Although this provides a favorable regulation of overall pulmonary blood flow, the distribution to right and left lungs is not symmetric. The usual 2:1 (ipsilateral:contralateral) distribution of blood flow that occurs following a Blalock-Taussig shunt is exaggerated by whatever degree of proximal left pulmonary artery obstruction is present. This combination of factors can lead to potential right pulmonary artery hypertension and left pulmonary artery hypoplasia. Once again, the adverse effects on a subsequent Fontan operation are apparent. A potential benefit of the right ventricular to pulmonary artery shunt as a source of pulmonary blood flow is the central location of the distal anastomosis; a more symmetric distribution of pulmonary blood flow is expected.

The Systemic Pulmonary Valve. Concern about the ability of the pulmonary valve to manage the systemic circulation seems to be unwarranted. There have been few recognizable problems.[24]

Management after Palliation

The initial palliation must allow the baby to survive surgery (Exhibit 41-1), to accommodate to the changes in pulmonary arteriolar resistance that occur during the first weeks of life, and to accommodate to the doubling or tripling of body size. Indeed, cardiopulmonary bypass (with or without a period of circulatory arrest), general anesthesia, and neuromuscular blockade, followed by a period of assisted ventilation, all have profound effects on the pulmonary vasculature. It is not unusual to have an anatomically large shunt appear to be physiologically small immediately following cardiopulmonary bypass. Within hours there may be a profound lowering of the pulmonary arteriolar resistance and the shunt that was *too small* an hour ago has suddenly become *too large*. The same modalities of treatment that were used before surgery are equally important immediately following surgery. Administration of high inspired oxygen, together with hyperventilation and alkalosis, may be necessary in the first hour after surgery, rapidly followed by a decrease in FiO_2 to room air, with controlled hypoventilation for the remainder of the period of assisted ventilation. The right ventricle may require some degree of inotropic support in the days following surgery.

Exhibit 41–1
Children's Hospital Boston Experience
1988-2002
Hypoplastic Left Heart Syndrome

A total of 402 patients with hypoplastic left heart syndrome was seen between 1988-2002—of these, 177 are known to have died. Of the 402, 330 underwent their initial surgery at Children's Hospital Boston, with 141 known deaths. A modified Fontan procedure has been carried out in 149 patients at Children's Hospital, with 7 deaths (5% mortality compared with 52% 1973-1987.)

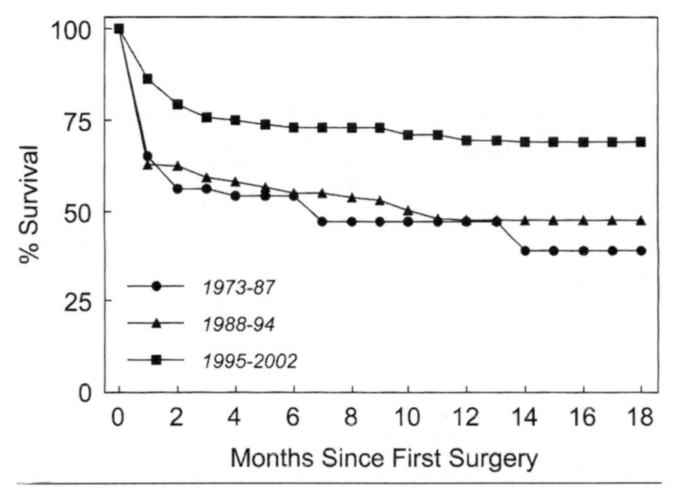

Survival curves for patients operated on at Children's Hospital Boston, showing considerable improvement in more recent group (1995-2002) compared to earlier groups (1988-1994, 1973-1987.)

Following hospital discharge, virtually all children require a cardiotonic regimen, of digoxin and diuretics for the period during which the shunt is relatively large. If all goes well, it will take several months for the child to *grow into the shunt*.

The status of the interatrial septum, right ventricular function, aortic arch reconstruction, and the pulmonary artery architecture should be monitored using oximetry and two-dimensional echocardiography. Cardiac catheterization or MRI is carried out some time before the child is 6 months old. Assuming an adequate atrial septectomy, good right ventricular and tricuspid valve function, an unobstructed pathway from the right ventricle around the aortic arch, and normal growth of the pulmonary arterial bed with a normal pulmonary arteriolar resistance. A bidirectional Glenn shunt, although others advocate a *hemi-Fontan* operation, is then carried out. If preoperative evaluation demonstrates a restrictive atrial septal defect, significant aortic arch obstruction, or hemodynamically significant aortic to pulmonary artery collaterals, these are usually addressed in the cardiac catheterization laboratory. Major pulmonary artery distortion or tricuspid regurgitation can be repaired at the time of the second stage procedure.

Fontan Operation

In earlier years, despite the initial success of the Fontan operation following palliative surgery for the hypoplastic left heart syndrome,[11] a number of problems subsequently occurred.[4,25] In part, these resulted from poor patient selection (Exhibit 41-1). Many of the problems that adversely affect the outcome of Fontan operation are the result of the near-lethal preoperative physiology and the complicated surgical manipulation required for survival. Today, with an eventual Fontan procedure in mind, every effort is made to avoid right ventricular injury, to assist the normal evolution of the pulmonary vasculature, and to avoid distortion of the pulmonary arteries. Current practice calls for aggressive catheter-directed treatment of residual structural defects following the initial stage I procedure, an *early* Glenn operation at 4 to 6 months to relieve the volume load on the single right ventricle, and a Fontan procedure, with a fenestration in the intra-atrial lateral tunnel wall, at two years of age. This strategy has resulted in a decrease in the mortality of the Fontan procedure to 5%.

Cardiac Transplantation

Cardiac transplantation is an alternative form of therapy for infants born with the hypoplastic left heart syndrome.[26,30] The technical feasibility of such a procedure has never been seriously questioned. Issues are the availability of donors[30] and the problems of rejection. The results of allotransplantation in newborns are good.[31] If issues of donor availability are resolved, and if the exceptionally low incidence of rejection reactions is confirmed over a longer period of observation, cardiac transplantation will remain as an alternative form of treatment.

Ethical Issues

The management of babies with hypoplastic left heart syndrome, whether by palliation leading to a Fontan procedure or by transplantation, has provoked vigorous ethical discussion. The scientific facts are as follows:

1. Untreated hypoplastic left heart syndrome is rapidly and virtually 100% fatal.
2. Surgical treatment (palliation followed by a Fontan procedure) has an improving mortality and unknown long-range outcome.
3. The initial mortality for transplantation may be better, provided a donor heart is found, but the long-range outcome is equally unknown.
4. Both approaches have produced children who appear and act normal.

It is clear that not all physicians would recommend either surgical route and not all parents would choose to risk the grief and expense associated with either form of treatment. The present standard of practice does not require that either form of treatment be recommended by the cardiologist or that the parents should agree.

The only ethical question remaining concerns the adequacy of the information available to all concerned in such decisions. A responsible physician may recommend against either approach, but no responsible physician would withhold his or her opinion or deny the information to anyone.

MITRAL ATRESIA WITH NORMAL AORTIC ROOT

Patients with mitral atresia and a normal aortic outflow[32] are not properly classified under the hypoplastic left heart syndrome; yet, by convention, this lesion complex appears in the hypoplastic left ventricle file of the Children's Hospital Boston.

Prevalence

In the period from January 1988 to January 2002, 58 children with mitral atresia and a normal aortic root were seen at Children's Hospital Boston. Of these, 41 had pulmonary outflow obstruction due to pulmonary atresia in 13 and pulmonary stenosis in 28. Coarctation of the aorta was present in five, and total anomalous pulmonary venous return in three. Of the 58 patients, 10 have died and 35 have undergone a Fontan procedure with 3 deaths (Exhibit 41-2).

Exhibit 41–2
Children's Hospital Boston Experience
1988-2002
Mitral Atresia

There were 58 patients with mitral atresia and an adequate aortic outflow. Of these 28 had pulmonary stenosis, 13 had pulmonary atresia, 5 had coarctation and 3 had total anomalous pulmonary venous return: 10 of these patients died. Of the 21 pulmonary banding procedures, 12 were at our hospital: among our 35 modified Fontan procedures there were 3 deaths (9%), much improved compared to the 33% of the 1973-1987 era.

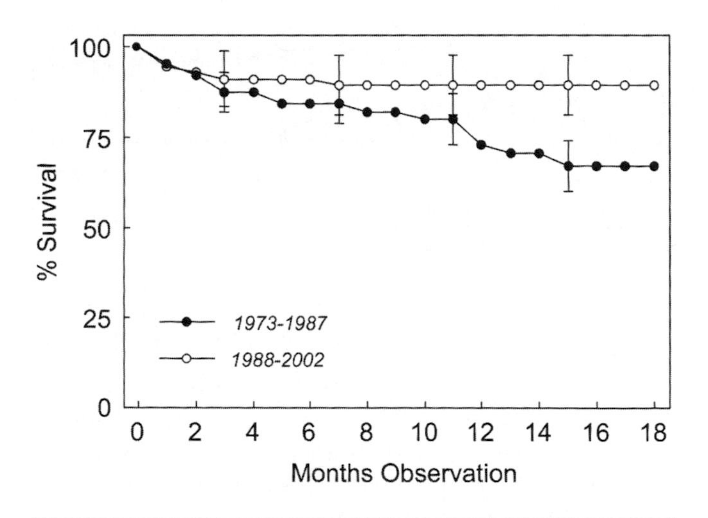

Survival curves showing considerable improvement in 1988-2002 group compared to 1973-1987 patients.

Pathophysiology

Mitral atresia with a good-sized left ventricle is associated with a ventricular septal defect if the aorta arises from the left ventricle. Sometimes the tricuspid valve is straddling. There may be a double-outlet right ventricle with the left ventricle being a blind pouch, or the ventricles may be inverted, with the physiology being that of tricuspid atresia. The great vessels may be transposed, the aorta arising from the right ventricle. A patent and incompetent foramen ovale is usually present, although egress from the left atrium may take other routes (i.e., via a sinoseptal defect). Often the orifice of the foramen ovale is small enough to raise left atrial pressure and the atrial septum is thickened. Most of our patients are classified as having a double-outlet right ventricle, the aorta arising from the right ventricle. Others use different terminology.[33] Sometimes the aorta arises from the left ventricle, in which case the size of the ventricular defect may have important hemodynamic consequences. Roughly half of these patients have pulmonary stenosis and occasionally one sees a patient who has pulmonary valve atresia. Coarctation of the aorta was noted in about 10% of our patients. Others have reported similar experience.[34,35]

Clinical Manifestations

All of these patients are cyanotic, although among those with excessive pulmonary blood flow this may not be apparent at first. Tachypnea is common because left atrial pressures are often high, causing pulmonary edema, or there is excessive pulmonary blood flow. When there is limited pulmonary blood flow because of pulmonary stenosis or atresia, cyanosis may be the chief complaint. Most are symptomatic in the first weeks of life with tachypnea or cyanosis.

Electrocardiography

In most cases, the electrocardiogram shows right ventricular hypertrophy.

Chest Radiography

Chest radiograph shows that the heart size is variably enlarged, depending on the amount of pulmonary blood flow, and the pulmonary vasculature may be prominent because of excess flow or may be diminished because of pulmonary stenosis. There may be evidence of pulmonary edema. Pulmonary edema is possible in the presence of pulmonary stenosis because the size of the foramen ovale determines left atrial pressure, and it may be very small even in the presence of normal or reduced amounts of pulmonary flow.

Echocardiography

The detailed anatomy can be documented by two-dimensional echocardiography using previously described techniques (see Chapter 13).

Cardiac Catheterization

Cardiac catheterization may be important to the successful management. If pulmonary artery flow, pressure, and resistance cannot be assessed by noninvasive imaging, then catheterization can measure these parameters. In addition, relief of an obstructive interatrial septum, likely critical for the development of the pulmonary vasculature, can be accomplished.

Management

With excessive pulmonary blood flow, pulmonary artery banding may be needed, or with diminished flow an arterial shunt may be helpful.[36] Enlargement of the atrial septal defect should be considered in all patients, particularly if a shunt procedure is being considered.[11] Recent experience with stent-augmented balloon septoplasty suggests that it may have longer lasting palliation than balloon septostomy alone. The goal is survival with anatomy and physiology that satisfy the requirements for a Fontan procedure at a later date (Exhibit 41-2).

AORTIC ATRESIA WITH NORMAL LEFT VENTRICLE

Aortic atresia with right and left ventricles of functionally normal capacity is an extremely rare anomaly and repair has been reported.[37]

REFERENCES

1. Noonan JA, Nadas AS. The hypoplastic left heart syndrome: an analysis of 101 cases. Pediatr Clin North Am 5:1029, 1959.
2. Botto LD, Correa A, Erickson JD. Racial and temporal variations in the prevalence of heart defects. Pediatr 107(3): 1, 2001.
3. Hoffman JE, Kaplan S. The incidence of congenital heart disease. J Am Coll Cardiol 39:1890, 2002.
4. Lang P, Norwood WI. Hemodynamic assessment after palliative surgery for hypoplastic left heart syndrome. Circulation 68: 104, 1983.
5. Von Reuden TJ, Knight L, Moller JH, et al. Coarctation of the aorta associated with aortic valvular atresia. Circulation 52:951, 1975.
6. Glauser TA, Rorke LB, Weinberg PW, et al. Congenital brain anomalies associated with the hypoplastic left heart syndrome. Pediatrics 85:984, 1990.
7. Ehrlich M, Bierman FZ, Ellis K, et al. Hypoplastic left heart syndrome: report of a unique survivor. J Am Coll Cardiol 7:361, 1986.
8. Weinberg PM, Chin AJ, Murphy JD, et al. Postmortem echocardiography and tomographic anatomy of hypoplastic left heart syndrome after palliative surgery. Am J Cardiol 58: 1228, 1986.
9. Jonas RA, Lang P, Hansen D, et al. First-stage palliation of hypoplastic left heart syndrome. J Thorac Cardiovasc Surg 92:6, 1986.
10. Vlahos A, Lock JE, McElhinney DB, et al. Hypoplastic left heart syndrome with intact or highly restrictive atrial septum: outcome after neonatal transcatheter atrial septostomy. Circulation 109:2326, 2004.
11. Norwood WI, Lang P, Hansen DD. Physiologic repair of aortic atresia-hypoplastic left heart syndrome. N Engl J Med 308:23, 1983.
12. Sano S, Ishino K, Kado H, et al. Outcome of right ventricle-to-pulmonary artery shunt in first-stage palliation of hypoplastic left heart syndrome: a multi-institutional study. Ann Thorac Surg, 78:1951, 2004.
13. Perry SB, Lang P, Keane JF, et al. Creation and maintenance of an adequate interatrial communication in left atrioventricular valve atresia or stenosis. Am J Cardiol 58:622, 1986.
14. Barber G, Helton JG, Aglira BA, et al. The significance of tricuspid regurgitation in hypoplastic left-heart syndrome. Am Heart J 116:1563, 1988.
15. Helton JG, Aglira BA, Chin AJ, et al. Analysis of potential anatomic and physiologic determinants of palliation surgery for hypoplastic left heart syndrome. Circulation 74 (Suppl): 1–70, 1986.
16. Lloyd TR, Evans TC, Marvin WJ. Morphologic determinants of coronary blood flow in the hypoplastic left heart syndrome. Am Heart J 112:666, 1986.
17. Lloyd TR, Marvin WJ. Age at death in the hypoplastic left heart syndrome: multivariate analysis and importance of the coronary arteries. Am Heart J 117:1337, 1989.

18. O'Connor WN, Cash JB, Cottrill CM. Ventriculo-coronary connections in hypoplastic left heart syndrome autopsy microscopic study. Circulation 66:1078, 1982.
19. Sauer U, Gittenberger-de Groot AC, Geishauser M, et al. Coronary arteries in the hypoplastic left heart syndrome: histopathologic and histometrical studies and implications for surgery. Circulation 80(Suppl I):I-168, 1989.
20. Murphy JD, Sands BL, Norwood WI. Intraoperative balloon angioplasty in aortic coarctation in infants with hypoplastic left heart syndrome. Am J Cardiol 59:949, 1987.
21. Saul JP, Keane JF, Fellows KE, et al. Balloon dilation angioplasty of post-operative aortic obstruction. Am J Cardiol 59: 943, 1987.
22. Alboliras ET, Chin AJ, Barber G, et al. Pulmonary artery configuration after palliative operations for hypoplastic left heart syndrome. J Thorac Cardiovasc Surg 97:878, 1989.
23. Pigott JD, Murphy JD, Barber G, et al. Palliative reconstructive surgery for hypoplastic left heart syndrome. Ann Thorac Surg 45:122, 1988.
24. Chin AJ, Barber G, Helton JG, et al. Fate of the pulmonic valve after proximal pulmonary artery-to-ascending aorta anastomosis for aortic outflow obstruction. Am J Cardiol 62: 435, 1988.
25. Ferrell PR, Chang AC, Murdison KA, et al. Outcome and assessment following modified Fontan repair for hypoplastic left heart syndrome (abstract). J Am Coll Cardiol 15:204A, 1990.
26. Bailey LL. Role of cardiac transplant in the neonate. J Heart Transplant 4:506, 1985.
27. Bailey LL, Assaad AN, Trim RF, et al. Orthotopic transplantation during early infancy as therapy for incurable congenital heart disease. Ann Surg 208:279, 1988.
28. Bailey L, Concepcion W, Shattuck H, et al. Method of heart transplantation for treatment of hypoplastic left heart syndrome. J Thorac Cardiovasc Surg 92:1, 1986.
29. Bailey LL, Nehlsen-Cannarella SL, Doroshow RW, et al. Cardiac allotransplantation in newborns as therapy for hypoplastic left heart syndrome. N Engl J Med 315:949, 1986.
30. Mavroudis C, Willias W, Min D, et al. Orthotopic cardiac transplantation for the neonate: the dilemma of the anencephalic donor. J Thorac Cardiovasc Surg 97:389, 1989.
31. Boucek MM, Kanakriyeh MS, Mathis CM, et al. Cardiac transplantation in infancy: donors and recipients. J Pediatr 116:171, 1990.
32. Moreno F, Quero M, Perez-Diaz L. Mitral atresia with normal aortic valve. Circulation 53:1004, 1976.
33. Thiene G, Daliento L, Frescura C, et al. Atresia of the left atrial orifice: anatomical investigation in 62 cases. Br Heart J 45:393, 1981.
34. Norwood WI. Hypoplastic left heart syndrome: a review. Cardiol Clin 7:377, 1989.
35. Rowe RD, Freedom RM, Mehrizi A, et al. The Neonate with Congenital Heart Disease. Philadelphia: WB Saunders, 1981.
36. Mickell JJ, Mathews RA, Park SC, et al. Left sided atrioventricular valve atresia: clinical management. Circulation 61: 123, 1980.
37. Austin EH, Jonas RA, Mayer JE, et al. Aortic atresia with normal left ventricle: single-stage repair in the neonate. J Thorac Cardiovasc Surg 97:392, 1989.

42

Pulmonary Atresia with Intact Ventricular Septum

JOHN F. KEANE AND DONALD C. FYLER

DEFINITION

In this condition, there is a complete obstruction of right ventricular outflow, an intact ventricular septum, and variable hypoplasia of the right ventricle and tricuspid valve.

PREVALENCE

In the New England Regional Infant Cardiac Program,[1] pulmonary atresia with intact ventricular septum was the tenth most common defect encountered among sick cardiac infants. The incidence rate was 0.069 to 0.074/1000 live births, with rates of 0.04 and 0.045 reported by others, with some decrease due to pregnancy terminations.[2,3] At the Boston Children's Hospital, over the past 14 years it was the 21st most common lesion among all ages, totaling 161 patients (Exhibit 42-1).

EMBRYOLOGY

The large pulmonary arteries, despite low pulmonary blood flow, the frequent observation of fused but well-formed valve leaflets, the absence of arterial collaterals to the pulmonary circulation, the variable size of the right ventricle, and the rarity of associated extracardiac anomalies, as well as the anatomic similarity to newborns with critical pulmonary valvar stenosis, all suggest that pulmonary atresia with intact ventricular septum is an acquired disease rather than an aberration of embryologic development. This is supported by the observation of progression of pulmonary stenosis to atresia in some on sequential fetal echocardiography.[2]

ANATOMY

The pulmonary valve is atretic. The valve ring is usually small, rarely tiny; the valve leaflets, although fused, are often identifiable, especially when the infundibulum is well developed.[4] The main pulmonary artery is present, usually somewhat smaller than normal, but only rarely is represented by a stringlike connection as is seen in patients with pulmonary atresia and ventricular septal defect. The right ventricle and its outflow tract and tricuspid valve vary from miniscule to near-normal size, a normal right ventricle consisting of inlet, apical, and infundibular segments. In a recent review of 189 infants, atresia was valvar in 75% and muscular in the others, the apical segment was absent in a third, and 58% had tripartite morphology.[5] Some decades ago, investigators using the tripartite classification made some surgical recommendations based on these findings.[6] In those with all three segments (tripartite) survival was best, being least satisfactory in those with absence of apical and infundibular components (unipartite). Some years later, reflecting echocardiographic and surgical advances, a more clinically useful classification by surgeons based on tricuspid valve size, which reflects right ventricular size and coronary artery abnormalities, was introduced.[7]

The tricuspid valve is invariably abnormal and small, with its annular size correlating with right ventricular size and is occasionally Ebstein-like, the latter usually with severe regurgitation.[7,8]

Coronary artery abnormalities including sinusoids between them and the right ventricle are very common,[6–9] as much as 70% at angiography.[9] These abnormalities include atresia of one or both aortic origins and one or more sites of obstruction or occlusion in either vessel, including abrupt

Exhibit 42–1
Children's Hospital Boston Experience: 1988–2002
Pulmonary Atresia with Intact Ventricular Septum

One hundred sixty-one patients were seen with pulmonary atresia and intact ventricular septum. In 16, the tricuspid valve was grossly incompetent, 9 of whom had Ebstein anomaly.
Compared with 1973 to 1987, the number seen from 1988 to 2002 has increased, with most having had their initial treatment elsewhere.

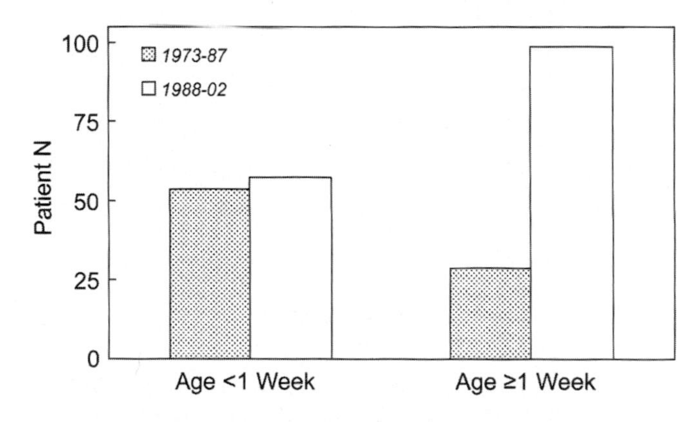

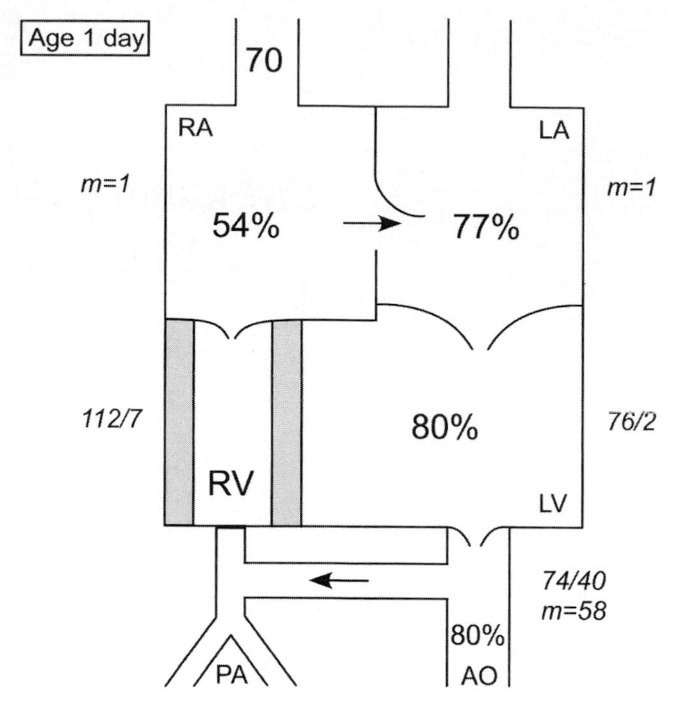

FIGURE 42–1 *Diagram of the hemodynamics in a patient with pulmonary atresia with intact ventricular septum. The tiny right ventricle most often has a higher pressure than the left ventricle; it is sometimes in excess of 200 mm Hg. The entire venous return (cardiac output) passes through the foramen ovale to the left atrium. The entire pulmonary blood flow is supplied by a patent ductus arteriosus.*
From Nadas' Pediatric Cardiology, ed Fyler DC, Hanley & Belfus, Philadelphia, 1992.

termination of the left anterior descending in one of the sinusoids. Abnormalities have also been identified even at the capillary level.[10] These sinusoids are (a) more common in those with smaller tricuspid valves and right ventricles (RVs) and (b) the major source of coronary perfusion (*RV dependent*) in 9% to 34%.[6,11–13]

Collateral circulation from the descending aorta to the lung via bizarre connecting vessels has been seen but is extremely rare, unlike in patients with pulmonary atresia and ventricular septal defect.

Associated cardiac or extracardiac anomalies are rare.

PHYSIOLOGY

The possible avenues of egress from the right ventricle are (a) the sinusoids to the coronary circulation and (b) the return to the right atrium through the tricuspid valve. Depending on the available egress, the right ventricle may develop pressures to very high levels during systole, up to 200 mm Hg (Fig. 42-1). The more opportunity for flow out of the ventricle, the lower the systolic pressure, and in the case of free tricuspid regurgitation the right ventricular systolic pressure may be near normal. With virtual absence of the tricuspid valve, flow in and out of the right ventricle may be sufficient to considerably enlarge the valve ring, the ventricle, and the right atrium (Fig. 42-2).

The venous return to the right atrium, except for that passing out of the right ventricle via sinusoids, goes through the foramen ovale to the left atrium and left ventricle. Restrictive foramina ovale have been described, but in our experience it has been rare to measure a pressure gradient between the right and left atrium of more than 2 or 3 mm Hg. After birth, blood flow to the lungs is initially supplied via the patent ductus arteriosus. Having been the source of pulmonary blood flow *in utero,* the ductus arteriosus is small compared with that in normal infants, whose ductus has supplied systemic blood flow to the descending aorta. Because the arterial oxygen saturation is determined by the amount of pulmonary blood flow, the arterial oxygen may be low. With closure of the ductus in the first few days of life, survival is no longer possible.

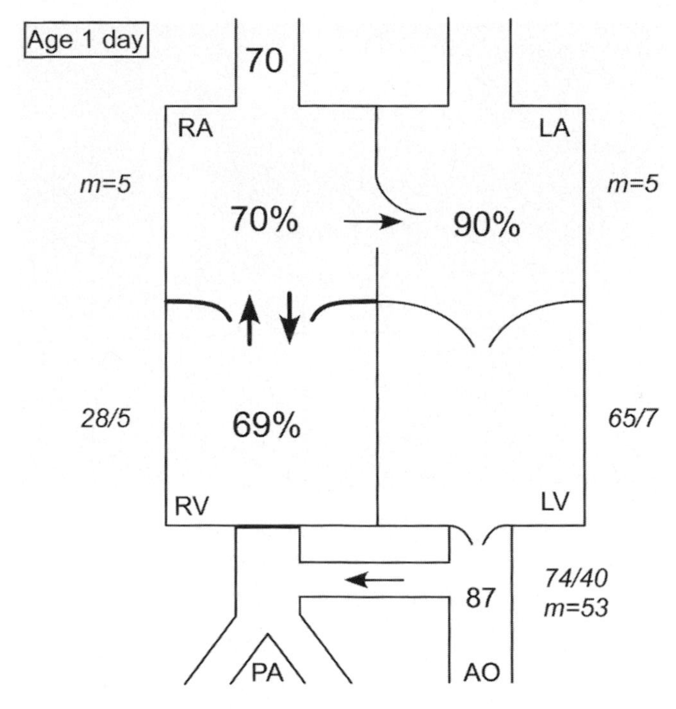

FIGURE 42–2 *Diagram of the hemodynamics in a patient with pulmonary atresia with intact ventricular septum and a grossly incompetent tricuspid valve. Although most patients with pulmonary atresia and intact ventricular septum have some tricuspid insufficiency, occasionally a patient has a grossly incompetent tricuspid valve incapable of supporting significant elevation of right ventricular pressure. Some of these patients have an Ebstein-like deformity of the tricuspid valve.*
From Nadas' Pediatric Cardiology, ed Fyler DC, Hanley & Belfus, Philadelphia, 1992.

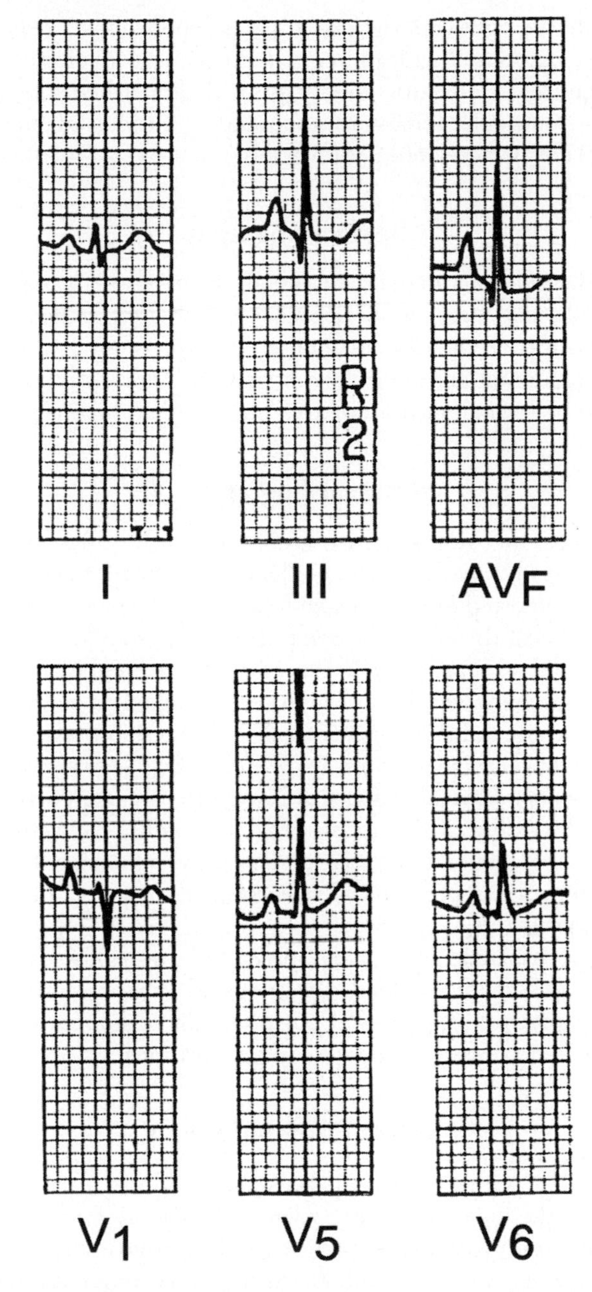

FIGURE 42–3 *The electrocardiogram of a patient with pulmonary atresia with intact septum at birth. Note right atrial enlargement and QRS axis of +60 degrees with decreased anterior right ventricular forces.*
From Nadas' Pediatric Cardiology, ed Fyler DC, Hanley & Belfus, Philadelphia, 1992.

CLINICAL MANIFESTATIONS

These infants are cyanotic at birth and because of their blueness, they are generally referred to a cardiac hospital within the first days of life. Frequently there may be a systolic murmur (tricuspid regurgitation), and rarely a continuous murmur (patent ductus arteriosus), but sometimes there is no murmur at all. Depending on the level of arterial oxygen, the infant may be in more or less distress with tachypnea or dyspnea.

Electrocardiography

The electrocardiogram shows a QRS axis between 0 and 120 degrees and decreased anterior right ventricular forces (Fig. 42-3). Other forms of right-sided obstruction can largely be distinguished by the electrocardiogram: a QRS axis to the right with right ventricular hypertrophy are most likely associated with pulmonary atresia and a ventricular defect; and a leftward-superior axis with diminished anterior right ventricular forces are associated with tricuspid atresia with normally related great vessels.

Chest Radiography

The chest radiograph shows the heart size is variable, usually not large, with normal or decreased pulmonary vascularity. In the rare situation in which there is free tricuspid regurgitation, the right ventricle and right atrium may both be large, contributing to a huge cardiac silhouette.

Echocardiography

Since the vast majority are seen shortly after birth, *windows* for viewing are excellent. With current echocardiographic and Doppler capabilities, virtually every cardiac anatomical detail can be seen. The study should include tricuspid valve anatomy and annulus size (including z score) and function, where the leaflets are attached as occasionally the apparatus may obstruct the small outflow tract, and the right ventricular inflow, apical and outflow segment sizes. The pulmonary valve and size can be readily identified, as can the extent of the atresia (Fig. 42-4). Other structures easily identified are the main and proximal pulmonary arteries, the atrial septum and defect size, and the patent ductus arteriosus.

The proximal coronary arteries and any sinusoids are very well seen[14]; indeed, the tricuspid valve z score has been shown to be an excellent predictor of sinusoids and right ventricular dependent coronary arteries.[9]

Cardiac Catheterization

As the primary diagnosis is established by echocardiography, the indications for cardiac catheterization are (a) to define coronary artery integrity and sinusoids, and (b) if pulmonary valve perforation using radiofrequency and dilation is being considered in the presence of valve atresia and an adequate outflow tract.[15–19] We avoid a balloon septostomy in this patient population because if the baby is to undergo shunt placement and an outflow patch, right ventricular cavity and tricuspid enlargement will not result since all venous return would then pass right to left across the lower resistance atrial hole rather than antegrade across the tricuspid valve. If catheterization is carried out, right ventricular angiography is initially done by injecting contrast (at most 1 mL/kg) via a side-hole catheter at low pressure to avoid muscle infiltration, in the frontal and lateral projections (Fig. 42-5). Coronary arteries can sometimes be well seen on antegrade aortography with balloon occlusion of the

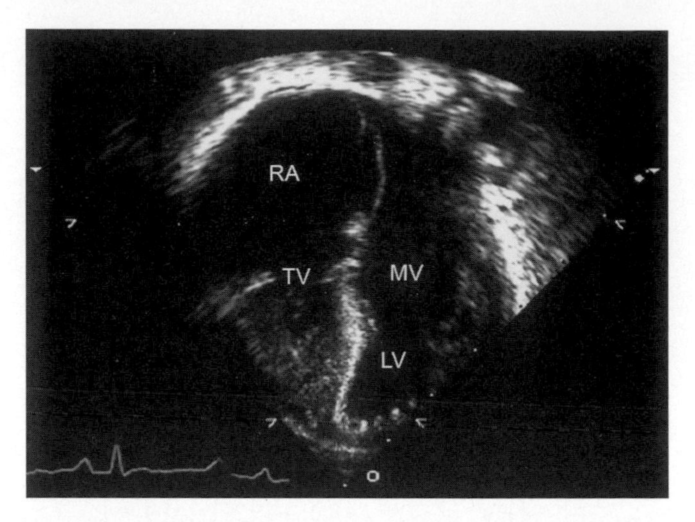

FIGURE 42–4 *Apical four chamber echocardiogram of pulmonary atresia with intact ventricular septum. The small tricuspid valve (TV) orifice connects the dilated right atrium (RA) to the small right ventricular chamber. The interatrial septum bows to the left and right-to-left atrial shunting is typical. The right ventricular walls are markedly thickened compared to those of the left ventricle (LV). The mitral valve (MV) diameter is more than twice that of the TV.*

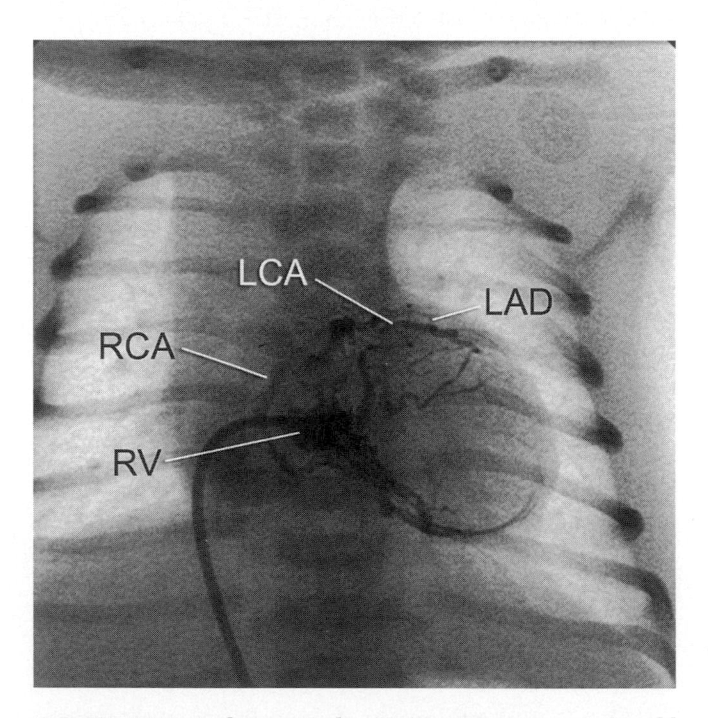

FIGURE 42–5 *Right ventricular (RV) angiogram in a 1-day-old neonate with pulmonary atresia and intact ventricular septum showing (A) tiny RV, (B) filling, via sinusoids from RV of right (RCA) and left (LCA) coronary arteries.*

distal ascending aorta—otherwise selective coronary arteriograms can be recorded using retrograde 3-French catheters via an umbilical artery.

MANAGEMENT

Initial Management

This is a very complex lesion with wide variations in the tricuspid, right ventricular, and coronary artery anatomy. However, all require immediately some form of pulmonary blood flow for survival. Initially, prostaglandin E_1 satisfies this need and stabilizes the patient. There is considerable variation in subsequent management from center to center. Most of our patients then undergo surgery usually consisting of a right ventricular outflow patch and placement of a modified Blalock-Taussig shunt. For those with right ventricular dependent coronary arteries, a shunt only is placed.[13,20,21] A select few undergo radiofrequency valve perforation and dilation.

Subsequent Management

Of those who have undergone an outflow patch and shunt placement, we catheterize those patients usually by age 2 years, at which time if temporary occlusion of the atrial septum is hemodynamically well tolerated, both shunt and atrial septum are occluded at that study. For those who do not tolerate this temporary occlusion, either a *1.5* ventricle repair or fenestrated Fontan is planned, the latter procedure sometimes preceded by a bidirectional Glenn shunt. Those with right ventricular dependent coronary flow also have a bidirectional Glenn shunt at age 6 months followed by a fenestrated Fontan at about age 2 years. Most of our small radiofrequency perforation group have required early shunt placement for cyanosis with or without an outflow patch for obstruction. Using the above approach, in recent years more than a third of the outflow patch and shunt group have had a biventricular repair so far (Exhibit 42-2) with an overall survival rate of 98% at 7 years[13] and a survival rate of 83% at 5 years in the right ventricular–dependent coronary flow group.[21] At a median of 2 years follow-up, our small group of 1.5 ventricle repair continue to do well.[22] Survival rates of 76% to 86% have been reported in other (some older) surgical series, including satisfactory outcomes from the Fontan group.[11,12,23] With regard to those with intact normal coronaries and some small sinusoids who had an outflow patch and shunt, it is our impression that these sinusoids have often closed or decreased in size spontaneously, and have not enlarged or resulted in a significant left to right coronary artery steal. On the other hand in the right ventricular dependent coronary flow group, progression of stenotic coronary artery lesions has occurred in some.

Exhibit 42–2

Children's Hospital Boston Experience: 1988–2002
Pulmonary Atresia with Intact Ventricular Septum
All Treatment at Children's Hospital Boston
149 Cardiac Procedures (62 Patients)

	N		*N*
BTS & RVP	34	2 V	30
BTS only	32	1.5 V	6
BDG	21	FF	21
RVP only	10	Others	5

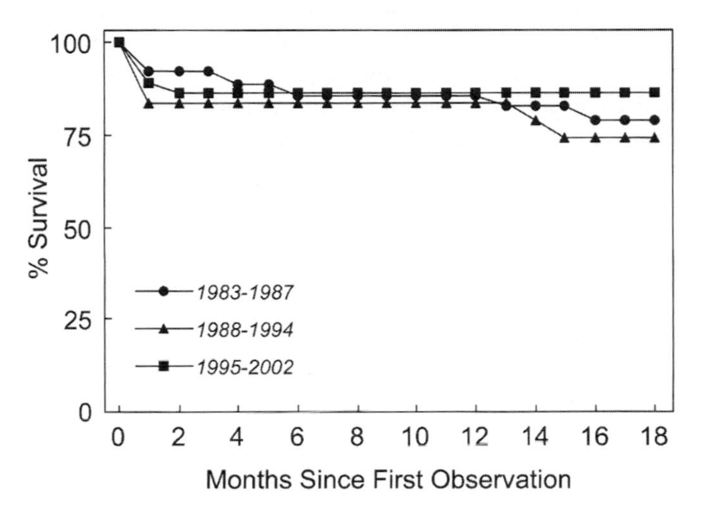

BTS, Blalock-Taussig shunt; RVP, right ventricular transannular outflow patch; BDG, bidirectional Glenn; 1.5V, 1.5 ventricle repair; 2V, two-ventricle circulation, 11 of whom had shunt and atrial defect closure at catheterization.
Life-table 18-month survival curves of pulmonary atresia with intact ventricular septum, of recent periods 1988–1094 (n = 26) and 1995 to 2002 (n = 36) and preceding 5-year period (1983 to 1987; n = 29); all similar other than modest improvement in most recent group.

Radiofrequency perforation and dilation is an evolving management technique in those selected patients with discrete valvar atresia and *mild* at most hypoplasia of the right ventricular cavity and tricuspid valve: ventricular dependent coronary supply is not seen in such patients. Among approximately 100 patients reported to date, there has been a mortality rate (early, late) of about 10%, about 33% have required early shunts, others have required outflow relief but, encouragingly, about 50% eventually have a biventricular heart.[15–19] These patients are, of course, at the most favorable end of the spectrum and would likely have had very satisfactory results from the outflow patch and shunt placement approach.

VARIATION

The rare patients with an unguarded severely regurgitant tricuspid valve, some with an Ebstein-like deformity, represent the worst cases of this disease.[8] The right atrium and right ventricle are large (Fig. 42-5). The right ventricular systolic pressure is minimally elevated, if at all (Fig. 42-2). Pulmonary valvotomy is not a realistic possibility; a Blalock shunt critically may allow survival, later followed by a cardiopulmonary shunt with or without right ventricular and tricuspid valve plication with a view to future fenestrated Fontan. Cardiac transplantation is another option in this extraordinarily difficult group.

REFERENCES

1. Fyler DC, Buckley LP, Hellenbrand WE, et al. Report of the New England Regional Infant Cardiac Program. Pediatrics 65(Suppl 2):387, 1980
2. Ekman Joelsson BM, Sunnegardh J, Hanseus K, et al. The outcome of children born with pulmonary atresia and intact ventricular septum in Sweden from 1980-1999. Scandinavian Cardiovasc J 35(3):192, 2001.
3. Daubeney PE, Sharland GK, Cook AC, et al. Pulmonary atresia with intact ventricular septum: impact of fetal echocardiography on incidence at birth and postnatal outcome. UK and Eire Collaborative Study of Pulmonary Atresia with Intact Ventricular Septum. Circulation 98(6):562, 1998.
4. Braunlin EA, Fomanek AG, Moller JH, et al. Angio-pathological appearances of pulmonary valve in pulmonary atresia with intact ventricular septum: interpretation of nature of right ventricle from pulmonary angiography. Br Heart J 47:281, 1982.
5. Daubeney PE, Delany DJ, Anderson RH, et al. Pulmonary atresia with intact ventricular septum: range of morphology in a population-based study. J Am Coll Cardiol 39(10):1670, 2002.
6. de Leval MR, Bull C, Stark J, et al. Pulmonary atresia and intact ventricular septum: management based on a revised classification. Circulation 66:272, 1982.
7. Hanley FL, Sade RM, Blackstone EH, et al. Outcomes in neonatal pulmonary atresia with intact ventricular septum: a multi-institutional study. J Thorac Cardiovasc Surg 105: 406, 1993.
8. Freedom RM, Nykanen DG. Pulmonary atresia and intact ventricular septum. In Allen HD, Gutgussell HP, Clark EB, Driscoll DG (eds). Moss and Adams Heart Disease in Infants Children and Adolescents. New York: Lippincott, Williams, & Wilkins, 2001, p 845–863.
9. Satou GM, Perry SB, Gauvreau K, et al. Echocardiographic predictors of coronary artery pathology in pulmonary atresia with intact ventricular septum. Am J Cardiol 85(11):1319, 2000.
10. Oosthoek PW, Moorman AF, Sauer U, et al. Capillary distribution in the ventricles of hearts with pulmonary atresia and intact ventricular septum. Circulation 91(6):1790, 1995.
11. Rychik J, Levy H, Gaynor JW, et al. Outcome after operations for pulmonary atresia with intact ventricular septum. J Thorac Cardiovasc Surg 116(6):924, 1998.
12. Najm HK, Williams WG, Coles JG, et al. Pulmonary atresia with intact ventricular septum: results of the Fontan procedure. Ann Thorac Surg 63(3):669, 1997.
13. Jahangiri M, Zurakowski D, Bichell D, et al. Improved results with selective management in pulmonary atresia with intact ventricular septum. J Thorac Cardiovasc Surg 118(6): 1046, 1999.
14. Sanders SP, Parness IA, Colan SD. Recognition of abnormal connections of coronary arteries with the use of Doppler color flow mapping. J Am Coll Cardiol 13:922, 1989.
15. Gibbs JL, Blackburn ME, Uzun O, et al. Laser valvotomy with balloon valvuloplasty for pulmonary atresia with intact ventricular septum: five years' experience. Heart 77(3):225, 1997.
16. Ovaert C, Qureshi SA, Rosenthal E, et al. Growth of the right ventricle after successful transcatheter pulmonary valvotomy in neonates and infants with pulmonary atresia and intact ventricular septum. J Thorac Cardiovasc Surg 115(5):1055, 1998.
17. Alwi M, Geetha K, Bilkis AA, et al. Pulmonary atresia with intact ventricular septum percutaneous radiofrequency-assisted valvotomy and balloon dilation versus surgical valvotomy and Blalock Taussig shunt. J Am Coll Cardiol 35(2): 468, 2000.
18. Humpl T, Soderberg B, McCrindle BW, et al. Percutaneous balloon valvotomy in pulmonary atresia with intact ventricular septum: impact on patient care. Circulation 108(7):826, 2003.
19. Agnoletti G, Piechaud JF, Bonhoeffer P, et al. Perforation of the atretic pulmonary valve. Long term follow up. J Am Coll Cardiol 41(8):1399, 2003.
20. Giglia TM, Mandell VS, Connor AR, et al. Right ventricular-dependent coronary circulation in pulmonary atresia with intact ventricular septum. Circulation 86:1516, 1992.
21. Powell AJ, Mayer JE, Lang P, et al. Outcome in infants with pulmonary atresia, intact ventricular septum, and right ventricle-dependent coronary circulation. Am J Cardiol 86(11): 1272, A9, 2000.
22. Gentles TL, Keane JF, Jonas, RA, et al. Surgical alternatives to the Fontan procedure incorporating a hypoplastic right ventricle. Circulation 90(Pt 2):11-1, 1994.
23. Mishima A, Asano M, Sasaki S, et al. Long-term outcome for right heart function after biventricular repair of pulmonary atresia and intact ventricular septum. Japanese J Thorac Cardiovasc Surg 48(3):145, 2000.

43

Double-Outlet Right Ventricle

JOHN F. KEANE AND DONALD C. FYLER

DEFINITION

Double-outlet right ventricle is said to be present when both great arteries arise completely above the right ventricle. This chapter relates to those with two adequate-sized ventricles.

PREVALENCE

Reported incidences of double-outlet right ventricle in infants range from 0.03 to 0.2/1000 live births.[1,2] The former value is from the New England Regional Program of primarily ill infants and the latter a more recent estimate recording all defects, aided by echocardiography, regardless of severity.

The diagnosis of double-outlet right ventricle depends greatly on how much one or the other great vessel overrides the right ventricle. The criteria for this diagnosis have varied over the years. The decision to use the term *double-outlet right ventricle* is, therefore, judgmental and its use has varied from time to time. Consequently, variation in prevalence from center to center and within one center over time is inherent in this diagnosis.

PATHOLOGY

Double-outlet right ventricle is not a single cardiac anomaly such as a ventricular septal defect. Rather, it is a term used to describe the position of the great arteries found in association with a variety of cardiac anomalies that can be viewed, physiologically, as ventricular septal defects, tetralogy of Fallot, transposition of the great arteries, single ventricle, or atrioventricular atresia (Exhibit 43-1). In most patients, the aorta and pulmonary artery are side by side with the former on the right (d-malposition) in the great majority.[3] In about a quarter they are in a d-transposition configuration, that is the pulmonary artery is posterior and leftward—it is often difficult, in the presence of a ventricular septal defect, to decide if this is a double outlet or transposition, and especially so when pulmonary atresia is present. Continuity between the mitral valve and the adjacent semilunar valve is absent and is thought by most to represent the sine qua non of this diagnosis. Conal musculature is usually seen under both great arteries, but it may be absent under one or the other, or both. In cases without bilateral conal tissue, there is usually continuity between the adjacent great artery and the tricuspid valve; most of these children have mitral atresia. Various types of pulmonary stenosis are common. A variety of atrioventricular valvar abnormalities, outflow valve and subvalvar obstructions, interrupted aortic arch, and coarctation of the aorta are often seen. Hypoplasia or stenosis of the aortic valve is often encountered when there is coarctation of the aorta, although subvalvar aortic stenosis may be seen in the absence of coarctation.

Any malfunction of the atrioventricular or semilunar valves may be present, with various types of pulmonary stenosis being the most common. A defect of the common atrioventricular canal is frequently present, with its associated mitral and tricuspid valve abnormalities (Exhibit 43-1).

There is a gradation of defects ranging from subaortic ventricular septal defect with subpulmonary stenosis, to tetralogy of Fallot, to double-outlet right ventricle with pulmonary stenosis. There is a similar range of clinical problems extending from subpulmonary ventricular septal

Exhibit 43–1
Boston Children's Hospital Experience
1988-2002

There were 300 patients who were categorized as having double-outlet right ventricle (compared to 213 patients 1973-1987). Additionally, 321 patients were categorized under "malpositions" who also had double-outlet right ventricle. Thirty-five children listed under the category of "single ventricle" were also listed as having a double-outlet right ventricle, all considered examples of single right ventricle, and 82 cases carried codes indicating double-outlet right ventricle but were categorized with the hypoplastic left heart group. Virtually all of these had mitral atresia with an unobstructed aortic outflow and, hence, were not true examples of hypoplastic left heart.

Diagnoses Associated with Double-Outlet Right Ventricle (DORV)

Associated Diagnoses	*DORV n=300*	*Malposition with DORV* n=321*	*Single Ventricle with DORV n=35*	*Hypoplastic Left Ventricle with DORV* n=82*
Single Ventricle	3	127	34	30
Hypoplastic Left Ventricle	42	113	9	63
D-Transposition Great Arteries	81	72	14	8
L-Transposition Great Arteries	13	47	8	1
Total Anomalous Pulmonary Veins	4	92	2	4
Endocardial Cushion Defect	45	202	7	4
Tetralogy of Fallot	25	12	0	1
Pulmonary Atresia	31	98	9	8
Pulmonary Stenosis	196	251	25	25
Aortic Stenosis	14	7	0	13
Subaortic Stenosis	101	37	8	32
Coarctation of Aorta	48	20	4	22
Mitral Atresia	1	35	0	67

Surgical Procedures

Operative Procedure	*DORV n=264*	*Malposition with DORV** n=260*	*Single Ventricle with DORV n=33*	*Hypoplastic Left Ventricle with DORV* n=64*
Fontan	54	159	29	41
Coarctation Repair**	40	13	2	10
Tetralogy of Fallot Repair	31	4	0	0
Double-Outlet Right Ventricle Repair†	115	19	0	1
Transposition of the Great Arteries Repair‡	70	14	2	13
Rastelli	36	10	0	0
Arterial-Pulmonary Shunt	68	155	19	39
Pulmonary Artery Band	72	47	10	22

*The majority of those categorized as having double-outlet right ventricle (a) within the context of malposition had asplenia or polysplenia and (b) with hypoplastic left heart had mitral atresia with unobstructed aortic flow.

**Includes patients with interrupted aortic arch.

†Repair of double-outlet right ventricle is, unfortunately, an acceptable code in our system that conveys little information and skews the figures in a table of this type.

‡Includes arterial and atrial (e.g., Senning and Mustard) repairs.

defect with varying degrees of overriding of the pulmonary artery (transposition of the great arteries) to double-outlet right ventricle. Another anatomic spectrum ranges from a single right ventricle with a hypoplastic left ventricle, to a double-outlet right ventricle with a small left ventricle that is, nevertheless, of sufficient size to permit a two-ventricle repair.

Ventricular Septal Defect

A ventricular septal defect is almost always present, although rarely there is none[4], in which case the pulmonary venous blood reaches the right ventricle by shunting left-to-right through an atrial septal opening. The ventricular defect is subaortic (about 50%), subpulmonary (about 30%), uncommitted (both subaortic and subpulmonary, or remote (muscular or endocardial cushion type) (Fig. 43-1).[3,5–10] The subaortic and subpulmonary defects rarely lie immediately below the corresponding semilunar valve without intervening conal tissue. Indeed, the case can be made that the subpulmonary and the subaortic ventricular defects have the same location and that it is the variation in distribution of conal tissue that determines the great artery with which the ventricular defect is associated. Because of variations in location of infundibular tissue (conal tissue), anteriorly or posteriorly, malalignment of the ventricular septal defect is directly related to the presence of subaortic stenosis on the one hand and pulmonary stenosis on the other.[5] As in most other complex groups of cardiac anomalies, some ventricular defects have a tendency to get smaller with time.

Pulmonary Stenosis

Almost three fourths of patients with double-outlet right ventricle have some degree of pulmonary stenosis and, even rarely, pulmonary atresia. The stenosis is usually subvalvar and is derived from conal tissue. Because extreme degrees of aortic override seen in patients with tetralogy of Fallot may resemble the anatomy seen in double-outlet right ventricle, at times it may not be possible to distinguish between the two. Usually, however, the presence of mitral–aortic valvar continuity establishes the diagnosis of tetralogy of Fallot, whereas absence of aortic–mitral continuity characterizes double-outlet right ventricle. The majority of patients in whom this question arises have tetralogy of Fallot, and the diagnosis of double-outlet right ventricle with subaortic ventricular septal defect and subvalvar pulmonary stenosis is most often not correct.

Transposition of the Great Arteries

When there is a subpulmonary ventricular defect that delivers left ventricular blood to the pulmonary artery, the hemodynamics and the anatomy resemble those of transposition of the great arteries and the latter is the diagnosis if there is mitral–pulmonary valvar continuity.

The **Taussig-Bing anomaly** is a specific variation of this problem, which includes the hemodynamics and usual anatomy of transposed great arteries but in which both arteries arise from the right ventricle. There is a subpulmonary ventricular septal defect, no pulmonary stenosis, and absence of mitral–pulmonary valve continuity. The level of the semilunar valves is the same and the great vessels are parallel.[6,7]

Other Associated Anomalies

Virtually every other cardiac anomaly can be found associated with double-outlet right ventricle. Mitral atresia, mitral stenosis, and straddling atrioventricular valves are common. Some babies with mitral atresia and a hypoplastic left ventricle do surprisingly well, because there may be no aortic valve obstruction and an aorta of normal size receives normal amounts of blood flow from the right ventricle. Superoinferior ventricles (upstairs–downstairs ventricles) are often associated with the origin of both great arteries from the upper right ventricle. Inverse ventricles are common, as are visceral heterotaxy, polysplenia, and asplenia (Exhibit 43-1).

PHYSIOLOGY

The relationship between the ventricular defect and the great arteries, the relative outflow obstruction, and the relative systemic-to-pulmonary artery resistance determine the hemodynamic situation. Double-outlet right ventricle may mimic ventricular septal defect, tetralogy of Fallot, single right ventricle, or transposition of the great arteries with or without pulmonary stenosis. Depending on the physiology, the child may have the problems of cyanosis, of congestive heart failure, or both. Some degree of arterial unsaturation is almost always present.

CLINICAL MANIFESTATIONS

The patient may have the symptoms of congestive heart failure, cyanosis, or no symptoms at all.

Electrocardiography

There is no characteristic electrocardiographic pattern, although virtually all have a pattern compatible with right ventricular hypertrophy.

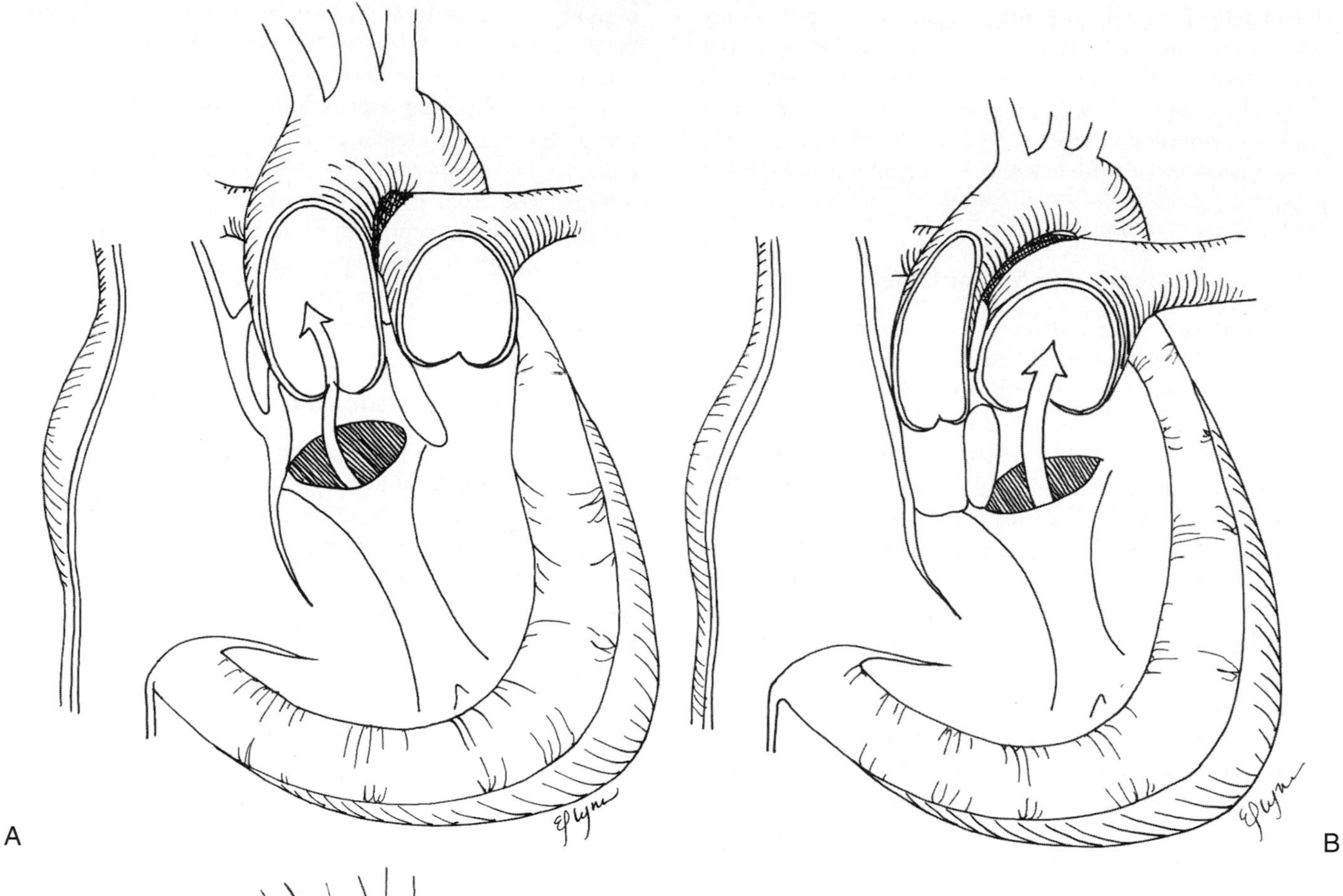

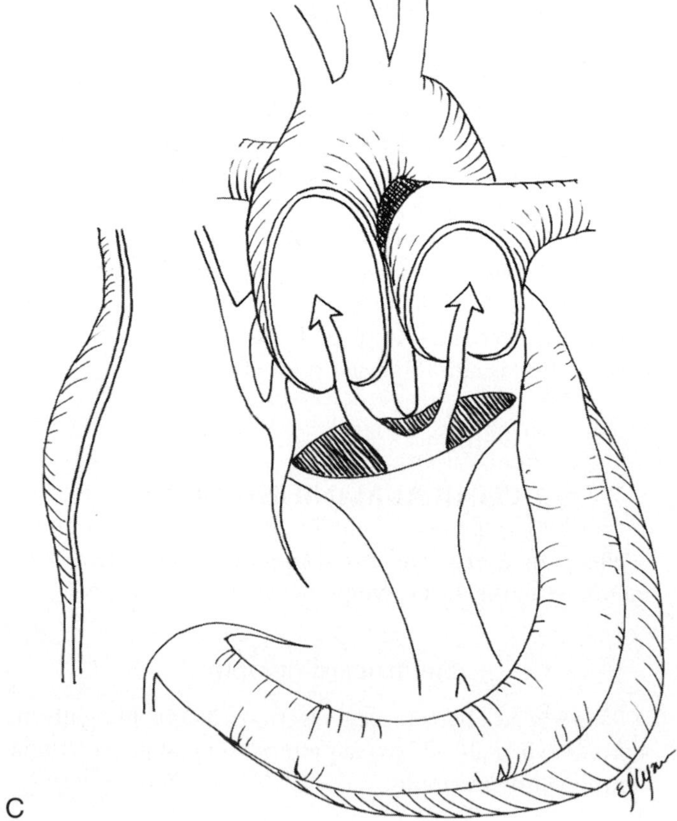

FIGURE 43–1 ***Three drawings of double-outlet right ventricle.*** *A, Subaortic ventricular septal defect. B, Subpulmonary ventricular defect. C, An uncommitted ventricular defect related equally to both great arteries. Not shown are ventricular defects of the atrioventricular canal type or one or more muscular ventricular defects that may be associated with the above anomalies or exist as the sole communication between the left and right ventricles. Additionally, double-outlet right ventricle with inverse ventricles and ventricular defects of comparable variety are encountered.*
From Nadas' Pediatric Cardiology. Ed, Fyler DC. Hanley & Belfus, Philadelphia 1992.

Chest Radiography

Similarly, there is no characteristic chest radiograph. The size of the heart and the amount of pulmonary vascularity are dependent on the hemodynamics and may range from a relatively small heart with decreased pulmonary vascularity to a large heart with increased pulmonary vascular markings.

Echocardiography

The criterion for diagnosis is alignment of both great arteries, totally or predominantly, with the right ventricle. Bilateral conus is often, but not invariably, present (Fig. 46-2). Because there are a large number of anatomic variations and associated intracardiac lesions, a thorough examination, including Doppler interrogation, of all segments of the heart is mandatory.

Cardiac Catheterization

Because of the precise anatomic information provided by echocardiography, together with Doppler estimations of obstructive lesions and regurgitant valves, cardiac catheterization is no longer necessary in all patients, particularly in infants (only 36% of our patients were catheterized preoperatively; Exhibit 43-2). It is indicated where anatomic and physiologic uncertainties exist, to evaluate pulmonary resistance in older patients and in those who have had prior palliative procedures. The patients catheterized usually have some degree of arterial oxygen unsaturation and have the hemodynamics of tetralogy of Fallot, single right ventricle, transposition of the great arteries, dominant left-to-right shunt, or pulmonary vascular obstructive disease. The information obtained from the echocardiogram may suggest the best positioning of the patient in order to demonstrate the origins of the great vessels and the location of the ventricular defects. Often these are seen best in a biplane angiogram in the anteroposterior and straight lateral views, since the great arteries often are side-by-side with the semilunar valves at the same level (Fig. 43-3).

Exhibit 43–2
Boston Children's Hospital Experience
1988–2002
Double-Outlet Right Ventricle

Of the 300 patients with double-outlet right ventricle, 154 had their first cardiac evaluation at Children's Hospital. Only 55 (36%) were catheterized preoperatively, most of whom were in the earlier years. 149 underwent surgery, 5 considered inoperable including a 49 year old with a ventricular septal defect and severe pulmonary vascular obstructive disease.

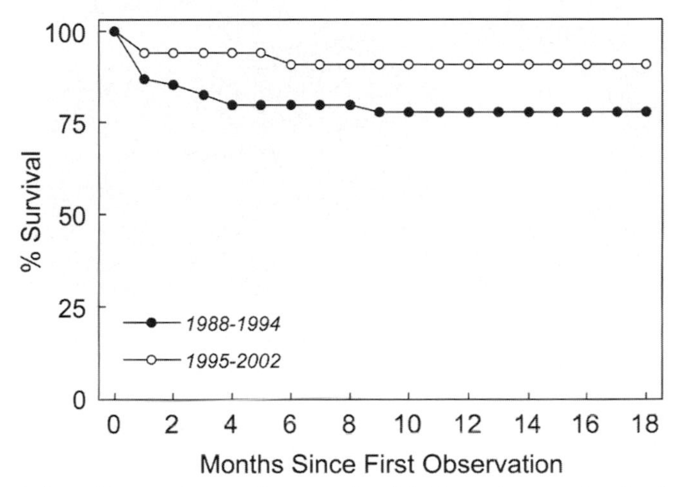

Life table analysis of survival of 149 patients who had initial operation at Children's Hospital. In recent era survival has improved compared to 1988.

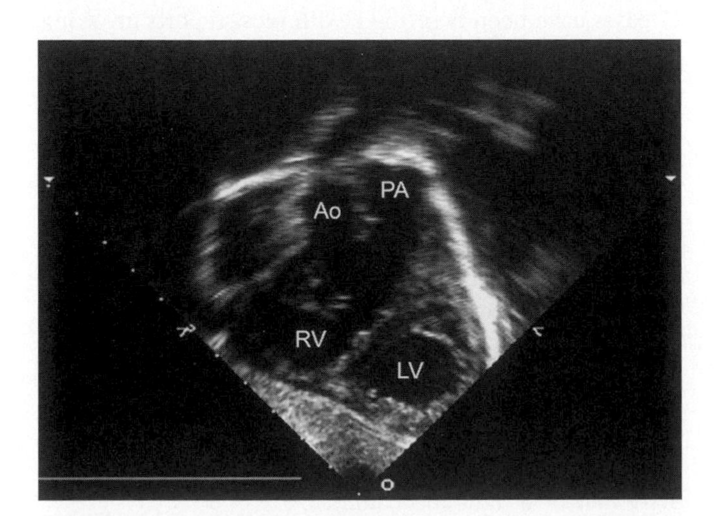

FIGURE 43–2 *Subxyphoid echocardiogram of a Taussig-Bing type of double-outlet right ventricle (RV). The apex of the left ventricle (LV) is seen with both the aorta (Ao) and pulmonary artery (PA) arising from the right ventricle, each from a subarterial infundibulum.*

MANAGEMENT

The initial decision concerns the ultimate goal and is dependent on sifting through and identifying those lesions present from the cacophony of potential associated lesions

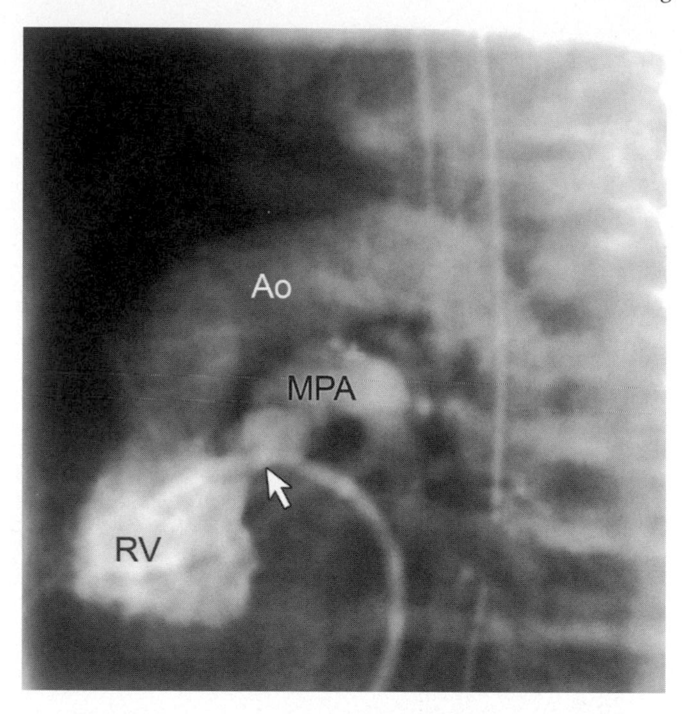

FIGURE 43–3 *Lateral right ventricular (RV) angiogram in a 1-day-old baby with a double-outlet right ventricle and subpulmonary stenosis (arrow). Note that both great vessels arise from the RV with the aorta (Ao) anterior to the main pulmonary artery (MPA).*

found with double-outlet right ventricle. The major questions to be answered include the following:

1. Are there two adequate sized ventricles present to accomplish a biventricular repair?
2. Where is (are) the ventricular septal defect(s), is it of adequate size and can it (they) be baffled to the future systemic great artery?
3. If pulmonary stenosis is present, can it be repaired or is a conduit necessary?
4. Can any associated lesions be repaired?

In the simplest case, namely an unrestrictive subaortic ventricular septal defect and d-malposed great vessels, baffling this defect to the aorta is all that is necessary.[9,10] If the defect is large and subpulmonary (Taussig-Bing anomaly), then baffling the left ventricle to the pulmonary artery together with an arterial switch operation repairs this lesion.[11–13] Some doubly or noncommitted ventricular defects have been baffled to the systemic great artery with or without an arterial switch.[14–17] At the single ventricle end of the spectrum, a modified stage 1 operation is often the initial surgery with a Fontan procedure to follow in the future. This approach is also an option in those in whom the ventricular septal defect location is a contraindication to baffling, such as in the inlet septum. A temporary modified Blalock-Taussig may be the initial procedure in some with pulmonary atresia.

COURSE

Early mortality rates in the past decade have ranged from 5% to 13%, with survival rates at 5 years or more ranging from 83% to 87%.[9,17] In simple uncomplicated patients, 96% survival at 15 years has been reported with lower rates in complicated patients.[9] Reoperations are necessary in about a third and include conduit replacement and relief of subaortic obstruction.

DOUBLE-OUTLET LEFT VENTRICLE

Double-outlet left ventricle is said to be present when both great arteries arise completely or nearly so from the left ventricle.

It is a very rare anomaly. We have seen only three such patients from 1988 to 2002: All had a ventricular septal defect (multiple in one) and infundibular pulmonary stenosis; a biventricular repair was undertaken in two (one of whom had preoperative device closure of an additional muscular defect) and the other, with severe tricuspid and right ventricular hypoplasia, had a fenestrated Fontan procedure. In the literature in the past decade only about 17 cases have been described, with most reports involving single patients. All had a ventricular septal defect, most had pulmonary stenosis, and most had a biventricular repair, some of these having the pulmonary artery relocated to the right ventricle. All but one (who also had a single left ventricle)[18] had situs solitus of the atria and viscera and atrioventricular concordance, in general comparable to the autopsy findings of Van Praagh et al.[19] In general about a third of the patients have lesions mimicking tetralogy of Fallot. Often, the similarity is so close that the presence of double-outlet left ventricle is only recognized by echocardiography. Once it is recognized that the pulmonary artery, as well as the aorta, originates from the left ventricle in a patient who otherwise seems to have tetralogy of Fallot, the diagnosis is made. Often the aorta appears to be overriding, and there may be a right aortic arch.

Management depends on the specific anatomy. If the anatomy is tetralogy-like, a two-ventricle repair connecting the right ventricle to the pulmonary artery with a patch or conduit is possible.

REFERENCES

1. Fyler DC, Buckley LP, Hellenbrand WE, et al. Report of the New England Regional Infant Cardiac Program. Pediatrics 65:375, 1980.
2. Botto LD, Correa A, Erickson J. Radial and temporal variations in the prevalence of heart defects. Pediatrics 107(3): 1, 2001.
3. Sridaromont S, Feldt RH, Ritter DG, et al. Double outlet right ventricle: hemodynamic and anatomic correlations. Am J Cardiol 38:85, 1976
4. Vairo U, Tagliente MR, Fasano ML, et al. Double outlet right ventricle with intact ventricular septum. Ital Heart J 2(5): 397, 2001.
5. Kurosawa H, Van Mierop LHS. Surgical anatomy of the infundibular septum in transposition of the great arteries with ventricular septal defect. J Thorac Cardiovasc Surg 91: 123, 1986.
6. Van Praagh R. What is the Taussig-Bing malformation? Circulation 38:445, 1968.
7. Yacoub MH, Radley-Smith R. Anatomic correction of the Taussig-Bing anomaly. J Thorac Cardiovasc Surg 88:380, 1984.
8. Beekman RP, Bartelings MM, Hazekamp MG, et al. The morphologic nature of noncommitted ventricular septal defects in specimens with double outlet right ventricle. J Thorac Cardiovasc Surg 124(5):984, 2002.
9. Brown JW, Ruzmetov M, Okada Y, et al. Surgical results in patients with double outlet right ventricle: a 20-year experience. Ann Thorac Surg 72(5):1630, 2001.
10. Belli E, Serraf A, Lacour-Gayet F, et al. Biventricular repair for double outlet right ventricle. Results and long term follow up. Circulation 98(19 Suppl):II360, 1998.
11. Masuda M, Kado H, Shiokawa Y, et al. Clinical results of arterial switch operation for double outlet right ventricle with subpulmonary VSD. Eur J Cardiothorac Surg 15(3): 283,1999.
12. Takeuchi K, McGowan FX, Jr., Moran AM, et al. Surgical outcome of double outlet right ventricle with subpulmonary VSD. Ann Thorac Surg 71(1):49, 2001.
13. Wetter J, Sinzobahamvya N, Blaschczok HC, et al. Results of arterial switch operation for primary total correction of the Taussig-Bing anomaly. Ann Thorac Surg 77(1):41, 2004.
14. Uemura H, Yagihara T, Kadohama T, et al. Repair of double outlet right ventricle with doubly-committed ventricular septal defect. Cardiology in the Young 11(4):415, 2001.
15. Lacour-Gayet F, Haun C, Ntalakoura K, et al. Biventricular repair of double outlet right ventricle with non-committed ventricular septal defect (VSD) by VSD rerouting to the pulmonary artery and arterial switch. (see comment). Eur J Cardiothorac Surg 21(6):1042, 2002.
16. Barbero-Marcial M, Tanamati C, Atik E, et al. Intraventricular repair of double outlet right ventricle with noncommitted ventricular septal defect: advantages of multiple patches. J Thorac Cardiovasc Surg 118(6):1056, 1999.
17. Belli E, Serraf A, Lacour-Gayet F, et al. Double outlet right ventricle with non-committed ventricular septal defect. Eur J Cardiothorac Surg 15(6):747, 1999.
18. Papagiannis J, Athanassopoulos G, Mavrogeni S, et al. Double inlet and double outlet left ventricle in situs inversus. Ped Cardiol 19(2):161, 1998.
19. Van Praagh R, Weinberg PM, Srebro JP. Double outlet left ventricle. In Adams FH, Emmanoulides GC, Riemenschneider TA (eds). Moss' Heart Disease in Infants, Children and Adolescents, 4th ed. Baltimore: Williams & Wilkins, 1989, p 461-485.

44

Single Ventricle

JOHN F. KEANE AND DONALD C. FYLER

DEFINITION

A single ventricle is defined as the presence of two atrioventricular valves with one ventricular chamber or a large dominant ventricle associated with a diminutive opposing ventricle.[1–3] The term *double-inlet ventricle* is also used to describe this group of anomalies.

While the term *univentricular* has been used interchangeably with single- and double-inlet ventricle and management strategies in the current era are very similar in all, we have not included patients with mitral or aortic atresia or those with malposition or asplenia in our single ventricle patient population.

PREVALENCE

The incidence of single ventricle in ill infants with congenital heart disease in New England ranged between 0.054 and 0.103 per 1000 live births[4] and in another study was found in 1.25% of infants with congenital heart disease.[5] At the Children's Hospital Boston, it was the eighteenth most common defect. If the idea of a univentricular heart is used, there are more than three times as many (Exhibit 44-1).[6]

Because all patients with malposed hearts are discussed elsewhere (see Chapter 39), some patients with dextrocardia or asplenia and single ventricle are not discussed here. Most notable, the patients who have single right ventricle with asplenia are not considered in this section.

EMBRYOLOGY

In early embryologic life, the atrioventricular canal, which later contributes to both the mitral and tricuspid valves, opens into the ventricular portion of the primitive heart tube, which later becomes the left ventricle (see Chapter 2). From the ventricular portion of the primitive heart tube, blood passes to the bulbus cordis, which later contributes to the development of the right ventricle. The arterial trunk, later to become both the aorta and the main pulmonary artery, arises from the bulbus cordis. With an arrest or a defect in interventricular septation, a double-inlet single left ventricle with a rudimentary right ventricle outflow chamber results,[7] most often in the context of L-looping of the ventricles (see Chapter 3).

ANATOMY

A single ventricular chamber can usually be recognized as being most like a left or a right ventricle because of the presence or absence of characteristic trabeculation, as well as by the position and anatomy of the atrioventricular valves. The most common form of single ventricle is a single left ventricle with L-transposition of the great arteries, with the aorta arising from a diminutive, leftward right ventricle and following the leftward, ascending pattern characteristic of *corrected transposition*. The pulmonary artery usually arises posteriorly; the mitral valve is right-sided and the tricuspid valve is to the left (Fig. 44-1). This form of single ventricle

Exhibit 44–1
Boston Children's Hospital Experience 1988-2002

There were 215 patients with single ventricle with levocardia. There were 212 others with single ventricle who had asplenia, polysplenia, abdominal heterotaxy, or dextrocardia (see Ch. 39).

Type of Single Ventricle
n = 215

Single Left Ventricle	150
Single Right Ventricle	16
Holmes' Heart	23
Unspecified	26

One hundred and twenty-two had pulmonary stenosis or atresia and 93 did not: 40 had coarctation of the aorta or interrupted aortic arch with mortality 13% (compared to 45% 1973-1987). Complete heart block

Univentricular Hearts
n = 786

	Not Malposed	*Malposition*	*Total*
Tricuspid Atresia	223	33	256
Mitral Atresia	58	45	103
Single Ventricle	215	212	427
Total	496	290	786

There were 786 patients who could be categorized as having univentricular hearts.

Surgical Treatment of Single Ventricle

Of the 215 patients, 161 (75%) underwent surgery (2.3 operations/patient): 134 underwent a Fontan operation (62% of all patients compared to 41% from 1973-1987) with 130 survivors.

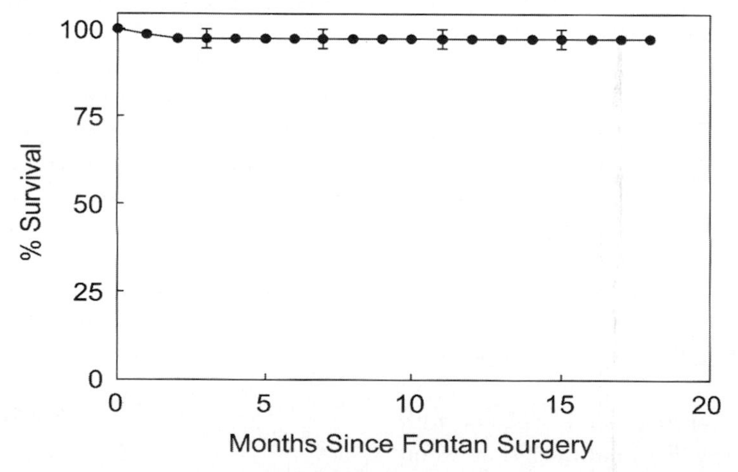

Initial Surgery

There were 87 patients who had their first ever surgical procedure at Boston Children's Hospital, at median age 44 days with an early mortality of 5%.

	N	*(%)*
Modified Stage I	27	(31)
Pulmonary Artery Band	19	(22)
Fenestrated Fontan	16	(19)
Blalock Taussig shunt	15	(17)
Bidirectional Glenn	8	(9)
Other	2	(2)

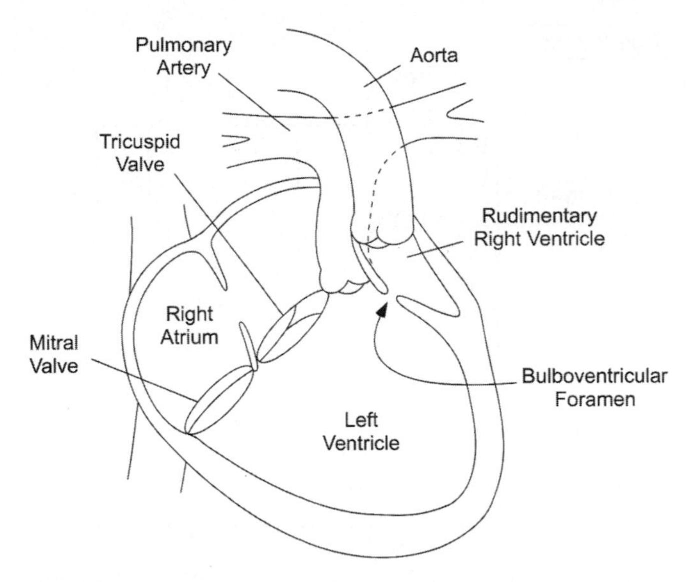

FIGURE 44–1 *Sketch of single left ventricle with transposed great arteries. There is a left-sided rudimentary right ventricle under the aortic valve. Entry to this chamber is through a bulboventricular foramen that tends to close spontaneously. The positions of the atrioventricular valves are reversed: the mitral is right-sided; the tricuspid is left-sided. The great vessels are transposed: the aorta is leftward and anterior; the pulmonary artery is rightward and posterior. This is the most common form of single ventricle. From Nadas AS, Fyler DC [eds]. Nadas' Pediatric Cardiology. Philadelphia, PA: Hanley and Belfus, 1992.*

accounts for the 74% of autopsied cases[3] and 70% of our clinical experience (Exhibit 44-1). In some cases, the ventricular septal defect between the large left ventricle and the rudimentary right ventricular outflow chamber (the bulboventricular foramen) may become progressively smaller with time, producing functional subaortic stenosis.[8,9] Pulmonary stenosis or atresia occurs in about 50% of patients; the remainder have unfettered flow to the pulmonary circuit. Coarctation of the aorta and interrupted aortic arch are common (Exhibit 44-1), as are abnormalities of the mitral or tricuspid valves.

The eponym *Holmes* heart[10] describes a rare double-inlet, single left ventricle without transposition and with pulmonary stenosis. In the remaining patients the types of single ventricle are less homogeneous; sometimes they appear to be derived from an anatomic right ventricle and are necessarily viewed case by case. Asplenia is common among those with single right ventricle.[3]

In earlier years, most data about patients with single ventricle were based on pathologic observations. Because most patients now survive (see Exhibit 44-1), some of the living patients have not been classified or the classification is debatable. This is particularly true when multiple observers from different disciplines (echocardiographers, angiographers, surgeons) are involved. Still the number of cases about which there is general agreement gradually increases as the years go by.

PHYSIOLOGY

The amount of pulmonary blood flow, as limited by pulmonary stenosis or pulmonary vascular resistance, determines the clinical course of babies with single ventricle. In the absence of pulmonary stenosis with regression of the fetal pulmonary vascular resistance, the pulmonary blood flow gradually increases, ultimately causing congestive heart failure (Fig. 44-2). It is not possible for pulmonary resistance to be reduced to normal levels and have the patient survive unless there is pulmonary stenosis. The balance point at which pulmonary resistance stabilizes varies from patient to patient, but usually is sufficiently low to result in congestive heart failure in a matter of days or weeks after birth.

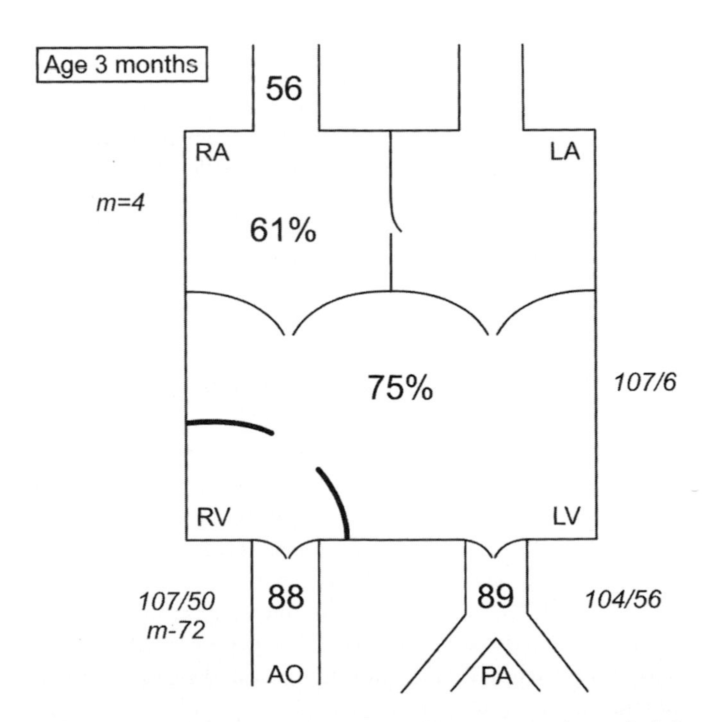

FIGURE 44–2 *Physiologic diagram of a patient with single left ventricle and transposed great arteries. Note the similarity of pulmonary, arterial and aortic oxygen saturation. In this case the rudimentary right ventricle has a large bulboventricular foramen and, therefore, systolic pressure in the left ventricle is equal to that in the aorta and pulmonary artery. A pulmonary artery band was placed. See later data Figure 44-5. RA, right atrium; LA, left atrium; AO, aorta; PA, pulmonary artery; %, percent oxygen saturation; italics, pressure in mm Hg.*
From Nadas AS, Fyler DC [eds]. Nadas' Pediatric Cardiology. Philadelphia, PA: Hanley and Belfus, 1992.

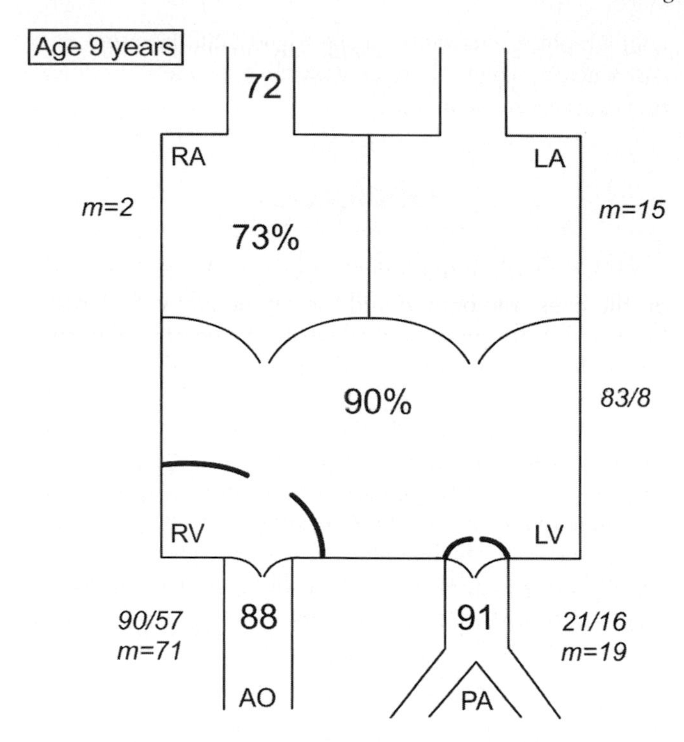

FIGURE 44–3 *Physiologic diagram of the circulation in a patient with single left ventricle, transposed great arteries, and pulmonary stenosis. Note the low pressure in the pulmonary artery and the similarity of pulmonary and aortic oxygen saturation. Abbreviations as in Figure 44-2.*
From Nadas AS, Fyler DC [eds]. Nadas' Pediatric Cardiology. Philadelphia, PA: Hanley and Belfus, 1992.

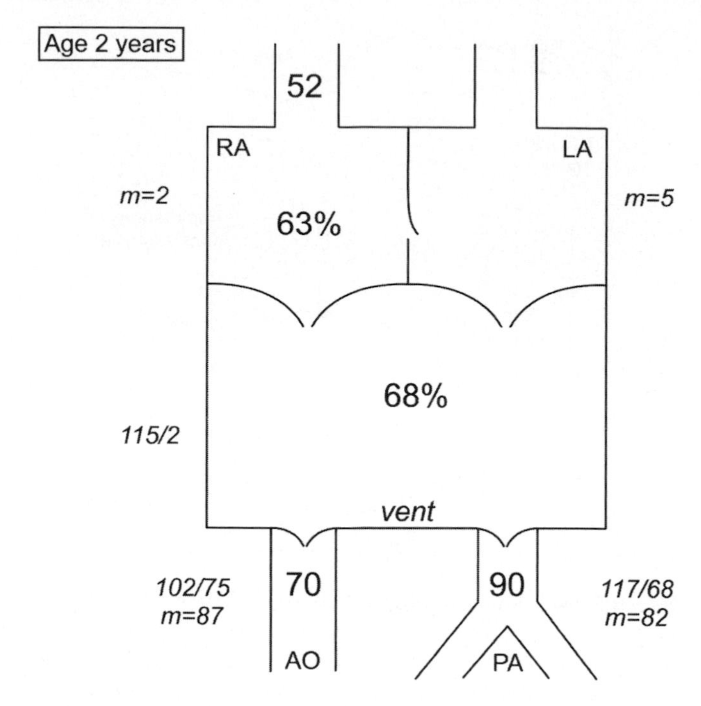

FIGURE 44–4 *Physiologic diagram of a patient with single ventricle and transposition of the great arteries. Note that the pulmonary artery and aortic saturations are dissimilar. This lack of complete mixing is seen in about 20% of patients with single ventricle. RA, right atrium; LA, left atrium; AO, aorta; PA, pulmonary artery; %, percent oxygen saturation; italics, pressure in mm Hg.*
From Nadas AS, Fyler DC [eds]. Nadas' Pediatric Cardiology. Philadelphia, PA: Hanley and Belfus, 1992.

Infants with single ventricle and pulmonary atresia are cyanotic at birth, the degree of cyanosis is determined by the amount of pulmonary flow supplied by the ductus arteriosus, persistent aortopulmonary collaterals, or bronchial circulation. Patients with severe pulmonary stenosis are comparable to those with pulmonary atresia. Those with moderate pulmonary stenosis may fare quite well (Fig. 44-3). Indeed, a few patients with pulmonary blood flow limited to about twice the systemic blood flow do very well for years and, despite recognizable cyanosis, grow and seem otherwise normal.

A single ventricle acts as a common mixing chamber in 80% of the patients, the aorta and pulmonary artery having identical oxygen saturation regardless of their anatomic location. Surprisingly, the remainder may have sufficient streaming of pulmonary and systemic venous return that mixing is incomplete (Fig. 44-4). It is possible for the pulmonary artery to receive dominantly pulmonary venous return and the aorta to receive dominantly systemic venous return despite the fact that both receive blood from the same ventricle. This is a variation on the circulation of transposition of the great arteries and clinical improvement was common following atrial septal defect creation or after an atrial venous switch operation (referred to as the palliative *Mustard operation*). For the most part, however, whether the great arteries are transposed or not had little influence on the hemodynamics.

An obstructed bulboventricular foramen, most often associated with a pulmonary artery band and rarely with pulmonary stenosis, may cause the single ventricle to pump at suprasystemic pressure (Fig. 44-5). Abnormalities of the mitral or tricuspid valve are common and occasionally they dominate the clinical picture (Fig. 44-6). Coarctation of the aorta and interrupted aortic arch cause high ventricular pressure if there is a pulmonary artery band, but, in the absence of pulmonary outflow obstruction, the pulmonary blood flow is forced to intolerable levels.

CLINICAL MANIFESTATIONS

Most infants with single ventricle are discovered in the first days or weeks of life.[4] They are seen earlier if there is severe pulmonary stenosis, because of cyanosis, and

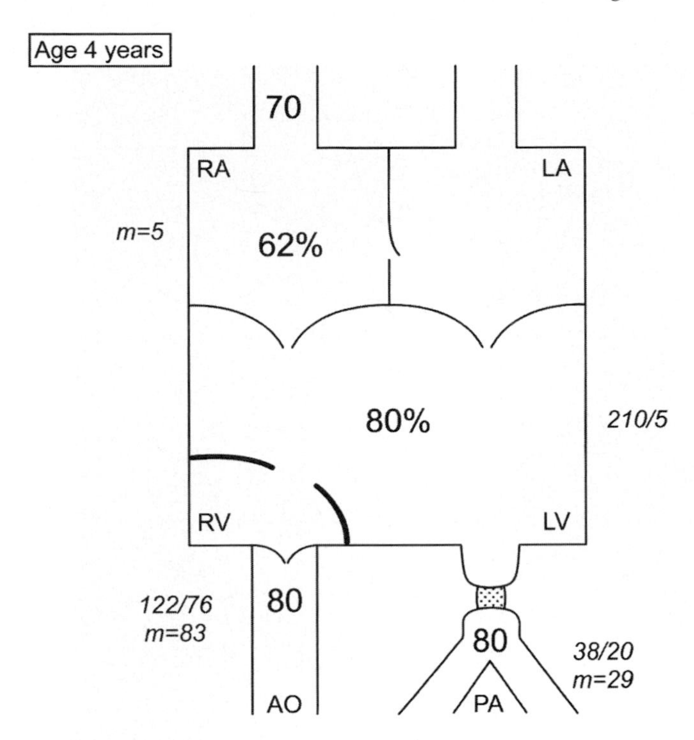

FIGURE 44–5 *Physiologic diagram of the circulation in a 4-year-old with single left ventricle and transposed great arteries. See prior data on this patient as an infant in Figure 44-2. Following the pulmonary artery banding procedure, there was spontaneous reduction in the size of the bulboventricular foramen sufficient to raise ventricular pressure to over 200 mm Hg. RA, right atrium; LA, left atrium; AO, aorta; PA, pulmonary artery; %, percent oxygen saturation; italics, pressure in mm Hg.*
From Nadas AS, Fyler DC [eds]. Nadas' Pediatric Cardiology. Philadelphia, PA: Hanley and Belfus, 1992.

later, in the absence of pulmonary stenosis, with congestive heart failure. Although all patients with single ventricle are cyanotic, among those with a large pulmonary flow, often in congestive heart failure, cyanosis may be so slight it is overlooked.

In patients with pulmonary stenosis there is an ejection systolic murmur; without a systolic murmur there can be no pulmonary stenosis. Right or left atrioventricular valvar regurgitation results in a pansystolic murmur. A continuous murmur suggests a patent ductus arteriosus or aortopulmonary collateral circulation. Coarctation of the aorta is discovered by a difference between arm and leg pulses or pressures.

Electrocardiography

The electrocardiogram is not especially helpful in recognizing ventricular hypertrophy, except that the tracing usually can be described as abnormal. Left ventricular hypertrophy is thought to be more common. Rhythm abnormalities are encountered in increasing numbers with advancing age; they include spontaneously occurring complete heart block and rhythms of junctional origin.[11,12]

Chest Radiography

If there is no pulmonary stenosis, the heart is enlarged on the chest radiograph and the pulmonary vascularity is increased. With pulmonary stenosis, the heart is of normal size or mildly enlarged and the pulmonary vasculature is normal or decreased. The more the pulmonary vascularity is increased, the more likely there will be gross congestive heart failure and, contrariwise, the more decreased the pulmonary vascularity the more cyanotic the patient will be.

Echocardiography

Fortunately, most of these patients are seen early in infancy when the most precise examinations by echocardiography are possible. Virtually every detail can be recognized if sufficient time is taken for a complete examination (Fig. 44-7). A systematic search is made for the missing ventricle, the origins of the great vessels documented, and the location, description, and competence of the atrioventricular valves established. The size of a bulboventricular orifice is measured, and pulmonary stenosis and associated defects are delineated. The type of single ventricle can usually be determined from the morphology of the chamber (see Chapter 13).

The large muscle bundles seen in a single right ventricle may mimic a septum, especially in the long axis view. In the short axis, however, the muscle bundle is surrounded by a cavity for a significant part of its length, whereas a true septum should connect with the anterior and/or posterior free wall for a significant portion of its length.

In patients with an L-loop single left ventricle, the left atrioventricular (tricuspid) valve is often regurgitant but may also be hypoplastic and stenotic: in a D-loop single left ventricle, the right atrioventricular valve (tricuspid) is often regurgitant. Doppler color flow mapping allows detection and quantitation of regurgitation, whereas pulsed or continuous-wave Doppler identifies and quantitates any stenosis. In the presence of a large atrial septal defect, however, a gradient may not be detectible across even a severely stenotic valve.

With normally related great arteries, the pulmonary artery is aligned with the outflow chamber and the aorta with the left ventricle; with transposition, the opposite is true. Rarely, a double-outlet infundibulum may occur when both great arteries are aligned with the outlet chamber.

Pulmonary stenosis in normally related great arteries is usually muscular, subvalvar, and/or valvar. When there is transposition of the great arteries, a small ventricular septal

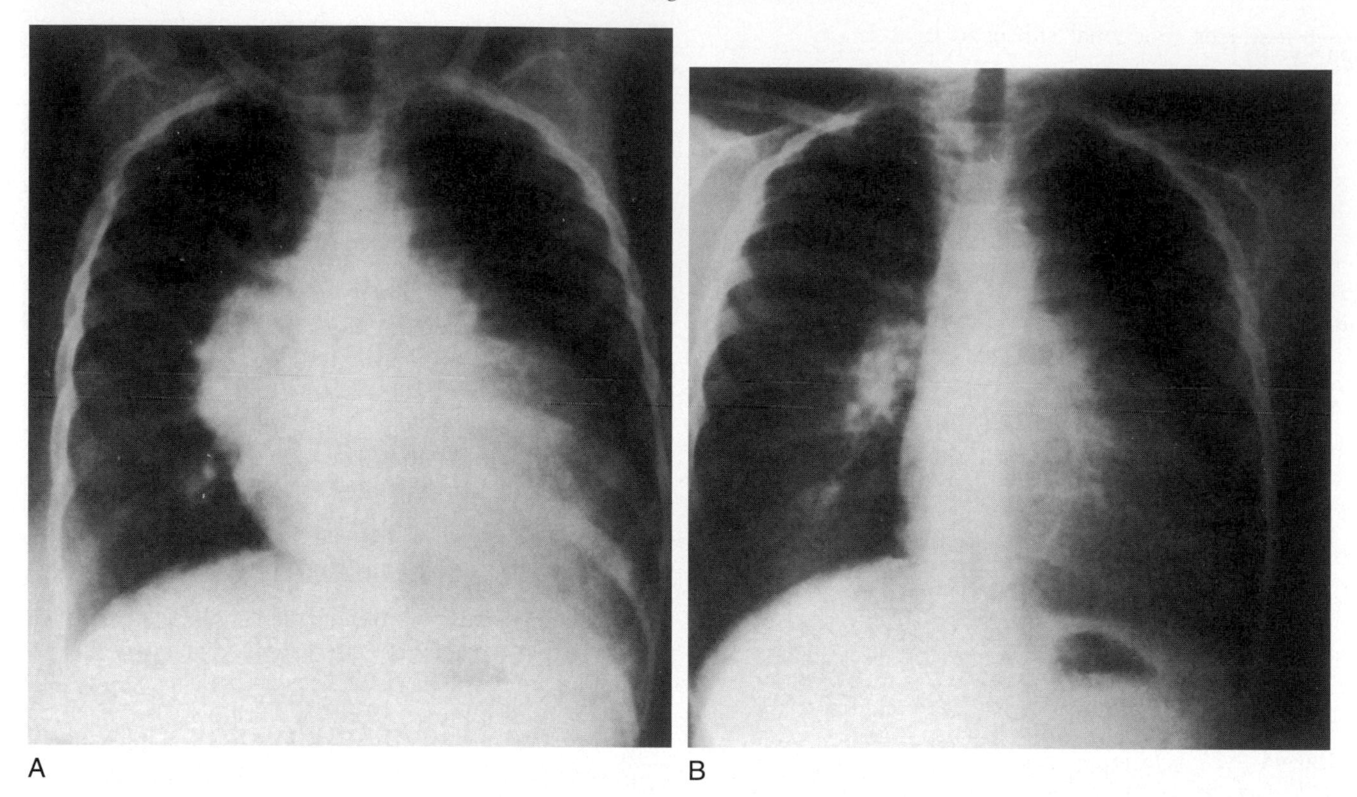

FIGURE 44–6 *Chest radiograph of a child who has a single left ventricle and developed progressively severe regurgitation of the right-sided mitral valve (A). Fortunately, there was an adequate left atrioventricular valve. At Fontan operation the mitral valve was occluded. One year later, the heart was much smaller (B).*
From Nadas AS, Fyler DC [eds]. Nadas' Pediatric Cardiology. Philadelphia, PA: Hanley and Belfus, 1992.

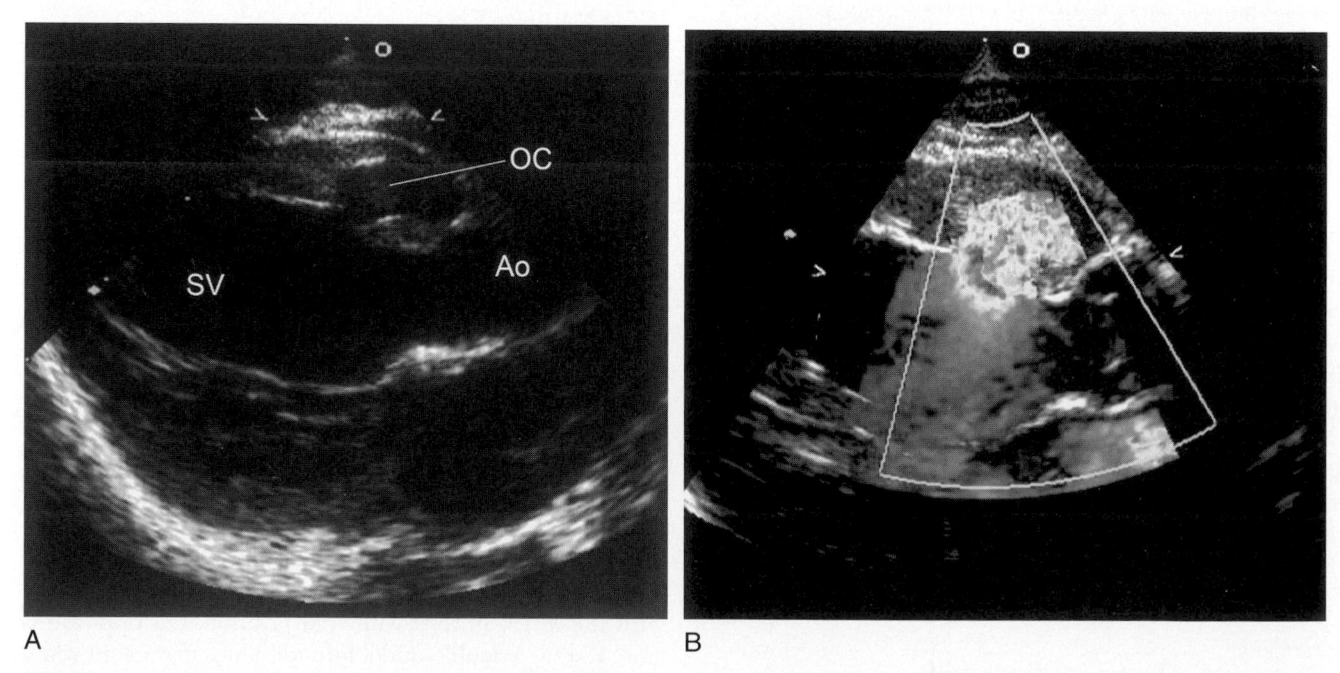

FIGURE 44–7 A, *Parasternal long-axis echocardiographic image of a large single ventricle of left ventricular morphology with an anterior subpulmonary outflow chamber (OC) and a posteriorly arising aorta (Ao).* B, *Color Doppler flow mapping with flow acceleration at the level of the inlet to the outflow chamber (so-called bulboventricular foramen) consistent with significant stenosis.*

defect produces functional subaortic stenosis. In a sick neonate, a gradient may not be detected despite a very small ventricular septal defect, and in such a patient, the appearance of the defect is more important than the absence of a pressure gradient.

At least two types of ventricular septal defects are seen. Subaortic defects, often associated with hypoplasia and/or malalignment of the infundibular septum, are immediately below the semilunar valves and often associated with pulmonary stenosis due to posterior deviation of the infundibular septum. The other type of defect is muscular, is close to the apex of the outflow chamber, is distant from the semilunar roots and is commonly obstructive. Coarctation is common with subarterial obstruction and may be long-segment or discrete juxtaductal or both.

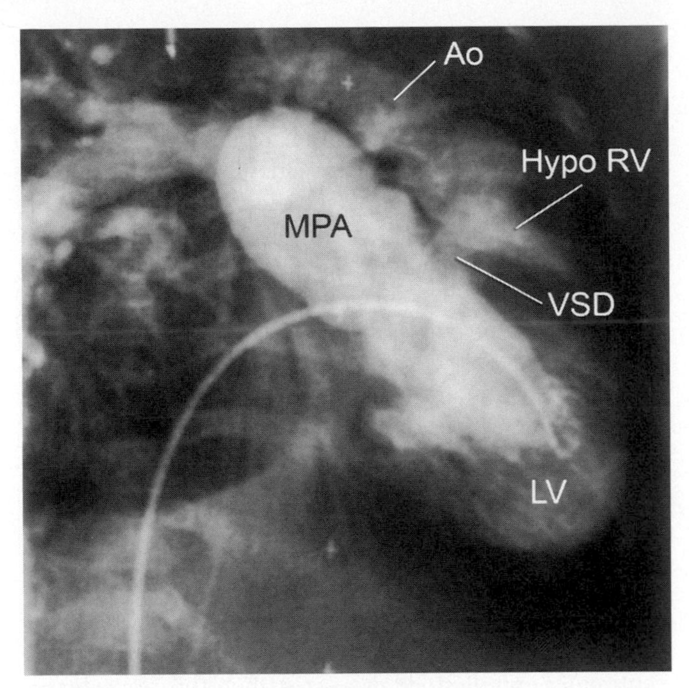

FIGURE 44–8 *Left ventricular (LV) cineangiogram in a 3-month-old baby, right anterior oblique view showing right-sided main pulmonary artery (MPA) arising from LV, contrast exiting via a restrictive ventricular septal defect (VSD) into a small right ventricle (Hypo RV) from which arises the leftward ascending aorta (Ao).*

Cardiac Catheterization

Routine preoperative catheterization before the initial operation is no longer a necessity. With the anatomical and physiological information provided by echocardiography, the majority of newborns are operated on without a study. Catheterization is reserved (a) for those in whom important anatomic and physiologic data are in doubt; (b) when an interventional procedure would be of benefit, such as atrial septal defect creation; and (c) probably in those with suspected pulmonary stenosis where medical follow-up for some time is being considered. In these patients, especially these with inverted ventricles (L-loop), induction of complete heart block, usually transient, by catheter manipulation is not uncommon: use of small balloon catheters guided to the posterior rightward pulmonary artery (Fig. 44-8) by tip-deflecting wires helps considerably. As an alternative to direct pulmonary artery pressure measurement, a pulmonary venous mean wedge if less than 18 mm Hg may be acceptable.[13] Postoperatively, catheterization is warranted in most patients before subsequent surgical procedures such as bidirectional Glenn shunts and Fontan operations.

MANAGEMENT

The ultimate goal is to accomplish a Fontan procedure with fully saturated systemic arterial blood. Because of the wide variety of associated lesions and the different ventricular morphologies of these single ventricles, a variety of management strategies will be utilized along the way.

Initially, management is concerned with lifesaving measures. Those newborns with pulmonary atresia require prostaglandins for survival, followed within days by a modified Blalock-Taussig shunt. Those in heart failure with no pulmonary stenosis and systemic arterial outflow obstruction may be managed initially with a pulmonary artery band recognizing that pulmonary artery deformity or progressive bulboventricular foramen narrowing may occur (subaortic stenosis in an L-loop).[9,14–16] Thus, those with an L-loop (the majority) who have any suggestion of restriction at the bulboventricular foramen are best managed with an initial modified stage I operation (Exhibit 44-1). This latter procedure includes an anastomosis between the ascending aorta and proximal divided main pulmonary artery, a modified Blalock-Taussig shunt and an atrial septectomy if necessary. Any arch obstruction can be managed at the same operation. Those stable neonates with an adequate amount of pulmonary stenosis and without subaortic obstruction can be followed medically initially.

Virtually all survivors require catheterization by the end of the first year. The main objectives of this study are to (a) evaluate pulmonary artery anatomy and resistance; (b) quantitate and delineate any intra- or extracardiac obstructions such as arch narrowing; (c) outline central venous anatomy for a subsequent bidirectional Glenn procedure; (d) occlude any potentially problematic venous collaterals such as a left superior vena cava to coronary sinus (which could result in significant right-to-left shunt after the Glenn procedure); and (e) balloon dilate any significant aortic arch/innominate artery/subclavian artery obstructions. In the future, if no interventions are deemed necessary by noninvasive evaluation (including physical examination, echocardiography, magnetic resonance imaging), catheterization may be omitted.[17] Many patients undergo a bidirectional Glenn-type procedure at this stage, this reducing volume load on the single ventricle at low surgical risk[18] and in some also decreasing accompanying atrioventricular valve regurgitation.[19] Significant degrees of the latter require complete closure or plasty of the involved valve. Leaving open any antegrade flow to the main pulmonary artery via a very stenotic ventricular outflow tract at this operation is debatable but it is clearly advantageous in some.[20,21]

Within a few years a modified fenestrated Fontan operation follows in most, preceded by catheterization, the latter for similar indications as for the pre-bidirectional Glenn procedure, this to include occlusion of any venous or arterial collateral flow if believed to be significant. If the requirements for the Fontan operation are fulfilled (including normal pulmonary artery resistance and anatomy and low ventricular end diastolic pressure), then this procedure is carried out which includes baffling of the inferior vena caval return to both pulmonary arteries via a fenestrated lateral intra-atrial tunnel or occasionally via an extracardiac conduit. After a year or more, if the fenestration remains significantly patent then it can be device-closed at catheterization. Other options which have been undertaken in small groups of patients with some success include heart transplantation[22] and septation.[23]

COURSE

Without treatment, survival is very poor (42% at age 1 year[4]) although rare patients with pulmonary stenosis can survive for many decades.[24] With surgery, survival has shown some improvement (48% to 60% at 10 years)[25,26] but remains very poor if total anomalous pulmonary venous return is an associated lesion (23% at 5 years).[27]

In our own recent experience (1988–2002), compared with 1973 to 1987, early survival has improved some and the number of Fontan procedures has increased considerably accompanied by a decrease in mortality rate (Exhibit 44-1). Some 62% of the patients first known to us after 1988 have survived to undergo a Fontan procedure with a mortality rate of 4% (compared with 41% and 19%, respectively from 1973 to 1987).

This population of patients is complex and difficult to manage. Surgery is clearly indicated in ill newborns (e.g., with pulmonary atresia or heart failure), and it is reasonable to follow the previously outlined management plan of catheterizations and surgeries (this being a variation of the hypoplastic left heart management plan; see Chapters 41 and 58). Patients whose circumstances create quite difficult clinical decisions include those who are very stable with a shunt or pulmonary stenosis (congenital or due to a pulmonary artery band), normal pulmonary artery pressure and anatomy, and a pulmonary/systemic flow ratio of 2:1 and aortic saturation about 85%. In these there is some evidence to suggest that an early bidirectional Glenn shunt/Fontan rather than continued medical follow-up may be better.[28,29] Adults followed up for long periods with an aortopulmonary or cavopulmonary shunt have a survival rate of only 52% at 10 and 20 years and an arrhythmia incidence of 50%.[30] Hopefully, earlier Fontan procedures will improve these values.

Atrioventricular valve regurgitation (right- or left-sided) is encountered and may be progressive: it does not preclude a Fontan operation, because the incompetent valve can be surgically closed and all pulmonary venous flow baffled toward the other valve. Complete heart block develops in 10% of patients with single left ventricle (Exhibit 44-1), is surprisingly well tolerated, and is managed with dual-chamber pacemaker implantation.

Atrial arrhythmias have been very common in our long-term survivors, particularly those who had an atriopulmonary anastomosis. It is hoped that the replacement of this by the fenestrated lateral tunnel will reduce this arrhythmia propensity although this is not obvious as yet. For the long term, in these patients the continued presence of an elevated central venous pressure remains a concern as does length of life. Nevertheless, the dramatic improvement in symptoms and physical activities which result and persist in the majority for the early postoperative decades is just remarkable.

REFERENCES

1. Van Praagh R, David I, Van Praagh S. What is a ventricle? The single ventricle trap. Pediatr Cardiol 2:79, 1982.
2. Van Praagh R, Ongley PA, Swan HJC. Anatomic types of single or common ventricle in man: morphologic and geometric aspects of 60 necropsied cases. Am J Cardiol 13:367, 1964.
3. Van Praagh R, Plett JA, Van Praagh S. Single ventricle: pathology, embryology, terminology and classification. Herx 4:113, 1979.
4. Fyler DC, Buckley LP, Hellenbrand WE, et al. Report of the New England Regional Infant Cardiac Program. Pediatrics 65(Suppl):376, 1980.
5. Steinberger EK, Ferencz C, Loffredo CA. Infants with single ventricle: a population based epidemiological study. Teratology 65(3):106, 2002.
6. Anderson RH, Macartney FJ, Tynan M, et al. Univentricular atrioventricular connection: the single ventricle trap unsprung. Pediatr Cardiol 4:273, 1983.
7. Streeter GL. Quoted by Van Praagh R, Plett JA, Van Praagh S.[3]
8. Barbar G, Hagler DJ, Edwards WD, et al. Surgical repair of univentricular heart (double-inlet left ventricle) with

obstructed anterior subaortic outlet chamber. J Am Coll Cardiol 4:771, 1984.
9. Freedom RM, Benson LN, Smallhorn JF, et al. Subaortic stenosis, the univentricular heart, and banding of the pulmonary artery: analysis of the courses of 43 patients with univentricular heart palliated by pulmonary artery banding. Circulation 73: 758, 1986.
10. Holmes WF. Case of malformation of the heart. Trans Med-Chir Soc Edinburgh 1:252, 1824.
11. Alboliras ET, Porter CJ, Danielson GK, et al. Results of the modified Fontan operation for congenital heart lesions in patients without preoperative sinus rhythm. J Am Coll Cardiol 6:228, 1985.
12. Gelatt M, Hamilton RM, McCrindle BW, et al. Risk factors for atrial tachyarrythmias after the Fontan operation. J Am Coll Cardiol 24(7):1735, 1994.
13. More Y, Nakarishi T, Ishii T, et al. Relation of pulmonary venous wedge pressures to pulmonary artery pressures in patients with single ventricle physiology. Am J Cardiol 91: 772, 2003.
14. Tchervenkov CI, Shum-tim D, Beland MJ, et al. Single ventricle systemic obstruction in early life: comparison of initial pulmonary artery banding versus the Norwood operation. Euro J Cardio-Thora Surg. 19(5):671, 2001.
15. Odim JN, Laks H, Drinkwater DC, Jr, et al. Staged surgical approach to neonates with aortic obstruction and single-ventricle physiology. Ann Thor Surg 68(3):962, 1999.
16. Bradley SM, Simsic JM, Atz AM, et al. The infant with single ventricle and excessive pulmonary blood flow: results of a strategy of pulmonary artery division and shunt. Ann Thor Surg 74(3):805, 2002.
17. Brown DW, Gauvreau K, Moran AM, et al. Clinical outcomes and utility of cardiac catheterization prior to superior cavopulmonary anastomosis. J Thor Cardiovasc Surg 126(1):272, 2003.
18. Jacobs ML, Rychik J, Rome JJ, at al. Early reduction of the volume work of the single ventricle: the hemi-Fontan operation. Ann of Thor Surg 62(2):456, 1996.
19. Mahle WT, Cohen MS, Spray TL, et al. Atrioventricular valve regurgitation in patients with single ventricle: impact of the bidirectional cavopulmonary anastomosis. Ann Thor Surg 72 (3):831, 2001.
20. Mainwaring RD, Lamberti JJ, Uzark K, et al. Effect of accessory pulmonary blood flow on survival after the bidirectional Glenn procedure. Circulation 100(19 Suppl):II151, 1999.
21. Caspi J, Pettit TW, Ferguson TB, Jr, et al. Effects of controlled antegrade pulmonary blood flow on cardiac function after bidirectional cavopulmonary anastomosis. Ann Thor Surg 76(6):1917, 2003.
22. Michielon G, Parisi F, Di Carlo D, et al. Orthotopic heart transplantation for failing single ventricle physiology. Euro J Cardio-Thor Surg 24(4):502, 2003.
23. Margossian RE, Solowiejczyk D, Bourlon F, et al. Septation of the single ventricle: revisited. J Thor Cardiovasc Surg 124(3):442, 2002.
24. Vitarelli A, Gabbarini F. Holmes heart in the adult: transesophageal echocardiographic findings and long-term natural survival. Int J Cardio 56(3):301, 1996.
25. Aeba R, Katogi T, Takeuchi S, et al. Long-term follow-up of surgical patients with single-ventricle physiology: prognostic anatomical determinants. Cardiovasc Surg 5(5):526, 1997.
26. Lee JR, Choi JS, Kang CH, et al. Surgical results of patients with a functional single ventricle. Euro J Cardio Thor Surg 24(5):716, 2003.
27. Gaynor JW, Collins MH, Rychik J, et al. Long-term outcome of infants with single ventricle and total anomalous pulmonary venous connection. J Thor Cardiovasc Surg 117(3):506, 1999.
28. Mahle WT, Wernovsky G, Bridges ND, et al. Impact of early ventricular unloading on exercise performance in preadolescents with single ventricle Fontan physiology. J Amer Coll Cardio 34(5):1637, 1999.
29. Milanesi O, Stellin G, Colan SD, et al. Systolic and diastolic performance late after the Fontan procedure for a single ventricle and comparison of those undergoing operation at <12 months of age and at >12 months of age. Am J Cardio 89(3):276, 2002.
30. Gatzoulis MA, Munk MD, Williams WG, et al. Definitive palliation with cavopulmonary or aortopulmonary shunts for adults with single ventricle physiology. Heart (British Cardiac Society) 83(1):51, 2000.

45

Tricuspid Atresia

JOHN F. KEANE AND DONALD C. FYLER

DEFINITION

Tricuspid atresia is characterized by absence of the tricuspid valve and hypoplasia of the right ventricle. By convention, patients are divided into groups, namely *type I*: those without transposition of the great arteries; *type II*: those with transposition; and *type III*: those with other complex anomalies (Exhibit 45-1). This chapter is confined to those with type I and type II lesions, some of which are depicted in Figure 45-1.

PREVALENCE

Tricuspid atresia occurred in 2.6% of infants hospitalized for congenital heart disease in New England, with a frequency of 0.057/1000[1] live births; comparable to other reports.[2]

ANATOMY

Atresia of the tricuspid valve occurs, and in most of these children there is no suggestion that a valve ever existed or that the atrium was ever aligned toward the right ventricle.[3] Blood passes from the right atrium through an atrial defect or, more often, a patent foramen ovale to the left atrium and from there to left ventricle. In patients with normally related great arteries (type I: about 80%; Exhibit 45-1) entry to the pulmonary circulation occurs through a ventricular defect and a hypoplastic right ventricle, and/or a patent ductus arteriosus. The latter is the only source of pulmonary blood in the rare patient with an intact ventricular septum or pulmonary atresia. The ventricular septal defect is usually perimembranous, less frequently muscular (single or multiple) in location. The right ventricle is variably small; in some patients it consists of no more than a channel from the left ventricle to the pulmonary artery. The passage through the ventricular defect to the pulmonary artery is usually restrictive; there may be pulmonary valvar stenosis, subvalvar obstruction, or pulmonary atresia. Usually, the ventricular defect is small, tends to get smaller with time, and may ultimately close. The ductus arteriosus usually has a small diameter and closes on schedule. In a few individuals (13%) the passage of blood to the main pulmonary artery is completely unobstructed.

When great arteries are transposed (type II), the ventricular defect carries blood to the aorta: thus restriction at this level results in subaortic stenosis. Aortic coarctation is more common in this group (about 33%) often in association with those with functional subaortic stenosis. Excessive pulmonary blood is more likely in these patients than in those with normally related great arteries (type I). Some minor cardiac anomalies such as right aortic arch, left juxtaposition of the atrial appendages, and persistent left superior vena cava and right aortic arch also occur among both types I and II.[2–4]

Patients with L-looped ventricles may have left-sided (tricuspid) atrioventricular valve atresia and a diminutive, left-sided right ventricle and have circulatory physiology comparable to mitral atresia.

PHYSIOLOGY

The entire cardiac output must pass through the foramen ovale; less than 6% of our patients with untouched foramina ovale have had pressure gradients of more than a few millimeters of mercury (mm Hg) between the two atria.

Exhibit 45–1
Children's Hospital Boston Experience
Tricuspid Atresia 1988–2002*

Types		N
Type 1	*Normally Related Great Arteries*	*161*
A - no VSD, PA	18%	
B - small VSD, PS	68%	
C - large VSD, no PS	14%	
Type 2 d-transposed great arteries		49
A - VSD, PA	12%	
B - VSD, PS	37%	
C - VSD, no PS	51%	
Type 3 Complex		23

VSD, ventricular septal defect; PA, pulmonary atresia; PS, pulmonary stenosis.
*There were 233 children with tricuspid atresia (compared with 154 patients from 1973–1987): 147 had their initial surgery elsewhere. With incomplete follow-up, 20 are known dead. Eighty-six patients, age 1 day to 15 years, 59 of whom were younger than 1 month had their first cardiac evaluation at our hospital.

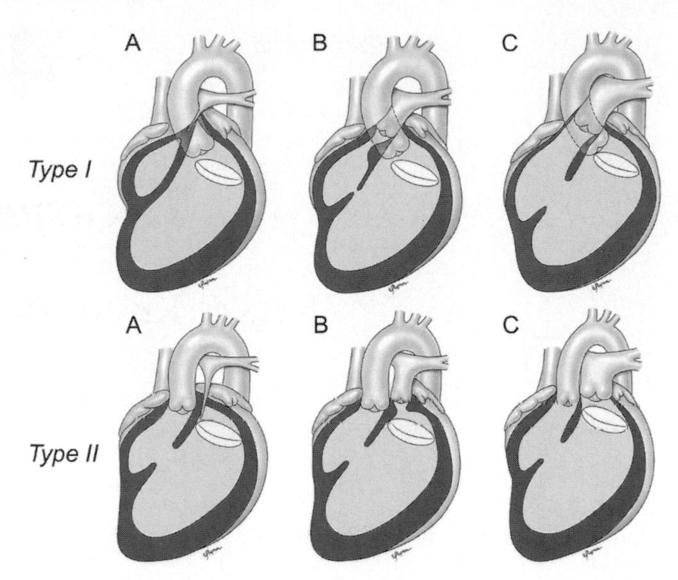

FIGURE 45–1 *Type 1: Normally related great arteries without a ventricular septal defect (VSD), with pulmonary atresia (PA) (A); small VSD and pulmonary stenosis (PS) (B) and large VSD, no PS (C). Type II: Transposed great arteries with a VSD and PA/PS (A); VSD and PS (B) and VSD and no PS (C). The VSD varies considerably in size and over time tends to get smaller. It may provide obstruction to pulmonary flow (type IB) or, in the presence of transposition, obstruct outflow to the aorta (functional subaortic stenosis).*
From Nadas' Pediatric Cardiology, ed Fyler DC, Hanley & Belfus, Philadelphia, 1992.

The streams of pulmonary venous return and systemic venous return join in the left atrium, passing to the left ventricle, which functions as a single ventricle. In those with normally related great vessels (type I), blood passes from the left ventricle to the aorta and, also via the ventricular septal defect, to the diminutive right ventricle and pulmonary artery (Fig. 45-2). Obstruction to flow by a restrictive ventricular defect, by right ventricular outflow, by the pulmonary valve and, in early infancy, by persistent elevation of fetal pulmonary resistance determines the amount of pulmonary blood flow. In general, the course of these patients is characterized by increasing cyanosis because of progressively diminishing pulmonary blood flow, most often because the ventricular defect gets smaller. Rarely, there is little obstruction, and pulmonary blood flow is excessive, to the point of producing congestive failure. The ductus arteriosus provides some blood flow to the pulmonary circulation after birth but most often it closes on schedule.

In those with transposition (type II), *subaortic stenosis* occurs because of an obstructive and closing ventricular septal defect (Fig. 45-2). As the ventricular defect gets smaller, there is increasing obstruction to outflow to the aorta. To provide adequate cardiac output, left ventricular pressure must rise. This increases pulmonary blood flow, ultimately resulting in congestive heart failure. When the pulmonary artery has been banded, the ventricular defect becomes more obstructive.[5]

CLINICAL MANIFESTATIONS

Most patients with tricuspid atresia are diagnosed by echocardiography in early infancy, having presented with cyanosis or a murmur. A few with excessive pulmonary blood flow have symptoms of congestive failure. Because the pulmonary blood flow is usually less than optimal, cyanosis is the most common presenting symptom. Those with maximal obstruction who are dependent on ductal blood flow become deeply cyanotic when the ductus closes, with some 50% being seen in the first week of life. Others gradually become more cyanotic as the months go by. When the cyanosis becomes intense, cyanotic spells may occur.

Hepatomegaly is rarely a notable observation in the more cyanotic children, although occasionally an obstructed foramen ovale is discovered by this means. Hepatomegaly is regularly seen in those with minimal cyanosis, tachypnea,

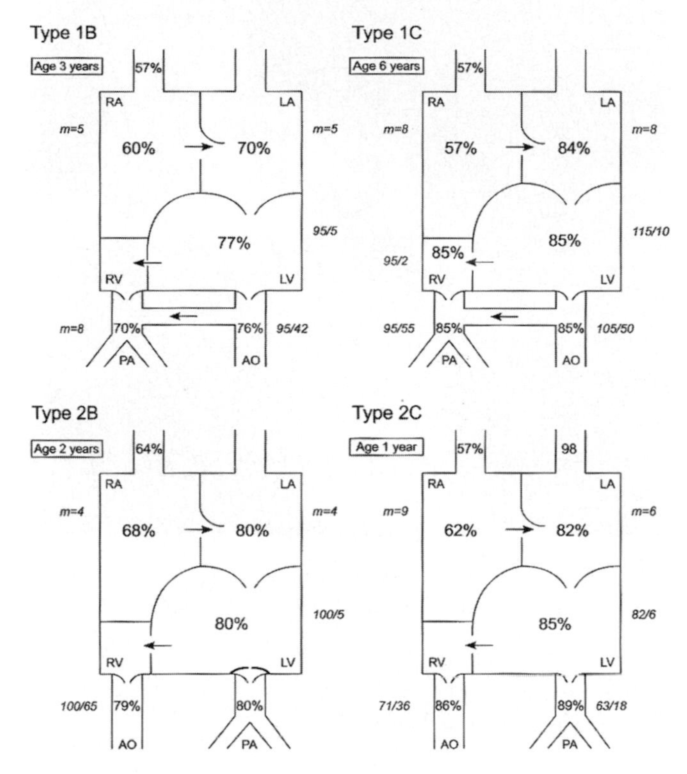

FIGURE 45–2 *Physiologic diagrams of patients with tricuspid atresia. Type 1B: Tricuspid atresia with normally related great arteries is usually associated with low pulmonary artery pressure either because of a small ventricular defect or, less often, because of pulmonary stenosis. Type 1C: Tricuspid atresia with normally related great arteries and a pulmonary artery pressure that approaches the systemic level is unusual. Type 2B: Tricuspid atresia and transposition of the great arteries may be associated with pulmonary stenosis or type 2C without pulmonary stenosis. Italics, mm Hg; %, oxygen saturation; RA, right atrium; RV, right ventricle, LA, left atrium; LV, left ventricle; PA, pulmonary artery; AO, aorta.*
From Nadas' Pediatric Cardiology, ed Fyler DC, Hanley & Belfus, Philadelphia, 1992.

hyperinflated lungs, and congestive heart failure because of unfettered pulmonary blood flow. There is usually, but not invariably, a moderate systolic murmur and the second heart sound is single and quite accentuated in those with transposed vessels.

Electrocardiography

Right atrial enlargement may be present, especially when older. The QRS axis is usually leftward and superior, right ventricular anterior forces are diminished, and left dominance is frequent. Some patients with transposition (type II) have a leftward inferior QRS axis and some may have left sided S-T and T-wave abnormalities. The frequent findings of left superior axis and diminished anterior right ventricular forces are clinically useful in distinguishing this lesion from pulmonary atresia with intact ventricular septum (left inferior axis and diminished right anterior ventricular forces) and pulmonary atresia with ventricular septal defect (right axis duration and right ventricular hypertrophy).

Chest Radiography

The heart size is proportionate to the pulmonary blood flow. Because the average patient has relatively limited blood flow, the heart size tends to be small or minimally enlarged; the resemblance to patients with tetralogy of Fallot is often striking. With increased pulmonary blood flow, the heart becomes proportionately enlarged.

Echocardiography

The anatomic features (Fig. 45-3) are readily demonstrable by echocardiography—these include the absence of a tricuspid valve, the atrial and ventricular septal defects and sizes, the diminutive right ventricle, the great vessels and patent ductus, and pulmonary stenosis if present. Doppler echocardiography quantitates the degrees of obstruction at atrial, ventricular septal, and pulmonary levels.

Usually the atrioventricular junction is filled with fibrous tissue. Occasionally the tricuspid valve is present but imperforate because of leaflet fusion. In such cases the valve leaflets may move with the cardiac cycle but Doppler examination determines if the valve is patent. An uncommon cause of tricuspid atresia is complete malalignment of a common atrioventricular valve over the left ventricle so that the tricuspid portion of the valve is atretic. The clue to this diagnosis is the presence of a primum atrial septal defect.

Pulmonary stenosis is common in infants with normally related great arteries (type I), and is usually due to subvalvar muscular hypertrophy and/or a small ventricular septal defect. The pulmonary valve is usually well formed and nearly normal in size. In patients with transposition of the great arteries (type II), a small ventricular septal defect or mid-cavity obstruction of the outflow chamber produces subaortic stenosis. If subaortic obstruction is seen on Doppler examination or if the ventricular septal defect and outflow chamber appear small by imaging, then coarctation should be suspected. If the ductus arteriosus is widely patent, coarctation may not be completely excluded: right to left shunting in the ductus may indicate a ductus-dependent systemic circulation.

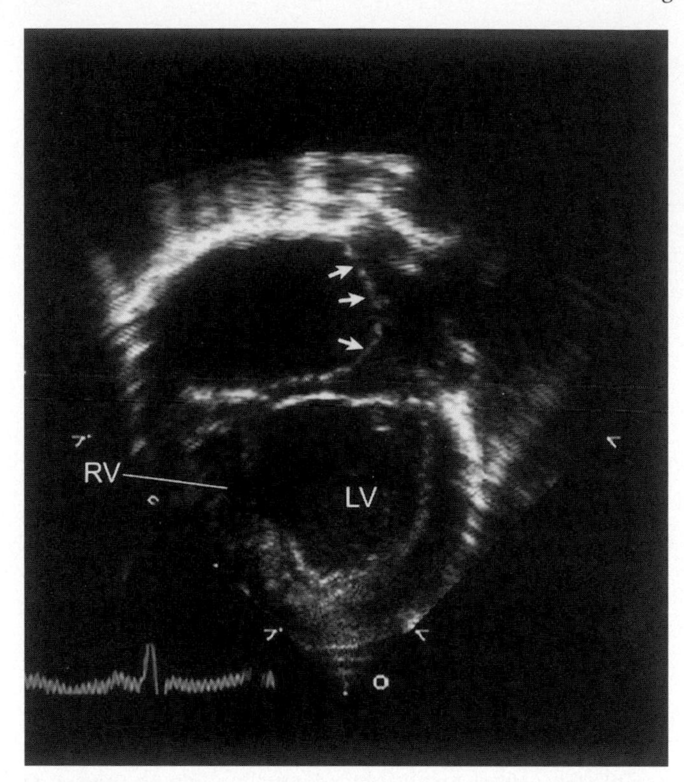

FIGURE 45–3 *Apical echocardiogram in a patient with tricuspid atresia. Note the small right ventricle (RV) with absence of a right atrioventricular connection. There is a muscular ventricular septal defect allowing the left ventricle (LV) to supply pulmonary blood flow. The atrial septum bows strikingly into the left atrium (arrows).*

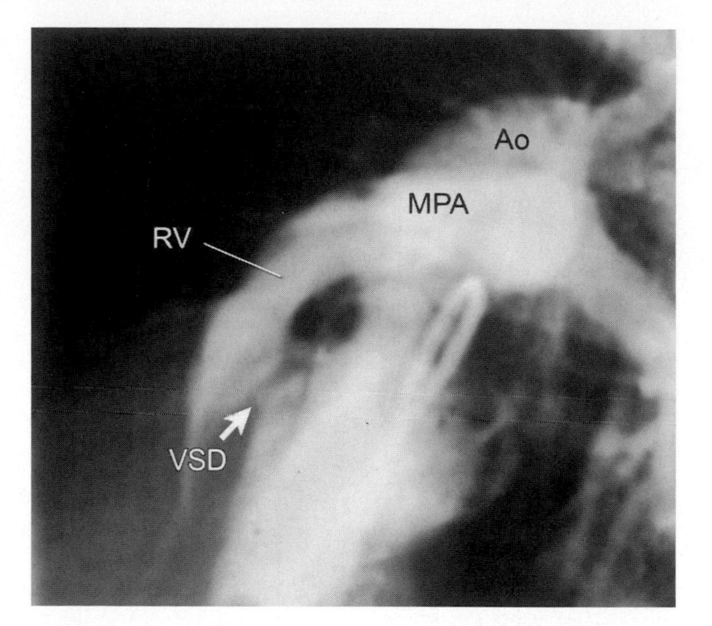

FIGURE 45–4 *Left ventricular angiogram, four-chambered view, in 2-month-old baby with tricuspid atresia (type 1B) with contrast passing via a small (arrow) ventricular septal defect (VSD) to a hypoplastic right ventricle (RV) and then to main pulmonary artery (MPA). The aorta (Ao) is normally located and fills directly from the left ventricle.*

Cardiac Catheterization

While catheterization in earlier years outlined precisely the anatomic details (Fig. 45-4), it is no longer necessary in the unoperated newborn as both anatomy and physiology are very well demonstrated by echocardiography. In the older patient who has not undergone surgical correction, and in those previously operated on, cardiac catheterization is necessary, particularly to visualize pulmonary arteries, measure arteriolar resistance, outline systemic venous return, and identify and coil occlude any unwanted channels such as a small left superior vena cava to coronary sinus or systemic–pulmonary venous collaterals.

MANAGEMENT

The goal of management for patients with tricuspid atresia is to achieve a successful Fontan operation.[6] To do this requires (a) no significant pulmonary arterial distortion from prior surgery (a potential problem because of prior shunting or banding operations), (b) normal pulmonary arteriolar vascular resistance (also a potential problem because of prior shunting procedures or inadequate pulmonary artery bands),[7] (c) good left ventricular function, and (d) a well-functioning mitral valve. Multivariate analysis has shown that elevated pulmonary resistance, distorted pulmonary arteries, and left ventricular dysfunction and hypertrophy are risk factors.[8,9]

Ideally, a Fontan operation is accomplished as early in life as possible, but, unfortunately, this operation is not tolerated well in early infancy. In the first months of life, there is pulmonary arteriolar muscle available to constrict and cause undesirable elevation of pulmonary resistance. The venous structures are small, and unobstructed flow to the lungs is difficult to achieve. Problems with recurrent pleural effusion are more common in this age group. The observed difficulties with Fontan surgery in infants decreases with age, so it is best to put off this intervention until the age of 2 years if things are going well clinically. Because of the many variations among patients and the ventricular septal defect size decreases in many with time, most patients require two catheterizations and two operations before the Fontan procedure. Because there is just one ventricle present, our current and evolving approach resembles that of the more common hypoplastic left heart syndrome (see Chapter 41). Briefly, in the latter following

Exhibit 45–2
Children's Hospital Boston Experience
Tricuspid Atresia 1988–2002

Fontan operation was carried out in 154 patients at Children's Hospital Boston, 111 of whom had normally related great arteries (type 1): four patients are known to have died. Life-table analysis of the first 18 months' survival after Fontan operations shows improvement in more recent era (1988–2002).

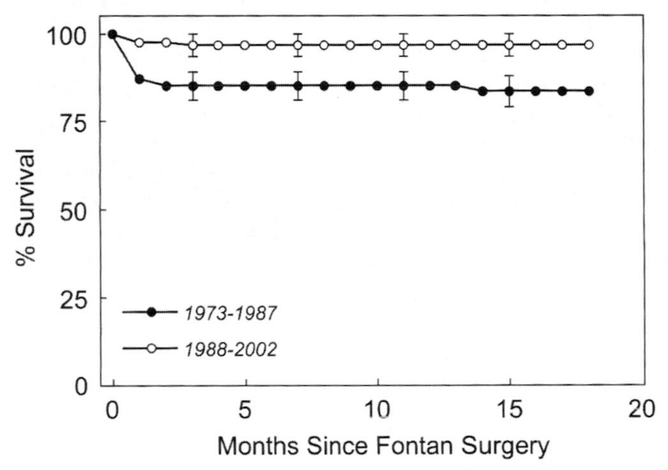

Life-table analysis of patients with and without d-transposition regardless of treatment, beginning with first observation at Children's Hospital Boston.

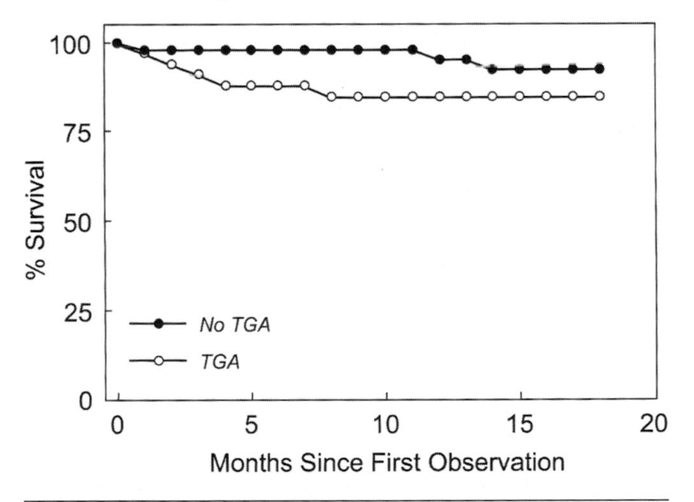

a neonatal modified Norwood operation, a bidirectional Glenn anastomosis is carried out at 6 months and a modified fenestrated Fontan by age 2 years, the latter two surgeries preceded by a catheterization with appropriate interventional procedures. In the tricuspid atresia population, some require immediate prostaglandin E_1 for pulmonary blood flow. In the neonatal period, an initial modified Norwood is usual in type 2B and type 2C[10] and in some type 1C (pulmonary artery band in others), a modified Blalock-Taussig shunt in types 1A and 2A, although medical follow-up is appropriate in type 1B patients if clinically well. Pulmonary artery banding because of its propensity for pulmonary distortion and ventricular septal defect size reduction[5] is avoided except in a few babies with type 1C.

All patients are catheterized at 6 months of age primarily to determine pulmonary artery anatomy, pressure, and resistance and to identify and coil occlude any venous channels such as a small left superior vena cava to coronary sinus, which because of the higher pressure following a bidirectional Glenn procedure will enlarge and produce significant right to left shunting. Most patients undergo a bidirectional Glenn shunt, which is better tolerated at this age than before age 2 months[11]; this has been shown to also reduce left ventricular volume.[12] The exceptions to this approach are the unusual patients who have a restrictive ventricular septal defect with normally related great vessels (type 1B) with normal pulmonary arteries, pressure, and resistance and an adequate arterial saturation.

At 2 years of age, all patients are again catheterized. This study again includes delineation of pulmonary artery anatomy, pressure and resistance together with detection of any pulmonary arteriovenous malformations, and coil occlusion of any systemic–pulmonary venous collaterals, which commonly result following the installation of the bidirectional Glenn shunt with its higher pressure and may produce significant right to left shunting. A fenestrated lateral tunnel modified Fontan operation then follows. The fenestration closes spontaneously in about 10% by the end of the first year and up to 26% at 34 months.[13] If it remains open and systemic saturation is 90% or less, it is closed with a double-umbrella device at catheterization—it is not uncommon to uncover additional sites of right-to-left shunting at this study (baffle suture line leaks, systemic–pulmonary venous collaterals), which can also be occluded at this procedure.

COURSE

Without treatment, patient survival to age 1 year is only 10% to 20%.[2,14,15] Our management plan, comparable to that at other institutions with similar patient populations, has been in effect just for several years. Since the Fontan procedure for tricuspid atresia was introduced more than three decades ago, it has undergone a number of modifications: artificial valves in the venous circuit were soon discontinued, as were the later right atrial ventricular conduits which invariably became obstructed with time.[16] Direct atriopulmonary anastomoses were used for many years with many survivors still continuing to lead satisfactory lives[17–19] but with increasing occurrences of complications such as severe right atrial enlargement, clot formation, right pulmonary vein compression, and atrial dysrhythmias necessitating conversion to lateral tunnels with atrial reduction or extra cardiac conduits.[20–22] The lateral tunnel modification, now standard for more than a decade, appears hemodynamically more satisfactory, and the addition of a fenestration has proven quite beneficial in reducing postoperative effusions.[23] Protein-losing enteropathy is another complication, very difficult to manage, that has appeared during follow up in some 2% to 11% of survivors. The etiology remains uncertain, although prolonged bypass time and single right ventricle anatomy have been implicated.[24] Although 5-year mortality rates to 54% have been reported, some limited success has been accomplished with long-term steroid[25,26] and heparin therapy.[27] Cardiac transplantation has been carried out in a few.

In general however, Fontan surgery has greatly helped these patients, many have a nearly normal life, and most are gainfully employed. Although some participate in sports, most are somewhat limited by the restricted cardiac output associated with this procedure. It is remarkable that these people with the equivalent of mild, chronic, right-sided congestive heart failure do so well for so long.

REFERENCES

1. Fyler DC, Buckley LP, Hellenbrand WE, et al. Report of the New England Regional Infant Cardiac Program. Pediatrics 65(Suppl):376, 1980.
2. Rowe RD, Freedom RN, Mehrizi A, et al. The Neonate with Congenital Heart Disease. Philadelphia: WB Saunders, 1981.
3. Van Praagh R, Ando, M, Dungan WT. Anatomic types of tricuspid atresia: clinical and developmental implications. Circulation 44:11, 1971.
4. Melhuish BPP, Van Praagh R. Juxtaposition of the atrial appendages: a sign of severe cyanotic heart disease. Br Heart J 30:269, 1968.
5. Freedom RM, Benson LN, Smallhorn JF, et al. Subaortic stenosis, the univentricular heart, and banding of the pulmonary artery: an analysis of the course of 43 patients with univentricular heart palliated by pulmonary artery banding. Circulation 73:758, 1986.
6. Fontan F, Baudet E. Surgical repair of tricuspid atresia. Thorax 26:240, 1971.
7. Juaneda E, Haworth SG. Pulmonary vascular structure in patients dying after Fontan procedure: the lung as a risk factor. Br Heart J 52;575, 1984.
8. Mayer JE, Helgason H, Jonas RA, et al. Extending the limits for modified Fontan procedures. J Thorac Cardiovasc Surg 92:1021, 1986.
9. Gentles TL, Mayer JE Jr, Gauvreau K, et al. Fontan operation in five hundred consecutive patients: factors influencing early and late outcome. J Thorac Cardiovasc Surg 114:376, 1997.
10. Mosca RS, Hennein HA, Kulik TJ, et al. Modified Norwood operation for single left ventricle and ventriculoarterial discordance: an improved surgical technique. Ann Thorac Surg 64(4):1126, 1997.
11. Reddy VM, McElhinney DB, Moore P, et al. Outcomes after bidirectional cavopulmonary shunt in infants less than 6 months old. J Am Coll Cardiol 29(6):1365, 1997.
12. Rychik J, Jacobs ML, Norwood WI Jr. Acute changes in left ventricular geometry after volume reduction operation. Ann Thorac Surg 60(5):1267, 1995.
13. Juneja R, Kothari SS, et al. Univentricular repair: is routine fenestration justified? Ann Thorac Surg 69(6): 1900, 2000.
14. Dick M, Fyler DC, Nadas AS. Tricuspid atresia: the clinical course in 101 patients. Am J Cardiol 36:327, 1975.
15. Keating P, Van der Shiptor M. Tricuspid atresia: profile and outcome. Cardiovasc J Southern Africa 12(4)202, 2001.
16. Dore A, Somerville J. Right atrioventricular extracardiac conduit as a Fontan modification: late results. Ann Thorac Surg 69(1)181, 2000.
17. Mair DD, Puga FJ, Danielson GK. The Fontan procedure for tricuspid atresia: early and late results of a 25-year experience with 216 patients. J Am Coll Cardiol 37(3):933, 2001.
18. Burkhart HM, Dearani JA, Mair DD, et al. The modified Fontan procedure: early and late results in 132 adult patients. J Thorac Cardiovasc Surg 125(6):1252, 2003.
19. Gates RN, Laks H, Drinkwater DC Jr, et al. The Fontan procedure in adults. Ann Thorac Surg 63(4):1085, 1997.
20. Kreutzer J, Keane JF, Lock JE, et al. Conversion of modified Fontan procedure to lateral atrial tunnel cavopulmonary anastomosis. J Thorac Cardiovasc Surg 111(6):1169, 1996.
21. van Son JA, Mohn FW, Hambsch J, et al. Conversion of atriopulmonary or lateral atrial tunnel cavopulmonary anastomosis to extracardiac conduit Fontan modification. Eur J Cardio-Thorac Surg 15(2):150, 1999.
22. Gelatt M, Hamilton RM, McCrindle BW, et al. Risk factors for atrial tachyarrhythmias after the Fontan operation. J Am Coll Cardiol 24(7):1735, 1994.
23. Bridges ND, Lock JE, Castaneda AR. Baffle fenestration with subsequent transcatheter closure: modification of the Fontan operation for patients at increased risk. Circulation 82:1681, 1990.

24. Powell AJ, Gauvreau K, Jenkins KJ, et al. Perioperative risk factors for development of protein-losing enteropathy following a Fontan procedure. Am J Cardiol 88:1206, 2001.
25. Rothman A, Snyder J. Protein-losing enteropathy following the Fontan operation: resolution with prednisone therapy. Am Heart J 121:618, 1991.
26. Rychik J, Riccoli DA, Barber G. Usefulness of corticosteroid therapy for protein-losing enteropathy after Fontan operation. Am J Cardiol 68:819, 1991.
27. Donnelly JP, Rosenthal A, Castle VP, et al. Reversal of protein-losing enteropathy with heparin therapy in three patients with univentricular hearts and Fontan palliation. J Pediatr 130:474, 1997.

46

Tricuspid Valve Problems

JOHN F. KEANE AND DONALD C. FYLER

Tricuspid valve problems (a somewhat vague title that Dr. Nadas would have likened to "a banker's aneurysm") may be anatomic, physiologic, primary or secondary, alone or in various combinations thereof, or even of no apparent significance (the largest group in our data base of tricuspid valve problems consists of more than 900 patients with the sole finding of echocardiographic mild or less regurgitation; see Chapter 19). Our most common primary anatomic abnormality is Ebstein anomaly, just over half of whom had other cardiac defects (Exhibit 46-1). Another group includes patients with tricuspid regurgitation secondary to annular dilatation in a variety of postoperative lesions with free pulmonary regurgitation and/or stenosis. Although tricuspid valve hypoplasia/stenosis/regurgitation is part and parcel of pulmonary atresia with intact septum (see Chapter 42), isolated tricuspid stenosis was absent in our population. Stenosis or regurgitation due to rheumatic fever is extremely rare in this country (see Chapter 24) and carcinoid heart disease occurs only in adults.

As a general rule, moderate degrees of tricuspid or pulmonary valve deformity (whether stenosis or regurgitation) are well tolerated; surgery is necessary. However if symptoms occur when both valves simultaneously are involved, symptomatic combinations of these lesions require surgery. Transient tricuspid incompetence does occur in newborns: The problem is presumed to result from major metabolic and hypoxic insults to the myocardium and usually results in death or complete recovery.

Recognition of tricuspid incompetence depends on the presence of a pansystolic (usually of high frequency) murmur audible at the lower left or right sternal border, and varies with respiration. Two-dimensional echocardiography readily establishes the diagnosis.

Tricuspid stenosis is clinically recognizable because of the presence of a diastolic rumbling murmur at the lower left sternal border, seeming to occur somewhat earlier in diastole than a mitral diastolic murmur. The diastolic murmur of tricuspid stenosis has been observed in rare patients with myxomas, rhabdomyomas, and extension of a Wilm tumor up the inferior vena cava.

EBSTEIN DISEASE

Definition

Ebstein disease characteristically involves the septal and posterior leaflets of the tricuspid valve. The leaflets are deformed, displaced, and variably adherent to the ventricular septum below the atrioventricular junction.

Prevalence

Ebstein disease is rare, with an incidence range from 0.012 to 0.06/1000 live births.[1,2] At Children's Hospital Boston, 245 patients were seen between 1988 and 2002 of whom 133 had other cardiac abnormalities (Exhibit 46-1).

Pathology

Although there is great variation in valve anatomy,[3] both septal and posterior leaflets are always involved to some degree. These leaflets are displaced toward the apex, are adherent to the ventricular septum, and may be redundant, contracted, or thickened, and even rarely atretic.

Exhibit 46–1
Children's Hospital Boston Experience
Ebstein Disease

	1973–1987		1988–2002	
	Pt. N.	*Deaths*	*Pt. N.*	*Deaths*
Ebstein, primary	75	14	112	7
Ebstein, secondary	45		133	
Dx				
Ventricular septal defect	4	0	12	2
Tetralogy of Fallot	4	1	16	4
Pulmonary stenosis	4	1	14	0
Malposition	4	0	12	4
Pulmonary atresia, intact ventricular septum	4	2	9	1
L-transposition	8	2	63	3
Other	17	9	63	3
TOTAL	120	29	245	24

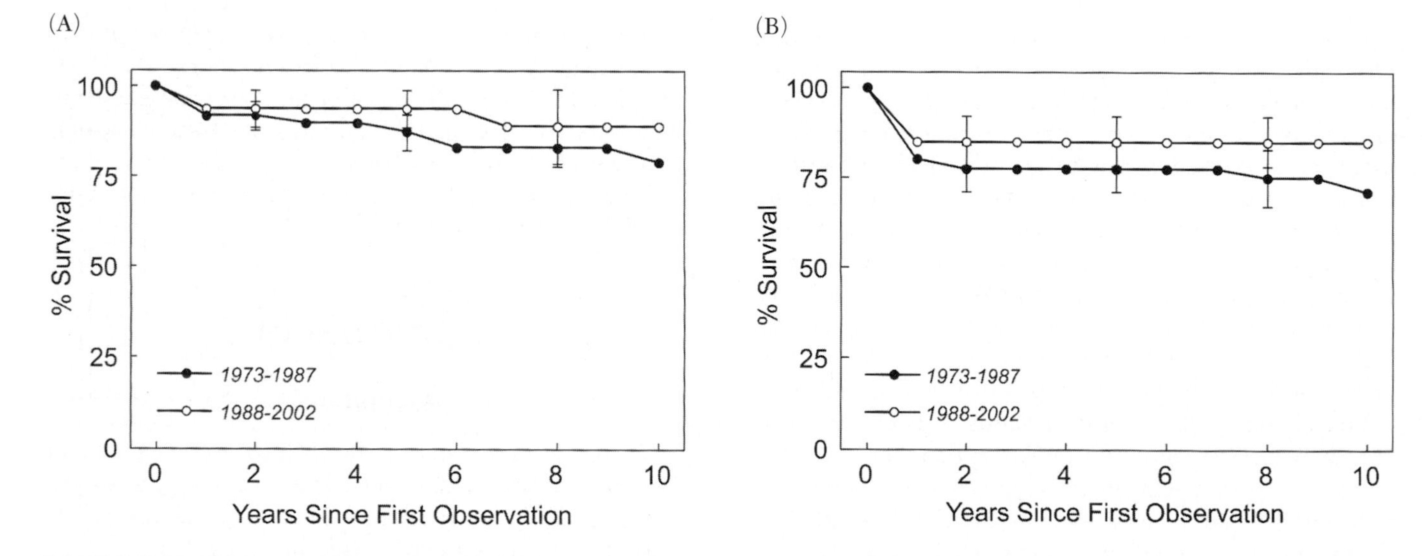

There were 245 patients with Ebstein seen 1988 to 2002 (compared to 120 from 1973 to 1987): 112 were uncomplicated whereas Ebstein was listed as a secondary diagnosis in the other 133. In 1988 to 2002 group (a) Wolfe-Parkinson-White syndrome was present in 36 (15%) (19% in primary 11% in secondary group), (b) overall mortality was 10% (vs. 24% for the 1973 to 1987 group), (c) only eight patients underwent tricuspid valve surgery (four plasty procedures; four replacements). Life tables comparing survival between 1973 to 1987 and current 1988 to 2002 period, for (A) Primary Ebstein diagnosis and (B) Ebstein as a secondary diagnosis: there has been a modest improvement in survival in both (A) and (B).

The part of the right ventricular wall proximal to the adherent valve leaflets is described as the *atrialized* portion of the right ventricle. The distal right ventricular chamber size ranges from small to large, the average length in one autopsy series was 0.9 that of the left ventricular value[4] whereas the right atrium is almost invariably enlarged, sometimes grossly so (Fig. 46-1). The tricuspid valve is usually incompetent, occasionally stenotic, with the orifice being displaced anterosuperiorly to varying degrees.[4] The proximal atrialized part of the ventricle may be paper thin with the distal portion unaffected.

There is virtually always a patent foramen ovale or an atrial septal defect. Pulmonary stenosis, pulmonary atresia, tetralogy of Fallot, ventricular septal defect, and other lesions are sometimes associated with Ebstein deformity. When the ventricles are inverse (as in corrected transposition), the left-sided tricuspid valve may have some of the features of Ebstein disease (see Chapter 51).

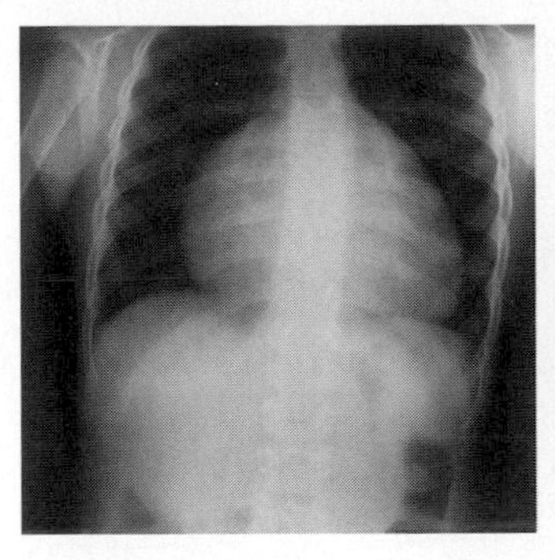
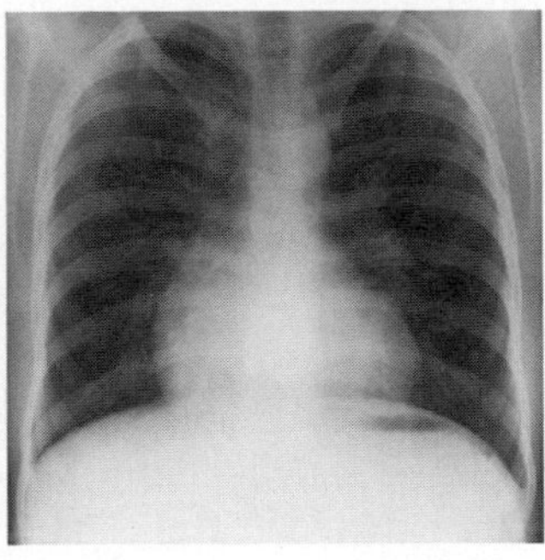

FIGURE 46–1 *Chest radiographs of two patients with Ebstein disease showing the great variation in heart size that may be encountered.*
From Fyler DC (ed) Nadas' Pediatric Cardiology, Hanley & Belfus, Philadelphia 1992.

Physiology

Whether there is tricuspid insufficiency or stenosis or both, the practical effect is limitation of passage of blood through the right heart. The right atrial pressure is higher than normal, and right-to-left shunting through a patent foramen ovale is usual. Occasionally, with minimal Ebstein disease, there is left-to-right shunting through an atrial defect. At birth, cyanosis may be extreme, gradually improving as pulmonary arterial resistance and right-to-left atrial shunting decrease over the first days and weeks of life. Attempts to define relative stenosis or regurgitation are unsuccessful when limited amounts of blood pass through the right ventricle, although magnetic resonance imaging may resolve this issue. The atrialized ventricular muscle and the remainder of the ventricle by contracting simultaneously (a) probably disrupt forward flow of blood and (b) likely oppose each other. It has been proposed that the distal attachments of the tricuspid valve subdivide the right ventricle into two chambers with deleterious effect on function.[5]

Replacement of the valve at or above the valve ring, or valve plasty, in association with closure of the atrial opening does help, although much of the symptomatic relief is due to elimination of the right-to-left shunt.

Clinical Manifestations

Infants

Infants with Ebstein disease are recognized because of cyanosis in the first days of life, the diagnosis in some being made by echocardiography even before birth. Cyanosis may vary from slight to severe and may be associated with tachypnea in direct proportion to the degree of cyanosis. The liver may be enlarged. There are no characteristic auscultatory findings and often there is no systolic murmur.

Children

After infancy, the child may or may not be cyanotic and is usually otherwise asymptomatic. Poor growth is rarely an issue. Older children may suffer the limitations of cyanosis and some may develop congestive heart failure. The cardiac impulse may be undulating. Both first and second heart sounds may be widely split and there may be a diastolic rumble. Triple and quadruple gallops and a systolic murmur are common.[6,7]

Electrocardiography

Just as the anatomic deformity varies greatly, so too does the electrocardiographic findings, which are normal in those with the mildest involvement and very abnormal in the most severely affected. Often there is right atrial enlargement and a bizarre right ventricular conduction delay (Fig. 46-2). The P-R interval is sometimes prolonged and 10% to 25% have Wolff-Parkinson-White syndrome.[8] Arrhythmias are

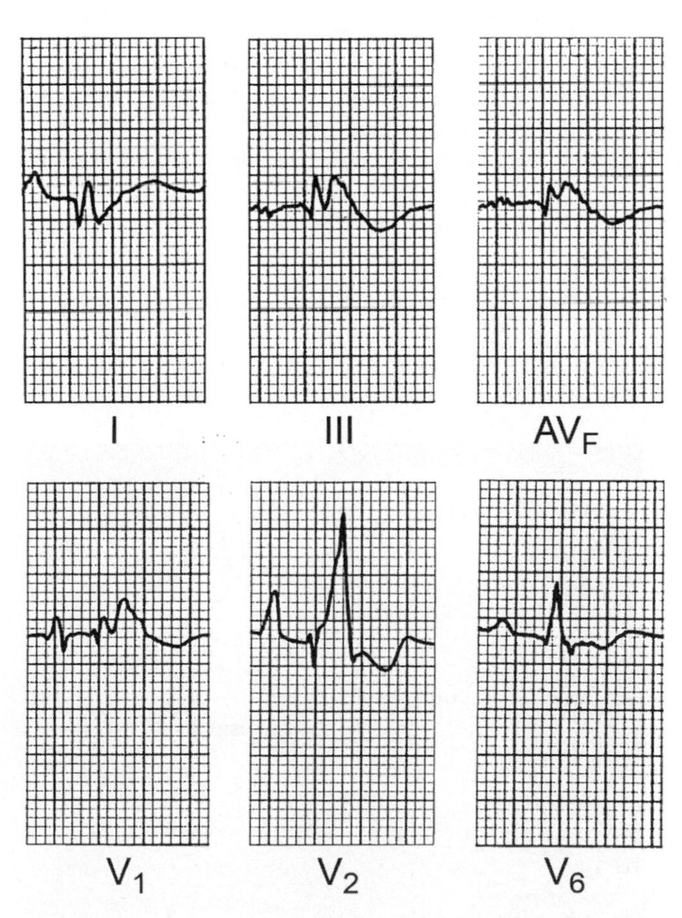

FIGURE 46–2 *An electrocardiogram from a patient with Ebstein disease. Note the large and bizarre P-waves and the wide and bizarre QRS complexes.*
From Fyler DC (ed) Nadas' Pediatric Cardiology, Hanley & Belfus, Philadelphia 1992.

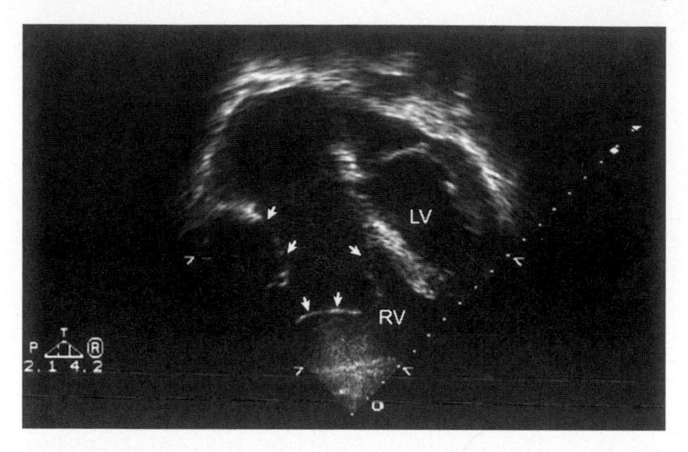

FIGURE 46–3 *Apical echocardiogram in Ebstein malformation of the tricuspid valve. The displacement of the tricuspid valve (arrows) into the right ventricle (RV) is apparent. Note that this is a systolic frame (the mitral valve is closed) indicating that the size of the atrialized RV is nearly the same as the size of the left ventricle (LV).*

common, increase with age, and include supraventricular tachycardia, atrial flutter, and atrial fibrillation.[7,9] Accessory conducting pathways when present are single in most (62%) and located in the right free wall, are right septal in 34%, atrioventricular nodal in location in a few, and multiple in 29%.[10]

Echocardiography

Using two-dimensional echocardiography, the degree of tricuspid valve deformity and right heart chamber sizes are readily seen and quantified (Fig. 46-3).[11] Non-Ebstein lesions causing regurgitation such as tricuspid valve dysplasia or prolapse or right ventricular dysplasia can usually be easily differentiated.[12] The degree of regurgitation and or stenosis is also readily evident on Doppler color flow and pulsed Doppler.

Magnetic Resonance Imaging

Magnetic resonance imaging, if necessary, provides excellent anatomic details and also functional information (Fig. 46-4).

Cardiac Catheterization

Because the two-dimensional echocardiographic and Doppler details are so informative, catheterization for anatomy and function has been unnecessary for some decades. Indications for catheterization are (a) electrophysiologic, namely to study arrhythmias and ablate if feasible underlying accessory pathways[10]; and (b) to device

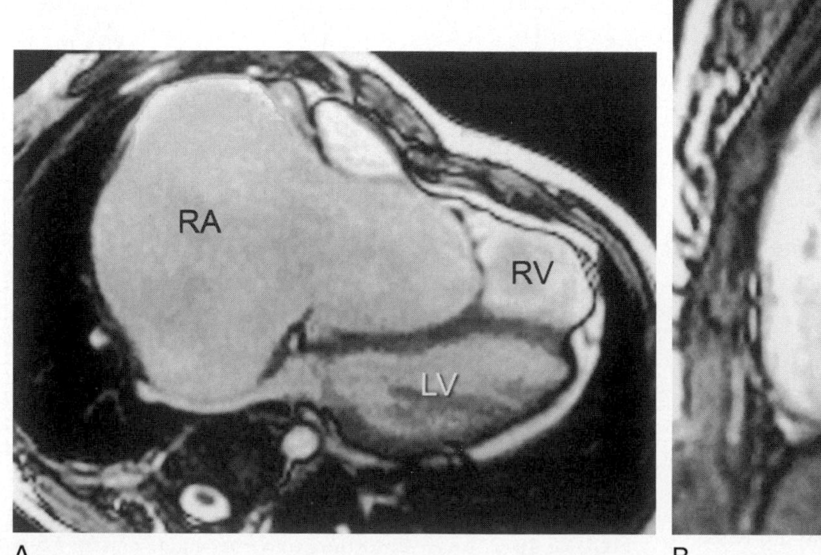

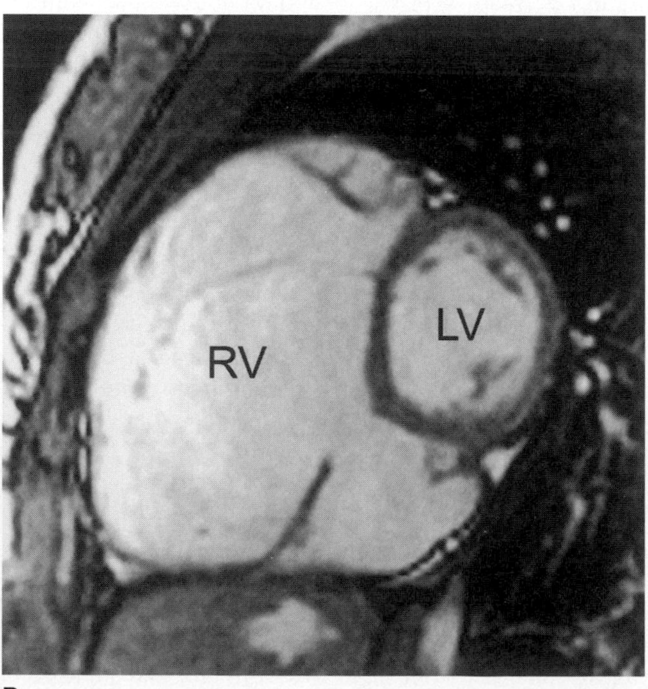

FIGURE 46–4 *Magnetic resonance images from patient with Ebstein anomaly showing (A) in four-chamber view, dilated right atrium (RA) apically displaced tricuspid valve (arrows) into right ventricle (RV) and (B) short-axis view, dilated RV much larger than left ventricle (LV) in this view (courtesy of Dr. T. Geva).*

close atrial septal defects if temporary balloon occlusion is hemodynamically tolerated and especially if a significant left-to-right shunt is present.

Management

In the newborn period, all efforts are made to support the infant through the period of transitional circulation, including prostaglandins and/or nitric oxide to increase pulmonary blood flow when the patient is dangerously cyanotic. Oxygen and correction of anemia may be helpful for those severely ill. Complex surgical procedures, including tricuspid valve plasty, atrial reduction and other defect repair and even tricuspid or pulmonary closure with a shunt, in small recent series seem to have some promise,[13–15] although in one large group over some decades mortality was some 47%.[16]

Older children generally can be followed medically. Rhythm problems however are common (≈30%), most are due to accessory connections (single or multiple), some are considered life threatening, and indeed sudden death is not uncommon.[17] Ablation of such pathways at catheterization is feasible in about 80% although recurrences are encountered in almost 30%.[10] Surgery is generally reserved for patients who are very symptomatic, deeply cyanosed, in heart failure, or with other associated anomalies. Increasing numbers are undergoing valve plasty (many with *wall* plication in addition, some including bidirectional Glenn procedures) with survival rates of 82% at 20 years.[18–20] In a large series of valve replacement only, at 10 years survival was 93% and freedom from reoperation 81%.[21] Some patients have undergone bypass tract ablation at the time of surgical valve plasty with a satisfactory outcome to date.[22,23]

Cyanosis, particularly if it is marked, or the appearance of congestive failure is ominous. The earlier these symptoms appear, the more likely life expectancy will be limited.

Course

Because modern echocardiographic techniques have revealed patients who formerly would have been unrecognized, a cadre of patients with mild forms of Ebstein disease has been added to the patient pool. These patients are expected to have a nearly normal life expectancy: Indeed survival at age 87 years has been reported.[24] Nevertheless, most of those who survive infancy are likely to have serious difficulties within a few decades, with survival rates of 59% at 10 years in one large series,[17] 81% in another, [25] and 89% of medically managed patients at 14 years in yet another.[9] The predictors that we and others feel are indicators of a poor outcome include heart failure, deterioration, cyanosis, other defects, and arrhythmias[25]; in the neonate echocardiographic right atrial and atrialized size exceeding that of the functional right ventricle and left heart chambers has been reported as ominous.[16] Brain abscess and endocarditis remain a threat.

REFERENCES

1. Fyler DC, Buckley LP, Hellenbrand WE, et al. Report of the New England Regional Infant Cardiac Program. Pediatrics 65(suppl): 453,1980.
2. Botto LD, Correa A, Erickson JD. Racial and temporal variations in the prevalence of heart defects. Pediatrics 107(3):1, 2001.
3. Anderson KR, Zuberbuhler JR, Anderson RH, et al. Morphologic spectrum of Ebstein's anomaly of the heart: a review. Mayo Clin Proc 54:174, 1979.
4. Schreiber C, Cook A, Ho SY, et al. Morphologic spectrum of Ebstein's malformation: revisitation relative to surgical repair. J Thorac Cardiovasc Surg 117(1):148, 1999.
5. Leung MP, Baker EJ, Anderson RH, et al. Cineangiographic spectrum of Ebstein's malformation: its relevance to clinical presentation and outcome. J Am Coll Cardiol 11:154, 1988.
6. Genton E, Blount Jr SG. The spectrum of Ebstein's anomaly. Am Heart J 73:395, 1967.
7. Kumar AE, Fyler DC, Miettinen OS, et al. Ebstein's anomaly: clinical profile and natural history. Am J Cardiol 28:84, 1971.
8. Smith WM, Gallagher JJ, Kerr CR, et al. The electrophysiologic basis and management of symptomatic recurrent tachycardia in patients. with Ebstein's anomaly of the tricuspid valve. Am J Cardiol 49:1223, 1982.
9. Jaiswal PK, Balakrishan KG, Saha A, et al. Clinical profile and natural history of Ebstein's anomaly of tricuspid valve. International J Cardiol 46(2):113, 1994.
10. Reich JD, Auld D, Hulse E, et al. The Pediatric Radiofrequency Registry's experience with Ebstein's anomaly. J Cardiovasc Electrophysiology 8(12):1370, 1998.
11. Shiina A, Seward JB, Edwards WB, et al. Two-dimensional echocardiographic spectrum of Ebstein's anomaly: detailed anatomic assessment. J Am Coll Cardiol 3:356, 1984.
12. Ammash NM, Warnes CA, Connoly HM, et al. Mimics of Ebstein's anomaly. Am Heart J 134(3):508, 1997.
13. Moura C, Guimaraes H, Areias JC, et al. Ebstein's anomaly in neonates. Revista Portuguesa de Cardiologia 20(9):865, 2001.
14. van Son JA, Falk V, Black MD, et al. Conversion of complex neonatal Ebstein's anomaly into functional tricuspid or pulmonary atresia. European J Cardiothorac Surg 13(3): 280, 1998.
15. Knott-Craig CJ, Overholt ED, Ward KE, et al. Repair of Ebstein's anomaly in the symptomatic neonate: an evolution of technique with 7-year follow up. Ann Thorac Surg 73(6): 1786, 2002.
16. Yetman AT, Freedom RM, McCrindle BW. Outcome in cyanotic neonates with Ebstein's anomaly. Am J Cardiol 81(6):749, 1998.

17. Celermajer DS, Bull C, Till JA, et al. Ebstein's anomaly: presentation and outcome from fetus to adult. J Am Coll Cardiol 23(1):170, 1994.
18. Augustin N, Schmidt-Habelmann P, Wottke M, et al. Results after surgical repair of Ebstein's anomaly. Ann Thorac Surg 63(6):1650, 1997.
19. Renfu Z, Zengwei W, Hongyu Z, et al. Experience in corrective surgery for Ebstein's anomaly in 139 patients. J Heart Valve Disease 10(3):396, 2001.
20. Chauvaud S, Berrebi A, d'Attellis N, et al. Ebstein's anomaly: repair based on functional analysis. European J Cardiothorac Surg 23(4):525, 2003.
21. Kiziltan HT, Theodoro DA, Warnes CA, et al. Late results of bioprosthetic tricuspid valve replacement in Ebstein's anomaly. Ann Thorac Surg 66(5):1539, 1998.
22. Pass RH, Williams MR, Quaegebeur JM, et al. Intraoperative radiofrequency linear catheter ablation of accessory pathways in children with Ebstein's anomaly undergoing tricuspid annuloplasty. Am J Cardiol 90(7):817, 2002.
23. Lazorishinets VV, Glagola MD, Stychinsky AS, et al. Surgical treatment of Wolff-Parkinson-White syndrome during plastic operations in patients with Ebstein's anomaly. European J Cardiothorac Surg 18 (4):487, 2000.
24. Hennebry TA, Calkins HG, Chandra-Strobos N. Successful interventional treatment of an octogenarian presenting with syncope and Ebstein's anomaly of the tricuspid valve. J Invasive Cardiol 14(1):44, 2002.
25. Attie F, Casanova JM, Zabal C, et al. Ebstein's anomaly. Clinical profile in 174 patients. Archivos del Instituto de Cardiologia de Mexico 69(1):17, 1999.

47

Truncus Arteriosus

JOHN F. KEANE AND DONALD C. FYLER

DEFINITION

Truncus arteriosus is characterized by a single arterial vessel that originates from the heart, overrides the ventricular septum, and supplies the systemic, coronary, and pulmonary circulations, all from the proximal ascending vessel. When the pulmonary circulation is supplied from the descending aorta by collateral vessels or a ductus arteriosus, the anatomy is considered to be that of tetralogy of Fallot with pulmonary atresia. There must be no remnant of a separate main pulmonary artery connected to the heart and no evidence of a separate pulmonary valve if one is to be confident of the presence of true truncus arteriosus.

PREVALENCE

Truncus arteriosus is a rare lesion. Reported incidence rates range from 0.006 to 0.043/1000 live births.[1,2] Overall, among all patients seen by us from 1988 to 2002, this was the major lesion in 0.3% (Exhibit 47-1). The common association with DiGeorge syndrome and deletion of chromosome 22q11 is well recognized and discussed in detail, together with recurrence risk data in Chapter 5.

EMBRYOLOGY

In the normal embryo, septation of the single truncus arteriosus into aorta and main pulmonary artery together with aortic and pulmonary valve formation occurs by the end of the fifth week. Shortly thereafter, conal septum formation is completed. It is thought that disturbances during these weeks, supported by experimental data[3–5] result in conotruncal abnormalities including truncus arteriosus.

ANATOMY

A single arterial trunk, larger in diameter than the normal aorta at a comparable age, arises from the heart. The trunk is positioned above the ventricular septum, being dominantly over either ventricle (the right in 42%, the left in 16%, and equally shared in 42%). The truncal valve is rarely normal, often having thickened and deformed leaflets (72%)[6] that are variably stenotic or, more often, incompetent (50%).[7] Valve anatomy is variable, with 42% tricuspid, 30% bicuspid, 24% quadricuspid, and 1% unicuspid in one study,[6] and 69%, 9%, 21%, and 1%, respectively, in a literature review.[7] A malalignment ventricular septal defect, which is rarely small, is present in almost all patients. This ventricular defect type, the overriding great artery and frequent right-sided aortic arch are reminiscent of tetralogy of Fallot, another conotruncal abnormality. The pulmonary arteries usually arise from the truncus within a short distance of the valve, as a single short vessel that divides into right and left pulmonary arteries (Fig. 47-1)[8,9] or as two separate vessels, usually without stenosis, from the posterior wall of the truncus. Occasionally, a pulmonary artery is absent.[10–12] An interrupted aortic arch is a common associated lesion in 11% to 14% of patients (Exhibit 47-1),[6] as are extracardiac anomalies (21% to 48%).[8,13] Coronary artery anomalies are frequent—these include a prominent right conal vessel, high or low origins of the vessels, greater than normal frequency of posterior descending origin from the left coronary artery, and a single coronary artery.[14–16]

Exhibit 47–1

Children's Hospital Boston Experience: Truncus Arteriosus Complicating Factors

Complicating Diagnoses	*1973–1987*		*1988–2002*	
	93 patients	Deaths %	171 patients	Deaths %
Interrupted aortic arch	10	70	24	25
Truncal stenosis	22	23	69	20
Truncal regurgitation	52	44	138	14
Mitral valve disease	13	31	83	12

There were 171 children with the diagnosis of truncus arteriosus: 62% were younger than 2 months when first seen: 22% were older than 6 months.

Some patients had more than one complicating diagnosis: survival with interrupted aortic arch has improved considerably. Life-table analysis of all 171 children with truncus arteriosus first seen between 1988 and 2002 compared with 49 seen 1983 to 1987, without respect to type of treatment. Late survival has improved.

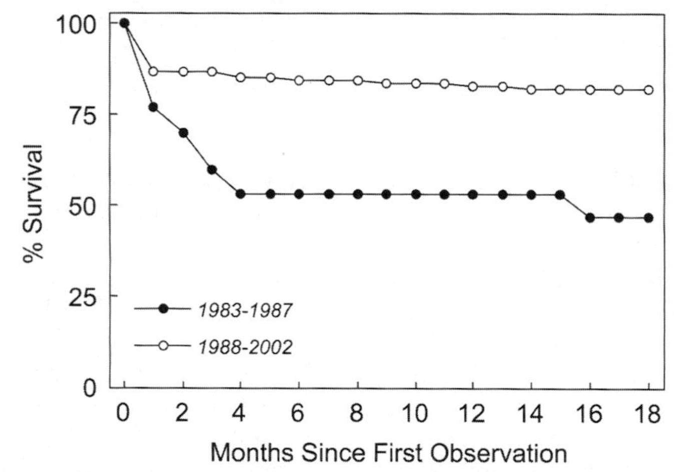

Life-table analysis of 131 children undergoing reparative surgery at Children's Hospital Boston (median age 19 days) 1988 to 2002 compared to 36 between 1983 and 1987. Survival is improving: The 14 early postoperative deaths included three in the interrupted aortic arch group and all three with severe truncal regurgitation and/or stenosis.

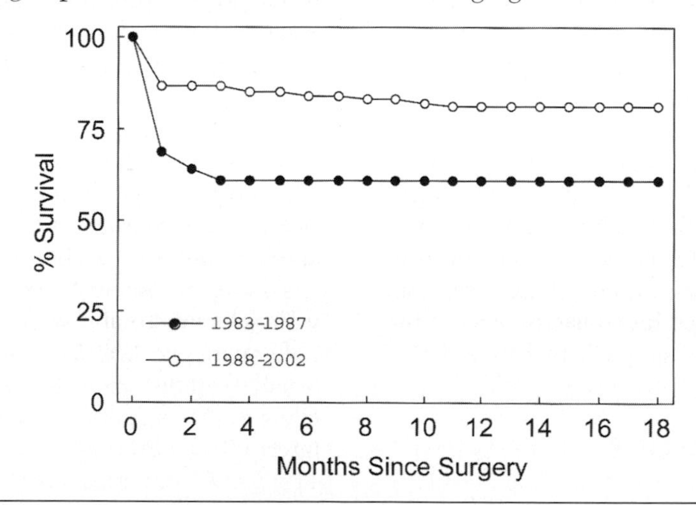

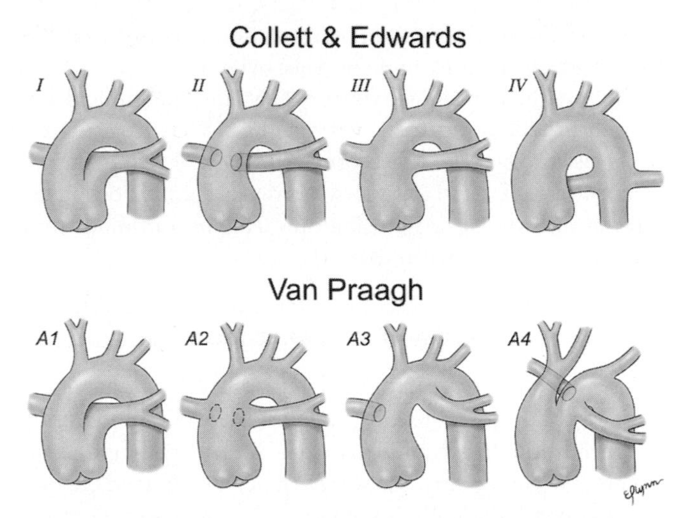

FIGURE 47–1 *There are similarities between the Collett and Edwards and the Van Praagh classifications of truncus. Type 1 is the same as A1. Types II and III are grouped as a single type A2, because they are not significantly distinct embryologically or therapeutically. Type A3 denotes unilateral pulmonary artery atresia with collateral supply to the affected lung. Type A4 is truncus associated with an interrupted aortic arch (13% of all cases of truncus arteriosus).*
From Hernanz-Schulman M, Fellows KE. Persistent truncus arteriosus: pathologic, diagnostic and therapeutic considerations. Semin Roentgenol 20:121–129, 1985, with permission.

PHYSIOLOGY

The truncus receives the output of both ventricles and, within a short distance, the blood destined for pulmonary circulation is diverted to the lungs (Fig. 47-2). In the absence of pulmonary stenosis, the pulmonary arterial pressure is equal to that in the truncus. The amount of pulmonary blood flow is determined by the presence of pulmonary stenosis or by the level of pulmonary arteriolar resistance. In the absence of pulmonary stenosis, the expected reduction in pulmonary resistance in the first days of life is not well tolerated; survival depends on persistence of some pulmonary arteriolar resistance to prevent flooding of the lungs. Pulmonary blood flows are greater than normal, the exact amount determining the systemic arterial saturation. When a main pulmonary artery arises immediately beyond the truncal valve, the pulmonary circulation may largely derive from the right ventricle, the pulmonary arterial oxygen saturation being less than that observed in the aorta. Truncal regurgitation of some degree is present in most patients, and when severe, the added burden of the regurgitant flow may be more than can be tolerated. The amount of blood passing through the truncal valve to supply the systemic blood flow and the pulmonary blood flow, as well as the regurgitant blood flow, is greatly excessive and often leads to early congestive heart failure. Because of the large pulmonary

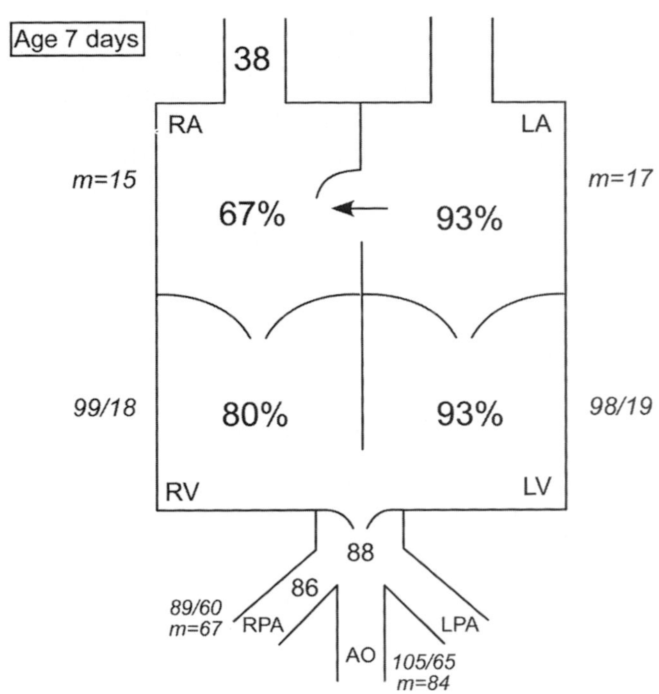

FIGURE 47–2 *Diagram of the hemodynamics in a patient with truncus arteriosus. Note the equilibration of systemic and pulmonary pressures; the complete mixing of systemic and pulmonary blood as evidenced by similar systemic and pulmonary oxygen concentrations; and the large left-to-right shunt as evidenced by high pulmonary oxygen saturation. Ao, aorta; LA, left atrium; LPA, left pulmonary artery; LV, left ventricle; RA, right atrium; RPA, right pulmonary artery; RV, right ventricle.*
From Nadas' Pediatric Cardiology, ed Fyler DC, Hanley & Belfus, Philadelphia, 1992.

blood flow, development of pulmonary vascular obstructive disease is common among survivors who have not undergone surgery: it can occur as early as 6 months of age.

CLINICAL MANIFESTATIONS

Most of these babies are found to have a cardiac problem within the first weeks of life, either because of a murmur or the appearance of tachypnea and/or costosternal retractions. The infants are sometimes visibly cyanotic, although tachypnea and even costal retractions are more common presenting symptoms and this evidence of congestive heart failure is usually readily apparent. The peripheral pulses are bounding. There is generally an easily palpable and often visible right ventricular impulse. There is usually a systolic murmur at the left sternal border, sometimes associated with the diastolic murmur of aortic regurgitation. There is frequently a prominent ejection click audible at the apex or the left sternal border, and the second heart sound is usually single although this may be difficult to detect in a small sick infant. An apical diastolic flow rumble due to relative mitral stenosis and a huge pulmonary blood flow is common. Once pulmonary vascular obstructive disease has developed, the clinical features reflect the elevated pulmonary vascular resistance (see Chapter 10).

Electrocardiography

The electrocardiogram may show left or right ventricular hypertrophy, with left or combined ventricular hypertrophy being more common.

Chest Radiography

Chest radiograph shows that the heart is large; pulmonary vasculature is increased. There may be a right aortic arch.

Echocardiography

From a subxiphoid long-axis view, the echocardiogram shows the overriding truncal root and its leftward posterior originating pulmonary artery is visualized atop a large conoventricular septal defect together with truncal valve thickness and mobility (Fig. 47-3). The atrial and ventricular septa, atrioventricular valves and truncal valve commissural details may be evaluated using a short-axis subxiphoid view. Truncal valve stenosis may be quantitated using Doppler from apical, suprasternal or right sternal border views, and regurgitation from parasternal or apical transducer locations. Coronary artery origins and branching details, including ostial to pulmonary artery origin measurements, are available from parasternal long and short-axis views.

The proximal pulmonary artery anatomy, including distal branches, that is the truncus type (Fig. 47-1) is displayed using parasternal short-axis and suprasternal notch views.

The ascending and transverse aortic arch, brachiocephalic arterial and ductal origin anatomy can be outlined on a suprasternal notch short-axis view.

Cardiac Catheterization

Given the precise anatomic details, together with truncal valve function information provided by echocardiography in these patients who are neonates when first seen (from which low pulmonary resistance may be inferred), there is little need for catheterization. The only preoperative indications for such a study would include (a) uncertainty about anatomic information (Fig. 47-4) or (b) suspicion of pulmonary vascular obstructive disease, which does occur even in infants with this lesion. The purpose of the study in the latter is to evaluate pulmonary resistance response to vasodilators such as oxygen and nitric oxide.

MANAGEMENT

Since (a) most of these patients will develop heart failure in the neonatal period, (b) pulmonary vascular obstructive disease is not uncommon by age 1 year,[17] and (c) surgical techniques have improved greatly, repair, including any associated lesions, is usually undertaken within days of diagnosis (Exhibit 47-1). In earlier years, palliative pulmonary artery banding was an initial approach but resulted frequently in

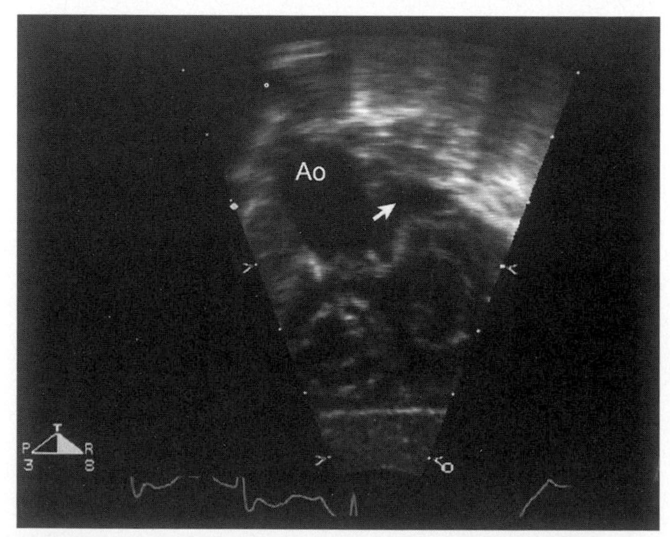

FIGURE 47–3 *Subxyphoid echocardiographic image showing the right and left ventricles connected by a large ventricular septal defect immediately below a thickened truncal valve. The pulmonary arteries (arrow) arise directly from the single arterial root, which continues to the ascending aorta (Ao).*

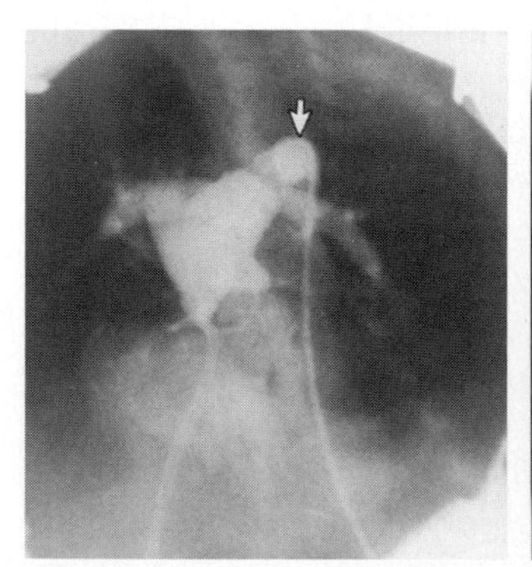

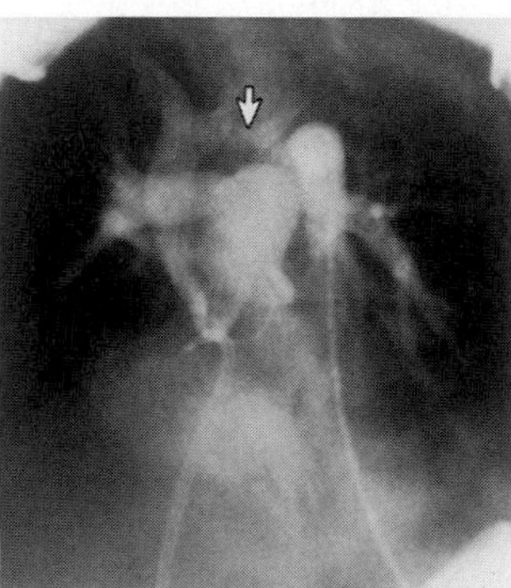

FIGURE 47–4 *A, Cineangiogram in the left anterior oblique view showing a truncus arteriosus 1. The descending aorta is supplied by a ductus arteriosus (arrow), through which the catheter entered the common truncus. B, the small transverse arch (arrow) ends in an interrupted aortic arch.*
From Nadas' Pediatric Cardiology, ed Fyler DC, Hanley & Belfus, Philadelphia, 1992.

severe obstruction/hypoplasia/atresia of vessels and even vascular obstructive disease in one or both lungs.[18]

Thus, where facilities (surgery, intensive care, cardiology) are available, after a brief period (days at most) of intensive medical treatment if necessary, surgical repair is undertaken. In the uncomplicated patient this includes ventricular septal defect closure and placement of a valved homograft from the right ventricle to the detached pulmonary arteries. Aortic arch interruption or coarctation is readily repaired (direct end-end anastomosis or patch plasty) at the same time. Early mortality rates for repair in recent years have ranged from 0% to 12.5%.[19–22]

The most difficult associated lesions to deal with are stenosis or regurgitation of the truncal valve. In general, mild degrees of either are left alone as these will likely remain unchanged or even improve postoperatively. Prosthetic valve placement at this age is often not possible, but a plasty procedure can be beneficial in some.[23]

These patients require life-long follow-up. All will need replacement of the right ventricular-pulmonary homograft because of increasing obstruction at least once. Replacement can be postponed for a period of some 2 years by stent placement at catheterization.[24] Pulmonary artery stenoses centrally are encountered, as is aortic obstruction following coarctation or interruption repair, all of which can be significantly improved by balloon dilation with or without stent placement at catheterization. Bacterial endocarditis prophylaxis is, of course, mandatory in all.

REFERENCES

1. Perry LW, Neill CA, Ferencz C, et al. Infants with congenital heart disease: the cases. In Ferencz C, Rubin JD, Loffredo CA, et al (eds) Perspectives in Pediatric Cardiology: Epidemiology of Congenital Heart Disease, the Baltimore-Washington Infant Study 1981-1989. Armonk, NY: Futura,1993, pp 33–62.
2. Fyler DC, Buckley LP, Hellenbrand WE, et al. Report of the New England Regional Infant Cardiac Program. Pediatrics 65(suppl 2):387, 1980.
3. Feiner L, Webber AL, Brown CB, et al. Targeted disruption of semaphorin 3C leads to persistent truncus arteriosus and aortic arch interruption. Development 128(16):3061, 2001.
4. Kirby ML. Nodose placode provides ectomesenchyme to the developing chick heart in the absence of cardiac neural crest. Cell Tissue Res 252:17, 1988,
5. Kirby ML, Gale TF, Stewart DE. Neural crest cells contribute to normal aorticopulmonary septation. Science 220:1059, 1983.
6. Butto F, Lucas RV, Edwards JE. Persistent truncus arteriosus: pathologic anatomy in 54 cases. Pediatr Cardiol 7:95, 1986.
7. Fuglestad SJ, Puga FJ, Danielson GK, et al. Surgical pathology of the truncal valve: a study of 12 cases. Am J Cardiovasc Pathol 2:39, 1988.
8. Van Praagh R, Van Praagh S. The anatomy of common aorticopulmonary trunk (truncus arteriosus communis) and its embryologic implications. Am. J. Cardiol 16:406, 1965
9. Collett RW, Edwards JE. Persistent truncus arteriosus: classification according to anatomic types. Surg Clin North Am 29:1245, 1949.
10. Fyfe DA, Driscoll DJ, DiDonato RM, et al. Truncus arteriosus with single pulmonary artery: influence of pulmonary vascular obstructive disease on early and late operative results. J Am Coll Cardiol 5:1168, 1985.
11. Mair DD, Ritter DG, Davis GD, et al. Selection of patients with truncus arteriosus for surgical correction: anatomic and hemodynamic considerations. Circulation 49:144, 1974.
12. Calder L, Van Praagh R, Van Praagh S, et al. Truncus arteriosus communis: clinical, angiocardiographic, and pathologic findings in 100 patients. Am Heart J 92:23, 1976.
13. Fyler DC, Buckley LP, Hellenbrand WE, et al. Report of the New England Regional Infant Cardiac Program. Pediatrics 65(suppl 2):392, 1980.
14. Dickinson DF, Arnold R, Wilkinson JL. Congenital heart disease among 160,480 liveborn children in Liverpool 1960-1969. Implications for surgical treatment. Br Heart J 46:55, 1981.
15. de la Cruz MV, Cayre R, Angelini P, et al. Coronary arteries in truncus arteriosus. Am J Cardiol 66:1482, 1990.
16. Shrivastava S, Edwards JE. Coronary arterial origin in persistent truncus arteriosus. Circulation 55:551, 1977.
17. Juaneda E, Haworth SG. Pulmonary vascular disease in children with truncus arteriosus. Am. J Cardiol 54:1314, 1984.
18. McFaul RC, Mair DD, Feldt RH, et al. Truncus arteriosus and previous pulmonary arterial banding: clinical and hemodynamic assessment. Am J Cardiol 38:626, 1976.
19. Elami A, Laks H, Pearl JM. Truncal valve repair: initial experience with infants and children. Ann Thoracic Surg 57(2):397, 1994.
20. Imamura M, Drummond-Webb JJ, Sarris CE, et al. Improving early and intermediate results of truncus arteriosus repair: a new technique of truncal valve repair. Ann Thoracic Surg 67(4):1142, 1999.
21. Ullmann MV, Gorenflo M, Sebening C, et al. Long-term results after repair of truncus arteriosus communis in neonates and infants. Thoracic & Cardiovasc Surgeon 51(4):175, 2003.
22. Rodefeld MD, Hanley FL. Neonatal truncus arteriosus repair: surgical techniques and clinical management. Sem Thoracic & Cardiovasc Surg, Pedi Card Surg Annual 5:212, 2002.
23. Mavroudis C, Backer CL. Surgical management of severe truncal insufficiency: experience with truncal valve remodeling techniques. Ann Thoracic Surg 72(2):396, 2001.
24. Powell AJ, Lock JE, Keane JF, et al. Prolongation of RV-PA conduit life-span by percutaneous stent implantation: intermediate term results. Circulation 92:3282, 1995.

48

Total Anomalous Pulmonary Venous Return

JOHN F. KEANE AND DONALD C. FYLER

DEFINITION

Drainage of the entire pulmonary venous circulation into systemic venous channels characterizes total pulmonary venous return.

PREVALENCE

Total anomalous pulmonary venous return as an isolated problem was the 12th most common cardiac defect among critically ill infants in the New England states (0.056 per 1000 live births), constituting 2.6% of the total experience.[1] This compares to the experience reported by others.[2,3] Because total anomalous pulmonary venous return is a disease of infancy, when it is listed as part of the entire experience of a cardiology department, it is a much less significant entity, with uncomplicated patients accounting for only 0.3% of our total experience. When patients with asplenia or polysplenia are included, the number of patients with total anomalous pulmonary venous return is increased by 48% (Exhibit 48-1).

EMBRYOLOGY

Normally, by the end of the first month, lung buds have developed within the splanchnic plexus. The latter has numerous connections with the cardinal and omphalovitelline systems. Shortly thereafter, a common pulmonary vein appears, connecting the pulmonary venous plexus and the sinoatrial portion of the heart, and later becomes incorporated into the left atrial wall, by which time the pulmonary–splanchnic venous connections have disappeared.[4] When failure of the common pulmonary vein to unite with the left atrium occurs, some of the pulmonary–splanchnic venous connections persist, allowing pulmonary venous return at various systemic venous–right atrial levels, such as the left innominate, portal, and coronary sinus levels.

ANATOMY

Any pulmonary vein, or combination of pulmonary veins, may drain anomalously into the systemic venous or right heart circulation, producing a left-to-right shunt. When all pulmonary veins return to the systemic venous circulation, the patient is said to have total anomalous pulmonary venous return (drainage, connection). There are several anatomic variations (Fig. 48-1; see Exhibit 48-1). Common to all types, other than mixed, is the presence of a common horizontal pulmonary vein, usually large and draining both lungs immediately posterior to the left atrium. This structure is more vertically oriented in infradiaphragmatic total veins and may vary somewhat in anomalous return to the coronary sinus, but it is this vein that allows the surgeon to cure this lesion by anastomosing it to the back of the left atrium.

1. **Supracardiac.** All the pulmonary veins return to the common pulmonary vein behind the left atrium, which then drains upward on the left side of the chest, usually in front of the pulmonary artery, into the left innominate vein. Sometimes the common pulmonary

Exhibit 48–1
Children's Hospital Boston Experience
Total Anomalous Pulmonary Venous Return

Between January 1988 and January 2002, 294 patients with total anomalous pulmonary venous return were seen. Of these patients, 152 had associated asplenia, polysplenia, malposition, or other major anomaly. When these patients were excluded, there were 142 patients with uncomplicated total anomalous pulmonary venous return.

30-Day Surgical Mortality by Age

	1973–1987		*1988–2002*	
Age (days)	*No. of Patients*	*Mortality (%)*	*No. of Patients*	*Mortality (%)*
0–14	27	11	61	5
15–60	25	16	22	4
61–180	28	4	16	5
181+	14	7	9	0
TOTAL	94	10	108	5

Three fourths of the patients first seen in 1988–2002 underwent corrective surgery before age 2 months, more than half in the first 2 weeks, the median age being 11 days. The overall mortality rate was 5%, improved compared with 10% in 1973–1987, and was unrelated to age.

30-Day Surgical Mortality by Type

	1973–1987		*1988–2002*	
Type	*No. of Patients*	*Mortality (%)*	*No. of Patients*	*Mortality (%)*
Supracardiac	43	7	44	5
Cardiac	23	0	13	0
Infracardiac	21	19	34	3
Mixed	7	20	17	12
TOTAL	94	10	108	5

The mortality rate was highest in the mixed type 1988–2002, but both it and the infracardiac rate were less than in the 1973–1987 era.

venous channel drains directly into the superior vena cava and occasionally into the azygous system.

2. **Cardiac.** All pulmonary veins drain into the common pulmonary vein, which then drains into the right atrium or, more often, into the coronary sinus.
3. **Infradiaphragmatic.** After collection by a common pulmonary vein behind the heart, the pulmonary venous blood passes down a venous channel shaped like an inverted Christmas tree, through the diaphragm to the portal vein, ductus venosus, or hepatic vein, reentering the heart through the left inferior vena cava.
4. **Mixed.** Any combination of anatomic entry of the pulmonary veins into the venous circulation is possible. For example, the right-sided veins may enter the right atrium, whereas the left veins travel upward to the left innominate.

Among large surgical series with available information, the averages of the return sites were supracardiac, 49%; cardiac, 25%; infradiaphragmatic, 18%; and mixed, 8%.[5–9]

The pulmonary venous system may be variably, absolutely, or relatively obstructed.[10,11] The point of obstruction may be caused by compression by adjacent structures; for example, the ascending channel to the left innominate vein may be compressed if it passes between the left bronchus and pulmonary artery, or it may be within the pulmonary venous system, almost always downstream from the common pulmonary vein. Veins draining below the diaphragm are almost always obstructed either at the diaphragm or at the ductus venosus. Those entering the coronary sinus are less often obstructed, whereas all other types may be obstructed in variable locations.[12] Often, increased pulmonary flow accentuates the obstruction. When there is obstruction, there is pulmonary venous hypertension and reflex pulmonary arterial hypertension, often at suprasystemic pressure levels.

Rarely, other isolated, simple, cardiac anomalies, such as ventricular septal defect, are associated with total anomalous veins; however, other major cardiac abnormalities are more likely to be present when there is asplenia and polysplenia (see Chapter 39).

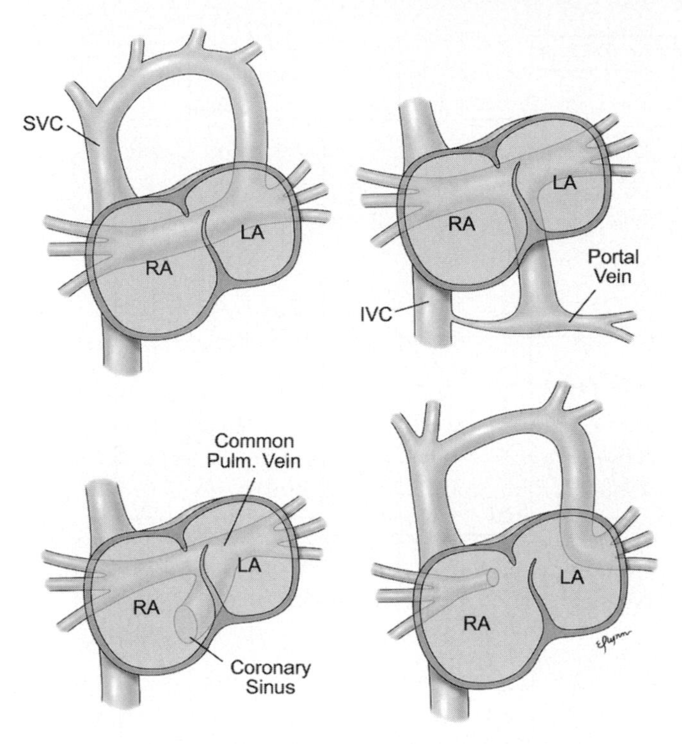

FIGURE 48–1 *A, Supracardiac total anomalous pulmonary venous return. All the pulmonary veins collect in a common channel behind the left atrium. From there, blood courses upward to the left innominate vein, then to the superior vena cava, and reenters the heart at the right atrium. All blood entering the left atrium passes from the right to the left atrium. B, Infradiaphragmatic total anomalous veins. All the pulmonary veins collect behind the left atrium and, through a common channel, proceed through the diaphragm to the portal or hepatic vein and ductus venosus, and from there to the inferior vena cava and to the right atrium. C, Total anomalous pulmonary venous return to the coronary sinus. All the pulmonary veins collect behind the left atrium and enter the coronary sinus. The pulmonary venous blood with coronary sinus blood drains into the right atrium. D, Mixed type of total anomalous pulmonary venous return. There are multiple variations of this anatomy. All pulmonary veins ultimately drain into the right atrium, with all blood entering the left atrium through the foramen ovale. In the example presented, the left veins course upward to the left innominate vein, and down the superior vena cava to the right atrium, whereas the right pulmonary veins drain directly into the right atrium. SVC, superior vena cava; IVC, inferior vena cava; RA, right atrium; LA, left atrium.*
From Fyler DC [ed]. Nadas' Pediatric Cardiology. Philadelphia: Hanley & Belfus, 1992.

PHYSIOLOGY

The entire pulmonary venous blood flow is returned to the systemic venous circulation, where there is mixing of the two venous returns. Characteristically, mixing is virtually complete, each chamber of the heart receiving blood of similar oxygen content (Fig. 48-2). The level of arterial oxygen saturation is dependent on the size of the pulmonary blood flow. When there is large pulmonary blood flow, the percent of arterial oxygen saturation may reach the high 80s, but with limited blood flow, it may be much lower.

The amount of pulmonary blood flow is governed by the pulmonary arteriolar resistance and by obstructions of the pulmonary veins. Although the obstruction may be severe, the entire pulmonary venous return is rarely completely obstructed: surprisingly, this latter anatomy is compatible with life for a few days or so (Fig. 48-3). When the obstruction is severe, the amount of pulmonary blood flow is small; when this is mixed with the systemic venous return, the result is a low arterial oxygen saturation. Pulmonary arterial pressure may be suprasystemic with severe obstruction, and because of this, in the first days of life, the ductus arteriosus may shunt right to left. Detection of the ductal right-to-left shunt is not possible by comparing the arterial oxygen saturation above and below the ductus because all oxygen saturations in the heart are identical, negating the value of this otherwise useful test.

Total anomalous pulmonary venous return below the diaphragm is characterized by severe obstruction (Fig. 48-4). Less often, there is obstruction in the tortuous pulmonary venous channels of the supracardiac types. Asymmetric obstructions in some pulmonary veins and not in others, in certain mixed varieties, forces increased blood flow to the least obstructed area of lung, thereby stimulating persistence of fetal pulmonary arteriolar vasculature, which may help the patient to survive.

With minimal obstruction, the pulmonary blood flow can be enormous; the patient may be pink and in congestive heart failure.

Generally, the left atrium and left ventricle seem to be relatively small compared with the very large right ventricle.[13,14] If the ductus arteriosus is patent, some of the cardiac output may bypass the left heart, further contributing to the impression of a small ventricle.

CLINICAL MANIFESTATIONS

Patients with totally anomalous pulmonary venous return range from those with maximally obstructed to those with completely unrestricted pulmonary blood flow. Although the extremes will be described in some detail, it must be recognized that most cases fall some place between them.

Obstructed Pulmonary Veins

When there is severe obstruction of the pulmonary venous return, the infant is discovered to be acutely ill within days after birth. Usually, there is rapid onset of tachypnea,

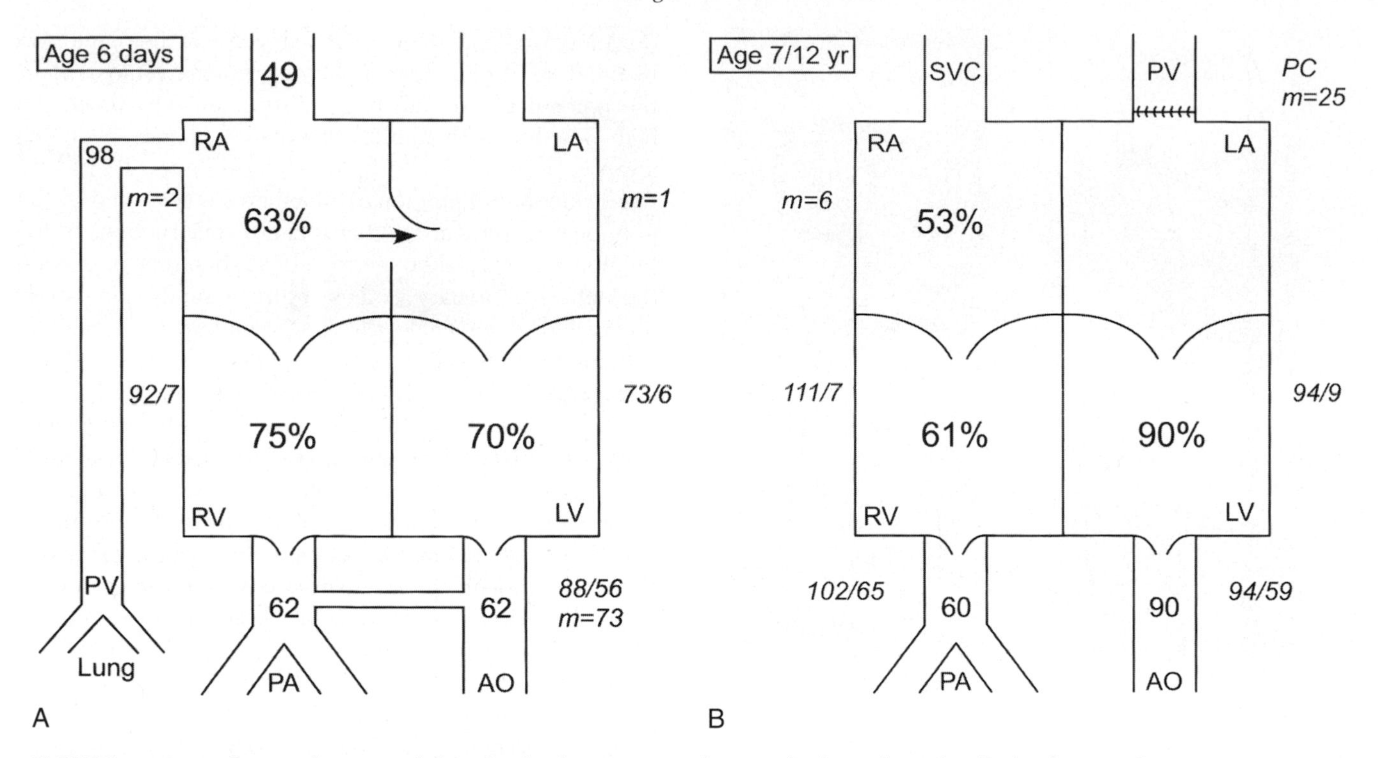

FIGURE 48–2 *Total anomalous veins below the diaphragm. A, At the age of 6 days, this infant had pulmonary hypertension approximately equal to systemic pressure. The difference in the percentage of oxygen saturation within the chambers of the heart and the great arteries was no greater than 13% by any comparison. The source of all blood entering the left heart was through the foramen ovale from the right atrium to the left. B, A surgical procedure was carried out, and 7 months later the infant was catheterized. On this occasion, there was pulmonary hypertension, some arterial oxygen desaturation, and an elevated pulmonary wedge pressure of 25 mm Hg. It was discovered that the original anastomotic site was obstructed, and this was subsequently repaired with complete recovery. RA, right atrium; LA, left atrium; RV, right ventricle; LV, left ventricle; AO, aorta; PA, pulmonary artery; PV, pulmonary vein; PC, pulmonary capillary wedge pressure; large bold numbers, arterial oxygen saturation; italics, pressure in mm Hg.*
From Fyler DC [ed]. Nadas' Pediatric Cardiology. Philadelphia: Hanley & Belfus, 1992.

gasping, and retractions indicative of pulmonary edema. The more severe the obstruction, the earlier the infant is symptomatic and discovered to have heart disease. Because the infradiaphragmatic return variety is invariably severely obstructed, it is not surprising that, although uncommon overall, it is the type most frequently found at autopsy among babies with total anomalous pulmonary venous return, many undiagnosed.[11]

Physical Examination

On physical examination, the infant often appears very ill. There is cyanosis, tachypnea, and hepatomegaly. Often there is no murmur, the only abnormality being a loud second heart sound.

Electrocardiography

The electrocardiogram shows right ventricular hypertrophy, but because these patients are usually neonates, it is difficult to be certain that this is abnormal. There is usually P pulmonale.

Chest X-ray

On chest x-ray, the heart is of normal size or slightly enlarged. There is evidence of pulmonary edema, sometimes marked (Fig. 48-5).

Echocardiography

The common collecting vein receiving all pulmonary veins is seen behind the heart, as is its connection to the systemic venous circulation.[15] Right ventricular and pulmonary hypertension are usually present, and if the ductus is open, right-to-left shunting may be visible. Each pulmonary vein is visualized, and Doppler techniques are used to assess the presence or absence of pulsatile pulmonary venous blood flow; absence suggests obstruction. The confluence and individual pulmonary veins are best seen from the suprasternal notch or high left sternal border. If the venous channel is obstructed, the confluence is usually dilated, and the velocity of blood flow is low. If at least four pulmonary veins are not identified, multiple drainage sites should be suspected.

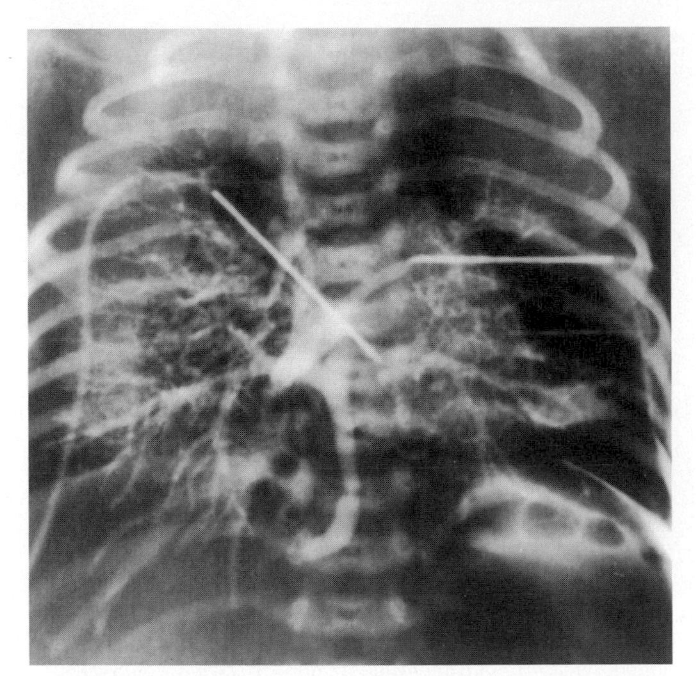

FIGURE 48–3 *Complete obstruction of infradiaphragmatic total anomalous pulmonary veins. This shows a postmortem injection of contrast material into the pulmonary venous system. There was no point of egress from the pulmonary veins into the systemic venous circulation at any point. This infant lived 3 days.*
From Fyler DC [ed]. Nadas' Pediatric Cardiology. Philadelphia: Hanley & Belfus, 1992.

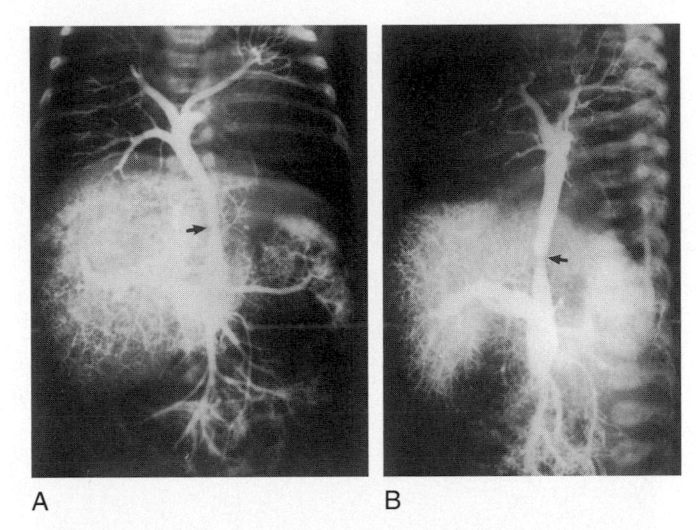

FIGURE 48–4 *A and B, Total anomalous veins below the diaphragm. This shows a postmortem injection of contrast material into the portal system, anteroposterior view (A) and lateral view (B), filling the pulmonary veins and portal drainage. Note the point of obstruction (arrow) at approximately the point where the common pulmonary venous channel pierces the diaphragm.*
From Fyler DC [ed]. Nadas' Pediatric Cardiology. Philadelphia: Hanley & Belfus, 1992.

Once the pulmonary venous confluence and individual pulmonary veins have been identified, the sites of communication with the systemic venous circuit are identified. The most common drainage site for obstructed anomalous venous connection is the portal-hepatic system. The descending vertical vein can be seen in a subxiphoid transverse view as a third vascular channel crossing the diaphragm between the inferior vena cava and the descending aorta (Fig. 48-6) and, using color-flow Doppler mapping, can be traced into the liver. Pulmonary venous flow returns to the right atrium through a dilated inferior vena cava.

Less commonly, obstruction occurs in supracardiac total anomalous pulmonary venous drainage (Fig. 48-7). One cause of obstruction in this type of drainage is compression of the vertical vein if it passes between the left pulmonary artery and the left main bronchus (unusual). The innominate vein and superior vena cava are usually dilated in relation to the severity of obstruction of pulmonary venous flow.

Rarely, total anomalous pulmonary venous return to the coronary sinus is obstructed,[12] either at the junction of the individual veins with the coronary sinus or by a short vertical connecting vein. Other sites of obstruction include the azygous vein and the right superior vena cava. Pulsed and continuous-wave Doppler echocardiography identifies

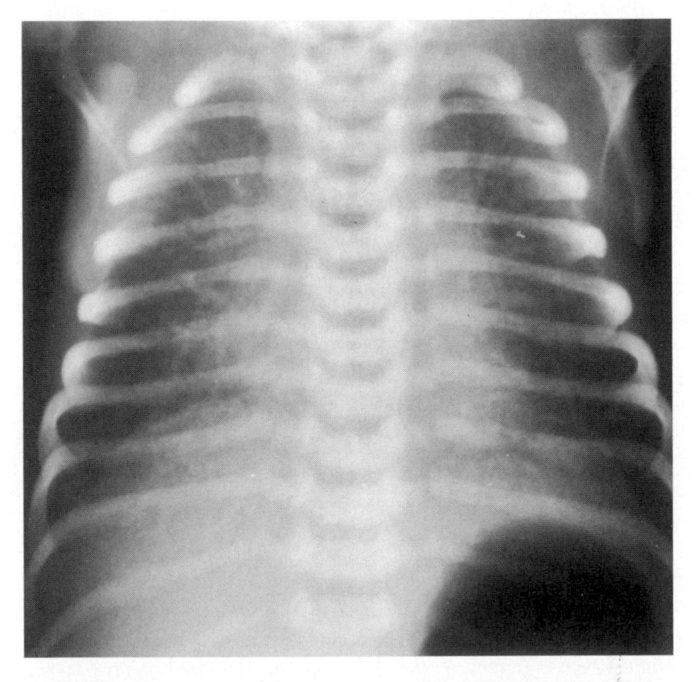

FIGURE 48–5 *This infant with obstructed total anomalous pulmonary veins has gross pulmonary edema with poorly visible pulmonary structures on chest x-ray. The heart is small.*
From Fyler DC [ed]. Nadas' Pediatric Cardiology. Philadelphia: Hanley & Belfus, 1992.

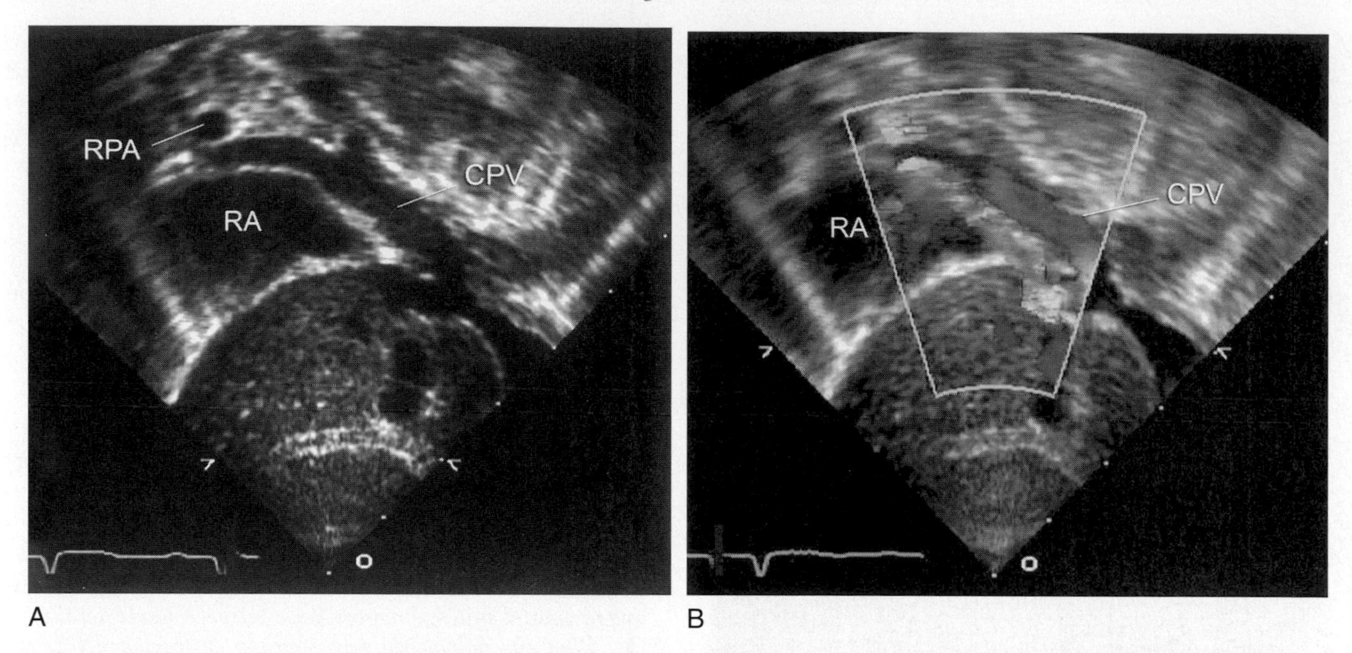

FIGURE 48–6 *Subxyphoid echocardiographic image of obstructed subdiaphragmatic totally anomalous pulmonary venous connection. A, The dilated common pulmonary vein (CPV) is located along the posterior aspect of the right atrium (RA). The connection of the right upper pulmonary vein is noted between the right pulmonary artery (RPA) and the RA. The connection to the inferior vena cava is noted within the liver. B, Color-flow mapping of the CPV shows flow toward the transducer (red) that turns anteriorly and reverses direction (blue) into the RA.*

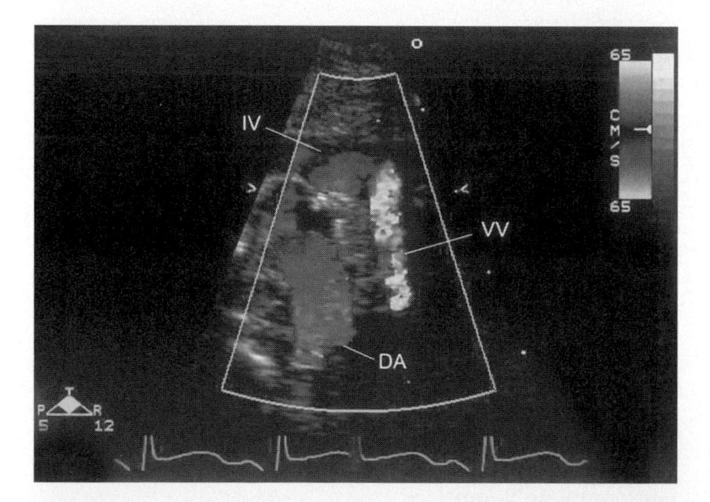

FIGURE 48–7 *Color-flow Doppler image of obstructed supracardiac totally anomalous pulmonary venous drainage. The four pulmonary veins join into a common pulmonary vein that connects to the systemic venous system by means of a vertical vein. The potential for obstruction exists at several levels. In this case, the vertical vein (VV) is the site of obstruction, as reflected by the turbulent flow seen ascending to the left of the descending aorta (DA) and connecting to the innominate vein (IV).*

nonpulsatile points of obstruction. The flow pattern should also be sampled in the individual veins, as well as in the venous confluence, because obstruction may occur at multiple sites.

Other findings with total anomalous pulmonary venous return include a right-to-left flow through the foramen ovale, a small left atrium, and an enlarged and hypertensive right ventricle. With severe obstruction, the right ventricular pressure is often suprasystemic, with posterior bowing of the ventricular septum. Tricuspid regurgitation, if present, allows estimation of the right ventricular pressure.

Magnetic Resonance Imaging

Magnetic resonance imaging (MRI) can provide excellent anatomic detail if echocardiographic information is incomplete (Fig. 48-8).

Cardiac Catheterization

Cardiac catheterization has been unnecessary in this lesion for many years.

Unrestricted Pulmonary Blood Flow

The neonate with unrestricted pulmonary blood flow is generally not very ill. In the current era, the diagnosis is frequently made within days as the detection of a heart

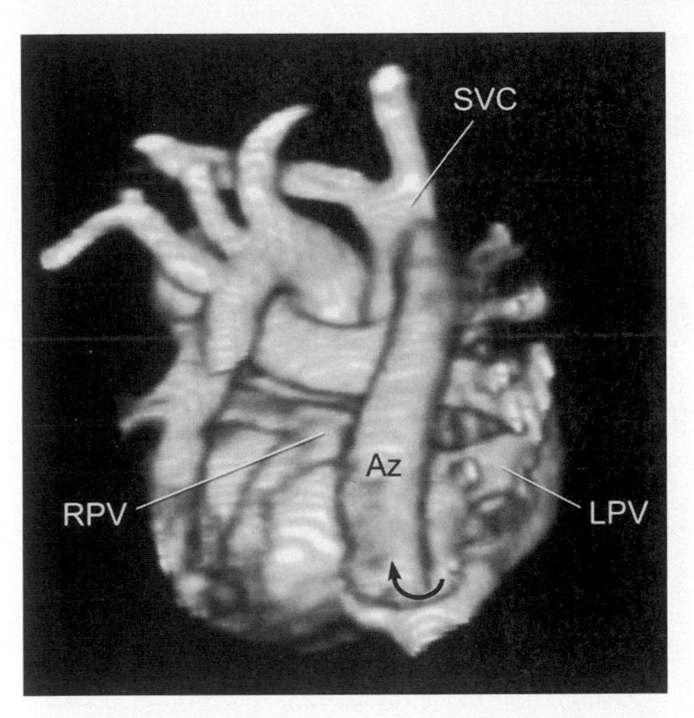

FIGURE 48–8 *Gadolinium-enhanced three-dimensional magnetic resonance angiogram showing total anomalous pulmonary venous return (arrow) to the azygos (Az) vein. SVC, superior vena cava; RPV, right pulmonary vein; LPV, left pulmonary vein.*

murmur or mild cyanosis leads to echocardiography. However, occasionally the diagnosis may be made after some years—we recently evaluated and surgically repaired unobstructed total anomalous pulmonary venous return to the azygous vein in a 16-year-old virtually asymptomatic patient.

Physical Examination

On physical examination, the infant may be thin, is often tachypneic, and has minimal or no visible cyanosis. Often there is hepatomegaly. There may be a prominence of the left side of the chest with a palpable right ventricular impulse, a gallop rhythm, and an accentuated pulmonary component of a widely split fixed second heart sound. A systolic ejection murmur, rarely more than grade 3, is audible at the left upper sternal border, followed by an early diastolic rumble at the lower sternal border. In the uncomplicated situation, the physical findings are similar to those of a large atrial septal defect. A loud systolic murmur suggests some additional cardiac anomaly.

Electrocardiography

The electrocardiogram shows abnormal right ventricular hypertrophy for age when the infant is more than a few weeks old. P pulmonale is usually present.

Chest X-ray

On chest x-ray, the heart is enlarged, and there is pulmonary vascular engorgement. Compared with the obstructive type, there is excessive pulmonary blood flow, often marked, but usually without pulmonary edema.

Laboratory Data

The level of oxygen saturation by skin oximetry is often only minimally reduced, at about 90%, a degree of desaturation often unappreciated by the naked eye.

Echocardiography

On echocardiographic examination, the common pulmonary vein is visible behind the left atrium, and each pulmonary vein can be identified. Pulmonary artery and right ventricular pressure can be determined when tricuspid regurgitation is present. If transthoracic imaging is unsatisfactory, transesophageal echocardiography can provide much better anatomic information.

Magnetic Resonance Imaging

Because precise anatomic details are outlined by echocardiography in the very young, there is little need for MRI in this age group, whether or not pulmonary venous obstruction is present. In the older, larger patients with poor windows, MRI can provide exquisite anatomic information.

Cardiac Catheterization

In these patients with uncomplicated total anomalous unrestricted pulmonary venous return, cardiac catheterization for anatomic reasons has not been necessary for many years. However, beyond infancy, it would be indicated when significant pulmonary hypertension or vascular obstruction was suspected, to quantitate resistance and study responses to vasodilators.

MANAGEMENT

Most patients with uncomplicated total anomalous pulmonary venous return have neither maximally obstructed nor completely unrestricted pulmonary blood flow and present clinical problems ranging from one extreme to the other. It is important to emphasize, however, that most patients with infradiaphragmatic return have severe obstruction and are very likely to become extremely ill rapidly within days after birth, particularly when the patent ductus arteriosus constricts (see Figs. 48-3 through 48-5).

Once the diagnosis is made, surgical repair is undertaken. Almost all patients have a large pulmonary venous confluence behind the left atrium. This structure is horizontal in those with supracardiac and cardiac anomalous return sites, and vertical in those with the infradiaphragmatic variety. The surgical procedure consists mostly of making as large an anastomosis as possible between this pulmonary venous confluence and the posterior wall of the left atrium. Perhaps the one exception to this management plan is in the group with mixed total anomalous return in whom the single large posterior pulmonary venous confluence is absent. In this group, if stable and without significant pulmonary hypertension or pulmonary venous obstruction, it is not unreasonable to follow these patients medically until such time when the individual anomalous veins are large enough to anastomose to the left atrium.

Early mortality has improved dramatically over the years, even as the age at surgery has decreased.[16] Among series of patients operated on in the past two decades, early mortality rates have ranged from 2% to 10% (median, 10%).[5–9,17–19]

COURSE

Most often, late follow-up shows an excellent result.[19] The major problem that survivors have encountered is pulmonary venous obstruction, either in individual veins or at the anastomotic site. It occurs in about 10% of patients, is often progressive, has required one or more operations or balloon dilations or stent placement, and is associated with high mortality rates, from 25% to 46%.[7,20–22] This has been reported by some to be more common after repair of infradiaphragmatic or mixed types.[20,22] Late postoperative arrhythmias, mostly supraventricular, have been reported in some patients.[23,24]

Total Anomalous Pulmonary Venous Return with Asplenia or Polysplenia

Total anomalous pulmonary venous return is either an isolated phenomenon or is associated with the complex cardiac abnormalities found in the asplenia-polysplenia syndromes.

The physiologic effect of the anomalous return may be negligible in this situation, in that these syndromes usually include other cardiac defects that allow common mixing, such as single ventricle, common atrium, and common atrioventricular canal. It is very common in asplenia patients, much less so in the polysplenia group (see Chapter 38). It is customary to repair the total veins at the initial surgery, whether it be shunt placement for pulmonary atresia or stenosis or a stage one procedure as a prelude to a later Fontan procedure. In the asplenia group, pulmonary vein stenosis is a common complication, occurring in 38% in our patients.

REFERENCES

1. Fyler DC, Buckley LP, Hellenbrand WE, et al. Report of the New England Regional Infant Cardiac Program. Pediatrics 65(Suppl):387, 1980.
2. Ferencz C, Rubin JD, McCarter RJ, et al. Congenital heart disease: Prevalence at live birth. The Baltimore-Washington Infant Study. Am J Epidemiol 121:31, 1984.
3. Dickinson DF, Arnold R, Wilkinson JL. Congenital heart disease among 160,480 live born children in Liverpool, 1960–1969. Br Heart J 46:55, 1981.
4. Geva T, VanPraagh S. Anomalies of the pulmonary veins. In Allen HD, Gutgesell HP, Clark EB, Driscoll DJ (eds). Moss and Adams: Heart Disease in Infants, Children, and Adolescents. Philadelphia: Lippincott, Williams & Wilkins, 2001:736–772.
5. Michielon G, DiDonato RM, Paquini L, et al. Total anomalous pulmonary venous connection: Long term appraisal with evolving technical solutions. Eur J Cardiothorac Surg 22(2):184, 2002.
6. Choudhary SK, Bhan A, Sharma R, et al. Total anomalous pulmonary venous connection: Surgical experience in Indians. Indian Heart J 53(6):754, 2001.
7. Hyde JA, Stumper O, Barth MJ, et al. Total anomalous pulmonary venous connection: Outcome of surgical correction and management of recurrent venous obstruction. Eur J Cardiothorac Surg. 15(6):735, 1999.
8. Sinzobahamvya N, Arenz C, Brecher AM, et al. Early and long-term results for correction of total anomalous pulmonary venous drainage (TAPVD) in neonates and infants. Eur J Cardiothorac Surg 10(6):433, 1996.
9. Lupinetti FM, Kulik TJ, Beekman RH 3rd, et al. Correction of total anomalous pulmonary venous connection in infancy. J Thorac Cardiovasc Surg. 106(5):880, 1993.
10. Lucas RV, Lock JE, Tandon R, et al. Gross and histologic anatomy of total anomalous pulmonary venous connection. Am J Cardiol 62:292, 1988.
11. James CL, Keeling JW, Smith NM, et al. Total anomalous pulmonary venous drainage associated with fatal outcome in infancy. J Thorac Cardiovasc Surg. 14(4):665, 1994.
12. Jonas RA, Smolinsky A, Mayer JE, et al. Obstructed pulmonary venous drainage with total anomalous pulmonary venous connection to the coronary sinus. Am J Cardiol, 59: 431, 1987.
13. Lima CO, Valdes-Cruz LM, Allen HD, et al. Prognostic value of left ventricular size by echocardiography in infants with total anomalous pulmonary venous drainage. Am J Cardiol 51:1155, 1983.
14. Rosenquist GC, Kelly JL, Chandra R, et al. Small left atrium and change in contour of the ventricular septum in total anomalous pulmonary venous connection: A morphometric analysis of 22 infant hearts. Am J Cardiol 55:777, 1985.
15. Chin AJ, Sanders SP, Sherman R, et al. Accuracy of subcostal two-dimensional echocardiography in prospective diagnosis of total anomalous pulmonary venous connection. Am Heart J 113:1153, 1987.

16. Bando K, Turrentine MW, Ensing GJ, et al. Surgical management of total anomalous pulmonary venous connection. Thirty-year trends. Circulation 94(9 Suppl):II12, 1996.
17. Anil Kumar D, Kumar RN, Narasinga Rao P, et al. Repair of total anomalous pulmonary venous connection in early infancy. Asian Cardiovasc Thorac Ann 11(1):18, 2003.
18. Cobanoglu A, Menashe VD. Total anomalous pulmonary venous connection in neonates and young infants: Repair in the current era [comment]. Ann Thorac Surg, 55(1):43, 1993.
19. Kirshbom PM, Myung RJ, Gaynor JW, et al. Preoperative pulmonary venous obstruction affects long-term outcome for survivors or total anomalous pulmonary venous connection repair. Ann Thorac Surg, 74(5):1616, 2002.
20. Ricci M, Elliott M, Cohen GA, et al. Management of pulmonary venous obstruction after correction of TAPVC: Risk factors for adverse outcome. Eur J Cardio Thorac Surg, 24(1):28, 2003.
21. Lacour-Gayet F, Zohgbi J, Serraf AE, et al. Surgical management of progressive pulmonary venous obstruction after repair of total anomalous pulmonary venous connection. J Thorac Cardiovasc Surg 117(4):679, 1999.
22. Caldarone CA, Najm HK, Katletz M. Relentless pulmonary vein stenosis after repair of total anomalous pulmonary venous drainage. Ann Thorac Surg 66(5):1514, 1998.
23. Korbmacher B, Buttgen S, Schulte HD, et al. Long-term results after repair of total anomalous pulmonary venous connection. Thorac Cardiovasc Surg 49(2):101, 2001.
24. Bhan A, Umre MA, Choudhary SK, et al. Cardiac arrhythmias in surgically repaired total anomalous pulmonary venous connection: a follow up study. Indian Heart J 52(4):427, 2000.

49

Aortopulmonary Window

JOHN F. KEANE AND DONALD FYLER

DEFINITION

An aortopulmonary window (aortopulmonary fenestration, aortopulmonary septal defect) is a hole between the ascending aorta and the main pulmonary artery. There must be two distinct and separate semilunar valves before this diagnosis can be made.

PREVALENCE

Aortopulmonary window is a rare anomaly; 34 patients have been seen in the past 14 years at Children's Hospital Boston (Exhibit 49-1).

EMBRYOLOGY

There is failure of aortopulmonary septation that, although in many ways reminiscent of truncus arteriosus communis, probably develops by a different mechanism.[1] In terms of associated lesions, among series with 10 or more patients reported in the past decade, an average of 57% had other defects, the most common being ventricular septal defect (13%), interrupted aortic arch (12%), and tetralogy of Fallot (8%).[2–8]

ANATOMY

An aortopulmonary window consists of an opening between the ascending aorta and the main pulmonary artery midway between the similar valves and the pulmonary artery bifurcation, distally at the bifurcation or encompassing both these areas.[1,9]

PHYSIOLOGY

The physiologic effects are those of a left-to right shunt, such as with ventricular septal defect or persistent patent ductus arteriosus. As pulmonary resistance drops in the days and weeks after birth, there is increasing left-to-right shunting, and ultimately, if the window is big, congestive heart failure develops in the first weeks of life. Because these defects are most often large, there is usually pulmonary hypertension at systemic levels. Without repair, pulmonary vascular disease develops later, possibly as early as the end of the first year of life.

CLINICAL MANIFESTATIONS

The clinical features in those without additional lesions are indistinguishable from those seen in a patient with a persistently patent ductus arteriosus. With a smaller opening, the murmurs are those of a classic patent ductus arteriosus (see Chapter 34). With larger defects, the murmurs are not necessarily continuous, and evidence of congestive heart failure or pulmonary hypertension may dominate the auscultatory findings. In those with an additional defect, the clinical features may be quite different; for example, with an interrupted aortic arch when the patent ductus becomes restrictive or closes, femoral pulses may be impalpable and the baby can become critically ill within hours.

Exhibit 49–1
Children's Hospital Boston Experience
Aortopulmonary Window

	1973–1987 N (%)	*1988–2002* N (%)
All Patients	19	34
All other lesions	10 (50)	22 (65)
IAA	1 (5)	8 (26)
TOF	4 (21)	5 (15)
VSD	8 (42)	4 (12)
Surgical mortality	2 (11)	2 (6)*

*Of our 31 surgical patients (median age, 15 days), 2 died, one a 1.9-kg baby in 1993 and the other a 7-year-old with severe pulmonary vascular obstructive disease (1998).
IAA, interrupted aortic arch; TOF, tetralogy of Fallot; VSD, ventricular septal defect.

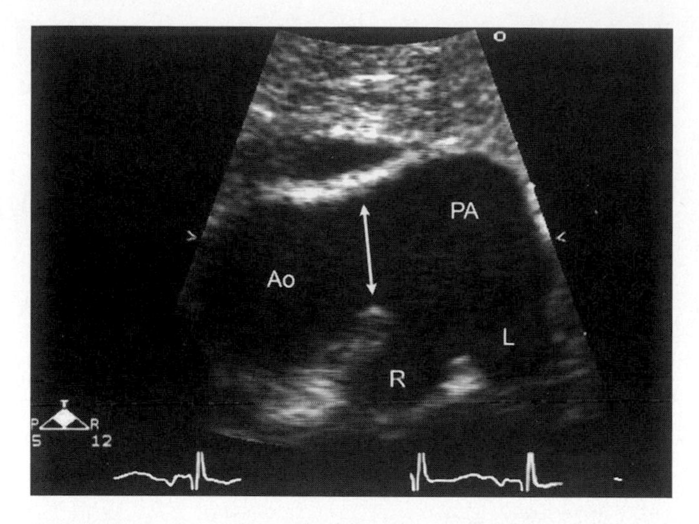

FIGURE 49–1 *Parasternal short-axis echocardiogram of an aortopulmonary window. The window (double-headed arrow) between the aorta (AO) and pulmonary artery (PA) is seen, as well as the relationship to the right (R) and left (L) pulmonary artery origins.*

Electrocardiography

The electrocardiographic patterns are the same as those seen in patients with patent ductus arteriosus.

Chest X-Ray

The chest x-ray shows evidence of left-to-right shunting and pulmonary hypertension indistinguishable from that seen in patients with patent ductus arteriosus.

Echocardiography

The hyperdynamic function and the enlarged chambers provide useful clues to the presence and location of a left-to-right shunt. The defect itself can be easily visualized and the shunting documented by Doppler examination (Fig 49-1). The diagnosis is made by scanning the aortopulmonary septum in multiple views (including subxiphoid, parasternal, and suprasternal notch). Imaging the defect in multiple views and detecting the flow through it by color-flow Doppler mapping (Fig. 49-2) allows confirmation of the true defect rather than false dropout. At the level of the defect, the joined vessels are elliptical in cross-section, whereas in contrast, false dropout is characterized by persistence of the normal circular contour of each vessel.

The distinguishing feature between aortopulmonary window and truncus arteriosus is the presence of two separate semilunar valves in the former. The aortopulmonary window is proximal to, or at the level of, the pulmonary artery branches, whereas a persistent ductus arteriosus is more distal and usually has some length.

Surgically important information that is readily derived from the echocardiogram includes the distance between the proximal border of the defect and the semilunar valves and coronary arteries, as well as the distance between the distal border and the pulmonary arteries. Although the

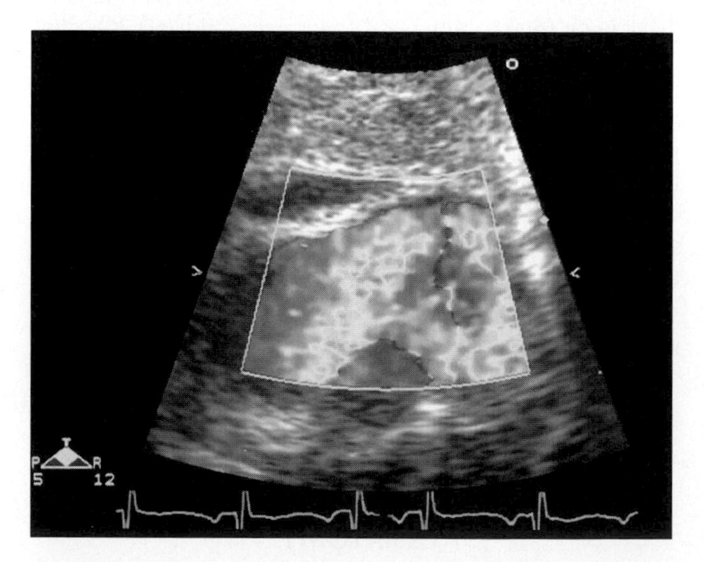

FIGURE 49–2 *Color-flow Doppler mapping of the aortopulmonary window in Fig. 49-1, showing flow toward the transducer (red signal) from the aorta into the pulmonary artery.*

Exhibit 49–2

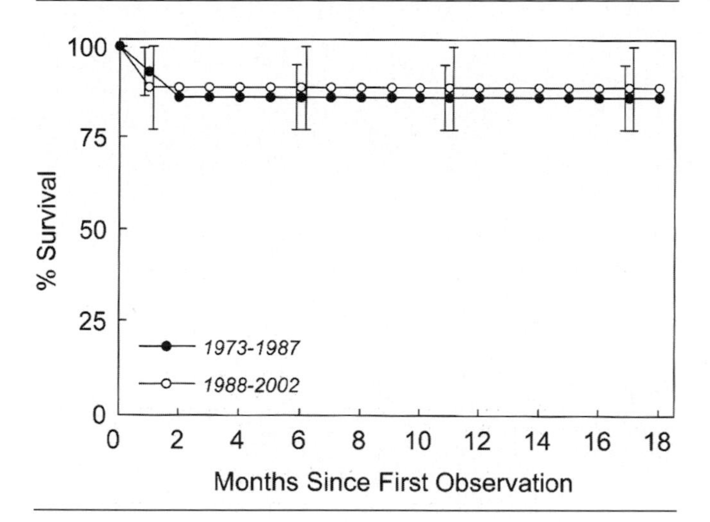

incidence of additional defects is quite high, these are all now readily identifiable by careful echocardiography.

Cardiac Catheterization

From an anatomic or hemodynamic standpoint, this is no longer necessary. The only indication at this time is if device closure is planned; there have been a few reports of such management with success in small defects without other lesions.[10,11]

MANAGEMENT

Catheter-delivered device closure of a small uncomplicated lesion is an option in a few. For most, surgical closure, including repair of any other lesions, should be undertaken with minimal delay after diagnosis in infants. A brief period of intensive anticongestive therapy is probably useful preoperatively, with prostaglandin E_1 treatment a necessity in those with interrupted aortic arch and ductal restriction. In a recent report from our hospital covering a 26-year period, among 38 patients operated on at median age of 5 weeks and weight of 3.9 kg, actuarial survival was 88% at 10 years, and patch closure through the aorta or defect rather than the pulmonary artery achieved the best outcome.[3] Surgical results are nowadays excellent (Exhibit 49-2), with only rare occurrences of right pulmonary artery stenosis or residual leaks, the latter in those either ligated or repaired through the pulmonary artery.

REFERENCES

1. Kutsche LM, Van Mierop LHS. Anatomy and pathogenesis of aorticopulmonary septal defect: Analysis of 286 reported cases. Am J Cardiol 59:443, 1987.
2. Backer CL, Mavroudis C. Surgical management of aortopulmonary window: A 40-year experience. Eur J Cardiothorac Surg 21(5):773, 2002.
3. Hew CC, Bacha EA, Zurakowski D, et al. Optimal surgical approach for repair of aortopulmonary window. Cardiol Young 11(4):385, 2001.
4. Tanoue Y, Sese A, Ueno Y, et al. Surgical management of aortopulmonary window. Jap J Thorac Cardiovasc Surg 48(9):557, 2000.
5. Soares AM, Atik E, Cortez TM, et al. Aortopulmonary window: Clinical and surgical assessment of 18 cases. Arq Bras Cardiol 7319, 1999.
6. Tkebuchava T, von Segesser LK, Vogt PR, et al. Congenital aortopulmonary window: Diagnosis, surgical technique and long-term results. Eur J Cardiothorac Surg 11(2):293, 1997.
7. Bertolini A, Dalmonte P, Bava GL, et al. Aortopulmonary septal defects: A review of the literature and report of ten cases. J Cardiovasc Surg 35(3):207, 1994.
8. van Son JA, Puga FJ, Danielson GK, et al. Aortopulmonary window: Factors associated with early and late success after surgical treatment. Mayo Clin Proc 68(2):128, 1993.
9. Blieden LC, Moller JH. Other left-to-right shunts. In Moller JH, Neal WS (eds). Fetal, neonatal and infant cardiac disease. 1989:443.
10. Tulloh RM, Rigby ML. Transcatheter umbrella closure of aortopulmonary window. Heart 77(5):479, 1997.
11. Naik GD, Chandra VS, Shenoy A, et al. Transcatheter closure of aortopulmonary window using Amplatzer device. Catheter Cardiovasc Interv 59(3):402, 2003.

50

Origin of a Pulmonary Artery from the Aorta (Hemitruncus)

JOHN F. KEANE AND DONALD C. FYLER

DEFINITION

The term *hemitruncus* is used when either pulmonary artery originates from the ascending aorta in the presence of a pulmonary valve and main pulmonary artery. The terminology "origin of the right (left) pulmonary artery from the aorta" may be more precise because there is no known relation of hemitruncus to true truncus arteriosus.

PREVALENCE

This is a rare anomaly, having been seen in 19 patients (13 females) at Children's Hospital Boston between 1988 and 2002 (Exhibit 50-1).

PATHOLOGY

The pathology is defined. Either the right or the left pulmonary artery arises from the ascending aorta, whereas the other arises from the main pulmonary trunk. Anomalous origin of the right pulmonary artery is much more common than the left; origin of both right and left pulmonary arteries from the ascending aorta in the presence of a pulmonary valve and main pulmonary artery has been reported in three patients.[1] In the usual case, a patent ductus arteriosus communicates with the pulmonary artery that derives its blood flow from the right ventricle. Associated cardiac anomalies are common, including ventricular septal defect and tetralogy of Fallot.[2,3] Anomalous origin of the right or left pulmonary artery may have a different etiology, and neither may be related to the pathogenesis of truncus arteriousus.[1,3,4]

PHYSIOLOGY

Before birth, one lung is supplied from the left ventricle and the ascending aorta, whereas the contralateral lung is supplied from the right ventricle and the main pulmonary artery. After birth, with falling pulmonary resistance, there is opportunity for excessive pulmonary flow into the lung supplied by the aorta. Blood flow to the opposite lung is excessive to the extent that it receives the entire venous return (cardiac output). The pulmonary artery pressure in both lungs is elevated (Fig. 50-1). A persistently patent ductus arteriosus may shunt left to right into the left lung. Congestive heart failure (a nearly universal phenomenon) occurs within the first weeks of life and is often severe.

CLINICAL MANIFESTATIONS

A systolic murmur is heard at birth. Within days or a week or so after birth, tachypnea, dyspnea, and the clinical syndrome of congestive heart failure become evident.

Exhibit 50–1
Origin of a Pulmonary Artery from Aorta

	1973–1987	*1988–2002**
No. of patients	10	19
RPA from Ao	10	17
LPA from Ao	0	2
Surgery	7	17
Mortality (surgical)	0	2†

*In the 1988–2002 group (68% female), median age at surgery was 10 days, the anomalous vessel was reimplanted in 94%, and associated lesions, including ventricular septal defect (26%) and tetralogy of Fallot (21%), were repaired.
†Surgical group deaths occurred 1 month after surgery in 1 (1990) and 2 months after surgery (1989) in the other.
RPA, right pulmonary artery; LPA, left pulmonary artery; Ao, ascending aorta.

The infant has the clinical picture of a large left-to-right shunt without cyanosis.

Electrocardiography

The electrocardiogram shows right ventricular hypertrophy.

Chest X-Ray

The heart is large, and the pulmonary vasculature is increased bilaterally. Sometimes the difference in vascularity between right and left lung is distinguishable, especially if tetralogy of Fallot is also present, but usually only in retrospect.

Echocardiography

The most difficult part of making the diagnosis is thinking of it. The pulmonary artery arising from the aorta (usually the right) is well seen in a parasternal long- or short-axis view (Fig. 50-2). Color-flow Doppler mapping or the pulsed Doppler examination demonstrates continuous flow into the pulmonary artery from the aorta. The other pulmonary artery (usually the left) connects normally with the main pulmonary trunk.

A persistent ductus arteriosus is commonly associated with hemitruncus. If the ductus is large, the pulmonary trunk may appear to bifurcate normally. This potential diagnostic pitfall is especially important if the left pulmonary artery connects abnormally with the aorta. It is essential to identify unequivocally both pulmonary artery branches and the ductus arteriosus or ligamentum arteriosum. If the ductus is small, a moderately high-velocity flow (>1.5 to 2 m/sec) may be detected from the pulmonary trunk and to the aorta because the pressure in the

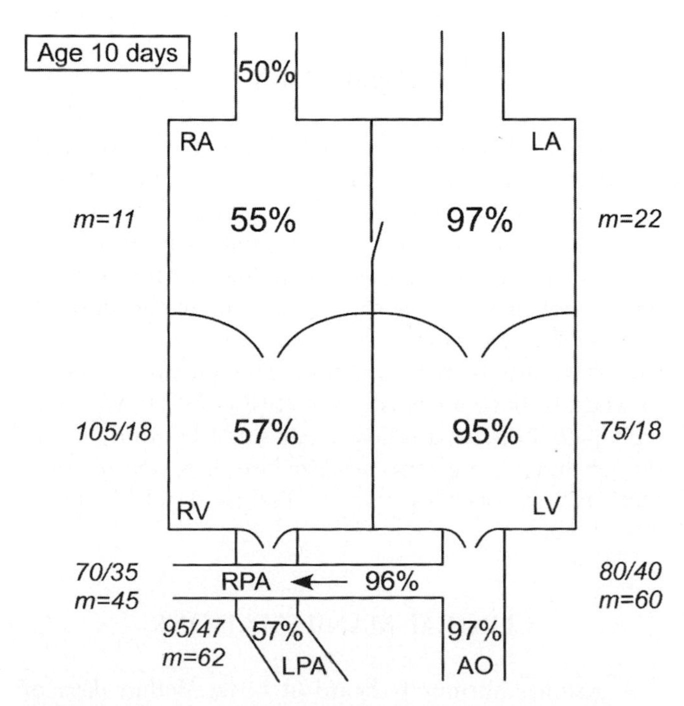

FIGURE 50–1 *Catheterization data in 10-day-old neonate with right pulmonary artery (RPA) arising from ascending aorta.*

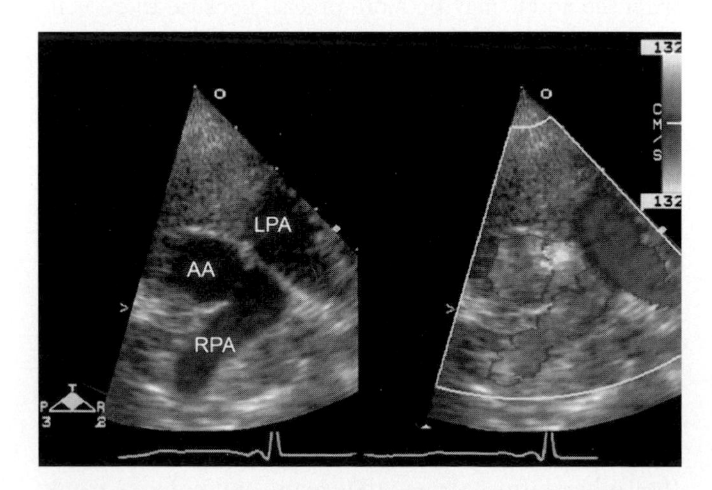

FIGURE 50–2 *Two-dimensional and color-flow Doppler images of origin of the right pulmonary artery (RPA) from the ascending aorta (AA). The left panel shows the anomaly, as well as the left pulmonary artery (LPA) that fails to connect with the RPA. The right panel shows the flow signal connecting the AA to the RPA and the absence of flow between the RPA and LPA. The area of red signal is due to flow acceleration and turbulence at the junction of the AA to the RPA.*

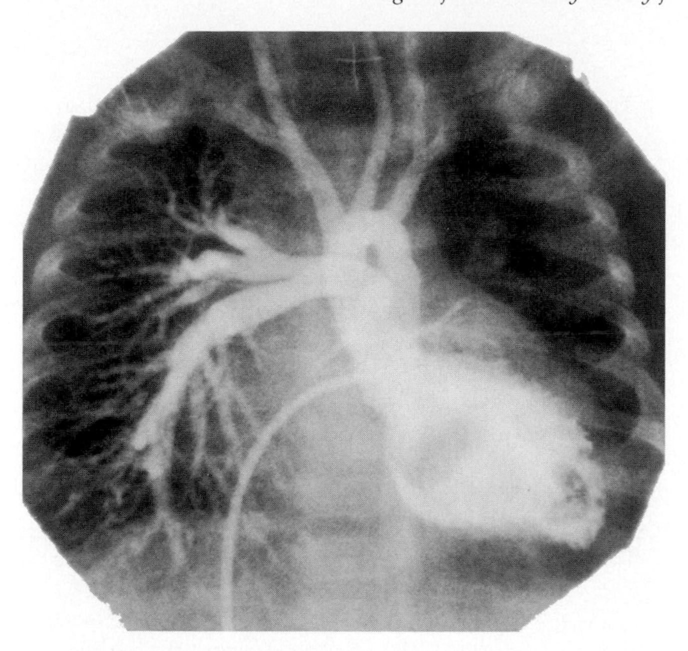

FIGURE 50–3 *Cineangiogram in left ventricle with catheter courses anterograde through a patent foramen ovale. In the anterior view, the right pulmonary artery arises from ascending aorta. The left pulmonary artery was earlier shown to arise from the right ventricle.*
From Fyler DC [ed]. Nadas' Pediatric Cardiology. Philadelphia: Hanley & Belfus.

pulmonary trunk and the normally connecting pulmonary artery branch are often suprasystemic.

Cardiac Catheterization

This is no longer necessary in the neonate because echocardiography provides all anatomic details. If considered necessary at a later age, the evaluation of right pulmonary resistance response to dilators may be necessary, at which time angiography in the left ventricle or ascending aorta may be done to confirm the diagnosis (Fig. 50-3).

MANAGEMENT

As soon as the diagnosis is established, the infant is stabilized on anticongestive medications, and cardiac surgery is carried out. Anastomosis of the pulmonary artery arising from the aorta to the contralateral pulmonary artery best normalizes the circulation. During follow-up, a hypoplastic or stenotic right pulmonary artery was evident in 7 of our 15 surgical survivors, and managed by balloon dilation without or with a stent. A very small supravalvar aortic gradient of 10 mmHg at the aortic repair site has not progressed in one patient during 14 years of follow-up.

The biggest difficulty in these children has been recognition of a very rare diagnosis. With modern superb echocardiography equipment, this anomaly should be clearly evident in all.

REFERENCES

1. Vizcaino A, Campbell J, Litovsky S, et al. Single origin of right and left pulmonary artery branches from ascending aorta with non branching main pulmonary artery: Relevance to a new understanding of truncus arteriosus. Pediatr Cardiol 23(2):230, 2002.
2. Abu-Sulaiman RM, Hashmi A, McCrindle BW, et al. Anomalous origin of one pulmonary artery from the ascending aorta: 36 Years experience from one centre. Cardiol Young 8(4):449, 1998.
3. Kutsche LM, Van Mierop LHS. Anomalous origin of a pulmonary artery from the ascending aorta: Associated anomalies and pathogenesis. Am J Cardiol 61:850, 1988.
4. Dodo H, Alejos JC, Perloff JK, et al. Anomalous origin of the left main pulmonary artery from the ascending aorta associated with DiGeorge syndrome. Am J Cardiol 75(17):1294, 1995.
5. Kim TK, Choe YH, Kim HS, et al. Anomalous origin of the right pulmonary artery from the ascending aorta: Diagnosis by magnetic resonance imaging. Cardiovasc Intervent Radiol 18(2):116, 1995.

51

"Corrected" Transposition of the Great Arteries

JOHN F. KEANE AND DONALD C. FYLER

DEFINITION

"Corrected" transposition of the great arteries is characterized by atrioventricular discordance and transposition of the great arteries (ventriculoatrial discordance). In such patients, systemic desaturated venous return passes from an atrium through a mitral valve to a left ventricle and from there to the pulmonary artery. The pulmonary artery venous blood then traverses the other atrium to cross a tricuspid valve into a right ventricle from which the aorta arises. Thus, because arterial oxygen saturation is normal in these patients in the absence of other cardiac lesions (rare), the term "corrected" has been given to this entity for physiologic reasons. In this chapter, only patients with two ventricles are considered; those with a single ventricle or with one atrioventricular valve are discussed elsewhere (see Chapters 41, 44, and 45).

PREVALENCE

Transposition of the great arteries with two functionally adequate but inverted ventricles and levocardia (also called *SLL*; see Chapter 4) is a rare anomaly, with an incidence ranging from 0.02 to 0.07 per 1000 live births.[1,2] At Children's Hospital Boston from 1988 to 2002, there were 83 new patients with this anomaly (Exhibit 51-1). In addition, there were 20 others seen during that time period with the next more common variety of "corrected transposition," that is, with dextrocardia and a "mirror image" of the above, referred to as *IDD* (see Chapter 4).

ANATOMY

The segmental anatomy (see Chapter 4) of this lesion is of two varieties: the more common is SLL and the other, its mirror image, IDD. In SLL, there is levocardia with situs solitus of the atria and viscera; the right-sided superior and inferior venae cavae drain into a right-sided atrium, which empties through a mitral valve with two papillary muscles into a finely trabeculated left ventricle (atrioventricular discordance or an L loop), which in turn exits through a right-sided posterior pulmonary valve. This great vessel arrangement (ventriculoarterial discordance) is also referred to as *L transposition*. The left atrium empties through a tricuspid valve into a coarsely trabeculated right ventricle, which in turn exits through a left-sided anterior aortic valve. The two outflow tracts are parallel to one another, in contrast to the crossed position in the normal heart, and the ventricular septum lies in a more anteroposterior position (Fig. 51-1). In IDD, "a mirror image," as it were, of the above, there is dextrocardia with inversion of the abdominal viscera; the superior and inferior venae cavae are left-sided and open into an atrium, which empties through a mitral valve into a left ventricle, which in turn connects to a left-sided posterior pulmonary artery. Pulmonary venous return is to a right-sided atrium, which empties through a tricuspid valve into a morphologic right ventricle ("D loop"), which in turn connects to a right-sided anterior aorta (D transposition).

Rarely, there are no associated cardiac defects, and survival in such patients to age 84 years has been reported.[3] However, most have other cardiac anomalies

Exhibit 51–1
Children's Hospital Boston Experience, 1988-2002
Corrected Transposition of the Great Arteries (SLL)

There were 83 patients with corrected transposition of the great arteries (SLL) as their primary problem: 54 were males (63%), and 29 (37%) were females; 45 patients had cardiac surgery; 5 had tricuspid valve replacement. Complete heart block developed in 24 patients.

Corrected transposition, or segmental description SLL, was mentioned in 396 patients listed under other diagnostic categories, mainly single ventricle and malposition. Of these, 71 developed complete heart block (18%) at some time.

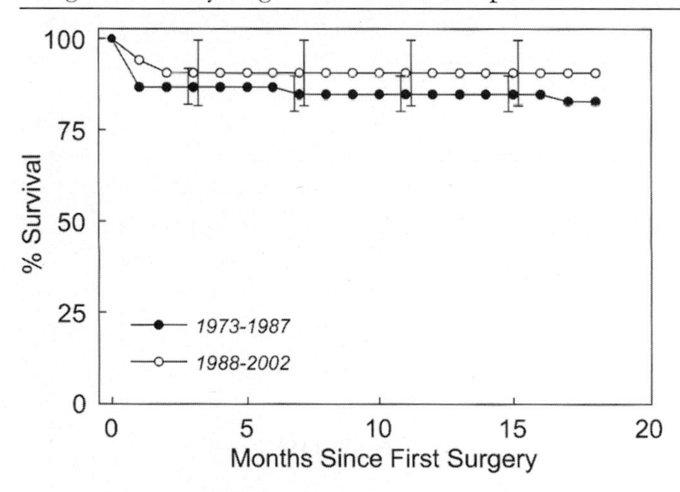

A. Life table plotted in 45 patients from date of first surgery of any type (38 other patients did not undergo cardiac surgery, one of whom, with pulmonary vascular obstructive disease, died the day after catheterization). Survival in recent period (1988–2002) was similar to that before the 1973–1987 period.

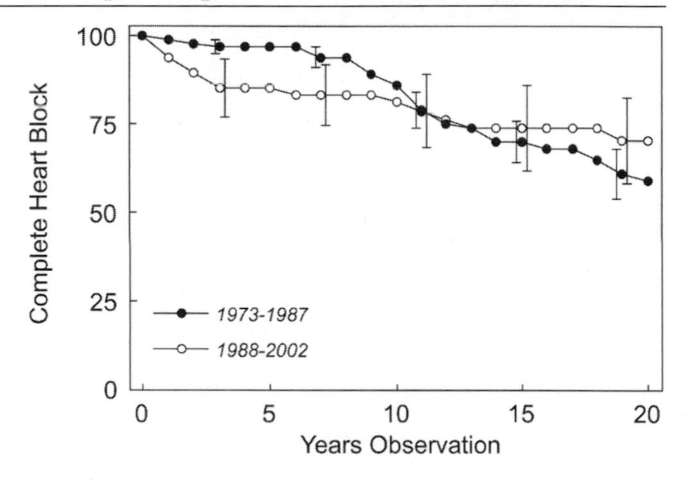

B. Curves calculated beginning with birth date and date of first-documented complete heart block (CHB) at Children's Hospital Boston as the end point. Because (a) heart block may have preceded time of first contact, curves may underestimate presence of heart block at any given age, and (b) heart block may have precipitated referral, true incidence may be overestimated: 4 patients developed heart block in association with cardiac surgery. Incidence in 1988–2002 (83 patients) was similar to that before 1973–1987 period.

Other Cardiac Problems Associated with "Corrected" Transposition of the Great Arteries

Other Diagnosis	*1973–1987 (%)*	*1988–2002 (%)*
Pulmonary stenosis	76	59
(with pulmonary atresia)	12	11
Ventricular septal defect	78	60
Tricuspid valve problems	56	83
(7 with Ebstein's anomaly)	8	20
Atrial septal defect	37	43
Mitral valve disease	37	54
Patent ductus arteriosus	11	13
Aortic stenosis	13	5
Pulmonary vascular disease	12	11
Endocardial cushion defect	3	6
Coarctation of the aorta	3	6
Complete heart block	32	29

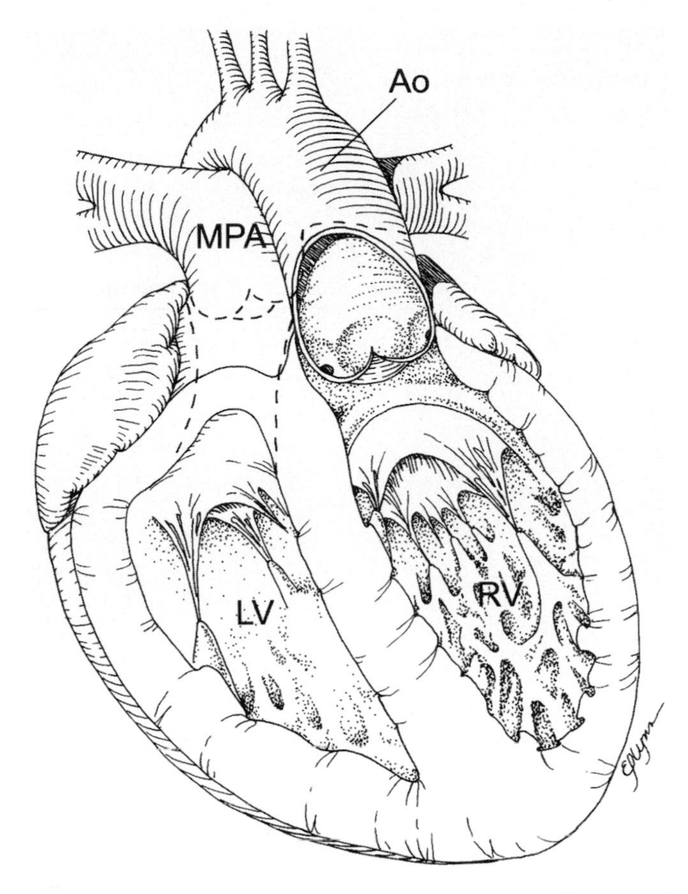

FIGURE 51–1 *Drawing of anteroposterior view of corrected transposition showing trabeculated right-sided left ventricle (LV) opening into posterior right-sided main pulmonary artery (MPA) and left-sided coarsely trabeculated right ventricle (RV) opening into anterior left-sided aorta (Ao). The anatomic LV has a mitral valve with two papillary muscles originating from the free wall, whereas the anatomic RV has a tricuspid valve, often "Ebstein-like" with at least one papillary muscle.*
From Fyler DC [ed]. Nadas' Pediatric Cardiology. Philadelphia: Hanley & Belfus, 1992.

(see Exhibit 51-1) that determine outcome.[4–7] Tricuspid valve abnormalities are common (97% in one autopsy series),[7] and regurgitation is frequent and often progressive.[5] The valve abnormality is commonly an Epstein's disease–like deformity, and dysfunction and failure of the systemic right ventricle,[8] also evident on exercise testing,[9] are common with increasing age.

Pulmonary outflow obstruction is common, is invariably subpulmonary; it is usually due to mitral valve apparatus or a diaphragm and rarely to isolated valvar stenosis. Most series include patients with pulmonary atresia, this diagnosis being mostly based on echocardiographic, angiographic, surgical, or autopsy observations, although it is sometimes uncertain to which ventricle the pulmonary artery was really related.

Ventricular septal defects may occur anywhere in the septum but are most commonly located in the membranous portion and adjacent areas. The pulmonary trunk may be substantially overriding in some, and straddling of the tricuspid or mitral valve associated with varying degrees of underdevelopment of either ventricle also occurs.

Conduction System

In the more common SLL variety, the sinus and atrioventricular nodes are in the usual location, but the distal conduction system is often superior to the ventricular septal defect. Complete heart block is sometimes present at birth and spontaneously occurs in many with time. In contrast, in those with the IDD variety, the conduction system is normally located, and spontaneous complete heart block is rare.

Coronary Anatomy

Variations are frequent[10,11] but in general in those with SLL, the arteries are a mirror image of normal in that the right-sided vessel is like a left coronary with a circumflex and anterior descending, and the left-sided vessel resembles a right coronary artery.[12] In those with IDD, the coronaries are usually normal.

PHYSIOLOGY

The physiologic problems presented by patients with corrected transposition of the great arteries are directly related to the associated defects.

The myocardial function of the systemic, but anatomic, right ventricle has been a matter of interest. Because the two ventricles have different geometric configurations, it is postulated that the right ventricle may not perform systemic pumping as well as an anatomic left ventricle. Right ventricular performance and coronary flow reserve are known to be decreased in both preoperative and postoperative patients.[13–17]

CLINICAL MANIFESTATIONS

The clinical features are, similarly, a direct function of the associated cardiac anatomy, although a relatively constant auscultatory finding regardless of associated lesions is the very loud (often palpable in the child) aortic valve closure component of the second heart sound at the upper left sternal border due to its proximity (see Fig. 51-1). The infant may suffer cyanosis or congestive heart failure, be discovered because of a murmur, or be found because

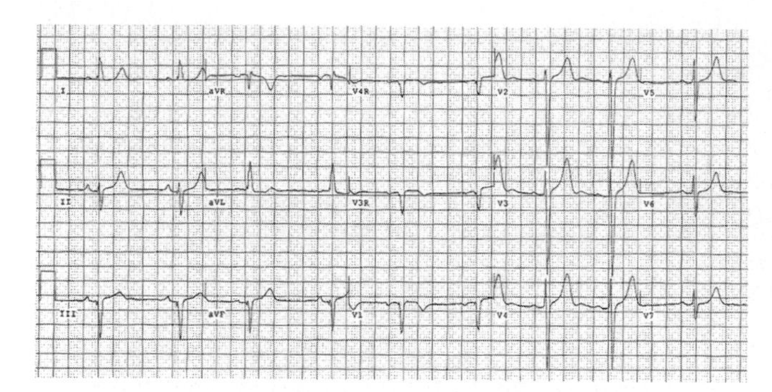

FIGURE 51–2 *Electrocardiogram of 17-year-old with corrected transposition and no other structural abnormality showing reversed septal ventricular depolarization with absent r in aVR, rsR pattern in aVL, small initial q wave in V_3R, V_1 and absent q wave in V_5, V_6.*

of an abnormality on a chest x-ray taken for some reason unrelated to the heart.

Electrocardiography

In the more common SLL variety, as the ventricular septum is depolarized from right to left (opposite of normal), an initial Q wave may be present in the right-sided chest leads and absent in the left (Fig. 51-2). Varying degrees of heart block, usually with a QRS complex of normal duration, are common—as many as 40% of patients are born with or develop complete heart block[6,18,19] (see Exhibit 51-1), apparently unrelated to associated anomalies.[20] In those with the IDD variety, because the sinus node is left sided, the P wave is negative in lead 1, but as the ventricular septum is normally depolarized, the right chest leads usually have an initial R wave and the left an initial Q.

Chest X-Ray

The anterior and leftward ascending aorta can often be recognized on the plain chest x-ray (Fig. 51-3).

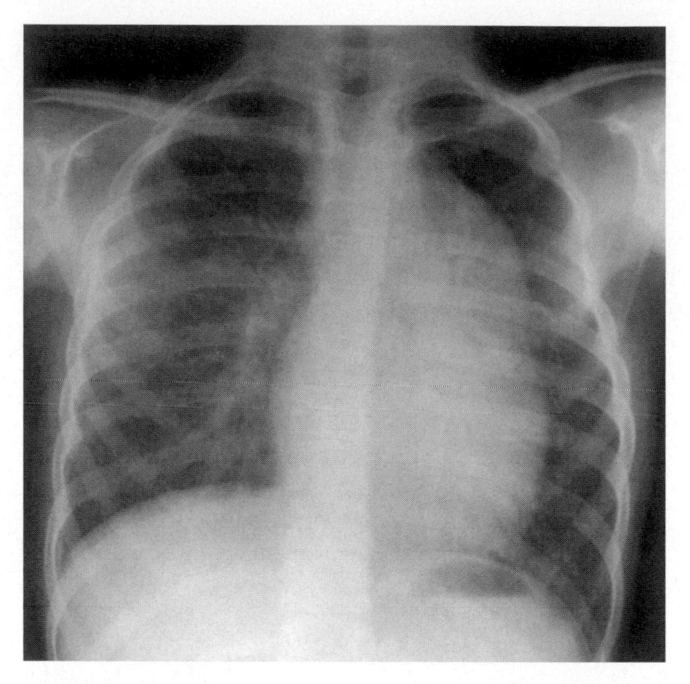

FIGURE 51–3 *Anteroposterior chest x-ray showing prominent left-sided ascending aorta in a patient with corrected transposition. From Fyler DC [ed]. Nadas' Pediatric Cardiology. Philadelphia: Hanley & Belfus, 1992.*

Echocardiography

Echocardiography is a highly reliable means of describing the anatomy. Inversion of the ventricles can be recognized by identification of the right-sided mitral valve and the left-sided tricuspid valve. The papillary muscles of the bicuspid mitral valve attach only to the free wall of the left ventricle, whereas the tricuspid valve attaches to the septal surface of the right ventricle. The fine trabeculations of the left ventricle may distinguish it from the coarse trabeculations of the right ventricle. Usually, the transposed aortic valve and main pulmonary artery are readily recognized. The function of the tricuspid valve should be evaluated because incompetence is common.[21,22]

The diagnosis is generally apparent from the initial subxiphoid long- and short-axis scans (Fig. 51-4). In SLL, the anterior and right-sided morphologic left ventricle is seen aligned with the pulmonary artery. Scanning more anteriorly displays the anterior and left-sided aorta aligned with the right ventricle. Because a ventricular septal defect is common, the septum should be scanned in multiple views with and without color-flow Doppler mapping. The tricuspid valve should be imaged using apical views to assess the location of the septal leaflet, and a Doppler examination should be performed to detect and grade regurgitation. A careful Doppler examination of the pulmonary outflow tract should be performed from subxiphoid and apical transducer locations because pulmonary stenosis is often present.

Magnetic Resonance Imaging

Magnetic resonance imaging, a rapidly developing promising technology, at the present time seems most useful in older patients primarily for assessment of right ventricular function and tricuspid valve competence.

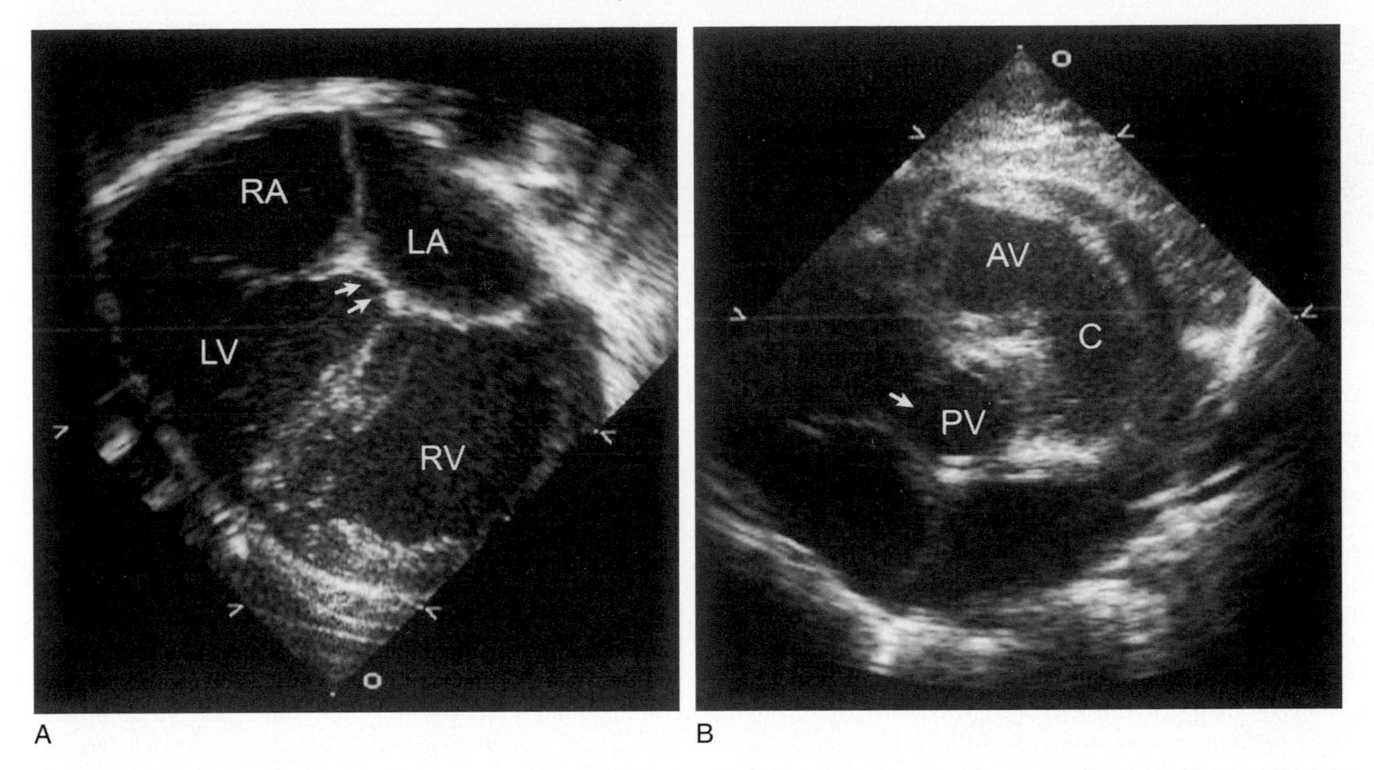

FIGURE 51–4 *Echocardiogram in SLL transposition of the great vessels. A, Apical four-chamber view. The ventricles are inverted, with the right atrium (RA) connecting to the right-sided left ventricle (LV), and the left atrium (LA) connecting to the left-sided right ventricle (RV). The atrioventricular septum (arrows) is positioned between the LV and LA, whereas in the normal heart, the atrioventricular septum separates the LV from the RA. B, Parasternal short-axis view at the level of the great vessels. The aortic valve (AV) is anterior and arises from a conus (C) that connects to the left-sided right ventricle. The pulmonary valve (PV) is posterior and is directly connected to the right sided left ventricle (arrow) without subarterial conus.*

Cardiac Catheterization

Because intracardiac anatomy and valve regurgitation can be delineated by echocardiography, catheterization is necessary only for specific reasons, including (1) pulmonary artery pressure and resistance determinations and anatomy, particularly in those who have had prior aortopulmonary shunt procedures; (2) interventional management (dilation or stent placement) of pulmonary artery stenoses or previously placed obstructed left ventricular–pulmonary artery conduits; or (3) device closure of surgically inaccessible ventricular septal defects; and (4) uncertain coronary artery anatomy or ventricular septal defect locations.

If ventricular angiography is necessary, because the ventricular septum is usually oriented in an anteroposterior plane, initial angiograms are best taken in the anteroposterior view with cranial angulation. For systemic right ventricular angiography, a retrograde transaortic approach is best because tricuspid regurgitation is so common in this condition (Figs. 51-5 and 51-6).

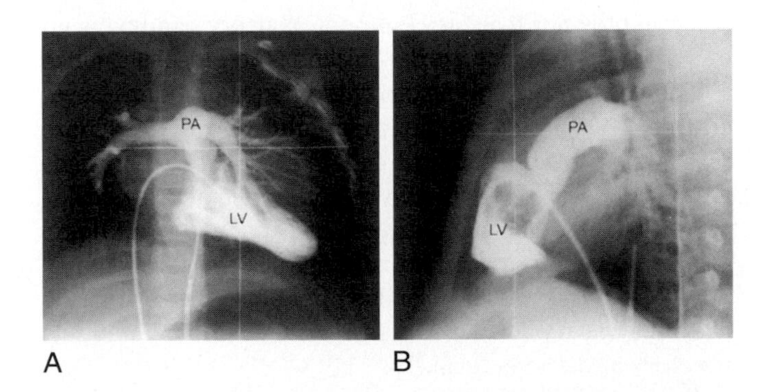

FIGURE 51–5 *Anteroposterior (A) and lateral (B) views from an angiogram of a patient with corrected transposition showing a right-sided left ventricle (LV). The finely trabeculated LV opens into a right-sided and posterior pulmonary artery (PA).*
From Fyler DC [ed]. Nadas' Pediatric Cardiology. Philadelphia: Hanley & Belfus, 1992.

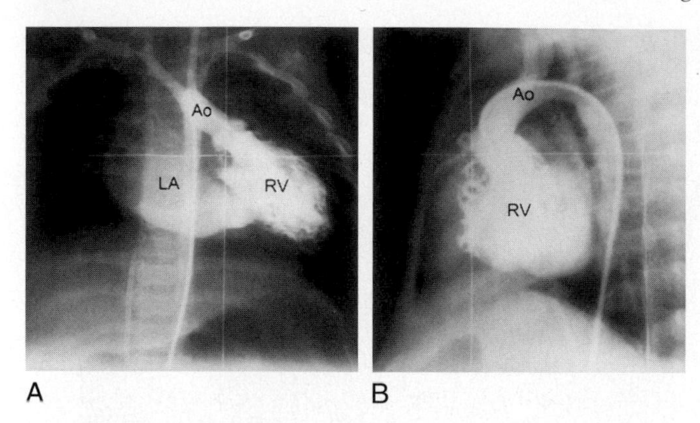

FIGURE 51–6 *Anteroposterior (A) and lateral (B) views from an angiogram in the same patient as in Fig. 51-5 showing a left-sided right ventricle (RV). The coarsely trabeculated RV opens into a left-sided and anterior aorta (Ao), and there is considerable tricuspid regurgitation into a dilated left atrium (LA).*

MANAGEMENT

Because of the wide range of associated defects and the tendency of many of these to progress with time, this group of patients is extraordinarily difficult to manage. In general, it is reasonable to follow medically (1) those with minor structural problems, (2) even some asymptomatic patients with significant but balanced lesions, and (3) even those with asymptomatic complete heart block because pacemaker placement alone is likely to result in increasing tricuspid regurgitation and right ventricular failure.

Palliative operations such as a modified Blalock-Taussig aortopulmonary shunt were a common procedure in the past for severe pulmonary stenosis or atresia but resulted in pulmonary artery distortion in many if left alone for years. Currently, it is reasonable to place such a shunt for a short time in an infant with pulmonary atresia when conduit placement is not feasible. Pulmonary artery banding is no longer carried out.

The earlier "repair" operation, which often included closure of a ventricular septal defect and relief of pulmonary stenosis, with or without conduit placement from left ventricle to pulmonary artery, was complicated by significant early mortality rates and heart block, later conduit obstruction, tricuspid regurgitation, right ventricular failure, and unsatisfactory long-term survival.[21–24] Isolated tricuspid valve plasty or replacement has also been unsatisfactory in the long term.[18]

Because of these problems, the current surgical approach is aimed at making the left ventricle the systemic and the right ventricle the pulmonary pumping chambers. This requires an atrial-level switch operation for venous return (Senning) in all, together with either an arterial switch operation (hence the designation "double switch") in those with an intact ventricular septum or a Rastelli procedure in those with a ventricular septal defect. A conduit from the right ventricle to the pulmonary artery is also necessary in some, and in others, prior placement of a pulmonary artery band to prepare a low-pressure left ventricle to assume systemic pumping function is required. Although long-term follow-up is as yet unavailable with this approach, preliminary results are encouraging, with low surgical mortality and heart block rates, improved tricuspid valve and right ventricular function, and 90% survival at 9 years, although the expected conduit obstruction has occurred in some.[25–27] When all else has failed, cardiac transplantation is another option.

COURSE

During follow-up, some of the associated defects, particularly tricuspid regurgitation and atrioventricular conduction abnormalities, are well known to progress and are significant risk factors for survival. With regard to regurgitation, increasing degrees of right ventricular failure commonly accompany this problem. Spontaneous complete heart block is also common, is present at birth in some, and progresses from first to second degree to complete in others, such that at least one third of patients will acquire this during follow-up (see Exhibit 51-1). In the earlier "repair" and in the current "double switch" approach, conduit obstruction is common, and temporary relief by transcatheter stent placement is feasible in many.

ANATOMICALLY CORRECTED MALPOSITION OF THE GREAT ARTERIES

This rare entity was initially described as "anatomically corrected transposition." As morphology understanding progressed, it was found to be distinctly different from the more common "corrected transposition" and hence was renamed "malposition."[28,29] The most common variety of this entity consists of normal atrioventricular and ventriculoarterial concordance (i.e., *normal*) but with the ascending aorta to the left of the pulmonary artery (i.e., malposed). Many have associated lesions such as ventricular septal defect or pulmonary or subaortic stenosis, which are amenable to surgical repair. The other extremely rare varieties in this entity usually have very complex defects, amenable only to palliative procedures.[30]

REFERENCES

1. Fyler DC. "Corrected" transposition of the great arteries. In Fyler DC (ed). Nadas' Pediatric Cardiology. Philadelphia: Hanley & Belfus, 1992:701–706.

2. Botto LD, Correa A, Erickson JD. Racial and temporal variations in the prevalence of heart defects. Pediatrics 107(3): 1, 2001.
3. Yamazaki I, Kondo J, Imoto K, et al. Corrected transposition of the great arteries diagnosed in an 84-year-old woman. J Cardiovasc Surg 42(2):201, 2001.
4. Beauchesne LM, Warnes CA, Connolly HM, et al. Outcome of the unoperated adult who presents with congenitally corrected transposition of the great arteries. J Am Coll Cardiol 40(2):285, 2002.
5. Prieto LR, Hordof AJ, Secic M, et al. Progressive tricuspid valve disease in patients with congenitally corrected transposition of the great arteries. Circulation 98(10):997, 1998.
6. Graham TP Jr, Bernard YD, Mellen BG, et al. Long term outcome in congenitally corrected transposition of the great arteries: A multi-institutional study. J Am Coll Cardiol 36(1):255, 2000.
7. VanPraagh R, Papagiannis J, Gruenfelder J, et al. Pathologic anatomy of corrected transposition of the great arteries: medical and surgical implications. Am Heart J 135(5 Pt 1): 772, 1998.
8. Piran S, Veldtman G, Siu S, et al. Heart failure and ventricular septal dysfunction in patients with single or systemic right ventricles. Circulation 105(10):1189, 2002.
9. Fredriksen PM, Chen SJ, Veldtman G. Exercise capacity in adult patients with congenitally corrected transposition of the great arteries. Heart (British Cardiac Society) 85(2):191, 2001.
10. Chiu IS, Wu SJ, Chen SJ, et al. Sequential diagnosis of coronary arterial anatomy in congenitally corrected transposition of the great arteries. Ann Thorac Surg 75(2):422, 2003.
11. Ismat FA, Baldwin HS, Karl TR, et al. Coronary anatomy in congenitally corrected transposition of the great arteries. Int J Cardiol 86(2–3):207, 2002.
12. Dabizzi RP, Barletta GA, Caprioli G, et al. Coronary artery anatomy in corrected transposition of the great arteries. J Am Coll Cardiol 12:486, 1988.
13. Benson LN, Burns R, Schwaiger M, et al. Radionuclide angiographic evaluation of ventricular function in isolated congenitally corrected transposition of the great arteries. Am J Cardiol 58:319, 1986.
14. Graham TP, Parrish MD, Boucek RJ, et al. Assessment of ventricular size and function in congenitally corrected transposition of the great arteries. Am J Cardiol 51:244, 1983.
15. Hauser M, Bengel FM, Hager A, et al. Impaired myocardial blood flow and coronary flow reserve of the anatomical right systemic ventricle in patients with congenitally corrected transposition of the great arteries. Heart (British Cardiac Society) 89(10):1231, 2003.
16. Parrish MD, Graham TP, Bender HW, et al. Radionuclide angiographic evaluation of right and left ventricular function during exercise after repair of transposition of the great arteries. Comparison with normal subjects and patients with congenitally corrected transposition. Circulation 67: 178, 1983.
17. Roest AA, Kunz P, Helbing WA, et al. Prolonged cardiac recovery from exercise in asymptomatic adults late after atrial correction of transposition of the great arteries: Evaluation with magnetic resonance flow mapping. Am J Cardiol 88(9):1011, 2001.
18. van Son JA, Danielson GK, Huhta JC, et al. Late results of systemic atrioventricular valve replacement in corrected transposition. J Thorac Cardiovasc Surg 109(4):642, 1995.
19. Westerman GR, Lang P, Castaneda AR, et al. Corrected transposition and repair of associated intracardiac defects. Circulation 66(Suppl I):I197, 1982.
20. Daliento L, Corrado D, Buja G, et al. Rhythm and conduction disturbances in isolated, congenitally corrected transposition of the great arteries. Am J Cardiol 51:244, 1983.
21. Hraska V, Duncan BW, Jonas RA, et al. Long-term outcome of surgically treated patients with corrected transposition of the great arteries. J Thorac Cardiovasc Surg 129:183, 2005.
22. Termignon JL, Leca F, Vouhe PR, et al. "Classic" repair of congenitally corrected transposition and ventricular septal defect. Ann Thorac Surg 62(1):199, 1996.
23. Biliciler-Denktas G, Feldt RH, Connoly HM, et al. Early and late results of operations for defects associated with corrected transposition and other anomalies with atrioventricular discordance in a pediatric population. J Thorac Cardiovasc Surg 122(2):234, 2001.
24. Rutledge JM, Nihill MR, Fraser CD, et al. Outcome of 121 patients with congenitally corrected transposition of the great arteries. Pediatr Cardiol 23(2):137, 2002.
25. Langley SM, Winlaw DS, Stumper O, et al. Midterm results after restoration of the morphologically left ventricle to the systemic circulation in patients with congenitally corrected transposition of the great arteries. J Thorac Cardiovasc Surg 125(6):1229, 2003.
26. Duncan BW, Mee RB, Mesia CI, et al. Results of the double switch operation for congenitally corrected transposition of the great arteries. Eur J Cardiothorac Surg 24(1):11, 2003.
27. Devaney EJ, Charpie JR, Ohye RG, et al. Combined arterial switch and Senning operation for congenitally corrected transposition of the great arteries: patient selection and intermediate results. J Thorac Cardiovasc Surg 125(3):500, 2003.
28. Van Praagh R, Van Praagh S. Anatomically corrected transposition of the great arteries. Br Heart J 29:112, 1967.
29. Van Praagh R. The story of anatomically corrected malposition of the great arteries. Chest 69:2, 1976.
30. Dalvi B, Sharma S. Anatomically corrected malposition: Report of six cases. Am Heart J 126:1229, 1993.

52

Vascular Fistulae

JOHN F. KEANE AND DONALD C. FYLER

DEFINITION

An arteriovenous fistula is any connection that bypasses the capillary circulation. The types of such connections are legion: this chapter is limited to descriptions of a few, the most commonly encountered, and includes coronary, pulmonary, and cerebral fistulae. Also included, albeit atypical, is aorto–left ventricular tunnel.

PREVALENCE

The total number of these lesions encountered by us has increased significantly, the most common now being a coronary artery fistula (Exhibit 52-1). This pattern has clearly been influenced by echocardiographic identification, catheterization, interventional treatment capabilities, and surgical procedures. In acyanotic patients such as those with coronary fistulae, small lesions are often expectedly encountered during echocardiography for other reasons,[1] whereas those with larger connections present with symptoms or murmurs.[2] In contrast, many with cerebral fistulae are severely compromised even before birth.[3] Pulmonary malformations, a cyanotic lesion, are currently more commonly secondary to surgical procedures such as a bidirectional Glenn shunt and are reversible.[4–6]

CORONARY FISTULAE

Definition

Fistulous connections occur between the coronary arteries and coronary veins, chambers of the right heart and pulmonary vessels.[7,8] Fistulous connections between the coronary arteries and the left ventricle have been described most often as aorto–left ventricular tunnels.

Prevalence

Although rare, coronary artery fistulae were seen in 79 patients at Children's Hospital Boston between 1988 and 2002 (see Exhibit 52-1).

Pathology

Origin of the fistula from the left coronary was more common than the right (75% versus 25%) in our patients, and entry sites were in the right heart in 92% (pulmonary artery, 33%; ventricle, 32%; atrium, 24%). Most often, the entry point was a single orifice, and only rarely multiple. The vessel as far as the exit site is generally dilated and tortuous when the fistula is large, even rarely aneurysmal.[9–11] These structures are thought of as having a congenital origin and enlarging gradually throughout life.

Physiology

The fistula acts as a shunt from the coronary artery to the right heart chambers. The shunt is often small and without symptoms, whereas those larger are often symptomatic even in infancy.[1,2,11,12] Because the fistula is present from an early stage and is only gradually thought to change, it rarely steals blood from the myocardium, such that evidence of myocardial ischemia or underperfusion is uncommon. Infective endocarditis is thought to occur in the fistula in as many as 5% of patients, and rupture has been reported.[10]

Exhibit 52–1
Children's Hospital Boston Experience
Vascular Fistulae

	1973–1987	*1988–2002*
Coronary	26	79
Pulmonary	6	60
Hepatic	5	8
Cerebral	7	7
Aorto–left ventricle tunnel	3	6
Ruptured sinus of Valsalva	3	0

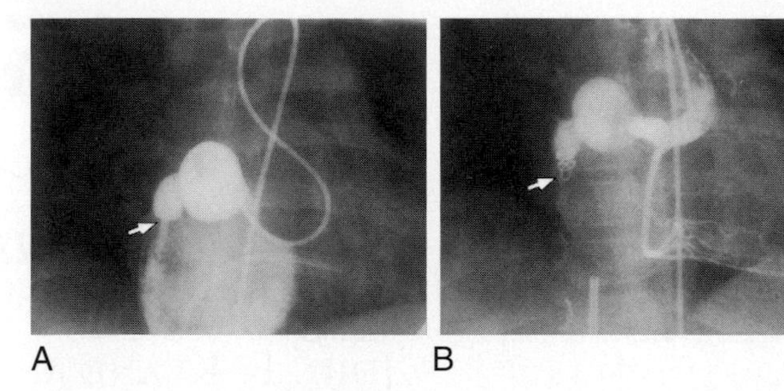

FIGURE 52–1 *Cineangiogram showing selective injection into right coronary artery with fistulous connection (arrow) to right atrium before (A) and after (B) closure with single Gianturco coil (arrow) in 4-year-old girl.*

Clinical Manifestations

Many of these patients are discovered during routine auscultation of an otherwise well child, whereas, increasingly, small silent fistulae are being identified unexpectedly during echocardiography. When a murmur is present, it is usually continuous, sounds like a patent ductus, but is in an atypical location usually to the right or left of the lower sternal region. The shunt is rarely sufficient to affect the pulse pressure.

Electrocardiography

Generally, there is no abnormality recognizable on the electrocardiogram unless the shunt is sufficiently large to overload the left or right heart circulation.

Chest X-Ray

Often, the chest x-ray is normal.

Echocardiography

The fistulous structures are readily identifiable at echocardiography; color-flow Doppler mapping is especially useful for documenting the connections with heart chambers.[13–15] Indirect evidence of shunt size can be recognized through chamber enlargement.

Cardiac Catheterization

Catheterization is indicated if intervention (transcatheter or surgical) is planned. Selective angiography best identifies the precise anatomy (Fig. 52-1), and if transcatheter occlusion is anticipated, balloon occlusion angiography is necessary to make sure there are no side branches at or distal to the location where device placement is planned.[2]

Management

It is reasonable to follow "silent" small fistulae without evidence of echocardiographic cardiac compromise medically because some 23% have been reported to close spontaneously.[1] In the others, and because endocarditis and aneurysm with rupture have been reported,[10] closure should be undertaken. Currently, this may be performed at catheterization using different devices[2,16,17] (see Fig. 52-1) or surgically,[18,19] with similar results in these small groups, in recent years, negligible mortality.

Course

Continued follow-up is necessary because recurrences or residual flow have been evident in some, and myocardial infarcts have been reported in two postoperative patients.[20,21]

PULMONARY ARTERIOVENOUS FISTULAE

Definition

Arteriovenous connections that bypass the pulmonary capillary circulation may take the form of multiple tiny angiomatous intercommunications (telangiectases) or may consist of large pulmonary artery–to–pulmonary vein communications.

Prevalence

The number of pulmonary arteriovenous fistulae has increased significantly in recent years (see Exhibit 52-1) largely because of surgical procedures such as the bidirectional Glenn shunt in which hepatic venous return is excluded from the pulmonary circulation. At Children's Hospital Boston from 1988 to 2002, of 60 patients listed with pulmonary fistulae in our files, 38 cases were secondary to such operations.

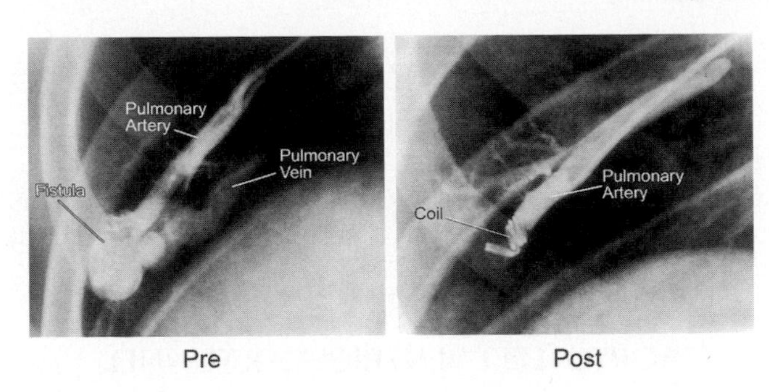

FIGURE 52–2 *Localized right lung pulmonary arteriovenous fistula in a 30-year-old man before and after closure with a Gianturco coil.*

Pathology

Lesions may be (1) multiple, tiny, and diffusely scattered throughout both lungs, as in Osler-Weber-Rendu syndrome or after Glenn shunting[4,22,23]; or (b) localized malformations confined to a single lobe (Fig. 52-2). The latter are likely congenital and get larger with time. The diffuse variety following surgical Glenn shunting result from exclusion of a hepatic factor directly reaching the pulmonary circulation, are also seen in patients with liver disease, and are reversible in both cases by connecting hepatic return to the lungs in the former[5] and liver transplantation in the latter.[24]

Physiology

The effect of a pulmonary arteriovenous fistula is to bypass the pulmonary capillaries. The consequence is that pulmonary venous oxygen content is less than normal in direct relation to the size of the shunt. Otherwise, there is little, if any, effect on the circulation. Pulmonary artery pressures are normal, and pulmonary arteriolar resistance is very low in the fistula itself, but calculates to a higher than normal number in that part of the lung that supplies the capillaries. The mechanism of increased shunting as the child grows older is not understood. Whether there is an increasing number of shunting connections or dilation of an existing connection,[25] these patients tend to become more cyanotic with time.

Clinical Manifestations

The patients without congenital heart disease are cyanotic in proportion to the amount of blood bypassing the pulmonary capillaries. They may have a continuous murmur over the fistula, although if multiple small lesions are present, murmurs are only rarely heard. In those with Glenn shunts and cyanotic heart lesions, and in some with multiple diffuse lesions, rapid progression of cyanosis may occur.

Electrocardiography

The electrocardiogram is normal in the absence of heart disease.

Echocardiography

A normal echocardiographic examination in a cyanotic child should suggest the possibility of this diagnosis. Echocardiography with bubble studies is exquisitely sensitive in demonstrating the right-to-left shunting, often identifying a much higher incidence of fistulae after Glenn shunts than angiography.[23,26]

Cardiac Catheterization

Cardiac catheterization shows a normal cardiac output and normal pressures. The arterial oxygen unsaturation can be traced to the pulmonary venous circulation, sometimes to the specific lobe involved. Angiography in multiple views identifies the defect and provides the anatomic detail needed to plan treatment (see Fig. 52-2). It is important to identify all intrapulmonary shunts. Balloon occlusion of pulmonary artery branches may provide clues to the precise anatomy of fistulae and the effect on arterial saturation in response to closure.

Management

Isolated single fistulae can usually be managed successfully by catheter-delivered devices (see Fig. 52-2) or surgery. Those secondary to Glenn shunts can be reversed by surgically channeling hepatic venous return directly to the pulmonary arteries, done usually as part of a Fontan procedure; on a few occasions, we have seen resolution of these fistulae after creation of an axillary artery-to-vein fistula. In those with bilateral diffuse fistulae and a normal heart, multiple coil occlusions of pulmonary artery branches may help initially, but progressive deterioration usually occurs, although improvement with nifedipine therapy has been reported.[27]

Course

Removal of a large single fistula, by whatever means, is likely to be successful permanently. Management of multiple tiny fistulae in patients without heart or liver disease has largely been unsuccessful. Neurologic complications are common.[28]

CEREBRAL FISTULAE

Definition

A cerebral fistula is a connection between a cerebral artery and a nearby vein; lesions are often multiple, the most common involving the vein of Galen.

Prevalence

These are very rare lesions; we have seen only seven from 1988 to 2002 (see Exhibit 52-1).

Pathophysiology

Left-to-right shunting occurs, adding increased volume to all heart chambers, and when very large, heart failure with fetal hydrops is not uncommon. Somewhat smaller shunts may be associated with the occurrence of rapid onset of severe congestive heart failure and death within days of birth in a well-nourished baby, probably related to the conversion of the fetal parallel circulation to the serial postdelivery one.

Clinical Manifestations

Many of these patients are identified during routine fetal echocardiography. After delivery, magnetic resonance imaging for brain assessment is usually done, and echocardiography is requested to determine whether any structural heart disease is present. The subsequent management of the patient, if treatment is planned, usually involves the neurosurgeon and interventional radiologist.

Clinically, if the shunt is large, severe congestive heart failure is common, with a hyperactive heart and prominent pulses initially. Cyanosis due to poor perfusion is common, and femoral pulses may be diminished.

Electrocardiography

Right or left ventricular hypertrophy may be evident depending on flow distribution before delivery.

Chest X-Ray

When ill, gross cardiomegaly and increased pulmonary blood flow are present.

Echocardiography

The cardiac chambers are enlarged, as is the superior vena cava, and the fistula is commonly identifiable.

Cardiac Catheterization

Again, this is no longer necessary.

Management

The only way to salvage these infants with gross heart failure, if treatment is to be undertaken, is to reduce the amount of shunting by catheter-delivered devices or surgically.[29–32]

AORTO–LEFT VENTRICULAR TUNNEL

Definition

An aorto–left ventricular tunnel is a rare, congenital communication between the aortic root and the left ventricle beneath the right side of the aortic valve, with some 80 cases, many single, reported in the literature to date.

Anatomy

The etiology of this lesion is uncertain, but because most infants with this condition are known to have a cardiac lesion at birth, it is thought to be congenital rather than acquired. The aortic end of the tunnel is usually in the right sinus of Valsalva and the left ventricular end just below the aortic valve. Some have aortic regurgitation and other associated lesions (in about 50%) include right coronary artery atresia and aortic valvar stenosis.

Physiology

The physiologic effect of this left-to-left shunt is comparable to aortic regurgitation. The burden on the circulation is proportionate to the amount of blood that flows retrograde from the aorta to the left ventricle.

Clinical Manifestations

In our experience, most present at birth with a diastolic murmur and bounding pulses, and eventually, congestive heart failure develops.[33]

Electrocardiography

Electrocardiograms show left ventricular hypertrophy.

Chest X-Ray

On chest x-ray, the heart is enlarged, but the pulmonary vasculature is not engorged.

Echocardiography

Echocardiography, with care, can establish the diagnosis, but with casual review of even the best data, the diagnosis may be missed (Fig. 52-3). Evidence suggesting aortic

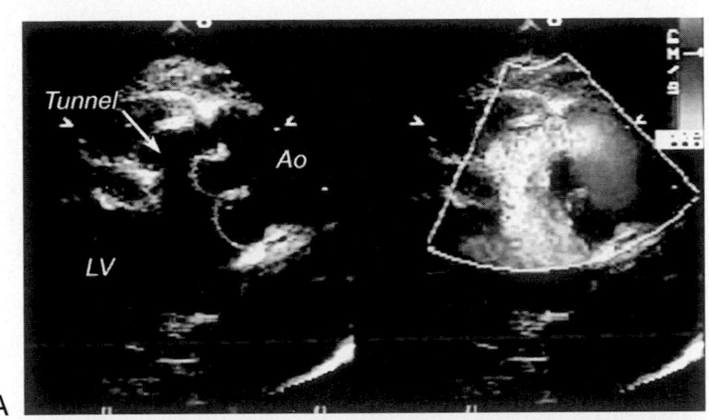

A

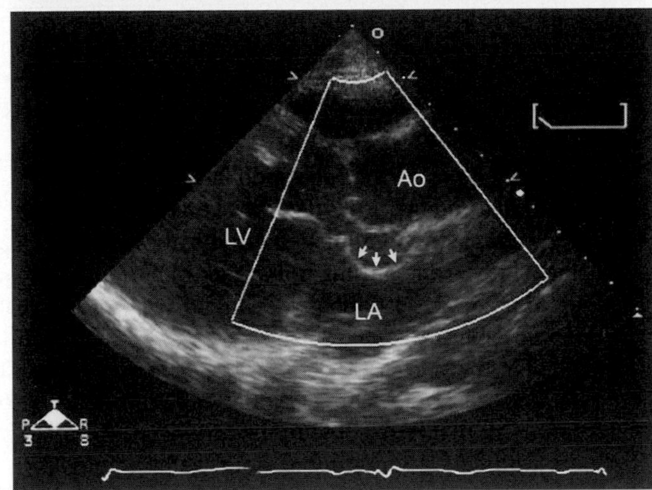

B

FIGURE 52–3 *A, Two-dimensional and color-flow Doppler images of a congenital aorta (Ao) to left ventricular (LV) tunnel. The tunnel connects the ascending aorta (above the sinuses of Valsalva) to the LV along the right and anterior aspect of the aorta (left panel). Flow through the tunnel is readily demonstrated by color Doppler (right panel). B, In contrast, a fistula (arrows) secondary to bacterial endocarditis connecting the ascending aorta (AO) to the left ventricle (LV) is seen to pass between the aortic root and the left atrium (LA).*

regurgitation associated with an abnormal structure between the septum and the right aortic sinus when there is no ventricular defect should raise the possibility of this diagnosis.

Cardiac Catheterization

Cardiac catheterization can confirm the diagnosis but is necessary only if uncertainty exists or if transcatheter closure is planned.

Management

For significant shunts, surgical closure, usually of the aortic end, remains our treatment of choice,[33,34] although catheter device closure has been reported in one patient.[35] A few lesions are small, and these may be followed medically because we have seen spontaneous closure occur in such a patient.[33]

Course

Although postoperatively a few have small residual shunts or mild aortic regurgitation, follow-up has been uneventful in our experience, even as long as 36 years.

REFERENCES

1. Sherwood MC, Rockenmacher S, Colan SD, et al. Prognostic significance of clinically silent coronary artery fistulas. Am J Cardiol 83:407,1999.
2. Armsby LR, Keane JF, Sherwood MC, et al. Management of coronary artery fistulae patient section and results of transcatheter closure. J Am Coll Cardiol 39:1026, 2002.
3. Johnson W, Berry JM, Einzig S, et al. Doppler findings in nonimmune hydrops fetalis and cerebral arteriovenous malformation. Am Heart J 115:1138, 1988.
4. Srivastava D, Preminger T, Jock LE, et al. Hepatic venous blood and the development of pulmonary arteriovenous malformations in congenital heart disease. Circulation 92(5):1217, 1995.
5. Angoletti G, Borghi A, Annecchine FP, Crupi G. Regression of pulmonary fistulas in congenital heart disease after redirection of hepatic venous flow to the lungs. Ann Thorac Surg 72(3):909, 2001.
6. Jacobs ML, Pourmoghadam KK, Geary EM. Pulmonary arteriovenous malformations after cavopulmonary connection. Ann Thorac Surg 69(2):634, 2000.
7. Baim DS, Kline H, Silverman JF. Bilateral coronary artery-pulmonary artery fistulas: Report of five cases and review of the literature. Circulation 65:810, 1982.
8. Thongtang V, Panchavinnin P, Chaithiraphan S, et al. Congenital coronary artery fistula: A report of 24 patients. J Med Assoc Thai 79(10):630, 1996.
9. Anne W, Bogaert J, Van de Werf F. A case report of a patient with a large aneurysmatic coronary artery fistula. Acta Cardiol 55(5):307, 2000.
10. Akashi H, Tayama E, Tayama K, et al. Rupture of an aneurysm resulting from a coronary artery fistula. Circulation 67(6):551, 2003.
11. Holzer R, Waller BR 3rd, Kahana M, et al. Percutaneous closure of a giant coronary arteriovenous fistula using multiple devices in a 12-day-old neonate. Catheter Cardiovasc Interv 12(2):291, 2003.
12. Starc TJ, Bowman FO, Hordof AJ. Congestive heart failure in a newborn secondary to coronary artery-left ventricular fistula. Am J Cardiol 58:366, 1986.
13. Sanders SP, Parness IA, Colan SD. Recognition of abnormal connections of coronary arteries with the use of

Doppler color flow mapping. J Am Coll Cardiol 13:922, 1989.

14. Barbosa MM, Katina T, Oliveira HG, et al. Doppler echocardiographic features of coronary artery fistula: report of 8 cases. J Am Soc Echocardiogr 12(2):149, 1999.
15. Nekkanti R, Nanda NC, Angsingkar KG, et al. Transesophageal three-dimensional echocardiographic assessment of left main coronary artery fistula. Echocardiography 18(4):305, 2001.
16. Alekyan BG, Podzolkov VP, Cardenas CE. Transcatheter coil embolization of coronary artery fistula. Asian Cardiovasc Thorac Ann 10:47, 2002.
17. McMahon CJ, Nihill MR, Kovalchin JP, et al. Coil occlusion. Tex Heart Inst J 28(1):287, 1997.
18. Schumacher G, Roithmaier A, Lorenz HP, et al. Congenital coronary artery fistula in infancy and childhood: Diagnostic and therapeutic aspects [comment]. Thorac Cardiovasc Surg 45(6):287, 1997.
19. Kamiya H, Yasuda T, Nagamine H, et al. Surgical treatment of congenital coronary artery fistulas: 27 Years' experience and a review of the literature. J Card Surg 17(2):173, 2002.
20. Mesko ZG, Damus PS. Myocardial infarction in a 14-year-old girl, ten years after surgical correction of congenital coronary artery fistula. Pediatr Cardiol 19(4):366, 1998.
21. Goldberg SL, Manchester J, Laks H. Late-term myocardial infarction after surgical ligation of a giant coronary artery fistula. J Invasive Cardiol 14(4):202, 2002.
22. Bernstein HS, Brook MM, Silverman NH, et al. Development of pulmonary arteriovenous fistulae in children after cavopulmonary shunt. Circulation 92(9 Suppl):11309, 1995.
23. Kim SJ, Bae EJ, Cho DJ, et al. Development of pulmonary arteriovenous fistulae in children after bidirectional cavopulmonary shunt. Ann of Thor Surg 70(6):1918, 2000.
24. Fewtrell MS, Noble-Jamieson G, Revell S, et al. Intrapulmonary shunting in the biliary atresia/polysplenia syndrome: Reversal after liver transplantation. Arch Dis Child 70(6):501, 1994.
25. Knight WB, Bush A, Busst CM, et al. Multiple pulmonary arteriovenous fistulas in childhood. Int J Cardiol 23:105, 1989.
26. Chang RK, Alejos JC, Atkinson D, et al. Bubble contrast echocardiography in detecting pulmonary arteriovenous shunting in children with univentricular heart after cavopulmonary anastomosis. J Am Coll Cardiol 33(7):2052, 1999.
27. Sands A, Dalzell E, Craig B, et al. Multiple intrapulmonary arteriovenous fistulas in childhood. Pediatr Cardiol 21(5):493, 2000.
28. Swanson KL, Prakash UB, Stanson AW. Pulmonary arteriovenous fistulas: Mayo Clinic experience, 1982–1997 [comment]. Mayo Clin Proc 74(7):671, 1999.
29. Tamburrini G, Caldarelli M, Iannelli A, Di et al. Two newborn children with large hemorrhages from arteriovenous malformations. Pediatr Neurosurg 37(3):164, 2002.
30. Hung PC, Wang HS. Successful endovascular treatment of cerebral arteriovenous fistula. Pediatric Neurol 27(4):300, 2002.
31. Chevret L, Durand P, Alvarez H, et al. Severe cardiac failure in newborns with VGAM. Intensive Care Med 28(8):1126, 2002.
32. Burrows PE, Lasjaunias PL, Ter Brugge KG, et al. Urgent and emergent embolization of lesions of the head and neck in children: Indications and results. Pediatrics 80:386, 1987.
33. Martins J, Sherwood M, Mayer JE, et al. Aortico left ventricular tunnel—35 year experience. J Am Coll Cardiol 44:446, 2004.
34. Turkey K, Silverman NH, Teital D, et al. Repair of aortico-left ventricular tunnel in the neonate: surgical, anatomic and echocardiographic considerations. Circulation 65:1015, 1982.
35. Chessa M, Chaudhari M, De Giovenni JV. Aorto-left ventricular tunnel: Transcatheter closure using an Amplatzer duct occluder device. Am J Cardiol 86(2):253, 2000.

53

Coronary Artery Anomalies

JOHN F. KEANE AND DONALD C. FYLER

DEFINITION

With increasing use and extraordinary sophistication of noninvasive imaging techniques such as echocardiography and magnetic resonance imaging (MRI), the number of coronary anomalies identified is increasing. The vast majority, such as minor degrees of origin eccentricity, separate origins of circumflex, and left anterior descending, are of no significance. This chapter discusses the significant anomalies: (1) origin of a coronary from a pulmonary artery, and (2) both coronary arteries from a single sinus, without other structural cardiac defects. Other anomalies, such as left anterior descending from the right coronary in tetralogy of Fallot, variations encountered in transposition, are described in the relevant chapters.

PREVALENCE

Among more than 1400 anomalies diagnosed by echocardiography between 1988 and 2002, there were 51 with origin of a coronary artery from a pulmonary artery, 7 with a single coronary, and a similar number with both from the same cusp (Exhibit 53-1). In three other patients, all with other cardiac defects, only the circumflex branch arose anomalously from the pulmonary artery.

ANOMALOUS CORONARY FROM A PULMONARY ARTERY

Of the 51 patients with this anomaly, the left originated from the pulmonary artery in 50 and the right in the other.

Pathology

The anomalous coronary artery arises from the low-pressure main pulmonary artery and follows its usual course over the heart. Because the other high-pressure coronary artery is the source of perfusion for the myocardium, it is bigger and takes over the other coronary circulation through collateral connections, and retrograde flow to the pulmonary artery occurs in most. Because the myocardium is generally poorly perfused, the heart may be dilated, and histologic evidence of inadequate myocardial perfusion may be found. At postmortem examination, there may be obvious myocardial infarction.

Physiology

Before birth, the pulmonary artery pressure is at systemic levels, allowing for satisfactory myocardial perfusion from the pulmonary artery through the anomalous coronary. With birth and falling pulmonary artery pressure, the antegrade perfusion of the anomalous coronary gradually decreases, the circulation being taken over by collateral vessels from the other coronary. In many patients, the flow in the anomalous coronary artery reverses, and, effectively, a coronary artery steal develops from the myocardium to the pulmonary artery. The size of this left-to-right shunt is rarely enough to be a significant hemodynamic burden except that it deprives the myocardium of perfusion. Sometime in the first week of reversed coronary flow, myocardial ischemia becomes sufficient to be recognizable on an electrocardiogram. The heart enlarges, and congestive heart failure becomes manifest. With ischemic damage to the left papillary muscles,

Exhibit 53–1
Children's Hospital Boston Experience
Coronary Artery Anomalies

	1973–1987	*1988–2002*
LCA from PA	29	50
RCA from PA	0	1
Female	55%	66%
Age at operation		
0–1 yr	36%	65%
1–10 yr	38%	23%
10 yr	26%	12%
Ligation	19%	0%
Takeuchi/implant/graft	81%	100%
Early deaths	8%	7%
Single RCA		3
Single LCA		4
RCA from left coronary sinus		6
LCA from right coronary sinus		1
LCA from noncoronary sinus		1

LCA, left coronary artery; PA, pulmonary artery; RCA, right coronary artery.

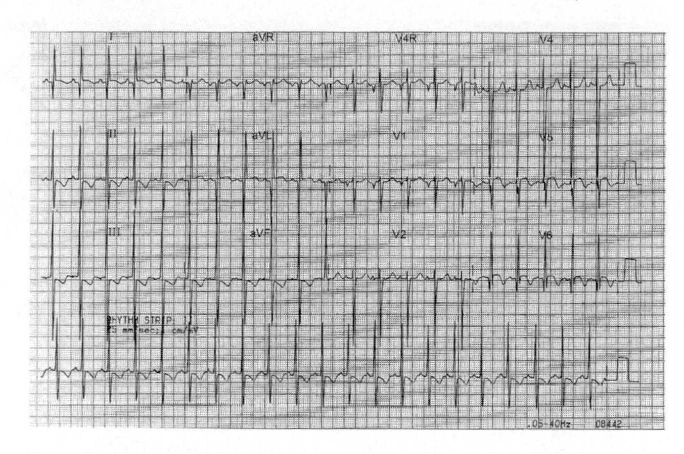

FIGURE 53–1 *Electrocardiogram from a 3-month-old infant with anomalous origin of left coronary artery from pulmonary artery showing evidence of extensive anterolateral infarction (deep Q waves leads 1, aVL, V_6; diminished anterior forces V_1–V_4; and left atrial enlargement V_1).*

mitral regurgitation is often added to an already deteriorating situation.

If, for any reason, the patient maintains systemic pressure in the pulmonary arteries, this sequence of events will not occur, and the anomalous coronary will be perfused by blood originating from the pulmonary artery. Despite the fact that this blood may have substantially lower oxygen saturation than that of the other coronary, evidence of myocardial ischemia is not seen.

Some patients with uncorrected anomalous origin from the main pulmonary artery survive to adulthood.[1] The right coronary artery arose from the pulmonary artery in 1 of our 51 patients; even more rarely, both coronary arteries may arise from the pulmonary artery.[2,3]

Clinical Manifestations

These patients appear to be normal at birth; approximately 60% of the patients seen at Children's Hospital Boston developed congestive heart failure weeks later. Occasionally, a history of irritability, perhaps related to angina, is elicited, but this is more of a retrospective explanation than a useful fact. Older patients are discovered because of symptoms, a systolic murmur of mitral regurgitation and cardiomegaly on chest x-ray, echocardiography, tomography, or angiography.[1,4]

The electrocardiogram almost always shows evidence of an anterolateral myocardial infarction (Fig. 53-1), even in the asymptomatic patient.

Chest X-Ray

The heart is enlarged, sometimes grossly, without an increase in pulmonary vascularity.

Echocardiography

Any patient with unexplained myocardial disease should have the origin of the coronary arteries identified. An enlarged, poorly functioning left ventricle is characteristic, as is mitral regurgitation. The anomalous origin of this coronary artery from the pulmonary artery is associated with an inequality of the coronary artery size.[5]

The parasternal short-axis view usually identifies the origins of the coronary arteries from the aorta (Fig. 53-2). Scanning in a parasternal, short- or long-axis view may identify clearly the orifice of the coronary artery in the pulmonary root (Fig. 53-3). Color-flow Doppler mapping is extremely valuable in demonstrating the direction of flow in the coronary, particularly into the pulmonary root when the pulmonary resistance is low.[5,6] Clearly, demonstration of antegrade flow in the coronary artery and branches by color-flow Doppler mapping excludes anomalous origin of that vessel.

Careful imaging and color-flow Doppler mapping allow accurate diagnosis in the majority such that surgery without cardiac catheterization can be undertaken. When the diagnosis is uncertain, cardiac catheterization with selective angiography is the usual option in the first few years of life, whereas MRI in the older child is currently an effective alternative.

Cardiac Catheterization

Cardiac catheterization is rarely necessary in the infant because echocardiographic anatomy details are excellent.

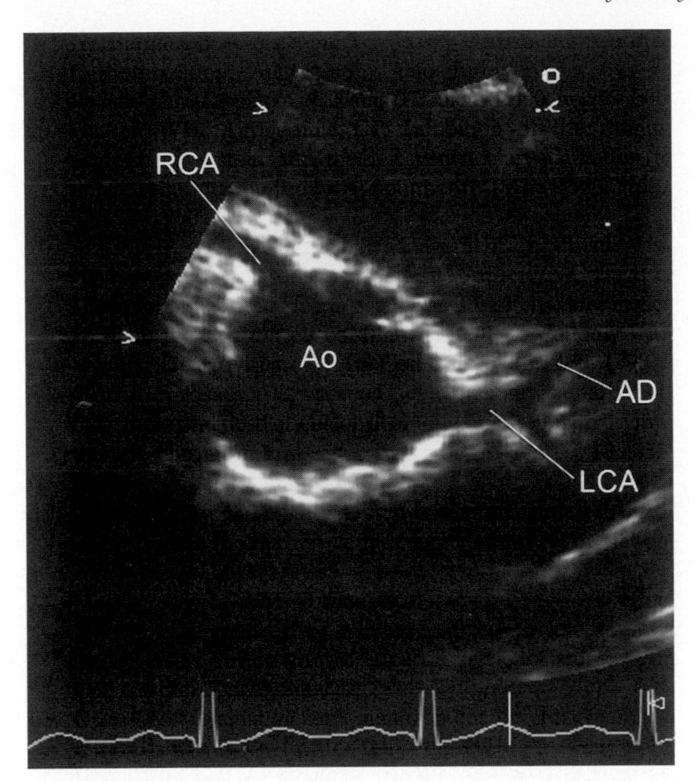

FIGURE 53–2 *Short-axis echocardiographic view at the level of the aortic root (Ao) demonstrating the normal origin of the right coronary artery (RCA), the left coronary artery (LCA), and anterior descending (AD) coronary artery.*

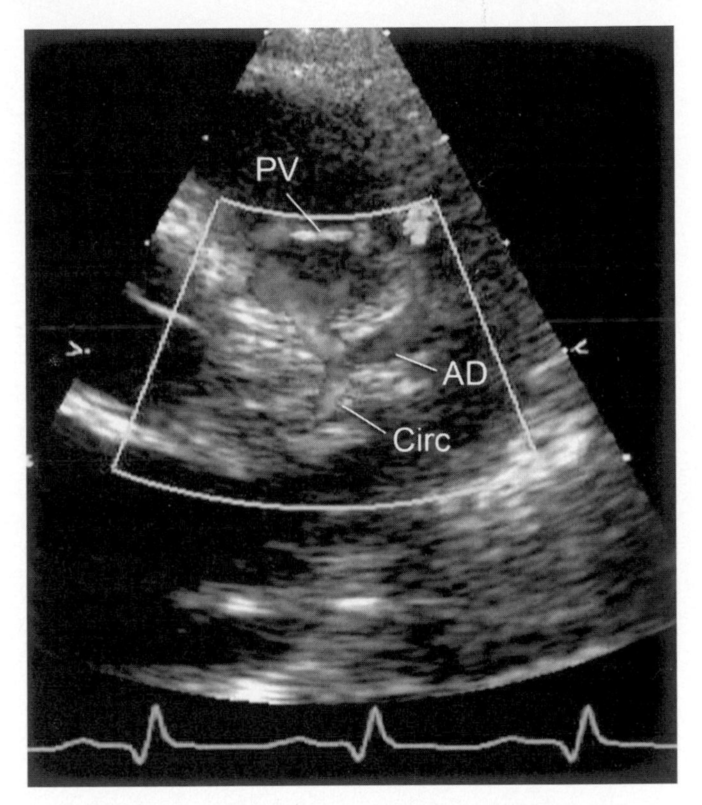

FIGURE 53–3 *Parasternal short-axis color Doppler echocardiogram of anomalous origin of the left coronary artery from the pulmonary artery. Flow in the anterior descending (AD) coronary artery is seen as a blue signal, indicating flow away from the transducer, which in this case is retrograde. Similarly, flow in the circumflex coronary artery (CIRC) is seen as a red signal, consistent with flow toward the transducer, which is also retrograde. The red jet entering the main pulmonary artery just above the level of the pulmonary valve (PV) is the flow signal from the left main coronary artery into the pulmonary root.*

If undertaken, the diagnosis is best established by injecting contrast in the ascending aorta or selectively in the normally originating coronary artery. The latter is seen to be large and often tortuous and fills through collaterals the left coronary artery, which in turn is seen to drain into the pulmonary artery (Fig. 53-4). In addition, findings of a dilated cardiomyopathy are usual with left ventricular dysfunction, as evidenced by an elevated left ventricular end-diastolic pressure and elevated left atrial pressure, usually demonstrable.

Management

After the diagnosis has been recognized and the infant stabilized with anticongestive medications, surgery is undertaken as soon as possible to provide a normal two-coronary circulation. Years ago, ligation of the anomalous artery was used to eliminate the left-to-right shunt to prevent a steal from the myocardium with some success but with significant early and late mortality. In the past couple of decades, a number of surgical techniques have been used to connect the anomalous artery to the aorta with considerable success. These include reimplanting, grafting, and especially the operation proposed by Takeuchi.[7] However it is accomplished, the desired effect is perfusion of the coronary from the aorta. Survival rates have improved significantly, and most patients become asymptomatic. The electrocardiogram generally improves, cardiomegaly on x-ray decreases, and striking left ventricular function improvement is seen echocardiographically.[8–13]

Course

The remarkable patient, electrocardiogram, and functional improvement are impressive, suggesting that the infant myocardium has a capacity for repair after ischemia and infarction that exceeds that seen in the adult. Continued observation is necessary because some require revision of operative connections or mitral regurgitation relief. At present, the future is very promising.

Among older patients, any evidence of cardiac embarrassment is a reason to connect the coronary artery to the aorta.

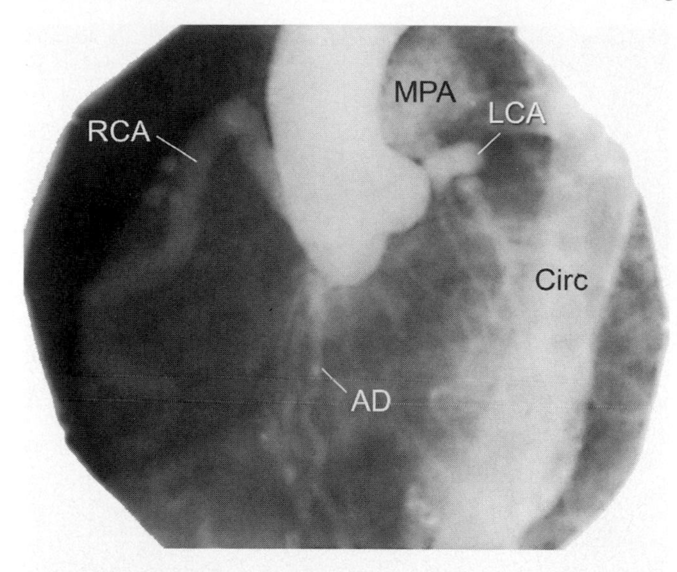

FIGURE 53–4 *Cineangiogram, lateral projection, showing dilated right coronary artery (RCA) arising normally from the aorta with contrast then passing retrograde into the anterior descending (AD) and circumflex (CIRC) branches to the main left coronary artery (LCA), which in turn empties through its anomalous origin into the main pulmonary artery (MPA).*

SINGLE SINUS CORONARY ARTERY ORIGIN

Abnormal origin of a coronary artery from another sinus or the other coronary artery remains an extremely rare anomaly, with only 15 being detected in our recent 14-year experience (see Exhibit 53-1). Sudden death, often with exercise, has been reported in some with this anomaly but does seem to occur only in those in whom the ectopic coronary (right or left) passes high between the aorta and pulmonary artery ("interarterial type")[14] (Figs. 53-5 and 53-6). Obstruction due to stenosis or intramural course may also be present and may be visualized by magnetic resonance imaging or intravascular ultrasound.[15] The passage of the ectopic left coronary artery from the right sinus through the conal septum ("septal type") is considered in some to be a benign anomaly.[16] Except for the latter, surgery is recommended for those with symptoms or whenever the interarterial type is identified.[17–19]

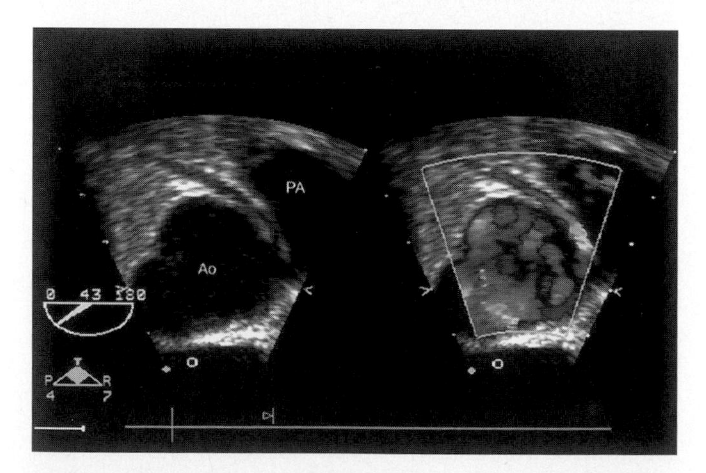

FIGURE 53–5 *Parasternal short-axis view of anomalous origin of the right coronary artery from the left sinus of Valsalva, obtained by transesophageal echocardiography. The right coronary is seen to pass between the aorta (Ao) and pulmonary artery (PA), and flow into the coronary is documented by color-flow mapping.*

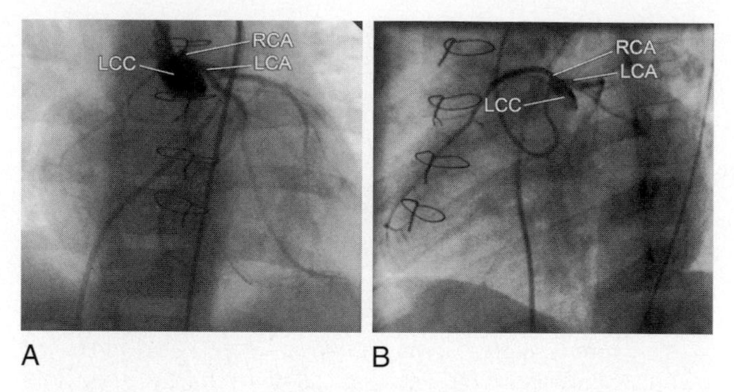

FIGURE 53–6 *Cineangiogram in the left coronary cusp (LCC) in anteroposterior (A) and long atrial oblique (B) projections, showing origin of both right (RCA) and left (LCA) coronary arteries arising from the LCC, with the RCA passing anteriorly between the aorta and main pulmonary artery.*

REFERENCES

1. Mesurolle B, Qanadli SD, Merad M, et al. Anomalous origin of the left coronary artery arising from the pulmonary trunk: Report of an adult case with long-term follow-up after surgery. Eur Radiol 9(8):1570, 1999.
2. Heiffetz SA, Robinowitz M, Muller KH, et al. Total anomalous origin of the coronary arteries from the pulmonary artery. Pediatr Cardiol 7:11, 2986.
3. Roberts WC. Anomalous origin of both coronary arteries from the pulmonary artery. Am J Cardiol 10:595, 1962.
4. Horisaki T, Yamashita T, Yokoyama H, et al. Three dimensional reconstruction of the computed tomographic images of anomalous origin of the left main coronary artery from the pulmonary trunk in an adult. Am J Cardiol 92:898, 2003.
5. Sanders SP, Parness IA, Colon SD. Recognition of abnormal connections of coronary arteries with the use of Doppler color flow mapping. J Am Coll Cardiol 13:922, 1989.
6. Karr SS, Parness IA, Spevak PJ, et al. Diagnosis of anomalous left coronary artery by Doppler color flow mapping: Distinction from other causes of dilated cardiomyopathy. J Am Coll Cardiol 19:1271, 1992.

7. Takeuchi S, Imamura H, Katsumoto K, et al. New surgical method for repair of anomalous left coronary artery from pulmonary artery. J Thorac Cardiovasc Surg 78:1, 1979.
8. Bunton R, Jonas RA, Lang P, et al. Anomalous origin of left coronary artery from pulmonary artery: Ligation versus establishment of a two coronary artery system. J Thorac Cardiovasc Surg 93:103, 1987.
9. Meahem S, Venables AW. Anomalous left coronary artery with the pulmonary artery: A 15 year sample. Br Heart J 58:378, 1987.
10. Schwartz ML, Jonas RA, Colan SD. Anomalous origin of left coronary artery from pulmonary artery: Recovery of left ventricular function after dual coronary repair. J Am Coll Cardiol 30(2):547, 1997.
11. Azakie A, Russell JL, McCrindle BW, et al. Anatomic repair of anomalous left coronary artery from the pulmonary artery by aortic reimplantation: Early survival, patterns of ventricular recovery and late outcome. Ann Thorac Surg. 74(5):1535, 2003.
12. Michielon G, Di Carlo D, Brancaccio G, et al. Anomalous coronary artery origin from the pulmonary artery: Correlation between surgical timing and left ventricular function recovery. Ann Thorac Surg 76(2):581, 2003.
13. Lambert V, Touchot A, Losay J, et al. Midterm results after surgical repair of the anomalous origin of the coronary artery. Circulation 94(9 Suppl):1138, 1996.
14. Liberthson RR. Nonatherosclerotic coronary artery disease. In: Eagle KA, ed. The Practice of Cardiology. Boston: Little, Brown and Company. 1989:614–651.
15. Angelini P, Velasco JA, Ott D, Khoshnevis GR. Anomalous coronary artery arising from the opposite sinus: descriptive features and pathophysiologic mechanisms, as documented by intravascular ultrasonography. J Invasive Cardiol. 15(9):507, 2003.
16. Yamanaka O, Hobbs R. Coronary artery anomalies in 126,595 patients undergoing coronary arteriography. Catheter Cardiovasc Diagn 21:28, 1990.
17. Steinburger J, Lucas RV, Edwards JE, Titus JL. Causes of sudden unexpected cardiac death in the first two decades of life. Am J Cardiol 77:992, 1996.
18. Barth CW, Roberts WC. Left main coronary artery originating from the right sinus of Valsalva and coursing between the aorta and pulmonary trunk. J Am Coll Cardiol 7:366, 1986.
19. Romp RL, Herlong JR, Landolfo CK, et al. Outcome of unroofing procedure for repair of anomalous aortic origin of left or right coronary artery. Ann Thorac Surg 76:[2]589, 2003.

54

Vascular Rings and Slings

ANDREW J. POWELL AND VALERIE S. MANDELL

Airway obstruction in children and its accompanying symptoms of stridor and respiratory distress can be caused by intrinsic abnormalities of the tracheobronchial tree and extrinsic compression of the airway. Among the causes of the latter are selected abnormalities in the embryologic development of the aorta or pulmonary arteries, which may be grouped together as vascular rings and slings.

VASCULAR RINGS

Definition

A vascular ring is an anomaly of aortic arch development that results in complete encirclement of the trachea and the esophagus by vascular structures. Some of the vascular components of the ring may not be patent but rather consist of fibrous remnants such as the ligamentum arteriosum.[1]

Embryologic Anatomy

Knowledge of the morphogenesis of the aortic arch system provides a framework for understanding and classifying the wide variety of vascular rings[2,3] (see Chapter 2). In the early embryo, six paired arches form to connect the truncus arteriosus of the embryonic heart tube to the paired dorsal aortae, which fuse to form the descending aorta (Fig. 54-1). In humans, the arches develop sequentially and persist or regress, but are never all present simultaneously. In normal development, the first arches contribute to the external carotid arteries (Table 54-1). The second arches regress rapidly, and only a portion remains to form the stapedial and hyoid arteries. The third arches become the common carotid arteries and the proximal portion of the internal carotid arteries. The left fourth arch forms that part of the definitive left aortic arch between the left carotid and left subclavian arteries. The right fourth arch is incorporated into the proximal right subclavian artery. The fifth arches regress. For the sixth arches, the proximal parts form the branch pulmonary arteries, and the distal portions join the pulmonary vascular tree to the descending aorta via bilateral ductus, with the right usually regressing completely to leave a left ductus arteriosus. Between the sixth arches (the ductus) and the descending aorta are the paired dorsal aortae, which connect to the descending aorta. The seventh intersegmental arteries arise from the dorsal aortae and become the left subclavian and distal right subclavian arteries. When the right dorsal aorta regresses, as is usual, the definitive left aortic arch is formed.

In conjunction with embryologic anatomy, the hypothetical double arch model originally introduced by Edwards,[4] and modified, simplified, and redrawn multiple times since, helps one to understand various arch anomalies (Fig. 54-2). In this model, the ascending aorta divides into two arches, one passing to the right of the trachea and esophagus and the other to the left. These arches join posteriorly to form the descending aorta. From each arch, there is a segment that gives rise to the right and left common carotids as the first branches on either side, and the right and left subclavian arteries as the second branches on either side. A ductus arises from the proximal aspect of each subclavian segment. This model allows anomalies of the aortic arch to be conceptualized as variations in regression of segments of the hypothetical double arch.

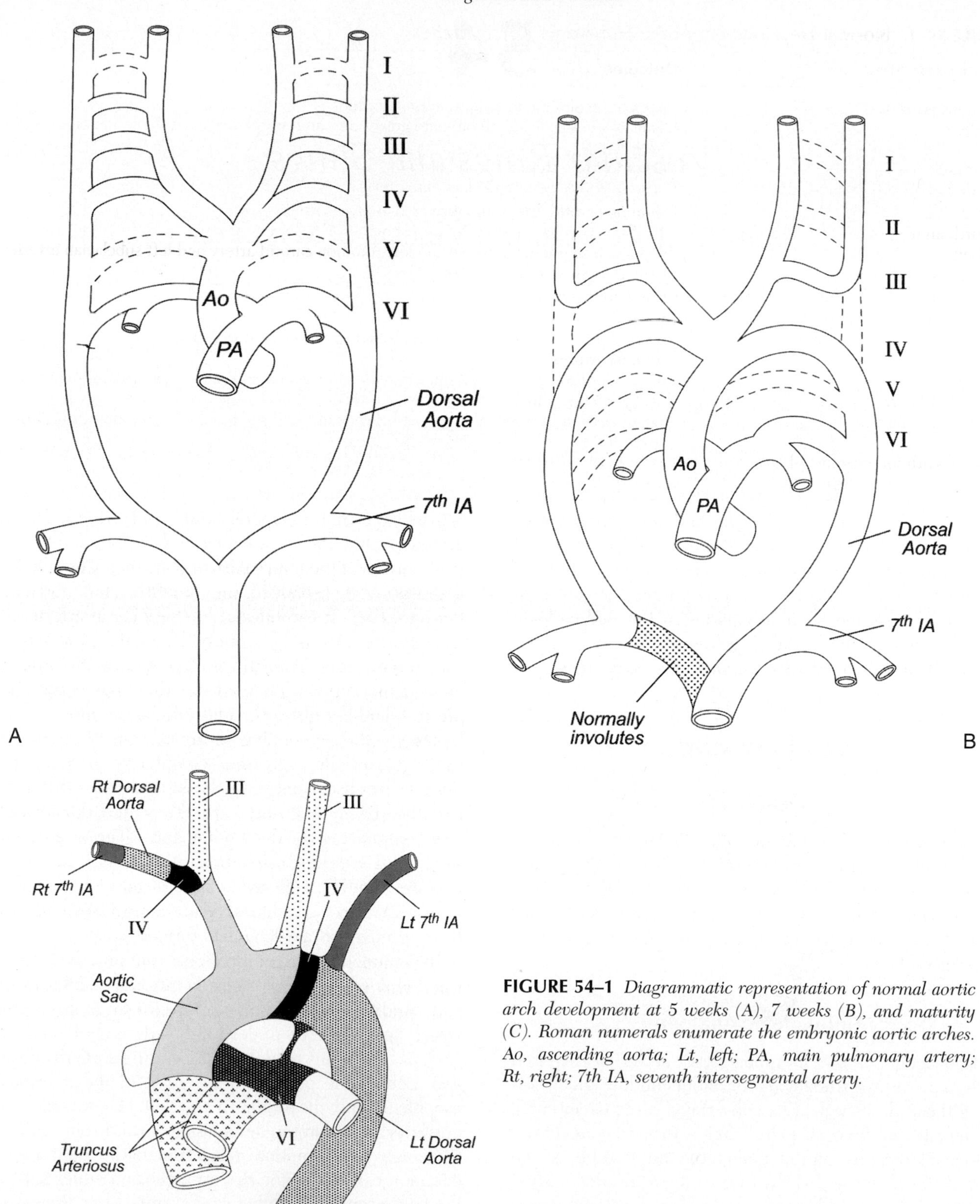

FIGURE 54–1 *Diagrammatic representation of normal aortic arch development at 5 weeks (A), 7 weeks (B), and maturity (C). Roman numerals enumerate the embryonic aortic arches. Ao, ascending aorta; Lt, left; PA, main pulmonary artery; Rt, right; 7th IA, seventh intersegmental artery.*

TABLE 54–1. Normal Development of the Embryonic Aortic Arches

Embryonic Structure	Outcome
Truncus arteriosus	Proximal ascending aorta and pulmonary root
Aortic sac	Distal ascending aorta, innominate artery, and arch to the origin of the left common carotid artery
First arch	Portion of the external carotid artery
Second arch	Portions of the hyoid and stapedial artery
Third arch	Common carotid artery and proximal internal carotid artery
Fourth arch	
Left	Aortic arch segments between the left common carotid artery and left subclavian arteries
Right	Proximal right subclavian artery
Fifth arch	Complete involution
Sixth arch	
Left	Proximal portion becomes the proximal left pulmonary artery; distal portion becomes the ductus arteriosus
Right	Proximal portion becomes the proximal right pulmonary artery; distal portion involutes
Left dorsal aorta	Aortic arch distal to the left subclavian artery
Right dorsal aorta	Cranial portion becomes the right subclavian artery distal to the contribution from the right fourth arch; distal portion involutes
Left seventh intersegmental artery	Left subclavian artery
Right seventh intersegmental artery	Distal right subclavian artery

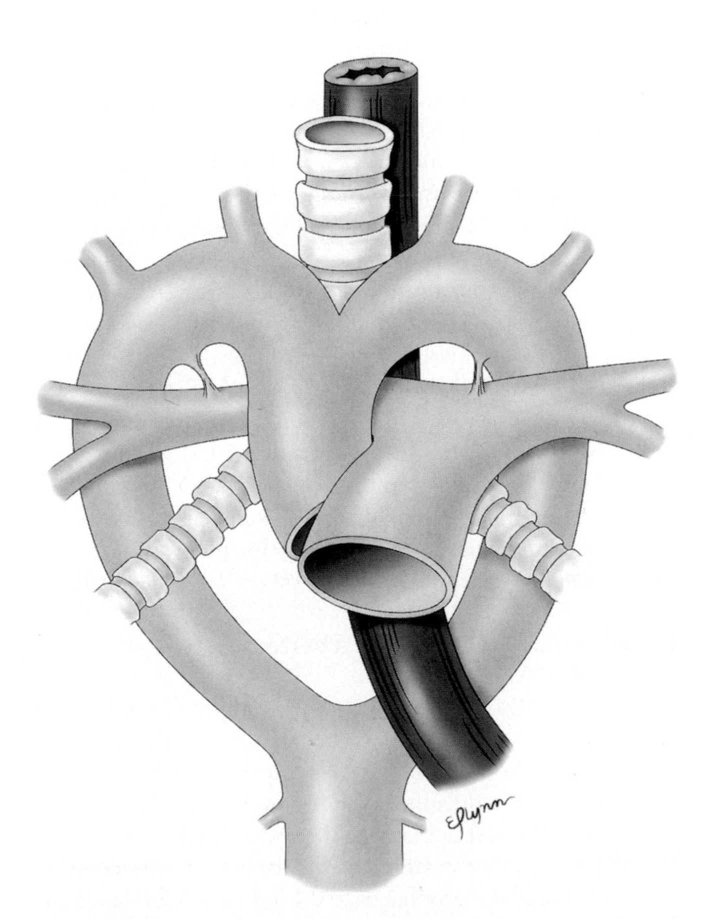

FIGURE 54–2 *Edwards' hypothetical double aortic arch with bilateral ducts.*

For example, beginning with the further simplified line drawing in Fig. 54-3*A*,[5] a number of anatomic situations can be visualized and illustrated. A normal left arch develops when the regression occurs between the right subclavian and the descending aorta (see Fig. 54-3*B*). Likewise, regression of the right arch between the right carotid artery and the origin of the right subclavian results in a left arch with an aberrant right subclavian artery arising as the fourth vessel from the arch (see Fig. 54-3*C*). Similarly, when regression occurs between the left subclavian and the descending aorta, a right arch with mirror-image branching is formed (see Fig. 54-3*D*). Regression between the left carotid and the left subclavian arteries results in a right arch with an aberrant left subclavian (see Fig. 54-3*E*). In the last instance, when the ductus arteriosus originates from the aberrant left subclavian artery (as it usually does), its insertion into the pulmonary artery creates a vascular ring. This model is easily sketched and can be used in daily practice to conceptualize almost every known arch anomaly.

Prevalence

Because some vascular rings may not cause symptoms, their true prevalence is difficult to ascertain. They are clearly a rare anomaly, and most evidence indicates that they represent about 1% to 3% of congenital cardiovascular anomalies.[6] Based on surgical case series, a double aortic arch is the most common vascular ring, followed by a right aortic arch with an aberrant left subclavian artery and a left ligamentum (ductus).[7–11] Together these two

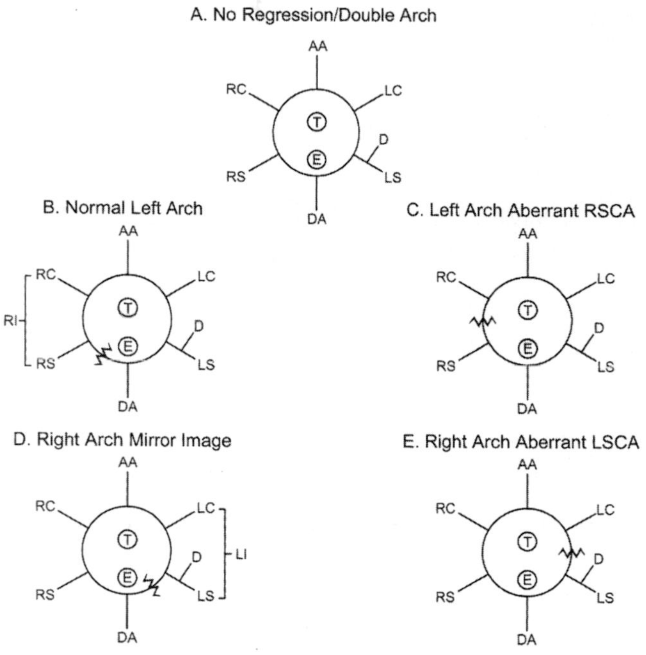

FIGURE 54–3 *Simple line drawings illustrating how anomalies of the aortic arch can be conceptualized as variations in regression of segments of the hypothetical double arch. The jagged line indicates regression of that arch segment. AA, ascending aorta; D, ductus; DA, descending aorta; E, esophagus; LC, left carotid; LS, left subclavian; LSCA, left subclavian artery; RC, right carotid; RS, right subclavian; RSCA, right subclavian artery; T, trachea.*

anomalies compose more than 90% of all complete vascular rings and thus will be the focus of this discussion. A description of the rare types of vascular rings such as left aortic arch with a right descending aorta and right ductus, right aortic arch with a left descending aorta and left ductus, and right aortic arch with mirror-image branching and left ductus can be found in more comprehensive reviews of aortic arch anomalies.[1,12,13]

Usually double aortic arch and right aortic arch with an aberrant left subclavian artery are isolated anomalies, although they may occur with other congenital heart disease, most commonly ventricular septal defect and tetralogy of Fallot[10] (Exhibit 54-1). In contrast, right arch with mirror-image branching occurs almost exclusively with congenital heart anomalies, most often tetralogy of Fallot. In right arch with mirror-image branching, the ductus or ligamentum typically arises from the base of the left subclavian artery anterior to the airways and, thus, does not form a ring. Chromosome band 22q11 deletions are associated with isolated aortic arch anomalies including vascular rings, as well as with conotruncal cardiac defects and noncardiac abnormalities.[14] Because this mutation is often sporadic and clinical manifestations may be subtle,

Exhibit 54–1

Children's Hospital Boston Experience, 1988–2002
Number of Patients with Vascular Rings and Slings

Total	83	223
Major lesion	33	64*
Other major lesion	50	159
Patients with TOF (%)	19	5
Patients with VSD (%)	16	14

In the 1988–2002 group, of the 223 patients, 195 had a vascular ring, 29 had a sling (1 patient had both), 77 had a vascular ring division (36 by video-assisted thoracoscopic surgery), and 20 had sling repair that included tracheal reconstruction/aortopexy in some.

*Of these 64 patients, 51 had surgery with no deaths.
TOF, tetralogy of Fallot; VSD, ventricular septal defect.

genetic testing of any patient with a vascular ring should be considered.

Anatomy

Double Aortic Arch

In a double aortic arch, both of the embryonic right and left arches persist, arising from the ascending aorta, passing on both sides of the trachea and esophagus, and joining posteriorly to form the descending aorta, thereby completely encircling the trachea and esophagus (Fig. 54-4). A ligamentum (ductus) arteriosum usually contributes to the ring and is most often left sided. The carotid and subclavian arteries arise separately from each arch and are usually symmetrically positioned around the trachea. The right arch is larger than the left in about 75% of cases, and typically higher as well.[13] Occasionally, a segment of an arch (usually the left) may be atretic with a fibrous cord either between the carotid and subclavian arteries, or distal to the left subclavian artery. In such cases, the aortic arch branching pattern evident on imaging studies may mimic other aortic anomalies.

Right Aortic Arch with an Aberrant Left Subclavian Artery

In the hypothetical double arch paradigm, a right aortic arch with an aberrant left subclavian artery is the result of regression of the left aortic arch segment between the left common carotid and subclavian segments (see Fig. 54-3*E*). As a result, the left subclavian artery originates as the last branch from the aortic arch, at a relatively posterior location, coursing behind the esophagus to the left arm. A left ligamentum (ductus) arteriosum originates from a bulbous dilation at the base of the left subclavian artery (the diverticulum

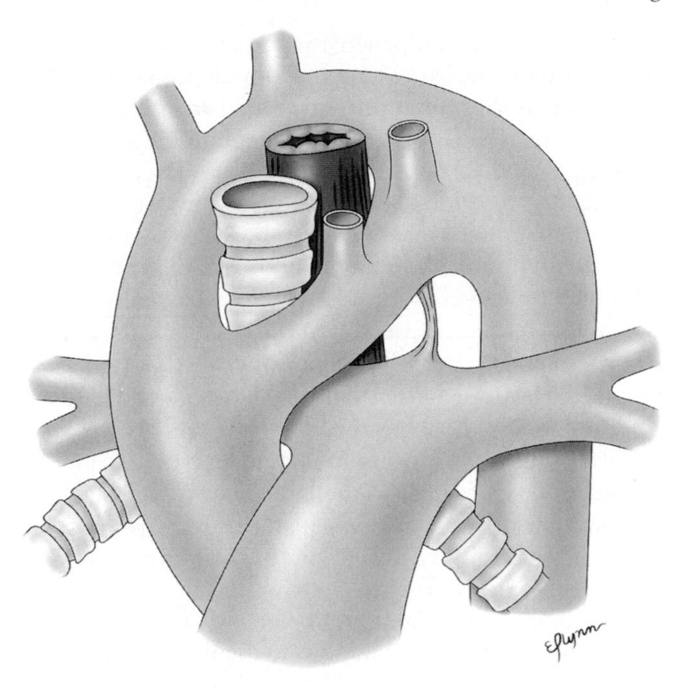

FIGURE 54–4 *Drawing of a double aortic arch. The ring encircling the trachea and esophagus is composed of the right and left aortic arches and the ductal ligament.*

of Kommerell) and attaches to the left pulmonary artery, effectively pulling the aorta and the diverticulum forward, compressing the esophagus and trachea, and forming a ring (Fig. 54-5). Rarely, the ductus arteriosus is right-sided and connects the right pulmonary artery to the right-sided aortic arch, and thus no vascular ring is formed. In such cases, there is no diverticulum of Kommerell, and the caliber of the left subclavian artery is uniform throughout.

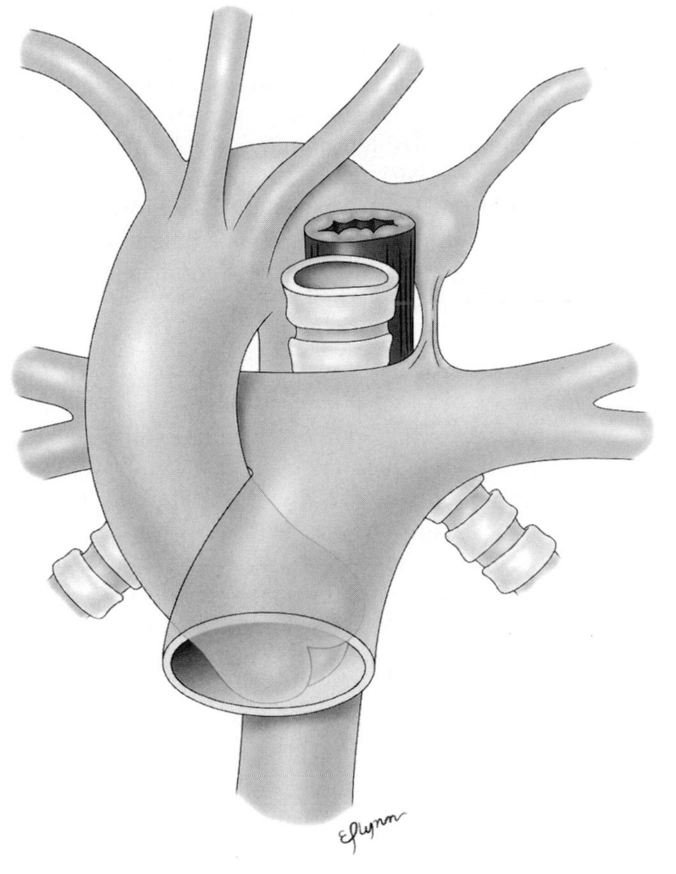

FIGURE 54–5 *Drawing of a right aortic arch with an aberrant origin of the left subclavian artery. The ring encircling the trachea and esophagus is composed of the right aortic arch, base of the left subclavian artery (diverticulum of Kommerell), and the left-sided ductal ligament.*

Clinical Manifestations

Symptoms

The symptoms of vascular rings are due to tracheal compression and, less commonly, to esophageal compression. Patients with double aortic arch usually present in early infancy with symptoms that include stridor, dyspnea, and a barking cough, all of which are worse during feeding or exertion.[8–11] "Reflex" apnea lasting seconds or even minutes may be triggered by feeding. Older children may have a history of chronic cough or wheezing misdiagnosed as asthma. Recurrent respiratory infections may be a result of aspiration or inadequate clearing of secretions. Symptoms related to esophageal compression are less frequent and less well defined. They include vomiting, choking, and nonspecific feeding difficulties in infants, and dysphagia and slow eating in older children.

In most patients with a right aortic arch, an aberrant left subclavian artery, and a left ligamentum, the ring is loose and causes no symptoms. The diagnosis is often discovered when imaging studies are performed for other reasons. However, in some cases, the ligamentum (ductus) arteriosum is short, or the diverticulum of Kommerell is especially large, and, thus, the ring may be tight. These patients have symptoms identical to those of patients with a double aortic arch. Occasionally, an older individual will complain of mild dysphagia as the aorta and left subclavian artery become larger and more tortuous and impinge on the posterior aspect of the esophagus because of tethering by the ligamentum. Similar symptoms may occur in older patients with a left arch and a retroesophageal aberrant right subclavian artery, even without a right-sided ligamentum. The latter condition has been referred to as *dysphagia lusoria* (from the Latin, *lusus naturae*, "prank of nature").

Physical Examination

Symptomatic infants show signs of increased respiratory work such as intercostal retractions and nasal flaring. Sometimes they lie with the back arched and the neck extended, which probably minimizes tracheal narrowing. Auscultation may reveal coarse upper airway sounds and wheezing. Mild intermittent cyanosis may be present. In patients with a right arch, an aberrant left subclavian, and a left ligamentum in whom the ring is loose, the physical examination will be completely normal.

Diagnostic Imaging

The diagnosis of vascular rings requires a high index of suspicion because of the relative infrequency of this entity compared with other conditions that cause respiratory distress in children, such as asthma, respiratory infection, and reflux. Once suspected, diagnostic imaging studies should be obtained with the goals of (1) identifying the cause of a patient's symptoms by demonstrating the relevant vascular and airway anatomy, and (2) preoperative planning. If video-assisted thoracoscopic surgery is available, it is important to determine whether the ring can be released by dividing ligamentous (nonpatent) or hypoplastic portions. This requires the diagnostician to have a high level of certainty regarding vessel caliber and patency throughout the ring. For both thoracoscopic and open surgery, the diagnosis must be established confidently enough to determine whether a right, left, or midline approach is appropriate.

Development of a single universal diagnostic imaging algorithm is complicated by varying ages and modes of presentation and the numerous specialists involved in such cases. There are no reported studies that rigorously compare different imaging strategies with respect to accuracy, patient safety, and cost-effectiveness. In practice, a center's diagnostic testing algorithm is tailored to fit local expertise, experience, costs, and available technology. The approach is then individualized to the patient, taking into account severity of symptoms, previous findings, age, and other medical conditions. It is important to note that no imaging modality except direct visualization can show ligamentous or atretic structures. Their presence is typically inferred based on anatomic patterns, the position of vessels, and the presence of a diverticulum.

Plain chest radiographs in posteroanterior and lateral views are a logical starting point for all cases.[15] Common findings suggesting the presence of a vascular ring are a right-sided aortic arch impression on the trachea on the posteroanterior view and anterior bowing of the airway on the lateral view (Fig. 54-6). The utility of chest radiographs in infants, however, is often limited because thymic tissue frequently obscures the superior mediastinum. Moreover, findings on radiographs are often nonspecific for the particular type of ring.

Barium contrast esophagograms reveal indentations on the esophagus caused by prominent arch segments.[16] This procedure is usually sufficient to determine whether a vascular ring is the likely cause of symptoms. A main drawback is its limited depiction of the vasculature and thus inability to determine the exact anatomy. It is clearly insufficient to determine whether a video-assisted thoracoscopic approach with division of a ligament can be offered. Bronchoscopy provides excellent visualization of the airway yet poor depiction of the vasculature. Because of this limitation, as well as its invasiveness and risk, it is not indicated for diagnosis if other tests suggest a vascular ring. It should be considered when primary tracheal abnormalities are suspected and noninvasive imaging is inconclusive. X-ray angiography can provide excellent visualization of the aortic vasculature, but care must be taken to avoid misdiagnosis from overlapping structures. Airway and vascular relationships, as well as the degree of airway compression, can be difficult to determine. Given its invasive nature and relatively high expense, x-ray angiography has been supplanted by noninvasive techniques. Echocardiography can provide good depiction of the relevant vasculature and in many cases is sufficient for diagnosis and surgical planning[17,18] (Fig. 54-7). It has the additional advantage of being able to define associated cardiovascular anomalies. Its principal weakness is poor visualization of the airway. In addition, some patients may have diminished acoustic windows, and portions of the dorsal aortic arch may be obscured by the trachea. In contrast, both magnetic resonance imaging and computer tomography clearly define the vasculature, the airway, and their three-dimensional relationship with high reliability and accuracy[19,20] (Figs. 54-8 and 54-9). The disadvantages of computer tomography are the rapid administration of an iodinated contrast bolus and the use of ionizing radiation. For echocardiography, magnetic resonance imaging, and computer tomography, younger patients typically require sedation to reliably obtain high-quality studies. Magnetic resonance examinations are currently longer and require more patient cooperation than computer tomography and echocardiography studies, and thus patients will usually have to be older (4 to 6 years) before these examinations can be performed without sedation.

Management

Surgical division of a vascular ring is the only definitive treatment. This was first performed in a patient with a double aortic arch by Dr. Robert Gross at Children's Hospital Boston in 1945.[21] Because in the current era the risk is small, prompt surgery is indicated for all patients with respiratory or dysphagic symptoms.[7–11,22,23] Asymptomatic patients, typically those with a relatively

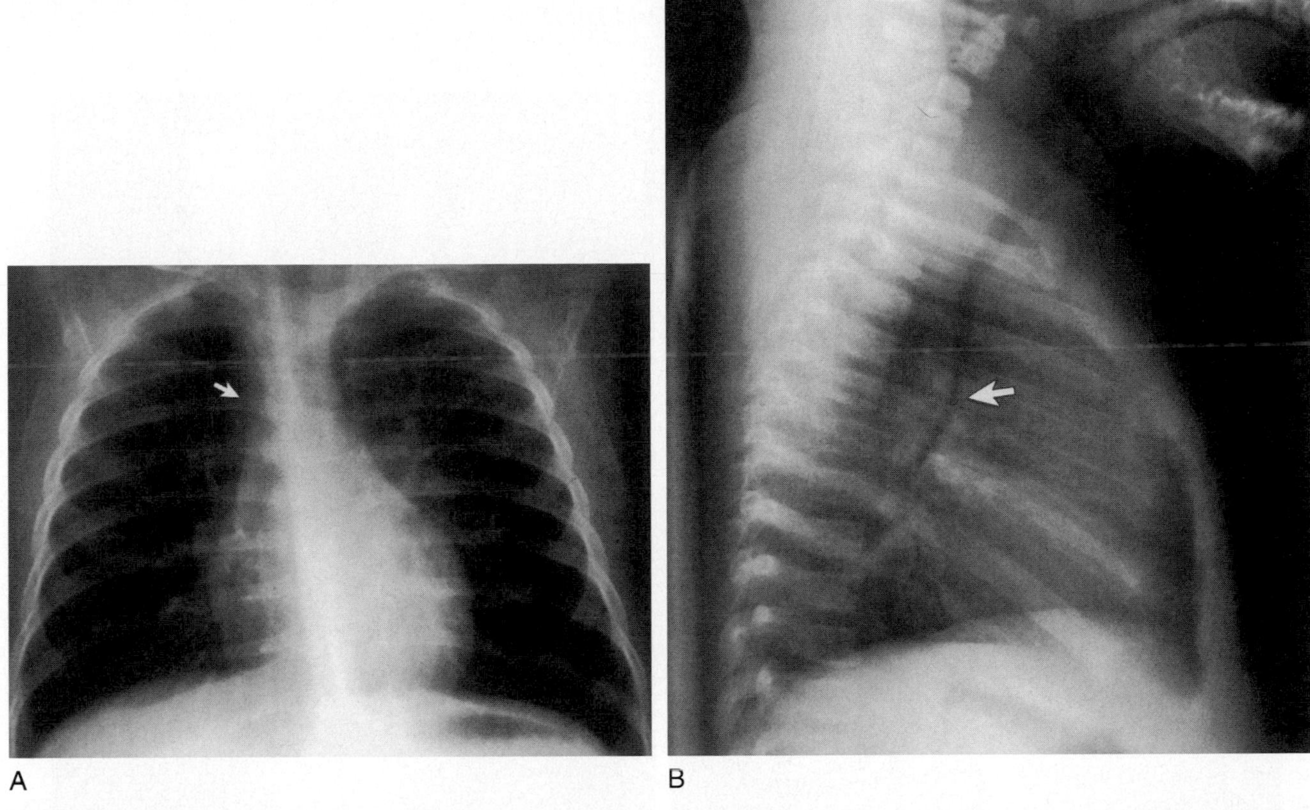

FIGURE 54–6 *A, Chest radiograph (posteroanterior projection) in a patient with a right aortic arch. Note the deviation of the trachea to the left caused by the right aortic arch (arrow). B, Chest radiograph (lateral projection) in a patient with a vascular ring composed of a right aortic arch and aberrant left subclavian artery. Note the anterior bowing of the tracheal air column (arrow).*

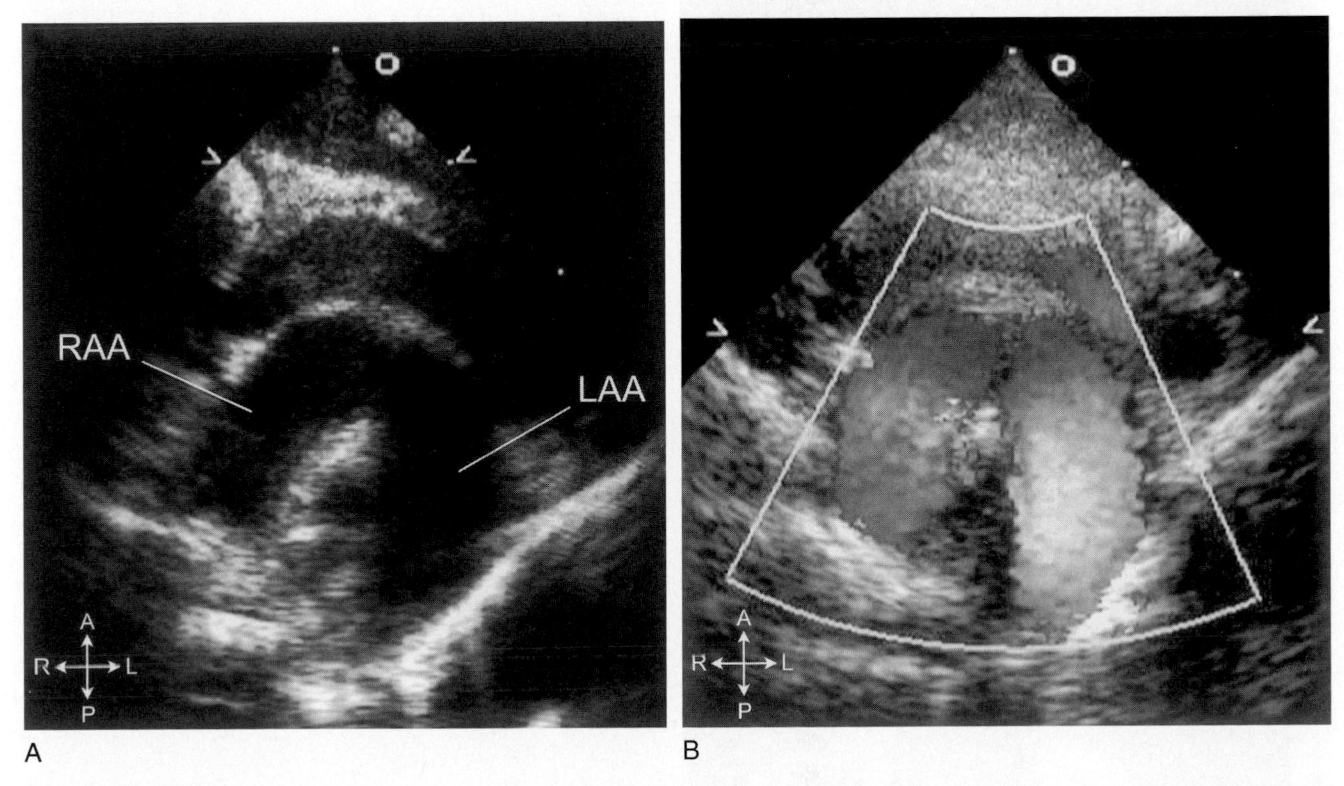

FIGURE 54–7 *Double aortic arch with both arches patent. Echocardiogram from a suprasternal notch view using two-dimensional (A) and color Doppler (B) imaging. LAA, left aortic arch; RAA right aortic arch.*

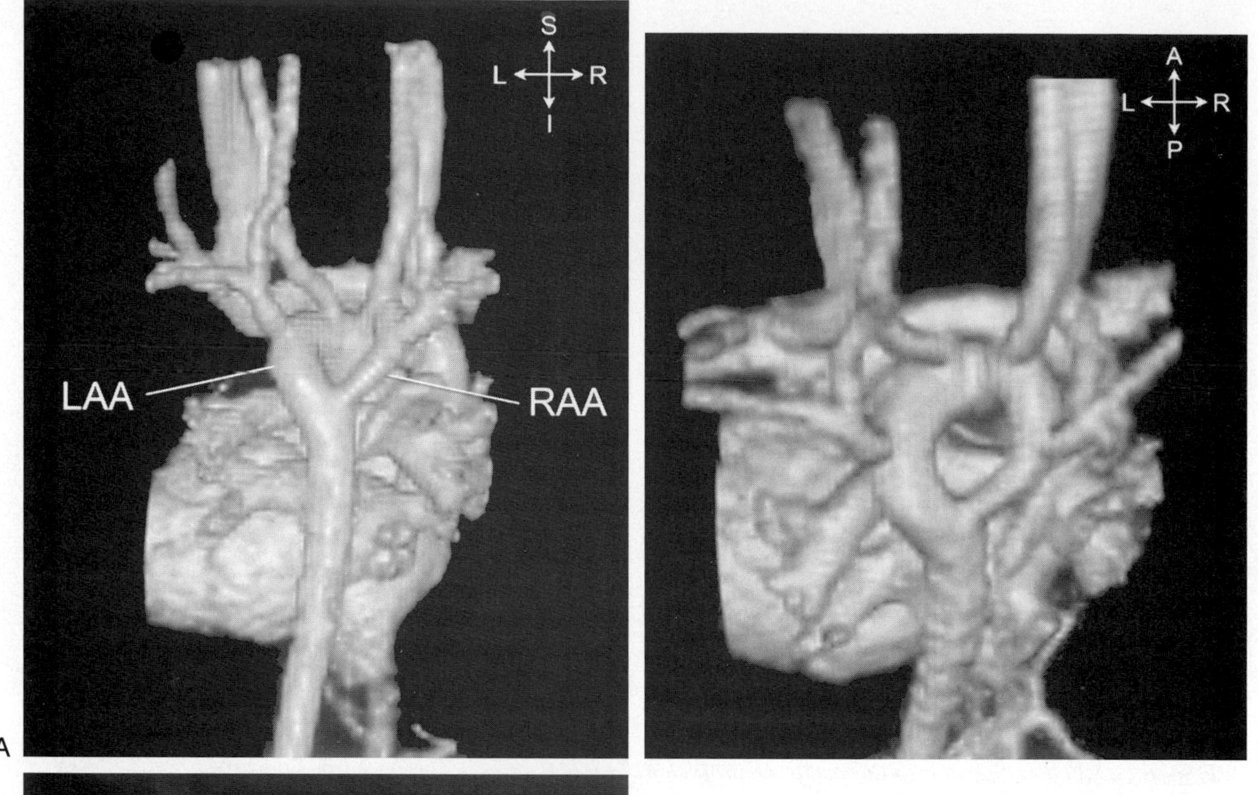

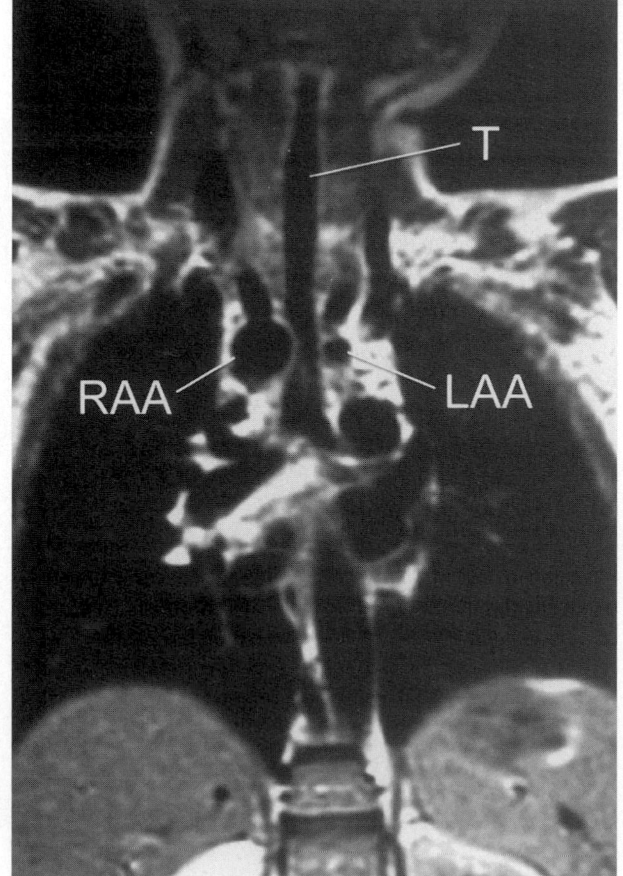

FIGURE 54–8 *Double aortic arch with both arches patent. Volume rendered three-dimensional magnetic resonance angiogram viewed from posterior (A) and superior (B) vantage points. C, MRI using fast spin echo imaging and blood signal suppression in an oblique coronal plane illustrating tracheal compression by the right and left aortic arches which are seen in cross-section. LAA, left aortic arch; RAA right aortic arch; T, trachea.*

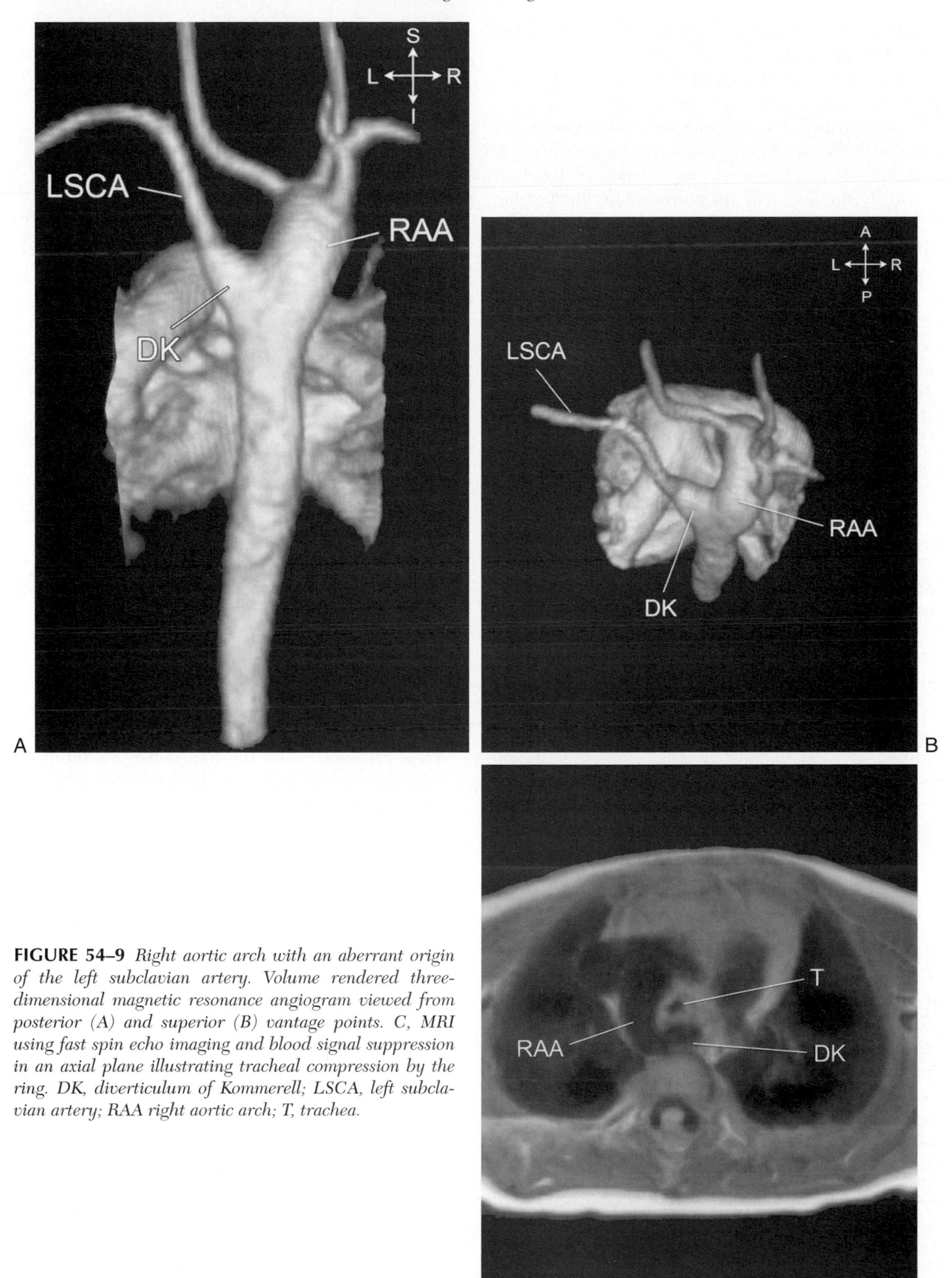

FIGURE 54–9 *Right aortic arch with an aberrant origin of the left subclavian artery. Volume rendered three-dimensional magnetic resonance angiogram viewed from posterior (A) and superior (B) vantage points. C, MRI using fast spin echo imaging and blood signal suppression in an axial plane illustrating tracheal compression by the ring. DK, diverticulum of Kommerell; LSCA, left subclavian artery; RAA right aortic arch; T, trachea.*

loose right aortic arch with an aberrant left subclavian artery, may be observed.

The traditional surgical approach for double arch, if the right arch is larger (as is usual), and for all cases of right arch with an aberrant left subclavian and a left ligamentum is a left posterolateral thoracotomy. In patients with a double aortic arch, division of the smaller of the two arches (usually the left) and any contributing ductal ligamentum is performed. In patients with a right arch and an aberrant left subclavian artery and a left ductal ligamentum, the ligamentum is divided, severing the ring and freeing the trachea and esophagus. Operative mortality is reported to be less than 5%, with most of the complications occurring either in earlier eras or in patients with additional intracardiac abnormalities[7–11,22,23] (see Exhibit 54-1). More recently, video-assisted thoracoscopic surgery has become the procedure of choice at Children's Hospital Boston to divide rings with ligamentous or small patent segments[24] (see Exhibit 54-1). Advantages of thoracoscopic surgery compared with open thoracotomy may include smaller incisions, improved visualization, reduced postoperative pain, lower risk for chest wall deformity, and earlier hospital discharge. Computer-assisted (robotic) thoracoscopic techniques for ring division are now being developed to overcome some of the limitations of conventional endoscopic instruments[25] (see Chapter 59).

Normally after vascular ring division, there is an uncomplicated postoperative course with immediate improvement of symptoms. Parents and care providers should be aware, however, that complete resolution of noisy respirations caused by tracheomalacia may take months or even years.[9,11] Longer-term follow-up studies indicate that most patients are asymptomatic, although abnormalities on pulmonary function tests may be present.[6,8,9,11,26,27]

PULMONARY ARTERY SLING

Definition

Pulmonary artery sling, also known as *anomalous left pulmonary artery from the right pulmonary artery*, is a vascular anomaly in which the left pulmonary artery arises aberrantly from the proximal part of the right pulmonary artery and courses posterior the trachea and anterior to the esophagus to reach the left hilum (Fig. 54-10). This arrangement creates a vascular "sling" surrounding and compressing the trachea but not the esophagus.

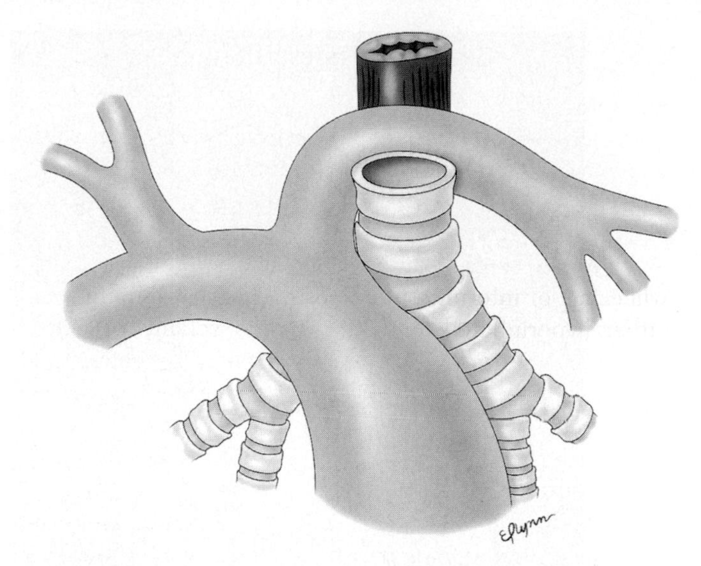

FIGURE 54–10 *Drawing of a left pulmonary artery sling. The left pulmonary artery arises aberrantly from the proximal right pulmonary artery and courses posterior the trachea and anterior to the esophagus toward the left hilum.*

Embryology and Anatomy

Normally, the distal pulmonary arteries arise from their respective lung buds and join the proximal pulmonary arteries, which have formed from the sixth aortic arch.[2] A pulmonary artery sling has been hypothesized to occur when the proximal part of the left sixth arch regresses or fails to develop its normal connections to the left lung bud and a "collateral" vessel to the left lung develops. This vessel originates from the transverse portion of the right pulmonary artery, just to the right of the trachea, and then curves posteriorly and sharply to the left, superior and posterior to the right main bronchus and trachea, but anterior to the esophagus in its course to the left hilum and lung. The ligamentum (ductus) arteriosum is positioned to the left of the trachea and connects the descending aorta to the distal main pulmonary artery. This anatomic arrangement causes constriction of the right main bronchus or trachea, or both. In at least half of the cases, there are associated complete cartilaginous tracheal rings in which the posterior membranous portion of the trachea and proximal bronchi is absent and the tracheal cartilage is circumferential, the so-called ring–sling complex.[28] The complete rings may be localized to the area adjacent to the sling or extend throughout the trachea. Complete rings are often but not always associated with significant airway narrowing and may be an important source of airway symptoms in addition to the sling itself. Other abnormalities associated with left pulmonary artery sling include a tracheal origin of the right upper lobe bronchus, hypoplastic left pulmonary artery, and atrial and ventricular septal defects[29] (see Exhibit 54-1).

Clinical Manifestations

Symptoms

Usually patients present in the first weeks of life with respiratory stridor and distress that is often severe.

Physical Examination

An affected infant may have stridor, dyspnea, tachypnea, wheezing, or intermittent cyanosis. The right lung may be either hyperinflated (and thus hyper-resonant) or partly atelectatic. Peripheral breath sounds may be decreased, and there may be signs of a mediastinal shift in either direction.

Diagnostic Imaging

Depending on the nature of right bronchus compromise, a chest radiograph may show right lung atelectasis or right lung hyperinflation from air-trapping. On a lateral chest x-ray, there may be anterior bowing of the lower trachea or right main bronchus, caused by the aberrant left pulmonary artery posterior to it. Barium contrast esophagograms often demonstrate an anterior indentation on the esophagus, in contrast to the posterior indentation seen in many vascular rings, but may be nondiagnostic.[16,30–32] Usually, echocardiography can demonstrate the abnormal origin of the left pulmonary artery as well as associated intracardiac abnormalities, and is sufficient to establish the diagnosis.[17,33] Because of the high incidence of tracheal anomalies other than simple compression by the sling, bronchoscopy is also warranted in most cases. This may be supplemented by computer tomography or magnetic resonance imaging as needed to ensure that the trachea, bronchi, and pulmonary arteries have been completely assessed[19,20,34] (Fig. 54-11). Angiography and bronchography are rarely indicated.

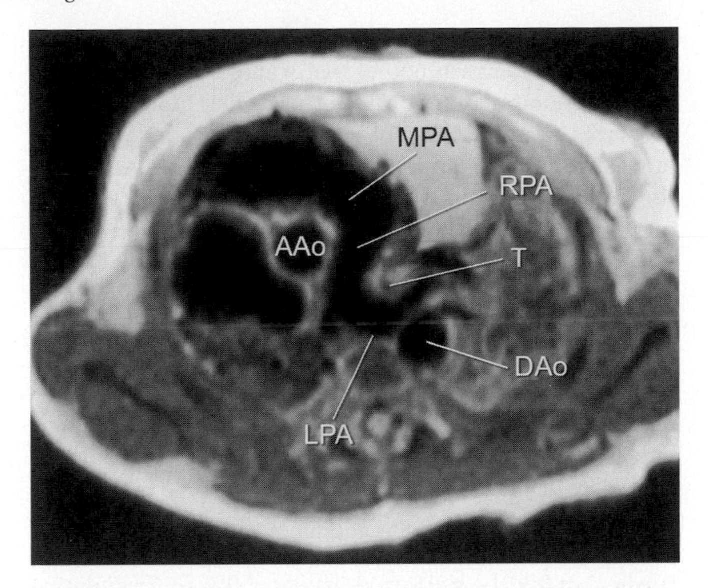

FIGURE 54–11 *Left pulmonary artery sling. MRI using fast spin echo imaging and blood signal suppression in an axial plane illustrating the left pulmonary artery arising from the right pulmonary artery and coursing posterior to the narrowed trachea. Note also the right lung hypoplasia and secondary dextrocardia. AAo, ascending aorta; DAo, descending aorta; LPA, left pulmonary artery; MPA, main pulmonary artery; RPA, right pulmonary artery; T, trachea.*

Management and Course

For the symptomatic patient, morbidity and mortality without surgical repair are high; therefore, prompt surgical intervention is indicated. If there is extrinsic tracheal compression without fixed stenosis, the left pulmonary artery is relocated from its right-sided origin and reanastomosed to the main pulmonary artery, anterior to the trachea.[35] Commonly, however, there is significant fixed tracheal stenosis, and the affected segment must be resected or a tracheoplasty procedure performed while on cardiopulmonary bypass support.[36,37] In this scenario with amenable anatomy, the undivided left pulmonary artery may be translocated anteriorly through the divided trachea before the airway is reanastomosed.[38] This technique avoids a vascular anastomosis and may therefore decrease the incidence of left pulmonary artery stenosis. Surgical outcome is primarily related to the extent of intrinsic airway stenosis and the severity of any associated cardiovascular disease.[27,35–37,39,40] Cases with mild airway involvement have minimal operative mortality and a good long-term outlook. Those requiring extensive tracheal reconstruction have higher mortality, may require prolonged mechanical ventilation, and often have residual airway symptoms. All patients should be followed longitudinally for the development of left pulmonary artery stenosis.

INNOMINATE ARTERY COMPRESSION SYNDROME

Innominate artery compression syndrome refers to children with symptoms of airway obstruction who are found to have significant tracheal narrowing where the innominate artery passes anteriorly to it.[41] Typically, localized tracheomalacia with dynamic airway narrowing is found, but it remains controversial whether this is primarily an intrinsic airway problem. Some reports have attributed the tracheal narrowing to a more distal, posterior, and leftward origin of the innominate artery from the aortic arch; however, careful studies have not found this to be a consistent finding.[42–44] Others have proposed that mediastinal crowding and an enlarged thymus gland contribute to the pathology. It is worth noting that some degree of anterior tracheal compression on a lateral chest radiograph is commonly seen in asymptomatic children and that it is normal for the innominate artery to originate slightly to the left of the trachea and to course immediately anterior to it.[42,45] Innominate artery compression syndrome is rarely associated with congenital heart disease.

Presentation is in infancy with stridor, which may be sufficiently severe to cause apnea or syncope. Feeding difficulties (e.g., poor weight gain, gastroesophageal reflux), as well as a history of esophageal atresia and tracheoesophageal fistulae, are common. The diagnosis can be made by a combination of bronchoscopy and computer tomography or magnetic resonance imaging (Fig. 54-12). On bronchoscopy, there is a characteristic anterior pulsatile indentation of the trachea 1 to 2 cm above the carina. The trachea should be narrowed at least 50% to 75% during spontaneous respiration to attribute symptoms to this diagnosis. Patients with mild symptoms should be managed conservatively because they usually improve over time.[46] Those with a history of apnea, severe stridor, or recurrent respiratory infections without an alternative explanation are candidates for surgery. The most favored surgical technique consists of an aortopexy procedure that lifts both the aortic arch and the innominate artery in an anterior and leftward direction by suturing them to the posterior aspect of the sternum, along with a partial thymectomy.[11,46] This low-risk procedure usually results in a dramatic decrease in stridor, although mild residual symptoms may remain because of tracheomalacia.

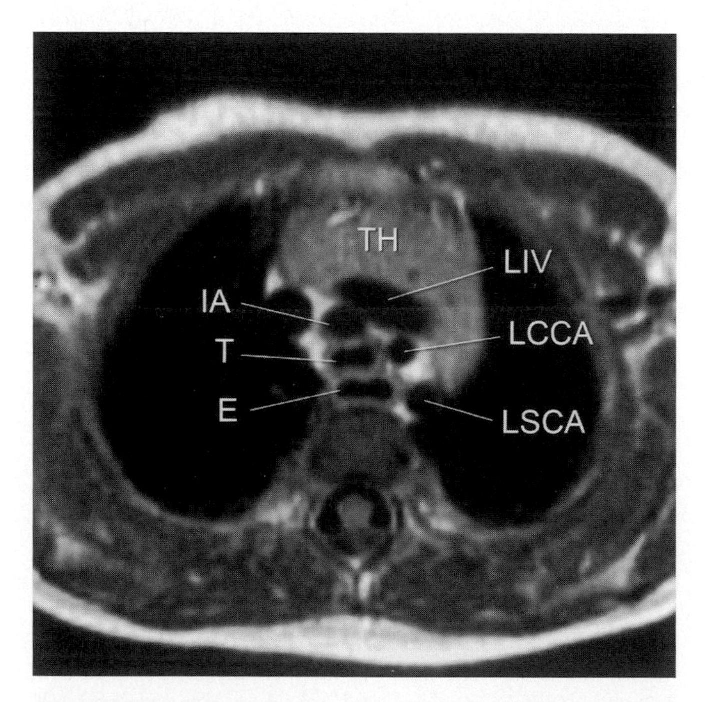

FIGURE 54–12 *Innominate artery compression syndrome. MRI using fast spin echo imaging and blood signal suppression in an axial plane illustrating a narrow trachea with the innominate artery located anteriorly. E, esophagus; IA, innominate artery; LCCA, left common carotid artery; LIV, left innominate vein; LSCA, left subclavian artery; T, trachea; TH, thymus.*

REFERENCES

1. Weinberg PM. Aortic arch anomalies. In Allen HD, Gutgesell HP, Clark EB, et al (eds). Moss and Adams' Heart Disease in Infants, Children, and Adolescents. Philadelphia: Lippincott Williams & Wilkins, 2001:707–735.
2. Larsen WJ. Human Embryology. New York: Churchill Livingstone, 1997.
3. Barry A. The aortic arch derivatives in the human adult. Anat Rec 111:221, 1951.
4. Edwards JE. Anomalies of the derivatives of the aortic arch system. Med Clin North Am 32:925, 1948.
5. VanZandt TF, Columbo CA, Danahy SA. Aortic arches simplified. Radiographics 10:126, 1990.
6. Marmon LM, Bye MR, Haas JM, et al. Vascular rings and slings: Long-term follow-up of pulmonary function. J Pediatr Surg 19:683, 1984.
7. Dodge-Khatami A, Tulevski II, Hitchcock JF, et al. Vascular rings and pulmonary arterial sling: From respiratory collapse to surgical cure, with emphasis on judicious imaging in the hi-tech era. Cardiol Young 12:96, 2002.
8. van Son JA, Julsrud PR, Hagler DJ, et al. Surgical treatment of vascular rings: The Mayo Clinic experience. Mayo Clin Proc 68:1056, 1993.
9. Bonnard A, Auber F, Fourcade L, et al. Vascular ring abnormalities: A retrospective study of 62 cases. J Pediatr Surg 38:539, 2003.
10. Woods RK, Sharp RJ, Holcomb GW, III, et al. Vascular anomalies and tracheoesophageal compression: A single institution's 25-year experience. Ann Thorac Surg 72:434, 2001.
11. Backer CL, Ilbawi MN, Idriss FS, et al. Vascular anomalies causing tracheoesophageal compression. Review of experience in children. J Thorac Cardiovasc Surg 97:725, 1989.
12. Steewart JR, Kincaid OW, Edwards JE. An Atlas of Vascular Rings and Related Malformations of the Aortic Arch System. Springfield, IL, Charles C Thomas, 1964.
13. Moes CAF. Vascular rings and related conditions. In Freedom RM, Mawson JB, Yoo SJ, et al (eds). Congenital Heart Disease: Textbook of Angiocardiography. Armonk, NY: Futura, 1997:947–983.
14. McElhinney DB, Clark BJ, III, Weinberg PM, et al. Association of chromosome 22q11 deletion with isolated anomalies of aortic arch laterality and branching. J Am Coll Cardiol 37:2114, 2001.
15. Neuhauser EB. The roentgen diagnosis of double aortic arch and other anomalies of the great vessels. AJR Am J Roentgenol 56:1, 1946.

16. Berdon WE, Baker DH. Vascular anomalies and the infant lungs: rings, slings, and other things. Semin Roentgenol 7:39, 1972.
17. Murdison KA, Andrews BA, Chin AJ. Ultrasonographic display of complex vascular rings. J Am Coll Cardiol 15:1645, 1990.
18. Lillehei CW, Colan S. Echocardiography in the preoperative evaluation of vascular rings. J Pediatr Surg 27:1118, 1992.
19. van Son JA, Julsrud PR, Hagler DJ, et al. Imaging strategies for vascular rings. Ann Thorac Surg 57:604, 1994.
20. Beekman RP, Hazekamp MG, Sobotka MA, et al. A new diagnostic approach to vascular rings and pulmonary slings: The role of MRI. Magn Reson Imaging 16:137, 1998.
21. Gross RE. Surgical relief for tracheal obstruction from a vascular ring. N Engl J Med 233:586, 1945.
22. Arciniegas E, Hakimi M, Hertzler JH, et al. Surgical management of congenital vascular rings. J Thorac Cardiovasc Surg 77:721, 1979.
23. Roesler M, de Leval M, Chrispin A, et al. Surgical management of vascular ring. Ann Surg 197:139, 1983.
24. Burke RP, Rosenfeld HM, Wernovsky G, et al. Video-assisted thoracoscopic vascular ring division in infants and children. J Am Coll Cardiol 25:943, 1995.
25. Mihaljevic T, Cannon JW, del Nido PJ. Robotically assisted division of a vascular ring in children. J Thorac Cardiovasc Surg 125:1163, 2003.
26. Bertrand JM, Chartrand C, Lamarre A, et al. Vascular ring: Clinical and physiological assessment of pulmonary function following surgical correction. Pediatr Pulmonol 2:378, 1986.
27. Anand R, Dooley KJ, Williams WH, et al. Follow-up of surgical correction of vascular anomalies causing tracheobronchial compression. Pediatr Cardiol 15:58, 1994.
28. Berdon WE, Baker DH, Wung JT, et al. Complete cartilage-ring tracheal stenosis associated with anomalous left pulmonary artery: The ring-sling complex. Radiology 152:57, 1984.
29. Tesler UF, Balsara RH, Niguidula FN. Aberrant left pulmonary artery (vascular sling): Report of five cases. Chest 66:402, 1974.
30. Capitanio MA, Ramos R, Kirkpatrick JA. Pulmonary sling: Roentgen observations. AJR Am J Roentgenol 112:28, 1971.
31. Rosenberg BF, Tantiwongse T, Witttenborg MH. Anomalous course of left pulmonary artery with respiratory obstruction. Radiology 67:339, 1956.
32. Backer CL, Idriss FS, Holinger LD, et al. Pulmonary artery sling. Results of surgical repair in infancy. J Thorac Cardiovasc Surg 103:683, 1992.
33. Yeager SB, Chin AJ, Sanders SP. Two-dimensional echocardiographic diagnosis of pulmonary artery sling in infancy. J Am Coll Cardiol 7:625, 1986.
34. Newman B, Meza MP, Towbin RB, et al. Left pulmonary artery sling: Diagnosis and delineation of associated tracheobronchial anomalies with MR. Pediatr Radiol 26:661, 1996.
35. Backer CL, Mavroudis C, Dunham ME, et al. Pulmonary artery sling: Results with median sternotomy, cardiopulmonary bypass, and reimplantation. Ann Thorac Surg 67:1738, 1999.
36. Backer CL, Mavroudis C, Dunham ME, et al. Intermediate-term results of the free tracheal autograft for long segment congenital tracheal stenosis. J Pediatr Surg 35:813, 2000.
37. Grillo HC, Wright CD, Vlahakes GJ, et al. Management of congenital tracheal stenosis by means of slide tracheoplasty or resection and reconstruction, with long-term follow-up of growth after slide tracheoplasty. J Thorac Cardiovasc Surg 123:145, 2002.
38. Jonas RA, Spevak PJ, McGill T, et al. Pulmonary artery sling: Primary repair by tracheal resection in infancy. J Thorac Cardiovasc Surg 97:548, 1989.
39. Cotter CS, Jones DT, Nuss RC, et al. Management of distal tracheal stenosis. Arch Otolaryngol Head Neck Surg 125:325, 1999.
40. Backer CL, Mavroudis C, Holinger LD. Repair of congenital tracheal stenosis. Semin Thorac Cardiovasc Surg Pediatr Card Surg Annu 5:173, 2002.
41. Gross RE, Neuhauser EB. Compression of the trachea by an anomalous innominate artery: An operation for its relief. Am J Dis Child 75:570, 1948.
42. Fletcher BD, Cohn RC. Tracheal compression and the innominate artery: MR evaluation in infants. Radiology 170:103, 1989.
43. Ardito JM, Ossoff RH, Tucker GF, Jr., et al. Innominate artery compression of the trachea in infants with reflex apnea. Ann Otol Rhinol Laryngol 89:401, 1980.
44. Mustard WT, Bayliss CE, Fearon B, et al. Tracheal compression by the innominate artery in children. Ann Thorac Surg 8:312, 1969.
45. Strife JL, Baumel AS, Dunbar JS. Tracheal compression by the innominate artery in infancy and childhood. Radiology 139:73, 1981.
46. Jones DT, Jonas RA, Healy GB. Innominate artery compression of the trachea in infants. Ann Otol Rhinol Laryngol 103: 347, 1994.

55

Cardiac Tumors

GERALD R. MARX AND DONALD C. FYLER

PREVALENCE

Primary cardiac tumors are extremely rare in children.[1–5] Fortunately, primary malignant cardiac tumors are even rarer. Recently, the incidence of primary cardiac tumors in the pediatric age group seems to be increasing[2,3,5,6] (Exhibit 55-1). However, this apparent increase is most probably related to increased diagnosis, especially as relates to the advent of echocardiography in the detection of cardiac tumors in the newborn, but also in the fetus.[5–8] Despite the low incidence, these tumors have been associated with significant mortality.[3,9] However, with recent advances in detection, diagnosis, and medical and surgical management, the outcome for children with primary cardiac tumors is improving.[1–3,7,10]

PATHOPHYSIOLOGY

General

By far, the most common primary tumor in the pediatric population is the rhabdomyoma. In most recent pediatric series, rhabdomyomas constitute 50% to 78% of such tumors.[1–5] In the fetus and newborn, the rhabdomyoma represents 70% to 90% of primary cardiac tumors.[1,2,5,6,8] Past studies have emphasized that fibroma was the second most common tumor.[2,4,5] However, in a more recent analysis at Children's Hospital Boston, the myxoma was as common as the fibroma (see Exhibit 55-1), each accounting for about 7% to 10% of tumors. The next tumor is even less frequent—the pericardial teratoma. In the fetus and patient younger than 1 year of age, the rhabdomyoma and fibroma are more prevalent, whereas in the older child and adolescent, the rhabdomyoma and myxoma are more prevalent. Other reported primary nonmalignant cardiac tumors include hemangiomas and lipomas. Malignant primary cardiac tumors include rhabdomyosarcomas, angiosarcomas, fibrosarcomas, fibrous histiocytomas, and leiomyosarcomas. Fortunately, malignant primary cardiac tumors are so rare that they are reported as isolated cases. Primary cardiac tumors have been detected in children with congenital heart defects.

Rhabdomyoma

Cardiac rhabdomyomas are benign tumors composed of cardiac myocytes and thus considered by certain experts to represent hamartomas.[11] These tumors are well-circumscribed, lobulated, tan-white masses with a glistening surface.[1,4,5] Rarely are these tumors hemorrhagic or calcified, and thus they appear rather homogenous in texture. Although these tumors are not encapsulated, they are well delineated from true myocardium. These tumor cells contain large vacuoles of glycogen and strands of cytoplasm extending from the nucleus to the cell membrane, the so-called spider cell. Rhabdomyomas are multiple in 75% to 90% of cases and have a marked predilection for the ventricles, the left ventricle greater than the right, but are also found in the atria. Most often these tumors are intramural, usually involving the interventricular septum. When large, these tumors may invade the cavitary space, culminating in right and left inflow or outflow tract obstruction. Pedunculated rhabdomyomas have been reported. Importantly, rhabdomyomas regress in size, or completely disappear, in more than half of cases.[12,13] The observation

Exhibit 55–1
Children's Hospital Boston Experience
CARDIAC TUMORS

Type	1973-1987	1988-2002
	No. of Patients	*No. of Patients*
Rhabdomyoma	21	33
Fibroma	2	7
Myxoma	4	9
Pericardial	4	5
Sarcoma	1	2
Carcinoid	1	0
Unspecified	2	35
Total	35	91
Intracardiac Thrombi	44	372

The increase in tumors in the 1988-2002 period is proportional to the increased patient population whereas the more than 8-fold increase in the intracardiac thrombi number seen largely reflects increased echocardiographic use and equipment improvement.

that these tumors resolve has been attributed to inability of tumor cell division.[11] Additionally, in a histologic study using intricate staining techniques, regression of tumors has been attributed to cell necrosis, apoptosis, and myxoid degeneration.[14] Autopsy and clinical studies previously reported that about half of patients with rhabdomyomas have tuberous sclerosis,[15] but with more widespread application of echocardiography, this association in the fetus and neonate is as high as 78% to 90% of patients.[12,13] This syndrome is an autosomal dominant disorder with widespread tumor involvement of other organ systems including the brain, skin, kidneys, and pancreas and is often associated with complex seizures and developmental delay. Recent genetic studies have implicated tuberous sclerosis with gene loci on 9q34 and 16p13.[16]

Fibroma

Cardiac fibromas are predominantly single tumors involving the left or right ventricular free walls.[1–5,9,10,17] They rarely involve the septum, bulging into the right and left ventricular cavities. These tumors are firm, gray-white, circumscribed, and noncapsulated and may have a bosselated external appearance. They often have a heterogeneous texture with regions of calcification, cystic degeneration, and focal necrosis. Fibromas may appear to invade the myocardium, entrapping regions of myocardial cells. Histologically, these tumors are composed of fibroblasts, collagen fibers, and minimal elastic tissue. They can be quite large, cause inflow and outflow tract obstruction, and may entrap the mitral or tricuspid valve apparatus or cause distortion in the position and course of the coronary arteries. In contrast to rhabdomyomas, these tumors are not known to regress in size or resolve completely. In a few patients, we have noted that the size remains unchanged as the heart undergoes normal growth. Some, however, have been reported to increase in size.[5,10]

Myxoma

The most common primary cardiac tumors in adults are myxomas,[18,19] but these are infrequent in the pediatric age group.[1–5] However, they have been diagnosed in children of all ages, including the neonate.[20] Because these tumors are increasingly detected with advancing age, in a pediatric practice, they are most commonly found in teenagers. Myxomas predominantly are found in the left atrium but can also occur in the right atrium and in the ventricular cavities, and may be multiple. They are thought to be derived from mesenchymal tissue, and as such, they may include histologic evidence of a variety of structures. The characteristic cell is eosinophilic, elongated to polygonal, with an oval nucleus with a speckled chromatin pattern.[4] The stalk of the myxoma often arises from the fossa ovalis, and the tumor may extend to the left atrium, right atrium, or both. The long pedicle can allow the tumor to extend across the atrioventricular valve during diastole, and prolapse retrograde into the atrium during systole. Myxomas have a propensity for embolization, this occurring in 70% of pediatric patients. About 5% of myxomas are familial. Cardiac myxomas can also be associated with Carney complex, an autosomal dominant disorder characterized by multiple lentigines, endocrine overactivity, myxomas, and schwannomas.[21] The gene defect for this complex has been mapped to two loci, one on chromosome 2p and the other on chromosome 17q.[21]

Pericardial Teratoma

Intrapericardial teratomas are single, bosselated, encapsulated, grayish tan tumors most often attached to the base of the great vessels—that is, aorta or pulmonary artery. Rarely these tumors may involve the cardiac chambers.[1–4] The intrapericardial tumor is diagnosed in the fetus or newborn. These tumors are derived from all three embryonic germinal layers and are nonhomogeneous, consisting of cyst formations and regions of calcification. They are often large and may cause external compression of the great vessels and cardiac chambers. Intrapericardial teratomas may be associated with a pericardial effusion and tamponade physiology, especially if the cysts rupture into the pericardial space. They are rarely malignant and usually do not recur after successful surgical extirpation.

Other Benign Primary Cardiac Tumors

Other primary cardiac tumors include lipomas, hemangiomas, Purkinje cell tumors, and "valvar excrescences." Cardiac hemangiomas most often are single; can involve the pericardium, myocardium, and cavitary space[22]; and consist of large blood vessels and vascular channels that interdigitate with the myocardium. When large and causing symptoms, these tumors have been removed. However, cardiac hemangiomas have been reported to regress with steroid or interferon therapy.[22] Valvar excrescences can occur as fairly discrete fibronodular masses (fibroelastomas) or as rather amorphous accessory endocardial cushion tissue. Such masses may interfere with valve function or significantly impede valvar flow. The very rare Purkinje cell tumors have been associated with intractable dysrhythmias.[5]

Primary Malignant Cardiac Tumors

Fortunately, primary malignant cardiac tumors are exceedingly rare in children[1,3,4] (see Exhibit 55-1). Even with the increased diagnosis of primary cardiac tumors seen in recent years, no similar increase in detection has been noted for primary malignant cardiac tumors.

Thrombi

At Children's Hospital Boston, a significant increase in diagnosis of intracardiac thrombi has occurred over the recent 14-year period (see Exhibit 55-1). This increase in detection is certainly related to application of noninvasive imaging technology including transthoracic echocardiography in postoperative newborns, infants, and children. Additionally, the application of transesophageal echocardiography in older adolescents and young adults with poor imaging windows has led to the increased detection of intracardiac thrombi. Despite improved imaging techniques, a significant increase in diagnosis is related to increased incidence. This increase has occurred as a result of the upsurge in critically and chronically ill children with the propensity for thromboembolic phenomenon. The propensity for thromboembolic phenomenon is exacerbated when such patients have indwelling central lines. Moreover, an increased incidence is certainly related to increased survival of specific substrates of patients with congenital heart disease, in particular those patients with single ventricle anatomy that have undergone various Fontan operations. Many patients operated on 20 to 30 years ago underwent direct anastomosis of the right atrium to pulmonary artery. Over time, these right atria have became markedly enlarged and hypocontractile and a site for thrombus formation, with swirling and stagnation of blood. This process is further exacerbated in patients with chronic atrial dysrhythmias. In addition to single ventricle patients, an alarming group of pediatric patients have recently been diagnosed with intracoronary thrombi. This includes patients with coronary artery aneurysms from Kawasaki disease, but also patients with hypoplastic left heart syndrome after various staged operations. The latter patients may have thrombus development within the native ascending aorta after the Stansel anastomosis, with thrombus propagation to the coronary arteries. Patients with dilated congestive cardiomyopathies are also at risk for development of left ventricular thrombi. In addition, thrombi are often noted early postoperatively in the vicinity of atrial suture lines or indwelling lines.

CLINICAL PRESENTATION

The clinical presentation of cardiac tumors has certain universal traits, owing to the conspicuous cardiac location. However, select tumors have more specific clinical presentations related to (1) predilection for anatomic region of the heart, (2) tissue composition, and (3) patient age.

Fetal

Cardiac tumors are increasingly diagnosed in the fetus; by far the most common tumors are rhabdomyomas. Many are detected by abnormal screening obstetric ultrasounds performed for a positive family history, especially as relates to tuberous sclerosis. Others masses are detected on a routine obstetric ultrasound with depiction of the mass on the standard four-chamber view. However, certain fetal primary cardiac tumors have been detected during evaluation of fetal dysrhythmias or pericardial effusions.

Neonate

When the tumors are large or multiple, they can obviously be associated with severe myocardial dysfunction and obstruction of flow across the atrioventricular or semilunar valves. This is often seen with the most prevalent tumors in this age group: rhabdomyomas, fibromas, and rare cases of pericardial teratomas and myxomas. Clinically, these cases may mimic hypoplastic left heart syndrome, with signs of congestive heart failure and low cardiac output. Right-sided tumors may mimic pulmonary or tricuspid atresia, and the neonate may present with extreme cyanosis. As in the fetus, severe atrial and ventricular dysrhythmias may prevail. Pericardial teratomas may present with tamponade physiology and the attendant physical findings.

Child and Adolescent

At initial presentation, the more likely tumors in this age group are myxomas and fibromas. Myxomas have a classic presentation triage of systemic symptoms, cardiac obstruction, and peripheral emboli. Systemic symptoms include chronic fever, malaise, weight loss, arthralgias, and myalgias. Embolic phenomenon can be systemic or pulmonary, depending on tumor site and presence of a cardiac communication. Embolic phenomenon has been attributed to tumor fragmentation, or embolization of thrombi on the tumor surface. In the adult or adolescent, myxomas or fibromas may present with heart failure, exercise intolerance, chest pain, or syncope. As noted earlier, myxomas may arise from a tumor pedicle and be highly mobile. Myxomas may prolapse across the mitral valve, culminating in sudden obstruction, and hence syncope. Fibromas, especially ventricular, may be associated with malignant ventricular dysrhythmias, and hence syncope. Occasionally the child and adolescent may present for evaluation of a murmur. Diastolic murmurs are evident when the tumors obstruct flow across the atrioventricular valves. Systolic murmurs occur with obstruction of flow across the semilunar valves. Certain tumors, especially fibromas, may envelop the entire mitral or tricuspid valve apparatus, culminating in a systolic murmur of insufficiency. Importantly, tumors may be detected during evaluation of patients with diseases such as tuberous sclerosis, Carney complex, or nevoid basal cell carcinoma syndrome.[23]

Obviously, any clinical manifestations may present in any age group, regardless of the tumor type. This is especially true for dysrhythmias, which have a fairly high association with rhabdomyomas,[7,13,24] and fibromas.[9,17] Significant morbidity and mortality related to dysrhythmias has been associated with primary cardiac tumors from the fetus to the adolescent. Obviously, the underlying cause of the dysrhythmias is due to the space-occupying nature of the tumor creating sinus node or atrioventricular node or bundle branch block. However, if tumors impede cardiac flow or cause myocardial dysfunction or extreme cyanosis, atrial and ventricular dysrhythmias may be a result of altered myocardial blood flow and oxygen delivery. Large rhabdomyomas and fibromas may directly compress, distort, or kink the coronary arteries. Preexcitation has been associated with rhabdomyoma, with the tumor itself serving as the alternate pathway.[24]

IMAGING MODALITIES

Electrocardiogram

The baseline electrocardiogram can display atrial or ventricular chamber enlargement. With large tumors, or tumors impeding coronary flow, S-T segment abnormalities may indicate myocardial ischemia. As mentioned, atrial or ventricular premature contractions or atrial or ventricular dysrhythmias may be encountered. Patients may have varying degrees of atrioventricular or bundle branch block patterns.

Chest X-Ray

Occasionally, a tumor may be discovered from an abnormal chest x-ray. The findings may depict an abnormal cardiac contour or cardiac enlargement (Fig. 55-1). Depending on the tumor, calcification maybe seen in the cardiac silhouette.

Echocardiography

Noninvasive two- and three-dimensional Doppler echocardiography has become the mainstay for the diagnosis of primary cardiac tumors in children (Figs. 55-2 and 55-3). Echocardiography certainly would be the most sensitive screening procedure when evaluating the pediatric patient because of a family history, a murmur, hemodynamic compromise, and an abnormal electrocardiogram or chest x-ray. Doppler echocardiography can demonstrate the presence of associated myocardial dysfunction, valvar insufficiency, and inflow or outflow tract obstruction. The echocardiographic depiction of the number, morphology, and location of the tumors may provide information to help differentiate the tumor type. For example, multiple tumors involving the ventricular chambers in the fetus and newborn would be

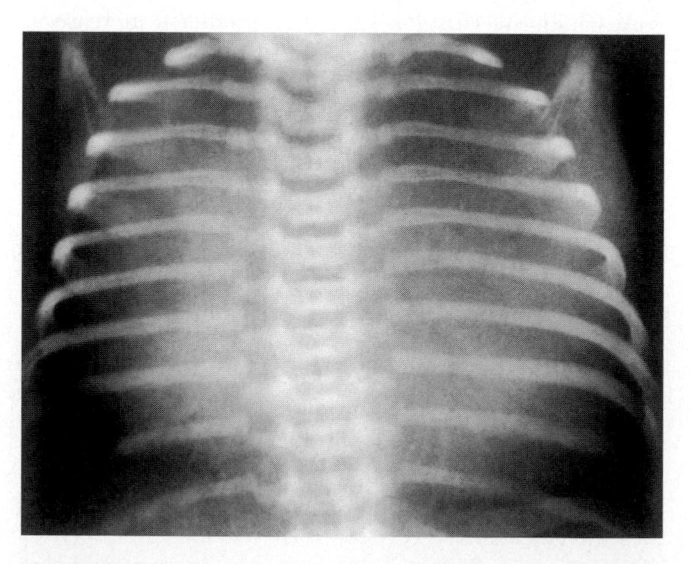

FIGURE 55–1 *Chest x-ray in a 2-week-old neonate demonstrating massive cardiomegaly. Initially the infant had multiple pericardiocenteses. Subsequently an intrapericardial teratoma was diagnosed and surgically removed.*
From Fyler DC [ed]. Nadas' Pediatric Cardiology. Philadelphia: Hanley & Belfus, 1992.

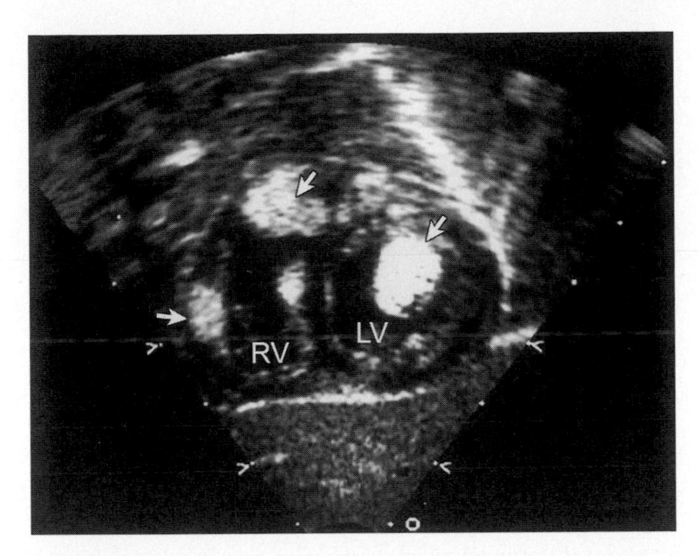

FIGURE 55–2 *Two-dimensional echocardiogram from a newborn infant with tuberous sclerosis and multiple rhabdomyomata (arrows) in right ventricle (RV) and left ventricle (LV).*

highly suggestive of rhabdomyoma. A single ventricular tumor in the fetus or newborn would suggest a rhabdomyoma or fibroma. Calcification, or variability of the tumor texture, would suggest a fibroma. In the fetus or newborn, a single intrapericardial tumor, arising from the base of the aorta or pulmonary artery, would be most consistent with an intrapericardial teratoma. An echolucent region of cystic necrosis, interspersed with areas of calcification, would help to confirm the appearance of an intrapericardial teratoma. A single atrial tumor arising from a pedicle attached to the fossa ovalis in the child or adolescent would be most consistent with a myxoma. However, it is important to note that considerable variability is encountered with all primary cardiac tumors in children.

Magnetic Resonance Imaging

Magnetic resonance imaging (MRI) can provide additional information as to the relationship of the tumors to the myocardium, great vessels, and adjacent structures, and also provide information about the tumor texture and encapsulation[2,22,25] (Fig. 55-4). Pediatric primary cardiac tumors can be differentiated on MRI signal intensity determination, and tumor tissue enhancement with gadolinium.[22]

Cardiac Catheterization

With present noninvasive imaging modalities, few patients undergo cardiac catheterization for determination of tumor presence or associated hemodynamic findings. Some centers advocate tumor biopsy at catheterization. In anticipating potential surgical intervention, angiography may provide important visualization of the relationship of the tumor mass to the coronary arteries. With improved gating and resolution, ultrafast computed tomography or MRI with contrast enhancement may provide optimal imaging of the coronary artery patterns in patients with large cardiac tumors.

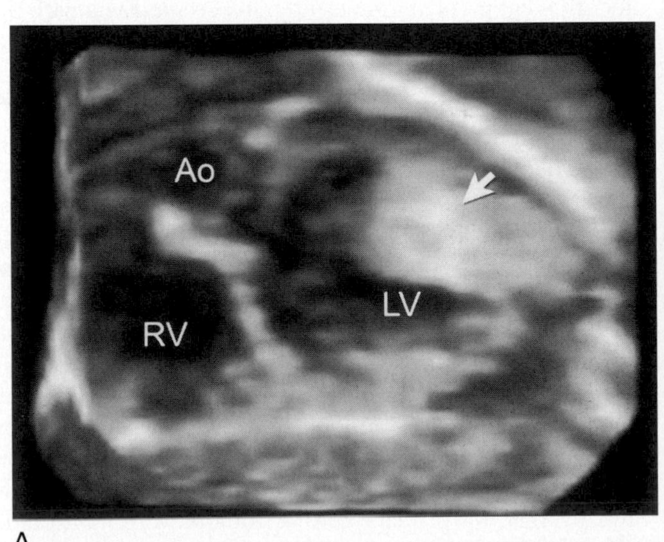

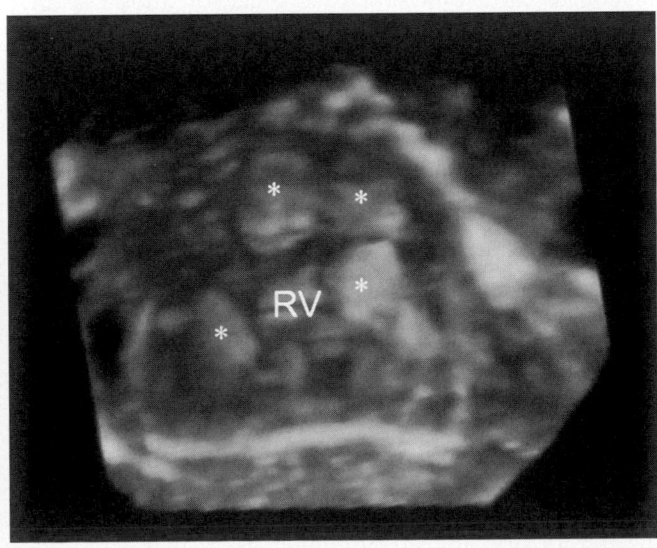

FIGURE 55–3 *A, Three-dimensional long-axis views of a massive left ventricular rhabdomyoma (arrow) in an infant with tuberous sclerosis. B, Three-dimensional short-axis view in the same patient showing multiple (asterisks) right ventricular rhabdomyomas. One was nearly occluding the right ventricular outflow tract. Surgery was not undertaken, and on follow-up, the infant had no cardiovascular compromise.*

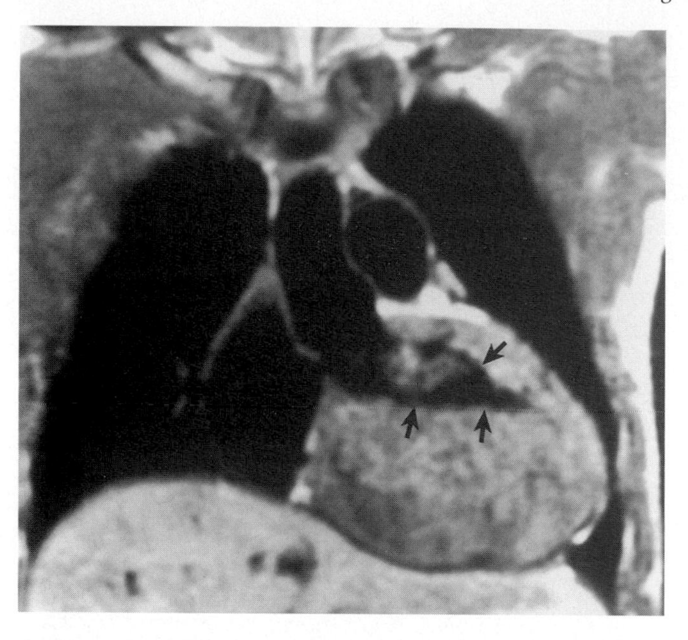

FIGURE 55–4 *MRI of a large intracardiac fibroma (arrows) from a 2-year-old infant.*
From Fyler DC [ed]. Nadas' Pediatric Cardiology. Philadelphia: Hanley & Belfus, 1992.

MANAGEMENT

The pivotal question concerning the management of primary cardiac tumors in children concerns surgical intervention. From a literature review and from our own experience, the following guidelines seem reasonable. Surgical resection of cardiac myxomas in pediatric patients at all ages is well established and supported by the universal propensity of these tumors to cause cardiac obstruction, systemic manifestations, and peripheral emboli. In addition, some pathologists have suggested potential for malignant transformation. Removal of all myxoma tissue is essential to prevent recurrence. Likewise, surgical removal, often on an emergency basis, is indicated for pericardial teratomas. Valvar excrescences should be removed when associated with significant valvar obstruction because these tumors do not regress. Presence of an aortic fibroelastoma may not cause significant obstruction but may be associated with serious embolic phenomena; hence, surgical removal is often undertaken. "Valvar excrescences" are usually easily removed.

Decision making concerning surgical intervention for cardiac rhabdomyomas and fibromas is more enigmatic. Certainly, consensus is fairly universal that surgery is indicated for primary cardiac tumors associated with life-threatening hemodynamic compromise. A large fibroma causing severe inflow or outflow tract obstruction and low cardiac output in a newborn, or syncope in an adolescent, should be removed. Although not encapsulated, the tumor is often well demarcated from ventricular myocardium allowing for "shelling out" of the tumor mass. Surgical intervention is generally accepted for a cardiac fibroma that impedes coronary flow that may lead to sudden death from ventricular dysrhythmias. The difficulty is that these fibromas might be massive, and surgical intervention could result in damage to the coronary arteries or valvar apparatus, or even culminate in serious myocardial dysfunction. Satisfactory results have been reported with debulking of the tumor mass. Ventricular tachycardia resolution has been noted after partial tumor excision.[10,17] Patients have undergone cardiac transplantation for massive cardiac fibromas.[5] Surgery is not generally indicated when the fibroma is small and not associated with ventricular dysrhythmias. However, fibromas have been reported to enlarge over time, and close follow-up is essential.

Many, if not most, cardiac rhabdomyomas regress in size or resolve completely over time. Hence, decision making concerning surgery for these primary cardiac tumors is more difficult. Again, if the tumors are associated with impending demise, surgical intervention should be undertaken. If the tumors are multiple and massive, tumor debulking with the potential for subsequent tumor regression might be advantageous. Cardiac dysrhythmias, such as preexcitation, have been treated successfully with radiofrequency ablation. Although surgical tumor removal for life-threatening dysrhythmias has been reported, even dysrhythmias have been noted to resolve with spontaneous regression. In general, however, in most pediatric centers, surgical intervention is deferred in noncomprising rhabdomyomas, even when massive and multiple.

In day-to-day clinical practice, however, the type of tumor identified at presentation is often uncertain. Even with the marked advances in noninvasive imaging, a specific diagnosis cannot be made in some. Surgical intervention decisions most often involve the newborn. Thus, knowledge of the prevalence of specific tumor types in this age group would aid clinical decision making, and several recent studies have been undertaken to shed some light on this issue. In a review of 14,000 echocardiograms performed over an 8-year period at seven centers, 17 primary cardiac tumors were identified in 19 pregnancies (0.14%)[6]; of these, 17 (90%) were rhabdomyomas, 1 was an atrial hemangioma, and the other a fibroma. Tuberous sclerosis was present in 10 patients (59%), 8 of whom had multiple tumors, all considered rhabdomyomas. Among those with a single tumor, 19% had tuberous sclerosis. In another recent echocardiographic review of fetal and age 3 months or less studies from five centers, 94 primary cardiac tumors were identified.[8] Of these, 84 (90%) were diagnosed as rhabdomyomas, and 68 (72%) of patients had tuberous sclerosis. All 64 multiple tumors were rhabdomyomas, 95% of which, and 23% of single tumors, were associated with tuberous sclerosis.

In another fetal study of patients with rhabdomyomas, 79% had tuberous sclerosis.[7]

Thus, in summary, of fetuses and newborns with a primary cardiac tumor, about 60% to 80% have tuberous sclerosis, and the tumors are most likely rhabdomyomas, especially if multiple. If the tumor is single, it is likely to be a rhabdomyoma in 20% to 25% of cases. In these patients, a complete evaluation for detection of rhabdomyomas in other organ systems is essential to establish the diagnosis of tuberous sclerosis. MRI can detect associated tumor involvement in the newborn and in the fetus, and the diagnosis of tuberous sclerosis usually means that a single tumor is a rhabdomyoma. Rhabdomyomas, especially in association with tuberous sclerosis, have a high propensity to regress or completely resolve. Some newborn infants with multiple large tumors creating hemodynamic compromise have been treated initially with prostaglandin E_1 to enable tumor regression over the next few weeks of life.[2]

Discussing the management of cardiac thrombi would entail a full chapter by itself. In general, surgery is rarely indicated except for embolic episodes, or when a massive thrombus impedes flow. The latter has been encountered in rare postoperative Fontan patients when a massive thrombus has occurred within the newly created lateral tunnel. Equally ominous are those patients with a fenestration, or tunnel leak, in whom a thrombus has been identified, leading to the possibility of systemic emboli. Thrombus formation has been encountered early postoperatively in patients with hypoplastic left heart syndrome, after the stage I or II procedures, and may be located in the pulmonary artery to native aortic connection, or in a coronary artery. In these early postoperative patients, thrombolytic therapy may be hazardous but is likely the first line of treatment in those chronically ill with an indwelling line. As mentioned, certain older Fontan patients are at risk for right atrial thrombus formation, especially with concomitant atrial dysrhythmias. These patients are often placed on long-term warfarin therapy. With high-resolution imaging or angiography, clot formation can be seen in the coronary arteries in Kawasaki patients. In such patients, medications to interfere with platelet aggregation might be most advantageous. At this time, it is reasonable to say that thromboembolic episodes are underdiagnosed as contributing to morbidity and mortality in children.

REFERENCES

1. Marx GR, Moran AR. Cardiac tumors. In Allen HD, Gutgesell HP, Clark EB, Driscoll DJ (eds). Moss and Adams' Heart Disease in Infants, Children, and Adolescents Including the Fetus and Young Adult Heart. Philadelphia: Lippincott Williams & Wilkins, 1995:1422–1445.
2. Beghetti M, Gow RM, Hanley I, et al. Pediatric primary benign cardiac tumors: A 15-year review. Am Heart J 134:1107, 1997.
3. Sallee D, Spector ML, van Heeckeren DW, et al. Primary pediatric cardiac tumors: A 17 year experience. Cardiol Young 9:155, 1999.
4. Becker AF. Primary heart tumors in the pediatric age group: A review of salient pathologic features relevant for clinicians. Pediatr Cardiol 21:317, 2000.
5. Freedom RM, Lee KJ, MacDonald C, et al. Selected aspects of cardiac tumors in infancy and childhood. Pediatr Cardiol 21:299, 2000.
6. Holley DG, Martin Gr, Brenner JI, et al. Diagnosis and management of fetal cardiac tumors: A multi-center experience and review of published reports. J Am Coll Cardiol 26:516, 1995.
7. Bader RS, Chitayat D, Kelly E, et al. Fetal rhabdomyoma: Prenatal diagnosis, clinical outcome, and incidence of associated tuberous sclerosis complex. J Pediatr 143:620, 2003.
8. Tworetzky W, McElhinney DB, Margossian R, et al. Association between cardiac tumors and tuberous sclerosis in the fetus and neonate. Am J Cardiol 92:487, 2003.
9. Verhaaren HA, Vanakker O, De Wolf DE, et al. Left ventricular outflow obstruction in rhabdomyoma of infancy: meta-analysis of the literature. J Pediatr 143:258, 2003.
10. Cho JM, Danielson GK, Puga FJ. Surgical resection of ventricular cardiac fibromas: Early and late results. Ann Thorac Surg 76:1929, 2003.
11. Fenoglio J, McAllister HA, Ferrans VJ. Cardiac rhabdomyoma: A clinicopathologic and electron microscopic study. Am J Cardiol 38:241, 1976.
12. Smythe JF, Dyck JD, Smallhorn JF, et al. Natural history of cardiac rhabdomyoma in infancy and childhood. Am J Cardiol 66:1247, 1990.
13. Bosi G, Linetermans JP, Pellegrino PA et al. The natural history of cardiac rhabdomyoma with and without tuberous sclerosis. Acta Paediatr 85:928, 1996.
14. Wu S, Collins MH, Chadarevian JP, et al. Study of the regression process in cardiac rhabdomyomas. Pediatr Dev Pathol 5:29, 2002.
15. Bass Jl, Breningstall GN, Swaiman KF. Echocardiographic incidence of cardiac rhabdomyoma in tuberous sclerosis. Am J Cardiol 55:1379, 1985.
16. Povey S, Burley MW, Attwood J. Two loci for tuberous sclerosis: One on 9q34 and one on 16p13. Ann Hum Genet 58:107, 1994.
17. Yamaguchi M, Hosokawa Y, Ohashi H, et al. Cardiac fibroma: Long-term fate after excision. J Thorac Cardiovasc Surg 103:140, 1992.
18. Miralles A, Bracamonte L, Soncul H, et al. Cardiac tumors: Clinical experience and surgical results in 74 patients. Ann Thorac Surg 52:886, 1991.
19. Fyke FE, Seward JB, Edwards W, et al. Primary cardiac tumors: Experience with 30 consecutive patients since the introduction of two-dimensional echocardiography. J Am Coll Cardiol 5:1465, 1985.
20. Van der Hauwaert LG. Cardiac tumors in infancy and childhood. Br Heart J 33:125, 1971.

21. Stratakis C, Kirshner LS, Carney JA. Carney complex: Diagnosis and management of the complex of spotty skin pigmentation, myxomas, endocrine overactivity and schwannomas. Am J Med Genet 80:183, 1998.
22. Kiaffas, MG, Powell AJ, Geva T. Magnetic resonance imaging evaluation of cardiac tumor characteristics in infants and children. Am J Cardiol 89:1229, 2002.
23. Cotton JL, Kavey RA, Palmier C. Cardiac tumors and the nevoid basal cell carcinoma syndrome. Pediatrics 87:725, 1991.
24. Mehta AV. Rhabdomyoma and ventricular preexcitation syndrome: A report of two cases and a review of literature. Am J Dis Child 147: 669, 1993.
25. Hoffman U, Globits S, Schima W, et al. Usefulness of magnetic resonance imaging of cardiac and paracardiac masses. Am J Cardiol 92:890, 2003.

56

Adult Congenital Heart Disease

MICHAEL J. LANDZBEG

In the early to mid 1970s, the establishment of the first units specifically designed to care for adults with congenital cardiac disease (Los Angeles, London) paved the way for future recognition of issues in management of congenital heart disease that can be more apparent in, and at times unique to, adolescent and adult survivors with congenital heart disease (CHD). Recognition of these complexities has led to awareness of new determinants of outcome, distinct from older anatomic considerations. The reader is referred elsewhere in this and other texts for the subacute natural and modified history of specific lesions observed into adulthood. This chapter will highlight some of the recent shifts in diagnosis and management paradigms facing the ever-expanding adult CHD population that now appears to have grown even larger in number than its pediatric counterpart. Initially under Heart Failure, a new paradigm with CHD, ventricular vascular coupling, pulmonary vascular disease, right ventricular dysfunction, and neurohormonal activation will be discussed and followed by a brief outline of current lesion management strategies in this population.

HEART FAILURE

Past assessment and review of the causes of heart failure in the adult with congenital heart disease largely focused on measures of ventricular systolic performance, typically emphasizing relationship with the "old baggage" of longstanding alterations of volume and anatomic loading conditions on ventricular function.[1,2] These issues not withstanding, there are a multitude of additional potentials for heart failure specific to, varying in, or first recognized in the aging patient with congenital heart disease.

Almost nowhere else in medicine does the categorization of a patient with "heart failure" carry so many pathophysiologic potentials as in the adult patient with CHD. Classic clinical definition of "failure of the heart (in whatever form it may be) to keep up with the demands of the body" is demonstrated by what may be considered premature senescence and decrement of not only cardiac function, but potentially by abnormalities and increased demand of nearly every organ system (Table 56-1). Increased potential for endocrinologic dysfunction, gas-exchanging and nonparenchymal lung disease, abnormalities of renal or hepatic function, and altered skeleton and muscle metabolism highlight the multitude of extracardiac conditions contributing to abnormal functional capacity or performance.

The adult with CHD objectively may be profoundly limited in aerobic functional capacity compared with normal controls.[3] Maximal achievable peak oxygen consumption (peak V_{O_2}) may be less than 50% of normal controls, with important reductions seen even in patients after repair of simple atrial level defects (Fig. 56-1). Restriction in ventilatory function (with respiratory volumes typically 75% to 85% normal predictions), whether due to developmental or acquired structural or physiologic changes, may contribute to fatigue and incapacity[3] (Fig. 56-2). Hepatitis-induced and "cardiac" cirrhosis, felt by many to be diseases of past medical generations, have found recapitulation in a patient population plagued by higher central venous pressures, potential for low systemic cardiac index, and continued exposure to blood products. The neurohormonal activation caused by portal hypertension may be profound, and it exacerbates volume retention and curbs functional ability.

TABLE 56–1. "Noncardiac" Potential Etiologies for "Heart Failure" in the Adult Patient with Congestive Heart Disease

Endocrinologic, neurohormonal
Hypothyroidism
Diabetes
Loss of adrenergic and vagal responsiveness
Pulmonary
Restrictive lung disease
Hypoventilation, obstructive sleep apnea
Arteriovenous malformations
Pulmonary vascular disease
Chronic parenchymal infection
Liver
Chronic hepatitis
Portal hypertension
Cirrhosis
Renal
Altered glomerular filtration
Altered water handling
Hyperuricemia
Hematologic
Iron deficiency
Erythrocytosis
Lymphopenia
Skeletal
Metabolically dependent poor muscle training
Volitional or iatrogenic poor muscle training
Kyphoscoliosis
Infectious
Chronic infectious potential
Neurologic
Cerebrovascular injury
Pregnancy

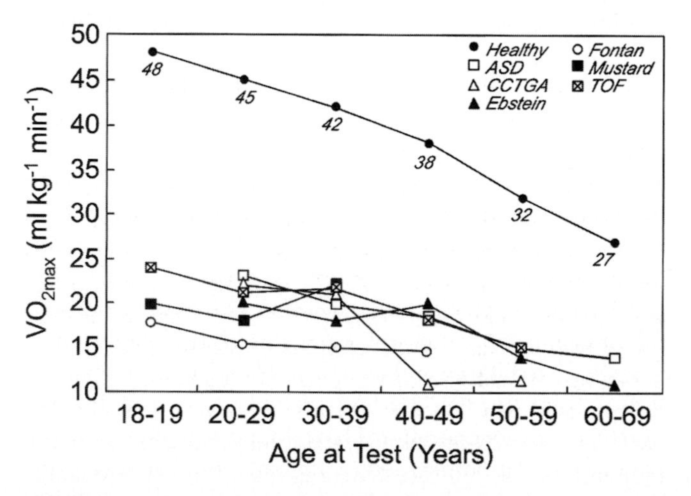

FIGURE 56–1 *Impaired maximal oxygen consumption in adult patients with congenital heart disease.*
From Fredriksen PM, Veldtman G, Hechter S, et al. Aerobic capacity in adults with various congenital heart diseases. Am J Cardiol 87:310, 2001.

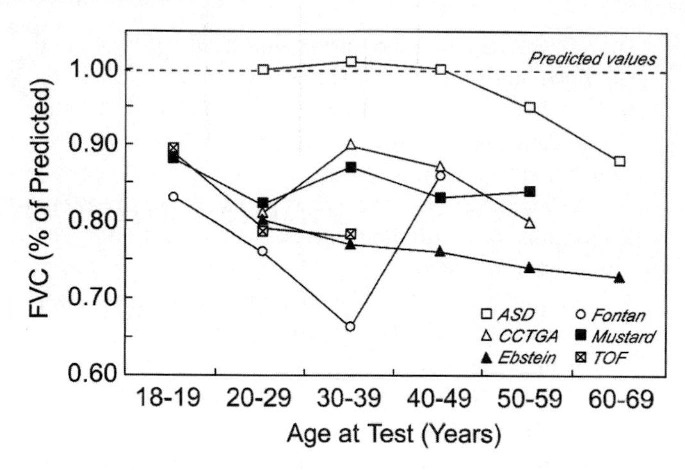

FIGURE 56–2 *Impaired vital capacity as a marker of restrictive lung disease in adult patients with congenital heart disease.*
From Fredriksen PM, Veldtman G, Hechter S, et al. Aerobic capacity in adults with various congenital heart diseases. Am J Cardiol 87:310, 2001.

Ventricular Vascular Coupling

Effective circulation within a ventricular-arterial system is designed as receipt of pulsatile flow and delivery of steady flow in a balance of forces that both preserves energy and minimizes stress relationships between ventricular myocardium and central and peripheral conduits, resistance vessels, and the microvasculature.[4–6] As well, balance of end-systolic and arterial elasticity allows for preservation of sensitivity to additional aspects of cardiac loading. Modern understanding of such ventricular-vascular coupling in health and disease suggests that determinants of systolic and diastolic ventricular performance as well as those of vascular function have direct and profound effects on each other, as well as on coronary perfusion.[7] Measures of the pulsatile hemodynamics of such coupling, including alterations in arterial stiffness and cushioning, pulse pressure, wave characteristics, and velocities, in both acquired systolic and nonsystolic heart failure, have been shown to correlate with changes in patient morbidity and mortality.[8–11] Demonstration of abnormal brachial arterial responsiveness to endothelium-dependent and -independent vasomediators in young adults after successful aortic coarctation repair led to investigation of conduit artery pulse wave velocity as a marker of arterial stiffness.[12,13] Delay of conduit artery pulse wave velocity correlated with alterations in vasodilation, pulse pressure, and development of increase in left ventricular (LV) mass, as well as abnormal baroreflex sensitivity and reduced inhibition of sympathetic drive.[14] Further investigation of similar pulse wave abnormalities in other congenital heart syndromes in the adult, and their relationship to heart failure syndromes, is expected.

There is increasing recognition that adult patients with CHD have additional cardiovascular abnormalities that directly affect key determinants of ventricular-vascular coupling. Changes in intrinsic heart rate (e.g., postoperative patients[14]), stroke volume (e.g., patients with intracardiac mixing and volume loading), pulse pressure (e.g., patients with nonpulsatile pulmonary blood flow, patients with systemic arterial diastolic runoff), systemic arterial impedance (e.g., patients with aortic coarctation[12–14]), neurohormonal or cardiac autonomic nervous system activity,[15,16] or salt and water control (e.g., erythrocytotic patients with focal glomerular sclerosis), seen in such patients, may have real and substantive effects on health and functional capacity for affected individuals. As such, adults with CHD may serve as prototypal models for evaluation of potential ventricular-vascular coupling changes and their effects in health and disease.

Compromise of effective circulation may result from intrinsic factors not typically considered within the cardiopulmonary tree (Table 56-2). For example, critical energy conservation within high-pressure nonpulsatile systemic venous inflow may be markedly diminished due to anatomic venous-atrial connections, jeopardizing forward output in atriopulmonary-type Fontan palliations.[17] As well, impaired atrial-ventricular transport, due to intrinsic functional or anatomic baffle abnormalities, may be, in part, responsible for limits in stroke volume augmentation in patients with atrial-level repair for (SDD) transposition of the great arteries[18] (Fig. 56-3).

Pulmonary Vascular Disease

Pulmonary endothelial dysfunction, worse in nonpulsatile atriopulmonary connection-type repairs and in pulmonary

TABLE 56–2. "Nonmyocardial" Potential Cardiopulmonary Etiologies for "Heart Failure" in the Adult Patient with Congestive Heart Disease

Alteration in
- Systemic venous-atrial transport
- Atrial-ventricular transport
- Ventricular transport
- Pulmonary vascular function
- Systemic arterial conduit function

Pericardial constriction
Residual
Anatomic obstruction
Shunting
Outflow tract aneurysm
Semilunar valve regurgitation
Intracardiac or vascular thrombosis

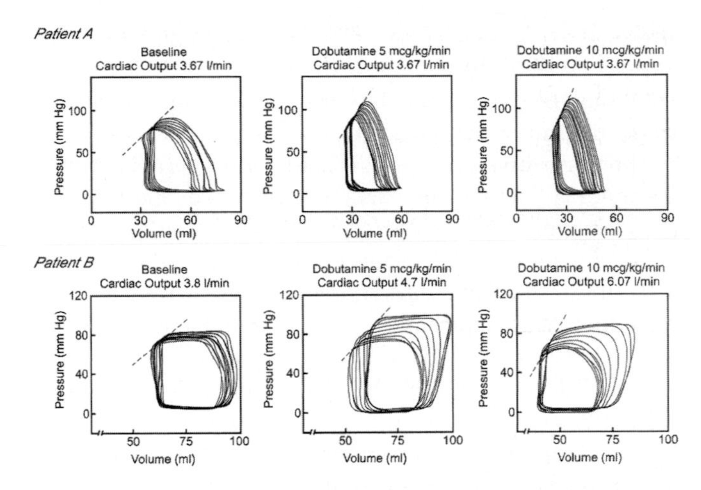

FIGURE 56–3 *Flow volume loops during preload reduction in patients with (SDD) transposition of the great arteries. Top panel, Failure to increase cardiac output with dobutamine yet preservation of rise of contractile indices. Bottom panel, Increase in both cardiac output and contractility is seen. In both patients, however, fall in stroke volume occurs.*
From Derrick GP, Narang I, White PA, et al. Failure of stroke volume augmentation during exercise and dobutamine stress is unrelated to load-independent indexes of right ventricular performance after the Mustard operation. Circulation 102[Suppl III]:154, 2000.

arteriolar hypertension (PAH), contributes to nonanatomic pulmonary ventricular afterload and, as such, potential for reduction in transpulmonary flow in patients with intracardiac mixing or lower systemic output in patients with Fontan palliation.[19] Given that presence of pulmonary hypertension may not necessarily imply presence of PAH, but rather can be indicative of any of a number of additional triggers for such (e.g., pulmonary venous hypertension, restrictive or hypoventilatory lung disease, thromboembolic pulmonary vascular occlusion), catheter-based hemodynamic assessment remains critical as the hallmark of diagnosis of PAH associated with CHD. Analyses of epidemiologic databases associated with patients with PAH have suggested similar untreated survival of patients with severe pulmonary hypertension, nearly universal regardless of etiology (with median survival between 2.8 and 3.4 years for the effected adult patient). Correlation of survival with variables relating to right ventricular function (typically assessed by hemodynamic measure of systemic cardiac output and mixed venous oxygen saturation and right atrial pressure) and physical capacity (typically measured by 6-minute walking capacity), emphasizes the delicate balance and direct relationships between pulmonary afterload, cardiac function, physical capacity, and life.[20] The improved survival outcomes seen in patients with severe PAH associated with Eisenmenger syndrome (10- to 20-year survival greater than 80%) suggest potential for improved response to increased pulmonary afterload when such is shared between right and left heart muscle.[20]

During the past decade, the "vasoconstriction" monolayer model of primary pulmonary hypertension has been replaced by the current vascular wall inflammation paradigm, with therapies reflecting this change in pathobiologic thought. Increasing evidence exists for genetically inherited abnormalities in endothelial cell apoptosis and growth potential, with links of familial and sporadic PAH to transforming growth factor-β superfamily bone morphogenetic protein receptor-2 (BMPR2), as well as angiopoietin-1, its specific endothelial cell receptor, BMPR1, and ALK1, encoding a BMPR receptor. In addition, increasing data suggest that the hallmark lesion of PAH, the plexiform lesion, is a response phenomenon to local hypoxia or inflammation and, in certain individuals with PAH, may represent a tumor-like proliferation of endothelial cells (monoclonal in PPH, polyclonal in secondary forms of PAH). Markers of cellular inflammation, matrix stimulation and cellular growth, and platelet and coagulant activity, including fractalkine, RANTES (*r*egulated upon *a*ctivation, *n*ormal T-cell *e*xpressed and *s*ecreted), interleukin 1β, interleukin-6, soluble intracellular adhesion molecule, soluble vascular cell adhesion molecule, soluble P-selectin, soluble electin, vascular endothelial growth factor, serum elastase, von Willebrand factors, serotonin plasminogen activator inhibitor, fibrinopeptide A, and thrombomodulin, have been noted in biopsy samples and circulation of patients with PAH.

For most affected patients, modern treatment, however indirectly, has begun to center on mediators of chemotaxis, cellular proliferation and differentiation, and regulation of vasoactive peptides and growth factors. These mediators currently include prostanoids (intravenous, inhaled, oral), endothelin antagonists, nitroso compounds, and phosphodiesterase inhibitors. At present, although phase III randomized controlled trials for many of these agents have included small numbers of patients with various types of CHD, we await results of trials specifically addressing safety and efficacy of these agents in adults.

Right Ventricular Dysfunction

The complex inter-relationships among aging, ventricular function, and outcome in adults with CHD is highlighted by long-term survival data in patients with tetralogy of Fallot (TOF) and transposition of the great arteries (SDD-TGA), where, linearly, continuous mortality appears to take a steeper drop-off in survival after the second postoperative decade.

Abnormalities in diastolic muscle function may correlate with functional capacity and survival. Most notable are those seen in patients after repair of TOF, in whom early postoperative echocardiographically demonstrable restrictive physiologic changes correlate with later similar restrictive markers, smaller chamber size, and narrower QRS duration.[21,22] Such physiology appears to limit the effects of pulmonary regurgitation, improving survival. Regional changes in not only systolic but also diastolic function in patients with TOF have been shown using echocardiographic tissue Doppler analyses.[23] Analysis of similar tissue Doppler characteristics has recently revealed regional variation and reduced early and late diastolic myocardial velocities, with prolonged isovolumic relaxation time and potential absence of A-wave myocardial velocities, independent of systolic abnormalities of the systemic right ventricle, in patients with SDD-TGA transposition of the great arteries.[24] These changes may reflect intrinsic muscle abnormalities, changes in electrical–mechanical coupling, or regional injury in affected patients.[25]

Native and postoperative anatomic sequelae (aside from residual shunts and obstructions) can contribute to abnormalities in cardiac output, functional capacity, and survival. The presence of right ventricular outflow aneurysm in patients with TOF correlates with magnetic resonance imaging–determined right ventricular dilation and hypertrophy and lower right ventricular (RV) and LV ejection fractions.[26] Strong potential for interventricular dependency for efficient systolic function is emphasized by these findings (Fig. 56-4). Although robust data from multicenter cohorts largely remain lacking, current risk stratification for survival in adult CHD patients with TOF emphasizes importance of preservation of LV function, in addition to

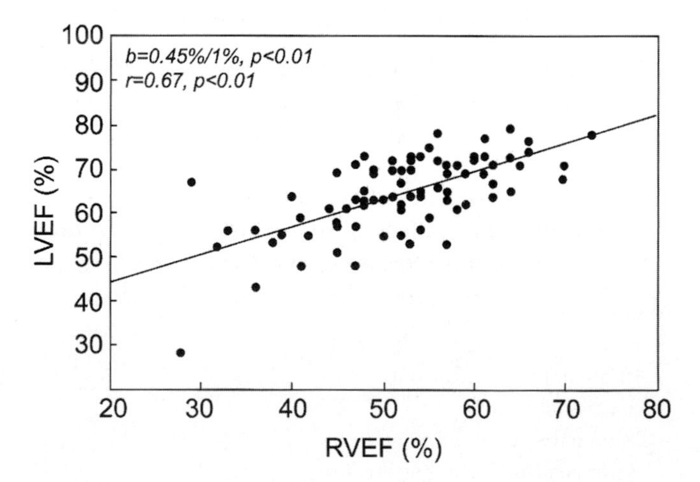

FIGURE 56–4 *Interdependence of right ventricular (RV) and left ventricular (LV) systolic function, as demonstrated by ejection fraction.*

From Davlouros PA, Kilner PJ, Hornung TS, et al. Right ventricular function in adults with tetralogy of Fallot assessed with cardiovascular magnetic resonance imaging. Detrimental role of right ventricular outflow aneurysms or akinesia and adverse right-left ventricular interaction. J Am Coll Cardiol 40:2044, 2002.

previously known markers of RV function, for continued survival with quality of life. Progressive aortic dilation or distortion, with or without associated aortic regurgitation, seen typically in bicuspid aortic valve disease and mixing lesions, including TOF and univentricular variants, carries potential for altering LV and ultimately RV contractile function, as well as ventricular–vascular coupling, and has been shown, on occasion, to eventuate in obstruction to coronary arterial origins or dissection.[27] Pulmonary arterial enlargement has been reported to encroach on the origins of the coronary arteries, causing acute ischemia or global myocardial stunning.

NEUROHORMONAL ACTIVATION

Abnormalities of cardiac autonomic nervous activity and elevations of neurohormones have been sought in the adult CHD population, owing, in part, to recognized heart rate reduction after surgery, effects of prior thoracic operations, and subsequent surgery-mediated denervation, alterations in gas exchange, and aging.[28,29] Such changes have been shown in chronic heart failure syndromes to correlate with degree of LV dysfunction, and with functional capacity and mortality, and have been incorporated into the definition of heart failure syndromes.[30–33]

Ohuchi and colleagues first demonstrated in primarily teenage postoperative (RV outflow tract reconstruction) patients that relatively severe postoperative sympathetic denervation of the ventricle was common (likely denervation rather than mediated by muscle dysfunction).[34] They confirmed in this population that exercise-mediated changes in heart rate, much related to parasympathetic nervous tone and postsynaptic β sensitivity (shown to correlate to functional ability) could be affected (directly related to cardiac autonomic nervous activity). Parasympathetic nervous activity early postsurgical repair appeared related to number of surgeries, significantly lowered with each, and had a tendency to recover in the first year after operation (likely related to recovery of sinus node ischemia). Postoperative β sensitivity was maintained, allowing for adequacy of augmentation of heart rate. Augmentation of heart rate correlated with maximal oxygen consumption (peak Vo_2) for postoperative patients without residual outflow tract stenosis, in contrast to patients with residual obstruction, in whom it did not. These results emphasized that surgically mediated changes in heart rate (parasympathetic nervous activity, baroreceptor sensitivity, postoperative β sensitivity) and their recovery were important determinants to functional ability. In addition, a relationship between abnormalities in cardiac autonomic nervous activity and arrhythmia genesis in the adult CHD patient was theorized.

A follow-up assessment of cardiac autonomic nervous activity in mostly teenage patients after Fontan palliation of single-ventricle physiology by this same group demonstrated similar global alterations in cardiac autonomic nervous activity, again excepting for preservation of postsynaptic β sensitivity, which was important for potential heart rate augmentation.[35] Cardiac autonomic nervous activity abnormalities correlated with reduction in augmentation of heart rate, but not with number of surgical procedures, age at time of Fontan operation, or length of follow-up. Similar to patients with residual RV outflow obstruction, heart rate augmentation in patients with Fontan physiology did not correlate with peak Vo_2. The authors theorized that, taken together, these changes suggested that the Fontan circulation (with attendant higher central filling pressures, lower resting systemic cardiac index, and lower resting systemic arterial blood pressure) and surgery-related direct or subclinical damage, per se, rather than specific hemodynamic abnormalities, led to changes in cardiac autonomic nervous activity. In a relatively small subset of studied patients, nonspecific use of angiotensin-converting enzyme inhibition for an average 6-month period did not correlate with altered cardiac autonomic nervous activity abnormalities.

These findings, in part, were challenged by Davos and colleagues, who assessed cardiac autonomic nervous activity in 22 adult Fontan patients.[36] Baroreceptor sensitivity was assessed, and heart rate variability was evaluated according to low- and high-frequency domains. Global depression of baroreceptor sensitivity and both domains of heart rate variability were noted, with a greater reduction in the low frequency (reduction in sympathetic modulation) range. In contrast to the findings of Ohuchi and colleagues[34] in younger patients, (1) reduction in low-frequency heart rate variability correlated with a marker of hemodynamic abnormality—increase in right atrial (RA) dimension; and (2) baroreceptor sensitivity was greater in patients with a history of sustained atrial tachyarrhythmia.

Bolger and colleagues measured resting neurohormones in 53 adults with a wide spectrum of congenital physiologies, and correlated findings with clinical patient variables, electrocardiographic indices, radiographic cardiothoracic ratio, and echocardiographic and exercise parameters.[15] Regardless of New York Heart Association (NYHA) functional class, neurohormones were elevated in all patients and correlated stepwise with worsening subjective functional ability. Atrial natriuretic peptide, brain natriuretic peptide, endothelin-1, norepinephrine, and epinephrine all correlated well with each other and with increases in QT interval and cardiothoracic ratio, all of which correlated with echocardiographically measured ventricular function and exercise peak Vo_2. Aldosterone and renin correlated only with each other and with RA and left atrial (LA) volumes, suggesting control mechanisms other than central pressure–volume relationships that are instrumental in control of natriuretic peptides and catecholamines. The authors theorized a global "phenotype of congenital heart disease" aligned with the syndrome of congestive heart failure. Neurohormonal abnormalities could persist even decades after surgical repairs, although the authors suggested potential for variation in abnormalities based, in part, on completeness of surgical correction. In a separate study, this same group showed elevation in circulating inflammatory cytokines, again correlating stepwise with adult congenital heart patient functional class.[37]

Ohuchi and colleagues[16] expanded on the results of Bolger and colleagues,[15] assessing both neurohormones as well as measures of cardiac autonomic nervous activity in 297 patients (pediatric 75%) with congenital heart disease. Stepwise increase in neurohormonal activation, correlating with subjective functional class regardless of asymptomatic state, was confirmed in pediatric and adult patients, with higher levels of natriuretic peptides seen in pediatric patients. Elevation of norepinephrine differentiated class II from III and IV adults, but not children. Baroreceptor sensitivity, heart rate variability, and vital capacity were related to functional capacity in NYHA I and II patients (but not class III and IV) of all ages, with adults having higher baroreceptor sensitivity and heart rate variability. The authors suggest that measure of both neurohormones and cardiac autonomic nervous activity are useful in categorizing patients with CHD, with measures of parasympathetic activity most helpful in the less symptomatic patients and neurohormones better in the more symptomatic patients (Fig. 56-5). Adults with a greater vital capacity (mitigating restrictive ventilatory reduction in heart rate variability) had lesser reduction of parasympathetic activity and a lesser rise in natriuretic hormones (with their own stimulatory ventilatory effects) than affected children. The authors theorized that exercise rehabilitation or other cardiac autonomic nervous activity, or neurohormonally targeted interventions, might lead to decrease in heart rate variability– and baroreceptor sensitivity–mediated arrhythmogenesis.

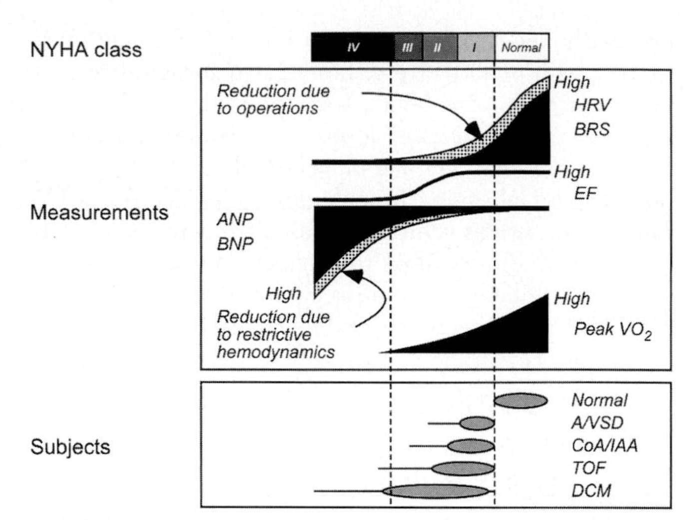

FIGURE 56–5 *Cartoon depicting utility of measures of neurohormonal activation (symptomatic end of spectrum) and cardiac autonomous nervous system activity (CANA), in particular PSNT (asymptomatic end of spectrum), in adult patients with congenital heart disease.*
From Ohuchi H, Takasugi H, Ohashi H, et al. Stratification of pediatric heart failure on the basis of neurohormonal and cardiac autonomic nervous activities in patients with congenital heart disease. Circulation 108:2368, 2003.

CONCLUSIONS

As suggested earlier, these past few decades have seen an increase in the population of adults with congenital heart disease to numbers now surpassing their pediatric counterparts. Indeed, in our own experience, by the early 1990s, 85% of all our patients (including those with hypoplastic left heart syndrome) were alive at age 17 years. Patients with increasing anatomic complexity, greater numbers of operative and catheter-based surgeries, alterations in pulmonary and systemic arterial and venous function, neurohormonal activation, and abnormalities in rhythm, coupled with changes of myocardial, vascular, and multiorgan "premature" senescence, are alive, functioning, and demanding our protection and care for today and for their future. The past number of years has seen an explosion in the understanding of heart failure syndromes in these patients, who, in their own existence, define a uniquely altered physiology. It is only through continued insights into these new paradigms of physiologic understanding, coupled with randomized clinical therapeutic trials in this growing population, that a future of optimal functioning can be best guaranteed for the adult patient with congenital heart disease.

LESION MANAGEMENT STRATEGIES

The improving survival of patients with congenital heart disease clearly reflects the remarkable surgical advances over the past few decades. The more widespread use of echocardiography continues to uncover lesions in adult patients, particularly atrial defects previously unrecognized, this also increasing the number of adults with CHD. In addition, increasing interventional catheter-based procedures, largely derived from pediatric experience, offer alternative treatment strategies to surgery in a variety of lesions (Exhibit 56-1).

Exhibit 56–1

Children's Hospital Boston Experience

1988-2002

Adults with Congenital Heart Disease

Total 2537 (64% F) > age 20 years

Lesion	*N*	*Lesion*	*N*	*Lesion*	*N*
Mitral	450	Pulmonary	126	DTGA	37
Tricuspid	289	Myocardial	118	Truncus Arteriosus	22
Aortic	273	Malposition	116	LTGA	16
ASD/PFO	176	Endocardial Cushion Defect	81	Single Ventricle	11
Ventricular septal defect	156	Coarctation	72	Double Outlet RV	9
Tetralogy of Fallot	139	Patent Ductus	53	Fistulas	8
		Other	385		

Catheter-based Intervention (641 patients)

Lesion	*N*		
ASD/PFO	246	Stent Placement (71 in 69 patients)	
Arrhythmia ablation	98	Coarctation	24
Peripheral pulmonary stenosis	80	Pulmonary Artery(PA)	23
Patent ductus arteriosus	53	RV-RA conduits	8
Ventricular septal defect	32	SVC/IVC stenosis s/p Mustard/Senning	7
Caorctation dilation	30	Other	9
Pulmonary valve dilation	25		
Aortic valve dilation	4		
Fenestration closure	4		

Abbreviations:
F = female
ASD = atrial septal defect
D/L TGA = D/L transposition of the great arteries
SVC/IVC = superior/inferior vena cava
N = number of patients
PFO = patent foramen ovale
RV = right ventricle

In terms of medical therapy of ventricular dysfunction and heart failure, without significant structural lesions, drugs remain the frontline approach (see Chapters 7 and 26).

Among those with structurally significant defects, whether unoperated or residual lesions, surgery remains the current treatment of choice in most. This is true for initial management of such lesions as tetralogy of Fallot, subaortic stenosis, mitral regurgitation, aortic valve disease, and endocardial cushion defects. It is also employed postoperatively for residual TOF ventricular defects, obstructed small RV–pulmonary artery conduits, revision of Fontan pathways, valve lesions, transposition pathway reconfigurations, and transplantation.

The variety, applicability, and effectiveness of interventional catheter-based procedures continue to expand. Balloon dilation is the initial management strategy for such lesions as pulmonary valvar and peripheral pulmonary artery stenosis. Stent placement in the latter and in aortic coarctation has become common. Occlusion, by coils usually, of most patent ductus arteriosi is effective, as is coil occlusion of the rare coronary arteriovenous fistula. Device closure of atrial defects (secundum, patent foramen ovale) is common (see Chapter 14) and the number of ventricular defects so closed, both congenital and residual, is increasing.[38,39] Although pulmonary valve replacement is currently largely surgical, transcatheter replacement is being evaluated and may become more widespread.[40] In addition, percutaneous aortic valve replacement has been reported, as has mitral valvular reduction for regurgitation.[41–43] As can be seen in Exhibit 56-1, electrophysiologic advances have been such that ablation procedures, for arrhythmias such as supraventricular tachycardias due to accessory pathways and atrial flutter and fibrillation, have become the second most common procedure in our adult population.

REFERENCES

1. Graham TP. Ventricular performance in congenital heart disease. Circulation 84:2259, 1991.
2. Perloff JK, Warnes CA. Challenges posed by adults with repaired congenital heart disease. Circulation 103:2637, 2001.
3. Fredriksen PM, Veldtman G, Hechter S, et al. Aerobic capacity in adults with various congenital heart diseases. Am J Cardiol 87:310, 2001.
4. Dell'Italia LJ, Blackwell GG, Thorn BT, et al. Time-varying wall stress: An index of ventricular vascular coupling. Am J Physiol 263:H597, 1992.
5. O'Rourke MF. Arterial Function in Health and Disease. Edinburgh: Churchill Livingstone, 1982.
6. O'Rourke MF, Safar ME, Dzau VJ. Arterial Vasodilation: Mechanisms and Therapy. Philadelphia: Lea & Febiger, 1993.
7. Smulyan H, Safar ME. Systolic blood pressure revisited. J Am Coll Cardiol 29:1407, 1997.
8. Mitchell GF, Tardif J-C, Arnold MO, et al. Pulsatile hemodynamics in congestive heart failure. Hypertension 38:1433, 2001.
9. Mitchell GF, Moye LA, Braunwald E, et al. Sphygmomanometrically-determined pulse pressure is a powerful independent predictor of recurrent events following myocardial infarction I patients with impaired left ventricular function. Circulation 96: 4254, 1997.
10. Domanski MJ, Mitchell GF, Norman J, et al. Independent prognostic information provided by sphygmomanometrically determined pulses pressure and mean arterial pressure in patients with left ventricular dysfunction. J Am Coll Cardiol 33:951, 1999.
11. Chae C, Pfeffer M, Glynn RJ, et al. Increased pulse pressure and risk of heart failure in the elderly. JAMA 281:634, 1999.
12. Gardiner HM, Celermajer DS, Sorensen KE, et al. Arterial reactivity is significantly impaired in normotensive young adults after successful repair of aortic coarctation in childhood. Circulation 89:1745, 1994.
13. de Devitiis M, Pilla C, Kattenhorn M, et al. Vascular dysfunction after repair of coarctation of the aorta. Circulation 104(Suppl I):165, 2001.
14. de Devitiis M, Pilla C, Kattenhorn M, et al. Ambulatory blood pressure, left ventricular mass, and conduit artery function late after successful repair of coarctation of the aorta. J Am Coll Cardiol 41:2259, 2003.
15. Bolger AP, Sharma R, Li W, et al. Neurohormonal activation and the chronic heart failure syndrome in adults with congenital heart disease. Circulation 106:92, 2002.
16. Ohuchi H, Takasugi H, Ohashi H, et al. Stratification of pediatric heart failure on the basis of neurohormonal and cardiac autonomic nervous activities in patients with congenital heart disease. Circulation 108:2368, 2003.
17. Be'eri E, Maier SE, Landzberg MJ, et al. In vivo evaluation of Fontan pathway flow dynamics by multidimension phase-velocity magnetic resonance imaging. Circulation 98:2873, 1998.
18. Derrick GP, Narang I, White PA, et al. Failure of stroke volume augmentation during exercise and dobutamine stress is unrelated to load-independent indexes of right ventricular performance after the Mustard operation. Circulation 102(Suppl III):154, 2000.
19. Khambadkone S, Li J, de Leval MR, et al. Basal pulmonary vascular resistance and nitric oxide responsiveness late after Fontan-type operation. Circulation 107:3204, 2003.
20. Oya H, Nagaya N, Uematsu M, et al. Poor prognosis and related factors in adults with Eisenmenger syndrome. Am Heart J 143(4):739, 2002.
21. Norgard G, Gatzoulis MA, Moraes F, et al. Relationship between type of outflow tract repair and postoperative right ventricular diastolic physiology in tetralogy of Fallot: Implications for long term outcome. Circulation 94:3276, 1996.
22. Norgard G, Gatzoulis MA, Josen M, et al. Does restrictive right ventricular physiology in the early postoperative period predict subsequent right ventricular restriction after repair of tetralogy of Fallot? Heart 79:481, 1998.
23. Vogel M, Sporing J, Cullen S, et al. Regional wall motion and abnormalities of electrical depolarization in patients after surgical repair of tetralogy of Fallot. Circulation 103:1660, 2001.
24. Vogel M, Derrick G, White PA, et al. Systemic ventricular function in patients with transposition of the great arteries after atrial repair: A tissue Doppler and conductance catheter study. J Am Coll Cardiol 43:100, 2004.
25. Chaturvedi RR, Shore DF, Lincoln C, et al. Acute right ventricular restrictive physiology after repair of tetralogy of Fallot: Association with myocardial injury and oxidative stress, Circulation 100:1540, 1999.
26. Davlouros PA, Kilner PJ, Hornung TS, et al. Right ventricular function in adults with tetralogy of Fallot assessed with cardiovascular magnetic resonance imaging. Detrimental role of right ventricular outflow aneurysms or akinesia and adverse right-left ventricular interaction. J Am Coll Cardiol 40:2044, 2002.
27. Niwa K, Siu SC, Webb GD, Gatzoulis MA. Progressive aortic root dilation in adults late after repair of tetralogy of Fallot. Circulation 106:1374, 2002.
28. Driscoll DJ, Danielson GK, Puga FJ, et al. Exercise tolerance and cardiorespiratory response to exercise after the Fontan operation for tricuspid atresia or functional single ventricle. J Am Coll Cardiol 7:1087, 1986.
29. Kondo C, Nazakawa M, Momma K, et al. Sympathetic denervation and reinnervation after arterial switch operation for complete transposition. Circulation 97:2414, 1998.
30. Cohn JN, Levine TB, Olivari MT, et al. Plasma norepinephrine as a guide to prognosis in patients with chronic congestive heart failure. N Engl J Med 311:819, 1984.
31. Gottlieb SS, Kukin ML, Ahern D, et al. Prognostic importance of atrial natriuretic peptide in patients with chronic heart failure. J Am Coll Cardiol 13:1534, 1989.
32. Eichorn EJ. Prognosis determination in heart failure. Am J Med 110;14S, 2001.
33. Remme WJ, Swedberg K, and the Task Force for the Diagnosis and Treatment of Chronic Heart Failure, European Society of Cardiology. Guidelines for the diagnosis and treatment of chronic heart failure. Eur Heart J 22:1527, 2001.

34. Ohuchu H, Suzuki H, Toyohara K, et al. Abnormal cardiac autonomic nervous activity after right ventricular outflow tract reconstruction. Circulation 102:2732, 2000.
35. Ohuchi H, Hasegawa S, Yasuda K, et al. Severely impaired cardiac autonomic nervous activity after the Fontan operation. Circulation 104:1513, 2001.
36. Davos CH, Francis DP, Leenarts MF, et al. Global impairment of cardiac autonomic nervous activity late after the Fontan operation. Circulation 108(Suppl II):180, 2003.
37. Sharma R, Bolger AP, Li W, et al. Elevated circulating levels of inflammatory cytokines and bacterial endotoxin in adults with congenital heart disease. Am J Cardiol 92:188, 2003.
38. Knauth AL, Lock JE, Perry SB, et al. Transcatheter device closure of congenital and post-operative residual ventricular septal defects. Circulation 110:501, 2004.
39. Holzer R, Balzer D, Cao DL, et al. Device closure of ventricular septal defects using the Amplatzer muscular ventricular septal defect occluder: Immediate and mid-term results of a U.S. registry. J Am Coll Cardiol 43(7), 2004.
40. Bonhoeffer P, Boudjemline Y, Qureshi SA, et al. Percutaneous insertion of the pulmonary valve. J Am Coll Cardiol 39:1664, 2002.
41. Cribier A, Eltchaninoff H, Bash A, et al. Percutaneous transcatheter implantation of an aortic valve prosthesis for calcific aortic stenosis: first human case description. Circulation 106:3006, 2002.
42. St. Goar FG, Fann JI, Komtebedde J, et al. Endovascular edge-to-edge mitral valve repair: Short-term results in a porcine model. Circulation 108:1990, 2003.
43. Kaye DM, Byrne M, Alferness C, et al. Feasibility and short-term efficacy of percutaneous mitral annular reduction for the therapy of heart failure-induced mitral regurgitation. Circulation 108:1795, 2003.

X

Surgical Considerations

57

Neonatal and Infant Cardiac Surgery

FRANK A. PIGULA AND PEDRO J. DEL NIDO

During the past 15 years, the practice of pediatric cardiac surgery has matured as a specialty. Among the most important changes that have occurred are those related to the surgical management of complex forms of congenital heart disease in the neonate and infant. There have been significant advances in our understanding of the physiology of congenital heart disease, particularly with respect to the management of the single-ventricle circulation. Furthermore, there has been a shift away from palliative surgical procedures to a more aggressive surgical stance with regard to neonatal surgical corrections. This approach, pioneered by Barratt-Boyes and Castenada, has changed the practice of congenital heart surgery (Table 57-1). It is within this context that we will discuss the current surgical treatment of the neonate and infant with heart disease, review the management strategies for palliation of the single ventricle, and describe the approach to the neonate with complex biventricular anatomy.

SINGLE-VENTRICLE PALLIATION

About 1 child in 5000 is born with congenital heart disease consisting of anatomy suitable for only single-ventricle circulations.[1] These lesions include, but are not limited to, hypoplastic left heart syndrome (HLHS), heterotaxy syndromes, unbalanced atrioventricular septal defects (ASDs), DILV, DORV, tricuspid atresia, and pulmonary atresia/intact ventricular septum. The unifying theme of these lesions is a circulation supported by a single pumping chamber. By examining the most common form of single-ventricle HLHS, we will illustrate specific management principles that may be generalized to other anatomic forms of the single ventricle.

HYPOPLASTIC LEFT HEART SYNDROME

HLHS is characterized by a generalized underdevelopment of the left ventricle and its dependent structures: the mitral valve, the aortic valve, and the preductal/ductal aorta. Males account for 57% to 67% of new cases, and the risk for sibling recurrence has been reported to be 0.5%.[2,3] No environmental risk factors associated with the diagnosis of HLHS have been identified.[4] In HLHS, the right ventricle must support both the systemic and pulmonary circulation. Pulmonary venous return must have access to the right atrium, through an ASD, PFO, or rarely, anomalous pulmonary venous connections to the systemic veins. Systemic output, delivered through the ductus arteriosus, is entirely dependent on ductal patency.

The treatment of HLHS has dramatically changed during the past two decades. With little to offer before Norwood's introduction of stage 1 palliation in 1983, treatment has developed into a three-stage progression to the Fontan operation. Although the 1-month mortality rate for untreated patients is 95%, the current 1-month survival rate among specialized centers approaches 80% to 90%.

Techniques

The "standard" Norwood operation involves incorporation of the pulmonary valve into the systemic circulation, with patch augmentation of the hypoplastic aortic arch. Because the pulmonary valve is now committed to the systemic circulation, an alternative source of pulmonary blood flow is required. This is usually provided by the placement of a Blalock-Taussig shunt between the innominate/right subclavian artery and the right pulmonary artery (Fig. 57-1).

TABLE 57–1. Survival after Neonatal or Infant Cardiac Surgery: Children's Hospital Boston Experience, 2001–2003

	30-Day Survival		1-Year Survival*	
	(%)	(N)	(%)	(N)
Hypoplastic Left Heart Syndrome				
Stage 1	91	(84/92)	88	(51/58)
Bidirectional Glenn	100	(139/139)	97	(73/75)
Repair Total Anomalous				
Pulmonary venous return	100	(41/41)	100	(27/27)
Truncus arteriosus	100	(22/22)	100	(15/15)
Tetralogy of Fallot				
Pulmonary stenosis	99	(125/126)	98	(78/80)
Pulmonary atresia	94	(32/34)	92	(23/25)
Arterial Switch Operation				
Intact ventricular septum	100	(72/72)	100	(51/51)
Ventricular septal defect	97	(57/59)	98	(40/41)
Repair Complete				
Atrioventricular canal	96	(86/88)	95	(57/60)

*One-year survival data reflect patients operated on in 2001–2002 only.

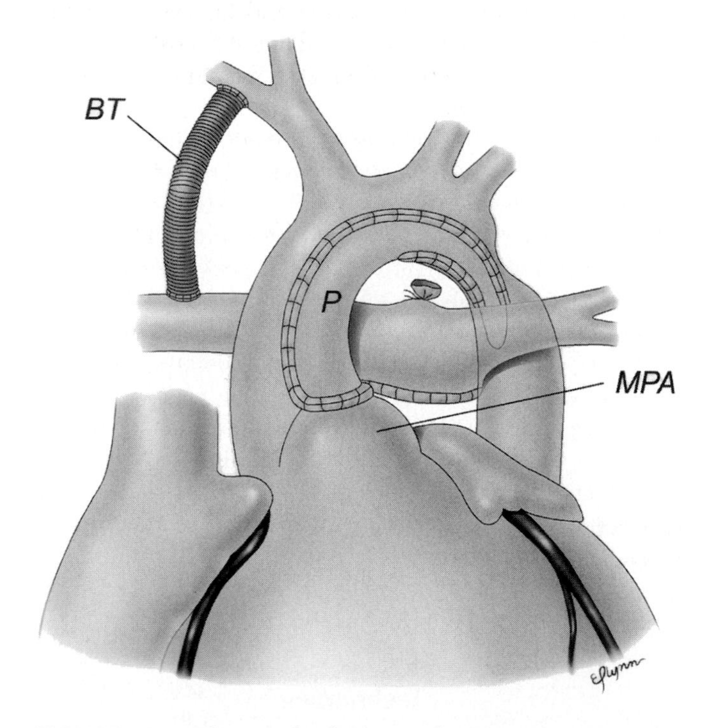

FIGURE 57–1 *The "standard" Norwood or stage 1 operation for hypoplastic left heart syndrome. The pulmonary valve and main pulmonary artery (MPA) are now committed to the systemic circulation, and the arch is augmented with a patch (P). Pulmonary blood flow is provided through the modified Blalock-Taussig shunt (BT). An atrial septectomy is also performed to assure unobstructed pulmonary venous drainage to the right ventricle. From Castaneda A. Cardiac Surgery of the Neonate and the Infant (p. 371). Philadelphia: WB Saunders, 1994.*

An atrial septectomy is performed to ensure unobstructed drainage of the pulmonary venous return to the right ventricle.

Although the goals of the Norwood operation remain unchanged, the methods employed to achieve them continue to evolve. Recently, pulmonary blood flow has been provided by the placement of a conduit between the right ventricle itself and the pulmonary arteries—the Sano modification (Fig. 57-2). Replacing the Blalock-Taussig shunt, the Sano modification has been reported to improve perioperative hemodynamic stability. This finding has not been a consistent finding among centers, and a multi-institutional trial comparing the two techniques is ongoing.

Surgical Results

Between 2001 and 2003, 100 children have undergone the stage 1 Norwood operation at Children's Hospital Boston, with a 92% 1-month survival rate (92 of 100). Although anatomic variables, such as caliber of the ascending aorta, have been implicated as determinants of mortality, this has not been a uniform finding.[5,6]

Management of Single-Ventricle Physiology

The surgical management of HLHS represents the paradigm from which a generalized approach to the shunted single ventricle has evolved. Simply stated, the cardiovascular system of the shunted single ventricle consists of a

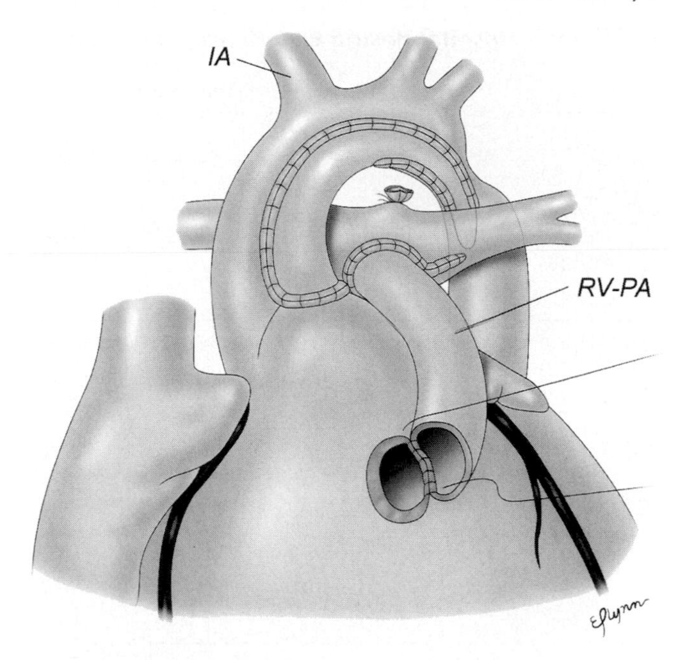

FIGURE 57–2 *Recent modifications of the stage 1 operation include the Sano modification. A right ventricle to pulmonary artery conduit (RV-PA, 5-mm Gore-Tex tube graft) provides pulmonary blood flow and replaces the Blalock-Taussig shunt. By virtue of pulmonary inflow arising proximal to the semilunar valves, the circulation is analogous to a banded circulation rather than a shunted circulation. Higher diastolic blood pressures, and presumably better coronary perfusion, are the result. A conduit is sewn to the innominate artery (IA) for use as a primary arterial cannulation site for regional perfusion of the brain during arch reconstruction.*

single pumping chamber supporting two parallel circulations. These parallel circulations are in competition with each other for blood flow. For any given cardiac output, the flow apportioned to each circulation is inversely proportional to the resistance of that circulation (i.e., high pulmonary vascular resistance, low pulmonary blood flow). Thus, efforts to control the circulation have focused on controlling the competing vascular resistances. These efforts have generally involved manipulation of the pulmonary vascular resistance using inspired gasses (O_2, CO_2, NO), and pressures.[7–10]

More recently, an alternative approach, one that targets manipulation of the systemic vascular resistance to maintain the balance between the pulmonary and systemic circulations, has been shown to be effective.

Manipulation of Pulmonary Vascular Resistance

CO_2

Inspired CO_2 has been suggested to improve the hemodynamic status after the Norwood operation. Clinically, Tabbutt and colleagues compared the use of hypoxia (17% FiO_2) to CO_2 in 10 neonates with HLHS before the Norwood operation under the conditions of fixed minute ventilation, anesthesia, and paralysis.[11]

Although both strategies reduced the Qp/Qs, CO_2 increased both superior vena cava (SVC) co-oximetry and cerebral oximetry, whereas hypoxia reduced these indices of oxygen delivery. Bradley and associates reported similar results among postoperative patients.[12] It is important to note, however, that these benefits were only realized when the *minute ventilation* remained constant.

Although thought to reflect a direct effect by some, there is evidence showing that the increase in peripheral vascular resistance is reversed by alkalinization, suggesting that the effect is mediated by H^+ and pH.[13]

O_2

Because the neonatal pulmonary vasculature is also sensitive to the concentration of inspired O_2, hypoxic mixtures incorporating nitrogen have also been used to control the circulation in patients with HLHS. Animal models have shown that nitrogen-induced hypoxic mixtures increase the pulmonary vascular resistance and increase systemic blood flow. However, the prolonged use of hypoxic mixtures has been shown to quickly induce anatomic changes in the pulmonary vasculature. In animals, changes in arterial wall thickness and muscularity can be seen within 24 hours, and fewer intra-acinar arteries are recruited into the circulation.[14–16]

Clinically, Day and associates have reported their experience using hypoxia to manipulate the peripheral vascular resistance in 20 neonates with single-ventricle, duct-dependent circulation awaiting heart transplantation.[17] Eight patients survived; of the 10 patients who underwent lung biopsy or autopsy, 9 showed medial hypertrophy in distal arterioles, and 7 of these 9 patients died. Although the outcome cannot be completely ascribed to hypoxic management, this strategy does suggest that prolonged supportive care of the neonatal single ventricle may expose these patients to significant risks.

Systemic Vascular Resistance

Manipulation of the systemic vascular resistance is a demonstrated means of controlling the shunted circulation. In fact, our ability to pharmacologically control the systemic vascular resistance probably exceeds our current ability to selectively manage the pulmonary vascular resistance. Clinically, this approach usually employs an irreversible α-adrenergic antagonist, phenoxybenzamine, to achieve systemic vasodilatation. The desired systemic vascular resistance, defined as that which optimizes the Qp/Qs and systemic oxygen delivery, is then obtained by titrating an α-adrenergic agonist, usually norepinephrine. Specifics of this approach have been reported in the literature.[18–20] A recent review of this strategy identified the use of phenoxybenzamine, continuous $S\dot{V}O_2$ monitoring, and the reduction of DHCA time as factors favoring survival to the bidirectional Glenn operation.[21]

To date, no studies directly comparing outcomes for these two fundamentally different management schemes have been performed.

Other Palliative Procedures for the Single Ventricle

The surgical strategy for the single ventricle is often dictated by the status of the pulmonary circulation. Patients with unobstructed systemic and pulmonary outflow tracts require pulmonary artery banding to balance the circulation, and protect the pulmonary vasculature. Patients with pulmonary stenosis or atresia require a procedure to provide reliable pulmonary blood flow, usually in the form of an arteriopulmonary shunt. Patients with moderate restriction to blood flow between the ventricle and the lungs may be well balanced ("autobanded") and require no immediate surgical intervention. These patients may go directly to the bidirectional Glenn operation within the first year of life.

Damus-Kaye-Stanzel Operation

Finally, an important group of children present with adequate great vessel dimensions, but with a real or potential intraventricular restriction of blood flow to the aorta. In lesions such as tricuspid atresia with transposition of the great arteries, the bulboventricular foramen may be restrictive. This anatomy should be viewed with caution because the natural history of the bulboventricular foramen is one of progressive restriction relative to somatic growth. In the setting of real or potential subaortic stenosis, pulmonary artery banding is to be avoided because biventricular outflow tract obstruction would result (Fig. 57-3). The Damus-Kaye-Stanzel (DKS) operation has been devised for these circumstances. Performed by transecting the main pulmonary artery at the bifurcation and sewing it to the side of the adjacent aorta, this operation is designed to circumvent obstruction of blood flow from the single ventricle to the systemic circulation. Pulmonary blood flow is then provided by an arteriopulmonary shunt (Fig. 57-4).

Arteriopulmonary Shunt

The arteriopulmonary shunt can be performed through a thoracotomy or a sternotomy. When performed through a thoracotomy, it is usually placed on the side of the innominate artery. In many cases, a sternotomy is preferable, especially in marginal patients who may require bypass support for the procedure. Sternotomy also allows direct access to the ductus arteriosus for ligation.

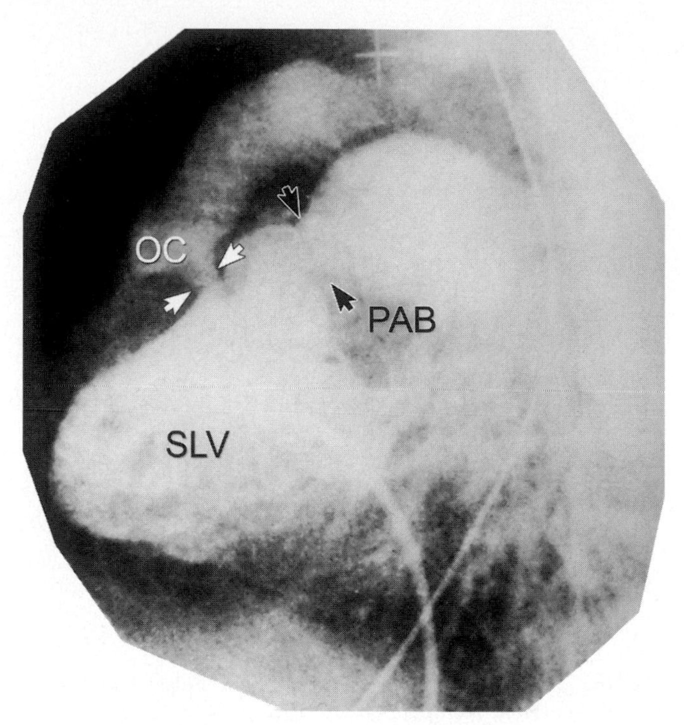

FIGURE 57–3 *Lateral view of a ventricular angiogram in a patient with double inlet left ventricle (SLV) with a subaortic outflow chamber (OC) after banding of the pulmonary artery (PAB, black arrows). Subaortic stenosis has developed because of a restrictive bulboventricular foramen (white arrows), resulting in biventricular outflow tract obstruction.*
From Jonas RA, Castaneda AR, Lang P. Single ventricle [single or double inlet] complicated by subaortic stenosis: Surgical options in infancy. Ann Thorac Surg 39:361, 1985. Reprinted with permission from the Society of Thoracic Surgeons, for Elsevier.

Pulmonary Artery Band

The role of the pulmonary band, traditionally employed to improve hemodynamics and to protect the pulmonary vasculature in a shunted circulation (such as a ventricular septal defect [VSD]), has also been reduced by the success of primary repair. At the present time it is reserved for children deemed poor candidates for repair because of comorbidities, such as pulmonary infection, sepsis, or contraindication to heparinization and cardiopulmonary bypass. Although pulmonary artery banding is usually performed through a sternotomy, a left parasternal (Chamberlain) incision provides suitable access for children with normally related great arteries.

Bidirectional Glenn Operation

The bidirectional Glenn operation (superior cavopulmonary anastomosis) is usually performed between 3 and 6 months of age. In this operation, the superior vena cava is amputated from the heart and sewn end to side into the right pulmonary artery. This is an intermediate step toward

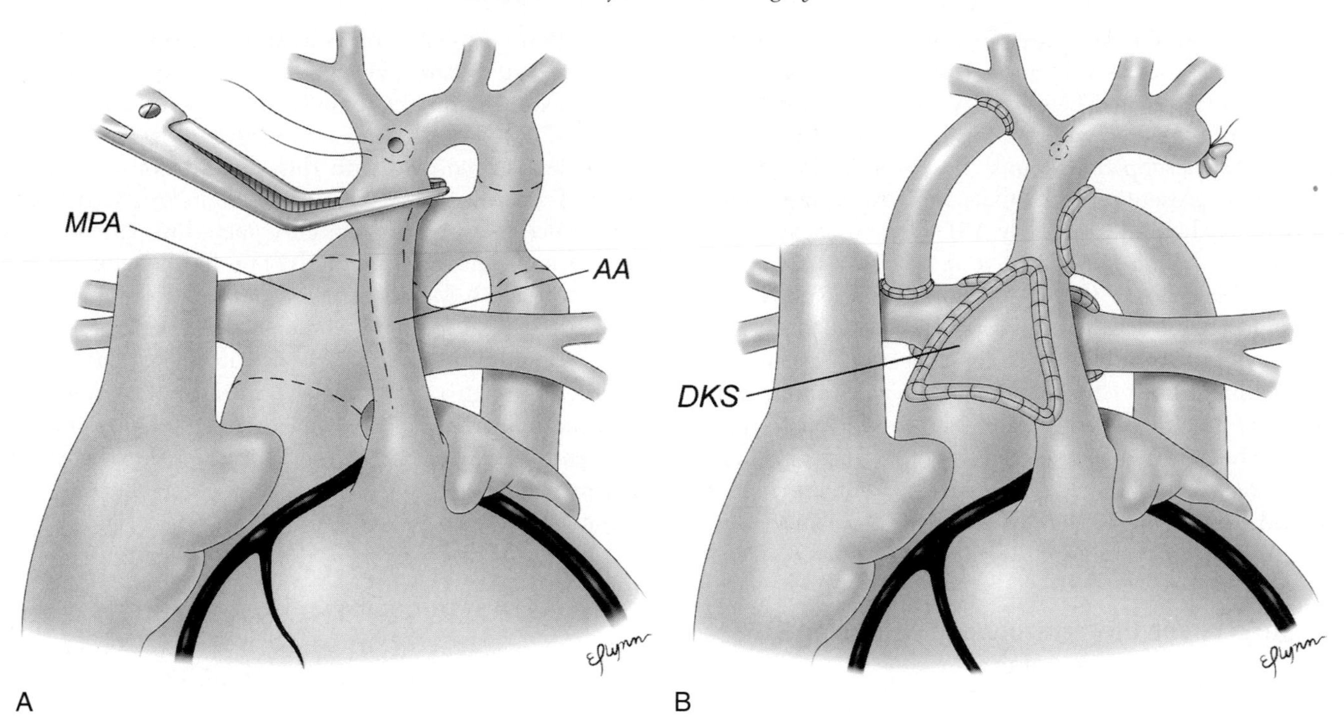

FIGURE 57–4 *A and B, In the single ventricle, the Damus-Kaye-Stanzel (DKS) anastomosis of the pulmonary artery (MPA) to the ascending aorta (AA) avoids systemic outflow obstruction resulting from aortic or subaortic obstruction. Concomitant lesions, such as coarctation or arch hypoplasia are common, and complicate the operation.*
From McElhinney DB, Reddy VM, Silverman N, et al. Modified Damus-Kaye-Stanzel procedure for single ventricle, subaortic stenosis, and arch obstruction in neonates and infants: Midterm results and techniques for avoiding circulatory arrest. J Thorac Cardiovasc Surg 114[5]:718, 1997. Reprinted with permission from the American Association for Thoracic Surgery for Elsevier.

completion of the Fontan procedure, and removal of the arteriopulmonary shunt serves to reduce the volume load on the single ventricle. This generally results in arterial saturations between 75% and 85%, an SVC pressure of 10 to 12 mmHg, and an atrial pressure of 5 to 6 mmHg. SVC pressure exceeding 16 mmHg or a transpulmonary gradient exceeding 8 to 10 mmHg should prompt critical appraisal of the anastomosis. The results of the bidirectional Glenn procedure are excellent, exceeding 95% in large series.[22,23]

BIVENTRICULAR REPAIR

To avoid the ongoing burden of an abnormal circulation, early anatomic correction is pursued whenever possible. Justification for early repair includes avoiding the chronic hemodynamic burden that palliation imposes on the developing myocardium, protection of the pulmonary vascular bed, and providing optimal support for the developing central nervous system. Furthermore, the palliated circulation is precarious and is associated with significant morbidity and measurable mortality.

However, it should be recognized that the "definitive" repair does not immunize the patient from future interventions. The use of nonvital vascular conduits and patches, as well as the underlying anatomy, often leads to subsequent procedures. In a large review, Lange and colleagues reported freedom from reoperation at 15 years to be 75% for tetralogy, 72% for complete ASDs, 73% for transposition of the great arteries, 45% for interrupted aortic arch, and 11% for truncus arteriosus.[24] Although these results do not detract from the rationale cited for early primary repair, they do help us understand the increasing population of adults presenting for surgical treatment for their congenital heart disease.

Surgery for the ASD in Infants

It has been observed that the repair of the isolated ASD in the infant is rarely indicated. In the unusual circumstances in which failure to thrive or signs and symptoms of congestive heart failure appear, other anatomic lesions or syndromes should be sought.

In a review at Children's Hospital Boston, symptomatic infants undergoing primum ASD closure had a high incidence of left-sided obstructive lesions, such as coarctation, subaortic stenosis, abnormal mitral valve, and left ventricular hypoplasia. The mortality rate for these patients was 36%, as compared with 1% for older patients.[25]

Although these patients must be carefully evaluated, rare patients presenting with otherwise inexplicable failure to thrive may benefit from early ASD closure.

It should also be noted that infants with anatomically small defects in both the interatrial and interventricular septum may require early repair. Even though either isolated lesion may not itself constitute an indication for surgical repair within infancy, the combination may lead to significant congestive heart failure. Even a modest left-to-right shunt at the ventricular level will tend to volume-load the left atrium, exaggerating the left-to-right shunt at the atrial level and exacerbating the total shunt. In these circumstances, surgical repair of both lesions is indicated.

Surgery for the Ventricular Septal Defect in Infants

Overall, surgical mortality for VSD closure has been reduced substantially during the past 15 years. Between 1973 and 1987, the 30-day mortality rate was 3%, and it decreased to 0.4% between 1988 and 2002, despite earlier surgical closure in marginal responders to medical management. At our institution, the proportion of children aged younger than 2 months undergoing VSD closure increased from 5% (1973–1987) to 15% (1988–2002). It is notable that the mortality rate for these two groups decreased from 20% to 0% over the same time period.

The overall morbidity of VSD closure during infancy may include injury to the conduction axis of the heart. This complication (complete heart block) is quite rare in the "usual" VSD (perimembranous, malalignment VSD [tetralogy or interrupted aortic arch, or IAA], or common arterioventricular canal defects) and occurs in about 1% to 2% cases.[26,27] Placement of a permanent pacing system is required in these patients.

Given these results, palliation, in the form of pulmonary artery banding, is reserved for patients with serious comorbidities (i.e., sepsis) and those with complex multiple VSDs that are surgically remote and in whom adequate closure cannot be assured.

Coarctation With and Without Ventricular Septal Defect

Aortic coarctation or hypoplasia is a common feature in congenital heart disease and is often found in combination with a ventricular septal defect. The surgical treatment of VSD/coarctation remains variable between institutions, however. Some programs prefer a staged approach, with coarctation repair (with or without pulmonary artery banding), followed by later VSD closure. This approach, however, leaves behind important hemodynamic residua, and primary repair of both lesions is favored. Between 1988 and 2002, 180 patients identified with this combination underwent surgical repair with a 30-day mortality rate of 7%. With the experience in aortic arch surgery gained in patients with HLHS, and with newer methods of perfusion management, even complicated arch repair can be performed in the newborn with little, if any, circulatory arrest time.

Neonates and infants with isolated coarctation are repaired through a left thoracotomy. In patients presenting with ventricular, hepatic, or renal dysfunction, preoperative resuscitation with assisted ventilation, inotropic support, and prostaglandins may be indicated. Surgical results are excellent, even in very small patients.[28]

SURGERY FOR THE INTERRUPTED AORTIC ARCH

There has been a progressive improvement in the outcomes for children born with IAA complex. A recent review of 472 neonates presenting with IAA between 1987 and 1997 was reported by McCrindle and colleagues and the Congenital Heart Surgeons Society (CHSS).[29] They reported an overall survival rate of 59% at 16 years, but noted improving survival over the time course of the study (Fig. 57-5). Low birth weight, type B IAA, and associated major cardiac anomalies place the patient at higher risk for death. The incidence of subsequent interventions remains high. Thirty-four percent of survivors required later left ventricular outflow tract (LVOT) intervention, whereas 29% required intervention for arch obstruction. Some authors have advocated staged repair of interrupted arch complex with severe subaortic LVOT. In these cases, Norwood palliation is performed, followed by subsequent VSD closure and the insertion of a right ventricle to pulmonary artery homograft. Although this is possible, we prefer to perform primary repair in the neonatal period. This approach has the advantage of comparable survival, with the additional benefit of a biventricular circulation in the perioperative period.

Staged approaches (establishment of aortic continuity with a synthetic or tissue conduit, followed by later VSD closure) are largely of historic interest.

TRUNCUS ARTERIOSUS

Since the first reported repair of truncus arteriosus by Behrent and colleagues in 1974, the surgical results have shown progressive improvement.[30] It was recognized by

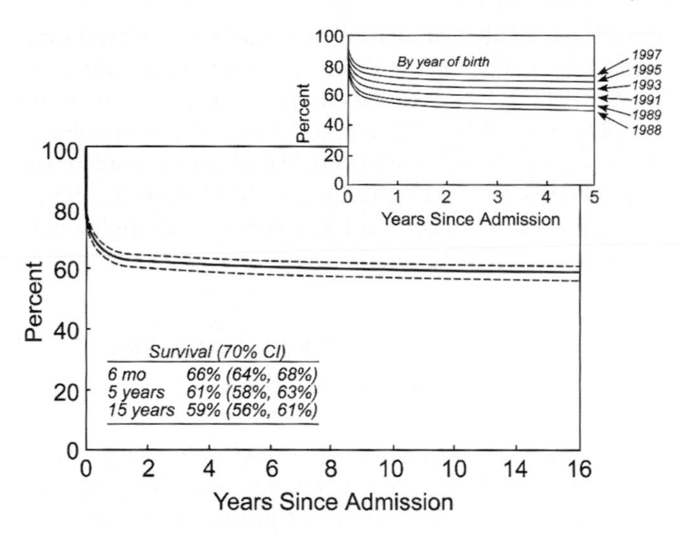

FIGURE 57–5 *Time-related survival of 472 neonates with interrupted aortic arch undergoing surgery at a Congenital Heart Surgeons Society (CHSS) institution between 1987 and 1997, with 70% confidence intervals. A, Overall survival. B, Predicted overall survival for the first 5 years after admission stratified by patient date of birth.*
From McCrindle BW, Tchervenkov CI, Konstantino IE, et al. Risk factors associated with mortality and interventions in 472 neonates with interrupted aortic arch: A Congenital Heart Surgeons Society study. J Thorac Cardiovasc Surgery 129(43):345, 2005. Reprinted with permission from the American Association for Thoracic Surgery for Elsevier.

Ebert and associates that early repair is important to avoid the morbidity and mortality of pulmonary vascular disease.[31] Further support for neonatal versus later repair is provided by reports from Children's Hospital Boston, demonstrating that children repaired at 2 weeks had lower mean pulmonary artery pressures than did children repaired at 3 months.

Because of this consideration, repair of truncus arteriosus is now typically performed in the neonatal period. Results with this approach are excellent, with mortality rates as low as 4% to 5%.[32–34] About 10% of patients with truncus arteriosus will present with important truncal valve disease, generally truncal regurgitation. When required, truncal valve repair is preferred over replacement and has met with good success.[33]

Because repair requires the creation of a right ventricle to pulmonary artery connection (usually with a small caliber homograft), future operations will be required. A risk factor for poor long-term survival is moderate to severe truncal valve insufficiency.

However, when patients present with the combination of truncus arteriosus with interrupted arch, the results are much poorer. Miyamoto and colleagues reported a 50% mortality rate for this combination of defects, and noted that truncal valve regurgitation was a common contributor of mortality. Reports such as this justify the aggressive repair of incompetent truncal valves during the primary procedure.[35]

TETRALOGY OF FALLOT

The goal of surgical treatment for tetralogy of Fallot is separation of the pulmonary and systemic circulations and relief of right ventricular outflow tract obstruction. Achievement of this goal depends on patient-specific anatomic substrate. Adopting the philosophy that early anatomic repair normalizes the circulation, early single-stage repairs of tetralogy of Fallot have been advocated by many groups. The major determinant on the suitability for primary single-stage repair rests on adequate development and distribution of the pulmonary vasculature.[36] Asymptomatic patients ("pink tetralogy") are analogous to VSD patients, and primary repair is deferred until 4 to 6 months of age.[37] For symptomatic (desaturated) patients presenting with adequate pulmonary arteries, prompt primary repair is performed. In these patients, complete repair includes VSD closure and relief of right ventricle to pulmonary artery obstruction (usually with a transannular patch). An atrial-level communication is intentionally left behind to allow right-to-left shunting at the atrial level during the postoperative period. This strategy has proven successful. In our review of 99 neonates and infants (age < 90 days) with tetralogy of Fallot with or without pulmonary atresia, early mortality was 3%. Patients with pulmonary atresia were found to require reintervention more frequently as a consequence of the homograft repair. Although the long-term impact of early repair on right ventricular function remains unclear, this is our preferred approach to the symptomatic neonate or infant with suitable pulmonary artery anatomy.[38] Palliation with a Blalock-Taussig shunt is reserved for patients with significant comorbidities and contraindications to open heart surgery.

Although primary repair is suitable for patients with adequate pulmonary arteries, these vessels may be diminutive, discontinuous, or even absent in some.

Whenever possible, we attempt to recruit the true pulmonary arteries by establishing antegrade flow from the right ventricle. Insertion of small aortic homografts (6 to 8 mm) into even very small pulmonary arteries (1 to 2 mm) is effective in stimulating pulmonary artery growth. In addition, this provides the interventional cardiologist access to the pulmonary circulation for the further rehabilitation of the pulmonary arteries. If these pulmonary arteries have adequate intraparenchymal distribution, the aortopulmonary collaterals become redundant and can be coil-occluded or ligated at surgery.

For patients dependent on aortopulmonary collaterals for pulmonary blood flow, the true pulmonary arteries are inadequate by virtue of their development, distribution, or both.

In these cases, staged reconstruction of the pulmonary vasculature is often required. This involves the unifocalization of the aortopulmonary collaterals to the available true pulmonary arteries, with connection to the right ventricle. In these cases, interventional rehabilitation of the pulmonary vasculature is indispensable in recruiting pulmonary vascular segments.

Because the approach for both scenarios must maintain and preserve right ventricular function, the VSD is closed when the pulmonary vasculature is deemed suitable. In questionable cases, we have found it helpful to fenestrate the VSD patch. In the case of inadequate pulmonary vascular bed, this allows the shunting of blood from the right ventricle to the left ventricle, avoiding suprasystemic right ventricular pressures. With further pulmonary artery rehabilitation, the fenestration can be closed electively with a device during catheterization. This approach has been successful in managing this difficult group of patients.[39]

ARTERIAL SWITCH OPERATION FOR D-TRANSPOSITION OF THE GREAT ARTERIES

The surgical treatment of transposition of the great arteries has undergone a dramatic shift during the past 20 years. Before the introduction of the arterial switch operation (ASO) by Jatene in 1975, atrial level repairs were the usual treatment. However, because late failure of the right ventricle and tricuspid valve in the systemic circulation was common, the ASO has become the procedure of choice. Whereas the atrial level switch was once reserved for difficult coronary artery patterns, even this indication has disappeared.[40] In fact, the boundaries for the arterial switch operation are continuing to be defined. Because of concerns about left ventricular deconditioning for transposition of the great arteries/intact ventricular septum (IVS) early operation (before 3 weeks of age) has been considered mandatory. Patients presenting later have been considered for atrial-level switch operation, or two-stage repair. The latter entails an initial operation to perform pulmonary artery banding (often in conjunction with a Blalock-Taussig shunt) followed by ASO 7 to 10 days later.[41] Although this approach has been successful, it has the disadvantage of two procedures, with an increased risk.

Recent data suggest that primary ASO/IVS can be performed, supplanting the two-stage approach, even in older children with a poorly prepared left ventricle. In a report by Kang and associates, 105 patients older than 3 weeks of age undergoing ASO, the mortality rate was 3.8%, and not different from the early (age younger than 3 weeks) group. Postoperative extracorporeal membrane oxygenation requirements were the same for both groups. These data would suggest that primary repair can be considered even for late presenting children with D-transposition of the great arteries/IVS.[42] A VSD is present in about 25% of children with D-transposition. When unrestrictive, deconditioning of the left ventricle does not occur. However, prompt repair of D-transposition of the great arteries/VSD is recommended because these patients tend to develop early pulmonary vascular occlusive disease.

ABNORMALITIES OF PULMONARY VENOUS RETURN

The surgical treatment of abnormal pulmonary venous return is very effective. The presentation of these children may vary greatly, from mild congestive heart failure at weeks or months of age, to true surgical emergencies requiring emergency surgery or immediate mechanical support. Most commonly, mild or moderate cyanosis after birth will prompt a cardiac workup, and the diagnosis is made by echocardiography.

Of the four types of the total anomalous pulmonary venous return, the supracardiac type is most common (45%), followed by the cardiac (25%), infracardiac (25%), and mixed type (5%).[43]

The goal of surgical treatment is identical for each form: an unobstructed connection between the pulmonary venous confluence and the left atrium. In a review of 123 patients from our institution, 68% of patients had biventricular anatomy, and 32% presented with a single ventricle.[44] Single-ventricle anatomy was a risk factor for death, with an early mortality rate of 36%, as compared with 7% for patients with biventricular anatomy. Postrepair pulmonary venous obstruction occurred in 11% of patients and was twice as common in the single-ventricle group. Recurrent stenosis in these patients can be a relentless and malignant process involving the intrapericardial and intraparenchymal pulmonary veins.[45] Despite all therapeutic attempts, including surgery, balloon dilation, and intravascular stents, the prognosis is poor. Because of this, some investigators are pursuing investigational therapies, including chemotherapy.

ENDOCARDIAL CUSHION DEFECTS

Complete Atrioventricular Septal Defect

The endocardial cushion defects, frequently associated with trisomy 21, result from lack of development of the central portion of the heart. Anatomically, this results in characteristic defects in the atrial septum and ventricular septum. As a consequence, these patients have one large atrioventricular valve spanning the atrioventricular connection.

The surgical goal is the removal of all significant intracardiac shunts, and conversion of the single large atrioventricular valve into two separate atrioventricular valves, each dedicated to one ventricle. This is accomplished using one of three techniques that have been well described elsewhere. Briefly, the one-patch technique, the two-patch technique, and the so-called Australian technique have been used to repair these defects.

Between 1988 and 2002, 332 children underwent surgical repair of the common atrioventricular canal. Of these, 233 (90%) were repaired within the first year of life and 63% at less than 6 months of age. After initial repair, 15% of children have required reoperation to address left atrioventricular valve repair. Valve repair was accomplished 75% of the time with the remainder requiring valve replacement.

These children typically present for surgery after a period of medical management, and surgical repair is usually performed within the first 3 months of life. Children demonstrating important or intractable congestive heart failure before this should undergo prompt repair. For the occasional patient who appears to thrive during early infancy, persistent elevation in the pulmonary vascular resistance should be suspected, and early operation is likewise recommended.

Ostium Primum Defect

When an isolated interatrial communication is the result of the endocardial cushion defect, it is known as a *primum defect*. Although the intracardiac shunting is isolated to the atrial level, it should be recognized that additional abnormalities exist. The left atrioventricular valve is typically cleft, with the cleft oriented toward the ventricular septum. This cleft is closed and is only left open if closure will result in important mitral stenosis. In addition, despite little or no shunting at the ventricular level, the interventricular septum is abnormal and demonstrates the same base-to-apex foreshortening seen in the complete defect. Because of this, the subaortic area remains at risk for later development of LVOT obstruction.

These patients occasionally require repair during infancy, but most often surgery can be deferred for several years. Only about 4% of patients will require reintervention for LAVV regurgitation, but these patients remain at risk for the late development of LVOT obstruction.

PULMONARY ATRESIA WITH INTACT VENTRICULAR SEPTUM

Pulmonary atresia with intact interventricular septum (PA/IVS) is characterized by absence of communication of the right ventricle to either the pulmonary or the systemic circulation. In addition, these patients often present with serious abnormalities of the tricuspid valve and the right ventricle. Abnormalities of the coronary circulation are also common, usually in the form of right ventricle to coronary fistulae. Because of the anatomic variability of this diagnosis, anatomic determinants of the most appropriate surgical pathway (single or biventricular repair) have been scrutinized.

Between 1991 and 1998, 47 patients with PA/IVS underwent surgery at our hospital.[46] Right ventricle–dependent coronary circulation (RVDCC) was identified in 34% and was associated with smaller tricuspid Z scores. When RVDCC is identified, decompression of the ventricle is contraindicated because it may result in vascular steal from the epicardial coronary circulation and cardiac ischemia.

Because RVDCC has been considered a risk for sudden death, primary heart transplantation has been advocated by some centers. However, our experience suggests that these patients do quite well in the single-ventricle pathway. Of the 32 patients identified with PA/IVS and RVDCC between 1989 and 2004, all received an initial arteriopulmonary shunt. Overall mortality was 19% (6 of 32 patients, including all 3 with aortocoronary atresia), with all deaths occurring within 3 months of shunt placement. Of the 26 survivors, 19 have been successfully staged to the Fontan operation, and there has been no mortality beyond 3 months of age.[47]

Although it seems that the majority of patients with PA/IVS and RVDCC can be successfully staged to single-ventricle circulations, patients presenting with aortocoronary atresia are an exception. Thus far, all 3 patients with this anatomy treated with arteriopulmonary shunting died before 3 months of age. The sole survivor was a recent patient treated with primary transplantation.

In a recent multi-institutional study of 408 neonates with PA/IVS, the 1-month survival rate was 77%, and the 15-year survival rate was 58%. By the end of the study, about half of patients had had a two-ventricle repair[48] (Fig. 57-6). Anatomic determinants of type of repair (single versus two ventricle) included tricuspid valve size and morphology and right ventricular size. Even when the anatomy is suitable for two-ventricle repair, patients often require an arteriopulmonary shunt after right ventricular decompression. This is related to the inability of the hypertrophic, poorly compliant right ventricle to provide adequate pulmonary blood flow during the perioperative period. Once right ventricular compliance improves, the shunt may be occluded in the catheterization laboratory

In general, patients presenting with a tricuspid valve Z score of less than −2.5, a poorly or undeveloped infundibulum, or RVDCC make poor candidates for biventricular repair.[49] Because of the high incidence of coronary abnormalities, angiography remains an important part of the evaluation in these patients.

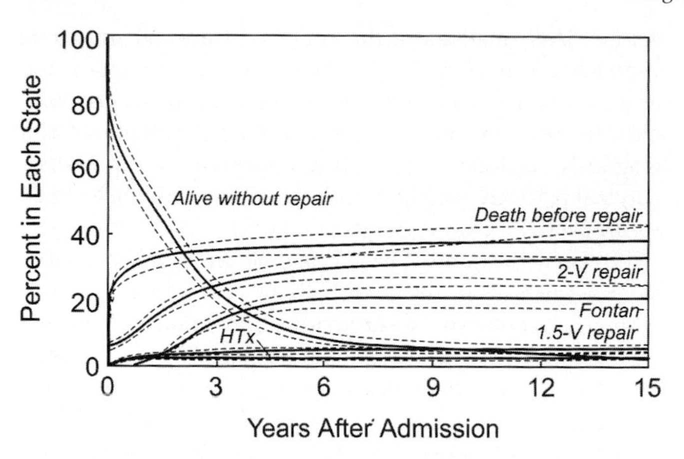

FIGURE 57–6 *Non–risk-adjusted competing risks. Depiction of treatment destination in 408 neonates with pulmonary atresia with intact interventricular septum treated at a Congenital Heart Surgeons Society institution between 1987 and 1997. Solid lines represent parametric estimates, with 70% confidence intervals. Anatomic characteristics as well as institutional protocols influence treatment destination. In the current era, 85% of neonates reach a treatment destination before death, with biventricular repair possible in about 50%. V, ventricle; HTx, heart transplant.*
From Ashburn DA, Blackstone EH, Wells WJ, et al, Determinants of mortality and type of repair in neonates with pulmonary atresia and intact ventricular septum. J Thorac Cardiovasc Surg 127: 4:1002, 2004. Reprinted with permission from the American Association for Thoracic Surgery for Elsevier.

PEDIATRIC VALVE REPLACEMENT

Valve replacement in children requires special consideration. Valve selection in this population is a compromise between size, durability, hemodynamic efficiency, anticoagulation, and growth potential (Table 57-2). Unfortunately, at the present time, no single valve adequately satisfies all these criteria.

The semilunar valves (aortic and pulmonary) require replacement more frequently than do the atrioventricular valves (tricuspid and mitral) in pediatric patients, and the options currently available include mechanical valves, xenograft valves (porcine, bovine), homografts (human valves obtained from cadavers), and autografts (Ross procedure).

Atrioventricular Valve Replacement

Mitral Valve Replacement

Mitral valve replacement is considered in children with adequate left-sided heart structures and in whom mitral valve repair is not possible. Replacement of an inadequate mitral valve in the setting of other marginal anatomic left heart structures is to be carefully avoided. In these patients, a single-ventricle approach should be pursued.

In those patients with an irreparable mitral valve, replacement can be life saving. The most suitable valve replacement is the mechanical tilting disc valve. It is preferred primarily for its size range (smallest size, 17 mm). These valves require systemic anticoagulation with warfarin sodium (Coumadin), the titration of which can be complicated by variations in dietary content of vitamin K. Regardless, the incidence of warfarin sodium–related morbidity remains relatively low.[50]

However, surgical morbidity and mortality in the youngest age group (younger than 2 years) undergoing mitral valve replacement is significant and is related to the mitral valve/body weight ratio. The 1-year survival rate in children with a ratio of 2 was 9%, with mortality increasing with greater mitral valve/body weight ratio mismatches.[51] Etrez and colleagues reported 52% mortality among 29 children younger than 2 years of age undergoing mitral valve replacement. Patients requiring mitral valve replacement after repair of ASDs, and those with Shone's syndrome fared less well than other groups.[52] Reoperations and complications in these patients were common, with a 5-year freedom-from-reoperation rate of 81% and with 16% of patients requiring permanent pacemakers.

Tricuspid Valve

Tricuspid valve replacement during infancy is rarely required. Important tricuspid regurgitation, as may be

TABLE 57–2. Relative Advantages and Disadvantages of Current Options for Valve Replacement

	Durability	Growth	Anticoagulation	Hemodynamics
Mechanical valve	++		+	
Xenograft valve		++		
Homograft valve (initially)		++	++	
Autograft valve		++	++	++

Note: The autograft replacement of the aortic valve (Ross operation) requires two valve replacements: the aortic valve with the autograft, and a homograft between the right ventricle and the pulmonary arteries to reestablish cardiopulmonary continuity. There is no ideal substitute at the present time, and valve replacement should be considered palliative.

encountered in the single right ventricle, can often be greatly improved by valvuloplasty.[53] When valve replacement must be performed, no clear superiority of mechanical versus xenograft valves has been reported, and factors described in Table 57-2 must be considered.

Atrioventricular Valve Replacement in the Single Ventricle

In the setting of the single ventricle, atrioventricular valve replacement is associated with significant morbidity and mortality.[54] On the other hand, valvuloplasty in this setting has been shown to be effective in reducing atrioventricular valve regurgitation and maintaining ventricular function, and is the procedure of choice whenever possible.[55]

Semilunar Valve Replacement

Pulmonary Valve

The pulmonary valve is the most commonly replaced valve during infancy. Often this is in the setting of congenital heart disease that includes pulmonary stenosis or atresia, and in this setting, the cryopreserved homograft has assumed predominance.[56] Although homografts are an invaluable source of appropriately sized conduits, they are nonviable, cannot grow, and eventually will require surgical revision.

Although durability and lack of growth potential of the homograft are major disadvantages, it is often the only appropriate-sized conduit for small patients. For larger patients, xenograft valves placed in the pulmonary position should be considered. Mechanical valves in the pulmonary position are avoided because of the increased risk for valve thrombosis, even with adequate anticoagulation.[57,58]

Aortic Valve

Mechanical versus tissue valves. All valve options (mechanical, xenograft, homograft, and autograft) can be considered for aortic valve replacement (AVR). A major decision point in valve selection for pediatric AVR is between mechanical and biologic (xenograft, homograft, autograft).

The early mortality rate of mechanical AVR has been reported at 0% to 13% and the late mortality rate at 0% to 11%. The incidence of reoperation on mechanical valves in the aortic position is between 6% and 16%, depending on the length of follow-up.[59–61] Patients receiving xenografts appear to have a lower mortality (early and late mortality rate, 0%), but a higher risk for reoperation; about half require replacement within 6 years.

Because of their tendency to degenerate, xenograft valves in the aortic position have generally been avoided in children. Turrentine and colleagues compared the results of mechanical versus biologic valves (autograft, homograft, xenograft) for AVR.[62] They reported a lower incidence of valve-related complications in the autograft group as compared with all other valve options. The homograft and xenograft types performed particularly poorly in terms of freedom from reoperation, with 70% (7 of 10) of xenografts and 50% (1 of 2) of homografts requiring replacement for deterioration within 9 years. Thus, in the absence of compelling indications for their use, homografts and xenografts in the aortic position in children should probably be avoided.

Autograft versus homograft. Comparisons between the autograft (Ross operation) and mechanical and xenograft valves for AVR have been reported. After the Ross operation, Elkins has reported an 89% rate of freedom from reoperation or death at 6 years, as compared with only 49% among children receiving a mechanical AVR. However, these populations were from different time periods, with the mechanical AVR being performed before 1986.[63]

In a more contemporary study, Alexiou and associates reported results more consistent with those obtained with the Ross operation.[64] They performed mechanical AVR on 56 children between 1972 and 1999. The rate of freedom from late events, including thrombosis, hemorrhage, and reoperation, was about 90% at 6 years. There were two major (valve thrombosis, stroke) and four minor (nose bleeds) complications related to anticoagulation.

In a review of 51 patients undergoing AVR (25 mechanical, 19 autografts, 6 homografts), Lupinetti and coworkers reported a significantly higher incidence of late complications in those receiving a mechanical valve.[61] The most common long-term complication reported in this group was the development of subaortic stenosis due to pannus ingrowth. Although these authors reported no serious complications related to anticoagulation, others have. Cabalka and colleagues reported six serious complications among 36 patients undergoing isolated AVR between 1982 and 1994, all occurring in the setting of supratherapeutic prothrombin times.[65] The rate of freedom from anticoagulation-related bleeding for isolated AVR was about 80% at 4 years.

Although homografts do not require anticoagulation, they do present other serious disadvantages. Besides a lack of growth potential, early degeneration of homografts has been documented, especially among young patients, and some authors have reported inferior hemodynamics as compared with autograft.[66,67] In the earliest and largest series comparing the autograft to the homograft in young patients, Gerosa and associates compared the results of 103 young patients receiving a homograft in the aortic position to those of 43 patients receiving an autograft.[68] The 15-year freedom-from-reoperation rate was 54% ± 8% versus 68% ± 11%; the rate of freedom from endocarditis was 97% ± 2% versus 75% ± 10%, and the rate of freedom from any complication was 41% ± 7% versus 50% ± 10%.

Primary tissue failure was identified in 19 homografts, but in none of the autografts.

Thus, although the homograft may provide excellent palliation among older patients, its lack of durability appears to be a serious disadvantage, especially among younger children. Under these circumstances, its use should probably be relegated to an option for children deemed unsuitable for the autograft or a mechanical valve.

Because of size constraints and anatomic requirements of neonates with LVOT lesions, the autograft can be particularly useful. At medium-term follow-up, Ohye and associates reported excellent durability and function, with appropriate growth, in neonates and infants undergoing autograft replacement of the aortic valve.[69]

LOW-BIRTH-WEIGHT SURGERY

Although low birth weight has been thought to increase the surgical risk, this must be placed in context. A treatment plan designed to provide time and support for the child to grow, thereby reducing the surgical risk, is undermined by the fact that these children cannot grow with the hemodynamic burdens of their heart disease. As a consequence, additional preoperative morbidities may be incurred for little return. In a review of 20 neonates weighing less than 1500 g, there were two early deaths (10%), and one late death.[70] Although the early surgical mortality of HLHS is increased, most centers advocate early surgical palliation in an attempt to reduce preoperative morbidity.[71]

Given these results, it appears that the prompt surgical treatment of even very small children with congenital heart disease should be performed. Low birth weight (less than 2.5 kg), consistently identified as a risk factor, was the subject of a subanalysis performed by Weinstein and coworkers.[72] These investigators reported a 47% survival among 67 patients weighing less than 2.5 kg undergoing the Norwood operation between 1990 and 1997. Although this survival rate is lower than the institution's overall stage 1 survival of 74%, these results are very similar to those reported by others.[73,74] The authors noted that, although patients were at higher risk, there was no appreciable weight gain in neonates awaiting surgery, and concluded that delaying surgery in the hope of somatic growth is unwarranted.

CIRCULATORY SUPPORT AND NEONATAL HEART SURGERY

Neonatal and infant cardiac surgery is often performed during a period of circulatory arrest. Circulatory arrest allows for a bloodless operative field devoid of obstructions produced by cannulae, and allows for precise surgical repairs. Unfortunately, extended periods of circulatory arrest have been shown to be deleterious, as shown by the Boston Circulatory Arrest Study.[75] This study, performed between 1988 and 1992, compared the outcomes of 171 neonates undergoing the arterial switch operation for D-transposition of the great arteries. Patients were randomized to repair during circulatory arrest or low-flow bypass. This longitudinal study has been of value in determining the neurocognitive and developmental impact of neonatal surgery.

Although there was little difference in the postoperative hemodynamic profiles between the two groups, patients assigned to circulatory arrest showed evidence of more severe neurological injury than did patients undergoing low flow bypass.[76,77] Incidence of clinical and electroencephalogram seizures was increased in the circulatory arrest group, and seizures were correlated with worse neurodevelopmental outcomes measured at ages 1 and 2½ years. Neurologic examination and brain magnetic resonance imaging at age 1 year also revealed more abnormalities. Developmental, neurologic, and speech outcomes measured at 8 years of age showed that neurodevelopmental outcomes were generally worse with longer durations of circulatory arrest.[78]

Because of these findings, surgeons have sought ways to reduce the exposure of the neonate to circulatory arrest during heart surgery. This has led to the development of techniques such as regional low-flow perfusion. These techniques are designed to provide circulatory support even during complex neonatal aortic surgery, such as the Norwood operation. By exploiting access to the cerebral circulation provided by the Blalock-Taussig shunt, regional perfusion allows nearly continuous circulatory support of the neonatal brain during arch surgery (Fig. 57-7). Although the Sano modification would somewhat undermine the rationale for this technique, a graft anastomosed to the innominate artery can still serve as the primary arterial cannulation.

Using this technique, the circulatory arrest time for the Norwood operation is drastically reduced, averaging about 6 minutes.[79] These techniques have taken advantage of the introduction of technologies such as near infrared spectroscopy (NIRS), which allows real-time, noninvasive monitoring of the cerebral circulation. Other modifications of bypass management that reduce the exposure of neonates to circulatory arrest during complex neonatal surgery have been described.[80]

Although intellectually attractive, no studies have documented the effect of regional perfusion on the neurodevelopmental outcomes of these neonates to date.

SUMMARY

In summary, the past 15 years have included a number of important developments in the surgical treatment of

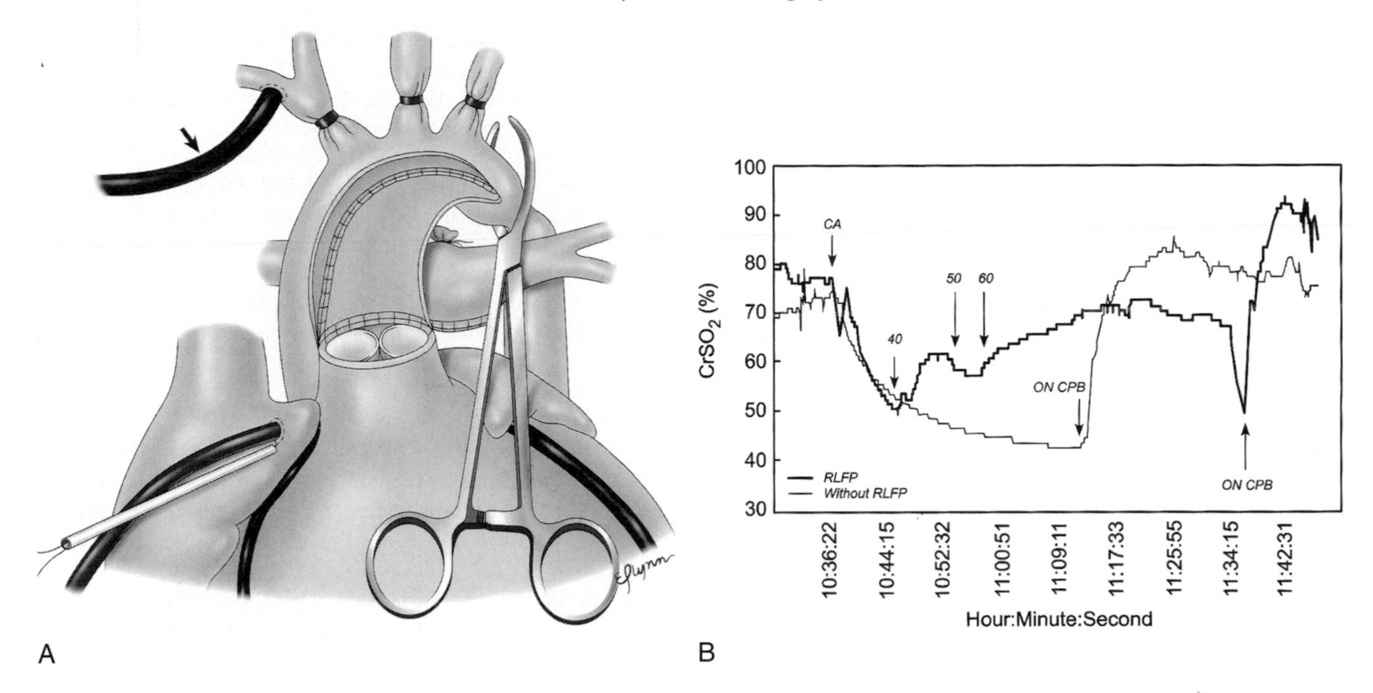

FIGURE 57–7 *A, Operative field during arch reconstruction using regional perfusion. Control of the brachiocephalic vessels and the descending aorta provide exposure of the aorta during augmentation. In the "standard" stage 1, the graft (arrow) is cut to the appropriate length and used as the arteriopulmonary shunt. When the "Sano modification" is performed, the graft is clipped and trimmed, and can be used in the event that postoperative mechanical circulatory support becomes necessary. B, Near infrared spectroscopy (NIRS) tracing of cerebral saturations ($CrSo_2$) of two neonates. The bold line represents a neonate undergoing "standard" stage 1 operation for hypoplastic left heart syndrome with regional perfusion (RLFP), and the thin line represents a neonate undergoing repair of total anomalous pulmonary venous return during circulatory arrest (CA). Although the rate of cerebral desaturation is similar between the 2 patients, regional perfusion restores $CrSo_2$ to near baseline. During circulatory arrest, $CrSo_2$ continues to decline in the patient undergoing veins repair during CA. 40, Initiation of regional perfusion at 40 mL/min; 50, 50 mL/min; 60, 60 mL/min.*

From Pigula FA, Nemoto EM, Griffith BP, et al. Regional low-flow perfusion provides cerebral circulatory support during neonatal aortic arch reconstruction. J Thorac Cardiovasc Surg 119:334, 2000. Reprinted with permission from Elsevier, Mosby division.

congenital heart disease in the neonate and infant. Greater understanding and improved management of the palliated circulation have undoubtedly contributed. Likewise, insights into the effects of cardiopulmonary bypass on the young child have improved our ability to perform complicated surgery on very small babies.

These achievements now allow for the early correction of complicated heart disease with low mortality. Because survival of surgical treatment of congenital heart disease has improved so much, other outcomes, such as quality of life and neurocognitive development, are assuming a new prominence in evaluating surgical outcomes.

REFERENCES

1. Anderson RH, Macartney FJ, Tynan M, et al. Univentricular atrioventricular connection: The single ventricle trap unsprung. Pediatr Cardiol 4:273, 1983.
2. Bridges ND, Mayer JE Jr, Lock JE, et al. Effect of baffle fenestration on outcome of the modified Fontan operation. Circulation 86:1762, 1992.
3. Nora JJ, Nora AH. Genetics and counseling in cardiovascular diseases. Springfield, IL: Charles C Thomas, 1978:155–185.
4. Tikkanen J, Heinonen OP. Risk factors for hypoplastic left heart syndrome. Tetratology 50(2):112, 1994.
5. Mahle WT, Spray TL, Wernovsky G, et al. Survival after reconstructive surgery for hypoplastic left heart syndrome: A fifteen-year experience from a single institution. Circulation 102(Suppl III):136, 2000.
6. Forbess JM, Cook N, Roth SJ, et al. Ten-year institutional experience with palliative surgery for hypoplastic left heart syndrome: Risk factors related to stage I mortality. Circulation 92(Suppl II):262, 1995.
7. Jobes DR, Nicholson SC, Stevens JM, et al. Carbon dioxide prevents pulmonary overcirculation in hypoplastic left heart syndrome. Ann Thorac Surg 54:150, 1992.
8. Riordan CJ, Randsbaek F, Storey JH, et al. Effect of oxygen, positive end-expiratory pressure, and carbon dioxide on

oxygen delivery in an animal model of the univentricular heart. J Thorac Cardiovasc Surg 112:644, 1996.
9. Mora GA, Pizzaro C, Jacobs ML, et al. Experimental model of single ventricle: Influence of carbon dioxide on pulmonary vascular dynamics. Circulation 90(Pt. 2):43, 1994.
10. Maegawa Y, Mizobe T, Yamagishi M, et al. The use of nitrogen and nitric oxide to control pulmonary blood flow in the Norwood operation. J Cardiothorac Vasc Anesth 16(2):264, 2002.
11. Tabbutt, Ramamoorthy C, Montenegro LM, et al. Impact of inspired gas mixtures on preoperative infants with hypoplastic left heart syndrome (HLHS) during controlled ventilation. Circulation 102(Suppl 2):469, 2000.
12. Bradley SM, Simsic JM, Atz AM. Hemodynamic effects of inspired carbon dioxide after the Norwood procedure. Ann Thorac Surg 72:2088, 2001.
13. Chang AC, Zucker HA, Hickey PR, et al. Pulmonary vascular resistance in infants after cardiac surgery: Role of carbon dioxide and hydrogen ion. Crit Care Med 23(3);568, 1995.
14. Hislop A, Reid L. New findings in pulmonary arteries of rat with hypoxia induced pulmonary hypertension. Br J Exp Pathol 57: 542, 1976.
15. Meyrick B, Reid L. The effect of continued hypoxia on rat pulmonary arterial circulation. Lab Invest 38: 188, 1978.
16. Haworth SG, Hislop. Effect of hypoxia on adaptation on the pulmonary circulation in the pig. Cardiovasc Research 16:293, 1982.
17. Day RW, Barton AJ, Pysher TJ, et al. Pulmonary vascular resistance of children treated with nitrogen during early infancy. Ann Thorac Surg 65:1400, 1998.
18. Tweddell JS, Hoffman GM, Federly RT, et al. Phenoxybenzamine improves systemic oxygen delivery after the Norwood procedure. Ann Thorac Surg 67:161, 1999.
19. Tweddell JS, Hoffman GM, Fedderly, et al. Patients at risk for low systemic oxygen delivery after the Norwood procedure. Ann Thorac Surg 69:1893, 2000.
20. Hoffman GM, Ghanayem NS, Kampine JM, et al. Venous saturation and the anaerobic threshold in neonates after the Norwood procedure for hypoplastic left heart syndrome. Ann Thorac Surg 70:1515, 2000.
21. Tweddell JS, Hoffman GM, Mussatto KA, et al. Improved survival of patients undergoing palliation of hypoplastic left heart syndrome: Lessons learned from 115 consecutive patients. Circulation 106(Suppl I):82, 2002.
22. Bove EL, Lloyd TR. Staged reconstruction for hypoplastic left heart syndrome. Ann Surg 224:387, 1996.
23. Cohen MI, Bridges ND, Gaynor JW, et al. Modifications to the cavopulmonary anastomosis do not eliminate early sinus node dysfunction. J Thorac Cardiovasc Surg 120:891, 2000.
24. Lange R, Schreiber C, Gunther T, et al. Results of biventricular repair of congenital cardiac malformations: Definitive corrective surgery? Eur J Cardiothorac Surg 20(6):1207, 2001.
25. Manning PB, Mayer JE Jr, Sanders SP, et al. Unique features and prognosis of primum ASD presenting in the first year of life. Circulation 90(5 Pt 2):30, 1994.
26. Bonatti V, Agnetti A, Squarcia U. Early and late postoperative complete heart block in pediatric patients submitted to open heart surgery for congenital heart disease. Pediatr Med Chir 20(3):181, 1998.
27. Weindling SN, Saul JP, Gamble WJ, et al. Duration of complete atrioventricular block after congenital heart disease surgery. Am J Cardiol 82(4):525, 1998.
28. Bacha EA, Almodovar M, Wessel DL, et al. Surgery for coarctation of the aorta in infants weighing less than 2 kg. Ann Thorac Surg 71(4):1260, 2001.
29. McCrindle BW, Tchervenkov CI, Konstantinov IE, et al. Risk factors associated with mortality and interventions in 472 neonates with interrupted aortic arch: A Congenital Heart Surgeons Society study. J Thorac Cardiovasc Surg 129:343, 2005.
30. Behrendt DM, Kirsch MM, Stern A, et al. The surgical therapy for pulmonary artery-right ventricular discontinuity. Ann Thor Surg 18:122, 1974.
31. Ebert PA, Turley K, Stanger P, et al. Surgical treatment of truncus arteriosus in the first six months of life. Ann Surg 200:451, 1984.
32. Lacour-Gayet F, Serraf A, Komiya T, et al. Truncus arteriosus repair: Influence of techniques of right ventricular outflow tract reconstruction. J Thorac Cardiovasc Surg 111:849, 1996.
33. Jahangiri M, Zurakowski D, Mayer JE, et al. Repair of truncal valve and associated interrupted arch in neonates with truncus arteriosus. J Thorac Cardiovasc Surg 119:508, 2000.
34. Thompson LD, McElhinney DB, Reddy VM, et al. Neonatal repair of truncus arteriosus: Continuing improvement in outcomes. Ann Thorac Surg 72:391, 2001.
35. Miyamoto T, Sinzobahamvya N, Kumpikaite D, et al. Repair of truncus arteriosus and aortic arch interruption: Outcome analysis. Ann Thorac Surg 79:2077, 2005.
36. Mulder TJ, Pyles LA, Stolfi A, et al. A multicenter analysis of the choice of initial surgical procedure in tetralogy of Fallot. Pediatric Cardiol 23(6):580, 2002.
37. Van Arsdell GS, Maharaj GS, Tom J, et al. What is the optimal age for repair of tetralogy of Fallot? Circulation 102(19 Suppl 3):123, 2000.
38. Pigula FA, Khalil PN, Mayer JE, et al. Repair of tetralogy of Fallot in neonates and young infants. Circulation 100 (Suppl II):157, 1999.
39. Marshall AC, Love BA, Lang P, et al. Staged repair of tetralogy of Fallot and diminutive pulmonary arteries with a fenestrated ventricular septal defect patch. J Thorac Cardiovas Surg 126(5):1427, 2003.
40. Scheule AM, Zurakowski D, Blume ED, et al. Arterial switch operation with a single coronary artery. J Thorac Cardiovasc Surg 123(6):1164, 2002.
41. Boutin C, Jonas RA, Sanders SP, et al. Rapid two-stage arterial switch operation. Acquisition of left ventricular mass after pulmonary artery banding in infants with transposition of the great arteries. Circulation 90(3):1304, 1994.
42. Kang N, de Leval MR, Eliot M, et al. Extending the boundaries of the primary arterial switch operation in patients with transposition of the great arteries and intact ventricular septum. Circulation 110(Suppl II):123, 1994.
43. Delisle G, Ando M, Calder AL, et al. Total anomalous pulmonary venous connection: Report of 92 autopsied cases

with emphasis on diagnostic and surgical considerations. Am Heart J 91:99; 1976.

44. Hancock Friesen C, Zurakowski D, Thiagarajan RR, et al. Total anomalous pulmonary venous connection: An analysis of current management strategies in a single institution. Ann Thorac Surg 79:596, 2005.
45. Sadr IM, Tan PE, Kieran MW, et al. Mechanism of pulmonary vein stenosis in infants with normally connected veins. Am J Cardiol 86:577, A10, 2000.
46. Jahangiri M, Zurakowski D, Bichell D, et al. Improved results with selective management in pulmonary atresia with intact ventricular septum. J Thorac Cardiovasc Surg 118:1046, 1999.
47. Guleserian KJ, Armsby LB, Thiagarajan RR, et al. Natural history of PA/IVS & RV-dependent coronary circulation managed by the single ventricle approach. Ann Thorac Surg (in press).
48. Ashburn DA, Blackstone EH, Wells WJ, et al. Determinants of mortality and type of repair in neonates with pulmonary atresia and intact ventricular septum. J Thorac Cardiovasc Surg 127(4):1000, 2004.
49. Pawade A, Capuani A, Penny DJ, et al. Pulmonary atresia with intact ventricular septum: surgical management based on right ventricular infundibulum. J Cardiac Surg 8(3):371, 1993.
50. Calderone CA, Raghuveer G, Hills CB, et al. Long-term survival after mitral valve replacement in children aged < 5 years: A multi-institutional study. Circulation 104(12 Suppl 1):143, 2001.
51. Raghuveer G, Calderone CA, Hills CB, et al. Predictors of prosthesis survival, growth, and functional status following mechanical valve replacement in children aged < 5 years, a multi-institutional study. Circulation 108(Suppl 1):174, 2003.
52. Etrez E, Kanter KR, Isom E, et al. Mitral valve replacement in children. J Heart Valve Dis 12(1):25, 2003.
53. Kanter KR, Forbess JM, Fyfe DA, et al. De Vega tricuspid annuloplasty for systemic tricuspid regurgitation in children with univentricular physiology. J Heart Valve Dis 13(1):86, 2004.
54. Mahle WT, Gaynor JW, Spray TL. Atrioventricular valve replacement in patients with a single ventricle. Ann Thorac Surg 72(1):182, 2001.
55. Freisen CL, Sherwood MC, Gavreau K, et al. Intermediate outcomes of atrioventricular valvuloplasty in lateral tunnel Fontan patients. J Heart Valve Dis 13(6):962, 2001.
56. Mayer JE Jr. Uses of homograft conduits for right ventricle to pulmonary artery connections in the neonatal period. Semin Thorac Cardiovasc Surg 7(3):130, 1995.
57. Kanter KR, Budde JM. Parks WJ, et al. One hundred pulmonary valve replacements in children after relief of right ventricular outflow tract obstruction. Ann Thorac Surg 73(6):1801, 2002.
58. Nurozler F, Bradley SM St. Jude medical valve in pulmonary position: Anticoagulation and thrombosis. Asian Cardiovasc Thorac Ann 10(2):181, 2002.
59. Mazzitelli DF, Guenther T, Schreiber C, et al. Aortic valve replacement in children: Are we on the right track? Eur J Cardiothorac Surg 13:565, 1998.
60. Champsaur G, Robin J, Tronc F, et al. Mechanical valve in aortic position is a valid option in children and adolescents. Eur J Cardiothorac Surg 11:117, 1997.
61. Lupinetti FM, Warner J, Jones TK, et al. Comparison of human tissues and mechanical prostheses for aortic valve replacement in children. Circulation 96:321, 1997.
62. Turrentine MW, Ruzmetov M, Vijay P, et al. Biological versus mechanical aortic valve replacement in children. Ann Thorac Surg 71:S356, 2001.
63. Elkins RC: Congenital aortic valve disease: Evolving management. Ann Thorac Surg 59:269, 1995.
64. Alexiou C, McDonald A, Langley SM, et al. Aortic valve replacement in children: Are mechanical prostheses a good option? Eur J Cardiothorac Surg 17:125, 2000.
65. Cabalka AK, Emery RW, Petersen RJ, et al. Long-term follow-up of the St. Jude medical prosthesis in pediatric patients. Ann Thorac Surg 60:S618, 1995.
66. Clarke DR, Campbell DN, Hayward AR, et al. Degeneration of aortic valve allografts in young recipients. J Thorac Cardiovasc Surg 103:934, 1993.
67. Ng SK, O'Brien MF, Harrocks S, et al. Influence of patient age and implantation technique on the probability of re-replacement of the homograft aortic valve. J Heart Valve Dis 11(2):217, 2002.
68. Gerosa G, McKay R, Davies J, et al. Comparison of the aortic homograft and the pulmonary autograft for aortic valve or root replacement in children. J Thorac Cardiovasc Surg 102:1, 1991.
69. Ohye RG, Gomez CA, Ohye BJ, et al. The Ross/Konno procedure in neonates and infants: Intermediate term survival and autograft function. Ann Thorac Surg 72:823, 2001.
70. Reddy VM, Hanley FL. Semin Pediatr Surg 9(2):91, 2000.
71. Pizzaro C, Davis DA, Galantowicz ME, et al. Stage I palliation for hypoplastic left heart syndrome in low birth weight neonates: can we justify it? Eur J Cardiothorac Surg 21(4):716, 2000.
72. Weinstein S, Gaynor JW, Bridges ND, et al. Early survival of infants weighing 2.5 kilograms or less undergoing first-stage reconstruction for hypoplastic left heart syndrome. Circulation 100(Suppl II):167, 1999.
73. Bove EL, Lloyd TR. Staged reconstruction for hypoplastic left heart syndrome. Ann Surg 224:387, 1996.
74. Rossi AF, Seiden HS, Sadeghi AM, et al. The outcome of cardiac operations in infants weighing two kilograms or less. J Thorac Cardiovasc Surg 116:28, 1998.
75. Newburger JW, Jonas RA, Wernovsky G, et al. A comparison of the perioperative neurologic effects of hypothermic circulatory arrest versus low-flow cardiopulmonary bypass in infant heart surgery. N Engl J Med 329(15):1057, 1993.
76. Wernovsky G, Wypij D, Jonas RA, et al. Postoperative course and hemodynamic profile after the arterial switch operation in neonates and infants. Circulation 92:2226, 1995.
77. Rappaport LA, Wypij D, Bellinger DC, et al. Relation of seizures after cardiac surgery in early infancy to neurodevelopmental outcome. Boston Circulatory Arrest Study Group. Circulation 97(8):773, 1998.

78. Wypij D, Newburger JW, Rappaport LA, et al. The effect of duration of deep hypothermic circulatory arrest in infant heart surgery on late neurodevelopment: The Boston Circulatory Arrest Trial. J Thorac Cardiovasc Surg 127(5):1256, 2004.
79. Pigula FA, Nemoto EM, Griffith BP, et al. Regional low-flow perfusion provides cerebral circulatory support during neonatal aortic arch reconstruction. J Thorac Cardiovasc Surg 119:331, 2000.
80. McElhinney DB, Reddy VM, Silverman N, et al. Modified Damus-Kaye-Stanzel procedure for single ventricle, subaortic stenosis, and arch obstruction in neonates and infants: Midterm results and techniques for avoiding circulatory arrest. J Thorac Cardiovasc Surg 114:718, 1997.

58

Surgical Management of the Patient with the Univentricular Heart

JOHN E. MAYER, JR.

Patients who are born with a single functional ventricle (including those with tricuspid atresia) have a dismal prognosis without surgical intervention,[1,2] and the results of the Fontan operation, which is currently the "definitive" procedure for these patients, are now quite good.[3–5] As a consequence, the management of these patients is directed toward making each patient an optimal candidate for the Fontan procedure,[6] and it is critically important that patient management begins at birth with this goal in mind. Most single-ventricle patients require palliative surgical procedures during the first few years of life to augment pulmonary blood flow to treat cyanosis, or to limit pulmonary blood flow to treat congestive heart failure. A variety of surgical procedures may be necessary to fulfill these short-term goals of relieving cyanosis and preventing congestive heart failure. The initial surgical procedures must not only achieve these short-term goals but also be carefully designed to achieve the longer-term goal of creating a suitable candidate for the "reparative" Fontan operation.

ANATOMY

The most common forms of functional single ventricle include tricuspid atresia, hypoplastic left heart syndrome, and several other anatomic variants in which there is functionally only a single ventricle of either right or left ventricular morphology. Each of these variants may be associated with normally related or transposed great vessels. The anatomic details of each of these anatomic subsets are covered in Chapters 41, 44, and 45. In general, most single-ventricle patients have valvar or subvalvar obstruction of blood flow to either the pulmonary or systemic circulation.[7,8] In uncommon circumstances, there may be no obstruction to either the pulmonary or systemic circulation. When there is obstruction to pulmonary blood flow, the patient will be cyanotic, and when there is obstruction to the systemic circulation, the patient will present with low systemic cardiac output. In the latter group with intracardiac obstruction to systemic blood flow, there is a high incidence of aortic arch obstruction.

NEONATAL SURGICAL INTERVENTIONS

Indications

In almost all anatomic single-ventricle situations, the patients can be temporarily palliated with prostaglandin E_1, which preserves or reestablishes patency of the ductus arteriosus, which in turn provides a pathway for blood flow to the circulation affected by the intracardiac obstruction. Use of prostaglandin E_1 thus allows patients to be resuscitated from the insult associated with initial ductal closure when the diagnosis of single ventricle is not made in the nursery. Adequate resuscitation with restoration of normal acid-base status and end-organ function is an important factor in achieving a satisfactory outcome after neonatal palliative procedures. The one situation in which patients cannot be successfully managed is when there is associated obstruction to pulmonary venous return, and in this situation, emergent relief of pulmonary venous obstruction in the catheterization laboratory or in the operating room is required. Because the goal of the neonatal interventions is to ensure appropriate anatomy and physiology for a Fontan procedure, pulmonary blood flow and pressure must be limited to prevent development of elevated pulmonary vascular resistance, central pulmonary architecture must be preserved, pulmonary venous drainage must be unobstructed, and obstruction to ventricular ejection and ventricular volume overload must be minimized to preserve ventricular function.

Single Ventricle with Obstruction to Pulmonary Blood Flow

In these situations, additional pulmonary blood flow must be provided, and a systemic–pulmonary artery shunt is placed. In newborns and children up to 3 months of age, we have most commonly carried out a modified Blalock-Taussig shunt procedure in which a 3.5-mm PTFE graft is interposed between the right innominate artery and the right pulmonary artery through a median sternotomy incision. The ductus arteriosus is generally ligated during the same operation to avoid excessive pulmonary blood flow. The advantage of using a prosthetic graft to augment pulmonary blood flow is that the amount of added pulmonary blood flow is controlled by the size of the graft. In addition, any pulmonary artery distortion developing as a result of the shunt procedure is readily accessible at subsequent operations carried out through a median sternotomy. In the case of hypoplastic left heart syndrome, there has been recent interest in placing a shunt between the single right ventricle and the pulmonary artery, but the long-term effects of the required ventriculotomy on the function of the single right ventricle remain unknown.

Single Ventricle with Obstruction to Systemic Blood Flow

In patients with valvar or subvalvar obstruction to the aorta and the systemic circulation, neonatal surgical palliation involves a much more extensive procedure. For these patients, there is no obstruction to pulmonary blood flow, and the initial surgical palliation involves a procedure to use this unobstructed pulmonary pathway as the pathway to the systemic circulation. This redirection is accomplished by a proximal main pulmonary artery–aorta anastomosis. Pulmonary blood flow is then restored with a modified Blalock-Taussig shunt (typically a 3.5-mm PTFE graft between a brachiocephalic artery and the pulmonary artery), or more recently a PTFE graft between the single ventricle and the pulmonary arteries. In most patients with obstruction to systemic blood flow, there is coexisting aortic arch obstruction. The paradigm for this type of procedure is the Norwood stage 1 procedure for hypoplastic left heart syndrome in which the hypoplastic aortic arch is augmented, the main pulmonary artery is anastomosed to the augmented aorta, and a modified Blalock-Taussig or ventricle–pulmonary artery shunt is inserted. However, a comparable procedure is carried out for other forms of single ventricle with obstruction to the systemic circulation.

There are anatomic situations in which there may not appear to be obstruction to either systemic or pulmonary blood flow, and in these patients, pulmonary blood flow will increase over the first few weeks of life as the normal postnatal fall in pulmonary vascular resistance occurs, and congestive heart failure ensues. There is a temptation to place a narrowing in the pulmonary artery (pulmonary artery band) to limit pulmonary blood flow, but the number of times when this procedure is appropriate for single-ventricle patients is very limited. In many single-ventricle situations in which there is no obstruction to pulmonary blood flow, the aorta is "transposed" and arises from a rudimentary infundibular chamber. In these cases, the pathway from the single ventricle to the aorta involves a bulboventricular foramen (BVF, a ventricular septal defect between the dominant ventricle and the rudimentary infundibular chamber), and even if this BVF is not obstructed at birth, it can be expected to become smaller in size over time.[9] As the BVF becomes restrictive, the functional effect is subaortic stenosis, which will result in ventricular hypertrophy and reduced compliance of the single ventricle. If there is a coarctation present, then it is very likely that the BVF will be restrictive in the newborn period.[9]

SURGICAL PROCEDURES AFTER THE NEWBORN PERIOD

The subsequent operative strategy for each patient is individualized based on the anatomy and physiology of that patient. After the first few months of life, pulmonary vascular resistance generally falls, and then the goals of subsequent surgical interventions should be to reduce the volume load on the single ventricle. This goal is met by eliminating systemic arterial–pulmonary artery shunts or eliminating connections between the single ventricle and the pulmonary circulation. Once these systemic–pulmonary artery connections are removed, pulmonary blood flow is reestablished by creating direct connections between the venous system and the pulmonary arteries by means of a bidirectional cavopulmonary artery shunt or the Fontan procedure. It has become relatively standard practice to carry out a bidirectional cavopulmonary shunt procedure as a preliminary procedure before the Fontan procedure, but use of this staged approach as opposed to proceeding directly to a Fontan procedure is made on an individual patient basis.

Any residual anatomic problems such as pulmonary artery distortion, intracardiac obstruction to systemic blood flow, or a restrictive atrial septal defect should be dealt with at the time of the bidirectional cavopulmonary shunt procedure to simplify the "definitive" Fontan procedure.

PREOPERATIVE EVALUATION OF PATIENTS FOR BIDIRECTIONAL CAVOPULMONARY SHUNT AND FONTAN PROCEDURES

These two procedures share the characteristic that pulmonary blood flow is passive (not directly propelled by a ventricle) and depends only on the difference between systemic venous pressure and left atrial pressure. Therefore, the critical issues for a satisfactory outcome after either of these procedures are low pulmonary vascular resistance, undistorted central pulmonary arteries of adequate caliber, and low pulmonary venous pressures (related to ventricular compliance). Cardiac catheterization provides the information on these parameters, although additional information can be obtained from echocardiography and magnetic resonance imaging. "Ideal" hemodynamic criteria for the Fontan procedure are a pulmonary vascular resistance (indexed to body surface area) of less than 2 Wood units, pulmonary artery mean pressures of less than 15 mmHg, undistorted large central pulmonary arteries, good ventricular function, and pulmonary venous atrial pressures of less than 5 mmHg.

BIDIRECTIONAL CAVOPULMONARY SHUNT OPERATION

Indications

The hemodynamic advantage of the bidirectional cavopulmonary artery shunt operation is that it allows the elimination of systemic–pulmonary artery shunts and elimination of connections between the systemic ventricle and the pulmonary arteries, thereby eliminating the volume load on the single ventricle and maintaining a viable level of oxygenation. In addition, the preoperative criteria associated with a successful bidirectional cavopulmonary shunt operation (BDCPS) are less stringent than for a Fontan procedure. We prefer to carry out this operation within the first 4 to 6 months of life in an attempt to reduce the volume load on the single ventricle and thereby preserve ventricular function for the subsequent Fontan operation. A calculated pulmonary vascular resistance as high as 3 to 4 Wood units (indexed to body surface area) or pulmonary artery mean pressures as high as 20 mmHg are compatible with a successful bidirectional cavopulmonary artery shunt operation.

An important question is how one makes the choice between a BDCPS and a Fontan operation in the young patient (usually between 9 and 18 months of age) who requires an intervention because of increasing cyanosis. Typically, this is the patient who has undergone a neonatal shunting or banding operation and develops increasing cyanosis. In our initial review of the Fontan operation, young age (younger than 4 years) was not found to be an independent risk factor for failure of the operation, but our subsequent analysis of a larger experience suggested that age younger than 3 years was a risk factor by multivariant analysis. Based on this experience, we have now adopted the approach that the younger patient is not excluded from consideration for a Fontan operation based on age alone, but must be an "ideal" candidate as previously outlined. It is our impression that younger patients tolerate elevated venous pressures less well than older patients, and therefore the criteria for carrying out a Fontan operation for these patients should be stricter. Otherwise, the young patient should undergo a BDCPS as an interval step. Conversely, we have also observed that the older patient is likely to have a lower arterial oxygen saturation after a BDCPS[10] and therefore may be better considered as a candidate for a "fenestrated" Fontan operation.

Operative Technique

The concept for the BDCPS is to create a functional end-to-side connection between the cranial end of the superior vena cava (SVC) and both pulmonary arteries. This operation is generally carried out using cardiopulmonary bypass with an ascending aortic cannula for arterial inflow and two venous cannulae in the innominate vein and in the right atrium. All systemic–pulmonary artery shunts are controlled before the start of bypass to prevent systemic pump flow from being "stolen" into the pulmonary circulation through an open shunt. Most commonly, this cavopulmonary connection is created by dividing the SVC at the level of the right pulmonary artery and then sewing the cranial end of the SVC into an incision in the superior aspect of the right pulmonary artery. It is necessary to divide the azygous vein to prevent decompression of the SVC blood away from the lungs and into the inferior vena cava.

An alternative approach, termed a *hemi-Fontan* procedure, is to create anastomoses between both the cranial and cardiac ends of the SVC and the pulmonary artery using arteriotomies in both the superior and inferior surfaces of the right pulmonary artery. To prevent SVC blood from reaching the right atrium and bypassing the lungs, the SVC–right atrial orifice must then be occluded with a patch of PTFE. Others use a prosthetic patch to both enlarge the central pulmonary arteries and occlude the connection with the right atrium. The advantage of the hemi-Fontan approach is that it simplifies the subsequent Fontan operation into a procedure in which the SVC–right atrial junction patch is removed and the intra-atrial baffle is placed. This approach thereby avoids dissection around the sinus node at the time of the Fontan operation.

In the presence of both left and right SVCs, both should be anastomosed to their respective pulmonary arteries unless one is clearly much smaller and can therefore be ligated. If one SVC is not connected to the pulmonary arterial system, then this SVC will decompress the contralateral SVC into either the inferior vena caval system or into the atrium directly, and there will be inadequate pulmonary blood flow.

Results

The results of the initial experience with the bidirectional cavopulmonary artery shunt operation are, in general, quite favorable. In one group of 28 patients undergoing this procedure as a second-stage operation in the management of their single-ventricle anatomy in our institution, 27 survived. The major sources of difficulty have been primarily related to either markedly elevated pulmonary vascular resistance or unrecognized venous collaterals from the SVC system to either the inferior vena cava or to the atrium, which will lead to decreased oxygen saturation.

FONTAN OPERATION

Indications

It is our current belief that most patients with single ventricle will be best served over the long term by undergoing a Fontan type of operation. However, the true long-term (lifetime) outcome of the Fontan operation is unknown, and at this time, the wisdom of adopting a treatment strategy of directing all single-ventricle patients toward a Fontan procedure as the "definitive" treatment remains unproved. However, if one accepts this treatment strategy as the preferred approach, the issue is not the indication for the operation, but rather the definition of the contraindications to this approach. Several studies have been undertaken to identify risk factors for this operation,[3–5,10] and the relative importance of the various risk factors has been in evolution over time. We currently view pulmonary vascular resistance greater than 2 Wood units (indexed to body surface area), significant pulmonary artery narrowings that cannot be repaired surgically, and pulmonary artery pressures greater than 15 mmHg as indicators of greater risk, although none of these variables should be viewed as absolute contraindications (Table 58-1). Each piece of data should be carefully evaluated for potential measurement errors, calculation errors, and physiologic conditions that might temporarily alter the patient's physiology and thereby convey an erroneous impression of the patient's ability to tolerate a Fontan operation. For example, calculation of pulmonary vascular resistance requires knowledge of both pulmonary artery mean pressure and pulmonary blood flow (PBF). Calculation of PBF by the Fick method depends on measurement of oxygen uptake and on accurate measurement of pulmonary artery and pulmonary venous oxygen content. If there is more than one source of PBF, and if the two sources do not have the same oxygen content, then calculation of pulmonary blood flow and resistance will not be reliable. Similarly, if the patient is hypoventilating with an elevated P_{CO_2} and low pH during the catheterization, then pulmonary resistance can be artificially elevated. When pulmonary resistance is measured in a nonpulsatile system, such as will be present after a bidirectional cavopulmonary shunt, it has been our impression that the calculated pulmonary vascular resistance tends to be higher (presumably owing to the nonpulsatile nature of the pulmonary blood flow), and we now do not view a pulmonary vascular resistance of up to 2.5 to 3 Wood units in this type of circulation as unacceptable for a Fontan operation. Ventricular function can be difficult to precisely quantify because of the variable geometry of many single ventricles. The presence of atrioventricular valvar regurgitation may occur as a consequence of volume loading of the single ventricle, if the patient has a systemic–pulmonary artery shunt or a persistent anatomic connection between the ventricle and the pulmonary circulation, and the regurgitation may improve when the volume load is removed. Also, we have at least a few patients who have been found to have atrioventricular valve regurgitation after the Fontan operation and who are tolerating this quite well. Finally, it must be emphasized that our loosening of the criteria for a Fontan operation is based on the fact that almost all of our patients now undergo a fenestrated Fontan operation, which we believe allows less "ideal" patients to tolerate this operation.[12]

TABLE 58–1. Multivariant Analysis: Preoperative Risk Factors for Early Failure, 1987–1991

Risk Factor	*P* Value
Younger age	.04
Higher pulmonary vascular resistance	.001
Pulmonary artery distortion	.04

Operative Technique

The technique of the Fontan operation has now become fairly standardized, and we routinely now use the

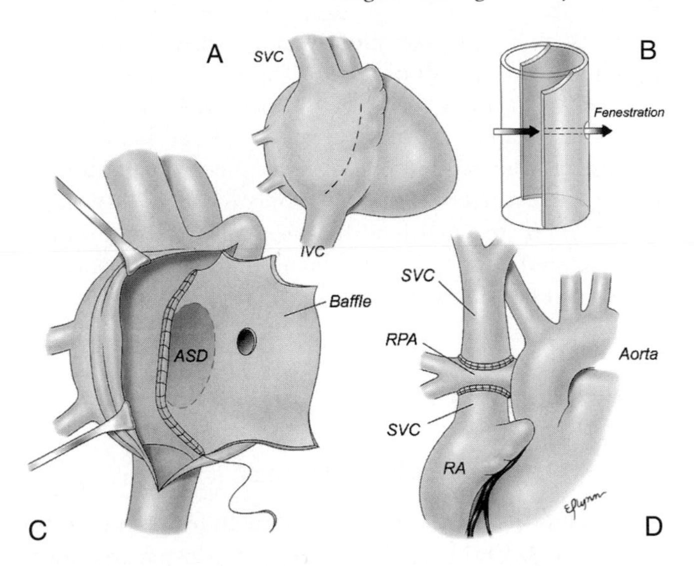

FIGURE 58–1 *Diagrammatic representation of components of lateral tunnel modified Fontan procedure. A, Right atrial (RA) incision (dotted line). SVC, superior vena cava; IVC, inferior vena cava. B, Polytetrafluoroethylene baffle construction with 4-mm fenestration (arrow). C, Posterior suture line of fenestrated baffle completed, anterior to surgically created atrial septal defect (ASD). D, Usual cavopulmonary anastomosis with divided ends of superior vena cava anastomosed to right pulmonary artery (RPA).*

"lateral tunnel" version with direct cavopulmonary anastomoses (Fig. 58-1). The operation is carried out using hypothermic cardiopulmonary bypass (24° to 28°C). All systemic–pulmonary artery shunts must be controlled before the institution of cardiopulmonary bypass to prevent runoff of systemic blood flow into the pulmonary circulation and to minimize volume loading of the single ventricle postoperatively. It is important to avoid ventricular distention once the heart has stopped having effective contractions, and a vent catheter is generally placed. Once the aorta is clamped and cardioplegia is given, the right atrium is opened with an incision parallel to the atrioventricular groove. The atrial septum should be inspected, and a large defect should be created to prevent any restriction to flow between the atria. The creation of a large ASD is particularly important when there is left atrioventricular valve atresia or stenosis because a restrictive ASD will cause pulmonary venous obstruction, which will virtually guarantee the failure of the Fontan operation. The location of all pulmonary and systemic venous connections must be confirmed. The lateral tunnel technique involves placement of a baffle along the lateral aspect of the right atrium, which conveys inferior vena cava blood to the SVC orifice. This baffle is cut in the form of a half cylinder of PTFE patch material, and a 4-mm fenestration (see Fig. 58-1) is made in the medial aspect of the baffle. The fenestration is placed in an attempt to prevent the systemic venous pressure from reaching intolerably high levels during the intraoperative and early postoperative period. In the presence of the fenestration, limited amounts of systemic venous blood are allowed to reach the pulmonary venous atrium and then the systemic circulation without being required to first pass through the lungs. Conceptually, this right-to-left shunt at the atrial level allows preservation of systemic cardiac output at the expense of some reduction in arterial oxygen saturation.[12] Initial experience with the use of the fenestration in Fontan patients indicated that it was associated with lower operative mortality and a lower incidence of postoperative pleural effusions.

Less common anatomic situations may require different approaches to achieve the goals of an unobstructed systemic venous pathway from the superior and inferior venae cavae to the pulmonary arteries and an unobstructed pathway for pulmonary venous blood to reach the atrioventricular valves and systemic ventricle. In the patients with a left SVC, the operation is modified by adding a left SVC–left pulmonary artery anastomosis, using the same technique as for a right SVC. In patients with heterotaxy-type heart disease, which may include anomalies of both systemic and pulmonary venous connections, it is preferable to use a complete tube (conduit) to convey inferior vena cava blood to the pulmonary arteries, and this conduit may lie either within or outside the atrium (extracardiac Fontan).

POSTOPERATIVE MANAGEMENT AFTER FONTAN AND BIDIRECTIONAL CAVOPULMONARY SHUNT OPERATIONS

After either of these operations, pulmonary blood flow will be driven by the difference between systemic venous pressure and the pulmonary venous pressure. Therefore, it is important to monitor these pressures and to employ measures to minimize pulmonary vascular resistance. In general, poor hemodynamics and a requirement for high levels of vasopressor support should prompt a thorough investigation for any residual anatomic problems with the operation. Echocardiography, or if necessary, a cardiac catheterization should be undertaken to identify residual problems. In the patient with a bidirectional cavopulmonary artery shunt, the arterial saturation will generally be in excess of 80%, although older patients will be more likely to have lower saturations because SVC return represents a smaller percentage of the total systemic venous return. More severe cyanosis may imply the presence of a venous connection, which decompresses the SVC into either the inferior vena cava (such as an azygous vein) or into the atrium. We have frequently observed systemic arterial hypertension after the BDCPS operation, which we believe is a reflex response to cerebral venous hypertension. It is generally treated acutely with systemic afterload reduction.

After the Fontan operation, it is again important to monitor systemic and pulmonary venous pressures and indicators of cardiac output such as strength of pulses, arterial blood pressure, urine output, and capillary refill time. An unfavorable hemodynamic course should result in prompt investigations, including an echocardiogram and catheterization to determine whether there are residual anatomic problems with the operation. Systemic venous hypertension, which is obligatory after a Fontan operation, seems to cause reflex arterial vasoconstriction, and this increased afterload may impair ventricular output. We liberally employ vasodilator agents in the postoperative period (e.g., milrinone, nitroprusside) to offset this vasoconstriction. In the absence of a correctable cause for a failing Fontan circulation, early takedown to a bidirectional cavopulmonary shunt offers the best hope for patient survival. Because it is relatively uncommon for there to be severe low cardiac output after a fenestrated Fontan operation, we regard low cardiac output that does not respond to low- to moderate-dose pharmacologic intervention and for which there is no correctable anatomic cause as an indication to take the Fontan procedure down, and we have found that takedown to a BDCPS is generally successful. In older patients, it may be necessary to add a small systemic–pulmonary artery shunt to provide adequate arterial saturation.

Atrial pacing wires are an essentially obligatory adjunct to postoperative management as well. There may be sinus node dysfunction due to surgical manipulation in this area, and patients after both Fontan and bidirectional cavopulmonary artery shunt operations seem to be quite sensitive to the loss of sinus rhythm. Atrial pacing in these situations can improve the hemodynamics quite remarkably by lowering the atrial filling pressures and augmenting cardiac output. Also, the atrial pacing wires allow the accurate diagnosis of arrhythmias in the postoperative patient.

Pleural effusions are the most common problem after a Fontan operation, and they have not been totally eliminated by the use of the fenestration. There is reasonably good evidence that the liver and mesenteric circulation are the source of the fluid that collects in the pleural or pericardial spaces. Complete drainage of effusions is generally advisable because a large fluid collection will compress the lung and can therefore raise the pulmonary vascular resistance. It is important to maintain adequate fluid replacement and nutrition for the patient who is having large chest tube losses for more than a few days after the operation. Fortunately, most patients with effusions stop draining within 1 to 3 weeks after the operation. For patients with persistent drainage, cardiac catheterization is advisable to rule out residual anatomic problems.

Occasionally, a fenestration spontaneously closes immediately or within days of surgery. Some of these patients have become acutely very ill with hypotension, renal failure, extensive edema, and fully saturated arterial blood. Such closure can be readily confirmed echocardiographically. Immediate catheterization is necessary for survival to either reopen or create a new fenestration, to allow cardiac output augmentation by right-to-left shunting and reduction of systemic venous hypertension.[13]

RESULTS OF FONTAN OPERATIONS

Early Outcomes

The early results of the entire Fontan experience from 1987 through 1991 at Children's Hospital Boston are shown in Table 58-2. In this experience, a number of techniques of carrying out the Fontan operation were used, with the lateral tunnel technique used by preference in the more recent years. The results have clearly improved over time when the entire experience with the first 500 patients up to 1991 is considered (Table 58-3). Importantly, during the 1987 to 1991 era, several factors that were associated with increased risk during earlier eras were no longer associated with adverse outcomes. In particular, the diagnosis of heterotaxy in association with functional single ventricle was no longer a risk factor, nor was the diagnosis of hypoplastic left heart syndrome. The improvements in treating these two patient groups were almost certainly a result of technical modifications of the Fontan procedure, which avoided the creation of pulmonary venous obstruction. The effects of the use of a fenestration are evident from a review of these same 500 patients, as shown in Table 58-3.

TABLE 58–2. Early Outcome of Fontan Operations, 1987–1991

Diagnosis	Success (*n*)*	Failed†	Success (%)
Single LV-NRGA	63	3	95.2
Single LV-TGA	81	3	96.3
Heterotaxy	22	1	95.5
Single RV	26	3	88.5
HLHS	15	3	80.0
Other	13	1	92.4
TOTAL	220	14	93.7

*Patients who survived Fontan operation.
†Patients who died or had or takedown of Fontan operation.
LV, left ventricle; RV, right ventricle; NRGA, normally related great arteries; TGA, transposed great arteries; HLHS, hypoplastic left heart syndrome.

TABLE 58–3. Effect of Date of Operation and Fenestration

Date of Operation	*N*	Success (*n*)	Failed	Success (%)
1973–84	133	98	35	73.7
1985–89	233	195	38	83.7
1990–91	134	125	9	93.3
Fenestration	***N***	**Success (*n*)**	**Failed**	**Success (%)**
Fenestrated	136	127	9	93.4
Nonfenestrated	361	289	72	80.0

Late Outcomes

Among those who survived the initial Fontan procedures carried out during the 1987 to 1991 era, there were 13 late failures consisting of 7 late deaths, 4 heart transplantations, and 2 Fontan procedure takedowns for chronic pleural or pericardial effusions. Of these patients, 6 had single ventricle with the aorta arising from an outlet chamber (transposed) and some degree of obstruction to the ventricle to aortic pathway ("subaortic stenosis"). Excluding the early failures, the freedom from late failure rates are 96% at 5 years and 92% at 10 years. The risk factors for late failure are shown in Table 58-4.

A significant source of late morbidity after Fontan procedures is the development of supraventricular tachyarrhythmias or bradyarrhythmias. Supraventricular tachycardia was noted in 12 patients during late follow-up. Freedom from symptomatic or documented postoperative supraventricular tachycardia was 94% at 5 years and 90% at 10 years. These dysrhythmias were frequently seen among those who had earlier Fontan modifications, especially direct tissue anastomoses such as right atrial appendage to pulmonary artery. Enormous enlargement of the right atrium was common, this sometimes even resulting in right pulmonary vein compression.[14] Conversion to the fenestrated lateral tunnel type has been carried out with varying success in some such patients. Bradyarrhythmias were noted in 32 patients, with rate of the freedom from new-onset bradyarrhythmia after the Fontan procedure equal to 88% at 5 years and 79% at 10 years. Pacemakers were implanted in 7 patients during the late follow-up period. The risk factors for late tachyarrhythmias and bradyarrhythmias by multivariant analysis are shown in Tables 58-5 and 58-6. Several of the factors are highly associated, such as the presence of a common atrioventricular valve and anomalies of systemic venous return in patients with heterotaxy-type heart disease.

TABLE 58–4. Risk Factors for Late Failure, 1987–1991

Prior systemic–pulmonary artery shunt, *P* = .008
Prior coarctation repair, *P* < .001

TABLE 58–5. Factors Associated with Supraventricular Tachycardia Early and Late After Fontan Procedures

Risk Factor	Early (*P* value)	Late (*P* value)
Heterotaxy syndrome	.01	
Prior PA band	.02	
Preoperative SVT	.0001	
Regurgitant AV valve		.03
Common AV valve		.006
Preoperative bradycardia		.001
Early postoperative SVT		.0001

AV, atrioventricular; PA, pulmonary artery; SVT, supraventricular tachycardia.

SUMMARY

The management of the single-ventricle patient clearly remains a challenge for both surgeons and cardiologists involved in their care. The current management, which is directed at attempting to create optimal candidates for a Fontan procedure, has resulted in remarkably good survival for periods of up to 10 to 15 years. The technical refinements to the Fontan operation outlined earlier have contributed to significant improvements in early patient outcome after this operation, particularly in the high-risk anatomic subgroups. However, the continuing appearance of both rhythm problems and the need for at least some of these patients to undergo heart transplantation suggest that the prognosis for the single-ventricle patient remains less than the normal population. Even longer-term follow-up is clearly necessary to determine whether this approach is optimal for all single-ventricle patients or for certain (as yet to be defined) physiologic or anatomic subsets of patients. Continued follow-up and reassessment of the "unnatural" history of the surgically treated patient with single ventricle

TABLE 58–6. Factors Associated with Bradyarrhythmias Early and Late after Fontan Procedures

Risk Factor	Early (*P* value)	Late (*P* value)
Anomalous systemic venous return	.05	
Preoperative bradycardia	.0001	
Prior PA band		.005
Prior PA-Ao anastomosis		.04
Preoperative bradyarrhythmia		.0001
Early postoperative bradyarrhythmia		.0001

Ao, aortic; PA, pulmonary artery.

beginning with neonatal and infant interventions and continuing through Fontan operations will be essential to refine the treatment of this difficult group of patients.

REFERENCES

1. Moodie DS, Ritter DG, Tajik AJ, et al. Long-term follow-up in the unoperated univentricular heart. Am J Cardiol 53:1124, 1984.
2. Franklin RCG, Spiegelhalter DJ, Anderson RH, et al. Double-inlet ventricle presenting in infancy. J Thorac Cardiovasc Surg 101:767, 1991.
3. Mayer JE Jr, Bridges ND, Lock JE, et al. Factors associated with marked reduction in mortality for Fontan operations in patients with single ventricle. J Thorac Cardiovasc Surg 103:444, 1992.
4. Stamm C, Friehs I, Mayer JE, et al. Long-term results of the lateral tunnel Fontan operation. J Thorac Cardiovasc Surg 121:28, 2001.
5. Gentles TL, Mayer JE, Gauvreau K, et al. Fontan operation in five hundred consecutive patients: Factors influencing early and late outcome. J Thorac Cardiovasc Surg 114:376, 1997.
6. Fontan F, Baudet E. Surgical repair of tricuspid atresia. Thorax 26:240, 1971.
7. Edwards JE. Congenital malformations of the heart and great vessels. C. Malformations of the Valves. In Gould SE (ed). Pathology of the Heart and Blood Vessels, 3rd ed. Springfield, IL: Charles C Thomas, 1968:312–351.
8. Van Praagh R, Ongley PA, Swan HJC. Anatomic types of single or common ventricle in man. Am J Cardiol 13:367, 1964.
9. Matitiau A, Geva T, Colan SD, et al. Bulboventricular foramen size in infants with double-inlet left ventricle or tricuspid atresia with transposed great arteries: Influence on initial palliative operation and rate of growth. J Am Coll Cardiol 19:142, 1992.
10. Gross GJ, Jonas RA, Castaneda AR, et al. Maturational and hemodynamic factors predictive of increased cyanosis following bidirectional cavopulmonary anastomosis. Am J Cardiol 74:705, 1994.
11. Mayer JE Jr, Helgason H, Jonas RA, et al. Extending the limits for modified Fontan procedures. J Thorac Cardiovasc Surg 92:1021, 1986.
12. Bridges ND, Mayer JE, Lock JE, et al. Effect of fenestration on outcome of Fontan repair. Circulation 84(Suppl II), 1991.
13. Kreutzer J, Lock JE, Jonas RA, et al. Transcatheter fenestration dilation and/or creation in postoperative Fontan patients. Am J Cardiol 79:228, 1996.
14. Kreutzer J, Keane JF, Lock JE, et al. Conversion of modified Fontan procedure to lateral atrial tunnel cavopulmonary anatomosis. J Thorac Cardiovasc Surg 111:1169, 1996.

59

Minimally Invasive and Robotically Assisted Cardiovascular Surgery, and Extracorporeal Membrane Oxygenation

PEDRO J. DEL NIDO

MINIMALLY INVASIVE AND ROBOTICALLY ASSISTED CARDIOVASCULAR SURGERY

With improved results in mortality and morbidity in cardiac surgery, even for corrective procedures in infants and children with complex heart defects, there has been a growing interest in developing alternative operative techniques that minimize postoperative recovery time and yield improved cosmetic results. In congenital cardiac surgery, alternative access techniques have been used to correct specific intracardiac defects for several years, primarily to avoid a full sternotomy and improve the cosmetic result. With few exceptions, the technique for intracardiac repair has not changed and follows the same principles as for the conventional full sternotomy approach. For extracardiac procedures, however, thoracoscopic techniques have changed not only the approach but also the technique for repair.

Thoracoscopic Approach for Noncardiac Procedures

Thoracoscopic procedures in children at present are, for the most part, confined to repairs of noncardiac defects or to provide access to the pericardium or epicardium. Examples include ligation of patent ductus,[1] division of vascular rings,[2] creation of a pericardial window, innominate artery or aortic suspension for tracheal compression, and more recently, pacer lead insertion for biventricular pacing. Much of the instrumentation has been adapted from other surgical applications, and the thoracoscopic procedures have been confined primarily to tissue dissection and ligation or division of small vessels with little reconstruction or suturing.

Surgical Approach

Positioning and location of port incisions follows the same principles of thoracoscopy or thoracotomy in adults. The patient's position needs to provide direct access to the intrathoracic target area, and the port positions need to cluster around the target area. For thoracoscopic ports, it is important to note that there must be a clear linear path between the port and the target structure, and there must be sufficient separation of the port sites to prevent interference of the instruments with the camera or each other. Usually four ports are required, two for the surgeon's instruments for the dissection, one port for the scope and camera, and the fourth port for the assistant to introduce lung retractors or occasionally a grasper or suction (Fig. 59-1). In procedures in which a surgical robot is used to assist, the same port position is used, but the port for the lung retractor and suction is placed at the mid-axillary line at the sixth or seventh intercostal space (Fig. 59-2).

Results

Thoracoscopic approaches to extracardiac lesions in children has only slowly gained acceptance among cardiac surgeons, at least in part owing to the lack of familiarity with thoracoscopic instrumentation and techniques, and the

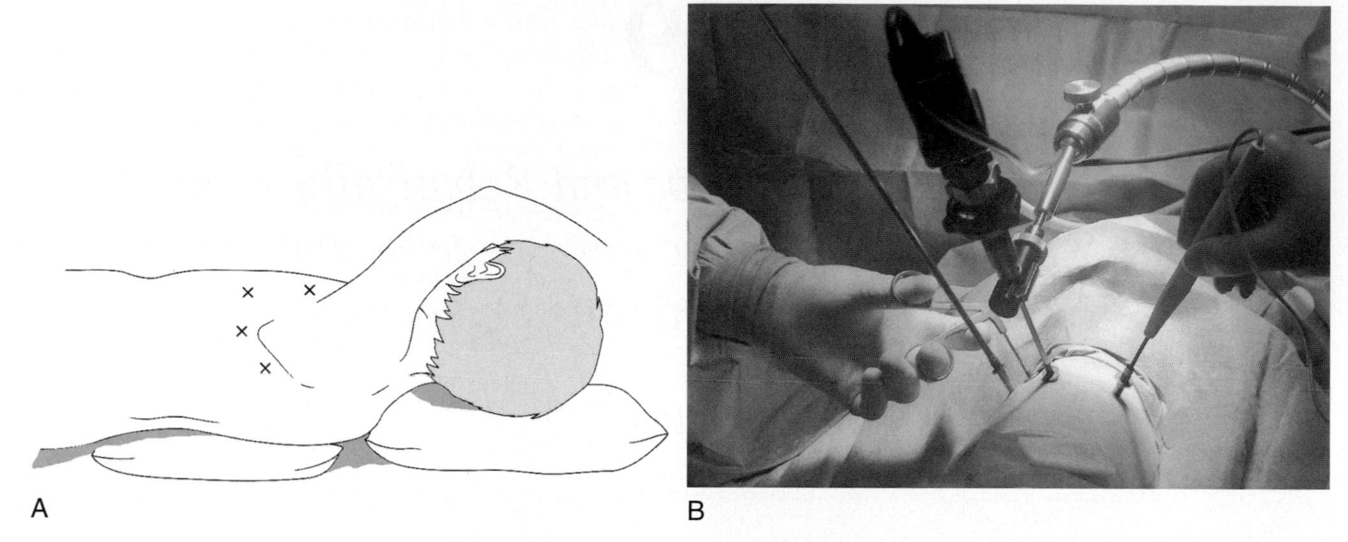

FIGURE 59–1 *Thoracoscopic approach that is most commonly used for ligation of patent ductus and division of vascular rings: schematics of patient position and port location (x marks the position of ports) (A) and a picture of instrument and camera position in a patient undergoing ligation of arterial duct (B).*
Courtesy of Dr. Barbara Robinson, Children's Hospital Boston.

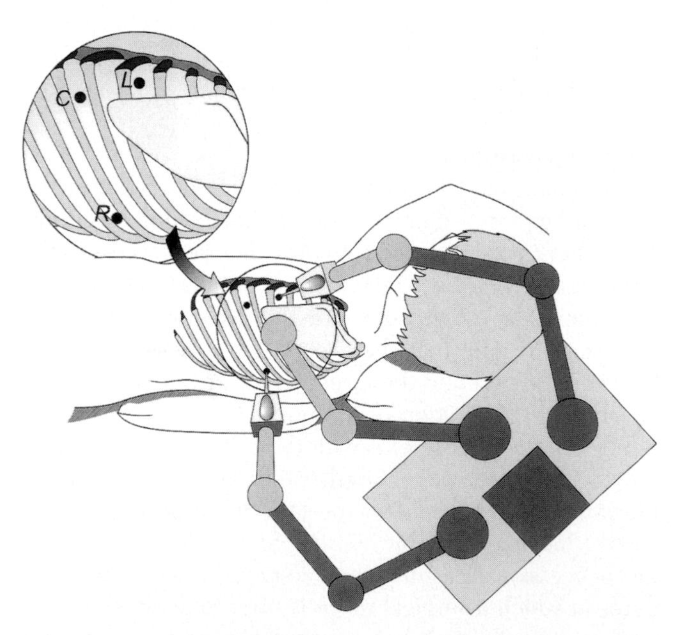

FIGURE 59–2 *Intraoperative setup for robot-assisted vascular ring division. The left instrument port (L) is placed in the third interspace along the anterior axillary line, whereas the camera port (C) is placed in the fifth intercostal space and the right instrument port (R) in the posterior sixth intercostal space behind the scapula.*
From Mihaljevic T, Cannon JW, del Nido PJ. Robotically assisted division of a vascular ring in children. J Thorac Cardiovasc Surg 125:1163, 2003.

widespread application of catheter-based methods particularly for occlusion of patent arterial duct. There is, however, a group of patients in whom catheter-based techniques are less desirable, such as small and premature infants, or children with a large duct for which a larger device is required or in whom the vessel has a short tubular shape. Thoracoscopic duct closure has a relatively low risk for serious complications, but these include bleeding requiring transfusion or conversion to open thoracotomy, recurrent nerve injury, and persistent pneumothorax or chylothorax.[3] The incidence of most of these is 1% or less, except for recurrent nerve injury, which occurs in 1% to 3% of patients, with most of these cases being transient injury.[4] Late recurrence of a patent duct has been reported after thoracoscopic closure, with an incidence varying from 0.6% to 3%.

Minimally Invasive Approach in Open-Heart Procedures

Cardiopulmonary bypass to support the circulation during repair of intracardiac defects by direct surgical techniques still remains a necessity in surgery for congenital heart defects. In children that require intracardiac repair, cannulation for bypass becomes an important limiting factor to application of minimally invasive techniques because of the small size of the femoral or axillary vessels and the potential for permanent occlusion. As a consequence, minimally invasive, port access, or thoracoscopic cardiac surgery, without a sternotomy or thoracotomy, has been done only rarely in children and primarily in adult-sized teenagers. Even in cases in which peripheral cannulation has been used in older children, the types of procedures performed have been confined mostly to low-risk and relatively simple repairs such as closure of atrial septal defects (ASDs) of the secundum type.[5] In most cases in which minimal incisions have been used in children, cannulation for bypass is done centrally through the mediastinum, cannulating the aorta and atrium or vena cavae directly. With increased experience, these techniques have been applied to more complex congenital defects in infants and children.[6]

Surgical Approaches

The approaches or types of incisions reported for minimally invasive repair of intracardiac defects in children vary from small anterior or inframammary thoracotomy, posterior thoracotomy, or limited inferior sternotomy, or the so-called trans-xyphoid approach. Each approach has its advocates; however, the advantages of a midline incision are avoidance of pericardial incisions near the phrenic nerve as with a thoracotomy, or the need to create myocutaneous flaps as often done with the inframammary incision, which may result in hematomas and skin denervation. Also, a midline incision with full or partial sternotomy is in general less painful and better tolerated than a lateral thoracotomy.

Because many of the intracardiac repairs in infants and children are accomplished through the right atrium, inferior partial sternotomy incisions can provide sufficient exposure for cannulation for cardiopulmonary bypass while giving direct access to the right atrium. Examples include repair of ASD, ventricular septal defect (VSD), complete atrioventricular canal defect, transatrial repair of tetralogy of Fallot, and mitral valve repair. This approach offers several advantages in that exposure to the great vessels can be accomplished in children of all ages with sufficient ease to permit safe cannulation for bypass. For most procedures, the skin incision extends from the level of the areola (midthorax) down to the tip of the xyphoid process (Fig. 59-3). A partial sternotomy can then be performed. Retraction of the sternum superiorly provides access to the upper thorax for aortic and superior caval cannulation.

A common alternative approach to a median sternotomy has been a right anterior thoracotomy. Other surgical approaches include a transverse inframammary skin incision with either a vertical sternotomy[7] or bilateral transverse anterior thoracotomy as described by Brom and modified

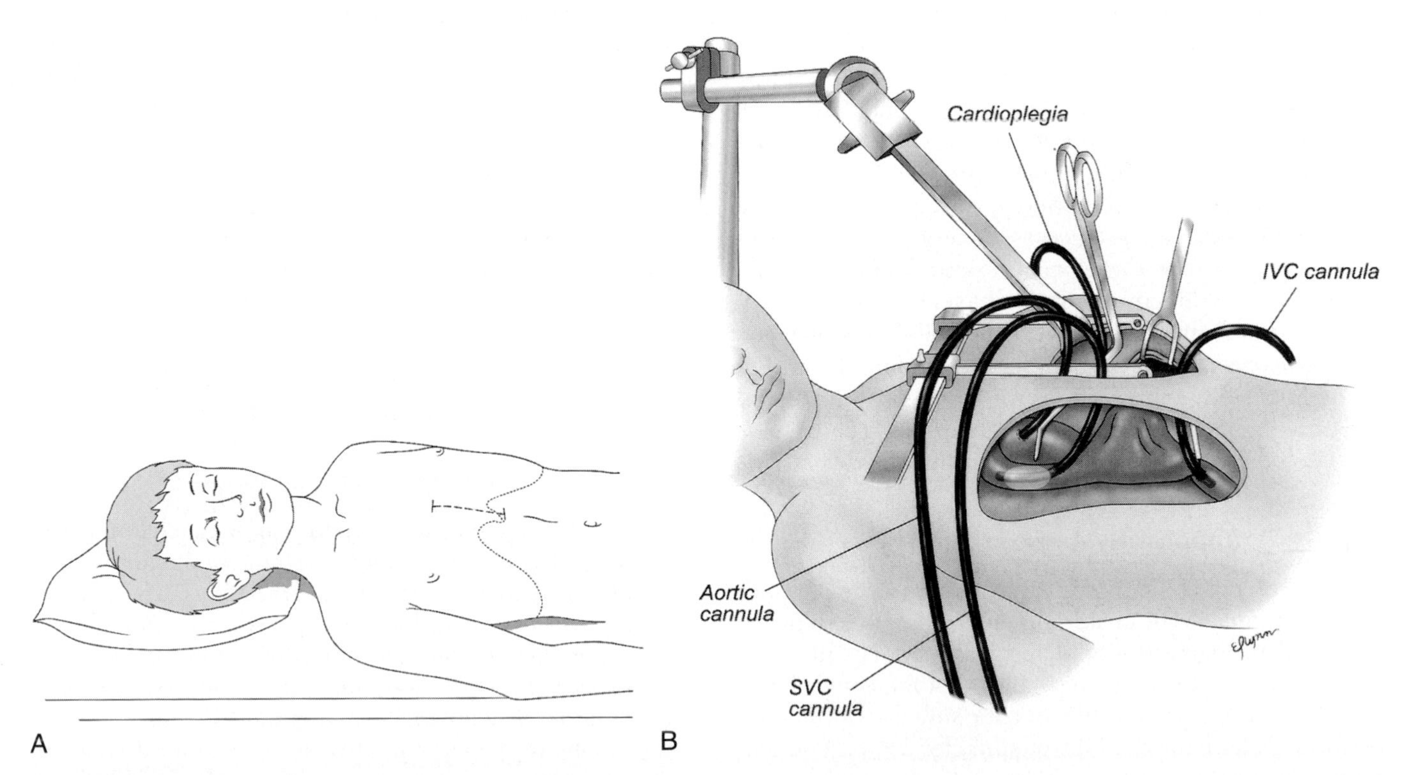

FIGURE 59–3 *Ministernotomy "trans-xyphoid" approach for open heart procedures. A, Low midline incision centered over xyphoid. B, Diagram of sternal retraction and cannulation for cardiopulmonary bypass. SVC, superior vena cava; IVC, inferior vena cava. From Bichell DP, Geva T, Bacha E, et al. Minimal access approach for the repair of atrial septal defect: Initial 135 patients. Ann Thorac Surg 70:115, 2000.*

by Willman and Hanlon.[8] These techniques have been recommended primarily for females older than 10 years in whom breast development is sufficient to permit accurate delineation of the extent of breast tissue. Although the cosmetic result with these alternative approaches have been satisfactory, complications related specifically to the incision have been noted. Phrenic nerve damage has been reported in as many as 16% of children who have ASD closure through an anterior right thoracotomy.[9] Breast and pectoral muscle maldevelopment has also been reported, along with paresthesia around the breast and even the right arm.[10]

Results

Our experience with the partial sternotomy or trans-xyphoid approach for repair of ASDs indicates that the procedure can be done safely, with similar bypass and cross-clamp times compared with a full sternotomy approach. Late follow-up also indicates that this approach is equally effective in achieving repair of the intracardiac defects equivalent to those achieved with full sternotomy. We have also used the trans-xyphoid or ministernotomy approach to repair other intracardiac defects, including isolated VSDs, partial arteriovenous canal (primum ASD) and complete arteriovenous canal defects and in selected patients with tetralogy of Fallot in whom a transatrial approach for complete repair was feasible.[6]

Whether other technologic advances such as surgical robotic instruments or device closure of septal defects will complement or replace these minimal access techniques is yet to be determined. More recently, surgeons have explored the use of catheter-based occluder devices to repair some types of VSDs that are less accessible through a right atriotomy approach. The device can be introduced through a sheath inserted directly into the right ventricle and navigation and positioning of the device guided by a combination of fluoroscopy and ultrasound. These procedures have been termed *hybrid* operations because they use both surgical and catheter-based techniques to accomplish reconstruction and also obviate the need for cardiopulmonary bypass.[11]

Robotically Assisted Surgery

Thoracoscopic procedures have the advantage of avoiding open thoracotomy or sternotomy but are limited by the restricted maneuverability of the instruments within the chest cavity and the relative simplicity of the conventional surgical instruments available. Robotic surgical instruments, however, do have the dexterity required for complex maneuvers, such as placing sutures and tying knots, and therefore hold the promise of facilitating truly thoracoscopic repair of cardiac defects even in children (for a complete review, see Suematsu and del Nido[12] and Cannon and associates[13]). Currently, two Food and Drug Administration–approved robotic systems have been used by surgeons in North America. Both are based on the teleoperation concept of a remote console with a master control system and surgeon interface, separated by cables that connect to the slave system of robotic arms and instrument manipulators at the patient's side. The DaVinci system (Intuitive Surgical Inc., Sunnyvale, CA) consists of a surgeon console and a surgical arm cart. Three or four robotic arms are mounted on the surgical arm cart, which can be moved over the surgical field. Two of these arms serve as detachable surgical EndoWrist instruments, each possessing small mechanical wrists with 7 degrees of freedom. The surgeon views the operative field through a binocular scope that provides a high-definition, full-color, magnified, three-dimensional image of the surgical site. The camera and instruments are both controlled by maneuvering the surgical instrument like master controllers on the console.

Although experience with robotic systems in cardiac surgery on adults is now widespread, application of these for congenital heart defects has been limited to adults or older teenagers with ASDs and to noncardiac thoracic procedures in children.[14] The main limitation to application of robotic systems in children has been the size of the available instruments (8 mm diameter) and endoscope (10 mm diameter), as well as the required working area for instrument task performance; however, 5-mm diameter instruments and scopes are now available and hold the promise of permitting application of robotic systems to smaller infants and children. Future advances in robotic use will likely include tactile feedback information and the ability to integrate images of the operative field with previously obtained images of the relevant anatomic structures to aid surgical navigation.

EXTRACORPOREAL MEMBRANE OXYGENATOR SUPPORT

Extracorporeal Life Support

Mechanical circulatory support to treat children with severe ventricular dysfunction is an important part of surgical management of congenital heart defects. The types of support systems available for application in children are more limited than the wide variety of systems available for adults. Nevertheless, the results with circulatory assistance in children are comparable, and in some cases superior, to the results reported in adult patients. The most common circulatory support system in use for pediatric patients is an extracorporeal life support (ECLS) system (also termed extracorporeal membrane oxygenation [ECMO], which is composed of a roller pump, oxygenator, and control systems to prevent cavitation or excessive negative pressure in the venous side and excessively high pressure on the arterial side, and inflow and outflow cannulae that attach to the patient and connect to the tubing diverting blood flow through the circuit.

Cannulae

Ideally, the cannula is thin walled (maximal inner to outer diameter ratio), reinforced to prevent kinking, and available in a variety of sizes to accommodate the large range of flow rates required for children.

Pumps

The most commonly used pump in cardiac surgery is a peristaltic pump that uses rollers to compress a length of tubing, thus forcing blood forward. Because these pumps are nearly occlusive, however, a regulation system is required to shut off the pump or decrease the pump speed to prevent cavitation. Most current ECMO circuits use a roller pump with a servo system to control pump speed, built into the control console. Other types of pumps used for ECLS are centrifugal pumps that are completely nonocclusive and depend on generation of a vortex to propel blood forward. Because of durability of the pump head (up to 48 hours), these systems have been more commonly used as ventricular assist devices without an oxygenator since they require little adjustment and are less prone to cavitation.

Oxygenators

Two types of membrane oxygenators are available for the bypass circuit, and although equally effective, there are fundamental differences in design that determine ease of priming and longevity. Hollow-fiber oxygenators consist of a large number of fibers with a central lumen and semiporous walls with holes large enough to let water through but small enough so that proteins, particularly plasma proteins, can cover these holes, creating a thin film or semipermeable membrane through which gas exchange occurs. Sheet-type membrane oxygenators do not have holes in the membrane wall and depend on the permeability of the plastic material that makes up the membrane to permit gas transfer. Because hollow-fiber membrane oxygenators have holes that can allow gas to escape, de-airing the fibers with the priming solution is easy and can be done rapidly. For this reason, they have been incorporated in some ECLS circuits for support after cardiac arrest as a rapid response system. Sheet membrane oxygenators require flushing the air out of the membrane with a very soluble gas, such as carbon dioxide, to prevent air trapping in the section that will contain the blood. Sheet membrane oxygenators have a much longer usable life span with approval for use up to 14 days, as compared with hollow-fiber oxygenators that require replacement within 6 to 12 hours in most cases.

Indications for Support

Most children placed on mechanical circulatory support require it for acute decompensation after a cardiac surgical procedure, or for acute decompensation of chronic heart failure.[15,16] In many of these, the expectation is that there will be recovery of contractile function, with the average duration of support being about 8 days. In children, indications for longer-term support (more than 10 days) have been primarily as a bridge to transplantation, with the exception of the acute myocarditis patients, in whom there is evidence that full recovery can occur late.

Postcardiotomy or Unexpected Cardiac Arrest

ECLS systems are used widely as a tool for resuscitation in children refractory to conventional cardiopulmonary resuscitation.[17,18] A key factor in the efficacy of this intervention is the ability to establish circulatory support quickly, before end-organ injury becomes irreversible. Centers that have developed rapid-response systems report long-term survival rates as high as 58% when ECMO-type systems are used as part of a rapid-response program.

Postcardiotomy Failure

Inability to wean from bypass represents the highest-risk group for children requiring mechanical circulatory support. The reasons for failure of the native heart to adequately support the systemic circulation after bypass are many but in most cases are due to either poor myocardial protection during the surgical procedure, inadequate hemodynamic repair with residual anatomic defects, or anatomic limitations preventing adequate ventricular function. Other, less frequent causes include severe hypoxemia and pulmonary hypertension.

Bridge to Transplantation

The most common indication in adults for the use of ventricular assist devices (VADs) is for long-term support as a bridge to transplantation. VAD support is viewed, in adults, as a way to improve patients who are candidates for transplantation and to decrease the morbidity and mortality in high-risk patients undergoing heart transplantation. In children, most of the experience with mechanical circulatory support as a bridge to transplantation has been with ECLS using a conventional ECMO circuit.[19,20] Although the experience is limited, reasonably good results have been reported, with about half of children listed for transplantation receiving an organ and surviving to hospital discharge. This is despite the fact that the ECMO circuit immobilizes the patient, requires full anticoagulation with heparin, and has many access ports where bacteria can be introduced. Thus, for many centers, conventional ECMO circuits provide adequate support for a significant number of children requiring circulatory support as a bridge to transplantation.

Acute Myocarditis

Acute fulminant myocarditis resulting in rapid hemodynamic deterioration is one indication for mechanical support for which recovery of contractile function can be expected in most children. The rate of recovery, however, can be quite slow, and therefore longer-term support may be required. In most cases, if significant recovery of contractile dysfunction is not seen within the first 4 to 5 days after initiation of ECMO, then it is likely that a long period of support will be required, potentially extending to 3 to 4 weeks. In older children, in whom VADs may be applicable, consideration should be given to converting to a true VAD system because in older teenagers, significant mobility is gained and anticoagulation is easier to manage.

Patient Management on Circulatory Support

Management of children placed on ECMO support evolves as the run progresses. In the first few hours after initiation of ECMO, the *stabilization phase*, the emphasis is on establishing adequate organ perfusion, decompression of the systemic ventricle if cardiac function is poor, and management of anticoagulation. Once stabilized on ECMO support, emphasis is placed on prevention of infection and optimizing nutrition, and a decision must be made regarding the likelihood of recovery versus the need to consider transplantation or longer-term circulatory support. An active search for potentially treatable causes of cardiac dysfunction must be sought. Initial evaluation with echocardiography is often sufficient, but cardiac catheterization may be required to fully evaluate surgical repair or to search for unsuspected residual defects. This is the *intermediate phase.* If a residual anatomic defect is detected by echocardiography or cardiac catheterization, then repair of the defect is imperative because without this, successful weaning from mechanical circulatory support is very unlikely. The timing of repair depends in great part on the nature of the residual defect and the degree of recovery of contractile function. In patients who recover cardiac function, the *weaning phase* requires accurate assessment of recovery, end-organ perfusion, and optimization of ventilation. With ECLS, weaning is usually done by gradually decreasing flow and monitoring end-organ perfusion and function, as well as cardiac contractile function, by echocardiography. Gradual weaning over several days may be required in cases in which recovery has been slow, such as with viral myocarditis, or when ventricular "retraining" is required.

Results

Rapid-response ECMO remains one of the most common indications for mechanical circulatory support. In centers with specialized teams and preprimed circuits that can be ready in 15 to 20 minutes, hospital survival rates of more than 60% have been reported by several groups,[17,18] and long-term outcomes are also very favorable.[21] These results reflect the fact that patients requiring ECMO for resuscitation often have reversible causes for the hemodynamic decompensation. Similar and even better results have been reported with ECMO support for acute viral myocarditis, with survival rates approaching 80%, albeit a significant portion required heart transplantation.[22] Survival in children with post–cardiac surgery heart failure is closely linked to the presence of residual defects. In most centers, survival in this group was low (less than 25%) if the residual defect was not corrected or transplantation was not available. In the patients who were able to undergo transplantation or have further surgery to correct the residual defects, survival is better than 60%.[15]

REFERENCES

1. Laborde F, Noirhomme P, Karam J, et al. A new video-assisted thoracoscopic surgical technique for interruption of patent ductus arteriosus in infants and children. J Thorac Cardiovasc Surg 105:278. 1993.
2. Burke R, Chang A. Video-assisted thoracoscopic division of a vascular ring in an infant: A new operative technique. J Cardiac Surg 8:537, 1993.
3. Villa E, Eynden FV, Le Bret E, et al. Paediatric video-assisted thoracoscopic clipping of patent ductus arteriosus: Experience in more than 700 cases. Eur J Cardiothorac Surg 25(3):387, 2004.
4. Odegard K, Kirse DJ, del Nido PJ, et al. Intraoperative recurrent laryngeal nerve monitoring during video assisted thoracoscopic surgery for patent ductus arteriosus. J Cardiothorac Vasc Anesth 14:562, 2000.
5. Bichell DP, Geva T, Bacha E, et al. Minimal access approach for the repair of atrial septal defect: The initial 135 patients. Ann Thorac Surg; 70:115, 2000.
6. Nicholson IA, Bichell DP, Bacha EA, et al. Minimal sternotomy approach for congenital heart operations. Ann Thorac Surg 71:469, 2001.
7. Brutel de la Riviere A, Brom A, Brom AG. Horizontal submammary skin incision for median sternotomy. Ann Thorac Surg 32:101, 1981.
8. Willman VL, Hanlon CR. Median sternotomy using a transverse submammary skin incision. Am J Surg 100:779, 1960.
9. Helps BA, Ross-Russel RI, Dicks-Mireaux C, et al. Phrenic nerve damage via a right thoracotomy in older children with secundum ASD. Ann Thorac Surg 56:328, 1993.
10. Bleiziffer S, Schreiber C, Burgkart R, et al. The influence of right anterolateral thoracotomy in prepubescent female patients on late breast development and on the incidence of scoliosis. J Thorac Cardiovasc Surg 127(5):1474, 2004.
11. Bacha EA, Hijazi ZM, Cao QL, et al. New therapeutic avenues with hybrid pediatric cardiac surgery. Heart Surg Forum 7:33, 2004.

12. Suematsu Y, del Nido PJ. Robotic pediatric cardiac surgery: Present and future perspectives. Am J Surg 188(4A Suppl): 98S, 2004.
13. Cannon JW, Howe RD, Dupont PE, et al. Application of robotics in congenital cardiac surgery. Semin Thorac Cardiovasc Surg Pediatr Card Surg Annu 6:72, 2003.
14. Mihaljevic T, Cannon JW, del Nido PJ. Robotically assisted division of a vascular ring in children. J Thorac Cardiovasc Surg 125:1163, 2003
15. Black MD, Coles JG, Williams WG, et al. Determinants of successes in pediatric cardiac patients undergoing extracorporeal membrane oxygenation. Ann Thorac Surg 60:133, 1995.
16. Kulik TJ, Moler FW, Palmisaro JM, et al. Outcome-associated factors in pediatric patients treated with extracorporeal membrane oxygenator after cardiac surgery. Circulation; 94(9 Suppl):63, 1996.
17. del Nido PJ, Dalton HJ, Thompson AE, et al. Extracorporeal membrane oxygenator rescue in children during cardiac arrest after cardiac surgery. Circulation 86(5 Suppl): 300, 1992.
18. Duncan BW, Ibrahim AE, Hraska V, et al. Use of rapid-deployment extracorporeal membrane oxygenation for the resuscitation of pediatric patients with heart disease after cardiac arrest. J Thorac Cardiovasc Surg; 116(2):305, 1998.
19. del Nido PJ, Armitage JM, Fricker FJ, et al. Extracorporeal membrane oxygenation support as a bridge to pediatric heart transplantation. Circulation 90(5 Pt 2):66, 1994.
20. Gajarski RJ, Mosca RS, Ohye RG, et al. Use of extracorporeal life support as a bridge to pediatric cardiac transplantation. J Heart Lung Transplant 22:28, 2003.
21. Ibrahim AE, Duncan BW, Blume ED, et al. Long-term follow-up of pediatric cardiac patients requiring mechanical circulatory support. Ann Thorac Surg 69:186, 2000.
22. Duncan BW, Bohn DJ, Atz AM, et al. Mechanical circulatory support for the treatment of children with acute fulminant myocarditis. J Thorac Cardiovasc Surg; 122:440, 2001.

60

Current and Future Cardiovascular Organ and Tissue Replacement Therapies

John E. Mayer, Jr. and Elizabeth D. Blume

Remarkable advances have been made in the treatment of most forms of congenital and acquired heart disease in children, but significant existing treatment strategies fall short of the ideal in two major areas. The first area is that of end-stage ventricular dysfunction when the heart cannot meet the body's demand for cardiac output on either an acute or chronic basis. The second area is that of malformed or absent cardiac valves or major conduit arteries that are not amenable to surgical repair or catheterization laboratory intervention. In each of these situations, *replacement therapies* are the only treatment strategies currently available. The intent of this chapter is to describe current cardiac transplantation practices at Children's Hospital Boston for the treatment of severe end-stage heart disease and to introduce the emerging discipline of cardiovascular tissue engineering, which offers the potential for construction of living replacement valves and conduit arteries for use in the cardiovascular system.

CARDIAC TRANSPLANTATION

"Inoperable" congenital heart disease was among the earliest indications for cardiac transplantation. The second reported clinical attempt at a human cardiac transplantation, albeit unsuccessful, was carried out by Kantrowitz in the 1960s for an infant with hypoplastic left heart syndrome.[1] The attractiveness of replacing a malformed heart with a structurally normal, four-chambered heart is obvious but is limited by the problems imposed by the recipient's immune response to the transplanted organ and by the shortage of human donors of appropriate size and blood type. However, transplantation for congenital heart disease and for certain forms of acquired heart disease in children has evolved to assume an accepted place in the therapeutic armamentarium for these disorders.

Indications

The indication for cardiac transplantation is an anticipated post-transplantation "natural history" that would be a significant improvement over that associated with the underlying congenital or acquired heart disease. With the currently imperfect ability to modulate the host immune response, the post-transplantation state must be viewed as one with ongoing risks that exceed those of children with normal hearts and immune systems. As a result, the indications for cardiac transplantation continue to remain a matter of judgment based on the individual patient's heart disease and its projected course with nontransplantation therapies. As a general rule, transplantation is considered when life expectancy from the underlying heart disease is less than 1 to 2 years.

Congenital Heart Disease

Almost all forms of congenital heart disease are amenable to some form of nontransplantation intervention that will improve the patient's prospects for survival and functional status. Results with palliative and reparative procedures have continued to improve, and therefore our institutional approach to almost all forms of congenital heart disease has not included transplantation as primary therapy. Other institutions continue to use a primary transplantation approach for certain conditions such as hypoplastic left heart syndrome.[2] Despite our institutional preference for initial nontransplantation therapies for congenital heart disease, more than half of patients transplanted in our institution have a primary diagnosis of congenital heart disease. Table 60-1 lists the types of congenital and acquired heart disease in our transplant recipients. All but two of the patients with congenital heart disease have undergone prior surgical procedures to palliate or repair their congenital heart defects. In these congenital heart disease patients, the indication for transplantation was not the structural heart disease but rather failure of the prior interventions to establish a durable cardiovascular physiology to allow survival of the patient.

Cardiomyopathy includes a diverse group of conditions in which there is a primary failure of the cardiac muscle with resulting reduction of cardiac output and elevation of cardiac filling pressures. Details of the cardiomyopathy variations and heart failure management are outlined in Chapters 7 and 26.

Pretransplantation Evaluation

Transplantation evaluation is directed at identification of comorbid disease that will increase the transplantation risk, delineation of cardiac and venous anatomy, and assessment of pulmonary vascular reactivity. Detailed venous and cardiac anatomy is critical in planning a successful transplantation procedure. From a surgical standpoint, there are almost no anatomic contraindications to transplantation. Patients with anomalies of systemic and pulmonary venous return,[3] cardiac malpositions,[4] or malpositions of the great arteries[5,6] have been successfully transplanted by using additional lengths of donor aorta, pulmonary artery, and systemic veins.[7]

The most important hemodynamic contraindication to transplantation in children is the presence of "fixed" pulmonary hypertension. In the presence of a significantly elevated pulmonary vascular resistance (PVR), the donor right ventricle, which has been exposed only to the low pulmonary vascular resistance of the normal circulation, is not physiologically "prepared" (hypertrophied) to overcome the afterload imposed by elevated pulmonary vascular resistance. Therefore, evaluation of the potential recipient's PVR at the pretransplantation cardiac catheterization is essential. This evaluation includes an assessment of the "reactiveness" of the pulmonary vasculature in response to ventilation with 100% oxygen, induction of hypocarbia and respiratory alkalosis, inhaled nitric oxide (NO), which acts as a selective pulmonary vasodilator, and administration of vasodilator agents, including calcium channel antagonists or prostacyclin. A PVR that remains greater than 4 to 5 Wood units (PVR indexed to body surface area) despite one or more of these interventions significantly raises the

TABLE 60–1. Etiology of Heart Disease Prior to Transplantation Children's Hospital Boston

Etiology of Heart Disease prior to Transplant (n=152)			
Congenital	**78**	**Cardiomyopathy**	**74**
• HLHS	18	• Dilated	57
• No Operation	1	• Restrictive	8
• After Stage 1	3	• Post Adriamycin	4
• After BDG	9	• Hypertrophic	3
• After Fontan	5	• Re-Transplant	2
• Other single ventricles	25		
• After palliation	13		
• After Fontan	12		
• d-TGA	11		
• Post Senning/Mustard	9		
• Post Rastelli	2		
• 1-TGA (2 vent repair)	5		
• TOF	2		
• Other	17		

Other congenital: Cong MR (1), Ebstein's (1), LV aneurysm(1), mult VSD (1), VSD (3), Shone (4). PS (1), VSD/CoAo (1), CAVC (1), ASD (1), Heterotaxy post Glenn, post ASO(1)

ABBREVIATIONS:

MR = mitral regurgitation; LV = left ventricular; VSD = ventricular septal defect; PS = pulmonary stenosis; CoAo = coarctation of aorta; CAVC = complete atrioventricular canal; HLHS = hypoplastic left heart syndrome; BDG = bidirectional Glenn; TGA = transposition of the great arteries; TOF = tetralogy of Fallot; ASD = atrial septal defect; ASO = atrial switch operation risk for donor right ventricular failure and patient survival. Patients with restrictive cardiomyopathy, chronically elevated left atrial pressures, and elevated PVR are a subgroup that has been at particular risk for donor right ventricular failure. A subgroup of patients with initially "nonreactive" pulmonary artery pressures have become "reactive" with aggressive tailored intravenous therapy for congestive heart failure over 1 to 3 months and then successfully transplanted.

Other medical conditions serve as relative contraindications to transplantation. A history of prior malignancy is a relative contraindication depending on the disease-free interval for the malignancy and the biology of the underlying neoplastic disease. Because immunosuppression is associated with an increased incidence of new malignancies after transplantation, and because there is some evidence for a role of immune surveillance in the "prevention" of primary malignancies under normal conditions, it has been generally assumed that immunosuppression in the presence of an existing malignancy will lead to a worsening of the course of the primary malignancy. We have one such case in which a leukemia was "reactivated" after transplantation. Typically cardiac failure in the postchemotherapy patient develops years after successful treatment of the neoplastic disease[8]; therefore, most of these patients can be candidates for transplantation.

Preexisting renal or hepatic dysfunction is an important consideration in the pretransplantation evaluation because of the important renal and hepatic toxicities of several of the immunosuppressive agents. Severe respiratory dysfunction is uncommon in pediatric patients, but pulmonary fibrosis with restrictive lung disease does occur in patients after certain chemotherapy regimens. Pulmonary function studies are carried out as part of pretransplantation evaluation when possible, but pulmonary dysfunction severe enough to preclude cardiac transplantation has been rare.

Preexisting psychiatric, neurodevelopmental, and psychosocial conditions of both patients and their families are also considered during the pretransplantation evaluation because the post-transplantation regimens for immunosuppression and surveillance for rejection require ongoing compliance. Assessments are made by a team of physicians, psychiatrists, nurse practitioners, and social workers. However, our ability to predict which patients and families will be able to comply with the complex post-transplantation medical regimens and to cope with the psychosocial challenges that they impose has been imperfect. Ongoing assessment and support for these patients and their families are essential.

In summary, there are relatively few absolute contraindications to cardiac transplantation in children other than a fixed severe elevation of PVR. Decisions regarding the listing of patients for heart transplantation therefore rest on development of a composite picture rather than considering each factor alone as an absolute contraindication to transplantation.

Allocation Process for Donor Organs

The U.S. organ transplant community has collectively agreed on a set of donor organ–sharing criteria, and an organization (United Network for Organ Sharing) has been created to match potential donors and recipients and to allocate each donor organ according to these criteria. Currently, the Federal government provides funding for the operation of this organization. Patients receive priority for each potential donor organ based on several criteria, including distance between donor and recipient, blood type compatibility, degree of recipient cardiovascular decompensation as reflected in levels of pharmacologic and mechanical support, and length of time on the waiting list. A range of donor size is defined for each individual recipient. In infants and small children, hearts from donors up to three times the weight of the recipient have been successfully implanted.[9]

The limited supply of donor organs for transplantation imposes another set of difficult considerations involving *allocation of a scarce resource*. In considering each individual recipient, the sometimes difficult question of whether transplantation of an organ or organs will do the "most good for the most patients" must be considered. The national allocation criteria that have been developed address this limited resource problem by giving priority to those patients who are judged to be at greatest risk for death in the short term. However, judgments regarding the impact of specific coexisting medical and psychosocial conditions on the likelihood of a successful transplantation for an individual patient remain with the individual transplantation program. The "allocation of a scarce resource" problem therefore imposes significant responsibilities on the transplant team when making the decision to list an individual patient for transplantation. We have adopted a shared responsibility/accountability approach to making these decisions involving all members of our transplant team, including physicians, surgeons, psychiatrists, nurse practitioners, and social workers.

Pretransplantation Management

After the decision is reached that transplantation is the optimal therapy for the individual patient's cardiac condition, management involves optimizing the cardiovascular and end-organ function until a donor heart becomes available. Some patients can be managed on an outpatient basis with combinations of pharmacologic and pacing therapies. Many patients require pretransplantation hospitalization for decompensated heart failure. Intravenous milrinone and dobutamine are the most commonly used agents because they have both positive inotropic and systemic vasodilator effects. Initial experience with nesiritide has been favorable. To reduce sensitization of the recipient to antigens expressed on the cell surface, transfusions are limited, and all blood products are leukocyte filtered. Optimizing nutritional status and maintaining overall conditioning are difficult in the end-stage cardiac population, but they remain important to the success of the pretransplantation and post-transplantation course. Comorbid disorders, such as protein-losing enteropathy and chronic liver and renal disease, may contribute to ongoing nutritional disorders. Malnutrition and growth failure are common due to anorexia and vomiting from high venous pressures and low cardiac output, worsened by malabsorption and the hypermetabolic state of heart failure. Because immunosuppressed patients have a less effective response to vaccines, immunizations should be given according to current recommendations.

Many new mechanical devices are being used in children to support the failing myocardium. Extracorporeal membrane oxygenation,[10,11] as well as several left ventricular assist devices,[12–14] have been successfully used as a bridge to transplantation in children (see Chapter 59).

Surgical Techniques

The fundamental techniques for implantation of a cardiac donor allograft were initially described by Lower and Shumway[15] and have changed relatively little since this initial description. Some modifications of the techniques of donor organ procurement and preservation and of implantation techniques in situations of venous and great arterial anomalies have been necessary.

Donor Selection and Procurement

The fundamental goal of the donor operation is to provide a donor heart that functions well after implantation. Donor selection is important in achieving this goal. Preexisting congenital or acquired cardiac disease (except for a secundum atrial septal defect) precludes heart donation in most situations. Other donor contraindications include active septicemia or malignancies outside the central nervous system. The remainder of the donor evaluation is centered on evaluation of the donor heart function. The circumstances under which donor brain death has occurred, particularly if there is a significant period of cardiac ischemia or a history of major blunt thoracic trauma, influence donor heart function. Measurement of markers of cardiac injury, including creatine phosphokinase MB and troponin, can indicate myocardial injury. Evaluation of cardiac function by echocardiogram and hemodynamic measurements of central venous pressure, pulmonary capillary wedge pressure, and levels of inotropic support are also important. The anticipated cardiac ischemic time between retrieval and implantation will affect donor heart function. We attempt to limit the ischemic time to less than 4 hours, but this limit has been exceeded, particularly when the condition of the recipient is critical and the condition of the donor is otherwise favorable.

The technique of donor heart procurement focuses on preservation of the donor heart for the period of ischemia required for transport of the donor organ but also includes acquisition of sufficient lengths of great artery and systemic vein to meet the anatomic requirements imposed by the recipient's anatomy. Important aspects of the donor cardiectomy are the rapid induction of hypothermic cardiac arrest with cold cardioplegia solution and the avoidance of cardiac distention by adequate venting of the right and left heart. Once the heart is excised, it is placed in a sterile container filled with additional cardioplegia solution, and then it is transported to the recipient institution at temperatures maintained near 4°C.

Recipient Operation

The recipient operation involves excision of the recipient heart and then the sequential construction of anastomoses of the donor and recipient venous and arterial structures. Donor and recipient teams must remain in close communication so that the recipient operation proceeds to minimize donor ischemic time and recipient cardiopulmonary bypass times.

The heart is approached through a median sternotomy incision, and cannulae for bypass are placed in the distal ascending aorta, the superior vena cava, and the inferior vena cava. In certain anatomic situations, cannulation of the femoral artery and vein may be necessary, and in infants, the carotid artery and internal jugular vein may be used for cannulation.

After the removal of the recipient's heart, sequential anastomoses are constructed between the donor and recipient left atria, superior and inferior venae cavae, pulmonary arteries, and aortae. In situations in which there are significant stenoses in the recipient's central pulmonary arteries, the donor branch pulmonary arteries can be used as onlay patches to enlarge the stenotic areas. If the recipient's aortic arch is stenotic, the donor aortic arch can be used for arch augmentation using a period of deep hypothermia and circulatory arrest. The technique of direct anastomoses between the donor and recipient venae cavae was used initially only in patients with a prior atrial-level repair of transposition, but is now used in most cases.[7] Monitoring catheters to measure right atrial, left atrial, and (in some cases) pulmonary artery pressures, and temporary atrial and ventricular pacing wires are placed. Pharmacologic support is used as necessary based on the hemodynamic parameters and on visual assessment of cardiac function. In certain situations, particularly those in which there is very marginal right ventricular function, primary closure of the sternotomy incision can be delayed and the mediastinal contents covered with a latex rubber sheet and an iodine-impregnated adhesive drape. Closure of the sternotomy incision is then accomplished within several days, after recovery of ventricular function and diuresis has occurred.

Postoperative Surgical Management

The immediate postoperative management of the cardiac transplant recipient closely resembles the management of other patients undergoing cardiac surgical procedures. Atrial filling pressures, pulmonary artery pressures, and systemic arterial pressure are monitored continuously using indwelling catheters. Assessment of cardiac output is made by monitoring of urine output, skin temperature, and strength of peripheral pulses. The most common cause for depressed cardiac output is the period of myocardial ischemia before implantation, although recipient immune responses to the donor organ must be considered. Generally, myocardial dysfunction is transient and can be managed with inotropic and vasodilation support. Because the donor heart is denervated, the initial cardiac rhythm after transplantation may be slow, and atrial pacing with temporary epicardial pacing wires is used to enhance cardiac output. The most serious problem following cardiac transplantation is right ventricular dysfunction, particularly when the recipient has preexisting elevations of PVR. The diagnosis of right ventricular failure can be difficult. Echocardiography can provide a qualitative assessment of right ventricular distention and contractility. Experimentally, right ventricular function in the face of elevated afterload is critically dependent on the coronary perfusion pressure, and therefore significant systemic hypotension should be avoided in situations of right ventricular failure.[16] Right ventricular afterload should also be minimized in situations of right ventricular dysfunction by induction of respiratory alkalosis and inhaled NO to reduce PVR. In severe cases, the circulation can be supported and the right ventricle decompressed with a venoarterial extracorporeal membrane oxygenation (ECMO) system. In most situations of significant right ventricular failure after transplantation, function recovers.

Survival

Improved life expectancy and improved quality of life compared with that resulting from the underlying heart disease are the two major goals of cardiac transplantation. Table 60-2 shows our results of cardiac transplantation since the program was initiated in 1986 and the results of pediatric cardiac transplantation nationwide. The Registry of the International Society for Heart and Lung Transplantation Fifth Official Pediatric Report[17] reported a 10-year actuarial survival for pediatric patients transplanted between 1982 and 2002 of more than 50% (Fig. 60-1). The early mortality has decreased significantly in the most recent era.[17] When analyzing survival by age, the infant group has a much higher early mortality risk after transplantation (see Fig. 60-1), but the long-term outcomes of patients who survive the first year after transplantation, is significantly better than older age groups. For infants, the incremental

TABLE 60–2. Survival at 30 days, 1, 3, 5, and 10 Years in Patients Transplanted at Children's Hospital Boston 1986-2003. National Data from UNOS are Included

	Childrens Hospital Boston		
	1986-1996	1997-2003	UNOS
30 Days	94%	96%	93%
1 Year	87%	90%	85%
3 Years	82%	87%	77%
5 Years	71%	84%	68%
10 Years	66%	NA	

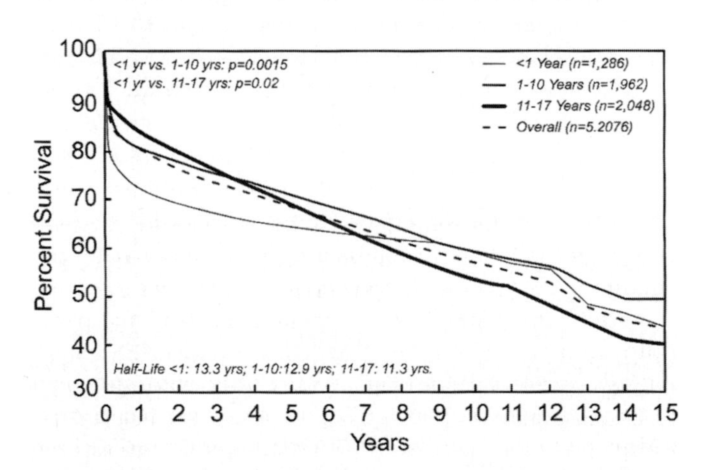

FIGURE 60–1 *Actuarial survival after pediatric heart transplantation between 1982 and 2001, by era of transplantation. Cumulative data from the International Society for Heart and Lung transplantation of more than 5000 pediatric recipients shows significantly improved survival over time.*
From Boucek MM, et al. The registry of the International Society for Heart and Lung Transplantation. J Heart Lung Transplant 23(8):933, 2004.

TABLE 60–3. Risk Factors for 1-year Mortality in Pediatric Heart Transplant Recipients (1996-2001)*

Variable	Odds Ratio	p Value
Diagnosis: congenital	2.01	<0.0001
Preop ventilator	1.92	0.001
Diagnosis: other[a]	1.92	0.009
VAD	1.85	0.04
Donor COD:other[b]	1.56	0.04

*Adapted with permission, Boucek et al Registry of the ISHLT, Pediatric report

[a]other: not congenital, cardiomyopathy, or re-transplant

[b]other: not head trauma, CVA, CNS tumor or anoxia

VAD: ventricular assist device, COD: cause of death, CVA: cerebral vascular accident, CNS: central nervous system.

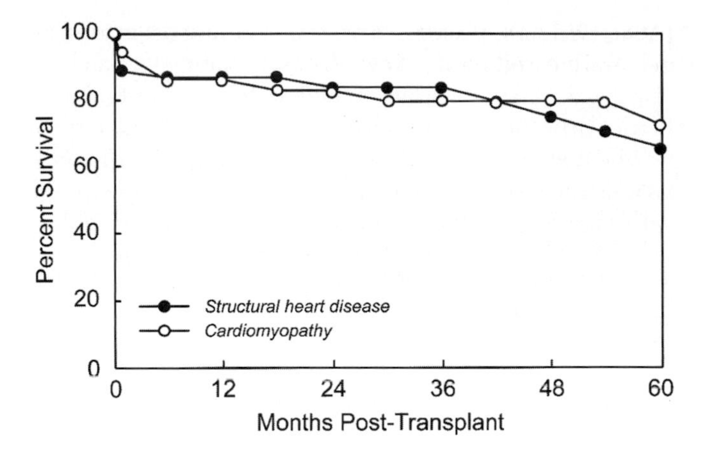

FIGURE 60–2 *Actuarial survival after pediatric heart transplantation between 1982 and 2001 shows the prominent early mortality risk of the younger age groups, with a possible survival benefit of this same group late in the follow-up.*

yearly mortality rate between 4 and 10 years after transplantation was less than 2% per year, whereas adolescent recipients have an annual survival decrement of 4% per year.[17] Risk factors for mortality include the need for ventilatory or mechanical support before transplantation, the need for retransplantation, and the diagnosis of congenital heart disease[2] (Table 60-3), although in institutions with high volume of congenital heart recipients such as ours, the effect of congenital heart disease seems to be lower (Fig. 60-2).

Causes of death after transplantation are summarized in Table 60-4. Acute failure of the transplanted heart is the most common cause of death in the first 30 days and occurs with greater frequency in infant recipients.[17] From 1 to 5 years after transplantation, acute cellular rejection and infection are the most common causes of death. Beyond 5 years, chronic rejection becomes the dominant cause of loss of either the heart or the patient.

Post-Transplantation Management Issues

Rejection

Modulation of the immune response remains the major challenge to organ transplantation, but the number of therapeutic agents available that alter the immune response has increased significantly in recent years. Aggressive monitoring for signs and symptoms of rejection is essential (Table 60-5). Although rejection may be manifested by the

TABLE 60–4. Pediatric Heart Transplant Recipients: Cause of Death (Deaths: January 1992 – June 2003)

Cause of Death	0-30 Days (N = 310)	31 Days-1 Year (N = 258)	>1 Year-3Years (N = 166)	>3 Years-5 Years (N = 106)	>5 Years (N = 199)
CAV	3 (1.0%)	25 (9.7%)	35 (21.1%)	42 (39.6%)	64 (32.2%)
Acute Rejection	26 (8.4%)	72 (27.9%)	45 (27.1%)	16 (15.1%)	24 (12.1%)
Lymphoma		5 (1.9%)	8 (4.8%)	2 (1.9%)	17 (8.5%)
Malignancy, other		4 (1.6%)	1 (0.6%)	1 (0.9%)	8 (4.0%)
CMV	1 (0.3%)	7 (2.7%)	1 (0.6%)		
Infection, non-CMV	40 (12.9%)	43 (16.7%)	12 (7.2%)	5 (4.7%)	12 (6.0%)
Primary Failure	55 (17.7%)	12 (4.7%)	5 (3.0%)	7 (6.6%)	11 (5.5%)
Graft Failure	78 (25.2%)	31 (12.0%)	31 (18.7%)	21 (19.8%)	40 (20.1%)
Technical	21 (6.8%)	3 (1.2%)	2 (1.2%)	1 (0.9%)	1 (0.5%)
Other	8 (2.6%)	8 (3.1%)	9 (5.4%)	4 (3.8%)	10 (5.0%)
Multiple Organ Failure	34 (11.0%)	26 (10.1%)	3 (1.8%)	1 (0.9%)	3 (1.5%)
Renal Failure	1 (0.3%)	1 (0.4%)			
Pulmonary	24 (7.7%)	14 (5.4%)	8 (4.8%)	5 (4.7%)	7 (3.5%)
Cerebrovascaular	19 (6.1%)	7 (2.7%)	6 (3.6%)	1 (0.9%)	2 (1.0%)

From Boucek MM, et al. The Registry of the International Society for Heart and Lung Transplantation. J Heart Lung Transplant 23(8):933, 2004.

TABLE 60–5. Signs and Symptoms of Acute Rejection in Children Following Heart Transplantation

Symptoms
• Fatigue
• Decreased appetite
• Nausea
• Abdominal pain
• Rapid increase in weight
• Fussiness, poor feeding (infants)
Signs
• Tachycardia
• Irregular rhythm, atrial flutter, ventricular tachycardia
• Fever
• Gallop (S3)
• Hepatomegaly

onset of atrial or ventricular arrhythmias[18] or reduced cardiac contractility, it also occurs in asymptomatic patients. Although changes in the electrocardiogram and the echocardiogram[19] can be useful warning signs of rejection, the endomyocardial biopsy[20] remains the most definitive diagnostic study. Tissue for histologic examinations is obtained with a biotome forceps introduced transvenously. Lymphocyte infiltration with myocardial necrosis is characteristic of cellular rejection, but a presumably humoral form of rejection also occurs in which there is myocardial edema and endothelial swelling without significant lymphocyte infiltration. Rejection identified by biopsy, particularly in the first year after transplantation, is aggressively treated with an increase in immunosuppression to minimize damage to the transplanted heart. Because acute rejection[21–26] is most frequently seen in the first 3 to 6 months after transplantation, "surveillance" biopsies are carried out at frequent intervals during this period. However, at any time there are indications that rejection may be occurring, the donor heart is biopsied immediately.

The immunosuppressive regimens currently in use in our institution are three-agent protocols that aim to affect multiple aspects of the immune response to the transplanted organ. The most common current regimen is a combination of a calcineurin inhibitor (cyclosporine or tacrolimus) to affect T-lymphocyte function, mycophenolate mofetil or azathioprine to reduce the proliferation of immune responsive leukocytes, and corticosteroids to reduce the inflammatory response and to reduce the numbers of circulating lymphocytes. Calcineurin inhibitors are begun in the postoperative period once hemodynamic stability and renal function are reestablished. Alternative regimens have also been used in specific circumstances. In highly sensitized patients, we have adopted a protocol of immediate pretransplantation and early post-transplantation plasmapheresis with nonspecific immunoglobulin G

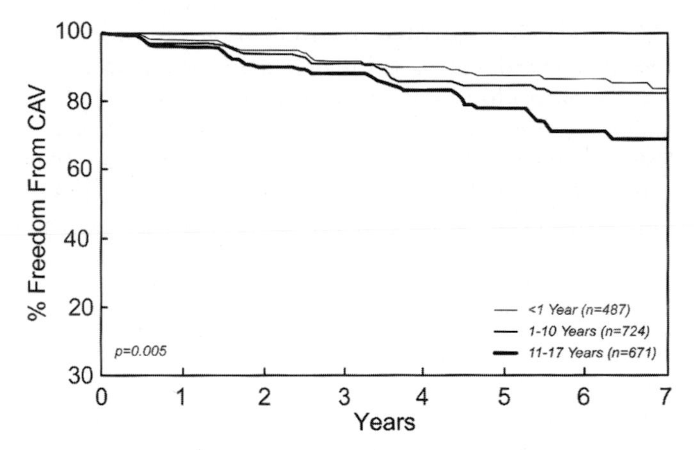

FIGURE 60–3 *Cumulative incidence of acute rejection and infection among 1114 primary transplantations in the Pediatric Heart Transplant Study (1993–2000). Freedom from coronary vasculopathy.*
From Boucek MM, et al. The registry of the International Society for Heart and Lung Transplantation. J Heart Lung Transplant 23(8):933, 2004.

infusion to reduce the levels of preformed antibodies. This protocol has been successfully used in seven highly sensitized patients with high levels of preformed antibodies, and hyperacute rejection of the donor heart has been avoided.

Coronary Vasculopathy

A more insidious and difficult problem occurs in the later post-transplantation period, which is characterized by the development of progressive narrowing of the coronary arteries leading to the development of myocardial ischemia, myocardial dysfunction, arrhythmias, and risk for sudden death. This post-transplantation coronary arteriopathy is generally thought to represent a form of chronic rejection and is the leading cause of death among late survivors of heart transplantation,[17,23] with an incidence in one series of almost 20% at 5 years (Fig. 60-3).

The diagnosis of coronary vasculopathy is difficult. Signs and symptoms are outlined in Table 60-6, although patients are often asymptomatic. Some transplanted hearts do become renervated, and chest pain can be of cardiac origin.

TABLE 60–6. Signs and Symptoms of Chronic Rejection Following Heart Transplantation in Children

- Ectopy/Atrial Flutter
- Presyncope
- Syncope
- Intermittent edema
- Exercise intolerance
- Chest pain (rare due to cardiac denervation)

Coronary angiography is a relatively insensitive marker of mild coronary vasculopathy but can identify severe disease.[27] Intravascular ultrasound suggests an overall prevalence in children studied more than 5 years after transplantation of 74%.[27] Myocardial perfusion scanning, dobutamine stress echocardiography,[28,29] and magnetic resonance imaging techniques are under investigation as more definitive diagnostic tools. At present, coronary angiography is recommended every 1 to 2 years to attempt to visualize the coronary vasculature.

The precise immune mechanisms involved in this chronic vasculopathy process are not well defined. Anecdotal reports, small clinical trials in adults, and experimental models in animals suggest that some agents may be useful in prevention of graft vasculopathy and coronary arterial events. In our institution, all patients are placed on angiotensin-converting enzyme inhibitors, a statin agent to lower lipids, aspirin, and an antiproliferative agent such as mycophenolate mofetil. Calcium channel blockers are also used frequently, and increased experience with rapamycin has been acquired in patients with renal dysfunction or early signs of vasculopathy. Rapamycin is of particular interest because it has been shown to prevent the development and progression of graft vasculopathy in a number of animal models. Retransplantation is considered for these patients with moderate to severe coronary vasculopathy.

Infection

Infection is an important issue in the post-transplantation patient because of the immunosuppression required to prevent rejection of the transplanted heart. The availability of effective antibacterial, antiviral, and antifungal agents has allowed many of these post-transplantation infections to be treated, but infection in the post-transplantation patient remains an important source of morbidity and potential mortality.

Prophylactic antibiotics are limited to the immediate preoperative and early postoperative period and usually involve antibiotics with gram-positive coverage such as cephalexin or vancomycin. Thereafter, antibiotic therapy is targeted only to treatment of specifically identified infections.

Viral infections represent a significant risk to the patient after transplantation, but the emergence of several antiviral therapies has mitigated these risks to some extent. The most common viral infection in the early post-transplantation period is caused by cytomegalovirus (CMV).[30] If either the donor or recipient has serologic evidence of prior infection with CMV, the recipient is prophylactically treated intravenously for 14 days with ganciclovir followed by 3 months of oral therapy. In recipient CMV-negative and donor CMV-positive situations, CMV immune globulin is given early postoperatively. Infection with Epstein-Barr virus is a later threat to the post-transplantation patient because of its association with post-transplantation lymphoproliferative disease (PTLD). In PTLD, there is rapid proliferation of B lymphocytes, generally in a single anatomic area, but these proliferating lymphocytes frequently behave in a malignant fashion. The occurrence of PTLD has been significantly associated with the use of monoclonal or polyclonal antilymphocyte globulins (rabbit antithymocyte globulin or the murine antilymphocyte antibody OKT-3). Therefore, the use of these antilymphocyte globulins has been reserved for treatment of rejection, which is refractory to other agents. The diagnosis is established by an excisional biopsy of the involved lymph nodes. The treatment of PTLD associated with Epstein-Barr viral infection includes reductions in the dosages of immunosuppressive agents and administration of ganciclovir. PTLD unresponsive to weaning of immunosuppression has been treated with rituximab (Rituxan), a CD20 antibody, with increasing success. The incidence of post-transplantation pulmonary pneumocystic infection has been effectively reduced by prophylactic administration of sulfonamides. Trimethoprim sulfa (Bactrim) is administered in prophylactic doses for 1 year after transplantation. Other infections, such as herpes zoster, parvovirus, and fungal infections, have been successfully treated but have a high risk for significant morbidity and mortality.

Long-Term Medical Management

Nephrotoxicity[31] is common after heart transplantation and results primarily from chronic calcineurin inhibitor therapy. Aggressive control of hypertension is crucial to aid in protecting the kidneys. Sixty percent of pediatric patients require antihypertensives 5 years after transplantation.[17] The addition of angiotensin-converting enzyme inhibition or diltiazem has been shown to be renal protective, and all our patients receive one for these medications. Other long-term issues, such as hypercholesterolemia,[32,33] osteoporosis, insulin-dependent diabetes,[34] and obesity, must be followed closely and treated.

Psychosocial Issues and Noncompliance

Although pediatric heart transplantation survivors are generally reported to return to good quality of life,[35,36] some level of adverse functioning has been reported.[37–40] This variability in reports on psychological functioning is reflective of the limited research as well as the paucity of longer-term or longitudinal follow-up studies. In a recent longitudinal study in a small group of patients from our institution,[40] most (73.3%) patients surviving almost a decade after heart transplantation show psychological functioning within the normal range and a significant improvement over their emotional functioning before transplantation. These patients maintained the same level of functioning that was described when the group averaged 2 years post-transplantation.[37] Similar to the previous study[37] of this group, post-transplantation medical severity was not correlated to post-transplantation functioning. Most children and adolescents have the capacity for healthy psychological functioning after heart transplantation. Nevertheless, there is a need for ongoing psychological assessment and intervention for patients and their families facing pediatric heart transplantation because more than 25% will likely present with emotional adjustment difficulties. In addition, the factors that may facilitate or hinder coping with pediatric heart transplantation have not been well defined and are in need of further study.

Nonadherence to complicated and life-sustaining therapy is even less well studied. Normal adolescent development, combined with the complex psychological issues surrounding heart transplantation, creates a large population of recipients at risk. Nonadherence has been linked to late rejection,[41] and higher mortality rates in the older adolescent group have been observed. Flippin and associates[42] suggest that high variability in trough drug levels (both high and low levels) is a sensitive marker for pediatric heart transplant recipients at greater risk for recurrent rejection and hospitalization after transplantation. Success of this treatment depends on the coordination and careful communication between the family, the primary care physician, and the transplant team.

Overall outcomes continue to improve for children awaiting and following pediatric heart transplantation. Newer immunosuppressive agents with lower side-effect profiles, and the possibility of immune tolerance, as well as close supervision of the health maintenance issues (Table 60-7), allow for a promising future for many of these patients.

TISSUE ENGINEERING

Organ transplantation has significant limitations as outlined previously, and currently available techniques for replacement of cardiovascular structures have similar limitations. Diseases of the heart valves and large "conduit" arteries account for about 60,000 cardiac surgical procedures each year in the United States, but the current replacement devices have well-known significant limitations. Ideally, any valve or artery substitute would function in similar fashion to the normal valve or artery to allow blood to pass through it without stenosis or regurgitation, but would also have the following characteristics: (1) durability, (2) growth potential, (3) compatibility with blood so that thrombus and emboli would not form on its surface, and (4) resistance to infection. None of the currently available devices constructed from prosthetic or biologic materials meet these criteria. In recent years, we and a number of other investigators have begun to use an approach termed *tissue engineering* to develop prototype cardiovascular replacement structures from their individual cellular components. These efforts in the cardiovascular field have focused on the development of semilunar valves, conduit arteries, and valved conduits, although there has been speculation about tissue-engineered organs, including the heart. Our concept has been that if valves or arteries could be made from autologous cells, then these new living tissues could potentially have these desirable characteristics. The potential for growth is of obvious importance to children.

TABLE 60–7. Optimizing Long Term Health

- Cholesterol management
- Routine exercise
- Smoking cessation/counseling
- Aggressive blood pressure control
- Optimize bone health and prevention
- Family support and counseling
- Adolescent noncompliance issues
- Neurocognitive and neuropsychiatric support

Tissue engineering is a developing discipline that brings together engineering and biology to develop replacement tissues from their individual cellular components. Much of the strength and flexibility in normal cardiovascular tissues are due to the specialized proteins and polysaccharide–protein complexes that form the extracellular matrix. The success of this approach depends on the ability of these cells to produce and remodel an appropriate extracellular matrix. Although it has been possible to grow individual types of cells in culture for some time, it is more difficult to induce these cells to assemble or organize into more complex structural forms found in normal tissues or to produce normal matrix proteins in an organized fashion. Our laboratory efforts to develop heart valves and large conduit arteries have used biodegradable polymers as scaffolds on which to have normal cells grow and proliferate. The scaffold also temporarily provides the structure and the mechanical stability, which are necessary for "tissues" to develop from their individual cellular components. Ideally, these polymer scaffolds then degrade during the time that the cells in the developing "tissue" are producing their own structural proteins and are becoming organized and oriented to replicate normal tissue structure.

Several projects have been undertaken in our laboratory aimed at constructing both heart valves and systemic and pulmonary arteries using the tissue-engineering approach. The initial studies[44–48] were carried out using a polyglycolic acid polymer as the scaffold. The source of the cells was from normal systemic arteries that were removed from the animal and separated into the various cell components. We found that it was important to use autologous tissue as the source of the cells to eliminate immune rejection of the engineered tissues once they were implanted.[46] The numbers of cells were "expanded" in culture, and then suspensions of the cells were seeded to the polymer scaffolds. These cell–polymer constructs were then incubated in culture for several more days and then implanted as a valve replacement or an artery replacement into the same animal from which the cells were originally removed. Valve leaflets[45–47] and segments of pulmonary artery[48] functioned well for periods of up to 4 months without structural failure and without formation of thrombus on their surfaces. Importantly, when these structures were implanted into growing animals, they demonstrated growth and complete degradation of the polymer by 6 weeks after implantation.[47,48] We were also able to demonstrate that cells from the wall of a systemic vein could be used to form a conduit artery for the pulmonary circulation.[48] The tissues appeared to have relatively normal structure and they produced the normal matrix proteins.

Despite these encouraging results, a significant number of problems remain to be resolved before application of these techniques for clinical use. First, all our published experiments to date have been carried out in animals, and it remains to be determined whether human cells could be used to develop tissues in the same way. We are currently engaged in studies with human cells to address this question. Second, the identification of an "ideal" polymer scaffold has not been accomplished. The PGA polymer used as the scaffold in the initial experiments is stiff and difficult to work with surgically. Our attempts (unreported) to create a three-leaflet valve yielded valve leaflets that were quite thick, and implantation of the valve was associated with intolerable pulmonary valvar stenosis. Experience with a more flexible polymer, polyhydroxyoctanoate (PHO), demonstrated that it was possible to construct a trileaflet valved conduit, which had good early function in vivo.[49,50] However, the prolonged degradation time of this material was associated with a less favorable outcome,[19] despite modification of the PHO by making it more porous by salt leaching.[50] Based on these experiments, we have concluded that a short degradation time for the polymer scaffold is preferable. More recently, we have used a composite material formed from PGA and poly-4-hydroxybutyrate (P4HB) with better early and intermediate-term results.[51] This composite polymer appears to completely degrade within 6 weeks after implantation but is more flexible than the PGA native polymer. Others have taken an approach in which native tissues are "decellularized" by incubation in trypsin/EDTA, leaving only the matrix proteins as a substrate to which donor cells are then added.[52] Steinhoff and colleagues reported that the recellularized valves showed "complete histological restitution of valve tissue and confluent endothelial surface coverage in all cases."[52] We continue to search for a biodegradable polymer or native scaffolding material that will have more acceptable initial strength and flexibility characteristics while still providing a hospitable environment for the cells to develop into tissues.

The ideal source of cells for the developing "tissues" has not been determined. In patients, the use of vascular wall cells for the engineered tissue is problematic, but veins would be preferable to arteries as the source of the cells. We have some evidence that heart valves developed using cells from the skin do not function as well as those developed using cells from the wall of the artery,[47] but vein wall cells seem to work reasonably well in conduit arteries.[48] We have recently begun to explore the use of circulating endothelial precursor cells (EPCs) and bone marrow mesenchymal stem cells as potential sources of cells for tissue engineered cardiovascular structures.[53] Using EPCs, we have been able to create tissue-engineered small-caliber arterial grafts that remained patent in sheep for periods of up to several months.[53] Histologically, these tissue-engineered vessels seem to form new matrix components in the wall of the neovessel. If similar results are obtained in creating tissue-engineered cardiac valves from these circulating endothelial cells (ongoing experiments), the sacrifice of native blood vessels for cells to seed scaffolds could be avoided. We have successfully isolated circulating endothelial cells from human cord blood (K. Guleserian, unpublished observations). Because it is now possible to diagnose many forms of congenital heart disease in fetal life, one might imagine using fetal cells to develop replacement valves or arteries while the gestation is continuing. These replacement valves or arteries, developed from the child's own cells, could be ready to be implanted when the child is born.

Finally, a number of questions remain regarding optimal *in vitro* conditions under which the tissue-engineered structures should be grown. One important area is that of the physical signals that are delivered to the developing tissues. We have recently completed initial studies, which assessed the effects of subjecting the developing valve leaflet tissue to physical signals (shear stress and hydrostatic pressure) provided by a pulse duplicator system.[51] These studies have shown that the developing tissue, grown on the PGA-P4HB polymer scaffold, does respond to imposed physical "signals" by increasing the amount of collagen produced and increasing the number of cells in the tissue.[51] The early function and the gross and histologic appearance of the tissue valves produced in this way are superior to those achieved by prior techniques, although there was some central valvar regurgitation after 4 months in vivo.[51] A variety of chemical or cytokine signals will likely also affect the development of these tissues *in vitro*. We anticipate that by controlling both the physical and biochemical environment of the developing tissue, it will be possible to more precisely guide the development of valve and arterial conduit tissues before implantation into the bloodstream.

Tissue engineering is a new approach to solving the problem of creating replacement tissues for use as heart valves or arteries. Although initial animal studies have been encouraging, numerous questions must be resolved before embarking on clinical trials.

REFERENCES

1. Kantrowitz A, Haller JD, Joos H, Cermti MM, Carstensen HE. Transplantation of the heart in an infant and an adult. Am J Cardiol 22:782, 1968.
2. Vricella LA, Razzouk AJ, del Rio M, Gundry SR, Bailey LL. Heart transplant for hypoplastic left heart syndrome: Modified technique for reducing circulatory arrest time. J Heart Lung Transplant 17:1167, 1998.
3. Hsu DT, Quaegebeur JM, Michler RE, et al. Heart transplantation in children with congenital heart disease. J Am Coll Cardiol 26:743, 1995.
4. Vricella LA, Razzouk AJ, Gundry SR, Larsen RL, Kuhn MA, Bailey LL. Heart transplantation in infants and children with situs inversus. J Thorac Cardiovasc Surgery 116:82, 1998.
5. Cooper M, Fuzesi L, Addonizio L, Hsu DT, Smith CR, Rose EA. Pediatric heart transplantation after operations involving the pulmonary arteries. J Thoracic Cardiovasc Surg 102:386, 1991.
6. Pigula FA, Gandhi S, Ristich J, et al. Cardiopulmonary transplantation for congenital heart disease in the adult. J Heart Lung Transplant 20:297, 2001.
7. Mayer JE Jr, Perry SB, O'Brien P, et al. Orthotopic Heart Transplantation for Complex congenital heart disease. J Thorac Cardiovasc Surg 99:484, 1990.
8. Ward KM, Canter CE, Webber SA, Chin C, Pahl E. Anthracycline cardiomyopathy and pediatric heart transplantation [abstract]. J Heart Lung Transplant 21:64, 2002.
9. Razzouk AJ, Johnston JK, Larsen RL, Chinnock RE, Fitts JA, Bailey LL. Effect of oversizing cardiac allografts on survival in pediatric patients with congenital heart disease. J Heart Lung Transplant, 24(2):195, 2005.
10. Del Nido PJ, Annitage JM, Fricker FJ, et al. Extracorporeal membrane oxygenation support as a bridge to pediatric heart transplantation. Circulation 90(2):66, 1994.
11. Weyand M, Kececioglu D, Kehl HG. Neonatal mechanical bridging to total orthotopic heart transplantation. Ann Thorac Surg 66:519, 1998.
12. Reinhartz O, Keith FM, El-Banayosy A, et al. Multi-center experience with the Thoratec ventricular assist device in children and adolescents. J Heart Lung Transplant 20:439, 2001.
13. Helman DN, Addonizio LJ, Morales DLS, et al. Implantable left ventricular assist devices can successfully bridge adolescent patients to transplant. J Heart Lung Transplant 16:121, 2000.
14. Blume ED, Naftel DC, Bastardi HJ, Duncan BW, Kirklin JK, Webber SA. Outcome of children ridged to transplant with ventricular assist device. J Heart Lung Transplant 24(25):575, 2005.
15. Lower RR, Shumway NE. Studies on the orthotopic nanotransplantation of the canine heart. Surg Forum 11:18, 1960.
16. Vlahakes GJ, Turley K, Hoffman JI. The pathophysiology of failure in acute right ventricular hypertension: hemodynamic and biochemical correlations. Circulation 63(1):87, 1981.
17. Boucek MM, Edwards LB, Keck BM, et al. The Registry of the International Society for Heart and Lung Transplantation: Fifth official pediatric report—2001 to 2002. J Heart Lung Transplant 21:826, 2001.
18. Collins KK, Thiagarajan RR, Chin C, et al. Atrial tachyarrhythmias and permanent pacing after pediatric heart transplantation. J Heart Lung Transplant 22(10):1126, 2003.
19. Boucek MM, Mathis CM, Boucek RJ Jr, et al. Prospective evaluation of echocardiography for primary rejection surveillance after infant heart transplantation: Comparison with endomyocardial biopsy. J Heart Lung Transplant 13(1 Pt 1):66, 1994.
20. Balzer DT, Moorhead S, Saffitz JE, Huddleston CB, Spray TL, Canter CE. Utility of surveillance biopsies in infant heart transplant recipients. J Heart Lung Transplant 14:1095, 1995.
21. Mills RM, Naftel DC, Kirklin JK, et al. Heart transplant rejection with hemodynamic compromise: A multi-institutional study of the role of endomyocardial infiltrate. J Heart Lung Transplant 16:813, 1997.
22. Pahl E, Naftel D, Kuhn M, et al. The incidence and impact of transplant coronary artery disease in pediatric recipients: A 9 year multi-institutional study. Circulation 106:396, 2002.
23. Webber SA, Naftel DC, Parker J, et al. Late rejection episodes more than 1 year after pediatric heart transplantation: risk factors and outcomes. J Heart Lung Transplant, In Press.
24. Chin C, Naftel DC, Singh TP, et al. Risk factors for recurrent rejection in pediatric heart transplantation: a multicenter experience. J Heart Lung Transplant, 23(3):323, 2004.
25. Rotondo K. Naftel rejection following cardiac transplantation in infants and children: A multi-institutional study. J Heart Lung Transplant 15:S80, 1996.
26. Kawauchi M, Gundry SR, de Begona JA, et al. Male donor into female recipient increases the risk of pediatric heart allograft rejection. Ann Thorac Surg 55(3):716, 1993.
27. Dent CL, Canter CE, Hirsch R, Balzer DT. Transplant coronary artery disease in pediatric heart transplant recipients. J Heart Lung Transplant 19:240, 2000.
28. Larsen RL, Applegate PM, Dyar DA, et al. Dobutamine stress echocardiography for assessing coronary artery disease after transplantation in children. J Am Coll Cardiol 32:515, 1998.

29. Pahl E, Crawford SE, Swenson JM, et al. Dobutamine stress echocardiography: Experience in pediatric heart transplant recipients. J Heart Lung Transplant 18:725, 1999.
30. Kanter K, Pahl E, Naftel DC, et al. Pediatric Heart Transplant Study Group. Preventing CMV Infection in Pediatric Heart Transplant Recipients: Does Prophylaxis Work [abstract]. J Heart Lung Transplant 17:59, 1998.
31. English RF, Pophal SA, Bacanu S, et al. Long-term Comparison of Tacrolimus and Cyclosporine Induced Nephrotoxicity in Pediatric Heart Transplant Recipients. Am J Transplant 2:769, 2002.
32. Chin C, Rosenthal D, Bernstein D. Lipoprotein abnormalities are highly prevalent in pediatric heart transplant recipients. Pediatr Transplant 4:193, 2000.
33. Penson MG, Winter WE, Fricker FJ, et al. Tacrolimus-based triple drug immunosuppression minimizes serum lipid elevations in pediatric cardiac transplant recipients. J Heart Lung Transplant 18:707, 1999.
34. First MR, Gerber DA, Hariharan S, Kauhan DB, Shapiro R. Posttransplant diabetes mellitus in kidney allograft recipients: incidence, risk factors, and management. Transplantation 73:379, 2002.
35. Uzark KC, Sauer SN, Lawrence KS, Miller J, Addonizio L, Crowley DC. The psychosocial impact of pediatric heart transplantation. J Heart Lung Transplant 11:1160, 1992.
36. Wray J, Pot-Mees C, Zeitlin H, Radley-Smith R, Yacoub M. Cognitive function and behavioural status in pediatric heart and heart-lung transplant recipients: the Harefield experience. BMJ 309:837, 1994.
37. DeMaso DR, Twente AW, Spratt EG, O'Brien P. The impact of psychological functioning, medical severity, and family functioning in pediatric heart transplantation. J Heart Lung Transplant 14:1102, 1995.
38. Wray J, Yacoub MH. Psychosocial evaluation of children after heart and heart-lung transplantation. In: Kapoor AS, Laks H, Schroeder JS, Yacoub MH, editors. Cardiomyopathies and heart-lung transplantation. New York: McGraw-Hill, 1991, p. 447-60.
39. Todaro JF, Fennell EB, Sears SF, Rodrigue JR, Roche AK. Review: Cognitive and psychological outcome of pediatric heart transplantation. J Pediatric Psychology 25:567, 2000.
40. DeMaso DR, Kelley SD, Bastardi H, OBrien P, Blume ED. The Longitudinal Impact of Psychological Functioning, Medical Severity, and Family Functioning in Pediatric Heart Transplantation. JofHeavt Lung Transplant, 23(4):473, 2004.
41. Ringewald JM, Gidding SS, Crawford SE, Backer CL, Mavroudis C, Pahl E. Nonadherence is associated with late rejection in pediatric heart transplant recipients. J Pediatr, 139:75, 2001.
42. Flippin MS, Canter CE, Balzer DT. Increased morbidity and high variability of cyclosporine levels in pediatric heart transplant recipients. Journal of Heart & Lung Transplantation. 19(4):343, 2000.
43. Schowengerdt KO, Ni J, Denfield SW, et al. Diagnosis, surveillance, and epidemiologic evaluation of viral infections in pediatric cardiac transplant recipients with the use of polymerase chain reaction. J Heart Lung Transplant 15:111, 1996.
44. Breuer C, Shin'oka T, Tanel RE, et al. Tissue engineering lamb heart valve leaflets. Biotechnol Bioeng 50:562, 1996.
45. Shin'oka T, Ma PX, Shum-Tim D, et al. Tissue engineered heart valves-autologous valve leaflet replacement study in a lamb model. Circulation 94:III64, 1996.
46. Shin'oka T, Breuer CK, Tanel RE, et al. Tissue engineering heart valves: valve leaflet replacement study in a lamb model. Ann Thorac Surg 60:S-513, 1995.
47. Shin'oka T, Shum-Tim D, Ma PX, et al. Tissue engineered valve leaflets: Does cell origin affect outcome? Circulation 96(Suppl II):II-102, 1997.
48. Shin'oka T, Shum-Tim D, Ma PX, et al. Creation of viable pulmonary artery autografts through tissue engineering. J Thorac Cardiovasc Surg 115:536. 1998.
49. Stock U, Nagashima M, Khalil PN, et al. Tissue engineered valved conduits in the pulmonary circulation. J Thoracic and Cardiovascular Surgery 119:732, 2000.
50. Sodian R, Hoerstrup SP, Sperling JS, et al. Early in vivo experience with tissue engineered trileaflet heart valves. Circulation 102:III-22, 2000.
51. Hoerstrup S, Sodian R, Daebritz S, Wang J, Bacha EA, Martin DP, Moran AM, Guleserian KJ, Sperling JS, Kaushal S, Vacanti JP, Schoen Fj, Mayer JE. Functional Living Trileaflet Heart Valves Grown in Vitro, Circulation, 102(Suppl III): III-44, 2000.
52. Steinhoff G, Stock U, Karim N, et al. Tissue Engineering of Pulmonary Heart Valves on Allograft Acellular Matrix Conduits. Circulation 102(Suppl III):III-50, 2000.
53. Kaushal S, Arniel G, Guleserian K, et al. Circulating Endothelial Cells for Tissue-Engineered Small Diameter Vascular Grafts (abstract) Circulation 102(Suppl II):II-766, 2000.

XI

The Future

61

Cardiac Excitability and Heritable Arrhythmias

DAVID E. CLAPHAM AND MARK T. KEATING

The heart is a complex electromechanical organ composed of cardiac myocytes, fibroblasts, and vascular cells. Myocytes range from sinoatrial (SA) nodal pacing cells with few contractile elements to paced ventricular cells packed with contractile muscle protein. The heart must contract unfailingly to provide the constant needs of the body's cells. The filling and subsequent contraction of atria and ventricles are electrically timed to efficiently pump blood to the periphery, and to respond to increasing or decreasing demands for blood supply (Fig. 61-1). Ion channels are the proteins responsible for the generation of the electrical signals traversing the heart. Skeletal muscle cells are a fused electrical syncytium, and contraction of functional units is initiated by neuronal release of acetylcholine. Individual cardiac cells make electrical continuity through low-resistance intercellular gap junctions.[1,2]

Each cell is a small battery with –50 to –90 mV across its plasma membrane. *Depolarization* is defined as a change in membrane potential to more positive voltages; *hyperpolarization* refers to changes to more negative potentials, regardless of the starting voltage. Cell voltage cannot hyperpolarize below about –98 mV or depolarize above +50 mV. Rapid voltage changes within this 150-mV range of large tissue masses are detected as 1- to 5-mV size changes in the surface electrocardiogram (ECG). The P, QRS, and T waves represent, respectively, atrial depolarization, ventricular depolarization, and ventricular repolarization. Arising in the SA node and transmitted sequentially throughout the atria, atrioventricular (AV) node, His-Purkinje system, and ventricles, the cardiac action potential is a summation of openings and closings of distinct populations of ion channels. Cardiac channelopathies are perturbations in ion channel function or structural malformations, which underlie heritable arrhythmia syndromes.

The predominant cation inside the cell is K^+ outside it is Na^+. Intracellular Ca^{2+} ($[Ca(2+)]_i$) is actively buffered, sequestered within organelles, or extruded to maintain free concentrations of about 100 nM, roughly 20,000-fold less than in the serum. Chloride anions are 4 to 20 times higher outside the cell than inside the cell with negatively charged amino acids and other molecules making up the difference. Thus, the extracellular solution is 140 mM NaCl, 4 mM KCl, 2 mM $CaCl_2$, and 1 mM $MgCl_2$. The intracellular cations are 155 mM K^+, about 10 mM Na^+, 1 mM Mg^{2+}, and about 100 nM free Ca^{2+}. These transmembrane concentration gradients are maintained by energy requiring ion pumps and exchangers. The electrogenic Na,K-ATPase pump maintains most of the monovalent cation gradient by transporting three Na^+ ions outward and two K^+ ions inward per adenosine triphosphate (ATP) hydrolyzed. Another major transporter is the Na/Ca exchanger, transporting Ca^{2+} in exchange for Na^+.

The direction of ion movement through channels is governed by the electrochemical gradient; at equilibrium, this is the Nernst potential. Equilibrium occurs when there is no chemical or electrical energy difference for an ion across the membrane. If a cell membrane contains only ion channels that are K^+ selective, the membrane potential at which no K^+ ions flow across the membrane is the Nernst potential for K^+ (E_K). Ions in solution diffuse from regions of higher concentration to lower concentration, dissipating their chemical energy and achieving the highest entropy.

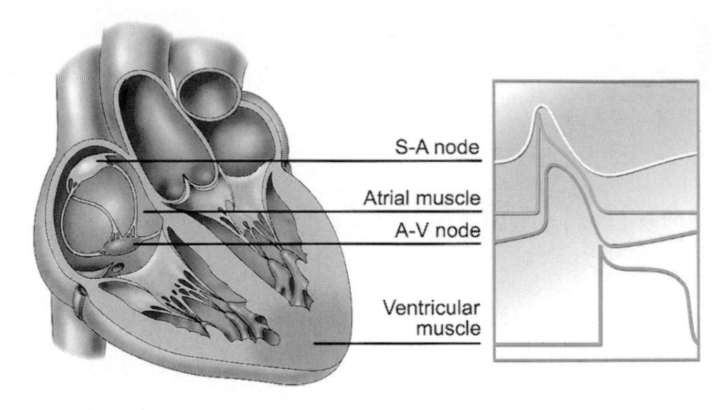

FIGURE 61–1 *Action potentials characteristic of various cardiac regions, as shown.*

Electrical energy arises from charge separation. Transmembrane voltage differences drive charged ions down an electrical gradient. When only K^+ selective channels are open in the membrane under physiologic conditions, 155 mM [K^+i (inside)] and 4 mM [K^+o (outside)], K^+ ions flow down their concentration gradients until there is a slight excess of cations in the more dilute solution. The excess K^+ ions are driven there by the concentration gradient across the membrane but forced to migrate alone by the selectivity filter of the ion channel. The slight excess of positive charge on the outside of the cell creates a negative membrane potential. (An important point is that ion exchange from ion channels is much too little to change the bulk concentrations of ions in either solution.) Equilibrium is reached when the electrical forces match and counteract the chemical forces. Thus, K^+ ions flow down their concentration gradient from inside to outside the cell until a sufficient excess of charge develops to repel the excess cations. At this point, where electrical and chemical energy are equal, no net current flows across the membrane. For a purely K^+ selective membrane, the Nernst potential is expressed as follows[3]:

$$E_K = \frac{RT}{F} \ln [K]_0 / [K]_i$$

where R is the gas constant, T is the absolute temperature in degrees Kelvin, and F is the Faraday constant. RT/F is approximately 27 mV at body temperature, so that for this example:

$$E_K = 27 \text{ mV} \ln (4/155) = -98 \text{ mV}$$

Thus, a cell with only K^+ selective channels would have an equilibrium, or resting membrane potential, equal to –98 mV. Other Nernst equilibrium potentials are E_{Na} (+70 mV), E_{Ca} (+150 mV), E_{Cl} (–45 to –65 mV), and E_{Mg} (0 mV). The membrane potential at any moment is determined by type, number, and individual conductances of the ion channels that are open.

Several features of the cardiac action potential can be appreciated with three of the Nernst potentials because for Cl^- and Mg^{2+} selective channels in the heart can be ignored for all practical purposes. First, because resting potentials of ventricular cells are closest to E_K, their highest permeability must be to K^+ ions. Also, there must be a relatively greater number of K^+ channels open at rest in the ventricular myocyte than in the nodal cell to maintain the ventricular cell in a more hyperpolarized (closer to E_K) state. Second, the ventricular myocyte depolarizes much more quickly than nodal cells, suggesting that faster, more numerous depolarizing channels are present in the ventricle (only Na^+ or Ca^{2+} channels can drive a cell to membrane potentials above 0 mV). Third, there must be a balance between depolarizing and repolarizing ion channels to account for the long plateau of the cardiac action potential.

CARDIAC ACTION POTENTIAL

The heart has its own independent rhythm; when removed from nervous system innervation and transplanted into another body, it continues to beat rhythmically. Nerves modulate the rate and rhythm of the heart but do not initiate or have fundamental control over heart rate. The duration of cardiac action potentials is 200 times longer than the about 1- to 2-msec duration of nerve and muscle. The long plateau phase around 0 mV provides the sustained depolarization and contraction needed to empty the heart's chambers. Cardiac action potentials vary from the simplest in the SA node to the most complex in the ventricle (see Fig. 61-1).

The SA node membrane potential dips to –50 to –60 mV during diastole but has no stable resting potential. After repolarization, the transmembrane potential spontaneously slowly depolarizes. The rate of rise of the upstroke of the action potential is slow (1 to 10 V/sec) in SA nodal cells, resulting in slow propagation of the impulse (less than 0.05 m/sec). In the atria, the upstroke is rapid (100 to 200 V/sec) from the steady resting potential (about –90 mV). The peak of the action potential occurs around +40 mV, and the action potential propagates at 0.3 to 0.4 m/sec (about 10 times faster than the nodal system). AV nodal action potentials are intermediate between the SA nodal and atrial action potentials. Slow conduction in the AV node is the result of a low rate of rise of the action potential and weak electrical coupling between AV nodal cells. In all remaining fibers of the heart, from the common bundle to ventricular muscle, the upstroke of the action potential is rapid (100 to 700 V/sec) and the action potential duration long (200 to 500 msec). Under normal conditions, ventricular cells do not undergo pacemaker depolarization but have resting membrane potentials (–85 mV) close to E_K. The impulse must spread rapidly throughout the myocardium and at the same time allow enough delay between impulses so that all fibers in the tissue have time to contract. Atrial and ventricular action potentials provide the time needed to wring the blood from their respective chambers.

SINOATRIAL NODAL ACTION POTENTIAL

There are 6 principal ion currents underlying the nodal action potential and 10 in the ventricle (Fig. 61-2). The properties of these inward and outward conductances are summarized in Tables 61-1 and 61-2. The SA node is paced by the I_{HCN} current (HCN for human, cyclic nucleotide gated) and by decreasing opposition to depolarization by the inwardly rectifying K^+ conductance, $I_{Kir2.1}$ (*KCNJ2*). I_{HCN} (*HCN2+HCN4*) is a nonselective inward current that is *inactive* at depolarized potentials where the action potentials are firing but is *activated* by hyperpolarization to the pacing range of potentials (–80 to –30 mV). Activation of I_{HCN} drives the membrane potential toward E_{HCN} (–20 mV). Thus, negative to its equilibrium voltage, I_{HCN} permits both K^+ and Na^+ into the cell, slowly depolarizing the membrane potential, and deactivates on continued depolarization (see Table 61-1). I_{HCN} is opposed by $I_{Kir2.1}$, resulting in a slow but carefully timed pacemaker depolarization to –40 mV. In addition, cyclic adenosine monophosphate (cAMP) causes a positive shift in the current–voltage relationship and accelerates channel activation of I_{HCN}, in part accounting for the adrenaline-mediated increase in heart rate.[4]

At –40 mV, Ca^{2+} channels begin to open, more rapidly depolarizing the membrane. The slow upstroke of the action potential in nodal cells results from a relative lack of Na^+ channels and dependence of depolarization on the fewer, slower, inward Ca^{2+} channels. Even if Na^+ channels

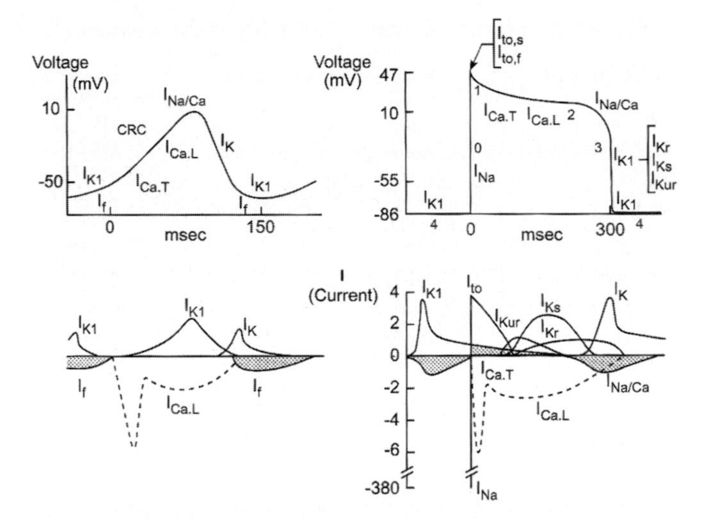

FIGURE 61–2 *Top, Principal currents responsible for the SA nodal (left) and ventricular (right) action potential. Bottom, Model of the magnitude and duration of the principal currents in the generation of the SA nodal and ventricular action potentials. Na, sodium; K, potassium; Ca, calcium; f, HCN pacemaking current; I_{to}, transient outward (K) currents; Na/Ca, sodium/calcium exchanger.*

were present, they would become inactivated by the depolarized resting membrane potentials of the SA node and therefore unable to participate significantly in depolarization. The first Ca^{2+} current to open is the transient Ca^{2+} current, $I_{CaV3.1}$ (*CACNA1H*). $I_{CaV3.1}$ drives the cell's membrane potential toward E_{Ca} and in the process triggers the activation of the L-type voltage-activated Ca^{2+} current ($I_{CaV1.2}$; *CACNA1C*) at –30 mV. Almost simultaneous with the activation of these inward currents, competing outwardly conducting delayed rectifying K^+ currents (I_{KVx}) are triggered at membrane potentials depolarized to –40 mV.

TABLE 61–1. Human Cardiac Ion Channels: Outward (Hyperpolarizing) Currents

Ion Current	Candidate Gene(s)	Gene Symbol	Chromosome Locus	Amino Acids (No.)
$I_{to,slow}$	Kv1.4	KCNA4	11p14	653
	hKvβ3	KCNAB1	3q26.1	401
$I_{to,fast}$	Kv4.2	KCND2	7q31	629
	±MiRP1	KCNE2	21q22.12	123
	±KChIP2	KCNIP2	10q24	252
	Or Kv4.3	KCND3	1p13.2	656
I_{Kr}	Kv11.1	KCNH2	7q35–q36	1,159
	(HERG) +MiRP1	KCNE2	21q22.12	123
I_{Ks}	Kv7.1 (KvLQT1)	KCNQ1	11p15.5	676
	+MinK	KCNE1	21q22.12	129
I_{Kur}	Kv1.5	KCNA5	12p13	611
$I_{K.ATP}$	Kir6.2 sulfonylurea	KCNJ11	11p15.1	390
	receptor 2A	SUR2A	12p12.1	1,407
$I_{K.ACh}$	Kir3.1 (GIRK1)	KCNJ3	2q24.1	501
	Kir3.4 (GIRK4)	KCNJ5	11q24	419

TABLE 61–2. Human Cardiac Ion Channels: Inward (Depolarizing) Currents

Ion Current	Candidate Gene(s)	Gene Symbol	Chromosome Locus	Amino Acids (No.)
I_f/I_h	$I_{f,fast}$	HCN2	19p13.3	889
	$I_{f,slow}$	HCN4	15q24–q25	1203
I_{Na}	$\alpha = Na_V1.5$	SCN5A	3p21	2015
	$+\beta 1 = Na_V\beta 1.1$	SCN1B	19q13.1	218
$I_{Ca.T}$	$\alpha 1H = Ca_VT.2$	CACNA1H	16p13.3	2353
$I_{Ca.L}$	$\alpha 1C = Ca_V1.2$	CACNA1C	12p13.3	2157
(DHPR)	$+\beta_{1\text{-}4}$	CACNB1-4	17q/10p12/	12q13/2q22
	$+\alpha 2/\delta$	CACNA2D1	7q21-q22	1091
$I_{Na/Ca}$	Na-Ca exchanger	NCX1 (SLC8A1)	2p21–p23	973

The result is again a balance between the inward conductances ($I_{CaV3.1}$, $I_{CaV1.2}$, and the Na^+/Ca^{2+} exchanger, $I_{Na/Ca}$ [*NCX1*] collectively the forces of depolarization) and the outwardly conducting (hyperpolarizing) K^+ currents, I_{KV}. The balance is reached at a peak depolarization of +10 mV before the outward K^+ current, I_{KV}, slowly overcomes the inward currents, is joined by $I_{K2.1}$, and repolarizes the cell back toward E_K.

As the membrane potential is driven hyperpolarized to –35 mV, I_{HCN} is activated again, and I_{KV} turns off. Thus, the membrane potential never reaches E_K. Rather, the depolarizing I_{HCN} pacemaker current gains the upper hand and slowly depolarizes the membrane potential away from the maximum diastolic potential. The inwardly rectifying behavior of $I_{Kir2.1}$ contributes significantly to this pacemaking activity. $I_{Kir2.1}$ has the unusual property that in the physiologic range of membrane potentials (above E_K), the net outward current has a negatively sloped I-V relation (negative conductance). Thus, $I_{Kir2.1}$ becomes smaller and smaller with depolarization (see Fig. 61-2). $I_{K2.1}$ is not very time dependent and does not inactivate significantly. If $I_{K2.1}$ were the only channel opening between –90 mV and –60 mV, any depolarization induced by an inward current of any kind results in *less* outward current. In essence, the membrane potential is unstable and driven in the depolarizing direction. The inward rectification of $I_{K2.1}$ ensures that a small inward current results in pacemaker depolarization.[5]

VENTRICULAR ACTION POTENTIAL

The cardiac action potential has been divided into five phases: phase 0, action potential upstroke or rapid depolarization; phase 1, early phase of repolarization; phase 2, the plateau; phase 3, the late phase of rapid repolarization; and phase 4, resting membrane potential and diastolic depolarization.[6]

Phase 0—The Action Potential Upstroke; Rapid Depolarization

In ventricular cardiocytes, the membrane potential at rest remains near E_K. Activation from pacemaker cells through the conduction system can stimulate the ventricular action potential. An excitatory stimulus or pacemaker potential that depolarizes the cell membrane beyond about –70 mV triggers a cascade of channel openings and closings that generate the ventricular action potential. The fast upstroke in atrial and ventricular cells is carried by Na^+ channels ($I_{NaV1.5}$). Once the threshold potential of –70 mV is reached, Na^+ channels are activated, resulting in an enormous, albeit brief (less than 5 msec) inward Na^+ current. The sodium current is 50 to 1000 times larger in net conductance than any other population of ion channels in heart. The depolarizing current carried by the influx of Na^+ drives the cell toward E_{Na}. Thus, the upstroke peaks at about +47 mV, short of the Na^+ equilibrium potential. The Na^+ conductance is short lived because the Na^+ channels are inactivated as a function of time and voltage. Inactivation causes the current to diminish almost as quickly as it turns on. The rapidity whereby Na^+ channels recover from this inactivation is a key determinant of the refractory period of the ventricle.[7]

Phase 1—The Early Phase of Repolarization

The activation of I_{Na} quickly depolarizes the membrane to the levels at which both inward Ca^{2+} currents and outward K^+ channels begin to open. The Ca^{2+} currents are substantially smaller than fully activated I_{Na} but also drive the membrane potential to very positive potentials (E_{Ca} = +150 mV). The whole point of the complex sequence of currents underlying the action potential is to deliver Ca^{2+} into the cytoplasm and sarcoplasmic reticulum where it triggers contraction. After the peak at +47 mV, there is rapid repolarization to +10 mV resulting from the rapid voltage-dependent inactivation of $I_{NaV1.5}$ and the activation of the Ca^{2+} independent transient outward K^+ current $I_{KV1.4+KV4.2/4.3}$ (*KCNA4+KCND2/KCND3*).[8] Notably, this current contributes outward current (efflux of K^+) well into the plateau (phase 2) of the action potential. Striking regional differences occur in the expression of this phase 1 repolarizing K^+ current with fivefold greater currents in epicardial layers compared with endocardial layers.[9] Heterogeneous expression not only accounts for regional variations in the action potential but also tunes repolarization throughout the ventricle and may enable regional modulation of cardiac contractility.[10]

Phase 2—The Action Potential Plateau

Cardiac action potentials have uniquely long periods of time during which the potential remains depolarized near 0 mV (plateau). Relatively few channels are open during the plateau, and thus the total membrane conductance is low. The high resistance of the membrane during the plateau acts like thick electrical insulation around a wire; it allows rapid propagation of the action potential with little dissipation. The plateau phase is maintained by a finely tuned balance between two types of inward Ca^{2+} currents and at least four types of outward K^+ currents. Ultimately, K^+ currents dominate, and the membrane potential is driven back toward E_K.

Two Ca^{2+} currents, the low voltage-activated, transient Ca^{2+} current ($I_{Ca.T}$, T-type, $I_{CaV3.2}$) and the high voltage-activated, long-lasting Ca^{2+} current ($I_{Ca.L}$, L-type, $I_{CaV1.2}$) admit the Ca^{2+} needed to initiate contraction. In the normal heart, $I_{CaV3.2}$ is found predominantly in atrial pacemaker cells, Purkinje fibers, and coronary artery smooth muscle. These Ca^{2+} channels rapidly activate at about –50 mV, peak at –20 mV, inactivate with time, are blocked by Ni^{2+} and a novel Ca^{2+} channel blocker, mibefradil, but are insensitive to dihydropyridines. $I_{CaV3.2}$ is only one fifth the size of $I_{CaV1.2}$ and thus contributes relatively little to the Ca^{2+} influx of excitation–contraction coupling.[11]

In contrast to $I_{CaV3.2}$, $I_{CaV1.2}$ is the dominant Ca^{2+} current found in virtually all cardiac cells in all species.[12] $I_{Ca.L}$ is activated at –30 mV, reaches its peak conductance at +10 mV within 3 to 5 msec, inactivates over hundreds of milliseconds, and is sensitive to block by dihydropyridines (nifedipine), benzothiazepines (diltiazem), and phenylalkylamines (verapamil).[6] These channels carry inward current throughout the plateau phase and are required for coupling membrane excitability to myocardial contraction.

The terminal portion of the plateau is sustained by inward current through the electrogenic Na^+/Ca^{2+} exchanger as Ca^{2+} is transported out of the cell at a ratio of 1 Ca^{2+} ion per 3 Na^+ ions.[13] This electrogenic current is capable of providing inward current up to 50% of the size of $I_{CaV1.2}$. During the action potential upstroke, the exchanger brings in Ca^{2+} ions, increasing contractility. As the chief means of extruding Ca^{2+} ions, the exchanger also modulates the Ca^{2+} content of the sarcoplasmic reticulum.[14]

Phase 3—Final Rapid Repolarization

At least four K^+ currents activated during the plateau compete with the inward currents. As the time-dependent inward currents inactivate at the end of the plateau, the outward K^+ currents rapidly drive the membrane potential toward E_K.[2] The K currents during the plateau consist of I_{Kr} (rapid; I_{KHERG}, *KCNH2*), I_{Ks} (slow; I_{KLVQT1}, *KCNQ1*), and I_{Kur} (ultra-rapid; $I_{KV1.5}$, *KCNA5*). I_{Kur} is more abundant in atria than in ventricle and activates 50 times faster than I_{Kr}.[15] I_{Kur} plays a major role in phase 3 repolarization of the atrial action potential.[2,6]

Phase 4—The Resting Membrane Potential and Diastolic Depolarization

The delayed rectifying K^+ channels repolarize the membrane potential to about –40 mV, where the various I_K currents deactivate. The inward rectifier $I_{Kir2.1}$, on the other hand, does not inactivate with time and continues to drive repolarization. During this repolarization, the heart cell cannot be triggered to fire another action potential (the absolute refractory period) because Na^+ channels remain inactivated. The voltage-dependent inactivation of Na^+ channels is a major mechanism for prevention of repetitive early firing; only hyperpolarization below about –70 mV can reprime Na^+ channels to enable them to open once again.

Because $I_{Kir2.1}$ predominantly sets the membrane potential, raising K^+o shifts the resting membrane potential to more depolarized potentials. At both low and high K^+o concentrations, the membrane potential is depolarized compared with that in 4-mm K^+o. Depolarization by high K^+o is explained by the shift of E_K and its effect on $I_{Kir2.1}$. At low K^+o, the Na,K-ATPase pump is slowly starved for K^+ substrate, K^+i, falls, and again E_K is shifted in the depolarized direction. Maintenance of serum K^+ levels in the 3.5- to 5-mM range is crucial to prevention of cardiac arrhythmias. Outside this range, heart cells are depolarized. Depolarization enhances pacing currents, decreases the size of Na^+ and Ca^{2+} currents through inactivation, and has broad effects on action potential duration.[16]

MODULATORY POTASSIUM CHANNELS

Other than the five principal K^+ currents, several other modulatory K^+ currents are found in heart. The most well-understood are I_{KACh} (Kir3.1 + Kir3.4; GIRK1 + GIRK4) and I_{KATP} (SUR + Kir6.2).

The vagus nerve, part of the parasympathetic nervous system, slows heart rate through activation of I_{KACh} (Kir3.1 + Kir3.4). Acetylcholine released onto the atria and pacing tissues binds to muscarinic m2 G-protein–coupled receptors. Receptor activation releases the G-protein βγ subunit that then directly binds the channel to increase its opening. $I_{K.ACh}$ is a heteromultimer of two inwardly rectifying K-channel subunits, GIRK1 (Kir3.1) and GIRK4 (Kir3.4). Native $I_{K.ACh}$ is the effector of vagally released Ach, but $I_{K.ACh}$ mediates a large part of the effect of intravenous adenosine. Adenosine binds to type 1 purinergic receptors in the heart, an autocrine G-protein–coupled receptor. The same steps occur as after activation of the muscarinic m2 receptor.

K_{ATP}, a heteromeric complex of SUR and Kir 6.2 proteins, may modulate action potential duration in response to metabolic status. I_{KATP} does not operate under normal physiologic conditions (ATP levels about 3 to 4 mM) because ATP blocks the channel. When intracellular ATP levels decrease to the point at which ATP-sensitive K^+ channels activate, there is a shorter plateau phase, early repolarization, and marked attenuation of the action potential duration. Activation of $I_{K.ATP}$ shortens the electrical and mechanical systole, perhaps reducing the loss of ATP. But the shortening of the action potential period duration decreases the refractory period and thus may also be proarrhythmic by enhancing reentry mechanisms.[2]

CARDIAC ARRHYTHMIAS

Although most hearts beat with remarkable fidelity, under certain circumstances the rhythm of the heart can fail. This is known as a cardiac arrhythmia. When the heartbeat is too slow (bradyarrhythmia or bradycardia) blood pressure cannot be maintained, leading to loss of consciousness and death. Bradyarrhythmias often result from disease or death of pacemaker and other specialized conducting cells and can be effectively treated with artificial, electronic pacemakers. Similarly, if the heart rhythm is too rapid (tachyarrhythmia or tachycardia), blood pressure cannot be maintained, leading to syncope and sudden death. The most dangerous tachyarrhythmias are focused in the ventricles and are known as ventricular tachycardia, torsades de pointes ventricular tachycardia, and ventricular fibrillation.

Cardiac arrhythmias are a leading cause of morbidity and mortality. More than 450,000 individuals in the United States die suddenly every year, and in most cases, it is assumed that the underlying cause of sudden death is ventricular tachyarrhythmia.[17,18] Despite their importance, at the time we began our research more than a decade ago, the understanding of the molecular mechanisms underlying life-threatening ventricular tachyarrhythmias was poor. Our ability to predict, prevent, and treat these disorders remains a major scientific and medical challenge.

LONG QT SYNDROME, A FAMILIAL CARDIAC ARRHYTHMIA

Long QT syndrome is a group of disorders characterized by syncope and sudden death due to episodic cardiac arrhythmias, particularly *torsades de pointes* ventricular tachycardia and ventricular fibrillation.[19,20] *Torsades de pointes* means twisting around the point, an allusion to the alternating axis of the QRS complex around the isoelectric line of the ECG during this arrhythmia.[21] Most individuals with long QT syndrome have no other symptoms or signs of disease, and arrhythmias are relatively rare except in severe cases. Some cases of long QT syndrome are associated with congenital deafness, and this disorder has also been associated with simple syndactyly.[22] Many individuals with this disorder have a subtle electrocardiographic abnormality known as prolonged QT interval.[23]

The long QT syndromes can be divided on clinical grounds into two main types: familial and acquired. There are at least two familial forms of long QT syndrome. One, which was described above, was believed to be inherited as an autosomal recessive trait and associated with congenital deafness, the Jervell and Lange-Nielsen syndrome.[24] A second, more common familial form is inherited as an autosomal dominant trait with no other phenotypic abnormalities. This form, which is sometimes referred to as the Romano-Ward syndrome,[25,26] is usually associated with less arrhythmia risk than the autosomal recessive form. The most common form of long QT syndrome is acquired. There are many different causes of acquired long QT syndrome, including heart diseases such as cardiomyopathy and cardiac ischemia, bradycardia, and metabolic abnormalities like reduced serum potassium concentration.[27] Treatment with many medications, including certain antibiotics, antihistamines, and antiarrhythmics, is the most common cause of acquired long QT syndrome.

When we began our molecular studies, there were two main theories invoked to explain the pathogenesis of long QT syndrome. One was the autonomic imbalance hypothesis. This theory was based on studies showing that manipulation of the autonomic nervous system in dogs could lead to QT prolongation and cardiac arrhythmias.[23] A second hypothesis, the cardiac ion channel hypothesis, suggested that inherited or acquired dysfunction of cardiac ion channels could lead to this disorder. In all studies reported to date, the cardiac ion channel hypothesis proved to be the primary mechanism of arrhythmia susceptibility. However, the autonomic imbalance hypothesis remains a viable theory, and it is clear that the autonomic nervous system plays a secondary role in many cardiac arrhythmias.

MUTATIONS IN CARDIAC ION CHANNEL GENES CAUSE ARRHYTHMIA SUSCEPTIBILITY

To define genes that contribute to arrhythmia susceptibility, we and others examined familial forms of this disorder, particularly long QT syndrome. During the past 10 years, seven arrhythmia susceptibility genes have been discovered: *KVLQT1*, *HERG*, *SCNA5A*, *minK*, *MiRP1*, *RyR2*, and *Kir2.1*[28–36] (Table 61-3). We discovered *KVLQT1* using positional cloning. *HERG*, *SCNA5A*, and *RyR2* were identified using the positional cloning–candidate gene approach, and *minK* and *MiRP1* were discovered using a candidate gene approach.[37] Additional locus heterogeneity was described, and several additional arrhythmia genes await discovery. These studies provided the first molecular insight into thc pathogenesis of cardiac arrhythmias.

Jervell and Lange-Nielsen syndrome was previously believed to be an autosomal recessive disorder. Phenotypic evaluation of families, however, revealed a more complicated picture.[32] Many family members, including proband's parents, had subtle prolongation of the QT interval with normal hearing. Some individuals gave a history of one or two syncopal episodes, but no cases of sudden death were noted. Furthermore, pedigree analyses revealed that some probands resulted from a consanguineous marriage. This led to the hypothesis that homozygous mutations of an autosomal dominant long QT syndrome gene might cause Jervell and Lange-Nielsen syndrome. This proved to be the case, and it is now clear that homozygous mutations of either *KVLQT1* or *minK* can cause this disorder.[32,38,39] The molecular genetics also helped to define the clinical picture. One aspect of Jervell and Lange-Nielsen syndrome, congenital deafness, is inherited as an autosomal recessive trait in that heterozygous carriers have no obvious hearing deficit. However, arrhythmia susceptibility is inherited as a semi-dominant trait. That is, heterozygotes and homozygotes both have arrhythmia susceptibility, but the risk for arrhythmia in homozygotes is much greater. Homozygous mutations of *HERG* have also been reported.[40] This condition

TABLE 61–3. Molecular and Cellular Mechanisms of Cardiac Arrhythmias

Disease	Inheritance	Gene (alternate name)	Protein	Mechanism
LQT	Autosomal dominant	*KVLQT1 (KCNQ1)*	I_{Ks} K^+ channel α-subunit	Repolarization
		HERG (KCNH2)	I_{Kr} K^+ channel α-subunit	Repolarization abnormality
		SCN5A	I_{Na} Na^+ channel α-subunit	Repolarization abnormality
		ANK2°	Anchor protein	Abnormal coordination of ion channels
		MinK (KCNE1)	I_{Ks} K^+ channel β-subunit	Repolarization abnormality
		MiRP1 (KCNE2)	I_{Kr} K^+ channel β-subunit	Repolarization abnormality
Andersen syndrome		*Kir2.1 (KCNJ2)*	I_{K1} K^+ channel α-subunit	Repolarization abnormality
LQT8	Autosomal recessive	*KVLQT1*	I_{Ks} K^+ channel α-subunit	Repolarization abnormality (with deafness)
		MinK	I_{Ks} K^+ channel β-subunit	Repolarization abnormality (syndactyly associated?)
	Acquired (drug induced)	*HERG*	I_{Kr} K^+ channel α-subunits	Repolarization abnormality
IVF	Autosomal dominant	*SCN5A*	I_{Na} Na^+ channel α-subunit	Conduction abnormality
IVF2				
CVT	Autosomal dominant	*RyR2*	Ryanodine receptor	Calcium overload
Ca^{2+} release channel	Autosomal recessive	*CASQ2*	Ca^{2+}-binding protein	Calcium overload

CVT, catecholaminergic ventricular tachycardia; IVF, familial idiopathic ventricular fibrillation; LQT, long QT syndrome.
°*ANK2* mutations cause atypical LQT; LQT8, IVF2: genes not identified.

also causes severe arrhythmia susceptibility but is not associated with other phenotypic abnormalities.

Autosomal dominant long QT syndrome genes became candidates for involvement in other familial arrhythmia susceptibility syndromes. Although the familial occurrence of virtually every arrhythmia has been reported, in most cases, the mode of inheritance is unclear. Familial ventricular fibrillation, by contrast, can be inherited as a clear, autosomal dominant trait. As in long QT syndrome, people with familial ventricular fibrillation often appear healthy.[41] Electrocardiographic evaluation of these individuals shows no evidence of QT interval prolongation. In some cases, subtle prolongation of the QRS complex can be demonstrated. A distinct electrocardiographic feature of elevation of the ST segment in leads V_1 through V_3, with or without right bundle branch block, has been described in some individuals and referred to as Brugada syndrome.[42] Some forms of familial ventricular fibrillation have also been associated with conduction abnormalities. In all cases, these individuals are at increased risk for episodic ventricular fibrillation, a particularly lethal arrhythmia. When ventricular fibrillation occurs, there is no cardiac output, and permanent brain damage and death ensue unless the arrhythmia is controlled. As noted earlier, *SCN5A* mutations can cause arrhythmia susceptibility in certain familial forms of long QT syndrome (see Table 61-3). Recent molecular genetic studies have demonstrated that *SCN5A* mutations can also cause familial ventricular fibrillation.[35] Thus, *SCN5A* mutations can cause several different forms of arrhythmia susceptibility.

The genetic basis for a third familial cardiac arrhythmia, catecholaminergic ventricular tachycardia, has recently become apparent. This disorder is characterized by syncope and sudden death in otherwise healthy young individuals due to episodic bidirectional ventricular tachycardia. Recent studies demonstrate that this disorder is caused by mutations in *RyR2*, the ryanodine receptor gene.[37]

In summary, the genetic basis of arrhythmia susceptibility has begun to emerge. Seven arrhythmia genes have been identified to date: *SCN5A*, *KVLQT1*, *minK*, *HERG*, *MiRP1*, *RyR2*, and *Kir2.1*. *SCNA5A* mutations can cause both long QT syndrome and familial ventricular fibrillation. *KVLQT1*, *minK*, *HERG* and *MIRP1* mutations have been implicated in long QT syndrome. *RyR2* mutations cause catecholaminergic ventricular tachycardia. *Kir2.1* mutations cause Andersen's syndrome. In general, arrhythmia susceptibility is more severe in homozygotes than in heterozygotes. Although some familial forms of arrhythmia susceptibility are associated with additional obvious phenotypic abnormalities (e.g. congenital neural deafness in Jervell and Lange-Nielsen syndrome), most of these individuals appear grossly normal and go undetected until their first arrhythmia strikes.

ION CHANNELS AND THE CARDIAC ACTION POTENTIAL

Like other excitable cells, including neurons, skeletal muscle, and smooth muscle, cardiac myocyte excitability results from action potentials. The cardiac myocyte action potential, however, is distinctive in its duration, which is much longer, at about 300 milliseconds. By contrast, the action potentials of neurons and skeletal muscle last a few milliseconds. The cardiac action potential consists of five phases, numbered 0 to 4. Phase 0 represents depolarization of the myocyte. This phase is initiated by the rapid opening (activation) of voltage-gated sodium channels. Depolarization of all ventricular myocytes is measurable as the QRS complex on the surface ECG. Phase 1 of the cardiac action potential occurs immediately after the peak of depolarization and is recognized as a partial repolarization of the membrane. This small repolarizing effect is due to the closure (inactivation) of cardiac sodium channels and activation of transient outward potassium current. Phase 2 of the action potential is the plateau phase. The relatively long duration of this phase is unique to ventricular and Purkinje fiber myocytes. The plateau is generated primarily by slowly decreasing inward calcium currents through L-type calcium channels and gradually increasing outward current through several types of potassium channels. The total amount of current during the plateau phase of the cardiac action potential is small. As a consequence, relatively small changes in ion current during this phase can have a major impact on action potential duration. At this point in the cardiac cycle, the ECG has returned to baseline. Phase 3 represents myocellular repolarization, an effect mediated by outward potassium currents. Physiologic and pharmacologic studies have defined two main repolarizing potassium currents, I_{Kr} and I_{Ks}, that sum to terminate the plateau phase and initiate final repolarization.[43] Other currents such as the plateau delayed rectifier K^+ current (I_{Kp}) and the inward rectifier K^+ current (I_{K1}) also contribute to repolarization. I_{Kr} is the rapidly activating delayed rectifier potassium current that is specifically blocked by methanesulfonanilide drugs. When I_{Kr} current is blocked by these drugs, I_{Ks}, the slowly activating delayed rectifier potassium current, remains. The repolarization phase correlates with the T wave on surface ECG. Phase 4 is the final phase of the action potential and signals a return of membrane potential to its baseline near –85 mV. This phase represents ventricular relaxation or diastole and is indicated on the ECG as a return to baseline. Thus, the coordinated opening and closing of ion channels mediates the cardiac action potential. Duration of the QT interval on surface ECG is related to the length of ventricular action potentials.

SODIUM CHANNEL DYSFUNCTION CAN CAUSE DIFFERENT TYPES OF ARRHYTHMIA

Investigators had previously demonstrated that *SCNA5A* encodes the α subunits of sodium channels that are responsible for initiating cardiac action potentials.[44] This gene is located on chromosome 3p21–p24 and encodes a protein with a predicted topology of four major domains, DI through DIV. Each of these domains is believed to have a structure similar to a voltage-gated potassium channel with six membrane spanning domains (S1 to S6) and pore domains located between S5 and S6. The α subunit can form functional channels, but accessory β subunits have also been identified that alter some biophysical properties of the channel. Mutational analyses have revealed 14 distinct mutations of *SCNA5A* associated with long QT syndrome.[45]

Based on the location of these mutations and the physiology of the disease, we hypothesized that gain-of-function mutations in *SCNA5A* would cause long QT syndrome. Normally, cardiac sodium channels open briefly in response to membrane depolarization. The channel is then inactivated and remains closed for the remainder of the action potential. Sodium channel inactivation is mediated by an intracellular domain located between DIII and DIV. This domain is referred to as the *inactivation gate* and is thought to physically block the inner mouth of the channel pore. Several *SCNA5A* mutations associated with long QT syndrome were identified in this region. Physiologic characterization of one of these mutants (Δ KPQ) led to the discovery that the mutations destabilized the inactivation gate.[46] Activation of these mutant sodium channels is normal, and the rate of inactivation appears slightly faster than normal, but mutant channels can also reopen during the plateau phase of the action potential. The net effect is a small, maintained depolarizing current that is modeled to be present during the plateau phase of the action potential.[46,47] This lengthens action potential duration. Other long QT syndrome–associated mutations of *SCNA5A* had slightly different effects on mutant channels at the single channel level, but all led to maintained depolarizing currents and action potential prolongation, setting up a substrate for arrhythmia.

SCNA5A mutations also cause familial ventricular fibrillation (see Table 61-3). In some cases, these mutations are clearly loss of function. For example, a nonsense mutation of *SCNA5A* has been associated with ventricular fibrillation in an otherwise healthy individual who has no obvious electrocardiographic abnormalities.[35] Other mutations that have been associated with this disorder are less clear-cut in terms of their physiologic consequences. It is also not yet clear exactly how reduction in the total number of functional sodium channels and expression of a heterogeneous population of sodium channels lead to arrhythmia. Clues may come from pharmacologic studies, which show that inhibition of sodium channel current can cause heterogeneous action potentials in the right ventricular epicardium, leading to marked dispersion of repolarization and refractoriness.[48] This creates a substrate for the development of reentrant arrhythmias. Some familial ventricular fibrillation mutations of *SCNA5A* may cause an abnormality of conduction, and in some cases, baseline ECGs in affected individuals show conduction abnormalities. In summary, both gain- and loss-of-function mutations of *SCNA5A* can cause arrhythmia susceptibility.

KVLQT1 AND *MinK* FORM CARDIAC I_{KS} POTASSIUM CHANNELS

KVLQT1 is located on chromosome 11p5.5[49] in a region associated with Beckwith-Weidemann syndrome.[50] Northern analyses indicate that *KVLQT1* is expressed in the heart, placenta, lung, kidney,[31] inner ear and pancreas, with greatest expression in the pancreas.[51] *KVLQT1* and other genes in the region are imprinted, with paternal silencing in most tissues. However, *KVLQT1* is not imprinted in the heart.[51] Two homologs of *KVLQT1* (*KCNQ2, KCNQ3*) have been identified in the brain and associated with benign familial neonatal seizures, an inherited form of epilepsy.[52–54]

The cDNA-predicted amino acid sequence of *KVLQT1* suggests that this gene encodes voltage-gated potassium channel α subunits. It has six putative membrane-spanning domains, S1 to S6, including a voltage sensor (S4) and a potassium channel pore signature sequence between S5 and S6. The intracellular N-terminal segment of *KVLQT1* is short. Mutational analyses have revealed 85 mutations of *KVLQT1* coding sequences, representing about 40% of known arrhythmia-associated mutations discovered to date. Most of these mutations are missense mutations located in membrane spanning regions as well as the pore region.

Heterologous expression of *KVLQT1* in mammalian cells and *Xenopus* oocytes revealed that this gene does encode α subunits that form voltage-gated potassium channels.[55,56] However, the biophysical properties of the induced current were unlike any potassium current identified in cardiac myocytes. This observation led to the hypothesis that *KVLQT1* subunits might assemble with subunits encoded by another gene to form a cardiac potassium channel.

MinK, which is located on chromosome 21, received this name because it was thought to encode the minimal potassium channel subunit. Only 130 amino acids long, this predicted amino acid sequence has room for one putative membrane-spanning domain. It contains no potassium channel pore signature sequence and no putative voltage-sensing domain. Although it is not a common cause of arrhythmia susceptibility, mutations in this gene have been associated with long QT syndrome and homozygous mutations cause Jervell and Lange-Nielson syndrome.[34,45,57] Ten arrhythmia-associated mutations of *minK* have been identified. This represents about 5% of long QT syndrome mutations identified to date.

MinK was initially cloned by functional expression in *Xenopus* oocytes.[58] The biophysical properties of the current elicited by expression of *minK* was similar to cardiac I_{Ks}, one of the main currents responsible for termination of the cardiac action potential. Thus, investigators concluded that *minK* encoded subunits that formed cardiac I_{Ks} channels. However, there were several problems with this hypothesis. First, as noted earlier, the structure of *minK* was unusual. The typical voltage-gated potassium channel has six membrane-spanning domains, and four subunits are required for assembly and formation of functional channels. Because *minK* was small and only had one putative membrane-spanning domain, investigators hypothesized many subunits might assemble to form functional channels. Some experiments, however, suggest that only two units were required for expression.[59,60] Second, physiologic studies indicated that expression of *minK* in mammalian cells failed to induce a current. Finally, expression of increasing amounts of *minK* in *Xenopus* oocytes did not lead to increasing current, indicating saturability.

It is now clear that *minK* β subunits assemble with *KVLQT1* α subunits to form cardiac I_{Ks} channels.[55,56] Heterologous expression of *minK* alone in mammalian cells produced no current. By contrast, heterologous expression of *KVLQT1* and *minK* together led to a large potassium current with the biophysical properties of cardiac I_{Ks}. Although the stoichiometry of coassembly is not yet known, it is likely that four *KVLQT1* α subunits assemble with four *minK* β subunits to form these channels.

How is it that *minK* alone can be functionally expressed in *Xenopus* oocytes? The explanation is that a homolog of *KVLQT1*, *XKVLQT1*, is constitutively expressed in *Xenopus* oocytes, but at a relatively low level.[56] This homolog can interact with *minK*, forming an I_{Ks}-like channel.

At least two molecular mechanisms account for reduced *KVLQT1* function in the long QT syndrome.[61,62] In the first, disease-associated intragenic deletions of one *KVLQT1* allele result in syntheses of abnormal subunits that do not assemble with normal subunits. As a result, only normal subunits form the functional tetrameric channels. This loss-of-function mechanism results in a 50% reduction in the number of functional channels. In the second mechanism, missense mutations result in synthesis of *KVLQT1* subunits with subtle structural abnormalities. Many of these subunits can assemble with normal subunits, forming heterotetramers with varying stoichiometry. Channels formed from the coassembly of normal and mutant subunits have reduced or no function. The net effect is a greater than 50% reduction in channel function, a dominant-negative effect. The severity of the dominant-negative effect varies considerably depending on the site and type of mutation. In some cases, the dominant-negative effect is relatively small, whereas in others, the effect is complete, leading to marked reduction of I_{Ks} even in heterozygotes. Missense mutations in the pore sequences seem to be particularly potent. The severity of the dominant-negative effect likely has an effect on the severity of arrhythmia susceptibility in individuals. However, there are many factors that affect arrhythmia susceptibility, and extensive phenotypic variability can be seen between family members carrying the same primary genetic mutations.

KVLQT1 and *minK* are both expressed in the inner ear. Here, the channel functions to produce a potassium-rich fluid known as *endolymph* that bathes the organ of Corti, the cochlear organ responsible for hearing. Individuals with Jervell and Lange-Nielsen syndrome have homozygous mutations of *KVLQT1* or *minK*, and therefore have no functional I_{Ks} channels. As noted earlier, these individuals have severe arrhythmia susceptibility and congenital neural deafness. The mechanism of deafness in these individuals is that the lack of I_{Ks} leads to inadequate endolymph production and deterioration of the organ of Corti.[63] Deafness can also result from mutations in *KCNQ4*, a gene that encodes a homolog of *KVLQT1* that is highly expressed within sensory outer hair cells of the inner ear.[64]

HERG ENCODES CARDIAC I_{KR} POTASSIUM CHANNELS

HERG, located on chromosome 7q35–q36, is expressed primarily in the heart.[28] *HERG* was originally identified from a human hippocampal cDNA library[65] and is also expressed in neural crest–derived neurons and microglia. Ninety-four distinct mutations of *HERG* have been identified.[45] These represent 45% of the total number of long QT syndrome mutations found to date.

Based on its predicted amino acid sequence, *HERG* was thought to encode a typical voltage-gated potassium channel α subunit with six membrane-spanning domains (S1 to S6), a voltage sensor (S4), and a K^+ selective pore between S5 and S6. *HERG* has a large intracellular C-terminal region containing a cyclic nucleotide–binding domain. *HERG* also has a large N-terminal domain, the first 135 amino acids of which are called the *eag domain* because it is highly conserved with comparable domains in related channels. The structure of the N-terminal domain has been solved and has structural similarity to PAS domains.[66] Proteins with

PAS domains are frequently involved in signal transduction. Analysis of long QT syndrome–associated missense mutations located in the eag domain of *HERG* revealed that the PAS domain is important in mediating the slow rate of channel deactivation.[67]

Expression of *HERG* in heterologous systems led to the discovery that this gene encodes alpha subunits that form cardiac I_{Kr} potassium channels, the second of the two channels primarily responsible for termination of the plateau phase of the action potential.[68,69] One of the unusual biophysical properties of I_{Kr} channels that was reproduced by *HERG* in *Xenopus* oocytes is the bell-shaped current–voltage relationship, a rectification caused by C-type inactivation.[70] This property accounts for the relative importance of I_{Kr} during phase 3 of the cardiac action potential. During repolarization of the action potential *HERG* channels rapidly recover from inactivation into the open state. This results in an increase in the magnitude of I_{Kr} during the first half of phase 3 repolarization despite a decrease in the electrochemical driving force for outward flux of K^+.[71]

Although many of the biophysical properties of *HERG* current in heterologous systems were nearly identical to cardiac I_{Kr}, two properties were out of line.[36,68] First, although deactivation of cardiac I_{Kr} was relatively slow, deactivation of *HERG* channels was much slower. Second, the kinetics and voltage-dependence of I_{Kr} block by methanesulfonanilide drugs were different than those of *HERG* channels. This problem led to the hypothesis that *HERG*, like *KVLQT1*, might assemble with an unknown β subunit to form cardiac I_{Kr} channels.

MiRP1, or *minK*-related protein 1, is located on chromosome 21, just 70 kb from *minK*.[36] The two genes have significant homology at the DNA and amino acid level and likely resulted from a recent duplication. Missense mutations of *MiRP1* have been associated with long QT syndrome, indicating that it is an arrhythmia-susceptibility gene. When *MiRP1* was expressed with *HERG* in heterologous systems, the biophysical and pharmacologic properties of the resultant current were nearly identical to I_{Kr} in cardiac myocytes.[36] Thus, *HERG* α subunits assemble with *MiRP1* β subunits to form cardiac I_{Kr} channels.

Many *HERG* mutations cluster around the membrane-spanning domains and the pore region. Some of these mutations, such as early nonsense mutations, have a pure loss-of-function effect. Often, the encoded mutant proteins misfold and are rapidly degraded,[72] leading to a dominant-negative effect or haploinsufficiency. However, many long QT syndrome–associated mutations in *HERG* are missense mutations. Because functional I_{Kr} channels are composed of heteromultimers with several *HERG* subunits, it is possible that many of these mutations have a dominant-negative effect on channel function. Heterologous expression studies indicate that this is a common effect and that different mutations lead to a spectrum of dominant-negative suppression of channel function.[27,73,74]

RyR2 ENCODES THE CALCIUM RELEASE CHANNEL

RyR2 encodes the ryanodine receptor, a calcium-induced calcium release channel located in cardiac sarcoplasmic reticulum. *RyR2* channels are activated by Ca^{2+} that transiently enters the cell through plasma membrane–bound L-type calcium channels during depolarization of the cardiac myocyte. This Ca^{2+} triggers the release of Ca^{2+} stored in the sarcoplasmic reticulum through *RyR2* channels, which in turn initiates activation of the contractile apparatus. The four mutations identified in *RyR2* to date are missense mutations. The functional consequences of these mutations are not yet known. A likely possibility, however, is episodic, stress-induced Ca^{2+} overload in cardiac myocytes, leading to a substrate for arrhythmia.

In summary, all known arrhythmia susceptibility genes encode cardiac ion channels. *SCNA5A* encodes sodium channels that are responsible for initiating cardiac action potentials. *HERG* encodes α subunits that assemble with *MIRP1* β subunits to form cardiac I_{Kr} potassium channels, whereas *KVLQT1* assembles with *minK* to form cardiac I_{Ks} potassium channels. I_{Kr} and I_{Ks} are responsible for termination of the plateau phase and contribute to final repolarization of the cardiac action potential. *RyR2* encodes the ryanodine receptor/calcium release channel crucial for excitation–contraction coupling. Mutations of *SCNA5A* associated with long QT syndrome destabilize the channel inactivation gate, resulting in repetitive reopening of mutant channels and abnormal depolarizing sodium current during the plateau phase of the action potential. Thus, gain-of-function mutations of the cardiac sodium channel cause long QT syndrome. By contrast, loss-of-function mutations of the cardiac sodium channel cause idiopathic ventricular fibrillation with or without baseline conduction abnormalities. Mutations of *KVLQT1*, *HERG*, *minK*, and *MiRP1* cause a loss of function, often with a dominant-negative effect that leads to a reduction in repolarizing current. *RyR2* mutations probably lead to abnormal intracellular calcium metabolism. Taken together, these studies demonstrate that mutations of cardiac ion channels cause arrhythmia susceptibility through multiple molecular mechanisms.

REENTRY, THE MECHANISM OF ARRHYTHMIA

Together with previous physiologic studies, recent genetic advances provide a picture of cardiac arrhythmias at the molecular, cellular, and organ levels. Gain-of-function mutations of cardiac sodium channels and loss-of-function mutations of potassium channels delay myocyte repolarization. Loss-of-function mutations of sodium channels cause conduction abnormalities. Calcium release channel dysfunction probably causes calcium overload. These channels are expressed at varying levels in different regions of the heart, so the effect of channel dysfunction has regional variability. Regional abnormalities of cardiac repolarization or conduction provide a substrate for arrhythmia. For example, during a prolonged action potential, myocytes are relatively refractory to electrical excitation by neighboring myocytes. Dispersion of refractoriness can lead to unidirectional block of a wave of electrical excitation. Thus, pockets of cells that are temporarily unable to conduct the normal flow of electrical activity in the heart create a substrate for arrhythmia.

Although the substrate of unidirectional block can increase the risk for arrhythmia, it is not sufficient; a triggering mechanism is still required. The trigger for arrhythmia in the long QT syndrome is believed to be spontaneous secondary depolarizations during the plateau phase of action potentials. These secondary depolarizations are mediated by depolarizing inward calcium currents through L-type calcium channels. This cellular mechanism predicts that the autonomic nervous system can have a significant impact on arrhythmia susceptibility. Heightened sympathetic tone can substantially increase spontaneous inward current through L-type calcium channels, increasing the likelihood that the spontaneous repolarization will trigger an arrhythmia. Once triggered, the arrhythmia is maintained by a regenerative circuit of electrical activity around relatively inexcitable tissue, a phenomenon known as *reentry*. The development of multiple reentrant circuits within the heart causes ventricular fibrillation, the arrhythmia of sudden death.

ION CHANNEL DYSFUNCTION UNDERLIES INHERITED AND ACQUIRED ARRHYTHMIAS

Abnormal cardiac repolarization, aberrant conduction, and arrhythmia susceptibility are most commonly acquired and not primarily genetic. Common acquired causes of arrhythmia include cardiac ischemia resulting from the sudden disruption of blood flow to a region of the heart, structural heart diseases like cardiomyopathy, developmental abnormalities of the heart such as arrhythmogenic right ventricular dysplasia, metabolic abnormalities like abnormal serum potassium, calcium or magnesium levels, and medications.

A common cause of acquired long QT syndrome is a side effect of numerous common medications of diverse therapeutic and structural classes. Examples of drugs associated with long QT syndrome include terfenadine, cisapride, erythromycin, amiodarone, quinidine, phenothiazines, tricyclic antidepressants, and certain diuretics (the latter mediated through drug-induced hypokalemia). Most of these medications block *HERG* channels, leading to reduced repolarizing potassium current and delayed myocellular repolarization. These findings show, therefore, that cardiac ion channel dysfunction underlies both inherited and acquired arrhythmias.

The problem of medication-induced long QT syndrome is a significant issue to the pharmaceutical industry and the Food and Drug Administration. Why are *HERG* channels so susceptible to nonspecific block by such a wide variety of medications, and why isn't acquired long QT syndrome commonly caused by block of potassium channels other than *HERG* that contribute to cardiac repolarization? The answer to these questions is just beginning to unfold through structural studies of *HERG* channels expressed in heterologous systems.[75,76] There are at least two important structural features that account for the unusual susceptibility of *HERG* channels to block by diverse drugs. First, the inner cavity of the *HERG* channel appears to be much larger than any other voltage-gated K^+ channel. Almost all voltage-gated K^+ channel α subunits, except *HERG*, have two proline residues in the S6 domains that line the inner cavity of the channel. These prolines cause a kink in the S6 and apparently reduce the volume of the inner cavity.[77] The large inner cavity of *HERG* channels can accommodate and trap large drugs that other K^+ channels cannot trap.[78] Second, the S6 domains of *HERG* channels, but not other voltage-gated K^+ channels, have two aromatic residues that face into the inner cavity that bind large aromatic drugs by a π-stacking interaction.[76] The two aromatic residues located in each subunit (Tyr652, Phe656) provide a total of 8 residues that can form a variable receptor site that can accommodate drugs from diverse therapeutic and structural classes. In addition, the binding affinity of drugs is enhanced by inactivation of the *HERG* channel.[79] The net effect of the structural peculiarities of *HERG* channels is heightened sensitivity of I_{Kr} to structurally diverse drugs. Continued structural analysis of *HERG* channels, coupled with structure–activity relationship analysis of medications, will help improve our ability to predict drugs that are likely to cause a significant risk for cardiac arrhythmia.

Genetic predisposition may play an important role in drug-induced long QT syndrome. For example, less than 5% of patients receiving a drug like quinidine have arrhythmia as a side effect, irrespective of dose and other risk factors such as hypokalemia. Recent studies indicate that drug-induced arrhythmia can be associated with sporadic mutations in *MiRP1*.[36] It is likely that mutations or polymorphisms in all the genes associated with the inherited forms of long QT syndrome will eventually be shown to increase the risk for the acquired form of this disease.

EPISODIC DISORDERS OF EXCITABLE CELLS

Studies of inherited and acquired arrhythmias have led us to hypothesize a multihit mechanism for this disease. It is clear that at least three things have to go wrong simultaneously for a life-threatening arrhythmia to occur. For example, most individuals carrying one mutant allele of an arrhythmia susceptibility gene have few, if any arrhythmias. By contrast, individuals carrying two mutant alleles (e.g., those with Jervell and Lange-Nielson syndrome) have many arrhythmias and usually die during childhood unless effective treatment is implemented. Nevertheless, these individuals who chronically carry two hits for arrhythmia susceptibility live into early childhood even if untreated. Thus, an additional event, such as the introduction of a medication, hypokalemia, or a sinus pause, is required for an arrhythmia. It is clear, however, that one need not invoke a genetic mechanism of arrhythmia. We know, for example, that arrhythmia can be induced in virtually anyone with the right combination of drug, hypokalemia, and a long sinus pause.

PREDICTION, PREVENTION, AND TREATMENT OF CARDIAC ARRHYTHMIAS

Despite recent advances, the fields of arrhythmia genetics, physiology, and therapy are still immature. Major problems that appear most prominent include the identification of all arrhythmia-susceptibility genes, the identification of common genetic variants that contribute to arrhythmia susceptibility in the general population and the implementation of reliable, cost-effective genetic testing. Genomics and the human genome project have already had a major impact on this field, and that influence will continue to grow in the near future. Early genetic studies involved cumbersome methods of positional cloning because relatively little of the human genome was mapped, genetically or physically, and few human genes were defined. Technology was also cumbersome a decade ago. The early genetics linkage studies, for example, required the use of restriction fragment-length polymorphisms (RFLPs) and Southern analysis. The situation is completely different today, and in the very near future, genomics and the human genome project will empower these fields to an even greater extent. Genetic maps will be at the limits of resolution, all human genes will be defined and available in online databases, and genetic technologies, particularly DNA sequence analysis, will be robust, reliable, and inexpensive. DNA sequence analysis, in particular, will greatly facilitate the implementation of effective genetic testing for large populations using existing information regarding arrhythmia susceptibility genes.

Although prospects for future research are promising, at least one significant hurdle remains—ascertainment and phenotypic characterization of individuals with arrhythmia susceptibility and appropriate controls. The identification of novel arrhythmia genes and common arrhythmia susceptibility variants will involve genetic epidemiology—the genotypic characterization of large numbers of carefully phenotyped individuals. For the most part, the process of ascertaining and phenotypically characterizing individuals has been slow to change, involving a great deal of one-on-one effort in a process that is not easily scalable. Even here, however, new technology holds the promise for significant improvement. The Internet revolution has connected populations of individuals separated by large distances to instantaneously and effortlessly meet and communicate about many subjects, including disease. Many for-profit and not-for-profit organizations have created websites aimed at unifying, organizing, empowering, and informing individuals with virtually every imaginable health concern. By creating and working with these websites, investigators may accelerate the rate-limiting step of the human molecular genetic process.

Functional genomics, thus far largely limited to expression and protein–protein interaction studies, will also have an impact on this field. It is already clear that by examining the expression of arrhythmia genes in tissues other than the heart, one can hypothesize the existence of pathology in other tissues that were not apparent from previous clinical studies. The clinical world tends to focus on the most severe, life-threatening, and obvious phenotypic features of the disorder. It is hard to ignore congenital deafness and sudden arrhythmic death. However, many of these genes are expressed in other tissues, and evidence of pathology in these tissues is beginning to emerge. *KVLQT1*, for example, is expressed in the pancreas, and we may discover that mutations in this gene cause a subtle risk factor for pancreatitis.

Because most ion channels are heteromultimers and may be modulated by interaction with signaling molecules, databases of protein–protein interactions will also be valuable. It is likely, however, that each interaction will require validation. We already know, for example, that *minK* can interact with *KVLQT1* and *HERG* when overexpressed in heterologous systems.[80] It is not clear, however, that the interaction of *minK* with *HERG* has any physiologic relevance.[36] Nevertheless, broad functional databases will have great value, at least as a starting point.

Recent molecular and cellular studies have important implications for the prevention and treatment of arrhythmias. Identification and characterization of arrhythmia susceptibility genes provide the foundation for prevention through genetic testing. The observation that *HERG* channel function is paradoxically sensitive to extracellular potassium concentrations highlights the importance of maintaining normal electrolyte levels and provides a new strategy for treatment.[81] The most important therapeutic consequence of this work, however, is the message it delivers to physicians and to the pharmaceutical industry: the observations that gain- and loss-of-function mutations of the cardiac sodium channel both cause arrhythmia susceptibility indicate that drugs that modulate cardiac ion channel function may reduce the risk for one type of arrhythmia but increase the risk of another. Thus, chronic use of cardiac ion channel blockers can be dangerous. The future of arrhythmia therapy may be devices that measure cardiac conduction and repolarization, deliver appropriate antiarrhythmic drugs when needed, and provide a safety net in the form of automatic internal defibrillation.[82]

REFERENCES

1. Roden DM, Balser JR, George AL, Jr., et al. Cardiac ion channels. Annu Rev Physiol 64:431, 2002.
2. Ackerman M, Clapham D. Normal cardiac electrophysiology. In Chien KR, Breslow JL, Leiden JM, Rosenberg RD, Seidman CE, Braunwald E (eds). The Molecular Basis of Heart Disease: Understanding the Action Potential in the Human Heart. Philadelphia: WB Saunders, 1998:281.
3. Hille B. Ion Channels of Excitable Membranes, 3rd ed. Sunderland, MA: Sinauer Associates, 2001.
4. Brown HF, DiFrancesco D, Noble SJ. How does adrenaline accelerate the heart? Nature 280:235, 1979.
5. Irisawa H, Brown HF, Giles W. Cardiac pacemaking in the sinoatrial node. Physiol Rev 73:197, 1993.
6. Carmeliet E. Cardiac ionic currents and acute ischemia: From channels to arrhythmias. Physiol Rev 79:917, 1999
7. Fozzard HA, Hanck DA. Structure and function of voltage-dependent sodium channels: Comparison of brain II and cardiac isoforms. Physiol Rev 76: 887, 1996.
8. Oudit GY, Kassiri Z, Sah R, et al. The molecular physiology of the cardiac transient outward potassium current [I(to) in normal and diseased myocardium. J Mol Cell Cardiol 33:851, 2001.
9. Liu DW, Antzelevitch C. Characteristics of the delayed rectifier current (I_{Kr} and I_{Ks}) in canine ventricular epicardial, midmyocardial, and endocardial myocytes: A weaker I_{Ks} contributes to the longer action potential of the M cell. Circ Res 76:351, 1995.
10. Volk T, Nguyen TH, Schultz JH, et al. Relationship between transient outward K+ current and Ca2+ influx in rat cardiac myocytes of endo- and epicardial origin. J Physiol 519(Pt 3): 841, 1999.
11. Balke CW, Gold MR. Calcium channels in the heart: an overview. Heart Dis Stroke 1:398, 1992.
12. Anderson ME. Ca2+-dependent regulation of cardiac L-type Ca2+ channels: Is a unifying mechanism at hand? J Mol Cell Cardiol 33:639, 2001.
13. Kang TM, Hilgemann DW. Multiple transport modes of the cardiac Na+/Ca2+ exchanger. Nature 427:544, 2004.
14. Bers DM. Calcium and cardiac rhythms: physiological and pathophysiological. Circ Res 90:14, 2002.
15. Wang Z, Fermini B, Nattel S. Sustained depolarization-induced outward current in human atrial myocytes: Evidence for a novel delayed rectifier K^+ current similar to Kv1.5 cloned channel currents. Circ Res 73:1061, 1993.
16. Tseng GN. I(Kr): The HERG channel. J Mol Cell Cardiol 33:835, 2001.
17. Kannel W, Cupples A, D'Agostino R. Sudden death risk in overt coronary heart diseases: The Framingham study. Am Heart J 113:799, 1987.
18. Willich S, Levy D, Rocco M, et al. Circadian variation in the incidence of sudden cardiac death in the Framingham heart study population. Am J Cardiol 60:801, 1987.
19. Vincent GM, Timothy K, Leppert M, et al. The spectrum of symptoms and QT intervals in carriers of the gene for the long QT syndrome. N Engl J Med 327:846, 1992.
20. Schwartz P, Moss A, Vincent G, et al. Diagnostic criteria for the long QT syndrome. Circulation 88:782, 1993.
21. Lazzara R. Twisting of the points. J Am Coll Cardiol 29:843, 1997.
22. Marks M, Whisler S, Clericuzio C, et al. A new form of long QT syndrome associated with syndactyly. J Am Coll Cardiol 25:59, 1995.
23. Abildskov J. The sympathetic imbalance hypothesis of QT interval prolongation. J Cardiovasc Electrophysiol 2:355, 1991.
24. Jervell A, Lange-Nielsen F. Congenital deaf-mutism, functional heart disease with prolongation of the QT interval, and sudden death. Am Heart J 54:59, 1957.
25. Romano C, Gemme G, Pongiglione R. Artimie cardiach rare dell'eta pediatrica. II. Accessi sincopali per fibrillazione ventricolare parossitica. Clin Pediatr 45:656, 1963.
26. Ward O. A new familial cardiac syndrome in children. J Ir Med Assoc 54:103, 1964.
27. Roden DM, Lazzara R, Rosen M, et al. Multiple mechanisms in the long-QT syndrome. Current knowledge, gaps, and future directions. The SADS Foundation Task Force on LQTS. Circulation 94, 1996.
28. Curran ME, Splawski I, Timothy KW, et al. A molecular basis for cardiac arrhythmia: HERG mutations cause long QT syndrome. Cell 80:795, 1995.
29. Wang Q, Shen J, Splawski I, et al. SCN5A mutations associated with an inherited cardiac arrhythmia, long QT syndrome. Cell 80:805, 1995.
30. Wang W, Shen J, Li Z, et al. Cardiac sodium channel mutations in patients with long QT syndrome, an inherited cardiac arrhythmia. Hum Mol Genet 4:1603, 1995.
31. Wang Q, Curran ME, Splawski I, et al. Positional cloning of a novel potassium channel gene: KVLQT1 mutations cause cardiac arrhythmias. Nat Genet 12:17, 1996.
32. Splawski I, Timothy KW, Vincent GM, et al. Molecular basis of the long-QT syndrome associated with deafness. N Engl J Med 336:1562, 1997.
33. Neyroud N, Tesson F, Denjoy I, et al. A novel mutation in the potassium channel gene KVLQT1 causes the Jervell

and Lange-Nielsen cardioauditory syndrome. Nat Genet 15: 186, 1997.
34. Splawski I, Tristani-Firouzi M, Lehmann MH, et al. Mutations in the hminK gene cause long QT syndrome and suppress IKs function. Nat Genet 17:338, 1997.
35. Chen Q, Kirsch GE, Zhang D, et al. Genetic basis and molecular mechanism for idiopathic ventricular fibrillation. Nature 392:293, 1998.
36. Abbott GW, Sesti F, Splawski I, et al. MiRP1 forms I_{Kr} potassium channels with HERG and is associated with cardiac arrhythmia. Cell 97:175, 1999.
37. Priori SG, Napolitano C, Tiso N, et al. Mutations in the cardiac ryanodine receptor gene (hRyR2) underlie catecholamine polymorphic ventricular tachycardia. Circulation 102:r49, 2000.
38. Jiang C, Atkinson D, Towbin J, et al. Two long QT syndrome loci map to chromosome 3 and 7 with evidence for further heterogeneity. Nat Genet 8:141, 1994.
39. Duggal P, Vesely MR, Wattanasirichaigoon D, et al. Mutation of the gene for IsK associated with both Jervell and Lange-Nielsen and Romano-Ward forms of Long-QT syndrome. Circulation 97:142, 1998.
40. Hoorntje T, Alders M, van Tintelen P, et al. Homozygous premature truncation of the HERG protein: The human HERG knockout. Circulation 100:1264, 1999.
41. Martini B. Ventricular fibrillation without apparent heart disease: Description of six cases. Am Heart J 118:1203, 1989.
42. Brugada J, Brugada R, Brugada P. Right bundle branch block, ST segment elevation in leads V1-V3: A marker for sudden death in patients without demonstrable structural heart disease. Circulation 96:1151, 1997.
43. Sanguinetti MC, Jurkiewicz NK. Two components of cardiac delayed rectifier K^+ current: Differential sensitivity to block by class-III antiarrhythmic agents. J Gen Physiol 96: 195, 1990.
44. Gellens M, George A, Chen L, et al. Primary structure and functional expression of the human cardiac tetrodotoxin-insensitive voltage-dependent sodium channel. Proc Natl Acad Sci USA 89:554, 1992.
45. Splawski I, Shen J, Timothy KW, et al. Spectrum of mutations in long-QT syndrome genes. KVLQT1, HERG, SCN5A, KCNE1, and KCNE2. Circulation 102:1178, 2000.
46. Bennett PB, Yazawa K, Makita N, et al. Molecular mechanism for an inherited cardiac arrhythmia. Nature 376:683, 1995.
47. Dumaine R, Wang Q, Keating MT, et al. Multiple mechanisms of sodium channel-linked long QT syndrome. Circ Res 78:914, 1996.
48. Krishnan SC, Antzelevitch C. Sodium channel block produces opposite electrophysiological effects in canine ventricular epicardium and endocardium. Circ Res 69:277, 1991.
49. Keating M, Atkinson D, Dunn C, et al. Linkage of a cardiac arrhythmia, the long QT syndrome, and the Harvey ras-1 gene. Science 252:704, 1991.
50. Lee MP, Hu RJ, Johnson LA, Feinberg AP. Human KVLQT1 gene shows tissue-specific imprinting and encompasses Beckwith-Wiedemann syndrome chromosomal rearrangements. Nat Genet 15:181, 1997.
51. Yang WP, Levesgue PC, Little WA, et al. KvLQT1, a voltage-gated potassium channel responsible for human cardiac arrhythmias. Proc Natl Acad Sci USA 94:4017, 1997.
52. Charlier C, Singh NA, Ryan SG, et al. A pore mutation in a novel KQT-like potassium channel gene in an idiopathic epilepsy family. Nat Genet 18:53, 1998.
53. Singh NA, Charlier C, Stauffer D, et al. A novel potassium channel gene, KCNQ2, is mutated in an inherited epilepsy of newborns. Nat Genet 18:25, 1998.
54. Yang WP, Levesque PC, Little WA, et al. Functional expression of two KvLQT1-related potassium channels responsible for an inherited idiopathic epilepsy. J Biol Chem 273:19419, 1998.
55. Barhanin J, Lesage F, Guillemare E, et al. KVLQT1 and IsK (minK) proteins associate to form the IKs cardiac potassium current. Nature 384:78, 1996.
56. Sanguinetti MC, Curran ME, Zou A, et al. Coassembly of KVLQT1 and minK (IsK) proteins to form cardiac IKs potassium channel. Nature 384:80, 1996.
57. Schulze-Bahr E, Wang Q, Wedekind H, et al. KCNE1 mutations cause Jervell and Lange-Nielsen syndrome. Nat Genet 17:267, 1997.
58. Takumi T, Ohkubo H, Nakanishi S. Cloning of a membrane protein that induces a slow voltage-gated potassium current. Science 242:1042, 1988.
59. Wang K, Goldstein S. Subunit composition of MinK potassium channels. Neuron 14:1303, 1995.
60. Tai KK, Wang KW, Goldstein SAN. MinK potassium channels are heteromultimeric complexes. J Biol Chem 272:1654, 1997.
61. Wollnik B, Schroeder BC, Kubisch C, et al. Pathophysiological mechanisms of dominant and recessive KVLQT1 K^+ channel mutations found in inherited cardiac arrhythmias. Hum Mol Genet 6:1943, 1997.
62. Wang Z, Tristani-Firouzi M, Xu Q, et al. Functional effects of mutations in KvLQT1 that cause long QT syndrome. J Cardiovasc Electrophysiol 10:817, 1999.
63. Vetter DE, Mann JR, Wangemann P, et al. Inner ear defects induced by null mutation of the isk gene. Neuron 17: 1251, 1996.
64. Kubisch C, Schroeder BC, Friedrich T, et al. KCNQ4, a novel potassium channel expressed in sensory outer hair cells, is mutated in dominant deafness. Cell 96:437, 1999.
65. Warmke J, Ganetzky B. A family of potassium channel genes related to eag in Drosophila and mammals. Proc Natl Acad Sci USA 91:3438, 1994.
66. Morais J, Lee A, Cohen S, et al. Crystal structure and functional analysis of the HERG potassium channel N terminus: A eukaryotic PAS domain. Cell 5:649, 1998.
67. Chen J, Zou A, Splawski I, et al. Long QT syndrome-associated mutations in the Per-Arnt Sim (PAS) domain of HERG potassium channels accelerate channel deactivation. J Biol Chem 274:10113, 1999.
68. Sanguinetti MC, Jiang C, Curran ME, et al. A mechanistic link between an inherited and an acquired cardiac arrhythmia: HERG encodes the IKr potassium channel. Cell 81: 299, 1995.
69. Trudeau MC, Warmke JW, Ganetzky B, et al. HERG, a human inward rectifier in the voltage-gated potassium channel family. Science 269:92, 1995.

70. Smith PL, Baukrowitz T, Yellen G. The inward rectification mechanism of the HERG cardiac potassium channel. Nature 379:833, 1996.
71. Spector P. Fast inactivation causes rectification of the IKr channel. J Gen Physiol 107:611, 1996.
72. Zhou Z, Gong Q, Epstein ML, January CT. HERG channel dysfunction in human long QT syndrome. Intracellular transport and functional defects. J Biol Chem 273:21061, 1998.
73. Sanguinetti MC, Curran ME, Spector PS, et al. Spectrum of HERG K^+ channel dysfunction in an inherited cardiac arrhythmia. Proc Natl Acad Sci USA 93:2208, 1996.
74. Li X, Xu J, Li M. The human delta1261 mutation of the HERG potassium channel results in a truncated protein that contains a subunit interaction domain and decreases the channel expression. J Biol Chem 272:705, 1997.
75. Lees-Miller JP, Duan Y, Teng GQ, et al. Molecular determinant of high-affinity dofetilide binding to HERG1 expressed in Xenopus oocytes: Involvement of S6 sites. Mol Pharmacol 57:367, 2000.
76. Mitcheson JS, Chen J, Lin M, Culberson C, Sanguinetti MC. A structural basis for drug-induced long QT syndrome. Proc Natl Acad Sci USA 97:12329, 2000.
77. del Camino D, Holmgren M, Liu Y, Yellen G. Blocker protection in the pore of a voltage-gated K^+ channel and its structural implications. Nature 403:321, 2000.
78. Mitcheson JS, Chen J, Sanguinetti MC. Trapping of a methanesulfonanilide by closure of the HERG potassium channel activation gate. J Gen Physiol 115:229, 2000.
79. Ficker E. Molecular determinants of dofetilide block of HERG K+ channels. Circ Res 82:386, 1998.
80. McDonald T, Yu Z, Ming Z, et al. A minK-HERG complex regulates the cardiac potassium current I-Kr. Nature 388: 289, 1997.
81. Compton SJ, Lux RL, Ramsey MR, et al. Gene derived therapy in inherited long QT syndrome: Correction of abnormal repolarization by potassium. Circulation 94:1018, 1996.
82. Moss AJ. Update on MADIT: The Multicenter Automatic Defibrillator Implantation Trial. The long QT interval syndrome. Am J Cardiol 79:16, 1997.

Appendix

Principal Drugs Used in Pediatric Cardiology

Dose regimens are based on our clinical use and provide guidelines that do not substitute for a formulary. In some clinical circumstances, higher or lower doses than those listed may be warranted. Dosages here are given on the assumption that they are being used in isolation. Drug interactions are common, and for some drugs, serum levels should be checked. Please consult appropriate computerized programs before prescribing any medication.

Principal Drugs Used in Pediatric Cardiology

Drug	Route	Dosage
RESUSCITATION		
Adenosine	IV	mg/kg (up to 6 mg) rapid IV push mg/kg for second dose (max, 12 mg)
Amiodarone	IV	Refractory pulseless VT/VF: 5 mg/kg rapid IV/IO push Perfusing tachycardias: 5 mg/kg over 20–60 min
Atropine	IV	0.02 mg/kg Minimum dose, 0.1 mg. Max single dose for child, 0.5 mg, for adolescent = 1 mg. May double for second dose.
Calcium chloride (10% solution)	IV	20 mg/kg slow IV bolus, central line preferred. Max, 2000 mg.
Dobutamine	IV	2.5 – 20 μg/kg/min
Dopamine	IV	2.5 – 20 μg/kg/min
Epinephrine 1:10,000	IV	Bolus: 0.01 mg/kg (0.1 mL/kg) every 3–5 min during CPR for pulseless arrest. Infusion: Initial at 0.05–1 μg/kg/min, titrate to desired effect (0.1–1 μg/kg/min)
Glucose	IV	0.5–1 g/kg (max, 2–4 mL/kg of 25% solution)
Lidocaine	IV	1 mg/kg slowly, then 20–50 μg/kg/min infusion
Magnesium sulfate	IV	25–50 mg/kg over 10–20 min. Max dose, 2g.
Naloxone	IV	If ≤ 5 years old or ≤ 20 kg, 0.01–0.1 mg/kg. If > 5 years old or > 20 kg, 2 mg. Titrate to desired effect.
Prostaglandin E_1	IV	0.01–0.05 μg/kg/min. Titrate. Monitor for apnea, hypotension, hypoglycemia, hypocalcemia.
Sodium bicarbonate	IV	1 mEq/kg infused slowly and only if ventilation is adequate.

(Continued)

Principal Drugs Used in Pediatric Cardiology—cont'd

Drug	Route	Dosage
CARDIAC MEDICATIONS		
Vasopressor and Inotropic Agents		
Digoxin	PO	8 μg/kg/day, divided bid
Dopamine	IV	2.5–20 μg/kg/min
Dobutamine	IV	2.5–20 μg/kg/min
Epinephrine	IV	0.05–2.0 μg/kg/min
Isoproterenol	IV	0.01–0.5 μg/kg/min
Fenoldopam	IV	0.05–1.6 μg/kg/min
Milrinone	IV	50 μg/kg load over 30–60 min, then 0.25–0.75 μg/kg/min
Natriuretic peptide (Nesiritide)	IV	0.01–0.03 μg/kg/min
Norepinephrine	IV	0.05–0.5 μg/kg/min
Phenylephrine	IV	0.01–0.5 μg/kg/min
Tri-iodothyronine (T_3)	IV	0.05–0.10 μg/kg/hr
Vasopressin	IV	0.0003–0.002 units/kg/min
Vasodilators		
Hydralazine	IV	0.1–0.5 mg/kg/dose, given q4–6h (max, 3.5 mg/kg/day)
	PO	0.25–1mg/kg/dose, given tid–qid (max daily dose 7 mg/kg/day or 200 mg)
Nitroglycerin	IV	0.5–10.0 μg/kg/min
Nitroprusside	IV	0.5–5.0 μg/kg/min. Check cyanide and thiocyanate levels if dosage > 4 μg/kg/min, renal dysfunction, or if used for > 3 days
Diuretic Agents		
Acetazolamide	PO/IV	IV: 5–10 mg/kg/dose (max, 1000 mg) given q12
Bumetanide	PO, IM, or IV	Neonates: 0.01–0.05 mg/kg/dose (max, 1 mg) qd Infants/children: 0.02–0.1 mg/kg/dose, given qd or qod (max, 10 mg) Adults: 2 mg qd–bid (max, 10 mg/day)
Chlorothiazide	PO	<6 mo: 10–20 mg/kg/dose (max, 188 mg) q12h ≥6 mo:10 mg/kg/dose, given bid (max daily dose, 1000 mg)
	IV	5–10 mg/kg/dose q12 hr (max, 500 mg dose)
Furosemide	IV	Bolus: 1–2 mg/kg/dose given q6–24h Infusion: 0.1 mg/kg bolus, then 0.05–0.1 mg/kg/hr starting rate, may titrate to 0.3 mg/kg/hr
	PO	1–2 mg/kg/dose, given q6–24h (max, daily dose 320 mg)
Hydrochlorothiazide	PO	<6 mo: 1–3 mg/kg/day, divided bid >6 mo: 1–2 mg/kg/day, divided bid Adolescent: 25–100 mg/day, given qd
Metolazone	PO	0.1–0.2 mg/kg/dose given qd–bid (max, 10 mg/day)
Spironolactone	PO	1.5 mg/kg/dose (max, 100 mg) PO q12h
β Blockers		
Atenolol	PO	1–2 mg/kg/dose, given qd (max, 2 mg/kg in 24 hr)
Esmolol	IV	100–500 μg/kg bolus over 1 min, then 50–250 μg/kg/min
Labetalol	IV	0.2–2 mg/kg/dose (usual max 20 mg) q4–6h Infusion: 0.25 – 1 mg/kg/h (max, 3 mg/kg/h)
Nadolol	PO	0.5–1 mg/kg/dose given qd
Propranolol	PO	0.5–4 mg/kg/day, divided tid or qid
Angiotensin-Converting Enzyme (ACE) Inhibitors		
Captopril	PO	Newborns: 0.1 mg/kg/dose given tid Children: 0.3–0.5 mg/kg/dose (max 2 mg/kg/dose) given tid Adolescents: 25 mg/dose given tid
Enalapril	PO	0.1–0.6 mg/kg/day, divided qd to bid (max 40 mg/day)
Enalaprilat	IV	5–10 μg/kg/dose (max, 1250 mg) every 8 to 24 hr
Lisinopril	PO	0.1–0.5 mg/kg/dose (max 40 mg) given qd

Principal Drugs Used in Pediatric Cardiology—cont'd

Drug	Route	Dosage
Calcium Channel Blockers		
Amlodipine	PO	0.1 mg/kg/dose (max, 10 mg) given qd–bid
Nifedipine	PO	Short-acting: 0.25–0.5 mg/kg/dose (max, 10 mg/dose), given q4–6h Extended release: 0.5–3 mg/kg/day (max, 120 mg) given qd
Verapamil	IV	0.1 mg/kg/dose over 2 min, may repeat one time after 30 min
	PO	3–4 mg/kg/day (max, 8 mg/kg or 480 mg/day), divided tid
Antiarrhythmic Agents Not Listed Above		
Adenosine	IV	0.1 mg/kg (max, 6 mg) rapid push; if not effective, repeat 0.2 mg/kg (max, 12 mg) rapid push
Amiodarone	PO	Initial: 10–20 mg/kg/day, given qd or q12h for 7–10 days Maintenance: 5 mg/kg/day for 1 to 2 months, then wean to lowest effective dose (min, 2.5 mg/kg/day)
Flecainide	PO	2–6 mg/kg/day, divided q8–12 h
Mexiletine	PO	5–10 mg/kg/day, divided q8h
Procainamide	IV	Bolus: 5–15 mg/kg (max, 1000 mg) over 30 min Infusion: 20–80 μg/kg/min (adjust to procainamide levels 4–10 μg/mL, drawing 2 hr after each drip rate change)
Propafenone	PO	150–300 mg/m²/day, divided q8h
Sotalol	PO	80–200 mg/m²/day, divided q8h in younger children to q12h in school-age children and adolescents
Ductal Manipulation		
Indomethacin	IV	2–7 days old: 0.2 mg/kg IV every 12–24 hr × 3 doses Over 7 days old: 0.2 mg/kg IV followed by 0.25 mg/kg every 12–24 hr × 2 doses If the ductus arteriosus reopens, a second course of 1–3 doses may be given
Prostaglandin E_1	IV	0.01–0.05 μg/kg/min
Miscellaneous		
Atropine	IV, SC, PO	0.02 mg/kg/dose (max, 1 mg), given q 4–6 h
Calcium gluconate 10%	IV/PO	**For resuscitation:** Neonates and infants: 100 mg/kg (1 mL/kg) IV bolus Adults: 10 mL or IgM IV bolus **For uses other than resuscitation:** Neonates: 200–250 mg/kg/day as a continuous infusion or in 4 divided doses Infants and children: 200–1000 mg/kg/day as a continuous infusion or in 4 divided doses Adolescents: 2–15 g/24 hr as a continuous infusion or in divided doses
Immune globulin	IV	2g/kg over 8–12 hr (more slowly for patients in congestive heart failure)
Nitric oxide	Inhaled	Initial: 20–80 ppm Maintenance range: 5–40 ppm, following methemoglobin levels When weaning, watch for rebound pulmonary hypertension.
NONCARDIAC MEDICATIONS		
Coagulation		
Abciximab	IV	Bolus: 0.25 mg/kg Infusion: 0.125 μg/kg/min for 12 hr.
Aminocaproic acid	IV	100 mg/kg × 1, then 30 mg/kg/hr (max, 18g/m²/day or plasma level 130 μg/mL)
Aprotinin	IV	Test dose: 5000–10,000 units × 1 over 10 min Infusion: 30,000 units/kg × 1, then 10,000 units/kg/hr
Aspirin	PO	Antiplatelet dose: 3–5 mg/kg qd
Clopidogrel	PO	1 mg/kg/day (max, 75 mg) given qd
Dipyridamole	PO	2–6 mg/kg/day, divided tid
Heparin, unfractionated	IV	Load: 50 units/kg Infusion: 20 units/kg/hr Adjust dose to achieve desired therapeutic level, usually plasma heparin level = 0.35 – 0.7 in terms of anti–factor Xa activity or activated partial thromboplastin time (aPTT) of 60 to 85 sec.

(Continued)

Principal Drugs Used in Pediatric Cardiology—cont'd

Drug	Route	Dosage
Heparin, low-molecular- weight heparin (enoxaparin sodium)	SC	**Infants < 12 mo** Treatment: 3 mg/kg/day, divided q12h Prophylaxis: 1.5 mg/kg/day, divided q12h **Children and adolescents** Treatment: 2 mg/kg/day, divided q12h Prophylaxis: 1 mg/kg/day, divided q12h Adjust dose to achieve desired therapeutic level, usually antifactor Xa = 0.5 – 1.0 units/mL
Streptokinase	IV	Bolus: 1000–4000 units/kg over 30 min Infusion: 1000–1500 units/kg/hr
Tissue plasminogen activator	IV	Bolus: 1.25 mg/kg Infusion: 0.1–0.5 mg/kg/hr for 6 hr, then reassess
Tranexamic acid	IV	Load: 100 mg/kg Continuous infusion: 10 mg/kg/hr for up to 6 hr
Urokinase	IV	Bolus: 4400 units/kg over 10 min Infusion: 4400 units/kg/hr
Warfarin	PO	0.1 mg/kg/day, given qd (range 0.05–0.34 mg/kg/day; adjust dose to achieve desired INR)
Intubation		
Etomidate	IV	0.3 mg/kg/dose
Ketamine	IV	1.0–2 mg/kg/dose
	IM	3–5 mg/kg/dose
Propofol	IV	1–3 mg/kg/dose
Fentanyl	IV	10–15 mg/kg/dose
Anesthetic/Sedatives/Analgesics		
Chloral hydrate	PO/PR	Sedation: 15–25 mg/kg/dose up to 1 g, or 50 mg/kg/day divided bid Hypnotic: 50 mg/kg/dose (max, 1000 mg) given once Conscious sedation for nonpainful procedure: 50–80 mg/kg given once
Fentanyl	IV	Infusion: 1–10 mcg/kg/hr, titrate as necessary
Lorazepam	IV/PO	0.05–0.1 mg/kg/dose, given q4–8h
Methadone	PO	0.1 mg/kg/dose, given q4–6h
Midazolam	IV	0.05–0.1 mg/kg/dose, given q1–2h, or Infusion: 0.5–0.1mg/kg/hr, titrate as necessary
Morphine	IV	0.05–0.2 mg/kg/hr, titrate as necessary
	IM/SC	0.1 mg/kg/dose, given q3–4h

Subject Index

A
Abciximab, 909
Abdominal pain, rheumatic fever with, 392
Ablation, 514–518
mapping for, 515–516
outcomes from, 517
positions for, 515
radiofrequency, 515–517
techniques for, 515–517
Abnormal automaticity, 478
Absent pulmonary valve, 561–567, 569, 572–573, 575–576
cardiac catheterization for, 568
chest X-ray for, 565
clinical manifestations of, 564
course for, 575–576
echocardiogram of, 566–567
management of, 572–573
MRI of, 569
pathology of, 561–562
physiology of, 563
Accessory endocardial cushion tissue, 590
ACEI. *See* Angiotensin-converting enzyme inhibitors
Acetazolamide, 908
Acid-based management, 104–105
Acidosis, 306
Acquired aortic regurgitation, 541–542
clinical manifestations of, 542
course for, 542
management of, 542
physiology of, 542
prevalence of, 541–542
Acquired complete AV block, 507
Acquired immune deficiency syndrome (AIDS), 428
Acquired valve disorders, 84
Action potential, 146
cardiac, 892–893
sinoatrial nodal, 893–894
ventricular, 894–895
diastolic depolarization in, 895
phase 0 depolarization in, 894
phase 1 early repolarization in, 894–895
phase 2 action potential plateau in, 895
phase 3 final repolarization in, 895
phase 4 resting membrane potential in, 895
Acute myocarditis, extracorporeal membrane oxygenation for, 874
Acute pericarditis, 459–460
electrocardiogram showing, 460
etiologies of, 460
Acute vasodilator testing, pulmonary hypertension therapy with, 121–122
Acyanotic tetralogy of Fallot, ventricular septal defect with, 544
Adenosine, 511, 907, 909
AIDS. *See* Acquired immune deficiency syndrome
Airway resistance, 317
Alagille syndrome, 67
Alcohol septal ablation, familial hypertrophic cardiomyopathy treated with, 439
Aldosterone escape, 89
Aldosterone-blocking agents, 89
Aminocaproic acid, 909
Amiodarone, 509–510, 907, 909
Amlodipine, 909
Analgesics, drug therapy with, 910
Anatomically corrected malposition of great arteries, 40, 45
Anatomy, morphologic, 27–37
atria in, 27–31
left, 28, 29–31
right, 27–29
ventricles in, 31–37
left, 34–37
right, 31–34
Anderson's syndrome, 168, 501
Anemia, 84
Anesthesia. *See* Sedation/anesthesia
Aneurysm of ductus arteriosus, 624
Angiographic evaluation, 118
angiocardiography in, 226–227
cardiac catheterization with, 223–227
congenital heart lesion anatomy views in, 229
contrast agents in, 225–226
equipment for, 223
image production in, 223–224
image recording/processing in, 224
radiation exposure in, 224–225
sedation/anesthesia with, 301
views, 227–229
Angiotensin receptor blockers (ARB), 89
Angiotensin-converting enzyme inhibitors (ACEI), 88–89
drug therapy with, 908
Anomalous drainage, 605, 606
Anthracycline-mediated cardiac injury, 426–427
Antiarrhythmics, familial hypertrophic cardiomyopathy treated with, 439–440
Antidromic reciprocating tachycardia (ART), 492, 494–496
WPW with, 494–496
Anti-inflammatory agents, 312
Antithrombotics, 406
Aortic arches. *See also* Interrupted aortic arch
development of, 18, 19, 23–24
double, 24
fifth, 23
first pair of, 18
second/third pairs of, 18
surgery for, 850
3,4, and 6, 22
Aortic atresia, 727
Aortic coarctation, stents in, 240–241
Aortic outflow abnormalities, 581–598
aortic regurgitation as, 595–598
bicuspid aortic valve as, 598
infant aortic stenosis as, 588–589
subaortic stenosis as, 589–593
supravalvar aortic stenosis as, 593–595
valvar aortic stenosis as, 581–589
Aortic regurgitation, 595–598
catheterization for, 597
chest X-ray for, 597
Children's Hospital Boston experience with, 582, 595
clinical manifestations of, 595–597
course of, 598
definition of, 595
echocardiogram of, 597, 598
electrocardiograph of, 597
management of, 597
pathology of, 596
physiology of, 596
prevalence of, 595–596
Aortic stenosis
coarctation of aorta with, 637–638
ventricular septal defect with, 543
Aortic valve annulus (AVA), 341, 342
Aortic valve replacement, 855

Aortic valve stenosis (AVS), 57, 84
Aorto-left ventricular tunnel, 802–803
anatomy of, 802
cardiac catheterization for, 803
chest X-ray for, 802
Children's Hospital Boston experience with, 800
clinical manifestations of, 802–803
course of, 803
definition of, 802
echocardiogram of, 802
electrocardiograph of, 802–803
management of, 803
physiology of, 802
Aortopulmonary vessels, coil embolization of, 242
Aortopulmonary window, 84, 783–785
anatomy of, 783
cardiac catheterization for, 785
chest X-ray for, 784
Children's Hospital Boston experience with, 784
clinical manifestations of, 783–785
definition of, 783
echocardiogram of, 770, 784–785
electrocardiograph of, 784
embryology of, 783
management of, 785
physiology of, 783
prevalence of, 783
Aprotinin, 909
Arachidonic acid metabolites, 113, 114
ARB. *See* Angiotensin receptor blockers
Arrhythmia, 84, 477–518, 891–904
atrioventricular conduction disorders with, 504–507
acquired complete AV block as, 507
congenital complete AV block as, 506–507
first-degree atrioventricular block as, 505
Mobitz I/Mobitz II, 505
second-degree atrioventricular block as, 505
third-degree atrioventricular block as, 506–507
block with, 479–480
bradycardia with, 479–480
cardiac ion channel mutations leading to, 897–898
cardiac ion channels with, ion channels and, 898
catheter ablation of, 514–518
mapping for, 515–516
outcomes from, 517
positions for, 515
radiofrequency, 515–517
techniques for, 515–517
episodic excitable cell disorders with, 903
evaluation, 143
familial hypertrophic cardiomyopathy with, 435
HERG encodes potassium channels with, 900–901
implantable defibrillators for, 511–515
ion channel dysfunction underlying, 902–903
Arrhythmia *(Continued)*
KVLQT1 form potassium channels with, 899–900
long QT syndrome with, 896–897
mechanism of, 901–902
MinK form potassium channels with, 899–900
molecular/cellular mechanisms of, 897
pacemakers for, 511–515
antibradycardia operation with, 512
class I indications for, 511
generators/pacing modes for, 512–513
implant techniques with, 513–514
leads with, 513–514
pathophysiology of, 477–480
abnormal automaticity in, 478
reentry in, 477–478
triggered automaticity in, 478–479
pharmacologic therapy for, 507–511, 909
adenosine in, 511
amiodarone in, 509–510
atenolol in, 508–509
digoxin in, 511
esmolol in, 508–509
flecainide in, 508
lidocaine in, 507–508
mexiletine in, 507–508
nadolol in, 508–509
procainamide in, 507
propafenone in, 508
propranolol in, 508–509
sotalol in, 509–510
verapamil in, 510–511
prediction/prevention/treatment of, 903–904
premature beats with, 477–481
atrial, 480
etiology of, 477–479
junctional, 480–481
ventricular, 481
reentry for, 901–902
Romano-Ward syndrome with, 896
RyR2 encodes calcium release channel with, 901
sinoatrial node dysfunction with, 504
sodium channel dysfunction causing, 899
susceptibility to, 897–898
tachycardia with, 477–479, 481–504
antidromic reciprocating, 492, 494–496
atrial fibrillation as, 483, 488–489
atrial flutter as, 483, 487–488
automatic supraventricular, 484–487
AV nodal reentrant, 489
bedside diagnosis of, 482
classification of, 482
differential diagnosis of QRS, 482–484
ectopic atrial, 483, 484–485
etiology of, 477–479
junctional ectopic, 483, 486–487
management of, 484–504
mechanisms for, 482
multifocal atrial, 483, 485–486
Arrhythmia *(Continued)*
orthodromic reciprocating, 491–494, 496
permanent form of junctional reciprocating, 483, 496–498
sinus, 483
SVA due to accessory pathways as, 490–492
SVA not involving accessory pathways as, 487–490
terminology with, 482
ventricular, 498–504
torsades de pointes with, 896
Arrhythmogenic right ventricular cardiomyopathy (ARVC), 444
Arrhythmogenic right ventricular dysplasia (ARVD), 165, 503
ART. *See* Antidromic reciprocating tachycardia
Arterial carbon dioxide tension, 104–105
Arterial switch procedures, 654
Arterial-pulmonary stenosis, HLHS surgical complications of, 724
Arteriopulmonary shunt, 848
Arteriovenous fistula, 84
ARVC. *See* Arrhythmogenic right ventricular cardiomyopathy
ARVD. *See* Arrhythmogenic right ventricular dysplasia
ASD. *See* Atrioventricular septal defects
Ashman's phenomenon, 489
Aspirin, 909
Asplenia, 676, 688, 692. *See also* Heterotaxy, visceral
associated anatomic findings in, 688
diagnosis of, 692
P-wave axis in electrocardiogram of, 691
Associations, 69
CHARGE, 69
VATER, 69
Atelectasis, 317
Atenolol, 508–509, 908
Atherosclerotic cardiovascular disease, risk from hypertension for, 377
Atrial dysrhythmias, atrial septal defect with, 610
Atrial enlargement, 156
Atrial fibrillation, 483, 488–489
Atrial flutter, 483, 487–488
Atrial isomerism, 30
Atrial premature beats, 480
Atrial septal defect, 603–613
anatomy of, 603–606
anomalous drainage in, 605
AV canal septum in, 603
common atrium in, 605
coronary sinus septal defect in, 605
inferior vena cava type defect in, 605
partial anomalous pulmonary venous connection in, 605
patent foramen ovale in, 604
Raghib syndrome in, 605
scimitar syndrome in, 605, 606
septum primum in, 603
septum secundum in, 603

Atrial septal defect (Continued)
sinus venosus defect in, 604
sinus venosus of right atrial type defect in, 605
sinus venosus septum in, 604
superior vena cava type defect in, 604
atrial dysrhythmias with, 610
catheterization for, 609
chest X-ray for, 608
Children's Hospital Boston experience with, 604
clinical manifestations of, 607–609
course of, 610
definition of, 603
device closure at catheterization for, 610
echocardiogram of, 608
electrocardiograph of, 607–608
management of, 609–610
MRI of, 609
physical examination of, 607–608
physiology of, 606–607
prevalence of, 603
pulmonary vascular obstructions with, 610
scimitar syndrome with, 605, 606, 612–613
secundum, 543
surgery for, 610
transcatheter closure of, 244–245
variations on, 610–613
inferior vena caval sinus venous defect in, 612
mitral valve prolapse in, 613
partial anomalous venous return in, 612
patent foramen ovale in, 611
scimitar syndrome in, 612–613
sinus venous defects in, 611–613
superior vena caval sinus venous defect in, 611
symptomatic infants in, 610–611
uncomplicated atrial defect with cyanosis in, 613
unroofed coronary sinus in, 611–612
Atrial situs ambiguus, 684
Atrial switch procedures, 654
Atriobiventricular pacing, 312
Atrioventricular canal (AVC), 603. *See also* Common atrioventricular canal
Down syndrome related defects in, 55
Tetralogy of Fallot with, 563–569, 573
Atrioventricular canal defects, 670–673
cardiac catheterization for, 671–673
chest X-ray for, 670
echocardiogram of, 670–671
electrocardiograph of, 670
history of, 670
management of, 673
physical examination for, 670
surgery for, 673
Atrioventricular conduction disorders, 504–507
acquired complete AV block as, 507
congenital complete AV block as, 506–507
first-degree atrioventricular block as, 505
Mobitz I/Mobitz II, 505
Atrioventricular conduction disorders (Continued)
second-degree atrioventricular block as, 505
third-degree atrioventricular block as, 506–507
Atrioventricular node and bundle, 29
Atrioventricular portion, 29
Atrioventricular septal defects (ASD). *See also* Endocardial cushion type of defects
surgery for, 849–850
Atrioventricular valve regurgitation, 84
Atrioventricular valve replacement, 854–855
advantages/disadvantages of, 854
mitral, 854
single ventricle, 855
tricuspid, 854–855
Atrium
left, 28, 29–31
external appearance of, 29
internal appearance of, 29
polysplenia syndrome with, 30
pulmonary veins of, 29
septum primum of, 29
situs ambiguus with, 30
morphologic anatomy of, 27–31
right, 27–29
anterior interatrial plica of, 27
atrioventricular node and bundle of, 29
atrioventricular portion of, 29
coronary sinus of, 27, 28
crista dividens of, 27, 28
crista terminalis of, 27
external appearance of, 27
internal appearance of, 27
interventricular portion of, 29
limbic ledge of, 27, 28
musculi pectinati of, 29
pars membranacea septi of, 29
penetrating bundle of, 29
septum secundum of, 27, 28
sinoatrial node of, 27
sulcus terminalis of, 27
superior vena cava of, 27, 28
tinea sagittalis of, 29
triangle of Koch of, 29
via dextra of, 27
via sinistra of, 27
situs, 30, 31
Atropine, 907, 909
Autograft, 855
Automatic supraventricular tachycardia, 484–487
AV canal septum, 603
AV nodal reentrant tachycardia (AVNRT), 489
AVA. *See* Aortic valve annulus
AVC. *See* Atrioventricular canal
AVNRT. *See* AV nodal reentrant tachycardia
AVS. *See* Aortic valve stenosis

B

Balloon angioplasty, 235–239
obstructed venous baffles in, 238–239
postoperative coarctation of aorta in, 237–238
pulmonary arteries in, 235–236
unrepaired coarctation of aorta in, 236–237
Balloon valvotomy, 228–234
mitral valvar stenosis in, 233–234
results with, 233–234
technique for, 233
prosthetic valvar stenosis in, 234
pulmonary atresia with intact septum in, 231–232
subaortic stenosis in, 233
valvar aortic stenosis in, 232–233
neonates with, 232–233
older patients with, 232
valvar pulmonary stenosis in, 228–231
neonates with, 230–231
older patients with, 229–230
Barth syndrome, 419
BAV. *See* Bicommissural aortic valve
BDCPS. *See* Bidirectional cavopulmonary shunt operation
Becker's muscular dystrophy, 168, 419, 426
Beckwith-Wiedemann syndrome, 432
Belhassen's tachycardia, 503
Beri-beri. *See* Thiamine deficiency
Biatrial enlargement, 156
Bicommissural aortic valve (BAV), 57
Bicuspid aortic valve, 598
Bidirectional cavopulmonary shunt operation (BDCPS), 863–864
indications for, 863
postoperative management after, 865–866
preoperative evaluation for, 863
results with, 864
technique in, 863–864
Bidirectional Glenn operation, 848–849
Birth defects, pediatric history with, 129–130
Biventricular repair, surgery for, 849–850
Blalock-Hanlon technique, 653
Blalock-Taussig shunt, 845–856
Block, cardiac electrical activation, 479–480
β-blockers, 90–91
drug therapy with, 908
familial hypertrophic cardiomyopathy treated with, 438
syncope treated with, 364
Blood chemistries, 141
Blood cultures, 141
Blood pressure, 133
exercise testing with, 285
hypertension defined by, 377–381
measurement of, 381
medication for, 383
normative values for children with, 378–380
Body surface area (BSA)
aortic valve annulus v., 341, 342
methods of calculating, 343
research methodology with, 340–343
Bone marrow mesenchymal stem cells, 886
Bosentan, 122
Boston Children's hospital. *See* Children's hospital Boston
BPEB. *See* British Pacing and Electrophysiology Group
Bradycardia, 479–480, 504
Brain abscess, hypoxemia with, 100

Breathing reserve, exercise testing with, 283–284
British Pacing and Electrophysiology Group (BPEB), 512
Bronchospasm, 317
Bruce protocol, 279
  endurance time on, 281
Brugada syndrome, 165, 168, 501
BSA. *See* Body surface area
Bumetanide, 908

C

Calcineurin inhibitor therapy, 884
Calcium channel, 146
Calcium channel blockers
  drug therapy with, 909
  familial hypertrophic cardiomyopathy treated with, 438
  pulmonary hypertension therapy with, 122
Calcium chloride, 907
Calcium gluconate, 909
Calcium release channel, RyR2 encodes, 901
Caloric supplementation, 132
Cantrell syndrome, 693
Captopril, 908
Cardiac catheterization, 213–247
  adult congenital heart disease in, 839
  angiographic evaluation with, 223–227
    angiocardiography in, 226–227
    congenital heart lesion anatomy views in, 229
    contrast agents in, 225–226
    equipment for, 223
    image production in, 223–224
    image recording/processing in, 224
    radiation exposure in, 224–225
    views, 227–229
  angiography with, 118
  aorto-left ventricular tunnel in, 803
  aortopulmonary window in, 785
  atrial septal defect in, 609
  atrioventricular canal defects in, 671–673
  balloon angioplasty with, 235–239
    obstructed venous baffles in, 238–239
    postoperative coarctation of aorta in, 237–238
    pulmonary arteries in, 235–236
    unrepaired coarctation of aorta in, 236–237
  balloon valvotomy with, 228–234
    mitral valvar stenosis in, 233–234
    prosthetic valvar stenosis in, 234
    pulmonary atresia with intact septum in, 231–232
    subaortic stenosis in, 233
    valvar aortic stenosis in, 232–233
    valvar pulmonary stenosis in, 228–231
  calculations in, 220–223
    cardiac output, 221
    Fick method for, 222
    shunts, 220–221
    thermodilution cardiac output, 221–222
    valve areas, 222–223
    vascular resistance, 222

Cardiac catheterization *(Continued)*
  cardiac tumors in, 829
  cerebral fistulae in, 802
  closure techniques for, 242–247
    atrial septal defects in, 244–245
    coil embolization of aortopulmonary vessels in, 242
    coil embolization of other vessels in, 242–243
    miscellaneous defects in, 246–247
    patent ductus arteriosus in, 243–244
    patent foramen ovale in, 245–246
    pulmonary valves in, 247
    ventricular septal defects in, 246
  coarctation of aorta in, 631, 636–638, 641
  complications of interventional, 215–216
  cor triatriatum in, 709
  coronary artery anomalies in, 806–807
  coronary fistulae in, 800
  corrected transposition great arteries in, 795–796
  database development influence by technology of, 333
  double-outlet right ventricle in, 739
  D-transposition of great arteries with, 652–653
  Ebstein disease in, 764–765
  familial hypertrophic cardiomyopathy with, 437
  fetal intervention with, 247
  hemitruncus in, 789
  hemodynamic evaluation with, 216–219
  history of, 213
  hypoplastic left heart syndrome in, 720
  indications for, 213–214
  interrupted aortic arch in, 641
  interventional, 227–228
    Children's Hospital Boston experience with, 230
  Kawasaki disease with, 405, 406
  mitral atresia in, 727
  mitral stenosis in, 705–706
  mitral valve prolapse in, 703
  myocardial biopsy with, 228
  nursing for, 349
  ostium primum defects in, 669–670
  oxygen content/saturation with, 219–220
  patent ductus arteriosus with, 620
  pressure measurements with, 216–219
    aortic, 219
    gradients, 219
    left atrial, 217
    left ventricular, 218, 219
    pulmonary artery, 218–219
    pulmonary artery wedge, 217–218
    pulmonary vein, 218
    pulmonary vein wedge, 218
    right atrial, 216–217
    right ventricular, 218
    superior/inferior vena caval, 217
  pulmonary atresia in, 732–733
  pulmonary hypertension in, 118, 119
  pulmonary vasodilator testing with, 118

Cardiac catheterization *(Continued)*
  pulmonary venous obstructions with, 239
    neonatal balloon atrial septostomy in, 239
  rheumatic fever with, 393, 397
  risks of, 214–216
    air emboli as, 215
    airway obstruction as, 215
    apnea as, 215
    arrhythmias as, 215
    arterial/venous complications as, 215
    death as, 215
    diagnostic, 215
    endocarditis as, 215
    myocardial stain/perforation as, 215
    transient fevers as, 215
  shunts with, 220
  single ventricle in, 749
  stents in, 239–242
    aortic coarctation with, 240–241
    other uses of, 241–242
    pulmonary arteries with, 240
    right ventricular conduits with, 241
  subaortic stenosis with, 592
  supravalvar aortic stenosis with, 595
  syncope evaluated with, 363
  tetralogy of Fallot with, 567–568
  total anomalous pulmonary venous return in, 778, 779
  tricuspid atresia in, 756
  truncus arteriosus in, 770
  valvar aortic stenosis in, 584–585
  valvar pulmonary stenosis in, 553, 555
  ventricular septal defect with, 535–537
  visceral heterotaxy in, 692
Cardiac loop formation, 13, 16
Cardiac malposition, 675–694. *See also* Congenital cardiovascular malformations
  asplenia with, 676, 688, 692
    associated anatomic findings in, 688
    diagnosis of, 692
  Cantrell syndrome as, 693
  Children's Hospital Boston experience with, 676
  classification of, 675
  clinical manifestations of, 676
  complete situs inversus as, 693
  definition of, 675
  dextrocardia with visceroatrial situs solitus as, 693–694
  ectopia cordis as, 693
  Kartagener syndrome as, 693
  pathology of, 675–676
  physiology of, 676
  polysplenia syndrome with, 676, 688, 692
    associated anatomic findings in, 688
    diagnosis of, 692
  prevalence of, 675
  thoracophagus twins with, 693
  visceral heterotaxy as, 676–693
    age at death with, 691
    cardiac catheterization for, 692
    characteristics of, 675
    chest X-ray for, 690

Cardiac catheterization (*Continued*)
clinical manifestations of, 688–692
definition of, 675
double rightness with, 677
echocardiogram of, 690–692
electrocardiograph of, 689–690
left lung isomerism with, 677
management of, 693
noncardiac anomalies in, 692–639
pathology of, 677–688
physical examination for, 688–689
prevalence of, 677
right atrial isomerism with, 677
right pulmonary isomerism with, 677
Cardiac resynchronization therapy (CRT), 91
Cardiac segments, 39–42
alignments v. connections with, 41–42
crisscross AV relations in, 40–41
malformations with, 42
segmental alignments with, 41
sets of, 39–41
types of heart in, 40
anatomically corrected malposition of great arteries as, 40, 45
double-outlet left ventricle as, 40, 45
double-outlet right ventricle as, 40, 45
isolated atrial noninversion as, 40, 43
isolated infundibuloarterial inversion as, 40, 43
isolated ventricular inversion as, 40, 43
isolated ventricular noninversion as, 40, 43
normal, 40, 42
transposition of great arteries as, 40, 43–45
Cardiac syncope, 360–361
Cardio-facial-cutaneous syndrome, 432
Cardiogenic crescent, development of, 13, 16
Cardio-inhibitory syncope, 360
Cardiomegaly, 306
Cardiomyopathy, 84, 415–445
arrhythmogenic right ventricular, 444
congestive, 416
dilated, 416–432
Becker muscular dystrophy as, 426
clinical presentation of, 416–418
definition of, 416
diagnostic evaluation of, 416–418
doxorubicin cardiomyopathy as, 426–428
Duchenne's muscular dystrophy as, 424–426
dystrophinopathies as, 423–424
endocardial fibroelastosis as, 422–423
epidemiology of, 416
HIV-associated cardiac disease as, 428–429
infective myocarditis as, 421–422
iron-overload cardiomyopathy as, 430–432
myotonic dystrophy as, 429–430
outcome for, 420–421
predictors of outcome in, 420
secondary forms of, 419
thalassemia as, 430–432
treatment of, 418–420
X-linked, 426
Cardiomyopathy (*Continued*)
echocardiography indications for, 184
history of classification as, 415
hypertrophic, 432–442
familial, 432–441
Friedreich ataxia as, 441–442
maternally inherited, 432
sarcomeric, 432
noncompaction of ventricular myocardium as, 444–445
of overload, 416
restrictive, 442–443
right ventricular, 444
ventricular tachycardia with, 502–503
Cardiomyopathy of overload, 84
Cardiopulmonary bypass, 104–105
acid-based management in, 104–105
arterial carbon dioxide tension in, 104–105
deep hypothermia in, 104
hemodilution in, 105
management of anesthesia with
after procedure, 299
during procedure, 298–299
minimally invasive approach to, 870–872
incisions for, 871
ministernotomy trans-xyphoid approach in, 871
results with, 872
total circulatory arrest in, 104
Cardiovascular magnetic resonance (CMR), 199–206
background, 199
black blood imaging in, 200
bright blood imaging in, 200–201
cardiac/respiratory gating in, 199
contrast-enhanced 3-dimensional MR angiography, 202
double inversion recovery in, 200
gradient echo in, 200–201
myocardial perfusion/viability with, 202
pulse sequences in, 199
spin echo in, 200
techniques, 199–202
velocity encoded cine, 202
ventricular function assessment with, 201–202
Carditis, rheumatic fever with, 391
CATCH 22, 53, 69
Catecholaminergic VT, 501
Catecholamines, 308–311
Cat-eye syndrome. *See* Tetrasomy 22p syndrome
Catheter ablation, 514–518
mapping for, 515–516
outcomes from, 517
positions for, 515
radiofrequency, 515–517
techniques for, 515–517
CCVM. *See* Congenital cardiovascular malformations
Cell death abnormalities, 56–57
abnormal targeted growth as, 56
immotile cilia syndrome with, 57
looping abnormalities as, 56–57
situs abnormalities as, 56–57
Central nervous system sequelae of CHD, 103–108
cardiac surgery for, 104–105
acid-based management in, 104–105
arterial carbon dioxide tension in, 104–105
cardiopulmonary bypass in, 104–105
deep hypothermia in, 104
hemodilution in, 105
total circulatory arrest in, 104
imaging for, 103–104
MRI for, 103–104
pathology of, 103
Cerebral fistulae, 802
cardiac catheterization for, 802
chest X-ray for, 802
Children's Hospital Boston experience with, 800
clinical manifestations of, 802
definition of, 802
echocardiogram of, 802
electrocardiograph of, 802
management of, 802
pathophysiology of, 802
prevalence of, 802
Cerebrovascular accidents, hypoxemia with, 100
Cervical venous hum, 359
Chagas' disease, 168
CHARGE association, 69
CHD. *See* Congenital heart disease
Chest examination, 139
Chest pain, 364–368
cardiac causes of, 366
aortic, 366
coronary, 366
myocardial, 366
pericardial, 366
rhythm abnormalities, 366
valvular, 366
chest X-ray for, 367
clinical evaluation of, 366–368
echocardiography for, 367–368
electrocardiogram for, 367
epidemiology of, 365
etiology of, 365–366
exercise testing for, 368
history in evaluation of, 366–367
noncardiac causes of, 365–366
chest wall, 365
gastrointestinal, 365
psychogenic, 365–366
pulmonary, 365
physical evaluation for, 367
Chest X-ray
for absent pulmonary valve, 565
aortic regurgitation in, 597
aorto-left ventricular tunnel in, 802
aortopulmonary window in, 784
atrial septal defect in, 608
atrioventricular canal defects in, 670
bicuspid aortic valve in, 598
cardiac tumors in, 828
cerebral fistulae in, 802
chest pain evaluated with, 367

Chest X-ray (Continued)
coarctation of aorta in, 631, 635, 637, 638, 640
cor triatriatum in, 708
coronary artery anomalies in, 806
coronary fistulae in, 800
corrected transposition great arteries in, 794
double-outlet right ventricle in, 739
D-transposition of great arteries in, 650
hemitruncus in, 788
hypoplastic left heart syndrome in, 719
interrupted aortic arch in, 640
mitral atresia in, 727
mitral regurgitation in, 699
mitral stenosis in, 705
mitral valve prolapse in, 703
ostium primum defects in, 668
patent ductus arteriosus in, 620, 623
pulmonary arteriovenous fistulae in, 801
pulmonary atresia in, 732
rheumatic fever in, 392–393
single ventricle in, 747
subaortic stenosis in, 591
tetralogy of Fallot in, 565
total anomalous pulmonary venous return in, 776, 777, 779
tricuspid atresia in, 755
truncus arteriosus in, 770
valvar aortic stenosis in, 584
valvar pulmonary stenosis in, 552
ventricular septal defect in, 534
visceral heterotaxy in, 690
Children's Hospital Boston
adult CHD experienced at, 839
aortic regurgitation experienced at, 582, 595
aortopulmonary window experienced at, 784
cardiac malposition experienced at, 676
cardiac transplantation experienced at, 878, 881
cardiac tumors experienced at, 826
cardiology at, 7–9
clinical care for, 7–8
collaboration with, 8–9
divisions of, 8
missions of, 7
research with, 8
sections of, 8
training for, 8
coarctation of aorta experienced at, 628, 630, 633
coronary artery anomalies experienced at, 806
corrected transposition great arteries experienced at, 792
Double-outlet right ventricle experienced at, 735, 739
D-transposition of great arteries experienced at, 645
Ebstein disease experienced at, 762
endocardial cushion defects experienced at, 666, 673
hypoplastic left heart syndrome experienced at, 725
Children's Hospital Boston (Continued)
intensive care unit at, 303–304
interrupted aortic arch experienced at, 639
interventional cardiac catheterization at, 230
mitral atresia experienced at, 726
mitral regurgitation experienced at, 698
mitral valve prolapse experienced at, 703
Nadas' work at, 3, 5, 7
nursing orientation program for, 348
patent ductus arteriosus experienced at, 618
postoperative management plans from, 351
pulmonary atresia experienced at, 730, 733
pulmonary stenosis at, 550, 554
rheumatic fever at, 388
single ventricle experienced at, 744
subaortic stenosis experienced at, 582, 591
supravalvar aortic stenosis experienced at, 582
surgery experienced at, 846
tetralogy of Fallot at, 560
total anomalous pulmonary venous return experienced at, 774
tricuspid atresia experienced at, 754, 757
truncus arteriosus experienced at, 768
valvar aortic stenosis experienced at, 582, 586
vascular fistulae experienced at, 800
ventricular septal defect experience at, 528, 529, 538
Chloral hydrate, 910
Chlorothiazide, 908
Chondroectodermal dysplasia. *See* Ellis-Van Creveld syndrome
Chorea, rheumatic fever with, 390–393
Chromosome 22q11 deletion syndrome, 53–54, 69
Chylomicrons, 374
Clark classification system, 51–53
Clicks, 136–137
Clinical practice guidelines (CPG), 352–353
Clopidogrel, 909
Clubbing, 139–140
hypoxemia with, 98, 99
CoA. *See* Coarctation of aorta
Coagulation, drug therapy with, 909–910
Coarctation of aorta (CoA), 57, 84, 627–642
anatomy of, 627–629, 634, 636, 637, 639
aortic stenosis with, 637–638
atypical, 642
balloon angioplasty for
postoperative, 237–238, 634
unrepaired, 236–237, 632–633
Children's Hospital Boston experience with, 628, 630, 633
clinical manifestations of, 629–631, 634–638, 640
complex heart disease with, 638
course of, 633–634, 636–638, 642
definition of, 627
D-transposition of great arteries with, 657
embryology of, 638–639
HLHS surgical complications of, 723–724
hypertension caused by, 382
interrupted aortic arch with, 638–642
management of, 631–633, 636–638, 641–642
Coarctation of aorta (CoA) (Continued)
mitral valve abnormalities with, 636–637
neonates/infants with, 634–636
physiology of, 629, 634, 636–638, 640
prevalence of, 627
stents in, 240–241
surgery for, 850
uncomplicated coarctation beyond infancy as, 627–634
anatomy of, 627–629
balloon angioplasty for, 632–634
cardiac catheterization for, 631
chest X-ray for, 631
clinical manifestations of, 629–631
course of, 633–634
echocardiogram of, 631
electrocardiograph of, 631
indications of intervention for, 631
management of, 631–633
MRI for, 631
natural history of, 633–634
physiology of, 629
postoperative course for, 634
surgery for, 631–632
ventricular septal defect with, 634–636
Common atrioventricular canal. *See also* Endocardial cushion type of defects
cardiac catheterization for, 568
chest X-ray for, 565
clinical manifestations of, 564
course for, 576
echocardiogram of, 567
electrocardiogram of, 565
management of, 573
MRI of, 569
pathology of, 563
physiology of, 563
Common atrioventricular orifices. *See* Endocardial cushion type of defects
Common atrium, 605
Computed tomography, 206
Computed tomography angiography (CTA), 206
Conal septum closure, 23
Concealed accessory pathways, 483
Conduction block, 479
Congenital cardiovascular malformations (CCVM), 49
pathogenetic classification of, 51–56
anatomic abnormality related to, 52
chromosome 22q11 deletion syndrome in, 53–54
Clark classification system in, 51–53
conotruncal malformations in, 53
disordered mechanisms in, 51–52
ectomesenchymal tissue migration abnormalities in, 53–54
etiology related to, 52
extracellular matrix abnormalities in, 55–56
intracardiac blood flow abnormalities in, 54
neural crest migration abnormalities in, 53–54

Congenital complete AV block, 506–507
Congenital heart disease (CHD), 49
adult, 833–839
catheter-based intervention for, 839
Children's Hospital Boston experience with, 839
heart failure as, 833–837
lesion management strategies for, 838–839
neurohormonal activation with, 837–838
pulmonary vascular disease as, 835–836
right ventricular dysfunction as, 836–837
ventricular vascular coupling as, 834–835
congestive heart failure with, 84
echocardiography indications for, 184
recurrence risks for, 59
ventricular tachycardia with, 502
Congestive cardiomyopathy, 416
Congestive heart failure, 83–91
adult v. child, 83
cardiomyopathy of overload with, 84
clinical presentation of, 86–87
childhood with, 86–87
infancy with, 86
diagnostic evaluation of, 87–88
epidemiology of, 83
etiology of, 83–85
congenital heart disease with, 84
normal heart, 84
management of, 88–91
aldosterone-blocking agents for, 89
angiotensin receptor blockers for, 89
angiotensin-converting enzyme inhibitors for, 88–89
β blockade for, 90–91
digitalis for, 90
diuretics for, 89
general measures for, 88
resynchronization therapy for, 91
myocardial failure with, 84
pathophysiology of, 85–86
severity classification of, 87
Conotruncal malformations, 53
Constrictive pericarditis, 462–464
MRI of, 463
square root sign with, 463
Continuous venovenous hemofiltration (CVVH), 318
Continuous-wave Doppler, 185
Contrast agents, angiographic, 225–226
adverse reactions to, 226
chemistry of, 225
physiology with, 225–226
toxicity, 226
Contrast-enhanced 3-dimensional MR angiography, 202
Conus arteriosus, 32, 34, 36, 37
anatomic variations in, 36, 37
Convulsive syncope, 361–362
Cor triatriatum, 707–709
cardiac catheterization for, 709
chest X-ray for, 708
clinical manifestations of, 708–709
definition of, 707
Cor triatriatum *(Continued)*
echocardiogram of, 708–709
electrocardiograph of, 708
management of, 709
pathology of, 707
physiology of, 707
prevalence of, 707
Coronary artery
left, 34
right, 34
Coronary artery anomalies, 805–808
anomalous coronary from pulmonary artery with, 805
cardiac catheterization for, 806–807
chest X-ray for, 806
Children's Hospital Boston experience with, 806
clinical manifestations of, 806–807
course of, 807
definition of, 805
echocardiogram of, 806
management of, 807
pathology of, 805
physiology of, 805–806
prevalence of, 805
single sinus origin of, 807
Coronary fistulae, 799–800
cardiac catheterization for, 800
chest X-ray for, 800
Children's Hospital Boston experience with, 800
clinical manifestations of, 800
course of, 800
definition of, 799
echocardiogram of, 800
electrocardiograph of, 800
management of, 800
pathology of, 799
physiology of, 799
prevalence of, 799
Coronary insufficiency, 656
Coronary sinus, 27, 28, 175
Coronary sinus septal defect, 605
Corrected transposition great arteries, 791–796
anatomically corrected malposition of, 796
anatomy of, 791–793
cardiac catheterization for, 795–796
chest X-ray for, 794
Children's Hospital Boston experience with, 792
clinical manifestations of, 793–796
conduction system with, 793
coronary anatomy with, 793
course of, 796
definition of, 791
echocardiogram of, 794–795
electrocardiograph of, 794
management of, 796
MRI of, 794
physiology of, 793
prevalence of, 791
Corrigan's pulse, 132
Corticosteroids, 406
Costello syndrome, 432
CPG. *See* Clinical practice guidelines
Creation of atrial septal defect, 653–654
Crista dividens, 27, 28
Crista terminalis, 27
CRT. *See* Cardiac resynchronization therapy
CTA. *See* Computed tomography angiography
CVVH. *See* Continuous venovenous hemofiltration
Cyanosis, 140
hypoxemia with, 97–98
pediatric history with, 130
uncomplicated atrial defect with, 613
Cyanotic spells, hypoxemia with, 100
Cytomegalovirus, 460

D

Damus-Kaye-Stanzel operation, 848, 849
DASH. *See* Dietary Approaches to Stop Hypertension
Database development, 323–335
analysis of outcomes in, 334–335
cardiac problems incidence in, 331
categorization of patients for, 327
coding and cardiac lesions in, 329–331
cost of current cardiovascular patient, 327
data analysis in textbook for, 327
data collection/coding for, 324–325
diagnosis ruled-out marker in, 326
error sources in, 326
hierarchical system for, 327–329
history of medical, 323–324
management of negative information in, 326
patient summary file with, 325–326
pediatric heart disease prevalence with, 327–329, 330
procedures per patient number in, 332
purpose for, 324
size of current, 327
survival in, 334–335
technology's influence on practice in, 331–334
cardiac catheterization, 333
echocardiography, 332–333
electrophysiologic procedures, 332–333
MRI, 332–233
noninvasive imaging modalities, 333
DCM. *See* Dilated cardiomyopathies
Dead space/tidal volume ratio, 277
Decremental conduction, 147, 479
Deep total circulatory arrest (DTCA), 104
Depolarization, 891
Detroit Children's hospital, Nadas' residency at, 3
Dextrocardia, 156, 168
with visceroatrial situs solitus, 693–694
Diagnosis, 39–49
cardiac segments in, 39–42
alignments v. connections with, 41–42
crisscross AV relations in, 40–41
malformations with, 42
segmental alignments with, 41
sets of, 39–41
types of heart in, 40

Diagnosis *(Continued)*
examples of, 42–45
anatomically corrected malposition of great arteries as, 40, 45
double-outlet left ventricle as, 40, 45
double-outlet right ventricle as, 40, 45
inverted normal heart as, 40, 42
isolated atrial noninversion as, 40, 43
isolated infundibuloarterial inversion as, 40, 43
isolated ventricular inversion as, 40, 43
isolated ventricular noninversion as, 40, 43
solitus normal heart as, 42
transposition of great arteries as, 40, 43–45
ventricular inversion with inverted normal arteries as, 40, 43
Diaphragmatic paresis, 316–317
Diastolic dysfunction, familial hypertrophic cardiomyopathy with, 434
Diastolic resting potential, 146
Dietary Approaches to Stop Hypertension (DASH), 382–383
DiGeorge sequence, 69
Digitalis, 90
Digoxin, 122, 511, 908
Dilated cardiomyopathies (DCM), ventricular tachycardia with, 503
Dilated cardiomyopathy, 164–165, 416–432
Becker muscular dystrophy as, 426
clinical presentation of, 416–418
definition of, 416
diagnostic evaluation of, 416–418
doxorubicin cardiomyopathy as, 426–428
Duchenne's muscular dystrophy as, 424–426
dystrophinopathies as, 423–424
endocardial fibroelastosis as, 422–423
epidemiology of, 416
HIV-associated cardiac disease as, 428–429
infective myocarditis as, 421–422
iron-overload cardiomyopathy as, 430–432
myotonic dystrophy as, 429–430
outcome for, 420–421
predictors of outcome in, 420
secondary forms of, 419
thalassemia as, 430–432
treatment of, 418–420
X-linked, 426
Dipyridamole, 909
Distal conal septum, 32, 34
Diuretic agents, drug therapy with, 908
Diuretics, 89, 122
Dobutamine, 907, 908
Dopamine, 907, 908
Doppler echocardiography, 185–187
color-coded flow mapping for, 186
continuous-wave, 185
high-pulse repetition frequency, 186
pulsed, 185–186
tissue, 186
Double rightness, 677
Double-chambered right ventricle, 544–545
Double-outlet left ventricle, 40, 45, 740
Double-outlet right ventricle, 40, 45, 735–740
anomalies associated with, 737
cardiac catheterization for, 739
chest X-ray for, 739
Children's Hospital Boston experience with, 735, 739
clinical manifestations of, 737–739
course of, 740
definition of, 735
echocardiogram of, 739
electrocardiograph of, 737, 739
management of, 739–740
pathology of, 735–737
physiology of, 737
prevalence of, 735
pulmonary stenosis with, 737
Taussig-Bing anomaly with, 737
transposition of great arteries with, 737
ventricular septal defect with, 737
Down syndrome (Trisomy 21), 61–62
atrioventricular canal defects in, 55
endocardial cushion defects with, 665–667
Doxorubicin cardiomyopathy, 426–428
characteristics of anthracycline-mediated cardiac injury with, 427
management of, 428
mechanism of anthracycline-mediated cardiac injury with, 426–427
prevention of, 427–428
risk factors for, 427
Drainage, 605, 606
Drug therapy
analgesics in, 910
angiotensin-converting enzyme inhibitors in, 908
arrhythmia treated with, 507–511, 909
adenosine in, 511
amiodarone in, 509–510
atenolol in, 508–509
digoxin in, 511
esmolol in, 508–509
flecainide in, 508
lidocaine in, 507–508
mexiletine in, 507–508
nadolol in, 508–509
procainamide in, 507
propafenone in, 508
propranolol in, 508–509
sotalol in, 509–510
verapamil in, 510–511
β-blockers in, 908
calcium channel blockers in, 909
cardiac medications in, 908–909
coagulation in, 909–910
diuretic agents in, 908
ductal manipulation in, 909
hypertension, 383
inotropic agents in, 908
intubation in, 910
noncardiac medications in, 909–910
resuscitation in, 907
sedative/anesthetic in, 910
syncope treated with, 364
Drug therapy *(Continued)*
vasodilators in, 908
vasopressor in, 908
DTCA. *See* Deep total circulatory arrest
D-transposition of great arteries, 20, 645–658
anatomy of, 646–647
mitral valve abnormalities in, 647
tricuspid abnormalities in, 647
ventricular defects in, 647
balloon atrial septostomy for, 652–653
cardiac catheterization for, 652–653
chest X-ray for, 650
Children's Hospital Boston experience with, 645
clinical manifestations of, 650 653
course following arterial switch repair for, 656–657
coronary insufficiency in, 656
left ventricular function in, 657
neoaortic regurgitation in, 657
rhythm abnormalities in, 656
supravalvar obstruction in, 656
course following atrial switch repair for, 655–656
baffle obstruction/leak in, 656
central nervous system injury in, 656
rhythm abnormalities in, 655–656
right ventricular function in, 656
tricuspid regurgitation in, 656
definition of, 645
echocardiogram of, 650–652
electrocardiograph of, 650
embryology of, 645–646
management of, 653–655
physical examination for, 650
physiology of, 647–650
large atrial defect with, 648
pulmonary stenosis with, 648
pulmonary vascular disease with, 649
ventricular septal defects with, 648
prevalence of, 645
surgery for, 653–655, 852
arterial switch procedures in, 654
atrial switch procedures in, 654
atrial switch to arterial switch conversion in, 655
Blalock-Hanlon technique in, 653
creation of atrial septal defect in, 653–654
Fontan procedure in, 655
palliative atrial baffle procedures in, 655
pulmonary artery banding in, 653
Rastelli procedure in, 654
staged physiologic repair in, 655
ventricular septal defect in, 654
variations on, 657–658
coarctation of aorta with, 657
overriding tricuspid valve and small right ventricle with, 658
pulmonary stenosis with, 657–658
ventricular defect with, 657–658
Duchenne's muscular dystrophy, 168, 419, 424–426
Ductal manipulation, drug therapy with, 909

Duke criteria, 470–471
Dyslipidemia, 374–377
genetic causes of, 376
lipids/lipoproteins description with, 374
lipids/lipoproteins measurement with, 375–376
management of, 376–377
normative lipid values with, 375
screening for, 374–376
secondary causes of, 376
Dysmorphology, 49–69
associations in, 69
CHARGE, 69
VATER, 69
cell death abnormalities in, 56–57
abnormal targeted growth as, 56
immotile cilia syndrome with, 57
looping abnormalities as, 56–57
situs abnormalities as, 56–57
chromosomal syndromes in, 61–64
Down syndrome as, 61–62
Tetrasomy 22p syndrome as, 63
Trisomy 13 syndrome as, 63
Trisomy 18 syndrome as, 62–63
Turner syndrome as, 63–64
contiguous gene deletion syndromes in, 68–69
CATCH 22 as, 53, 69
chromosome 22q deletions as, 53, 69
DiGeorge sequence as, 69
velocardiofacial syndrome as, 69
Williams syndrome as, 68
defined, 49
developmental approach to child in, 49–51
fetal alcohol syndrome in, 65, 66
genetic counseling with, 57–60
cardiovascular gene defects and, 58, 60
CHD recurrence risks in, 59
known cardiovascular gene defects in, 58, 60
allelic/nonallelic heterogeneity as, 60
arrhythmias as, 60
familial cardiomyopathy as, 60
malformation syndromes as, 58, 60
mitochondrial disorders as, 60
nonsyndromic defects as, 60
multiple malformation syndromes in, 50–51, 60–61
congenital heart defects with, 60
Hurler syndrome as, 51
retinoic acid embryopathy as, 50
syndromic congenital cardiovascular patterns of, 61
pathogenetic malformation classification with, 51–56
anatomic abnormality related to, 52
chromosome 22q11 deletion syndrome in, 53–54
Clark classification system in, 51–53
conotruncal malformations in, 53
disordered mechanisms in, 51–52
ectomesenchymal tissue migration abnormalities in, 53–54
etiology related to, 52
Dysmorphology *(Continued)*
extracellular matrix abnormalities in, 55–56
intracardiac blood flow abnormalities in, 54
neural crest migration abnormalities in, 53–54
patterns of cardiovascular malformation in, 61
defect pathognomonic for specific syndrome with, 61
defect required for diagnosis with, 61
increased risk for specific defect with, 61
nonspecific increased risk with, 61
single gene disorders in, 65–68
Alagille syndrome as, 67
Ellis-Van Creveld syndrome as, 68
Holt-Oram syndrome as, 67
Marfan syndrome as, 65–66
Noonan syndrome as, 66–67
structurally defective child in, 49–51
prenatal v. postnatal onset of, 49
teratogens in, 64–65
Dysplastic pulmonary valves, 555, 561–562
Dystrophinopathies, 423–424

E

Early tracheal extubation, 298
EAT. *See* Ectopic atrial tachycardia
Ebstein disease, 761–765
cardiac catheterization for, 764–765
Children's Hospital Boston experience with, 762
clinical manifestations of, 763–765
course of, 765
definition of, 761
echocardiogram of, 764
electrocardiograph of, 763–764
management of, 765
MRI for, 764
pathology of, 761–763
physiology of, 763
prevalence of, 761
Echocardiogram
of absent pulmonary valve, 566–567
aortic regurgitation in, 597, 598
aorto-left ventricular tunnel in, 802
aortopulmonary window in, 784–785
atrial septal defect in, 608
atrioventricular canal defects in, 670–671
bicuspid aortic valve in, 598
cardiac tumors in, 828–829
cerebral fistulae in, 802
coarctation of aorta in, 631, 635–638, 640–641
cor triatriatum in, 708–709
coronary artery anomalies in, 806
coronary fistulae in, 800
corrected transposition great arteries in, 794–795
double-outlet right ventricle in, 739
D-transposition of great arteries in, 650–652
Ebstein disease in, 764
Echocardiogram *(Continued)*
familial hypertrophic cardiomyopathy in, 436
fetal, 667
hemitruncus in, 788–789
hypoplastic left heart syndrome in, 719–720
infective endocarditis in, 469–471
interrupted aortic arch in, 640–641
Kawasaki disease with, 404–405
mitral atresia in, 727
mitral regurgitation in, 699–700
mitral stenosis in, 705
mitral valve prolapse in, 703
ostium primum defects in, 668–669
patent ductus arteriosus in, 620, 623
pulmonary arteriovenous fistulae in, 801
pulmonary atresia in, 732
rheumatic fever in, 392–393, 397
single ventricle in, 747–749
subaortic stenosis in, 591–592
supravalvar aortic stenosis in, 594
tetralogy of Fallot in, 565–567
total anomalous pulmonary venous return in, 776, 779
tricuspid atresia in, 575–756
truncus arteriosus in, 770
valvar aortic stenosis in, 584
valvar pulmonary stenosis in, 552–553
ventricular septal defect in, 534–536
visceral heterotaxy in, 690–692
Echocardiography, 183–199
anesthesia monitoring with, 294–295
chest pain evaluated with, 367–368
complications with, 198–199
contrast, 187–188
database development influence by technology of, 332–333
Doppler, 185–187
color-coded flow mapping for, 186
continuous-wave, 185
high-pulse repetition frequency, 186
pulsed, 185–186
tissue, 186
equipment for, 188
examination objectives for, 188
examination technique with, 188
fetal, 195–198
indications for, 184
M-mode, 184
pulmonary hypertension in, 117–118
quantitative analysis for, 191–193
Doppler evaluation of pressure gradients in, 193
pressure gradient calculations in, 193
technique in, 191–192
ventricular function in, 192–193
safety for, 198–199
sedation with, 188
special procedures for, 193–195
syncope evaluated with, 363
technical background on, 183–184
three-dimensional, 185
transesophageal, 193–195

Echocardiography (Continued)
two-dimensional, 184–185
views, 188–191
apical, 189, 190
four-chamber, 188
interpretations of, 191
parasternal, 189–191
reporting of, 191
standard imaging planes for, 188–189
subcostal, 189, 190
subxiphoid, 189, 190
suprasternal notch, 190, 191
ECLS. *See* Extracorporeal life support
ECMO. *See* Extracorporeal membrane oxygenation
Ectomesenchymal tissue migration abnormalities, 53–54
Ectopia cordis, 693
Ectopic atrial tachycardia (EAT), 483–485
Edema, 139
EFE. *See* Endocardial fibroelastosis
Effective refractory period (ERP), 147
Eisenmenger's complex. *See* Pulmonary vascular disease
Ejection murmur, diagram of, 583
Electrocardiograph
aortic regurgitation in, 597
aorto-left ventricular tunnel in, 802–803
aortopulmonary window in, 784
atrial septal defect in, 607–608
atrioventricular canal defects in, 670
bicuspid aortic valve in, 598
cardiac tumors in, 828
cerebral fistulae in, 802
chest pain evaluated with, 367
coarctation of aorta in, 631, 635, 637, 638, 640
cor triatriatum in, 708
coronary fistulae in, 800
corrected transposition great arteries in, 794
double-outlet right ventricle in, 737, 739
D-transposition of great arteries in, 650
Ebstein disease in, 763–764
familial hypertrophic cardiomyopathy in, 436
hemitruncus in, 788
hypoplastic left heart syndrome, 719
interrupted aortic arch in, 640
Kawasaki disease with, 404
mitral atresia in, 727
mitral regurgitation in, 699
mitral stenosis in, 705
mitral valve prolapse, 703
ostium primum defects in, 668
patent ductus arteriosus in, 620, 623
pericardial disease in, 460
pericardial effusion in, 461
pulmonary arteriovenous fistulae in, 801
pulmonary atresia in, 731–732
rheumatic fever in, 392
single ventricle in, 747
subaortic stenosis in, 591
supravalvar aortic stenosis in, 594
tetralogy of Fallot in, 564–565
Electrocardiograph (Continued)
total anomalous pulmonary venous return in, 776, 779
tricuspid atresia in, 755
truncus arteriosus in, 770
valvar aortic stenosis in, 583–584
valvar pulmonary stenosis in, 552, 553
ventricular septal defect in, 534
visceral heterotaxy in, 689–690
Electrocardiography, 145–180
abnormal, 155
rhythm/rate in, 155
atrial enlargement in, 156
autonomic testing with, 170–171
basic electrophysiology for, 145–151
cell-to-cell conduction in, 146–147
cellular action potential in, 145–146
conduction through intact heart in, 147–149
depolarization in, 149–151
graphic recording of activity in, 149–151
ventricular cycle in, 150
cardiac malpositions in, 155–156
L-looped ventricles as, 156
situs inversus as, 156
diagnostic maneuvers with, 175–180
ancillary tests in, 179–180
AV node in, 176–177
baseline recordings in, 175–176
His-Purkinje conduction in, 177
SA node in, 176
supraventricular tachycardia evaluation in, 177–178
ventricular arrhythmias evaluation in, 178–179
ventricular tissue in, 177
exercise testing with, 168–170, 285–286
intracardiac electrophysiologic studies with, 173–175
coronary sinus in, 175
equipment for, 174–175
high right atrium in, 175
His bundle electrogram in, 175
right ventricular apex in, 175
intraventricular conduction abnormalities in, 160–163
bifascicular block as, 162
complete left bundle branch block as, 161–162
complete right bundle branch block as, 160, 161
incomplete right bundle branch block as, 160
left anterior hemiblock as, 160–161
left posterior hemiblock as, 161
preexcitation as, 162–163
lead system in, 151–152
normal, 152–155
axis in, 152–154
normal range/mean values of measurements in, 153
P wave in, 154
PR interval in, 154
Electrocardiography (Continued)
QRS complex in, 154
QT interval in, 155
rhythm/rate in, 154
ST segment in, 154–155
T wave in, 155
T_A wave in, 154
U wave in, 155
pulmonary hypertension in, 117
signal averaging with, 171–172
ST segment/T wave changes with, 163–167
arrhythmogenic right ventricular dysplasia in, 165
Brugada syndrome in, 165
dilated cardiomyopathy in, 164–165
electrolyte abnormalities in, 166–167
hyperkalemia in, 166
hypertrophic cardiomyopathy in, 164
ischemia in, 165–166
long QT syndrome in, 165
myocarditis in, 164
pathognomonic electrocardiographic patterns in, 167, 168
pericarditis/pericardial effusion in, 164
short QT syndrome in, 165
syncope evaluated with, 363
technique in, 151–152
transesophageal recording/pacing with, 172–173
ventricular hypertrophy in, 156–160
left, 158–159
right, 156–158
single, 159–160
Ellis-Van Creveld syndrome (Chondroectodermal dysplasia), 68
Embroyology, 13–25
aortic arches development in, 18, 19, 23–24
cardiac loop formation in, 13, 16
cardiogenic crescent development in, 13, 16
defined, 13
fifth week of life in, 19–23
first week of life in, 13, 14
forth week of life in, 15–19
horizons in, 15, 20
intra-embryonic celom development in, 13, 17
mesoderm development in, 13, 15
second week of life in, 13, 14
sixth/seventh week of life in, 23
straight heart tube development in, 13, 16
third week of life in, 13–15, 16, 17
ventricle formation in, 17
Emery-Dreifuss muscular dystrophy, 419
Enalapril, 88, 908
Enalaprilat, 908
Endocardial cushion type of defects, 529, 540, 663–674
anatomy of, 663–666
atrioventricular defect in, 664–665
ventricular defect in, 664
atrioventricular canal defects as, 670–673
cardiac catheterization for, 671–673
chest X-ray for, 670

Endocardial cushion type of
defects *(Continued)*
echocardiogram of, 670–671
electrocardiograph of, 670
history of, 670
management of, 673
physical examination for, 670
surgery for, 673
Children's Hospital Boston experience with, 666, 673
clinical manifestations of, 667–673
definition of, 663
embryology of, 663
fetal echocardiogram of, 667
genetics of, 663
ostium primum defects as, 667–670
cardiac catheterization for, 669–670
chest X-ray for, 668
course for, 670
echocardiogram of, 668–669
electrocardiograph of, 668
history of, 667
management of, 670
physical examination for, 667–668
physiology of, 666–667
summary of, 673–674
surgery for, 852–853
Endocardial fibroelastosis (EFE), 419, 422–423
Endocarditis. *See also* Infective endocarditis
cardiac catheterization risks of, 215
Endocrinopathies, 84
Endothelial precursor cells (EPC), 886
Endothelin, 314
Endothelin receptor antagonists, pulmonary hypertension therapy with, 122, 123
Endothelin-1, 113, 114
Entrance block, 479
EPC. *See* Endothelial precursor cells
Epinephrine, 907, 908
Erythema marginatum, rheumatic fever with, 391
Erythrocyte sedimentation rate (ESR), 141
Esmolol, 508–509, 908
ESR. *See* Erythrocyte sedimentation rate
Etomidate, 910
Excitability, cardiac, 891–904
cardiac action potential with, 892–893
ion channels and, 898
cardiac arrhythmias and, 896
cardiac ion channels with, 893, 894
depolarization with, 891
episodic excitable cell disorders with, 903
HERG encodes potassium channels with, 900–901
hyperpolarization with, 891
ion channel dysfunction with, 902–903
KVLQT1 form potassium channels with, 899–900
long QT syndrome with, 896–897
mechanism of arrhythmia with, 901–902
MinK form potassium channels with, 899–900
modulatory potassium channels with, 895–896
Excitability, cardiac *(Continued)*
Romano-Ward syndrome with, 896
RyR2 encodes calcium release channel with, 901
sinoatrial nodal action potential with, 893–894
sodium channel dysfunction with, 899
torsades de pointes with, 896
ventricular action potential with, 894–895
diastolic depolarization in, 895
phase 0 depolarization in, 894
phase 1 early repolarization in, 894–895
phase 2 action potential plateau in, 895
phase 3 final repolarization in, 895
phase 4 resting membrane potential in, 895
Exercise intolerance
familial hypertrophic cardiomyopathy with, 434
hypoxemia with, 100
valvar aortic stenosis with, 587
Exercise testing, 275–268
bicycle v. treadmill in, 278
Bruce protocol in, 279
central hemodynamics with, 277–278
chest pain evaluated with, 368
clinical questions for, 278
conduct of, 278–279
electrocardiography evaluation with, 168–170
interpretation of physiology tests with, 279–286
blood pressure in, 285
breathing reserve in, 283–284
end-tidal P_{CO2} in, 284–285
exercise electrocardiogram in, 285–286
heart rate in, 282
minute ventilation in, 283–284
V_{O2} max in, 279–280
oxygen pulse in, 282–283
peak work rate in, 280–281
respiratory exchange ratio in, 282
respiratory rate in, 284
tidal volume in, 284
ventilatory anaerobic threshold in, 281–282
physiology with, 275–277
dead space/tidal volume ratio in, 277
heart rate in, 275
oxygen extraction in, 276–277
respiratory rate in, 277
stroke volume in, 275–276
tidal volume in, 277
syncope evaluated with, 363
valvar aortic stenosis in, 584
Exit block, 479
Extracorporeal life support (ECLS), 872–873
Extracorporeal membrane oxygenation (ECMO), 872–874
cannulae in, 873
contraindications for, 316
indications for, 315, 873–874
acute myocarditis as, 874
bridge to transplantation as, 873–874
postcardiotomy failure as, 873
unexpected cardiac arrest as, 873
Extracorporeal membrane oxygenation (ECMO) *(Continued)*
intensive care unit with, 315
oxygenators in, 873
patient management with, 874
pumps in, 873
results with, 874
stabilization phase in, 874
weaning phase in, 874

F

Fainting, 360. *See also* Syncope
Familial cardiomyopathy, 60
Familial hyperlipidemia (FH), 376
Familial hypertrophic cardiomyopathy (FCM), 432–441
alcohol septal ablation for, 439
antiarrhythmics for, 439–440
arrhythmias with, 435
β blockers for, 438
calcium channel blockers for, 438
cardiac catheterization for, 437
clinical course for, 440–441
clinical description of, 435–437
diastolic dysfunction with, 434
differential diagnosis for, 437–438
echocardiogram for, 436
electrocardiogram for, 436
exercise intolerance with, 434
exercise restriction for, 440
exercise testing for, 436–437
genetics of, 432–433
ischemia with, 434–435
magnetic resonance imaging for, 437
management of, 438–440
myocardial bridging with, 435
pacemaker therapy for, 439
pathology of, 433–434
pathophysiology of, 434–435
physical examination for, 435–436
risk stratification for, 440
sudden death with, 435
surgical myectomy for, 439
systemic bacterial endocarditis prophylaxis for, 439
vasodilators for, 438–439
Fast response, 146
Fenoldopam, 908
Fentanyl, 910
Fetal alcohol syndrome, 65, 66
Fetal arrhythmia, 197–198
Fetal circulation, 75–78. *See also* Transitional circulation
blood oxygen content with, 75, 76
congenital heart disease consequences for, 77–78
inferior vena cava return with, 75
lamb, 76, 77
placenta blood return with, 75
umbilical venous return with, 75
Fetal echocardiography, 195–198
CHD detection with, 195–196
clinical implications with, 198

Fetal echocardiography *(Continued)*
counseling with, 198
fetal arrhythmia in, 197–198
fetal circulation in, 196
history, 195
indications for, 197
limitations of, 198
technique with, 196–197
views, 196
FH. *See* Familial hyperlipidemia
Fibroma, 826
Fistula, between coronary artery and cardiac chamber, 620
Fistulae, vascular, 799–803
aorto-left ventricular tunnel, 802–803
cerebral, 802
coronary, 799–800
definition of, 799
prevalence of, 799
pulmonary arteriovenous, 800–801
Flecainide, 508, 909
Fick method, 222
Fludrocortisone, syncope treated with, 364
Fontan procedure, 655
components modified by, 865
Hypoplastic left heart syndrome treated with, 725
indications for, 864
postoperative management after, 865–866
results with, 866–867
early outcome, 866–867
late outcome, 867
risk factors for, 864, 867
single ventricle treated with, 744, 749
technique in, 864–865
tricuspid atresia treated with, 756
univentricular heart managed with, 864–867
Friedreich ataxia, 168, 441–442
Furosemide, 908

G

Gene defects, cardiovascular, 58, 60
allelic/nonallelic heterogeneity as, 60
arrhythmias as, 60
familial cardiomyopathy as, 60
malformation syndromes as, 58, 60
mitochondrial disorders as, 60
nonsyndromic defects as, 60
Glenn operation, bidirectional, 848–849
Glucose, 907
Glycogenosis, 419
Gradients, 219

H

HCM. *See* Hypertrophic cardiomyopathy
HDL. *See* High-density lipoprotein
Head-up tilt (HUT), 170
Head-up tilt testing, syncope evaluated with, 363
Heart failure
adult congenital heart disease with, 833–837
impaired oxygen consumption in, 834
impaired vital capacity in, 834
noncardiac etiologies for, 834

Heart failure *(Continued)*
pulmonary vascular disease as, 835–836
right ventricular dysfunction as, 836–837
ventricular vascular coupling as, 834–835
Heart failure with normal systolic function, 83
Heart rate, 275
exercise testing with, 282
Heart sounds
clicks, 136–137
first, 135
fourth, 136
murmurs, 137–138
opening snap, 136
pericardial friction rub, 137
second, 135–136
third, 136
HEB. *See* His bundle electrogram
Helicobacter pylori infection, 365
Hematocrit, 140
Hematology tests, 140–141
erythrocyte sedimentation rate in, 141
hematocrit in, 140
Howell-Jolly bodies in, 141
leukocytosis in, 140
platelets in, 140–141
Hemitruncus, 787–789
cardiac catheterization for, 789
chest X-ray for, 788
clinical manifestations of, 787–789
definition of, 787
echocardiogram of, 788–789
electrocardiograph of, 788
management of, 789
pathology of, 787
physiology of, 787
prevalence of, 787
Hemodialysis, 318
Hemodilution, 105
Heparin, 909–910
Hereditary hemorrhagic telangiectasia (HHT), 115
HERG, 900–901
Heterotaxy syndrome, 141
Heterotaxy, visceral, 676–693
age at death with, 691
anatomic findings in asplenia with, 688
anatomic findings in polysplenia syndrome with, 688
cardiac catheterization for, 692
characteristics of, 675
chest X-ray for, 690
clinical manifestations of, 688–692
definition of, 675
double rightness with, 677
echocardiogram of, 690–692
electrocardiograph of, 689–690
left lung isomerism with, 677
management of, 693
noncardiac anomalies in, 692–639
pathology of, 677–688
anatomically left atrium, 684
anatomically right atrium, 684
atrial septum, 682, 686

Heterotaxy, visceral *(Continued)*
atrial situs, 682–684
atrial situs ambiguus in, 684
atrioventricular valves, 684–686
bilateral superior venae cavae, 680
coronary sinus septum, 679
hepatic veins, 678–679
inferior vena cava, 678, 679
linkages between anomalies in, 687–688
liver, 677
lungs, 677
mesentery, 677
pulmonary veins, 680–682
segmental combinations in, 687
spleen, 677
superior vena cava, 679–680
systemic veins, 677, 679
ventricles, 685–686
ventricular outflow tract obstruction in, 686–687
physical examination for, 688–689
prevalence of, 677
right atrial isomerism with, 677
right pulmonary isomerism with, 677
HHT. *See* Hereditary hemorrhagic telangiectasia
Hibernoma, 465
High right atrium (HRA), 175
High-density lipoprotein (HDL), 373–374
High-pulse repetition frequency Doppler (HPRF), 186
His bundle electrogram (HBE), 175
His-Purkinje conduction, 177
Histiocytoid cardiomyopathy, 500
History, pediatric, 129–131
birth defects in, 129–130
chest pain evaluated with, 367
chest pain in, 130–131
common issues in, 130–131
cyanosis in, 130
endurance in, 130
family history in, 130
growth/development in, 130
initial murmur detection in, 130
palpitations in, 131
perinatal history in, 129
pregnancy history in, 129
prenatal testing for, 129
pulmonary hypertension in, 120–124
syncope in, 131
HIV. *See* Human immunodeficiency virus
HLHS. *See* Hypoplastic left heart syndrome
Holmes heart, 745
Holter monitoring/event recording, 167–168
Holt-Oram syndrome, 67
Homograft, 855–856
Horizons, developmental, 15, 20
Howell-Jolly bodies, 141
HPRF. *See* High-pulse repetition frequency Doppler
HRA. *See* High right atrium

Human immunodeficiency virus (HIV), 460
cardiac disease associated with, 428–429
Hunter syndrome, 432
Hurler syndrome, 51
HUT. *See* Head-up tilt
Hydralazine, 908
Hydrochlorothiazide, 908
Hyperkalemia, 166, 168
Hyperlipidemia. *See* Dyslipidemia
Hyperoxia test, 141–142
Hyperpolarization, 891
Hypersensitive xiphoid, 365
Hypertaurinuria, 419
Hypertension, 84, 377–383. *See also* Pulmonary hypertension
atherosclerotic cardiovascular risk from, 377
blood pressure defining, 377–381
causes for secondary, 382
central nervous system causing, 382
coarctation of aorta causing, 382
diagnostic evaluation for, 381–382
dietary approaches to, 382–383
endocrine disorders causing, 382
management algorithm for, 381
management of, 382–383
measurement of, 381
medication for, 383
white-coat, 377
Hyperthermia, 168
Hyperthyroidism, 168
Hypertrophic cardiomyopathy (HCM), 164, 168, 432–442
classification of, 432
familial, 432–441
Friedreich ataxia as, 441–442
maternally inherited, 432
sarcomeric, 432
ventricular tachycardia with, 502
Hypertrophic osteoarthropathy, hypoxemia with, 98, 99
Hypertrophic subaortic stenosis, 590
Hypoglycemia, 84
Hypokalemia, 167, 168
Hypoplastic left heart syndrome (HLHS), 57, 715–726
anatomy of, 715, 716
cardiac catheterization for, 720
cardiac transplantation for, 725
chest X-ray for, 719
Children's Hospital Boston experience with, 725
clinical manifestations of, 719–720
definition of, 715
echocardiogram of, 719–720
electrocardiograph of, 719
Fontan operation for, 725
management of, 720–726
controlled hypoventilation in, 720–721
ethical issues in, 725–726
after palliation, 724–725
physiology of, 715–719
closing ductus in, 717
Hypoplastic left heart syndrome (HLHS) *(Continued)*
force feeding of pulmonary circulation in, 717
honeymoon period in, 717
ideal preoperative, 715
overview, 715–716
transitional circulation in, 716–719
prevalence of, 715
surgery for, 721–724, 845–857
arteriopulmonary shunt in, 848
bidirectional Glenn operation in, 848–849
Blalock-Taussig shunt for, 845–856
Damus-Kaye-Stanzel operation in, 848, 849
inspired CO_2 in, 847
inspired O_2 in, 847
pulmonary artery band in, 848
pulmonary vascular resistance manipulation in, 847–848
results with, 846
single-ventricle physiology in, 846–847
standard Norwood operation for, 845–856
systemic vascular resistance in, 847–848
techniques for, 845–856
surgical complications in treatment of, 721–724
arterial-pulmonary shunts with, 724
arterial-pulmonary stenosis with, 724
atrial septum with, 721–722
coarctation of aorta with, 723–724
peripheral pulmonary stenosis with, 724
pulmonary vascular disease with, 724
right ventricular myocardial problems with, 723
stenosis of pulmonary veins with, 722
systemic pulmonary valve with, 724
tricuspid regurgitation with, 722–723
Hypotension, 306
Hypothermia, deep, 104
Hypothyroidism, 84, 168
Hypoxemia, 97–100
brain abscess with, 100
cerebrovascular accidents with, 100
clinical correlates of, 97–100
clubbing with, 98, 99
cyanosis with, 97–98
cyanotic spells with, 100
defined, 97
exercise intolerance with, 100
hypertrophic osteoarthropathy with, 98, 99
hypoxic spells with, 100
polycythemia with, 98–99
squatting with, 99–100
transitional circulation with, 79
Hypoxic ischemic injury, 84
Hypoxic spells, hypoxemia with, 100

I

IART. *See* Intra-atrial reentrant tachycardia
ICD. *See* Implantable cardioverter defibrillators
Idiopathic dilation of pulmonary artery, 555
Idiopathic VT, 503
IDL. *See* Intermediate-density lipoprotein
Imaging techniques, 183–206
computed tomography, 206
database development influence by technology of, 332–333
echocardiography, 183–199
apical view in, 189, 190
complications with, 198–199
contrast, 187–188
Doppler, 185–187
equipment for, 188
examination objectives for, 188
examination technique with, 188
fetal, 195–198
four-chamber view in, 188
indications for, 184
interpretations of, 191
M-mode, 184
parasternal views in, 189–191
quantitative analysis for, 191–193
reporting of, 191
safety for, 198–199
sedation with, 188
special procedures for, 193–195
standard imaging planes for, 188–189
subcostal view in, 189, 190
subxiphoid view in, 189, 190
suprasternal notch view in, 190, 191
technical background on, 183–184
three-dimensional, 185
two-dimensional, 184–185
views, 188–191
MRI, 199–206
anesthesia for, 205–206
background, 199
black blood imaging in, 200
bright blood imaging in, 200–201
cardiac/respiratory gating in, 199
CHD evaluation with, 202–205
contraindications for, 205
contrast-enhanced 3-dimensional MR angiography, 202
double inversion recovery in, 200
gradient echo in, 200–201
indications for, 203–205
myocardial perfusion/viability with, 202
pulse sequences in, 199
safety for, 205
sedation for, 205–206
spin echo in, 200
techniques, 199–202
velocity encoded cine, 202
ventricular function assessment with, 201–202
Immotile cilia syndrome, 57
Immune globulin, 909
Implantable cardioverter defibrillators (ICD), 440, 511–515
chest x-ray showing, 515
functions of, 514
leads/implant techniques for, 514–515
operation of, 514
Incisional atrial reentrant tachycardia, 487
Indomethacine, 909

Infant aortic stenosis, 588–589
Infection, 84, 319
  helicobacter pylori, 365
  post-transplantation management with, 884
Infective endocarditis, 395, 467–475
  cardiac conditions associated with, 473
  complications with, 472
  definition of, 470–471
  diagnosis of, 468–469
  Duke criteria for, 470–471
  echocardiogram with, 469–471
  epidemiology of, 467–468
  laboratory diagnosis of, 469
  pathophysiology of, 468
  prophylaxis for, 472–475
  treatment for, 471–472
  valvar aortic stenosis with, 587
Infective myocarditis, 421–422
Inferior vena cava type defect, 605
Inferior vena caval sinus venous defect, 612
Inflammatory bowel disease, 460
Infundibular defects, 529, 539
Infundibulum, 32, 34
Innocent heart murmurs, 357–360
  cervical venous hum as, 359
  clinical manifestations of, 357–359
  diagnostic testing for, 359
  general characteristics of, 357–358
  innocent pulmonic systolic murmur as, 359
  laboratory findings on, 359
  management of, 359–360
  physiologic ejection murmur as, 359
  physiologic pulmonary artery branch stenosis of newborn as, 359
  prevalence of, 357
  prognosis for, 360
  Still's murmur as, 358
  supraclavicular arterial bruit as, 359
Innocent pulmonic systolic murmur, 359
Innominate artery compression syndrome, 821–822
Inotropic agents, drug therapy with, 908
Intensive care unit, 303–319
  cardiovascular interactions with other organs in, 315–319
    atelectasis with, 317
    bronchospasm with, 317
    central nervous system with, 317–318
    diaphragmatic paresis with, 316–317
    fluid management with, 318
    gastrointestinal issues with, 318–319
    heart-lung, 315–317
    increased airway resistance with, 317
    infection with, 319
    pleural effusions with, 317
    pneumonia with, 317
    postextubation stridor with, 317
    pulmonary edema with, 317
    renal function with, 318
    respiratory function with, 315–317
  diastolic dysfunction with, 312–313
  history of, 303
  multidisciplinary care at, 304
Intensive care unit *(Continued)*
  newborn considerations for, 304–305
  nursing orientation program for, 348
  postoperative care with, 305–312
    afterload-reducing agents for, 312
    anti-inflammatory agents for, 312
    assessment during, 305–306
    atriobiventricular pacing for, 312
    catecholamines for, 308–311
    elevated left atrial pressure causes for, 307
    low cardiac output during, 305
    low cardiac output syndrome during, 306, 307–308
    monitoring during, 306–307
    oxygen saturation causes for, 307
    pharmacologic support for, 308–312
    phosphodiesterase III inhibitors for, 311
    thyroid hormone for, 311–312
  preoperative care with, 305
  pulmonary hypertension managed in, 313–315
    critical care strategies for, 313
    mechanical circulatory support for, 315
    pulmonary vasodilators for, 313–315
  staff/patients, Children's Hospital Boston, 303–304
  tetralogy of Fallot postoperative care at, 570
Intermediate-density lipoprotein (IDL), 374
Interrupted aortic arch, 638–642
  anatomy of, 639
  cardiac catheterization for, 641
  chest X-ray for, 640
  Children's Hospital Boston experience with, 639
  clinical manifestations of, 640
  course of, 642
  definition of, 638
  echocardiogram of, 640–641
  electrocardiograph of, 640
  management of, 641–642
  physiology of, 640
  prevalence of, 638
  surgery for, 850
Interatrial plica, anterior, 27
Interventricular portion, 29
Intra-atrial reentrant tachycardia (IART), 487
Intra-embryonic celom, development of, 13, 17
Intravenous gamma globulins (IVIG), 406
Intraventricular conduction abnormalities, 160–163
  bifascicular block as, 162
  complete left bundle branch block as, 161–162
  complete right bundle branch block as, 160, 161
  incomplete right bundle branch block as, 160
  left anterior hemiblock as, 160–161
  left posterior hemiblock as, 161
  preexcitation as, 162–163
  ST segment changes with, 163–167
Intubation, drug therapy with, 910
Inverted normal heart, 40, 42
Ion channel
  cardiac, 893, 894
  dysfunction underlying arrhythmia from, 902–903
Iron-overload cardiomyopathy, 430–432
Ischemia, 165–166
  familial hypertrophic cardiomyopathy with, 434–435
Isolated atrial noninversion, 40, 43
Isolated infundibuloarterial inversion, 40, 43
Isolated ventricular inversion, 40, 43
Isolated ventricular noninversion, 40, 43
Isometric atrial appendages, 30
Isoproterenol, 313, 908
IVIG. *See* Intravenous gamma globulins

J

JET. *See* Junctional ectopic tachycardia
Joint diseases, 395
Jones criteria, 393–394
Junctional ectopic tachycardia (JET), 483, 486–487
Junctional premature beats, 480–481

K

Kartagener syndrome, 57, 693
Kawasaki disease, 84, 401–409, 419, 460
  antithrombotics for, 406
  cardiac catheterization with, 405, 406
  chest radiography with, 404
  clinical manifestations of, 402–404
  coronary aneurysms with, 407–408
  coronary arterial changes with, 407
  corticosteroids for, 406
  course of, 407
  course without detectable lesions of, 408–409
  definition of, 401
  echocardiogram with, 404–405
  electrocardiogram with, 404
  etiology of, 401–402
  intravenous gamma globulins for, 406
  laboratory data on, 404
  management of, 405–407
  myocardial infarction with, 407
  pathogenesis of, 401–402
  pathology of, 402
  prevalence of, 401
  salicylates for, 405
  spontaneous regression of aneurysm with, 408
  surgical management of, 407
  thrombolytics for, 406–407
Kearns-Sayre syndrome, 60, 168, 419
Keshan disease. *See* Selenium deficiency
Ketamine, 910
KVLQT1 form, potassium channels with, 899–900

L

Labetalol, 908
Laboratory tests, routine, 140–143
  arrhythmia evaluation as, 143
  chest radiograph, 142–143
  hematology, 140–141

Laboratory tests, routine *(Continued)*
erythrocyte sedimentation rate in, 141
hematocrit in, 140
Howell-Jolly bodies in, 141
leukocytosis in, 140
platelets in, 140–141
radioisotope scans, 142–143
urinalysis, 141–142
blood chemistries in, 141
blood cultures in, 141
hyperoxia test in, 141–142
oxygenation level in, 141–142
Laplace, law of, 254
Large atrial defect, D-transposition of great arteries with, 648
LDL. *See* Low-density lipoprotein
Left atrial enlargement, 156
Left atrial problems, 706–710
cor triatriatum as, 707–709
pulmonary vein stenosis as, 709–710
supravalvar mitral membrane as, 706–707
Left lung isomerism, 677
Left posterior fascicular tachycardia, 503
Left ventricular noncompaction (LVNC), 444–445
LEOPARD syndrome, 432
Leukocytosis, 140
Lidocaine, 507–508, 907
Limbic ledge, 27, 28
Lipoma, 465
Lipoproteins, 373–376
chylomicrons, 374
high-density, 373–374
intermediate-density, 374
low-density, 373–374
management of, 376–377
normative lipid values with, 375–376
very low-density, 374
Lisinopril, 908
L-loop ventricles, 168
Long QT syndrome, 500–501, 896–897
Lorazepam, 910
Low cardiac output syndrome, 306, 307–308
right-to-left shunts for, 308
signs of, 306
volume adjustments with, 308
Low-density lipoprotein (LDL), 373–374
Lupus erythematosis, 419
LVNC. *See* Left ventricular noncompaction
Lyme disease, 168

M

Magnesium sulfate, 907
Magnetic resonance imaging (MRI), 199–206
anesthesia for, 205–206, 301
atrial septal defect in, 609
background, 199
black blood imaging in, 200
bright blood imaging in, 200–201
cardiac tumors in, 829–830
cardiac/respiratory gating in, 199
central nervous system sequelae in, 103–104
CHD evaluation with, 202–205
Magnetic resonance imaging (MRI) *(Continued)*
coarctation of aorta in, 631
constrictive pericarditis in, 463
contraindications for, 205
contrast-enhanced 3-dimensional MR angiography, 202
corrected transposition great arteries in, 794
database development influence by technology of, 332–333
double inversion recovery in, 200
Ebstein disease in, 764
familial hypertrophic cardiomyopathy with, 437
gradient echo in, 200–201
indications for, 203–205
myocardial perfusion/viability with, 202
pulse sequences in, 199
safety for, 205
sedation for, 205–206
spin echo in, 200
supravalvar aortic stenosis in, 595
techniques, 199–202
tetralogy of Fallot in, 568–569
velocity encoded cine, 202
ventricular function assessment with, 201–202
ventricular septal defect in, 535
Mahaim fiber, 168
Marfan syndrome, 65–66
MAT. *See* Multifocal atrial tachycardia
Maternal lupus, 168
Maternal rubella, 624
Maternally inherited hypertrophic cardiomyopathy, 432
Maternally inherited myopathy and cardiomyopathy. *See* MIMyCA
Mechanical heart, cow implant of, 4
Mediastinitis, 319
MELAS (Mitochondrial myopathy, encephalopathy, lactacidosis, stroke syndrome), 60, 419
Membranous defects, 528–529, 539
MERFF (Myoclonic epilepsy and ragged-red fibers syndrome), 60, 419
Mesoderm, development of, 13, 15
Mesothelioma, 465
Methadone, 910
Metolazone, 908
Mexiletine, 507–508, 909
Midazolam, 910
Midodrine hydrochloride, syncope treated with, 364
Milrinone, 908
MIMyCA (Maternally inherited myopathy and cardiomyopathy), 60
MinK form, potassium channels with, 899–900
Minute ventilation, exercise testing with, 283–284
Mitochondrial myopathy, encephalopathy, lactacidosis, stroke syndrome. *See* MELAS
Mitral atresia, 726–727
cardiac catheterization for, 727
chest X-ray for, 727
Children's Hospital Boston experience with, 726
clinical manifestations of, 726–727
echocardiogram of, 727
electrocardiograph of, 727
management of, 727
pathophysiology of, 726
prevalence of, 726
Mitral regurgitation, 697–701
cardiac catheterization for, 700
chest X-ray for, 699
Children's Hospital Boston experience with, 698
clinical manifestations of, 698–700
echocardiogram of, 699–700
electrocardiograph of, 699
management of, 700–701
pathology of, 697
physiology of, 697–698
prevalence of, 697
Mitral stenosis, 84, 704–706
cardiac catheterization for, 705–706
chest X-ray for, 705
clinical manifestations of, 704–706
coarctation of aorta with, 636–637
echocardiogram of, 705
electrocardiograph of, 705
management of, 706
pathology of, 704
physiology of, 704–705
prevalence of, 704
Mitral valvar stenosis, balloon valvotomy for, 233–234
results with, 233–234
survival following, 234
technique in, 233
Mitral valve, 35
Mitral valve abnormalities, D-transposition of great arteries with, 647
Mitral valve disease. *See also* Mitral regurgitation; Mitral stenosis; Mitral valve prolapse
ventricular septal defect with, 545
Mitral valve prolapse, 701–704
atrial septal defect with, 613
cardiac catheterization for, 703
chest X-ray for, 703
Children's Hospital Boston experience with, 703
clinical manifestations of, 702–703
definition of, 701
echocardiogram of, 703
electrocardiograph of, 703
management of, 703–704
pathology of, 702
physiology of, 702
prevalence of, 701–702
Mitral valve replacement, 854
M-mode echocardiography, 184
Mobitz I, 505

Morphine, 910
MPS I. *See* Mucopolysaccharidosis type I
MRI. *See* Magnetic resonance imaging
Mucopolysaccharidoses, 419
Mucopolysaccharidosis type I (MPS I), 51
Multifocal atrial tachycardia (MAT), 483, 485–486
Murmurs, heart, 137–138. *See also* Innocent heart murmurs
  continuous, 138
  diastolic, 137
  initial detection of, 130
  intensity of, 137
  location of, 138
  phonocardiogram of, 583
  quality of, 138
  radiation of, 138
  rheumatic fever with, 397
  shape of, 138
  systolic, 137
  timing of, 137–138
Muscle relaxants, 298
Muscular defects, 529, 539
Muscular dystrophy, 168
Musculi pectinati, 29
Myocardial bridging, 435
Myocardial disease, 394–395
Myocardial failure, 84
Myocardial infarction, Kawasaki disease with, 407
Myocardial performance. *See* Performance assessment, myocardial/ventricular
Myocarditis, 164
Myoclonic epilepsy and ragged-red fibers syndrome. *See* MERFF
Myotonic dystrophy, 419, 429–430
Myotubular dystrophy, 419
Myxedema, 460
Myxoma, 826

N

Nadas, Sandor Alexander, 3–5
  birth of, 3
  Boston Children's hospital work of, 3, 5, 7
  death of, 5
  Detroit Children's hospital residency of, 3
  Greenfield, Massachusetts practice of, 3
  honors conferred on, 5
  Natural History Study with, 4
  pediatric cardiology in years of, 4–5
  retirement of, 5
  studies of, 3
  success of, 5
Nadolol, 508–509, 908
Naloxone, 907
NASPE. *See* North American Society of Pacing and Electrophysiology
Natriuretic peptide, 908
Natural History Study, 4
Necrotizing enterocolitis, 319
Nemaline myopathy, 419
Neoaortic regurgitation, 657
Neonatal balloon atrial septostomy, 239
Nephrotoxicity, 884
Neural crest migration abnormalities, 53–54
Neurally mediated syncope, 360, 361
Neurohormonal activation, adult congenital heart disease with, 837–838
Neurologic function. *See* Central nervous system sequelae of CHD
New York Heart Association (NYHA), 87
Nifedipine, 122, 909
Nitric oxide, 113–114, 314, 909
  pulmonary hypertension therapy with, 123
Nitroglycerine, 908
Nitroprusside, 313, 908
Node reentry, 483
Noonan syndrome, 66–67, 555
Norepinephrine, 908
North American Society of Pacing and Electrophysiology (NASPE), 512
Norwood operation, 845–856
Nothing by mouth guidelines (NPO), 293
NPO. *See* Nothing by mouth guidelines
Nuclear lung perfusion scanning, tetralogy of Fallot with, 568
Nursing, pediatric cardiovascular, 347–353
  advanced practice nurses in, 349
  conclusion on, 353
  fundamentals of, 350–353
    care coordination in, 352
    clinical practice guidelines in, 352–353
    managing complex therapies in, 352
    optimizing nutrition in, 352
    pain management in, 350
    patient-technology interface in, 352
    providing comfort in, 350–352
    sedation management in, 352
  importance of, 347
  intensive care unit orientation program for, 348
  leadership in, 347–349
  Master's degree holding nurses in, 349
  nurse-patient relationship with, 349–350
    developmentally appropriate care in, 350
    family-centered care in, 349–350
  organizational structure with, 347–349
  postoperative management plans with, 351
  specialty units with, 348
Nutrition, nursing in management of, 352
NYHA. *See* New York Heart Association

O

Obstructed pulmonary veins, 775–778
Obtuse margin, 34
Oliguria, 306, 318
Opening snap, 136
Opoids, 297
Orthodromic reciprocating tachycardia (ORT), 491–494, 496
  concealed accessory pathway with, 496
  WPW with, 492–494
Osteogenesis imperfecta, 419
Ostium primum closure, 22
Ostium primum defects, 667–670
  cardiac catheterization for, 669–670
  chest X-ray for, 668
  Children's Hospital Boston, experience with, 666
  course for, 670
  echocardiogram of, 668–669
  electrocardiograph of, 668
  history of, 667
  management of, 670
  physical examination for, 667–668
  surgery for, 853
Oxygen content, 219–220
Oxygen extraction, 276–277
Oxygen pulse, exercise testing with, 282–283
Oxygen saturation, 219–220
  causes for abnormal, 307
Oxygenation level, 141–142

P

P wave, 154
Pacemakers, 511–515
  antibradycardia operation with, 512
  class I indications for, 511
  familial hypertrophic cardiomyopathy treated with, 439
  generators/pacing modes for, 512–513
  implant techniques for, 513–514
  leads for, 513–514
Pain management, nursing for, 350
PA/IVS. *See* Pulmonary atresia with intact ventricular septum
Palliative atrial baffle procedures, 655
Pallid breath-holding spells, 360, 362
Palpation, cardiac examination with, 134
Palpitations, pediatric history with, 131
Pancuronium, 298
Papillary muscles, 31–32, 35
Parietal band, 32–33
Pars membranacea septi, 29
Partial anomalous pulmonary venous connection, 605
Partial anomalous venous return, 612
Patent ductus arteriosus, 84, 617–624
  anatomy of, 617–618, 623
  cardiac catheterization for, 620
  catheter closure of, 243–244
  chest X-ray for, 620, 623
  Children's Hospital Boston experience with, 618
  clinical manifestations of, 619–620
    fistula between coronary artery and cardiac chamber as, 620
    ruptured sinus of Valsalva as, 620
    tetralogy of Fallot with pulmonary atresia as, 620
    venous hum as, 620
  course of, 622–623
  definition of, 617
  echocardiogram of, 620, 623
  electrocardiograph of, 620, 623
  management of, 620–622
  physiology of, 618–619
  prevalence of, 617
  surgery for, 621

Patent ductus arteriosus *(Continued)*
variations on, 623–624
aneurysm of ductus arteriosus as, 624
maternal rubella as, 624
premature infants, 623–624
ventricular septal defect with, 543–544
Patent foramen ovale, 604
transcatheter closure of, 245–246
Pathobiological Determinants of Atherosclerosis in Youth (PDAY), 373
PDAY. *See* Pathobiological Determinants of Atherosclerosis in Youth
PEEP. *See* Positive end expiratory pressure
Penetrating bundle, 29
Penicillin, 395, 471
Performance assessment, myocardial/ventricular, 251–269
cardiac v. myocardial function in, 251–252
diastolic, 263–265
ventricular relaxation in, 263–265
fiber shortening factors in systolic, 253–263
afterload as, 254–257
contractility as, 257–263
Laplace, law of, with, 254
length-dependent activation as, 253–254
preload as, 253
preload-adjusted dP/dt in, 259
preload-adjusted maximal ventricular power in, 259
preload-recruitable stroke work in, 259
pressure-volume relationship in, 257–259
shortening deactivation in, 257
stress-shortening/stress-velocity analysis in, 259–263
wall stress v. fiber stress in, 257
systolic, 252–263
endocardial/mid-wall/global fiber shortening in, 252–253
fiber shortening factors in, 253–263
ventricular relaxation in diastolic, 263–265
factors affecting relaxation in, 264–265
indices of relaxation in, 264
ventricular/myocardial compliance with, 265–269
clinical interpretation of diastolic indices in, 268–269
diastolic filling in, 267–269
indices of myocardial compliance in, 265–266
overlap of active/passive periods of diastole in, 266–267
rate of ventricular flow propagation in, 268
tissue-Doppler diastolic indices in, 268
Pericardial cysts/tumors, 465
Pericardial disease, 459–465
absence of pericardium as, 463–465
acute pericarditis as, 459–460
electrocardiogram showing, 460
etiologies of, 460
constrictive pericarditis as, 462–464
definition of, 459
echocardiography indications for, 184
Pericardial disease *(Continued)*
pericardial cysts/tumors as, 465
pericardial effusion as, 460, 461–462
electrocardiogram showing, 461
etiologies of, 460
postpericardiotomy syndrome as, 460–461
pulsus paradoxus as, 461–462
tamponade as, 461–462
Pericardial effusion, 460, 461–462
electrocardiogram showing, 461
etiologies of, 460
Pericardial friction rub, 137
Pericardial hypertension, echocardiography indications for, 184
Pericarditis, 164
Pericardium, absence of, 463–465
Peripartum cardiomyopathy, 419
Peripheral pulmonary stenosis, 555–556
HLHS surgical complications of, 724
Peritoneal dialysis, 318
Permanent form of junctional reciprocating tachycardia (PJRT), 483, 496–498
Pharmacologic support, postoperative care with, 308–312
anti-inflammatory agents in, 312
catecholamines in, 308–311
phosphodiesterase III inhibitors in, 311
thyroid hormone in, 311–312
Pharmacologic therapy. *See* Drug therapy
Pharyngitis, 388–389
Phenoxybenzamine, 313
Phenylephrine, 908
Phosphodiesterase III inhibitors, 311
Phosphodiesterase inhibitors, pulmonary hypertension therapy with, 122, 123
Physical examination, 131–140
abdomen, 139
atrial septal defect in, 607–608
atrioventricular canal defects in, 670
blood pressure in, 133
caloric supplementation with, 132
cardiac, 134–138
auscultation in, 134–135
clicks in, 136–137
first heart sound in, 135
fourth heart sound in, 136
inspection in, 134
murmurs in, 137–138
opening snap in, 136
palpation in, 134
pericardial friction rub in, 137
second heart sound in, 135–136
third heart sound in, 136
chest, 139
chest deformity in, 139
chest wall examination in, 139
pulmonary auscultation in, 139
extremities, 139–140
clubbing in, 139–140
differential cyanosis in, 140
edema in, 139
familial hypertrophic cardiomyopathy in, 435–436
Physical examination *(Continued)*
general, 131–132
ostium primum defects in, 667–668
pulmonary hypertension in, 117
pulse in, 132–133
prominence of, 132–133
rate of, 132
rhythm of, 132
variation in, 133
respirations in, 133
total anomalous pulmonary venous return in, 776, 779
vascular rings in, 816
venous pressure in, 133–134
ventricular septal defect in, 532–534
visceral heterotaxy in, 688–689
vital signs in, 132–133
Physiologic ejection murmur, 359
Physiologic pulmonary artery branch stenosis of newborn, 359
PJRT. *See* Permanent form of junctional reciprocating tachycardia
Platelets, 140–141
Pleural effusions, 317
Pneumonia, 317, 460
Polyarteritis nodosa, 419
Polyarthritis, rheumatic fever with, 390–391
Polycythemia, 140
hypoxemia with, 98–99
Polymyositis, 419
Polysplenia syndrome, 30, 676, 688, 692. *See also* Heterotaxy, visceral
associated anatomic findings in, 688
diagnosis of, 692
Pompe's disease, 168
Portsmann plug, 243
Positive end expiratory pressure (PEEP), 316
Postextubation stridor, 317
Postnatal onset, 49
Postpericardiotomy syndrome, 460–461
Postural orthostatic tachycardia syndrome, 360, 362
Potassium channels
HERG encodes, 900–901
KVLQT1 form, 899–900
minK form, 899–900
modulatory, 895–896
PR interval, 154
Pregnancy history, 129
Premature beats, 477–481
atrial, 480
etiology of, 477–479
abnormal automaticity in, 478
reentry in, 477–478
triggered automaticity in, 478–479
junctional, 480–481
ventricular, 481
Premature infants, patent ductus arteriosus with, 623–624
Prenatal onset, 49

Preventive heart disease, 373–383
autopsy studies on, 373
dyslipidemia as, 374–377
genetic causes of, 376
lipids/lipoproteins description for, 374
lipids/lipoproteins measurement with, 375–376
management of, 376–377
normative lipid values with, 375
screening for, 374–376
secondary causes of, 376
hypertension as, 377–383
atherosclerotic cardiovascular risk from, 377
blood pressure defining, 377–381
causes for secondary, 382
central nervous system causing, 382
coarctation of aorta causing, 382
diagnostic evaluation for, 381–382
dietary approaches to, 382–383
endocrine disorders causing, 382
management algorithm for, 381
management of, 382–383
measurement of, 381
medication for, 383
white-coat, 377
risk factors with, 373
Primary ciliary dyskinesia, 57
Procainamide, 507, 909
Propafenone, 508, 909
Prophylaxis
for genitourinary procedures, 474
infective endocarditis recommended, 472–475
cardiac conditions associated with, 473
regimens, 473, 474
Propofol, 910
Propranolol, 508–509, 908
Prostacyclin, 113, 114, 313
pulmonary hypertension therapy with, 122, 123
Prostaglandin E_1, 907, 909
Proximal conal septum, 32–33
Psychogenic syncope, 362
Pulmonary arteries. *See also* Hemitruncus
balloon angioplasty for, 235–236
stents in, 240
Pulmonary arteriovenous fistulae, 800–801
chest X-ray for, 801
Children's Hospital Boston experience with, 800
clinical manifestations of, 801
course of, 801
definition of, 800
echocardiogram of, 801
electrocardiograph of, 801
management of, 801
pathology of, 801
physiology of, 801
prevalence of, 800
Pulmonary artery banding, 653, 848
Pulmonary artery sling, 820–821
anatomy of, 820
clinical manifestations of, 821
symptoms in, 821
course of, 821
definition of, 820
embryology of, 820
management of, 821
physical examination with, 821
Pulmonary atresia
cardiac catheterization for, 567–568
chest X-ray for, 732
clinical manifestations of, 564
course for, 575
echocardiogram of, 566, 732
management of, 571–572
MRI of, 569
pathology of, 561
physiology of, 563
tetralogy of Fallot with, 561, 563–564, 566–569, 571–572, 575
Pulmonary atresia with intact ventricular septum (PA/IVS), 729–734
anatomy of, 729–730
cardiac catheterization for, 732–733
Children's Hospital Boston experience with, 730, 733
clinical manifestations of, 731–733
definition of, 729
electrocardiograph of, 731–732
embryology of, 729
management of, 733–734
physiology of, 730–731
prevalence of, 729
surgery for, 853–854
variation with, 734
Pulmonary auscultation, 139
Pulmonary edema, 317
Pulmonary hypertension, 113–124
cardiac evaluation for, 117–118
cardiac catheterization in, 118, 119
echocardiography in, 117–118
cardiac transplantation contraindicated by, 878
chest radiograph for, 117, 118
clinical classification of, 116
clinical presentation of, 116–118
diagnostic evaluation of patients with, 118–120
electrocardiogram for, 117
evaluation of patients with, 116–120
functional classification of, 117
genetic causes of, 115–116
intensive care unit for, 313–315
mediators of, 113–114
arachidonic acid metabolites as, 113, 114
Endothelin-1 as, 113, 114
nitric oxide as, 113–114
prostacyclin as, 113, 114
natural history for, 120–124
pathophysiology of, 113–115
physical examination for, 117
pulmonary vascular development with, 113
Pulmonary hypertension *(Continued)*
refractory, 124
symptoms with, 116–117
therapy for, 120–124
acute vasodilator testing with, 121–122
agents in, 122
anticoagulation in, 123
calcium channel blockers in, 122
endothelin receptor antagonists in, 122, 123
general supportive care in, 123–124
inhaled nitric oxide in, 123
oxygen in, 123–124
patient survival with, 120–121
phosphodiesterase inhibitors in, 122, 123
prophylaxis measures in, 124
prostacyclin in, 122, 123
refractory pulmonary hypertension in, 124
right heart failure management in, 124
warfarin in, 122, 123
Pulmonary regurgitation, 555
Pulmonary stenosis, 549–556. *See also* Valvar pulmonary stenosis
anatomy of, 549, 550
Children's Hospital Boston experience with, 550, 554
critical in neonate, 553–554
definition of, 549
double-outlet right ventricle with, 737
D-transposition of great arteries with, 648, 657–658
dysplastic pulmonary valves with, 555
peripheral, 555–556
physiology with, 549–551
prevalence of, 549, 550
pulmonary regurgitation with, 555
valvar, 551–553
ventricular septal defect with, 544–545
Pulmonary valve replacement, 855
Pulmonary valves, transcatheter implantation of, 247
Pulmonary vascular disease
adult congenital heart disease with, 835–836
D-transposition of great arteries with, 649
HLHS surgical complications of, 724
ventricular septal defect with, 540–541
Pulmonary vascular obstructions, atrial septal defect with, 610
Pulmonary vascular resistance (PVR), 878
Pulmonary vasodilator
endothelin as, 314
hypertension managed with, 313–315
isoproterenol as, 313
nitric oxide as, 314
nitroprusside as, 313
phenoxybenzamine as, 313
prostacyclin as, 313
testing, 118
tolazaline as, 313
Pulmonary vein stenosis, 709–710
clinical manifestations of, 709–710
Pulmonary veins, 29

Pulmonary venous obstructions
cardiac catheterization for, 239
surgery for, 852
Pulmonary venous stenosis, 84
Pulse, 132–133
Corrigan's, 132
prominence of, 132–133
rate of, 132
rhythm of, 132
Takayasu's arteritis with, 132
variation in, 133
water hammer, 132
Pulsed Doppler, 185–186
Pulseless disease, 132
Pulsus paradoxus, 461–462
PVR. *See* Pulmonary vascular resistance

Q

QRS complex, 154
QT interval, 155
QT syndrome, 60, 165, 168, 500–501

R

RACHS-1. *See* Risk Adjustment for Congenital Heart Surgery
Radiofrequency (RF), 515–517
Radiography, chest, 142–143. *See also* Chest X-ray
Kawasaki disease with, 404
pulmonary hypertension in, 117, 118
Radioisotope scans, 142–143
Raghib syndrome, 605
RALES. *See* Randomized Aldosterone Evaluation Study
Randomized Aldosterone Evaluation Study (RALES), 89
Rapid incessant VT in infancy, 500
Rashkind device, 243
Rastelli procedure, 654
Reentry, 477–478
Reflex anoxic seizures, 360, 362
Refractory period, 147
Regional Infant Cardiac Program, 5
Repolarization, 146
Research, methodological issues in, 337–345
age/size related issues of, 340–343
AVA v. BSA with, 341
indexing for, 340–341
normalization for, 340–341
per-BSA method for, 340–341
transformation for, 342
z scores for, 342–343
anatomic diversity related issues of, 343–345
analytical techniques with, 344
RACHS-1 method for, 344–345
research tools with, 344–345
study group choice with, 344
hypothesis-driven analytical studies with, 337
pediatric cardiology with, 337
small study populations with, 337–340
alternative analytical strategies in, 339–340
informative patients in, 337–338
outcome variable choice in, 338
study design in, 338–339
Respiration, 133
Respiratory exchange ratio, exercise testing with, 282
Respiratory rate, 277
exercise testing with, 284
Restrictive cardiomyopathy, 442–443
causes of, 443
Resuscitation, drug therapy for, 907
Resynchronization therapy, 91
Retinoic acid embryopathy, 50
Reye syndrome, 419
RF. *See* Radiofrequency
Rhabdomyoma, 825–826
Rheumatic fever, 387–399, 460
abdominal pain with, 392
acute attack treatment with, 395–396
ancillary studies for, 392–393
cardiac catheterization for, 393, 397
carditis with, 391
chest X-ray for, 392–393
Children's Hospital Boston experience with, 388
chorea with, 390–393
clinical manifestations of, 390–392
course of, 396–397
definition of, 387
developing countries with, 387
diagnosis of, 393–394
differential diagnosis of, 394–395
infective endocarditis in, 395
joint diseases in, 395
myocardial disease in, 394–395
rheumatoid arthritis in, 395
sickle cell disease in, 395
echocardiogram for, 392–393, 397
electrocardiogram for, 392
erythema marginatum with, 391
genetic factors with, 389
group A streptococcal pharyngitis with, 388–389
Jones criteria for, 393–394
laboratory tests for, 392
management of, 395–396
penicillin in, 395
salicylates in, 395
murmurs with, 397
pathogenesis of, 388–389
pathogenetic hypothesis for, 389
pathology of, 389–390
polyarthritis with, 390–391
poverty-stricken populations with, 388
prevalence of, 387–388
primary prevention of, 398
probable, 393
pure chorea with, 392
recurrent, 396–398
secondary prevention of, 398–399
subcutaneous nodules with, 391
Rheumatic heart disease, echocardiography indications for, 184
Rheumatoid arthritis, 395, 460
Rhythm abnormalities, D-transposition of great arteries with, 655–656
Right atrial enlargement, 156
Right atrial isomerism, 677
Right pulmonary isomerism, 677
Right ventricle-dependent coronary circulation (RVDCC), 853
Right ventricular apex (RVA), 175
Right ventricular cardiomyopathy, 444
Right ventricular conduits, stents in, 241
Right ventricular dysfunction, adult congenital heart disease with, 836–837
Right ventricular myocardial problems, HLHS surgical complications of, 723
Risk Adjustment for Congenital Heart Surgery (RACHS-1), 344–345
Rocuronium, 298
Romano-Ward syndrome, 896
Roussey-Levy polyneuropathy, 419
Ruptured sinus of Valsalva, 620
RVA. *See* Right ventricular apex
RVDCC. *See* Right ventricle-dependent coronary circulation
Ryanodine receptor, 501
RyR2 encodes, calcium release channel with, 901

S

SAECG. *See* Signal averaged electrocardiogram
Salicylates, 395
Kawasaki disease treated with, 405
Sarcoidosis, 419
Sarcomeric hypertrophic cardiomyopathy, 432
SBE. *See* Infective endocarditis; Systemic bacterial endocarditis
Scapulohumeral muscular dystrophy, 419
Scimitar syndrome, 605, 606, 612–613
Secundum atrial septal defect, ventricular septal defect with, 543
Sedation/anesthesia, 291–301
angiography using, 301
cardiac arrest risk in surgery with, 292
cardiac surgery with, 292–295
cardiopulmonary bypass with
management after, 299
management during, 298–299
catheterization with, 299–301
anesthesia for, 299
general anesthesia for, 301
laboratory environment for, 299–300
sedation for, 300–301
drug therapy for, 910
early tracheal extubation with, 298
induction of, 295–296
inhalation, 296
intravenous, 295–296
maintenance of, 296–297
factors determining technique for, 296
inhalational anesthesia in, 296–297
opioid-based anesthesia in, 297
monitoring with, 294–295
intracardiac pressure measurement in, 294
intraoperative echocardiography in, 294–295
standard, 294

Sedation/anesthesia *(Continued)*
MRI using, 205–206, 301
nothing by mouth guidelines for, 293
nursing in management of, 352
overview, 291–292
premedication for surgery with, 293–294
preoperative assessment for, 292–293
preparation for, 292–293
stress response to surgery/bypass with, 297–298
muscle relaxants for, 298
structure of service in, 292
Segmental approach. *See* Diagnosis
Selenium deficiency (Keshan disease), 419
Semilunar valve replacement, 855–856
aortic, 855
autograft v. homograft for, 855–856
mechanical v. tissue valves for, 855
pulmonary, 855
Sepsis infection, 319
Septal band, 32–33
Septum primum, 29, 603
Septum secundum, 27, 28, 603
Sickle cell disease, 395
Signal averaged electrocardiogram (SAECG), 171–172
Sildenafil, 122
Single ventricle, 743–750
anatomy of, 743–745
cardiac catheterization for, 749
chest X-ray for, 747
Children's Hospital Boston experience with, 744
clinical manifestations of, 746–749
course of, 750
definition of, 743
echocardiogram of, 747–749
electrocardiograph of, 747
embryology of, 743
Fontan procedure for, 744, 749
Holmes heart with, 745
management of, 749–750
physiology of, 745–746
prevalence of, 743
surgical treatment of, 744
Sinoatrial node, 27
Sinoatrial node dysfunction, 504
Sinus node recovery time (SNRT), 176
Sinus tachycardia, 483
Sinus venosus defect, 604
Sinus venosus of right atrial type defect, 605
Sinus venosus septum, 604
Situational syncope, 362
Situs ambiguus, 30, 31
Situs inversus, 31, 168, 693
Situs solitus, 31
Slow response, 146
Slow transient VT in infancy, 500
SNRT. *See* Sinus node recovery time
Sodium bicarbonate, 907
Sodium channel, 146
Solitus normal heart, 42
Sotalol, 509–510, 909
Spinal muscular dystrophy, 419
Spironolactone, 89, 908
Square root sign, 463
Squatting, hypoxemia with, 99–100
ST segment, 154–155
St. Vitus' dance. *See* Sydenham's chorea
Stages, 15, 20
Standing wave effect, 582, 583
Stem cells, 886
Stenosis of pulmonary veins, HLHS surgical complications of, 722
Stents
aortic coarctation with, 240–241
cardiac catheterization with, 239–242
other uses of, 241–242
pulmonary arteries with, 240
right ventricular conduits with, 241
Still's murmur, 358
Straight heart tube, development of, 13, 16
Streptococcal pharyngitis, rheumatic fever with, 388–389
Streptokinase, 910
Stress testing. *See* Exercise testing
Stroke volume, 275–276
Subacute bacterial endocarditis (SBE). *See* Infective endocarditis
Subaortic stenosis, 84, 589–593
accessory endocardial cushion tissue type of, 590
cardiac catheterization for, 592
chest X-ray of, 591
Children's Hospital Boston experience with, 582, 591
clinical manifestations of, 590–592
course of, 593
definition of, 589
echocardiogram of, 591–592
electrocardiograph of, 591
hypertrophic type of, 590
management of, 592–593
pathogenesis of, 590
pathology of, 590
physiology of, 590
prevalence of, 582, 589
tricuspid atresia with, 754
tunnel type of, 590
Subclavian artery, aberrant, 24
Subcutaneous nodules, rheumatic fever with, 391
Subpulmonary defects, 529, 539
Succinylcholine, 298
Sulcus terminalis, 27
Superior vena cava, 27, 28
Superior vena cava type defect, 604
Superior vena caval sinus venous defect, 611
Supraclavicular arterial bruit, 359
Supravalvar aortic stenosis, 593–595
cardiac catheterization for, 595
Children's Hospital Boston experience with, 582
clinical manifestations of, 594–595
course of, 595
definition of, 593
Supravalvar aortic stenosis *(Continued)*
echocardiogram of, 594
electrocardiograph of, 594
management of, 595
MRI of, 595
physiology of, 593–594
prevalence of, 593
Supravalvar mitral membrane, 706–707
Supravalvar obstruction, 656
Supraventricular tachycardia (SVT), 177–178, 482, 484–498
automatic, 484–487
ectopic atrial tachycardia as, 483, 484–485
junctional ectopic tachycardia as, 483, 486–487
multifocal atrial tachycardia as, 483, 485–486
reentrant with accessory pathways, 490–498
antidromic reciprocating tachycardia as, 492, 494–496
orthodromic reciprocating tachycardia as, 491–494, 496
reentrant without accessory pathways, 487–490
atrial fibrillation as, 483, 488–489
atrial flutter as, 483, 487–488
AV nodal reentrant tachycardia as, 489
Surgery. *See also* Transplantation, cardiac
ASD in infants managed with, 849–850
atrial septal defect managed with, 610
atrioventricular canal defects managed with, 673
bidirectional cavopulmonary shunt, 863–864
indications for, 863
postoperative management after, 865–866
preoperative evaluation for, 863
results with, 864
technique in, 863–864
biventricular repair in, 849–850
central nervous system sequelae with, 104–105
acid-based management in, 104–105
arterial carbon dioxide tension in, 104–105
cardiopulmonary bypass in, 104–105
deep hypothermia in, 104
hemodilution in, 105
total circulatory arrest in, 104
Children's Hospital Boston experience in, 846
circulatory support in neonatal heart, 856
coarctation of aorta managed with, 631–632, 850
congestive heart failure managed with, 91
D-transposition of great arteries managed with, 653–655, 852
arterial switch procedures in, 654
atrial switch procedures in, 654
atrial switch to arterial switch conversion in, 655
Blalock-Hanlon technique in, 653
creation of atrial septal defect in, 653–654
Fontan procedure in, 655
palliative atrial baffle procedures in, 655
pulmonary artery banding in, 653

Surgery *(Continued)*
Rastelli procedure in, 654
staged physiologic repair in, 655
ventricular septal defect in, 654
endocardial cushion defects managed with, 852–853
extracorporeal membrane oxygenator support for, 872–874
cannulae in, 873
indications for, 873–874
oxygenators in, 873
patient management with, 874
pumps in, 873
results with, 874
stabilization phase in, 874
weaning phase in, 874
Fontan operation, 864–865
components modified by, 865
indications for, 864
postoperative management after, 865–866
results with, 866–867
risk factors for, 864, 867
technique in, 864–865
hypoplastic left heart syndrome managed with, 721–724, 845–857
arterial-pulmonary shunts complicating, 724
arterial-pulmonary stenosis complicating, 724
arteriopulmonary shunt in, 848
atrial septum complicating, 721–722
bidirectional Glenn operation in, 848–849
Blalock-Taussig shunt for, 845–856
coarctation of aorta complicating, 723–724
complications from, 721–724
Damus-Kaye-Stanzel operation in, 848, 849
inspired CO_2 in, 847
inspired O_2 in, 847
peripheral pulmonary stenosis complicating, 724
pulmonary artery band in, 848
pulmonary vascular disease complicating, 724
pulmonary vascular resistance manipulation in, 847–848
results with, 846
right ventricular myocardial problems complicating, 723
single-ventricle physiology in, 846–847
standard Norwood operation for, 845–856
stenosis of pulmonary veins complicating, 722
systemic pulmonary valve complicating, 724
systemic vascular resistance in, 847–848
techniques for, 845–856
tricuspid regurgitation complicating, 722–723
interrupted aortic arches managed with, 850
low-birth-weight, 856
minimally invasive, 869–872
incisions for, 871
ministernotomy trans-xyphoid approach in, 871
open-heart with, 870–872
results with, 872
thoracoscopic procedures for, 872

Surgery *(Continued)*
neonatal/infant, 845–857
ostium primum defect managed with, 853
patent ductus arteriosus managed with, 621
pediatric valve replacement in, 854–856
advantages/disadvantages of, 854
aortic, 855
atrioventricular, 854–855
autograft v. homograft for, 855–856
mechanical v. tissue valves for, 855
mitral, 854
pulmonary, 855
semilunar, 855–856
tricuspid, 854–855
pulmonary atresia with IVS managed with, 853–854
pulmonary venous obstructions managed with, 852
robotically assisted, 869–872
vascular ring division with, 870
sedation/anesthesia with, 292–295
single-ventricle palliation managed with, 845
stress response to, 297–298
technology's influence on, 333
tetralogy of Fallot managed with, 851–852
thoracoscopic approach to, 869–870, 872
port incisions in, 869–870
positioning in, 869–870
results with, 869–870
truncus arteriosus managed with, 850–851
univentricular heart managed with, 861–868
anatomy in, 861
neonatal interventions in, 861–862
after newborn, 862–863
pulmonary blood flow obstruction in, 862
systemic blood flow obstruction in, 862
ventricular septal defect in infants managed with, 850
Surgical myectomy, familial hypertrophic cardiomyopathy treated with, 439
SVT. *See* Supraventricular tachycardia
Sydenham's chorea (St. Vitus' dance), 391
Syncope, 360–364
cardiac, 360–361
cardiac catheterization for, 363
cardio-inhibitory, 360
clinical manifestations of, 361–362
common fainting as, 360
convulsive, 361–362
course for, 364
definition of, 360
diagnostic evaluation for, 362–363
drug therapy for, 364
echocardiography for, 184, 363
electrocardiography for, 363
exercise-induced, 362
head-up tilt testing for, 363
incidence of, 360
management of, 363–364
neurally mediated, 360, 361
nonpharmacologic, nondevice therapy for, 364
pallid breath-holding spells as, 360, 362

Syncope *(Continued)*
pediatric history with, 131
physiology of, 360–361
postural orthostatic tachycardia syndrome as, 360, 362
premonitory symptom frequency for, 358
psychogenic, 362
reflex anoxic seizures as, 360, 362
situational, 362
toddler, 362
treadmill exercise testing for, 363
vasodepressor, 360
vasovagal, 360
white, 362
Systemic bacterial endocarditis (SBE), 439
Systemic inflow obstruction, 84
Systemic lupus erythematosus, 460
Systemic outflow obstruction, 84
Systemic pulmonary valve, HLHS surgical complications of, 724

T

T wave, 155
T_A wave, 154
Tachy-brady syndrome, 504
Tachycardia, 306, 477–479, 481–504
antidromic reciprocating, 492, 494–496
atrial fibrillation as, 483, 488–489
atrial flutter as, 483, 487–488
automatic supraventricular, 484–487
AV nodal reentrant, 489
bedside diagnosis of, 482
classification of, 482
differential diagnosis of QRS, 482–484
ectopic atrial, 483, 484–485
etiology of, 477–479
abnormal automaticity in, 478
reentry in, 477–478
triggered automaticity in, 478–479
junctional ectopic, 483, 486–487
management of, 484–504
mechanisms for, 482
multifocal atrial, 483, 485–486
orthodromic reciprocating, 491–494, 496
permanent form of junctional reciprocating, 483, 496–498
sinus, 483
SVA due to accessory pathways as, 490–492
SVA not involving accessory pathways as, 487–490
terminology with, 482
ventricular, 498–504
Takayasu's arteritis, 132
Tamponade, 461–462
TAPVC. *See* Total anomalous pulmonary venous connection
Taussig-Bing anomaly, Double-outlet right ventricle with, 737
Taussig-Bing malformation, 20
TEE. *See* Transesophageal echocardiography
Teratogens, 64–65
cardiovascular abnormalities caused by, 65
fetal alcohol syndrome with, 65, 66

Teratoma, 465
  pericardial, 826–827
Tetralogy of Fallot, 20, 43, 559–576
  anatomy of, 559–560
  cardiac catheterization for, 567–568
    absent pulmonary valve with, 568
    common atrioventricular canal with, 568
    pulmonary atresia with, 567–568
  chest X-ray of, 565
    absent pulmonary valve with, 565
    pulmonary atresia with, 565
  Children's Hospital Boston experience with, 560, 573
  clinical manifestations of, 563–564
    absent pulmonary valve with, 564
    common atrioventricular canal with, 564
    pulmonary atresia with, 564
  course for, 573–576
    absent pulmonary valve with, 575–576
    common atrioventricular canal with, 576
    pulmonary atresia with, 575
  definition of, 559
  drugs for vasodilation for, 570
  echocardiogram of, 565–567
    absent pulmonary valve with, 566–567
    common atrioventricular canal with, 567
    pulmonary atresia with, 566
  electrocardiogram of, 564–565
    common atrioventricular canal with, 565
  intensive care unit for, 570
  management of, 569–573
    absent pulmonary valve with, 572
    common atrioventricular canal with, 573
    pulmonary atresia with, 571–572
  MRI of, 568–569
    absent pulmonary valve with, 569
    common atrioventricular canal with, 569
    pulmonary atresia with, 567–569
  nuclear lung perfusion scanning for, 568
  patent ductus arteriosus with, 620
  pathology of, 559–562
    absent pulmonary valve with, 561–562
    common atrioventricular canal with, 562
    pulmonary atresia with, 561
  phonocardiogram of, 563
  physiology of, 562–563
    absent pulmonary valve with, 563
    common atrioventricular canal with, 563
    pulmonary atresia with, 563
  prevalence of, 559
  surgery for, 851–852
  surgical repair of, 570
Tetrasomy 22p syndrome (Cat-eye syndrome), 63
Thalassemia, 430–432
Thiamine deficiency (Beri-beri), 419
Thoracophagus twins, 693
Thoracoscopic procedures, 869–870, 872
  cardiopulmonary bypass with, 872
Threshold potential, 146
Thrombi, 827
Thrombocytopenia, 140
Thrombolytics, 406–407
Thyroid hormone, 311–312
Tidal volume, 277
  exercise testing with, 284
Tinea sagittalis, 29
Tissue Doppler, 186
Tissue engineering, 885–887
  bone marrow mesenchymal stem cells for, 886
  current replacement devices and, 885
  endothelial precursor cells for, 886
  laboratory projects with, 885–886
  need for, 885
  problems with, 886
Tissue plasminogen activator, 910
Toddler syncope, 362
Tolazaline, 313
Torsades de pointes, 896
Total anomalous pulmonary venous connection (TAPVC), 314
Total anomalous pulmonary venous return, 773–780
  anatomy of, 773–775
  cardiac catheterization for, 778, 779
  chest X-ray for, 776, 777, 779
  Children's Hospital Boston experience with, 774
  clinical manifestations of, 775–779
  course of, 780
  definition of, 773
  echocardiogram of, 776, 779
  electrocardiograph of, 776, 779
  embryology of, 773
  management of, 779–780
  obstructed pulmonary veins with, 775–778
  physical examination for, 776, 779
  physiology of, 774
  prevalence of, 773
  unrestricted pulmonary blood flow with, 778–779
Total circulatory arrest, 104
Totally anomalous pulmonary veins, 84
Trabeculae carneae, 31
Tranexamic acid, 910
Transesophageal echocardiography (TEE), 172–173, 193–195
  equipment for, 194
  indications for, 193–194
  patient selection for, 194
  safety for, 194
  technique for, 194
  views, 195
Transitional circulation, 78–79
  hypoxemia with, 79
Transplantation, cardiac, 877–885
  allocation process for, 879
  cardiomyopathy with, 878
  cause of death following, 882
  Children's Hospital Boston experience with, 878, 881
  congenital heart disease with, 877–878
  contraindications for, 878–879
    malignancy as, 879
    pulmonary hypertension as, 878
    renal/hepatic dysfunction as, 879
Transplantation, cardiac *(Continued)*
  donor selection/procurement with, 880
  evaluation for, 878–879
  extracorporeal membrane oxygenation for, 873–874
  health maintenance following, 885
  hypoplastic left heart syndrome treated with, 725
  indications for, 877
  noncompliance with therapy following, 884–885
  outcome following, 885
  postoperative management for, 881
  post-transplantation management issues for, 882–884
    coronary vasculopathy as, 883–884
    infection as, 884
    long-term management as, 884
    nephrotoxicity as, 884
    rejection as, 882–883
  pretransplantation management for, 879–880
  psychosocial issues with, 884–885
  surgical techniques for, 880–881
    recipient operation in, 880–881
  survival following, 881–882
Transposition of great arteries, 40, 43–45. *See also* Corrected transposition great arteries
  double-outlet right ventricle with, 737
Triangle of Koch, 29, 147, 148
Tricuspid abnormalities, D-transposition of great arteries with, 647
Tricuspid atresia, 168, 753–758
  anatomy of, 753
  cardiac catheterization for, 756
  chest X-ray for, 755
  Children's Hospital Boston experience with, 754, 757
  clinical manifestations of, 754–756
  course of, 757–758
  definition of, 753
  echocardiogram of, 575–756
  electrocardiograph of, 755
  Fontan procedure for, 756
  management of, 756–757
  physiology of, 753–754
  prevalence of, 753
  subaortic stenosis with, 754
Tricuspid regurgitation, 656
  HLHS surgical complications of, 722–723
Tricuspid valve, 32. *See also* Ebstein disease
  problems, 761–765
  replacement, 854–855
Triggered automaticity, 478–479
Tri-iodothyronine, 908
Trisomy 13 syndrome, 63
Trisomy 18 syndrome, 62–63
Trisomy 21. *See* Down syndrome
Truncal valve stenosis, 84

Truncus arteriosus, 84, 767–771
anatomy of, 767–769
cardiac catheterization for, 770
chest X-ray for, 770
Children's Hospital Boston experience with, 768
clinical manifestations of, 769–770
definition of, 767
echocardiogram of, 770
electrocardiograph of, 770
embryology of, 767
management of, 770–771
physiology of, 769
prevalence of, 767
surgery for, 850–851
Tumors, cardiac, 825–831
benign primary, 827
cardiac catheterization for, 829
chest X-ray of, 828
Children's Hospital Boston experience with, 826
clinical manifestations of, 827–828
child/adolescent, 828
fetal, 827
neonate, 827
echocardiogram of, 828–829
electrocardiogram of, 828
fibroma as, 826
imaging modalitics for, 828–830
management of, 830–831
MRI for, 829–830
myxoma as, 826
pathophysiology of, 825–827
pericardial teratoma as, 826–827
prevalence of, 825
primary malignant, 827
rhabdomyoma as, 825–826
thrombi as, 827
Turner syndrome, 63–64
TWA. *See* T-wave alternans
T-wave alternans (TWA), 171

U
U wave, 155
Uhl anomaly, 444
Ulcer, 319
Unifocalization, 572
Unrestricted pulmonary blood flow, 778–779
Unroofed coronary sinus, 611–612
Untwisting of arteries, 20
Urinalysis, 141–142
blood chemistries in, 141
blood cultures in, 141
hyperoxia test in, 141–142
oxygenation level in, 141–142
Urokinase, 910

V
Valvar aortic stenosis
balloon dilation with, 586–587
balloon valvotomy for, 232–233
neonates with, 232–233
older patients with, 232
cardiac catheterization for, 584–585
chest X-ray of, 584
Valvar aortic stenosis *(Conntinued)*
Children's Hospital Boston experience with, 582, 586
clinical manifestations of, 582–583
course of, 586–588
definition of, 581
echocardiogram of, 584
ejection murmur diagram with, 583
electrocardiogram of, 583–584
exercise intolerance with, 587
exercise testing for, 584
infant aortic stenosis as, 588–589
infective endocarditis with, 587
management of, 585–586
pathology of, 581
phonocardiogram of, 583
physiology of, 581–582
prevalence of, 581
rhythm abnormalities with, 587
sudden death with, 587
Valvar pulmonary stenosis, 551–553
balloon valvotomy for, 228–231
neonates with, 230–231
older patients with, 229–230
cardiac catheterization for, 553, 555
chest X-ray for, 552
Children's Hospital Boston, experience with, 550
clinical manifestations of, 551–552
echocardiogram for, 552–553
electrocardiogram for, 552, 553
Valve replacement, pediatric, 854–856
advantages/disadvantages of, 854
aortic, 855
atrioventricular, 854–855
autograft v. homograft for, 855–856
mechanical v. tissue valves for, 855
mitral, 854
pulmonary, 855
semilunar, 855–856
tricuspid, 854–855
Vascular rings, 23, 811–820
anatomy of, 814–815
double aortic arch in, 814
right arch with aberrant left subclavian artery in, 814–815
chest X-ray for, 816, 817
clinical manifestations of, 815–816
symptoms in, 815–816
definition of, 811
embryologic anatomy of, 811–813
management of, 816–820
physical examination with, 816
prevalence of, 813–814
Vasculopathy, coronary, post-transplantation management with, 883–884
Vasodepressor syncope, 360
Vasodilators
drug therapy with, 908
familial hypertrophic cardiomyopathy treated with, 438–439
Vasopressin, 908
Vasopressor, drug therapy with, 908
Vasovagal syncope, 360
VATER association, 69
Velocardiofacial syndrome, 69
Velocity encoded cine MRI, 202
Venous baffles, obstructed, balloon angioplasty for, 238–239
Venous pressure, 133–134
Ventilatory anaerobic threshold, exercise testing with, 281–282
Ventral-septal defect (VSD), 54
Ventricles
formation of, 17
left, 34–37
conduction system of, 35
external appearance of, 34
four anatomic components of, 35–36
internal appearance of, 35
mitral valve of, 35
obtuse margin of, 34
papillary muscles of, 35
morphologic anatomy of, 31–37
right, 31–34
acute margin of, 31
conduction system of, 34
conus arteriosus of, 32, 34
distal conal septum of, 32, 34
external appearance of, 31
four anatomic components of, 32, 34
inflow tract of, 32, 34
infundibulum of, 32, 34
internal appearance of, 31–32
outflow tract of, 32, 34
papillary muscles of, 31–32
parietal band of, 32–33
proximal conal septum of, 32–33
septal band of, 32–33
trabeculae carneae of, 31
tricuspid valve of, 32
ventricular septal defects of, 34
Ventricular arrhythmias, 178–179
Ventricular defects, D-transposition of great arteries with, 647, 657–658
Ventricular hypertrophy, 156–160
left, 158–159
abnormal lateral Q-wave in, 159
lateral T-wave inversion in, 158–159
left axis deviation in, 159
R-wave amplitude in, 158
right, 156–158
abnormal R/S ratio in, 158
abnormal T-wave direction in, 157
QR pattern in, 158
right axis deviation in, 158
RSR pattern in, 158
R-wave amplitude in, 157
S-wave depth in, 157–158
single, 159–160
Ventricular performance. *See* Performance assessment, myocardial/ventricular
Ventricular premature beats, 481
Ventricular septal defect, 84, 527–545, 654
acquired aortic regurgitation with, 541–542
clinical manifestations of, 542

Ventricular septal defect *(Continued)*
course for, 542
management of, 542
physiology of, 542
prevalence of, 541–542
acyanotic tetralogy of Fallot with, 544
anatomy of, 527–529
endocardial cushion type of defects in, 529, 540
infundibular defects in, 529, 539
membranous defects in, 528–529, 539
muscular defects in, 529, 539
subpulmonary defects in, 529, 539
angiogram for, 536–537
aortic stenosis with, 543
cardiac catheterization for, 535–537
chest X-ray for, 534
Children's Hospital Boston experience with, 528, 529, 538
clinical manifestations of, 532–537
coarctation of aorta with, 634–636
course for, 540–542
pulmonary vascular disease with, 540–541
spontaneous diminution in size with, 540
definition of, 527
discovery of, 532
double-chambered right ventricle with, 544–545
double-outlet right ventricle with, 737
D-transposition of great arteries with, 648
echocardiogram for, 534–536
electrocardiogram for, 534
embryology with, 527
laboratory tests for, 537
magnetic resonance imaging for, 535
management of, 538–540
size of defect influencing, 538
type of defect influencing, 539–540
mitral valve disease with, 545
Ventricular septal defect *(Continued)*
patent ductus arteriosus with, 543–544
physical examination for, 532–534
physiology of, 529–532
prevalence of, 527
pulmonary stenosis with, 544–545
secundum atrial septal defect with, 543
surgery for, 850
symptoms of, 532
transcatheter closure of, 246
vulvar pulmonary stenosis with, 544
Ventricular tachycardia (VT), 498–504
acute treatment of, 499
chronic management of, 499–500
definition of, 499
specific forms in children of, 500–504
arrhythmogenic right ventricular dysplasia with, 503
Belhassen's tachycardia as, 503
Brugada syndrome as, 501
cardiomyopathies with, 502–503
catecholaminergic VT as, 501
congenital heart disease with, 502
dilated cardiomyopathies with, 503
hypertrophic cardiomyopathies with, 502
idiopathic VT as, 503
left posterior fascicular tachycardia as, 503
long QT syndrome as, 500–501
rapid incessant VT in infancy as, 500
slow transient VT in infancy as, 500
verapamil-sensitive VT as, 503
Ventricular vascular coupling, adult congenital heart disease with, 834–835
Verapamil, 510–511, 909
Verapamil-sensitive VT, 503
Very low-density lipoprotein (VLDL), 374
Via dextra, 27
Via sinistra, 27
Visceroatrial situs solitus, dextrocardia with, 693–694
Vital signs, 132–133
blood pressure as, 133
exercise testing with, 275–277
dead space/tidal volume ratio in, 277
heart rate in, 275
oxygen extraction in, 276–277
respiratory rate in, 277
stroke volume in, 275–276
tidal volume in, 277
pulse as, 132–133
respirations as, 133
venous pressure as, 133–134
VLDL. *See* Very low-density lipoprotein
VSD. *See* Ventral-septal defect
VT. *See* Ventricular tachycardia
Valvar pulmonary stenosis, ventricular septal defect with, 544

W

Warfarin, 122, 123, 910
Water hammer pulse, 132
Wenckebach periodicity, 147, 148, 479
White syncope, 362
White-coat hypertension, 377
Williams syndrome, 68
Wolff-Parkinson-White syndrome (WPW), 162, 163, 168, 478, 488
antidromic reciprocating tachycardia in, 494–496
orthodromic reciprocating tachycardia with, 492–494

X

X-linked dilated cardiomyopathy, 426

Z

Z scores, 342–343